The Complete Directory
for
Pediatric Disorders

2008
Fourth Edition

The Complete Directory
for
Pediatric Disorders

- Disorder Descriptions
- Body Systems Descriptions
- National & State Associations
- Libraries & Resource Centers
- Support Groups & Hotlines
- Books & Periodicals
- Research Centers
- Web Sites

A SEDGWICK PRESS Book

Grey House
Publishing

PUBLISHER:	Leslie Mackenzie
EDITORIAL DIRECTOR:	Laura Mars-Proietti
PRODUCTION MANAGER:	Karen Stevens
PRODUCTION ASSISTANTS:	Alysia Giglio, Jael Powell, Erica Schneider
MEDICAL EDITOR:	Sarah Zarbock
MARKETING DIRECTOR:	Jessica Moody

A Sedgwick Press Book
Grey House Publishing, Inc.
185 Millerton Road
Millerton, NY 12546
518.789.8700
FAX 518.789.0545
www.greyhouse.com
e-mail: books @greyhouse.com

Complete directory for pediatric disorders – 1st ed. (2000)-
v.;27.5 cm.
Includes index.
ISSN: 1537-7180
1.   Pediatric—Directories. 2. Children—Diseases—Treatment—Directories. 3. Pediatrics—Periodicals. 4. Children—Diseases—Treatments—Periodicals. 5. Pediatrics—United States—Directory. 6. Child Health Services—United States—Directory. 7. Information Services—United States—Directory. 8. Self-Help Groups—United States—Directory. I. Grey House Publishing, Inc. II. Title: Directory for pediatric disorders.
RJ61.C728
618.92

ISBN: 159237-150-7
ISSN: 1537-7180

Table of Contents

Introduction

Disorders by Biologic System

SECTION I: PEDIATRIC DISORDERS

Each disorder chapter includes a description and all or some of the following:

National Associations & Support Groups	Conferences
State Agencies & Support Groups	Media Resources
Libraries & Resource Centers	Camps
Research Centers	Web Sites

Each disorder chapter includes a description and all or some of the following:

National Associations & Support Groups	Conferences
State Agencies & Support Groups	Media Resources
Libraries & Resource Centers	Camps
Research Centers	Web Sites

Each disorder chapter includes a description and all or some of the following:

National Associations & Support Groups	Conferences
State Agencies & Support Groups	Media Resources
Libraries & Resource Centers	Camps
Research Centers	Web Sites

Each disorder chapter includes a description and all or some of the following:

National Associations & Support Groups	Conferences
State Agencies & Support Groups	Media Resources
Libraries & Resource Centers	Camps
Research Centers	Web Sites

Each disorder chapter includes a description and all or some of the following:

National Associations & Support Groups	Conferences
State Agencies & Support Groups	Media Resources
Libraries & Resource Centers	Camps
Research Centers	Web Sites

SECTION II: GENERAL RESOURCES

SECTION III: THE HUMAN BODY

SECTION IV: GLOSSARY

SECTION V: GUIDELINES FOR ADDITIONAL RESOURCES

SECTION VI: INDEXES

Introduction

Welcome to the fourth edition of *The Complete Directory for Pediatric Disorders*. It provides current, understandable medical information, resources and support services on pediatric disorders for not only parents and the support network of an afflicted child, but also for professionals such as physician assistants and social workers who are in a position to provide concerned caregivers vital information.

This directory includes 209 disorders that are most prevalent in the pediatric population, ages 0-18. They include both physical and mental conditions, and range from life threatening childhood cancers to less serious disorders such as learning disabilities, allergies and bed wetting.

The Complete Directory for Pediatric Disorders includes several articles following this introduction that discuss new treatment guidelines for several conditions, including **AIDS, Epilepsy, Hypertension, Asthma, Gastroenteritis, ADD, Ear Infections** and **Autism.**

This edition includes 8,511 listings – 1,478 more than last edition. Each listing has updated contact data – address, phone, fax, web site, e-mail -- and helpful descriptions. You will find 5,615 fax numbers, 4,580 e-mail addresses, 6,720 web sites and 4,134 key executives – **4,810 more pieces of contact data than last edition**.

This Directory is a one-stop resource, enabling professionals and the families they serve to obtain immediate, important information from one comprehensive source. It is organized in the following six sections:

Section I – Disorders

This section includes 209 major disorder chapters, that comprise more than 260 specific disorders, diseases, or conditions. They are arranged in alphabetical order, from Achondroplasia to Wilson Disease. Each chapter begins with an extensive description, written in understandable language. All disorder descriptions in this fourth edition have been carefully reviewed and revised by medical professionals to include the most up-to-date methods of diagnoses and treatment. Each description includes the following:

Disorder name and synonyms
Physical findings
Cause
Standard treatment

Primary symptoms
Related disorders
Body system affected

Following each description are *disorder-specific resources*, including Associations, Federal and State Agencies, Support Groups, Libraries, Resource Centers, Research Centers, Web sites, Media Resources and Camps. The more prevalent a disorder is, the more resources there are available.

The Complete Directory of Pediatric Disorders also includes the many hospitals, medical organizations, and advocacy groups that offer extended information on a great variety of conditions. These combined resources offer the most comprehensive coverage available of the 209 most prevalent pediatric disorders being diagnosed in pediatrician's offices around the country.

Section II – General Resources

This section includes 1,016 resources, including Government Agencies, National Associations, State Agencies, Support Groups, Newsletters, Books, Magazines, Camps and

Wish Foundations. These may not be limited to a specific disorder, but offer information and support for categories of disorders.

Users will find resources on not only physical pediatric disorders, but also on mental and emotional conditions that affect our younger population. There are also resources that deal with multi-disorder conditions.

Section III – The Human Body

This educational element is comprised of 14 detailed descriptions of body systems or medical categories. It is designed to provide a comprehensive overview of the human body, enabling the user to broaden his or her understanding of how a particular disorder affects a specific body system(s). This information enables the reader to broaden his or her understanding of how the disorders relate to the body, and ranges from the structure and function of human cells and tissues to child growth and development.

Section IV – Glossary

This guide to medical terminology provides important navigational tips and more than 200 commonly used medical prefixes, roots, and suffixes to help readers decipher terms they may encounter in the disorder descriptions, or in other resources they are using.

Section V – Guidelines for Obtaining Additional Information and Resources

These guidelines assist parents and caregivers who are interested in obtaining more information on such diverse topics as physicians who specialize in certain pediatric disorders, accredited hospitals, approved drugs or medical devices for certain pediatric conditions, or current clinical trials that are investigating possible new therapies for particular diseases.

Section VI – Indexes

The Complete Directory for Pediatric Disorders contains three indexes to help readers access the information from several places:

- **Entry Index** is an alphabetical listing of all entry names.
- **Geographic Index** groups listings by state.
- **Subject Index** includes an alphabetical list of pediatric disorders, condition names, synonyms, and related disorders.

Disorders by Biologic System Affected

Cardiovascular Disorders; see also *Cardiovascular System,* page 1004.
Aortic Stenosis
Arrhythmias
Atrial Septal Defects
Coarctation of the Aorta
Hypertrophic Cardiomyopathy
Hypoplastic Left Heart Syndrome (HLHS)
Kawasaki Disease
Marfan Syndrome
Noonan's Syndrome
Patent Ductus Arteriosus
Pulmonary Hypertension
Pulmonary Valve Stenosis
Syncope
Tetralogy of Fallot
Transposition of the Great Arteries
Ventricular Septal Defects
Williams Syndrome

Connective Tissue Disorders; see also *Cells,* page 1006.
Childhood Dermatomyositis
Ehlers-Danlos Syndrome
Sarcoidosis
Scleroderma

Dental Disorders; see also *Digestive System,* page 1012.
Dental Conditions
Ectodermal Dysplasia
Microdontia

Dermatologic Disorders; see also *Dermatologic System,* page 1010.
Albinism
Alopecia Areata
Burn Injuries
Childhood Dermatomyositis
Cleft Lip and Cleft Palate
Ectodermal Dysplasia
Eczema
Epidermolysis Bullosa
Hemangiomas and Lymphangiomas
Icthyosis
Keloids
Neurofibromatosis
Pemphigus
Photosensitivity
Pityriasis Rosea
Tuberous Sclerosis
Psoriasis
Telangiectasia
Urticaria

Developmental, Behavioral and Psychiatric Disorders; see also *Growth and Development*, page 1018.
Asperger Syndrome
Attention Deficit Hyperactivity Disorder
Autistic Disorder
Bipolar Disorder
Childhood Schizophrenia
Conduct Disorder
Depression
Eating Disorders
Encopresis
Lead Poisoning
Learning Disability, Reading Disability Dyslexia
Mental Retardation
Migraine Headaches
Nightmares
Night Terrors
Nocturnal Enuresis
Obesity
Obsessvie-Compulsive Disorder
Oppositional Defiant Behavior
Passive-Aggressive Behavior
Phobias
Physical and Sexual Abuse
PICA
Post-Traumatic Stress Disorder
Sleepwalking
Stuttering
Thumbsucking

Endocrinologic Disorders; see also *Endocrine System*, page 1015.
Congenital Adrenal Hyperplasia
Cushing's Syndrome
Diabetes Mellitus
Growth Hormone Deficiency
Hypothyroidism
McCune-Albright Syndrome
Obesity
Prader-Willi Syndrome
Precocious Puberty

Gastrointestinal Disorders; see also *Digestive System*, page 1012.
Acute Gastrointestinal Infections
Alpha-1-Antitrypsin Deficiency
Anorectal Malformations
Biliary Atresia
Celiac Disease
Colic
Congenital Diaphragmatic Hernia
Crohn's Disease
Encopresis
Esophageal Atresia
Galactosemia
Hepatitis

Hirschsprung Disease
Milk Protein Allergy and Lactose Intolerance
Omphalocele
Pyloric Stenosis
Ulcerative Colitis
Wilson's Disease

Genetic/Chromosomal/Syndrome/Metabolic Disorders; see also *Growth and Development*, page 1018.
Achondroplasia
Albinism
Alpha-1-Antitrypsin Deficiency
Asperger Syndrome
Congenital Cataracts
Cornelia de Lange Syndrome
DiGeorge Syndrome
Down Syndrome
Familial Dysautonomia
Fetal Alcohol Syndrome
Fragile X Syndrome
Galactosemia
Gaucher's Disease
Hereditary Fructose Intolerance
Homocystinuria
Klinefelter Syndrome
Klipple-Feil Syndrome
Leukodystrophies
Maple Syrup Urine Disease
Marfan Syndrome
McCune-Albright Syndrome
Mucolipidoses
Mucopolysaccharidoses
Noonan's Syndrome
Osteogenesis Imperfecta
Phenylketonuria
Polydactyly
Prader-Willi Syndrome
Tay-Sachs Disease
Trisomy 18 Syndrome
Trisomy 13 Syndrome
Turner Syndrome
Williams Syndrome

Hematologic and Oncologic Disorders; see also *Hematologic System*, page 1021.
Acute Lymphoblastic Leukemia
Acute Myeloid Leukemia
Ewing's Sarcoma
Hemolytic Disease of the Newborn
Hemophilia
Histiocytosis
Hodgkins Disease
Neuroblastoma
Neutropenia
Non-Hodgkins Lymphoma

Porphyria
Protein C Deficiency
Retinoblastoma
Sickle Cell Disease
Thalasemias
Thrombocytopenias
Wilm's Tumor

Immunologic and Rheumatologic Disorders; see also *Immune System,* page 1023.
Alopecia Areata
DiGeorge Syndrome
HIV Infection
Juvenile Rheumatoid Arthritis
Kawasaki Disease
Subacute Sclerosing Panencephalitis (SSPE)
Systemic Lupus Erythematosus

Infectious Diseases; see also *Immune System,* page 1023.
Acute Gastrointestinal Infections
Conjunctivitis
Cytomegalovirus
Erythema Infectiosum
HIV Infection
Hepatitis
Herpes Simplex
Lyme Disease
Meningitis
Neonatal Herpes Simplex
Otitis Media
Pinworm
Pityriasis Rosea
Pneumonia
Preventable Childhood Infections
Respiratory Syncytial Virus Infection
Toxoplasmosis
Tuberculosis

Neonatal and Infant Disorders; see also *Growth and Development,* page 1018.
Apnea of Prematurity
Bronchopulmonary Dysplasia
Colic
Congenital Dysplasia of the Hip
Hemolytic Disease of the Newborn
Interventricular Hemorrhage
Kernicterus
Neonatal Herpes Simplex
Neonatal Jaundice
Omphalocele
Prematurity
Respiratory Distress Syndrome of the Newborn
Retinopathy of Prematurity
Sudden Infant Death Syndrome

Neurologic Disorders; see also *Nervous System*, page 1026.
Anencephaly
Arnold-Chiari Malformation
Asperger Syndrome
Ataxia
Brain Tumors
Cerebral Palsy
Autistic Disorder
Bell's Palsy
Chorea
Dyslexia
Dystonia
Encephalocele
Erb's Palsy
Familial Dysautonomia
Guillain-Barre Syndrome
Head Injuries
Hearing Impairment/Deafness
Hydrocephalus
Interventricular Hemorrhage
Lead Poisoning
Leukodystrophies
Lissencephaly
Macrocephaly
Meningitis
Mental Retardation
Microcephaly
Muscular Dystophies
Narcolepsy
Nystagmus
Ptosis
Seizures
Speech Impairment
Spina Bifida
Spinal Muscular Atrophies
Strabismus
Stuttering
Subacute Sclerosing Panencephalitis (SSPE)
Tics
Tourette Syndrome
Tuberous Sclerosis

Ophthalmologic Disorders; see also *Sensory Organs*, page 1034.
Aniridia
Congenital Cataracts
Congenital Glaucoma
Conjunctivitis
Nystagmus
Ptosis
Refraction Disturbances
Retinitis Pigmentosa
Retinoblastoma
Retinopathy of Prematurity
Strabismus

Orthopedic and Muscle Disorders; see also *Musculoskeletal System,* page 1025.
Achondroplasia
Ankylosing Spondylitis
Arthorogryposis Mutiplex Congenita
Cerebral Palsy
Charcot-Marie-Tooth Disease
Childhood Dermatomyositis
Cleft Lip and Cleft Palate
Clubfoot
Congenital Dysplasia of the Hip
Craniosynostosis
Dystonia
Ewing's Sarcoma
Legg-Calve-Perthes Disease
Marfan Syndrome
Muscular Dystophies
Neurofibromatosis
Osteogenesis Imperfecta
Polydactyly
Scoliosis
Spina Bifida
Spinal Muscular Atrophies
Strabismus
Syndactyly

Renal and Urologic Disorders; see also *Urologic System,* page 1036
Cryptorchidism
Nephrotic Syndrome
Nocturnal Enuresis

Respiratory Disorders; see also *Respiratory System,* page 1032.
Alpha-1-Antitrypsin Deficiency
Apnea of Prematurity
Asthma
Bronchopulmonary Dysplasia
Congenital Diaphragmatic Hernia
Cystic Fibrosis
Pneumonia
Pulmonary Hypertension
Respiratory Distress Syndrome of the Newborn
Respiratory Syncytial Virus Infection
Sleep Apnea
Tuberculosis

New Treatment Guidelines for HIV-Positive Children

By Tim Horn

October 31, 2006 (AIDSmeds.com)—The U.S. Department of Health and Human Services (DHHS) has completely revised its treatment guidelines for HIV-positive children. The October 26 edition of the Guidelines for the Use of Antiretroviral Agents in Pediatric HIV Infection contains significant changes to its recommendations regarding when to begin therapy and which agents to use, along with a major overhaul of the discussion sections to improve their organization and readability.

Since the pediatric guidelines were first developed in 1993, there have been a number of dramatic advances in the treatment of HIV-positive children. AIDS-related deaths have dropped by 70% since the introduction of combination HIV treatment, and opportunistic infections have also significantly decreased in HIV-positive children with access to antiretroviral therapy. What's more, advances from clinical trials and studies exploring laboratory monitoring – such as drug-resistance testing and therapeutic drug monitoring – have enabled physicians to more carefully choose very effective first-time treatment regimens while preserving other important drugs for subsequent regimens.

Treating HIV-positive children is not without its challenges. While fewer children are being diagnosed with HIV today, thanks to highly successful preventive treatment during pregnancy, there are still a sizable number of HIV-positive children in the United States. As a group, these children are growing older, bringing new challenges of dosing, adherence, drug resistance, and management of multiple drugs.

Much like the Guidelines for the Use of Antiretroviral Agents in HIV-1-Infected Adults and Adolescents (last updated October 10, 2006), the experts responsible for maintaining the pediatric guidelines meet regularly to discuss changes that are necessary to meet the treatment needs and challenges of HIV-positive children and their healthcare providers.

The October 26 version of the pediatric guidelines involves a major rewrite of previous editions. Much of the rewrite, the authors say, was intended to make the document more accessible to clinicians and to help better organize the information.

One of the most significant changes, with respect to recommendations, involves the initiation of treatment in HIV-positive children. Deciding when to begin treatment, the panelists say, greatly depends on the age of the child. There are now specific recommendations for children under 12 months of age, between one and four years of age, four to 12 years of age, and 13 years of age and older. (See Table 6 on page 57 of the revised guidelines for more information.)

The October pediatric guidelines also contain revisions to a table highlighting the preferred medications choices for HIV-positive children starting therapy for the first time (see Table 7 on page 58). For example, Sustiva® (efavirenz) plus two nucleoside reverse transcriptase inhibitors (NRTIs) is the preferred non-nucleoside reverse transcriptase inhibitor (NNRTI)-based option for children three years of age or older. For those younger than three years of age, or those unable to swallow pills, the pediatric formulation of Viramune® (nevirapine) is the preferred NNRTI choice. As for protease inhibitors, Kaletra® (lopinavir plus ritonavir) remains the preferred choice.

Also of note are revised recommendations for adolescents, including issues related to dosing, use of birth control, pregnancy, and transition into adult care.

The revised pediatric guidelines can be accessed at: http://aidsinfo.nih. gov/ContentFiles/PediatricGuidelines.pdf. Source: POZ.com, October 2006. Reprinted with permission. ©2006 CDM Publishing, LLC.

New Treatment Guidelines for Epilepsy

By Melissa Schorr

April 27, 2004 (San Francisco) — Physicians who prescribe medication for epileptic patients must take into account which drugs will be most suited to patients' particular needs, considering medical history, age, sex, potential long-term adverse effects, and the benefits of newer drugs, according to new guidelines issued here by the American Academy of Neurology (AAN) and the American Epilepsy Society at the AAN annual meeting.

"There has been an explosion in the number of epilepsy drugs, which is a lot for physicians to come to terms with," said Jacqueline French, MD, a professor in the department of neurology at the University of Pennsylvania in Philadelphia. "We wanted to explain the advantages and disadvantages of the new drugs and where physicians should use them."

The new guidelines, which are published in the April 27 issue of Neurology, offer physicians guidance on seven new antiepileptic medications released in the past 10 to 15 years, divided into recommendations for newly diagnosed and refractory patients.

The guidelines include specific advice for patients with refractory epilepsy, which makes up 30% to 40% of all patients with epilepsy. Physicians treating adult patients with partial epilepsy were advised to consider topiramate, oxcarbazepine, or lamotrigine as monotherapy, Dr. French said.

A major problem for unresponsive patients has been the lag time in aggressively receiving treatment of medications or progressing to surgery, said Jerome Engel, Jr., MD, a professor of neurology and chief of epilepsy at the University of California in Los Angeles. "If you can stop the seizures early, you can rescue patients from a lifetime of disability."

For patients with newly diagnosed epilepsy, physicians should consider trying newer antiepileptic drugs from the outset, despite the higher cost, because once a drug is prescribed, a patient is often highly reluctant to switch, despite known adverse effects of many of the older antiepileptic medications. Some of the older antiepileptic drugs, which include phenobarbital and primidone, have been found to elevate homocysteine levels, increase the risk of osteoporosis, and interfere with the metabolism of other drugs, such as birth control pills, Dr. Engel said.

"These drugs have long-term effects," he said. "It's better not to be on them an entire lifetime if you don't have to be."

For newly diagnosed adults and adolescents with partial or mixed seizure disorders, the guidelines suggest oxcarbazepine, which is approved by the U.S. Food and Drug Administration for monotherapy, as well as gabapentin, lamotrigine, and topiramate, which are approved in the United States for adjunctive therapy but have been studied in Europe.

"The choice of an initial drug is extremely important, so you have to make the proper choices," said Dr. French. "There are advantages of the new drugs."

The newer antiepileptic drugs are better tolerated, have less effect on homeostasis, and there is a lower rating for the risk of birth defects, she noted.

Physicians also need to take into consideration the needs of specific subgroups when prescribing, Dr. French added.

For example, most old antiepileptic drugs, as well as topiramate and oxcarbazepine, have been found to interfere with the effectiveness of oral contraceptives for women, putting them at increased risk of unintended pregnancies.

For newly diagnosed children with absence seizures, gabapentin and lamotrigine were recommended for having less of an effect on neuropsychosocial measures, said Andres Kanner, MD, professor of neurological sciences at Rush University Medical Center in Chicago, Illinois.

Eric Hargis, president of the Epilepsy Foundation, a patient advocacy group, pointed out that health insurance providers and formularies must offer coverage of all the new drugs, despite the higher short-term cost. "Epilepsy isn't a cookie-cutter disease, there is no best epilepsy medicine. Physicians must have access to all drug options," he said.

"Cost savings by restricting access is often illusory in epilepsy," Dr. Hargis added. "If a patient has a seizure on the wrong medication, it can cost thousands of dollars in hospital costs and visits to the emergency room."

AAN 56th Annual Meeting: Special Media Briefing. Presented April 27, 2004. Reviewed by Gary D. Vogin, MD. Melissa Schorr is a freelance writer for Medscape. Reprinted with permission from Medscape Medical News 2004.
http://www.medscape.com/viewarticle/474657 © 2004 Medscape.

New Guidelines for Children Suggest More Aggressive Hypertension Strategy

By Peggy Peck

May 21, 2004 (New York) — The latest report from the National High Blood Pressure Education Program Working Group on Hypertension Control in Children and Adolescents identifies a new area of clinical concern — prehypertension — in children and recommends lifestyle interventions for children with this condition.

Bonita Falkner, MD, chair of the guidelines committee and professor of medicine at Jefferson Medical School in Philadelphia, Pennsylvania, previewed them here at the American Society of Hypertension 19th annual scientific meeting. The full guidelines will be published in the July issue of Pediatrics.

The guidelines define prehypertension as blood pressure levels in the 90th to 95th percentile. In addition, the new guidelines suggest that an adolescent with blood pressure of 120/80 mm Hg, which JNC-VII used as the threshold for prehypertension in adults, should also be considered prehypertensive regardless of percentile rank.

Dr. Falkner told Medscape that lifestyle interventions — such as a diet rich in fruits and vegetables and low in sodium as well as a regular exercise program — should be initiated in all children with prehypertension.

She said the guidelines spell out what in the past has been considered merely theoretical, that "hypertension in children is real."

The guidelines also suggest changes in the way these children are evaluated. In the past "the clinician would always look for an underlying cause [for hypertension], for example, a problem in the kidneys," Dr. Falkner said. "We will still do that evaluation, but in addition we will be evaluating for target organ damage because children can suffer from pressure injury just as adults. Since the best place to evaluate for pressure injuries is the heart, we are recommending echocardiography for children with hypertension."

The guidelines recommend regular blood pressure screening beginning at age three years, but some children such as those born preterm or children with congenital heart defects should be screened earlier "and if hypertension is identified earlier, it should be treated."

The guidelines identify stage 1 hypertension as blood pressures that "are higher than the 95th percentile to 5 mm Hg above the 99th percentile. Stage II hypertension is at least 5 mm Hg above the 99th percentile," she said. Dr. Falkner estimated that "1% to 3% of children have hypertension."

Lifestyle intervention should also be the first intervention for these children, Dr. Falkner said. But if six months of diet and exercise fail to control blood pressure, "a pharmacologic approach is needed."

The guidelines contain a complete listing of antihypertensive drugs that have been tested in children and can be used as first-line agents. "There are about 15 drugs in which we have clinical data in children," Dr. Falkner said. "This includes all the classes of antihypertensives except diuretics." She noted that the choice of agent in children is similar to the choice in adults. For example, an angiotensin-converting enzyme inhibitor or an angiotensin receptor blocker should be considered for children with diabetes. Likewise, nonselective beta-blockers should be avoided in children with asthma and beta-blockers as a class should be avoided in children who are competitive athletes.

ASH 19th Annual Scientific Meeting: Themes II and III — Hypertension in Children and Adolescents. Presented May 20, 2004. Reviewed by Gary D. Vogin, MD. Reprinted with permission from Medscape Medical News 2004.
http://www.medscape.com/viewarticle/478598 © 2004 Medscape.

Experts Provide New Consensus on Childhood Asthma

New international guidelines from the PRACTALL Pediatric Asthma Group have emphasized the importance of asthma management strategies that are specifically tailored for children. The guidelines, which will be presented on 10 June 2007 at the XXVI Congress of the European Academy of Allergology and Clinical Immunology (EAACI), recommend strategies that include not only pharmacological treatment, but also allergen and trigger avoidance and asthma education.

Professor Ulrich Wahn, PRACTALL Chairman and Head of the Department of Paediatric Pneumology and Immunology, at Charité-Humboldt University, Berlin, Germany said: "Children with asthma are fundamentally different from adults with asthma. Their lungs are still developing, their immune systems are immature and they have smaller airways that get obstructed more easily. The new PRACTALL guidelines address these issues and offer clinicians practical recommendations for diagnosis, management and monitoring of asthma in children."

The guidelines include a new treatment algorithm for asthmatic children over 2 years of age that recommends either inhaled corticosteroids (ICS) or leukotriene receptor antagonists (LTRAs) as first-line treatment. If the child's asthma is not sufficiently controlled, the ICS dose can be increased or LTRA can be combined with ICS. Treatment can be stepped up further to achieve control by adjusting ICS doses and adding other medications, such as long-acting ß2 agonists. The guidelines recommend that treatment should subsequently be stepped down to the lowest dose at which good control can be maintained.

Treatment of children 2 years of age and under is addressed in a separate section in the new guidelines. Professor Wahn commented: "The 0-2 year age group is the most difficult to diagnose and treat because so few studies have been done. Persistent asthma often begins at this age and any changes in lung structure and function that occur will likely have a major effect on asthma status throughout childhood."

In addition to pharmacological treatment, the guidelines recommend that children avoid allergens and other potential triggers of an asthma attack. These include pets, house-dust mites, food allergens and, most importantly, passive tobacco smoke. Although exercise will trigger an asthma attack in many asthmatic children, the guidelines highlight the need for children to be well controlled so that they can participate fully in exercise and sporting activity.

Education should be a key aspect of the asthma management strategy. Ideally, the guidelines recommend a three-tier education program that considers disease severity, stage of development, and the need for information. Education should target not only children, but also parents, caregivers and healthcare professionals including primary care physicians, nurses and pharmacists.

Professor Wahn commented: "A good asthma education programme should increase knowledge of the disease, allay any fears about medication and increase communication between children, caregivers and healthcare providers. Parents need to be aware of the benefits as well as the potential risks of all therapies so that they can make informed choices for their children."

The new PRACTALL guidelines were developed to address the lack of up-to-date international guidelines that focus exclusively on paediatric asthma. They were developed by the PRACTALL Paediatric Asthma Group, which consists of approximately 40 international experts in paediatric allergy and asthma. The guidelines are part of the PRACTALL initiative, which is endorsed by EAACI and the American Academy of Allergy, Asthma and Immunology (AAAAI). They will be published in both Europe and North America in future issues of journals published by the two academies.

Article URL: http://www.medicalnewstoday.com/articles/73845.php.
Source: www.medicalnewstoday.com

Merck HPV Vaccine Effective in Preventing Infection With Four Strains Linked to Genital Warts, Cervical Cancer, Study Says

Merck's experimental vaccine targeting the four strains of the sexually transmitted disease human papillomavirus that are most likely to cause cervical cancer or genital warts was 89% effective in preventing infection with the viral strains and 100% effective in preventing cervical cancer, precancerous lesions or genital warts, according to a study published in the April issue of the journal Lancet Oncology, Reuters Health reports. Luisa Villa, a biologist at the Ludwig Institute for Cancer Research in Sao Paulo, Brazil, and colleagues conducted the Phase II trial of the vaccine among 552 women ages 16 to 23 in the United States, Europe and Brazil. None of the participants were pregnant, had a history of abnormal Pap tests or had more than four sexual partners (Reuters Health, 4/7). Participants who had tested positive for HPV antibodies in the past were not excluded from the study. Of the 552 study participants, 277 received three shots of the vaccine — known as Gardasil — and 275 women received placebo injections over a six-month period (Rubin, USA Today, 4/6). Over three years, study participants underwent routine pelvic exams, Pap testing, serum testing for HPV antibodies and cervicovaginal sampling for HPV DNA (Villa et al., Lancet Oncology, 4/1).

Results

Among the women who received the placebo, 36 either contracted HPV or developed one of the diseases associated with it (Johnson, AP/Long Island Newsday, 4/6). Of those, three developed genital warts and three developed pre-cancerous cervical lesions (USA Today, 4/6). Among the women who received the vaccine, four contracted HPV, but none of them developed any of the diseases associated with the virus. Overall, the researchers found that the experimental vaccine led to approximately 90% fewer cases of persistent infection or disease due to HPV types 16 and 18, which cause about 70% of cervical cancer cases, or types 6 and 11, which cause about 90% of all cases of genital warts, AP/Newsday reports (AP/Long Island Newsday, 4/6). Although HPV antibodies dropped at the end of the study period among women who had received the experimental vaccine, their antibody levels were still higher than in women naturally infected with HPV (USA Today, 4/6).

Reaction

"It's the first time we show efficacy for the most broad-coverage vaccine in development," Eliav Barr, head of Merck's HPV vaccine development program, said (AP/Long Island Newsday, 4/6). "If (larger) Phase III studies demonstrate the vaccine is as effective as this, I'm sure that it will change the history of cervical cancer," Villa said in a phone interview (Hirschler, Reuters, 4/6). The researchers believe the vaccine would be most effective if administered to girls ages 10 to 13 because they likely would not have been exposed to the virus previously (BBC News, 4/7). Christopher Crum, director of women's and perinatology pathology at the Brigham and Women's Hospital in Boston, said he is "cautiously optimistic" that the vaccine's protective effects would last throughout a woman's reproductive years, according to USA Today (USA Today, 4/6).

Other Ongoing Trials

GlaxoSmithKline also is developing a vaccine against HPV that is being tested in thousands of women around the world to confirm the effectiveness and safety of the vaccines (Kaiser Daily Reproductive Health Report, 4/5). The newly released results of the Merck study are "almost identical" to the findings of a study testing the effectiveness of GSK's experimental HPV vaccine targeting strains 16 and 18, Reuters reports (Reuters, 4/6). Currently, the companies are competing to get their products approved. GSK plans to file for regulatory approval for its vaccine, called Cervarix, in Europe in 2006. Merck plans to apply for FDA approval for its expanded HPV vaccine in late 2005 (Kaiser Daily Reproductive Health Report, 4/5).

AAP Endorses New Treatment Guidelines for Gastroenteritis

CHICAGO — Acute gastroenteritis is a common illness in children in the United States, resulting in 1.5 million outpatient visits, 200,000 hospitalizations, approximately 300 deaths, as well as costing approximately $1 billion per year. In developing countries, an estimated 2 million children under 5 years old die from acute diarrhea each year. A worldwide campaign by the World Health Organization to treat acute diarrhea with oral rehydration therapy (ORT) is credited with reducing the death toll from 5 million deaths in 1982 to 3 million deaths in 1992 to 2 million in 2003.

In the fall of 2003, a panel of specialists convened by the Centers for Disease Control and including Christopher Duggan, MD, Director, Clinical Nutrition Service at Children's Hospital Boston, updated the 1992 CDC guidelines based on recent developments in the science of gastroenteritis management. The data reported by the expert panel agreed with the recent change by the World Health Organization concerning the composition of oral rehydration solutions, the first such change in 30 years. On August 2, the American Academy of Pediatrics (AAP) adopted the guidelines for use in the care of children in the United States.

The new guidelines incorporate a number of findings, including that zinc supplementation can reduce the incidence and severity of acute diarrhea; the effectiveness of a new oral rehydration solution (ORS) with reduced osmolarity (the proportionally reduced concentrations of sodium and glucose in the solution); and the recognition that the combination of oral rehydration and early nutritional support that has proven effective throughout the world should be incorporated into practice in developed countries. ORT protocols designed for developing countries are now recommended as the standard of care for children in the United States and other industrialized countries, where intravenous therapy has become the first line treatment for acute diarrhea and dehydration. In the U.S., approximately 30 percent of pediatricians shy away from oral rehydration therapy for children with vomiting or moderate dehydration. In addition, continued feeding of children during diarrheal episodes has been difficult to establish as a standard of care. The new CDC report and recommendations, which are hoped to change the way pediatricians in the United States manage acute diarrhea in children, can be found at www.cdc.gov/mmwr/preview/mmwrhtml/rr5216a1.htm'.

The AAP's Managing Acute Gastroenteritis Among Children: Oral Rehydration, Maintenance, and Nutritional Therapy states that the American Academy of Pediatrics "endorses the Centers for Disease Control and Prevention updated recommendations concerning diarrhea management in children. Oral rehydration therapy (ORT), which includes timely use of oral rehydration solutions (ORS) and early nutritional support, has been proven to be safe and effective therapy for almost all cases of acute diarrhea. Recent clinical trials have also documented improved outcomes with an ORS of reduced concentrations of sodium and glucose. Educating physicians and parents about ORT is urged in order to avoid unnecessary clinic visits, hospitalizations and in some cases, death."

Children's Hospital Boston is home to the world's largest research enterprise based at a pediatric medical center, where its discoveries have benefited both children and adults for over 100 years. More than 500 scientists, including seven members of the National Academy of Sciences, nine members of the Institute of Medicine and nine members of the Howard Hughes Medical Institute comprise Children's research community. Founded in 1869 as a 20-bed hospital for children, Children's Hospital Boston today is a 300-bed comprehensive center for pediatric and adolescent health care grounded in the values of excellence in patient care and sensitivity to the complex needs and diversity of children and families. It is also the primary pediatric teaching affiliate of Harvard Medical School. For more information about the hospital visit: www.childrenshospital.org

The American Academy of Pediatrics is an organization of 57,000 primary care pediatricians, pediatric medical subspecialists and pediatric surgical specialists dedicated to the health, safety and well-being of infants, children, adolescents and young adults.

The Centers for Disease Control and Prevention (CDC) is recognized as the lead federal agency for protecting the health and safety of people - at home and abroad, providing credible information to enhance health decisions, and promoting health through strong partnerships. CDC serves as the national focus for developing and applying disease prevention and control, environmental health, and health promotion and education activities designed to improve the health of the people of the United States.

Reprinted with permission. Children's Hospital Boston and American Academy of Pediatrics.

Treatment Guidelines for Children with ADD

Guidelines from American Academy of Pediatrics

The American Academy of Pediatrics, released recommendations for primary care physicians in treating children diagnosed with ADHD. Prior to any treatment, a thorough evaluation and diagnosis of ADHD is needed.

Research included children, aged 6-12, without additional co-existing conditions.

Many of the recommendations can be applied to children with related conditions such as depression, anxiety, bi-polar disorder, and other disorders, however, there would need to be further research in order to provide specific recommendations for treatment of ADHD with additional conditions.

The guidelines have 5 major points:
- Accepting ADHD as a chronic disorder
- Specification of targeted outcomes
- Recommendation of stimulant medication and/or behavior modification
- Re-evaluation for non-effective treatments
- Continued monitoring and follow up care.

1) Primary care clinicians should establish a treatment program that recognizes ADHD as a chronic condition.

According to the guidelines, accepting and treating ADHD as a chronic condition would include the following:
- Providing information about the condition
- Updating and monitoring family knowledge and understanding on a periodic basis
- Counseling about family response to the condition
- Developmentally appropriate education of the child about ADHD, with updates as the child grows
- Availability to answer family questions
- Ensuring coordination of health and other services
- Helping families set specific goals in areas related to the child's condition and its effects on daily activities
- Linking families with other families with children who have similar chronic conditions as needed

2) The treating clinician, parents, and child, in collaboration with school personnel, should specify appropriate target outcomes to guide management.

The recommendations for treatment specify that physicians, with the aid of feedback from parents, teachers and other involved school personnel, should target 3-6 specific desired changes in determining the treatment plan. These targets can be and often will be different in each child. Each area should have a specific outcome. These targets should become the basis for the initial treatment plan.

Examples:
- Improvements in relationships with parents, siblings, teachers, and peers
- Decreased disruptive behaviors
- Improved academic performance, particularly in volume of work, efficiency, completion, and accuracy
- Increased independence in self-care or homework
- Improved self-esteem
- Enhanced safety in the community, such as in crossing streets or riding bicycles.

3) The clinician should recommend stimulant medication and/or behavior therapy as appropriate to improve target outcomes in children with ADHD.

80% of children with ADHD respond favorably to stimulant medication treatment. However, family circumstances, family beliefs and other factors such as co-existing conditions should go into the consideration of a plan of treatment. Previous studies have shown that stimulant medication together with a behavior modification plan seems to be the best approach for the majority of children with ADHD.

Behavior modification has proved beneficial and is many times the main treatment option. The targets, as previously discussed, should be kept in mind when determining the best type of treatment.

For additional information on the American Academy of Pediatrics research and statement on stimulant medication and behavior medication, read abstract.

Note: For children on stimulants, if one stimulant does not work at the highest feasible dose, the clinician should recommend another.

Research has shown that children who do not respond to a certain stimulant medication, will many times respond favorably to a different medication. Before disregarding stimulant medication, the doctor should recommend a trial of at least 2-3 different stimulant medications.

4) When the selected management for a child with ADHD has not met target outcomes, clinicians should evaluate the original diagnosis, use of all appropriate treatments, adherence to the treatment plan, and presence of coexisting conditions.

During follow up, if it is determined that the treatment plan is not working, the physician should first discover if the family/school is adhering to the specified plan. If not, adjustments should be made to allow for following the plan. Family situations, school cooperation and other factors can influence whether a treatment plan is being followed. Setting up a plan that takes such factors into consideration will have the best chance of success.

Once it is determined that treatment is being followed but goals of treatment have not been met, (if the child can not tolerate stimulant medication, has not been able to reach the targets set or there is co-existing conditions), the physician should refer the family to mental health specialists for further evaluation.

5) The clinician should periodically provide a systematic follow-up for the child with ADHD. Moni- toring should be directed to target outcomes and adverse effects, with information gathered from parents, teachers, and the child.

Consistent communication between the parents and the physician is essential to providing the best medical care. A regular office visit, every 3-6 months for assessment of the treatment plan is recommended. Weight and growth can be consistently monitored at this time, as well as re-evaluation of targets.

In addition, requests for refills of medication can provide the doctor and the parents to have ongoing communication as to the progress of the child.

If at any time, the treatment plan does not seem to be working, Recommendation #4 should begin.

Ongoing communication, with not only the parents, but also with school personnel is recommended.

Social activities can also be a source of problems for children with ADHD, therefore, the physician should be knowledgeable of their community, age-appropriate activities and services that are available.

Ear Infections Treatment Guidelines

From Vincent Iannelli, M.D., Your Guide to Pediatrics

Ear infections are the most common bacterial infection in kids, and one of the most common reasons for children to go see their Pediatrician and be prescribed antibiotics. With the current concerns about the overuse of antibiotics and that they may not work as well because of resistance, cutting back on antibiotic prescribing for kids with ear infections is likely a good idea. The latest clinical practice guideline from the American Academy of Pediatrics on the Diagnosis and Management of Acute Otitis Media offers help to parents and pediatricians who want to avoid giving kids antibiotics when they aren't needed.

To understand the guideline, it is important to first understand what it doesn't say. The guideline specifically do not say that antibiotics can't be used to treat ear infections anymore. Instead, they offer guidelines so that you can choose which children may not need antibiotics to treat their ear infection and may be simply observed instead.

The most clear part of the guidelines is that children under six months of age should always be treated with antibiotics when they have an ear infection. For children between six months and two years of age, they should also be prescribed antibiotics if your Pediatrician is sure of their diagnosis, or if they are unsure, but your child has severe symptoms, like severe ear pain or a fever at or above 102.2 degrees Fahrenheit. Older children, over 2 years of age, usually don't need antibiotics at first, unless they have severe symptoms, and can instead be managed using an 'observation option'.

The Observation Option

If your child meets the criteria described above and does not have any other medical problems, like Down syndrome, immune system problems, cleft palate, or a cochlear implant, then they may qualify to be observed without being treated with antibiotics. If these children do not improve or worsen over the next 48 to 72 hours, then they should be prescribed antibiotics. This may mean a return visit to your Pediatrician in some cases, but this may also be done over the phone, or by use of a 'safety-net' antibiotic prescription which your doctor gives you to fill just in case.

This method of observation instead of prescribing antibiotics right away has been working successfully in many other countries and has few risks. It works because most kids with ear infections will likely get better on their own anyway. These children aren't simply left in pain though. The guidelines strongly recommend steps be taken to reduce the child's pain using acetaminophen or ibuprofen.

If your child has had an ear infection in the previous 30 days or has chronic fluid in their ears, then they will need antibiotics and won't qualify for the 'observation option'.

Diagnosis of Ear Infections

For parents who read the full guidelines, one of the most surprising things is going to be the talk about the 'uncertain diagnosis' of ear infections. It should seem like a clear cut thing. You look inside a child's ear and you can tell if it is infected or not, right?

It isn't always that simple though. Younger children's ears can be difficult to see, especially for health professionals who don't treat a lot of children. The doctor may mistake fluid in the ear for an infection, not even see the ear drum because of ear wax, or they may confuse an ear that is red from fever or crying to be from an infection.

If your doctor has said things like 'it looks a little red' or 'I see a little fluid' then they may not have been making a 'certain' diagnosis of an ear infection. This is especially true if the diagnosis was made when your child had no other symptoms at all. With a true ear infection, in addition to having fluid in their ear, your child should instead have the more classic symptoms of 'a history of rapid onset of signs and symptoms such as otalgia (or pulling of the ear in an infant), irritability in an infant or toddler, otorrhea, and/or fever.'

User's Guide

Below is a sample listing illustrating the kind of information that is or might be included in an Association entry, with additional fields that apply to publication and trade show listings. Each numbered item of information is described in the paragraphs on the following page.

1. 12345

2. **American Board of Pediatrics**
3. **555 Lake Avenue**
    Anytown, NY 00000

4. 999-555-1212
5. 999-555-1211
6. 400-555-1212
7. TDD: 400-555-1211
8. ambope@disorders.com
9. www.ambope/4/dis

10. **Anthony Parsons, Executive Director**
    Angelina Marino, Public Relations Specialist
    Cass Conte, MD, Medical Consultant
    Rosemary Gabriel, Publications Director

11. **The American Board of Pediatric Disorders is dedicated to the support and education of children and families afflicted by disorders whose onset typically occurs before 21 years of age, including congenital conditions. Offers information on hospitals, medical assistance, educational workshops and seminars. Hundreds of publications are available at no cost, and many more through an extensive lending library. Also available is access to a database of information and resources, and a variety of audio visual aids.**

12. **2M Members**

13. **Founded: 1984**

14. **Monthly**

15. **$64.00**

16. **110,000**

User's Key

1. **Record Number:** Entries are listed alphabetically within each category and numbered sequentially. The entry number, rather than the page number, are used in the indexes to refer to listings.

2. **Title:** Formal name of association or publication. Where names are completely capitalized, the listing will appear at the beginning of the section. If listing is a publication or trade show, the publisher or sponsoring organization will appear below the title.

3. **Address:** Location or permanent address of the association.

4. **Phone Number:** The listed phone number is usually for the main office of the association, but may also be for the sales, marketing, or public relations office as provided.

5. **Fax Number:** This is listed when provided by the association.

6. **Toll-Free Number:** This is listed when provided by the association.

7. **TDD:** This is listed when provided by the association. It refers to Telephone Device for the Deaf.

8. **E-Mail:** This is listed when provided by the association.

9. **Web Site:** This is listed when provided by the association and is also referred to as an URL address. These web sites are accessed through the Internet by typing http:// before the URL address.

10. **Key Executives:** Lists key contacts of the association, publication or sponsoring organization.

11. **Description:** This paragraph contains a brief description of the association, their purpose and services.

12. **Members:** Total number of association members.

13. **Founded:** Year association was founded.

14. **Frequency,** if listing is a publication.

15. **Subscription price,** if listing is a publication.

16. **Circulation,** if listing is a publication.

DESCRIPTION

1   **ACHONDROPLASIA**

Synonyms: Chondrodystrophy, Fetal rickets

Involves the following Biologic System(s):

Genetic/Chromosomal/Syndrome/Metabolic Disorders, Orthopedic and Muscle Disorders

Achondroplasia is a disorder of the skeletal system that belongs to a group of diseases known as chondrodystrophies. These disorders involve a disturbance in the development of cartilage of the long bones (e.g., arms and legs). They frequently cause a disproportionately short stature (dwarfism). Achondroplasia is a result of a spontaneous change in one gene (mutation) and is transmitted as an autosomal dominant trait. It occurs in approximately 1 out of every 40,000 births. In anchondroplasia, there is an abnormality in the conversion of cartilage into bone at the growing ends (epiphyses) of the long bones. This process prevents the bones from further growth which ceases at a relatively early age. Symptoms and characteristic findings include a disproportionately large head with protruding or prominent forehead (frontal bossing); a flattened nasal bridge; an underdeveloped upper jaw and prominent lower jaw (prognathism); a well-developed, shortened trunk; and short, bowed arms and legs. The upper portion of arms and legs are proportionately shorter than other parts of the limbs; the elbows may have a limited range of motion. In addition, the fingers and toes are usually short with a v-shaped space or gap between the third and fourth fingers; however, the hands are relatively wide. As children with achondroplasia grow, the pelvis tilts forward, resulting in a pronounced spinal curvature (lumbar lordosis) characterized by a prominent abdomen and buttocks. Diagnosis is made based on physical examination and skeletal radiograph findings.

Complications associated with achondroplasia may include dental problems such as malocclusion as well as chronic and severe middle ear infections (otitis media) that may lead to conductive hearing loss. Potentially life-threatening complications include the temporary cessation of breathing during sleep (sleep apnea) due to obstruction of the airway as a result of certain craniofacial abnormalities or compression of the spinal cord at its entrance to the vertebral column (foramen magnum). In addition, hydrocephalus, which is a condition characterized by an abnormal accumulation of cerebrospinal fluid around the brain, may also have life-threatening implications. Hydrocephalus may also result from obstruction of the foramen magnum.

The availability of somatropin (recombinant human growth hormone) has revolutionized the treatment of short stature. Growth hormone is currently being used to augment the height of patients with achondroplasia. Other treatment for achondroplasia is directed toward prevention or correction of complications. Monitoring head growth during infancy to ensure that it is within established guidelines is effective to determine the presence of hydrocephalus and the need for surgical intervention or other measures.

To avoid further complications, dental irregularities, ear infections, and some skeletal irregularities may respond to physiotherapy as well as the use of orthopedic appliances such as braces. In addition, emotional and psychologic support may be provided through appropriate counseling.

See also **General Resources** on page 917

Government Agencies

2   **NIH/National Institute of Arthritis and Mu sculoskeletal and Skin Diseases**
1 AMS Circle
Bethesda, MD 20892

301-402-4484
Fax: 301-718-6366
e-mail: ord@od.nih.gov
rarediseases.info.nih.gov

The mission of the National Institute of Arthritis and Musculoskeletal and Skin Diseases is to support research into the causes, treatment, and prevention of arthritis and musculoskeletal and skin diseases, the training of basic and clinical scientists to carry out this research, and the dissemination of information on research progress in these diseases.

Stephen I Katz MD PhD, Director

3   **NIH/National Institute of Environmental He alth Sciences (NIEHS)**
111 T.W. Alexander Drive
Research Triangle Park, NC 27709

301-496-3511
www.niehs.nih.gov

NIEHS reduces the burden of human illness and dysfunction from environmental causes by defining how environmental exposures, genetics and age interact to affect an individual's health.

4   **NIH/National Institute on Drug Abuse (NIDA)**
6001 Executive Boulevard/Room 5213
Bethesda, MD 20892

301-443-1124
e-mail: information@nida.nih.gov
www.nida.nih.gov

NIDA leads the nation in bringing the power of science to bear on drug abuse and addiction through support and conduct of research across all disciplines and rapid and effective dissemination of results of that research to improve drug abuse and addiction prevention and treatment.

National Associations & Support Groups

5   **Human Growth Foundation**
997 Glen Cove Avenue, Suite 5
Glen Head, NY 11545

800-451-6434
Fax: 516-671-4055
e-mail: hgf1@hgfound.org
www.hgfound.org

A voluntary, nonprofit organization whose mission is to help children and adults with disorders of growth and growth hormones through research, education, support and advocacy. The foundation is dedicated to helping medical science to better understand the process of growth. It is composed of concerned parents and friends of children and adults with growth problems; and interested health professionals.

Frank Diamond, President
Emily Germain, Vice President

6   **Little People of America**
5289 NE Elam Young Parkway, Suite F-100
Hillsboro, OR 97124

503-846-1562
888-572-2001
Fax: 503-846-1590
e-mail: info@lpaonline.org
www.lpaonline.org

A nonprofit organization that provides support and information to people of short stature and their families.

Billy Barty, Founder
Lois Gerage-Lamb, President

7   **MAGIC Foundation: Major Aspects of Growth in Children**
6645 W North Avenue
Oak Park, IL 60302

708-383-0808
800-362-4423
Fax: 708-383-0899
e-mail: mary@magicfoundation.org
www.magicfoundation.org

A national nonprofit organization providing support and education regarding growth disorders in children and related adult disorders. Provides educational information, networking, a national conference, a kids' program and an extensive medical library.

10,000 members

Dianne Tamburrino, Executive Director
Susan Smith, Director Medical Education

State Agencies & Support Groups

Indiana

8   **Neurofibromatosis, Inc - Indiana**
1173 Hague Court
Franklin, IN 46131

317-736-7577
www.nfinc.org

Dottie Whitehurst, Chapter President

Libraries & Resource Centers

9   **NIH/National Library of Medicine (NLM)**
8600 Rockville Pike
Bethesda, MD 20894

www.nlm.nih.gov

NLM collects, organizes and makes avialiable biomedical science information to scientists, health professionals and the public. The library's databases, including PubMed/Medline and MedlinePlus, and used extensively around the world. NLM conducts and supports research in biometric communications; creates information resouces for molecular biology, biotechnology, toxicology, and environmental health; and provides grant support for training, medical library resources, and biomedical informatics.

Research Centers

10   **Little People's Research Fund**
616 Old Edmondson Avenue
Catonsville, MD 21228

410-747-1100
800-232-5773
Fax: 410-747-1374
e-mail: lprf@LPRF.org
www.LPRF.org

Only health organization established to serve people with skeletal dysplasia (dwarfism), providing research, consultation, medical care and family respite.

Web Sites

11   **Achondroplasia UK**
www.achondroplasia.co.uk

Offers information on health supervision for children of all ages, divided into the following growth stages: newborn; infancy; early childhood; late childhood; and adolescence to early adulthood.

12   **Dysmorphic Syndromes**
www.hgmp.mrc.ac.uk/dhmhd-bin/hum-look-up

13   **Human Growth Foundation**
www.hgfound.org

Information for parents and friends of children and adults with growth problems, as well as interested health professionals.

14   **Little People of America**
www.lpaonline.org

Offers resources pertaining to dwarfism and Little People of America, medical data, instructions on how to join an e-mail discussion group, and links to numerous other dwarfism-related sites.

15   **MAGIC Foundation: Major Aspects of Growth in Children**
www.magicfoundation.org

Provides educational information regarding growth disorders.

16   **Medical College of Wisconsin**
www.mcw.edu

A private, academic institution dedicated to leadership and excellence in education, research, patient care, and service.

17   **Online Mendelian Inheritance in Man**
www.ncbi.nlm.nih.gov

This database is a catalog of human genes and genetic disorders.

18   **Restricted Growth Association**
www.rgaonline.org.uk

Provides medical advice, welfare and counseling services with the support of Regional Coordinators, and offers contact with others and the sharing of helpful information through an information magazine, advisory booklets, meetings, social events and conventions.

Pamphlets

19   Achondroplasia
Human Growth Foundation
977 Glen Cove Avenue, Suite 5
Glen Head, NY 11545

516-671-4041
800-451-6434

Signs, causes, and prevention of achondroplasia.

DESCRIPTION

20 ACUTE GASTROINTESTINAL INFECTIONS
Covers these related disorders: Acute infectious diarrhea, Gastroenteritis
Involves the following Biologic System(s):
Gastrointestinal Disorders, Infectious Disorders

Acute gastrointestinal infections are conditions of the gastrointestinal tract caused by various microorganisms such as certain bacteria, viruses, and parasites (a more common cause outside the U.S.) and are usually characterized by diarrhea and vomiting. Such microorganisms may be transmitted through fecal-oral contamination or contamination of food or water. Bacterial gastrointestinal infection may result from the release of toxins by bacteria or by bacterial growth inside or outside the walls of the intestines. Viral infection by gastroenteritis viruses, especially the rotavirus, is a major source of diarrhea-causing infection in the United States. Although infectious gastroenteritis often resolves on its own (spontaneously), some patients experience acute or prolonged symptoms that may require treatment as well as identification of the causative agent.

Symptoms and findings associated with infectious gastroenteritis depend upon the cause of the infection and the age and general health of the patient. The most common manifestation of infection is watery or bloody diarrhea that usually appears suddenly and lasts from a few days to two weeks or longer. Other symptoms may include nausea, vomiting, loss of appetite, and abdominal cramping or distress. Infants and those with compromised immune systems are at risk for potentially severe illness. Diarrhea and vomiting in infants younger than six months, or in older children if severe, may result in a potentially life-threatening and excessive fluid loss (dehydration) as well as the loss of essential substances, known as electrolytes, in the fluid portion of the blood (e.g., sodium, potassium, and calcium). Symptoms associated with dehydration may include fever, thirst, less-than-average urinary output, dry mouth, and poor feeding. In addition, severely dehydrated infants and older children may become weak, listless, or sleepy and their eyes may have a sunken, dry appearance. Bacteria associated with gastroenteritis sometimes cause infection outside the gastrointestinal tract and may involve the urinary tract, the eyes, the vulva and vaginal areas in females, as well as inflammation of the membranes surrounding the brain and spinal cord (meningitis), the liver (hepatitis), the lungs (pneumonia), the bone and bone marrow (osteomyelitis), and other tissues. In addition, certain foodborne or waterborne infections caused by bacterial or other toxins may produce severe, sudden, and potentially life-threatening symptoms including neurologic involvement such as numbness and paralysis.

Acute infectious diarrhea symptoms are similar to those associated with infectious gastroenteritis. In addition, a temporary inability to properly digest milk may result from damage to the mucosal lining of the small intestine.

Prevention of some types of infectious gastroenteritis may include vaccination against certain infectious diseases when traveling to countries in which these illnesses are widespread. In addition, care in handling and preparing foods may help to alleviate certain types of foodborne illness. Treatment for both infectious gastroenteritis and acute infectious diarrhea is first directed toward the replacement of body fluids and electrolytes through oral preparations or, in the case of more severe dehydration, through intravenous administration. Once dehydration is corrected, nursing infants may resume breast-feeding, while other infants may resume feedings with a lactose-free formula, gradually followed by their regular formula. If indicated, identification of the cause may then be established through evaluation of family history including recent travels, foods eaten, other similar family illness as well as physical examination and testing of stool specimens. Although some cases of acute infectious diarrhea will resolve spontaneously, other treatment may be directed at the underlying cause. Bacterial infections may be treated with appropriate antibiotics. Prevention of this potentially severe condition may often be accomplished by attention to good hygienics such as frequent hand washing, etc. Other treatment is symptomatic and supportive.

See also **General Resources** on page 917

Government Agencies

21 Centers for Disease Control
1600 Clifton Road
Atlanta, GA 30333

404-639-3311
www.cdc.gov

Mission is to promote health and quality of life by preventing and controlling disease, injury, and disability.

22 NIH/National Institute of Allergy and Infectious Diseases
6610 Rockledge Drive, MSC 6612
Bethesda, MD 20892

301-496-5717
Fax: 301-402-3573
TDD: 800-877-8339
www.niaid.nih.gov

Conducts and supports basic and applied research to better understand, treat, and ultimately prevent infectious, immunologic, and allergic diseases.

Anthony S Fauci MD, Director

National Associations & Support Groups

23 American College of Gastroenterology
PO Box 342260
Bethesda, MD 20827

301-263-9000
www.acg.gi.org

The American College of Gastroenterology was founded in 1932 to advance the scientific study and medical practice of diseases of the GI tract.

Jack A DiPalma, President
Amy E Foxx-Orenstein, Vice President

24 American Gastroenterological Association
4930 Del Ray Avenue
Bethesda, MD 20814

301-654-2055
Fax: 301-654-5920
e-mail: member@gastro.org
www.gastro.org

Society of physicians, surgeons, scientists and other individuals within the healthcare community interested in the functions and disorders of the digestive system.

Robert B Greenberg, JD, Executive Vice President
Stacie Gallice, Director Information & Planning Svs

25 Digestive Disease National Coalition
507 Capitol Court NE, Suite 200
Washington, DC 20002

202-544-7497
Fax: 202-546-7105
www.ddnc.org

Advocacy organization comprised of 22 voluntary and professional societies concerned with the many diseases of the digestive tract and liver.

Nancy Norton, Chairperson
Dr. Maurice Cerulli, President

26 International Foundation for Functional Gastrointestinal Disorders
PO Box 170864
Milwaukee, WI 53217

414-964-1799
888-964-2001
Fax: 414-964-7176
e-mail: iffgd@iffgd.org
www.iffgd.org

The organization offers responses to those commonly asked questions for families and individuals whose lives have been touched with the disorder.

Nancy J Norton, Founder
William Norton, VP

27 Intestinal Disease Foundation
100 W Station Square Drive
Pittsburgh, PA 15219

412-261-5888
877-587-9606
Fax: 412-471-2722
e-mail: info@intestinalfoundation.org
www.intestinalfoundation.org

Nonprofit organization whose mission is to improve the quality of life of adults and children affected by chonic digestive illness through information, guidance and support. IDF offers a quarterly newsletter, Intestinal Fortitude, educational seminars, volunteer phone network, and Pittsburgh area support groups.

Linda Schurr, MS Ed. NCC, Executive Director
Harriet Gibbs, LPN, Client Services Manager

28 North American Society for Pediatric Gastroenterology/Hepatology/Nutrition
PO Box 6
Flourtown, PA 19031

215-233-0808
Fax: 215-233-3918
e-mail: naspghan@naspghan.org
www.naspghan.org

Strives to improve the care of infants, children and adolescents with digestive disorders by promoting advances in clinical care of children with chronic abdominal pain, diarrhea, constipation, vomiting, bleeding from the GI tract, inflammatory bowel disease, liver diseases, diseases of the pancreas, poor weight gain and nutritional problems.

Philip Sherman, President
Margaret K Stallings, Executive Director

29 Oley Foundation
214 Hun Memorial, MC-28, Albany Medical Center
Albany, NY 12208

518-262-5079
800-776-6539
Fax: 518-262-5528
e-mail: info@oley.org
www.oley.org

Helping people whose daily survival depends on home intravenous or tube-fed nutrition.

Joan Bishop, Executive Director
Roslyn Dahl, Director, Communications & Develop

30 World Health Organization
Avenue Appia 20
CH-1211 Geneva 27,
Switzerland

www.who.int

WHO is the directing and coordinating authority for health within the United Nations system.

Dr Margaret Chan, Director General

Libraries & Resource Centers

31 National Digestive Diseases Information Clearinghouse
2 Information Way
Bethesda, MD 20892

301-654-3810
800-891-5389
Fax: 703-738-4929
e-mail: nddic@info.niddk.nih.gov
www.digestive.niddk.nih.gov

The National Institute of Diabetes and Digestive and Kidney Diseases conducts and supports research on many of the most serious diseases affecting public health. The Institute supports much of the clinical research on the diseases of internal medicine and related subspecialty fields as well as many basic science disciplines.

Kathy Kranzfelder, Project Officer

Computer Software

32 Digestive Diseases Self-Education Program (DDSEP 5.0)
American Gastroenterological Association
4930 Del Ray Avenue
Bethesda, MD 20814

301-654-2055
Fax: 301-654-5920
e-mail: member@gastro.org
www.gastro.org

Available in January 2007. Provides an in-depth review of core topics in gastroenterology and hepatology. gastroenterologists use this software to assess and update their knowledge and earn CME credit.

Eugene Chang, MD, Editor
John F Kuemmerle, MD, Associate Editor

Web Sites

33 American Gastroenterological Association
www.gastro.org

Information regarding prevention, treatment and cure of digestive diseases.

34 Ask NOAH About: Stomach and Intestinal (Gastrointestinal) Disorders
noah-health.org/english/illness/gastro/gastro.html

Information on many conditions, including colic, celiac disease, ulcerative colitis, Crohn's disease, diarrhea, hernia and Hirschsprung's disease.

35 Baby Center
www.babycenter.com

The Academy is committed to the attainment of optimal physical, mental and social health for all infants, children, adolescents, and young adults. To this end, the members of the Academy dedicate their efforts and resources.

36 Child Health Research Project
www.childhealthresearch.org

To help achieve USAID's strategic objectives to reduce childhood mortality and morbidity, the Child Health Research Project (CHR) conducts applied research in: diarrheal and respiratory diseases, infectious diseases, neonatal health, and malnutrition.

37 Health Research Project (HaRP)
www.harpnet.org

A program by USAID, the project strives to improve the health status of infants, children, mothers and families through the development and research of new tools, technologies, policies and approaches.

38 National Digestive Diseases Information Clearinghouse
www.digestive.niddk.nih.gov

Information regarding Digestive and Kidney Diseases.

Book Publishers

39 Digestive Diseases Dictionary
Nat'l Digestive Diseases Information Clearinghouse
2 Information Way
Bethesda, MD 20892

301-654-3810
Fax: 301-907-8906
e-mail: nddic@info.niddk.nih.gov
www.niddk.nih.gov

Defines words that are often used when talking or writing about digestive diseases.

40 Digestive Diseases in the United States: Epidemiology and Impact
NDDIC
2 Information Way
Bethesda, MD 20892

301-654-3810
800-891-5389
Fax: 301-907-8906
e-mail: nddic@info.niddk.nih.gov
www.niddk.nih.gov

Answers hundreds of questions about the scope and impact of the major infectious, chronic, and malignant digestive diseases. Provides information about prevalence, incidence, medical care, disability, mortality, and research needs regarding specific digestive diseases.

800 pages

41 Directory of Digestive Diseases Organizations for Professionals
Nat'l Digestive Diseases Information Clearinghouse
2 Information Way
Bethesda, MD 20892

301-654-3810
Fax: 301-907-8906
e-mail: nddic@info.niddk.nih.gov
www.niddk.nih.gov

Lists organizations that represent health professionals involved in the study and treatment of digestive disease. The organizations do not provide medical services or advice.

42 Research Opportunities & Programs in the Digestive Diseases & Nutrition
Nat'l Digestive Diseases Information Clearinghouse
2 Information Way
Bethesda, MD 20892

301-654-3810
Fax: 301-907-8906
e-mail: nddic@info.niddk.nih.gov
www.niddk.nih.gov

43 What I Need To Know About Hepatitis A
NDDIC
2 Information Way
Bethesda, MD 20892

301-654-3810
800-891-5389
Fax: 301-907-8906
e-mail: nddic@info.niddk.nih.gov
www.niddk.nih.gov

Explains the prevention, causes, symptoms, modes of transmission, and treatment of Hepatitis A.

16 pages

44 What I Need To Know About Hepatitis B
NDDIC
2 Information Way
Bethesda, MD 20892

301-654-3810
800-891-5389
Fax: 301-907-8906
e-mail: nddic@info.niddk.nih.gov
www.niddk.nih.gov

Explains the prevention, causes, symptoms, modes of transmission, and treatment of Hepatitis B.

16 pages

45 What I Need To Know About Hepatitis C
NDDIC
2 Information Way
Bethesda, MD 20892

301-654-3810
800-891-5389
Fax: 301-907-8906
e-mail: nddic@info.niddk.nih.gov
www.niddk.nih.gov

Explains the prevention, causes, symptoms, modes of transmission, and treatment of Hepatitis C.

16 pages

46 Why Do I Have Gas?
Nat'l Digestive Diseases Information Clearinghouse
2 Information Way
Bethesda, MD 20892

301-654-3810
Fax: 301-907-8906
e-mail: nddic@info.niddk.nih.gov
www.niddk.nih.gov

Magazines

47 Digestive Health & Nutrition
American Gastroenterological Association
4930 Del Ray Avenue
Bethesda, MD 20814

301-654-2055
Fax: 301-654-5920
www.dhn-online.org

Up-to-date news, tips and treatment information.

Daniel K Podolsky, President
David A Peura, VP

Journals

48 American Journal of Gastroenterology
American College of Gastroenterology
Po Box 342260
Bethesda, MD 20827

301-263-9000
www.acg.gi.org

Publishes scientific papers relevant to the practice of clinical gastroenterology, Features outstanding original research, review articles and consensus papers related to new drugs and therapeutic modalities.

Joel E Richter, Editor-In-Chief
Nicholas J Talley, Editor-In-Chief

49 Journal of Pediatric Gastroenterology and Nutrition
NASPGHAN, author

Lippincott Williams & Wilkins
530 Walnut Street
Philadelphia, PA 19106

215-521-8300
Fax: 215-521-8902
www.lww.com

Provides a forum for original papers and reviews dealing with nutrition in normal and abnormal functions of the alimentary tract and its associated organs including the salivary glands, pancreas, gallbladder, and liver. Particular emphasis is on development and its relation to infant and childhood nutrition.

Newsletters

50 Intestinal Fortitude
Intestinal Disease Foundation
100 W Station Square Drive
Pittsburgh, PA 15219

412-261-5888
877-587-9606
Fax: 412-471-2722
e-mail: info@intestinalfoundation.org
www.intestinalfoundation.org

Quarterly newsletter of the Intestinal Disease Foundation. News of seminars, volunteers and Pittsburgh area support groups.

51 NASPGHAN News
PO Box 6
Flourtown, PA 19031

215-233-0808
Fax: 215-233-3939
e-mail: naspghan@naspghan.org
www.naspgn.org

Publication of the North American Society for Pediatric Gastroenterolgy, Hepatology and Nutrition, which strives to improve the care of infants, children and adolescents with digestive disorders by promoting advances in clinical care of children with chronic abdominal pain, diarrhea, constipation, vomiting, bleeding from the GI tract, inflammatory bowel disease, liver diseases, diseases of the pancreas, poor weight gain and nutritional problems.

Pamphlets

52 Bleeding in the Digestive Tract
NDDIC
2 Information Way
Bethesda, MD 20892

301-654-3810
800-891-5389
Fax: 301-907-8906
e-mail: nddic@info.niddk.nih.gov
www.niddk.nih.gov

Includes information on the causes of bleeding in the digestive tract and how the bleeding is recognized, diagnosed, and treated.

6 pages

53 Cyclic Vomiting Syndrome
NDDIC
2 Information Way
Bethesda, MD 20892

301-654-3810
800-891-5389
Fax: 301-907-8906
e-mail: nddic@info.niddk.nih.gov
www.niddk.nih.gov

Describes the four phases of cyclic vomiting syndrome and the current treatment options available. outlines the complications asociated with the disorder and provides additional resources.

4 pages

54 Diagnostic Tests
NDDIC
2 Information Way
Bethesda, MD 20892

301-654-3810
800-891-5389
Fax: 301-907-8906
e-mail: nddic@info.niddk.nih.gov
www.niddk.nih.gov

Contains patient education fact sheets on seven diagnostic tests for gastrointestinal disorders (Colonoscopy, Sigmoidoscopy, Upper Endoscopy, Lower GI Series, ERCP, Liver Biopsy). Designed to be photocopy masters for health professionals to copy and distribute to patients.

55 Diarrhea
NDDIC
2 Information Way
Bethesda, MD 20892

301-654-3810
800-891-5389
Fax: 301-907-8906
e-mail: nddic@info.niddk.nih.gov
www.niddk.nih.gov

Includes general on diarrhea and what can cause it. Also provides information about diagnosis, treatment, and prevention.

6 pages

56 Diverticulosis & Diverticulitis
NDDIC
2 Information Way
Bethesda, MD 20892

301-654-3810
800-891-5389
Fax: 301-907-8906
e-mail: nddic@info.niddk.nih.gov
www.niddk.nih.gov

Provides clear definitions of diverticulosis and diverticulitis, along with information on symptoms, causes, complications, and treatments.

6 pages

57 Facts & Fallacies About Digestive Diseases
NDDIC
2 Information Way
Bethesda, MD 20892

301-654-3810
800-891-5389
Fax: 301-907-8906
e-mail: nddic@info.niddk.nih.gov
www.niddk.nih.gov

Provides information about common digestive disorders, including ulcers, inflammatory bowel disease, and constipation, in true/false format.

4 pages

58 Gallbladder and Biliary Tract Diseases
Nat'l Digestive Diseases Information Clearinghouse
2 Information Way
Bethesda, MD 20892

301-654-3810
Fax: 301-907-8906
e-mail: nddic@info.niddk.nih.gov
www.niddk.nih.gov

59 Gallstones
NDDIC
2 Information Way
Bethesda, MD 20892

301-654-3810
800-891-5389
Fax: 301-907-8906
e-mail: nddic@info.niddk.nih.gov
www.niddk.nih.gov

Provides general information on gallstones, including what causes them, who is at risk, and how they are diagnosed and treated.

6 pages

60 Gas in the Digestive Tract
NDDIC
2 Information Way
Bethesda, MD 20892

301-654-3810
800-891-5389
Fax: 301-907-8906
e-mail: nddic@info.niddk.nih.gov
www.niddk.nih.gov

Describes what causes gas, discusses the symptoms and the problems they cause, and provides information on treatment.

8 pages

61 Gastritis
Nat'l Digestive Diseases Information Clearinghouse
2 Information Way
Bethesda, MD 20892

301-654-3810
Fax: 301-907-8906
e-mail: nddic@info.niddk.nih.gov
www.niddk.nih.gov

62 Gastroesophageal Reflux Disease in Children
NDDIC
2 Information Way
Bethesda, MD 20892

301-654-3810
800-891-5389
Fax: 301-907-8906
e-mail: nddic@info.niddk.nih.gov
www.niddk.nih.gov

Describes gastroesophageal reflux (GER) in children and adolescents, including information about the causes, symptoms, and diagnosis of this condition, as well as its treatment.

4 pages

63 Heart Burn, Hiatal Hernia, and Gastroesophageal Reflux Disease
NDDIC
2 Information Way
Bethesda, MD 20892

301-654-3810
800-891-5389
Fax: 301-907-8906
e-mail: nddic@info.niddk.nih.gov
www.niddk.nih.gov

Defines gastroesophageal reflux disease (GERD) and describes the role of hiatal hernia. Provides general information on heartburn, as well as treatments for GERD, including surgery.

6 pages

64 Helicobacter Pylori and Peptic Ulcer
NDDIC
2 Information Way
Bethesda, MD 20892

301-654-3810
800-891-5389
Fax: 301-907-8906
e-mail: nddic@info.niddk.nih.gov
www.niddk.nih.gov

6 pages

65 Hemochromatosis
NDDIC
2 Information Way
Bethesda, MD 20892

301-654-3810
800-891-5389
Fax: 301-907-8906
e-mail: nddic@info.niddk.nih.gov
www.niddk.nih.gov

Provides information about the causes, risk factors, symptoms, diagnosis, treatment, diagnostic tests for, and current research about hemochromatosis. Includes a list of additional resources.

6 pages

66 Indigestion (Dyspepsia)
Nat'l Digestive Diseases Information Clearinghouse
2 Information Way
Bethesda, MD 20892

301-654-3810
Fax: 301-907-8906
e-mail: nddic@info.niddk.nih.gov
www.niddk.nih.gov

67 Irritable Bowel Syndrome
NDDIC
2 Information Way
Bethesda, MD 20892

301-654-3810
800-891-5389
Fax: 301-907-8906
e-mail: nddic@info.niddk.nih.gov
www.niddk.nih.gov

Describes causes, symptoms, tests to rule out more serious intestinal diseases, and lifestyle and medical approaches to syptom management.

4 pages

68   Irritable Bowel Syndrome (IBS) in Children
Nat'l Digestive Diseases Information Clearinghouse
2 Information Way
Bethesda, MD 20892

301-654-3810
Fax: 301-907-8906
e-mail: nddic@info.niddk.nih.gov
www.niddk.nih.gov

69   NDDIC News
NDDIC
2 Information Way
Bethesda, MD 20892

301-654-3810
800-891-5389
Fax: 301-907-8906
e-mail: nddic@info.niddk.nih.gov
www.niddk.nih.gov

Published twice a year by the clearinghouse. Features news from NDDIC, including new publications and reports on scientific meetings.

70   NSAIDs and Peptic Ulcer
Nat'l Digestive Diseases Information Clearinghouse
2 Information Way
Bethesda, MD 20892

301-654-3810
Fax: 301-907-8906
e-mail: nddic@info.niddk.nih.gov
www.niddk.nih.gov

71   Overview of Digestive Diseases
Nat'l Digestive Diseases Information Clearinghouse
2 Information Way
Bethesda, MD 20892

301-654-3810
Fax: 301-907-8906
e-mail: nddic@info.niddk.nih.gov
www.niddk.nih.gov

72   Short Bowel Syndrome
Nat'l Digestive Diseases Information Clearinghouse
2 Information Way
Bethesda, MD 20892

301-654-3810
Fax: 301-907-8906
e-mail: nddic@info.niddk.nih.gov
www.niddk.nih.gov

73   Travelers' Diarrhea
Nat'l Digestive Diseases Information Clearinghouse
2 Information Way
Bethesda, MD 20892

301-654-3810
Fax: 301-907-8906
e-mail: nddic@info.niddk.nih.gov
www.niddk.nih.gov

74   Ulcerative Colitis
NDDIC
2 Information Way
Bethesda, MD 20892

301-654-3810
800-891-5389
Fax: 301-907-8906
e-mail: nddic@info.niddk.nih.gov
www.niddk.nih.gov

Outlines the symptoms, diagnostic procedures, and risks and benefits of several drugs and kinds of surgery to treat this disease.

6 pages

75   Your Digestive System & How it Works
NDDIC
2 Information Way
Bethesda, MD 20892

301-654-3810
800-891-5389
Fax: 301-907-8906
e-mail: nddic@info.niddk.nih.gov
www.niddk.nih.gov

Provides general information about the organs of the digestive system, the digestive process, and the absorption of nutrients. Includes a list of additional readings.

6 pages

76   Zollonger-Ellison Syndrome
Nat'l Digestive Diseases Information Clearinghouse
2 Information Way
Bethesda, MD 20892

301-654-3810
Fax: 301-907-8906
e-mail: nddic@info.niddk.nih.gov
www.niddk.nih.gov

DESCRIPTION

77   ACUTE LYMPHOBLASTIC LEUKEMIA
Synonyms: Acute lymphocytic leukemia, ALL
Involves the following Biologic System(s):
Hematologic and Oncologic Disorders

Acute lymphoblastic leukemia (ALL) is a malignant disease characterized by excessive production of immature white blood cells known as lymphoblasts. ALL is the most common type of leukemia in children with a slightly higher incidence in boys. Although this type of leukemia may develop in adolescents or occasionally in adults, ALL occurs most commonly in children between 3 and 7 years of age.

Lymphoblasts are immature white cells that normally develop into lymphocytes primarily responsible for fighting infection.However, uncontrolled lymphoblast production associated with ALL results in their accumulation in the bone marrow, thus impairing the ability of the bone marrow to produce normal blood cells. In addition, lymphoblasts also proliferate in organs other than the marrow, particularly the liver, spleen, and lymph nodes. Children and young adults present with symptoms related to either direct infiltration of the marrow or other organs by leukemic cells or to the decreased production of normal marrow elements.These symptoms include loss of appetite (anorexia) and a generalized feeling of ill health (malaise), followed by fatigue and weakness resulting from decreased levels of circulating red blood cells (anemia). Bleeding from the gums or nose, easy bruising, and the development of small red or purple spots on the skin (petechiae) result from decreased levels of blood platelets (responsible for clotting); and infection and fever result from decreased levels of mature white blood cells. In addition, children with ALL may appear pale, experience headache and have bone or joint pain. Other findings include swollen lymph glands and an enlarged spleen (splenomegaly).

Acute lymphoblastic leukemia is believed to result from lymphoid precursor cells (ie, lymphoblasts) that are arrested in an early stage of development. This arrest is caused by a chromosomal change or genetic mutation resulting in uncontrolled cell division and subsequent overproduction of leukemic blood cells. Certain factors may place children at increased risk for developing ALL including Trisomy 21 (the chromosomal abnormality responsible for Down syndrome), certain genetic disorders such as Fanconi's anemia, exposure to radiation, some chemotherapy drugs, and certain chemicals such as benzene.

The diagnosis of ALL is established by demonstrating the presence of lymphoblasts in a bone marrow sample obtained through biopsy. Treatment for this type of leukemia is directed toward the destruction of leukemic cells through the administration of chemotherapy. Treatment for the presence of leukemic cells in the brain or the membranes surrounding the brain and spinal cord (meninges) may require the direct injection of the chemotherapy agent methotrexate through the spinal cord (intrathecal injection) into the cerebrospinal fluid. In addition, radiation may sometimes be administered to the brain. Supportive measures may include blood transfusions to alleviate anemia and bleeding irregularities, as well as the administration of antibiotics to treat infections resulting from the white cell abnormalities associated with both the disease and its treatment. Relapse after successful initial remission of ALL usually results from lymphoblastic infiltrates of the bone marrow and brain, and may necessitate the administration of an additional chemotherapeutic regimen. In addition, boys with recurring leukemic cells in the testes may require radiation therapy in addition to systemic chemotherapy. Bone marrow transplantation is used in patients with poor response to treatment. Greater than 50% of children with ALL can be cured with chemotherapy. Prognosis is related to age and white cell count at diagnosis.

See also **General Resources** on page 917

Government Agencies

78   NIH/National Cancer Institute
6116 Executive Boulevard, Room 3036A
Bethesda, MD 20892

800-422-6237
www.cancer.gov

The National Cancer Institute coordinates the National Cancer Program, which conducts and supports research, training, health information dissemination, and other programs with respect to the cause, diagnosis, prevention, and treatment of cancer, rehabilitation from cancer, and the continuing care of cancer patients and the families of cancer patients.

John E Niederhuber MD, Director

79   NIH/National Heart, Lung and Blood Institu te
National Institute of Health
31 Center Dr MSC 2486, Bldg 31, Room 5A48
Bethesda, MD 20892

301-592-8573
Fax: 240-629-3246
TTY: 240-629-3255
e-mail: NHLBIinfo@nhlbi.nih.gov
www.nhlbi.nih.gov

Primary responsibility of this organization is the scientific investigation of heart, blood vessel, lung and blood disorders. Oversees research, demonstration, prevention, education, control and training activities in these fields and emphasizes the prevention and control of heart diseases.

Elizabeth G Nabel, MD, Director
Susan Shurin, MD, Deputy Director

National Associations & Support Groups

80 B.A.S.E. Camp Children's Cancer Foundation
7501 Glenmoor Lane
Winter Park, FL 32792

407-673-5060
Fax: 407-673-5095
e-mail: email@basecamp.org
basecampcf.org

Provides a year round base of support for children and families facing the challenge of living with cancer, hemophilia and other blood related illnesses.

Terri Jones, Executive Director

81 Believe In Tomorrow- National Children's Foundation
6601 Frederick Road, PO Box 21243
Baltimore, MD 21228

410-744-1032
800-933-5470
Fax: 410-744-1984
e-mail: info@believeintomorrow.org
www.believeintomorrow.org

Provides exceptional hospital and retreat housing services to critically ill children and their families.

Brian Morrison, Founder & CEO
Michael R Murphy, President

82 Cancer Fund of America
2901 Breezewood Lane
Knoxville, TN 37921

865-938-5281
800-578-5284
www.cfoa.org

A nonprofit organization set up to help cancer patients, hospices and other healthcare providers by way of sending products free of charge directly to them.

James T Reynolds, President

83 CancerCare
275 7th Avenue
New York, NY 10001

212-712-8400
800-813-4673
Fax: 212-712-8495
e-mail: info@cancercare.org
www.cancercare.org

Dedicated to providing emotional support, information, and practical help to people with cancer and their loved ones. CancerCare is the oldest, largest, nonprofit agency devoted to offering professional services.

Diane S Blum, ACSW, Executive Director
Paul Friedman, Board President

84 Candlelighters Childhood Cancer Foundation
PO Box 498
Kensington, MD 20895

301-962-3520
800-366-2223
Fax: 310-962-3521
e-mail: staff@candlelighters.org
www.candlelighters.org

The Candlelighters Childhood Cancer Foundation National Office was founded in 1970 by concerned parents of children with cancer. Today our membership of over 50,000 members of the national office and more than 100,000 members across the across the country, including Candlelighters affiliate groups, includes, parents of children who are being treated or have been treated for cancer.

Ruth Hoffman, Executive Director

85 Child Life Council
11820 Parklawn Drive, Suite 240
Rockville, MD 20852

301-881-7090
Fax: 301-881-7092
e-mail: clcstaff@childlife.org
www.childlife.org

Professionals who strive to reduce the impact of stressful or traumatic life events and situations which affect the development, health and well being of infants, children, youth and families. They embrace the value of play as a healing modality while working to enhance the normal growth and development of children through assessment, intervention, prevention, advocacy and education. The council offers publications, annual conferences, professional certification and more.

Susan Krug, CMP, CAE, Executive Director

86 Childhood Cancer Foundation Candlelighters Canada
1300 Yonge Street, Suite 405
Toronto, Ontario,
Canada

416-489-6440
Fax: 416-489-9812
e-mail: info@childhoodcancer.ca
www.candlelighters.ca

The Childhood Cancer Foundation Candlelighters Canada is a national, volunteer governed, charitable organization dedicated to improving the quality of life for children with cancer and their families.

David Stones, President/CEO

87 Children's Blood Foundation
333 E 38th Street, Suite 830
New York, NY 10016

212-297-4336
Fax: 212-297-4340
e-mail: info@childrensbloodfoundation.org
www.childrensbloodfoundation.org

The foundation's major emphasis is on blood diseases affecting children: leukemia, thalassemia, hemophilia, sickle cell amenia, platelet disorders, retinoblastoma and AIDS.

John Calicchio, Chairman

88 Children's Leukemia Association
National Leukemia Research Association
585 Stewart Avenue, Suite 18
Garden City, NY 11530

516-222-1944
Fax: 516-222-0457
e-mail: info@childrensleukemia.org
www.childrensleukemia.org

A not-for-profit organization dedicated to raising funds to support research efforts towards finding the causes and cure for Leukemia.

Peter H Wiernik MD, Chairman

89 Dreams Come True Emery Clinic-Peds
1365 Clifton Road NE
Atlanta, GA 30322

778-248-3496

Serves any child with cancer or chronic blood disease treated at Emory University Homo/Onc Clinic. Dreams submitted by children.

90 Hair Club for Kids: Hair Club for Men
270 Farmington Avenue, Suite 232
Farmington, CT 06032

860-674-0202
888-888-8986
Fax: 860-676-0805
www.hairclub.com/kids

If your child expresses an interest in wearing a wig, send pictures prior to hair loss with snippets of hair for a good match of original color and texture. The cost of the wig may be covered by insurance.

Lydia Caffarino, Regional Manager

91 Just In Time
PO Box 27693
Philadelphia, PA 19118

215-247-8777
Fax: 215-247-0956
www.softhats.com

All cotton headwear for girls and women who have experienced hair loss.

92 Leukemia & Lymphoma Society
1311 Mamaroneck Avenue, Suite 310
White Plains, NY 10605

914-949-5213
Fax: 914-949-6691
www.lls.org

Largest voluntary health organization dedicated to funding blood cancer research, education and patient services.

Dwayne Howell PhD, President & CEO
Larry Hausner, Chief Operating Officer

93 National Bone Marrow Transplant Link
20441 W 12 Mile Road, Suite 108
Southfield, MI 48076

248-358-1886
800-546-5268
www.nbmtlink.org

Publications designed to help you understand and deal with the logistics of bone marrow transplantation, finances and medical insurance, information about the National Bone Marrow Transplant Link and its peer support program, and a celebration of BMT survivor stories.

Myra Jacobs, Executive Director
Tiffany Rowe, Director of Operations

94 National Childhood Cancer Foundation
4600 East West Highway, Suite 600
Bethesda, MD 20814

800-458-6223
e-mail: info@curesearch.org
www.curesearch.org

CureSearch unites the world's largest childhood cancer research organization, the Children's Oncology Group, and the National Childhood Cancer Foundation through our mission to cure childhood cancer. Research is the key to the cure.

95 National Coalition for Cancer Survivorship
1010 Wayne Road, Suite 770
Silver Spring, MD 20910

301-650-9127
877-622-7937
Fax: 301-565-9670
e-mail: info@canceradvocacy.org
www.canceradvocacy.org

Furnishes information about legal rights and advocacy services for cancer survivors of all ages. Publications include: Health Insurance and Cancer: What You Need to Know; Working It Out: Your Employment Rights As a Cancer Survivor; and Charting the Journey: An Almanac of Practical Resources for Cancer Survivors.

Ellen Stovall, President & CEO
Michael Bergin, Chief Operating Officer

State Agencies & Support Groups

North Carolina

96 Leukemia Society of America - North Carolina Chapter
Leukemia Society of America
5950 Fairview Road, Suite 250
Charlotte, NC 28210

704-998-5012
800-888-9934
Fax: 704-998-5010
www.leukemia.org

Dedicated to finding cures for leukemia and related cancers and to improving the quality of life for patients and their families.

Selena Rogers, Executive Director

Ohio

97 Leukemia Society of America - Central Ohio Chapter
Leukemia Society of America
2225 Citygate Drive, Suite E
Columbus, OH 43219

614-476-7194
800-686-CURE
Fax: 614-476-7189
www.leukemia.org

Dedicated to finding cures for leukemia and related cancers and to improving the quality of life for patients and their families.

William Carnes, Executive Director

98 Leukemia Society of America - Northern Ohio Chapter
Leukemia Society of America
902 Westpoint Parkway, Suite 300
Cleveland, OH 44145

440-617-2873
800-589-5721
Fax: 440-617-2879
www.leukemia.org

Dedicated to finding cures for leukemia and related cancers and to improving the quality of life for patients and their families.

Ann Stover, Executive Director

99 Leukemia Society of America - Southern Ohio Chapter
Leukemia Society of America
2300 Wall Street, Suite H
Cincinnati, OH 45212

513-361-2100
Fax: 513-361-2109
www.leukemia.org

Dedicated to finding cures for leukemia and related cancers and to improving the quality of life for patients and their families. This chapter serves a 22-county geographic area that includes Adams, Brown, Butler, Clermont, Clinton, Darke, Gallia, Greene, Hamilton, Highland, Jackson, Lawrence, Meigs, Miami, Montgomery, Pike, Preble, Scioto and Warren counties in Ohio and Boone, Campbell and Kenton counties in Kentucky.

Tonya S Blythe, Executive Director

Oklahoma

100 Leukemia Society of America - Oklahoma Chapter
Leukemia Society of America
500 N Broadway, Suite 250
Oklahoma City, OK 73102

405-943-8888
888-828-4572
Fax: 405-945-8355
www.leukemia.org

Dedicated to finding cures for leukemia and related cancers and to improving the quality of life for patients and their families.

Susan Walters, Executive Director

Oregon

101 Leukemia Society of America - Oregon Chapter
Leukemia Society of America
9320 SW Barbur Blvd, Suite 140
Portland, OR 97219

503-245-9866
800-466-6572
Fax: 503-245-9865
www.leukemia.org

Dedicated to finding cures for leukemia and related cancers and to improving the quality of life for patients and their families.

Gregory Knox, Executive Director

Pennsylvania

102 Leukemia Society of America - Western Pennsylvania/West Virginia Chapter
Leukemia Society of America
333 E Carson Street, Suite 441
Pittsburgh, PA 15219

412-263-2873
800-726-2873
Fax: 412-395-2888
www.leukemia.org

George Omiros, Executive Director

Tennessee

103 Leukemia & Lymphoma Society, Tennessee Chapter
404 BNA Drive, Suite 102
Nashville, TN 37217

615-331-2980
800-332-2980
Fax: 615-331-2941
e-mail: llstennchap@netscape
www.leukemia-lymphoma.org

To better serve the needs of Tennesseans - offers contribution-funded community services, family support groups, free educational materials and financial assistance for those affected by leukemia, Hodgkin's disease, myeloma and the lymphomas.

Karen Rudzinski, Executive Director
Barbara Burk

Texas

104 Leukemia Society of America - North Texas Chapter
Leukemia Society of America
8111 LBJ Freeway, Suite 425
Dallas, TX 75251

972-239-0959
800-800-6702
Fax: 972-239-0892
www.leukemia.org

Dedicated to finding cures for leukemia and related cancers and to improving the quality of life for patients and their families.

Richard Reader, Executive Director

105 Leukemia Society of America - South/West Texas Chapter
Leukemia Society of America
950 Isom Road
San Antonio, TX 78216

210-377-1775
800-683-2458
www.leukemia.org

Dedicated to finding cures for leukemia and related cancers and to improving the quality of life for patients and their families.

Cindy Atmar, Executive Director

106 Leukemia Society of America - Texas Gulf Coast Chapter
Leukemia Society of America
5005 Mitchelldale, Suite 115
Houston, TX 77092

281-680-8088
Fax: 281-683-9504

Dedicated to finding cures for leukemia and related cancers and to improving the quality of life for patients and their families.

Joan Jarrett, Executive Director

Virginia

107 Leukemia Society of America - National Capital Area Chapter
Leukemia Society of America
5845 Richmond Highway, Suite 800
Alexandria, VA 22303

703-960-1100
Fax: 703-960-0920
www.leukemia.org

Serves the greater Washington DC metropolitan area, including Northern Virginia, Prince George's and Montgomery counties.

David Timko, Executive Director

Wisconsin

108 Leukemia Society of America - Wisconsin Chapter
Leukemia Society of America
4125 North 124th Street, No A
Brookfield, WI 53005

262-790-4701
800-261-7399
Fax: 262-790-4706
www.leukemia.org

To serve Wisconsites touched by leukemia, lymphoma, Hodgkin's disease and myeloma.

Libraries & Resource Centers

South Carolina

109 Children's Center for Cancer and Blood Disorders
University of South Carolina School of Medicine
5 Richland Memorial Park
Columbia, SC 29203

803-777-7000

Joint clinical and basic research of juvenile cancer and blood disorders.

Dr. Robert S Ettinger, Director

Research Centers

110 International Bone Marrow Transplant Registry
Medical College of Wisconsin
8701 Watertown Plank Road, PO Box 26509
Milwaukee, WI 53226

414-456-8325
Fax: 414-456-6530
e-mail: cibmtr-contact@nmdp.org
www.ibmtr.org

Objectives are to develop and maintain databases of comprehensive clinical information regarding use and outcome of allogeneic and autologous bone marrow and peripheral blood transplants for cancer, to use this data for scientific studies addressing important issues in transplantation and to serve as an information resource for scientists, clinicians, patients and others involved in cancer treatment.

Sherry L Fisher, Associate Director, Development
Kim R Jackson, Senior Administrative Assistant

Audio Video

111 Childhood Cancer: Today's Crisis
Children's Hospital Medical Center
Elland Avenue
Cincinnati, OH 45229

513-559-4266

Video of how one family coped with their son's diagnosis of leukemia.

112 Coping with Childhood Cancer
Films for the Humanities and Sciences
PO Box 2053
Princeton, NJ 08543

800-257-5126
Fax: 609-275-3767
www.films.com

Presents open and honest interviews with five family members of childhood cancer patients. The stress on the family is intense; often, the brothers and sisters of children with cancer or any chronic life-threatening illness are most severely affected emotionally. The program provides caretakers and concerned adults with an insight into the coping mechanisms, and provides those who are themselves subject to such stress with a model of coping.

28 minutes
ISBN: B-VL2519- -

113 My Hair's Falling Out...Am I Still Pretty?
Necessary Pictures
7 W 20th Street, Suite 2F
New York, NY 10011

212-675-1809
800-221-3170

Moving film about two children with cancer who are hospital roommates. Using dance, animation and music, the video explores the feelings of the patients, families, and friends while it sensitively informs and educates the viewers about the emotional and physical aspects of childhood cancer. The child with leukemia grows up to become a doctor, while her roommate with a tumor dies. For school-age children and their families. Purchase is $25 for families and $79 for professionals.

22 minutes
ISBN: 0-965083-20-9

Web Sites

114 ALL Kids
www.all-kids.org/
ALL Kids is an Internet mailing list providing support for families and caregivers of children with Acute Lymphoblastic Leukemia.

115 CancerCare
www.cancercare.org
Provides information, and practical help to people with cancer and their loved ones.

116 CancerNet
cancernet.go
A part of the National Cancer Institute, offering information on types of cancer, cancer treatment, cancer prevention, genetics, and causes, and how to cope with cancer.

117 Children's Cancer Web
www.cancerindex.org/ccw
An independent nonprofit site, established to provide a directory of childhood cancer resources.

118 Leukemia and Lymphoma Society of America
www.leukemia.org
Is the largest voluntary health organization dedicated to funding blood cancer research, education and patient services. The mission is to cure leukemia, lymphoma, Hodgkin's disease and myeloma, and to improve the quality of life of patients and their families.

Book Publishers

119 Blood & Circulatory Disorders Sourcebook 2nd Edition
Omnigraphics
PO Box 625
Holmes, PA 19043

800-234-1340
Fax: 800-875-1340
e-mail: info@omnigraphics.com
www.omnigraphics.com

Basic consumer health information on blood and its components, anemias, leukemias, bleeding disorders, and circulatory disorders, including aplastic anemia, thalassemia, sickle-cell disease and hemophilia.

659 pages
ISBN: 0-780817-46-4

120 Childhood Leukemia: A Guide for Families, Friends & Caregivers
O'Reilly & Associates
1005 Gravenstein Highway North
Sebastopol, CA 95472

707-827-7000
800-998-9938
Fax: 707-829-0104
e-mail: patientguides@oreilly.com
www.oreilly.com

Features a wealth of tools to help parents become strong advocates for their child, detailed and precise medical information, and day-to-day practical advice to help cope with procedures, hospitalization, family and friends, schools, social, emotional and financial issues.

528 pages Softcover
ISBN: 0-596500-15-7

121 Draw Me a Picture
Cancervive
11636 Chayote Street
Los Angeles, CA 90049

310-203-9232
800-486-2873
Fax: 310-471-4618
e-mail: cancervivr@aol.com
www.cancervive.org

A fun coloring book for children with cancer (ages three to six). Marty Bunny talks about how it was when he was in the hospital for cancer and invites readers to draw about their experiences.

122 Going to the Hospital
Child Life Council
11820 Parklawn Drive, Suite 202
Rockville, MD 20852

301-881-7090
Fax: 301-881-7092
www.childlife.org

Describes what happens during a stay in the hospital, including some of the common forms of medical treatment.

123 Having Leukemia Isn't So Bad, of Course, It Wouldn't Be My First Choice
Sargasso Enterprises
18 Ginn Road
Winchester, MA 01890

781-729-9037
Fax: 781-729-2726
e-mail: cak@krumme.com

Personal story of Catherine Krumme, diagnosed with leukemia at age four, relapsed at age seven, finished treatment at age ten. Catherine graduated from college in 1998 and is a graduate student. The book is a supportive resource for families with cancer, for their friends, and for teachers working with children with health issues.

149 pages Softcover
ISBN: 0-963555-44-8

Ann Combs

124 Kathy's Hats: A Story of Hope
Albert Whitman and Company
6340 Oakton Street
Morton Grove, IL 60053

847-581-0033
800-255-7675
Fax: 847-581-0039
e-mail: mail@awhitmanco.com
www.awhitmanco.com

A charming book for ages five to ten about chemotherapy and the loss of Kathy's hair.

32 pages Hardcover
ISBN: 0-807541-16-8

Trudy Krisher, Author

125 Late Effects of Treatment for Childhood Cancer
John Wiley & Sons
1 Wiley Drive
Somerset, NJ 08875

732-469-4400
Fax: 732-302-2300
e-mail: custserv@wiley.com
www.wiley.com

Medical text for oncologists, radiologists, students.

200 pages
ISBN: 0-471561-66-5

126 Let's Talk About Going to the Hospital
Rosen Publishing Group's PowerKids Press
29 E 21st Street
New York, NY 10010

212-777-3017
800-237-9932
Fax: 888-436-4643
e-mail: rosenpub@tribeca.ios.com
www.powerkidspress.com

If a child has to check into the hospital, chances are he or she is already upset about being ill. Knowing how a hospital functions and what the procedures are, such as when family members can visit, will help in what is already a stressful situation. Grades K-5.

24 pages
ISBN: 0-823950-36-0

127 Non-Chew Cookbook
Wilson Publishing
PO Box 2190
Glenwood Springs, CO 81602

970-945-5600
Fax: 970-945-5600
e-mail: randyw@rof.net
www//.rof.net/yp/randyw

Contains recipes for patients unable to chew due to the side effects of chemotherapy and/or radiation.

200 pages

128 Pediatric Cancer Sourcebook
Omnigraphics
PO Box 625
Holmes, PA 19043

800-234-1340
Fax: 800-875-1340
e-mail: info@omnigraphics.com
omnigraphics.com

Basic consumer health information about leukemias, brain tumors, sarcomas, lymphomas and other cancers in infants, children and adolescents.

587 pages
ISBN: 0-780802-45-4

129 Surviving Childhood Cancer: A Guide for Families
New Harbinger Publications
5674 Shattuck Avenue
Oakland, CA 94609

510-652-0215
800-748-6273
Fax: 510-652-5472
e-mail: customerservice@newharbinger.com
newharbinger.com

Cancer in a child is an overwhelming experience for a family. This book explains common medical procedures and offers readers practical advice about how to cope with emotions and stress during this time.

1998 232 pages
ISBN: 1-572241-02-0

Magazines

130 Coping with Cancer Magazine
PO Box 682268
Franklin, TN 37068

615-790-2400
Fax: 615-794-0179
e-mail: info@copingmag.com
www.copingmag.com

A bimonthly publication devoted to people whose lives have been touched by cancer.

Newsletters

131 Friends Network
PO Box 4545
Santa Barbara, CA 93140

805-693-1017
e-mail: info@cancerfunletter.com
www.cancerfunletter.com

A national nonprofit organization which distributes an activities newsletter printed in color, called The Funletter, to children with cancer. We service all major cancer treatment centers throughout the United States.

Pamphlets

132 Resource Center for the American Alliance of Cancer - Pain Initiatives
Wisconsin Cancer Pain Initiative
1300 University Avenue, Room 4720
Madison, WI 53706

608-265-4013
Fax: 608-265-4014
e-mail: aacpi@mailplus.wisc.edu
www.aacpi.org

A booklet that helps parents determine if their child is in pain and provides methods to manage the pain. Single copy free. Also available, a Handbook of Cancer Pain Management, 5th edition.

12 pages Paperback

133 What Everyone Should Know About Leukemia
Leukemia and Lymphoma Society

800-955-4572

Written in easy-to-read terms with explanatory line drawings, this booklet explains leukemia, its symptoms, treatment and its probable causes.

16 pages

DESCRIPTION

134 ACUTE MYELOID LEUKEMIA
Synonyms: Acute granulocytic leukemia, Acute myeloblastic leukemia, Acute myelocytic leukemia, Acute myelogenous leukemia, Acute myelomonocytic leukemia, AML
Involves the following Biologic System(s):
Hematologic and Oncologic Disorders

Acute myeloid leukemia (AML), also called granulocytic, myelocytic, myeloblastic or myeloid leukemia — accounts for about 20 percent of childhood leukemias. It is a malignant disease characterized by excessive production in the bone marrow of certain cells called granulocytes, a type of white cell that normally fights infection. Although AML is primarily a disease of adulthood (median age at onset is 60 years), this disease accounts for approximately 20 percent of all childhood leukemias.

The symptoms and characteristic findings associated with acute myeloid leukemia result from the accumulation of myelocytes in the bone marrow, eventually impairing the bone marrow's ability to produce mature blood cells. In addition, myelocytes are released into the general blood circulation and carried to other organs where they continue to grow at a rapid rate. Children and young adults present with fatigue, abrupt onset of fever, lethargy, headache and bone and/or joint pain. Older adults have a slow, progressive onset, with lethargy, loss of appetite and shortness of breath. Other findings may include enlargement of the liver and spleen (hepatosplenomegaly) and swollen lymph glands. Some children may also exhibit swollen gums as well as swelling of the salivary glands in front of the ears. In addition, small leukemic cell tumors (chloromas) may develop under the skin or on the membranes surrounding the brain and spinal cord leading to inflammation of these membranes (meningitis). Most children with AML develop blood irregularities such as abnormally low levels of circulating red blood cells (anemia) and platelets (thrombocytopenia), although the white blood cell count may range from low to high.

Acute myeloid leukemia is thought to result from a chromosomal change or mutation in the genetic material of white blood cells. This mutation is thought to cause uncontrolled cell division and subsequent rapid increase in numbers of leukemic blood cells. Certain factors may place children and adults at increased risk for developing AML. Such factors include genetic disorders such as trisomy 21 (the chromosome abnormality responsible for Down syndrome), Bloom syndrome (small red lesions and sensitivity to light), Fanconi anemia, and certain other inherited disorders as well as a history of chemotherapy or radiation for earlier malignancies.

The diagnosis of AML is confirmed through the evaluation of a bone marrow sample obtained through biopsy. Treatment for this type of leukemia is directed initially toward the destruction of leukemic cells through the administration of combinations of chemotherapeutic drugs, followed with more chemotherapy to destroy any remaining leukemic cells. However, these potent drugs also suppress white blood cell production, thus increasing susceptibility to infection; therefore, antibiotic therapy is often given prophylactically and when a specific causative agent is identified. In some patients, transfusions of red bloodcells and platelets may also be indicated to alleviate anemia and bleeding irregularities. Additional chemotherapy may be initiated to destroy leukemic cells affecting the central nervous system or to prevent their recurrence. This type of treatment requires direct injection of medication into the spinal canal (intrathecal injection). Radiation may sometimes be administered directly to the central nervous system. Greater than 70% of adults younger than 60 achieve complete remission with treatment for AML; additional chemotherapy leads to cure in 30-40% of patients. For some patients, a bone marrow or cord blood transplant may offer the best chance for a long-term remission.

See also **General Resources** on page 917

Government Agencies

135 NIH/National Cancer Institute
6116 Executive Boulevard, Room 3036A
Bethesda, MD 20892

800-422-6237
www.cancer.gov

The National Cancer Institute coordinates the National Cancer Program, which conducts and supports research, training, health information dissemination, and other programs with respect to the cause, diagnosis, prevention, and treatment of cancer, rehabilitation from cancer, and the continuing care of cancer patients and the families of cancer patients.

John E Niederhuber MD, Director

136 NIH/National Heart, Lung and Blood Institu te
National Institute of Health
31 Center Dr MSC 2486, Bldg 31, Room 5A48
Bethesda, MD 20892

301-592-8573
Fax: 240-629-3246
TTY: 240-629-3255
e-mail: NHLBIinfo@nhlbi.nih.gov
www.nhlbi.nih.gov

Primary responsibility of this organization is the scientific investigation of heart, blood vessel, lung and blood disorders. Oversees research, demonstration, prevention, education, control and training activities in these fields and emphasizes the prevention and control of heart diseases.

Elizabeth G Nabel, MD, Director
Susan Shurin, MD, Deputy Director

National Associations & Support Groups

137 B.A.S.E. Camp Children's Cancer Foundation
7501 Glenmoor Lane
Winter Park, FL 32792

407-673-5060
Fax: 407-673-5095
e-mail: email@basecamp.org
basecampcf.org

Provides a year round base of support for children and families facing the challenge of living with cancer, hemophilia and other blood related illnesses.

Terri Jones, Executive Director

138 Cancer Fund of America
2901 Breezewood Lane
Knoxville, TN 37921

865-938-5281
800-578-5284
www.cfoa.org

A nonprofit organization set up to help cancer patients, hospices and other healthcare providers by way of sending products free of charge directly to them.

James T Reynolds, President

139 CancerCare
275 7th Avenue
New York, NY 10001

212-712-8400
800-813-4673
Fax: 212-712-8495
e-mail: info@cancercare.org
www.cancercare.org

Dedicated to providing emotional support, information, and practical help to people with cancer and their loved ones. CancerCare is the oldest, largest, nonprofit agency devoted to offering professional services.

Diane S Blum, ACSW, Executive Director
Paul Friedman, Board President

140 Candlelighters Childhood Cancer Foundation
PO Box 498
Kensington, MD 20895

301-962-3520
800-366-2223
Fax: 310-962-3521
e-mail: staff@candlelighters.org
www.candlelighters.org

The Candlelighters Childhood Cancer Foundation National Office was founded in 1970 by concerned parents of children with cancer. Today our membership of over 50,000 members of the national office and more than 100,000 members across the across the country, including Candlelighters affiliate groups, includes, parents of children who are being treated or have been treated for cancer.

Ruth Hoffman, Executive Director

141 Child Life Council
11820 Parklawn Drive, Suite 240
Rockville, MD 20852

301-881-7090
Fax: 301-881-7092
e-mail: clcstaff@childlife.org
www.childlife.org

Professionals who strive to reduce the impact of stressful or traumatic life events and situations which affect the development, health and well being of infants, children, youth and families. They embrace the value of play as a healing modality while working to

enhance the normal growth and development of children through assessment, intervention, prevention, advocacy and education. The council offers publications, annual conferences, professional certification and more.

Susan Krug, CMP, CAE, Executive Director

142 Children's Blood Foundation
333 E 38th Street, Suite 830
New York, NY 10016

212-297-4336
Fax: 212-297-4340
e-mail: info@childrensbloodfoundation.org
www.childrensbloodfoundation.org

The foundation's major emphasis is on blood diseases affecting children: leukemia, thalassemia, hemophilia, sickle cell anemia, platelet disorders, retinoblastoma and AIDS.

John Calicchio, Chairman

143 Children's Leukemia Association
National Leukemia Research Association
585 Stewart Avenue, Suite 18
Garden City, NY 11530

516-222-1944
Fax: 516-222-0457
e-mail: info@childrensleukemia.org
www.childrensleukemia.org

A not-for-profit organization dedicated to raising funds to support research efforts towards finding the causes and cure for leukemia.

Peter H Wiernik MD, Chairman

144 Dreams Come True Emery Clinic-Peds
1365 Clfton Road NE
Atlanta, GA 30322

778-248-3496

Serves any child with cancer or chronic blood disease treated at Emory University Homo/Onc Clinic. Dreams submitted by children.

145 Grant-A-Wish, The Children's Promise Foundation
PO Box 21211
Baltimore, MD 21228

410-744-1032
800-933-5470
Fax: 410-744-1984
e-mail: grant-a-wish@worldnet.att.net

Provides a variety of special services and programs (such as beach and mountain retreats or attending Orioles games) to any child up to 18 years of age who is being treated for cancer. Services are provided free of charge and are available on an ongoing basis throughout treatment.

146 Hair Club for Kids: Hair Club for Men
270 Farmington Avenue, Suite 232
Farmington, CT 06032

860-674-0202
888-888-8986
Fax: 860-676-0805
www.hairclub.com/kids

If your child expresses an interest in wearing a wig, send pictures prior to hair loss with snippets of hair for a good match of original color and texture. The cost of the wig may be covered by insurance.

Lydia Caffarino, Regional Manager

147 ICARE
International Cancer Alliance
4853 Cordell Avenue, Suite 14
Bethesda, MD 20814

301-656-3461
800-422-7361
www.icare.org

The International Care Alliance for Research and Education (ICARE) is a nonprofit organization which provies high-quality, focused, user-friendly, cancer information to each patient as well as their physician on an on-going, and person to person basis.

148 Just In Time
PO Box 27693
Philadelphia, PA 19118

215-247-8777
Fax: 215-247-0956
www.softhats.com

All cotton headwear for girls and women who have experienced hair loss.

149 Leukemia & Lymphoma Society
1311 Mamaroneck Avenue, Suite 310
White Plains, NY 10605

914-949-5213
Fax: 914-949-6691
www.lls.org

Largest voluntary health organization dedicated to funding blood cancer research, education and patient services.

Dwayne Howell PhD, President & CEO
Larry Hausner, Chief Operating Officer

150 National Bone Marrow Transplant Link
20441 W 12 Mile Road, Suite 108
Southfield, MI 48076

248-358-1886
800-546-5268
www.nbmtlink.org

Publications designed to help you understand and deal with the logistics of bone marrow transplantation, finances and medical insurance, information about the National Bone Marrow Transplant Link and its peer support program, and a celebration of BMT survivor stories.

Myra Jacobs, Executive Director
Tiffany Rowe, Director of Operations

151 National Coalition for Cancer Survivorship
1010 Wayne Road, Suite 770
Silver Spring, MD 20910

301-650-9127
877-622-7937
Fax: 301-565-9670
e-mail: info@canceradvocacy.org
www.canceradvocacy.org

Furnishes information about legal rights and advocacy services for cancer survivors of all ages. Publications include: Health Insurance and Cancer: What You Need to Know; Working It Out: Your Employment Rights As a Cancer Survivor; and Charting the Journey: An Almanac of Practical Resources for Cancer Survivors.

Ellen Stovall, President & CEO
Michael Bergin, Chief Operating Officer

State Agencies & Support Groups

New York

152 Leukemia Society of America - Westchester/ Hudson Valley Chapter
Leukemia Society of America
1311 Mamaroneck Avenue, Suite 130
White Plains, NY 10603

914-949-0084
Fax: 914-949-0391
www.leukemia.org

Dedicated to finding cures for leukemia and related cancers and to improving the quality of life for patients and their families.

Rochelle Kaufman, Executive Director

153 Leukemia Society of America - Western New York & Finger Lakes Chapter
Leukemia Society of America
4053 Maple Road, Suite 110
Amherstsville, NY 14226

716-834-2578
Fax: 716-837-0335
www.leukemia.org

Dedicated to finding cures for leukemia and related cancers and to improving the quality of life for patients and their families.

Nancy Hails, Executive Director

North Carolina

154 Leukemia Society of America - North Carolina Chapter
Leukemia Society of America
5950 Fairview Road, Suite 250
Charlotte, NC 28210

704-998-5012
800-888-9934
Fax: 704-998-5010
www.leukemia.org

Dedicated to finding cures for leukemia and related cancers and to improving the quality of life for patients and their families.

Selena Rogers, Executive Director

Ohio

155 Leukemia Society of America - Central Ohio Chapter
Leukemia Society of America
2225 Citygate Drive, Suite E
Columbus, OH 43219

614-476-7194
800-686-CURE
Fax: 614-476-7189
www.leukemia.org

Dedicated to finding cures for leukemia and related cancers and to improving the quality of life for patients and their families.

William Carnes, Executive Director

156 Leukemia Society of America - Northern Ohio Chapter
Leukemia Society of America
902 Westpoint Parkway, Suite 300
Cleveland, OH 44145

440-617-2873
800-589-5721
Fax: 440-617-2879
www.leukemia.org

Dedicated to finding cures for leukemia and related cancers and to improving the quality of life for patients and their families.

Ann Stover, Executive Director

157 Leukemia Society of America - Southern Ohio Chapter
Leukemia Society of America
2300 Wall Street, Suite H
Cincinnati, OH 45212

513-361-2100
Fax: 513-361-2109
www.leukemia.org

Dedicated to finding cures for leukemia and related cancers and to improving the quality of life for patients and their families. This chapter serves a 22-county geographic area that includes Adams, Brown, Butler, Clermont, Clinton, Darke, Gallia, Greene, Hamilton, Highland, Jackson, Lawrence, Meigs, Miami, Montgomery, Pike, Preble, Scioto and Warren counties in Ohio and Boone, Campbell and Kenton counties in Kentucky.

Tonya S Blythe, Executive Director

Oklahoma

158 Leukemia Society of America - Oklahoma Chapter
Leukemia Society of America
500 N Broadway, Suite 250
Oklahoma City, OK 73102

405-943-8888
888-828-4572
Fax: 405-945-8355
www.leukemia.org

Dedicated to finding cures for leukemia and related cancers and to improving the quality of life for patients and their families.

Susan Walters, Executive Director

Oregon

159 Leukemia Society of America - Oregon Chapter
Leukemia Society of America
9320 SW Barbur Blvd, Suite 140
Portland, OR 97219

503-245-9866
800-466-6572
Fax: 503-245-9865
www.leukemia.org

Dedicated to finding cures for leukemia and related cancers and to improving the quality of life for patients and their families.

Gregory Knox, Executive Director

Pennsylvania

160 Leukemia Society of America - Western Pennsylvania/West Virginia Chapter
Leukemia Society of America
333 E Carson Street, Suite 441
Pittsburgh, PA 15219

412-263-2873
800-726-2873
Fax: 412-395-2888
www.leukemia.org

George Omiros, Executive Director

Tennessee

161 Leukemia & Lymphoma Society, Tennessee Chapter
404 BNA Drive, Suite 102
Nashville, TN 37217

615-331-2980
800-332-2980
Fax: 615-331-2941
e-mail: llstennchap@netscape
www.leukemia-lymphoma.org

To better serve the needs of Tennesseans - offers contribution-funded community services, family support groups, free educational materials and financial assistance for those affected by leukemia, Hodgkin's disease, myeloma and the lymphomas.

Karen Rudzinski, Executive Director
Barbara Burk

Texas

162 Leukemia Society of America - North Texas Chapter
Leukemia Society of America
8111 LBJ Freeway, Suite 425
Dallas, TX 75251

972-239-0959
800-800-6702
Fax: 972-239-0892
www.leukemia.org

Dedicated to finding cures for leukemia and related cancers and to improving the quality of life for patients and their families.

Richard Reader, Executive Director

163 Leukemia Society of America - South/West Texas Chapter
Leukemia Society of America
950 Isom Road
San Antonio, TX 78216

210-377-1775
800-683-2458
www.leukemia.org

Dedicated to finding cures for leukemia and related cancers and to improving the quality of life for patients and their families.

Cindy Atmar, Executive Director

164 Leukemia Society of America - Texas Gulf Coast Chapter
Leukemia Society of America
5005 Mitchelldale, Suite 115
Houston, TX 77092

281-680-8088
Fax: 281-683-9504

Dedicated to finding cures for leukemia and related cancers and to improving the quality of life for patients and their families.

Joan Jarrett, Executive Director

Virginia

165 Leukemia Society of America - National Capital Area Chapter
Leukemia Society of America
5845 Richmond Highway, Suite 800
Alexandria, VA 22303

703-960-1100
Fax: 703-960-0920
www.leukemia.org

Serves the greater Washington DC metropolitan area, including Northern Virginia, Prince George's and Montgomery counties.

David Timko, Executive Director

Wisconsin

166 Leukemia Society of America - Wisconsin Chapter
Leukemia Society of America
4125 North 124th Street, No A
Brookfield, WI 53005

262-790-4701
800-261-7399
Fax: 262-790-4706
www.leukemia.org

To serve Wisconsites touched by leukemia, lymphoma, Hodgkin's disease and myeloma.

Libraries & Resource Centers

South Carolina

167 Children's Center for Cancer and Blood Disorders
University of South Carolina School of Medicine
5 Richland Memorial Park
Columbia, SC 29203

803-777-7000

Joint clinical and basic research of juvenile cancer and blood disorders.

Dr. Robert S Ettinger, Director

Audio Video

168 Childhood Cancer: Today's Crisis
Children's Hospital Medical Center
Elland Avenue
Cincinnati, OH 45229

513-559-4266

Video of how one family coped with their son's diagnosis of leukemia.

Web Sites

169 CancerCare
www.cancercare.org

Provides information, and practical help to people with cancer and their loved ones.

170 Children's Cancer Web
www.cancerindex.org/ccw

An independent nonprofit site, established to provide a directory of childhood cancer resources.

171 ICARE
www.icare.org

Provies high-quality, focused, user-friendly, cancer information.

172 Leukemia and Lymphoma Society of America
www.leukemia.org

Is the largest voluntary health organization dedicated to funding blood cancer research, education and patient services. The mission is to cure leukemia, lymphoma, Hodgkin's disease and myeloma, and to improve the quality of life of patients and their families.

173 Mediconsult
www.mediconsult.com

We are committed to provide excellent and professional services to our business partners. Through a team approach we will develop, provide and continuously improve our knowledge and competency. We work towards the betterment of healthcare delivery systems for the community.

Book Publishers

174 Blood & Circulatory Disorders Sourcebook 2nd Edition
Omnigraphics
PO Box 625
Holmes, PA 19043

800-234-1340
Fax: 800-875-1340
e-mail: info@omnigraphics.com
www.omnigraphics.com

Basic consumer health information on blood and its components, anemias, leukemias, bleeding disorders, and circulatory disorders, including aplastic anemia, thalassemia, sickle-cell disease and hemophilia.

659 pages
ISBN: 0-780817-46-4

175 Let's Talk About Going to the Hospital
Rosen Publishing Group's PowerKids Press
29 E 21st Street
New York, NY 10010

212-777-3017
800-237-9932
Fax: 888-436-4643
e-mail: rosenpub@tribeca.ios.com
www.powerkidspress.com

If a child has to check into the hospital, chances are he or she is already upset about being ill. Knowing how a hospital functions and what the procedures are, such as when family members can visit, will help in what is already a stressful situation. Grades K-5.

24 pages
ISBN: 0-823950-36-0

176 Let's Talk About when Kids Have Cancer
Rosen Publishing Group's PowerKids Press
29 E 21st Street
New York, NY 10010

212-777-3017
800-237-9932
Fax: 888-436-4643
e-mail: customerservice@rosenpub.com
www.powerkidspress.com

In a straightforward yet comforting way, this book explains what cancer is, what kinds of treatments surround the disease and how to cope if a child has cancer.

24 pages
ISBN: 0-823951-95-2

177 Pediatric Cancer Sourcebook
Omnigraphics
PO Box 625
Holmes, PA 19043

800-234-1340
Fax: 800-875-1340
e-mail: info@omnigraphics.com
omnigraphics.com

Basic consumer health information about leukemias, brain tumors, sarcomas, lymphomas and other cancers in infants, children and adolescents.

587 pages
ISBN: 0-780802-45-4

178 Surviving Childhood Cancer: A Guide for Families
New Harbinger Publications
5674 Shattuck Avenue
Oakland, CA 94609

510-652-0215
800-748-6273
Fax: 510-652-5472
e-mail: customerservice@newharbinger.com
newharbinger.com

Cancer in a child is an overwhelming experience for a family. This book explains common medical procedures and offers readers practical advice about how to cope with emotions and stress during this time.

1998 232 pages
ISBN: 1-572241-02-0

Pamphlets

179 Acute Lymphocytic Leukemia
Leukemia and Lymphoma Society
1311 Mamaroneck Avenue, Suite 310
White Plains, NY 10605

914-949-5213
Fax: 914-949-6691
www.lls.org

Information about acute lymphocytic leukemia for patients and their families and a glossary of terms to help readers understand technical terms.

16 pages

180 What Everyone Should Know About Leukemia
Leukemia and Lymphoma Society

800-955-4572

Written in easy-to-read terms with explanatory line drawings, this booklet explains leukemia, its symptoms, treatment and its probable causes.

16 pages

181 Let's Talk About when Kids Have Cancer
Rosen Publishing Group's PowerKids Press
29 E 21st Street
New York, NY 10010

212-777-3017
800-237-9932
Fax: 888-436-4643
e-mail: customerservice@rosenpub.com
www.powerkidspress.com

In a straightforward yet comforting way, this book explains what
cancer is, what kinds of treatments surround the disease and how to
cope if a child or the friend of a child has cancer.

24 pages
ISBN: 0-823951-95-2

DESCRIPTION

182 ALBINISM

Covers these related disorders: Tyrosinase negative albinism, Oculocutaneous albinism, Waardenburg syndrome

Involves the following Biologic System(s):
Dermatologic Disorders,
Genetic/Chromosomal/Syndrome/Metabolic Disorders

Albinism refers to a condition that is present at birth (congenital) and results when the body is unable to produce and distribute the pigment melanin, because of one of several possible genetic defects. This pigment is responsible for the coloration of the hair, skin, and eyes. Albinism occurs in about one in 20,000 individuals worldwide. Although there are many different types of albinism, two major forms known as tyrosinase negative and tyrosinase positive oculocutaneous (referring to the eyes and skin) albinisms have been identified.

Tyrosinase negative (type I albinism), the most severe form of generalized oculocutaneous albinism, results from the reduced or absent activity of the enzyme tyrosinase. This enzyme is essential to the proper metabolism of the pigment melanin. It is characterized by the absence of melanin in the hair, skin, and eyes. Other findings include white hair, pink or white skin, and eyes that may appear pink or bluish-gray. In addition, individuals with type I albinism often have other eye irregularities such as involuntary, flickering-type movements of the eyes (nystagmus), nearsightedness (myopia), sensitivity or intolerance to bright light (photophobia), or other visual abnormalities. Tyrosinase negative oculocutaneous albinism is due to a genetic defect in tyrosinase and is inherited as an autosomal recessive trait. A specific mutation of this gene is thought to cause a milder form of this type of albinismthat is prevalent among Amish communities in the United States. Individuals with this typealbinism have hair, skin, and eyes that tend to darken somewhat with age. In addition, eye irregularities are usually less severe.

Tyrosinase positive (type II) albinism is more common and less severe than type I. This type of albinism is thought to result from an inborn error in the transport of tyrosine, a chemical precursor of melanin. Newborns with this disorder may have little to no melanin at birth, but pigment may accumulate as these children grow, thus darkening the skin color during the course of childhood. In addition, visual improvements may become apparent as individuals mature. Tyrosinase positive albinism is inherited as an autosomal recessive trait. The gene for this type of albinism is located on chromosome 15. Several other types of tyrosinase positive albinism are thought to be caused by mutations of this gene. In addition, tyrosinase positive albinism may be present in association with several other disorders such as Hermansky-Pudlak syndrome, Chediak-Higashi syndrome, and Cross-McKusick-Breen syndrome.

Other forms of albinism may include ocular albinism that mainly affects the pigment of the eyes and is characterized by photophobia; nystagmus; and decreased visual acuity. The hair and eyes may be light although not excessively light in color. Ocular albinism may be inherited as an X-linked trait as in Nettleship-Falls type ocular albinism and Forsius-Eriksson syndrome, or as an autosomal dominant or autosomal recessive trait. In addition, some individuals may have partial albinism, sometimes called piebaldism that is characterized by the appearance of patchy, unpigmented areas of hair or skin. In some individuals, this type of albinism may only have a lock of white hair near the forehead. Piebaldism is inherited as an autosomal dominant trait and may be part of Waardenburg syndrome, which is associated with hearing impairment.

Treatment for albinism is dependent upon the severity of the physical findings. People with albinism are at increased risk for skin cancer resulting from sun exposure; therefore, appropriate sunscreen (SPF = 15) or avoidance of direct sunlight on the skin is crucial. In addition, lack of pigment in the eyes may indicate the need for tinted or dark glasses to help reduce light sensitivity. Early evaluation and treatment for other visual irregularities is necessary so that affected children may overcome potential difficulties in school. Other treatment is symptomatic and supportive.

See also **General Resources** on page 917

Government Agencies

183 NIH/National Institute of Child Health and Human Development
31 Center Drive, Building 31
Bethesda, MD 20892

301-496-5133
Fax: 301-496-1104
www.nichd.nih.gov

Established in 1962 by congress, today the institute conducts and supports research on topics related to the health of children, adults, families and populations. Some of these topics include: developmental disabilities, growth and development, infant death, reproductive health and birth defects.

Nancy D Wirth, Director
Lisa Kaeser, Program & Public Liaison

National Associations & Support Groups

184 American Council of the Blind
1155 15th Street, NW, Suite 1004
Washington, DC 20005

202-467-5081
800-424-8666
Fax: 202-467-5085
www.acb.org

The council strives to improve the well being of all blind and visually impaired people by serving as a representative national organization of blind people, elevating the social, ecomonic and cultural levels of blind people, improving educational and rehabilitation facilities and opportunities and cooperating with the public and private institutions and organizations concerned with blind services.

Melanie Brunson, Executive Director

185 American Foundation for the Blind
11 Penn Plaza, Suite 300
New York, NY 10001

212-502-7600
800-232-5463
Fax: 212-502-7777
e-mail: arbinfo@afb.net
www.afb.org

The Amcican Foundation of the Blind, has been eliminating barriers the prevent people who are blind or visually impaird from reaching their potential. AFB is dedicated to addressing the most critical issues of facing this growing population: independent living, literacy, employment, and technology.

Carl R Augusto, President & CEO

186 Genetic Alliance
4301 Connecticut Avenue NW
Washington, DC 20008

202-966-5557
800-336-4363
Fax: 202-966-8553
e-mail: info@geneticalliance.org
www.geneticalliance.org

A coalition of voluntary genetic support groups, consumers and professionals addressing the needs of individuals and families affected by genetic disorders from a national perspective.

Sharon Terry, President/CEO

187 Hermansky-Pudlak Syndrome Network
One South Road
Oyster Bay, NY 11771

516-922-3440
800-789-9477
Fax: 516-922-4022
e-mail: appell@worldnet.att.net
www.medhelp.org/web/hpsn.htm

A volunteer, nonprofit, self-help support group for persons and families dealing with the syndrome. Assists in networking families and doctors, maintains a bibliography of materials and promotes research.

Donna Jean Appell, Founder & President

188 Natalie's Way Foundation
16 Lyle Court
Staten Island, NY 10306

718-351-0806
e-mail: admin@natalieswayfoundation.com
www.ourwebpage.org/nwf

Conducts fundraising for research into albinism and children's eye disorders.

Robert Stasi, President
Annette Stasi, VP

189 National Mental Health Consumers' Self-Help Clearinghouse
1211 Chestnut Street, Suite 1207
Philadelphia, PA 19107

215-751-1810
800-553-4539
Fax: 215-636-6312
e-mail: info@mhselfhelp.org
www.mhselfhelp.org

Offers information, support and appropriate referrals; and promotes public and professional education. Provides networking for those with special interests related to albinism. Promotes and supports research and funding that will improve diagnosis and management of albinism and hypopigmentation.

Joseph Rogers, Executive Director & Founder

190 National Organization for Albinism and Hypopigmentation
PO Box 959
East Hampstead, NH 03826

603-887-2310
800-473-2310
Fax: 800-648-2310
e-mail: info@albinism.org
www.albinism.org

Presents data for individuals and their families for the commonly asked questions through several media options.

Mike McGowan, President

191 Positive Exposure
Rick Guidotti
43 E 20th Street, 6th Floor
New York, NY 10003

212-420-1931
Fax: 212-228-0592
e-mail: rick@positiveexposure.org
www.rickguidotti.com

Utilizes photography and video interviews to investigate the social and psychological experiences of people with albinism of all ages and ethnocultural heritages. This innovative program challenges the stigma associated with difference, attacks public fears about difference and celebrates the richness of genetic variation.

Rick Guidotti, Director & Photographer

192 Society for Pediatric Dermatology
8365 Keystone Crossing, Suite 107
Indianapolis, IN 46240

317-202-0224
Fax: 317-205-9841
e-mail: spd@hp-assoc.com
www.pedsderm.net

The objective of the Society is to promote, develop and advance education, research and care of skin disease in all pediatric age groups.

Kent Lindeman, Executive Director

193 Vision of Children Foundation
12671 High Bluff Drive, Suite 300
San Diego, CA 92130

858-799-0810
Fax: 858-794-2348
e-mail: sdurso@visionofchildren.org
www.visionofchildren.org

Provides information, promotes research and assists the families of blind and visually impaired children, including those with ocular albinism, in locating organizations and service providers who can give support.

Samuel A Hardage, Chairman & Co-Founder
Vivian L Hardage, Chairman & Co-Founder

Conferences

194 Annual World Symposium on Ocular Albinism
12671 High Bluff Drive, Suite 300
San Diego, CA 92130

858-799-0810
Fax: 858-794-2348
e-mail: sdurso@visionofchildren.org
www.visionofchildren.org

The Vision of Children Foundation's team of doctors, scientists and researchers will collaborate on their research efforts in Ocular Albinism.

March

Samuel A Hardage, Chairman & Co-Founder
Vivian L Hardage, Chairman & Co-Founder

195 Hermansky-Pudlak Syndrome Network Annual Family Conference
One South Road
Oyster Bay, NY 11771

516-922-3440
800-789-9477
Fax: 516-922-4022
e-mail: appell@worldnet.att.net
www.medhelp.org/web/hpsn.htm

A volunteer, nonprofit, self-help support group for persons and families dealing with the syndrome. Assists in networking families and doctors, maintains a bibliography of materials and promotes research.

Donna Jean Appell, Founder & President

196 National Organization for Albinism and Hypopigmentation Bi-Annual Conference
PO Box 959
East Hampstead, NH 03826

603-887-2310
800-473-2310
Fax: 800-648-2310
e-mail: info@albinism.org
www.albinism.org

To be held in Las Vegas.

July 2008

Audio Video

197 Assistive Media
400 Maynard Street, Suite 404
Ann Arbor, MI 48104

734-332-0369
e-mail: info@assistivemedia.org
www.assistivemedia.org/

The mission of Assistive Media is to heighten the educational, cultural, and quality-of-living standard for people with disabilites and help achieve independence and become better integrated within the mainstream of society and community life in general. Assistve Media accomplishes this by providing free-of-charge, copyright-approved, high caliber audio literary works to the world-wide disability community via the internet effectively, inexpensively, and efficiently.

David Henry Erdody, Founder

Web Sites

198 International Albinism Center
www.cbc.umn.edu/iac/

Is a team of dedicated research professionals interested in understanding the basis of albinism in humans. We are a munlti-disciplinary group of researchers that include interests in clinical genetics, molecular biology, ophthalmology, dermatology, and biochemistry, all with a central theme of understnading the cause and effect of albinism and other forms of pigment loss in humans.

Newsletters

199 Hermansky-Pudlak Syndrome Network Newsletter
One South Road
Oyster Bay, NY 11771

516-922-3440
800-789-9477
Fax: 516-922-4022
e-mail: appell@worldnet.att.net
www.medhelp.org/web/hpsn.htm

A volunteer, nonprofit, self-help support group for persons and families dealing with the syndrome. Assists in networking families and doctors, maintains a bibliography of materials and promotes research.

Donna Jean Appell, Founder/President

DESCRIPTION

200 ALOPECIA AREATA

Synonyms: Alopecia circumscripta, Androgenetic alopecia, Pelade

Involves the following Biologic System(s):

Dermatologic Disorders, Immunologic and Rheumatologic Disorders

Alopecia is partial or complete loss of hair (baldness) and may result from genetic factors, aging or local or systemic disease. Alopecia areata is characterized by the sudden, localized loss of patches of scalp hair and other areas of hair growth, such as the eyelashes and eyebrows. These patches are usually well-defined, round or oval in shape, and most often appear on the scalp or beard area. On rare occasions, progression of hair loss may result in the total loss of scalp hair in a condition called alopecia totalis. If the disease progresses to include the total loss of both scalp and body hair, the condition is called alopecia universalis. Another uncommon form of alopecia areata called ophiasis involves the loss of hair in a continuous band around the head. If hair loss associated with alopecia areata is not widespread, the condition is usually reversible, with most patients exhibiting new hair growth within a few months to a year; however, recurrences are quite common. Children who develop this condition at a very young age, patients who experience recurring episodes, and those who have extensive involvement are less likely to experience spontaneous remission. Although this disease occurs most commonly in the adult population, approximately 20 percent of those affected develop the disorder between birth and 20 years of age. This type of hair loss is different than male pattern baldness, an inherited condition.

Although the skin in the area of hair loss may appear unremarkable, microscopic examination may reveal the presence of inflammation. In addition, some individual hairs that appear at the margins of the bald, patchy areas may be easily removed and, upon microscopic examination, reveal a lightly-pigmented, tapered hair shaft that ends in a hair root that is reduced in size (exclamation hairs). Symptoms or characteristic findings sometimes associated with alopecia areata include the development of irregularities such as nail pitting and ridging, allergic or hypersensitivity reactions, and opacities of the lenses of the eye (cataracts). Alopecia areata may also be associated with certain autoimmune diseases such as Addison disease, Hashimoto thyroiditis, vitiligo, and others. In addition, approximately seven percent of children with Trisomy 21 exhibit the symptoms associated with alopecia areata.

The exact cause of alopecia areata is not known; however, approximately 25 percent of those affected are believed to inherit the disease through autosomal dominant transmission. Other suggested causes include autoimmune responses or emotional factors related to stress. Because alopecia areata so often resolves spontaneously, treatment for this disease in young children may simply include ongoing observation. A variety of treatments can be tried. Steroid injections and cream to the scalp have been used for many years. Other medications include minoxidil, irritants (anthralin or topical coal tar), and topical immunotherapy (cyclosporine), each of which are sometimes used in different combinations. The use of hairpieces and other cosmetic considerations may be beneficial to the emotional well-being of children, especially adolescents, with alopecia areata.

See also **General Resources** on page 917

National Associations & Support Groups

201 Alopecia Areata Research Foundation

PO Box 150760
San Rafael, CA 94915

415-472-3780
Fax: 415-472-5343
e-mail: info@naaf.org
www.naaf.org

To support research to find a cure or acceptable treatment for alopecia areata and to support those with the disease and to educate the public about alopecia areata.

Sandy Frum, Chairman
Vicki Kalabokes, President & CEO

202 National Alopecia Areata Foundation

PO Box 150760
San Rafael, CA 94915

415-472-3780
Fax: 415-472-5343
www.alopeciaareata.com

Funds research, provides local support and education for people with alopecia areata and their families, informs the public about alopecia areata and advocates for people affected by alopecia areata.

Sandy Frum, Chairman
Vicki Kalabokes, President & CEO

203 Society for Pediatric Dermatology

8365 Keystone Crossing, Suite 107
Indianapolis, IN 46240

317-202-0224
Fax: 317-205-9841
e-mail: spd@hp-assoc.com
www.pedsderm.net

National organization dedicated to promote, develop and advance education, research and care of skin disease in all pediatric age groups.

Kent Lindeman, Executive Director

DESCRIPTION

204 ALPHA-1-ANTITRYPSIN DEFICIENCY
Involves the following Biologic System(s):
Gastrointestinal Disorders,
Genetic/Chromosomal/Syndrome/Metabolic Disorders,
Respiratory Disorders

Alpha-1-antitrypsin (AAT) deficiency is a hereditary metabolic disorder characterized by deficiency of alpha-1-antitrypsin, an enzyme that is produced by the liver and inhibits the actions of other enzymes that break down certain proteins. Deficiency of alpha-1-antitrypsin may result in emphysema, a progressive destructive change in the lungs. In addition, some patients may experience liver disease that is thought to result from abnormal retention of the alpha-1-antitrypsin enzyme in liver cells. Alpha-1-antitrypsin deficiency is caused by certain changes (mutations) of a gene known as Pi (protease inhibitor). Alpha-1-antitrypsin deficiency is typically inherited as an autosomal recessive trait due to inheritance of two deficiency-causing genes (homozygosity).

The specific symptoms associated with alpha-1-antitrypsin deficiency as well as the age of onset vary from patient to patient. Shortly after birth, a small percentage of affected children may develop suppression or cessation of the flow of bile (neonatal cholestasis). Bile, a liquid secreted by the liver, carries waste products away from the liver and assists in the digestion of fats in the small intestine. During the first week of life, affected infants may have yellowish discoloration of the skin, whites of the eyes, and mucous membranes (jaundice); abnormal enlargement of the liver (hepatomegaly); and the presence of unabsorbed fat in the feces. Jaundice often spontaneously resolves within two to four months after birth. Affected infants and children may appear to have no further associated symptoms (asymptomatic), may have chronic liver disease, or, in the most severe cases, may experience scarring of the liver and gradual impairment of liver function (cirrhosis). Older children may develop chronic liver disease or cirrhosis and associated high blood pressure within veins from the spleen and intestines to the liver (portal hypertension). In some patients with portal hypertension, there may be a diversion of portal circulation to veins in the walls of the stomach and esophagus, causing abnormal widening of such blood vessels (esophageal varices). Without treatment, some patients with liver disease may experience potentially life-threatening complications.

In general, AAT deficiency leads to emphysema, progressive degeneration of and destructive changes in the air sacs (alveoli) of the lungs in the fourth decade of life in smokers and a decade later in nonsmokers. (emphysema).

In children with alpha-1-antitrypsin deficiency, the treatment of associated liver disease is primarily symptomatic and supportive. AAT deficiency is the main cause of liver transplantation in children. Preventing or slowing the progression of lung disease is the major goal of AAT deficiency management. No treatment for emphysema has a greater effect on survival than quitting smoking. Other options include prompt, aggressive treatment of respiratory infections and provision of oxygen therapy. Medications are available to improve lung function. In addition, patients should avoid exposure to tobacco smoke, aerosol sprays, and other lung irritants. Alpha-1-antitrypsin enzyme replacement therapy (e.g., prolastin therapy) is also available. Two surgical approaches may help selected patients with AAT deficiency - volume-reduction surgery and lung transplantation.

See also **General Resources** on page 917

National Associations & Support Groups

205 Alpha-1 Association
2937 SW 27 Avenue, Suite 106
Miami, FL 33133

305-648-0088
800-521-3025
Fax: 305-648-0089
e-mail: info@alpha1.org
www.alpha1.org

Founded to identify those affected and to improve the quality of their lives through support, education, advocacy, and research

Marlene Erven, Exutive Director

206 American Liver Foundation
75 Maiden Lane, Suite 603
New York, NY 10038

212-668-1000
800-465-4837
Fax: 212-483-8179
e-mail: info@liverfoundation.org
www.liverfoundation.org

The American Liver Foundation is the nation's leading nonprofit organization promoting liver health and disease prevention. ALF provides research,education and advocacy for those affecte by liver-related diseases, incluing hepatitis.

Frederick G. Thompson, President/CEO
Gerald Jeglinski, Chief Operating Officer

207 American Lung Association
61 Broadway, 6th Floor
New York, NY 10006

212-315-8700
800-586-4872
www.lungusa.org

The American Lung Association fights lung disease in all its forms, with special emphasis on asthma, tobacco control and environmental health. The American Lung Association is funded with contributions from the public, along with gifts and grants from corporations, foundations and government agencies. The association achieves its many successes through the work of thousands of committed volunteers and staff.

Terri E Weaver, PhD RN CS FAAN, Chairman

208 Children's Liver Alliance
3835 Richmond Avenue, Suite 190
Staten Island, NY 10312

718-987-6200
Fax: 718-987-6200
www.liverkids.tk

Aids in easing the physical and emotional strains that the child is experiencing, so they can better deal with the disorder, through different media resources that are also available to both family and friends.

Kathie DeLuca, Office Manager

209 Children's Liver Association for Support Services
27023 McBean Parkway, #126
Valencia, CA 91355

661-263-9099
877-679-8256
Fax: 661-263-9099
e-mail: supportsru@aol.com
www.classkids.org

CLASS is an all volunteer, nonprofit organization dedicated to serving the emotional, educational and financial needs of families coping with childhood liver disease and transplantation. Our goal is to be both a service to families and a valuable resource for the medical community.

Diane Sumner, President
Ann Whitehead, VP

210 Genetic Alliance
4301 Connecticut Avenue NW
Washington, DC 20008

202-966-5557
800-336-4363
Fax: 202-966-8553
e-mail: info@geneticalliance.org
www.geneticalliance.org

A coalition of voluntary genetic support groups, consumers and professionals addressing the needs of individuals and families affected by genetic disorders from a national perspective.

Sharon Terry, President/CEO

211 March of Dimes Birth Defects Foundation
1275 Mamaroneck Avenue
White Plains, NY 10605

914-428-7100
888-663-4637
Fax: 914-428-8203
e-mail: resourcecenter@modimes.org
www.marchofdimes.com

Partnership of volunteers and professionals dedicates to improving the health of babies by preventing birth defects and infant mortality. Over 100 chapters are located across the country and can be located through the National Office.

Dr Jennifer Howse, President

Web Sites

212 Children's Liver Alliance
www.livertx.org

213 Children's Liver Association for Support Services
www.classkids.org

Information for families coping with childhood liver disease and transplantation.

214 Online Mendelian Inheritance in Man
www.ncbi.nlm.nih.gov

This database is a catalog of human genes and genetic disorders.

Book Publishers

215 Let's Talk About Going to the Hospital
Rosen Publishing Group's PowerKids Press
29 E 21st Street
New York, NY 10010

212-777-3017
800-237-9932
Fax: 888-436-4643
e-mail: rosenpub@tribeca.ios.com
www.powerkidspress.com

If a child has to check into the hospital, chances are he or she is already upset about being ill. Knowing how a hospital functions and what the procedures are, such as when family members can visit, will help in what is already a stressful situation. Grades K-5.

24 pages
ISBN: 0-823950-36-0

Newsletters

216 Children's Liver Alliance Newsletter
3835 Richmond Avenue, Suite 190
Staten Island, NY 10312

718-987-6200
Fax: 718-987-6200

Aids in easing the physical and emotional strains that the child is experiencing, so they can better deal with the disorder, through different media resources that are also available to both friends and family.

4-12 pages

Kathie DeLuca, Office Manager

DESCRIPTION

217 ANENCEPHALY

Involves the following Biologic System(s):

Neurologic Disorders

Anencephaly is an abnormality that is present at birth (congenital) and belongs to a group of birth defects known as neural tube defects. This condition is characterized by the absence of a major portion of the brain, skull, and scalp. Approximately one of 1,000 infants is born with anencephaly.

During the early stages of pregnancy, a specialized layer of tissue extends along the back portion of the developing embryo. As the embryo grows, this tissue, known as the neural plate, forms a groove that is bordered by folds. This groove eventually deepens and closes to form the neural tube. Later in development, the neural tube gives rise to tissue that later forms the brain and spinal cord. The neural tube is surrounded and protected by the bones of the back (vertebrae). Failure in this sequence of developmental events results in a neural tube defect.

Anencephaly represents a type of neural tube defect that is incompatible with life. Infants with this disorder are born without a forebrain, the largest part of the brain consisting mainly of the cerebral hemispheres which are responsible for higher level cognition, i.e., thinking. The remaining brain tissue is often exposed - not covered by bone or skin. Infants born with anencephaly are usually blind, deaf, unconscious, and unable to feel pain. Additional physical findings associated with this abnormality include folded ears, incomplete closure of the palate (cleft palate), and congenital heart defects. The cause of anencephaly is unknown, although it is thought to occur as the result of genetic or environmental factors, alone or in combination. Neural tube defects do not follow direct patterns of heredity. However, the theory of a genetic predisposition to anencephaly is supported by the fact that the risk of additional children being born with this defect rises with each pregnancy.

Supplementation with high-dose folic acid, initiated before and given during pregnancy, reduces the risk of neural tube defects to 1%.

See also **General Resources** on page 917

Government Agencies

218 NIH/National Institute of Child Health and Human Development
31 Center Drive, Building 31
Bethesda, MD 20892

301-496-5133
Fax: 301-496-1104
www.nichd.nih.gov

Established in 1962 by congress, today the institute conducts and supports research on topics related to the health of children, adults, families and populations. Some of these topics include: developmental disabilities, growth and development, infant death, reproductive health and birth defects.

Nancy D Wirth, Director
Lisa Kaeser, Program & Public Liaison

National Associations & Support Groups

219 Anencephaly Support Foundation
30827 Sifton
Spring, TX 77386

281-364-9222
888-206-7526
e-mail: info@asfhelp.com
www.asfhelp.com

A nonprofit religious foundation dedicated to serving parents, families and educational communities. Offered are information, personal stories and medical articles regarding the neural tube defect of anencephaly, support and encouragement to parents who have chosen to carry an anencephalic pregnancy to term, and information regarding possible causations, prevention theories, and support group referrals.

220 Birth Defect Research for Children
930 Woodcock Road, Suite 225
Orlando, FL 32803

407-895-0802
Fax: 407-895-0824
e-mail: staff@birthdefects.org
www.birthdefects.org

Organization that helps families with free birth defect information, parent matching that links families of children with similar defects and research through the National Birth Defect Registry to discover the causes of birth defects. Support group information and newsletter on Internet.

Betty Mekdeci, Executive Director

221 Fighters for Encephaly Support Group
332 Brereton Street
Pittsburgh, PA 15219

412-261-5363

222 Genetic Alliance
4301 Connecticut Avenue NW
Washington, DC 20008

202-966-5557
800-336-4363
Fax: 202-966-8553
e-mail: info@geneticalliance.org
www.geneticalliance.org

A coalition of voluntary genetic support groups, consumers and professionals addressing the needs of individuals and families affected by genetic disorders from a national perspective.

Sharon Terry, President/CEO

223 March of Dimes Birth Defects Foundation
1275 Mamaroneck Avenue
White Plains, NY 10605

914-428-7100
888-663-4637
Fax: 914-428-8203
e-mail: resourcecenter@modimes.org
www.marchofdimes.com

Partnership of volunteers and professionals dedicates to improving the health of babies by preventing birth defects and infant mortality. Over 100 chapters are located across the country and can be located through the National Office.

Dr Jennifer Howse, President

224 National Dissemination Center for Children with Disabilities
PO Box 1492
Washington, DC 20013

202-884-8200
800-695-0285
Fax: 202-884-8441
e-mail: nichcy@aed.org
www.nichcy.org

A national information and referral center for families, educators and other professionals on: disabilities in children and youth; programs and services; IDEA, the nation's special education law; and research-based information on effective practices.

Suzanne Ripley, Executive Director

Web Sites

225 Online Mendelian Inheritance in Man
www.ncbi.nlm.nih.gov

This database is a catalog of human genes and genetic disorders.

226 Rare Genetic Diseases in Children (NYU)
www.med.nyu.edu/rgdc/homenow.htm

We target issues arising from rare genetic diseases affecting children. And to assist in the endeavor to bring knowledge and hope to those for whom there is, at present, so little.

DESCRIPTION

227   ANIRIDIA

Synonym: Hypoplasia of iris

Involves the following Biologic System(s):

Ophthalmologic Disorders

Aniridia is a birth defect characterized by absence of all or a portion of the colored area of the eye (iris). Both eyes are typically affected (bilateral aniridia). The term aniridia may be a misnomer, since an undeveloped (vestigial) portion of the iris is usually present (i.e., apparent upon slit-lamp examination or gonioscopy). The iris is an involuntary circular muscle that is visible through the transparent, front portion of the eye (cornea). When certain fibers in the iris contract, the hole in the center of the iris (pupil) either widens or constricts, allowing in additional or less light.

In some infants with aniridia, the corneas of the eyes are also abnormally small. In addition, many affected infants and children experience loss of transparency of the lenses of the eyes (cataracts) or displacement of the lenses, which are located behind the pupils. Aniridia is often associated with underdevelopment (hypoplasia) of the macula, the central portion of the retina that distinguishes detail in the central field of vision.

Additional eye abnormalities often associated with aniridia include rapid, involuntary movements of the eyes (nystagmus); reduced fields of vision; abnormally increased sensitivity to light (photophobia); and progressively increased fluid pressure within the eyes (glaucoma). In most cases, glaucoma is not apparent during the first month of life (neonatal period).

Depending upon the range and severity of associated eye abnormalities, children with aniridia may have varying levels of visual impairment. However, in most cases, affected children may have visual acuity of approximately 20/200 or even further reductions in vision. The clearness or sharpness of vision (i.e., visual acuity) is typically measured on a scale comparing a patient's vision at 20 feet with that of an unaffected individual with full visual acuity. Thus, a person with 20/200 vision sees at 20 feet what someone with full visual acuity sees at 200 feet.

Aniridia may be an isolated condition or may occur in association with certain syndromes, such as WAGR syndrome, a rare disorder characterized by kidney tumors (Wilms tumor), aniridia, genitourinary anomalies (abnormalities of the reproductive and urinary tracts, due to spontaneous genetic changes (mutations), and retardation. WAGR is inherited as an autosomal dominant trait; in very rare cases, aniridia is inherited as an autosomal recessive trait (e.g., aniridia-cerebellar ataxia-mental deficiency). Medical care for aniridia is directed toward prevention of glaucoma and control of intraocular pressure (fluid pressure inside the eye. Other measures focus on specific problems, such as nystagamus, sensitivity to light (photophobia)and supportive measures, such as removal of cataracts. Visual aids, such asartificial pupil contact lenses, may also be used.

See also **General Resources** on page 917

Government Agencies

228   NIH/National Eye Institute
31 Center Drive MSC 2510
Bethesda, MD 20892

301-496-5248
e-mail: 2020@nei.nih.gov
www.nei.nih.gov

Conducts and supports research that helps prevent and treat eye diseases and other disorders of vision. This research leads to sight-saving treatments, reduces visual impairment and blindness, and improves the quality of life for people of all ages. NEI-supported research has advanced our knowledge of how the eye functions in health and disease.

Paul A Sieving M.D., Ph.D., Director

National Associations & Support Groups

229   Genetic Alliance
4301 Connecticut Avenue NW
Washington, DC 20008

202-966-5557
800-336-4363
Fax: 202-966-8553
e-mail: info@geneticalliance.org
www.geneticalliance.org

A coalition of voluntary genetic support groups, consumers and professionals addressing the needs of individuals and families affected by genetic disorders from a national perspective.

Sharon Terry, President/CEO

230   March of Dimes Birth Defects Foundation
1275 Mamaroneck Avenue
White Plains, NY 10605

914-428-7100
888-663-4637
Fax: 914-428-8203
e-mail: resourcecenter@modimes.org
www.marchofdimes.com

Partnership of volunteers and professionals dedicates to improving the health of babies by preventing birth defects and infant mortality. Over 100 chapters are located across the country and can be located through the National Office.

Dr Jennifer Howse, President

231 National Association for Visually Handicapped
22 W 21st Street, 6th Floor
New York, NY 10010

212-889-3141
Fax: 212-727-2931
e-mail: navh@navh.org
www.navh.org

NAVH is the only nonprofit health organization in the world solely dedicated to providing assistance to the partially sighted.

Dr Lorraine Marchi, Founder & CEO

232 National Eye Research Foundation
910 Skokie Boulevard, Suite 207A
Northbrook, IL 60062

847-564-4652
800-621-2258
Fax: 847-564-0807
e-mail: info@nerf.org
www.nerf.org

Devoted to the enhancement of care and study of eye related diseases.

Web Sites

233 Aniridia Network
www.clubs.yahoo.com/clubs/aniridianetwork

We are an international support group which aims to bring people with aniridia closer together as well as providing practical support and information.

234 Aniridia Web Site
www.aniridia.org

The Aniridia Network is an international nonprofit organization dedicated to supporting people with aniridia and their families, increasing awareness of aniridia and improving the quality of information about aniridia around the world.

235 National Association for Visually Handicapped
www.navh.org

Provides information on large print books, textbooks and educational tools.

236 Online Mendelian Inheritance in Man
www.ncbi.nlm.nih.gov

This database is a catalog of human genes and genetic disorders.

Book Publishers

237 Children with Visual Impairments: A Parents' Guide
Peytral Publications
PO Box 1162
Minnetonka, MN 55345

952-949-8707
877-739-8725
Fax: 952-906-9777
www.peytral.com

Covers visual impairments ranging from low vision to total blindness. Offers authoritative information and empathy, parental insight on diagnosis and treatment, orientation and mobility, literacy, legal issues and more. Valuable to parents, educators and support staff.

395 pages

M Cay Holbrook PhD, Editor

238 Let's Talk About Going to the Hospital
Rosen Publishing Group's PowerKids Press
29 E 21st Street
New York, NY 10010

212-777-3017
800-237-9932
Fax: 888-436-4643
e-mail: rosenpub@tribeca.ios.com
www.powerkidspress.com

If a child has to check into the hospital, chances are he or she is already upset about being ill. Knowing how a hospital functions and what the procedures are, such as when family members can visit, will help in what is already a stressful situation. Grades K-5.

24 pages
ISBN: 0-823950-36-0

DESCRIPTION

239 ANKYLOSING SPONDYLITIS
Synonyms: AS, Marie-Strumpell spondylitis
Involves the following Biologic System(s):
Orthopedic and Muscle Disorders

Ankylosing spondylitis (AS) is a chronic, progressive, inflammatory disease that affects joints of the spine and results in pain, stiffness, and possible loss of spinal mobility. In most patients, the joints between the spine and the hip-bones (sacroiliac joints) are affected. In addition, joints in the spinal column of the lower back (lumbosacral spine) and the neck (cervical spine) may be involved to varying degrees. Although the disease usually becomes apparent during young adulthood or middle age, it may also begin during childhood. Males are more commonly affected than females.

In most cases, children initially present with periodic inflammation and discomfort in the joints of the arms and legs (transient peripheral arthritis), particularly the large joints of the legs. Many also experience arthritis in the shoulders, the lower jaw bone (i.e., temporomandibular joints), and the feet. Such inflammation results in swelling, pain, abnormal warmth (erythema), and possible limited movement of affected joints. In children with AS, involvement of the sacroiliac joints may be apparent at the disorder's onset or may develop over several months or years. The different regions of the spine may then be progressively affected, usually beginning in the spinal column of the lower back (lumbar spine) and eventually involving the upper back (thoracic spine) and the cervical spine. Children with the disease experience periodic pain and stiffness that may be alleviated by movement. Many have hip, thigh, and lower back pain that is more severe at night and experience stiffness of affected areas in the mornings. In addition, some children have involvement of the joints that connect the ribs to the spine (costovertebral joints). The resulting inflammation, pain, and stiffness may limit expansion of the chest when taking deep breaths. Disease progression may spontaneously cease at any stage; however, in some cases, all regions of the spine may gradually be affected, potentially resulting in severely impaired spinal mobility.

Other symptoms associated with ankylosing spondylitis include fatigue, low-grade fever, lack of appetite (anorexia), low levels ofred blood cells (anemia), growth retardation, and repeated inflammation of the colored region of the eye (iritis) and its muscle (iridocyclitis). Inflammation of the aorta, the largest artery of the body (aoritis), is a finding that is often seen in adults with ankylosing spondylitis, but is rarely seen in affected children.

Research has shown that approximately 95 percent of affected individuals have a specific human leukocyte antigen or HLA. Antigens are proteins that stimulate the body to produce certain antibodies in response to invading microorganisms or foreign tissues. Most individuals with ankylosing spondylitis have a specific genetically determined HLA known as HLA-B27. The possible role of HLA-B27 in predisposing an individual to the disorder has not been determined. Anklosing spondylitis is thought to be an autosomal dominant disorder. In some cases, individuals with a defective gene for AS may not experience symptoms and findings associated with the disorder (reduced penetrance). AS is thought to have a higher penetrance among males.

Although HLA-B27 is present in most individuals with ankylosing spondylitis, it is not considered diagnostic for the disorder. AS is typically diagnosed based upon a complete patient and family history, characteristic physical findings, and specialized x-ray techniques. Treatment of children is primarily directed toward relieving pain and ensuring proper posture to help preserve spinal mobility. Certain medications may be prescribed to help alleviate or manage pain (e.g., indomethacin or other nonsteroidal antiinflammatory medications [NSAIDs]). Special exercises may be recommended to help strengthen back muscles and maintain proper posture. In addition, certain lifestyle changes may be suggested, including avoiding thick pillows and using a firm mattress. Additional treatment is usually symptomatic and supportive.

See also **General Resources** on page 917

Government Agencies

240 NIH/National Institute of Arthritis and Mu sculoskeletal and Skin Diseases
1AMS Circle
Bethesda, MD 20892

301-402-4484
Fax: 301-718-6366
e-mail: ord@od.nih.gov
rarediseases.info.nih.gov

The mission of the National Institute of Arthritis and Musculoskeletal and Skin Diseases is to support research into the causes, treatment, and prevention of arthritis and musculoskeletal and skin diseases, the training of basic and clinical scientists to carry out this research, and the dissemination of information on research progress in these diseases.

Stephen I Katz MD PhD, Director

National Associations & Support Groups

241 American Autoimmune Related Diseases Association
22100 Gratiot Avenue
E Detroit, MI 48021

586-776-3900
www.aarda.org

The American Autoimmune Related Diseases Association is dedicated to the eradication of autoimmune diseases and the alleviation of suffering and the socioeconomic impact of autoimmunity through fostering and facilitating collabration in the areas of education, public awareness, research,and patient in an effective, ethical and efficient manner.

Virginia Ladd, Director

242 American Juvenile Arthritis Organization
2970 Peachtree Road NW, Suite 200
Atlanta, GA 30305

404-237-8771
800-933-7023
Fax: 404-237-8153
e-mail: info.ga@arthritis.org
www.arthritis.org

Devoted to serving the special needs of children, teens, and young adults with childhood rheumatic diseases and their families. Offers both support and information through national and local programs that serve the needs of families, friends and health professionals. Serves as a clearinghouse of information, sponsors an annual national conference, monitors and promotes legislation, sponsors research, and offers training to both parents and health professionals.

Sage Rhodes, President

243 Arthritis Foundation
PO Box 7669
Atlanta, GA 30357

404-872-7100
800-568-4045
Fax: 404-872-0457
www.arthritis.org

The only nonprofit organization that supports the more than 100 types of arthritis and related conditions with advocacy, programs, services and research.

John H Klippel MD, President & CEO

244 March of Dimes Birth Defects Foundation
1275 Mamaroneck Avenue
White Plains, NY 10605

914-428-7100
888-663-4637
Fax: 914-428-8203
e-mail: resourcecenter@modimes.org
www.marchofdimes.com

Partnership of volunteers and professionals dedicates to improving the health of babies by preventing birth defects and infant mortality. Over 100 chapters are located across the country and can be located through the National Office.

Dr Jennifer Howse, President

245 Spondylitis Association of America
PO Box 5872
Sherman Oaks, CA 91413

818-981-1616
800-777-8189
e-mail: info@spondylitis.org
www.spondylitis.org

A nonprofit volunteer organization dedicated to the eradication of ankylosing spondylitis and related diseases through education, advocacy, awareness and research.

Katherine Culpepper, Executive Director
Laurie Savage, Associate Executive Director

Web Sites

246 AS Web
www.asweb.com/home.html

247 Online Mendelian Inheritance in Man
www.ncbi.nlm.nih.gov

This database is a catalog of human genes and genetic disorders.

Pamphlets

248 Ankylosing Spondylitis
Arthritis Foundation
PO Box 7669
Atlanta, GA 30357

404-872-7100
800-568-4045
Fax: 404-872-0457
www.arthritis.org

An informative pamphlet published by the Arthritis Foundation.

DESCRIPTION

249   ANORECTAL MALFORMATIONS

Covers these related disorders: Anal atresia, Anal fistula, Anal stenosis, Ectopic anus, Imperforate anus

Involves the following Biologic System(s):
Gastrointestinal Disorders

Anorectal malformations are a group of birth defects affecting the rectum, the anus, or both. The rectum is the final straight portion of the large intestine that terminates at an external opening known as the anus. Anorectal malformations are birth defects in which the anus and rectum do not develop normally and vary in severity. For example, the anal opening may be in its normal location but may be unusually small or narrow (e.g., anal stenosis or imperforate anus). Some anorectal malformations may not be apparent upon physical examination (e.g., imperforate anus or anal atresia). In infants with imperforate anus, the anal opening is partially or completely closed due to the presence of a thin membrane (i.e., cloacal membrane). In anal atresia, the rectum may end blindly due to absence (atresia) of the anal canal. In addition, in many affected infants, an abnormal channel (fistula) may be present between the rectum and certain other unusual locations. Anorectal malformations affect approximately one in 4,000 newborns.

Most newborns with anorectal malformations experience lower intestinal obstruction within 24 hours after birth due to incomplete passage of meconium, the thick, darkish green material that accumulates in the fetal intestines and forms a newborn's first stool. Newborns normally pass meconium during the first 24 to 48 hours after birth. Affected infants may also have incomplete or infrequent bowel movements or experience difficulty passing stools (constipation) within days or weeks after birth. Associated findings may include rectal bleeding; periodic episodes of diarrhea following constipation and associated abrasions of the skin (e.g., of the perineum and the buttocks); and abnormal enlargement of a segment of the large intestine (megacolon). In affected males with a channel between the rectum and the urinary tract, there can be passage of gas (pneumaturia) and meconium in the urine.

When newborns are diagnosed with anorectal malformations, physicians may consider surgical measures to prevent intestinal or urinary obstruction. Therapies for affected newborns or infants depend upon the nature and location of the anorectal malformation and, in some cases, other associated birth defects that may be present. Treatment measures, which may be conducted during the newborn period or later during infancy, may include surgical correction of anorectal malformations (e.g., anoplasty) and widening (dilatation) of the anal opening or other supportive measures; a colostomy is often needed.

Anorectal malformations are thought to result from abnormalities in the development of the embryonic structures that form the rectum and portions of the urinary tract. In cases in which anorectal malformations occur as isolated findings, such malformations are thought to result from abnormal changes (mutations) of one or several different genes, possibly in association with certain environmental factors (multifactorial). However, familial cases have also been reported that appear to have autosomal dominant, autosomal recessive, X-linked, or multifactorial inheritance. In approximately 50 percent of affected infants, anorectal malformations occur in association with other birth defects or underlying malformation syndromes, such as VACTERL association, a rare disorder that may be characterized by (V)ertebral abnormalities, (A)nal atresia, (C)ardiac defects, (T)racheo(E)sophageal fistula, (R)enal malformations, and (L)imb defects. Therefore, it is essential that newborns diagnosed with anorectal malformations are thoroughly examined and carefully monitored to ensure the detection and appropriate treatment of associated abnormalities.

See also **General Resources** on page 917

National Associations & Support Groups

250   American College of Gastroenterology
PO Box 342260
Bethesda, MD 20827

301-263-9000
www.acg.gi.org

The American College of Gastroenterology was founded in 1932 to advance the scientific study and medical practice of diseases of the GI tract.

Jack A DiPalma, President
Amy E Foxx-Orenstein, VP

251   Digestive Disease National Coalition
507 Capitol Court NE, Suite 200
Washington, DC 20002

202-544-7497
Fax: 202-546-7105
www.ddnc.org

Advocacy organization comprised of 22 voluntary and professional societies concerned with the many diseases of the digestive tract and liver.

Nancy Norton, Chairperson
Dr. Maurice Cerulli, President

252 International Foundation for Functional Gastrointestinal Disorders
PO Box 170864
Milwaukee, WI 53217

414-964-1799
888-964-2001
Fax: 414-964-7176
e-mail: iffgd@iffgd.org
www.iffgd.org

The organization offers responses to those commonly asked questions for families and individuals whose lives have been touched with the disorder.

Nancy J Norton, Founder
William Norton, VP

253 Intestinal Disease Foundation
100 W Station Square Drive
Pittsburgh, PA 15219

412-261-5888
877-587-9606
Fax: 412-471-2722
e-mail: info@intestinalfoundation.org
www.intestinalfoundation.org

Nonprofit organization whose mission is to improve the quality of life of adults and children affected by chonic digestive illness through information, guidance and support. IDF offers a quarterly newsletter, Intestinal Fortitude, educational seminars, volunteer phone network, and Pittsburgh area support groups.

254 March of Dimes Birth Defects Foundation
1275 Mamaroneck Avenue
White Plains, NY 10605

914-428-7100
888-663-4637
Fax: 914-428-8203
e-mail: resourcecenter@modimes.org
www.marchofdimes.com

Partnership of volunteers and professionals dedicated to improving the health of babies by preventing birth defects and infant mortality. Over 100 chapters are located across the country and can be located through the National Office.

Dr Jennifer Howse, President

255 National Dissemination Center for Children with Disabilities
PO Box 1492
Washington, DC 20013

202-884-8200
800-695-0285
Fax: 202-884-8441
e-mail: nichcy@aed.org
www.nichcy.org

A national information and referral center that provides information on disabilities and disability-related issues for families, educators and other professionals.

Suzanne Ripley, Executive Director

256 North American Society for Pediatric Gastroenterology/Hepatology/Nutrition
PO Box 6
Flourtown, PA 19031

215-233-0808
Fax: 215-233-3918
e-mail: naspghan@naspghan.org
www.naspghan.org

Strives to improve the care of infants, children and adolescents with digestive disorders by promoting advances in clinical care of children with chronic abdominal pain, diarrhea, constipation, vomiting, bleeding from the GI tract, inflammatory bowel disease, liver diseases, diseases of the pancreas, poor weight gain and nutritional problems.

Philip Sherman, President
Margaret K Stallings, Executive Director

257 Oley Foundation
214 Hun Memorial, MC-28, Albany Medical Center
Albany, NY 12208

518-262-5079
800-776-6539
Fax: 518-262-5528
e-mail: info@oley.org
www.oley.org

Helping people whose daily survival depends on home intravenous or tube-fed nutrition.

Joan Bishop, Executive Director
Roslyn Dahl, Director, Communications & Develop

258 Pull-Thru Network
2312 Savoy Street
Hoover, AL 35226

205-978-2930
e-mail: info@pullthrough.org
www.pullthrough.org

A chapter of the United Ostomy Association. Nonprofit service organization dedicated to the support of children and adults with anorectal malformations. Provides information, parent networking, medical supplies, financial assistance for parents needing to travel to obtain medical care for their child and a lending library and article reprint service.

Bonnie McElroy, President

Libraries & Resource Centers

259 National Digestive Diseases Information Clearinghouse
2 Information Way
Bethesda, MD 20892

301-654-3810
800-891-5389
Fax: 703-738-4929
e-mail: niddc@info.niddk.nih.gov
www.digestive.niddk.nih.gov

The National Institute of Diabetes and Digestive and Kidney Diseases conducts and supports research on many of the most serious diseases affecting public health. The Institute supports much of the clinical research on the diseases of internal medicine and related subspecialty fields as well as many basic science disciplines.

Kathy Kranzfelder, Project Officer

Web Sites

260 Baby Center
www.babycenter.com

The Academy is committed to the attainment of optimal physical, mental and social health for all infants, children, adolescents, and young adults. To this end, the members of the Academy dedicate their efforts and resources.

261 Child Health Research Project
www.childhealthresearch.org

To help achieve USAID's strategic objectives to reduce childhood mortality and morbidity, the Child Health Research Project (CHR) conducts applied research in: diarrheal and respiratory diseases, infectious diseases, neonatal health, and malnutrition.

262 Health Research Project (HaRP)
www.harpnet.org

A program by USAID, the project strives to improve the health status of infants, children, mothers and families through the development and research of new tools, technologies, policies and approaches.

263 National Digestive Diseases Information Clearinghouse
www.digestive.niddk.nih.gov

Supports clinical research on the diseases of internal medicine and related subspecialty fields as well as many basic science disciplines.

Journals

264 Journal of Pediatric Gastroenterology and Nutrition

NASPGHAN, author

Lippincott Williams & Wilkins
530 Walnut Street
Philadelphia, PA 19106

215-521-8300
Fax: 215-521-8902
www.lww.com

Publication of the North American Society for Pediatric Gastroenterolgy, Hepatology and Nutrition, which strives to improve the care of infants, children and adolescents with digestive disorders by promoting advances in clinical care of children with chronic abdominal pain, diarrhea, constipation, vomiting, bleeding from the GI tract, inflammatory bowel disease, liver diseases, diseases of the pancreas, poor weight gain and nutritional problems.

Newsletters

265 NASPGHAN News
PO Box 6
Flourtown, PA 19031

215-233-0808
Fax: 215-233-3939
e-mail: naspghan@naspghan.org
www.naspgn.org

Publication of the North American Society for Pediatric Gastroenterolgy, Hepatology and Nutrition, which strives to improve the care of infants, children and adolescents with digestive disorders by promoting advances in clinical care of children with chronic abdominal pain, diarrhea, constipation, vomiting, bleeding from the GI tract, inflammatory bowel disease, liver diseases, diseases of the pancreas, poor weight gain and nutritional problems.

266 PTN News
2312 Savoy Street
Hoover, AL 35226

205-978-2930
e-mail: info@pullthrough.org
www.pullthrough.org

Newsletter of the Pull-thru Network, a chapter of the United Ostomy Association and a nonprofit service organization dedicated to the support of children and adults with anorectal malformations.

Quarterly

Pamphlets

267 Anorectal Malformations- A Parent's Guide
2312 Savoy Street
Hoover, AL 35226

205-978-2930
e-mail: info@pullthrough.org
www.pullthrough.org

Brochure distributed free to physicians, nurses and hospitals by the Pull-thru Network, a chapter of the United Ostomy Association and a nonprofit service organization dedicated to the support of children and adults with anorectal malformations.

Quarterly

DESCRIPTION

268 AORTIC STENOSIS

Synonym: Aortic stenosis

Involves the following Biologic System(s):

Cardiovascular Disorders

Aortic stenosis is a condition characterized by the abnormal narrowing (stenosis) of the valve through which blood flows from the left ventricle of the heart to the aorta, the majory artery of the body. The normal aortic valve is comprised of three leaflets (cusps) that open when the heart contracts and permits the flow of blood into the aorta. A bi-cuspid aortic valve, a congenital (from birth) abnormality is one in which there are two cusps instead of three, and while many of these valves work reasonably well, there is a higher incidence of narrowing at the level of the valve. In infants with aortic valve stenosis, it is common for the aortic valve to be bicuspid. In some patients, the aortic valve leaflets may be fused together or may form an unusual funnel shape. This results in narrowing of the valve and inhibiting of the normal rate and pressure of blood flow. In addition, an irregular valve may not grow as the heart grows with advancing age. In these patients, the opening is not large enough to accommodate the larger volumes of blood pumped by the heart. The heart muscle may become thicker (hypertrophied) as it has to develop a higher pressure to eject blood across this thickened, narrowed valve. Eventually the heart muscle may sustain damage from working against elevated pressure further decreasing its ability to pump sufficiently.

Aortic stenosis may be present as an isolated finding, or in association with other congenital heart defects or other disorders such as Turner syndrome, a chromosomal abnormality. In adults, aortic valve stenosis may result from scarring or the accumulation of calcium on the aortic valve. Symptoms of aortic valve stenosis depend upon the severity of the abnormality. Valve obstruction that occurs in early infancy may be characterized by enlargement of the heart (cardiomegaly), congestive heart failure, abnormal accumulation of fluid in the lungs (pulmonary edema), weak pulses, and a low output of urine. Children with less severe stenosis may have no symptoms other than a heart murmur on physical examinations, while those with more severe involvement may experience fatigue, dizziness, and chest pain. Some severe cases of aortic valve stenosis may become life-threatening.

Treatment for aortic valve stenosis is dependent upon the severity of the obstruction. Initial therapy includes catheterization (valvuloplasty), a procedure in which a thin hollow tube (catheter) with a small balloon attached at its tip is threaded across the valve. Once in place, the balloon is inflated, thus increasing the size of the valve's opening. According to recent treatment guidelines, balloon valvuloplasty is not to be recommended, except for certain adolescent congenital defects. The preferred alternative, if available, is aortic valve replacement.

See also **General Resources** on page 917

Government Agencies

269 NIH/National Heart, Lung and Blood Institu te
National Institute of Health
31 Center Dr MSC 2486, Bldg 31, Room 5A48
Bethesda, MD 20892

301-592-8573
Fax: 240-629-3246
TTY: 240-629-3255
e-mail: NHLBIinfo@nhlbi.nih.gov
www.nhlbi.nih.gov

Primary responsibility of this organization is the scientific investigation of heart, blood vessel, lung and blood disorders. Oversees research, demonstration, prevention, education, control and training activities in these fields and emphasizes the prevention and control of heart diseases.

Elizabeth G Nabel, MD, Director
Susan Shurin, MD, Deputy Director

270 NIH/National Institute of Child Health and Human Development
31 Center Drive, Building 31
Bethesda, MD 20892

301-496-5133
Fax: 301-496-1104
www.nichd.nih.gov

Established in 1962 by congress, today the institute conducts and supports research on topics related to the health of children, adults, families and populations. Some of these topics include: developmental disabilities, growth and development, infant death, reproductive health and birth defects.

Nancy D Wirth, Director
Lisa Kaeser, Program & Public Liaison

National Associations & Support Groups

271 American Heart Association
7272 Greenville Avenue
Dallas, TX 75231

214-373-6300
800-242-8721
Fax: 214-706-1341
e-mail: inquire@amhrt.org
www.amhrt.org

Supports research, education and community service programs with the objective of reducing premature death and disability from cardiovascular diseases and stroke; coordinates the efforts of health professionals, and others engaged in the fight against heart and circulatory disease.

M Cass Wheeler, CEO

272 Genetic Alliance
4301 Connecticut Avenue NW
Washington, DC 20008

202-966-5557
800-336-4363
Fax: 202-966-8553
e-mail: info@geneticalliance.org
www.geneticalliance.org

A coalition of voluntary genetic support groups, consumers and professionals addressing the needs of individuals and families affected by genetic disorders from a national perspective.

Sharon Terry, President/CEO

273 March of Dimes Birth Defects Foundation
1275 Mamaroneck Avenue
White Plains, NY 10605

914-428-7100
888-663-4637
Fax: 914-428-8203
e-mail: resourcecenter@modimes.org
www.marchofdimes.com

Partnership of volunteers and professionals dedicates to improving the health of babies by preventing birth defects and infant mortality. Over 100 chapters are located across the country and can be located through the National Office.

Dr Jennifer Howse, President

Web Sites

274 Southern Illinois University School of Medicine
www.siumed.edu/peds/index.htm

Mission is to meet the health care needs of children and their families in Central and Southern Illinois through the provision of high quality, coordinated care of children with acute and chronic conditions with inpatient, ambulatory, and community-based programs.

275 Yale University School of Medicine
www.info.med.yale.edu/intmed/cardio/chd

Information on congential heart conditions, including Aortic Stenosis — symptoms, treatments and support.

Book Publishers

276 Congenital Disorders Sourcebook 2nd Edition
Omnigraphics
PO Box 625
Holmes, PA 19043

800-234-1340
Fax: 800-875-1340
e-mail: info@omnigraphics.com
www.omnigraphics.com

Provides basic consumer health information about the most common types of nonhereditary birth defects and disorders related to prematurity, gestational injuries, congenital infections, and birth complications, including disorders of the heart, brain, gastrointestinal tract, musculoskeletal system, urinary tract, and reproductive system, craniofacial disorders, cerebral palsy, spina bifida, and fetal alcohol syndrome, and detailing the causes, diagnostic tests, and treatments for each.

650 pages
ISBN: 0-780809-45-9

277 Heart Disease
Franklin Watts
90 Old Sherman Turnpike
Danbury, CT 06816

203-797-3500
800-621-1115
Fax: 203-797-3197
www.grolier.com

Using diagrams, this book discusses strokes and other blood vessel disorders, as well as their treatment and prevention.

112 pages Grades 7-12
ISBN: 0-531108-84-8

278 Living with Heart Disease
Franklin Watts
90 Old Sherman Turnpike
Danbury, CT 06816

203-797-3500
800-621-1115
Fax: 203-797-3197
www.grolier.com

Shows how persons with heart disease can overcome their illness and lead productive lives.

32 pages Grades 5-7
ISBN: 0-531108-45-7

DESCRIPTION

279   APNEA OF PREMATURITY
Synonym: Idiopathic apnea of prematurity
Involves the following Biologic System(s):
Neonatal and Infant Disorders, Respiratory Disorders

Apnea is a condition characterized by a temporary cessation of breathing. Newborns may experience episodes of apnea due to several underlying disorders or conditions, including certain respiratory, neurologic, digestive, cardiovascular, metabolic, or infectious diseases. However, in newborns with apnea of prematurity, apneic episodes occur in the absence of identifiable, underlying disorders (idiopathic). The condition primarily affects premature infants who are born before 34 weeks of pregnancy (gestation). In general, the greater the degree of prematurity, the greater the frequency of the condition.

Apnea of prematurity is thought to occur due to immaturity of the region of the brain that controls breathing (respiratory centers of the medulla), causing failed stimulation of respiratory muscles. Resulting episodes of apnea, which are referred to as central apnea, are characterized by an absence of airflow as well as of chest wall movements. Apnea of prematurity may also be caused by obstruction of the upper airways due to improper coordination of the tongue and upper airway muscles, instability of the throat (pharynx), or other factors. Resulting episodes of apnea, known as obstructive apnea, are characterized by absence of airflow but ongoing chest wall movements. Most infants with apnea of prematurity experience both central and obstructive apnea.

With infant apnea, more appropriately called an apparent life-threatening event, initial episodes of apnea typically occur on the second to the seventh day of life. Such episodes are defined as serious if breathing spontaneously ceases for more than 15 to 20 seconds or if they result in decreased levels of oxygen in the blood and associated bluish discoloration of the skin and mucous membranes (cyanosis) and slowing of the heart rate (bradycardia).

The frequency of apnea episodes typically increases during the cycle of sleep that is associated with rapid eye movements (REMs), dreaming, increased levels of brain activity, and involuntary muscle jerks. During REM sleep, infants are more likely to experience abnormal chest wall movements during breathing, such as relaxation of the chest muscles while inhaling rather than exhaling. Abnormal chest wall movements as well as inhibition of muscle tone (particularly of the throat) during REM sleep contribute to the increased frequency of apneic episodes.

Infants at risk for episodes of apnea should be monitored with devices that detect abnormal changes in chest wall movements, heart rate, and respiratory activity. These devices, known as apnea monitors, sound an alarm when spontaneous breathing temporarily ceases. In infants who experience mild, occasional episodes of apnea, supportive measures may be sufficient, such as gentle skin stimulation and massage. In patients with severe, prolonged, and recurrent apnea episodes, treatment should include close monitoring, immediate measures to assist breathing (e.g., bag and maskentilation) and oxygen therapy to ensure sufficient oxygen supply to body tissues. Infants with apnea may be monitored at home which can have a significant impact on caregivers. In general, as the child matures, the cause of the ALTE is diagnosed and treated or spontaneously resolves.

See also **General Resources** on page 917

See also **General Resources** on page 917

Government Agencies

280   NIH/National Institute of Child Health and Human Development
31 Center Drive, Building 31
Bethesda, MD 20892

301-496-5133
Fax: 301-496-1104
www.nichd.nih.gov

Established in 1962 by congress, today the institute conducts and supports research on topics related to the health of children, adults, families and populations. Some of these topics include: developmental disabilities, growth and development, infant death, reproductive health and birth defects.

Nancy D Wirth, Director
Lisa Kaeser, Program & Public Liaison

281   NIH/National Institute of Neurological Dis orders and Stroke (NINDS)
PO Box 5801
Bethesda, MD 20824

301-496-5751
800-352-9424
Fax: 301-496-0296
TTY: 301-468-5981
www.ninds.nih.gov

Works to reduce the burden of neurological disease by conducting, fostering, coordinating and guiding research on the causes, prevention, diagnosis and treatment of neurological disorders and stroke, while supporting basic research in related scientific areas.

Story C Landis Ph.D., Director
Audrey S Penn M.D., Deputy Director

National Associations & Support Groups

282 American Sleep Apnea Association
1424 K Street NW, Suite 302
Washington, DC 20005

202-293-3650
Fax: 202-293-3656
e-mail: asaa@sleepapnea.org
www.sleepapnea.org

Dedicated to reducing injury, disability and death from sleep apnea and to enhancing the well-being of those affected by this common disorder. They promote education and awareness. Network of voluntary mutual support groups, research, and continuous improvement of care.

Rochelle Goldberg, MD, President & CMO
Dave Hargett, Chair

283 National Sleep Foundation
1522 K Street NW, Suite 500
Washington, DC 20005

202-347-3471
Fax: 202-347-3472
e-mail: nsf@sleepfoundation.org
www.sleepfoundation.org

Works to improve the quality of life for millions of Americans who suffer from sleep disorders, and to prevent the catastrophic accidents that are related to poor or disordered sleep through research, education and the dissemination of information towards the cause of the Narcolepsy Project. Seeks patients to aid new research project targeting the cause of the disorder.

Richard Gelula, CEO

284 Tri-State Sleep Disorders Center Center for Research in Sleep Disorders
1275 E Kemper Road
Cincinnati, OH 45246

513-671-3101
800-838-4322
Fax: 513-671-4159
e-mail: web@tristatesleep.com
www.tristatesleep.com

Provides diagnostics and treatment services to thousands of people in Cincinnati and throughout the country at our state-of-the-art sleep clinic through cutting edge research efforts.

Dr Martin Scharf, Director

Web Sites

285 Apnea of Prematurity
www.emedicine.com/ped/topic1157.htm

Provides information on how to tell if an unborn baby has sleep apnea.

DESCRIPTION

286 ARNOLD-CHIARI MALFORMATION

Synonyms: ACM, Arnold-Chiari deformity, Arnold-Chiari syndrome, Chiari malformation

Covers these related disorders: Arnold-Chiari malformation type I, Arnold-Chiari malformation type II

Involves the following Biologic System(s):

Neurologic Disorders

Arnold-Chiari malformation is a developmental abnormality characterized by malformations at the base of the brain that are present at birth (congenital). Such deformities typically include abnormal elongation of a portion of the cerebellum (cerebellar tonsils) and the lowest region of the brain stem (medulla oblongata), resulting in protrusion of these regions through the large opening (foramen magnum) in the base of the skull into the upper spinal canal (cervical canal). The cerebellum is a region of the brain that plays an essential role in coordinating voluntary movement and maintaining posture and balance. The brain stem, which is the lowest section of the brain, helps to relay motor and sensory impulses between other regions of the brain and the spinal cord and connects with most of the cranial nerve pairs, which send impulses involved in such functions as taste, vision, swallowing, facial expressions, and tongue, head, and shoulder movements.

In some affected newborns, Arnold-Chiari malformation occurs in association with myelomeningocele, a developmental abnormality characterized by protrusion (herniation) of a portion of the spinal cord and its protective membrane (meninges) through an abnormal opening in the spinal column. Arnold-Chiari malformation without a myelomeningocele is termed Arnold-Chiari malformation type I. Patients with a myelomeningocele have Arnold-Chiari malformation type II. In both types, the foramen magnum is abnormally large. The base of the skull is also flattened and may appear pushed upward by the upper vertebrae (cervical vertebrae) surrounding the spinal cord.

Affected infants and children with Arnold-Chiari malformation type II experience progressive hydrocephalus, a condition characterized by abnormal accumulation of cerebrospinal fluid (CSF) in the brain. In infants and children with hydrocephalus, obstruction or impaired absorption of the CSF causes it to abnormally accumulate and results in an increase in pressure within cavities (ventricles) of the brain. Other findings may include abnormal enlargement of the ventricles, potential enlargement of the head, and other associated symptoms and findings. Some infants with Arnold-Chiari malformation type II may also experience abnormalities due to impairment of lower cranial nerves. Such abnormalities, which vary in range and severity, include uncontrollable twitching (fasciculations) of the tongue, a high-pitched sound upon inhalation (i.e., laryngeal stridor), facial weakness, hearing impairment, lagging of the head (sternomastoid paralysis), or weakness or impaired control of muscles that turn the eyes outward (bilateral abducens palsies). During later childhood, some patients may experience increased stiffness (rigidity), causing restriction of movement (spasticity); abnormalities in walking (abnormal gait); and progressive lack of coordination. During later childhood or adolescence, individuals may also experience symptoms and findngs often associated with Arnold-Chiari malformation type I.

However, these symptoms may not develop until adolescence or adulthood and often do not include hydrocephalus. Associated symptoms and findings may include recurrent headaches; neck pain; impaired control of voluntary movements (ataxia); or progressive muscle weakness, degeneration (atrophy), spasticity, and potential sensory loss affecting the lower and, in some cases, the upper limbs.

Treatment of individuals with Arnold-Chiari malformation depends upon the severity of the malformation and associated symptoms and findings. If symptoms are only mild, treatment includes regular monitoring and symptomatic and supportive measures as required. However, in more severe cases, surgery is required. The basic operation is one of uncrowding the area at the base of the cerebellum where it is pushing against the brainstem and spinal cord. This is done by removing a small portion of bone at the base of the skull deep to the neck muscles as well as often removing a part of the back of the first and occasionally additional spinal column segments, e.g., upper cervical laminectomy). Although the exact cause of Arnold-Chiari malformation is unknown, researchers have suggested that it may result from the interaction of several genes, environmental influences, or both (multifactorial inheritance).

See also **General Resources** on page 917

Government Agencies

287 NIH/National Institute of Child Health and Human Development
31 Center Drive, Building 31
Bethesda, MD 20892

301-496-5133
Fax: 301-496-1104
www.nichd.nih.gov

Established in 1962 by congress, today the institute conducts and supports research on topics related to the health of children, adults, families and populations. Some of these topics include: developmental disabilities, growth and development, infant death, reproductive health and birth defects.

Nancy D Wirth, Director
Lisa Kaeser, Program & Public Liaison

National Associations & Support Groups

288 Arnold-Chiari Family Network
67 Spring Street
Weymouth, MA 02188

614-334-2368

289 Genetic Alliance
4301 Connecticut Avenue NW
Washington, DC 20008

202-966-5557
800-336-4363
Fax: 202-966-8553
e-mail: info@geneticalliance.org
www.geneticalliance.org

A coalition of voluntary genetic support groups, consumers and professionals addressing the needs of individuals and families affected by genetic disorders from a national perspective.

Sharon Terry, President/CEO

290 March of Dimes Birth Defects Foundation
1275 Mamaroneck Avenue
White Plains, NY 10605

914-428-7100
888-663-4637
Fax: 914-428-8203
e-mail: resourcecenter@modimes.org
www.marchofdimes.com

Partnership of volunteers and professionals dedicates to improving the health of babies by preventing birth defects and infant mortality. Over 100 chapters are located across the country and can be located through the National Office.

Dr Jennifer Howse, President

291 Spina Bifida Association of America
4590 MacArthur Boulevard NW, Suite 250
Washington, DC 20007

202-944-3285
800-621-3141
Fax: 202-944-3295
e-mail: sbaa@sbaa.org
www.sbaa.org

Serves as the national office representing approximately 80 chapters of parents and other members of families having children born with Spina Bifida, individuals with Spina Bifida, and health professionals who work with them. Operates a national information clearinghouse, an information and referral toll-free number, periodic public awareness, scholarships and related efforts and an annual meeting.

Cindy Brownstein, CEO
Christine Poward, COO

292 World Arnold-Chiari Malformation Association
31 Newtown Woods Road
Newtown Square, PA 19073

610-353-4737
www.pressenter.com/~wacma/

Staffed by volunteers, we are committed to providing support, current information, and understanding to those affected by the Arnold Chiari malformation and syringomyelia. It is also our goal to raise the awareness of, and educate the medical community as to the complex nature of this disease and how it affects the lives of those who have it.

Chip Vierow, Manager/Moderator
Sally Reusser, Manager/Moderator

Web Sites

293 National Institute of Health NINDS Information Page
www.ninds.nih.gov

The mission is to reduce the burden of neurological disease — a burden born by every age group, by every segment of society, by people all over the world.

294 Online Mendelian Inheritance in Man
www.ncbi.nlm.nih.gov

This database is a catalog of human genes and genetic disorders.

295 Rare Genetic Diseases in Children (NYU)
www.med.nyu.edu/rgdc/homenow.htm

We target issues arising from rare genetic diseases affecting children. And assist in the endeavor to bring knowledge and hope to those for whom there is, at present, so little.

Book Publishers

296 Let's Talk About Going to the Hospital
Rosen Publishing Group's PowerKids Press
29 E 21st Street
New York, NY 10010

212-777-3017
800-237-9932
Fax: 888-436-4643
e-mail: rosenpub@tribeca.ios.com
www.powerkidspress.com

If a child has to check into the hospital, chances are he or she is already upset about being ill. Knowing how a hospital functions and what the procedures are, such as when family members can visit, will help in what is already a stressful situation. Grades K-5.

24 pages
ISBN: 0-823950-36-0

DESCRIPTION

297 ARRHYTHMIAS

Covers these related disorders: Supraventricular Tachycardia (SVT), Wolff-Parkinson-White Syndrome (WPW)

Involves the following Biologic System(s): Cardiovascular Disorders

The term arrhythmia refers to an abnormality in the heart beat or electrical conduction system of the heart. Arrhythmia may describe an irregularity in the rhythm, either abnormally slow or abnormally fast. Supraventricular Tachycardia (SVT), also known as paroxysmal SVT, is the most common significant arrhythmia in children. The term supraventricular describes the area of the heart above the ventricles and generally refers to the tissue of the atria (upper chambers) and the conduction tissue such as the Atrioventricular Node (AVN) and junctional cells that connect the upper chambers to the lower chambers. Tachycardia refers to a heart rate that is increased; this may be normal, such as a sinus tachycardia, or abnormal as in the Supraventricular Tachycardias.

The electrocardiogram (ECG) is a diagnostic test that utilizes small adhesive leads placed in precise and predetermined positions on the arms, legs and chest to determine the electrical conduction of energy through the heart. It is, in essence, a road map of how the electrical impulse of the heart is transmitted. Supraventricular Tachycardia describes a group of arrhythmias with similar findings on the ECG, but different pathologic mechanisms by which they lead to a fast heart rate.

Among the various types of Supraventricular Tachycardia are those that use accessory or bypass tracts of conduction tissue to deliver the electrical impulse from the top of the heart to the ventricles, and those that have abnormal collections of electrically generating cells in the atria, AVN and junction. These different types of Supraventricular Tachycardia yield subtly distinct patterns on the ECG, which is the basis for the diagnosis in most patients.

Wolff-Parkinson-White Syndrome (WPW) is a type of Supraventricular Tachycardia that has, as its hallmark, a specific finding on the ECG when the patient *is not* experiencing Supraventricular Tachycardia. This finding is referred to as pre-excitation and results from the ventricle receiving its electrical stimulus from a specialized accessory pathway that connects the atrium to the ventricle without going through the normal relay point in the junction between the upper and lower chambers (AV node). As a result, the ventricle receives its signal to beat early and this pre-excitation is visible on the routine ECG.

Symptoms in children with Supraventricular Tachycardia include palpitations or intermittent irregularities in their heart rate. They may complain of a racing heart, as the typical Supraventricular Tachycardia heart rate is often well into the mid 200/minute range (normal heart rate ranges between 60 and 100 bpm). In some infants and children, symptoms may include pallor, easy fatigue, sweating, dizziness or fainting. If Supraventricular Tachycardia goes unrecognized, symptoms may be more severe, and include shortness of breath, respiratory distress, poor appetite and lethargy.

Treatment of Supraventricular Tachycardia is based on the exact mechanism of the arrhythmia and the age of the patient. There are a variety of medications(anti-arrhythmia agents) that can be used to control and prevent Supraventricular Tachycardia. These medications have side effects, some of which require close monitoring. Many of the Supraventricular Tachycardias are amenable to a procedure called radio-frequency ablation, in which specialized catheters are placed into the veins. These catheters can then be advanced into the heart and precisely measure the heart's conduction system. Often the generating site of the arrhythmia or the accessory tract that is used during the arrhythmia can be identified and isolated. When this is accomplished, the catheters can be used to deliver radio-frequency energy to disable the arrhythmia site, return the patient to a normal heart rhythm and essentially prevent recurrence of the Supraventricular Tachycardia. In general, these procedures are remarkably successful.

See also **General Resources** on page 917

National Associations & Support Groups

298 American College of Cardiology
9111 Old Georgetown Road
Bethesda, MD 20814

301-897-5400
800-253-4636
Fax: 301-897-9745
e-mail: resource@acc.org
www.acc.org

The mission of the American College of Cardiology is to advocate for quality cardiovascular care, through education, research promotion, development and applicatin of standards and guidelines, and to influence health care policy.

Steven E Nissen, MD FACC, President

299 American Heart Association
7272 Greenville Avenue
Dallas, TX 75231

214-373-6300
800-242-8721
Fax: 214-706-1341
e-mail: inquire@amhrt.org
www.amhrt.org

Our mission is to reduce disability and death from cardiovascular diseases and stroke. Parents will find education and support to you better care for a child with arrhythmias.

M Cass Wheeler, CEO

300 Heart Failure Society of America
2550 University Avenue W
Saint Paul, MN 55114

651-642-1633
Fax: 651-642-1502
e-mail: info@hfsa.org
www.hfsa.org

Provides a forum for all those interested in heart function, heart failure and congestive heart failure research.

Gary S Francis MD, President

301 Rush Children's Heart Center
1653 W Congress Parkway
Chicago, IL 60612

312-942-6003
e-mail: KidsHeart@rpslmc.edu
www.rush.edu

Dedicated to compassionate, state of the art and convenient delivery of care to children and young adults with heart problems. We strive for excellence in eduation and research to enhance our patient care efforts.

Andrew Griffin MD, Director

302 Sudden Arrhythmia Death Syndromes Foundation
508 E South Temple, Suite 20
Salt Lake City, UT 84102

801-531-0937
800-786-7723
Fax: 801-531-0945
e-mail: sads@sads.org
www.sads.org

Our mission is to save lives of chilren and young adults who are genetically predisposed or otherwise susceptible to sudden death due to cardiac arrhythmias and to provide education and support to families and the medical community who are dealing with these disorders.

Alice Lara, Executive Director
Jennifer Zimmerman, Development Director

Research Centers

303 Cardiovascular Research Foundation
55 E 59th Street
New York, NY 10022

212-851-9300
www.crf.org

A nonprofit organization dedicated to research, education and patient care. Promotes advances in cardiovascular medicine, specifically interventional cardiology, and through diagnosis and treatment of endovascular disorders.

Victor W Yick, President
Roni Amiel, Director, Information Technology

Conferences

304 International Sudden Arrhythmia Death Syndrome Conference
503 E South Temple, Suite 20
Salt Lake City, UT 84102

801-531-0937
800-786-7723
Fax: 801-531-0945
e-mail: sads@sads.org
www.sads.org

Annual conference for all those who care for those with arrhythmias, including exhibitors and educational workshops.

August

Alice Lara, Executive Director

Web Sites

305 Heart Center Online
www.heartcenteronline.com

The mission of the Heart Center Online is to be the premier cardiovascular specialized health care site on the Internet, to provide cardiovascular patients, their families and site visitors with tools they need to better understand the complex nature of heart-related conditions, treatments and preventive care, and to provide services and applications that deliver value to cardiovascullar practices.

306 Rush Children's Heart Center
www.rush.edu

Provides complete clinical services for the diagnosis and treatment of congenital and acquired heart disease in children and young adults.

307 Yale University School of Medicine
www.info.med.yale.edu/intmed/cardio/chd

Information on heart conditions, including arrhythmias.

Book Publishers

308 Clinical Pediatric Arrhythmias
Elsevier-Health Sciences Division
225 Wildwood Avenue
Woburn, MA 01801

617-928-2500
800-366-2665
Fax: 800-446-6520

The purpose of this new edition is to assist the clinician in evaluating and understanding arrhythmias in children as a reference for determining appropriate treatment strategies.

hardcover
ISBN: 0-721666-29-9

309 Practical Management of Pediatric Cardiac Arrhythmias
Futura Publishing Company
6770 Bertner Avenue
Houston, TX 77030

832-355-4011
e-mail: pubcentral@nih.gov
www.pubmedcentral.nih.gov

A concise, practical, up-to-date resource for the diagnosis and management of pediatric arrhythmias.

2001 422 pages
ISBN: 0-879934-66-2

Journals

310 Journal of Cardiac Failure
Cardiac Heart Failure Society of America
2550 University Avenue W
Saint Paul, MN 55114

651-642-1633
Fax: 651-642-1502
www.hfsa.org

Contains review articles on clinical research, basic human studies, animal studies, and bench research with potential clinical applications to heart failure, pathogenesis, etiology, epidemiology, pathophysiological mechanisms, assessment, prevention and treatment.

6x year

311 Texas Heart Institute Journal
Texas Heart Institute
6770 Bertner Avenue
Houston, TX 77030

832-355-4011
Fax: 832-355-3714
www.texasheartinstitute.org

The purpose of the Texas Heart Institute Journal is to educate, with emphasis on the dissemination of information to physicians in practice.

Quaterly

Newsletters

312 Heart Failure Society Newsletter
2550 University Avenue W
Saint Paul, MN 55114

651-642-1633
Fax: 651-642-1502
www.hfsa.org

Provides information on the society and also on different aspects of heart failure.

Quaterly

DESCRIPTION

313 ARTHROGRYPOSIS MULTIPLEX CONGENITA
Synonym: AMC
Covers these related disorders: Amyoplasia
Involves the following Biologic System(s):
Orthopedic and Muscle Disorders

Arthrogryposis multiplex congenita (AMC) refers to a group of disorders present at birth (congenital) that are characterized by limited movement or immobility of multiple joints and partial or complete replacement of involved muscle with fibrous or fatty tissue. Affected joints may be permanently flexed or extended in various fixed postures (joint contractures). Approximately 150 syndromes have been identified that are characterized by the presence of congenital multiple contractures. The most common form of arthrogryposis multiplex congenita is known as amyoplasia. This classic form of AMC affects approximately one in 10,000 newborns.

In newborns with amyoplasia, multiple congenital contractures are present that typically affect the upper and lower extremities. In most newborns who are affected, such contractures include abnormal flexion or extension of the elbows; flexion of the wrists toward either the thumb side or pinky side of the hands(radial or ulnar deviation); cupping of the hands; and internal rotation of the shoulders. Many newborns with amyoplasia also have severe deformities of the feet (clubfoot or talipes equinovarus) in which the heels are turned inward and the soles of the feet are flexed (plantar flexion). Additional musculoskeletal deformities are also typically present including abnormal rigidity of the joints between the bones of the thumbs and other fingers (interphalangeal joints); deformities of the palms of the hands; fixed flexion or extension of the knees; and abnormal flexion, extension, rotation, and possible dislocation of the hips. These abnormalities are usually similar from one side of the body to the other (symmetric). Amyoplasia is also characterized by a susceptibility to bone fractures (i.e., perinatal fractures) and progressive abnormal sideways curvature of the spine (scoliosis) that varies in severity and in age at onset. Most newborns with amyoplasia also have distinctive facial abnormalities including short, upturned (anteverted) nostrils; a rounded face; a slightly small jaw (mild micrognathia); and a benign, reddish, purple growth in the midportion of the face (midline frontal hemangioma). Amyoplasia appears to occur randomly for unknown reasons (sporadically), and the underlying causes of amyoplasia and other forms of AMC are not fully understood.

All newborns with multiple congenital joint contractures should receive a thorough neuromuscular evaluation to help detect, confirm, or rule out potential underlying muscular or neurologic abnormalities. The treatment of infants and children with amyoplasia includes symptomatic and supportive measures. The presence of fractures should be ruled out or confirmed (e.g., with x-ray studies) and treated as necessary (e.g., with appropriate immobilization) before physical therapy is begun. Other treatment measures for congenital contractures and associated abnormalities include physical therapy (e.g., passive range of motion exercises) and splinting of extremities to improve the range of motion; the use of casts or other orthopedic appliances; and possible surgical interventions. In addition, orthopedic appliances may be used to help slow the progression of scoliosis. In most patients with severe scoliosis, surgical measures may also be required.

See also **General Resources** on page 917

Government Agencies

314 NIH/National Institute of Arthritis and Mu sculoskeletal and Skin Diseases
1AMS Circle
Bethesda, MD 20892

301-402-4484
Fax: 301-718-6366
e-mail: ord@od.nih.gov
rarediseases.info.nih.gov

The mission of the National Institute of Arthritis and Musculoskeletal and Skin Diseases is to support research into the causes, treatment, and prevention of arthritis and musculoskeletal and skin diseases, the training of basic and clinical scientists to carry out this research, and the dissemination of information on research progress in these diseases.

Stephen I Katz MD PhD, Director

National Associations & Support Groups

315 Genetic Alliance
4301 Connecticut Avenue NW
Washington, DC 20008

202-966-5557
800-336-4363
Fax: 202-966-8553
e-mail: info@geneticalliance.org
www.geneticalliance.org

A coalition of voluntary genetic support groups, consumers and professionals addressing the needs of individuals and families affected by genetic disorders from a national perspective.

Sharon Terry, President/CEO

316 Human Growth Foundation
997 Glen Cove Avenue, Suite 5
Glen Head, NY 11545

516-671-4041
800-451-6434
Fax: 516-671-4055
e-mail: hgfl@hgfound.org
www.hgfound.org

A voluntary, nonprofit organization whose mission is to help children and adults with disorders of growth and growth hormones through research, education, support and advocacy. The foundation is dedicated to helping medical science to better understand the process of growth. It is composed of concerned parents and friends of children and adults with growth problems and interested health professionals.

Patricia D Costa, Executive Director

317 MAGIC Foundation: Major Aspects of Growth in Children
6645 W North Avenue
Oak Park, IL 60302

708-383-0808
800-362-4423
Fax: 708-383-0899
e-mail: mary@magicfoundation.org
www.magicfoundation.org

A national nonprofit organization providing support and education regarding growth disorders in children and related adult disorders. Provides educational information, networking, a national conference, a kids' program and an extensive medical library.

Dianne Tamburrino, Executive Director
Susan Smith, Director Medical Education

318 March of Dimes Birth Defects Foundation
1275 Mamaroneck Avenue
White Plains, NY 10605

914-428-7100
888-663-4637
Fax: 914-428-8203
e-mail: resourcecenter@modimes.org
www.marchofdimes.com

Partnership of volunteers and professionals dedicates to improving the health of babies by preventing birth defects and infant mortality. Over 100 chapters are located across the country and can be located through the National Office.

Dr Jennifer Howse, President

Web Sites

319 Online Mendelian Inheritance in Man
www.ncbi.nlm.nih.gov

This database is a catalog of human genes and genetic disorders.

320 Wheeless' Textbook of Orthopaedics
www.wheelessonline.com

Comprehensive, unparalleled, dynamic online medical textbook that is updated daily.

Book Publishers

321 Let's Talk About Going to the Hospital
Rosen Publishing Group's PowerKids Press
29 E 21st Street
New York, NY 10010

212-777-3017
800-237-9932
Fax: 888-436-4643
e-mail: rosenpub@tribeca.ios.com
www.powerkidspress.com

If a child has to check into the hospital, chances are he or she is already upset about being ill. Knowing how a hospital functions and what the procedures are, such as when family members can visit, will help in what is already a stressful situation. Grades K-5.

24 pages
ISBN: 0-823950-36-0

DESCRIPTION

322 ASPERGER SYNDROME

Involves the following Biologic System(s):
Developmental/Behavioral/Psychiatric Disorders,
Genetic/Chromosomal/Syndrome/Metabolic Disorders,
Neurologic Disorders

Asperger syndrome is a condition that many researchers consider a high-functioning form of autism. However, others indicate that the disorder is more appropriately considered a nonverbal learning disability. According to those who classify the condition as a higher functioning form of autism, Asperger syndrome may be differentiated from autistic disorder by a later age at onset and lack of major language delays. The symptoms associated with Asperger syndrome typically become apparent after the age of 30 months and vary in range and severity.

Children with Asperger syndrome typically have a normal intelligence quotient (I.Q.), but have deficient communication and social skills, and exhibit autistic-like behaviors. Ironically, many affected children appear to have normal language development and even develop rich vocabularies. However, they often experience difficulties with the subtleties of language, such as the slight variations in rhythm and pitch that help to communicate different shades of meaning (prosody). In addition, many children with the disorder have poor motor skills; they may be clumsy, avoid eye contact, experience varying levels of difficulty processing information, and have impairments in the use and comprehension of certain nonverbal cues and behaviors (e.g., facial expressions, gestures, etc.). Affected children also typically adopt certain routines or rituals; have difficulties with change; may be abnormally preoccupied with one or more areas of interest; and have deficient social skills. For example, many children with Asperger syndrome are socially withdrawn; lack awareness of others' thoughts or feelings; and are unusually sensitive to certain sights, sounds, or tastes. Some affected children may possess an extraordinary talent or skill in a particular area.

Children with Asperger syndrome are typically educated in the mainstream setting but usually require special education services. These children often have difficulty making friends and are often teased or bullied by their peers. The management and treatment of children with Asperger syndrome may include integrated, multidisciplinary techniques, such as therapy to teach practical and social skills. Medications may be used to treat specific behavioral symptoms associated with Asperger syndrome, such as anxiety and depression. The cause of Asperger syndrome is unknown. However, as is the case with autistic disorder, researchers indicate that genetic factors may play some role in causing or resulting in susceptibility for the disorder.

See also **General Resources** on page 917

Government Agencies

323 NIH/National Institute of Mental Health
6001 Executive Boulevard, Room 8184, MSC 9663
Bethesda, MD 20892

301-443-4513
866-615-6464
Fax: 301-443-4279
TTY: 301-443-8431
e-mail: nimhinfo@nih.gov
www.nimh.nih.gov

Conducts strategic planning for specific research areas as well as for the Institute as a whole.

Dr Thomas R Insel, Director

324 NIH/National Institute of Neurological Dis orders and Stroke (NINDS)
PO Box 5801
Bethesda, MD 20824

301-496-5751
800-352-9424
Fax: 301-496-0296
TTY: 301-468-5981
www.ninds.nih.gov

Works to reduce the burden of neurological disease by conducting, fostering, coordinating and guiding research on the causes, prevention, diagnosis and treatment of neurological disorders and stroke, while supporting basic research in related scientific areas.

Story C Landis Ph.D., Director
Audrey S Penn M.D., Deputy Director

325 NIH/National Institute on Deafness and Oth er Communication Disorders (NIDCD)
31 Center Drive, MSC 2320
Bethesda, MD 20892

800-241-1044
TTY: 800-241-1055
e-mail: nidcdinfo@nidcd.nih.gov
www.nidcd.nih.gov

Conducts and supports biomedical research and research training on normal mechanisms, as well as diseases and disorders of hearing, balance, smell, taste, voice, speech and language.

Dr James F Battey Jr, Director
Judith A Cooper PhD, Deputy Director

National Associations & Support Groups

326 American Juvenile Arthritis Organization
2970 Peachtree Road NW, Suite 200
Atlanta, GA 30305

404-237-8771
800-933-7023
Fax: 404-237-8153
e-mail: info.ga@arthritis.org
www.arthritis.org

Devoted to serving the special needs of children, teens, and young adults with childhood rheumatic diseases and their families. Offers both support and information through national and local programs that serve the needs of families, friends and health professionals. Serves as a clearinghouse of information, sponsors an annual national conference, monitors and promotes legislation, sponsors research, and offers training to both parents and health professionals.

Sage Rhodes, President

327 Asperger Syndrome Education Network (ASPEN)
9 Aspen Circle
Edison, NJ 08820

732-321-0880
www.aspennj.org

A regionally based nonprofit organization headquartered in New Jersey, with 12 local chapers, providing for families and those individuals affected with Asperger Syndrome, PDD-NOS, High Functioning Autism, and other related disorders.

Lori Shery, President

328 Autism Network International
PO Box 35448
Syracuse, NY 13235

315-476-2462
e-mail: jisincla@mailbox.syr.edu
http://ani.autistics.org

Supported by individuals who want to make a difference for the sufferers, the foundation provides a variety of support and educational references to inform on the latest changes in the field.

Jim Sinclair, Coordinator

329 Autism Society of America
7910 Woodmont Avenue, Suite 300
Bethesda, MD 20814

301-657-0881
800-328-8476
e-mail: info@autism-society.org
www.autism-society.org

A national charitable organization with the mission of providing as much information as possible about autism and the various options, approaches, methods and systems available to parents of children with autism, family members and those professionals who work with them.

Lee Grossman, President & CEO
Cathy Pratt PhD, Chair

330 Center for Outreach and Services for the Autism Community
1450 Parkside Avenue, Suite 22
Ewing, NJ 08638

609-883-8100
800-428-8476
Fax: 609-883-5509
e-mail: information@njcosac.org
www.njcosac.org

Nonprofit agency providing information and advocacy, services, family and professional education, and consultation to New Jersey's autism community.

Paul A Potito, Executive Director

331 MAAP Services for Autism, Asperger's Syndrome and PDD
PO Box 524
Crown Point, IN 46307

219-662-1311
Fax: 219-662-0638
e-mail: chart@netnitco.net
www.maapservices.org

Nonprofit organization dedicated to providing information and advice to families of more advanced individuals with Autism, Asperger's sundrome, and Pervasive developmental disorder.

Susan Moreno, Founder & President

332 National Mental Health Consumers' Self-Help Clearinghouse
1211 Chestnut Street, Suite 1207
Philadelphia, PA 19107

215-751-1810
800-553-4539
Fax: 215-636-6312
e-mail: info@mhselfhelp.org
www.mhselfhelp.org

Offers information, support and appropriate referrals; and promotes public and professional education. Provides networking for those with special interests related to albinism. Promotes and supports research and funding that will improve diagnosis and management of albinism and hypopigmentation.

Joseph Rogers, Executive Director & Founder

Web Sites

333 AS Support Network
home.vincent.net.au/~asperger

To give mutual support, provide relevant information, support research about the syndrome, and providing services to members.

334 Asperger's Association of New England
http://aane.autistics.org

The immediate goal of austistic.org is to build a global database of information and resouces by and for persons on the autistic spectrum.

335 Autism Resources
www.autism-resources.com

Offers information and links regarding the developemental disabilities autism and Asperger's Syndrom.

336 Family Village
www.familyvillage.wisc.edu

A global community that integrates information, resources and communication opportunities on the Internet for persons with cognitive and other disabilities, for their families and for those that provide them services and support.

337 Online Asperger Syndrome Information and Support
www.udel.edu/bkirby/asperger/

Provides parents, professionals and person with the links they need to research anything.

338 University Students with Autism and Asperger's Syndrome Web Site
www.users.dircon.co.uk/~cns/

Helps to develop an understanding of the difficulties people with Asperger Syndrome may face. We also work on a one to one basis with the student and liase with staff and peers. Help is also given in setting up support networks such as mentors and providing effective strategies to aid independent learning.

Book Publishers

339 Asperger Syndrome
Guilford Publications
72 Spring Street
New York, NY 10012

212-431-9800
800-365-7006
Fax: 212-966-6708
e-mail: info@guilford.com
www.guilford.com

Brings together preeminent scholars and practitioners to offer a definitive statement of what is currently known about Asperger syndrome and to highlight promising leads in research and clinical practice. Sifts through the latest developments in theory and research, discussing key diagnostic and conceptual issues and reviewing what is known about behavioral features and neurobiology. The effects of Asperger syndrome on social development, learning and communication are examined.

484 pages
ISBN: 1-572305-34-7

340 Asperger Syndrome and Your Child: A Parent's Guide
Autism Society of North Carolina Bookstore
505 Oberlin Road, Suite 230
Raleigh, NC 27605

919-743-0204
Fax: 919-743-0208
e-mail: books@autismsociety-nc.org
www.autismbookstore.com

Written primarily for parents, this book provides a clinician's view of Asperger Syndrome.

341 Asperger Syndrome: A Practical Guide for Teachers
ADD WareHouse
300 NW 70th Avenue, Suite 102
Plantation, FL 33317

954-792-8100
800-233-9273
Fax: 954-792-8545
www.addwarehouse.com

A clear and concise guide to effective classroom practice for teachers and support assistants working with children with Asperger Syndrome in school. The authors explain characteristics of children with Asperger Syndrome, discuss methods of assessment and offer practical strategies for effective classroom interventions.

90 pages
ISBN: 1-853464-99-6

342 Asperger Syndrome: Guide for Educators and Parents, Second Edition
Pro-Ed
8700 Shoal Creek Boulevard
Austin, TX 78757

512-451-3246
800-897-3202
Fax: 800-397-7633
e-mail: info@proedinc.com
www.proedinc.com

A ground-breaking resource on Asperger Syndrome, this text outlines, in lay terms, the characteristics of the syndrome sometimes referred to as higher-functioning autism.

215 pages
ISBN: 0-890798-98-2

343 Asperger's Syndrome: A Guide for Parents and Professionals
ADD WareHouse
300 NW 70th Avenue, Suite 102
Plantation, FL 33317

954-792-8100
800-233-9273
Fax: 954-792-8545
addwarehouse.com

Providing a description and analysis of the unusual characteristics of Asperger's Syndrome, with strategies to reduce those that are most conspicuous or debilitating. This guide brings together the most relevant and useful information on all aspects of the syndrome, from language and social behavior to motor clumsiness.

240 pages
ISBN: 1-853025-77-1

344 Autism and Asperger Syndrome
Autism Society of North Carolina Bookstore
505 Oberlin Road
Raleigh, NC 27605

919-743-0204
Fax: 919-743-0208
www.austismsociety-nc.org

Chapters include topics such as the relationship of autism and Asperger Syndrome, living with the syndrome and Asperger Syndrome in adulthood.

247 pages

345 Can I Tell You About Asperger Syndrome?: A Guide for Friends and Family
Autism Society of North Carolina Bookstore
505 Oberlin Road, Suite 230
Raleigh, NC 27605

919-743-0204
Fax: 919-743-0208
e-mail: books@autismsociety-nc.org
www.autismbookstore.com

Written for young people so that they can better understand the challenges faced by a sibling, friend, or classmate who has Asperger Syndrome. For readers ages 7-15.

346 Oasis Guide to Asperger Syndrome
Autism Society of North Carolina Bookstore
505 Oberlin Road, Suite 230
Raleigh, NC 27605

919-743-0204
Fax: 919-743-0208
e-mail: books@autismsociety-nc.org
www.autismbookstore.com

Combining the most current information about Asperger Syndrome (AS) diagnosis and treatment with hundreds of practical tips and reosurce listings, this guide is comprehensive in scope.

347 Out-of-Sync Child: Recognizing and Coping with Sensory Processing Disorder
Autism Society of North Carolina Bookstore
505 Oberlin Road, Suite 230
Raleigh, NC 27605

919-743-0204
Fax: 919-743-0208
e-mail: books@autismsociety-nc.org
www.autismbookstore.com

The author provides, readers with information on the symptoms and diagnosis of sensory processing disorder (SPD), as well as treatment approach based on early intervention.

348 To Be Me: Understanding What It's Like to Have Asperger's Syndrome
Autism Society of North Carolina Bookstore
505 Oberlin Road, Suite 230
Raleigh, NC 27605

919-743-0204
Fax: 919-743-0208
e-mail: books@autismsociety-nc.org
www.autismbookstore.com

Colorfully illustrated book is about a boy named David, who has Asperger Syndrome (AS). Told from David's point of view, the story focuses on his social difficulties, as he struggles to fit in with his classmates at school. For readers ages 9-12.

Pamphlets

349 Asperger Syndrome
NINDS
PO Box 5801
Bethesda, MD 20824

301-496-5751
800-352-9424
www.ninds.nih.gov

Information sheet.

350 Autism Fact Sheet
NINDS
PO Box 5801
Bethesda, MD 20824

301-496-5751
800-352-9424
TTY: 301-468-5981
www.ninds.nih.gov

Also available in Spanish.

DESCRIPTION

351 ASTHMA

Synonym: Bronchial asthma
Involves the following Biologic System(s):
Respiratory Disorders

Asthma is a chronic respiratory disorder in which abnormal sensitivity (hyperresponsiveness) to certain stimuli causes inflammation and associated narrowing of the lungs' large and small airways, resulting in shortness of breath and other symptoms. Approximately 14 million adults and 6 million children have asthma. It is the primary cause of chronic illness in children. Up to 10 percent of girls and 15 percent of boys are affected by asthma at some point during childhood. Initial symptoms occur during the first year of life in about 30 percent of patients and before the age of four to five years in approximately 80 to 90 percent.

Episodes may be triggered by exposure to many different stimuli, such as certain foreign substances (allergens) including pollen, mold, house dust, or animal hair. Asthma attacks may also be triggered by respiratory infections or exposure to smoke, certain chemicals or medications, strong odors, cold air, vigorous exercise, or stress. Exposure to such stimuli or precipitating factors may prompt certain cells within the lungs' airways (e.g., mast cells) to release particular substances that may cause spasms of the smooth muscles lining the airways, inflammation and swelling of the airway walls, excessive secretion of mucus, and associated airway narrowing (bronchoconstriction) and obstruction.

Asthma episodes may vary greatly in frequency, severity, and duration. For example, attacks may subside after minutes or have a duration of hours or even days. Some patients may have only occasional, mild episodes of shortness of breath. Others may regularly cough and produce a high-pitched whistling sound while breathing (wheezing) and experience severe asthma episodes upon exposure to certain triggering stimuli. Most children with asthma have only periodic episodes that are mild to moderate in severity. However, a small percentage of children have severe asthma that interferes with regular daily functioning. Interestingly, most patients become relatively free of symptoms within 10 to 20 years after disease onset; however, many may have recurrences at some time during adulthood. Children with severe asthma may experience chronic disease through adulthood.

Asthma episodes may begin suddenly or gradually and are initially characterized by signs of air hunger, such as sighing, yawning, wheezing that may be most apparent while exhaling. Other symptoms include shortness of breath and a hacking, nonproductive cough. As mucus secretions increase, exhaling may become abnormally prolonged; however, this finding may not be obvious in infants and young children. Shortness of breath may become so severe that patients have difficulty walking and become unable to speak other than in a panting manner. These patients may assume a hunched over position in an attempt to make breathing easier. Additional symptoms may include chest tightness, profuse sweating due to exertion and anxiety, nausea, and vomiting. During extremely severe episodes, wheezing may diminish due to lack of airflow in the airways; breathing may become irregular and shallow; and patients may become listless (lethargic), appear confused due to lack of oxygen, and develop abnormal bluish discoloration of the skin and mucous membranes (cyanosis) due to abnormally diminished oxygen levels in the blood. Without immediate treatment, such patients may experience life-threatening complications.

Asthma is classified according to frequency of symptoms and the result of lung (pulmonary) tests. Classification and monitoring assists with the management of asthma and includes minimizing exposure to possible precipitating factors, such as avoiding rapid changes in humidity or temperature and reducing exposure to tobacco smoke, pollen, strong odors, fumes, or other possible irritants. In some cases, specialized tests may help to determine specific triggering stimuli that should be avoided. Asthma medications can be divided into long-term control and quick relief medications. Treatment choices are based on the severity of the patient's underlying asthma and the severity of asthma exacerbations. Treatment should be administered as quickly a|s possible to open the airways and restore normal breathing and proper oxygen levels in the blood. Drug therapy may include medications that relax and widen the airways (bronchodilators), such as albuterol. Depending upon the specific drugs prescribed or the severity of an episode, such medications may be administered by a metered dose inhaler with a spacer, or by a nebulizer, which produces a mist for inhalation. Inhaled steroids are the most effective anti-inflammatory medications for management of chronic asthma. Intravenous medications may be used in the hospitalized patient. If a patient is unable to be managed at home, or has progression of symptoms requiring intervention more often than every 4 hours, they should seek emergency care. Emergency treatment may include IV corticosteroids, IV bronchodilators, continuous nebulizer treatments and, in the most severe cases, possibly intubation with mechanical ventilation.

See also **General Resources** on page 917

See also **General Resources** on page 917

Government Agencies

352 NIH/National Heart, Lung and Blood Institu te Information Center
NHLBI Information Center
PO Bo 30105
Bethesda, MD 20824

301-592-8573
Fax: 301-629-3246
TTY: 240-629-3255
e-mail: nhlbinfo@nhlbi.nih.gov
www.nhlbi.nih.gov

The National Heart, Lung and Blood Institute, provides leafership for a national program in diseases of the heart, blood vessles, lung, and blood; blood resources; and sleep disorders.

Elizabeth Nabel, MD, Director

353 NIH/National Institute of Allergy and Infectious Diseases
6610 Rockledge Drive, MSC 6612
Bethesda, MD 20892

301-496-5717
Fax: 301-402-3573
TDD: 800-877-8339
www.niaid.nih.gov

Conducts and supports basic and applied research to better understand, treat, and ultimately prevent infectious, immunologic, and allergic diseases.

Anthony S Fauci MD, Director

354 National Advisory Allergic and Infectious Disease Council
6610 Rockledge Drive MSC 6612
Bethesda, MD 20892

301-496-5717
Fax: 301-402-3573
www.niaid.nih.gov/ncn

The principal advisory board of the NIAID. The council is composed of physicians, scientists and representatives of the public and advises on the conduct and support or research, training and dissemination of health information regarding allergies and infectious diseases.

Anthony S Fauci MD, Director

National Associations & Support Groups

355 Allergy & Asthma Network Mothers of Asthmatics
2751 Prosperity Avenue, Suite 150
Fairfax, VA 22031

800-878-4403
800-878-4403
Fax: 703-573-7794
e-mail: info@aanma.org
www.aanma.org

A nonprofit association dedicated to educating families with asthma and allergies. Facilitates communication of accurate information among patients, parents, physicians and industry. Provides an important communication link among the home, school, physician and the pharmaceutical industry in an effort to help families create a management program for those with asthma and allergies. Provides accurate guidance and clearly written resources on asthma and allergies.

Nancy Sander, President/Founder
Pamela Mason, Chairman

356 American Academy of Allergy, Asthma and Immunology
555 East Wells Street, Suite 1100
Milwaukee, WI 53202

414-272-6071
800-822-2762
e-mail: info@aaaai.org
www.aaaai.org

Represents allergists, clinical immunologists, allied health professionals, and others with a special interest in treating and researching diseases such as allergic rhinitis, asthma, atopic dermatitis/eczema, and anaphylaxis.

Steve Folstein, Managing Director

357 American College of Allergy, Asthma and Immunology
85 W Algonquin Road, Suite 550
Arlington Heights, IL 60005

847-427-1200
800-842-7777
Fax: 847-427-1294
e-mail: mail@acaai.org
www.acaai.org

An information and news service for patients, parents of patients, members, the news media, and purchasers of health care programs.

William K Dolen, MD, President

358 American Lung Association
61 Broadway, 6th Floor
New York, NY 10006

212-315-8700
800-586-4872
www.lungusa.org

The American Lung Association fights lung disease in all its forms, with special emphasis on asthma, tobacco control and environmental health. The American Lung Association is funded with contributions from the public, along with gifts and grants from corporations, foundations and government agencies. The association achieves its many successes through the work of thousands of committed volunteers and staff.

Terri E Weaver, PhD RN CS FAAN, Chairman

359 Asthma and Allergy Foundation of America
1233 20th Street NW, Suite 402
Washington, DC 20036

202-466-7643
800-727-8462
Fax: 202-466-8940
e-mail: info@aafa.org
www.aafa.org

The Foundation was formed to alleviate suffering and loss from asthma and allergy disorders. The Foundation offers a nationwide network of chapters and support groups, and provides education and emotional support for persons with allergies and asthma. Also funds research for improved treatments and ultimately a cure.

Chris Ward, President
William McLin, Executive Director

360 Genetic Alliance
4301 Connecticut Avenue NW
Washington, DC 20008

202-966-5557
800-336-4363
Fax: 202-966-8553
e-mail: info@geneticalliance.org
www.geneticalliance.org

A coalition of voluntary genetic support groups, consumers and professionals addressing the needs of individuals and families affected by genetic disorders from a national perspective.

Sharon Terry, President/CEO

361 Get a Grip on Asthma Programs
Allergy and Asthma Network/Mothers of Asthmatics
2751 Prosperity Avenue, Suite 150
Fairfax, VA 22031

703-641-9595
Fax: 703-573-7794
e-mail: info@aanma.org
www.aanma.org

Programs designed to broaden the awareness among the inner-city asthma population of what asthma is, what triggers asthma, and how to recognize the symptoms. Facts and information about the use of medications and holding chambers are discussed as well. Program is conducted in five major cities across the United States.

Nancy Sander, President/Founder

362 Support for Asthmatic Youth (SAY) Support Groups
Asthma and Allergy Foundation of America
1080 Glen Cove Avenue
Glen Head, NY 11545

516-625-5735
Fax: 516-625-2976
e-mail: reneeTheo1@aol.com

A network of educational/support groups for adolescents between the ages of nine and seventeen. All meetings are free and feature guest speakers, informational programs, games and other fun activities.

Renee Theodorakis, MA

363 Support for Asthmatic Youth Pals-Pen Pals
Asthma and Allergy Foundation of America
1080 Glen Cove Avenue
Glen Head, NY 11545

516-625-5735
Fax: 516-625-2976
e-mail: reneeTheo1@aol.com

A pen pal program that matches adolescents ages 9 to 17 who share similar interests and also happen to have asthma and/or allergies.

Renee Theodorakis, MA, Adolescent Services

State Agencies & Support Groups

Alabama

364 Asthma and Allergy Foundation of America - Alabama Chapter
150 Inverness Corners
Birmingham, AL 35242

205-408-9077
Fax: 205-408-4377
e-mail: aafaal@aol.com
www.AsthmaAndAllergy.org

Provides education to those who have asthma or allergies, their families and others, through community resources, support groups and educational programs. Programs include Asthma Camp at U.S. Space Camp in Huntsville.

Karen Brennan, Executive Director

Alaska

365 Alaska Chapter of Asthma and Allergy Foundation of America
Po Box 201927
Anchorage, AK 99520

907-696-4810
Fax: 800-651-4914
e-mail: aafaalaska@gci.net
www.aafaalaska.com

Dedicated to improving the quality of life for people affected by asthma and allergies through education, collaboration and with communit resources, support and research.

Suzi Jackson, RN, Executive Director
Sheila Arkell, Associate Director

California

366 Northern California Chapter of Asthma and Allergy Foundation of America
2269 Chestnut Street, Suite 481
San Francisco, CA 94123

415-339-8880
800-727-8462
Fax: 415-339-8881
www.aafa.org

AAFA is a not-for-profit, voluntary health organization dedicated to improving the quality of life for people with asthma and allergies, and their caregivers, through education, research and advocacy. Publishes educational pamphlets and a bimonthly patient newsletter with timely asthma and allergy information.

Linda Christopher, Executive Director

367 Southern California Chapter of Asthma and Allergy Foundation of America
5900 Wilshire Boulevard, Suite 2330
Los Angeles, CA 90036

323-937-7859
800-624-0044
Fax: 323-937-7815
e-mail: info@aafasocal.com
www.aafasocal.com

AAFA is a not-for-profit, voluntary health organization dedicated to improving the quality of life for people with asthma and allergies, and their caregivers, through education, research and advocacy. Publishes educational pamphlets and a bimonthly patient newsletter with timely asthma and allergy information.

Francene Lifson, Executive Director

Florida

368 Florida Chapter of Asthma and Allergy Foundation of America
200 Orangewood Drive
Dunedin, FL 34698

727-736-4484
800-727-8462
Fax: 727-738-1146
e-mail: cherylsmall@aafaflorida.org
www.aafaflorida.org

AAFA is a not-for-profit, voluntary health organization dedicated to improving the quality of life for people with asthma and allergies and their caregivers, through education, research and advocacy. Publishes educational pamphlets and a bimonthly patient newsletter with timely asthma and allergy information.

Cheryl Small, Executive Director

Georgia

369 Asthma and Allergy Foundation of America - Georgia Chapter
5850 Dovnick Drive SW
Lilburn, GA 30047

770-717-8377
Fax: 770-717-8377

Marie Schuster, Executive Director

Maryland

370 Maryland-Greater Washington, DC Chapter of Asthma and Allergy Foundation of America
1777 Reisterstown Road, Suite 290
Baltimore, MD 21208

410-653-2880
800-727-9333
Fax: 410-653-9611
e-mail: info@aafa-md.org
www.aafa-md.org

AAFA MD-DC is a not-for-profit organization dedicated to improving the quality of life for people with asthma and allergies, and their caregivers through education, research and advocacy. We publish pamphlets and a bimonthly patient newsletter with timely asthma and allergy information.

Linda R Boyer, Executive Director

Massachusetts

371 Asthma & Allergy Foundation of America New England Chapter
109 Highland Avenue
Needham, MA 02494

> 781-444-7778
> 800-2AS-THMA
> Fax: 781-444-7718
> e-mail: aafane@aafane.org
> www.aafa.org

AAFA is a not-for-profit, voluntary health organization dedicated to improving the quality of life for people with asthma and allergies, and their caregivers, through education, research and advocacy. Publishes educational pamphlets and a patient newsletter with timely asthma and allergy information.

Elaine Erenrich Rosenburg, Executive Director

Michigan

372 Michigan Chapter of Allergy and Asthma Foundation of America
17520 W 12 Mile Road, Suite 102
Southfield, MI 48076

> 248-557-8050
> 888-444-0333
> Fax: 248-557-8768
> e-mail: aafamich@sbcglobal.net
> www.aafamich.org

AAFA is a not-for-profit, voluntary health organization dedicated to improving the quality of life for people with asthma and allergies, and their caregivers, through education, research and advocacy. Publishes educational pamphlets with timely asthma and allergy information.

Kathleen Felice Slonager, Executive Director

Missouri

373 Allergy and Pulmonary Medicine
Saint Louis Children's Hospital
One Children's Place
Saint Louis, MO 63110

> 314-454-6000
> Fax: 314-454-2515
> www.stlouischildrens.org

Evaluating and treating a child's allergy or pulmonary disorder is only part of the care provided by the professionals at St. Louis Children's Hospital. Many of the difficulties children endure also require extensive treatment at home, therefore, educating parents and caregivers about home care and progress monitoring is a primary concern for the Allergy and Pulmonary Medicine staff. In most cases, the staff works with other team members throughout the hospital.

Alan Schwartz, Chief of Staff

374 Asthma and Allergy Foundation of America Greater Kansas City Chapter
9140 Ward Parkway, Suite 120
Kansas City, MO 64114

> 816-333-6608
> 888-542-8252
> Fax: 816-333-6684
> e-mail: info@aafaks.org
> www.aafakc.org

Provides education, support and aid for people with asthma and allergies (and their families) in the Greater Kansas City area. Some major programs include Smoke-Free Dining Guide, Annual Family

Asthma Education Day, Asthma Camp, Asthma Coalition and support groups. Most of our programs are offered free to the public. The few that have a small fee also have scholarships available.

Noel Albert, Executive Director

375 Asthma and Allergy Foundation of America - Saint Louis Chapter
1500 South Big Bend, Suite 18
Saint Louis, MO 63117

> 314-645-2422
> Fax: 314-645-2022
> e-mail: aafa@aafastl.org
> www.aafastl.org

Serves Saint Louis, E Saint Louis and surrounding counties through education, support and medical resources. Some major activities include Project Concern for low-income children with asthma, annual asthma screening and education health line.

Robert Novelly, Executive Director

New Jersey

376 Asthma and Allergy Foundation of America - Southeast Pennsylvania Chapter
PO Box 115, 32 Caspertown St
Gibbstown, NJ 08027

> 856-224-9547
> 800-778-2232
> Fax: 856-224-5893
> e-mail: aafasepa@prodigy.net
> www.aafa.org

Serves southeastern Pennsylvania and portions of New Jersey. Program highlights include the Children at Risk program.

Debi Maines, Executive Director

New York

377 New York Chapter of Asthma and Allergy Foundation of America
984 N Village Avenue
Rockville Center, NY 11570

> 540-370-0016
> 800-727-8462
> Fax: 540-370-0015
> e-mail: aafany@aol.com
> www.aafa.org

AAFA is a not-for-profit, voluntary health organization dedicated to improving the quality of life for people with asthma and allergies, and their caregivers, through education, research and advocacy. Publishes educational pamphlets and a bimonthly patient newsletter with timely asthma and allergy information.

Peggy McElgunn, Executive Director

Oregon

378 Asthsma and Allergy Foundation of America Oregon Chapter
14530 SW 144th Avenue
Tigard, OR 97224

> 503-579-8375
> e-mail: hensches@teleport.com

Pennsylvania

379 SE Pennsylvania Chapter of Asthma and Allergy Foundation of America
PO Box 115
Gibbstown, NJ 08027

> 856-224-9547
> 800-727-8462
> Fax: 856-224-5893
> e-mail: aafasepa@prodigy.net
> www.aafa.org

AAFA is a not-for-profit, voluntary health organization dedicated to improving the quality of life for people with asthma and allergies, and their caregivers, through education, research and advocacy. Publishes educational pamphlets and a bimonthly patient newsletter with timely asthma and allergy information.

Debi Maines, Executive Director

Texas

380 Asthma and Allergy Foundation of America - North Texas Chapter
9101 Quarterhouse Ln
Ft Worth, TX 76123

817-297-3132
888-933-AAFA
Fax: 817-297-6564
e-mail: aafantx1@hotmail.com
www.aafa.org

Offers many educational programs and services that touch patients, caregivers, physicians and allied health professionals.

Joan Hart, Executive Director

Washington

381 Washington State Chapter of Asthma and Allergy Foundation of America
3400 Harbor Avenue, SW, #113
Seattle, WA 98126

206-368-2866
800-778-2232
Fax: 206-368-2941
e-mail: aafawa@aafawa.org
www.aafawa.org

AAFA is a not-for-profit, voluntary health organization dedicated to improving the quality of life for people with asthma and allergies, and their caregivers, through education, research and advocacy. Publishes educational pamphlets and a bimonthly patient newsletter with timely asthma and allergy information.

Penny Nelson, Executive Director

Libraries & Resource Centers

382 Lung Line Information Service
National Jewish Center for Immunology
1400 Jackson Street
Denver, CO 80206

303-388-4461
800-222-5864
Fax: 303-270-2162
www.nationaljewish.org

A free information service answering questions, sending literature and giving advice to patients with immunologic or respiratory illnesses. The Line is an educational service and not a substitute for medical care. Diagnosis or suggested treatment will not be provided for a caller's specific condition. The Line does suggest topics that a patient might want to discuss with his or her doctor.

Michael Salem MD, Vice President & CEO

383 Physician Referral and Information Line
American Academy of Allergy, Asthma and Immunology
555 East Wells Street, Suite 1100
Milwaukee, WI 53202

414-272-6071
800-822-2762
Fax: 414-272-6070
e-mail: info@aaaai.org
www.aaaai.org

Referral line offering information on allergy and asthma, referral to an allergy/immunology specialist.

Michele Martinez, Director, Communications

Research Centers

384 Brigham and Women's Hospital, Asthma and Allergic Disease Research Center
75 Francis Street
Boston, MA 02115

617-732-5500
Fax: 617-432-0979
TTY: 617-732-6458
e-mail: bwhinfo@partners.org
www.brighamandwomens.org

Integral unit of the hospital focusing research attention on asthma and allergy related disorders.

K Frank Austen, MD, Director

385 Center for Interdisciplinary Research on Immunologic Diseases
Children's Hospital Medical Center
300 Longwood Avenue
Boston, MA 02115

617-355-6000
Fax: 617-730-0310
www.childrenshospital.org

Organizational research unit of the Children's Hospital that focuses on the causes, prevention and treatments of asthma, infections and allergies.

Fred S Rosen, MD, Principal Investigator

386 Duke University Asthma and Allergic Disease Center
School of Medicine
Box 2898
Durham, NC 27710

919-684-2922
www.2mc.duke.edu/son

Rebecca H Buckley, Director

387 Johns Hopkins University, Asthma and Allergy Center
5501 Hopkins Bayview Circle
Baltimore, MD 21224

410-550-2101
Fax: 410-550-2090
e-mail: jhuallergy@jhmi.edu
www.hopkinsmedicine.org

Studies of allergic diseases and individuals with allergic disease, pulmonary diseases and diseases involving inflammation and immunological processes.

Dr. Lawrence Lichtenstein, Director

388 National Jewish Center for Immunology and Respiratory Medicine
1400 Jackson Street
Denver, CO 80206

303-388-4461
www.nationaljewish.org

The only medical center in the country whose research and patient care resources are dedicated to respiratory and immunologic diseases.

Michael Salem MD, President & CEO
David H Engleberg, Chair

389 National Jewish Medical & Research Center
1400 Jackson Street
Denver, CO 80206

303-388-4461
800-222-5864
Fax: 303-270-2162
www.njc.org

A world renowned institute devoted to the treatment and study of respiratory and allergic diseases.

Michael Salem MD, President/CEO

390 Northwestern University Asthma and Allergy Disease Center
303 E Chicago Avenue
Chicago, IL 60611

312-908-8107
Fax: 312-908-0205

Roy Patterson, MD, Head

391 Tulane University Clinical Immunology Section
1700 Perdido Street
New Orleans, LA 70112

504-988-5578
800-355-7944
Fax: 504-988-3686
www.som.tulane.edu/medciar/index.html

Mauel Lopez, MD, Director

392 University of Texas Southwestern Medical Center/Asthma & Allergic Diseases
5323 Harry Hines Boulevard
Dallas, TX 75390

214-648-8074
Fax: 214-688-8275

Paul Bergstresser, MD, Principal Investor

393 University of Virginia General Clinical Research Center
PO Box 800787
Charlottesville, VA 22908

434-924-2394
Fax: 434-924-9960
e-mail: gcrc@virginia.edu
www.healthsystem.virginia.edu

Focuses on asthmatic disorders.

Eugene J Barrett, Program Director

394 University of Wisconsin Asthma and Allergic Disease Center
600 Highland Avenue
Madison, WI 53792

608-263-1530

Professor Richard Hong, Head

Audio Video

395 A Regular Kid
American Lung Association
1740 Broadway
New York, NY 10019

212-315-8700
800-586-4872
Fax: 212-765-7876
e-mail: info@lungusa.org
www.lungusa.org

This film shows how families and children cope with asthma problems. Proven asthma management strategies are presented through the experiences of four children with asthma, ranging in age from toddler to teenager.

Film

396 Allergy Control Begins at Home: House Dust Allergy
Allergy Control Products
96 Danbury Road
Ridgefield, CT 06877

888-222-6837
Fax: 203-431-8963
e-mail: info@allergycontrol.com
www.allergycontrol.com

Shows simple steps to decrease your level of dust mite exposure.

1993 35 minutes

397 Asthma Management
American Academy of Allergy, Asthma and Immunology
611 E Wells Street
Milwaukee, WI 53202

414-272-6071
Fax: 414-272-6070
www.aaaai.org

Although there is currently no cure for asthma, attacks can be controlled by appropriate asthma management. This video describes what happens during an asthma attack, how your allergists diagnoses asthma, and ways your allergist can help you to manage your condition.

10-13 minutes

398 Baby Breath
Allergy and Asthma Network/Mothers of Asthmatics
2751 Prosperity Avenue
Fairfax, VA 22031

703-641-9595
Fax: 703-573-7794
www.aanma.org

Shows babies and toddlers taking a nebulizer treatment.

2003 Video

399 Environmental Control Measures
American Academy of Allergy, Asthma and Immunology
611 E Wells Street
Milwaukee, WI 53202

414-272-6071
Fax: 414-272-6070
www.aaaai.org

By conrtolling your environment, you can reduce your exposure to substances called allergens that trigger your allergic symptoms. This program depicts common outdoor and indoor allergens, methods an allergist uses to diagnose which substances you're allergic to, and how to reduce your exposure to allergic triggers.

10-13 minutes

400 Immunotherapy
American Academy of Allergy, Asthma and Immunology
611 E Wells Street
Milwaukee, WI 53202

414-272-6071
Fax: 414-272-6070
www.aaaai.org

Immunotherapy, with allergy shots is a long-term allergy and asthma treatment program that helps control allergic symptoms and reduces the need for medications. Learn more about immunotherapy through this video, which includes information on allergy testing and how your allergist determines if immunotherapy is right for you.

10-13 minutes

401 Managing Childhood Asthma
American Lung Association
Box 596-COL
New York, NY 10001

212-245-8000
Fax: 312-440-9374
e-mail: webmaster@ala.org
www.ala.org

What parents need to know to manage asthma. 22 minutes.

Video

402 Mastering Asthma
Aquarius Health Care Videos
18 North Main Street
Sherborn, MA 01770

508-650-1616
888-440-2963
Fax: 508-650-1665
e-mail: info@aquariusproductions.com
www.aquariusproductions.com

Mastering Asthma, so it doesn't master you, is an entertaining and informative video for both parents and children that takes viewers into the lives of three different families learning about and living with childhood asthma. Learn what is Asthma and what causes it. Everything from allergens and triggers to peak flow meters and bronchodilators and more is discussed. Closed captioned.

ISBN: 1-581402-93-7

403 Pharmacologic Therapy of Pediatric Asthma
American Lung Association
1740 Broadway
New York, NY 10019

212-315-8700

A Learning Resource Program developed by a joint committee of the American Thoracic Society and the ALA.

Film

404 Super Asthma Kids: We Take Control
Association for the Care of Children's Health
7910 Woodmont Avenue
Bethesda, MD 20814

301-654-6549
Fax: 301-986-4553

The latest video from the acclaimed Mount Sinai Medical Center production shop, young people with asthma talk about how, despite having asthma, they enjoy life to the fullest.

1997 26 minutes

405 What School Personnel Should Know About Asthma
American Lung Association
1740 Broadway
New York, NY 10019

212-315-8700

Professionally produced videotape discussing the triggers, symptoms and management of childhood asthma.

Videotape

Web Sites

406 Allergy & Asthma Network Mothers of Asthmatics
www.aanma.org

A national nonprofit network of families whose desire is to overcome not to cope with allergies and asthma.

407 Allergy and Asthma Network/Mothers of Asthmatics
www.mothersofasthmatics.org

A national nonprofit network of families whose desire is to overcome not to cope with allergies and asthma.

Jennifer M Miller, Executive Director

408 American Academy of Allergy, Asthma and Immunology
www.aaaai.org

The mission of the American Academy of Allergy, Asthma and Immunology, is the advancement of the knowledge and practice of allergy, asthma and immunology for optimal patient care: by discussion at meetings, by fostering the education of students and the public, by encouraging union and cooperation among those engaged in the field, and by promoting and stimulating research and study in allergy, asthma and immunology.

409 American Lung Association
www.lungusa.org

Information regarding lung disease in all its forms, with special emphasis on asthma, tobacco control and environmental health.

410 Asthma Triggers
www.aaaai.org

Offers a world of information on allergy, asthma, and immunology.

411 Asthma and Allergy FAQs
www.cs.unc.edu/~kupstas/FAQ.html

The Allergy and Asthma FAQ is an informal gathering of the net wisdom on allergies and asthma. It uncludes links to various (Web and non-Web) sources of information. This started as the misc.kids Allergy and Asthma FAQ, so a certain amount of this information is geared towards parents, but there is plenty of information for adults, too.

412 Asthma and Allergy Foundation of America
www.aafa.org

Provides information, support and referrals through a national network of chapters and educational support groups.

413 Gazoontite
www.gazoontite.com

We are an employee-owned company of allergy sufferers, dedicated to providing you with the very best allergen control products.

414 NIH/National Insitute of Allergy and Infectious Diseases
www.niaid.nih.gov/

The National Institute of Allergy and Infectous Diseases is a component of the National Institutes of Health. NIAID conducts and supports research that strives to understand, treat, and ultimately prevent the myriad infectious, immunologic, and allergic diseases that threaten hundreds of millions of people worldwide.

415 National Eczema Association for Science and Education
www.nationaleczema.org

Information and education works to improve the health and the quality of life of persons living with atopic dermatists/eczema, including those who have the disease as well as their loved ones.

416 Online Mendelian Inheritance in Man
www.ncbi.nlm.nih.gov

This database is a catalog of human genes and genetic disorders.

Book Publishers

417 101 Ways to Reduce Allergens In Your Home
Allergy and Asthma Network/Mothers of Asthmatics
2751 Prosperity Avenue, Suite 150
Fairfax, VA 22031

703-641-9595
Fax: 703-573-7794
e-mail: info@aanma.org
www.aanma.org

If you're feeling overwhelmed by all the things you've been told you need to do to control your allergies, this is the book for you. Helps prioritize the tasks in removing allergens from your home.

Nancy Sander, President/Founder

418 A Parent's Guide to Allergies and Asthma
National Allergy and Asthma Network
3554 Chain Bridge Road, Suite 200
Fairfax, VA 22030

703-385-4403
Fax: 703-352-4354
TTY: 123-019-99

A up-to-date, easy-to-read resource offering essential information on asthma and allergies.

419 Aaron's Awful Allergies
Allergy and Asthma Network/Mothers of Asthmatics
2751 Prosperity Avenue, Suite 150
Fairfax, VA 22031

703-641-9595
Fax: 703-573-7794
e-mail: info@aanma.org
www.aanma.org

5-year-old Aaron's allergies are so severe, he is told he must part with his pets. He is very sad until he discovers a solution to his problem - one that might work for you too.

420 Allergies & Asthma for Dummies

Allergy and Asthma Network/Mothers of Asthmatics
2751 Prosperity Avenue, Suite 150
Fairfax, VA 22031

703-641-9595
Fax: 703-573-7794
e-mail: info@aanma.org
www.aanma.org

An entertaining and highly useful book on a difficult subject.

Nancy Sander, President/Founder

421 Allergy, Asthma & Immunology from Infancy to Adulthood

WB Saunders Company
Independence Square W
Philadelphia, PA 19106

215-238-7800
www.wbsanders.com

1995 (3rd) 784 pages
ISBN: 0-721655-87-4

422 Asthma

Franklin Watts c/o Grolier
90 Old Sherman Turnpike
Danbury, CT 06816

203-797-3500
Fax: 203-797-3197
http://librarypublishing.scholastic.com

This book offers vital information on causes and treatments, plus advice on how to prevent flare-ups.

128 pages Grades 9 12
ISBN: 0-531113-31-0

423 Asthma In the School: Improving Control With Peak Flow Monitoring

National Allergy and Asthma Network
3554 Chain Bridge Road, Suite 200
Fairfax, VA 22030

703-385-4403
Fax: 703-352-4354
TTY: 123-019-99

Comprehensive and practical guide to help the school nurse monitor and assist students with asthma.

424 Asthma Self Help Book

Allergy Control Products
PO Box 793
Ridgefield, CT 06877

203-438-9580
800-422-3878
Fax: 203-431-8963
TTY: 123-019-99
www.allergycontrol.com

A comprehensive manual on the management of asthma for parents of asthmatic children, adult asthmatics, and for health professionals.

Softcover

425 Asthma and Exercise

Henry Holt and Company
3554 Chain Bridge Road, Suite 200
Fairfax, VA 22030

703-385-4403
Fax: 703-352-4354
TTY: 123-019-99

This book offers clear and detailed advice on how adults and children with asthma can participate in exercise and sports activities.

1990

426 Best of Superstuff Activity Booklet

American Lung Association
1740 Broadway
New York, NY 10019

212-315-8700

For young children with asthma featuring a series of activities designed to help youngsters cope with asthma.

32 pages Ages 6-8

427 Children with Asthma: A Manual for Parents

Allergy Control Products
PO Box 793
Ridgefield, CT 06877

203-438-9580
Fax: 203-431-8963
www.allergycontrol.com

Known as the asthma bible, this second edition is sprinkled with anecdotes by patients and their parents.

296 pages Paperback

428 Consumer Update on Asthma

Allergy and Asthma Network/Mothers of Asthmatics
2751 Prosperity Avenue, Suite 150
Fairfax, VA 22031

703-641-9595
Fax: 703-573-7794
e-mail: info@aanma.org
www.aanma.org

Addresses the diagnosis and treatment of all levels of asthma severity in people from infancy to elder years. Includes information on pregnancy, occupational asthma, and environmental control.

429 Determined to Win: Children Living with Allergies & Asthma

Gareth Stevens
1555 N Rivercenter Drive
Milwaukee, WI 53212

414-225-0333
Fax: 414-225-0377
www.gsinc.com

1994 48 pages
ISBN: 0-836810-75-9

430 Go Blow Your Nose, Robert

Allergy and Asthma Network/Mothers of Asthmatics
2751 Prosperity Avenue, Suite 150
Fairfax, VA 22031

703-641-9595
Fax: 703-573-7794
e-mail: info@aanma.org
www.aanma.org

A runny nose causes all sorts of trouble for Robert, until a friend helps him. Colorful illustrations and funny rhymes teach parents and children how to stop the symptoms of rhinitis.

431 How Asthma Makes Me Feel

Allergy and Asthma Network/Mothers of Asthmatics
2751 Prosperity Avenue, Suite 150
Fairfax, VA 22031

703-641-9595
Fax: 703-573-7794
e-mail: info@aanma.org
www.aanma.org

Essays written by and for children about living with Asthma.

432 I'm Tougher Than Asthma!

Albert Whitman & Company
6340 Oakton Street
Morton Grove, IL 60053

847-581-0033
800-255-7675
Fax: 847-581-0039
www.albertwhitman.com

Eight year old Siri loves to sing, play baseball, and catch toads. She won't let her asthma stop her. In her own words (with a little help from Dad), she tells how she was first diagnosed with asthma at age three and how she is learning to understand and manage her disease.

32 pages Hardcover
ISBN: 0-807534-74-9

Caity Anast, Promotion Coordinator
Joe Campbell, Customer Service

433 Let's Talk About Going to the Hospital
Rosen Publishing Group's PowerKids Press
29 E 21st Street
New York, NY 10010

212-777-3017
800-237-9932
Fax: 888-436-4643
e-mail: rosenpub@tribeca.ios.com
www.powerkidspress.com

If a child has to check into the hospital, chances are he or she is already upset about being ill. Knowing how a hospital functions and what the procedures are, such as when family members can visit, will help in what is already a stressful situation. Grades K-5.

24 pages
ISBN: 0-823950-36-0

434 Let's Talk About Having Asthma
Rosen Publishing Group's PowerKids Press
29 E 21st Street
New York, NY 10010

212-777-3017
800-237-9932
Fax: 888-436-4643
e-mail: rosenpub@tribeca.ios.com
www.powerkidspress.com

This book talks about the cause and treatments for asthma as well as the precautions sufferers should take. Recommended for grades K-4.

1997 24 pages
ISBN: 0-823950-32-8

435 Living with Asthma
Walker & Company
104 Fifth Avenue
New York, NY 10011

212-727-8300
Fax: 212-727-0984
www.walkeryoungreaders.com

Dispels the myths surrounding this disease and introduces readers to famous athletes and public figures who deal with it on a daily basis. Explains what asthma is, how to cope with it, what triggers an attack, and what to do if you or somone you are with is having an attack.

2000 112 pages
ISBN: 0-802775-85-3

436 Luke Has Asthma Too
Allergy Control Products
PO Box 793
Ridgefield, CT 06877

Fax: 203-431-8963

This gentle book will make for good reading with children, whether they have asthma or not.

437 Lung Disorders Sourcebook
Omnigraphics
615 Griswold
Detroit, MI 48226

800-234-1340
Fax: 800-875-1340
e-mail: info@omnigraphics.com
omnigraphics.com

Basic consumer health information on lung disorders including tuberculosis, asthma and cystic fibrosis.

2002 678 pages
ISBN: 0-780803-39-6

438 National Asthma Education and Prevention Program Expert Panel Report
NHLBI
PO Box 30105
Bethesda, MD 20824

301-592-8573
Fax: 301-592-8563
TTY: 240-629-3255
www.nhlbi.nih.gov

Guidelines for management and diagnosis of asthma. Outlines clinical practice guidelines, treatment and diagnosis, written for physicians, however should be in every health collection.

146 pages

439 Parent's Guide to Allergies and Asthma
Allergy and Asthma Network/Mothers of Asthmatics
2751 Prosperity Avenue, Suite 150
Fairfax, VA 22031

703-641-9595
800-878-4403
Fax: 703-573-7794
e-mail: info@aanma.org
www.aanma.org

An up-to-date, easy to read resource offering essential information on asthma and allergies.

263 pages

440 Peak Flow Meter Book & Asthma Tracker
Allergy and Asthma Network/Mothers of Asthmatics
2751 Prosperity Avenue, Suite 150
Fairfax, VA 22031

703-641-9595
Fax: 703-573-7794
e-mail: info@aanma.org
www.aanma.org

Two of our most popular resources, these are now sold together in one breathe-easy package. Step by step, the flow meter book explains how to use a peak flow meter in user friendly, fill in the blanks, workbook style. Use the Asthma Tracker symptom diary a few short minutes each morning and evening to track symptoms, peak expiratory rates, and medication use. Over time, you'll see emerging patterns and be able to document important information your physician needs.

Price each

441 School Information Packet
Allergy and Asthma Network/Mothers of Asthmatics
2751 Prosperity Avenue, Suite 150
Fairfax, VA 22031

703-641-9595
Fax: 703-573-7794
e-mail: info@aanma.org
www.aanma.org

Practical, medical, and legal information for school administrators and parents of students with asthma.

442 Understanding Asthma
University Press of Mississippi
3825 Ridgewood Road
Jackson, MS 39211

601-432-6205
800-737-7788
Fax: 601-432-6217
e-mail: press@ihl.state.ms.us
www.upress.state.ms.us

Noting that understanding and education are key to halting the rise in numbers of asthma cases, Dr. Phil Lieberman has written this book for families and the individual sufferer. Subjects include lungs of an asthmatic, allergies which trigger the disease, and measures used to control asthma. A Choice outstanding book for 2000, and American Journal of Nursing Book of the Year award for 2001.

120 pages Hardcover/Ppbck
ISBN: 1-578061-42-3

443   Understanding Asthma: The Blueprint for Breathing
Asthma & Allergy Foundation of America
11700 N 58th Street
Tampa, FL 33617

813-983-0244
www.aafaflorida.org

A layman's guide to asthma facts.

444   You Can Control Asthma - Books for the Family & Kids
Asthma and Allergy Foundation of America
1233 20th Street NW, Suite 402
Washington, DC 20036

202-466-7643
800-727-8462
Fax: 202-466-8940
e-mail: info@aafa.org
www.aafa.org

Here is a set of easy to read workbooks, one for the family and one for children, ages 6-12, to help learn everything one needs to know about asthma. Learn how to keep asthma episodes from starting, what to do when an asthma episode starts, how to use flow meters, spacers, and inhalers through the use of pictures, captions and activities. Kids have their own workbook that helps them to make choices and to feel more in control of their asthma. Workbooks are available in English or Spanish.

45-61 pages

Magazines

445   Allergy & Asthma Today
Allergy and Asthma Network/Mothers of Asthmatics
2751 Prosperity Avenue, Suite 150
Fairfax, VA 22031

703-641-9595
Fax: 703-573-7794
e-mail: info@aanma.org
www.aanma.org

Communicates practical advice and support for the benefit of all people affected by allergies, asthma and related conditions. Seeks to improve health outcomes by providing information in a consumer-friendly format with strategies for implementing behavior changes. Free to AANMA members.

Quarterly

446   Controlling Asthma
American Lung Association
1740 Broadway
New York, NY 10019

212-315-8700

For parents of children with asthma, this newsmagazine tells how parents can help their child deal with the many problems presented by asthma.

16 pages

447   Coping with Allergies and Asthma
PO Box 682268
Franklin, TN 37068

615-790-2400
Fax: 615-794-0179
e-mail: info@copingmag.com
www.copingmag.com

A bimonthly publication devoted to people whose lives are affected by difficult breathing conditions.

Newsletters

448   Asthma and Allergy Health
Allergy and Asthma Network/ Mothers of Asthmatics
2751 Prosperity Avenue, Suite 150
Fairfax, VA 22031

800-878-4403
e-mail: aanma@aol.com

Provides in-depth reporting on new products, medications, and complementary and alternative therapies.

1999

449   MA Report
Allergy and Asthma Network Mothers of Asthmatics
2751 Prosperity Avenue, Suite 150
Fairfax, VA 22031

800-878-4403
Fax: 703-573-7794
e-mail: aanma@aol.com
www.aanma.org

Practical allergy and asthma management information along with the latest allergy and asthma news, recalls, medical updates, product reviews and advocacy initiatives.

8 pages free w/member

Pamphlets

450   Asthma and Allergy Answers: Patient Education Library
Asthma and Allergy Foundation of America
1233 20th Street NW, Suite 402
Washington, DC 20036

202-466-7643
800-727-8462
Fax: 202-466-8940
www.aafa.org

This resource tool has information on more than forty topics of interest to patients. These reproducible camera ready answers are written in a patient friendly question and answer format. There is space to personalize the handy patient education materials with your practice or facility information. Topics covered are adult onset of asthma and allergies, food allergies, latex allergies, asthma medications, peak flow meters and managing your asthma.

In binder form

451   Asthma and the School Child
American Academy of Allergy, Asthma and Immunology
611 E Wells Street
Milwaukee, WI 53202

414-272-6071
Fax: 414-272-6070
www.aaaai.org

452   Childhood Asthma
American Academy of Allergy, Asthma and Immunology
611 E Wells Street
Milwaukee, WI 53202

414-272-6071
Fax: 414-272-6070
www.aaaai.org

Providees information on what to look for in children with asthma.

453   Childhood Asthma: A Matter of Control
American Lung Association
1740 Broadway
New York, NY 10019

212-315-8700

A guide for parents of children with asthma, this booklet covers topics such as identifying asthma signs and symptoms as well as controlling the condition.

28 pages

454   Living with Asthma and Allergies Brochure Series
Asthma and Allergy Foundation of America
1233 20th Street NW, Suite 402
Washington, DC 20036

202-466-7643
800-727-8462
Fax: 202-466-8940
www.aafa.org

This informative series was developed to provide up-to-date, accurate information on common topics. Written in easy to understand language, with helpful illustrations, the brochures covers some of the most commonly asked questions about asthma and allergies. Perfect for individuals, whether newly diagnosed or more experienced, and for distribution to patients. Titles include, Allergy Basics, Seasonal Allergies: Pollens and Molds, Asthma Basics, Exercise and Asthma, and more.

455   Superstuff
American Lung Association
1740 Broadway
New York, NY 10019

212-315-8700

Kit specifically designed to help the elementary school child with asthma to learn how to manage the condition. The kit contains teaching tools, puzzles, riddles, stories and games.

456   Teens Talk to Teens About Asthma
Asthma and Allergy Foundation of America
1233 20th Street NW, Suite 402
Washington, DC 20036

202-466-7643
Fax: 202-466-8940
www.aafa.org

This brochure is a great gift of support to a teen you care about. Includes quotes and thoughts from teens that capture the essence of what it feels like to live with asthma. Perfect for newly diagnosed teens. Single copies free with two first class stamps on a business-sized, self-addressed envelope.(Order #P-012) Quantities available, please call for prices.

457   There are Solutions for the Student with Asthma
American Lung Association
1740 Broadway
New York, NY 10017

212-315-8700

Leaflet telling how parents and school personnel can work together to make life easier for children with asthma.

4 pages

458   Your Child and Asthma
National Jewish Center for Immunology
1400 Jackson Street
Denver, CO 80206

303-388-4461
www.nationaljewish.org

A booklet offering information to parents and family about their child with asthma. Offers information on diagnosis, treatments, triggers and family concerns.

DESCRIPTION

459 ATAXIA

Involves the following Biologic System(s):
Neurologic Disorders

Ataxia is a neuromuscular condition characterized by an impaired ability to coordinate voluntary movements. The condition is caused by abnormalities of or damage to the region of the brain known as the cerebellum, nerve pathways that transmit messages to and from the cerebellum, or certain regions of the spinal cord. The cerebellum plays an essential role in regulating the maintenance of normal postures, sustaining balance, and producing smooth and coordinated movements. The spinal cord conducts sensory and motor impulses to and from the brain. The symptoms associated with ataxia vary, depending upon the specific regions of the brain that are affected; however, symptoms may often include imbalance and an abnormal staggering manner of walking (gait). Ataxia may be the result of certain infection, malformations of the cerebellum of spinal cord that are present at birth (congenital), head injury, brain tumors, exposure to particular medications, or certain genetic disorders. The primary infectious causes of ataxia during childhood include the formation of pus-filled pockets of infection in the cerebellum (cerebellar abscesses); sudden, severe inflammation of the passages within the inner ear (acute labyrinthitis): or acute cerebellar ataxia. Acute labyrinthitis typically occurs due to middle ear infections and may be characterized by vomiting and a sense that one's body or environment is spinning (vertigo). Acute cerebellar ataxia occurs subsequent to certain viral infections, such as chicken pox, and is thought to result from an abnormal immune response causing inflammation of the brain. Acute cerebellar ataxia typically occurs suddenly and may be characterized by impaired control of voluntary movements of the torso (truncal ataxia) and difficulties sitting or standing; involuntary, rapid eye movements (nystagmus); and severe slurring of speech or an inability to speak. Although the condition typically improves within a few weeks, it sometimes is present for up to two months. Most children have a complete recovery; however, some may have residual speech abnormalities and lack of coordination.

Abnormalities present at birth (congenital) that may cause ataxia include absence of the region of the brain between the two sides or hemispheres of the cerebellum (agensis of cerebellar vermis); protrusion of part of the brain through an opening in the skull (encephalocele); or protrusion of certain, malformed regions of the brain through the opening at the base of the skull (foramen magnum) into the upper spinal canal (Arnold-Chiari malformation). Infants and children with such birth defects develop ataxia due to malformation of or damage to certain regions of the cerebellum.

Ataxia may also be an initial symptom associated with certain brain tumors, including tumors affecting the cerebellum or a particular area of the cerebrum where it joins with the cerebellum (i.e., frontal lobe). In addition, brain tumors known as neuroblastomasmay result in progressive ataxia. Neuroblastomas are solid, malignant tumors that may originate in any part of the sympathetic nervous system, which is that part of the nervous system that regulates certain involuntary activities during times of stress, such as raising blood pressure and increasing the heart rate.

In some children, ataxia may result from the administration of certain drugs, such as anticonvulsant medications, particularly phenytoin. In addition, the condition may be caused by exposure to a household pesticide that is commonly used as a rat poison (thallium).

Ataxia may also occur in association with certain inborn errors of metabolism and is a primary feature of many hereditary degenerative disorders of the brain and spinal cord. These degenerative disorders, which may be referred to as hereditay ataxias, include ataxia-telangiectasia and Friedreich's ataxia.

Ataxia-telangiectasia (AT) is a multisystem disorder that is inherited as an autosomal recessive trait. Affected children typically develop ataxia at approximately two years of age, eventually leading to an inability to walk. Friedreich's ataxia is a genetic disorder that is usually inherited as an autosomal recessive trait. The disorder is characterized by degenerative changes of certain regions of the spinal cord and is categorized as a spinocerebellar ataxia. Children with Friedreich's ataxia typically develop ataxia before age 10. The ataxia is slowly progressive and usually affects the legs and feet more severely than the arms and hands. Patients develop unusual high arching and severe muscle weakness of the feet and progressive difficulties walking, typically resulting in the need of a wheelchair. Additional hereditary spinocerebellar ataxia of childhood, such as Roussy-Levy syndrome, cause symptoms and findings similar to those associated with Friedreich's ataxia. Roussy-Levy syndrome often becomes apparent during infancy and is characterized by loss of joint position sensation (sensory ataxia), causing poorly judged, uncoordinated movements. Such ataxia initially affects the legs, causing difficulty walking, and later progresses to affect the hands. Roussy-Levy syndrome is transmitted as an autosomal dominant trait.

Another group of hereditary disorders, known as the olivopontocerebellar atrophics (OPCAs) are associated with ataxia. These disorders are characterized by progressive degeneration of the cerebellum as well as other areas of the brain. Although associated symptoms of most forms of OPCA become apparent during adolescence or adulthood, one form of the disorder is known to occur during infancy (OPCA of neonatal onset). Symptoms may include severely diminished muscle tone; rapidly progressive ataxia; involuntary, rapid eye movements; episodes of abnormally increased electrical activity in the brain (seizures); failure to grow and gain weight at the expected rate (failure to thrive); abnormalities in the structure and function of heart muscle (hypertrophic cardiomyopathy); and other symptoms and findings. Methods used in the management of ataxia may vary and depend upon the condition's underlying cause, the specific form of ataxia present, and other factors. Such measures are typically symptomatic and supportive.

See also **General Resources** on page 917

Government Agencies

460 NIH/National Institute of Neurological Dis orders and Stroke (NINDS)
PO Box 5801
Bethesda, MD 20824

301-496-5751
800-352-9424
Fax: 301-496-0296
TTY: 301-468-5981
www.ninds.nih.gov

Information and advocacy resources for families and professionals. Includes listings of organizations providing general information and organizations focusing on more specific areas of concern to families and young adults who have disabilities.

Story C Landis Ph.D., Director
Audrey S Penn M.D., Deputy Director

National Associations & Support Groups

461 National Ataxia Foundation
2600 Fernbrook Lane N
Minneapolis, MN 55447

763-553-0020
Fax: 763-553-0167
e-mail: naf@ataxia.org
www.ataxia.org

Objectives of this organization are to make an early diagnosis of ataxia by locating all potential victims and encouraging them to

have an examination, public information and professional education materials and basic research on the disease.

State Agencies & Support Groups

Alabama

462 Birmingham Support Group
National Ataxia Foundation
16 The Oaks Circle
Birmingham, AL 35244

205-987-2883
Fax: 763-553-0167
e-mail: donnelly613b@aol.com
www.ataxia.org

The primary mission is to encourage and support research into Hereditary Ataxia, a group of neurological disorders which are chronic and progressive conditions affecting coordination.

Fred Donnelly, Contact
Becky Donnelly, Contact

Arizona

463 Arizona Ataxia Support Group
National Ataxia Foundation
2322 W Sagebrush Drive
Chandler, AZ 85224

480-726-3579
Fax: 763-553-0167
e-mail: naf@ataxia.org
www.ataxia.org

The primary mission is to encourage and support research into Hereditary Ataxia, a group of neurological disorders which are chronic and progressive conditions affecting coordination.

Rita Garcia, Contact

California

464 Central California Support Group
National Ataxia Foundation
28767 Sequoia Court
Coarsegold, CA 93614

559-658-8675
Fax: 763-553-0167
e-mail: naf@ataxia.org
www.ataxia.org

The primary mission is to encourage and support research into Hereditary Ataxia, a group of neurological disorders which are chronic and progressive conditions affecting coordination.

Ree Howell

465 Greater North Valley California Support Group
National Ataxia Foundation
4335 Bourdeaux Drive
Oakley, CA 94561

925-625-0738
www.geocites.com/hotsprings/

The primary mission is to encourage and support research into Hereditary Ataxia, a group of neurological disorders which are chronic and progressive conditions affecting coordination.

Debra Kellerman

466 Los Angeles Ataxia Support Group
National Ataxia Foundation
339 W Palmer, Apartment A
Glendale, CA 91204

818-246-5758
Fax: 763-553-0167
e-mail: harryluther@sbcglobal.net
www.geocities.com/hotsprings/falls/6629/

The primary mission is to encourage and support research into Hereditary Ataxia, a group of neurological disorders which are chronic and progressive conditions affecting coordination.

Sid Luther, President

467 Northern California Support Group
National Ataxia Foundation
26840 Edridge Ave
Hayward, CA 94544

510-783-3190
Fax: 763-553-0167
e-mail: rsisbig@aol.com

The primary mission is to encourage and support research into Hereditary Ataxia, a group of neurological disorders which are chronic and progressive conditions affecting coordination.

Deborah Omictin, Contact

468 Orange County Support Group
National Ataxia Foundation
15202 Clemente Street
Westminster, CA 92683

714-892-8468
Fax: 763-553-0167
e-mail: mahyatt@social.rr.com
www.geocities.com/ocasg

The primary mission is to encourage and support research into Hereditary Ataxia, a group of neurological disorders which are chronic and progressive conditions affecting coordination.

Margeret Hyatt, Contact

469 Pacific Southwest Regional Genetics Group
2151 Berkeley Way
Berkeley, CA 94704

510-540-2696
Fax: 510-540-2966

Coordinates genetic services; promotes communication among genetic professionals and consumers through network newsletter, meetings, and other events; share resources; and promote education and awareness of genetic disorders,

George C Cunningham, Director

470 San Diego Support Group
National Ataxia Foundation
2087 Granite Hills Drive
El Cajon, CA 92019

619-447-3753
Fax: 763-553-0167
e-mail: emclaugh@cox.net
www.geocities.com/ataxia_sdasg

The primary mission is to encourage and support research into Hereditary Ataxia, a group of neurological disorders which are chronic and progressive conditions affecting coordination.

Earl McLaughlin, Contact

471 San Fernando Valley Support Group
National Ataxia Foundation
19450 Turtle Ridge Lane
Northridge, CA 91326

818-363-5335

The primary mission is to encourage and support research into Hereditary Ataxia, a group of neurological disorders which are chronic and progressive conditions affecting coordination.

Darneal J Myers

Colorado

472 Denver Colorado Support Group
National Ataxia Foundation
5902 W Marlewood Drive
Littleton, CO 80123

303-794-6357
e-mail: tom.sathre@acm.org

The primary mission is to encourage and support research into Hereditary Ataxia, a group of neurological disorders which are chronic and progressive conditions affecting coordination.

Donna Sathre, Contact
Tom Sathre, Contact

473 Mountain States Regional Genetics Services Network
4300 Cherry Creek Drive S
Denver, CO 80222

303-692-2423
Fax: 303-782-5576

Coordinates genetic services; promotes communication among genetic professional and consumers through network newsletters, meetings, and other events; share resources; and promote education and awareness of genetic disorders.

474 Northern Colorado Area Support Group
National Ataxia Foundation
1416 Antero Drive
Loveland, CO 80538

970-898-4390
Fax: 763-553-0167
e-mail: kittel@webaccess.net
www.fortnet.org/ncsg

The primary mission is to encourage and support research into Hereditary Ataxia, a group of neurological disorders which are chronic and progressive conditions affecting coordination.

Joe Kittel

475 Pikes Peak Area Support Group
National Ataxia Foundation
730 Elkgen Court
Colorado Springs, CO 80906

719-576-4772
Fax: 763-553-0167
e-mail: naf@ataxia.org
www.ataxia.org

The primary mission is to encourage and support research into Hereditary Ataxia, a group of neurological disorders which are chronic and progressive conditions affecting coordination.

Jacquie Gray

Connecticut

476 Connecticut Area Support Group
National Ataxia Foundation
23 Cobb's Mill Lane
Glastonbury, CT 06033

203-659-8855
Fax: 763-553-0167
e-mail: pstrong96@peoplepc.com
www.ataxia.org

The primary mission is to encourage and support research into Hereditary Ataxia, a group of neurological disorders which are chronic and progressive conditions affecting coordination.

Peter Strong

Florida

477 Broward County Support Group
National Ataxia Foundation
10603 NW 49th Place
Coral Springs, FL 33076

954-341-8565
Fax: 954-753-6761
e-mail: pathamilto@aol.com
community.insidecentralflorida.com/bcfasg/

The primary mission is to encourage and support research into Hereditary Ataxia, a group of neurological disorders which are chronic and progressive conditions affecting coordination.

20 members

Patricia B Hamilton

478 Clearwater, FL Support Group
National Ataxia Foundation
2363 Mary Lane
Clearwater, FL 33763

727-799-2852
e-mail: joyous7@mciworld.com

The primary mission is to encourage and support research into Hereditary Ataxia, a group of neurological disorders which are chronic and progressive conditions affecting coordination.

Joyce Robbins

479 NE Florida Support Group
National Ataxia Foundation
9 Arborclub Drive, #21-107
Ponte Vedra, FL 32082

904-273-4644
Fax: 763-553-0167
e-mail: naf@ataxia.org
www.ataxia.org

The primary mission is to encourage and support research into Hereditary Ataxia, a group of neurological disorders which are chronic and progressive conditions affecting coordination.

June McGrane, Contact

480 Orlando Support Group
National Ataxia Foundation
3212 Lee Shore Loop
Orlando, FL 32820

407-568-9092
Fax: 763-553-0167
www.ataxia.org

The primary mission is to encourage and support research into Hereditary Ataxia, a group of neurological disorders which are chronic and progressive conditions affecting coordination.

Jim Henderson, Contact

481 Tampa Support Group
National Ataxia Foundation
306 Caloosa Palm St
Son City Center, FL 33573

e-mail: charlie@flataxia1.org

The primary mission is to encourage and support research into Hereditary Ataxia, a group of neurological disorders which are chronic and progressive conditions affecting coordination.

Charlie Kirchner, Contact

Georgia

482 Georgia Ataxia Support Group
National Ataxia Foundation
320 Peters Street, Unit 12
Atlanta, GA 30313

404-822-7457
e-mail: rooksgj@yahoo.com

The primary mission is to encourage and support research into Hereditary Ataxia, a group of neurological disorders which are chronic and progressive conditions affecting coordination.

Greg Rooks, Contact

483 Greater Atlanta Area Support Group
National Ataxia Foundation
320 Peters Street, Unit 12
Atlanta, GA 30313

404-822-7451
e-mail: rookssgj@yahoo.com
www.geocities.com/atlantaataxia

The primary mission is to encourage and supportt research into Hereditary Ataxia, a group of neurological disorders which are chronic and progressive conditions affecting coordination.

Greg Rooks, Contact

484 Macon Support Group
National Ataxia Foundation
116 Summerfield Drive
Macon, GA 31210

912-757-9454

The primary mission is to encourage and support research into Hereditary Ataxia, a group of neurological disorders which are chronic and progressive conditions affecting coordination.

Millard H McWhorter III, MD

485 Southeast Regional Genetics Group
PO Box 1642
Decatur, GA 30031

404-778-8551
Fax: 404-778-8562
e-mail: mlane@sergginc.org
www.sergginc.org

Coordinates genetic services; promotes communication among genetic professionals and consumers through network newsletters, meeting, and other events; share resources; and promote education and awareness of genetic diseases.

Jess G Thoene MD, President
Mary Rose Lane BS, Secretary/Treasurer

Illinois

486 Chicago, IL Area Ataxia Support Group
National Ataxia Foundation
3400 Wellington Court, #302
Rolling Meadows, IL 60008

847-797-9398
e-mail: caasgz@aol.com
www.ataxia.org

The primary mission is to encourage and support research into Hereditary Ataxia, a group of neurological disorders which are chronic and progressive conditions affecting coordination.

Craig Lisack, Contact

487 Southern, IL Support Group
National Ataxia Foundation
36 Lindorf Drive
Belleville, IL 62223

618-397-3259
Fax: 763-553-0167
e-mail: elainedante@yahoo.com
www.ataxia.org

The primary mission is to encourage and support research into Hereditary Ataxia, a group of neurological disorders which are chronic and progressive conditions affecting coordination.

Elaine Dante

Indiana

488 Central Indiana Support Group
National Ataxia Foundation
5716 N 225 W
W Lafayette, IN 47906

765-463-3973
Fax: 765-463-3972
e-mail: turtle23@mindspring.com

The primary mission is to encourage and support research into Hereditary Ataxia, a group of neurological disorders which are chronic and progressive conditions affecting coordination.

Judy Marten

489 NE Indiana Support Group
National Ataxia Foundation
4522 Shenandoah Circle W
Fort Wayne, IN 46835

219-485-0965
Fax: 763-553-0167
e-mail: naf@ataxia.org
www.ataxia.org

The primary mission is to encourage and support research into Hereditary Ataxia, a group of neurological disorders which are chronic and progressive conditions affecting coordination.

Don & Jenny Roemke

Iowa

490 Great Plains Genetic Service Network
University of Iowa
Division of Medical Genetics
Iowa City, IA 52242

319-356-2674
Fax: 319-356-3347

Dolores Nesbitt, PhD, Coordinator

491 Iowa Support Group
Finley Hospital-National Ataxia Foundation
350 N Grandview Avenue
Dubeque, IA 52001

319-589-2372
Fax: 763-553-0167
e-mail: theraspeecher@MWCI.net
www.ataxia.org

The primary mission is to encourage and support research into Hereditary Ataxia, a group of neurological disorders which are chronic and progressive conditions affecting coordination.

Elizabeth Burke

492 Sioux County Iowa Chapter
National Ataxia Foundation
209 2nd Street NE
Orange City, IA 51041

763-553-0020
Fax: 763-553-0167
e-mail: naf@ataxia.org
www.ataxia.org

The primary mission is to encourage and support research into Hereditary Ataxia, a group of neurological disorders which are chronic and progressive conditions affecting coordination.

Joan Vande Brake, President

Louisiana

493 Louisiana Chapter
National Ataxia Foundation
PMB 51056, 2250 Gause Blvd
Slidell, LA 70461

985-643-0783
e-mail: ataxia1@earthlink.net
www.angelfire.com

The primary mission is to encourage and support research into Hereditary Ataxia, a group of neurological disorders which are chronic and progressive conditions affecting coordination.

Carla Hagler, Contact

494 Louisiana Support Group
National Ataxia Foundation
3113 Roosevelt Boulevard
Kenner, LA 70065

504-467-0610
Fax: 763-553-0167
e-mail: DD3@peodigy.net
www.angelfire.com/la/ataxiachapter

The primary mission is to encourage and support research into Hereditary Ataxia, a group of neurological disorders which are chronic and progressive conditions affecting coordination.

Denise Drake, President

Maine

495 Maine Support
National Ataxia Foundation
56 Ten Penny Street
Freeport, ME 04032

207-865-4969
Fax: 763-553-0167
e-mail: info@ataxiame.com
www.ataxia.org

The primary mission is to encourage and support research into Hereditary Ataxia, a group of neurological disorders which are chronic and progressive conditions affecting coordination.

June West, Contact

496 New England Regional Genetics Group
PO Box 920288
Needham, MA 02492

781-444-0126
Fax: 781-444-0127
e-mail: mfgnergg@verizon.net
www.nergg.org

Human genetic services and educational planning pertaining to birth defects.

Mary-Frances Garber, Coordinator

Maryland

497 Chesapeake Chapter
National Ataxia Foundation
5938 Rossmore Drive
Bethesda, MD 20814

301-530-4989
Fax: 301-530-2480
e-mail: carljlauter@erols.com
www.geocities.com/Hotsprings/Oasis/4988/

The primary mission is to encourage and support research into Hereditary Ataxia, a group of neurological disorders which are chronic and progressive conditions affecting coordination.

Carl J Lauter, President

Massachusetts

498 Boston Area Support Group
National Ataxia Foundation
45 Juliette Street
Andover, MA 01810

978-475-8072

The primary mission is to encourage and support research into Hereditary Ataxia, a group of neurological disorders which are chronic and progressive conditions affecting coordination.

Donna Gozzela, Contact
Rich Gozzela, Contact

499 Marshfield, MA Support Group
National Ataxia Foundation
100 Hancock Street
Marshfield, MA 02050

617-834-7374
Fax: 763-553-0167
e-mail: naf@ataxia.org
www.ataxia.org

The primary mission is to encourage and support research into Hereditary Ataxia, a group of neurological disorders which are chronic and progressive conditions affecting coordination.

Joan C Terra

500 New England Support Group
National Ataxia Foundation
17 Highland Avenue
Lexington, MA 02421

781-862-1979
Fax: 763-553-0167
e-mail: naf@ataxia.org
www.ataxia.org

The primary mission is to encourage and support research into Hereditary Ataxia, a group of neurological disorders which are chronic and progressive conditions affecting coordination.

Michael Martignetti

Michigan

501 Detroit Michigian Ataxia Support Group
National Ataxia Foundation
1062 Stafford Place
Detroit, MI 48207

313-393-3799
Fax: 763-553-0167
e-mail: babcockj@assess.cl.detroit.mi.us
www.ataxia.org

The primary mission is to encourage and support research into Hereditary Ataxia, a group of neurological disorders which are chronic and progressive conditions affecting coordination.

Jill Babcock

Minnesota

502 Chisago County, MN Support Group
National Ataxia Foundation
10600 282 Street, Apartment 5
Chisago City, MN 55013

612-257-6014
Fax: 763-553-0167
e-mail: naf@ataxia.org
www.ataxia.org

The primary mission is to encourage and support research into Hereditary Ataxia, a group of neurological disorders which are chronic and progressive conditions affecting coordination.

Roxanne Hippe

503 Minneapolis, MN Support Group
National Ataxia Foundation
2549 32nd Avenue S
Minneapolis, MN 55406

612-724-3784
Fax: 763-553-0167
e-mail: lschultz@bitstream.net
www.geocities.com/twincitiesataxia

The primary mission is to encourage and support research into Hereditary Ataxia, a group of neurological disorders which are chronic and progressive conditions affecting coordination.

Lenore Healays, Contact

504 Southwestern Minnesota Support Group
National Ataxia Foundation
218 Cashuin Drive
Luverne, MN 56156

763-553-0020
Fax: 763-553-0167
e-mail: naf@ataxia.org
www.ataxia.org

The primary mission is to encourage and support research into Hereditary Ataxia, a group of neurological disorders which are chronic and progressive conditions affecting coordination.

Julie Schuur

Mississippi

505 Mississippi Chapter
National Ataxia Foundation
PO Box 17005
Hattiesburg, MS 39404

763-553-0020
Fax: 763-553-0167
e-mail: daglio@c-gate.net
www.ataxia.org

The primary mission is to encourage and support research into Hereditary Ataxia, a group of neurological disorders which are chronic and progressive conditions affecting coordination.

Camille Daglio, President

Missouri

506 Central Missouri Area Support Group
National Ataxia Foundation
12 Jackson
Jefferson City, MO 65101

573-659-4759
Fax: 763-553-0167
e-mail: dr-susie@plnet.net
www.geocities.com/HotSprings/Resort/2999/

The primary mission is to encourage and support research into Hereditary Ataxia, a group of neurological disorders which are chronic and progressive conditions affecting coordination.

Susie Strode, PhD

507 Kansas City, Missouri Support Group
National Ataxia Foundation
6605 N Holmes
Gladstone, MO 64118

816-468-7260
Fax: 763-553-0167
e-mail: clarkstone9348@sbcglobal.net
www.ataxia.org

The primary mission is to encourage and support research into Hereditary Ataxia, a group of neurological disorders which are chronic and progressive conditions affecting coordination.

Jim Clark, Contact

508 Saint Louis, MO Support Group
National Ataxia Foundation
1306 Cypress
Pacific, MO 63069

636-271-6432
Fax: 763-553-0167
e-mail: Mbel400@aol.com
www.stlataxia.org

The primary mission is to encourage and support research into Hereditary Ataxia, a group of neurological disorders which are chronic and progressive conditions affecting coordination.

Mark Bellamy

509 Springfield Area Support Group
National Ataxia Foundation
Route 6, Box 235-7B
Ozark, MO 65721

417-581-8697

The primary mission is to encourage and support research into Hereditary Ataxia, a group of neurological disorders which are chronic and progressive conditions affecting coordination.

Patty Humbert

Nebraska

510 Omaha, NE Support Group
National Ataxia Foundation
5904 Henninger Drive, Apartment 104
Omaha, NE 68104

402-573-5838
Fax: 763-553-0167
e-mail: naf@ataxia.org
www.ataxia.org

The primary mission is to encourage and support research into Hereditary Ataxia, a group of neurological disorders which are chronic and progressive conditions affecting coordination.

Lavonne Randolph

New Jersey

511 Fairlawn, NJ Support Group
National Ataxia Foundation
31-04 Heywood Avenue
Fairlawn, NJ 07410

201-797-6657
Fax: 763-553-0167
e-mail: naf@ataxia.org
www.ataxia.org

The primary mission is to encourage and support research into Hereditary Ataxia, a group of neurological disorders which are chronic and progressive conditions affecting coordination.

Hortense Oberndorf

New York

512 Genetic Network of the Empire State
Laboratory of Human Genetics
Empire State Plaza
Albany, NY 12201

518-474-7148
Fax: 518-474-8590

Coordinates genetic services; promotes communication among genetic professionals and consumers through network newsletters, meetings, and other events; share resources; and promote education and awareness of genetic disorders.

Karen Greendale, Coordinator

513 New York City Area Support Group
National Ataxia Foundation
460 Brielle Avenue
Staten Island, NY 10314

718-317-3802

The primary mission is to encourage and support research into Hereditary Ataxia, a group of neurological disorders which are chronic and progressive conditions affecting coordination.

Mary Ann Costa, Contact

514 New York Support Group
National Ataxia Foundation
460 Brielle Avenue
Staten Island, NY 10314

718-317-3802
www.ataxia.org

Primary mission is to encourage and support research into Hereditary Ataxia, a group of neurological disorders which are chronic and progressive conditions affecting coordination.

Mary Ann Costa, Contact

515 Western New York Area Support Group
National Ataxia Foundation
210 E Utica Street
Buffalo, NY 14208

716-881-0677
Fax: 763-553-0167
e-mail: naf@ataxia.org
www.ataxia.org

The primary mission is to encourage and support research into Hereditary Ataxia, a group of neurological disorders which are chronic and progressive conditions affecting coordination.

Diane P Hall

Ohio

516 Ohio Support Group
National Ataxia Foundation
7852 Country Court
Mentor, OH 44060

440-255-8584
e-mail: iksnabru@earthlink.net

The primary mission is to encourage and support research into Hereditary Ataxia, a group of neurological disorders which are chronic and progressive conditions affecting coordination.

Cecelia Urbanski, Contact

Oklahoma

517 North Central Oklahoma Support Group
National Ataxia Foundation
1704 Surrey Lane
Enid, OK 73703

405-233-1837

The primary mission is to encourage and support research into Hereditary Ataxia, a group of neurological disorders which are chronic and progressive conditions affecting coordination.

Jeannie Howard

Oregon

518 Pacific Northwest Regional Genetics Group
PO Box 574
Portland, OR 97207

503-494-8342
Fax: 503-494-4447

Coordinates genetics services; promotes communationa among genetic professional and consumers through network newsletters, meetings, and other events; share resources; and promote education and awareness of genetic disorders.

Jonathan Zonana, MD, Director

519 Willamette Valley Ataxia Support Group
Albany General Hospital-National Ataxia Foundation
1046 6th Avenue SW
Albany, OR 97321

541-812-4162
Fax: 541-812-4614
e-mail: malindam@samhealth.org
www.ataxia.org

The primary mission is to encourage and support research into Hereditary Ataxia, a group of neurological disorders which are chronic and progressive conditions affecting coordination.

Melinda Moore, CCC-SLP

Pennsylvania

520 Central Pennsylvania Area Support Group
National Ataxia Foundation
51/12 Nichols Street
Weilsboro, PA 16901

763-553-0020
e-mail: bronson1@epix.net
www.geocities.com/hotsprings/sauna/7081

The primary mission is to encourage and support research into Hereditary Ataxia, a group of neurological disorders which are chronic and progressive conditions affecting coordination.

Susan Bronson

521 Mid-Atlantic Regional Human Genetics Network
260 S Broad Street
Philadelphia, PA 19102

215-456-7910
Fax: 215-456-7911

Coordinates genetics services; promotes communication among genetic professional and consumers through network newsletters, meeting, and other events; share resources; and promote education and awareness of genetic disorders.

Deborah Eunpu, MS, President

522 Southeast Pennsylvania Support Group
National Ataxia Foundation
220 Beechwood Road
Norristown, PA 19401

610-277-7722
e-mail: lizout@aol.com
www.ataxia.org

The primary mission is to encourage and support research into Hereditary Ataxia, a group of neurological disorders which are chronic and progressive conditions affecting coordination.

Liz Nussear

Rhode Island

523 Rhode Island Support Group
National Ataxia Foundation
11 Orchard Avenue
Warren, RI 02885

401-245-8587

The primary mission is to encourage and support research into Hereditary Ataxia, a group of neurological disorders which are chronic and progressive conditions affecting coordination.

Geraldine DeBlois

South Carolina

524 Carolinas Support Group
National Ataxia Foundation
1305 Cely Road
Easley, SC 29642

864-220-3395
e-mail: cecerussell@hotmal.com

The primary mission is to encourage and support research into Hereditary Ataxia, a group of neurological disorders which are chronic and progressive conditions affecting coordination.

Cece Russell, Contact

Texas

525 Golden Triangle Area Support Group
National Ataxia Foundation
2801 W Sunset Drive
Orange, TX 77630

409-883-5570

The primary mission is to encourage and support research into Hereditary Ataxia, a group of neurological disorders which are chronic and progressive conditions affecting coordination.

Dana Leblanc, Contact

526 Houston Support Group
National Ataxia Foundation
9405 Hwy 65
Houston, TX 77083

281-693-1826

The primary mission is to encourage and support research into Hereditary Ataxia, a group of neurological disorders which are chronic and progressive conditions affecting coordination.

Angela Cloud, Contact

527 North Texas Support Group
National Ataxia Foundation
7 Wentworth Court
Trophy Club, TX 76262

903-785-7058
e-mail: chevelle@sbcglobal.net
www.northtexasataxia.info

The primary mission is to encourage and support research into Hereditary Ataxia, a group of neurological disorders which are chronic and progressive conditions affecting coordination.

David Henry Jr, Contact

Utah

528 Utah Support Group
National Ataxia Foundation
Moran Eye Center, 50 N Medical Drive
Salt Lake City, UT 84132

801-585-2213
e-mail: juliakleinschmidt@hsc.utah.edu

The primary mission is to encourage and support research into Hereditary Ataxia, a group of neurological disorders which are chronic and progressive conditions affecting coordination.

Julia Kleinschmidt, Contact

Washington

529 Seattle Area Support Group
National Ataxia Foundation
14104 107th Avenue NE
Kirkland, WA 98037

425-823-6239
e-mail: mmlewendon@comcast.net

The primary mission is to encourage and support research into Hereditary Ataxia, a group of neurological disorders which are chronic and progressive conditions affecting coordination.

Milly Lewendon, Contact

Wisconsin

530 Appleton Support Group
National Ataxia Foundation
256 N Campbell Road
Oshkosh, WI 54902

920-232-8295

The primary mission is to encourage and support research into Hereditary Ataxia, a group of neurological disorders which are chronic and progressive conditions affecting coordination.

Jerry Last

531 GLaRGG BLuRBB
Great Lakes Regional Genetics Group
1500 Highland Avenue
Madison, WI 53705

608-265-2907
Fax: 608-263-3496
NMCHC@circsol.com

The primary mission is to encourage and support research into Hereditary Ataxia, a group of neurological disorders which are chronic and progressive conditions affecting coordination.

Louise Elbaum, Coordinator

532 Madison, WI Area Support Group
National Ataxia Foundation
1404 Marthys Road
Monona, WI 53716

608-221-1742
e-mail: pflast@itis.com

The primary mission is to encourage and support research into Hereditary Ataxia, a group of neurological disorders which are chronic and progressive conditions affecting coordination.

Carolyn Pflasterer

Research Centers

533 Ataxia Telangiectasia Children's Project
668 S Military Trail
Deerfield Beach, FL 33442

954-481-6611
800-543-5728
Fax: 954-725-1153
e-mail: info@atcp.org
www.atcp.org

Formed to raise funds through events and contributions from corporations, foundations and friends. Theses funds are used to accelerate first-rate, international scientific research aimed at finding a cure and improving the lives of all children with ataxia-telagiectasia.

Brad Margus, President
Jennifer Thornton, Executive Director

534 Ataxia Telangiectasia Medical Research Foundation
5241 Round Hills Meadow Road
Hidden Hills, CA 91302

818-704-8146
Fax: 818-704-8310
e-mail: becca4435@aol.com

Private nonprofit organization dedicated to finding a cure for ataxia-telangiectasia.

535 Ataxia Telangiectasia Project
3002 Enfield Road
Austin, TX 78703

512-472-4892
e-mail: A-TProject@austin.rr.com
www.atproject.org

Nonprofit foundation that supports basic scientific research into treatments for neurological deterioration and cancer in children with ataia-telangiectasia.

Audio Video

536 Diagnostic Approach to the Dysmorphic Patient
Southeastern Resgional Genetics Group, Inc SERGG
PO Box 1642
Decatur, GA 30031

404-778-8551
Fax: 404-778-8562
e-mail: mlane@sergginc.org
www.sergginc.org

This 2-hour video focuses on learning how to approach, categorize, and conceptualize the patient with multiple congenital anomalies (MCA). Critical terminology is illustrated. Patients are seen in hospital and clinic settings. Emphasis is placed in prioritizing clinical features and weighing each feature's value in reaching a diagnosis. An outline is included with time frames and detailed explanations of what each statement, definition and categorization means.

537 Pearls of Dysmorphology
Southeastern Resgional Genetics Group, Inc SERGG
PO Box 1642
Decatur, GA 30031

404-778-8551
Fax: 404-778-8562
e-mail: mlane@sergginc.org
www.sergginc.org

This 1 1/2-hour video which contains 87 individual features considered 'pearls' or 'semi-pearls' relative to their value in reaching or suspecting a specific diagnosis. Many additional features are commented on as the formal 'pearls' are presented. There is an exercise at the end of the tape for helping viewers understand how dysmorphology pearls can be used to prioritize the diagnostic value of individual features. A handout accompanies this tape, to help make this exercise fun and educational.

538 Syndromes Associated with Multiple Congenital Anomalies
Southeastern Resgional Genetics Group, Inc SERGG
PO Box 1642
Decatur, GA 30031

404-778-8551
Fax: 404-778-8562
e-mail: mlane@sergginc.org
www.sergginc.org

This 2-hour video includes 30 of the more common malformation syndromes within the categories of single gene, chromosomal, teratogens, associations, and sequences. Each disorder is preceded by a Table of Features and each disorder is shown at different ages and often includes some verbal interaction. The vast majority of the cases are within the hospital or clinic setting. There is minimal use of slides.

539 Together...There Is Hope
National Ataxia Foundation
2600 Fernbrook Lane N
Minneapolis, MN 55447

763-553-0020
Fax: 763-553-0167
e-mail: naf@ataxia.org
www.ataxia.org

A video discussing ataxias genetic patterns of inheritance and the National Ataxia Foundation and its research efforts.

Web Sites

540 Gene Clinics
www.geneclinics.org/profiles/ataxias

By providing current, authoritative information on genetic testing and its use in diagnosis, management, and genetic counseling, GeneTests promotes the appropriate use of genetic services in patient care and personal decision making.

541 Health Answers
www.healthanswers.com

HealthAnswers offers a breadth of services in medical education, sales force training, patient support solutions, professional promotion and consumer solutions.

542 International Network of Ataxia Friends
www.internaf.org

Website mailing list which is maintained by volunteers who have some form of ataxia.

543 National Ataxia Foundation
www.ataxia.org

Information regarding support, education, and research for dominant ataxia, recessive ataxia, and sporatic ataxia.

Book Publishers

544 A Balancing Act: Living with Spinal Cerebellar Ataxia
Describes living with Spinocerebellar Ataxia. Available from Amazon.com only.

ISBN: 1-889826-00-6

Patricia B Hamilton

545 Directory of National Genetic Voluntary Organizations
Genetic Alliance
4301 Connecticut Avenue NW
Washington, DC 20008

202-966-5557
Fax: 202-966-8553
e-mail: info@genticalliance.org
www.genticalliance.orgtm

Lists hundreds of organizations and associations dealing with genetic conditions.

Sharon F. Terry, President
Donna Foster, Director Of Administration

546 Hereditary Ataxia: A Guidebook for Managing Speech & Swallowing
National Ataxia Foundation
2600 Fernbrook Lane N
Minneapolis, MN 55447

763-553-0020
Fax: 763-553-0167
e-mail: naf@ataxia.org
www.ataxia.org

547 Living with Ataxia
National Ataxia Foundation
2600 Fernbrook Lane N
Minneapolis, MN 55447

763-553-0020
Fax: 763-553-0167
e-mail: naf@ataxia.org
www.ataxia.org

A compassionate resource for people who have or may be at risk of having ataxia, and for their families. This book explains the nature and causes of ataxia, the basic genetics that underlie many kinds of ataxia, discusses medical management of ataxia, provides practical advice for everyday living, points the way to many useful resources and assures that living a good life is an entirely reasonable aspiration, even with ataxia.

112 pages

548 Ten Years to Live
National Ataxia Foundation
2600 Fernbrook Lane N
Minneapolis, MN 55447

763-553-0020
Fax: 763-553-0167
e-mail: naf@ataxia.org
www.ataxia.org

Struggles of the Schut family with hereditary ataxia.

ISBN: 0-962716-63-1

Newsletters

549 A-TMRF Newsletter
A-T Medical Research Foundation
5241 Round Meadow Road
Hidden Hills, CA 91302

818-704-8146
Fax: 818-704-8310

Reports on the two major labs that are supported and funded by us.

550 Alert
Alliance of Genetic Support Groups
4301 Connecticut Avenue NW
Washington, DC 20008

301-652-5553
e-mail: alliance@capaccess.org
medhelp.org/www/agsg.htm

Functions as a vehicle of communication between the Alliance and its constituency. Provides timely and useful information on genetics research.

Monthly

551 GENES Information Services
Genetic Network of the Empire State
Empire State Plaza
Albany, NY 12201

518-474-7148
Fax: 518-473-1733

Investigates the mechanism of action of genes and how this rapidly evolving information base may be applied to the prevention, diagnosis and treatment of disease.

552 Generations
National Ataxia Foundation
2600 Fernbrook Lane N
Minneapolis, MN 55447

763-553-0020
Fax: 763-553-0167
e-mail: naf@ataxia.org
www.ataxia.org

Contains reports on the organization and its chapters, offers research, advice and guides to other resources available.

553 Genetically Speaking
Pacific Southwest Regional Genetics Network
2151 Berkeley Way
Berkeley, CA 94704

510-540-2696
Fax: 510-540-2966
www.psrgn.org

A genetics newsletter for California, Hawaii and Nevada.

554 Genexus
Great Plains Genetic Service Network
The University of Iowa
Iowa City, IA 52242

319-356-2674
Fax: 319-356-3347

555 Great Lakes Genetic News
Great Lakes Regional Genetics Group
1500 Highland Avenue
Madison, WI 53705

608-266-2907
Fax: 608-263-3496

556 MARGIN
Mid-Atlantic Regional Human Genetics Network
260 S Broad Street
Philadelphia, PA 19102

215-456-7910
Fax: 215-456-7911

557 MSRGSN Newsletter
Mountain States Regional Genetics Service Network
4300 Cherry Creek Drive S
Denver, CO 80222

303-692-2423
Fax: 303-782-5576

Joyce Hooker, Coordinator

558 NERG News
New England Regional Genetics Group
PO Box 670
Mount Desert, ME 04660

207-288-2701
Fax: 207-288-2705

559 SERGG Regional News
Southeast Regional Genetics Group
PO Box 1642
Decatur, GA 30031

404-775-8551
Fax: 404-775-8562
e-mail: mlane@sergginc.org
www.sergginc.org

Provides information on genetics services, public health departments, consumers, and related laboratory services.

Pamphlets

560 Alliance Brochure
Alliance of Genetic Support Groups
4301 Connecticut Avenue NW
Washington, DC 20008

301-652-5553
Fax: 202-966-8553
e-mail: alliance@capaccess.org
medhelp.org/www/agsg.htm

Explains the services and programs offered by the Alliance.

561 Ataxia Fact Sheet
National Ataxia Foundation
2600 Fernbrook Lane N
Minneapolis, MN 55447

763-553-0020
Fax: 763-553-0167
e-mail: naf@ataxia.org
www.ataxia.org

Describes ataxia as a symptom and its association with other medical problems as well as the hereditary types.

562 Consumer Indicators of Quality Genetic Services
Alliance of Genetic Support Groups
4301 Connecticut Avenue NW, #404
Washington, DC 20008

202-966-5557
800-336-4363
Fax: 202-966-8553
e-mail: info@geneticalliance.org
www.geneticalliance.org

Describes the Alliance of Genetic Support Groups Partnership Program, which strives to increase provider awareness of the unique needs and resources of genetic consumers, improve provider access to quality, consumer-oriented support group resources, and develop replacable educational materials for other programs.

Nachama Wilker, Director Partnership Program

563 Facts About Friedreich's Ataxia
Muscular Dystrophy Association
3300 E Sunrise Drive
Tucson, AZ 85718

520-529-2000
800-572-1717
Fax: 520-529-5300
www.mda.org/publications/fa-fried.html

Explains Friedreich's ataxia in layman's terms and answers commonly asked questions about the disease.

Carol Sowell, Director Publications

564 Familial Spastic Paraplegia
National Ataxia Foundation
2600 Fernbrook Lane N
Minneapolis, MN 55447

763-553-0020
Fax: 763-553-0167
e-mail: naf@ataxia.org
www.ataxia.org

Defines this disorder and notes symptoms, causes and treatments.

565 Frenkel's Exercises
National Ataxia Foundation
2600 Fernbrook Lane N
Minneapolis, MN 55447

763-553-0020
Fax: 763-553-0167
e-mail: naf@ataxia.org
www.ataxia.org

Describes an exercise program designed for those with ataxia.

566 Friedrich's Ataxia
National Ataxia Foundation
2600 Fernbrook Lane N
Minneapolis, MN 55447

763-553-0020
Fax: 763-553-0167
e-mail: naf@ataxia.org
www.ataxia.org

Describes symptoms, diagnosis, genetics and hints on coping.

567 Gene Testing for Ataxia
National Ataxia Foundation
2600 Fernbrook Lane N
Minneapolis, MN 55447

763-553-0020
Fax: 763-553-0167
e-mail: naf@ataxia.org
www.ataxia.org

Describes the latest information about who should consider it and where to have it done.

568 Health Insurance
National Ataxia Foundation
2600 Fernbrook Lane N
Minneapolis, MN 55447

612-553-0020
Fax: 612-553-0167
e-mail: naf@mr.net
www.ataxia.org

Offers health insurance advice for persons with ataxia.

569 Hereditary Ataxia: The Facts
National Ataxia Foundation
2600 Fernbrook Lane N
Minneapolis, MN 55447

612-553-0020
Fax: 612-553-0167
e-mail: naf@mr.net
www.ataxia.org

Describes recessive and dominant ataxias, information on how hereditary ataxia is transmitted and explanations of the NAF's role in education, service and prevention.

570 Incorporating Consumers into Regional Genetics Networks
Alliance of Genetic Support Groups
4301 Connecticut Avenue NW, Suite 404
Washington, DC 20008

301-652-5553
Fax: 202-966-8553
e-mail: alliance@capaccess.org
medhelp.org/www/agsg.htm

571 Informed Consent: Participation in Genetic Research Studies
Alliance of Genetic Support Groups
4301 Connecticut Avenue NW, Suite 404
Washington, DC 20008

202-966-5557
800-336-4363
Fax: 202-966-8553
e-mail: info@geneticalliance.org
www.geneticalliance.org

This booklet explains the nature of genetic research with its benefits and risks.

Lois O Lender, Helpline/Resources Coordinator

572 Pen-Pal Directory
National Ataxia Foundation
2600 Fernbrook Lane N
Minneapolis, MN 55447

763-553-0020
Fax: 763-553-0167
e-mail: naf@ataxia.org
www.ataxia.org

National, state and international directory of others who are affected by ataxia. Available to NAF Pen-Pal members only.

573 Students with Friedreich's Ataxia
National Ataxia Foundation
2600 Fernbrook Lane N
Minneapolis, MN 55447

763-553-0020
Fax: 763-553-0167
e-mail: naf@ataxia.org
www.ataxia.org

Worksheet for teachers, parents and others who need to understand
the physical constraints of ataxia.

DESCRIPTION

574 ATRIAL SEPTAL DEFECTS

Synonyms: ASD, Atrioseptal defects

Involves the following Biologic System(s):

Cardiovascular Disorders

The term atrial septal defect, or ASD, refers to a group of congenital abnormalities characterized by the presence of a hole in the wall (septum) that separates the two upper chambers of the heart (atria). Atrial septal defects are classified according to their location and may occur as a single anomaly or in association with other heart (cardiac) defects. These types of abnormalities occur in approximately 2000 of every 100,000 births.

The upper left chamber of the heart (left atrium) receives blood that is rich with oxygen (oxygenated) from the lungs. The blood then passes into the lower left chamber (left ventricle) from which it is then pumped through the arteries of the body into the general circulation. The right atrium receives blood that has been depleted of oxygen (deoxygenated) that then passes into the right ventricle and is pumped to the lungs where it once again receives oxygen. Atrial septal defects may allow the passage of some oxygenated blood from the upper left side of the heart into the upper right side of the heart where it mixes with blood that is oxygen depleted. In some patients, this results in a reduced oxygen supply to the body and an increase in blood flow to the lungs. Physical findings associated with ASDs may include enlargement of the right atrium, the right ventricle, or both, and characteristic heart sounds. In some patients, symptoms may be completely absent, especially in early childhood. ASDs are often discovered during routine physical examination by the pressure of a systolic heart murmur. Some affected individuals may experience fatigue upon exertion or exercise. Other findings or symptoms may become apparent after the age of 30 years or when an affected woman becomes pregnant. In these patients, symptoms may include fatigue upon exercise (exercise intolerance), valve insufficiencies, and other, more serious problems such as heart failure and or arrhythmias.

The standard method for closure of atrial septal defects has been open-heart surgery. However, a new nonsurgical procedure has been developed and is done in the heart catheterization laboratory, thus avoiding the need for surgery. A patch, usually resembling a small umbrella, is inserted into the damaged area through a catheter. It is then put into place to close the hole.

See also **General Resources** on page 917

Government Agencies

575 NIH/National Heart, Lung and Blood Institute

National Institute of Health
31 Center Dr MSC 2486, Bldg 31, Rm 5A48
Bethesda, MD 20892

301-592-8573
Fax: 240-629-3246
TTY: 240-629-3255
e-mail: nhlbiinfo@nhlbi.nih.gov
www.nhlbi.nih.gov

Primary responsibility of this organization is the scientific investigation of heart, blood vessel, lung and blood disorders. Oversees research, demonstration, prevention, education, control and training activities in these fields and emphasizes the prevention and control of heart diseases.

Elizabeth G Nabel, MD, Director
Susan Shurin, MD, Deputy Director

576 NIH/National Institute of Child Health and Human Development

31 Center Drive, Building 31
Bethesda, MD 20892

301-496-5133
Fax: 301-496-1104
www.nichd.nih.gov

Established in 1962 by congress, today the institute conducts and supports research on topics related to the health of children, adults, families and populations. Some of these topics include: developmental disabilities, growth and development, infant death, reproductive health and birth defects.

Nancy D Wirth, Director
Lisa Kaeser, Program & Public Liaison

National Associations & Support Groups

577 American Heart Association

7272 Greenville Avenue
Dallas, TX 75231

214-373-6300
800-242-8721
Fax: 214-706-1341
e-mail: inquire@amhrt.org
www.amhrt.org

Supports research, education and community service programs with the objective of reducing premature death and disability from cardiovascular diseases and stroke; coordinates the efforts of health professionals, and others engaged in the fight against heart and circulatory disease.

M Cass Wheeler, CEO

578 Genetic Alliance

4301 Connecticut Avenue NW
Washington, DC 20008

202-966-5557
800-336-4363
Fax: 202-966-8553
e-mail: info@geneticalliance.org
www.geneticalliance.org

A coalition of voluntary genetic support groups, consumers and professionals addressing the needs of individuals and families affected by genetic disorders from a national perspective.

Sharon Terry, President/CEO

579 March of Dimes Birth Defects Foundation
1275 Mamaroneck Avenue
White Plains, NY 10605

914-428-7100
888-663-4637
Fax: 914-428-8203
e-mail: resourcecenter@modimes.org
www.marchofdimes.com

Partnership of volunteers and professionals dedicates to improving the health of babies by preventing birth defects and infant mortality. Over 100 chapters are located across the country and can be located through the National Office.

Dr Jennifer Howse, President

Web Sites

580 Southern Illinois University School of Medicine
www.siumed.edu/peds/index.htm

Mission is to meet the health care needs of children and their families in Central and Southern Illinois through provision of high quality, coordinated care of children with acute and chronic conditions with inpatient, ambulatory, and community-based programs.

581 Yale University School of Medicine
www.info.med.yale.edu/intmed/cardio/chd

Offers information on congential heart conditions such as Atrial Septal Defects, including symptoms, causes and treatments.

Book Publishers

582 Congenital Disorders Sourcebook 2nd Edition
Omnigraphics
PO Box 625
Holmes, PA 19043

800-234-1340
Fax: 800-875-1340
e-mail: info@omnigraphics.com
www.omnigraphics.com

Provides basic consumer health information about the most common types of nonhereditary birth defects and disorders related to prematurity, gestational injuries, congenital infections, and birth complications, including disorders of the heart, brain, gastrointestinal tract, musculoskeletal system, urinary tract, and reproductive system craniofacial disorders, cerebral palsy, spina bifida, and fetal alcohol syndrome, and detailing the causes, diagnostic tests, and treatments for each.

650 pages
ISBN: 0-780809-45-9

583 Heart Disease
Franklin Watts
90 Old Sherman Turnpike
Danbury, CT 06816

203-797-3500
800-621-1115
Fax: 203-797-3197
www.grolier.com

Using diagrams, this book discusses strokes and other bloodvessel disorders, as well as their treatment and prevention.

112 pages Grades 7-12
ISBN: 0-531108-84-8

584 Living with Heart Disease
Franklin Watts
90 Old Sherman Turnpike
Danbury, CT 06816

203-797-3500
800-621-1115
Fax: 203-797-3197
www.grolier.com

Shows how persons with heart disease can overcome their illness and lead productive lives.

32 pages Grades 5-7
ISBN: 0-531108-45-7

DESCRIPTION

585 ATTENTION DEFICIT HYPERACTIVITY DISORDER

Synonyms: ADHD, Hyperactive child syndrome, Hyperkinetic syndrome

Involves the following Biologic System(s):
Developmental/Behavioral/Psychiatric Disorders

Attention deficit hyperactivity disorder, or ADHD, is a syndrome of childhood and adolescence characterized by impulsive behavior, motor-related overactivity (hyperactivity), and inattention. The short attention span results in a decreased ability or inability to complete chores, assignments, or other tasks. ADHD is four to six times more prevalent among boys than it is in girls. In approximately 50 percent of cases, this disorder develops before the age of four years, while in others it appears before seven years of age. Over the last decade, it has been increasingly diagnosed in adults. Some behavioral symptoms associated with this disorder may be present at times in children with ADHD or in children with certain other disorders (e.g., conduct disorder, learning disabilities, hearing impairment, etc.). Therefore, specialists often base their diagnosis on the frequent presence of eight or more characteristic findings. Among these are restlessness, difficulty in remaining seated, difficulty in waiting for a turn in group activities, inclination to be easily distracted, impulsively answering questions before they are completed, difficulty following instructions, inability to sustain concentration while performing tasks or playing, shifting to other tasks before completing others, talking excessively, poor ability to play quietly, interrupting or butting in on others, not appearing to listen when others speak, losing things, and frequently taking part in dangerous physical activities.Evaluation of an individual with ADHD involves taking a detailed family and medical history, paying careful attention to such things as activity level, behavior, and temperament during the early years of the life of the affected child. Obtaining this information may be helpful in determining the extent of the disorder and the presence of additional difficulties (e.g., learning disabilities, anxiety disorders, conduct disorders, etc.).

ADHD is currently considered to be a persistent and chronic condition for which no medical cure is available. Although the cause of ADHD is not known, genetic influences may be a factor in the development of this disorder. In addition, children with neurological disorders and other abnormalities related to the central nervous system may be predisposed to the development of ADHD. Treatment of attention deficit hyperactivity disorder may include an ongoing behavioral and psychosocial therapeutic plan that includes the cooperation of school personnel, the child, and the child's parents or caregivers. In addition, psychostimulant drugs or other medications may be prescribed and carefully monitored. Affected children may also benefit from a structured environment at home and in school. Studies show that, in many phases children who receive multifaceted treatment are better able to cope with ADHD through their adolescent years and into adulthood. Other treatment is supportive.

See also **General Resources** on page 917

Government Agencies

586 NIH/National Institute of Mental Health
6001 Executive Boulevard, Room 8184, MSC 9663
Bethesda, MD 20892

301-443-4513
866-615-6464
Fax: 301-443-4279
TTY: 301-443-8431
e-mail: nimhinfo@nih.gov
www.nimh.nih.gov

Conducts strategic planning for specific research areas as well as for the Institute as a whole.

Dr Thomas R Insel, Director

587 NIH/National Institute of Neurological Dis orders and Stroke (NINDS)
PO Box 5801
Bethesda, MD 20824

301-496-5751
800-352-9424
Fax: 301-496-0296
TTY: 301-468-5981
www.ninds.nih.gov

Works to reduce the burden of neurological disease by conducting, fostering, coordinating and guiding research on the causes, prevention, diagnosis and treatment of neurological disorders and stroke, while supporting basic research in related scientific areas.

Story C Landis Ph.D., Director
Audrey S Penn M.D., Deputy Director

National Associations & Support Groups

588 AD-IN: Attention Deficit Information Network
475 Hillside Avenue
Needham, MA 02194

781-455-9895
Fax: 781-444-5466
e-mail: adin@gis.net
www.addinfonetwork.com

Provides information on training programs and speakers for those who work with individuals with ADD.

589 ADHD Challenge
PO Box 488
West Peabody, MA 01985

978-535-3276
800-233-2322
TDD: 508-535-3276

Provision of data and emotional assistance to both sufferers and medical professionals.

590 ARC of the United States
1010 Wayne Avenue, Suite 650
Silver Spring, MD 20910

301-565-3842
Fax: 301-565-5342
e-mail: info@thearc.org
www.thearc.org

The ARC of the United States advocates for the rights and full participation of all children and adults with intellectual and developmental disabilities. Together with our network of members and affiliated chapters, we improve systems of supports and services; connect families; inspire communities an influence public policy.

Michael Coburn, Assistant Executive Director
Adam Aaronson, Public Inquiries Director

591 Attention Deficit Disorder Association
15000 Commerce Parkway, Suite C
Mount Laurel, NJ 08054

856-439-9099
Fax: 856-439-0525
e-mail: mail@add.org
www.add.org

Provides children, adolescents and adults with ADD information, support groups, publications, videos, and referrals.

Linda S Anderson MA MCC, President

592 CHADD: Children and Adults with Attention Deficit Disorders
8181 Professional Place, Suite 150
Landover, MD 20785

301-306-7070
800-233-4050
Fax: 301-306-7090
e-mail: national@chadd.org
www.chadd.org

Many children and/or adults have a disorder characterized by deficits in attention span and impulse control, which is frequently accompanied by hyperactivity. C.H.A.D.D. (Children and Adults with Attention Deficit Disorders) provides parents, professionals and adults diagnosed with ADD information, support and educational material dealing with this disorder. C.H.A.D.D. has over 600 chapters across the country and over 28,000 active members.

E Clarke Ross, CEO
Ann Teeter Ellison Ed.D, President

593 Children and Adults with AD/HD
8181 Professional Plaza Suite 150
Landover, MD 20785

301-306-7070
800-233-4050
Fax: 301-306-7090
chadd.org

National nonprofit organization representing children and adults with attention deficit/hyperactivity disorder (AD/HD).Works to improve the lives of people affected by AD/HD through leadership, advocacy, research, education and support.

594 Feingold Association of the US
554 East Main Street, Suite 301
Riverhead, NY 11901

631-369-9340
800-321-3287
Fax: 631-369-2988
e-mail: help@feingold.org
www.feingold.org

Helps families of children with learning and behavior problems, including attention deficit disorder. Also helps chemically-sensitive and salicylate-sensitive adults. Program is based upon a diet which primarily eliminates certain synthetic food additives.

595 Genetic Alliance
4301 Connecticut Avenue NW
Washington, DC 20008

202-966-5557
800-336-4363
Fax: 202-966-8553
e-mail: info@geneticalliance.org
www.geneticalliance.org

A coalition of voluntary genetic support groups, consumers and professionals addressing the needs of individuals and families affected by genetic disorders from a national perspective.

Sharon Terry, President/CEO

596 Learning Disabilities Association of Ameri ca
4156 Library Road
Pittsburgh, PA 15234

412-341-1515
888-300-6710
Fax: 412-344-0224
e-mail: info@LDAAmerica.org
www.LDAAmerica.org

Helps families of the affected individual through information and referral to professionals in their area. A membership organization with affiliates in 43 states.

Sheila Buckley, Executive Director

597 March of Dimes Birth Defects Foundation
1275 Mamaroneck Avenue
White Plains, NY 10605

914-428-7100
888-663-4637
Fax: 914-428-8203
e-mail: resourcecenter@modimes.org
www.marchofdimes.com

Partnership of volunteers and professionals dedicates to improving the health of babies by preventing birth defects and infant mortality. Over 100 chapters are located across the country and can be located through the National Office.

Dr Jennifer Howse, President

598 National ADD Association
PO Box 543
Pottstown, PA 19464

484-945-2101
Fax: 610-970-7520
e-mail: mail@add.org
add.org

An organization dedicated to children with attention deficit disorder and their families. Provides workshops, training, referrals, and resources materials.

599 National Alliance for the Mentally Ill
2107 Wilson Blvd, Ste 300, Colonial Place Three
Arlington, VA 22201

703-524-7600
800-950-6264
Fax: 703-524-9094
TDD: 703-516-7227
e-mail: info@nami.org
www.nami.org

NAMI is a nonprofit, grassroots, self-help, support and advocacy organization of consumers, families and friends of people with severe mental illness, such as schizophrenia, bipolar disorder, major despressive disorder, obsessive compulsive disorder, anxiety disorders, autism and other severe and persistent mental illnesses that affect the brain.

Suzanne Vogel-Scibilia MD, President

600 National Attention Deficit Disorder Association
1788 2nd Street Suite 2000
Highland Park, IL 60035

847-432-2332
Fax: 847-432-5874
e-mail: mail@add.org
add.org

An organization focused on the needs of adults and young adults with ADD/ADHD, as well as their children and families. Seeks to serve individuals with ADD, as well as those who love, live with, teach, counsel and treat them. ADDA is a growing organization built on a foundation of service to its members, the public and the professional community. ADDA is a nonprofit organization, staffed by unpaid volunteers.

601 National Center for Learning Disabilities
381 Park Avenue S, Suite 1401
New York, NY 10016

212-545-7510
888-575-7373
Fax: 212-545-9665
www.ncld.org

The mission of the NCLD is to increase opportunities for all individuals with learning disabilities to achieve their potential. NCLD accomplishes this by increasing public awareness and understanding of learning disabilities, conducting educational programs and services that promote research-based knowledge and providing national leadership in shaping public policy.

Sheldon Horowitz, MD, Director, Professional Services
James H Wendorf, Executive Director

602 National Mental Health Association
2000 N Beauregard Street, 6th Floor
Alexandria, VA 22311

703-684-7722
800-969-6642
Fax: 703-684-5968
TTY: 800-433-5959
www.nmha.org

Addresses all aspects of mental health and mental illness. NMHA with over 340 affiliates works to improve the mental health of all Americans.

David L Shern PhD, President & CEO

603 National Mental Health Consumers' Self-Help Clearinghouse
1211 Chestnut Street, Suite 1207
Philadelphia, PA 19107

215-751-1810
800-553-4539
Fax: 215-636-6312
e-mail: info@mhselfhelp.org
www.mhselfhelp.org

Offers information, support and appropriate referrals; and promotes public and professional education. Provides networking for those with special interests related to albinism. Promotes and supports research and funding that will improve diagnosis and management of albinism and hypopigmentation.

Joseph Rogers, Executive Director & Founder

604 Option Institute: Son Rise Program
Autism Treatment Center of America
2080 S Undermountain Road
Sheffield, MA 01257

413-229-2100
800-714-2779
Fax: 413-229-3202
e-mail: information@son-rise.org
www.son-rise.org

Describes an effective, loving and respectful method for treating children with autism. It teaches parents and healing professionals how to set up a home based program using the child's motivation to reach their special child.

Barry Neil Kaufman, Co-Founder/Co-Creator
Samahria Lyte Kaufman, Co-Founder/Co-Creator

605 The Council For Exceptional Children
1110 North Glede Road Suite 300
Arlington, VA 22201

703-620-3660
888-232-7733
Fax: 703-264-9494
TTY: 866-915-5000
e-mail: service@cec.sped.org
www.ccbd.net

wide mission of the Council for Exceptional Children is to improve educational outcomes for individuals with exceptionalities.

Bruce Ramirez, Executive Director

Audio Video

606 ADD From A To Z-Understanding The Diagnosi s & Treatment of ADD in Children & Adult
Connecticut Association for Children with LD
25 Van Zant Street, Suite 15-5
East Norwalk, CT 06855

203-838-5010
Fax: 203-866-6108
e-mail: cacld@optonline.net
www.cacld.org

Provides a comprehensive overview of this complicated and often misunderstood subject. Informative, authorative, and entertaining, this video will be useful to anyone who wants a clear understanding of what ADD is and what is not.

107 Minutes

607 ADD, Stepping Out of the Dark
ADD Videos
PO Box 622
New Paltz, NY 12561

845-255-3612
Fax: 845-883-6452

A powerful, effective video, ideal for health professionals, educators and parents providing a visual montage designed to promote an understanding and awareness of attention deficit disorder. Based on actual accounts of those who have ADD, including a neurologist, an office worker, and parents of children with ADD. The video allows the viewer to feel the frustration and lack of attention that ADD brings to many.

Video

Lenae Madonna, Producer

608 ADHD: What Can We Do?
ADD WareHouse
300 NW 70th Avenue, Suite 102
Plantation, FL 33317

954-792-8100
800-233-9273
Fax: 954-792-8545
www.addwarehouse.com

Can serve as a companion to ADHD: What Do We Know. This video focuses on the most effective ways to manage ADHD, both in the home and in the classroom. Scenes depict the use of behavior management at home and accommodations and interventions in the classroom which have proven to be effective in the treatment of ADHD. Thirty seven minutes.

1993
ISBN: 0-898629-82-1

609 ADHD: What Do We Know?
Guilford Publications
72 Spring Street
New York, NY 10012

212-431-9800
Fax: 212-966-6708

An introduction for teachers and special education practitioners, school psychologists and parents of ADHD children. Topics outlined in this video include the causes and prevalence of ADHD, ways children with ADHD behave, other conditions that may accompany ADHD and long-term prospects for children with ADHD.

Video

610 Around the Clock
Guilford Publications
72 Spring Street
New York, NY 10012

212-431-9800
Fax: 212-966-6708

This videotape provides both professionals and parents a helpful look at how the difficulties facing parents of ADHD children can be handled.

611 Attention Deficit Disorder
Pro-Ed
8700 Shoal Creek Boulevard
Austin, TX 78757

512-451-3246
Fax: 800-897-7633
e-mail: marketing@proedinc.com
www.proedinc.com

A video and book providing helpful suggestions for both home and classroom management of students with attention deficit disorder.

216 pages Paperback
ISBN: 0-890797-42-0

612 Attention Deficit Disorder: Children
Aquarius Health Care Videos
18 North Main Street
Sherborn, MA 01770

508-650-1616
888-440-2963
Fax: 508-650-1665
e-mail: info@aquariusproductions.com
www.aquariusproductions.com

Everyone has been impulsive or easily distracted for different periods of time, so these symptoms that are hallmarks of Attention Deficit Disorder (ADD) have also led to criticism that too many people are being diagnosed with this biochemical brain disorder. This program examines who is being diagnosed, and what treatments are working. An innovative private school specializing in alternate education is profiled, and tips on structuring the school and home environment are included.

Video

Donna Kaufman

613 Concentration Video
Learning disAbilities Resources
PO Box 716
Bryn Mawr, PA 19010

610-525-8336
Fax: 610-525-8337

An instructional video which provides a perspective about attention problems, possible causes and solutions.

Video

614 Diagnosis & Treatment of Attention Deficit Disorder in Children
Fanlight Productions
4196 Washington Street, Suite 2
Boston, MA 01230

617-469-4999
Fax: 617-469-3379
e-mail: fanlight@fanlight.com
www.fanlight.com

Follows several children with ADD, and includes suggestions about ways to restructure home and school environments to support such children. Dartmouth Hitchcock Medical Center Series, The Doctor is In...

28 minutes

615 Educating Inattentive Children
ADD WareHouse
300 NW 70th Avenue, Suite 102
Plantation, FL 33317

954-792-8100
800-233-9273
Fax: 954-792-8545
www.addwarehouse.com

An excellent resources for teachers who encounter inattention and hyperactivity in the classroom. It helps teachers distinguish deliberate misbehavior from the incompetent, nonpurposeful behavior of the inattentive child.

1990 Video

616 How to Help Your Child Succeed in School
Peytral Publications
PO Box 1162
Minnetonka, MN 55345

952-949-8707
877-739-8725
Fax: 952-906-9777
www.peytral.com

In this deeply powerful video, Sandra Reif presents the essential information needed by those who work with ADHD and/or Learning Disabilities to help children in school. The focus is on the key for success, a strong partnership in education between home and school.

56 Minutes

Donna Kaufman

617 It's Just Attention Disorder
Western Psychological Services
12031 Wilshire Boulevard
Los Angeles, CA 90025

310-478-2061
Fax: 310-478-7838

This ground-breaking videotape takes the critical first steps in treating attention-deficit disorder: enlisting the inattentive or hyperactive child as an active participant in his or her treatment.

Video

618 Medication for ADHD
ADD WareHouse
300 NW 70th Avenue, Suite 102
Plantation, FL 33317

954-792-8100
800-233-9273
Fax: 954-792-8545
www.addwarehouse.com

This comprehensive DVD program addresses the critical questions regarding the use of medicati in the treatment of ADD or ADHD. WGN-TV medical reporter Dina Bair interviews two long-time ADHD experts: psychiatrist Dr Jonathan Bloomberg and clinical psychologist Dr Thomas Phelan.

ISBN: 1-889140-18-X

619 Understanding Attention Deficit Disorder
Connecticut Association for Children with LD
25 Van Zant Street, Suite 15-5
East Norwalk, CT 06855

203-838-5010
Fax: 203-866-6108
e-mail: cacld@optonline.net
www.cacld.org

A video in an interview format for parents and professionals providing the history, symptoms, methods of diagnosis and three approaches used to ease the effects of attention deficit disorder.

45 minutes

620 Understanding Hyperactivity
Psychiatric Support Services

Houston, TX
281-580-0046

Designed for parents and teachers, a video explaining the symptoms and consequences of attention deficit hyperactivity disorder.

Video

621 Why Can't Michael Pay Attention?
Active Parenting Publishers
1955 Vaughn Road NW, Suite 108
Kennesaw, GA 30144
770-429-0565
800-825-0060
Fax: 770-429-0334
e-mail: cservice@activeparenting.com
www.activeparenting.com

Watch a first-grade boy receive a thorough assessment for ADHD. See techniques used to help organize Michael's behavior.

19 minutes

622 Why Won't My Child Pay Attention?
Wiley Publishing Inc
10475 Crosspoint Boulevard
Indianapolis, IN 46256
317-572-3000
877-762-2974
Fax: 800-597-3299
e-mail: consumer@wiley.com
www.wiley.com

Practical and reassuring videotape. Noted child psychologist tells parents about two of the most common and complex problems of childhood: inattention and hyperactivity.

1993 Video
ISBN: 0-471303-19-4

Web Sites

623 American Academy of Pediatrics Practice Guidelines
aappolicy.aappublications.org

The mission of the American Academy of Pediatrics in to attain optional physical, mental and social health and well-being for all infants, children, adolescents and young adults. To this purpose, the AAP and its members dedicate their effors and resources.

624 Attention Deficit Disorder Association
www.add.org

Provides children, adolescents and adults with ADD information, support groups, publications, videos, and referrals.

625 Attention Deficit Disorder and Parenting Site
www.LD-ADD.com

Website has been created for parents to help them recognize and manage ADHD/LD in children.

626 Attention Deficit Information Network
www.addinfonetwork.com

Nonprofit volunteer organization. We offer support and information to families of children with ADD and adults with ADD, professionals through a network of AD-IN chapters.

627 CHADD: Children and Adults with Attention Deficit Disorders
www.chadd.org

Many children and/or adults have a disorder characterized by deficits in attention span and impulse control, which is frequently accompanied by hyperactivity. C.H.A.D.D. (Children and Adults with Attention Deficit Disorders) provides parents, professionals and adults diagnosed with ADD information, support and educational material dealing with this disorder. C.H.A.D.D. has over 600 chapters across the country and over 28,000 active members.

628 Feingold Association of the US
www.feingold.org

Helps families of children with learning and behavior problems, including attention deficit disorder. Also helps chemically-sensitive and salicylate-sensitive adults. Program is based upon a diet which primarily eliminates certain synthetic food additives.

629 Health Answers
www.healthanswers.com

HealthAnswers offers a breadth of services in medical education, sales force training, patient support solutions, professional promotion and consumer solutions.

630 Learning Disabilities Association of Ameri ca
www.LDAAmerica.org

Helps families of the affected individual through information and referral to professionals in their area. A membership organization with affiliates in 43 states.

631 National Center for Learning Disabilities
www.ncld.org

The mission of the NCLD is to increase opportunities for all individuals with learning disabilities to achieve their potential. NCLD accomplishes this by increasing public awareness and understanding of learning disabilities, conducting educational programs and services that promote research-based knowledge and providing national leadership in shaping public policy.

632 Option Institute: Son Rise Program
www.son-rise.org

Describes an effective, loving and respectful method for treating children with autism. It teaches parents and healing professionals how to set up a home based program using the child's motivation to reach their special child.

Book Publishers

633 ADD & Learning Disabilities
Bantam Doubleday Dell Publishing
1745 Broadway
New York, NY 10019
212-782-9000
Fax: 212-782-9700
www.randomhouse.com

For parents of children with learning disabilities and attention deficit disorder - and for educational and medical professionals who encounter these children - two experts in the field have devised a handbook to help identify the very best treatments.

256 pages
ISBN: 0-385469-31-4

634 ADD: Helping Your Child
Warner Books
1271 Avenue of the Americas
New York, NY 10020
212-484-2900
Fax: 617-263-2854

1994 224 pages Paperback
ISBN: 0-446670-13-8

635 ADHD Parenting Handbook: Practical Advice for Parents from Parents
Taylor Publishing
1550 W Mockingbird Lane
Dallas, TX 75235
214-637-2800
Fax: 214-819-8141

Provides guidelines, suggestions, and advice to help parents interact with their children who have ADHD.

1994 224 pages Paperback
ISBN: 0-878338-62-4

636 ADHD Survival Guide for Parents and Teachers
Hope Press
PO Box 188
Duarte, CA 91009

818-303-0644
800-321-4039
Fax: 818-358-3520
hopepress.com

Guide for parents and teacher and other caretakers of ADHD children.

ISBN: 1-878267-43-4

637 ADHD in Schools: Assessment and Intervention Strategies
Guilford Publications
72 Spring Street
New York, NY 10012

212-431-9800
Fax: 212-966-6708

This landmark volume emphasizes the need for a team effort among parents, community-based professionals and educators. Provides practical information for educators that is based on empirical findings. Chapters focus on: how to identify and assess students who might have ADHD; the relationship between ADHD and learning disabilities; how to develop and implement classroom-based programs; communication strategies to assist physicians; and the need for community-based treatments.

269 pages Hardcover
ISBN: 0-898622-45-0

638 ADHD in the Young Child
ADD WareHouse
300 NW 70th Avenue, Suite 102
Plantation, FL 33317

954-792-8100
800-233-9273
Fax: 954-792-8545
www.addwarehouse.com

The authors sensitively and effectively describe what life is like living with a young child with ADHD. With the help of over 75 cartoon illustrations they provide practical solutions to common problems found at home, in school and elsewhere.

2006 202 pages
ISBN: 1-886941-32-7

639 ADHD: Handbook for Diagnosis & Treatment
Guilford Press
72 Spring Street
New York, NY 10012

800-365-7006
Fax: 212-966-6708
e-mail: info@guilford.com
www.guilford.com

This second edition helps clinicians diagnose and treat Attention Deficit Hyperactivity Disorder. Written by an internationally recognized authority in the field, it covers the history of ADHD, its primary symptoms, associated conditions, developmental course and outcome, and family context. A workbook companion manual is also available.

2005 770 pages
ISBN: 1-593852-10-8

640 All Kinds of Minds
ADD WareHouse
300 NW 70th Avenue, Suite 102
Plantation, FL 33317

954-792-8100
800-233-9273
Fax: 954-792-8545
www.addwarehouse.com

Primary and elementary students with learning disorders can now gain insight into the difficulties they face in school. This book helps all children understand and respect all kinds of minds and can encourage children with learning disorders to maintain their motivation and keep from developing behavior problems stemming from their learning disorders.

1993 283 pages
ISBN: 0-838820-90-5

641 Alphabet Soup: A Recipe for Understanding & Treating ADD
Minerva Books
137 W 14th Street
New York, NY 10011

212-343-6100
Fax: 212-343-6934

1994 50 pages Paperback
ISBN: 0-934695-00-8

642 Attention Deficit Disorder ADHD and ADD Syndromes
8700 Shoal Creek Boulevard
Austin, TX 78757

800-897-3202
Fax: 800-397-7633
e-mail: info@proedinc.com
www.proedinc.com

Always up-to-date, this book enters its third edition with even more complete explanations of how ADHD and ADD interfere with classroom learning, behavior at home, job performance, and social skills development. New chapters explain the critical roles that emotions and feelings play in perception, comprehension, and decision making. Plus, this is the first book about ADHD and ADD to describe in detail the shadow syndromes that tend to accompany ADHD and ADD.

216 pages Softcover
ISBN: 0-890797-42-0

643 Attention Deficit Disorder and Learning Disabilities
Random House
1745 Broadway
New York, NY 10019

212-782-9000
www.randomhouse.com

Realities, myths, and controversial treatments. Section I tries to dispel the myths and discusses proven treatments for ADHD and LD. Section II explains how the scientific community evaluates new treatment methods, and Section III summarizes alternative treatments and discusses scientific evidence pertaining to its usefulness.

256 pages
ISBN: 0-385469-31-4

644 Attention Deficit Disorder in Children and Adolescents
Charles C Thomas Publishing
2600 S 1st Street
Springfield, IL 62704

217-789-8980
800-258-8980
Fax: 217-789-9130
e-mail: books@ccthomas.com
www.ccthomas.com

Presents an analysis of case studies of children and adolescents with attentional deficits and hyperactivity, demonstrating causal factors in these disorders and suggesting treatment strategies both in psychological and medical practice. Written as a review and summary of twenty years of private practice.

1992 292 pages Paperback
ISBN: 0-398061-12-2

645 Attention Deficit Disorder: Concise Source of Information for Parents
Temeron Books
210, 1220 Kensington Road NW
Calgary, Alberta,
Canada

403-283-0900
Fax: 403-283-6947
e-mail: temeron@telusplanet.net
www.temerondetselig.com

Help with a frustrating situation that many parents face.

2006 112 pages
ISBN: 1-550590-82-0

TE Giles, President

646 Attention Deficit Disorders: Assessment & Teaching
Brooks/Cole Publishing Company
511 Forest Lodge Road
Pacific Grove, CA 93950

408-373-0728
Fax: 408-375-6414
e-mail: bc-info@brookscole.com
www.brookscole.com

A handy resource that offers teachers, school psychologists, councelors, social workers, administrators and parents practical advice for working with children who have attention deficit disorders.

1995 258 pages Paperback
ISBN: 0-534250-44-0

647 Attention Deficit Hyperactivity Disorder in Children: Medication Guide
Madison Institute of Medicine
7617 Mineral Point Road
Madison, WI 53717

608-827-2470
Fax: 608-827-2479
e-mail: mim@miminc.org
www.miminc.org

Written for parents, this explains the various medications used commonly to treat ADHD/ADD. It includes a review of the symptoms of ADHD, medication therapy, commonly asked questions, and side effects of medications.

54 pages Paperback
ISBN: 1-890802-31-X

Bette Hartley

648 Attention Deficit Hyperactivity Disorder: What Every Parent Wants to Know
Paul H Brookes & Company
PO Box 10624
Baltimore, MD 21285

301-337-9580
Fax: 410-337-8539
e-mail: custserv@brookspublishing.com
www.brookespublishing.com

The new edition breaks down the complex issues surrounding ADHD today into easy-to-understand, non-technical terms. Now you can quickly get the information you need to help your child with ADHD, without taking the time to wade through heavy research or statistics.

2000 304 pages Paperback
ISBN: 1-557663-98-X

649 Attention Deficit/Hyperactivity Disorder
Guilford Publications
72 Spring Street
New York, NY 10012

212-431-9800
Fax: 212-966-6708

A second edition that is the handbook on the diagnosis and treatment of ADHD in the 1990s. A companion workbook is also available with forms that may be photocopied.

747 pages Hardcover
ISBN: 0-898624-43-6

650 Attention-Deficit Hyperactivity Disorder
Guilford Publications
72 Spring Street
New York, NY 10012

212-431-9800
800-365-7006
Fax: 212-966-6708
e-mail: info@guilford.com
www.guilford.com

A second edition that is the handbook on the diagnosis and treatment of ADHD in the 1990s. A companion workbook is also available with forms that may be photocopied.

747 pages Hardcover
ISBN: 0-898624-43-6

651 Beyond Ritalin: Facts About Medication and Other Strategies for Helping Children
ADD WareHouse
300 NW 70th Avenue, Suite 102
Plantation, FL 33317

954-792-8100
800-233-9273
Fax: 954-792-8545
www.addwarehouse.com

The authors respond to concerns all parents and individuals have about using medication to treat disorders such as ADHD, explain the importance of a treatment program for those with this condition and discuss fads and fallacies in current treatments.

1996 272 pages
ISBN: 0-060977-25-6

652 Coping with ADD/ADHD
Rosen Publishing Group
29 E 21st Street
New York, NY 10010

212-777-3017
Fax: 212-777-0277
e-mail: rosenpub@tribeca.ios.com

At least 3.5 million American youngsters suffer from attention deficit disorder. This book defines the syndrome and provides specific information about treatment and counseling.

ISBN: 0-823920-70-4

653 Distant Drums, Different Drummers: A Guide for Young People with ADHD
ADD WareHouse
300 NW 70th Avenue, Suite 102
Plantation, FL 33317

954-792-8100
800-233-9273
Fax: 954-792-8545
www.addwarehouse.com

This book presents a positive perspective of ADHD - one that stresses the value of individual differences. Written for children and adolescents struggling with ADHD, it offers young readers the opportunity to see themselves in a positive light and motivates them to face challenging problems. Ages 8-14.

1995 39 pages
ISBN: 0-964854-80-5

Barbara Ingersoll, PhD

654 **Don't Give Up Kid**
ADD WareHouse
300 NW 70th Avenue, Suite 102
Plantation, FL 33317

954-792-8100
800-233-9273
Fax: 954-792-8545
www.addwarehouse.com

Alex, the hero of this book, is one of two million children in the US who have learning disabilities. This book gives children with reading problems and learning disabilities a clear understanding of their difficulties and the necessary courage to learn to live with them. Ages 5-12.

ISBN: 1-884281-10-9

655 **Driven to Distraction**
National Alliance for the Mentally Ill
PO Box 753
Waldorf, MD 20604

703-524-7600
Fax: 703-524-9094

A practical book discussing adult, as well as child attention deficit disorder (ADD). Non-technical, realistic and optimistic, it is an informative how-to manual for parents and consumers.

1994

656 **Eagle Eyes A Child's View od Attention Deficit Disorder**
Connecticut Association for Children with LD
25 Van Zant Street, Suite 15-5
East Norwalk, CT 06855

203-838-5010
Fax: 203-866-6108
e-mail: cacld@optonline.net
www.cacld.org

Story about a boy with ADHD. A valuable tool for parents and teachers to use with elementary school age children with ADHD, their siblings and classmates to help them understand the strengths as well as weaknesses of this population.

30 pages

657 **Eagle Eyes: A Child's View of Attention Deficit Disorder**
ADD WareHouse
300 NW 70th Avenue, Suite 102
Plantation, FL 33317

954-792-8100
800-233-9273
Fax: 954-792-8545
www.addwarehouse.com

This book helps readers of all ages understand ADD and gives practical suggestions for organization, social cues and self calming. Expressive illustrations enhance the book and encourage reluctant readers. Ages 5-12.

ISBN: 1-884281-11-7

Jeanne Gehret

658 **Eukee the Jumpy, Jumpy Elephant**
ADD WareHouse
300 NW 70th Avenue, Suite 102
Plantation, FL 33317

954-792-8100
800-233-9273
Fax: 954-792-8545
www.addwarehouse.com

A story about a bright young elephant who is not like all the other elephants. Eukee moves through the jungle like a tornado, unable to pay attention to the other elephants. He begins to feel sad, but gets help after a visit to the doctor who explains why Eukee is so jumpy and hyperactive. With love, support and help, Eukee learns

ways to help himself and gain renewed self-esteem. Ideal for ages 3-8.

1995 22 pages
ISBN: 0-962162-98-1

Cliff Corman, MD
Esther Trevino

659 **First Star I See**
ADD WareHouse
300 NW 70th Avenue
Plantation, FL 33317

954-792-8944
800-233-9273
Fax: 954-792-8545
addwarehouse.com

This entertaining and funny look at ADD without hyperactivity is a must-read for middle grade girls with ADD, their teachers and parents.

150 pages

Jaye Andras Caffrey

660 **Getting a Grip on ADD: A Kid's Guide to Understanding & Coping with ADD**
Educational Media Corporation
6021 Wish Avenue
Encino, CA 91316

818-708-0962

1994 64 pages Paperback
ISBN: 0-932796-60-3

661 **Give Your ADD Teen a Chance: A Guide for Parents of Teenagers with ADD**
ADD WareHouse
300 NW 70th Avenue, Suite 102
Plantation, FL 33317

954-792-8100
800-233-9273
Fax: 954-792-8545
www.addwarehouse.com

Parenting teenagers is never easy, especially if your teen suffers from ADD. This book provides parents with expert help by showing them how to determine which issues are caused by 'normal' teenager development and which are caused by ADD.

1996 299 pages
ISBN: 0-891099-77-8

Lynn Weiss, PhD

662 **Grandma's Pet Wildebeast Ate My Homework (and other suspect stories)**
ADD WareHouse
300 NW 70th Avenue
Plantation, FL 33317

954-792-8944
800-233-9273
Fax: 954-792-8545
addwarehouse.com

Parents and teachers dealing with hyperactive or daydreaming kids will find this book outstanding. As an ADHD adult himself, Quinn draws upon his own experience, making use of straightforward, creative behavioral management techniques, along with a keen sense of humor. A highly informative and enlightened book.

272 pages

Tom Quinn

663 Handbook of Childhood Impulse Disorders and ADHD: Theory and Practice
Charles C Thomas Publishing
2600 S 1st Street
Springfield, IL 62704

217-789-8980
800-258-8980
Fax: 217-789-9130
e-mail: books@ccthomas.com
www.ccthomas.com

This handbook responds to the controversy over diagnosis, use and abuse of pharmacology and offers effectively proven practical treatment typically overlooked in traditional medical treatise.

252 pages Softcover
ISBN: 0-398058-44-X

664 Hyperactive Child, Adolescent, and Adult: ADD Through the Lifespan
Connecticut Association for Children with LD
25 Van Zant Street, Suite 15-5
East Norwalk, CT 06855

203-838-5010
Fax: 203-866-6108
e-mail: cacld@optonline.net
www.cacld.org

Comprehensive general review. Update on previous research by the author, offering a basic text.

162 pages

665 Hyperactivity: Why Won't My Child Pay Attention?
John Wiley & Sons
1 Wiley Drive
Somerset, NJ 08875

732-469-4400
Fax: 732-302-2300
e-mail: custserv@wiley.com
www.wiley.com

Deals with children who experience problems paying attention, controlling their emotions and physical actions and acting without forethought. Helps parents and professionals to accept the hyperactive child's behavior and find ways to help the child succeed. Provides and accurate understanding of the current state of science concerning the cause, developmental course, evaluation and outcome of this problem.

224 pages
ISBN: 0-471533-07-6

666 It's So Much Work to Be Your Friend
Active Parenting Publishers
1955 Vaughn Road NW, Suite 108
Kennesaw, GA 30144

770-429-0565
800-825-0060
Fax: 770-429-0334
e-mail: cservice@activeparenting.com
www.activeparenting.com

Offers practical strategies to help learning disabled children ages six through seventeen navigate the treacherous social waters of their school, home, and community.

448 pages

667 Jumpin' Johnny Get Back to Work! A Child's Guide to ADHD/Hyperactivity
Connecticut Association for Children with LD
25 Van Zant Street, Suite 15-5
East Norwalk, CT 06855

203-838-5010
Fax: 203-866-6108
e-mail: cacld@optonline.net
www.cacld.org

Written primarily for elementary age youngsters with ADHD to help them understand their disability. Also valuable as an educa-

tional tool for parents, siblings, friends, and classmates. Includes two pages on medication.

24 pages

668 Kids With Incredible Potential Parent's Guide
Active Parenting Publishers
1955 Vaughn Road NW, Suite 108
Kennesaw, GA 30144

770-429-0565
800-825-0060
Fax: 770-429-0334
e-mail: cservice@activeparenting.com
www.activeparenting.com

The guide for parents of ADHD children is designed as an add-on to the Active Parenting Now video and discussion program. Adds an ADHD emphasis that makes the parenting information more immediate and practical for these parents' special needs.

669 Kids with Incredible Potential Leader's Guide
Active Parenting Publishers
1955 Vaughn Road NW, Suite 108
Kennesaw, GA 30144

770-429-0565
800-825-0060
Fax: 770-429-0334
e-mail: cservice@activeparenting.com
www.activeparenting.com

Allows the facilitator to give parents specialized information that is more immediate and practical to these parents' needs.

670 Learning To Slow Down and Pay Attention
Connecticut Association for Children with LD
25 Van Zant Street, Suite 15-5
East Norwalk, CT 06855

203-838-5010
Fax: 203-866-6108
e-mail: cacld@optonline.net
www.cacld.org

Written for elementary school age children with ADHD to read with their parents. A checklist helps families decide if attention and concentration are problems. Interventions are given for parents, doctors and teachers. Includes practical strategies for paying better attention, getting more organized and problem solving.

62 pages

671 Managing Attention Deficit Hyperactivity Disorder in Children
John Wiley & Sons
1 Wiley Drive
Somerset, NJ 08875

732-469-4400
Fax: 732-302-2300
e-mail: custserv@wiley.com
www.wiley.com

This book explores symptoms of ADHD, the crossover into adulthood with such a disorder, and the latest and most controversial treatments.

1998 896 pages
ISBN: 0-471121-58-4

672 Managing Attention Disorders in Children: A Guide for Practitioners
Books on Special Children
PO Box 305
Congers, NY 10920

845-638-1236

Offers information about human personality, structure and dynamics, assessment and adjustment.

214 pages

673 Maybe You Know My Kid: A Parent's Guide to Identifying ADHD
Birch Lane Press
120 Enterprise Avenue S
Secaucus, NJ 07094

The author writes about her family experiences with their son, David, who has attention deficit disorder. Contains a comprehensive review of important issues plus descriptions of some helpful management techniques.

222 pages

674 Medications for Attention Disorders and Related Medical Problems
Specialty Press
300 NW 70th Avenue
Plantation, FL

954-792-8100
Fax: 954-792-8545
e-mail: sales@addwarehouse.com
www.addwarehouse.com

A comprehensive handbook covering the history, characteristics, and causes of ADHD. The equal importance of appropriate academic programming, counseling, and medication are stressed throughout.

415 pages Hardcover

675 My Brother's a World Class Pain: A Sibling's Guide To ADHD/Hyperactivity
Connecticut Association for Children with LD
25 Van Zant Street, Suite 15-5
East Norwalk, CT 06855

203-838-5010
Fax: 203-866-6108
e-mail: cacld@optonline.net
www.cacld.org

A young girl tells what it's like to have a little brother with ADHD. She expresses the frustration, anger, embarrassment and resentment that often develop living with a sibling who has attention deficit. Her parents seek professional help to understand the disability and enlisted in trying to bring about positive changes in the family.

34 pages

676 Otto Learns About His Medicine A Story About Medication for Hyperative Children
Connecticut Association for Children with LD
25 Van Zant Street, Suite 15-5
East Norwalk, CT 06855

203-838-5010
Fax: 203-866-6108
e-mail: cacld@optonline.net
www.cacld.org

A book about Otto, a young, hyperactive car. Otto has difficulty paying attention in school, so his parents take him to a mechanic who prescribes medication that will help him control his behavior.

28 pages

677 Parenting Children with ADHD: Lessons That Medicine Cannot Teach
Active Parenting Publishers
1955 Vaughn Road NW, Suite 108
Kennesaw, GA 30144

770-429-0565
800-825-0060
Fax: 770-429-0334
e-mail: cservice@activeparenting.com
www.activeparenting.com

Gives parents a framework for building a successful parenting program at home. Presents a series of ten lessons that are essential for promoting the success of kids with ADHD.

261 pages

678 Parents Helping Parents: A Directory of Support Groups for ADD
CibaGelgy, Pharmaceuticals Division
External Communications
Summit, NJ 07901

908-277-5000
Fax: 973-781-2601

679 Parents' Hyperactivity Handbook: Helping the Fidgety Child
Plenum Press
233 Spring Street
New York, NY 10013

212-620-8000
Fax: 212-463-0742
e-mail: info@plenum.com

1993 306 pages
ISBN: 0-306444-65-8

680 Putting On The Brakes - Young People's Guide To Understanding ADHD
Connecticut Association for Children with LD
25 Van Zant Street, Suite 15-5
East Norwalk, CT 06855

203-838-5010
Fax: 203-866-6108
e-mail: cacld@optonline.net
www.cacld.org

Written from both a medical and educational perspective. Reviews what it is like to have ADHD. It explains what's going on in the brain, discusses feelings and tries to help children gain some control of their lives.

64 pages

681 Putting on the Brakes
Courage To Change
PO Box 486
Wilkes-Barres, PA 18703

800-440-4003
Fax: 800-772-6499
www.couragetochange.com

This book written for kids ages eight to thirteen tells all they need to know about ADHD. Also available is a companion activity book that teaches organizing, setting priorities, problem solving, maintaining control and other life management skills. The activity book is 88 pages and sells for $14.95.

682 Rethinking Attention Deficit Disorders
Brookline Books
34 University Road
Brookline, MA 02445

617-734-6772
800-666-2665
Fax: 617-734-3952
www.brooklinebooks.com

Gives the classroom teacher useful information that provides ideas and strategies for working with children suffering from ADD.

ISBN: 1-571290-37-0

683 Ritalin is Not the Answer
Jossey-Bass
111 River Street
Hoboken, NJ 07030

201-748-6000
800-956-7739
Fax: 201-748-6088
www.josseybass.com

A healthy, drug-free alternative to Ritalin and an absolute must read for every physician before prescribing it.

224 pages
ISBN: 0-787945-14-5

684 Self-Control Games & Workbook
Western Psychological Services
12031 Wilshire Boulevard
Los Angeles, CA 90025

310-478-2061
Fax: 310-478-7838

This game is designed to teach self-control in academic and social situations. Addresses a total of 24 impulsive, inattentive and hyperactive behaviors. The companion workbook reinforces the use of positive self-statements, and problem-solving techniques, instead of expressing anger.

Game

685 Shelley The Hyperactive Turtle
Connecticut Association for Children with LD
25 Van Zant Street, Suite 15-5
East Norwalk, CT 06855

203-838-5010
Fax: 203-866-6108
e-mail: cacld@optonline.net
www.cacld.org

Delightful picture book for use with very young children. Sensitive text and wonderful colored illustrations help little ones understand ADHD.

20 pages

686 Shelley, the Hyperactive Turtle
Woodbine House
6510 Bells Mill Road
Bethesda, MD 20817

800-843-7323
Fax: 301-897-5838

Entertaining picture book for use with very young children. Sensitive text and colorful illustrations help children understand ADHD.

20 pages

Carol Schwartz, Illustrator

687 Taking Charge of ADHD
Courage To Change
PO Box 1268
Newburgh, NY 12551

800-440-4003
Fax: 800-772-6499

Learn positive strategies for meeting the challenges of raising children with Attention Deficit Hyperactivity Disorder. This excellent resource teaches you how to prevent ADHD from becoming a major obstacle in your child's life. Provides techniques for managing behavior, information on the latest medications and much more.

294 pages Soft Cover

688 Taking Charge of ADHD: The Complete, Authoritative Guide for Parents
Guilford Press
72 Spring Street
New York, NY 10012

800-365-7006
Fax: 212-966-6708
www.guilford.com

Provides a guide to understanding attention-deficit/hyperactivity disorder and relating to the children whose behavior can be frustrating and confusing.

2005 331 pages
ISBN: 1-572305-60-6

689 Teach and Reach Students with Attention Deficit Disorders
MultiGrowth Resources
12345 Jones Road
Houston, TX 77070

281-890-5334
Fax: 281-894-8611

Handbook and resource guide for parents and educators of ADD students.

1994 200 pages
ISBN: 0-963084-70-4

690 The 'putting On The Brakes' Activity Book For Young People With ADHD
Connecticut Association for Children with LD
25 Van Zant Street, Suite 15-5
East Norwalk, CT 06855

203-838-5010
Fax: 203-866-6108
e-mail: cacld@optonline.net
www.cacld.org

A companion to the book 'Putting On The Brakes: Young People's Guide To Understanfing Attention Deficit Hyperactivity Disorder (ADHD)'. Offers various exercises to help children with ADHD learn to deal with their problems in a positive way. Some activities can be done independently, others need the collaboration of an adult.

88 pages

691 The ADHD Book of Lists
Courage To Change
PO Box 486
Wilkes-Barres, PA 18703

800-440-4003
Fax: 800-772-6499
www.couragetochange.com

Presented in list format and created for parents, school psychologists, and mental health professionals. A reliable source of answers, strategies, tools, interventions, support, and additional resources.

692 The LD Child and the ADHD Child: Ways Parents and Professionals Can Help
John F Blair Publishers
1406 Plaza Drive
Winston-Salem, NC 27103

336-768-1374
800-222-9796
Fax: 336-768-9194
e-mail: blairpub@aol.com
www.blairpub.com

The author recommends other options that can be explored to treat LD and ADHD children without drugs.

261 pages Paperback
ISBN: 0-895871-42-4

693 You and Your ADD Child
Nelson Publications
1 Gateway Plaza
Port Chester, NY 10573

914-937-8400
Fax: 914-937-8676

1995 252 pages Paperback
ISBN: 0-785278-95-8

Magazines

694 Attention
Children & Adults with Attention Deficit Disorder
8181 Professional Place
Landover, MD 20785

301-306-7070
Fax: 301-306-7090
TTY: 301-429-0641

Available with membership.

Quarterly

Newsletters

695 ADHD Report
Guilford Publications
72 Spring Street
New York, NY 10012

212-431-9800
Fax: 212-966-6708

Presents the most up-to-date information on the evaluation, diagnosis and management of ADHD in children, adolescents and adults. This important newsletter is an invaluable resource for all professionals interested in ADHD.

Bimonthly
ISBN: 1-065802-5 -

696 Chadder
Children & Adults with Attention Deficit Disorder
8181 Professional Place
Landover, MD 20785

301-306-7070
Fax: 301-306-7090
TTY: 301-429-0641

Quarterly

697 Pure Facts
Feingold Association of the US
554 East Main Street, Suite 301
Riverhead, NY 11901

631-369-9340
800-321-3287
Fax: 631-369-2988
www.feingold.org

Monthly newsletter with articles on nutrition and behavior and lists of approved brand-name foods.

Pamphlets

698 ADHD
Learning Disabilities Association of America
4156 Library Road
Pittsburgh, PA 15234

412-341-1515
Fax: 412-344-0224

A booklet for parents offering information on Attention Deficit-Hyperactivity Disorders and learning disabilities.

699 Attention Deficit Disorders and Hyperactivity
ERIC Clearinghouse on Disabled and Gifted Children
1920 Association Drive
Reston, VA 20191

703-620-3660
Fax: 703-620-2521

Dedicated to improving educational outcomes for individuals with exceptionalities, students with disabilities, and/or the gifted.

700 Attention Deficit-Hyperactivity Disorder: Is it a Learning Disability?
Georgetown University, School of Medicine
3800 Reservoir Road NW
Washington, DC 20007

202-687-2000
Fax: 202-687-2387

Offers information on learning disabilities and related disorders.

701 COGREHAB
Life Science Associates
1 Fennimore Road
Bayport, NY 11705

631-472-2111
Fax: 631-472-8146
e-mail: lifesciassoc@pipeline.com
www.lifesciassoc.home.pipeline.com

Divided into six groups for diagnosis and treatment of attention, memory and perceptual disorders to be used by and under the guidance of a professional.

$95 - $1,950

702 Children with ADD: A Shared Responsibility
Council for Exceptional Children
1100 N Glebe Road
Arlington, VA 22201

703-264-9494
e-mail: service@cec.sped.org
www.cec.sped.org

This book represents a consensus of what professionals and parents believe ADD is all about and how children with ADD may best be served. Reviews the evaluation process under IDEA and 504 and presents effective classroom strategies.

35 pages
ISBN: 0-865862-33-8

703 Coping with Your Inattentive Child
Connecticut Association for Children with LD
25 Van Zant Street, Suite 15-5
East Norwalk, CT 06855

203-838-5010
Fax: 203-866-6108
e-mail: cacld@optonline.net
www.cacld.org

Lists signs of ADHD and discusses managing the problems of children with ADHD from infancy through elementary school.

13 pages

704 Helping Your Child with Attention Deficit Hyperactivity Disorder
Learning Disabilities Association of America
4156 Library Road
Pittsburgh, PA 15234

412-341-1515
Fax: 412-344-0224

705 How to Own and Operate an Attention Deficit Disorder
Learning Disabilities Association of America
4156 Library Road
Pittsburgh, PA 15234

412-341-1515
Fax: 412-344-0224

Clear, informative and sensitive introduction to ADHD. Packed with practical things to do at home and school, the author offers her own insight, being a professional and mother of a son with ADHD.

43 pages

706 Hyperactivity, Attention Deficits, and School Failure: Better Ways
Learning Disabilities Association of America
4156 Library Road
Pittsburgh, PA 15234

412-341-1515
Fax: 412-344-0224

707 Identification and Treatment of Attention Deficit Disorders
Therapro
225 Arlington Street
Framingham, MA 01701

508-872-9494
800-257-5376
Fax: 508-875-2062

This handbook contains information that is based on research and offers practical suggestions for parents, teachers and other professionals.

708 Management of Children and Adolescents with AD-HD
Learning Disabilities Association of America
4156 Library Road
Pittsburgh, PA 15234

412-341-1515
Fax: 412-344-0224

709 Out of Darkness
Connecticut Association for Children with LD
25 Van Zant Street, Suite 15-5
East Norwalk, CT 06855

203-838-5010
Fax: 203-866-6108
e-mail: cacld@optonline.net
www.cacld.org

Article by an adult who discovers at age 30 that he has ADD.

4 pages

710 Parenting Attention Deficit Disordered Teens
Connecticut Association for Children with LD
25 Van Zant Street, Suite 15-5
East Norwalk, CT 06855

203-838-5010
Fax: 203-866-6108
e-mail: cacld@optonline.net
www.cacld.org

Detailed outline of the various problems of adolescents with ADHD.

14 pages

711 School Based Assessment of Attention Deficit Disorders
National Clearinghouse of Rehabilitation Materials
5202 N Richmond Hill Drive
Stillwater, OK 74078

405-624-7650
800-223-5219
Fax: 405-624-0695
TDD: 405-624-3156
www.nchrtm.okstate.edu

The 1992 OSEP ruling, placing more responsibility on schools for the assessment of students who may have attention deficit disorders, has raised questions concerning the assessment process. This guide was developed to help states formulate new policies. The paper seeks to: present an overview of current thoughts concerning ADD from an educational perspective, contrast traditional assessment strategies with an alternative model, and describe phases of evaluation.

David Brooks, Director
Carolyn Cain

Camps

712 Camp Buckskin
8700 W 36th Street Suite 6w
Saint Louis Park, MN 55426

952-930-3544
Fax: 952-938-6996
e-mail: buckskin@spacestar.net
www.campbuckskin.com

LD and ADD/ADHD youth have often experienced frustration and a lack of success. Buckskin assists these individuals to realize and develop the potentials and abilities which they possess. Teaches a combination of academic and camp activities, so the campers experience success in many areas. By necessity fairly structured, the 1:3 staff ratio ensures the program is individualized to meet each camper's needs. Parents report that their children benefit from the experience in many ways.

Thomas R Bauer, CCD, Camp Director

713 Camp Nuhop
404 Hillcrest Drive
Ashland, OH

419-289-2227
Fax: 419-289-2227
e-mail: cnuhop@bright.net
www.campnuhop.org

A summer residential program for any youngster from 6 to 18 with a learning disability, behavior disorder or Attention Deficit Disorder. Sixty two campers and 35 staff members live on site in groups of 7 campers to every 3 counselors. Activities focus on positive self-concept and behaviors and teach children to learn how to find their strengths, abilities and talents from a positive, yet realistic viewpoint.

Jerry Dunlap, Director

714 Dallas Academy
950 Tiffany Way
Dallas, TX

214-324-1481
Fax: 214-327-8537
e-mail: mail@dallas-academy.com
www.dallas-academy.com

7-week summer session for students who are having difficulty in regular school classes.

Jim Richardson, Director

715 Developmental Center
6710 86th Avenue N
Pinellas Park, FL

Specifically designed for the learning disabled child and other children with difficulties in concentration, strategy, social skills, impulsivity, distractibility and study strategies. Programs offered include: attention training, visual-motor remediation, socialization skills training, relaxation training, horseback riding and more. The day camp meets weekdays from 9-3 for 3,4 or 5 week sessions.

Dr. Eric Larson

716 Eagle Hill School - Summer Program
242 Old Petersham Road
Hardwick, MA 01037

413-477-6000
Fax: 413-477-6837
e-mail: admission@eaglehillschool.com
www.chs1.org

For the child, age 9-19, with a specific learning disability or Attention Deficit Disorder, this summer program offers a structured curriculum designed to build a basic foundation of academic competence. Extracurricular and outdoor activities complement the educational program.

Erin E Wynne, Dean of Admission

717 Groves Learning Center
3200 Highway 100 S
Saint Louis Park, MN

A nonprofit day school in Minnesota designed especially for children with learning differences. The Center has a full day academic program from September through June, as well as an 8 week summer program. Groves also offers community services such as: psychoeducational testing for children and adults, consulting services, workshops on learning disabilities and other special learning needs, and afternoon/evening tutorial services for children and adults.

Sue Kirchhoff, Head of School

718 Hill School of Fort Worth
4817 Odessa Avenue
Fort Worth, TX

817-923-9482
Fax: 817-923-4894
e-mail: admission@hillschool.org
www.hillschool.org

Provides an alternative learning environment for students having average or above-average intelligence with learning differences. Hill school is an established leader in North Texas with a 25 year history of effectively serving LD children. Beginning in 1961 as a tutorial service, Hill became a formal school in 1973. Our mission is to help those who learn differently develop skills and strategies to succeed. We do this by developing academic/study skills, and self-discipline.

Lucille H Helton, Principal
Cathy Allen, Admissions Director

719 Lab School of Washington
4759 Reservoir Road NW
Washington, DC 20007

202-965-6600
Fax: 202-965-5106
www.labschool.org

The Lab School six week summer session includes individualized reading, spelling, writing, study skills, and math programs. A multisensory approach addresses the needs of bright learning disabled children. Related services such as speech/language therapy and occupational therapy are integrated into the curriculum. Elementary/Intermediate; Junior High/High School.

Sally Smith, Founder
Susan Ferley, Admissions Director

720 Maplebrook School
5142 Route 22
Amenia, NY

845-373-8191
Fax: 845-373-7029
e-mail: mbsecho@aol.com

A coeducational boarding school for students with learning differences and ADD. A New York State registered high school servicing ages 11-18. Post secondary options offered to 18-21.

Donna M Konkolios, Head of School
Jennifer Scully, Director Admissions

721 Round Lake Camp
21 Plymouth Street
Fairfield, NJ

973-575-3333
Fax: 973-575-4188
e-mail: rlc@njycamps.org
www.njycamps.org

For ages 7-18, this camp provides individualized academics in reading, language development and math for children with mild learning disabilities, Round Lake also offers therapeutic recreation and Jewish cultural values to its participants.

Sheira Director, Asst. Director

DESCRIPTION

722 AUTISTIC DISORDER

Synonyms: Infantile autism, Kanner's syndrome
Involves the following Biologic System(s):
Developmental/Behavioral/Psychiatric Disorders,
Neurologic Disorders

Autistic disorder, also known as infantile autism, is classified as a developmental disability that results from a disorder of the human central nervous system. It usually
becomes apparent by three years of age. It is thought to affect approximately four in 10,000 children and is about
three to four times more common in males than females.
Autistic disorder is characterized by deficient verbal and
nonverbal communication, impaired social interactions, and
a restricted range of interests and activities.

Children with autistic disorder may fail to acquire or have
poorly developed verbal and nonverbal communication
skills. If children do communicate verbally, abnormal
speech patterns are typically present, such as repetition of
another's words or phrases (echolalia); reversal of the
proper use of pronouns, such as use of the term "you"
rather than "I" when referring to themselves; and nonsensi-
cal rhyming. In addition, affected children may be withdrawn, make little or no eye contact, resist cuddling, lack
awareness of others' thoughts or feelings, or fail to seek
comfort when distressed. Children also typically engage in
solitary play for hours, perform ritualistic behaviors and repeated body movements (e.g., rocking, flicking fingers) and
have a strong need for a predictable, consistent environment. Certain behaviors (e.g., rubbing an object or surface)
may demonstrate a heightened awareness of particular stimuli, whereas others, such as a lack of reaction to sudden,
loud noises, may indicate a lowered sensitivity to other
stimuli. In many children with autistic disorder, disruptions
of rituals or routines may result in tantrum-like outbursts or
rages. In addition, some children may exhibit self-injurious
or outwardly aggressive behaviors. Because of impairment
of language and socialization skills, it may be difficult to
obtain accurate estimates of overall intelligence levels and
potential. Although such testing often demonstrates functional retardation, some affected children perform adequately in nonverbal areas, such as spatial and motor skills,
and those with speech skills may perform adequately in all
test areas.

In most patients, the symptoms and findings associated
with autistic disorder continue to affect them throughout
life. The Food and Drug Administration (FDA) recently approved the use of an antipsychotic, risperidone, for the
treatment of irritability associated with autistic disorder, including symptoms of aggression, deliberate self-injury,
temper tantrums, and quickly changing moods. This is the
first time the FDA has approved any medication for use in
children and adolescents with autism. In addition, the management and treatment of affected children may include integrated, multidisciplinary techniques, such as language
therapy, structured play and interpersonal exercises, and
other behavioral therapies. Some patients, particularly those
with speech development, may lead somewhat independent
lives with proper support. However, other individuals with
autistic disorder may require special, ongoing care.

The cause of autistic disorder is unknown. However, according to the medical literature, several underlying neurologic, infectious, and other disorders are known to produce
or to increase a predisposition toward autistic-like behaviors in children. Genetic abnormalities are also thought to
play some role in causing or resulting in susceptibility for
the disorder. For example, some researchers theorize that
autistic disorder may result from certain brain abnormalities during infancy (e.g., particular biochemical abnormalities, brain injury, etc.), potentially in combination with a
genetic predisposition for the condition (multifactorial).

See also **General Resources** on page 917

Government Agencies

**723 NIH/National Institute of Neurological Dis orders and
Stroke (NINDS)**
PO Box 5801
Bethesda, MD 20824

301-496-5751
800-352-9424
Fax: 301-496-0296
TTY: 301-468-5981
www.ninds.nih.gov

America's focal point for support of research on brain and nervous
system disorders.

Story C Landis Ph.D., Director
Audrey S Penn M.D., Deputy Director

**724 NIH/National Institute on Deafness and Oth er
Communication Disorders (NIDCD)**
31 Center Drive, MSC 2320
Bethesda, MD 20892

800-241-1044
TTY: 800-241-1055
e-mail: nidcdinfo@nidcd.nih.gov
www.nidcd.nih.gov

Conducts and supports biomedical research and research training
on normal mechanisms, as well as diseases and disorders of hearing, balance, smell, taste, voice, speech and language.

Dr James F Battey Jr, Director
Judith A Cooper, Deputy Director

National Associations & Support Groups

725 ARRISE
9238 Parklane Avenue
Franklin Park, IL 60131

847-451-2740
Fax: 847-451-4008
e-mail: akiehn@arrise.org

Provides information about autism.

726 Association for Science in Autism Treatment
389 Main Street, Suuite 202
Malden, MA 02148

781-397-8943
e-mail: info@asatonline.org

To disseminate accurate information about autism and treatments, and to improve access to effective, science-based treatments for all people with autism.

David Celiberti PhD BCBA, President
Sharon A Reeve PhD BCBA, Vice President

727 Autism National Committee
PO Box 6175
North Plymouth, MA 02362

800-378-0386
e-mail: SusanG1961@aol.com
www.autcom.org

Organzation dedicated to social justice for all citizens with autism through a shared vision and a commitment to positive approaches.

728 Autism Network International
PO Box 35448
Syracuse, NY 13235

315-476-2462
e-mail: jisincla@mailbox.syr.edu
http://ani.autistics.org

Supported by individuals who want to make a difference for the sufferers, the foundation provides a variety of support and educational references to inform on the latest changes in the field.

Jim Sinclair, Coordinator

729 Autism Network for Hearing and Visually Impaired Persons
7510 Ocean Front Avenue
Virginia Beach, VA 23451

757-428-9036
Fax: 757-428-0019

Provides communication, education, research and advocacy for persons with autism combined with a hearing or visual disability, their families, and professionals. Sharing of educational materials, phone help, support groups, refferrals and conferences.

Dolores Bartel, Contact
Alan Bartel, Contact

730 Autism Research Foundation
C/O Moss-Rosene Lab, W701
715 Albany Street
Boston, MA 02118

617-414-7012
Fax: 617-414-7207
e-mail: tarf@ladders.org
www.ladders.org

The Autism Research Founation, is a nonprofit, tax-exempt organization dedicated to researching the neurological underpinnings of atuism and other related developmental brain disorders.

Claudia Persico, Project Manager/Coordinator

731 Autism Research Institute
4182 Adams Avenue
San Diego, CA 92116

619-281-7165
Fax: 619-563-6840
e-mail: media@autismresearchinstitute.com
www.autismresearchinstitute.com

A clearinghouse for research on autism and related disorders. Conducts and compiles research findings to provide people with the latest research available. Sponsors conferences and think tanks to advance research.

Matt Kabler, Director

732 Autism Services Center
PO Box 507
Huntington, WV 25710

304-525-8014
Fax: 304-525-8026
www.autismservicescenter.org

Provides educational information to the public and professional communities on autism, provides case management activities and referrals for persons afflicted with autism and their families.

Ruth Christ Sullivan, Director

733 Autism Society of America
7910 Woodmont Avenue, Suite 300
Bethesda, MD 20814

301-657-0881
800-328-8476
e-mail: info@autism-society.org
www.autism-society.org

A national charitable organization with the mission of providing as much information as possible about autism and the various options, approaches, methods and systems available to parents of children with autism, family members and those professionals who work with them.

Lee Grossman, President & CEO
Cathy Pratt PhD, Chair

734 Autism Speaks
2 Park Avenue, 11th Floor
New York, NY 10016

212-252-8584
Fax: 212-252-8676
e-mail: contactus@autismspeaks.org
www.autismspeaks.org

Goal is to give a voice to an entire community, to every family dealing with the hardshipsod autism. Joined forces with the National Alliance for Autism Research (NAAR), creating the largest single organization devoted to autism in the nation.

Mark Roithmayr, President
Bob Wright, Co-Founder

735 Autism Treatment Center of America: The Son-Rise Program
Option Institute
2080 S Undermountain Road
Sheffield, MA 01257

413-229-2100
800-714-2779
Fax: 413-229-8931
e-mail: information@son-rise.org
www.son-rise.org

Since 1983 the Center has provides innovative training programs for parents and professionals caring for children challenged by Autism and Autism Spectrum Disorders, Pervasive Developmental Disorder and other developmental difficulties. Teaches a specific yet comprehensive system of treatment and education designed to help families and caregivers enable their children to dramatically improve in all areas of learning, development, communication and skill aquisition.

William Hogan, Executive Director of Programs

736 Autistic Services
4444 Bryant Stratton Way
Williamsville, NY 14221

716-631-5777
888-288-4764
Fax: 716-631-9234
www.autisticservices.org

Agency exclusively dedicated to serving the unique lifelong needs of autistic individuals. Also a regional resource for parents, school districts, physicians and other professionals.

Veronica Federiconi, Executive Director

737 CANDLE
4414 McCampbell Drive
Montgomery, AL 36106

334-271-3947
Fax: 334-271-3947

738 Center for Outreach and Services for the Autism Community
1450 Parkside Avenue, Suite 22
Ewing, NJ 08638

609-883-8100
800-428-8476
Fax: 609-883-5509
e-mail: information@njcosac.org
www.njcosac.org

Nonprofit agency providing information and advocacy, services, family and professional education, and consultation to New Jersey's autism community.

Paul A Potito, Executive Director

739 Center for Study of Autism
PO Box 4538
Salem, OR 97005

503-363-9110
Fax: 503-363-9110
e-mail: autism@euphora.com
www.autism.org/

Provides information about autism to parents and professionals, and conducts research on the efficacy of various therapeutic interventions.

740 Children and Adults with Autism
Autism Society of America
7910 Woodmont Avenue, Suite 300
Bethesda, MD 20814

301-657-0881
800-328-8476
e-mail: info@autism-society.org
www.autism-society.org

The Autism Society of America (ASA) is a charitable organization with the mission of providing as much information as possible about autism and about the various options, approaches, methods and systems available to parents of autistic children, family members, and those professionals who work with them. ASA also advocates for the rights and needs of autistic individuals and their families.

741 Community Services for Autistic Adults & Children (CSAAC)
751 Twinbrook Parkway
Rockville, MD 20851

301-762-1650
Fax: 301-762-5230
e-mail: csaac@csaac.org
www.csaac.org

Private nonprofit agency dedicated to serving persons disabled by autism.

Ian Paregol, Executive Director

742 Community Services for People with Autism
751 Twinbrook Parkway
Rockville, MD 20851

301-762-1650
Fax: 301-762-5320

743 Cure Autism Now Foundation
5455 Wilshire Boulevard, Suite 2250
Los Angeles, CA 90036

323-549-0500
888-828-8476
Fax: 323-549-0547
e-mail: info@cureautismnow.org
www.cureautismnow.org

Organization of parents, clinicians and leading scientists committed to accelerating the pace of biomedical research in autism through raising money for research projects, education and outreach.

Peter Bell, CEO

744 Developmental Delay Resources (DDR)
5801 Beacon Street
Pittsburgh, PA 15217

800-497-0944
Fax: 412-422-1374
e-mail: devdelay@mindspring.com
www.devdelay.org

Dedicated to meeting the needs of those working with children who have developmental delays in sensory, motor, language, social, and emotional areas. Publicizes research into determining identifiable factors that would put a child at risk and maintains a registry, tracking possible trends.

Patricia Lemer, Executive Director

745 Facilitated Communication Institute at Syracuse University
307 Huntington Hall
Syracuse, NY 13244

315-443-9657
Fax: 315-443-2274
e-mail: fcstaff@sued.syr.edu
http://suedweb.syr.edu/thefci

College offering facilitated learning research into communication with persons who have autism or severe disabilities. Offers books, videos and public awareness information on the research projects.

746 Families for Early Autism Treatment
PO Box 255722
Sacramento, CA 95865

916-843-1536
Fax: 916-381-5029
e-mail: info@feat.org
feat.org

A nonprofit organization of parents and professionals, designed to help families with children who are diagnosed with autism or pervasive developmental disorder. It offers a network of support for families. FEAT has a Lending Library, with information on autism and also offers Support Meetings on the third Wednesday of each month.

Nancy Fellmeth, President
Kathleen Berry, VP

747 Federation of Families for Children's Mental Health
9605 Medical Center Drive, Suite 280
Rockville, MD 20850

240-403-1901
Fax: 240-403-1909
e-mail: ffcmh@ffcmh.org
www.ffcmh.org

The National family run organization is dedicated exclusively to helping children with mental health needs and their families achieve a better quality of life.

Sandra Spencer, Executive Director

748 Genetic Alliance
4301 Connecticut Avenue NW
Washington, DC 20008

202-966-5557
800-336-4363
Fax: 202-966-8553
e-mail: info@geneticalliance.org
www.geneticalliance.org

A coalition of voluntary genetic support groups, consumers and professionals addressing the needs of individuals and families affected by genetic disorders from a national perspective.

Sharon Terry, President/CEO

749 MAAP Services for Autism, Asperger's Syndrome and PDD
PO Box 524
Crown Point, IN 46307

219-662-1311
Fax: 219-662-0638
e-mail: chart@netnitco.net
www.maapservices.org

Nonprofit organization dedicated to providing information and advice to families of more advanced individuals with autism, asperger's syndrome, and pervasive developmental disorde.

Susan Moreno, Founder & President

750 March of Dimes Birth Defects Foundation
1275 Mamaroneck Avenue
White Plains, NY 10605

914-428-7100
888-663-4637
Fax: 914-428-8203
e-mail: resourcecenter@modimes.org
www.marchofdimes.com

Partnership of volunteers and professionals dedicates to improving the health of babies by preventing birth defects and infant mortality. Over 100 chapters are located across the country and can be located through the National Office.

Dr Jennifer Howse, President

751 More Advanced Autistic People
PO Box 524
Crown Point, IN 46307

219-662-1311
Fax: 219-662-0638
e-mail: chart@netnitco.net
www.maapservices.org

Dedicated to providing information and advice to families of More Advanced individuals with Autism, Asperger Syndrome, and Pervasive developmental disorder (PDD).

752 National Autism Hotline - Autism Services Center
605 Ninth Street Prichard Bldg PO Box 507
Huntington, WV 25710

304-525-8014
Fax: 304-525-8026

Service agency for individuals with autism and developmental disabilities, and their families. Assists families and agencies attempting to meet the needs of individuals with autism and other developmental disabilities. Makes available technical assistance in designing treatment programs and more. The hotline provides informational packets to callers re: autism and assists via telephone when possible.

Ruth Sullivan, Director

753 National Dissemination Center for Children with Disabilities
PO Box 1492
Washington, DC 20013

202-884-8200
800-695-0285
Fax: 202-884-8441
e-mail: nichcy@aed.org
www.nichcy.org

A national information and referral center that provides information on disabilities and disability-related issues for families, educators and other professionals.

Suzanne Ripley, Executive Director

754 National Mental Health Association
2000 N Beauregard Street, 6th Floor
Alexandria, VA 22311

703-684-7722
800-969-6642
Fax: 703-684-5968
TTY: 800-433-5959
www.nmha.org

Addresses all aspects of mental health and mental illness. NMHA with over 340 affiliates works to improve the mental health of all Americans.

David L Shern PhD, President & CEO

755 National Mental Health Consumers' Self-Help Clearinghouse
1211 Chestnut Street, Suite 1207
Philadelphia, PA 19107

215-751-1810
800-553-4539
Fax: 215-636-6312
e-mail: info@mhselfhelp.org
www.mhselfhelp.org

Offers information, support and appropriate referrals; and promotes public and professional education. Provides networking for those with special interests related to albinism. Promotes and supports research and funding that will improve diagnosis and management of albinism and hypopigmentation.

Joseph Rogers, Executive Director & Founder

756 New England Center for Children
33 Turnpike Road
Southborough, MA 01772

508-481-1015
Fax: 508-485-3421
e-mail: info@necc.org
www.necc.org

Serving students between the ages of 3 and 22 diagnosed with autism, learning disabilities, language delays, mental retardation, behavior disorders and related disabilities; educational curriculum encompasses both the teaching of functional life skills and traditional academics; communication skills are taught throughout all activities in the school, residence, and community. Tuition and fees are set by the state. Consulting services also available.

L Vincent Strully Jr, Executive Director & Founder

757 Oak-Leyden Developmental Services
411 Chicago Avenue
Oak Park, IL 60302

708-524-1050
Fax: 708-524-2469
e-mail: webmaster@oakleyden.org
www.oakleyden.org

The mission of Oak-Leyden Developmental Services is to serve people with developmental disabilities and their families in a manner which recognizes their dignity, is supportive of their personal choices and promotes their inclusion in the larger community.

Bob Atkinson, President & CEO
Michelle Stopka, Director of Development

758 Option Institute: Son Rise Program
Autism Treatment Center of America
2080 S Undermountain Road
Sheffield, MA 01257

413-229-2100
800-714-2779
Fax: 413-229-3202
e-mail: information@son-rise.org
www.son-rise.org

Describes an effective, loving and respectful method for treating children with autism. It teaches parents and healing professionals how to set up a home based program using the child's motivation to reach their special child.

Barry Neil Kaufman, Co-Founder/Co-Creator
Samahria Lyte Kaufman, Co-Founder/Co-Creator

759 Raleigh TEACCH Center
University of North Carolina at Chapel Hill
1418 Aversboro Road
Garner, NC 27529

919-662-4625
Fax: 919-662-4634
e-mail: raleighteacch@med.unc.edu
www.teacch.com

This organization is the division for the treatment and education of Autistic and related communication handicapped children.

Eric Schopler, Founder & Co-Director

760 Society for Autistic Children
NYS Society for Autistic Children
879 Madison Avenue
Albany, NY 12208

518-459-1418

An organization of people concerned about the welfare of children with severe disorders of communication and behavior. Provides a directory of services and programs for autistic children.

State Agencies & Support Groups

Alabama

761 Autism Society of Alabama
Autism Society of America
4778 Overton Road
Irondale, AL 35210

205-951-1364
877-428-8476
Fax: 205-951-1366
e-mail: al-alabama@autismsocietyofamerica.org
www.autism-alabama.org

Helps approximately 600 individuals with autism spectrum disorders, their parents, and their service providers (doctors, therapists, teachers, etc).

Jennifer Muller MPH, Executive Director

762 Autism Society of North Alabama
Autism Society of America
PO Box 2902
Huntsville, AL 35804

256-776-0505
e-mail: al-northalabama@autismsocietyofamerica.o
www.autism-society.org/chapter101

Provides information on autism spectrum disorder.

Kay Burns, President

Arizona

763 Autism Society of America Greater Phoenix Chapter
PO Box 10543
Phoenix, AZ 85064

480-940-1093
e-mail: az-phoenix@autismsocietyofamerica.org
www.phxautism.org

Dedicated to the welfare of children and adults with autism and related disorders.

Jim Adams, President

764 Autism Society of America Northern Arizona Chapter
PO Box 2014
Flagstaff, AZ 86003

928-779-9948
e-mail: az-northernarizona@autismsocietyofameric
www.nazasa.org

Supports the options policy adopted by the National Autism Society of America. Dedicated to increasing public awareness and providing support to family members and individuals with autism spectrum disorders within the Northern Arizona region.

Brent Morrison, Co-President
Lynn Morrison, Co-President

765 Autism Society of America Pima County Chapter
PO Box 44156
Tucson, AZ 85733

520-770-1541
Fax: 520-319-5979
e-mail: az-pimacounty@autismsocietyofamerica.org
www.tucsonautism.org

Volunteer organization of parents, professionals, and friends of persons with autism, designed to promote the general welfare of persons with autism.

Peter Earhart, President

Arkansas

766 Autism Society of America Arkansas Chapter
2001 Pershing Circle F-13
North Little Rock, AR 72114

501-626-9048
e-mail: ar-arkansas@autismsocietyofamerica.org

Offers information and support.

California

767 Autism Society of America Coachella Valley
Autism Society of America
PO Box 11052
Palm Desert, CA 92255

760-779-0012
e-mail: info@coachellavalleyautism.org
www.coachellavalleyautism.org

Helps you to become educated about autism spectrum disorder, network with other parents and professionals, and realize you are not alone in your search for answers and support.

Beverly Viramontes, Co-President
Dianne Russom, Co-President

768 Autism Society of America Greater Long Beach/South Bay Chapter
Autism Society of America
8620 Portafino Place
Whittier, CA 90603

562-943-3335
562-941-1931
Fax: 562-943-3335
e-mail: ca-longbeach@autismsocietyofamerica.org
www.greaterlongbeach-asa.org

Holds family support meetings monthly, featuring speakers and topics of interest. Sponsors several workshops and conferences throughout the year. Publishes a quarterly newsletter containing a list of upcoming events, conference highlights from around the country, information on diagnosis, treatment and more.

Rita Rubin, Co-President
Gloria McNeil, Co-President

769 Autism Society of America Inland Empire Chapter
Autism Society of America
PO Box 2886
Corona, CA 92878

909-578-7005
e-mail: ca-inlandempire@autismsocietyofamerica.o

Provides support and information to families of persons with an autism spectrum disorder in the Inland Empire area.

770 Autism Society of America Los Angeles Chapter
Autism Society of America
PO Box 8600
Long Beach, CA 90808

562-804-5556
Fax: 562-425-4940
e-mail: ca-losangeles@autismsocietyofamerica.org
www.asalosangeles.org

Volunteer parent organization committed to improving the lives of those affected by autism and their families through education, advocacy, public awareness and support.

Caroline Wilson, President

771 Autism Society of America North California Chapter
Autism Society of America
976 Mangrove Avenue
Chico, CA 95926

530-897-0900
Fax: 530-897-0100

Provides information and support.

772 Autism Society of America North San Diego County Chapter
Autism Society of America
PO Box 131161
Carlsbad, CA 92013

760-295-9774
760-295-9774
www.nccasa.atomicshops.com/page/page/2337088.htm

Offers chapter meetings, local groups for support and information, family events, and a lending library.

Julie Klingsberg, Co-President
Nora George, Co-President

773 Autism Society of America Orange County Chapter
Autism Society of America
5591 Yuba Avenue
Westminster, CA 92683

714-318-7571
www.asaoc.org

Promotes lifelong access and opportunities for persons within the autistic spectrum and their families, to be fully included, participating members of their communities through advocacy, public awareness, education, and research related to autism.

774 Autism Society of America San Diego Chapter
Autism Society of America
PO Box 420908
San Diego, CA 92142

619-298-1981
e-mail: ca-sandiego@autismsocietyofamerica.org
www.sd-sutism.org

Promotes lifelong access and opportunities for persons within the autism spectrum and their families, to be fully included, participating members of their communities through advocacy, public awareness, education, and research related to autism.

John VanBrabant, President

775 Autism Society of America San Francisco Bay Chapter
Autism Society of America
1360 Sixth Avenue
Belmont, CA 94002

650-637-7772
http://sfautismsociety.virtualave.net

776 Autism Society of America San Gabriel Valley Chapter
Autism Society of America
PO Box 1755
Glendora, CA 91740

626-388-2134

Penne Fode, President

777 Autism Society of America Santa Barbara Chapter
Autism Society of America
PO Box 30364
Santa Barbara, CA 93130

805-560-3762
e-mail: sdshove@cox.net
www.asasb.org

Promote lifelong access and opportunity for all individuals within the autism spectrum, and their families, to be fully participating, included members of their community. Support, education, advocacy, and an active public awareness from the cornerstones of ASA SAnta Barbara's efforts to carry forth its mission.

Marcia Eichelberger, Co-President
Patti Gaultney, Co-President

778 Autism Society of America Tulare County Chapter
Autism Society of America
3201 West Payson Avenue
Visalia, CA 93291

559-747-2126
e-mail: lori10677@aol.com

Promote lifelong access and opportunity for all individuals within the autism spectrum, and their families, to be fully participating, included members of their community. Support, education, advocacy, and an active public awareness from the cornerstones of ASA SAnta Barbara's efforts to carry forth its mission.

Lori Collins, President

779 Autism Society of California
Autism Society of America
PO Box 8600
Long Beach, CA 90808

800-700-0037
e-mail: ca-california@autismsocietyofamerica.org
www.autismsocietyca.org

The mission of the Autism Society of California is to promote lifelong access and opportunities for persons within the autism spectrum and their families, and to be fully included, participating members of their communities through advocacy, public awareness, education and research related to autism.

Dean Wilson, President

780 Kern Autism Network
Autism Society of America
15401 Lake Berryessa Court
Bakersfield, CA 93314

661-588-4235
661-762-7528
Fax: 661-762-7449
e-mail: ca-bakersfield@autismsocietyofamerica.or
www.kernautism.org

Provides information and support, holds an annual conference in February.

Ramona Puget, President
Carl Twisselman, Vice President

Colorado

781 Autism Society of America Colorado Chapter
701 S Logan Street #103
Denver, CO 80209

720-214-0794
Fax: 720-274-2744
www.autismcolorado.org

Promote quality of life for people in Colorado with Autism Spectrum Disorders and their families.

Val Saiz, President

782 Autism Society of America Larimer County Chapter
6221 Treestead Court
Fort Collins, CO 80528

970-377-9640
e-mail: aslc@autismlarimer.org
www.autismlarimer.org

Mission is to serve as a resource for individuals and families affected by autism spectrum disorder by providing information, advocacy, public awareness activities and promoting the development of services and reosurces.

Darla Beuerman, President

783 Autism Society of America Pikes Peak Chapter
918 Crown Ridge Drive
Colorado Springs, CO 80920

719-630-7072
e-mail: co-pikespeak@autismsocietyofamerica.org
www.asappr.org

Sponsors training opportunities for educators and parents in Southern Colorado to learn best practice strategies that will help students with autism be successful in inclusive classrooms and communities.

Alison Seyler, President

784 Autism Society of American Boulder County Chapter
194 Mesa Ct
Louisville, CO 80027

720-272-8231
Fax: 303-604-6656
www.autismboulder.org

Provide education, timely information and resource referral regarding Autism Spectrum Disorder for our affected community and community at large within Boulder and Broomfield Counties.

Theresa Wrangham, President

Connecticut

785 Autism Society of America Connecticut Chapter
PO Box 1404
Guilford, CT 06437

888-453-4975
e-mail: ct-connecticut@autismsocietyofamerica.or
www.autismsocietyofct.org

Worked with parents, educators, state government, and therapeutic and medical professionals to enhance the lives of those touched by Autism Soectrum Disorders. ASCONN serves the entire autism spectrum, across specific diagnosis, needs, challenges, and age ranges.

Sara Reed, President

Delaware

786 Autism Society of Delaware
Autism Society of America
5572 Kirkwood Highway
Wilmington, DE 19808

302-472-2638
302-472-2639
Fax: 302-472-2640
e-mail: de-delaware@autismsocietyofamerica.org
www.delautism.org

The Autism Society of Delaware is a chapter of the Autism Society of America. We are family members and friends of people with autism, and professionals who work in the autism field. Our mission is to improve the lives of people with autism and those of their families through education, advocacy, and public awareness, and to promote lifelong opportunity and acceptance for people with autism in their communities. We serve the entire state of Delaware.

Theda M Ellis, Co-President
Cheryl Kelley, Co-President

District of Columbia

787 Autism Society of America District of Columbia Chapter
5167 7th Street NE
Washington, DC 20011

202-561-5300
202-561-8634
www.autism-society.org/chapter130

Provides information and referrals for families affected by autism and related disabilities. Advocate for appropriate services in education, medical and other areas.

Sondra Cunningham, President

Florida

788 Autism Society of America Broward Chapter
PO Box 450476
Sunrise, FL 33345

954-577-4141
954-474-5333
www.asabroward.org

Dedicated to the education and welfare of children and adults with autism spectrum disorders. Monthly meetings held on the third Wednesday of each month at 7:30 pm at ARC Broward located at 10250 NW 53st, Sunrise, FL.

Stacy Hoaglund, President

789 Autism Society of America Emerald Coast Chapter
916 Lido Circle East
Niceville, FL 32578

850-897-2252
e-mail: ecautism@aol.com

Provides information and support.

790 Autism Society of America Florida Chapter
PO Box 970646
Pompano Beach, FL 33097

954-349-2820
Fax: 954-571-2136
e-mail: fl-florida@autismsocietyofamerica.org
www.autismfl.com

791 Autism Society of America Jacksonville Chapter
1526 University Blvd W #235
Jacksonville, FL 32217

904-399-4490
www.autism-society.org/chapter1003

Mission is to support, inform and empower the families of Jacksonville.

Jeenifer Nunes, President

792 Autism Society of America Manasota Chapter
PO Box 18934
Sarasota, FL 34276

941-426-3885
941-780-5237

Purpose is to provide support and education.

793 Autism Society of America Panhandle Chapter
4148 N Cambridge Way
Milton, FL 32571

850-995-0003
www.autismpensacola.org

A nonprofit, tax-exempt association of parents, professionals and other concerned community members dedicated to the education and welfare of children and adults with autism and related disorders of communication and behavior.

Susan Byram, President

794 Autism Society of Greater Orlando
Autism Society of America
4743 Hearthside Drive
Orlando, FL 32837

407-855-0235
Fax: 407-240-0318
e-mail: contact@asgo.org
www.asgo.org

Our mission is to promote lifelong access and opportunity for all individuals in the Autism spectrum, and their families and to be fully included, participating members of our community.

Donna Lorman, President

Georgia

795 Autism Society of America Greater Georgia Chapter
2971 Flowers Road S, Suite 140
Atlanta, GA 30341

770-451-0954
Fax: 678-935-1152
e-mail: office@asaga.com
www.asaga.com

Chapter of ASA, we offer resource info to individuals and their families and to professionals about autism, add, adhd and othe developmental disabilities

Tiffany Fleming, President

Hawaii

796 Autism Society of Hawaii
Autism Society of America
PO Box 2995
Honolulu, HI 96802

808-282-3676
808-228-0122
e-mail: hi-hawaii@autismsocietyofamerica.org
www.autismhawaii.org

Committed to educating service providers and the community about autism spectrum disorders, as well as advocating for supporting individuals with autism spectrum disorders and their families.

Naomi Grossman, Contact
Evelyn Akamine, Contact

Idaho

797 Autism Society of America Treasure Valley Chapter
7842 Rainbow Place
Nampa, ID 83687

208-336-5676
e-mail: info@asatvc.org
www.asatvc.org

Top provide advocacy, support and information to individuals with autism, their families, professionals, and communities throughout Treasure Valley Chapter.

Illinois

798 Autism Society of Illinois
Autism Society of America
2200 South Main Street, #317
Lombard, IL 60148

630-691-1270
888-691-1270
Fax: 630-932-5620
e-mail: il-illinois@autismsocietyofamerica.org
www.autismillinois.org

Mission is to promote through advocacy, public awareness, education and research, lifelong access and opportunities for persons within the autism spectrum disorder and their families in order that they may be fully included, participating members of their communities.

Kimberly Maddox, Executive Director

Indiana

799 Autism Society of Indiana
Autism Society of America
PO Box 1064
Carmel, IN 46082

317-695-0252
www.autismindiana.org

The Autism Society of Indiana is dedicated to Autism Advocacy and Awareness, Support (for individuals with autism, their parents and families, and the professionals that work with them), and to provide information about autism to anyone interested.

Susan Pieples, President

Iowa

800 Autism Society of Iowa
Autism Society of America
4549 Waterford Drive
West Des Moines, IA 50265

515-327-9075
888-722-4799
e-mail: autism50ia@aol.com
www.autismia.org

To provide advocacy, support and information to individuals with autism, their families, professionals, and communities throughout the state of Iowa.

801 The Link
Autism Society of Iowa
4549 Waterford Drive
West Des Moines, IA 50265

515-327-9075
888-722-4799
e-mail: autism50ia@aol.com
www.autismia.org

Provides information for parents, professionals and care givers on autism spectrum disorders.

Kansas

802 Autism Society of Kansas
Autism Society of America
2250 N Rock Road
Wichita, KS 67226

316-943-1191
e-mail: arkansas@att.net
www.ask.hostrack.net

To provide advocay, support and information to individuals with autism, their families, professionals, and communities throughout state Kansas.

Kentucky

803 Autism Society of America Bluegrass Chapter
Autism Society of America
243 Shady Lane
Lexington, KY 40503

859-299-9000
e-mail: ky-lexington@autismsocietyofamerica.org
www.asbg.org

A resource and support group for families and professionals in the Central kentucky area who are involved with autism.

Sara Spragens, President

Louisiana

804 Autism Society of Louisiana
Autism Society of America
5430 South Woodchase Court
Baton Rouge, LA 70808

800-955-3760
www.lastateautism.org

Provides information and referrals, advocacy, and training for parents, teachers, and service providers. Help families identify qualified professional and service providers in their community and assist them in securing benefits and services provided by law.

Pat Giamanco, President

Maine

805 Autism Society of Maine
Autism Society of America
72B Main Street
Winthrop, ME 04364

800-273-5200
e-mail: info@asmonline.org
www.asmonline.org

Advocates for improved services for people with autism and their families by lending library and educational materials and holding workshops for parents, educators and providers.

Maryland

806 Autism Society of America Baltimore Chesapeake Chapter
PO Box 10822
Parkville, MD 21234

410-655-7933
e-mail: questions@bcc-asa.org
www.bcc-asa.org

Serves families of children and adults with autism spectrum disorders in Baltimore County, Maryland, Baltimore City, and the State of Maryland by providing information, advocacy, and support for families and individuals with autism.

Massachusetts

807 Autism Society of America Massachusetts Chapter
Autism Society of America
47 Walnut Street
Wellesley Hills, MA 02481

781-237-0272
Fax: 781-237-5020
e-mail: asamasschapter@hotmail.com
www.geocities.com/asamasschapter

Mission is to promote lifelong access and opportunity for all individuals within the autism spectrum and their families to be fully participating, included members of their community.

Barry Neil Kaufman, Co-Founder/Co-Creator
Samahria Lyte Kaufman, Co-Founder/Co-Creator

808 Option Institute: Son Rise Program
Autism Treatment Center of America
2080 S Undermountain Road
Sheffield, MA 01257

413-229-2100
800-714-2779
Fax: 413-229-3202
e-mail: information@son-rise.org
www.son-rise.org

Since 1983, the Autism Treatment Center of America has provided innovative training programs for parents and professionals caring for children challenged by Autism, Autism Spectrum Disorders, Pervasive Developmental Disorder (PDD) and other developmental difficulties. The Son-Rise Program teaches a specific yet comprehensive system of treatment and education designed to help families and caregivers enable their children to dramatically improve in all areas of learning.

Barry Neil Kaufman, Co-Founder/Co-Creator
Samahria Lyte Kaufman, Co-Founder/Co-Creator

Michigan

809 Autism Society of Michigan
Autism Society of America
6035 Executive Drive, #109
Lansing, MI 48911

517-882-2800
800-223-6722
Fax: 517-862-2816
e-mail: autism@autism-mi.org
www.autism-mi.org

The Autism Society of Michigan is committed to empowering individuals with autism and their families by offering educational resources and materials, workshops, seminars and other services. ASM advocates that making human connections in a supportive, integrated community is a right of all persons.

Bob Opsommer, President

Minnesota

810 Autism Society of Minnesota
Autism Society of America
2380 Wycliff Street, Suite 102
Saint Paul, MN 55114

651-647-1083
Fax: 651-642-1230
e-mail: info@ausm.org
www.ausm.org

To enhance the lives of individuals with autism spectrum disorders.

Mary Powell, Executive Director

Mississippi

811 Autism Society of Mississippi
Autism Society of America
5908 Tolar Road
Moss Point, MS 39562

e-mail: ms-mississippi@autismsocietyofamerica.or

Offers information, referrals, and support to parents, professionals and caregivers.

Missouri

812 Autism Society of America Gateway Chapter
Autism Society of America
7777 Bonhomme Avenue, Suite 1501
St Louis, MO 63105

314-863-0077
314-821-3656
Fax: 314-863-7494
e-mail: pegisues@aol.com

Provides information and support.

Pegi Price, President

Nebraska

813 Autism Society of Nebraska
Autism Society of America
1540 Arapohoe
Lincoln, NE 68502

402-472-4346
e-mail: gglenn2@unl.edu
www.autismnebraska.org

Supports and advocates for individuals with autism and their families through increasing education and awareness, fundraising, and facilitating community involvment for persons with autism spectrum disorders to achieve their potential by becoming a productive, accepted, and integral part of society.

Greta Glenn, President

Nevada

814 Autism Society of Northern Nevada Chapter
Autism Society of America
3490 Southampton Drive
Reno, NV 89509

775-786-9315
Fax: 775-786-0984
www.autism-society.org/chapter547

Promote and advocate for the general welfare of persons with autism. To further the education and training of parents and professional personnel for training, educating, and caring for persons with autism.

Paul Deane, Vice President

New Hampshire

815 Autism Society of New Hampshire
Autism Society of America
PO Box 68
Concord, NH 03302

603-679-2424
Fax: 301-657-0869
e-mail: info@nhautism.com
www.nhautism.com

The Autism Society of New Hampshire is dedicated to individuals with Autism and Pervasive Developmental Disorders.

Stacey Shannon, President

New Jersey

816 New Jersey Center for Outreach & Services for the Autism Community (COSAC)
1450 Parkside Avenue, Suite 22
Ewing, NJ 08638

609-883-8100
800-428-8476
Fax: 609-883-5509
e-mail: information@njcosac.org
www.njcosac.org

Purpose is to assist families, individuals and agencies concerned with the welfare and education of children and adults with autism and pervasive development disorder not otherwise specified.

Paul A Potito, Executive Director

New Mexico

817 New Mexico Autism Society
Autism Society of America
PO Box 30955
Albuquerque, NM 87190

505-332-0306
www.nmautismsociety.org

Our mission is to promote lifelong access and opportunities for persons within the autism spectrum, and their families, to be fully included participating members of their communities.

New York

818 Center for Family Support
333 7th Avenue, 9th Floor
New York, NY 10001

212-629-7939
Fax: 212-239-2211
www.cfsny.org

The Center for Family (CFS) is a not-for-profit human service agency providing support and assistance to individuals with developmental disabilities and traumatic brain injuries throughout New York City, Long Island, the lower Hudson Valley region and New Jersey.

Steven Vernickofs, Executive Director

819 New York Autism Network
Autism Society of America
PO Box 3847
Schenectady, NY 12303

518-355-2191
Fax: 518-355-2191
www.albanyautism.org

Provide ongoing support to families and professionals, develop regional networks, provide technical assistance, and conduct conferences related to pervasive developmental disorders.

Cindy Barkowski, President

North Carolina

820 Autism Society of North Carolina
Autism Society of America
505 Oberlin Road
Raleigh, NC 27605

919-743-0204
Fax: 919-743-0208
www.autismsociety-nc.org

The Autism Society of North Caorlina is committed to improving the lives of individuals and families affected by autism through the provision of advocacy, information and referral services and a wide variety of individualized, community based programs.

Ohio

821 Autism Society of Greater Cincinatti
Autism Society of America
PO Box 43027
Cincinnati, OH 45243

513-561-2300
Fax: 513-561-4748
www.autismcincy.org

The mission of the Autism Society of Greater Cincinatti is to improve the quality of life for all people with autism spectrum disorders and their families.

822 Autism Society of Ohio Tri-County Chapter
Autism Society of America
PO Box 313
Canfield, OH 44406

320-799-7523
www.triautism.com

To improve the quality of life for all people with autism spectrum disorders and their families.

Frank Aiello, President

Oklahoma

823 Autism Society of Oklahoma
Autism Society of America
PO Box 720103
Norman, OK 73070

405-370-3220
www.asofok.org

Dedicated to the education and welfare of all people with autism and other pervasive developmental disorders.

Oregon

824 Autism Society of Oregon
Autism Society of America
PO Box 396
Marylhurst, OR 97306

503-636-1676
888-288-4761
Fax: 503-636-1696
www.oregonautism.com

Promote mutual communication, autism awareness and better service delivery across Oregon.

Pennsylvania

825 Autism Society of America Greater Harrisburg Area Chapter
PO Box 101
Enola, PA 17112

717-732-8400
800-244-2425
www.autism-hbgpa.org

To promote opportunities for individuals with autism spectrum disorders, to participate in the same value life experiences as do other citizens.

Nancy Richey, President
Lori Klein, VP

Rhode Island

826 Autism Society of Rhode Island
Autism Society of America
PO Box 16603
Rumford, RI 02916

401-595-3241

Provides information and support.

Lisa Rego, President

South Carolina

827 Autism Society of South Carolina
Autism Society of America
652 Bush River Road, Suite 203
Columbia, SC 29210

803-750-6988
800-438-4790
Fax: 803-750-8121
e-mail: scas@scautism.org
www.scautism.org

Services include Family Support; Information and Referral and Advocacy; Autism and Informed Response (first responder training program); Parent School Partnership; Developmental disability awareness training; and Service Coordination (must be DDSN eligable).

Craig Stoxen, President & CEO

South Dakota

828 Autism Society of South Dakota Black Hills Chapter
Autism Society of America
1818 W Fulton Street #101
Rapid City, SD 57702

605-737-0377
e-mail: burnsinsd@aol.com
www.autismsd.com

Enables families and others associated with an autistic, Asperger's or Pervasive Developmental Disorder individual to have access to support groups, meetings, additional information and resources.

Tennessee

829 Autism Society of America East Tennessee Chapter
PO Box 30015
Knoxville, TN 37930

865-637-3914
http://asaetc.org

To promote lifelong access and opportunity fo all individuals within the autism spectrum, and their families, to be fully participating, included members of their community.

Cheri Howlett, President

Texas

830 Autism Society of America Greater Austin Chapter
Autism Society of America
PO Box 50315
Austin, TX 78716

512-479-4199
e-mail: tx-austin@autismsocietyofamerica.org
www.autism-society.org/chapter244

Mission is to promote lifelong access and opportunities for person within the autism spectrum, and their families, to be fully included, participating members of their communities through advocacy, public awareness, education, and research related to Autism.

Vermont

831 Autism Society of Vermont
Autism Society of America
PO Box 978
White River Junction, VT 05001

800-559-7398
e-mail: vt-vermont@autismsocietyofamerica.org
www.autism-society.org

Organization of parents, professionals, and friends of persons with autism, designed to promote the welfare of persons with autism in Vermont

Virginia

832 Autism Society of America Northern Virginia Chapter
PO Box 1334
Vienna, VA 22183

703-495-8444
Fax: 703-495-8445
e-mail: info@asanv.org
www.asanv.org

Provides information and support to individuals with autism and their families in Northern Virginia area.

Andrea Kramer, Executive Director

Washington

833 Autism Society of Washington
Autism Society of America
1403 S Grand Blvd, Suite 203 South
Spokane, WA 99203

888-ASW-4YOU
Fax: 253-503-1557
e-mail: wa-washington@autismsocietyofamerica.org
www.autismsocietyofwa.org

The mission of the Autism Society of Washington is to promote lifelong access and opportunities for persons within the autism spectrum and their families, and to be fully included, participating members of their communities through advocacy, public awareness, education, and research related to autism.

Chanda Davis, Treasurer

West Virginia

834 Autism Society of West Virginia
RD #4 Box 133
New Cumberland, WV 26047

304-748-3103
www.geocities.com/autismsocietyofwv/

Our mission is to promote and advocate for the general welfare of persons with autism; to develop a better understanding of the problems of persons with autism in Hancock County; to further the education and training of parents and professional personnel for training, educating and caring for persons with autism; to promote the establishment of adequate diagnostic, therapeutic, educational and recreational facilities for persons with autism.

Luann Decker, President

Wisconsin

835 Autism Society of Wisconsin
Autism Society of America
PO Box 165
Two Rivers, WI 54241

920-553-0278
888-428-8476
Fax: 920-553-0034
e-mail: wi-wisconsin@autismsocietyofamerica.org
www.asw4autism.org

To promote lifelong opportunities for persons within the autism spectrum and their families to be fully included, participating members of their communties through information and referral, advocacy, public awareness, and education and support for local Autism Society of America chapters, professionals and others who support individuals with autism in Wisconsin.

Jane Pribek, President

Libraries & Resource Centers

Georgia

836 Emory Autism Resource Center
Emory University
718 Gatewood Road
Atlanta, GA 30322

404-727-3360
Fax: 404-727-3969

Offers online bulletin boards which are relevant to autism.

Indiana

837 Indiana Resource Center for Autism
Inst. for the Study of Developmental Disabilities
2853 E 10th Street
Bloomington, IN 47408

812-855-6508
Fax: 812-855-9630
TTY: 812-855-9396
www.iidc.indiana.edu

Conducts outreach training and consultation, engage in research, and develops and disseminate information on behalf of individuals across the autism spectrum, including autism, asperger's syndrome, and other pervasive developmental disorders.

Dr. Cathy Pratt, Director

Michigan

838 Burger School for the Autistic
30922 Beechwood Street
Garden City, MI 48135

734-762-8420
Fax: 734-762-8533
www.resa.net/gardencity/burger.htm

Committed to maximizing the potential of each student to gain independence and self-fulfillment.

Mary O'Neill, Director

Missouri

839 Judevine Center for Autism
1101 Olivette Executive Parkway
Saint Louis, MO 63132

314-432-6200
Fax: 314-849-2721
e-mail: judevine@judevine.org
www.judevine.org

Rooted in principles of applied behabior analysis within a social exchange framework, th Judevine Center has provided effective training and treatment to thousands of families locally, nationally and globally.

New Jersey

840 New Jersey Center for Outreach and Services for the Autism Community(COSAC)
1450 Parkside Avenue, Suite 22
Ewing, NJ 08648

609-883-8100
800-428-8476
Fax: 609-883-5509
e-mail: information@njcosac.org
www.njcosac.org

Nonprofit agency providing information and advocacy, services, family and professional education and consultation. COSAC encourages responsible basic and applied research that would lead to a lessening of the effects and potential prevention of autism. COSAC is dedicated to ensuring that all people with autisim receive appropriate, effective services to maximize their growth potential and to enhance the overall awareness of autism in the general public.

Paul A Potito, Executive Director

New York

841 Institute for Basic Research in Developmental Disabilities
1050 Forest Hill Road
Staten Island, NY 10314

718-494-0600
Fax: 718-494-0833
www.omr.state.ny.us/ws/ws_ibr_resources.jsp

To conduct basic and clinical research in order to further the prevention and early detection and treatment of mental retardation and developmental disabilities.

Dr. Piotr B Kozlowski, Director

842 State University of New York Health Sciences Center
450 Clarkson Avenue, Box 32
Brooklyn, NY 11203

718-778-5332
Fax: 718-778-5397

Child psychiatry research programs.

Adolf Christ, Director

North Carolina

843 Autism Society of North Carolina
505 Oberlin Road, Suite 230
Raleigh, NC 27605

919-743-0204
800-442-2762
Fax: 919-743-0208
e-mail: books@autismsociety-nc.org
www.autismbookstore.com

Offers a library that carries one of the largest selections of books about autism.

West Virginia

844 Autism Services Center
605 9th Street, PO Box 507
Huntington, WV 25710

304-525-8014
Fax: 304-525-8026
www.autismservicescenter.org

Works to improve appropriate and professional training, advocacy, consulting and information for individuals responsible for the welfare and care of autistic individuals and others with developmental disabilities.

Ruth Christ Sullivan, Director

845 Autism Training Center
Marshall University
1 John Marshall Drive, Suite 316
Huntington, WV 25755

304-696-2332
800-344-5115

To provide education, training and treatment programs for West Virginians who have autism, pervasive developmental disorders or Asperger's disorders and have been formally registered with the center.

Research Centers

846 Autism Research Foundation
C/O Moss-Rosene Lab, W701
715 Albany Street
Boston, MA 02118

617-414-7012
Fax: 717-414-7207
e-mail: tarf@ladders.org
ladders.org

A nonprofit, tax-exempt organization dedicated to researching the neurological underpinnings of autism and other related developmental brain disorders. Seeking to rapidly expand and accelerate research into the pervasive developmental disorders. To do this, time and effort goes into investigating the neuropathology of autism in their laboratories, collecting and redistributing brain tissue to promising research groups for use by projects approved by the Tissue Resource Committee.

Claudia Persico, Project Manager/Coordinator

847 Autism Research Institute
4182 Adams Avenue
San Diego, CA 92116

619-281-7165
Fax: 619-563-6840
e-mail: media@autismresearchinstitute.com
www.autismresearchinstitute.com

A clearinghouse for research on autism and related disorders. Conducts and compiles research findings to provide people with the latest research available. Sponsors conferences and think tanks to advance research.

Matt Kabler, Director

848 Autism Speaks
2 Park Avenue, 11th Floor
New York, NY 10016

212-252-8584
Fax: 212-252-8676
e-mail: contactus@autismspeaks.org
www.autismspeaks.org

Helping to find a cure for autism by raising the funds that will facilitate and quicken the pace of research, to raise public awareness of autism, and to give hope to all those who suffer from this disorder.

Bob Wright, Co-Founder
Suzanne Wright, Co-Founder

849 Children's Center for Neurodevelopmental Studies
5430 West Glenn Drive
Glendale, AZ 85301

623-915-0345
Fax: 623-937-5425
e-mail: info@thechildrenscenteraz.org
www.thechildrenscenteraz.org

Effective treatment methods for autism and developmental disabilities are subjects researched and studied at the Center.

850 Facilitated Communication Institute at Syracuse University
370 Huntington Hall
Syracuse, NY 13244

315-443-9657
Fax: 315-443-2340
e-mail: scstaff@sued.syr.edu
http://suedweb.syr.edu/thefci

College offering facilitated learning research into communication with persons who have autism or severe disabilities. Offers books, videos and public awareness information on the research projects.

851 State University of New York Health Sciences Center
450 Clarkson Avenue
Brooklyn, NY 11203

718-778-5332
Fax: 718-778-5397

Child psychiatry research programs.

Adolf Christ, Director

852 University of North Carolina at Chapel Hill, Brain Research Center
CB 7250
Chapel Hill, NC 27599

919-966-2405
Fax: 919-966-1844

Kunihiko Suzuki, MD, Director

Audio Video

853 A Sense of Belonging: Including Students with Autism in their School Community
Indiana Resource Center for Autism
2853 E 10th Street
Bloomington, IN 47408

812-855-6508
Fax: 812-855-9630
TTY: 812-855-9396
e-mail: prattc@indiana.edu
www.iidc.indiana.edu

Highlights the efforts of two elementary and one middle school in Indiana in teaching students with autism in general education settings. Truly involving students in their school community requires teamwork, the adoption of effective instructional practices, and a school committed to supporting a diverse range of students.

854 Autism
Fanflight Productions
4196 Washington Street
Boston, MA 02130

617-469-4999
800-937-4113
Fax: 617-469-3379
e-mail: fanflight@fanflight.com
www.fanflight.com

The stories of three families show us waht the textbooks and studies cannot — what it's really like to love and care for children with autism.

28 minutes

Kelli English, Publicity Coordinato

855 Autism Is a World
Syracuse University, Institute on Communication
370 Huntington Hall
Syracuse, NY 13244

315-443-9657
Fax: 315-443-2274
http://suedweb.syr.edu/thefci

Documentary that takes the viewer on a journey into the mind of 13 year old girl, into her world and her obsessions. Explores Sue's world world, her writings, and the remarkable friendships she has created while in college.

Videotape

856 Autism: A Strange, Silent World
Filmakers Library
124 E 40th Street
New York, NY 10016

212-808-4980
Fax: 212-808-4983
e-mail: info@filmakers.com
filmakers.com

British educators and medical personnel offer insight into autism's characteristics and treatment approaches through the cameos of three children.

52 Minute

Sue Oscar, Co-President

857 Autism: A World Apart

Fanlight Productions
4196 Washington Street, Suite 2
Boston, MA 02131

617-469-4999
800-937-4113
Fax: 617-469-3379
e-mail: fanlight@tiac.net
www.fanlight.com

In this documentary, three families show us what the textbooks and studies cannot, what it's like to live with autism day after day, raise and love children who may be withdrawn and violent and unable to make personal connections with their families.

29 Minutes Video
ISBN: 1-572950-39-0

858 Autism: Being Friends

Indiana Resource Center for Autism
2853 East 10th Street
Bloomington, IN 47408

812-855-6508
800-280-7010
Fax: 812-855-9630
TTY: 812-855-9396
e-mail: prattc@indiana.edu
iidc.indiana.edu

This autism awareness videotape was produced specifically for use with young children. The program portrays the abilities of the child with autism and describes ways in which peers can help the child to be a part of the everyday world.

859 Autism: Learning to Live

Indiana Institute on Disability and Community
Indiana University
Bloomington, IN 47408

812-855-6508
800-280-7010
Fax: 812-855-9630
TTY: 812-855-9396
e-mail: uap@indiana.edu
iidc.indiana.edu

Filmed throughout the state of Indiana, this public television documentary focuses on children and young adults with autism as they learn in community settings. Sites vary from a family home, to a bakery, to a classroom. Teachers, friends, a principal, a speech clinician, a job coach, and parents talk about the ways they have helped specific individuals with autism learn, and about what they have learned from these individuals.

860 Autism: The Unfolding Mystery

Aquarius Health Care Videos
18 North Main Street
Sherborn, MA 01770

508-650-1616
888-440-2963
Fax: 508-650-1665
www.aquariusproductions.com

Explores what it means to be autistic, how you can recognize the signs of autism in your child, and hear about new tretments and programs to help children learn to deal with the disorder.

26 Minutes

861 Behind the Glass Door: Hannah's Story

Fanlight Productions
4196 Washington Street
Boston, MA 02131

617-469-4999
Fax: 617-469-3379
e-mail: fanlight@fanlight.com
www.fanlight.com

Giving hope and inspiration to those who are determined to bring their children out from behind the glass door of autism.

52 minutes

862 Children and Autism Time is Brain

Aquarius Health Care Videos
18 North Main Street
Sherborn, MA 01770

508-650-1616
888-440-2963
Fax: 508-650-1665
www.aquariusproductions.com

A mother of an autistic child implores parents who suspect their child may be autisitc not to 'wait and see.' Don't wait, don't be afraid of that diagnosis, siagnosis is a tool, not a stigma. the term 'time is brain' is absolutely accurate for children with autism, because the sooner diagnosed, the sooner they can get excellent care.

27 Minutes
ISBN: 1-581404-44-1

863 Come Back Jack

Aquarius Health Care Videos
18 North Main Street
Sherborn, MA 01770

508-650-1616
888-440-2963
Fax: 508-650-1665
e-mail: info@aquariusproductions.com
www.aquariusproductions.com

Not long after he celebrated his first birthday, Jack Micheal Parish began to slowly slip away from his family. Persistant ear infections, medically misguided over-treatment with antibiotics, and other myterious physiological factors sent Jack's mind spinning. This and other troubles sent Jack's terrified parents searching for answers when their son was diagnosed as moderately to severly autistic. Chronicles the ups and downs of a family's journey which eventually leads them to help.

55 minutes
ISBN: 1-581400-95-0

864 Developing Friendships: Wonderful People to Get to Know

Indiana Resource Center for Autism
2853 E 10th Street
Bloomington, IN 47408

812-855-6508
Fax: 812-855-9630
TTY: 812-855-9396
e-mail: prattc@indiana.edu
www.iidc.indiana.edu

Individuals discuss the various social difficulties they experience, such as being bullied, missing subtle social cues, and following and maintaining conversations. Strategies for supporting social interactions are highlighted.

865 Developing and Writing IEPs Under the New IDEA

LRP Publications
747 Dresher Road, Suite 500, PO Box 980
Horsham, PA 19044

215-784-0860
Fax: 215-784-9639
TTY: 215-658-0938
e-mail: custserve@lrp.com
www.lrp.com

Addresses the new IEP content and IEP team requirements by explaining the new provisions, providing context and background to the changes, and predicting their potential impact on special education programs.

2005 90 minutes

866 Discipline Under the New Idea: Practical Methods and Procedures

LRP Publications
747 Dresher Road
Horsham, PA 19044

Fax: 215-784-9639
e-mail: custserve@lrp.com
www.lrp.com

Provides a practical explanation of the discipline methods and procedures school officials are permitted to use for students with disabilities.

26 minutes

867 Educating Students with Autism: Implementa tion of Applied Bahavior Analysis

LRP Publications
747 Dresher Road, Suite 500, PO Box 980
Horsham, PA 19044

215-784-0860
Fax: 215-784-9639
TTY: 215-658-0938
e-mail: custserve@lrp.com
www.lrp.com

During this taped audio conference, behavior and autism consultant Dr Susan Catlett discusses the practical aspects of using ABA in your public school programs for students with autism spectrum disorders.

2006 90 Minutes

868 Getting Started with Facilitated Communication

Syracuse University, Institute On Communication
370 Huntington Hall
Syracuse, NY 13244

315-443-9657
Fax: 315-443-2274
e-mail: fastaff@sued.syr.edu
http://suedweb.syr.edu/thefci

Describes in detail how to help individuals with autism and/or severe communication difficulties to get started with facilitated communication.

Videotape

869 I Want My Little Boy Back

Option Institute
2080 S Undermountain Road
Sheffield, MA 01257

413-229-2100
800-714-2779
Fax: 413-229-8931
e-mail: information@son-rise.org
www.son-rise.org

This BBC documentary follows an English family with a child with autism before, during and after their time at the Son Rise Program. It uniquely captures the heart of the Son Rise Program and is extremely useful in understanding our techniques.

1981 379 pages Video
ISBN: 0-449201-08-2

William Hogan, Executive Director of Programs

870 Sense of Belonging: Including Students with Autism in Their School Community

Indiana Resource Center for Autism
2853 E 10th Street
Bloomington, IN 47408

812-855-9630
Fax: 812-855-6508
www.iidc.indiana.edu

Highlights the efforts of two elementary and one middle school in Indiana in teaching students with autism in general education settings.

20 minutes

Clerta Bowman

871 Teaching Nontraditional Communicative Behavior

Indiana Resource Center for Autism
2853 E 10th Street
Bloomington, IN 47408

812-855-9630
Fax: 812-855-6508
www.iidc.indiana.edu

Focuses on gestural communication, an often overlooked type of augmentative communication. Discusses several assessment and intervention strategies which can be used with individuals with autism who do not effectively use oral speech as their primary means of communication.

19 minutes

Cleta Bowman

872 The Different Shades of Autism: Produced by Veronica Bird Charitable Foundation

American Academy of Pediatrics
141 Northwest Point Boulevard
Elk Grove Village, IL 60007

847-434-4000
Fax: 847-434-8000
www.aap.org

The American Academy of Pediatrics recognizes that it serves a broad and diverse constituency comprised of individuals from many different backgrounds. The Academy respects and values diversity among its constituency and emploees.

33 minutes

873 Understanding Autism

Fanlight Productions
4196 Washington Street, Suite 2
Boston, MA 02131

617-469-4999
800-937-4113
Fax: 617-469-3379
e-mail: fanlight.com
www.fanlight.com

Parents of children with autism discuss the nature and symptoms of this lifelong disability, and outline a treatment program based on behavior modification principles.

19 minutes
ISBN: 1-572951-00-1

Kelli English, Publicity Coordinator

874 We've Climbed Mountains: Increasing Our Un derstanding of Autism Spectrum Disorders

Indiana Resource Center for Autism
2853 E 10th Street
Bloomington, IN 47408

812-855-6508
Fax: 812-855-9630
TTY: 812-855-9396
e-mail: prattc@indiana.edu
www.iidc.indiana.edu

Provides general information about autism spectrum disorders with the hope of increasing overall awareness, especially about those with high-functioning autism/Asperger's syndrome. Specific topics addressed include sensory challenges, social understanding, and responses to the diagnosis.

Web Sites

875 Asperger Syndrome Education Network
www.aspennj.org

Regionally based nonprofit organization headquartered in NJ, with 12 local chapters, providing for families and those individuals affected with Asperger Syndrome, PDD-NOS, High Function Autism, and related disorders.

876 Autism Network International
http://ani.autistics.org

An autistic-run self-help and advocacy organization for autistic people.

877 Autism Network for Dietary Intervention
www.autismndi.com

Providing help and support for families using a gluten and casein free diet in the treatment of autism and related developmental disabilities.

878 Autism Research Institute
www.autismresearchinstitute.com

Provides information based on research to parents and professionals throughout the world.

879 Autism Resources
www.autism-resources.com

Offers information and links regarding the developmental dsabilities of autism and aspergers syndrome.

880 Autism Society of America
www.autism-society.org

Information regarding autism.

881 Autism Speaks
www.autismspeaks.org

Information about Autism Research.

882 Center for the Study of Autism
www.autism.org

Information about autism to parents and professionals.

883 Center for the Study of Autism Website
www.autism.org

Provides information about autism to parents and professionals.

884 Community Services for Autistic Adults & Children (CSAAC)
www.csaac.org

Information about autism to parents and professionals.

885 Facilitated Communication Institute at Syracuse University
http://suedweb.syr.edu/thefci

Is an alternatice means of expession for people who cannot speak, or whose speech is highly limites, and who cannot point reliably. The method has been ised as a means to communicate for individuals with sever disabilities, including persons with labes of mental retardation, austism, down syndrome and other developmental disabilities.

886 Families for Early Autism Treatment
www.feat.org

Information about autism.

887 Online Mendelian Inheritance in Man
www.ncbi.nlm.nih.gov

This database is a catalog of human genes and genetic disorders.

888 University Students with Autism and Asperger's Syndrome Web Site
www.users.dircon.co.uk/~cns

Helps to develop and understanding of the difficulties people with Asperger Syndrome may face. We also work on a one to one basis with the student and liase with staff and peers. help is also given in setting up support networks such as mentors and providing effective strategies to aid independent learning.

Book Publishers

889 ABA Program Companion
Autism Society of North Carolina Bookstore
505 Oberlin Road, Suite 230
Raleigh, NC 27605

919-743-0204
800-442-2762
Fax: 919-743-0208
e-mail: books@autismsociety.org
www.autismbookstore.com

A guide developed to help educational teams organize an implement Applied Behavior Analysis (ABA) programs, including home, school, and center-based programs.

890 Activity Schedules for Children with Autism
Autism Society of North Carolina Bookstore
505 Oberlin Road, Suite 230
Raleigh, NC 27605

919-743-0204
Fax: 919-743-0208
e-mail: books@autismsociety-nc.org
www.autismbookstore.com

Written to help parents and professionals utilize activity schedules to promote independence in children in a variety of settings.

891 Al Capone Does My Shirts: A Novel
Autism Society of North Carolina Bookstore
505 Oberlin Road, Suite 230
Raleigh, NC 27605

919-743-0204
Fax: 919-743-0208
e-mail: books@autismsociety-nc.org
www.autismbookstore.com

Set in 1935, this colorful novels tells the story of Matthew 'Moose' Flanagan, a 12-year-old boy who moves with his family (including sister with autism) to Alcatraz Island. For readers age 12 and up.

892 Autism Acceptance Book: Being A Friend to Someone With Autism
Autism Society of North Carolina Bookstore
505 Oberlin Road, Suite 230
Raleigh, NC 27605

919-743-0204
Fax: 919-743-0208
e-mail: books@autismsociety-nc.org
www.autismbookstore.com

Colorfully illustrated activity book was created to help neurotypical children learn about autism spectrum disorder (ASD) and the characteristics that make kids with ASD unique. For readers age 6 and up.

893 Autism Spectrum Disorders: The Complete Guide
Autism Society of North Carolina Bookstore
505 Oberlin Road, Suite 230
Raleigh, NC 27605

919-743-0204
Fax: 919-743-0208
e-mail: books@autismsociety-nc.org
www.autismbookstore.com

Written to help parents, professionals, and other members of the community learn more about autism spectrum disorder (ASD), and it presents a thorough overview of the disorder, from diagnosis through adulthood.

894 Autism and Learning
David Fulton Publishers
2 Park Square, Milton Park
Abingdon, 0X14 4RN,
United Kingdom

207-017-7913
Fax: 207-017-6707
e-mail: mail@fultonpublisher.co.uk
http://catalogue.fultonpublishers.co.uk

This book is about how a cognitive perception on the way in which individuals with autism think and learn may be applied to particular curriculum areas.

1997 180 pages Paperback
ISBN: 1-853464-21-X

895 Autism and the Family: Problems, Prospects and Coping with the Disorder
Charles C Thomas Publishing
2600 S 1st Street
Springfield, IL 62704

217-789-8980
800-258-8980
Fax: 217-789-9130
e-mail: books@ccthomas.com
www.ccthomas.com

Examination of certain issues such as stress, coping and stigma. Contains 33 interviews with parents whose children attended an autistic treatment center. An excellent resource text.

1998 210 pages Softcover
ISBN: 0-398068-43-7

896 Autism as an Executive Director
Oxford University Press
2001 Evans Road
Cary, NC 27513

919-677-0977
Fax: 919-677-1303
www.us.oup.com

Provides a new and conroversial perspective from some of the leading researchers in this field.

1998 328 pages
ISBN: 0-198523-49-1

897 Autism: Effective Biomedical Treatments
Autism Society of North Carolina Bookstore
505 Oberlin Road, Suite 230
Raleigh, NC 27605

919-743-0204
Fax: 919-743-0208
e-mail: books@autismsociety-nc.org
www.autismbookstore.com

Written for clinicians, professionals, and parents who would like to understand more about specific biomedical treatments for autism spectrum disorder (ASD).

898 Autism: From Tragedy to Triumph
Branden Publishing Company
17 Station Street
Brookline Village, MA 02447

617-734-2045
Fax: 617-734-2046
e-mail: branden@branden.com
www.branden.com

A book that deals with the Lovaas method and includes a foreward by Dr. Ivar Lovaas. The book is broken down into two parts — the long road to diagnosis and then treatment.

ISBN: 0-828319-65-0

899 Autism: Information and Resources for Parents, Families, and Professionals
Pro-Ed
8700 Shoal Creek Boulevard
Austin, TX 78757

512-451-3246
800-897-3202
Fax: 512-451-8542
e-mail: info@proedinc.com
www.proedinc.com

Addresses the frustation and concern of parents and family members by answering questions about autism and summarizing what is known.

188 pages Softcover
ISBN: 0-890795-38-X

900 Autism: Mind and Brain
Oxford University Press
2001 Evans Road
Cary, NC 27513

919-677-0977
Fax: 919-677-1303
www.us.oup.com

An important work describing the latest advances in autism research.

2004 320 pages
ISBN: 0-198529-24-4

901 Autism: The Facts
Oxford University Press
2001 Evans Road
Cary, NC 27513

919-677-0977
800-451-7556
Fax: 919-677-1303
www.us.oup.com

Contains valuable information for families and those afflicted with this condition.

1994 124 pages
ISBN: 0-192623-27-3

902 Behavioral Intervention for Young Children with Autism
Pro-Ed
8700 Shoal Creek Boulevard
Austin, TX 78757

512-451-3246
800-897-3202
Fax: 512-451-8542
e-mail: info@proedinc.com
www.proedinc.com

This manual, inspired by research which shows benefits from early intervention based on the principles of Applied Behavior Analysis gives concrete information on how to differentiate between fads and scientifically validated interventions.

1996 400 pages
ISBN: 0-890796-83-1

903 Beyond the Autism Diagnosis: A Professiona l's Guide to Helping Families
Autism Society of North Carolina Bookstore
505 Oberlin Road, Suite 230
Raleigh, NC 27605

919-743-0204
Fax: 919-743-0208
e-mail: books@autismsociety-nc.org
www.autismbookstore.com

Helps to change the way professionals communicate with parents of children with autism spectrum disorder (ASD), making the experience more effective and meaningful for all involved.

904 Breakthroughs: How to Reach Students with Autism
Pro-Ed
8700 Shoal Creek Boulevard
Austin, TX 78757

512-451-3246
800-897-3202
Fax: 512-451-8542
e-mail: info@proedinc.com
www.proedinc.com

Hands-on approach for teachers of students with autism: suggestions, activities, materials, lesson plans and closed-captioned video.

243 pages manual & video

905 Children With Autism: A Parents Guide
Peytral Publications
P.O. Box 1162
Minnetonka, MN 55345

952-949-8707
877-739-8725
Fax: 952-906-9777
www.peytral.com

Informative handbook for parents of children and teens; covers medical, educational, legal, family life, daily care, emotional issues and more.

456 pages

906 Children wIth Starving Brains
Autism Society of North Carolina Bookstore
505 Oberlin Road, Suite 230
Raleigh, NC 27605

919-743-0204
800-442-2762
Fax: 919-743-0208
e-mail: books@autismsociety-nc.org
www.autismbookstore.com

Written by an experienced physician who is the grandmother of a child with autism spectrum disorder (ASD), this book takes a biomedical approach toward the treatment of ASD.

Eric Schopler, Editor
Gary Mesibov, Co-Editor

907 Children with Autism and Asperger Syndrome A Guide for Practitioners and Carers
John Wiley & Sons
10475 Crosspoint Blvd
Indianapolis, IN 46256

877-762-2974
Fax: 800-597-3299
www.wiley.com

Covers the disorders of autism, understanding the causes and the different approaches of treatment for autistic children.

1999 342 pages
ISBN: 0-471983-28-4

908 Children with Autism: A Developmental Perspective
Harvard University Press
79 Garden Street
Cambridge, MA 02138

401-531-2800
800-405-1619
Fax: 401-531-2801
e-mail: hup@harvard.edu
www.hup.harvard.edu

Offers a rare close look at the mysterious condition that afflicts approximately 350,000 Americans and millions more.

1997
ISBN: 0-674053-13-3

909 Children with Autism: Parents' Guide
Woodbine House
6510 Bells Mill Road
Bethesda, MD 20817

301-897-3570
800-843-7323
Fax: 301-897-5838
e-mail: info@woodbinehouse.com
woodbinehouse.com

Recommended as the first book parents should read, this completely revised volume offers information and a complete introduction to autism, while easing the family's fears and concerns as they adjust and cope with their child's disorder.

456 pages
ISBN: 1-890627-04-6

910 Developmental Therapy for Young Children with Autistic Characterisics
8700 Shoal Creek Boulevard
Austin, TX 78757

800-897-3202
Fax: 800-397-7633

This methods book for teachers and parents describes a complete program of developmental therapy for young children with autistic characteristics. It includes samples of techniques and materials, routines and environments, activity periods, learning experiences, and home programs designed specifically for the young child with autism functioning developmentally from birth to three years.

185 pages Large Format
ISBN: 0-890795-87-8

911 Diagnosis Autism: Now What? 10 Steps to Improve Treatment Outcomes
Autism Society of North Carolina Bookstore
505 Oberlin Road, Suite 230
Raleigh, NC 27605

919-743-0204
Fax: 919-743-0208
e-mail: books@autismsociety-nc.org
www.autismbookstore.com

Practical guide was written to help parents of children with autism spectrum disorder (ASD) form successful pediatric partnerships with physicians and other healthcare practitioners involved in their child's diagnosis and treatment.

912 Different Like Me: My Book of Autism Heroe s
Autism Society of North Carolina Bookstore
505 Oberlin Road, Suite 230
Raleigh, NC 27605

919-743-0204
Fax: 919-743-0208
e-mail: books@autismsociety-nc.org
www.autismbookstore.com

This beautifully illustrated children's book tells the tales of many famous people throughout history who all had on thing in common: they didn't fit in. It's also possible they may have had autism spectrum disorder (ASD). For readers ages 7-12.

913 Does My Child Have Autism?
Autism Society of North Carolina Bookstore
505 Oberlin Road, Suite 230
Raleigh, NC 27605

919-743-0204
Fax: 919-743-0208
e-mail: books@autismsociety-nc.org
www.autismbookstore.com

Written for parents of children age three and younger who have concerns about their child's development.

914 Educating Children and Youth with Autism
Pro-Ed
8700 Shoal Creek Boulevard
Austin, TX 78757
512-451-3246
800-897-3202
Fax: 512-451-8542
e-mail: info@proedinc.com
www.proedinc.com

A best-practices text that explains and critiques a number of approaches to autism in children with information based on current research literature and the authors' personal expertise.

915 Effective Teaching Methods for Autistic Children
Charles C Thomas Publishing
2600 S 1st Street
Springfield, IL 62704
217-789-8980
800-258-8980
Fax: 217-789-9130
e-mail: books@ccthomas.com
www.ccthomas.com

124 pages 20.95 Softcover
ISBN: 0-398028-58-3

916 Everybody is Different: A Book for Young People
Autism Society of North Carolina Bookstore
505 Oberlin Road, Suite 230
Raleigh, NC 27605
919-743-0204
800-442-2762
Fax: 919-743-0208
e-mail: books@autismsociety-nc.org
www.autismbookstore.com

Written for brothers and sisters of young persons with autism spectrum disorder (ASD). It not only explains the basic characterisitics of ASD, but also answers the questions often asked by a sibling of a child with ASD. For readers ages 8-16.

Hardbound

917 Everyday Solutions: A Practical Guide for Families of Children with Autism
Autism Society of North Carolina Bookstore
505 Oberlin Road, Suite 230
Raleigh, NC 27605
919-743-0204
Fax: 919-743-0208
e-mail: books@autismsociety-nc.org
www.autismbookstore.com

Presents 37 everyday situations that may present difficulties for a child with autism spectrum disorder (ASD), along with recommendations and strategies.

918 Functional Behavior Assessment for People with Autism
Autism Society of North Carolina Bookstore
505 Oberlin Road, Suite 230
Raleigh, NC 27605
919-743-0204
Fax: 919-743-0208
e-mail: books@autismsociety-nc.org
www.autismbookstore.com

provides and introduction to functional behavior assessment (FBA). FBA is a valuable tool that can be used by parents and professionals to understand and address the challenging behaviors of persons with autism spectrum disorder (ASD).

919 Handbook Of Autism and Pervasive Developmental Disorders
Autism Society of North Carolina Bookstore
505 Oberlin Road, Suite 230
Raleigh, NC 27605
919-743-0204
Fax: 919-743-0208
e-mail: books@autismsociety-nc.org
www.autismbookstore.com

Two-volume scholarly resource presents the latest scientific research on autism spectrum disorders (ASD).

920 Healthcare for Children on the Autism Spectrum
Autism Society of North Carolina Bookstore
505 Oberlin Road, Suite 230
Raleigh, NC 27605
919-743-0204
800-442-2762
Fax: 919-743-0208
e-mail: books@autismsociety-nc.org
www.autismbookstore.com

The first publication of its kind to focus on the health and medical care of children with autism spectrum disorder (ASD).

921 Helping Children with Autism Learn
Oxford University Press
2001 Evans Road
Cary, NC 27513
919-677-0977
Fax: 919-677-1303
www.us.oup.com

A leading authority on autism offers practical, reliable advice on coping with learning disorders associated with autism.

2003 512 pages
ISBN: 0-195138-11-2

922 Hidden Child: The Linwood Method for Reaching the Autistic Child
Woodbine House
6510 Bells Mill Road
Bethesda, MD 20817
301-897-3570
Fax: 301-897-5838
e-mail: info@woodbinehouse.com
www.woodbinehouse.com

Chronicle of the Linwood Children's Center's successful treatment program for autistic children.

286 pages Paperback
ISBN: 0-933149-06-9

923 Higher Functioning Adolescents and Young Adults with Autism
Pro-Ed
8700 Shoal Creek Boulevard
Austin, TX 78757
512-451-3246
800-897-3202
Fax: 512-451-8542
e-mail: info@proedinc.com
www.proedinc.com

Practical strategies for teaching and supporting higher functioning students with autism, elementary school through college situations.

924 Ian's Walk: A Story About Autism
Autism Society of North Carolina Bookstore
505 Oberlin Road, Suite 230
Raleigh, NC 27605
919-743-0204
Fax: 919-743-0208
e-mail: books@autismsociety-nc.org
www.autismbookstore.com

In this moving fictional story, a young girl named Julie realizes how much she cares for her brother, Ian, who has autism spectrum disorder (ASD). For readers ages 4-8.

925 Incredible 5-Point Scale
Autism Society of North Carolina Bookstore
505 Oberlin Road, Suite 230
Raleigh, NC 27605

919-743-0204
Fax: 919-743-0208
e-mail: books@autismsociety-nc.org
www.autismbookstore.com

Shows parents and professionals how to implement a simple 5-point scale to help students with sutism spectrum disorder (ASD) understand and control their emotional responses and behavior.

926 Inner Life of Children with Special Needs
Taylor & Francis
325 Chestnut Street
Philadelphia, PA 19106

215-625-8900
Fax: 215-625-2940
www.taylorandfrancis.com

Paperback
ISBN: 1-897635-43-5

Rebecca Rich, Marketing Associate

927 Just Take a Bite: Easy, Effective Answers to Food Aversions and Eating Challenges
Autism Society of North Carolina Bookstore
505 Oberlin Road, Suite 230
Raleigh, NC 27605

919-743-0204
Fax: 919-743-0208
e-mail: books@autismsociety-nc.org
www.autismbookstore.com

A much-need resource that specifically addresses the eating challenges of children who may have autism spectrum disorder (ASD), sensory processing disorder (SPD), or other developmental delays.

928 Kids In the Syndrome Mix
Autism Society of North Carolina Bookstore
505 Oberlin Road, Suite 230
Raleigh, NC 27605

919-743-0204
Fax: 919-743-0208
e-mail: books@autismsociety-nc.org
www.autismbookstore.com

Children with autism spectrum disorder (ASD) often have coexisting neuropsychiatric diagnoses, and this handbook focuses on the most common neuropsychiatric disorders and their symptoms.

929 Looking After Louis
Autism Society of North Carolina
505 Oberlin Road, Suite 230
Raleigh, NC 27605

919-743-0204
800-442-2762
Fax: 919-743-0208
e-mail: books@autismsociety-nc.org
www.autismbookstore.com

Colrfully illustrated fictional story introduces readers to Louis, a new boy in school who has autism spectrum disorder (ASD). Told from the perspective of a female classmate, the story describes how Louis plays and interacts with students and teachers in a general education classroom. For readers ages 4-8.

930 Mindblindness: An Essay on Autism & Theory of Mind
MIT Press
100 Maple Ridge Drive
Cumberland, RI 02864

401-658-4226
800-405-1619
Fax: 401-658-4193
e-mail: mitpress-order-inq@mit.edu
http://mitpress.mit.edu

Interpretations and research into the theory of mindblindness in children with autism.

1995 208 pages
ISBN: 0-262023-84-9

931 Miracle to Believe In
Fawcett

A group of people from all walks of life come together and are transformed as they reach out, under the direction of the Kaufmans, to help a little boy the medical world has given up as hopeless. The heartwarming journey of loving a child back to life will not only inspire you, the reader, but presents a compelling new way to deal with life's traumas and difficulties.

1982 384 pages
ISBN: 0-449201-08-2

932 My Brother Sammy
Autism Society of North Carolina Bookstore
505 Oberlin Road, Suite 230
Raleigh, NC 27605

919-743-0204
Fax: 919-743-0208
e-mail: books@autismsociety-nc.org
www.autismbookstore.com

Filled with beautiful watercolor illustrations, this book tells the fictional story of Sammy, a young boy with autism spectrum disorder (ASD). The story is told from the perspective of Sammy's older brother, who is sometimes frustrated by Sammy's behavior. For readers ages 4-8.

933 My Friend With Autism
Autism Society of North Carolina Bookstore
505 Oberlin Road, Suite 230
Raleigh, NC 27605

919-743-0204
Fax: 919-743-0208
e-mail: books@autismsociety-nc.org
www.autismbookstore.com

Created for teachers and students in her son's elementary school class. The book is a valuable tool for helping typical children understand the traits and behaviors of their classmates with autism spectrum disorder (ASD). For readers ages 4-10.

934 My Social Stories Book
Autism Society of North Carolina Bookstore
505 Oberlin Road, Suite 230
Raleigh, NC 27605

919-743-0204
Fax: 919-743-0208
e-mail: books@autismsociety-nc.org
www.autismbookstore.com

The Social Stones in this book are written for children with autism spectrum disorder (ASD) ages 2 to 6, and they include over 150 everyday situations that are frequently encountered in early childhood.

935 Neurobiology of Autism
Johns Hopkins University Press
2715 N Charles Street
Baltimore, MD 21218

410-516-6900
Fax: 410-516-6998
www.press.jhu.edu

This book discusses recent advances in scientific research that point to a neurobiological basis for autism and examines the clinical implications of this research.

2006 424 pages
ISBN: 0-801880-47-5

936 News From the Border: A Mother's Memoir of Her Autistic Son
Houghton Mifflin Company/Order Processing
222 Berkeley Street
Boston, MA 02116

617-351-5000
www.hmco.com

A searingly honest account of the author's family experiences with autism. Raising an autistic child is the central, ongoing drama of her married life and this riveting account of acceptance and coping.

1993 384 pages Cloth

937 Parenting Across the Autism Spectrum
Autism Society of North Carolina Bookstore
505 Oberlin Road, Suite 230
Raleigh, NC 27605

919-743-0204
Fax: 919-743-0208
e-mail: books@autismsociety-nc.org
www.autismbookstore.com

Two mothers who have children on the opposite ends of the autism spectrum wrote this poignant and insightful book, and the book also provides a look at what lies beyond the early intervention and elementary school years.

938 Preschool Education Programs for Children with Autism
8700 Shoal Creek Boulevard
Austin, TX 78757

512-451-3246
800-897-3202
Fax: 512-451-8542
e-mail: info@proedinc.com
www.proedinc.com

Written for special education teachers, school administrators, child-study team members, psychologists, speech therapists, and advocates and parents who are concerned about the education of preschool-age children with autism. It will be especially helpful to persons who are considering creating a classroom to serve these children or persons interested in ensuring that the services they currently offer meet state-of-the-art criteria.

939 Preschool Issues in Autism
Plenum Publishing Corporation
233 Spring Street
New York, NY 10013

212-620-8000
Fax: 212-463-0742
e-mail: info@plenum.com
plenum.com

Combines some of the most important theory and data related to the early identifiction and intervention in autism and related disorders. Addresses clinical aspects, parental concerns and legal issues. Helps professionals understand and implement state-of-the-art services for young children and their families.

294 pages
ISBN: 0-306444-40-2

940 Prescription for Success
Autism Society of North Carolina Bookstore
505 Oberlin Road, Suite 230
Raleigh, NC 27605

919-743-0204
Fax: 919-743-0208
e-mail: books@autismsociety-nc.org
www.autismbookstore.com

Written for medical professionals who work with patients who have autism spectrum disorder.

941 Reaching the Autistic Child: A Parent Training Program
Brookline Books/Lumen Editions
34 University Road
Brookline, MA 02445

617-734-6772
800-666-2665
Fax: 617-734-3952
www.brooklinebooks.com

Detailed case studies of social and behavioral change in autistic children and their families show parents how to implement the principles for improved socialization and behavior.

1998 Softcover
ISBN: 1-571290-56-7

942 Riddle of Autism: A Psychological Analysis
Jason Aronson
4501 Forbes Blvd, Suite 200
Lanham, MD 20706

301-459-3366
800-462-6420
Fax: 301-429-5748
e-mail: custserv@rowman.com
www.aronson.com

Dr. Victor examines the myths that cloud an understanding of this disorder and describes the meanings of its specific behavioral symptoms.

356 pages Softcover
ISBN: 1-568215-73-8

943 Russell Is Extra Special
Autism Society of North Carolina Bookstore
505 Oberlin Road
Raleigh, NC 27605

919-743-0204
Fax: 919-743-0208
e-mail: ASNC@aol.com

A sensitive portrayal of an autistic boy written by his father.

1992 Hardcover

944 Siblings of Children with Autism: A Guide for Families
Autism Society of North Carolina Bookstore
505 Oberlin Road
Raleigh, NC 27605

919-743-0204
Fax: 919-743-0208
e-mail: ASNC@aol.com

Offers information on the needs of a child with autism.

1994

945 Social Skills Picture Book
Autism Society of North Carolina Bookstore
505 Oberlin Road, Suite 230
Raleigh, NC 27605

919-743-0204
Fax: 919-743-0208
e-mail: books@autismsociety-nc.org
www.autismbookstore.com

(Teaching Play, Emotions, and Communication to Children with Autism). Through photographs and conversation bubbles, the author demonstrates approximately 30 social skilld in the areas of communication, play, and emotion.

946 Solving Behavior Problems in Autism
Autism Society of North Carolina Bookstore
505 Oberlin Road, Suite 230
Raleigh, NC 27605

919-743-0204
Fax: 919-743-0208
e-mail: books@autismsociety-nc.org
www.autismbookstore.com

In this guide, the author explains how to use effective communication techniques to reduce problem behaviors in persons with autism spectrum disorder (ASD).

947 Son-Rise: The Miracle Continues

Describes an effective, loving and respectful method for treating children with autism. It documents the development of the Son Rise Program throught the record of Raun Kaufman's astonishing development from a lifeless, autistic, retarded child into a highly verbal, loveable youngster with no traces of his former condition. It further details Raun's extraordinary progress from the age of four into young adulthood. It also shares moving accounts of five families who successfully used the program.

1995 384 pages
ISBN: 0-915811-61-8

948 Stress and Coping in Autism

Oxford University Press
2001 Evans Road
Cary, NC 27513

919-677-0977
Fax: 919-677-1303
www.us.oup.com

Provides a theoretical framework for the usefukness of the stress construct in understanding and treating autism.

2006 472 pages
ISBN: 0-195182-26-X

949 Taking Autism to School

Autism Society of North Carolina Bookstore
505 Oberlin Road, Suite 230
Raleigh, NC 27605

919-743-0204
Fax: 919-743-0208
e-mail: books@autismsociety-nc.org
www.autismbookstore.com

A fictional story about a girl named Angel and her friendship woth Sam, a classmate who has autism spectrum disorder (ASD). From her own point of view, Angel explains how Sam thinks and behaves in school and at home. For readers ages 5-10.

950 Teach Me Language

Autism Society of North Carolina Bookstore
505 Oberlin Road
Raleigh, NC 27605

919-743-0204
Fax: 919-743-0208

Language manual for children with autism, asperger's syndrome and related developmental disorders.

951 Teaching Children with Autism

Books on Special Children
PO Box 305
Congers, NY 10920

845-638-1236

Contributions from people in the field regarding communication and language use. Support for families, parent education, school placement, IEP process and other topics relating to many levels of abilites of the autistic child. Good book to help understand symptoms and intervention for improving skills in autistic children.

1995 236 pages Softcover
ISBN: 4-557661-80-4

952 Teaching Children with Autism - Strategies to Enhance Communication

Autism Society of North Carolina Bookstore
505 Oberlin Road
Raleigh, NC 27605

919-743-0204
Fax: 919-743-0208
e-mail: ASNC@aol.com

This valuable new book describes teaching strategies and instructional adaptations which promote communication and socialization in children with autism.

953 Teaching Children with Autism to Mind-Read A Pratical Guide for Teachers & Parents

John Wiley & Sons
10475 Crosspoint Blvd
Indianapolis, IN 46256

877-762-2974
Fax: 800-597-3299
www.wiley.com

This book explains the Theory of Mind, which is the ability to infer other's mental states and then interpret their speech and actions based on this information. The author applies this theory to autistic children to help their social and communicative abnormalities.

1999 302 pages
ISBN: 0-471976-23-7

954 Teachinjg Coversations to Children With Autism: Scripts and Script Fading

Autism Society of North Carolina Bookstore
505 Oberlin Road, Suite 230
Raleigh, NC 27605

919-743-0204
Fax: 919-743-0208
e-mail: books@autismsociety-nc.org
www.autismbookstore.com

Uses the principles of Apllied Behavior Analysis (ABA) to create strategies that facilitate communication in children who have autism spectrum disorder.

955 Ten Things Every Child With Autism Wishes You Know

Autism Society of North Carolina Bookstore
505 Oberlin Road, Suite 230
Raleigh, NC 27605

919-743-0204
Fax: 919-743-0208
e-mail: books@autismsociety-nc.org
www.autismbookstore.com

Describes how children with autism spectrum disorder (ASD) function and what they are trying to say to the world when they cannot always express it in a conventional way.

956 The Neurology of Autism

Oxford University Press
2001 Evans Road
Cary, NC 27513

919-677-0977
Fax: 919-677-1303
www.us.oup.com

A valuable resource for both the latest information from basic-science research and its application to the diagnosis and treatment of autism.

2005 272 pages
ISBN: 0-195182-22-7

957 Toilet Training for Individuals with Autism and Related Disorders

Autism Society of North Carolina Bookstore
505 Oberlin Road, Suite 230
Raleigh, NC 27605

919-743-0204
Fax: 919-743-0208
e-mail: books@autismsociety-nc.org
www.autismbookstore.com

Comprehensive guide for parents and professionals provides over 200 toilet training tips and more than 40 helpful case examples.

958 Treasure Chest of Behavioral Strategies for Individuals with Autism
Autism Society of North Carolina Bookstore
505 Oberlin Road, Suite 230
Raleigh, NC 27605

919-743-0204
Fax: 919-743-0208
e-mail: books@autismsociety-nc.org
www.autismbookstore.com

Comprehensive resource manual provides parents and teachers with numerous behavior management strategies for individuals with autism spectrum disorder (ASD).

959 Ultimate Stranger: The Autistic Child
Autism Society of North Carolina Bookstore
505 Oberlin Road
Raleigh, NC 27605

919-743-0204
Fax: 919-743-0208

Delacato's thesis is that autism is neuro-genic and not psy-cho-genic in origin.

1974

960 Understanding and Treating Children with Autism
John Wiley & Sons
10475 Crosspoint Blvd
Indianapolis, IN 46256

877-762-2974
Fax: 800-597-3299
www.wiley.com

Aimed at those concerned with the education and welfare of the children with autism, particularly at teachers in Special education and the psychologists and care professionals who work with teachers and parents of children with autism.

1995 188 pages
ISBN: 0-471958-88-3

961 Understanding the Nature of Autism
Autism Society of North Carolina Bookstore
505 Oberlin Road
Raleigh, NC 27605

919-743-0204
Fax: 919-743-0208
e-mail: ASNC@aol.com

Guide to autism spectrum disorders.

962 Until Tomorrow: A Family Lives with Autism
Autism Society of North Carolina Bookstore
505 Oberlin Road
Raleigh, NC 27605

919-743-0204
Fax: 919-743-0208

The central theme of this book is an effort to show what it is like to live with a child who cannot communicate.

1988

963 Visual Strategies for Improving Communication
Autism Society of North Carolina Bookstore
505 Oberlin Road, Suite 230
Raleigh, NC 27605

919-743-0204
Fax: 919-743-0208
e-mail: books@autismsociety-nc.org
www.autismbookstore.com

This how-to manual describes a communication intervention strategy for teaching persons with autism spectrum disorder (ASD) that evolved from learning style research.

964 Visually Structured Tasks
Autism Society of North Carolina Bookstore
505 Oberlin Road
Raleigh, NC 27605

919-743-0204
Fax: 919-743-0208
e-mail: ASNC@aol.com

Independent activites for students with autism and other visual learners.

965 When Snow Turns to Rain
Woodbine House
6510 Bells Mill Road
Bethesda, MD 20817

301-897-3570
Fax: 301-897-5838
e-mail: info@woodbinehouse.com
www.woodbinehouse.com

A gripping personal account of one family's experiences with autism. Chronicles a family's journey from parental bliss to devastation, as they learn that their son has autism. This book delves into diagnosis, treatments and attitudes toward persons with autism.

1993 250 pages Paperback
ISBN: 0-933149-63-8

966 Winter's Flower
Autism Society of North Carolina Bookstore
505 Oberlin Road
Raleigh, NC 27605

919-743-0204
Fax: 919-743-0208

The story of Ranae Johnson's quest to rescue her son from a world of silence. A story of love, patience and dedication.

1992

967 World of the Autistic Child
Oxford University Press
2001 Evans Road
Cary, NC 27513

919-677-0977
800-451-7556
Fax: 919-677-1303
www.us.oup.com

Comprehensive guide for parents with children diagnosed or suspected of being autistic. Includes current thinking on causes, diagnosis, and treatment, using illustrative case studies.

1998 368 pages
ISBN: 0-195119-17-7

Magazines

968 Autism Advocate
Autism Society of America
7910 Woodmont Avenue, Suite 300
Bethesda, MD 20814

301-657-0881
800-328-8476
www.autism-society.org

Gathers a diverse collection of the latest autism news, chapter highlights, first-person accounts of families living with and growing with autism, and tips from paretns and professionals. Published 5 times a year.

969 Newslink
Autism Society Ontario
1179A King Street West, Suite 004
Toronto, ON
M6K 3C5

416-246-9592
Fax: 416-246-9417
e-mail: mail@autismsociety.on.ca
autismsociety.on.ca

Covers society activities and contains information on autism. Recurring features include news of research, a calendar of events, reports of meetings, and book reviews.

10 pages

Journals

970   Focus on Autism and Other Developmental Disabilities
8700 Shoal Creek Boulevard
Austin, TX 78757

512-451-3246
800-897-3202
Fax: 512-451-8542
e-mail: info@procdinc.com
www.procdinc.com

Practical elements of management, treatment, planning, and education for persons with autism or other pervasive developmental disabilities. Published quarterly, Focus publishes articles representing diverse philosophical and theoretical positions and reflecting a wide range of disciplines, including education, psychology, psychiatry, medicine, physical therapy, occupational therapy, speech/language pathology and related areas.

Quarterly

Newsletters

971   Autism Research Review International
Autism Research Institute
4182 Adams Avenue
San Diego, CA 92116

619-281-7165
Fax: 619-563-6840
www.autismresearchinstitute.com

Discusses current research and provides information about the causes, diagnosis, and treatment of autism and related disorders.

8 pages Quarterly

972   Autism Society News
Autism Society of Utah
668 S 13th E
Salt Lake City, UT 84102

801-583-7049
Fax: 801-581-0193

Presents news, research information, and legislative updates regarding autism. Recurring features include a calendar of events and columns titled Parent Meetings, What's On in the News, Research News, Parent Corner, Legislative Summary, and A Big Thank You!

8 pages

Kim Moody, Director

973   MAAP Newsletter
PO Box 524
Crown Point, IN 46308

219-662-1311
Fax: 219-662-0638
e-mail: chart@netnitco.net
www.maapservices.org

Shares information that are not find in textbooks or read in other sources.

974   Queens Services for Autistic Children Newsletter
12055 Queens Boulevard
Jamaica, NY 11424

718-793-7202
Fax: 718-268-1308

Offers information on books and resources, meetings and support groups, chapter information and more for parents and families affected by autism.

Monthly

Pamphlets

975   Autism Fact Sheet
NINDS
PO Box 5801
Bethesda, MD 20824

301-496-5751
800-352-9424
TTY: 301-468-5981
www.ninds.nih.gov

Also available in Spanish.

976   Autism Society of America, General Information on Autism
7910 Woodmont Avenue, Suite 300
Bethesda, MD 20814

301-657-0881
800-328-8476
e-mail: info@autism-society.org
www.autism-society.org

Offers a definition and introduction to autism, offers reading material and suggested resources pertaining to autism and points out the educational implications of students with autism.

977   Autism Spectrum Disorders in Children and Adolescents
Center for Mental Health Services
PO Box 42490
Washington, DC 20015

800-789-2647
Fax: 301-984-8796
e-mail: ken@mentalhealth.org
mentalhealth.org

This fact sheet defines autism, describes the signs and causes, discusses types of help available, and suggests what parents or other caregivers can do.

2 pages

978   Fact Sheet: Autism
Autism Society of America
7910 Woodmont Avenue, Suite 300
Bethesda, MD 20814

301-657-0881
800-328-8476
e-mail: info@autism-society.org
www.autism-society.org

Offers information on autism. What it is, symptoms, causes, diagnosis, treatments and research.

979   Facts About Autism
Indiana Institute on Disability and Community
Indiana University
Bloomington, IN 47408

812-855-6508
800-280-7010
Fax: 812-855-9630
TTY: 812-855-9396
e-mail: uap@indiana.edu
iidc.indiana.edu

Provides concise information describing autism, diagnosis, needs of the person with autism from diagnosis through adulthood. Information on the Autism Society of America chapters in Indiana is listed in the back, along with a description of the Indiana Resource Center for Autism and suggested books to look for in the local library. Also available in Spanish.

17 pages

Marci Wheeler
Suzie Rimstidt

980 Parents as Trainers of Legislators, Other Parents and Researchers
Autism Services Center
101 Richmond Street
Huntington, WV 25702

304-525-8014
Fax: 304-525-8026

Reprint offering information on parents of autistic children that learn early in their child's life how little professionals know about autism.

981 Pervasive Developmental Disorders
National Inst. of Neurological Disorders/Stroke
31 Center Drive, MSC 2540, Building 31, Room 8A06
Bethesda, MD 20892

301-496-5751
800-352-9424

Detailed booklet that describes symptoms, causes, and treatments, with information on getting help and coping.

982 What Is Autism
Autism Society of America
7910 Woodmont Avenue, Suite 300
Bethesda, MD 20814

301-657-0881
800-328-8476
e-mail: info@autism-society.org
www.autism-society.org

Offers a definition and introduction to autism, produces autism information written for kids only.

Camps

983 Beech Brook
3737 Lander Road
Cleveland, OH

216-831-2255
Fax: 216-831-0436

A year-round residential and day treatment center, accepts summer residents when there are openings in the regular enrollment. The program is designed for emotionally disturbed, learning disabled and autistic children, providing therapeutically oriented teaching and programming techniques in a camp setting.

Don Harris, Director

984 Big Crystal Camp
8533 Williams Road
DeWitt, MI

517-669-9367

One week residential camp sponsored by Lansing Area Chapter of Michigan Association for Children with Learning Disabilities.

Florence Curtis

985 Camp Buckskin
8700 W 36th Street Suite 6w
Saint Louis Park, MN 55426

952-930-3544
Fax: 952-938-6996
e-mail: buckskin@spacestar.net
www.campbuckskin.com

LD and ADD/ADHD youth have often experienced frustration and a lack of success. Buckskin assists these individuals to realize and develop the potentials and abilities which they possess. Teaches a combination of academic and camp activities, so the campers experience success in many areas. By necessity fairly structured, the 1:3 staff ratio ensures the program is individualized to meet each camper's needs. Parents report that their children benefit from the experience in many ways.

Thomas R Bauer, CCD, Camp Director

986 Camp Nuhop
404 Hillcrest Drive
Ashland, OH

419-289-2227
Fax: 419-289-2227
e-mail: cnuhop@bright.net
www.campnuhop.org

A summer residential program for any youngster from 6 to 18 with a learning disability, behavior disorder or Attention Deficit Disorder. Sixty two campers and 35 staff members live on site in groups of 7 campers to every 3 counselors. Activities focus on positive self-concept and behaviors and teach children to learn how to find their strengths, abilities and talents from a positive, yet realistic viewpoint.

Jerry Dunlap, Director

987 Dallas Academy
950 Tiffany Way
Dallas, TX

214-324-1481
Fax: 214-327-8537
e-mail: mail@dallas-academy.com
www.dallas-academy.com

7-week summer session for students who are having difficulty in regular school classes.

Jim Richardson, Director

988 Developmental Center
6710 86th Avenue N
Pinellas Park, FL

Specifically designed for the learning disabled child and other children with difficulties in concentration, strategy, social skills, impulsivity, distractibility and study strategies. Programs offered include: attention training, visual-motor remediation, socialization skills training, relaxation training, horseback riding and more. The day camp meets weekdays from 9-3 for 3,4 or 5 week sessions.

Dr. Eric Larson

989 Eagle Hill School - Summer Program
242 Old Petersham Road
Hardwick, MA 01037

413-477-6000
Fax: 413-477-6837
e-mail: admission@eaglehillschool.com
www.chs1.org

For the child, age 9-19, with a specific learning disability or Attention Deficit Disorder, this summer program offers a structured curriculum designed to build a basic foundation of academic competence. Extracurricular and outdoor activities complement the educational program.

Erin E Wynne, Dean of Admission

990 Groves Learning Center
3200 Highway 100 S
Saint Louis Park, MN

A nonprofit day school in Minnesota designed especially for children with learning differences. The Center has a full day academic program from September through June, as well as an 8 week summer program. Groves also offers community services such as: psychoeducational testing for children and adults, consulting services, workshops on learning disabilities and other special learning needs, and afternoon/evening tutorial services for children and adults.

Sue Kirchhoff, Head of School

991 Hill School of Fort Worth
4817 Odessa Avenue
Fort Worth, TX

817-923-9482
Fax: 817-923-4894
e-mail: admission@hillschool.org
www.hillschool.org

Provides an alternative learning environment for students having average or above-average intelligence with learning differences.

Hill school is an established leader in North Texas with a 25 year history of effectively serving LD children. Beginning in 1961 as a tutorial service, Hill became a formal school in 1973. Our mission is to help those who learn differently develop skills and strategies to succeed. We do this by developing academic/study skills, and self-discipline.

Lucille H Helton, Principal
Cathy Allen, Admissions Director

992 Lab School of Washington
4759 Reservoir Road NW
Washington, DC 20007

202-965-6600
Fax: 202-965-5106
www.labschool.org

The Lab School six week summer session includes individualized reading, spelling, writing, study skills, and math programs. A multisensory approach addresses the needs of bright learning disabled children. Related services such as speech/language therapy and occupational therapy are integrated into the curriculum. Elementary/Intermediate; Junior High/High School.

Sally Smith, Founder
Susan Ferley, Admissions Director

993 Maplebrook School
5142 Route 22
Amenia, NY

845-373-8191
Fax: 845-373-7029
e-mail: mbsecho@aol.com

A coeductional boarding school for students with learning differences and ADD. A New York State registered high school servicing ages 11-18. Post secondary options offered to 18-21.

Donna M Konkolios, Head of School
Jennifer Scully, Director Admissions

994 Round Lake Camp
21 Plymouth Street
Fairfield, NJ

973-575-3333
Fax: 973-575-4188
e-mail: rlc@njycamps.org
www.njycamps.org

For ages 7-18, this camp provides individualized academics in reading, language development and math for children with mild learning disabilities, Round Lake also offers therapeutic recreation and Jewish cultural values to its participants.

Sheira Director, Asst. Director

DESCRIPTION

995 BELL'S PALSY

Involves the following Biologic System(s):

Neurologic Disorders

Bell's palsy is the most common form of facial nerve paralysis and may affect children at any age from infancy through adolescence. The facial nerve, also known as the seventh cranial nerve, arises from a certain area of the brain (i.e., brainstem) and divides into several branches that supply (innervate) the forehead, scalp, eyelids, cheeks, jaws, and muscles of facial expression. The facial nerve also conveys taste sensations from the front two thirds of the tongue. Bell's palsy is a temporary form of facial paralysis that usually develops suddenly approximately two weeks after a widespread viral infection, such as Epstein-Barr virus, herpesvirus, or mumps virus. It is thought to represent a postinfectious demyelination of the facial nerve (neuritis) due to allergic or immune responses.

Bell's palsy typically affects one side of the face and may involve upper and lower areas on the affected side. Symptoms of Bell's palsy usually begin suddenly and reach their peak within 48 hours. Children with the condition may experience weakness or slight paralysis of the upper and lower face; drooping of the corner of the mouth; an inability to close the eye; loss of taste sensations from the front two thirds of the tongue; or abnormal sensitivity to loud sounds (hyperacusis). Because the affected eye may be overexposed to the air, some patients may develop inflammation (exposure keratitis) of the transparent, front region of the eye (cornea). In addition, saliva may dribble from the corner of the mouth and food may tend to collect between the teeth and lips.

There is no cure or standard course of treatment for Bell's palsy. Some cases are mild and do not require treatment since the symptoms usually subside on their own within 2 weeks. For others, treatment may include medications such as acyclovir, used to fight viral infections, combined with an anti-inflammatory drug such as the steroid prednisone, used to reduce inflammation and swelling. Pain medications, such as aspirin, acetaminophen, or ibuprofen may be helpful. Other treatment of children with Bell's palsy is supportive, including eye drops to lubricate the cornea, particularly at night. In over 85 percent of affected children, Bell's palsy spontaneously resolves with no remaining facial weakness. About 10 percent may have mild longstanding weakness, and approximately five percent may experience severe, permanent facial weakness.

See also **General Resources** on page 917

Government Agencies

996 NIH/National Institute of Neurological Dis orders and Stroke (NINDS)
PO Box 5801
Bethesda, MD 20824

301-496-5751
800-352-9424
Fax: 301-496-0296
TTY: 301-468-5981
www.ninds.nih.gov

The mission is to reduce the burden of neurological disease - a burden borne by every age group, by every segment of society, by people all over the world.

Story C Landis Ph.D., Director
Audrey S Penn M.D., Deputy Director

National Associations & Support Groups

997 American Academy of Otolaryngology-Head and Neck Surgery
1 Prince Street
Alexandria, VA 22314

703-836-4444
Fax: 703-683-5100
TTY: 703-519-1585
e-mail: webmaster@entnet.org
www.entnet.org

The missions of the AAO-HNS and its foundation are to advance the art and science of otolaryngology-head and neck surgery through state-of-the-art education, research and learning; and to unite, serve and represent the interests of its members and their patients to the public, government, other medical specialists and related organizations. Founded in 1896, the AAO-HNS is the world's largest organization of otolaryngologist-head and neck surgeons.

11,600 Members

C Ron Cannon, President

998 March of Dimes Birth Defects Foundation
1275 Mamaroneck Avenue
White Plains, NY 10605

914-428-7100
888-663-4637
Fax: 914-428-8203
e-mail: resourcecenter@modimes.org
www.marchofdimes.com

Partnership of volunteers and professionals dedicates to improving the health of babies by preventing birth defects and infant mortality. Over 100 chapters are located across the country and can be located through the National Office.

Dr Jennifer Howse, President

999 National Centers for Facial Paralysis
18403 Woodfield Road, Suite D
Gaithersburg, MD 20879

301-330-3223
Fax: 301-330-9075
e-mail: lgamliel@targangroup.com
www.bellspalsy.com

Strives to evaluate, inform and assist patients with past and/or current history of Facial Palsy, Bell's Palsy, Ramsey-Hunt Syndrome, or Facial Paralysis from surgery, trauma, pregnancy, lyme disease, or other causes.

Research Centers

1000 Bell's Palsy Research Foundation
19550 Club House Road
Montgomery Village, MD 20886

301-651-9605
Fax: 301-216-2477
e-mail: drtargan@erols.com
www.bellspalsy.com

An online support foundation for facial palsy patients, providing informations and support to patients worldwide; also functions to educate the medical community about facial paralysis and to advance research and development in all aspects of facial palsy and facial pain.

Bob Targen, MD, Director

Web Sites

1001 American Academy of Otolaryngology Head an d Neck Surgery
www.entnet.org

Mission is to advance the art and science of otolaryngology-head and neck surgery through state-of-the-art education, research and learning.

1002 Bell's Palsy Network
www.bellspalsy.net/

Provides information on facial paralysis, Bell's Palsy, Ramsey Hunt Syndrome and other forms of facial paralysis. We were the first dedicated web portal for Bell's palsy and facial paralysis informaton and host the largest and most popular forum about bell's palsy and facial palsy information.

1003 Bell's Palsy Research Foundation
www.bellspalsyresearch.com

Online support foundation for facial palsy patients, providing information and supprt to patients worldwide.

1004 NIH/National Institute of Neurological Dis orders and Stroke (NINDS)
www.ninds.nih.gov

Mission is to reduce the burden of neurological disease-a burden borne by every age group, by every segment of society, by people all over the world.

DESCRIPTION

1005 BILIARY ATRESIA

Involves the following Biologic System(s):

Gastrointestinal Disorders

Biliary atresia is a rare condition that is present at birth (congenital) in approximately 1 in 12,500 births, and is characterized by the absence of or the abnormal or incomplete development (hypoplasia) of the bile ducts. These ducts carry bile from the liver and gallbladder into the small intestine. Bile, which is secreted by the liver, is a yellowish or greenish fluid that aids in the digestion of fats. Bile passes through the common bile duct and into the upper portion of the small intestine (duodenum). Absence or underdevelopment of the bile ducts interferes with or prevents the passage of bile into the intestine and, as a result, characteristic findings and symptoms may be noticed within the first few weeks of life.

Symptoms may include progressively darkening urine; pale stools (acholic); a persistent yellowing of the skin, eyes, and mucous membranes (jaundice); and enlargement of the liver (hepatomegaly). If untreated, additional symptoms and findings may become apparent within two or three months. These may include growth retardation, increased irritability, and itching (pruritus). A potential complication of biliary atresia involves an increase in pressure in the vein that conveys blood from the spleen, stomach, pancreas, and intestine to the liver (portal hypertension). In addition, untreated biliary atresia may result in a life-threatening condition known as biliary cirrhosis, in which the liver's function is impaired and, eventually, the liver becomes irreversibly damaged.

Treatment for biliary atresia is often determined by the site of the obstruction and includes various surgical procedures. In some infants, surgery may be performed as a means to help postpone cirrhosis and growth retardation until liver transplantation is feasible.

See also **General Resources** on page 917

National Associations & Support Groups

1006 American Association for the Study of Liver Diseases
1729 King Street, Suite 200
Alexandria, VA 22314

703-299-9766
Fax: 703-299-9622
e-mail: aasld@aasld.org
www.aasld.org

AASLD is the catalyst for the investigation and treatment of liver diseases. Offers scientific educational symposia developed by leading hepatolgist.

John M Vierling, MD FACP, President

1007 CHARGE Syndrome Foundation
409 Vandiver Drive
Columbia, MO 65202

573-499-4694
800-442-7604
Fax: 573-499-4694
e-mail: marion@chargesyndrome.org
www.chargesyndrome.org

CHARGE (Coloboma, Heart Malformations, Atresia Choanae, Retardation, Genital Abnormalities, Ear Abnormalities)

Marion Norbury, Executive Director

1008 Children's Liver Alliance
3835 Richmond Avenue, Suite 190
Staten Island, NY 10312

718-987-6200
Fax: 718-987-6200

Aids in easing the physical and emotional strains that the child is experiencing, so he or she can better deal with the disorder through different media resources that are also available to both family and friends.

Kathie DeLuca, Office Manager

1009 Children's Liver Association for Support Services
27023 McBean Parkway, #126
Valencia, CA 91355

661-263-9099
877-679-8256
Fax: 661-263-9099
e-mail: supportsru@aol.com
www.classkids.org

CLASS is an all volunteer, nonprofit organization dedicated to serving the emotional, educational and financial needs of families coping with childhood liver disease and transplantation. Our goal is to be both a service to families and a valuable resource for the medical community.

Diane Sumner, President
Ann Whitehead, VP

1010 Genetic Alliance
4301 Connecticut Avenue NW
Washington, DC 20008

202-966-5557
800-336-4363
Fax: 202-966-8553
e-mail: info@geneticalliance.org
www.geneticalliance.org

A coalition of voluntary genetic support groups, consumers and professionals addressing the needs of individuals and families affected by genetic disorders from a national perspective.

Sharon Terry, President/CEO

Research Centers

1011 Clinical Research Center, Pediatrics
Children's Hospital Research Foundation
3333 Burnett Avenue
Cincinnati, OH 45229

513-636-4200
800-344-2462
Fax: 513-636-7151
TTY: 513-636-4900
www.cincinnatichildrens.org

A pediatric research institute serving infants to adolescents. A medical center in pediatric health care, research and education.

James Heubi, MD, Director

1012 Univ. of Texas-Southwestern Med. Ctr. at Dallas - Clinical Ctr. for Liver Disease
5323 Harry Hines Boulevard
Dallas, TX 75235

214-648-3323
Fax: 214-648-3715
e-mail: LIVER@UTSouthwestern.edu

To achieve optimal outcomes for patients with a variety of liver disorders, including but not limited to Hepatitis B, C, and acute liver failure.

Dr. William Lee, Director

Conferences

1013 CHARGE Syndrome Conference
409 Vandiver Drive, 5-104
Columbia, MO 65202

573-499-4694
800-442-7604
e-mail: conference@chargesyndrome.org
www.chargesyndrome.org

Annual conference sponsored by CHARGE (Coloboma, Heart Malformations, Atresia Choanae, Retardation, Genital Abnormalities, Ear Abnormalities). Includes exhibitors, workshops, and networking for professionals, patients and parents. July 27-29, 2007, in Costa Mesa, California.

July

Marilyn Ogan, Chairperson, Conference Committee

Web Sites

1014 Children's Liver Alliance
www.liverkids.org.au

1015 Children's Liver Association for Support Services
www.classkids.org

Information regarding education and financial needs of families coping with childhood liver disease and transplantation.

1016 Online Mendelian Inheritance in Man
www.ncbi.nlm.nih.gov

This database is a catalog of human genes and genetic disorders.

Book Publishers

1017 Liver Disease in Children
Lippincott Williams & Wilkins
530 Walnut Street
Philadelphia, PA 19106

215-521-8300
Fax: 215-521-8902
www.lww.com

This is a difinitive book on pediatric liver disease, providing extensive, well-edited information that is not easily accessible or avail-

able in other textbooks. A must-have for those interested in this rapidly growing subspecialty in pediatrics.

2000 1008 pages
ISBN: 0-781720-98-2

1018 Liver Disorders in Childhood
Elsevier Science Health Science Division
225 Wildwood Avenue
Woburn, MA 01801

617-928-2500
800-366-2665
Fax: 800-446-6520

1999 432 pages
ISBN: 0-750642-00-9

Newsletters

1019 Children's Liver Alliance Newsletter
3835 Richmond Avenue, Suite 190
Staten Island, NY 10312

718-987-6200
Fax: 718-987-6200

Aids in easing the physical and emotional strains that the child is experiencing, so they can better deal with the disorder through different media resources that are also available to both friends and family.

4-12 pages

Kathie DeLuca, Office Manager

Pamphlets

1020 Biliary Atresia
American Liver Foundation
1425 Pompton Avenue
Cedar Grove, NJ 07009

973-857-2626
www.liverfoundation.org

Pamphlet with information and symptoms on biliary atresia

1021 Facts on Liver Transplantation
American Liver Foundation
1425 Pompton Avenue
Cedar Grove, NJ 07009

973-256-2550
800-223-0179
www.liverfoundation.org

Provides information on liver transplantation, and the effects.

DESCRIPTION

1022 BIPOLAR DISORDER

Synonyms: Manic-depressive disorder, Manic-depressive illness, Manic-depressive psychosis

Involves the following Biologic System(s):
Developmental/Behavioral/Psychiatric Disorders

Bipolar disorder, also known as manic-depressive disorder, is a condition characterized by alternating depression and mania or, in rare cases, mania alone. The disorder is thought to affect less than two percent of the general population. Although bipolar disorder usually becomes apparent during the third or fourth decade of life, a significant proportion of individuals are initially affected in childhood, adolescence, or early adulthood. Individuals with bipolar disorder may initially experience either a depressive or a manic episode. In some affected children and adolescents, manic episodes may be more frequent than depressive episodes during the first years of their illness. However, as the disease progresses, episodes of depression may become more frequent than manic episodes. Bipolar disorder is often further classified as unipolar in cases in which only depression is experienced and bipolar when mania occurs, with or without depression. In addition, mixed affected states are characterized by the occurrence of depressive and manic symptoms during a single episode.

In children and adolescents with bipolar disorder, associated symptoms resemble those seen in affected adults. Depressive states usually emerge gradually and may be characterized by feelings of sadness, despair, hopelessness, and discouragement; loss of self-esteem; physical and emotional exhaustion; and lack of interest of formerly enjoyed activities. In severe cases, affected individuals may have suicidal tendencies, and hospitalization in a pediatric, general, or psychiatric facility may be essential. In such cases, consultation with child psychiatrists is important for ongoing support and decision-making regarding treatment options.

In affected children and adolescents, manic states may be characterized by overactivity (hyperactivity); excessive talking; inability to sleep (insomnia); impulsive behavior and impaired judgment that may result in reckless spending; elation that may quickly change to irritability and anger; personal neglect that may result in poor hygiene; and, in some cases, delusions of grandeur and persecution (paranoid delusions). Initial episodes of depression or mania often last approximately six months without treatment. Although most manic or depressive episodes usually cease in months, some individuals may be affected for longer periods.

Adolescents with bipolar disorder may be misdiagnosed, e.g., with a psychotic disorder characterized by disturbances in behavior, cognition, and emotional reactions (schizophrenia) or a maladjusted reaction to a stressful life event (adjustment disorder). However, most affected individuals are correctly diagnosed with bipolar disorder during adulthood. According to reports in the literature, the earlier the onset of bipolar disorder, the more susceptible affected individuals may be to frequent episodes, rapid cycling between depressive and manic states, and severe episodes that may result in suicidal tendencies. In addition, earlier onset of the disorder is often associated with an increased incidence of depression and bipolar disorder in immediate (first-degree) relatives.

The treatment of children and adolescents with bipolar disorder may include therapy with certain medications (e.g., lithium carbonate, carbamazepine) and integrated, multidisciplinary management (e.g., behavioral therapy; individual, family, or group psychodynamic therapy; etc.). In children and adolescents with the disorder, thorough patient and family histories and specific medical evaluations are typically conducted before medications are prescribed. Pretreatment evaluation for lithium may include assessment of electrolyte levels, and kidney (renal) and thyroid function. Pretreatment evaluation for tricyclic antidepressants may include a cardiovascular examination including electrocardiography. If such medications are prescribed, regular blood levels should be taken until an adequate dose is determined.

Other treatment options include antipsychotics or tranquilizers if agitation or psychotic symptoms are present, especially at the initiation of treatment when acute manic episodes are likely. Recent studies have shown that about 80% of patients treated with electroconvulsive therapy (ECT) experienced improvement, and for some, it was the only treatment that worked. The exact cause of bipolar disorder is unknown. However, many researchers agree that genetic abnormalities may playsome role in the etiology of the disorder.

See also **General Resources** on page 917

Government Agencies

1023 Center for Mental Health Services Knowledge Exchange Network
US Department of Health and Human Services
PO Box 42557
Washington, DC 20015

800-789-2647
Fax: 240-747-5470
TDD: 866-889-2647
http://mentalhealth.samhsa.gov

Supplies the public with responses to their commonly asked questions about mental health issues and services.

1024 NIH/National Institute of Mental Health
6001 Executive Boulevard, Room 8184, MSC 9663
Bethesda, MD 20892

301-443-4513
866-615-6464
Fax: 301-443-4279
TTY: 301-443-8431
e-mail: nimhinfo@nih.gov
www.nimh.nih.gov

Conducts strategic planning for specific research areas as well as for the Institute as a whole.

Dr Thomas R Insel, Director

National Associations & Support Groups

1025 Bipolar Disorders Treatment Information Center
Madison Institute of Medicine
7617 Mineral Point Road
Madison, WI 53717

608-827-2470
Fax: 608-827-2479
e-mail: mim@miminc.org
www.miminc.org

Provides information on mood stabilizers other than lithium for bipolar disorder. With more than 4,000 references on file, the Center collects and disseminates information about all medications and other forms of treatment of bipolar disorder, including divalproex sodium (valproate), carbamazepine, lamotrigine, gabapentin and topiramate.

Margaret Baudhuin, Coordinator

1026 Depression and Bipolar Support Alliance
730 N Franklin Street, Suite 501
Chicago, IL 60610

312-642-0049
800-826-3632
Fax: 312-642-7243
www.dbsalliance.org

Patient-directed organization focusing on the most prevelant mental illnesses- depression and bipolar disorder. Fosters an understanding about the impact and management of these life-threatning illnesses by providing up-to-date, scientifically-based tools and information written in language the general public can understand.

Susan Bergeson, President

1027 Federation of Families for Children's Mental Health
9605 Medical Center Drive, Suite 280
Rockville, MD 20850

240-403-1901
Fax: 240-403-1909
e-mail: ffcmh@ffcmh.org
www.ffcmh.org

The National family run organization is dedicated exclusively to helping children with mental health needs and their families achieve a better quality of life.

Sandra Spencer, Executive Director

1028 National Alliance for the Mentally Ill
2107 Wilson Blvd, Ste 300, Colonial Place Three
Arlington, VA 22201

703-524-7600
800-950-6264
Fax: 703-524-9094
TDD: 703-516-7227
e-mail: info@nami.org
www.nami.org

NAMI is a nonprofit, grassroots, self-help, support and advocacy organization of consumers, families and friends of people with severe mental illness, such as schizophrenia, bipolar disorder, major despressive disorder, obsessive compulsive disorder, anxiety disorders, autism and other severe and persistent mental illnesses that affect the brain.

Suzanne Vogel-Scibilia MD, President

1029 National Mental Health Association
2000 N Beauregard Street, 6th Floor
Alexandria, VA 22311

703-684-7722
800-969-6642
Fax: 703-684-5968
TTY: 800-433-5959
www.nmha.org

Addresses all aspects of mental health and mental illness. NMHA with over 340 affiliates works to improve the mental health of all Americans.

David L Shern PhD, President & CEO

State Agencies & Support Groups

1030 Center for Family Support
333 7th Avenue, 9th Floor
New York, NY 10001

212-629-7939
Fax: 212-239-2211
www.cfsny.org

The Center for Family (CFS) is a not-for-profit human service agency providing support and assistance to individuals with developmental disabilities and traumatic brain injuries throughout New York City, Long Island, the lower Hudson Valley region and New Jersey.

Steven Vernickofs, Executive Director

1031 Depressive and Manic-Depressive Assocation of Mount Sinai
100 LaSalle Street, Suite 5A
New York, NY 10027

917-445-2399
e-mail: jgg17@columbia.edu
www.columbia.edu/~jgg17/DMDA/PAGE_1.html

The NYC Depressive and Manic-Depressive Group is a support group for persons with mood disorders, depression and bipolar disorder, as well as their family members and friends.

Research Centers

1032 Information Centers for Bipolar Disorders
Madison Institute of Medicine
7617 Mineral Point Road, Suite 300
Madison, WI 53717

608-827-2470
Fax: 608-827-2479
e-mail: mim@miminc.org
www.miminc.org

The center provides information on mood stabilizers other than Lithium for bipolar disorder. With more than 4,000 references already on file, the Center collects and disseminates information about all medications and other forms of treatment of bipolar disorder, including divalprolex sodium (valproate), carbmazepine, lamotrigine, and topiramate.

Margaret Baudhuin, MLS, Coordinator

1033 National Alliance for Research on Schizophrenia and Depression
60 Cutter Mill Road, Suite 404
Great Neck, NY 11021

516-829-0091
800-829-8289
Fax: 516-487-6930
e-mail: info@narsad.org
www.narsad.org

NARSAD raises and distributes funds for scientific research into the causes, cures, treatments, and prevention of severe mental illnesses, primarily schizophrenia.

Stephen G Doochin, Executive Director

Audio Video

1034 Families Coping with Mental Illness
Mental Illness Education Project
PO Box 470813
Brookline Village, MA 02247
USA

617-562-1111
800-343-5540
Fax: 617-779-0061
e-mail: info@miepvideos.org
miepvideos.org

Ten family members share their experiences of having a family member with schizophrenia or bipolar disorder. Designed to provide insights and support to other families, the tape also profoundly conveys to professionals the needs of families when mental illness strikes. In two versions: a 22-minute version ideal for short classes and workshops, and a richer 43-minute version with more examples and details. Discounted price for families/consumers.

Video

Michael M Faenza, Executive Director

Web Sites

1035 Bipolar Disorders Information Center
www.mhsource.com

We specialize in providing high-quality information and continuing medical education opportunities for primary care physicians, psychiatrists, neurologists, nurses, pharmacists and other healthcare progessionals.

1036 Bipolar Kids Homepage
www.geocities.com/EnchantedForest/1068

This page has been developed to educate and support parents, guardians, doctors, teachers, and those who live with childhood bipolar in their lives.

1037 Bipolar World
www.bipolarworld.net

A support and educational web site for individuals diagnosed with Bipolar Affective Disorder and for the families and friends who care for them.

1038 CyberPsych
www.cyberpsych.org

CyberPsych presents information about psychoanalysis, psychotherapy, and special topics such as anxiety disorder, the problematic use of alcohol, homophobia, and the traumatic effects of racism. CyberPsych is a nonprofit network which offers free web hosting and technical support for internet communication to nonprofit groups and individuals.

1039 Internet Mental Health
www.mentalhealth.com

Our goal is to improve understanding, diagnosis, and teatment of mental illness throughout the world.

1040 Mental Health Net
www.mentalhelp.net

We wish to provide the following: to discuss, develop and debate in an open forum the future of the mental health field in America and throughout the world. To help coordinate various components of the mental health field so as to bring about greater communication between them.

1041 Planetpsych
www.planetpsych.com

Online resource for mental health information.

Book Publishers

1042 Bipolar Disorders: A Guide to Helping Children & Adolescents
O'Reilly and Associates
1005 Gravenstein Highway N
Sebastopol, CA 95472

707-827-7000
800-998-9938
Fax: 707-829-0104
e-mail: patientguides@oreilly.com
www.patientcenters.com

A million children and adolescents in the US may have childhood-onset bipolar disorder, including an estimated 23 percent of those currently diagnosed with ADHD. Bipolar Disorders helps parents and professionals recognize, treat, and cope with bipolar disorders in children and adolescents. It covers diagnosis, family life, medications, talk therapies, other interventions (improving sleep patterns, diet, preventing seasonal mood swings), insurance and school.

1999 460 pages
ISBN: 1-565926-56-0

1043 Bipolar Disorders: Clinical Course and Outcome
American Psychiatric Press
1000 Wilson Boulevard, Suite 1825
Arlington, VA 22209

703-907-7322
800-368-5777
Fax: 703-907-1091
e-mail: appi@psych.org
www.appi.org

This book relates empirical data on outcome with practical information on the prognosis, course and potential complications of bipolar disorders in the modern era.

1999 344 pages

1044 Bipolar Puzzle Solutions
Taylor & Francis
325 Chestnut Street, Suite 800
Philadelphia, PA 19106

800-821-8312
Fax: 215-625-8914
e-mail: corey.gray@taylorandfrancis.com
www.taylorandfrancis.com

187 answers to questions asked by support group members about living with manic depressive illness.

ISBN: 1-560324-93-7

1045 Covert Modeling and Reinforcement

New Harbinger Publications
5674 Shattuck Avenue
Oakland, CA 94609

510-652-0215
800-748-6273
Fax: 510-652-5472
e-mail: customreservice@newharbinger.com
www.newharbinger.com

Audio programs based on our essential book of cognitive behavioral techniques for effecting change in your life, Thoughts & Feelings. Listeners learn step-by-step protocols for controlling destructive behaviors such anxiety, obessional thinking, uncontrolled anger, and depression.

ISBN: 0-934986-29-0

1046 Guideline for Treatment of Patients with Bipolar Disorder

American Psychiatric Press
1000 Wilson Boulevard, Suite 1825
Arlington, VA 22209

703-907-7322
800-368-5777
Fax: 703-907-1091
e-mail: appi@psych.org
www.appi.org

Provides guidance to psychiatrists who treat patients with bipolar I disorder. Summarizes the pharmacologic, somatic and psychotherapeutic treatments used for patients.

74 pages Softcover
ISBN: 0-890423-02-4

1047 Management of Bipolar Disorder -Pocketbook

Martin Dunitz Ltd, Taylor & Francis Group
325 Chestnut Street, Suite 800
Philadelphia, PA 19106

800-354-1420
Fax: 215-625-8914
www.dunitz.co

Contains the need for treatment, what defines bipolar disorders, spectrum of the disorder, getting the best out of the treatment of mania and bipolar depression, preventing new episodes, special problems in treatment, mood stabilizers, and case studies.

96 pages
ISBN: 1-833172-74-X

1048 Manic Depressive Illness

National Alliance for the Mentally Ill
200 N Glebe Road, Suite 1015
Arlington, VA 22203
USA

703-524-7600
800-950-6264
Fax: 703-524-9094
TDD: 703-516-7227
www.nami.org

A definitive overview of bipolar disorder.

1049 Touched with Fire-Manic Depressive Illness & the Artistic Temperament

Free Press
866 3rd Avenue
New York, NY 10022
USA

212-832-2101
800-323-7445
Fax: 800-943-9831
www.simonsays.com

Describing and discussing the markedly increased rates of severe mood disorders and suicides among the artistically creative and the reasons why.

384 pages
ISBN: 0-684831-83-X

Newsletters

1050 Outreach

Depression and Bipolar Support Alliance
730 N Franklin Street, Suite 501
Chicago, IL 60610

800-826-3632
Fax: 312-642-7243
www.dbsalliance.org

Quarterly publication serving members and constituents of the organization. National DMDA educates patients, families, professionals, and the public concerning the nature of depressive and manic-depressive illnesses as treatable medical diseases; fosters self-help for patients and families; eliminates discrimination and stigma; improves access to care; advocates for research toward the elimination of these illnesses.

Lydia Lewis, Executive Director
Gloria Pope, External Relations Director

Pamphlets

1051 Bipolar Disorder

National Institutes of Health
5600 Fishers Lane, Room 7C-02
Rockville, MD 20857

301-443-3706
Fax: 301-443-6349
www.nih.gov

A short booklet offering a concise description of this disorder, which is also called manic-depressive illness.

1052 Child and Adolescent Bipolar Disorder

Child and Adolescent Bipolar Foundation
1000 Skokie Blvd, Suite 570
Wilmette, IL 60091

847-256-8525
Fax: 847-920-9498
e-mail: CABF@bpkids.org
www.bpkids.org

To educate families, professsionals and the public about early onset bipolar disorder.

1053 Mood Disorders

Center for Mental Health Services
PO Box 42557
Washington, DC 20015

800-789-2647
Fax: 240-747-5470
TDD: 866-889-2647
e-mail: nmhic-info@samhsa.hhs.gov
http://mentalhealth.samhsa.gov

This fact sheet provides basic information on the symptoms, formal diagnosis, and treatment for bipolar disorder.

3 pages

DESCRIPTION

1054 BRAIN TUMORS

Involves the following Biologic System(s):

Neurologic Disorders

Brain tumors are abnormal growths in or on the brain that may be cancerous (malignant) or noncancerous (benign). In addition, these growths may be classified as primary tumors that arise directly from brain tissue or as secondary tumors, which are almost always malignant and have spread or metastasized to the brain from other parts of the body. Space-occupying benign tumors may also present complications resulting from increasing intracranial pressure. Symptoms and characteristic findings associated with brain tumors depend upon their location as well as their size and rate of growth. However, many symptoms are common to most types of brain tumors and may include recurrent or constant headache, irregularities of vision, difficulties in balance and the coordination of voluntary movements, muscle weakness, speech difficulties, and sometimes seizures. Nausea, vomiting, fever, and fluctuations in pulse rate, breathing rate, and blood pressure may be later and more foreboding manifestations. Although there are many different types of brain tumors, children are most commonly affected by primary tumors, especially those that develop toward the back of the brain (posterior fossa tumor).

The most common of the posterior fossa tumors in children is the cerebellar astrocytoma. This type of tumor may be fluid-filled (cystic) or relatively solid and may often have a low grade of malignancy. However, cerebellar astrocytomas may sometimes invade the fibers on each side of the cerebellum that connect with other areas of the brain as well as the spinal cord (cerebellar peduncles). Symptoms and findings may include an abnormal accumulation of cerebrospinal fluid, often under increased pressure, within the skull (hydrocephalus) that is characterized by an increase in head size in infants as well as irritability, vomiting, lethargy, irregular reflex action, and leg rigidity followed by drowsiness and seizures. Older children may have a headache and may vomit, lose coordination, and exhibit deteriorating mental capabilities. Effective treatment for low-grade cerebellar astrocytoma includes surgical removal. Radiation treatment may be indicated for children with cerebellar astrocytoma of high-grade malignancy or in children who exhibit evidence of tumor growth after surgery.

Medulloblastoma is the second most common of the posterior fossa tumors in children and, in children younger than seven years of age, is the most common brain tumor. This type of malignant tumor usually grows relatively fast and spreads to other parts of the brain, the spinal cord, and sometimes other areas of the body. Symptoms associated with medulloblastoma may include headache, recurrent vomiting, and frequent falling. Diagnosis is achieved through imaging studies such as magnetic resonance imaging (MRI) or computer tomography (CT scan) which give a detailed picture of the size and extent of the tumor. Treatment may include surgical excision. In addition, children older than four years of age may receive radiation therapy, especially if the tumor is small and has not yet spread. Children who have evidence of some remaining tumor growth after surgery and those whose tumor has spread may benefit from chemotherapy in addition to further surgery and radiation therapy. Due to the possibility of adverse effects on the brain, radiation is delayed in very young children with medulloblastoma.

Craniopharyngioma is a tumor that appears most often in children and adolescents, and arises from the pituitary, an endocrine gland that is located at the base of the skull. This type of tumor may sometimes interfere with pituitary gland and other endocrine functions as well as cause compression resulting in hydrocephalus and its associated symptoms. Other findings may include headache, vomiting, irregularities in vision, and short stature resulting from hormonal irregularities. Treatment for craniopharyngioma includes surgical excision. Additional treatment with radiation may be indicated for those children whose tumor is not able to be completely removed through surgery or who experience a recurrence. Subsequent to surgery, some children may develop such hormonal abnormalities as an underactive thyroid (hypothyroidism), growth hormone deficiency, diabetes insipidus, and other problems. Evaluation for these hormonal disorders is indicated and treatment is dependent upon the particular abnormality.

See also **General Resources** on page 917

Government Agencies

1055 NIH/National Cancer Institute

6116 Executive Boulevard, Room 3036A
Bethesda, MD 20892

800-422-6237
www.cancer.gov

The National Cancer Institute coordinates the National Cancer Program, which conducts and supports research, training, health information dissemination, and other programs with respect to the cause, diagnosis, prevention, and treatment of cancer, rehabilitation from cancer, and the continuing care of cancer patients and the families of cancer patients.

John E Niederhuber MD, Director

1056 NIH/National Institute of Neurological Dis orders and Stroke (NINDS)
PO Box 5801
Bethesda, MD 20824

301-496-5751
800-352-9424
Fax: 301-496-0296
TTY: 301-468-5981
www.ninds.nih.gov

Works to reduce the burden of neurological disease by conducting, fostering, coordinating and guiding research on the causes, prevention, diagnosis and treatment of neurological disorders and stroke, while supporting basic research in related scientific areas.

Story C Landis Ph.D., Director
Audrey S Penn M.D., Deputy Director

National Associations & Support Groups

1057 American Brain Tumor Association
2720 River Road
Des Plaines, IL 60018

847-827-9910
800-886-2282
Fax: 847-827-9918
e-mail: info@abta.org
www.abta.org

Services include over 20 publications which address brain tumors, their treatment, and coping with the disease. Materials address brain tumors in all age groups. Provides free social service consultations; a mentorship program for new brain tumor support group leaders; a nationwide database of established support groups; the Connections pen-pal program; networking with organizations that provide services to patients and families; a resource listing of physicians offering investgative treatments.

John Hipchen, President
Naomi L Berkowitz, Executive Director

1058 American Brain Tumor Association Patient Line
2720 River Road
Des Plaines, IL 60018

847-827-9910
800-886-2282
Fax: 847-827-9918
e-mail: info@abta.org
www.abta.org

Offers emergency support, information and referrals for patients and their families.

1059 American Cancer Society
Brain Tumor Support Group
ACS Building, 8900 Carpenter Freeway
Dallas, TX 75247

214-819-1200
800-227-2345
Fax: 214-631-3869
www.cancer.org

Attacks the support aspect of this disease from every angle including data on lowering risks to dealing with grief.

Maria Clarke, Executive Director

1060 Brain Tumor Foundation - National
National Brain Tumor Foundation
22 Battery Street, Suite 612
San Francisco, CA 94111

415-834-9970
800-934-2873
Fax: 415-834-9980
e-mail: nbtf@braintumor.org
www.braintumor.org

Nonprofit organization that was founded in 1981 by a group of brain tumor patients, their families and friends. NBTF has two major goals: raising funds for research to treat and cure brain tumors and providing information, education and support to patients, family members and friends. We offer a patient support line, support groups, a newsletter, national and regional conferences, a medical advice nurse, fact sheets and other printed information and special patient and caregiver programs.

Rob Tufel, MSW MPH, Executive Director
Nancy Gaggioli-Medeiros, Deputy Director

1061 Brain Tumor Foundation for Children
6065 Roswell Road NE, Suite 505
Atlanta, GA 30328

404-252-4107
Fax: 404-252-4108
www.braintumorkids.org

The BFTC provides information and emotional support for families of children with brain tumors. They also raise funds for brain tumor research and provide a telephone network system of parents who offer emotional support.

Mary Campbell, Executive Director

1062 Brain Tumor Society
124 Watertown Street, Suite 3H
Watertown, MA 02472

617-924-9997
800-770-8287
Fax: 617-924-9998
e-mail: info@tbts.org
www.tbts.org

The Brain Tumor Society exists to find a cure for brain tumors. It strives to improve the quality of life of brain tumor patients and their families. It disseminates educational information and provides access to psychosocial support. It raises funds to advance carefully selected scientific research projects, improve clinical care and find a cure.

Neal P Levitan Esq, Executive Director

1063 CancerCare
275 7th Avenue
New York, NY 10001

212-712-8400
800-813-4673
Fax: 212-712-8495
e-mail: info@cancercare.org
www.cancercare.org

Dedicated to providing emotional support, information, and practical help to people with cancer and their loved ones. CancerCare is the oldest, largest, nonprofit agency devoted to offering professional services.

Diane S Blum, ACSW, Executive Director
Paul Friedman, Board President

1064 Candlelighters Childhood Cancer Foundation
PO Box 498
Kensington, MD 20895

301-962-3520
800-366-2223
Fax: 310-962-3521
e-mail: staff@candlelighters.org
www.candlelighters.org

The Candlelighters Childhood Cancer Foundation National Office was founded in 1970 by concerned parents of children with cancer. Today our membership of over 50,000 members of the national office and more than 100,000 members across the across the country, including Candlelighters affiliate groups, includes, parents of children who are being treated or have been treated for cancer.

Ruth Hoffman, Executive Director

1065 Childhood Brain Tumor Foundation
20312 Watkins Meadow Drive
Germantown, MD 20876

301-515-2900
877-217-4166
Fax: 301-540-8367
e-mail: cbtf@childhoodbraintumor.org
www.childhoodbraintumor.org

A major service this organization provides is the Childhood Cancer Ombudsman Program, a free service consisting of volunteers trained in the disiplines of medicine, law, and education who provide assistance in : 1) seeking second opinions, 2) access to healthcare, and 3) combating discrimination. The foundation also funds research, has a hotline and publishes a newsletter three times a year.

Jeanne Young, President

1066 Children's Brain Tumor Foundation
274 Madison Avenue, Suite 1004
New York, NY 10016

212-448-9494
866-228-4673
Fax: 212-448-1022
e-mail: info@cbtf.org
www.cbtf.org

CBTF is a nonprofit organization, founded in 1988 by dedicated parents, physicians and friends. Our mission is to improve the treatment, quality of life and the long term outlook for children with brain and spinal cord tumors through research, support, education and advocacy to families and survivors.

Judy Hurley, Executive Director

1067 Heads Up Brain Tumor Support Group
Dominican Hospital
1555 Soquel Drive
Santa Cruz, CA 95065

831-462-7700

1068 Healing Exchange Brain Trust
186 Hampshire Street
Cambridge, MA 02139

617-876-2002
Fax: 617-876-2332
e-mail: info@braintrust.org
www.braintrust.org

Shares information and support about brain tumor and related conditions.

Samantha J Scolamiero, President & Founding Director

1069 National Brain Research Association
1439 Rhode Island Avenue NW
Washington, DC 20005

202-483-6272

Also provides support groups for parents.

1070 National Brain Tumor Foundation
22 Battery Street, Suite 612
San Francisco, CA 94111

415-834-9970
800-934-2873
e-mail: nbtf@braintumor.org
www.braintumor.org

NBTF is a national nonprofit health organization dedicated to providing information and support for brain tumor patients, family members, and healthcare professionals, while supporting innovative research into better treatment options and a cure for brain tumors.

Rob Tufel, MSW MPH, Executive Director

1071 National Childhood Cancer Foundation
4600 East West Highway, Suite 600
Bethesda, MD 20814

800-458-6223
e-mail: info@curesearch.org
www.curesearch.org

CureSearch unites the world's largest childhood cancer research organization, the Children's Oncology Group, and the National Childhood Cancer Foundation through our mission to cure childhood cancer. Research is the key to the cure.

1072 Preuss Foundation
2223 Avenida de la Playa, Suite 220
La Jolla, CA 92037

619-454-0200
Fax: 619-454-4449

Foundation that provides information on support groups, brochures and pamphlets.

Peter Preuss, President

State Agencies & Support Groups

Alabama

1073 Pediatric Brain Tumor Support Group
Children's Hospital
1600 7th Avenue S
Birmingham, AL 35233

205-939-9090
Fax: 205-939-9010

Groups for parents and siblings of brain tumor patients. Related to Children's Hospital of Alabama. Babysitting available.

Paul Byrd

Arizona

1074 Brain Tumor Support Group at NovaCare Rehabilitation Institute of Tucson
2650 N Wyatt Drive
Tucson, AZ 85726

520-293-8040

Scott Gulbrandsen

1075 Brain Tumor Support Group at Phoenix
Saint Joseph's Hospital and Medical Center
350 W Thomas Road
Phoenix, AZ 85026

602-873-2757

Steve Westerhoff

California

1076 Brain Tumor Patient & Family Support Group
Saint Jude Medical Center
2151 N Harbor Blvd, St Jude Medical Plaza, Rm 2266
Fullerton, CA 92635

714-446-7182
www.stjudemedicalcenter.org

Periodic guest presentations.

Robert Merlino

1077 Brain Tumor Support Group at Newport Beach
Hoag Cancer Center Auditorium
4000 Pacific Coast Highway
Newport Beach, CA 92658

949-760-5542

Speakers once a month, education materials available.

Kris O'Neal

1078 Brain Tumor Support Group at San Diego
UC San Diego Complex
132 Dickinson Street, Camelot Room
San Diego, CA 92199

619-543-5540

Donna Gilpatrick RN, MS, FNP

1079 Brain Tumor Support Group at San Luis Obispo
1911 Johnson Avenue
San Luis Obispo, CA 93401

805-461-3989

Becky Nunez

1080 Brain Tumor Support Group at Santa Monica
Wellness Community
2200 Colorado Boulevard
Santa Monica, CA 90406

310-453-2200

Michael Slater, Program Director

1081 Brain Tumor Support Program Cedars-Sinai Neurosurgical Inst. & Wellness Community
8631 W 3rd Street, Suite 800 E
Los Angeles, CA 90048

310-855-7900
Fax: 310-423-0777

Last Wednesday of month 6-7:30 pm with an RSVP.

Jennice Vilhauer, Contact

1082 Fresno Brain Tumor Support Group
1303 E Herndon
Fresno, CA 93720

559-449-3452
Fax: 559-449-3990

Paula Jordan

1083 Inland Empire Brain Tumor Support Group
Medical Annex Building
Kaiser, Fontana Neurosurgery Waiting Room
Fontana, CA 92324

909-877-4923

First Tuesday of month at 6:30pm.

Sue Melton, Contact

1084 Neuroscience Institute Brain Tumor Support Group
Hospital of the Good Samaritan
637 S Lucas Avenue, Suite 501
Los Angeles, CA 90052

213-977-2234
800-762-1692

Claudia Perdices, MSW

1085 Northridge Hospital: Leavey Cancer Center
18300 Roscoe Boulevard
Northridge, CA 91328

818-885-8500

David Antelman

1086 Palo Alto Brain Tumor Support Group
Palo Alto Medical Foundation Bldg, Urgent Care Ctr
920 Bryant Street, 2nd Floor Room B
Palo Alto, CA 94303

415-284-0208

Joanie Taylor, RN

1087 Peninsula Support & Education Group for Parents of Children with Brain Tumors
Parents Helping Parents
3041 Olcott
Santa Clara, CA

650-325-4523

Sheri Sobrato, MA, MFC

1088 Sacramento Area Brain Tumor Support Group
Lawrence J Ellison Ambulatory Care Ctr
UC Davis Medical Center, Camellia Cottage
4860 Y Street Room 3015
Sacramento, CA 95813

916-734-5613

First Thursday of month 6:30-8:30 pm.

Karen Smith RN

1089 San Francisco Brain Tumor Support Group
UC San Francisco, Clinical Sciences Building
521 Parnassus Avenue, Room C130
San Francisco, CA 94188

415-284-0208

Contact is National Brain Tumor Foundation. Holiday potluck with other Bay Area support groups, lending library (books audio and visual tapes). First Wednesday of each month 7:00-8:30 pm. Call to Confirm.

Sharon Lamb RN, Contact

1090 Santa Barbara Brain Tumor Support Group
Cancer Foundation of Santa Barbara
300 W Pueblo Conference Room
Santa Barbara, CA 93102

805-682-7300

Second Thursday of each month, 5:30-7:00 pm.

Cathie Nelson MSW, Contact

1091 Santa Cruz County Brain Tumor Support Group
3031 Main Street
Soquel, CA 95073

831-438-8344

Gregory Valki-Tarsy

1092 Santa Rosa Brain Tumor Support Group
North Coast Rehab Hospital Fulton Campus Conf Room
1287 Fulton
Santa Rosa, CA 95402

415-353-2966

Last Wednesday of each month, 6:30-8:00 pm.

Jane Rabbitt RN, Contact

1093 South Bay Brain Tumor Support Group
667 Chapman Street
San Jose, CA 95101

650-725-8630

Genny See-Tho RN

1094 Southern California Pediatric Brain Tumor Network
UCLA Medical Center
10833 LeConte Avenue, Suite 501
Los Angeles, CA

818-362-3428

For parents of children with brain tumors, and for teenagers with brain tumors.

Kathy Riley

1095 Support Group for Caregivers of Brain Tumor Patients
UCLA Medical Center
UCLA Medical Plaza Building
Los Angeles, CA 90052

310-206-6731

Guest speakers on occasion.

Pamela Hoff, LCSW

1096 Support Group for Parents of Children with Brain Tumors
Oakland Children's Hospital
747 52nd Street, Auditorium Sd II
Oakland, CA 94623

510-428-3885

Contact can be reached at extension 2161.

Trish Murphy

1097 Vital Options
4419 Coldwater Canyon
Studio City, CA 91604

818-508-5657

Support group for young adult cancer patients.

1098 Wellness Community San Francisco/East Bay
3276 McNutt Avenue
Walnut Creek, CA 94596

925-933-0107

Many general support groups, workshops, classes, etc. offered.
Calendar available.

Erika Maslan MFCC

1099 West Los Angeles Brain Tumor Support Group
2716 Ocean Park Boulvard, Suite 1040
Santa Monica, CA 90406

310-314-2555

Michael States, Program Director

Colorado

1100 Brain Tumor Patient & Family Support Group
Swedish Medical Center Conference Center
701 E Hampden Avenue #330
Englewood, CO 80113

303-806-7420
e-mail: lgibson@thecni.org

Sponsored by Colorado Neurological Institute Center for Brain and
Spinal Tumors. First Wednesday of month, 6:30-8:00 pm.

Lorre Gibson, Contact

1101 Brain Tumor Patient/Family Group
Anchutz Cancer Pavillion, University of Colorado
Fitzsimons Campus, 1635 Ursula Street
Aurora, CO 80045

303-315-6635
e-mail: amy.ebert@uchsc.edu

First Wednesday of each month, 5:00-7:00 pm. call to confirm location.

Amy Ebert, Contact

1102 Brain Tumor Support Group
Poudre Valley Hospital
1024 S Lemay, Neuroscience Floor
Ft. Collins, CO 80521

970-495-8320
e-mail: ryjj@aol.com

Second Thursday of each month at 5:00 pm. Call to confirm location.

Georgie Knaub, Contact

Connecticut

1103 Brain Tumor Support Group
Cancer Program
80 Seymour Street
Hartford, CT 06102

860-545-5000
860-545-2318
Fax: 860-545-5066

First Thursday of each month, 5:30-7:00 pm. Call in advance to
RSVP.

Hillary Keller, Contact

1104 Connecticut Brain Tumor Support Group (Adult)
Yale New Haven Hospital, Children's Hospital
20 York Street, Room 201
New Haven, CT 06050

203-688-7528

Second Tuesday of each month, 2:00-3:30 pm (please call to confirm date and time).

Betsy D'Andrea, Contact
Angela Thomas MSW, Contact

Delaware

1105 Pediatric Brain Tumor Support Group
Ronald McDonald House
1901 Rockland Road
Wilmington, DE

302-995-0938

Cathy Francisco

District of Columbia

1106 Washington DC Metropolitan Area Support Group
George Washington University
2121 Eye Street, NW
Washington, DC 20052

202-994-1000

Florida

1107 Angels in the Sun Brain Tumor Support Group
Health South Rehabilitative Hospital
3251 Proctor Road
Sarasota, FL 34230

941-364-9105

Anna Browder

1108 Brain Tumor Support Group
American Cancer Society
1703 W Colonial Drive
Orlando, FL 32862

407-740-0007

David Cox, MD

1109 Brain Tumor Support Group at Miami
Miami Children's Hospital Foundation
3000 SW 62nd Avenue, Founders Lounge
Miami, FL 33152

305-662-8386

Call to confirm time and date.

Maria Penate RN, Contact

1110 Brain Tumor Support Group at St. Petersburg
Saint Anthony's Hospital
Saint Petersburg, FL 33730

813-825-1100

Contact can be reached at extension 4231.

Karen McGough

1111 Brain Tumor Support Group at Tampa
Moffitt Cancer Ctr, Dept. Psychosocial Onocology
12902 Magnolia Drive
Tampa, FL 33630

813-979-7258
800-456-3434

Inez Rodriquez

1112 Cancer Support Group for Children
Memorial Hospital Children's Center
3501 Johnson Street, 4th Floor
Hollywood, FL

954-987-2000

Sub-groups for children with brain tumors and their parents. Contact at ext. 4193.

Suzanne Baxter RN

1113 South Florida Brain Tumor Association Lynn Regional Cancer Center
Boca Raton Community Hospital
800 Meadows Road, Education Center
Boca Raton, FL 33431

561-955-5658
561-955-5897

Neuropsychologist Dr. Laurence Miller and therapist Marjorie
O'Sullivan are present to facilitate the meetings. Second and
Fourth Thursdays of each month, 7:30-8:30 pm.

Debbie Yudenfriend, Contact
Laura Moon, Contact

1114 Tampa Bay Area Brain Tumor Support Group
St Joseph's Hospital, Medical Arts Building
3000 West Martin Luther King Boulevard
Tampa Bay, FL 33630

813-870-4101

Third Tuesday of each month, 6:30-7:30 pm.

Georgia

1115 All Ages Support Group
1835 Savoy Drive, Suite 316
Atlanta, GA 30341

770-458-5554
e-mail: btfc@bellsouth.net
www.braintumorkids.org

Contact for details.

Mary Campbell, Contact

1116 Brain Tumor Foundation for Children
6065 Roswell Road NE, Suite 505
Atlanta, GA 30328

404-252-4107
Fax: 404-252-4108
www.braintumorkids.org

The BFTC provides information and emotional support for families of children with brain tumors. They also raise funds for brain tumor research and provide a telephone network system of parents who offer emotional support.

Mary Campbell, Executive Director

1117 Brain Tumor Support Group
Emory Clinic, Neurosurgery Conference Room
1365 Clifton Road, Building B, 2nd Floor
Atlanta, GA 30341

404-778-4153
404-778-3091

First Thursday of each month, 12:30-2:30 pm. Please RSVP to attend.

Karen Shires, Contact
Linda Phillips, Contact

1118 Cancer Support Group
University Hospital Healthcare Systems
1350 Walton Way
Augusta, GA 30901

706-774-2843

Meets second Tuesday each month at 6:00 pm. Call to register.

1119 Southeastern Brain Tumor Foundation Brain Tumor Support Group
Wellness Community, Peachtree Dunwoody Pavillion
5775 Peachtree Dunwoody Rd, Building C, Room 225
Atlanta, GA 30342

678-584-6781
e-mail: sbtfatlanta@aol.com
www.sbtf.org

Second Monday of each month, 7:00-8:30 pm.

Amy Glover, Contact

Hawaii

1120 Brain Tumor Support Group
Saint Christopher's Episcopal Church, Choir Room
93 N Kainalu, Kailu
Oahu, HI

808-254-1989

Chuck Rogers
Kari Rogers

Idaho

1121 Treasure Valley Brain Injury Support Group
Idaho Elks Rehabilitation Hospital
600 North Robbins Road
Boise, ID 83702

208-489-4558
www.idahoelksrehab.org

Fourth Tuesday of each month 7:00-9:00 pm.

Kathy Smith, Contact
Katie McCurdy, Brain Injury Program Director

Illinois

1122 Brain Tumor Resource & Support Group
Central DuPage Hospital, Neuro-Spine Unit
25 North Winfield Road
Winfield, IL 60190

630-933-6955
e-mail: debbie_brunelle@cdh.org

Second and Fourth Wednesday of each month, 7:30-9:00 pm.

Deborah Brunelle RN, Contact

1123 Brain Tumor Support Group
Northwestern Memorial Hospital
303 E Superior
Chicago, IL 60607

312-908-8177

Mary Ellen Maher Deleon

1124 Brain Tumor Support Group at Northwestern Memorial Hospital
251 East Huron, Suite 3-520
Chicago, IL 60611

312-695-8143

Educational program offered at each meeting by members of the professional committee. Third Monday of each month, 5:00-6:00 pm.

Mary Ellen Maher Deleon, Contact

1125 Brain Tumor Support Group at Park Ridge
Lutheran General Hospital, Cancer Care Center
1700 Luther Lane, 2nd Floor Conference Room
Park Ridge, IL 60068

847-920-1356

Third Wednesday of each month, 7:30-9:00 pm.

Syril Gilbert LCSW, Contact

1126 Caregiver Brain Tumor Support Group

847-570-2043
e-mail: habramowitz@cnh.org

Fourth Wednesday of each month, 7:00-8:30 pm. Contact for location.

Helane Abramowitz MSW LCSW, Contact

1127 Parents of Children with Brain Tumors (PCBT)
Children's Memorial Hospital
2300 Children's Plaza
Chicago, IL 60614

773-880-4316

Monthly newsletter. Library available at meetings (at CMH). Educational speakers and family functions. Call to confirm meetings.

Rebecca West-Sibbett, Contact

Indiana

1128 Benign Brain Tumor Support Group
Howard Regional Health Systems
322 North Main Street
Kokomo, IN 46901

765-455-2613

Third Wednesday of each month, 5:00-6:30 pm. Meet in southeast corner of the building, enter at set of double doors on corner of North Main and Taylor Street.

Marsha Mahoney, Contact

1129 Brain Tumor Support Group
First Christian Church
205 E Kirkwood Avenue
Bloomington, IN 47408

812-332-4459
Fax: 812-332-4479

Jean Bauer

1130 Brain Tumor Support Group at Indianapolis
Community Hospital North
Regional Cancer Center
Indianapolis, IN 46256

317-485-6616
317-842-1229
e-mail: m.w.kempf@sbcglobal.net

Third Wednesday of each month, 6:3-7:30 pm. The Regional Cancer Center is in a building just to the south of the main hospital, across Clearvista Drive.

Lisa Peters RN, Contact
Michael Kempf, Contact

1131 Primary Brain Cancer Support Group
Women's Cancer Center at Lutheran Hospital
7910 W Jefferson Boulevard, Suite 112
Fort Wayne, IN 46804

260-435-7959

First Tuesday of every month, 6:00 pm.

Linda Jordan RN, Contact

Iowa

1132 Brain Tumor Support Group
University Of Iowa Hospitals
200 Hawkins Drive
Iowa City, IA 52242

319-356-3000
319-356-2301

First Tuesday of each month with exception of July, August, January. Meeting held at the Cancer Center Waiting Room from 7-8:30 pm.

Lori Gingerich, Contact
Sue May, Contact

1133 Quad Cities Brain Tumor Support Group
Genesis Medical Center
1401 W Central Park
Davenport, IA 52804

563-421-1905

Fourth Monday of each month, 6:30-8:00 pm.

Pat Christy RN, Contact

Kansas

1134 Headstrong Brain Tumor Support Group
Victory in the Valley
917 N Market
Witchita, KS 67276

316-262-7559

Second Wednesday of each month at 7pm. Call for information.

Diana Thomi, Contact

Kentucky

1135 Brain Injury Support Group
2050 Versailles Road
Lexington, KY 40504

859-254-5701

First Thursday of each month at 6:00 pm. Meeting will be held in Conference Room A or B in the Center of Learning.

Tonia Wells, Contact

Louisiana

1136 Brain Injury Support And Education Group
Touro Infirmary
1401 Foucher Street
New Orleans, LA 70115

504-897-8560

Second and fourth Wednesday and families are every Third Monday. Offers outreach programs for survivors of brain injuries as well as their family members and caregivers.

1137 Brain Injury Support Group
West Jefferson Medical Center
1101 Medical Center Boulevard
Marrero, LA 70072

504-349-1343

Second Wednesday, 2:00 pm.

1138 Brain Tumor Support Group
3939 Houma Boulevard, Doctor's Row, Suite 6
Metairie, LA 70006

504-835-5715

Third Sunday of each month, 1:30 pm, call to confirm.

Gayle Johnson, Contact

1139 Cancer Support Group
Ochsner Clinic Foundation
1516 Jefferson Highway
New Orleans, LA 70121

800-231-5257

First Thursday of each month.

1140 Tlane Cancer Center
150 S Liberty Street
New Orleans, LA 70112

504-988-6313
e-mail: tpearman@tulane.edu

Every other Wednesday, 6-8 pm.

Tim Pearman, Contact

Maine

1141 Brain Tumor Support Group
9 Spring Street
East Millinocket, ME 04430

207-746-5863

Joan Gordon

1142 Brain Tumor Support Group of Maine
Maine Medical Center
22 Bramhall Street
Portland, ME 04102

207-662-4527

Second Tuesday of each month, 7:00-9:00 pm.

Nancy Fortier LCSW, Contact

1143 Open Support Group-All Kinds of Cancer Care of Maine

800-987-3005

Wednesdays at 10:30 AM - 12 Noon. For families and patients.

Linda Murphy, Contact

Maryland

1144 Brain Tumor Networking Group

410-832-2719

Fourth Monday of each month, 7:00-8:30 pm.

Carol Sharp, Contact

1145 Johns Hopkins Brain Tumor Education Group
Weinberg Building
401 N Broadway
Baltimore, MD 21231

410-955-8371

First Wednesday of the month, 10:30-11:30 am. All are welcome at this group. Each meeting includes a speaker followed by discussion.

Ashley Varner LCSW-C, Contact

Massachusetts

1146 Brain Center Brain Tumor Support Group
Promontory Point
Mashpee, MA 02649

508-477-5300

Last Sunday of each month, 3:00 pm. Call to confirm.

Eleanor Grace, Contact
Dick Grace, Contact

1147 Brain Tumor Support Group
Dana Farber Cancer Center
Dana Building, 16th Floor, Room D-1635
Boston, MA 02155

617-632-3769
617-732-6826

First and Third Thursday of each month, 12:00-1:30 pm. Free parking is available in the Smith Garage at Dana Farber.

Nancy Olson RN, MBA, Contact
Genevieve Mason LCSW, Contact

1148 Brain Tumor Support Group at Burlington
Lahey Clinic Medical Center
41 Mall Road
Burlington, MA 01805

617-726-1061

First and Third Monday of each month, 7:00-9:00 pm. 5 Central Clinic Conference Room.

Michele Lucas MSW LICSW, Contact

1149 Brain Tumor Support Group at Worcester
University of Massachusetts Medical Center
Dept of Surgery Waiting Area, 55 Lake Avenue N
Worcester, MA 01605

508-334-3515

This group meets for 2 hours once a month and occasionally has speakers. Second Tuesday of every month, 6:00-8:00 pm.

Alexis Van Horn RN, Contact

1150 Brain Tumor Survivor Support Group
196 Main Street
Andover, MA 01810

617-543-1709
e-mail: ddemella@hotmail.com

Second Saturday of the month, 10:00 am - 12 Noon. This is a Mutual Help support group that is peer led. It is an informal opportunity to share experiences, information, resources, and challenges as we learn to LIVE with brain tumors.

Debbie DeMella, Contact

1151 Headstrong
81 Highland Avenue
Salem, MA 01970

Maryanne Ferry MSW

1152 Long Term Survivors Support Group
Brain Tumor Society
84 Seattle Street
Boston, MA 02134

617-783-0340
800-770-8287
Fax: 617-783-9715
e-mail: info@tbts.org
www.tbts.org

Our support mission is to be involved in support issues to help patients and families better deal with the catastrophic problem of a brain tumor.

Robert D Calhoun, ACSW, LICSW

1153 Neurological Support Group of St. Luke's Hospital
101 Page Street
New Bedford, MA 02741

508-997-1515

Contact can be reached at extension 2764.

Diane Robinson RN

1154 Parent Education/Support Group
Dana Farber Cancer Institute, Smith Family Room
44 Binney Street
Boston, MA

617-632-4271
617-632-4386

For parents of children with brain tumors. Call for details.

Kelly Birdsey, Contact

1155 Support Group for Brain Tumor Patients & Family
Massachusetts General Hosiptal
55 Fruit Street
Boston, MA 02114

617-726-2000

Sarah Murphy LICSW

Michigan

1156 Brain Tumor Networking Club
Gilda's Club Metropolitan Center
3517 Rochester Road
Royal Oak, MI 48073

248-577-0800

Second Monday of each month 6:00-8:00 pm.

Christin Bernat, Contact

1157 Brain Tumor Support Group
Henry Ford Hospital
6777 West Maple
West Bloomfield, MI 48322

313-916-1796

Third Saturday of each month, 10:00 am - 12 Noon. Call for location.

Sandy Remer, Contact

1158 Brain Tumor Support Group at Ann Arbor
St Joseph Mercy Hospital, Cancer Care Center
5301 E Huron River Drive
Ann Arbor, MI 48106

734-712-3658

Fourth Tuesday of each month, 7:00-8:30 pm.

Paula Nedela RN, Contact

1159 Brain Tumor Support Group at Grand Rapids
Blodgett Memorial Medical Ctr
1840 Wealthy SE
Grand Rapids, MI 49506

616-774-7449

Guest speaker each month focusing on relevant topics.

Deb Hansen RN

1160 Brain Tumor Support Group for Patients & Families: University of Michigan Med Ctr
De Jong Neuro-Oncology Library, Taubman Ctr
1500 E Medical Center Dr, Reception Area C, 1st Lv
Ann Arbor, MI 48109

734-936-7910

Third Tuesday of each month, 7:00-8:30 pm.

Michaelyn Page MS RN OCN CNS, Contact

1161 Spectrum Brain Tumor Support Group
Spectrum Health East
1840 Wealthy SE
Grand Rapids, MI 49501

616-774-7278

Second Monday of each month, 7:00-9:00 pm.

Nancy Rude, Contact

1162 West Michigan Cancer Center Support Group
Lower Level Resource Room
200 N Park Street
Kalamazoo, MI 49003

616-373-7446

First Thursday of each month, 2:30-4:00 pm. Call to confirm.

Cindy Murray MSW, Contact

Minnesota

1163 Abbott Northwestern Brain Tumor Support Group at Abbott Northwestern Hospital
913 E 26th Street
Minneapolis, MN 55407

612-863-3732

Second and Fourth Thursday of each month, 5:30-8:00 pm. Call to verify time.

Kathy Gilliland RN, Contact

1164 Brain Injury Support Group at Abbott Northwestern Hospital
Abbott Northwestern Board Room 1st Floor
913 E 26th Street
Minneapolis, MN 55407

612-863-3339
e-mail: susan.newman@allinia.com

Second Wednesday of the month, 6:30-8:00 pm. This group has speakers that address group concerns. New members always welcome.

Sue Newman, Contact

1165 Brain Tumor Support Group at Duluth
St Mary's Medical Center
407 E 3rd Street, Michiras Room
Duluth, MN 55806

218-726-4230

Third Monday of the month at 6:30 pm.

Jan Stevens RN, Contact

1166 Brain Tumor Support Group at Robbinside
North Memorial Medical Center North Ed Ctr
3300 Oakdale Avenue N
Robbinside, MN 58422

612-520-5158

Facilitated by Radiation RN, social worker, rehab staff, chaplain and physician. Third Wednesday of each month, 7:00-8:30 pm.

Judy Zak, Contact

1167 Brain Tumor Support Group at United Hospital
St Luke's Room, Conference B & C
310 N Smith Avenue, Suite 300
Saint Paul, MN 55101

651-241-8575

Second Monday each month, 7:00-8:30 pm.

Sharon Mason MA, Contact
Cathy Maiers RN, Contact

1168 Non-Malignant Brain Tumor Support Group
800 East 28th Street
Minneapolis, MN 55407

612-775-4681

Second Thursday, 7:00-8:30 pm.

Jerry , Contact

Mississippi

1169 Brain Tumor Support Group
Special Olympics Building
Madison
Jackson, MS 39205

601-957-8517

Tammy Wellington

Missouri

1170 AMOR - A Cancer Support Group for Patients & Their Families
Brain Tumor Institute of Kansas City
2316 E Meyers Boulevard, Dining Room 3
Kansas City, MO 64141

816-235-5960

Every other Wednesday, 2:00-3:00 pm.

Peggy Smith MS, RN, Contact

1171 Brain Cancer Support Group at Mid-America Cancer Center
Saint John's Regional Health Center
2055 S Fremont, Room 116, 1st Floor
Springfield, MO 65801

417-885-3324
800-432-2273
Fax: 417-888-8761

Primary and metastatic brain tumors; patients, families, and friends welcome. Second and Fourth Tuesday of each month, 2:00-3:30 pm. Light refreshments provided.

Connie Zimmerman, Contact

1172 Brain Tumor Support Group
Saint Luke's Hospital of Kansas City
44th & Wornall Road, Spencer Bldg, 2nd Floor
Kansas City, MO 64141

816-932-6220

Educational materials, telephone help line, newsletter, lectures, bereavement support group. Second Tuesday of each month, 7:00-8:30 pm.

1173 Brain Tumor Support Group of Greater St Louis
The Wellness Community of Greater St Louis
1058 Old Des Peres Road
Saint Louis, MO 63131

314-238-2000
e-mail: aeilers@wellnesscommunitystl.org

Third Thursday of each month, 6:30-8:30 pm.

Amy Eilers MSW LCSW, Program Director

1174 Pediatric Brain Tumor Support Network
Saint Louis Children's Hospital
1 Children's Place, 3rd Floor
Saint Louis, MO

314-454-6103

Occasional guest speakers. Affiliated with the Brain Tumor Support Network which produces newsletter.

Sally Koesterer, MSW, LCSW

Montana

1175 Brain Tumor Support Group
Deconess Medical Center
2800 Tenth Avenue N
Billings, MT 59101

406-657-4165

Lottie Harris RN

Nebraska

1176 Brain Tumor Support Group at the Nebraska Medical Center
981130 Nebraska Medical Center
Omaha, NE 68198

402-559-4420

Meets monthly. Call for more information. Please contact the Social Work Department at The Nebraska Medical Center for further information regarding this monthly support group.

Sue Stensland, Contact

Nevada

1177 Southern Nevada 'Grey Matters' Valley Hospital Medical Center
Medical Executive Conference Room
620 Shadow Lane
Las Vegas, NV 89106

702-204-1907

Third Tuesday of each month, 5:30-7:00 pm.

Janet Leinen RN, Contact

New Hampshire

1178 Angels of Hope
Derry Public Library
64 East Broadway
Derry, NH 03038

603-425-2822
e-mail: angelsofhope@comcast.net

Second Monday of each month, 5:30-7:00 pm. Downstairs in the Paul Collette Conference Room A.

Urszula Mansur, Contact

1179 Portsmouth Regional Home
Health and Hospice Services
333 Borthwick Avenue
Portsmouth, NH 03801

603-436-5110
888-870-6952

Pam Sollenberger BSW

New Jersey

1180 Brain Tumor Support Group
Saint Barnabas Medical Center
94 Old Short Hills Road
Livingston, NJ 07039

973-322-5859

Third Wednesday of each month, 6:30-8:00 pm.

Elaine Downs, Contact

1181 Brain Tumor Support Group at Plainfield Muhlenberg Medical Center, Neuroscience
Saint Luke's Roman Catholic Church
300 Clinton Avenue
North Plainfield, NJ 07060

732-321-7000
e-mail: info@njbt.org

First Thursday of each month, 7:00-8:30 pm.

Patty Anthony RN, Contact
Virginia Shrodo, Contact

1182 Brain Tumor Support Group of Monmouth County
Hazlet Township Library
251 Middle Road
Hazlet, NJ 07730

732-739-2657

Darren Eagan

New Mexico

1183 NM Alliance for the Neurologically Impaired
531 Harkle Road, Suite B
Santa Fe, NM 87501

505-992-3126
505-670-0274

traumatic brain injury program but no support group.

Terry Lucero, Contact

1184 People Living Through Cancer
3939 San Pedro NE, Building C-8
Albuquerque, NM 87110

888-441-4439

Many groups; also peer counseling. Call for more information.

New York

1185 Brain Tumor Support Group
Albany Medical Center
47 New Scotland Avenue, D Building, Room D105
Albany, NY 12212

518-262-6696

First Monday of the month, 5:30-7:30 pm.

Susan Weaver MD, Contact

1186 Brain Tumor Support Group at South Nassau Community Hospital
One Healthy Way

Oceanside, NY 11752

516-632-3310
e-mail: maddybrisman@aol.com

Third Wednesday of each month at 7:00 pm. We have just started this support group. We welcome patients, family members, and friends to join us and share feelings, concerns, and wuestions about brain tumors and treatments available.

Maddy Singer CSW, Contact
Kathy Garizio RN, Contact

1187 Goodays Brain Tumor Support Group
Holiday Inn - Henrietta 111 Jefferson Road
Courtyrd Marriott, 33 Corp
Rochester, NY

716-334-4502

For parents/children or caregivers of individuals with brain tumor/spinal cord tumors.

Sue Allen

1188 Long Island Adult Brain Tumor Support Group
Plainview-Old Bethpage Public Library
999 Old Country Road
Plainview, NY 11803

516-747-8749

First Thursday of the month, 7:00-9:00 pm, but call for information.

Billie Wilczek, Contact

1189 Long Island Brain Tumor Support Group
Emma Clark Library
120 Main Street
Setauket, NY 11733

516-747-8749

Billie Wilczek

1190 Making Headway Foundation-Family Support Program
115 King Street
Chappaqua, NY 10514

914-238-8384
Fax: 914-238-1693
www.makingheadway.org

Call for scheduling. Dedicated to the Care, Comfort and Cure of Children with Brain and Spinal Cord Tumors. The program offers free, short-term individual counseling, educational remediational services and ongoing support groups.

1191 New York Brain Tumor Support Group
525 East 68th Street, Room 5-106
New York, NY 10021

212-746-3986
e-mail: wem9011@nyp.org

First Wednesdady of the month, 6:00 pm. Open to patients with brain tumors of any kind and their families, caregivers, and friends.

Wendy Mitchell LMSW, Contact

1192 People Treated for Brain Tumors and Their Caregivers
Memorial Sloan-Kettering Cancer Center
Rockefeller Research Lab, 430 East 67th Street
New York, NY 10021

212-717-3527

Fourth Wednesday of each month, 6:00-7:30 pm.

Clarissa Potter, Contact

1193 People Treated for Brain Tumors and their Caregivers
Memorial Sloan-Kettering Cancer Center
215 E 68th Street, Ground Floor
Manhattan, NY

212-717-3527

The Post-Treatment Resource Program (PTRP) offers support groups, lectures, and open house meetings. Newsletter, lending library, and special counseling also available.

Melinda Friedrich CSW

1194 Support for Parents of Children with Brain Tumors, Siblings and Young Adults
19 E 88 Street, Suite 1D
New York, NY 10128

212-534-8877

Call for specific times.

Marcia Greenleaf MD, Contact

1195 WNY Brain Tumor Support Group
3980 Sheriddan Drive
Amherst, NY 14226

716-824-1761
e-mail: cjh99@adelphia.net

Third Tuesday of the month, 6:30 pm. This group has been in existence since 2000(We also facilitate the Orchard Park, NY group). We have at least 3 speakers a year, usually doctors, and we focus on positive ways to sope with living with a brain tumor or caring for a loved one with a brain tumor.

Cheri Hodgson, Contact

North Carolina

1196 Brain Tumor Support Group of the Carolinas and Virginia Cancer Services
Wake Forest University-Baptist Medical Center
3175 Maplewood Avenue
Winston-Salem, NC 27157

336-716-4137
www.wfubmc.edu

Second Tuesday of each month, 6:30-8:00 pm.

Rayetta Johnson RN, MSN, Contact

1197 Duke Brain Tumor Support Group
Duke University Medical Center
3000 Erwin Road
Durham, NC 27710

919-681-1687
e-mail: calho006@mc.duke.edu

First Wednesday of the month, 3:00-4:00 pm.

Roberta Calhoun-Eagan LCSW, Clinical Social Worker

1198 Duke Pediatric Brain Tumor Family Support Program
Duke University Medical Center
Durham, NC 27710

919-684-2913

First and Third Tuesday, Second and Fourth Thursday, 12:00-1:00 pm. Teen group meets on the 1st Thursday of the month from 5:00-6:30 pm.

Jean Hartford-Todd, Contact

1199 Raleigh Area Brain Tumor Support Group
Raleigh Community Hospital
3400 Wake Forest Road
Raleigh, NC 27626

919-876-1856

Lectures, educational materials, newsletter. Home and hospital visitation.

Barbara Brookshire

1200 Western North Carolina Brain Tumor Support Group
West Asheville Presbyterian Church
690 Haywood Road
Asheville, NC 28806

828-253-0726
e-mail: wncbt@cs.com

Third Thursday of each month, 6:15-8:00 pm. We will have guest speakers occasionally. This group os for adults and their caregivers/family. Please call for location and details. Refreshments provided.

George Plym, Contact

Ohio

1201 Brain Tumor Support Group
Cleveland Clinic Foundation
9500 Euclid Avenue, Conference Room R3-003
Cleveland, OH 44101

216-445-6910
800-223-2273
Fax: 216-444-9170

Fourth Wednesday of each month, 5:00-6:30 pm.

Kathy Lupica RN, MSN, Contact

1202 Central Ohio Brain Tumor Support Group
Arthur James Cancer Hospital & Research Institute
300 W 10th Avenue, Room 518
Columbus, OH 43216

614-293-3440

Call for times.

Diana Blue MSW

1203 Cleveland Brain Tumor Patient Network - Adult and Pediatric
Univ Hospitals of Cleveland, Neurosurgery Conf Rm
2065 Abington, Lakeside Room, 5218
Cleveland, OH 44101

216-932-8510
e-mail: info@clevelandclinic.org
www.clevlandclinic.org

This group does not currently meet, but does offer support through networking. Please call and leave a message.

Lynn Szakacs, Contact

1204 Neuro-Oncology Support Group
Wellness Community of Greater Cincinnati
8044 Montgomery Road, Suite 385
Cincinnati, OH 45214
513-791-4060

Don Smith
Sherry Wethers

1205 Southwest Ohio Brain Tumor Support Group
Kettering Hospital
3535 Southern Boulevard, Dining Room 2B
Dayton, OH 45401
937-687-3325
937-298-4331

Second Monday each month, 7:00-8:30 pm.

Darlene Carroll, Contact
Jean Ruppert, Contact

1206 Support Group for Parents of Children with a Brain Tumor
Children's Hospital Medical Center
Cincinnati, OH 45229
513-559-4726

Call for specific times.

Karen Burkett CNS, Contact
Susan Mcgee CNS, Contact

Oregon

1207 Bend Support Group
St Charles Medical Center
2500 NE Neff Road
Bend, OR 97701
541-388-7730

Second Saturday of every month.

1208 Brain Tumor Education & Support Group
Comprehensive Cancer Center
1130 NW 22nd Avenue, 2nd Floor, Conference Room
Portland, OR 97208
503-413-7921

First and Third Wednesday of each month, 4:00-5:30 pm. Parking is available in the garage #3-enter between NW 21st and NW 22nd on NW Marshall.

Dawn Brucker LCSW, Contact

1209 Klamath Falls Support Group
415 Main Street
Klamath Falls, OR 97601
541-883-7547
e-mail: info@spokeunlimited.org
www.spokeunlimited.org

Third week of every month. Meets at the office, with a monthly fliar, and focuses on traumatic brain injuries.

Dann Lytle, Contact

Pennsylvania

1210 Brain Tumor Support Group
Bradford Regional Medical Center
116 Interstate Parkway
Bradford, PA 16701
814-362-8329

Debby Abrams

1211 Brain Tumor Support Group at Lancaster
Lancaster Regional Medical Center
250 College Avenue
Lancaster, PA 17603
717-392-4512

Betty Greider

1212 Brain Tumor Support Group at Philadelphia
Hospital of University of Pennsylvania Hospital
3400 Spruce Street, 1 Rhoads Conference Room
Philadelphia, PA 19104
215-746-7742

Third Tuesday of each month, 6:30-8:00 pm.

Stacy Oppleman, Contact

1213 Brain Tumor Support Group at Pittsburgh
Cancer Caring Center
4117 Liberty Avenue
Pittsburgh, PA 15224
412-662-1212
Fax: 412-622-1216
e-mail: cancercr@sgi.net

Rebecca Whitlinger

1214 Brain Tumor Support Group of Philadelphia Hospital of Univ. of PA Cancer Center
3400 Spruce Street, Bridge Level, Penn Town Hotel
Philadelphia, PA 19104
215-662-4485

Nancy O'Conner, RN, MSN

1215 Brain Tumor Support Group of Pittsburgh
Pittsburgh Cancer Institute
Monte Fiore Hospital, 7 Main Lounge
Pittsburgh, PA 15260
412-624-1115
800-237-4724

Contact is the Cancer Info and Referral Services.

1216 Brain Tumor Support Group of the Lehigh Valley
Saint John's Lutheran Church
5th and Chestnut Street
Emmaus, PA 18049
610-830-0659

Second Tuesday of each month, 7:30 pm.

Dolores Fioriglio, Contact

1217 C-Brain (Cranial Base Resource & Information Network)
230 Lothrop Street
Pittsburgh, PA 15219
412-683-4273

Liz Odoroff

1218 Camelot For Children
Pediatric Cancer Foundation of the Lehigh Valley
2354 W Emmaus Ave
Allentown, PA 18103
610-264-7026
www.cancersupportgroup.org

Fourth Tuesday of each month at 6:30 pm.

Nicole Ronco, Contact

1219 Pittsburgh Area Brain Tumor Support Group
Allegheny General Hospital
320 E North Avenue, Magoven Conference Center
Pittsburgh, PA 15212
800-448-0904

Separate meetings for people with advanced disease and benign tumors, and post-acute patients.

Stacy Lang

1220 Presbyterian Hospital/Pittsburgh Cancer Center
DeSoto at O'Hara Street
Pittsburgh, PA 15213
412-647-3475

Susan Chamberlin-Downie

1221 Support Group for Parents and Children with Brain Tumors

Children's Hospital of Philadelphia
34th & Civic Center Boulevard
Philadelphia, PA 19104

609-924-7367

Six newsletters each year, informal meetings alternate with guest speakers.

Marion Roemner

1222 Wills Eye Brain Tumor Support Group

900 Walnut Street
Philadelphia, PA 19104

215-928-7045

Ann Marie DiBona

Rhode Island

1223 Brain Tumor Support Group at Providence

Brown University Campus
BioMedical Center
Providence, RI 02940

401-789-0126
401-647-2935

First and Third Tuesday of each month, 6:30-8:00 pm.

Judy Allenson, Contact
Betty Bentley, Contact

South Carolina

1224 Newberry County Memorial Hospital Brain Tumor Support Group

2669 Kinard Street, Education Room
Newberry, SC 29108

803-276-5290
e-mail: info@newberryhospital.org
www.angelfire.com/sc2/sctumor/

First Thursday of each month, 7:00-8:30 pm.

Tina Doran, Contact

Tennessee

1225 Memphis Regional Brain Tumor Survivors Group

Colonial Park United Methodist Church
5330 Park Avenue
Memphis, TN 38119

901-757-0806
e-mail: midsouth-brain@hotmail.com

First THursday of every month at 6:30 pm.

Robert Lowery, RN, BSN

1226 Nashville Brain Tumor Support Group

Southern Hills Medical Center
391 Wallace Road
Nashville, TN 37202

615-781-4190

Ronnie Gammons

Texas

1227 Brain Tumor Support Group at Dallas

American Cancer Society
8900 Carpenter Freeway
Dallas, TX 75260

214-977-7969

Second Wednesday of each month, 7:00-8:30 pm.

Alice Anderson, Contact

1228 Brain Tumor Support Group at Plano

Health South Rehab Hospital
SE Corner of Independence Pkwy and 15th Street
Plano, TX 75075

972-335-4948
972-867-3431
http://community.dallasnews.com/dmn/greymatters

Second Tuesday of each month, 7:00-9:00 pm.

Colleen Balcer, Contact

1229 Brain Tumor Support Group for Families of Children with Brain and Spinal Tumors

Methodist Hospital, Hodges Care Center
3615 19th Street, Conference Room
Lubbock, TX

806-792-1011
800-687-5437

Jim Powell

1230 Central Texas Brain Tumor Support Group

Health South Rehab Hospital
1215 Red River
Austin, TX 78710

512-636-3015
e-mail: tennistoml@hotmail.com

Second Thursday of the month, 6:30 pm.

Thomas Lewman, Contact
Joam Lewman, Contact

1231 HOPE (Helping Oncology Parents Endure) Brain Tumor Foundation of the Southwest

Children's Medical Center of Dallas
1935 Motor Street
Dallas, TX

214-456-6139

Call for meeting times.

Shane Valles, Contact

1232 Houston Area Brain Tumor Network

University of Texas MD Anderson Cancer Center
Place of Wellness, 1515 Holcombe Boulevard
Houston, TX 77030

713-794-1777
800-392-1611

First Tuesday of each month, 6:00-8:00 pm.

Susana Lee, Contact

1233 Shirvers Cancer Center Brain Tumor Support Group

University of Texas Nursing School
1215 Red River, Cafeteria
Austin, TX 78710

512-469-7378

Ann Harris
Karen Martin

1234 We've Just Begun to Live Brain Tumor Support Group

Audie Murphy VA Hospital
7400 Merton Minter, 2nd Floor, Room 234
San Antonio, TX 78265

210-617-5300

Diane Johnson

1235 West Texas Brain Tumor Support Group

Abilene Regional Medical Center
1680 Antilley Road, 2nd Floor, Room 270
Abilene, TX 79604

915-698-7566

Jana Boss RN

Utah

1236 Peer-Led Brain Tumor Support Group
University of Utah Hospital and Clinics
50 N Medical Drive, 2nd Floor
Salt Lake City, UT 84119

801-581-2584

Karen Elliott

Virginia

1237 Brain Tumor Support Group
Saint Mary's Hospital
5801 Bremo Road, Room 159
Richmond, VA 23261

877-284-3905
e-mail: curebt@hotmail.com
www.curebt.org

Second Tuesday of the month, 7:00-9:00 pm.

Carol Roberts RN MS, Contact

Washington

1238 Adult Brain Tumor Support Group
Virginia Mason Medical Center
1201 Terry Ave, Lindeman Pavillion, 10th Floor
Seattle, WA 98109

206-341-0420

Third Tuesday of every month, 2:30-4:00 pm.

Rick Edwards, Contact

1239 Brain Tumor Support Group University of Washington Medical Center
1959 NE Pacific Street, Box 356043
Seattle, WA 98105

206-598-4108

Meets first Wednesday of each month, 5:30-7:30 pm.

Stephanie Martin MSW LICSW, Contact

1240 Northwest Hospital Brain Tumor Support Group
Northwest Hospital
1560 N 115th Street, Building 4, Lower G Level
Seattle, WA 98109

206-368-1304

Mark Filler SW

1241 Northwest Hospital Brain Tumor Group Support Hotline
Northwest Hospital
1560 N 115th Street, Building 4, Lower G Level
Seattle, WA 98644

206-368-1606

West Virginia

1242 Southern West Virginia Brain Tumor Support Group
First Presbyterian Church
16 Broad Street, Room A-204
Charleston, WV 25301

304-744-0393

Jeri McDonald

Wisconsin

1243 Brain Tumor Support Group
Luther Hospital
1221 Whipple Street, Conference Rooms 2 & 3
Eau Claire, WI 54703

715-838-1900

Second Tuesday of the Month, 6:30-7:30 pm.

Karen Snoble, Contact

1244 Brain Tumor Support Group at Milwaukee
St Lukes Medical Center
2900 W Oklahoma Avenue
Milwaukee, WI 53201

414-649-7200
800-252-2990

Second Wednesday of the month, 5:00-6:30 pm.

Linda Piacentine RN, MS, CNRN

1245 Brain Tumor Support Group at Wauwatosa Froederdt Memorial Lutheran Hospital
Administrative Board Room
9200 W Wisconsin Avenue
Wauwatosa, WI 53226

414-805-2629

Third Tuesday of each month, 6:30-8:30 pm.

Celeste Volcesek, Contact

1246 John Sierzant Brain Tumor Support Group
Gunderson Lutheran Medical Center
John Netti Mooney Resource Ctr, 1836 S Ave, 3rd Fl
LaCrosse, WI 54601

608-782-7300

First Tuesday of each month, 7:00-9:00 pm.

Polly Davenport-Fortune NP

1247 LODAT (Living One Day at a Time) Brain Tumor Support Group
Children's Hospital of Wisconsin
900 W Wisconsin Avenue, PO Box 1997
Milwaukee, WI 53201

414-266-2000
www.chw.org

Parent support group for families of children with cancer. Monthly newsletter, informational meetings, social activities for families, and bereavement support.

Frances Swigart

Libraries & Resource Centers

1248 Brain Tissue Resource Center
McLean Hospital
115 Mill Street
Belmont, MA 02178

781-855-2400

Edward D Bird, Director

Research Centers

1249 Brain Research Center
Children's Hospital National Medical Center
111 Michigan Avenue NW
Washington, DC 20010

202-884-2070
800-787-0021
www.cnmc.org

Barbara Herman, Chief

1250 Brain Research Foundation
5812 S Ellis Ave MC 7112 Room J-141
Chicago, IL 60637

773-834-6750
Fax: 773-834-6751
e-mail: info@brainresearchfdn.org
www.brainresearchfdn.org

Provides support to scinetists who are working to undersatnd the functioning of the brain. It establishes and provides financial assistance for research at the Brain Research Foundation. It also funds professional and scientific education.

Patricia Koldyke, Vice President Executive Committee

1251 National Family Brain Tumor Registry
The Johns Hopkins Oncology Center
600 N Wolfe Street
Baltimore, MD 21287

301-955-3071
Fax: 301-448-1022
www.childrensneuronet.org

This Registry is currently participating in a study that is researching the genetic and environmental aspects of brain tumors.

Medhat Osman, MD

1252 University of California, San Francisco Brain Tumor Research Center
1001 Portero Road
San Francisco, CA 94110

415-206-8313

Research done on brain tumors.

Lawrence H Pitts, MD

Audio Video

1253 National Brain Tumor Conference Audiotapes
National Brain Tumor Foundation
414 13th Street, Suite 700
Oakland, CA 94612

510-839-9777
800-934-2873
Fax: 510-839-9779
e-mail: nbtf@braintumor.org
www.braintumor.org

Audiotapes of keynote addresses and conference workshops from NBTF's biennial National Brain Tumor Conferences. Leading researchers, physicians and health professionals address a wide range of issues affecting brain tumor survivors, such as new approaches to radiation and surgery, research and coping skills for families.

Web Sites

1254 American Brain Tumor Association
www.abta.org

Information about brain tumors.

1255 CancerCare
www.cancercare.org

Provides information, and practical help to people with cancer and their loved ones.

1256 Online Mendelian Inheritance in Man
www.ncbi.nlm.nih.gov

This database is a catalog of human genes and genetic disorders.

1257 Pediatric Brain Tumor Foundation of the United States
www.ride4kids.org

Our mission is in support of the efforts of the Pediatric Brian Tumor Foundation of the United States, a nonprofit chariable foundation.

1258 Starting Point: To Connect with Resources Related to Pediatric Neuro-oncology
www.med.miami.edu/neurosurgery/start_intro.htm

Specializes in the management of patients with surgically treatable neurological diseases. The scope of practice includes the care of patients with disorders of the brain, spinal cord and nerves including cerebrovascular disease, intracranial and spinal tumors, disorders of the spinal cord and vertebral column, pediatric neurosurgical problems, movement disorders, medically intractable seizure disorders, and head and spinal injuries.

Book Publishers

1259 Alex's Journey: The Story of a Child with a Brain Tumor
American Brain Tumor Association
2720 River Road, Suite 146
Des Plaines, IL 60018

847-827-9910
800-886-2282
Fax: 847-827-9918
e-mail: info@abta.org
www.abta.org

Available in DVD or Cassette.

1260 Let's Talk About Going to the Hospital
Rosen Publishing Group's PowerKids Press
29 E 21st Street
New York, NY 10010

212-777-3017
800-237-9932
Fax: 888-436-4643
e-mail: rosenpub@tribeca.ios.com
www.powerkidspress.com

If a child has to check into the hospital, chances are he or she is already upset about being ill. Knowing how a hospital functions and what the procedures are, such as when family members can visit, will help in what is already a stressful situation. Grades K-5.

24 pages
ISBN: 0-823950-36-0

1261 Let's Talk About when Kids Have Cancer
Rosen Publishing Group's PowerKids Press
29 E 21st Street
New York, NY 10010

212-777-3017
800-237-9932
Fax: 888-436-4643
e-mail: customerservice@rosenpub.com
www.powerkidspress.com

In a straightforward yet comforting way, this book explains what cancer is, what kinds of treatments surround the disease and how to cope if a child or the friend of a child has cancer.

24 pages
ISBN: 0-823951-95-2

1262 Pediatric Cancer Sourcebook
Omnigraphics
PO Box 625
Holmes, PA 19043

800-234-1340
Fax: 800-875-1340
e-mail: info@omnigraphics.com
omnigraphics.com

Basic consumer health information about leukemias, brain tumors, sarcomas, lymphomas and other cancers in infants, children and adolescents.

587 pages
ISBN: 0-780802-45-4

Newsletters

1263 Childhood Brain Tumor Foundation Newsletter
20312 Watkins Meadow Drive
Germantown, MD 20876

301-515-2900
877-217-4166
Fax: 301-540-8367
www.childhoodbraintumor.org

Seeking second opinions, access to healthcare, and combating discrimination.

3x/year

1264 Message Line

American Brain Tumor Association
2720 River Road, Suite 146
Des Plaines, IL 60018

847-827-9910
800-886-2282
Fax: 847-827-9918
e-mail: info@abta.org
www.abta.org

Describes research advances and announces updates to publications.

Booklet

1265 SEARCH

National Brain Tumor Foundation
22 Battery Street, Suite 612
San Francisco, CA 94111

415-834-9970
800-934-2873
Fax: 415-834-9980
e-mail: nbtf@braintumor.org
www.braintumor.org

Newsletter that covers topics of current interest to brain tumor survivors and their families.

Quarterly

Pamphlets

1266 A Brain Tumor- Sharing Hope

American Brain Tumor Association
2720 River Road, Suite 146
Des Plaines, IL 60018

847-827-9910
800-886-2282
Fax: 847-827-9918
e-mail: info@abta.org
www.abta.org

Also available in Spanish.

Pamphlet

1267 A Primer of Brain Tumors

American Brain Tumor Association
2720 River Road, Suite 146
Des Plaines, IL 60018

847-827-9910
800-886-2282
Fax: 847-827-9918
e-mail: info@abta.org
www.abta.org

A patient's reference manual offering information on brain tumors.

Pamphlet

1268 About Ependymoma

American Brain Tumor Association
2720 River Road, Suite 146
Des Plaines, IL 60018

847-827-9910
800-886-2282
Fax: 847-827-9918
e-mail: info@abta.org
www.abta.org

Pamphlet

1269 About Glioblastoma Multiforme and Anaplastic Astrocytoma

American Brain Tumor Association
2720 River Road, Suite 146
Des Plaines, IL 60018

847-827-9910
800-886-2282
Fax: 847-827-9918
e-mail: info@abta.org
www.abta.org

Pamphlet

1270 About Medulloblastoma/PNET (Medulloblastoma)

American Brain Tumor Association
2720 River Road, Suite 146
Des Plaines, IL 60018

847-827-9910
800-886-2282
Fax: 847-827-9918
e-mail: info@abta.org
www.abta.org

Pamphlet

1271 About Meningioma

American Brain Tumor Association
2720 River Road, Suite 146
Des Plaines, IL 60018

847-827-9910
800-886-2282
Fax: 847-827-9918
e-mail: info@abta.org
www.abta.org

Pamphlet

1272 About Metastatic Tumors to the Brain and Spine

American Brain Tumor Association
2720 River Road, Suite 146
Des Plaines, IL 60018

847-827-9910
800-886-2282
Fax: 847-827-9918
e-mail: info@abta.org
www.abta.org

Pamphlet

1273 About Oligodendroglioma and Mixed Glioma

American Brain Tumor Association
2720 River Road, Suite 146
Des Plaines, IL 60018

847-827-9910
800-886-2282
Fax: 847-827-9918
e-mail: info@abta.org
www.abta.org

Pamphlet

1274 About Pituitary Tumors

American Brain Tumor Association
2720 River Road, Suite 146
Des Plaines, IL 60018

847-827-9910
800-886-2282
Fax: 847-827-9918
e-mail: info@abta.org
www.abta.org

Pamphlet

1275 About the American Brain Tumor Association

American Brain Tumor Association
2720 River Road, Suite 146
Des Plaines, IL 60018

847-827-9910
800-886-2282
Fax: 847-827-9918
e-mail: info@abta.org
www.abta.org

Pamphlet

1276 Brain Tumor Resource Directory

NBTF Publications and Items
414 13th Street, Suite 700
Oakland, CA 94612

510-839-9777
800-934-2873
Fax: 510-839-9779

A comprehensive reference for health care providers. The directory contains the names and phone numbers of various organizations that offer services and products of particular interest to brain tumor patients and their families.

1277 Brain Tumor Support Groups in North America

NBTF
414 13th Street, Suite 700
Oakland, CA 94612

510-839-9777
800-934-2873
Fax: 510-839-9779

A listing of over 170 groups for patients and families.

1278 Brain Tumors: A Guide

National Brain Tumor Foundation
414 13th Street, Suite 700
Oakland, CA 94612

510-839-9777
800-934-2873
Fax: 510-839-9779
www.braintumor.org

Published by the National Brain Tumor Foundation, this easy-to-read booklet about brain tumors contains valuable information for newly diagnosed patients, long term survivors, family members and health professionals. Current information on treatment, patient rights, nutrition, research and more. Also contains a glossary of terms, plus information on support groups and other resources.

56 pages

1279 Brain Tumors: Understanding Your Care

National Brain Tumor Foundation
22 Battery Street, Suite 612
San Francisco, CA 94111

415-834-9970
800-934-2873
Fax: 415-834-9980
e-mail: nbtf@braintumor.org
www.braintumor.org

Easy-to-read, 24-page brochure that describes brain tumor diagnosis, surgery, radiation therapy options, chemotherapy, continuing care and adjusting to daily life.

1280 Chemotherapy of Brain Tumors

American Brain Tumor Association
2720 River Road, Suite 146
Des Plaines, IL 60018

847-827-9910
800-886-2282
Fax: 847-827-9918
e-mail: info@abta.org
www.abta.org

Provides information that will help you understand and participate in your chemotherapy treatment.

1281 Clinical Trial for Brain Tumors

National Brain Tumor Foundation
22 Battery Street, Suite 612
San Francisco, CA 94111

415-834-9970
800-934-2873
Fax: 415-834-9980
e-mail: nbtf@braintumor.org
www.braintumor.org

Lists of clinical trials by state, tumor type and/or treatment type.

1282 Conventional Radiation Therapy

American Brain Tumor Association
2720 River Road, Suite 146
Des Plaines, IL 60018

847-827-9910
800-886-2282
Fax: 847-827-9918
e-mail: info@abta.org
www.abta.org.

1283 Coping with Your Loved One's Brain Tumor

National Brain Tumor Foundation
22 Battery Street, Suite 612
San Francisco, CA 94111

415-834-9970
800-934-2873
Fax: 415-834-9980
e-mail: nbtf@braintumor.org
www.braintumor.org

A 12-page brochure that describes important coping strategies for caregivers and family members of a loved one with a brain tumor.

1284 Coping with a Brain Tumor Part I: From Diagnosis to Treatment

American Brain Tumor Association
2720 River Road, Suite 146
Des Plaines, IL 60018

847-827-9910
800-886-2282
Fax: 847-827-9918
e-mail: info@abta.org
www.abta.org

1285 Coping with a Brain Tumor Part II: During and After Treatment

American Brain Tumor Association
2720 River Road, Suite 146
Des Plaines, IL 60018

847-827-9910
800-886-2282
Fax: 847-827-9918
e-mail: inffo@abta.org
www.abta.org

1286 Dictionary for Brain Tumor Patients

American Brain Tumor Association
2720 River Road, Suite 146
Des Plaines, IL 60018

847-827-9910
800-886-2282
Fax: 847-827-9918
e-mail: info@abta.org
www.abta.org

Offers a dictionary of terms used in the diagnosis and everyday living with brain tumors.

128 pages

1287 National Brain Tumor Foundation Fact Sheets
National Brain Tumor Foundation
22 Battery Street, Suite 612
San Francisco, CA 94111

415-834-9970
800-934-2873
Fax: 415-834-9980
e-mail: nbtf@braintumor.org
www.braintumor.org

Titles include: Health Insurance Coverage and Brain Tumors, Overview of Complementary and Alternative Medicine Therapies, How Tumors Affect the Mind, Emotion and Personality, Healing Power of your Fork: A Brain Tumor Survivor's Eating Plan, Pilocytic Astrocytoma in the Adult, Childhood Brain Tumors Occuring in Adults, Who Gets Brain Tumors and Why?, How to Choose a Treatment Center and Issues to Consider, Clinical Trials for Brain Tumors and How to Get Access, and many others.

1288 Organizing and Facilitating a Support Group
American Brain Tumor Association
2720 River Road, Suite 146
Des Plaines, IL 60018

847-827-9910
800-886-2282
Fax: 847-827-9918
e-mail: info@abta.org
www.abta.org

1289 Stereotactic Radiosurgery
American Brain Tumor Association
2720 River Road, Suite 146
Des Plaines, IL 60018

847-827-9910
800-886-2282
Fax: 847-827-9918
e-mail: info@abta.org
www.abta.org

1290 Understanding Glioblastoma Multiforme
National Brain Tumor Foundation
22 Battery Street, Suite 612
San Francisco, CA 94111

415-834-9970
800-934-2873
Fax: 415-834-9980
e-mail: nbtf@braintumor.org
www.braintumor.org

A 16 page brochure to help patients and care-givers understand more about the diagnosis and treatment of the glioblastoma multiforme.

1291 Understanding and Coping with Your Child's Brain Tumor
National Brain Tumor Foundation
785 Market Street
San Francisco, CA 94103

510-839-9777
Fax: 510-839-9779
e-mail: nbtf@braintumor.org
www.braintumor.org

Published by the National Brain Tumor Foundation, this guide for families and resource for hope contains information for parents of children with brain tumors. Provides information about diagnosis, tumor types, treatment methods, social and emotional support and more. Also contains a glossary and listings of organizations and resources.

1292 Using a Medical Library
American Brain Tumor Association
2720 River Road, Suite 146
Des Plaines, IL 60018

847-827-9910
800-886-2282
Fax: 847-827-9918
e-mail: info@abta.org
www.abta.org.

1293 What You Need to Know About Brain Tumors
National Cancer Institute
Building 31, Room 10A24
Bethesda, MD 20892

800-422-6237

Offers factual information about brain tumors, possible causes, primary and secondary tumors, symptoms, diagnosis, treatment, side effects, follow up care, support and medical terms.

1294 When Your Child is Ready to Return to School
American Brain Tumor Association
2720 River Road, Suite 146
Des Plaines, IL 60018

847-827-9910
800-886-2282
Fax: 847-827-9918
e-mail: info@abta.org
www.abta.org

Guides parents and teachers through a successful return to school when a child has had a brain tumor.

Paperback

Camps

1295 Association for Neurologically Impaired Brain Injured Children
212-12 26th Avenue
Bayside, NY

718-423-9550
Fax: 718-423-9838
e-mail: info@anibic.org

ANIBIc is a voluntary, multi-service organization that is dedicated to serving individuals with severe learning disabilities, neurological impairments and other developmental disabilities. Services include: residential, vocational, family support services, recreation (children and adults), respite (adult), summer day camp, counseling, and tramatic brain injury services (adults).

Jeanne Parisi, Executive Director
Lisa Eisenberg, Director Family Support Services

DESCRIPTION

1296 BRONCHOPULMONARY DYSPLASIA

Synonym: BPD

Involves the following Biologic System(s):

Neonatal and Infant Disorders, Respiratory Disorders

Bronchopulmonary dysplasia (BPD) is a chronic lung disease of infancy that is characterized by injury to the lung's airways, causing abnormal tissue changes, inflammation, and eventual scarring of lung tissue. BPD often affects infants who have become dependent on the long-term use of ventilators to mechanically assist their breathing. In these infants with BPD, lung injury is thought to result from prolonged breathing of high concentrations of oxygen under abnormally high pressure and volume (oxygen toxicity, barotrauma, and volutrauma). BPD affects infants who are born prior to 37 weeks of pregnancy (premature newborns) and are affected by severe respiratory distress syndrome of the newborn (RDS). RDS is characterized by insufficient production of a substance (surfactant) that is produced as the lungs mature during fetal development. Surfactant reduces the surface tension of fluids lining the air sacs (alveoli) of the lungs, enabling the air sacs to remain open between breaths. Due to insufficient surfactant in premature newborns with RDS, greater pressure is required to expand the lungs' airways and air sacs. As a result, the air sacs may collapse and the lungs may become unable to properly provide oxygenated blood to the body. Within minutes or hours after birth, newborns with RDS experience increasing difficulty breathing (dyspnea), characterized by rapid, labored, shallow breaths (tachypnea); grunting upon exhalation; drawing in of the chest wall during inhalation; and bluish discoloration of the skin and mucous membranes (cyanosis) due to lack of sufficient oxygen supply to bodily tissues (hypoxia). In infants with severe RDS, treatment typically includes prolonged support with a ventilator to keep the aveoli open (positive pressure ventilator). BPD is said to exist if lung disease persists, usually with an oxygen requirement, beyond the first month of life.

Despite receiving increasing concentrations of oxygen and other treatment measures, newborns with RDS and subsequent bronchopulmonary dysplasia continue to experience severe respiratory symptoms rather than improve as expected. These infants have ongoing respiratory distress associated with hypoxia, abnormally high levels of carbon dioxide in the blood (hypercarbia), a reduced ability of the right side of the heart to pump blood efficiently (right-sided heart failure), and continued oxygen dependency. Approximately two to three weeks after continued ventilation support, x-ray examination and other diagnostic techniques may demonstrate the abnormal tissue changes (bronchiolar metaplasia) and scarring of lung tissue associated with bronchopulmonary dysplasia.

The treatment of infants with BPD may include gradual weaning off mechanical ventilation; prescription of corticosteroid medications (e.g., dexamethasone) to reduce inflammation, administration of medications to helpexpand the airways of the lungs (bronchodilators) and drugs to promote the excretion of fluid from the body (diuretics); restriction of fluid intake; and therapies to help prevent or treat certain respiratory infections (e.g., respiratory syncytial virus). Maturation of the lungs is the most important treatment and most patients recover by approximately six to 12 months. However, these children may have an increased susceptibility to inflammation and infection of the lungs (pneumonia) or other potential complications, such as temporary growth failure. In some patients with severe BPD, prolonged hospitalization may be necessary.

See also **General Resources** on page 917

Government Agencies

1297 NIH/National Heart, Lung and Blood Institu te

National Institute of Health
31 Center Dr MSC 2486, Bldg 31, Room 5A48
Bethesda, MD 20892

301-592-8573
Fax: 240-629-3246
TTY: 240-629-3255
e-mail: NHLBIinfo@nhlbi.nih.gov
www.nhlbi.nih.gov

Primary responsibility of this organization is the scientific investigation of heart, blood vessel, lung and blood disorders. Oversees research, demonstration, prevention, education, control and training activities in these fields and emphasizes the prevention and control of heart diseases.

Elizabeth G Nabel, MD, Director
Susan Shurin, MD, Deputy Director

1298 NIH/National Institute of Child Health and Human Development

31 Center Drive, Building 31
Bethesda, MD 20892

301-496-5133
Fax: 301-496-1104
www.nichd.nih.gov

Established in 1962 by congress, today the institute conducts and supports research on topics related to the health of children, adults, families and populations. Some of these topics include: developmental disabilities, growth and development, infant death, reproductive health and birth defects.

Nancy D Wirth, Director
Lisa Kaeser, Program & Public Liaison

National Associations & Support Groups

1299 American Lung Association
61 Broadway, 6th Floor

New York, NY 10006

212-315-8700
800-586-4872
www.lungusa.org

The American Lung Association fights lung disease in all its forms, with special emphasis on asthma, tobacco control and environmental health. The American Lung Association is funded with contributions from the public, along with gifts and grants from corporations, foundations and government agencies. The association achieves its many successes through the work of thousands of committed volunteers and staff.

Terri E Weaver, PhD RN CS FAAN, Chairman

1300 Genetic Alliance
4301 Connecticut Avenue NW
Washington, DC 20008

202-966-5557
800-336-4363
Fax: 202-966-8553
e-mail: info@geneticalliance.org
www.geneticalliance.org

A coalition of voluntary genetic support groups, consumers and professionals addressing the needs of individuals and families affected by genetic disorders from a national perspective.

Sharon Terry, President/CEO

1301 March of Dimes Birth Defects Foundation
1275 Mamaroneck Avenue
White Plains, NY 10605

914-428-7100
888-663-4637
Fax: 914-428-8203
e-mail: resourcecenter@modimes.org
www.marchofdimes.com

Partnership of volunteers and professionals dedicates to improving the health of babies by preventing birth defects and infant mortality. Over 100 chapters are located across the country and can be located through the National Office.

Dr Jennifer Howse, President

Web Sites

1302 American Lung Association
www.lungusa.org

The American Lung Association fights lung disease in all its forms, with special emphasis on asthma, tobacco control and environmental health. The American Lung Association is funded with contributions from the public, along with gifts and grants from corporations, foundations and government agencies. The association achieves its many successes through the work of thousands of committed volunteers and staff.

DESCRIPTION

1303 BURN INJURIES

Involves the following Biologic System(s):

Dermatologic Disorders

Burn injuries account for approximately 6,000 deaths per year in the United States. Among children, it follows only automobile accidents as a leading cause of accidental fatalities. Burns may be caused by heat, chemicals, or electrical current and are classified as first degree burns, second degree burns, or third degree burns, according to the severity and depth of the injury.

First degree burns, the least severe, affect the surface of the skin (superficial) and are characterized by a sensitive or painful reddened area of skin that sometimes swells and, in some cases, peels off. These types of burns affect only the top layer of skin (epidermis), do not blister, and, in most cases, heal spontaneously with no complications.

Second degree burns affect both the upper layer of skin and varying degrees of the underlying layer (dermis). This type of burn causes blistering. Even if the burn is relatively superficial, the pain may be intense as a result of exposed nerve endings. Superficial second degree burns usually heal within one to two weeks with no residual effects. Deeper second degree burns may actually be less painful and, if kept clean and free of infection, also heal with no complications. Second degree burns that cover more than 30 percent of the body surface area are considered critical.

Third degree burns destroy the upper layer of the skin and the underlying tissues; therefore, this type of burn typically requires skin grafting or other special treatment. Third degree burns are usually characterized by either a white or charred appearance; however, the burned area may appear bright red. Third degree burns that cover more than 10 percent of the body surface area or that involve the face or extremities are considered critical.

Burns that are chracterized by significant charring and exposure of muscle and bone are sometimes referred to as fourth degree burns. Hospitalization for first and second degree burn injuries is largely determined by the amount of the body surface area that is affected. As a general rule, if there is less than 10 percent involvement, treatment may be provided at home or on an outpatient basis. Treatment may include thorough cleansing of the wounds and topical application of antibacterial ointments to small burn areas. Blister management may be provided through cream dressings. If blisters break, thorough cleansing (debridement) to prevent infection is indicated. Bandage or gauze dressings may be applied to keep the injured areas clean to avoid infection. Skin grafting may be indicated for extensive second degree burns. Other treatment may include the administration of antibiotics and analgesics, aswell as injection of a tetanus booster, if necessary.

Third degree or other severe burns may be life-threatening and usually require hospitalization. Smoke and injury due to inhalation can be severe yet go unrecognized. Facials burns should raise the suspicion that there may be damage to the respiratory tract, requiring special vigilance. Emergency intervention may include the administration of oxygen and use of a ventilator to assist in breathing. Vital signs are routinely checked. To prevent kidney failure and other serious complications such as shock, other treatment usually includes intravenous replacement of proteins, body fluids, and essential elements in the fluid portion of the blood (electrolytes such as sodium, potassium, and calcium) lost as a result of extensive injury. The wounds are meticulously cleaned and dressed, and antibiotics are usually administered intravenously to prevent infection. As with less severe burns, tetanus immunization is updated. Extreme vigilance is required in order to preserve the integrity of surrounding tissue, sometimes necessitating the surgical removal of crusted dead skin (escharotomy) that may interfere with circulation. If injured, arms or legs are elevated. In order to help avoid the tightening and contracting of skin and muscles, the limbs may be splinted. Temporary skin grafting may be performed until permanent grafting is possible. In addition, nutritional considerations may necessitate the administration of supplements or, in the case of those unable to eat or drink, insertion of a tube through the nose to deliver nutrition directly into the stomach. Burns sustained through chemical and electrical influences may involve other systems of the body and, as such, are treated symptomatically. Psychological support by a team of professionals is an extremely important element in the recovery of individuals with burn injuries. Other treatment is symptomatic and supportive.

See also **General Resources** on page 917

National Associations & Support Groups

1304 Burn Institute
8825 Aero Drive, Suite 200
San Diego, CA 92123

858-541-2277
Fax: 858-541-7179
www.burninstitute.org

A nonprofit health agency dedicated to reducing burn injuries and deaths through fire and burn prevention education, burn survivor support programs and the funding of burn care research and treatment.

James A Floros, Executive Director/CEO

1305 Burn Prevention Foundation
236 N 17th Street
Allentown, PA 18104

610-969-3930
800-207-3090
Fax: 610-969-3940
e-mail: info@burnprevention.org
www.burnprevention.org

The mission of the Burn Foundation is to provide burn injury prevention education and advocacy for those at greatest risk. Our primary service area is in Eastern Pennsylvania, although many of our programs and products are utilized worldwide.

B Daniel Dillard, Executive Director

1306 Burn Survivors Throughout the World
650 N Beneva Road, #305
Sarasota, FL 34232

941-364-8457
800-503-8058
Fax: 941-364-8441
e-mail: info@burnsurvivorsttw.org
www.burnsurvivorsttw.org

An international nonprofit organization working to rebuild the lives of the current and future burn survivors worldwide. Offers membership, a peer support team, education, advocacy, medical referrals, a free medical treatment program, medical equipment, legal referrals, healing weekends, and public awareness for the burn survivor community and the public worldwide.

Michael Appleman, CEO

1307 International Society for Burn Injuries
55 Fruit Street
Boston, MA 02114

617-726-3447
Fax: 617-367-8936
e-mail: rtompkins@partners.org
www.worldplasticsurgury.org.isbi.html

Our society acknowledges the importance of all of these specialists in burn care and had intelligently admitted those professionals as members since its foundation. We must mention there are very few, in fact almost no other medical societies like ours which bring together such a number of different specialists, including nurses. One of the main purposes and aims of our society is to disseminate knowledge and to stimulate prevention in the field of burns.

1308 National Burn Victim Foundation
246A Madisonville Road
Basking Ridge, NJ 07920

www.nbvf.com

The National Burn Victim Foundation is a nonprofit service agency that addresses the problems associated with burn injuries and their prevention through consultation and education. The NBVF also serves as an advocate for burn survivors and their families. The foundation has provided free emergency services to more than 3,000 New Jersey burn survivors since 1976.

1309 National Fire Protection Association
1 Batterymach Park
Quincy, MA 02169

617-770-3000
800-344-3555
Fax: 617-770-0700
www.nfpa.org

The mission of the international nonprofit NFPA is to reduce the worldwide burden of providing and advocating scientifically-based consensus codes and standards, research, training and education.

James M Shannon, President & CEO

1310 Society for Pediatric Dermatology
8365 Keystone Crossing, Suite 107
Indianapolis, IN 46240

317-202-0224
Fax: 317-205-9841
e-mail: spd@hp-assoc.com
www.pedsderm.net

The objective of the society is to promote, develop and advance education, research and care of skin disease in all pediatric age groups. The society has an international membership comprised of physicians, scientists and professionals in training who have an interest in pediatric skin and its diseases.

Kent Lindeman, Executive Director

Web Sites

1311 Burn Institute
www.burninstitute.org

Burn prevention education, burn survivor support.

1312 Burn Prevention Foundation
www.burnprevention.org

Provides burn injury prevention education and advocacy for those at greatest risk.

1313 Burn Survivors Throughout the World
www.burnsurvivorsttw.org

Offers a support team, e-lists, articles, stories, pictures, poems, polls, newsletters, message boards and links, as well as weekly scheduled, emergency, and public chats.

1314 Consumer Products Safety Commission
www.cpsc.gov

The U.S. Comsumer Product Safety Commission is committed to providing access to its web pages for individuals with disabilities.

1315 Cool the Burn
www.regionshospital.com

Cool the Burn is a unique resource for children whose lives have been affected by a burn injury. Whether you, a family member or a friend have been burned, this section will help you better understand burn unjuries.

1316 International Society for Burn Injuries
www.worldplasticsurgury.org.isbi.html

Information on prevention of burn injuries.

1317 National Burn Victim Foundation
www.nbvf.com

Addresses the problems associated with burn injuries and their prevention through consultation and education.

1318 National Fire Protection Association
www.nfpa.org

Providing and advocating scientifically-based consensus codes and standards, research, training and education.

1319 Society for Pediatric Dermatology
www.pedsderm.net

Promotes, develop and advance education, research and care of skin disease in all pediatric age groups.

Book Publishers

1320 Burns Sourcebook
Omnigraphics
PO Box 625
Holmes, PA 19043

800-234-1340
Fax: 800-875-1340
e-mail: info@omnigraphics.com
www.omnigraphics.com

Basic consumer health information on various types of burns and scalds.

604 pages
ISBN: 0-780802-04-7

DESCRIPTION

1321 CELIAC DISEASE

Synonyms: CD, Celiac sprue, Gluten-sensitive enteropathy, GSE, Nontropical sprue

Involves the following Biologic System(s):

Gastrointestinal Disorders

Celiac disease (CD) is a digestive disorder in which the lining of the small intestine is damaged by gluten, a protein that is found in wheat, barley, rye, and oats. People with CD are thought to have an abnormal immune response to dietary gluten, causing degeneration (atrophy) and flattening of the tiny projections that line the small intestine (villi). Flattening of the surface area of the intestinal villi seriously impairs their ability to absorb fats and other nutrients from food products (malabsorption). Although the specific underlying cause of CD is unknown, the disorder is thought to result from the interactions of many genes (polygenic) in association with certain environmental factors (multifactorial). CD may affect young children as well as adults. The frequency of the disorder varies greatly in different countries and among different populations, and more cases occur in Europe than in the United States. Approximately one in 10,000 infants is thought to be affected by CD in the U.S.

The symptoms associated with celiac disease do not become apparent until gluten is introduced into the diet. In most children with the disorder, symptoms begin to occur between the ages of one to five years. Although symptoms and findings may be variable, many children initially have diarrhea, and the stools become abnormally bulky, pale, frothy, and offensive smelling due to an abnormally increased fat content (steatorrhea). Additional abnormalities may include excessive gas (flatulence), a failure to grow and gain weight at the expected rate (failure to thrive), lack of appetite (anorexia) and weight loss, vomiting, and swelling (distension) of the abdomen. Many children also experience muscle wasting, are unusually clingy and irritable, and have abnormally pale skin (pallor). Due to malabsorption of fats and other nutrients, children typically have deficiencies of certain vitamins, and some patients may have abnormally reduced levels of the oxygen-carrying protein of the blood (hemoglobin) due to iron deficiency (iron-deficiency anemia). Diagnosis is made by a gastroenterologist and will include special testing.

The treatment of celiac disease requires the elimination of gluten from the diet. Wheat and rye products must be completely excluded; however, many children with CD may be able to tolerate some barley and oat products. Because gluten is widely used in various food products, parents and children may initially require the assistance and guidance of an experienced dietitian. In addition, specially manufactured, gluten-free food products are available commercially, such as gluten-free pasta, bread, and flour. Treatment may also include iron and vitamin supplementation as required.

See also **General Resources** on page 917

See also **General Resources** on page 917

National Associations & Support Groups

1322 American Celiac Society
PO Box 23455
New Orleans, LA 70183

504-737-3293
Fax: 504-737-3283
e-mail: info@americanceleacsociety.org
http://williamshaffer.org/acs

Nonprofit, tax exempt organization that supports efforts in education, research and natural support. Helps to set up support groups, sponsors conferences, seeks funding for education and research, identifies ingredients in foods and educates the public about problems facing its members.

Annette Bentley, President
Jim Bentley, VP

1323 American Dietetic Association
120 South Riverside Plaza, Suite 2000
Chicago, IL 60606

800-877-1600
www.eatright.org

Nation's largest organization of food and nutrition professionals.

Judith A Gilbride PhD RD CDN FADA, President

1324 Celiac Disease Foundation
13251 Ventura Boulevard, #1
Studio City, CA 91604

818-990-2354
Fax: 818-990-2379
e-mail: cdf@celiac.org
www.celiac.org

Provides services and support to persons with celiac disease and dermatitus herpetiformis, through programs of awareness, education, advocacy and research; telephone information and referral services; medical advisory board; and special educational seminars and quarterly meetings.

1325 Celiac Sprue Association/USA
PO Box 31700
Omaha, NE 68131

402-558-0600
877-272-4272
Fax: 402-558-1347
e-mail: celiacs@csaceliacs.org
www.csaceliacs.org

National support organization that provides information and referral services for persons with celiac sprue and dermatitis herpetiformis and parents of celiac children. Made up of six regions in the United States, with 84 chapters and 36 resource units.

Tom Sullivan, President
Mary Schuluckebier, Executive Director

1326 Gluten Intolerance Group of North America (GIG)
31214 124th Ave SE
Auburn, WA 98092

206-246-6652
Fax: 206-246-6531
e-mail: info@gluten.net
www.gluten.net

Provides instructional and general information materials, as well as counseling and access to gluten-free products and ingredients to persons with celiac sprue and their families; operates telephone information and referral service; conducts educational seminars for health professionals; conducts and supports research; and offers leadership and assistance to contacts, provide for a gluten-free kids camp.

Cynthia Kupper, CRD, Executive Director

Audio Video

1327 Adjustment to Long-Term Health Problems
Gluten Intolerance Group of North America
1833 Broadway
Seattle, WA 98122

206-246-6652
Fax: 206-246-6631
e-mail: gig@accessone.com

1328 Autoimmune Disorders Genetically Related to Celiac Disease
Gluten Intolerance Group of North America
1833 Broadway
Seattle, WA 98122

206-246-6652
Fax: 206-246-6631
e-mail: gig@accessone.com

1329 Celiac Disease in the USA-Where We Are vs. Where We Need to Be
Gluten Intolerance Group of North America
1833 Broadway
Seattle, WA 98122

206-246-6652
Fax: 206-246-6631
e-mail: gig@accessone.com

Question and answer session.

1330 Great Gluten-Free Baking Ideas
Gluten Intolerance Group of North America
1833 Broadway
Seattle, WA 98122

206-246-6652
Fax: 206-246-6631
e-mail: gig@accessone.com

1331 Pathologist's View of Celiac Sprue
Gluten Intolerance Group of North America
1833 Broadway
Seattle, WA 98122

206-246-6652
Fax: 206-246-6631
e-mail: gig@accessone.com

1332 Unmarking Celiac Disease
American Celiac Society
PO Box 23455
New Orleans, LA 70183

504-737-3293
Fax: 504-737-3283
e-mail: amerceliacsoc@onebox.com

1333 Well-Plan Foods Demonstration
Gluten Intolerance Group of North America
1833 Broadway
Seattle, WA 98122

206-246-6652
Fax: 206-246-6631
e-mail: gig@accessone.com

Web Sites

1334 Ask NOAH About: Stomach and Intestinal (Gastrointestinal) Disorders
noah-health.org/english/illness/gastro/gastro.html

Information on many conditions, including colic, celiac disease, ulcerative colitis, Crohn's disease, diarrhea, hernia and Hirschsprung's disease.

1335 Celiac Disease Foundation
www.celiac.org

Provides support, information and assistance to people affected by Celiac Disease/Dermatitis Herpetiformis.

1336 Celiac Support Page
www.celiac.com

To help as many people as possibe with celiac disease get diagnosed and living happy, healthy gluten-free life.

1337 Gluten-Free Page
www.panix.com/~donwiss

Offers links about Gluten Free Pages about the Celiac Disease/ Gluten Intolerance, gluten free food vendors, and other types of gluten free food sites.

1338 Health Answers
www.healthanswers.com

The vision was to provide a breadth of services to clients through the formation of a network of companies. Each company plays a key role in meeting out clients' needs.

Book Publishers

1339 Digestive Diseases & Disorders Sourcebook
Omnigraphics
PO Box 625
Holmes, PA 19043

610-461-3548
800-234-1340
Fax: 610-532-9001
e-mail: info@omnigraphics.com
www.omnigraphics.com

Basic consumer health information including celiac disease, Crohn's disease, diarrhea, hernias, irritable bowel syndrome and ulcers.

2000 335 pages
ISBN: 0-780803-27-2

1340 GIG Cookbook
Gluten Intolerance Group of North America
PO Box 23035
Seattle, WA 98122

206-325-6980
Fax: 206-320-1172
e-mail: gig@accessone.com

225 recipes.

1341 Gluten Intolerance
American Dietetic Association
1120 Connecticut Avenue, NW
Washington, DC 20036

202-775-8277
www.eatright.org

Resource and recipe book.

Newsletters

1342 GIG Quarterly
Gluten Intolerance Group of North America
31214 124th Avenue SE
Auburn, WA 98092

253-833-6655
Fax: 253-833-6675

Offers updated medical and technological information for patients with celiac sprue, their families and health care professionals.

Quarterly

Cynthia Kupper, Director

1343 Lifeline
Celiac Sprue Association/USA
PO Box 31700
Omaha, NE 68131

402-558-0600
877-272-4272
Fax: 402-558-1347
e-mail: celiacs@csaceliacs.org
www.csaceliacs.org

Quarterly newsletter for celiacs with membership forms, chapter information, resource unit information and promotion brochure.

1344 Whoo's Report
PO Box 23455
New Orleans, LA 70183

504-737-3293
Fax: 504-737-3283

Provides practical assistance to members and individuals with celiac disease and information about the disease to the public.

Pamphlets

1345 A Diet Management
Celiac Sprue Association/USA
PO Box 31700
Omaha, NE 68131

402-558-0600
Fax: 402-558-1347
www.csaceliacs.org

A personalized chart that shows how to make your diet work.

1346 A Success Story
Celiac Sprue Association/USA
PO Box 31700
Omaha, NE 68131

402-558-0600
Fax: 402-558-1347
www.csaceliacs.org

Tells about the history of CSA. Also provides the information of how the CSA Gluten-Free Product Listing Book came about.

1347 American Celiac Society
PO Box 23455
New Orleans, LA 71083

504-737-3293
Fax: 504-737-3283
e-mail: info@americanceliacsociety.org
http://williamshaffer.org/acs

Information package on American Celiac Society, a national support organization that provides information on celiac disease and related disorders. Provides information on local support groups throughout the US and the world.

1348 Basics for the Gluten-free Diet
Celiac Sprue Association/USA
PO Box 31700
Omaha, NE 68131

402-558-0600
Fax: 402-558-1347
www.csaceliacs.org

Information sheets by the Celiac Sprue Association/USA Inc, a national support organization that provides information and referral services for persons with celiac sprue and dermatitis herpetiformis and parents of celiac children. Made up of 6 regions in the United States, with 84 chapters and 36 resource units.

1349 Celiac Sprue
Celiac Sprue Association/USA
PO Box 31700
Omaha, NE 68131

402-558-0600
Fax: 402-558-1347
www.csaceliacs.org

Information sheets by the Celiac Sprue Association/USA Inc, a national support organization that provides information and referral services for persons with celiac sprue and dermatitis herpetiformis and parents of celiac children. Made up of 6 regions in the United States, with 84 chapters and 36 resource units.

1350 Celiac Sprue Resource Guide
Gluten Intolerance Group of North America
1833 Broadway
Seattle, WA 98122

206-325-6980
Fax: 206-320-1172

1351 Diet Instruction
Gluten Intolerance Group of North America
31214 124th Avenue SE
Auburn, WA 98092

253-833-6655
Fax: 253-833-6675

1352 Gluten-free Commercial Products
Celiac Sprue Association/USA
PO Box 31700
Omaha, NE 68131

402-558-0600
877-272-4272
Fax: 402-558-1347
e-mail: celiacs@csaceliacs.org
www.csaceliacs.org

Information sheets by the Celiac Sprue Association/USA.

1353 Introductory Packet Brochure
Gluten Intolerance Group of North America
31214 124th Avenue SE
Auburn, WA 98092

253-833-6655
Fax: 253-833-6675

Offers facts and statistics on celiac sprue and dermatitis herpetiformis.

1354 Living a Full Life with Celiac Sprue
Celiac Sprue Association/USA
PO Box 31700
Omaha, NE 68131

402-558-0600
Fax: 402-558-1347
www.csaceliacs.org

Provides information on celiac-symptoms, treatments and where it was derived from.

1355 On the Celiac Condition

Celiac Sprue Association/USA
PO Box 31700
Omaha, NE 68131

402-558-0600
Fax: 402-558-1347
www.csaceliacs.org

Handbook with information on celiac sprue and dermatitis herpetiformis.

1356 Patient Packets For Celiac Disease

Gluten Intolerance Group of North America
31214 124th Avenue SE
Auburn, WA 98092

253-833-6655
Fax: 253-833-6675

Includes various brochures and research reports on celiac sprue, recipes, diet instruction and more.

DESCRIPTION

1357 CEREBRAL PALSY

Synonym: CP

Covers these related disorders: Ataxic cerebral palsy, Choreoathetoid cerebral palsy, Mixed cerebral palsy, Spastic cerebral palsy

Involves the following Biologic System(s):

Neurologic Disorders, Orthopedic and Muscle Disorders

Cerebral palsy (CP) is a nonprogressive condition characterized by stiff, rigid, and awkward movements (spasticity); involuntary, slow writhing movements (athetosis); and poor balance and coordination of voluntary movement (ataxia). Approximately two of every 1,000 infants are affected with cerebral palsy. Both premature and low birth weight infants are particularly at risk for this condition. Cerebral palsy may occur as the result of an injury to the brain during pregnancy, birth, or the early childhood years. Such brain injuries may be caused by a decrease in the supply of oxygen to the brain during the birthing period; an infection passed from the mother to the fetus during pregnancy; or an excess of bile pigment (bilirubin) in the developing fetus, usually arising from a blood incompatibility between mother and child. After birth, cerebral palsy may result from head trauma, an infection of the brain (e.g., encephalitis,), an infection of the membranes surrounding the brain (meningitis), or other insult to the brain or surrounding tissue.

This condition is divided into four main types, based on the movement disorder. These include spastic, choreoathetoid, ataxic, and mixed cerebral palsy. Spastic cerebral palsy is the most common type of this condition and is characterized by stiff and weak muscles in the arms and legs on one or both sides of the body. Choreoathetoid cerebral palsy is characterized by poorly controlled, spontaneous slow movements of the muscles and accounts for approximately 20 percent of affected children. Ataxic cerebral palsy affects approximately 10 percent of all those with cerebral palsy and is characterized by poor coordination and shaky movements. Mixed cerebral palsy is a combination of two or more types of this abnormality and is characterized by the physical characteristics of the types. Although some children with cerebral palsy have below-average intelligence or are mentally retarded, others are of average or above-average intelligence.

There is no cure for cerebral palsy, but the disabilities associated with CP can be reduced. The type and extent of treatment depends upon the degree and type of disability experienced by the individual child. Medications are prescribed to reduce spasticity and abnormal movements and to prevent seizures. Surgery can also be used to reduce spasticity. Occupational and physical therapy may aid affected children with walking and muscle coordination and control. Some children may benefit from the use of braces or other orthopedic intervention. Speech therapy may be useful for improvement of speech and eating difficulties. Physical and emotional stimulation and support are very important aspects of treatment and will aid in helping children with cerebral palsy to realize their full potential.

See also **General Resources** on page 917

Government Agencies

1358 NIH/National Institute of Child Health and Human Development
31 Center Drive, Building 31
Bethesda, MD 20892

301-496-5133
Fax: 301-496-1104
www.nichd.nih.gov

Established in 1962 by congress, today the institute conducts and supports research on topics related to the health of children, adults, families and populations. Some of these topics include: developmental disabilities, growth and development, infant death, reproductive health and birth defects.

Nancy D Wirth, Director
Lisa Kaeser, Program & Public Liaison

1359 NIH/National Institute of Neurological Dis orders and Stroke (NINDS)
PO Box 5801
Bethesda, MD 20824

301-496-5751
800-352-9424
Fax: 301-496-0296
TTY: 301-468-5981
www.ninds.nih.gov

Works to reduce the burden of neurological disease by conducting, fostering, coordinating and guiding research on the causes, prevention, diagnosis and treatment of neurological disorders and stroke, while supporting basic research in related scientific areas.

Story C Landis Ph.D., Director
Audrey S Penn M.D., Deputy Director

National Associations & Support Groups

1360 ADA Technical Assistance Program
6959 Old Dominion Drive, Suite 250
McLean, VA 22101

703-448-6155
800-949-4232
Fax: 703-442-9015
TTY: 703-448-3079
e-mail: adata@adata.org
www.adata.org

A federally funded network of grantees which provides information, training and technical assistance to businesses and agencies with duties and responsibilities under the ADA (American with Disabilities Act) and to people with disabilities with rights under the ADA. Materials-the ADA and newsletters are available.

Lyn Sowdon, Project Director

1361 American Academy for Cerebral Palsy and Developmental Medicine
555 E Wells Street, Suite 1100
Milwaukee, WI 53202

414-918-3014
Fax: 414-276-2146
e-mail: tdurr@aacpdm.org
www.aacpdm.org

The American Academy for Cerebral Palsy and Developmental Medicine is a multidisciplinary scientific society devoted to the study of cerebral palsy and other childhood onset disabilities, to promoting professional education for the treatment and management of these conditions, and to improving the quality of life for people with these disabilities.

Tracy Durr, Executive Director

1362 Children's Neurobiological Solutions Foundation
1726 Franceschi Road
Santa Barbara, CA 93103

805-965-8838
866-267-5580
Fax: 805-965-8838
e-mail: info@cnsfoundation.org
www.cnsfoundation.org

Children's Neurobiological Solutions Foundation (CNS), is a national, nonprofit, 501(c)(3) organization, whose mission is to orchestrate cutting-edge, collaborative research with the goal of expediting the creation of effective treatments and therapies for children with neurodevelopmental abnormalities, birth injuries to the nervous system, and related neurological problems.

Carol Abrams JD, President

1363 Easter Seals
230 West Monroe Street, Suite 1800
Chicago, IL 60606

312-726-6200
Fax: 312-726-1494
TTY: 312-726-4258
www.easterseals.com

Easter Seals offers a variety of services to help people with disabilities address life's challenges and achieve personal goals.

1364 Easter Seals Disability Services
230 West Monroe Street, Suite 1800
Chicago, IL 60606

312-726-6200
800-221-6827
Fax: 312-726-1494
TTY: 312-726-4258
e-mail: info@easterseals.com
www.easterseals.com

Easter Seals has been helping individuals with disabilities and special needs, and their families, live better lives for more then 80 years. From child development centers to physical rehabilitation and jobs training for peoplewith disabilities, Easter Seals offers a variety of services to help people with disabilities address life's challenges and achieve personal goals.

1365 Epilepsy Foundation
8301 Professional Place
Landover, MD 20785

301-459-3700
800-332-1000
Fax: 301-577-2684
e-mail: postmaster@efa.org
www.epilepsyfoundation.org

A toll free information and referral service staffed by specially trained people who will answer questions and discuss concerns about seizure disorders and their treatment. Staff will direct callers to local affiliates of the foundation and provide information about a broad range of services that respond to the needs of people with seizure disorders.

18,000 members

Eric R Hargis, President & CEO

1366 Family Support Network
Tuberous Sclerosis Alliance
801 Roeder Road, Suite 750
Silver Spring, MD 20910

301-562-9890
800-225-6872
Fax: 301-562-9870
e-mail: info@tsalliance.org
www.tsalliance.org

The Support Network is an organized partnership of individuals whose lives have been affected by tuberous sclerosis. Across the nation, the Support Network is providing the latest medical information, education and support to those individuals who are seeking understanding about the genetic disease and offering them words of encouragement and empowerment.

Nancy L Taylor, CEO

1367 March of Dimes Birth Defects Foundation
1275 Mamaroneck Avenue
White Plains, NY 10605

914-428-7100
888-663-4637
Fax: 914-428-8203
e-mail: resourcecenter@modimes.org
www.marchofdimes.com

Partnership of volunteers and professionals dedicated to improving the health of babies by preventing birth defects and infant mortality. Over 100 chapters are located across the country and can be located through the National Office.

Dr Jennifer Howse, President

1368 National Disability Sports Alliance
25 W Independence Way
Kingston, RI 02882

401-792-7130
Fax: 401-792-7132
e-mail: info@ndsaonline.org
www.ndsaonline.org

Nonprofit organization. Coordinates sports, recreation and fitness activities for individuals with physical disabilities. Main focus is on cerebral palsy, traumatic brain injury and stroke.

Jerry McCole, Executive Director

1369 National Dissemination Center for Children with Disabilities
PO Box 1492
Washington, DC 20013

202-884-8200
800-695-0285
Fax: 202-884-8441
e-mail: nichcy@aed.org
www.nichcy.org

A national information and referral center that provides information on disabilities and disability-related issues for families, educators and other professionals.

Suzanne Ripley, Executive Director

1370 United Cerebral Palsy Associations
1660 L Street NW, Suite 700
Washington, DC 20036

202-776-0406
800-872-5827
Fax: 202-776-0414
TTY: 202-973-7197
e-mail: ucpnatl@ucp.org
www.ucp.org

A network of approximately 119 state and local voluntary agencies which provide services, conduct public and professional education programs and support research in cerebral palsy.

Thomas O'Donnell, Chair

1371 WE MOVE (Worldwide Education and Advocacy for Movement Disorders)
Mt. Sinai Medical Center
204 W 84th Street
New York, NY 10024

212-241-8567
800-437-6682
Fax: 212-875-8389
e-mail: wemove@wemove.org
www.wemove.org

WE MOVE provides movement disorder information and educational materials to physicians, patients and families, the media, and the public via its comprehensive Web sites, training courses, and more. Its goal is to make early diagnosis, up-to-date treatment and patient support a reality for all people living with movement disorders.

Susan Bressman MD, President

State Agencies & Support Groups

Alabama

1372 United Cerebral Palsy of Alabama a
C/O UCP of East Central Alabama
301 EA Darden Drive, Box 694
Anniston, AL 36202

256-237-8203
Fax: 256-235-2388
e-mail: executivedirector@ecaucp.org
www.ecaucp.org

United Cerebral Palsy provides information, advocacy, referral services for persons with disabilities and/or their families. UCP also operates an equipment loan program, conducts parent workshops, disseminates written literature on topics of interest to people with disabilities.

Linda Johns, Executive Director

1373 United Cerebral Palsy of Greater Birmingham
120 Oslo Circle
Birmingham, AL 35211

205-944-3900
Fax: 205-944-3933
e-mail: lindab@ucpbham.com
www.ucpbham.com

United Cerebral Palsy provides information, advocacy, referral services for persons with disabilities and/or their families. UCP also operates an equipment loan program, conducts parent workshops, disseminates written literature on topics of interest to people with disabilities.

Dr Gary Edwards, Executive Director

1374 United Cerebral Palsy of Huntsville & Tennessee Valley
2075 Max Luther Drive
Huntsville, AL 35810

256-852-5600
256-852-5673
Fax: 256-852-6722
e-mail: csmith@ucphuntsville.org
www.ucphuntsville.org

United Cerebral Palsy provides information, advocacy, referral services for persons with disabilities and/or their families. UCP also operates an equipment loan program, conducts parent workshops, disseminates written literature on topics of interest to people with disabilities.

C Smith, Executive Director

1375 United Cerebral Palsy of Mobile
3058 Dauphin Square Connector
Mobile, AL 36607

334-479-4900
Fax: 334-479-4998
e-mail: info@ucpmobile.org
www.ucpmobile.org

United Cerebral Palsy provides information, advocacy and referral services for persons with disabilities and/or their families. UCP also operates an equipment loan program, conducts parent workshops, disseminates written literature on topics of interest to people with disabilities and provides early intervention, supported employment, pre-school, therapy, and inclusive camp and adolescent services.

Glenn Harger, President & CEO

1376 United Cerebral Palsy of Northwest Alabama
4212 Jackson Highway
Sheffield, AL 35660

256-381-4310
Fax: 256-381-4378
e-mail: alison@ucpshoals.org
www.ucpshoals.org

United Cerebral Palsy provides information, advocacy, referral services for persons with disabilities and/or their families. UCP also operates an equipment loan program, conducts parent workshops, disseminates written literature on topics of interest to people with disabilities.

1377 United Cerebral Palsy of West Alabama
1100 UCP Parkway
Northport, AL 35476

205-345-3031
Fax: 205-345-3035
e-mail: tfrankucp@comcast.net
www.ucpwa.org

Provides early intervention for birth through age 3, preschool services, afternoon and summer CARE services, (child and adult respite/education), Start on Success Alabama (high school transition to work program), Adult Day Habilitation Program (adults with mental retardation), UCP Miracle Riders (equestrian physical therapy program).

Toni Franklin, Executive Director

Alaska

1378 United Cerebral Palsy of Alaska/PARENTS
4743 E Northern Lights Boulevard
Anchorage, AK 99508

907-337-7678
Fax: 907-337-7671
e-mail: sanja@parentsinc.org
www.parentsinc.org

United Cerebral Palsy provides information, advocacy, referral services for persons with disabilities and/or their families. UCP also operates an equipment loan program, conducts parent workshops, disseminates written literature on topics of interest to people with disabilities.

Sanja Bolling, Executive Director

Arizona

1379 United Cerebral Palsy of Central Arizona
1802 W Parkside Lane
Phoenix, AZ 85027

602-943-5472
888-943-5472
Fax: 602-943-4936
e-mail: info@ucpofaz.org
www.ucpofaz.org

United Cerebral Palsy provides information, advocacy, referral services for persons with disabilities and/or their families. UCP also operates an equipment loan program, conducts parent workshops, disseminates written literature on topics of interest to people with disabilities.

1380 United Cerebral Palsy of Southern Arizona
4002 East Grant Road
Tucson, AZ 85712

520-795-3108
Fax: 520-795-3196
e-mail: staff@ucpsa.org
www.ucpasa.org

United Cerebral Palsy provides information, advocacy, referral services for persons with disabilities and/or their families. UCP also operates an equipment loan program, conducts parent workshops, disseminates written literature on topics of interest to people with disabilities.

Cindy Mars, Executive Director

Arkansas

1381 United Cerebral Palsy of Central Arkansas
9720 N Rodney Parham Road
Little Rock, AR 72227

501-224-6067
Fax: 501-227-5591
e-mail: info@ucpcark.org
www.ucpcark.org

United Cerebral Palsy provides information, advocacy, referral services for persons with disabilities and/or their families. UCP also operates an equipment loan program, conducts parent workshops, disseminates written literature on topics of interest to people with disabilities.

1382 United Cerebral Palsy of Northeast Arkansas
Box 4081
Jonesboro, AR 72403

870-972-6711
Fax: 870-932-7050
e-mail: ucpofnea@fastdate.net
www.ucpa.org

United Cerebral Palsy provides information, advocacy, referral services for persons with disabilities and/or their families. UCP also operates an equipment loan program, conducts parent workshops, disseminates written literature on topics of interest to people with disabilities.

1383 United Cerebral Palsy of South Arkansas
714 W Grove
El Dorado, AR 71730

870-863-8194
Fax: 870-881-4600
www.ucpa.org

United Cerebral Palsy provides information, advocacy, referral services for persons with disabilities and/or their families. UCP also operates an equipment loan program, conducts parent workshops, disseminates written literature on topics of interest to people with disabilities.

California

1384 United Cerebral Palsy of Central California
4224 N Cedar Avenue
Fresno, CA 93726

559-221-8272
Fax: 559-221-9347
e-mail: jamiem@ccucp.org
www.ccucp.org

United Cerebral Palsy provides information, advocacy, referral services for persons with disabilities and/or their families. UCP also operates an equipment loan program, conducts parent workshops, disseminates written literature on topics of interest to people with disabilities.

Laurie Alves, Executive Director

1385 United Cerebral Palsy of Greater Sacramento
191 Lathrop Way, Suite N
Sacramento, CA 95815

916-565-7700
Fax: 916-565-7773
e-mail: ucp@ucpsacto.org
www.ucpsacto.org

UCP provides programs and services for people with all types of developmental disabilities. These services include: day programs for adults, an in-home respite service, transportation, independent living services, information and referral services, a toy lending library, a recreational program for children, and advocacy at the State and National levels. UCP will, upon request, furnish written literature regarding their programs and services or information regarding a variety of disabilities.

Doug Bergman, President & CEO

1386 United Cerebral Palsy of Los Angeles, Ventura and Santa Barbara Counties
6430 Independence Avenue
Woodland Hills, CA 91367

818-782-2211
Fax: 818-909-9106
e-mail: mail@ucpla.org
www.ucpla.com

Serving Los Angeles, Ventura and Santa Barbara counties. Serves hundreds of adults and children with disabilities every day with housing, education programs and professional and personal support for people with disabilities and their families. In addition to the high volume of people assisted, UCP is known for a caring, personal approach to each family's individual situation and choices.

Kevin McCarthy, Chairman
Ellen Kessler, President

1387 United Cerebral Palsy of Orange County
230 Commerce, Suite 190
Irvine, CA 92602

714-200-2600
Fax: 714-200-2640
e-mail: ppulver@ucp-oc.org
www.ucp-oc.org

United Cerebral Palsy of Orange County operaptes an infant stimulation program with physical, occupational and speech therapy consultation. Aditionally, UCP provides information and referral services for the families of children having developmental disabilities as well as an equiptment loan program, Respitality program, parent support groups and individulized support, respite/babysitter programs, and consultation/training to childcare providers.

Paul Pulver, Executive Director

1388 United Cerebral Palsy of San Diego County
8525 Gibbs Drive, #100
San Diego, CA 92123

858-571-7803
Fax: 858-571-0919
e-mail: ucp@ucpsd.org
www.ucpsd.org

United Cerebral Palsy provides information, advocacy, referral services for persons with disabilities and/or their families. UCP also operates an equipment loan program, conducts parent workshops, disseminates written literature on topics of interest to people with disabilities.

1389 United Cerebral Palsy of San Joaquin, Calaveras & Amador Counties
333 W Benjamin Holt Drive, Suite 1
Stockton, CA 95207

209-956-0290
Fax: 209-956-0294
e-mail: jschumacher@ucpsj.org
www.ucpsj.org

United Cerebral Palsy provides information, advocacy, referral services for persons with disabilities and/or their families. UCP also operates an equipment loan program, conducts parent workshops, disseminates written literature on topics of interest to people with disabilities.

1390 United Cerebral Palsy of San Luis Obispo
3620 Sacramento Drive, Suite 201C
San Luis Obispo, CA 93401

805-543-2039
Fax: 805-543-2045
e-mail: shaftmt@aol.com
www.ucp-slo.org

United Cerebral Palsy provides information, advocacy, referral services for persons with disabilities and/or their families. UCP also operates an equipment loan program, conducts parent workshops, disseminates written literature on topics of interest to people with disabilities.

Mark Shaffer, Executive Director

1391 United Cerebral Palsy of Santa Barbara County
423 W Victoria Street
Santa Barbara, CA 93101

805-966-1112
800-761-1112
Fax: 805-962-7201
e-mail: ucpsbl@aol.com
www.ucpa.org

United Cerebral Palsy provides information, advocacy, referral services for persons with disabilities and/or their families. UCP also operates group homes, independent living apartments and supportive living and work services.

Ron Cohen, Executive Director
Marty Kinrosel, Associate Director

1392 United Cerebral Palsy of Santa Clara & San Mateo Counties
512 E Maude Avenue
Sunnyvale, CA 94085

408-737-7112
650-917-6900
Fax: 650-948-8503
e-mail: ucp@ucpscsm.org
www.ucpscsm.org

United Cerebral Palsy provides information, advocacy, referral services for persons with disabilities and/or their families. UCP also operates an equipment loan program, conducts parent workshops, disseminates written literature on topics of interest to people with disabilities.

1393 United Cerebral Palsy of Stanislaus County Stanislaus
1213 13th Street, PO Box 3443
Modesto, CA 95353

209-577-2122
Fax: 209-577-2392
e-mail: rlonczak@ucpstan.org
www.ucpstan.org

United Cerebral Palsy provides information, advocacy, referral services for persons with disabilities and/or their families. Conducts parent workshops, disseminates written literature on topics of interest to people with disabilities.

Bobert S Lonczak, Executive Director

1394 United Cerebral Palsy of the Golden State
1970 Broadway, Suite 115
Oakland, CA 94612

510-832-7430
Fax: 510-839-1329
e-mail: info@ucpgg.org
www.ucpgg.org

United Cerebral Palsy provides information, advocacy, referral services for persons with disabilities and/or their families. UCP also operates an equipment loan program, conducts parent workshops, disseminates written literature on topics of interest to people with disabilities.

Mary Jo Bernardo, Executive Director

1395 United Cerebral Palsy of the Inland Empire
35-325 Date Palm Drive, Suite 136
Cathedral City, CA 92234

760-321-8184
Fax: 760-321-8284
e-mail: ucpie@dc.rr.com
www.ucpie.org

United Cerebral Palsy provides information, advocacy, referral services for persons with disabilities and/or their families. UCP conducts parent workshops, disseminates written literature on topics of interest to people with disabilities.

Jeffrey Snyder, Executive Director

1396 United Cerebral Palsy of the North Bay
PO Box 124
Penngrove, CA 94951

707-664-2660
e-mail: mchughe@sonoma.edu
www.ucpa.org

United Cerebral Palsy provides information, advocacy, referral services for persons with disabilities and/or their families. UCP also operates an equipment loan program, conducts parent workshops, disseminates written literature on topics of interest to people with disabilities.

Colorado

1397 United Cerebral Palsy Colorado
2200 S Jasmine Street
Denver, CO 80222

303-691-9339
Fax: 303-691-0846
e-mail: jham@ucpco.org
www.ucpa.org

United Cerebral Palsy provides information, advocacy, referral services for persons with disabilities and/or their families. UCP also operates an equipment loan program, conducts parent workshops, disseminates written literature on topics of interest to people with disabilities.

Connecticut

1398 United Cerebral Palsy of Eastern Connecticut
42 Norwich Road
Quaker Hill, CT 06375

860-443-3800
Fax: 860-443-8272
e-mail: mmorisson@ucpect.org
www.ucpect.org

United Cerebral Palsy provides information, advocacy, referral services for persons with disabilities and/or their families. UCP also operates an equipment loan program, conducts parent workshops, disseminates written literature on topics of interest to people with disabilities.

Margaret (Peg) Morrison, Executive Director

1399 United Cerebral Palsy of Greater Hartford
80 Whitney Street
Hartford, CT 06105

860-236-6201
Fax: 860-218-2454
e-mail: jmcmahon@sunrisegroup.org
www.ucpa.org

United Cerebral Palsy provides information, advocacy, referral services for persons with disabilities and/or their families. UCP also operates an equipment loan program, conducts parent workshops, disseminates written literature on topics of interest to people with disabilities.

1400 United Cerebral Palsy of Southern Connecticut
94-96 South Turnpike Road
Wallingford, CT 06492

203-269-3511
Fax: 203-269-7411
e-mail: ucpasouthernct@yahoo.com
www.ucpasouthernct.com

United Cerebral Palsy provides information, advocacy, referral services for persons with disabilities and/or their families. UCP also operates an equipment loan program, conducts parent workshops, disseminates written literature on topics of interest to people with disabilities.

Maureen Linderfelt, Executive Director

Delaware

1401 United Cerebral Palsy of Delaware
700A River Road
Wilmington, DE 19809

302-764-2400
Fax: 302-764-8713
e-mail: wmccool@ucpde.org
www.ucpde.org

United Cerebral Palsy provides information, advocacy, referral services for persons with disabilities and/or their families. UCP also operates an equipment loan program, conducts parent workshops, disseminates written literature on topics of interest to people with disabilities.

District of Columbia

1402 United Cerebral Palsy of Washington DC & Northern Virginia
1818 New York Avenue NE, Suite 101
Washington, DC 20002

202-526-0146
Fax: 202-526-0519
e-mail: webmaster@ucpdc.org
www.ucpdc.org

United Cerebral Palsy provides information, advocacy, referral services for persons with disabilities and/or their families. UCP also operates an equipment loan program, conducts parent workshops, disseminates written literature on topics of interest to people with disabilities.

Ted Bergeron, Executive Director

Florida

1403 Cerebral Palsy of Northeast Florida
3311 Beach Boulevard
Jacksonville, FL 32207

904-396-1462
Fax: 904-396-1199
e-mail: agency@cpnef.org
www.cpnef.org

United Cerebral Palsy provides information, advocacy, referral services for persons with disabilities and/or their families. UCP also operates an equipment loan program, conducts parent workshops, disseminates written literature on topics of interest to people with disabilities, and provides individual and family counseling. Locations also in Kissimme, Winter Garden, Sanford and East Orange.

1404 United Cerebral Palsy of Central Florida
3305 S Orange Avenue
Orlando, FL 32806

407-852-3300
Fax: 407-852-3301
e-mail: lwilkins@ucpcdc.org
www.ucpcdc.org

United Cerebral Palsy provides information, advocacy, referral services for persons with disabilities and/or their families. UCP also operates an equipment loan program, conducts parent workshops, disseminates written literature on topics of interest to people with disabilities, and provides individual and family counseling. Locations also in Kissimme, Winter Garden, Sanford and East Orange.

Ilene Wilkins, President & CEO

1405 United Cerebral Palsy of East Central Florida
1100 Jimmy Ann Drive
Daytona Beach, FL 32117

386-274-6474
Fax: 386-274-6532
e-mail: info@ucpecf.org
www.ucpecf.org

United Cerebral Palsy provides information, advocacy, referral services for persons with disabilities and/or their families. UCP also operates an equipment loan program, conducts parent workshops, disseminates written literature on topics of interest to people with disabilities, and provides individual and family counseling. Locations also in Kissimme, Winter Garden, Sanford and East Orange.

1406 United Cerebral Palsy of Florida
1830 Buford Court
Tallahassee, FL 32308

850-878-2141
Fax: 850-922-1258
e-mail: rsanders@sunrisegroup.org
www.ucpa.org

United Cerebral Palsy provides information, advocacy, referral services for persons with disabilities and/or their families. UCP also operates an equipment loan program, conducts parent workshops, disseminates written literature on topics of interest to people with disabilities.

1407 United Cerebral Palsy of North Florida/ Tender Loving Care
1241 N East Avenue
Panama City, FL 32401

850-769-7960
Fax: 850-769-1060
e-mail: ucpstlc@aol.com
www.ucpa.org

United Cerebral Palsy provides information, advocacy, referral services for persons with disabilities and/or their families. UCP also operates an equipment loan program, conducts parent workshops, disseminates written literature on topics of interest to people with disabilities.

1408 United Cerebral Palsy of Northwest Florida
2912 North E Street
Pensacola, FL 32501

850-432-1596
Fax: 850-432-1930
e-mail: information@ucpnwfl.org
www.ucpnwfl.org

The number one service provider in Northwest Florida for individuals with cerebral palsy and other developmental disabilities, UCP provides information, advocacy and referral services for persons with disabilities and/or their families. Additionally, UCP offers individuals assistance with daily living skills training, computer training, basic education, speech, physical and occupational therapy, residential, supported living and finding long-term employment.

1409 United Cerebral Palsy of Sarasota-Manatee
1090 S Tamiami Trail
Sarasota, FL 34236

941-957-3599
Fax: 947-957-3499
e-mail: ucpwendy@aol.com
www.ucpsarasota.org

United Cerebral Palsy provides information, advocacy, referral services for persons with disabilities and/or their families. UCP also operates an equipment loan program, conducts parent workshops, disseminates written literature on topics of interest to people with disabilities.

1410 United Cerebral Palsy of South Florida
2700 West 81 Street
Hialeah, FL 33016

305-325-1080
Fax: 305-325-1313
e-mail: info@ucpsouthflorida.org
www.ucpsouthflorida.org

United Cerebral Palsy provides information, advocacy, referral services for persons with disabilities and/or their families. UCP also operates an equipment loan program, conducts parent workshops, disseminates written literature on topics of interest to people with disabilities.

1411 United Cerebral Palsy of Tallahassee
1830 Buford Court
Tallahassee, FL 32308

850-922-5630
Fax: 850-922-1258
e-mail: gator1@netally.com
www.ucpa.org

United Cerebral Palsy provides information, advocacy, referral services for persons with disabilities and/or their families. UCP also operates an equipment loan program, conducts parent workshops, disseminates written literature on topics of interest to people with disabilities.

1412 United Cerebral Palsy of Tampa Bay
2215 E Henry Avenue
Tampa, FL 33610

813-239-1179
Fax: 813-237-3091
e-mail: kryals@achievetampabay.org
www.achievetampabay.org

United Cerebral Palsy provides information, advocacy, referral services for persons with disabilities and/or their families. UCP also operates an equipment loan program, conducts parent workshops, disseminates written literature on topics of interest to people with disabilities.

Georgia

1413 United Cerebral Palsy of Georgia
3300 Northeast Expressway, Building 9
Atlanta, GA 30341

770-676-2000
Fax: 770-455-8040
e-mail: info@ucpga.org
www.ucpga.org

United Cerebral Palsy provides information, advocacy, referral services for persons with disabilities and/or their families. UCP also operates an equipment loan program, conducts parent workshops, disseminates written literature on topics of interest to people with disabilities.

Ouida Spencer, Chairperson

Hawaii

1414 United Cerebral Palsy of Hawaii
414 Kuwili Street, Suite 105
Honolulu, HI 96817

808-532-6744
Fax: 808-532-6747
e-mail: ucpa@ucpahi.org
www.ucpahi.org

United Cerebral Palsy provides information, advocacy, referral services for persons with disabilities and/or their families. UCP also operates an equipment loan program, conducts parent workshops, disseminates written literature on topics of interest to people with disabilities.

Idaho

1415 United Cerebral Palsy of Idaho
5420 W Franklin, Suite A
Boise, ID 83705

208-377-8070
Fax: 208-322-7133
e-mail: info@ucpidaho.org
www.ucpidaho.org

United Cerebral Palsy provides information, advocacy, referral services for persons with disabilities and/or their families.

Kim Kane, Executive Director
Kathy Griffen, Program Director

Illinois

1416 United Cerebral Palsy Land of Lincoln
101 North 16th Street
Springfield, IL 62703

217-525-6522
Fax: 217-525-9017
e-mail: ucpll@hotmail.com
www.ucpll.org

United Cerebral Palsy provides information, advocacy, referral services for persons with disabilities and/or their families. UCP also operates an equipment loan program, conducts parent workshops, disseminates written literature on topics of interest to people with disabilities.

Leo Zappa, Chairman

1417 United Cerebral Palsy of East Central Illinois
1023 N Water
Decatur, IL 62523

217-428-5033
Fax: 217-428-5094
www.ucpa.org

United Cerebral Palsy provides information, advocacy, referral services for persons with disabilities and/or their families. UCP also operates an equipment loan program, conducts parent workshops, disseminates written literature on topics of interest to people with disabilities.

1418 United Cerebral Palsy of Greater Chicago
7550 West 183rd Street
Tinley Park, IL 60477

708-444-8460
Fax: 708-429-3981
e-mail: pdulle@ucpnet.org
www.ucpnet.org

United Cerebral Palsy provides information and referral services for persons with disabilities and/or their families. UCP also operates an equipment loan program, conducts parent workshops, disseminates written literature on topics of interest to people with disabilities.

Paul J Dulle, President & CEO

1419 United Cerebral Palsy of Illinois
310 East Adams
Springfield, IL 62701

217-528-9681
Fax: 217-528-9739
e-mail: ucpillinois.org
www.ucpillinois.org

United Cerebral Palsy provides information, advocacy, referral services for persons with disabilities and/or their families. UCP also operates an equipment loan program, conducts parent workshops, disseminates written literature on topics of interest to people with disabilities.

Don Moss, Executive Director

1420 United Cerebral Palsy of Southern Illinois
9 Cusumano Professional Pplaza Drive
Mt Vernon, IL 62864

618-244-2505
800-332-9745
Fax: 618-244-3568
e-mail: ucpsi@onemain.com
http://home.onemain.com/~ucpsi

United Cerebral Palsy provides information, advocacy, referral services for persons with disabilities and/or their families. UCP also operates an equipment loan program, conducts parent workshops, disseminates written literature on topics of interest to people with disabilities.

1421 United Cerebral Palsy of Will County
311 South Reed Street
Joliet, IL 60436

815-744-3500
Fax: 815-744-3504
e-mail: ucpwill@ucpwill.org
www.ucpwill.org

United Cerebral Palsy provides information, advocacy, referral services for persons with disabilities and/or their families. UCP also operates an equipment loan program, conducts parent workshops, disseminates written literature on topics of interest to people with disabilities.

Thomas R Osterberger, President

1422 United Cerebral Palsy of the Blackhawk Region
7399 Forest Hills Road
Rockford, IL 61111

815-636-7132
Fax: 815-282-8835
e-mail: accessni@aol.com
www.ucpa.org

United Cerebral Palsy provides information, advocacy, referral services for persons with disabilities and/or their families. UCP also operates an equipment loan program, conducts parent workshops, disseminates written literature on topics of interest to people with disabilities.

Indiana

1423 United Cerebral Palsy of Greater Indiana
1915 W 18th Street, Suite C
Indianapolis, IN 46202

317-632-3561
800-732-7620
Fax: 317-632-3338
e-mail: donnar@ucpaindy.org
www.ucpa.org

United Cerebral Palsy provides information, advocacy, referral services for persons with Cerebal Palsy and/or their families. UCP also provides funding for equipment and operates an equipment loan program, disseminates written literature on topics of interest to people with disabilities.

1424 United Cerebral Palsy of the Wabash Valley
621 Poplar Street
Terre Haute, IN 47807

812-232-6305
Fax: 812-234-3683
e-mail: ucp.wv@verizon.net
www.ucpwv.org

United Cerebral Palsy provides information, advocacy, referral services for persons with disabilities and/or their families. UCP also operates an equipment loan program, conducts parent workshops, disseminates written literature on topics of interest to people with disabilities.

Jacquie Denehie, Executive Director

Iowa

1425 Center for Disabilities and Development
University of Iowa Hospitals and Clinics
100 Hawkins Drive
Iowa City, IA 52242

319-353-6900
877-686-0031
e-mail: cdd-webmaster@uiowa.edu
www.healthcare.uiowa.edu/cdd

A trusted resource for healthcare, training, research and information for people with disabilities that include: behavior disorders, brain injury, cerebral palsy, diabetes, down syndrome, learning disabilities, mental retardation, sleep disorders and spina bifida.

Elayne Sexsmith, Administrator
Amy Mikelson, Supervisor Info Resource Service

Kansas

1426 United Cerebral Palsy of Greater Kansas City
1044 Main Street, Suite 600
Kansas City, KS 64105

816-531-4454
Fax: 816-531-3383
e-mail: bscott@ucpkc.org
www.ucpa.org

United Cerebral Palsy provides information, advocacy, referral services for persons with disabilities and/or their families. UCP also operates an equipment loan program, conducts parent workshops, disseminates written literature on topics of interest to people with disabilities.

1427 United Cerebral Palsy of Kansas
5111 E 21st Street
Wichita, KS 67208

316-688-1888
Fax: 316-688-5687
e-mail: davej@cprf.org
www.ucpa.org

United Cerebral Palsy provides information, advocacy, referral services for persons with disabilities and/or their families. UCP also operates an equipment loan program, conducts parent workshops, disseminates written literature on topics of interest to people with disabilities.

Louisiana

1428 United Cerebral Palsy of Baton Rouge McMains Children's Developmental Center
1805 College Drive
Baton Rouge, LA 70808

225-923-3420
Fax: 225-922-9316
e-mail: cdcjanet@gmail.com
www.ucpa.org

United Cerebral Palsy provides information, advocacy, referral services for persons with disabilities and/or their families. UCP also operates an equipment loan program, conducts parent workshops, disseminates written literature on topics of interest to people with disabilities.

1429 United Cerebral Palsy of Greater New Orleans
2200 Veterans Memorial Boulevard, Suite 103
New Orleans, LA 70062

504-461-4266
Fax: 504-461-9976
e-mail: info@ucpgno.com
www.ucpgno.org

United Cerebral Palsy provides information, advocacy, referral services for persons with disabilities and/or their families. UCP also operates an equipment loan program, conducts parent workshops, disseminates written literature on topics of interest to people with disabilities.

Maine

1430 United Cerebral Palsy of Northeastern Maine
700 Mount Hope Avenue, Suite 320
Bangor, ME 04401

207-941-2952
Fax: 207-941-2955
e-mail: bobbijo.yeager@ucpofmaine.org
www.ucpofmaine.org

United Cerebral Palsy provides information, advocacy, referral services for persons with disabilities and/or their families. UCP also operates an equipment loan program, conducts parent workshops, disseminates written literature on topics of interest to people with disabilities.

Bobbi Jo Yeager, Executive Director

Maryland

1431 United Cerebral Palsy of Central Maryland
1700 Reistertown Road, Suuite 226
Baltimore, MD 21208

410-484-4540
Fax: 410-484-1807
TTY: 800-451-2452
e-mail: info@ucp-cm.org
www.ucp-cm.org

United Cerebral Palsy provides information, advocacy, referral services for persons with disabilities and/or their families. UCP also operates an equipment loan program, conducts parent workshops, disseminates written literature on topics of interest to people with disabilities.

1432 United Cerebral Palsy of Prince Georges & Montgomery Counties
4409 Forbes Boulevard
Lanham, MD 20706

301-459-0566
Fax: 301-459-7691
TTY: 301-262-4982
e-mail: ucppgmc@aol.com
www.ucppgmc.com

United Cerebral Palsy provides information, advocacy, referral services for persons with disabilities and/or their families. UCP also operates an equipment loan program, conducts parent workshops, disseminates written literature on topics of interest to people with disabilities.

1433 United Cerebral Palsy of Southern Maryland
211 Chinquapin Round Road
Annapolis, MD 21401

410-280-2003
Fax: 410-269-5757
e-mail: ucpinfo@ucpsm.org
www.ucpsm.org

United Cerebral Palsy provides information, advocacy, referral services for persons with disabilities and/or their families. UCP also operates an equipment loan program, conducts parent workshops, disseminates written literature on topics of interest to people with disabilities.

Massachusetts

1434 United Cerebral Palsy of Berkshire County
208 West Street
Pittsfield, MA 01201

413-442-1562
Fax: 413-499-4077
e-mail: info@ucpberkshire.org
www.upcberkshire.org

United Cerebral Palsy provides information, advocacy, assistive technology, referral services for persons with disabilities and/or their families. UCP also operates an equipment loan program, conducts parent workshops, disseminates written literature on topics of interest to people with disabilities.

1435 United Cerebral Palsy of MetroBoston
71 Arsenal Street
Watertown, MA 02472

617-926-5480
Fax: 617-926-3059
e-mail: upcbost@aol.com
www.ucpboston.org

United Cerebral Palsy provides information, advocacy, referral services for persons with disabilities and/or their families. UCP also operates an equipment loan program, conducts parent workshops, disseminates written literature on topics of interest to people with disabilities.

1436 United Cerebral Palsy of the North Shore
103 Johnson Street
Lynn, MA 01902

781-593-2727
Fax: 781-593-2542
e-mail: ucpans@aol.com
www.ucpa.org

United Cerebral Palsy provides information, advocacy, referral services for persons with disabilities and/or their families. UCP also operates an equipment loan program, conducts parent workshops, disseminates written literature on topics of interest to people with disabilities.

Michigan

1437 United Cerebral Palsy Michigan
3401 E Saginaw, Suite 216
Lansing, MI 48912

517-203-1200
800-828-2714
Fax: 517-203-1203
e-mail: ucp@ucpmichigan.org
www.ucpmichigan.org

United Cerebral Palsy provides information, advocacy, referral services for persons with disabilities and/or their families. UCP also operates an equipment loan program, conducts parent workshops, disseminates written literature on topics of interest to people with disabilities.

1438 United Cerebral Palsy of Metropolitan Detroit
23077 Greenfield, Suite 205
Southfield, MI 48075

248-557-5070
Fax: 248-557-4456
e-mail: main@ucpdetroit.org
www.ucpdetroit.org

United Cerebral Palsy provides information, advocacy, referral services for persons with disabilities and/or their families. UCP also operates an equipment loan program, conducts parent workshops, disseminates written literature on topics of interest to people with disabilities.

Minnesota

1439 United Cerebral Palsy of Central Minnesota
510 25th Avenue N
Saint Cloud, MN 56303

320-253-0765
Fax: 320-253-6753
e-mail: info@ucpcentralmn.org
www.ucpcentralmn.org

United Cerebral Palsy provides information, advocacy, referral services for persons with disabilities and/or their families. UCP also operates an equipment loan program, conducts parent workshops, disseminates free newsletter. Computers Go Round recycles quality used computers to persons with disabilities.

1440 United Cerebral Palsy of Minnesota
1821 University Avenue W #219 South
Saint Paul, MN 55104

651-646-7588
800-328-4827
Fax: 651-646-3045
e-mail: ucpmn@cpinternet.com
www.ucpmn.org

United Cerebral Palsy provides information, advocacy, referral services for persons with disabilities and/or their families. UCP also operates an equipment loan program, conducts parent workshops, disseminates written literature on topics of interest to people with disabilities.

Missouri

1441 United Cerebral Palsy of Greater Kansas City
1044 Main Street, Suite 600
Kansas City, MO 64105

816-531-4454
Fax: 816-531-3383
e-mail: bscott@ucpkc.org
www.ucpa.org

United Cerebral Palsy provides information, advocacy, referral services for persons with disabilities and/or their families. UCP also operates an equipment loan program, conducts parent workshops, disseminates written literature on topics of interest to people with disabilities.

1442 United Cerebral Palsy of Greater St. Louis
8645 Old Bonhomme Road
Saint Louis, MO 63132

314-994-1600
Fax: 314-994-0179
e-mail: forkoshr@ucpstl.org
www.ucpstl.org

Offers skill development and training programs in the areas of independent living, human relations, social and leisure activities, assistive technology, sensory and tactile stimulation, community integration, career exploration, job placement, and functional academics to individuals eighteen years of age and older with developmental disabilities.

1443 United Cerebral Palsy of Missouri
8645 Old Bonhomme Road
Saint Louis, MO 63132

314-994-1600
Fax: 314-994-0179
www.ucpa.org

United Cerebral Palsy provides information, advocacy, referral services for persons with disabilities and/or their families. UCP also operates an equipment loan program, conducts parent workshops, disseminates written literature on topics of interest to people with disabilities.

1444 United Cerebral Palsy of Northwest Missouri
3303 Frederick Avenue
Saint Joseph, MO 64506

816-634-3836
Fax: 816-390-8546
e-mail: ucp@ucpnwmo.org
www.ucpnwmo.org

United Cerebral Palsy provides information, advocacy, referral services for persons with disabilities and/or their families. UCP also operates an equipment loan program, conducts parent workshops, disseminates written literature on topics of interest to people with disabilities.

Nebraska

1445 United Cerebral Palsy of Nebraska
10730 Pacific Street, Suite 43
Omaha, NE 68114

402-502-3572
800-729-2556
Fax: 402-502-6791
e-mail: ucp@ucpnebraska.org
www.ucpa.org

United Cerebral Palsy provides information, advocacy, referral services for persons with disabilities and/or their families. UCP also operates an equipment loan program, conducts parent workshops, disseminates written literature on topics of interest to people with disabilities.

Nevada

1446 United Cerebral Palsy of Northern Nevada
4068 S McCarran Boulevard
Reno, NV 89502

775-331-3323
Fax: 775-331-7913
e-mail: upcnn@ucpnn.org
www.ucpa.org

United Cerebral Palsy provides information, advocacy, referral services for persons with disabilities and/or their families. UCP also provides employment and supported living services and disseminates written literature on topics of interest to people with disabilities.

Russ Rougeau, Executive Director
Jennifer Culbert

New Jersey

1447 United Cerebral Palsy of Hudson County
721 Broadway
Bayonne, NJ 07002

201-436-2200
Fax: 201-436-6642
e-mail: hudsonucp@aol.com
www.geocities.com/ucpofhudsoncty

United Cerebral Palsy provides information, advocacy, referral services for persons with disabilities and/or their families. UCP also operates an equipment loan program, conducts parent workshops, disseminates written literature on topics of interest to people with disabilities.

1448 United Cerebral Palsy of New Jersey
354 S Broad Street
Trenton, NJ 08608

609-392-4004
Fax: 609-392-3505
e-mail: info@ucpanj.org
www.ucpa.org

United Cerebral Palsy provides information, advocacy, referral services for persons with disabilities and/or their families. UCP also operates an equipment loan program, conducts parent workshops, disseminates written literature on topics of interest to people with disabilities.

1449 United Cerebral Palsy of Northern, Central & Southern New Jersey
245 Main Street Suite 113
Chester, NJ 07930

908-879-2243
Fax: 908-879-8363
e-mail: info@ucpncsnj.org
www.ucpncsnj.org

United Cerebral Palsy provides information, advocacy, referral services for persons with disabilities and/or their families. UCP also operates an equipment loan program, conducts parent workshops, disseminates written literature on topics of interest to people with disabilities.

New York

1450 Aspire of WNY
2356 N Forest Road
Getzville, NY 14068

716-505-5510
Fax: 716-897-8257
e-mail: info@aspirewny.org
www.aspirewny.org

Aspire of WNY is a provider of comprehensive programs and services for developmentally disabled children and adults in Western New York. Services areas include residential, bocational, therapeutic, clinical, habilitative and educational services amoung others. Aspire also offers advocacy, case management, work shops and referral services for the disabled and their families.

Thomas Sy, Executive Director
Janet Hansen-Moyes, Associate Executive Director

1451 Center for the Disabled
314 S Manning Boulevard
Albany, NY 12208

518-453-2273
Fax: 518-437-5554
www.centercares.org

Center Health Care offers a wide variety of medical dental and therapy services provided in an outpatient practice setting, serving individuals with developmental disabilities and chronic disabling conditions. In addition, educational diagnostic and evaluation services are offered to children of different ages. parent workshops and support groups are conducted throughout the year.

Daniel Silverman MD, Medical Director
Alan Krafchin, President/CEO

1452 Inspire - Cerebral Palsy Center
2 Fletcher Street
Goshen, NY 10924

845-294-8806
Fax: 845-294-8650
e-mail: ggengel@hotmail.com

An affiliate of Cerebral Palsy Associations of New York, provides information, advocacy, referral services for persons with disabilities and/or their families. Inspire runs a rehabilitative clinic and special needs preschool, conducts parent workshops, disseminates written literature on topics of interest to people with disabilities.

Gehe Gengel, Executive Director

1453 UCP of Greater Suffolk
250 Marcus Boulevard, PO Box 18045
Hauppauge, NY 11788

631-232-0011
Fax: 631-232-4422
e-mail: info@ucp-suffolk.org
www.ucp-suffolk.org

UCP Suffolk provides information, advocacy, referral services for persons with disabilities and/or their families. UCP also operates an equipment loan program, conducts parent workshops, disseminates written literature on topics of interest to people with disabilities.

Stephen H Friedman, Executive Director

1454 United Cerebral Palsy Associations of New York State
330 W 34th Street
New York, NY 10001

212-947-5770
Fax: 212-356-0746
e-mail: ucpofnys@aol.com
www.ucpa-nys.org

Cerebral Palsy provides information, advocacy, referral services for persons with disabilities and/or their families. CP also operates an equipment loan program, conducts parent workshops, disseminates written literature on topics of interest to people with disabilities.

Michael Parker, Executive Director

1455 United Cerebral Palsy of Chemung County
PO Box 1554
Elmira, NY 14902

607-734-7107
Fax: 607-734-7334
www.ucpa.org

United Cerebral Palsy provides information, advocacy, referral services for persons with disabilities and/or their families. UCP also operates an equipment loan program, conducts parent workshops, disseminates written literature on topics of interest to people with disabilities.

1456 United Cerebral Palsy of Fulton & Montgomery Counties
67 Division Street
Amsterdam, NY 12010

518-842-3511
Fax: 518-843-6042
www.ucpa.org

United Cerebral Palsy provides information, advocacy, referral services for persons with disabilities and/or their families. UCP also operates an equipment loan program, conducts parent workshops, disseminates written literature on topics of interest to people with disabilities.

1457 United Cerebral Palsy of Nassau County
380 Washington Avenue
Roosevelt, NY 11575

516-378-2000
Fax: 516-868-4089
e-mail: info@ucpn.org
www.ucpn.org

United Cerebral Palsy provides information, advocacy, referral services for persons with disabilities and/or their families. UCP also operates an equipment loan program, conducts parent workshops, disseminates written literature on topics of interest to people with disabilities.

Robert Masterson, President

1458 United Cerebral Palsy of New York City
80 Maiden Lane, 8th Floor
New York, NY 10038

212-683-6700
Fax: 212-685-8394
e-mail: info@ucpnyc.org
www.ucpnyc.org

United Cerebral Palsy provides information, advocacy, referral services for persons with disabilities and/or their families. UCP also operates an equipment loan program, conducts parent workshops, disseminates written literature on topics of interest to people with disabilities.

1459 United Cerebral Palsy of Niagara County
9812 Lockport Road
Niagara Falls, NY 14304

716-297-0798
Fax: 716-297-0998
e-mail: niagaraucp@aol.com
www.ucpa.org

United Cerebral Palsy provides information, advocacy, referral services for persons with disabilities and/or their families. UCP also operates an equipment loan program, conducts parent workshops, disseminates written literature on topics of interest to people with disabilities.

1460 United Cerebral Palsy of Putnam & Southern Dutchess Counties
40 John Barret Road
Patterson, NY 12563

845-878-9078
Fax: 845-878-3203
e-mail: hvcs@aol.com
www.ucpa.org

United Cerebral Palsy provides information, advocacy, referral services for persons with disabilities and/or their families. UCP also operates an equipment loan program, conducts parent workshops, disseminates written literature on topics of interest to people with disabilities.

1461 United Cerebral Palsy of Queens
81-15 164th Street
Jamaica, NY 11432

718-380-3000
Fax: 718-380-0483
e-mail: info@ucp-queens.org
www.ucpa.org

United Cerebral Palsy provides information, advocacy, referral services for persons with disabilities and/or their families. UCP also operates an equipment loan program, conducts parent workshops, disseminates written literature on topics of interest to people with disabilities.

1462 United Cerebral Palsy of Westchester County
King Street & Lincoln Avenue
Purchase, NY 10577

914-937-3800
Fax: 914-937-0967
e-mail: ucpwest@aol.com
www.ucpa.org

United Cerebral Palsy provides information, advocacy, referral services for persons with disabilities and/or their families. UCP also operates an equipment loan program, conducts parent workshops, disseminates written literature on topics of interest to people with disabilities.

1463 United Cerebral Palsy of the North Country
101 Main Street
Canton, NY 13617

315-379-9667
Fax: 315-379-9388
e-mail: ucpa@imcnet.net
www.ucpa.org

United Cerebral Palsy provides information, advocacy, referral services for persons with disabilities and/or their families. UCP also operates an equipment loan program, conducts parent workshops, disseminates written literature on topics of interest to people with disabilities.

1464 United Cerebral Palsy of the Tri-Counties
133 Aviation Road
Queensbury, NY 12804

518-798-0170
Fax: 518-798-0533
www.ucpa.org

United Cerebral Palsy provides information, advocacy, referral services for persons with disabilities and/or their families. UCP also operates an equipment loan program, conducts parent workshops, disseminates written literature on topics of interest to people with disabilities.

North Carolina

1465 United Cerebral Palsy of North Carolina
2315 Myron Drive
Raleigh, NC 27607

919-783-8898
800-662-7119
Fax: 919-782-5486
e-mail: info@nc.eastersealsucp.com
www.nc.eastersealsucp.com

United Cerebral Palsy provides information, advocacy, referral services for persons with disabilities and/or their families. UCP also operates an equipment loan program, conducts parent workshops, disseminates written literature on topics of interest to people with disabilities.

Ohio

1466 United Cerebral Palsy of Central Ohio
440 Industrial Mile Road
Columbus, OH 43228

614-279-0109
Fax: 914-279-2527
e-mail: gthorpe@ucpofcentralohio.org
www.ucpofcentralohio.org

United Cerebral Palsy provides information, advocacy, referral services for persons with disabilities and/or their families. UCP also operates an equipment loan program, conducts parent workshops, disseminates written literature on topics of interest to people with disabilities.

1467 United Cerebral Palsy of Cincinnati
3601 Victory Parkway
Cincinnati, OH 45229

513-221-4606
Fax: 513-872-5262
e-mail: info@ucp-cincinnati.org
www.ucp-cincinnati.org

United Cerebral Palsy provides information, advocacy, referral services for persons with disabilities and/or their families. UCP also operates an equipment loan program, conducts parent workshops, disseminates written literature on topics of interest to people with disabilities.

1468 United Cerebral Palsy of Greater Cleveland
1011 Euclid Avenue
Cleveland, OH 44106

216-791-8363
Fax: 216-721-3372
e-mail: wmorgan@ucpcleveland.org
www.ucpcleveland.org

United Cerebral Palsy provides information, advocacy, referral services for persons with disabilities and/or their families. UCP also operates an equipment loan program, conducts parent workshops, disseminates written literature on topics of interest to people with disabilities.

Susan A Dean EdD, Executive Director

Oklahoma

1469 United Cerebral Palsy of Oklahoma
10400 Greenbriar Place, Suite 101
Oklahoma City, OK 73159

405-917-7080
800-827-2289
Fax: 405-917-7082
e-mail: info@ucpok.org
www.ucpok.org

United Cerebral Palsy provides information, advocacy, referral services for persons with disabilities and/or their families. UCP also operates an equipment loan program, disseminates written literature on topics of interest to people with disabilities.

Oregon

1470 United Cerebral Palsy of Oregon & SW Washington
11731 Northeast Glenn Widing Drive
Portland, OR 97220

503-777-4166
800-473-4581
Fax: 503-771-8048
e-mail: ucpa@ucpaorwa.org
www.ucpaorwa.org

United Cerebral Palsy provides information, advocacy, referral services for persons with disabilities and/or their families. UCP also operates an equipment loan program, conducts parent workshops, disseminates written literature on topics of interest to people with disabilities.

Pennsylvania

1471 United Cerebral Palsy Central PA
44 South 38th Street
Camp Hill, PA 17011

717-975-0611
Fax: 717-975-0839
e-mail: kidscenter@ucpcentralpa.org
www.ucpcentralpa.org

United Cerebral Palsy provides information, advocacy, referral services for persons with disabilities and/or their families. UCP also operates an equipment loan program, conducts parent workshops, disseminates written literature on topics of interest to people with disabilities.

1472 United Cerebral Palsy of Northeastern Pennsylvania
425 Wyoming Avenue
Scranton, PA 18503

570-347-3357
877-827-8324
Fax: 570-341-5308
TTY: 570-347-3117
e-mail: ucpnepa@epix.net
www.ucpnepa.com

United Cerebral Palsy provides information, advocacy, referral services for persons with disabilities and/or their families. UCP also operates an equipment loan program, conducts parent workshops, disseminates written literature on topics of interest to people with disabilities.

1473 United Cerebral Palsy of Northwestern Pennsylvania
3745 W 12th Street
Erie, PA 16505

814-836-9113
Fax: 814-833-3919
e-mail: leaton@mecaucp.com
www.mecaucp.com

United Cerebral Palsy provides information, advocacy, referral services for persons with disabilities and/or their families. UCP also operates an equipment loan program, conducts parent workshops, disseminates written literature on topics of interest to people with disabilities.

1474 United Cerebral Palsy of Pennsylvania
908 North Second Street
Harrisburg, PA 17102

717-441-6049
866-761-6129
Fax: 717-236-2046
e-mail: info@ucpofpa.org
www.ucpofpa.org

United Cerebral Palsy provides information, advocacy, referral services for persons with disabilities and/or their families. UCP also operates an equipment loan program, conducts parent workshops, disseminates written literature on topics of interest to people with disabilities.

1475 United Cerebral Palsy of Philadelphia & Vicinity
102 E Mermaid Lane
Philadelphia, PA 19118

215-242-4200
Fax: 215-247-4229
e-mail: ucpkravitz@aol.com
www.ucpphila.org

United Cerebral Palsy provides information, advocacy, referral services for persons with disabilities and/or their families. UCP also operates an equipment loan program, conducts parent workshops, disseminates written literature on topics of interest to people with disabilities.

Willis A Dibble, Executive Director

1476 United Cerebral Palsy of Pittsburgh
4638 Centre Avenue
Pittsburgh, PA 15213

412-683-7100
Fax: 412-683-4160
e-mail: info@ucppittsburgh.org
www.ucppittsburgh.org

United Cerebral Palsy provides information, advocacy, referral services for persons with disabilities and/or their families. UCP also operates an equipment loan program, conducts parent workshops, disseminates written literature on topics of interest to people with disabilities.

1477 United Cerebral Palsy of South Central Pennsylvania
788 Cherry Tree Court
Hanover, PA 17331

717-632-5552
Fax: 717-632-2315
e-mail: phoughton@ucpsouthcentral.org
www.ucpsouthcentral.org

United Cerebral Palsy provides information, advocacy, referral services for persons with disabilities and/or their families. UCP also operates an equipment loan program, conducts parent workshops, disseminates written literature on topics of interest to people with disabilities.

1478 United Cerebral Palsy of Southern Allegenies Region
119 Jari Drive
Johnstown, PA 15904

814-262-9600
877-371-1110
Fax: 814-262-9650
e-mail: info@ucpsar.org
www.ucpsar.org

United Cerebral Palsy provides information, advocacy, referral services for persons with disabilities and/or their families. UCP also operates an equipment loan program, conducts parent workshops, disseminates written literature on topics of interest to people with disabilities.

1479 United Cerebral Palsy of Southwestern Pennsylvania
Washington Federal Square
190 North Main Street, Suite 306
Washington, PA 15301

724-229-0851
Fax: 724-229-9252
e-mail: info@ucpswpa.org
www.ucpswpa.org

United Cerebral Palsy provides information, advocacy, referral services for persons with disabilities and/or their families. UCP also operates an equipment loan program, conducts parent workshops, disseminates written literature on topics of interest to people with disabilities.

1480 United Cerebral Palsy of Western Pennsylvania
2904 Seminary Drive
Greensburg, PA 15601

724-832-8272
Fax: 724-837-8278
e-mail: ucp@ucpofwesternpa.org
www.ucpofwesternpa.org

United Cerebral Palsy provides information, advocacy, referral services for persons with disabilities and/or their families. UCP also operates an equipment loan program, conducts parent workshops, disseminates written literature on topics of interest to people with disabilities.

Debra Forsha, Children's Services Director

Rhode Island

1481 United Cerebral Palsy of Rhode Island
200 Main Street, Suite 210, PO Box 36
Pawtucket, RI 02862

401-728-1800
Fax: 401-728-0182
e-mail: ucprisupport@ucpri.org
www.ucpri.org

United Cerebral Palsy provides information, advocacy, referral services for persons with disabilities and/or their families. UCP also operates an equipment loan program, conducts parent workshops, disseminates written literature on topics of interest to people with disabilities.

South Carolina

1482 United Cerebral Palsy of South Carolina a
342 Riverchase Way, Suite C
Lexington, SC 29072

803-926-8878
888-827-7277
Fax: 803-926-1272
e-mail: info@ucpsc.org
www.ucpsc.org

United Cerebral Palsy provides information, advocacy, referral services for persons with disabilities and/or their families. UCP also operates an equipment loan program, conducts parent workshops, disseminates written literature on topics of interest to people with disabilities.

Tennessee

1483 United Cerebral Palsy of Middle Tennessee
1200 9th Avenue Northm Suite 110
Nashville, TN 37208

615-242-4091
Fax: 615-242-3582
e-mail: info@ucpnashville.org
www.ucpnashville.org

United Cerebral Palsy provides information, advocacy, referral services for persons with disabilities and/or their families. UCP also operates an equipment loan program, conducts parent workshops, disseminates written literature on topics of interest to people with disabilities.

1484 United Cerebral Palsy of the Mid-South
4189 Leroy Avenue
Memphis, TN 38108

901-761-4277
Fax: 901-761-7876
e-mail: ucp@ucpmemphis.org
www.ucpmemphis.org

United Cerebral Palsy provides information, advocacy, referral services for persons with disabilities and/or their families. UCP also operates an equipment loan program, conducts parent workshops, disseminates written literature on topics of interest to people with disabilities.

Texas

1485 United Cerebral Palsy of Greater Houston
4500 Bissonet, Suite 340
Bellaire, TX 77401

713-838-9050
Fax: 713-838-9098
e-mail: ucp@ucphouston.org
www.ucphouston.org

United Cerebral Palsy provides information, advocacy, referral services for persons with disabilities and/or their families. UCP also operates an equipment loan program, conducts parent workshops, disseminates written literature on topics of interest to people with disabilities.

1486 United Cerebral Palsy of Metropolitan Dallas
8802 Harry Hines Boulevard
Dallas, TX 75235

214-351-2500
800-999-1898
Fax: 214-351-2610
e-mail: billknudsen@ucpdallas.org
www.ucpdallas.org

United Cerebral Palsy provides information, advocacy, referral services for persons with disabilities and/or their families. UCP also operates an equipment loan program, conducts parent workshops, disseminates written literature on topics of interest to people with disabilities.

Eddy Herrera, Executive Director
Rebecca Adams

1487 United Cerebral Palsy of Tarrant County
1555 Merrimac Circle
Fort Worth, TX 76107

817-332-7171
Fax: 817-332-7601
e-mail: mprather@ucptc.org
www.ucpa.org

United Cerebral Palsy provides information, advocacy, referral services for persons with disabilities and/or their families. UCP also operates an equipment loan program, conducts parent workshops, disseminates written literature on topics of interest to people with disabilities.

1488 United Cerebral Palsy of Texas
1016 La Posada Drive, Suite 145
Austin, TX 78752

512-472-8696
800-798-1492
Fax: 512-472-8026
e-mail: info@ucptexas.org
www.ucptexas.org

United Cerebral Palsy provides information, advocacy, referral services for persons with disabilities and/or their families. UCP also operates an equipment loan program, conducts parent workshops, disseminates written literature on topics of interest to people with disabilities.

Utah

1489 United Cerebral Palsy of Utah
PO Box 65219
South Salt Lake, UT 84165

801-266-1805
Fax: 801-266-2404
e-mail: shellyp@ucputah.org
www.ucputah.org

United Cerebral Palsy provides information, advocacy, referral services for persons with disabilities and/or their families. UCP also operates an equipment loan program, conducts parent workshops, disseminates written literature on topics of interest to people with disabilities.

Virginia

1490 United Cerebral Palsy of Southern & Central Virginia
5291 Greenwich Road
Virginia Beach, VA 23462

757-497-7474
Fax: 757-497-0868
e-mail: ucpofva@pilot.infi.net
www.ucpa.org

United Cerebral Palsy provides information, advocacy, referral services for persons with disabilities and/or their families. UCP also operates an equipment loan program, conducts parent workshops, disseminates written literature on topics of interest to people with disabilities.

1491 United Cerebral Palsy of Washington DC & Northern Virginia
1818 New York Avenue NE, Suite 101
Washington, DC 20002

202-526-0146
Fax: 202-526-0519
e-mail: webmaster@ucpdc.org
www.ucpdc.org

United Cerebral Palsy provides information, advocacy, referral services for persons with disabilities and/or their families. UCP also operates an equipment loan program, conducts parent workshops, disseminates written literature on topics of interest to people with disabilities.

Washington

1492 United Cerebral Palsy of South Puget Sound
633 North Mildred Street, Suite C
Tacoma, WA 98406

253-565-1463
Fax: 253-565-0153
e-mail: info@ucp-sps.org
www.ucp-sps.org

United Cerebral Palsy provides information, advocacy, referral services for persons with disabilities and/or their families. UCP also operates an equipment loan program, conducts parent workshops, disseminates written literature on topics of interest to people with disabilities.

Wisconsin

1493 United Cerebral Palsy of Greater Dane County
1502 Greenway Cross
Madison, WI 53713

608-273-4434
Fax: 608-273-3426
e-mail: ucpgdc@ucpdane.org
www.ucpdane.org

United Cerebral Palsy provides information, advocacy, referral services for persons with disabilities and/or their families. UCP also conducts parent workshops and disseminates written literature on topics of interest to people with disabilities.

1494 United Cerebral Palsy of North Central Wisconsin
108 Scott Street
Wausau, WI 54401

715-842-8700
800-472-4408
e-mail: glamping@ucp-wausau.org
www.ucpa.org

United Cerebral Palsy provides information, advocacy, referral services for persons with disabilities and/or their families. UCP also operates an equipment loan program, conducts parent workshops, disseminates written literature on topics of interest to people with disabilities.

Glenn J Lamping, Executive Director

1495 United Cerebral Palsy of Southeastern Wisconsin
7519 W Oklahoma Avenue
Milwaukee, WI 53219

414-329-4500
888-482-7739
Fax: 414-329-4510
TTY: 414-329-4511
e-mail: info@ucpsew.org
www.ucpsew.org

United Cerebral Palsy provides information, advocacy, referral services for persons with disabilities and/or their families. UCP also operates an equipment loan program, conducts parent workshops, disseminates written literature on topics of interest to people with disabilities.

1496 United Cerebral Palsy of West Central Wisconsin
206 Water Street
Eau Claire, WI 54703

715-832-1782
Fax: 715-832-8203
e-mail: ucpwcw@charterinternet.com
www.ucpwcw.org

United Cerebral Palsy provides information, advocacy, referral services for persons with disabilities and/or their families. UCP also operates an equipment loan program, conducts parent workshops, disseminates written literature on topics of interest to people with disabilities.

Libraries & Resource Centers

1497 National Rehabilitation Information Center
4200 Forbes Blvd, Suite 202
Lanham, MD 20706

301-459-5900
800-346-2742
Fax: 301-459-4263
TTY: 301-459-5984
e-mail: naricinfo@heitechservices.com
www.naric.com

Committed to providing direct, personal and high quality information services to anyone interested in disability rehabilitation issues; Committed to serving consumers, researchers, family members, health professionals, educators, counselors, students, librarians and the administrators throughout the country.

Mark Odum, Director

Research Centers

1498 Orthopaedic Biomechanics Laboratory
Shriners Hospital for Crippled Children
1701 19th Avenue
San Francisco, CA 94122

415-665-1100
Fax: 415-661-3615

Offers research and studies into cerebral palsy.

Stephen R Skinner, Clinical Director

1499 United Cerebral Palsy Research and Educational Foundation
1660 L Street NW, Suite 700
Washington, DC 20036

202-973-7140
800-872-5827
Fax: 202-776-0414
e-mail: national@ucp.org
www.ucpresearch.org

Provides research grants to prevent cerebral palsy and to improve treatment, management and functioning of persons with cerebral palsy.

Audio Video

1500 Accidents of Nature
Random House
1745 Broadway
New York, NY 10019

212-782-9000
www.randomhouse.com

About a girl who goes to a camp and has experiences that will change her life forever. Audio book feature.

2006
ISBN: 0-739335-30-8

1501 I Am Not What You See
Filmakers Library
124 E 40th Street
New York, NY 10016

212-808-4980
Fax: 212-808-4983
e-mail: inf@filmmakers.com
www.filmmakers.com

Sondra Diamond was born with cerebral palsy. The result of that syndrome was that Sondra became a quadriplegic with limited ability to care for herself.

Films

Web Sites

1502 American Academy for Cerebral Palsy and Developmental Medicine
www.aacpdm.org

Organization of professionals involved in the care of people with Cerebral Palsy, developmental disorders, and related diseases.

1503 Cerebral Palsy Support Network
www.home.aone.net.au/cpsn/

We aim to promote the principles of community inclusion for individuals with Cerebral Palsy, and their families, offers support to members by linking them together, as well as liking members to services and programs that are relevant and sensitive to their needs, to help empower people with cerebral palsy, and thier families, by providing regular relevant information. To raise community awareness of Cerebral Palsy.

1504 Children's Neurobiological Solutions Foundation
www.cnsfoundation.org

Children's Neurobiological Solutions Foundation (CNS), is a national, nonprofit, 501(c)(3) organization, whose mission is to orchestrate cutting-edge, collaborative research with the goal of expediting the creation of effective treatments and therapies for children with neurodevelopmental abnormalities, birth injuries to the nervous system, and related neurological problems.

1505 Easter Seals Disability Services
www.easterseals.com

For more than 80 years, Easter Seals has helped people with disabilities in communities nationwide. From creating the first national voluntary act on behalf of children with disabilities in the 1920's to leading the creation and implementation of the Americans with Disabilities Act in the 1990's. Easter Seals child development services build strong foundations for children of all abilities.

1506 Family Support Network
www.tsalliance.org

The Support Network is an organized partnership of individuals whose lives have been affected by tuberous sclerosis. Across the nation, the Support Network is providing the latest medical information, education and support to those individuals who are seeking understanding about the genetic disease and offering them words of encouragement and empowerment.

1507 Health Answers
www.healthanswers.com

The vision was to provide a breadth of services to clients through the formation of a network of companies. Each company plays a key role in meeting out clients' needs.

1508 Infinitec
www.infinitec.org

The mission of Infinitec is to advance independence and promote inclusive opportunities for children and adults with disabilities throught technology.

1509 National Dissemination Center for Children with Disabilities
www.nichcy.org

A national information and referral center that provides information on disabilities and disability-related issues for families, educators and other professionals.

1510 Scope (UK)
www.scope.org.uk/

Our aim is that disabled people achieve equality: a society in which they are as valued and have the same human and civil rights as everyone else.

1511 United Cerebral Palsy Associations
www.ucp.org

The UCP is the leading source of information on cerebral palsy and is a pivitol advocate for the rights of persons with any disability. As one of the largest health charities in America, UCP's mission is to advance the independence, productivity and full citizenship of people with Cerebral Palsy and other diabilities.

1512 WE MOVE (Worldwide Education and Advocacy for Movement Disorders)
www.wemove.org

WE MOVE provides movement disorder information and educational materials to physicians, patients and families, the media, and the public via its comprehensive Web sites, training courses, and more. Its goal is to make early diagnosis, up-to-date treatment and patient support a reality for all people living with movement disorders.

Book Publishers

1513 A Mother's Touch: The Tiffany Callo Story
United Cerebral Palsy Associations
1660 L Street NW, Suite 700
Washington, DC 20005

202-776-0406
800-872-5823
Fax: 202-776-0414
e-mail: ucpnatl@ucpa.org
www.ucpa.org

A vivid portrayal of a woman with cerebral palsy who faced discrimination because of her disability.

1514 After the Tears: Parents Talk About Raising a Child with a Disability
United Cerebral Palsy Associations
1522 L Street NW, Suite 700
Washington, DC 20036

202-776-0406
800-872-5823
Fax: 202-776-0414
e-mail: ucpnatl@ucpa.org
www.ucpa.org

Book draws on stories of parents who have struggled, learned and grown in the years since their child was born with a disability.

89 pages Softcover

1515 An Introduction to Your Child Who Has Cerebral Palsy
Medic Publishing Company
PO Box 89
Redmond, WA 98073

425-881-2883

Information and answers to questions for parents of children with cerebral palsy.

1516 Breaking Ground: Ten Families Building Opportunities Through Integration

United Cerebral Palsy Associations
1522 L Street NW, Suite 700
Washington, DC 20036

202-776-0406
800-872-5823
Fax: 202-776-0414
e-mail: ucpnatl@ucpa.org
www.ucpa.org

Gives examples of strategies families have used to integrate the children fully into their schools and communities.

75 pages Softcover

1517 Can't You be Still?

Gemma B Publishing
Box 713-776 Corydon Avenue
Winnipeg, Manitoba,
Canada

204-452-7566
Fax: 204-475-9903
e-mail: gernpub@mts.net
www.gemmab.mb.ca

This wonderfully written children's book features a heroine, Ann, with cerebral palsy going to school for the first time. First in a trilogy, written in first person, since Ann cannot speak out loud.

28 pages Softcover

Sarah Yates
Anne Allan

1518 Cerebral Palsy

Franklin Watts c/o Grolier
90 Old Sherman Turnpike
Danbury, CT 06816

203-797-3500
Fax: 203-797-3197
www.grolier.com

A look at the causes, detection, prevention, effects and treatment of Cerebral Palsy.

112 pages Grades 7-12
ISBN: 0-531125-29-7

1519 Children With Cerebral Palsy: A Parents Guide

Peytral Publications
PO Box 1162
Minnetonka, MN 55345

952-949-8707
877-739-8725
Fax: 952-906-9777
www.peytral.com

Informative handbook for parents of children and teens; covers medical, educational, legal, family life, daily care, emotional issues and more.

470 pages

1520 Children with Cerebral Palsy

Woodbine House
6510 Bells Mill Road
Bethesda, MD 20817

301-897-3570
Fax: 301-897-5838
e-mail: info@woodbinehouse.com
www.woodbinehouse.com

Explains what Cerebral Palsy is and discusses its diagnosis and treatment. Also offers information and advice concerning daily care, early intervention, therapy, educational options and family life.

1998 470 pages Paperback
ISBN: 0-933149-82-4

1521 Congenital Disorders Sourcebook 2nd Edition

Omnigraphics
PO Box 625
Holmes, PA 19043

800-234-1340
Fax: 800-875-1340
e-mail: info@omnigraphics.com
www.omnigraphics.com

Provides basic consumer health information about the most common types of nonhereditary birth defects and disorders related to prematurity, gestational injuries, congenital infections, and birth complications, including disorders of the heart, brain, gastrointestinal tract, musculoskeletal system, urinary tract, and reproductive system, craniofacial disorders, cerebral palsy, spina bifida, and fetal alcohol syndrome, and detailing the causes, diagnostic tests, and treatments for each.

650 pages
ISBN: 0-780809-45-9

1522 Connecting Students: A Guide to Thoughtful Friendship Facilitation

United Cerebral Palsy Associations
1522 L Street NW, Suite 700
Washington, DC 20036

202-776-0406
800-872-5823
Fax: 202-776-0414
e-mail: ucpnatl@ucpa.org
www.ucpa.org

Contains helpful strategies on real-life experiences on building friendships.

48 pages Softcover

1523 Discovery Book

United Cerebral Palsy Association
959 Transport Way, A-1
Petaluma, CA 94952

707-765-6770

Created within a United Cerebral Palsy group for children with physical disabilities, The Discovery Book is an exploration of social and psychological aspects of childhood disability. Accompanied by their artwork, children speak in their own words about important areas of life such as: What about friends?; Doctors and hospitals; Problems and challenges; and Goals, wishes & dreams.

96 pages

1524 Each of Us Remembers: Parents of Children With Cerebral Palsy

United Cerebral Palsy Associations
1522 L Street NW, Suite 700
Washington, DC 20036

202-776-0406
800-872-5823
Fax: 202-776-0414
e-mail: ucpnatl@ucpa.org
www.ucpa.org

Parents of children with cerebral palsy answer questions that people really need to know.

1525 Handling the Young Cerebral Palsied Child at Home

United Cerebral Palsy Associations
1522 L Street NW, Suite 700
Washington, DC 20036

202-776-0406
800-872-5823
Fax: 202-776-0414
e-mail: ucpnatl@ucpa.org
www.ucpa.org

Offers chapters on bathing, feeding, dressing and play for parents of children with cerebral palsy.

337 pages Softcover

1526 Here's What I Mean to Say
Gemma B Publishing
Box 713-776 Corydon Avenue
Winnipeg, Manitoba,
Canada

204-452-7566
Fax: 204-475-9903
e-mail: gernpub@mts.net
www.gemmab.mb.ca

Third in the Ann trilogy. Ann's father gets her a computer and with Jay and Mum's help, she explores and uncovers the world of literacy, fantasy and reality.

24 pages
ISBN: 0-969647-72-7

Sarah Yates
Anne Allan

1527 Karen
Dell Publishing
666 5th Avenue
New York, NY 10103

212-765-6500

After seeing many doctors, the family found that Karen had cerebral palsy. The parents developed many ways to deal with Karen's problems and spent all their time and money to figure out simulation activities.

286 pages Paperback
ISBN: 0-440943-76-0

1528 Mine for Keeps
Little, Brown & Co.
34 Beacon Street
Boston, MA 02108

617-227-0730

Sarah Jean Copeland was born with cerebral palsy. At four years of age she was placed in a school for handicapped children but made such good progress that she could return home. Coming home for Sarah meant a new school, and new adjustments to her parents, two sisters and her brother. At first Sarah was scared and didn't think she could do all the things she needed to do, but she soon learned her fears were not well-founded.

186 pages Hardcover

1529 My Brother, Matthew
Woodbine House
6510 Bells Mill Road
Bethesda, MD 20817

301-468-8800
800-843-7323
Fax: 301-897-5838
e-mail: info@woodbinehouse.com
www.woodbinehouse.com

A book written from the point of view of David, the brother of Matthew, who has multiple disabilities. David describes the incidents characterizing how life in his family changes.

28 pages Grades K-5

Sarah Strickler

1530 Natural Supports in School/Work/Community for the Severely Disabled
United Cerebral Palsy Associations
1522 L Street NW, Suite 700
Washington, DC 20036

202-776-0406
800-872-5823
Fax: 202-776-0414
e-mail: ucpnatl@ucpa.org
www.ucpa.org

Promotes the position that assistance must be defined by the needs of individuals rather than the requirements of the service systems.

361 pages Softcover

1531 No Time for Jello: One Family's Experience
Brookline Books
34 University Road
Brookline, MA 02445

617-734-6772
Fax: 617-734-3952
http://brooklinebooks.com

One family's story of their attempts to remediate and cure the effects of cerebral palsied condition the oldest son was born with. The Bratts traveled traditional routes, through distinguished medical centers in Boston, and nontraditional routes in a search for treatments that would help their son.

Softcover
ISBN: 0-253363-65-9

1532 Nobody Knows
Gemma B Publishing
Box 713-776 Corydon Avenue
Winnipeg, Manitoba,
Canada

204-452-7566
Fax: 204-475-9903
e-mail: gernpub@mts.net
www.gemmab.mb.ca

Childrens book with heroine Ann, who is very frustrated when no one can understand the words inside her head. With her friend Jay, she sets out to find someone who will understand what she wants. Second in a trilogy, written in first person, since Ann cannot speak out loud.

24 pages
ISBN: 0-969647-71-9

Sarah Yates
Anne Allan

1533 Opening Doors: Strategies for Including All Students in Regular Education
United Cerebral Palsy Associations
1522 L Street NW, Suite 700
Washington, DC 20036

202-776-0406
800-872-5823
Fax: 202-776-0414
e-mail: ucpnatl@ucpa.org
www.ucpa.org

Contains practical information for including and supporting all students in regular classes.

55 pages Softcover

1534 Teaching Motor Skills to Children with Cerebral Palsy & Similar Movement Disorders
Woodbine House
6510 Bells Mill Road
Bethesda, MD 20817

301-897-3570
Fax: 301-897-5838
e-mail: info@woodbinehouse.com
www.woodbinehouse.com

The resource that parents, therapists, and other caregivers can consult to help children with gross motor delays learn and practice motor skills outside of therapy sessions.

2006 275 pages
ISBN: 1-890627-72-0

1535 Walk with Me
United Cerebral Palsy Associations
1522 L Street NW, Suite 700
Washington, DC 20036

202-776-0406
800-872-5823
Fax: 202-776-0414
e-mail: ucpnatl@ucpa.org
www.ucpa.org

A story written by eight-year-old Eric Grimm covering his thoughts on living with cerebral palsy.

Newsletters

1536 Family Support Bulletin

United Cerebral Palsy Associations
1522 L Street NW, Suite 700
Washington, DC 20036

202-776-0406
800-872-5823
Fax: 202-776-0414
e-mail: ucpnatl@ucpa.org
www.ucpa.org

A detailed quarterly journal that takes a comprehensive look at the latest policies, resources and legislative information enacted in Washington and state capitals.

Quarterly

1537 Networker

United Cerebral Palsy Associations
1522 L Street NW, Suite 700
Washington, DC 20036

202-776-0406
800-872-5823
Fax: 202-776-0414
e-mail: ucpnatl@ucpa.org
www.ucpa.org

Offers the latest information on the newest technology available for persons with cerebral palsy.

Quarterly

Pamphlets

1538 Cerebral Palsy-Facts & Figures

United Cerebral Palsy Associations
1660 L Street NW
Washington, DC 20036

Fax: 202-776-0414
www.ucp.org

Offers information on what cerebral palsy is, the effects, causes, types, and prevention.

Camps

1539 Cerebral Palsy Center Summer Program

7 Sanford Avenue
Belleville, NJ

201-751-0200
www2.kidscamps.com

DESCRIPTION

1541 CHARCOT-MARIE-TOOTH DISEASE

Charcot-Marie-Tooth (CMT) disease belongs to a group of disorders known as hereditary motor-sensory neuropathies or HMSNs. The HMSNs are progressive disorders of nerves outside of the central nervous system that extend from the brain and spinal cord to particular areas of the body (peripheral nervous system). Symptoms and findings associated with these disorders are primarily the result of involvement of motor nerve fibers (those that affect motion). These nerves transmit various nerve impulses away from the brain and spinal cord to their termination (e.g., muscle tissue). As these disorders progress, affected individuals may experience some symptoms due to sensory and autonomic involvement. Sensory nerve fibers carry impulses to the brain and spinal cord. The autonomic nervous system is the portion of the peripheral nervous system that regulates involuntary functioning of particular tissues and organs.

There are different types of Charcot-Marie-Tooth disease that have varying modes of inheritance. Charcot-Marie-Tooth disease (in all its forms) is the most prevalent hereditary peripheral neuropathy, affecting approximately one in 2,500 individuals. The most common form of the disease, known as Charcot-Marie-Tooth disease type 1A or CMT1A, is inherited as an autosomal dominant trait. A disease gene for CMT1A is located on the short arm of chromosome 17.

Children with CMT type 1A usually do not have associated symptoms until late childhood or early adolescence. However, some may experience abnormalities in their manner of walking (gait disturbances) as early as the second year of life. In other, rare instances, associated symptoms may not become apparent until middle adulthood. CMT1A initially affects muscles supplied by nerves of the lower legs (peroneal and tibial nerves), causing muscle degeneration (atrophy) in the lower legs and feet. This is accompanied by muscle weakness and a distinctive stork-like contour of the legs. Bending movements of the ankles become progressively weaker, eventually resulting in footdrop, a condition in which the foot does not flex or bend upward. In addition, the arch of the foot becomes unusually increased in height (pescavus deformities). An unstable gait may develop, and children may appear clumsy, easily tripping or falling. Although muscles of both legs are affected, disease progression and associated findings usually differ slightly from one side of the body to the other.

As the disorder progresses, individuals with CMT1A also usually develop a loss of muscle tissue mass and weakness in the forearms and hands. These areas seem to be less severely affected than the lower legs. However, patients may eventually develop permanent fixation of certain joints in a bend position. This typically occurs in the fingers and wrists. Some patients also experience gradual sensory involvement, such as abnormal burning or tingling sensations (paresthesias) in the feet. Associated autonomic abnormalities may include unusual paleness (pallor) or blotching of the skin, especially of the feet. In individuals with CMT1A, specialized testing typically reveals a marked reduction in the transmission of motor and sensory nerve signals to affected muscles (reduced conduction velocities).

Although CMT1A is progressive, most affected individuals maintain the ability to walk. However, the use of special orthopedic appliances, such as stiff boots that reach to the midcalf, plastic splints, or light leg braces, are typically necessary to help stabilize the ankles. Surgical measures may be considered, such as surgical fusion of the ankles. In addition, certain medications may help to alleviate burning sensations in the feet (e.g., carbamazepine or phenytoin). Other treatment is symptomatic and supportive.

In addition to Charcot-Marie-Tooth disease type 1A, additional autosomal dominant, autosomal recessive, and X-linked forms of the disease have been identified. Specific symptoms and findings and the nature of the disorder progression may vary, depending upon the specific form of the disease.

See also **General Resources** on page 917

State Agencies & Support Groups

New York

1542 CMTA Chapter - New York (Greater)
CMT Association
400 E 34th Street
Manhattan, NY 10016

212-535-4314
Fax: 212-535-4314
e-mail: david.younger@med.nyu.edu
www.cmtnyc.org

Every other month (Third Saturday from 1:00 - 3:00 p.m.) - check website

Dr David Younger, Contact

Ohio

1543 CMTA Chapter - Ohio
CMT Association
405 Wagner Avenue
Greenville, OH 45331

937-548-3963
e-mail: Greenville-Ohio-CMT@who.rr.com
www.charcot-marie-tooth.org

Fourth Thursday, April - October

Dot Cain, Contact

Pennsylvania

1544 CMTA Chapter - Pennsylvania
CMT Association
2700 Chestnut Street
Chester, PA 19013

610-499-9264
800-606-2682
Fax: 610-499-9267
e-mail: cmtassoc@aol.com
www.charcot-marie-tooth.org

Bi-monthly (3rd Saturday, 10:00 a.m. - 12:00 p.m.)

Dana Schwertfeger, Contact
Pat Dreibelbis, Contact

Audio Video

1545 Charcot-Marie-Tooth Disease: A Brief Overview
CMT International
One Springbank Drive
Saint Catharines, Ontario, L2S

905-687-3630
Fax: 905-687-8753
e-mail: cmtint@vaxxine.com
www.cmtint.org

Profiles of five people who have various degrees of CMT.

17 minutes

Linda Crabtree, Founder/Executive Director

Web Sites

1546 CMT Net
www.ultranet.com/~smith/CMTnet.html

CMTNet is intended to provide information for both the medical and non-medical communities.

1547 Charcot-Marie-Tooth Association
www.charcot-marie-tooth.org

Information regarding patient support, public education, promotion of research and ultimately the treatment and cure of CMT.

1548 Charcot-Marie-Tooth International
www.cmtint.org

A support group for people who are affected by Charcot-Marie-Tooth Disease.

1549 Health Answers
www.healthanswers.com

The vision was to provide a breadth of services to clients through the formation of a network of companies. Each company plays a key role in meeting our clients' needs.

1550 Muscular Dystrophy Association
www.mdausa.org/publications/fa-cmt.html

Information regarding neuromuscular diseases through programs of worldwide research, comprehensive medical and community services, and far-reaching professional and public health education.

Book Publishers

1551 Charcot-Marie-Tooth Disorders: A Handbook for Primary Care Physicians
Charcot-Marie-Tooth Association
2700 Chestnut Street
Chester, PA 19013

610-499-9264
800-606-2682
Fax: 610-499-9267
e-mail: info@charcot-marie-tooth.org
www.charcot-marie-tooth.org

Excellent source of information about the causes, symptoms, and treatment/management of CMT.

1995 130 pages

1552 Let's Talk About Going to the Hospital
Rosen Publishing Group's PowerKids Press
29 E 21st Street
New York, NY 10010

212-777-3017
800-237-9932
Fax: 888-436-4643
e-mail: rosenpub@tribeca.ios.com
www.powerkidspress.com

If a child has to check into the hospital, chances are he or she is already upset about being ill. Knowing how a hospital functions and what the procedures are, such as when family members can visit, will help in what is already a stressful situation. Grades K-5.

24 pages
ISBN: 0-823950-36-0

Magazines

1553 MDA/ALS Newsmagazine
Muscular Dystrophy Association
3300 E Sunrise Drive
Tucson, AZ 85718

800-344-4863
www.mdausa.org

provides information about ALS.

1554 Quest
Muscular Dystrophy Association
3300 E Sunrise Drive
Tucson, AZ 85718

800-344-4863
www.mdausa.org

Contains stories about vital concerns of people with neuromuscular diseases, their friends, families and caregivers.

Bi-Monthly

Newsletters

1555 CMT Newsletter
CMT International
One Springbank Drive
Saint Catharines, Ontario, L2S

905-687-3630
Fax: 905-687-8753
e-mail: cmtint@vaxxine.com
www.cmtint.org

Offers information on all facets of CMT, articles by doctors, research reports, drugs that can make the disorder worse, and many letters and articles from readers who have CMT or HNPP.

32 pages 6 times a year

Linda Crabtree, Founder/Executive Director

1556 CMTA Report

CMT Association
2700 Chestnut Street
Chester, PA 19013

610-499-9264
Fax: 610-499-9267
e-mail: info@charcot-marie-tooth.org
www.charcot-marie-tooth.org

Contains articles on CMT topics, research news and patient pro-files. Free with membership.

Bi-Monthly

Patricia Dreibelbis, Editor

Pamphlets

1557 Accepting CMT: The Grieving Process and You

CMT International
One Springbank Drive
Saint Catharines, Ontario, L2S

905-687-3630
Fax: 905-687-8753
e-mail: cmtint@vaxxine.com
www.cmtint.org

1558 Basics of Charcot-Marie-Tooth Disease

CMT International
One Springbank Drive
Saint Catharines, Ontario, L2S

905-687-3630
Fax: 905-687-8753
e-mail: cmtint@vaxxine.com
www.cmtint.org

Questions answered and what you need to know to look after your-self. This information is sent out to every new member in their in-troductory kit.

Linda Crabtree, Founder/Executive Director

1559 Bracing Available for CMT Feet and Ankles

CMT International
One Springbank Drive
Saint Catharines, Ontario, L2S

905-687-3630
Fax: 905-687-8753
e-mail: cmtint@vaxxine.com
www.cmtint.org

1560 CMT & Exercise

CMT International
One Springbank Drive
Saint Catharines, Ontario, L2S

905-687-3630
Fax: 905-687-8753
e-mail: 194int@vaxxine.com
www.cmtint.org

Excerpts from the CMT Newsletter, plus how to test to see if you are exercising muscles served by CMT affected nerves.

1561 CMT Brochure

Charcot-Marie-Tooth Association
2700 Chestnut Street
Chester, PA 19013

610-499-9264
800-606-2682
Fax: 610-499-9267
e-mail: info@charcot-marie-tooth.org
www.charcot-marie-tooth.org

Provides a quick overview of CMT.

2005 8 pages

1562 CMT Facts I

Charcot-Marie-Tooth Association
2700 Chestnut Street
Chester, PA 19013

610-499-9264
Fax: 610-499-9267
e-mail: info@charcot-marie-tooth.org
www.charcot-marie-tooth.org

Offers information on the neurotrophic drugs, genetics and thera-pies for CMT, surgical options and an overview of the disorder.

1993 16 pages

1563 CMT Facts II

Charcot-Marie-Tooth Association
2700 Chestnut Street
Chester, PA 19013

610-499-9264
Fax: 610-499-9267
e-mail: info@charcot-marie-tooth.org
www.charcot-marie-tooth.org

Offers information on adaptive devices, feature specialists and the Americans with disabilities act.

1993 24 pages

1564 CMT Facts III

Charcot-Marie-Tooth Association
2700 Chestnut Street
Chester, PA 19013

610-499-9264
Fax: 610-499-9267
e-mail: info@charcot-marie-tooth.org
www.charcot-marie-tooth.org

Offers information on neurotrophic drugs, neuromuscular disor-ders, genetic news and doctor's questions and answers.

1995 24 pages

1565 CMT Facts IV

Charcot-Marie-Tooth Association
2700 Chestnut Street
Chester, PA 19013

610-499-9264
800-606-2682
Fax: 610-499-9267
e-mail: info@charcot-marie-tooth.org
www.charcot-marie-tooth.org

Provides information for Charcot-Marie-Tooth patients.

1998 32 pages

1566 CMT Facts V

Charcot-Marie-Tooth Association
2700 Chestnut Street
Chester, PA 19013

610-499-9264
800-606-2682
Fax: 610-499-9267
e-mail: info@charcot-marie-tooth.org
www.charcot-marie-tooth.org

Source for information on orthotics, pain, emotional, HNPP, physi-cal and occupational therapy, Social Security Disability and more.

2002 56 pages

1567 CMT Feet

CMT International
One Springbank Drive
Saint Catharines, Ontario, L2S

905-687-3630
Fax: 905-687-8753
e-mail: cmtint@vaxxine.com
www.cmtint.org

1568 CMT Hands
CMT International
One Springbank Drive
Saint Catharines, Ontario, L2S

905-687-3630
Fax: 905-687-8753
e-mail: cmtint@vaxxine.com
www.cmtint.org

1569 CMT and Alternate Therapies
CMT International
One Springbank Drive
Saint Catharines, Ontario, L2S

905-687-3630
Fax: 905-687-8753
e-mail: cmtint@vaxxine.com
www.cmtint.org

Some experiences of members and good books.

Linda Crabtree, Founder/Executive Director

1570 CMT and Coping with the Pain
CMT International
One Springbank Drive
Saint Catharines, Ontario, L2S

905-687-3630
Fax: 905-687-8753
e-mail: cmtint@vaxxine.com
www.cmtint.org

Linda Crabtree, Founder/Executive Director

1571 CMT and Dentistry
CMT International
One Springbank Drive
Saint Catharines, Ontario, L2S

905-687-3630
Fax: 905-687-8753
e-mail: cmtint@vaxxine.com
www.cmtint.org

1572 CMT, Children and Youth
CMT International
One Springbank Drive
Saint Catharines, Ontario, L2S

905-687-3630
Fax: 905-687-8753
e-mail: cmtint@vaxxine.com
www.cmtint.org

Linda Crabtree, Founder/Executive Director

1573 Charcot-Marie-Tooth Disease and Anesthetics
CMT International
One Springbank Drive
Saint Catharines, Ontario, L2S

905-687-3630
Fax: 905-687-8753
e-mail: cmtint@vaxxine.com
www.cmtint.org

Linda Crabtree, Founder/Executive Director

1574 Charcot-Marie-Tooth Disease and Wellness
CMT International
One Springbank Drive
Saint Catharines, Ontario, L2S

905-687-3630
Fax: 905-687-8753
e-mail: cmtint@vaxxine.com
www.cmtint.org

The signs and symptoms of CMT and how to keep yourself as well as possible.

Linda Crabtree, Founder/Executive Director

1575 Charcot-Marie-Tooth Disorders: A Guide abo ut Genetics for Patients
Charcot-Marie-Tooth Association
2700 Chestnut Street
Chester, PA 19013

610-499-9264
800-606-2682
Fax: 610-499-9267
e-mail: info@charcot-marie-tooth.org
www.charcot-marie-tooth.org

Illustrated with easy-to-understand diagrams, this booklet outlines the basics of genetics inheritance and CMT.

2000 21 pages

1576 Diagnosing CMT
CMT International
One Springbank Drive
Saint Catharines, Ontario, L2S

905-687-3630
Fax: 905-687-8753
e-mail: cmtint@vaxxine.com
www.cmtint.org

How a diagnosis is made.

Linda Crabtree, Founder/Executive Director

1577 Facts About Charcot-Marie-Tooth Disease an d Dejerine-Sottas
Muscular Dystrophy Association
3300 E Sunrise Drive
Tucson, AZ 85718

520-529-2000
800-572-1717
Fax: 520-529-5300
e-mail: publications@mdausa.org
www.mda.org/publications/fa-cmt.html

Covers the basic knowledge of both diseases in order to prepare patents for present and future challanges. It outlines the character-istics and genetic patterns of the CMTs. Research efforts aimed at finding the causes, treatments, and cures are also described. Also available in Spanish and online.

15 pages Paperback

1578 MDA Fact Sheet
Muscular Dystrophy Association
3300 E Sunrise Drive
Tucson, AZ 85718

800-344-4863
e-mail: mda@mdausa.org
www.mdausa.org

Provides information about the association, how it got started, and what muscular dystrophy can affect the body.

1579 When You Fall
CMT International
One Springbank Drive
Saint Catharines, Ontario, L2S

905-687-3630
Fax: 905-687-8753
e-mail: cmtint@vaxxine.com
www.cmtint.org

How to prepare yourself for the inevitable.

DESCRIPTION

1580 CHILDHOOD DERMATOMYOSITIS

Synonym: Juvenile dermatomyosis (JDMS)

Involves the following Biologic System(s):

Connective Tissue Disorders, Dermatologic Disorders, Orthopedic and Muscle Disorders

Dermatomyosis is a connective tissue disorder characterized by inflammatory and degenerative changes of the muscles and distinctive lesions of the skin. Although the disorder may become apparent at any time, it most commonly occurs in children between five to 15 years of age or adults between the ages of 40 to 60 years. In children, the average age at onset is eight or nine years. More females than males are affected by dermatomyosis.

The cause of dermatomyosis is unknown. However, immune, genetic, and environmental factors are thought to play some role. Many researchers suggest that dermatomyosis is an autoimmune disorder resulting from abnormal immune responses directed against the body's own tissues.

The symptoms and findings associated with childhood dermatomyosis are similar to those seen in the adult form of the disease. However, involvement of the gastrointestinal (GI) tract and the development of abnormal calcium deposits (calcifications) within skin and muscle tissues are more frequent and widespread in childhood dermatomyosis. Affected children usually have widespread inflammation of small blood vessels (vasculitis) within connective tissues of the skin, muscles, tissues beneath the skin (subcutaneous tissues), and tissues underlying the nails (nail beds). In addition, cancerous growths (malignancies) occur in approximately 20 percent of affected adults; malignancies are rarely seen in those with childhood dermatomyosis.

In most patients with childhood dermatomyosis, the onset of symptoms is relatively gradual and subtle. Children initially experience slowly progressive muscle weakness affecting the upper arms, shoulders, hips, and thighs (proximal muscles) as well as the trunk. Involved muscles tend to be sore, stiff, tender, or abnormally hard. Affected children may develop an awkward manner of walking and gradually lose the ability to perform certain tasks, such as lifting the arms above the shoulders, combing their hair, dressing, climbing stairs, or rising from the floor unassisted. Involved muscles may eventually show varying degrees of degeneration (atrophy) and, in severe cases, permanent bending or extension in various fixed postures

(joint contractures). Although muscles of the upper arms or legs are typically most severely affected, any muscle may become involved. In severe cases, affected muscles may include those of the roof of the mouth and those involved in respiration, resulting in a nasal quality to the voice; breathing difficulties; hyperventilation; inadvertent breathing of foreign materials into the respiratory passages (bronchial aspiration); and potentially life-threatening complications. In addition, involvement of muscles of the gastrointestinal tract may cause difficulties swallowing; abdominal pain; passage of dark, tarry stools containing digested blood (melena); and infrequent bowel movements or difficulty passing stools (constipation). In severe cases, gastrointestinal bleeding (hemorrhage) or other associated abnormalities (e.g., intestinal perforations) may cause potentially life-threatening conditions .

Patients with childhood dermatomyosis also develop characteristic skin changes, such as a reddish-purple rash of the upper eyelids (heliotrope rash); an abnormal accumulation of fluid in body tissues surrounding the eyes and in other facial areas (periorbital and facial edema); a reddish rash across the skin of the nose and cheeks (butterfly rash); and reddish-purple, raised, scaling skin lesions (papules) on the surfaces of certain joints, particularly the knuckles (Gottron's sign), elbows, and knees. These scaling lesions develop a central area of tissue loss (atrophy) that lacks color (vitiligo) or has increased pigmentation (hyperpigmentation). Patients may also have a dusky reddish rash covering the upper arms and legs and the upper trunk.

Approximately 20 to 50 percent of affected children also develop abnormal calcium deposits (calcifications) within muscle, skin, and subcutaneous tissues. These deposits may contribute to localized areas of muscle loss or the freezing of joints in permanently bent positions. Some patients may also experience additional symptoms and findings, such as a low-grade fever, joint inflammation (arthritis), enlargement of the liver and spleen (hepatosplenomegaly), or other abnormalities. In most patients, childhood dermatomyosis gradually becomes inactive over several years.

The treatment of patients with childhood dermatomyosis requires early, aggressive measures to help prevent potentially life-threatening complications. Such measures include evaluation to detect possible involvement of the respiratory or gastrointestinal systems and provision of ongoing nursing care for those with such involvement. Such care may include mechanical suctioning of the throat by way of the nose (nasopharyngeal suction), the creation of a temporary opening in the throat to ease breathing difficulties (tracheostomy), or mechanical breathing support (e.g., endotracheal intubation or respirator). In addition, the treatment of patients typically includes the use of corticosteroids (e.g., prednisone) to help suppress the inflammatory process of the disease. Blood levels of certain muscle enzymes are regularly measured to help gauge the effectiveness of such therapy. Once such enzyme levels are reduced to normal ranges, the steroid dosage may gradually be decreased to as low as possible while still being effective, owing to the numerous problems associated with prolonged administration or high-dose steroids. After about two years, such treatment may be discontinued without the reemergence of symptoms. In patients who do not respond to steroid therapy, certain immunosuppressant drugs such as methotrexate, azathioprine, or cyclosporine or, in some patients, intravenous immunoglobulin therapy may be beneficial. In addition, treatment may include surgical removal of calcium deposits. Physical therapy (e.g., passive exercises, eventual progression to active exercises) is important in helping to rebuild muscle strength and prevent permanent, disabling contractures. Splints may be required to help ensure proper positioning of certain limbs. Proper skin hygiene is also important in patients with childhood dermatomyositis.

See also **General Resources** on page 917

National Associations & Support Groups

1581 American Autoimmune Related Diseases Association
22100 Gratiot Avenue
E Detroit, MI 48021

586-776-3900
www.aarda.org

Dedicated to the eradication of autoimmune diseases and the alleviation of suffering and the socio-economic impact of autoimmunity through fostering and facilitating collaboration in the areas of education, public awareness, research and patient services in an effective, ethical and efficient manner.

Virginia Ladd, Director

1582 American Osteopathic College of Dermatology
1501 E Illinois Street, PO Box 7525
Kirksville, MO 63501

660-665-2184
800-449-2623
Fax: 660-627-2623
e-mail: info@aocd.org
www.aocd.org

Strives to improve the standards of the practice of dermatology, to stimulate the study and extend knowledge in the field of dermatology, and to promote a more general understanding of the nature and scope of services rendered by osteopathic dermatologists to other divisions of practice, hospitals, clinics and the public.

Rebecca A Mansfield, Executive Director

1583 Arthritis Foundation
PO Box 7669
Atlanta, GA 30357

404-872-7100
800-568-4045
Fax: 404-872-0457
www.arthritis.org

The only nonprofit organization that supports the more than 100 types of arthritis and related conditions with advocacy, programs, services and research.

John H Klippel MD, President & CEO

1584 Juvenile Dermatomyositis
Arthritis Foundation
PO Box 7669
Atlanta, GA 30357

404-872-7100
800-283-7800
Fax: 404-872-0457
e-mail: info@jdfcure.com
www.atrhritis.org

1585 Myositis Association of America
1233 20th Street NW, Suite 402
Washington, DC 20036

202-887-0088
Fax: 202-466-8940
e-mail: tma@myositis.org
www.myositis.org

The mission of The Myositis Association is to find a cure for inflammatory and other related myopathies, while serving those affected by these diseases.

Bob Goldberg, Executive Director

1586 New Onset Juvenile Dermatomytosis Registry
Children's Memorial Hospital
2300 Children's Plaza Center
Chicago, IL 60614

773-880-3333
Fax: 773-880-4179
e-mail: e-mendez@nwu.edu

Registry firm on giving children and their families the proper outlets to deal with this disorder.

1587 Society for Pediatric Dermatology
8365 Keystone Crossing, Suite 107
Indianapolis, IN 46240

317-202-0224
Fax: 317-205-9841
e-mail: spd@hp-assoc.com
www.pedsderm.net

National organization dedicated to promote, develop and advance education, research and care of skin disease in all pediatric age groups.

Kent Lindeman, Executive Director

Libraries & Resource Centers

California

1588 University of California, San Francisco Dermatology Drug Research
515 Spruce
San Francisco, CA 94143

415-476-2001
Fax: 415-476-6014
cc.ucsf.edu/people

Conducts clinical testing of new or existing pharmalogic agents used in the treatment of skin disorders.

John Koo, MD, Director

Delaware

1589 Delaware Division of Libraries for the Blind and Physically Handicapped
43 S Dupont Highway
Dover, DE 19901

302-736-4748
800-282-8676
Fax: 302-736-6787
TDD: 302-739-4748
e-mail: bedpg@lib.de.us

Braille readers receive service from Philadelphia and Pennsylvania, summer reading program, braille writer and cassettes.

Beth Landon, Librarian

Illinois

1590 Dermatology Information Network (DERMINFONET)
American Academy of Dermatology
PO Box 4014
Schaumburg, IL 60168

847-330-0230
Fax: 847-330-0050

Consists of a collection of dermatologic databases that are available to members on a subscription and/or purchase basis. These databases are designed to run on a wide variety of personal computers.

1591 National Library of Dermatologic Teaching Slides
American Academy of Dermatology
930 N Meacham Road
Shaumburg, IL 60173

847-330-0230
Fax: 847-330-0050
www.aad.org

A collection of dermatologic teaching slides offering the most comprehensive series ever assembled. Each set offers a realistic presentation of classic clinical skin conditions encountered by the dermatologist.

New York

1592 Laboratory of Dermatology Research
Memorial Sloan-Kettering Cancer Center
1275 York Avenue
New York, NY 10021

212-639-2000
Fax: 212-639-3576
www.mskcc.org

Specific studies on the identification of skin disorders and dermatology.

Biijan Safai, MD, Head

1593 Rockefeller University Laboratory for Investigative Dermatology
1230 York Avenue
New York, NY 10021

212-327-7458
Fax: 212-327-7459

Research into skin disorders and the whole specialty of dermatology in general.

D Martin Carter, MD, PhD, Head

Research Centers

1594 University of California, San Francisco Dermatology Drug Research
515 Spruce
San Francisco, CA 94143

415-476-2001
Fax: 415-221-4751

Conducts clinical testing of new or existing pharmacologic agents used in the treatment of skin disorders.

John Koo, MD, Director

Web Sites

1595 American Autoimmune Related Diseases Association
www.aarda.org

Dedicated to the eradication of autoimmune diseases and the alleviation of suffering and the socioeconomic impact of autoimmunity through fostering and facilitating collaboration in the areas of education, public awareness, research and patient services in an efective, ethical and efficient manner.

1596 American Osteopathic College of Dermatology
www.aocd.org

Improving the standards of the practice of dermatology, to stimulate the study and extend knowledge in the field of dermatology, and to promote a more general understanding of the nature and scope of services rendered by osteopathic dermatologists to other divisions of practice, hospitals, clinics and the public.

1597 Arthritis Foundation
www.arthritis.org

Supports more than 100 types of arthritis and related conditions with advocacy, programs, services and research.

1598 Myositis Association of America
www.myositis.org

Mission is to find a cure for inflammatory and other related myopathies, while serving those affected by these diseases.

1599 Society for Pediatric Dermatology
www.pedsderm.net

Objective is to promote, develop and advance education, research and care of skin disease in all pediatric age groups.

Book Publishers

1600 Let's Talk About Going to the Hospital
Rosen Publishing Group's PowerKids Press
29 E 21st Street
New York, NY 10010

212-777-3017
800-237-9932
Fax: 888-436-4643
e-mail: rosenpub@tribeca.ios.com
www.powerkidspress.com

If a child has to check into the hospital, chances are he or she is already upset about being ill. Knowing how a hospital functions and what the procedures are, such as when family members can visit, will help in what is already a stressful situation. Grades K-5.

24 pages
ISBN: 0-823950-36-0

Magazines

1601 International Journal of Dermatology
International Society of Dermatology
138 Palm Coast Parkway, NE No 333
Palm Coast, FL 32137

386-437-4405
Fax: 386-437-4427
e-mail: info@intsocdermatol.org
www.intsocderm.org

Focuses on information for dermatologists and the whole specialty of dermatology research and education.

10 times a year

1602 JM Companion

The Myositis Association
1233 20th St NW, Suite 402
Washington, DC 20036

202-887-0088
Fax: 202-466-8940
e-mail: tma@myositis.org
www.myositis.org

Focuses on special concerns and also has an 'Ask the doctor' column with answers from leading JM physicians, a special insert for children, and clinical trial listings for JM patients.

Quarterly

1603 Journal of Dermatologic Surgery and Oncology

International Society for Dermatologic Surgery
930 N Meachan Road
Schaumburg, IL 60173

847-330-9830
Fax: 847-330-1135

Focuses on medical updates and information on dermatology.

Monthly

Newsletters

1604 Awareness

NAPVI
PO Box 317
Watertown, MA 02471

617-972-7441
800-562-6265
Fax: 617-972-7444
www.spedex.com/napvi

Newsletter offering regional news, sports and activities, conferences, camps, legislative updates, book reviews, audio reviews, professional question and answer column and more for the visually impaired and their families.

Quarterly

1605 DVH Quarterly

University of Arkansas at Little Rock
2801 S University Avenue
Little Rock, AR 72204

Fax: 501-663-3536

Offers information on upcoming events, conferences and workshops on and for visual disabilities. Book reviews, information on the newest resources and technology, educational programs, want ads and more.

Quarterly

Bob Brasher, Editor

1606 Dermatology Focus

Dermatology Foundation
1560 Sherman Avenue
Evanston, IL 60201

847-328-2256
Fax: 847-328-0509
dermatologyfoundation.org

Includes membership activities, research articles and lists recipients of foundation awards.

Quarterly

1607 Dermatology World

American Academy of Dermatology
PO Box 94020
Palatine, IL 60094

847-330-0230
Fax: 847-330-0050

Offers Academy members information outside the clinical realm. It carries news of government actions, reports of socioeconomic issues, societal trends and other events which impinge on the practice of dermatology.

Monthly

1608 Keep In Touch (KIT) Forum

The Myositis Association
1233 20th Street NW, Suite 402
Washington, DC 20036

202-887-0088
Fax: 202-466-8940
e-mail: tma@myositis.org
www.myositis.org

Allows KIT leaders to share information about what their groups are doing to support one another and raise awareness of myositis in their own communities; provide a forum for members to exchange information and ideas for day-to-day living

1609 Progress in Dermatology

Dermatology Foundation
1560 Sherman Avenue
Evanston, IL 60201

847-328-2256
Fax: 847-328-0509
dermatologyfoundation.org

Bulletin offering information on research reports and clinical trials.

Quarterly

1610 The OutLook

The Myositis Association
1233 20th Street NW, Suite 402
Washington, DC 20036

202-887-0088
Fax: 202-466-8940
e-mail: tma@myositis.org
www.myositis.org

Newsletter featuring articles for patients with polymyositis, dermatomyositis, inclusion-body myositis, and juvenile forms of myositis.

Quarterly

Pamphlets

1611 Arthritis in Children

Arthritis Foundation
PO Box 7669
Atlanta, GA 30357

404-872-7100
800-568-4045
www.arthritis.org

Includes definitions of nine types of juvenile arthritis and related conditions, diagnosis, treatment options, emotional coping, school issues, federal laws and financial assistance.

28 pages

1612 Juvenile Dermatomyositis

Arthritis Foundation
PO Box 7669
Atlanta, GA 30357

404-872-7100
Fax: 404-872-0457
e-mail: info@jdfcure.com
www.jdfcure.com

DESCRIPTION

1613 CHILDHOOD SCHIZOPHRENIA

Involves the following Biologic System(s):
Developmental/Behavioral/Psychiatric Disorders

Childhood schizophrenia is characterized by disturbances in behavior, thought, and emotional reactions. These changes initially become apparent between approximately seven years of age and the onset of adolescence. Affected children may become increasingly withdrawn, have flat or blunted emotions that do not appear to change in response to environmental or external stimuli, experience episodes of unexplained silliness (hebephrenic silliness), exhibit aggressive behaviors, and have distortions in thinking. For example, some children may regularly repeat the same responses to different questions; experience sudden blockages in thought; perceive sights, sounds, or other sensations in the absence of external stimuli (hallucinations); and hold false beliefs in spite of evidence to the contrary (psychotic delusions), such as delusions of persecution (paranoid delusions). Affected children often appear to be chaotic in their emotions, thought, and behavioral patterns.

The relationship of childhood schizophrenia and adult schizophrenia remains unclear. Because schizophrenia typically becomes apparent during late adolescence or early adulthood and affects approximately one percent of the general population, only a small percentage of children exhibit symptoms that meet the criteria for a diagnosis of schizophrenia. In addition, many children who are diagnosed with schizophrenia before puberty are later diagnosed with mood disorders, such as bipolar disorder, or other conditions, such as mental retardation or a metabolic disorder. Although there is no clear relationship between childhood and adult schizophrenia, childhood symptoms that most likely predict adult psychotic disorders appear to include social withdrawal, disturbed interpersonal relationships, and blunted emotions. Though the specific underlying abnormalities that may contribute to childhood schizoid behaviors are unknown, genetic factors and certain biochemical abnormalities of the brain play some role in their development.

The treatment of children with schizoid behaviors may include therapy with certain medications known as neuroleptics to manage psychotic delusions, hallucinations, and severe agitation. In addition, an integrated, multidisciplinary approach may include individual therapy or parental training to help modify the child's behavior. In severe cases, hospitalization may be required to ensure appropriate medication adjustments, to prevent children from harming themselves, or to prevent them from hurting others if they exhibit aggressive or violent behavior.

Although certain medications can help treat children with schizoid behaviors, these drugs should be prescribed with great caution due to the potential for side effects. For example, such therapy may result in tardive dyskinesia (TD), a usually nonreversible condition characterized by tics or spasms of facial muscles and involuntary, rapid or writhing movements of the limbs (choreoathetoid movements). In other cases, therapy may cause abnormally slow movement (bradykinesis); involuntary hand movements; abnormal twisting of the neck (torticollis); drooling; and other findings. If TD develops, treatment with other medications may be indicated and the neuroleptic medication may be decreased or discontinued.

See also **General Resources** on page 917

Government Agencies

1614 Center for Mental Health Services Knowledge Exchange Network
US Department of Health and Human Services
PO Box 42557
Washington, DC 20015

800-789-2647
Fax: 240-747-5470
TDD: 866-889-2647
http://mentalhealth.samhsa.gov

Develops national mental health policies that promote Federal/State coordination and benefit from input from consumers, family members and providers. Ensures that high quality mental health services programs are implemented to benefit seriously mentally ill populations, disasters or those involved in the criminal justice system.

Irene S Levine, PhD, Deputy Director

1615 NIH/National Institute of Mental Health
6001 Executive Boulevard, Room 8184, MSC 9663
Bethesda, MD 20892

301-443-4513
866-615-6464
Fax: 301-443-4279
TTY: 301-443-8431
e-mail: nimhinfo@nih.gov
www.nimh.nih.gov

Conducts strategic planning for specific research areas as well as for the Institute as a whole.

Dr Thomas R Insel, Director

National Associations & Support Groups

1616 American Mental Health Foundation
191 Presidential Boulevard, Suite 3-W, PO Box 345
Bala Cynwyd, PA 19004

212-639-1561
Fax: 212-737-9027

Dedicated to the extensive and intensive research in the theories and techniques of treatment of emotional illness and to the implementation of reforms in the mental health system. Efforts have resulted in development of better and less expensive treatment methods. Findings are disseminated in English and other major languages.

Monroe W Spero MD

1617 American Schizophrenia Association
900 N Federal Highway, Suite 300
Boca Raton, FL 33432
561-393-6167

1618 Federation of Families for Children's Mental Health
9605 Medical Center Drive, Suite 280
Rockville, MD 20850
240-403-1901
Fax: 240-403-1909
e-mail: ffcmh@ffcmh.org
www.ffcmh.org

The National family run organization is dedicated exclusively to helping children with mental health needs and their families achieve a better quality of life.

Sandra Spencer, Executive Director

1619 Mental Health Clinical Research Center for Schizophrenia/Psychiatry
VA Medical Center
Wilshire and Sawtelle Boulevards
Los Angeles, CA 90073
213-824-6620

Offers research into the various facets of schizophrenia and mental illness.

Robert Liberman, MD, Director

1620 NADD: National Association for the Dually Diagnosed
132 Fair Street
Kingston, NY 12401
845-331-4336
800-331-5362
Fax: 845-331-4569
e-mail: info@thenadd.org
www.thenadd.org

Nonprofit organization designed to promote the interests of professional and parent development with resources for individuals who have the coexistence of mental illness and mental retardation. Provides conferences, educational services and training materials to professionals, parents, concerned citizens and service organizations.

Dr Robert Fletcher, CEO

1621 National Alliance for Research on Schizophrenia and Depression
60 Cutter Mill Road, Suite 404
Great Neck, NY 11021
516-829-0091
800-829-8289
Fax: 516-487-6930
e-mail: info@narsad.org
www.narsad.org

Largest private 501 (c) (3) not for profit corporation and registered public charity. Raises and distributes funds for scientific research into the causes, cures, treatments and prevention of brain disorders.

Stephen G Doochin, Executive Director

1622 National Alliance for the Mentally Ill
2107 Wilson Blvd, Ste 300, Colonial Place Three
Arlington, VA 22201
703-524-7600
800-950-6264
Fax: 703-524-9094
TDD: 703-516-7227
e-mail: info@nami.org
www.nami.org

NAMI is a nonprofit, grassroots, self-help, support and advocacy organization of consumers, families and friends of people with severe mental illness, such as schizophrenia, bipolar disorder, major despressive disorder, obsessive compulsive disorder, anxiety disorders, autism and other severe and persistent mental illnesses that affect the brain.

Suzanne Vogel-Scibilia MD, President

1623 National Mental Health Association
2000 N Beauregard Street, 6th Floor
Alexandria, VA 22311
703-684-7722
800-969-6642
Fax: 703-684-5968
TTY: 800-433-5959
www.nmha.org

Addresses all aspects of mental health and mental illness. NMHA with over 340 affiliates works to improve the mental health of all Americans.

David L Shern PhD, President & CEO

1624 National Mental Health Consumers' Self-Help Clearinghouse
1211 Chestnut Street, Suite 1207
Philadelphia, PA 19107
215-751-1810
800-553-4539
Fax: 215-636-6312
e-mail: info@mhselfhelp.org
www.mhselfhelp.org

Disperses information to the families and friends of individuals diagnosed with a mental illness.

Joseph Rogers, Executive Director & Founder

1625 National Schizophrenia Foundation
403 Seymour Avenue, Suite 202
Lansing, MI 48933
517-485-7168
Fax: 517-485-7180
e-mail: inquiries@nsfoundation.org
www.nsfoundation.org

Mission is to develop and maintain support groups for individuals, and their friends and family members, affected by schizophrenia and related disorders; and to be broad resource for all persons regarding schizophrenia and related disorders through education, information, and public awareness services.

Eric Hufnagel, President & CEO
Sharon Pederson, Director of Programs

1626 North American Society for Childhood Onset Schizophrenia - NACOS
88 Briarwood Drive East
Berkeley Heights, NJ 07922
www.nascos.org

Non-profit, internet based group formed to provide a Web site devoted solely to childhood onset schizophrenia (COS). Families, caregivers and medical professionals will be able to locate and contact each other in order to access and share information related to this rare, devastating disease.

Karen Sniezek, Director
Meredith Morgan, Director

1627 Schizophrenia Schizoaffective Disorder Institute
Western Psychiatric Institute and Clinic
3811 O'Hara Street
Pittsburgh, PA 15213
412-624-2100
Fax: 412-624-0446
e-mail: nimca@pitt.edu
wpic.upmc.com

Dedicated to supporting and serving those suffering from schizophrenic disorders, as well as their friends and families.

Dr Val Nimcaenkar, Associate Professor/Psychiatry

1628 Schizophrenics Anonymous Forum
Mental Health Association in Michigan
30233 Southfield Road, Suite 220
Southfield, MI 48076

248-647-1711
Fax: 248-647-1732
e-mail: schizanon@aol.com
schizophrenia.org

Self-help organization sponsored by American Schizophrenia Association. Groups are comprised of dignosed schizophrenics who meet to share experiences, strengths and hopes in an effort to help each other cope with common problems and recover from the disease. Rehabilitation program follows the 12 principles of Alcoholics Anonymous. Publications: Newsletter, semi-annual. Monthly support group meeting.

State Agencies & Support Groups

1629 Center for Family Support
333 7th Avenue, 9th Floor
New York, NY 10001

212-629-7939
Fax: 212-239-2211
www.cfsny.org

The Center for Family (CFS) is a not-for-profit human service agency providing support and assistance to individuals with developmental disabilities and traumatic brain injuries throughout New York City, Long Island, the lower Hudson Valley region and New Jersey.

Steven Vernickofs, Executive Director

Libraries & Resource Centers

1630 National Alliance for Research on Schizophrenia and Depression
60 Cutter Mill Road, Suite 404
Great Neck, NY 11021

516-829-0091
800-829-8289
Fax: 516-487-6930
e-mail: info@narsad.org
www.narsad.org

Largest private 501 (c) (3) not for profit corporation and registered public charity. Raises and distributes funds for scientific research into the causes, cures, treatments and prevention of brain disorders.

Stephen G Doochin, Executive Director

Research Centers

1631 National Alliance for Research on Schizophrenia and Depression
60 Cutter Mill Road, Suite 404
Great Neck, NY 11021

516-829-0091
800-829-8289
Fax: 516-487-6930
e-mail: info@narsad.org
www.narsad.org

Largest private 501 (c) (3) not for profit corporation and registered public charity. Raises and distributes funds for scientific research into the causes, cures, treatments and prevention of brain disorders.

Stephen G Doochin, Executive Director

1632 Schizophrenia Research Branch: Division of Clinical and Treatment Research
Chief, 500 Fishers Lane
Parklawn Building, Room 18
Rockville, MD 20857

301-443-4707
Fax: 301-443-6000

Plans, supports and conducts programs of research, research training and resource development of schizophrenia and related disorders. Reviews and evaluates research developments in the field and recommends new program directors. Collaborates with organizations in and outside of the National Institute of Mental Health to stimulate work in the field through conferences and workshops.

1633 Suncoast Residential Training Center/Developmental Services Program
Goodwill Industries-Suncoast
10596 Gandy Boulevard
Saint Petersburg, FL 33702

727-523-1512
888-279-1988
Fax: 727-563-9300
TTY: 727-579-1068
www.goodwill-suncoast.org

A large group home which serves individuals diagnosed as mentally retarded with a secondary diagnosis of psychiatric difficulties as evidenced by problem behavior. Providing residential, behavioral and instructional support and services that will promote the development of adaptive, socially appropriate behavior. Each individual is assessed to determine, socialization, basic academics and recreation. The primary intervention strategy is applied behavior analysis.

Martin Gladysz, Chairman
R Lee Waits, President & CEO

Audio Video

1634 Bonnie Tapes
Mental Illness Education Project
PO Box 470813
Brookline Village, MA 02447

617-562-1111
800-343-5540
Fax: 617-779-0061
e-mail: info@miepvideos.org
www.miepvideos.org

Bonnie's account of coping with schizophrenia will be a relevation to people whose view of mental illness has been shaped by the popular media. She and her family provide an intimate view of the frequently feared, often misrepresented and much stigmatized illness and the human side of learning to live with a psychiatric disability. Tape 1: Mental Illness in the Family (26 minutes); Tape 2: Recovering from Mental Illness (27 minutes); Tape 3: My Sister Is Mentally Ill (22 minutes) $99.95 each

1997 $143.88 for 3

1635 Families Coping with Mental Illness
Mental Illness Education Project
PO Box 470813
Brookline Village, MA 02247

617-562-1111
800-343-5540
Fax: 617-779-0061
e-mail: info@miepvideos.org
miepvideos.org

10 family members share their experiences of having a family member with schizophrenia or bipolar disorder. Designed to provide insights and support to other families, the tape also profoundly conveys to professionals the needs of families when mental illness strikes. In two versions: a twenty two minute version ideal for short classes and workshops, and a richer forty three min-

ute version with more examples and details. Discounted price for families/consumers.

Michael M Faenza, Executive Director

1636 Living with Schizophrenia

Guilford Press
72 Spring Street
New York, NY 10012

800-365-7006
Fax: 212-966-6708
e-mail: info@guilford.com
www.guilford.com

Offers essential information and huidance for individuals and families coping with schizophrenia diagnosis. Features illuminating first-hand accounts from three people with schizophrenia and one person with schizoaffective disorder, along with commentary from treatment expert Dr Andy Campbell. Learn clear steps to take to lead fuller, more successful lives. Available on VHS or DVD 39 minutes.

2006
ISBN: 1-593853-86-6

1637 Pharmacotherapy of Schizophrenia

American Psychiatric Publishing
1000 Wilson Boulevard, Suite 1825
Arlington, VA 22209

703-907-7322
800-368-5777
Fax: 703-907-1091
e-mail: appi@psych.org
www.appi.org

Presented by John M Kane MD, Chairman of Psychiatry at LI Jewish Medical Center, and Professor of Psychiatry at Albert Einstein College of Medicine. Illustrates the major issues and treatment considerations, and the latest findings on the effectiveness as well as on the side effects of the many and varied psychopharmacological agents are carefully illustrated and discussed. 75 minutes. ISBN # 9780880483803

1995

John M Kane MD, Author

Web Sites

1638 CyberPsych

www.cyberpsych.org

CyberPsych presents information about psychoanalysis, psychotherapy, and special topics such as anxiety disorder, the problematic use of alcohol, homophobia, and the traumatic effects of racism. CyberPsych is a nonprofit network which offers free web hosting and technical support for internet communication to nonprofit groups and individuals.

1639 Internet Mental Health

www.mentalhealth.com

Our goal is to improve understanding, diagnosis, and treatment of mental illness throughout the world.

1640 Mental Health Net

www.mentalhelp.net

We wish to provide the following: to discuss, develope and debate in an open forum the future of the mental health field in America and throughout the world. To help coordinate various components of the mental health field so as to bring about greater communication between them. To educate the public about mental health issues, to promote active collaboration between professionals in all segments of mental health development, implementation and policy.

1641 Mental Wellness

www.mentalwellness.com

Mental Wellness is an online resource for bipolar disorder, schizophrenia and general mental health information.

1642 Online Mendelian Inheritance in Man

www.ncbi.nlm.nih.gov

This database is a catalog of human genes and genetic disorders.

1643 Planetpsych

www.planetpsych.com

Planetpsych is an online resource for mental health information.

1644 Psych Central

www.psychcentral.com

Offers free informational and educational articles and resources on psychology, support and mental health online.

1645 Schizophrenia Support Organizations

www.members.aol.com/leonardjk/USA.htm

Contains a listing of support organizations for people with schizophrenia and their families.

1646 Schizophrenia.com

www.schizophrenia.com

Is a leading web commuity dedicated to providing high quality information, support and education to the family members, caregivers and individuals who's lives have been impacted by schizophrenia.

1647 Schizophrenia.com Home Page

www.schizophrenia.com/discuss/Disc3.html

On-line support for patients and families.

1648 Schizophrenia.com Newsletter

www.schizophrenia.com/newsletter

Comprehensive psychoeducational site on schizophrenia.

1649 Schizophrenia: Handbook for Families

www.mentalhealth.com/book/p40-sc01.html

This handbook is dedicated to the families and to their loved ones who carry the burden of schizophrenia, a major psychiatric disorder.

Book Publishers

1650 Biology of Schizophrenia and Affective Disease

American Psychiatric Publishing
1000 Wilson Boulevard, Suite 1825
Arlington, VA 22209

703-907-7322
800-368-5777
Fax: 703-907-1091
e-mail: appi@psych.org
www.appi.org

Provides a state-of-the-art look at the biological bases of severe mental illness from the perspective of the researchers making these exceptional discoveries. ISBN # 9780880487467

1995 560 pages

Stanley J Watson PhD MD, Author

1651 Breakthroughs in Antipsychotic Medications A Guide for Consumers, Families, Clinics

National Alliance for the Mentally Ill
200 N Glebe Rd, Suite 1015
Arlington, VA 22203

703-524-7600
800-950-6264
Fax: 703-524-9094
www.nami.org

Helps consumers and their families weigh the pros and cons of switching from older antipsychotics to newer ones. Answers frequently asked questions about antipsychotics and guides readers through the process of switching. Includes fact sheets on the new medications and their side affects.

1999 200 pages

1652 Contemporary Issues in the Treatment of Schizophrenia
American Psychiatric Press
1000 Wilson Boulevard, Suite 1825
Arlington, VA 22209

703-907-7322
800-368-5777
Fax: 703-907-1091
e-mail: appi@psych.org
www.appi.org

Covers approaches to the patient by investigating biological, pharmacological, and psychological treatments. ISBN #: 9780880486811

1995 889 pages

Christian L Shriqui, MD, Editor
Henry A Nasrallah, MD, Editor

1653 Coping with Schizophrenia: A Guide for Families
New Harbinger Publications
5674 Shattuck Avenue
Oakland, CA 94609

510-652-2002
800-748-6273
Fax: 510-652-5472
e-mail: customerservice@newharbinger.com
newharbinger.com

Provides detailed, step by step strategies for preventing relapses, regulating medications, establishing household rules, dealing with depression and anxiety, overcoming alcohol and drug abuse, responding to crises, improving quality of life, and planning for the patient's future.

368 pages
ISBN: 1-879237-78-4

1654 Diagnosis Schizophrenia: A Comprehensive Resource
Columbia University Press
61 W 62nd Street
New York, NY 10023

212-459-0600
Fax: 212-459-3678
www.columbia.edu/cu/cup

Has alot of consumers' stories in the first person and sketches of their faces sprinkled throughout.

2002

Rachel Miller, Author
Susan E Mason, Author

1655 Encyclopedia of Schizophrenia and the Psychotic Disorders
Facts on File
11 Penn Plaza
New York, NY 10001

212-290-8090
800-322-8755
Fax: 212-678-3633

This volume details recent theories and research findings on schizophrenia and psychotic disorders, together with a complete overview of the field's history.

368 pages

1656 Family Care of Schizophrenia: A Problem- Solving Approach...
Guilford Publications
72 Spring Street
New York, NY 10012

212-431-9800
800-365-7006
Fax: 212-966-6708
e-mail: info@guilford.com
guilford.com

Falloon and his colleagues have developed a model for the broad-based community treatment of schizophrenia and other severe forms of mental illness that taps this underutilized potential.

The goal of their program is not merely the reduction of stress that can trigger florid episodes, but also the restoration of the patient to a level of social functioning that permits employment and socialization with people outside the family.

451 pages
ISBN: 0-898629-23-3

1657 First Episode Psychosis
American Psychiatric Publishing
1400 K Street NW
Washington, DC 20005

202-682-6262
800-368-5777
Fax: 202-789-2648
e-mail: appi@psych.org
appi.org

160 pages
ISBN: 1-853174-35-1

Katie Duffy, Marketing Assistant

1658 Getting Your Life Back Together When You Have Schizophrenia
New Harbinger Publications
5674 Shattuck Ave
Oakland, CA 94609

800-748-6273
Fax: 510-652-5472
e-mail: customerservice@newharbinger.com
www.newharbinger.com

Provides good information for someone who has just been diagnosed with schiophrenia.

2002

Roberta Temes PhD, Author

1659 Group Therapy for Schizophrenic Patients
American Psychiatric Publishing
1400 K Street NW
Washington, DC 20005

202-682-6262
800-368-5777
Fax: 202-789-2648
e-mail: appi@psych.org
appi.org

Acquaints mental health practitioners with this cost-effective method of treatment.

192 pages
ISBN: 0-880481-72-2

Katie Duffy, Marketing Assistant

1660 Guidelines for the Treatment of Patients with Schizophrenia
American Psychiatric Publishing
1400 K Street NW
Washington, DC 20005

202-682-6262
800-368-5777
Fax: 202-789-2648
e-mail: appi@psych.org
appi.org

Provides therapists with a set of patient care strategies that will aid their clinical decison making. Describes the best and most appropriate treatments available to patients.

160 pages
ISBN: 0-890423-09-1

Katie Duffy, Marketing Assistant

1661 How to Cope with Mental Illness In Your Family: Guide for Siblings and Offspring
Health Source
1404 K Street NW
Washington, DC 20005

202-789-7303
800-713-7122
Fax: 202-789-7899
e-mail: healthsource@appi.org
healthsourcebooks.org

Illnesses such as schizophrenia, manic depression and major depression are discussed. Also provides the tools to overcome the devastating effects of growing up or living in a family where these disorders exist. Covers the essential stages of recovery and how to reclaim your life.

240 pages
ISBN: 0-874779-23-5

1662 Innovations in the Psychological Management of Schizophrenia
John Wiley & Sons
605 3rd Avenue
New York, NY 10058

212-850-6000
Fax: 212-850-6008
e-mail: info@wiley.com
www.wiley.com

Innovations in the Psychological Management of Schizophrenia: Assessment, Treatment and Services.

1992 338 pages

1663 Medical Illness and Schizophrenia
American Psychiatric Publishing
1000 Wilson Boulevard, Suite 1825
Arlington, VA 22209

703-907-7322
800-368-5777
Fax: 703-907-1091
e-mail: appi@psych.org
www.appi.org

Examines the links between medical conditions and severe chronic mental illness, with a focus on the need for better medical assessment and treatment to improve outcomes in patients; links between schizophrenia and conditions such as obesity, cardiovascular disease, diabetes, HIV and hepatitis C, endocrine-related diorders, and others; the association between therapy with certain antipsychotics and adverse health outcomes; the importance of improving community health. ISBN # 9781585621064

2003 256 pages

Jonathan M Meyer MD, Author
Henry A Nasrallah MD, Author

1664 Negative Symptom and Cognitive Deficit Tre atment Response in Schizophrenia
American Psychiatric Publishing
1000 Wilson Boulevard, Suite 1825
Arlington, VA 22209

703-907-7322
800-368-5777
Fax: 703-907-1091
e-mail: appi@psych.org
www.appi.org

Addresses the complex issues-issues rarely confronted in empirical studies of patients with schizophrenia-and controversial research surrounding the assessment of negative symptoms and cognitive deficits in patients with schizophrenia. ISBN # 9780880487856

2001 216 pages

Richard S E Keefe PhD, Author
Joseph P McEvoy MD, Author

1665 New Pharmacotherapy of Schizophrenia
American Psychiatric Press
1000 Wilson Boulevard, Suite 1825
Arlington, VA 22209

703-907-7322
800-368-5777
Fax: 703-907-1091
e-mail: appi@psych.org
www.appi.org

Discusses the new class of antipsychotic agents that promises superior efficiency and more favorable side-effects; offers an improved understanding of how to employ exsisting pharmachotherapeutic agents. ISBN # 9780880484916

1996 264 pages

1666 Plasma Homovanillic Asid in Schhizophrenia
American Psychiatric Publishing
1000 Wilson Boulevard, Suite 1825
Arlington, VA 22209

703-907-7322
800-368-5777
Fax: 703-907-1091
e-mail: appi@psych.org
www.appi.org

Provides the most comprehensive and current collection of information on plasma HVA levels to be found anywhere. Provides a consice synthesis and critique of current data as well as interesting proposals for future research. ISBN # 9780880484893

1997 216 pages

Arnold J Friedhoff MD, Author
Farooq Amin MD, Author

1667 Prenatal Exposures in Schizophrenia
American Psychiatric Press
1000 Wilson Boulevard, Suite 1825
Arlington, VA 22209

703-907-7322
800-368-5777
Fax: 703-907-1091
e-mail: appi@psych.org
www.appi.org

Considers a range of epigenetic elements thought to interact with abnormal genes to produce the onset of illness. Attention to the evidence implicating obstetric complications, prenatal infection, autoimmunity and prenatal malnutrition in brain disorders. ISBN # 9780880484992

1999 296 pages Hardcover

Ezra S Susser MD, Author
Alan S Brown MD, Author

1668 Psychoses and Pervasive Development Disorders in Childhood and Adolescence
American Psychiatric Press
1400 K Street NW
New York, NY 20005

202-682-6262
800-368-5777
Fax: 202-789-2648
e-mail: order@appi.org
www.appi.org

Provides a concise summary of current knowledge of psychosis and pervasive developmental disorders of childhood and adolescence. Discusses recent range changes in aspects of diagnosis and the definition of these disorders, advances in knowledge and aspects of treatment.

1996 368 pages

1669 Schizophrenia
American Psychiatric Publishing
1000 Wilson Boulevard, Suite 1825
Arlington, VA 22209

703-907-7322
800-368-5777
Fax: 703-907-1091
e-mail: appi@psych.org
www.appi.org

Ideas in treating the disease, and how many patients can lead productive lives without relapse. ISBN # 9780880489508

1994 294 pages

Nancy C Andleasen MD, Author

1670 Schizophrenia Into Later Life: Treatment, Research, and Policy
American Psychiatric Publishing
1000 Wilson Boulevard, Suite 1825
Arlington, VA 22209

703-907-7322
800-368-5777
Fax: 703-907-1091
e-mail: appi@psych.org
www.appi.org

Multidisciplinary reference on this important topic-a landmark work for researchers, service providers, and policy makers. ISBN # 9781585620371

2003 344 pages

Carl I Cohen MD, Author

1671 Schizophrenia Revealed: From Neurons to Social Interactions
W.W. Norton
500 Fifth Avenue
New York, NY 10110

212-354-5500
Fax: 212-869-0856
www.wwnorton.com

Educational, informational, scientific and yet readable.

2003

1672 Schizophrenia and Comorbid Conditions Diagnosis and Treatment
American Psychiatric Publishing
1000 Wilson Boulevard, Suite 1825
Arlington, VA 22209

703-907-7322
800-368-5777
Fax: 703-907-1091
e-mail: appi@psych.org
www.appi.org

Lays diagnostic oversimplification of schizophrenia to rest once and for all. Editors are criticizing the reductionist view of schizophrenia as a single unitary disorder- a view that has led many psychiatrists and mental health care professionals to overlook potentially important syndromes. ISBN # 9780880487719

2001 256 pages

1673 Schizophrenia and Genetic Risks
National Alliance for the Mentally Ill
200 N Glebe Road
Arlington, VA 22203

703-524-7600
800-950-6264
Fax: 703-524-9094
nami.org

Provides basic facts about schizophrenia and its familial distribution so consumers and mental health workers can become informed enough to initiate appropriate actions. Includes suggested resources.

1674 Schizophrenia: Straight Talk for Family an d Friends
William Morrow & Company
1350 Avenue of the Americas
New York, NY 10019

212-261-6500
Fax: 212-261-6549
williammorrow.com

Lists more than 150 local chapters of the National Alliance for the Mentally Ill.

1675 Scizophrenia in a Molecular Age
American Psychiatric Publishing
1000 Wilson Boulevard, Suite 1825
Arlington, VA 22209

703-907-7322
800-368-5777
Fax: 703-907-1091
e-mail: appi@psych.org
www.appi.org

Reviews neuroscience mechanisms and analyzes genetic determinants. ISBN # 9780880489614

1999 204 pages

Carol A Tamminga MD, Author

1676 Surviving Schizophrenia: A Manual for Families, Consumers and Providers
Harper Collins
10 E 53rd Street
New York, NY 10022

212-207-7000
800-242-7737
Fax: 212-207-2271
harpercollins.com

The third edition of this indispensable manual throughly details everything patients, families and mental health professionals need to know about one of the most widespread and misunderstood illnesses. Paperback.

464 pages
ISBN: 0-060950-76-5

1677 The American Psychiatric Publishing Text book of Schizophrenia
American Psychiatric Publishing
1000 Wilson Boulevard, Suite 1825
Arlington, VA 22209

703-907-7322
800-368-5777
Fax: 703-907-1091
e-mail: appi@psych.org
www.appi.org

Offers broad coverage that encompasses the current state of knowledge the cause, nature, and treatment of schizophrenia. ISBN # 9781585621910

2006 453 pages

Jeffrey A Lieberman MD, Author
T Scott Stroup MD MPH, Author

1678 The Complete Family Guide to Schizophrenia
Guilford Press
72 Spring Street
New York, NY 10012

800-365-7006
Fax: 212-966-6708
e-mail: info@guilford.com
www.guilford.com

Walks readers through a range of treatment and support options that can lead to a better life for the entire family.

2006 486 pages
ISBN: 1-593852-73-8

Kim T Mueser, Author
Susan Gingerich, Author

1679 The Early Stages of Schizophrenia
American Psychiatric Publishing
1000 Wilson Boulevard, Suite 1825
Arlington, VA 22209

703-907-7322
800-368-5777
Fax: 703-907-1091
e-mail: appi@psych.org
www.appi.org

Divided into three major parts: Early Intervention, Epidemiology, and Natural History of Schizophrenia; Management of the Early Stages of Schizophrenia; and Neurobiological Investigations of the Early Stages of Schizophrenia. ISBN # 9780880488402

2002 280 pages

Robert B Zipursky MD, Author
S Charles Schulz MD, Author

1680 The Natural History of Mania, Depression, and Schizophrenia
American Psychiatric Publishing
1000 Wilson Boulevard, Suite 1825
Arlington, VA 22209

703-907-7322
800-368-5777
Fax: 703-907-1091
e-mail: appi@psych.org
www.appi.org

Takes an unusual look at the course of mental illness, based on data from the Iowa 500 Research Project. This project involved the long-term (30-40 yrs) follow-up of patients diagnosed with schizophrenia, depression, and bipolar illness. ISBN # 9780880487269

1996 384 pages

George Winokur MD, Author
Ming T Tsuang MD PhD, Author

1681 Water Balance in Schizophrenia
American Psychiatric Publishing
1000 Wilson Boulevard, Suite 1825
Arlington, VA 22209

703-907-7322
800-368-5777
Fax: 703-907-1091
e-mail: appi@psych.org
www.appi.org

Represents the first attempt to provide clinicians with a consolidated guide to polydipsia-hyponatremia, associated with schizophrenia. ISBN # 9780880484855

1996 360 pages

David B Schnur MD, Author
Darrell G Kirch MD, Author

Magazines

1682 Schizophrenia Research
PO Box 945
New York, NY 10159

212-633-3730
888-437-4636
Fax: 212-633-3680
elsevier.nl/locate/schres

Newsletters

1683 NADD Bulletin
132 Fair Street
Kingston, NY 12401

845-331-4336
800-331-5362
Fax: 845-331-4569
e-mail: info@thenadd.org
www.thenadd.org

Official publication of the National Association for the Dually Diagnosed. It features articles that address clinical, programmatic, research or family oriented issues concerning mental health aspects in persons with disabilities.

20 pages Bimonthly

Pamphlets

1684 Schizophrenia
National Institute of Mental Health
6001 Executive Boulevard, Room 8184, MSC 9663
Bethesda, MD 20892

301-443-4513
866-615-6464
Fax: 301-443-4279
TTY: 866-415-8051
e-mail: nimhinfo@nih.gov
www.nimhinfo@nih.gov

This booklet answers many common questions about schizophrenia, one of the most chronic, severe and disabling mental disorders. Current research-based information is provided for people with schizophrenia, their family members, friends and the general public about the symptoms and diagnosis of schizophrenia, possible causes, treatments and treatment resources.

2006 28 pages

1685 Schizophrenia Fact Sheet
Center for Mental Health Services
PO Box 42557
Washington, DC 20015

800-789-2647
Fax: 240-747-5470
TDD: 866-889-2647
http://mentalhealth.samhsa.gov

This fact sheet provides information on the symptoms, diagnosis, and treatment for schizophrenia.

2 pages

1686 Understanding Schizophrenia
National Alliance on Mental Illness
Colonial Place Three, 2107 Wilson Place, Suite 300
Arlington, VA 22201

703-524-7600
Fax: 703-524-9094
TDD: 703-516-7227
www.nami.org

An excellent introduction to schizophrenia. Appropriate for supprt groups, physicians offices, coventions, health fairs, and the workplace.

DESCRIPTION

1687 CHOREA

Covers these related disorders: Benign familial chorea, Drug-induced chorea, Sydenham's chorea

Involves the following Biologic System(s):
Neurologic Disorders

Chorea is a neuromuscular condition characterized by irregular, rapid, jerky movements that may appear to be well coordinated but actually occur involuntarily. These movements may be simple or highly complex. In addition, the arms and legs may have abnormally diminished muscle tone (hypotonia) and therefore may be abnormally loose or slack. Choreic movements are often subtle. However, if several of these movements are present, they may essentially flow into one another, causing them to appear relatively slow, sinuous, and writhing in nature (athetosis).

The specific underlying cause of chorea is unknown. However, some researchers suspect that it may result due to overactivity of certain neurotransmitters (dopamine) in the brain. Neurotransmitters are naturally produced chemicals that regulate the transmission of messages between certain nerve cells (neurons). In some children, chorea may result from the use of particular drugs, such as certain antiseizure medications, particularly phenytoin, or antipsychotic (neuroleptic) drugs, such as haloperidol or phenothiazines. Chorea may also occur in association with certain underlying disorders, such as systemic lupus erythematosus (lupus) or Wilson's disease, a disorder of copper metabolism. In addition, chorea is a primary feature of a rare genetic disorder known as benign familial chorea in which nonprogressive chorea begins in infancy or early childhood in the absence of other neurologic abnormalities. Associated symptoms and findings include delays in attaining certain motor milestones during childhood and poorly coordinated movements of the arms and legs. Benign familial chorea is likely inherited as an autosomal dominant trait.

In addition, chorea is the dominant feature of a disorder known as Sydenham's chorea. This disorder is the most common cause of acquired chorea during childhood. Sydenham's chorea occurs in association with rheumatic fever, which is an inflammatory disease following throat infection with certain strains of streptococcal bacteria. Patients with rheumatic fever may experience fever, inflammation and swelling of one or more large joints, or inflammation of the heart (carditis), potentially causing thickening, scarring, and associated disease of heart valves. If rheumatic fever affects the nervous system, Sydenham's chorea may result. Although Sydenham's chorea previously occurred in as many as half of those with rheumatic fever, recent studies suggest that it more likely affects approximately 10 percent of rheumatic patients in the United States.

Sydenham's chorea most commonly occurs in children between ages five and 15. The condition may begin subtly and gradually, sometimes as long as several months after other symptoms associated with rheumatic fever have resolved. Patients may initially experience increasing clumsiness. As symptoms progress, involuntary movements may become prominent in the face, trunk, and arms and legs; move from one muscle group to another; and eventually affect all motor movements, including walking and speech. In some patients, chorea may be restricted to one side of the body (hemichorea). If children have severe chorea and abnormally diminished muscle tone (hypotonia), they may become unable to dress, feed themselves, or walk. Many children with the condition also experience rapid mood swings and episodes of uncontrollable crying (emotional lability).

Sydenham's chorea is usually a self-limited disorder that subsides in weeks or months. However, in some patients, the condition may persist for up to one to two years. In approximately 20 percent of children, the condition may recur within two years of the initial episode. If patients experience mild symptoms, treatment may include symptomatic and supportive measures, including minimizing stress as much as possible. In children with more severe symptoms, treatment may be attempted with the drug diazepam.

See also **General Resources** on page 917

Government Agencies

1688 NIH/National Institute of Neurological Disorders and Stroke (NINDS)
PO Box 5801
Bethesda, MD 20824

301-496-5751
800-352-9424
Fax: 301-496-0296
TTY: 301-468-5981
www.ninds.nih.gov

Works to reduce the burden of neurological disease by conducting, fostering, coordinating and guiding research on the causes, prevention, diagnosis and treatment of neurological disorders and stroke, while supporting basic research in related scientific areas.
Story C Landis Ph.D., Director
Audrey S Penn M.D., Deputy Director

National Associations & Support Groups

1689 American Academy of Child and Adolescent Psychiatry
3615 Wisconsin Avenue NW
Washington, DC 20016

202-966-7300
Fax: 202-966-2891
www.aacap.org

The AACAP (American Academy of Child and Adolescent Psychiatry) is the leading national professional medical association dedicated to treating and improving the quality of life for children, adolescents, and families affected by these disorders.

Robert L. Hendren, D.O., President
Gregory Fritz, Secretary

1690 Genetic Alliance
4301 Connecticut Avenue NW
Washington, DC 20008

202-966-5557
800-336-4363
Fax: 202-966-8553
e-mail: info@geneticalliance.org
www.geneticalliance.org

A coalition of voluntary genetic support groups, consumers and professionals addressing the needs of individuals and families affected by genetic disorders from a national perspective.

Sharon Terry, President/CEO

1691 March of Dimes Birth Defects Foundation
1275 Mamaroneck Avenue
White Plains, NY 10605

914-428-7100
888-663-4637
Fax: 914-428-8203
e-mail: resourcecenter@modimes.org
www.marchofdimes.com

Partnership of volunteers and professionals dedicates to improving the health of babies by preventing birth defects and infant mortality. Over 100 chapters are located across the country and can be located through the National Office.

Dr Jennifer Howse, President

1692 Muscular Dystrophy Association
3300 E Sunrise Drive
Tucson, AZ 85718

520-529-2000
800-572-1717
Fax: 520-529-5300
e-mail: mda@mdausa.org
www.mdausa.org

Voluntary health agency aimed at conquering nucromuscular diseases that affect more than 1,000,000 Americans. The diseases in MDA's program include nine forms of muscular dystrophy, amyotrophic lateral sclerosis (Lou Gehrig's disease), spinal muscular atrophy, Charcot-Marie-Tooth disease, and other neuromuscular conditions. With over 200 offices across the country, MDA conducts research, medical and community services, clinics, support groups, summer camps for youngsters and much more.

Bob Mackle, Director Public Information
Carol Sowell, Director Publications

1693 WE MOVE (Worldwide Education and Advocacy for Movement Disorders)
204 W 84th Street
New York, NY 10024

212-241-8567
800-437-6682
Fax: 212-987-7363
e-mail: wemove@wemove.org
www.wemove.org

Gives the general public the knowledge that they desire regarding any disorder involving movement difficulties.

Susan Bressman MD, President

Web Sites

1694 Online Mendelian Inheritance in Man
www.ncbi.nlm.nih.gov

This database is a catalog of human genes and genetic disorders.

Book Publishers

1695 Diagnostic and Statistical Manual of Mental Disorders
American Psychiatric Association
1000 Wilson Boulevard, Suite 1825
Arlington, VA 22209

703-907-7300
e-mail: apa@psych.org
www.psych.org

Includes updated information on diagnoses, etiology, and research on mental illness.

1696 Merck Manual of Diagnosis and Therapy 18th Edition
Wiley Publishers
10475 Crosspoint Boulevard
Indianapolis, IN 46256

317-572-3000
877-762-2974
Fax: 800-597-3299
e-mail: consumer@wiley.com
www.wiley.com

Packed with essential information on diagnosing and treating medical disorders to help health care professionals and medical students deliver the best care.

2006
ISBN: 0-911910-18-2

1697 Neuroanatomy: Text and Atlas 3rd Edition
McGraw-Hill Medical
2 Penn Plaza
New York, NY 10121

877-833-5524
http://books.mcgraw-hill.com

Comprehensive appraoch to neuroanatomy from both functional and regional perspective! Examines how parts of the nervous system work together to regulate body systems and produce behavior.

2003 532 pages
ISBN: 0-071381-83-X

Pamphlets

1698 Huntington's Disease Information Page
National Inst. of Neurological Disorders/Stroke
NIH, 31 Center Drive, MSC 2540, Bldg. 31, Rm 8A06
Bethesda, MD 20892

301-496-5751
800-352-9424
www.ninds.nih.gov/disorders/huntington/

1699 Huntington's Disease: Hope Through Research
National Inst. of Neurological Disorders/Stroke
NIH, 31 Center Drive, MSC 2540, Bldg. 31, Rm 8A06
Bethesda, MD 20892

301-496-5751
800-352-9424

1700 Sydenham Chorea Information Page
National Inst. of Neurological Disorders/Stroke
PO Box 5801
Bethesda, MD 20824

301-496-5751
800-352-9424
TTY: 301-468-5981
www.ninds.nih.gov/disorders/sydenham/sydenham.html

Provides information on the disease, treatment options, and the prognosis, as well as provides some research centers regarding the disease.

DESCRIPTION

1701 CLEFT LIP AND CLEFT PALATE

Involves the following Biologic System(s):

Dermatologic Disorders, Orthopedic and Muscle Disorders

Cleft lip and cleft palate are birth defects that may occur together or as isolated conditions. Newborns with cleft lip have a groove in the upper lip that may be a small notch or, in more severe cases, may be deep and extend up to the nose. Cleft palate is characterized by incomplete closure of the roof of the mouth (palate). In affected newborns, an abnormal gap runs along the midline of the soft, fleshy area of the palate (soft palate) and, in some patients, extends into one or both sides of the bony, front region of the palate (hard palate). As a result, the nasal cavity may open into the palate. Cleft lip with or without cleft palate affects approximately one in 600 newborns, whereas cleft palate alone occurs in about one in 1,000 births.

In newborns with cleft lip, the defect may occur on one or both sides of the upper lip and typically affects the bony ridge of the upper jaw (upper alveolar ridge). This ridge contains the sockets in which the roots of the teeth are held (dental alveoli). As a result, affected children often experience improper development of certain teeth, potentially resulting in absent, malformed, improperly positioned, or extra teeth and increased risk of dental decay (dental caries). In addition, infants with cleft lip and cleft palate typically have feeding difficulties associated with poor suckling capability and excessive swallowing of air. Affected children with cleft palate are also prone to repeated infections of the middle ear (otitis media) that, in some cases, may contribute to associated hearing loss. Many children also experience speech defects that may be due to inadequate functioning of certain muscles of the throat and palate (pharyngeal and palatal muscles).

In affected newborns, treatment initially consists of measures to ensure improved feeding and proper intake of nutrients. In many patients, a plastic device (a prosthetic known as an obturator) may be fitted that covers the gap in the palate, thereby improving suction and intake of fluids, milk, and or formula. The obturator is typically replaced every few weeks due to rapid growth during infancy. In addition, in those with cleft palate, modified artificial nipples may help to improve feeding. In many cases, cleft lip may be surgically closed by approximately two months of age and additional corrective surgery may be performed later during childhood. If affected children do not have associated physical abnormalities, surgical correction of cleft palate may be performed before the age of one year to help improve normal speech development. However, if surgery is delayed until the age of three years or later, a device (such as a contoured speech bulb) may be used to help close off the uppermost portion of the throat (nasopharynx) during the production of certain sounds. This helps children to develop understandable speech. Treatment may also include dental procedures to correct improperly positioned teeth or to replace absent teeth (e.g., with prosthetic devices). Speech therapy may be beneficial for some affected children. Additional treatment for infants and children with cleft lip and cleft palate is symptomatic and supportive.

Cleft lip and cleft palate may occur as isolated conditions or in association with several underlying chromosomal disorders or malformation syndromes. Isolated cleft lip and/or cleft palate may potentially result due to certain environmental factors, occur randomly for unknown reasons (sporadically), or be familial. Many cases have been reported in which several individuals in multigenerational families (kindreds) have been affected by isolated cleft lip and cleft palate. In such cases, the specific modes of inheritance are not understood. The frequent association of cleft lip and cleft palate is thought to result from certain developmental abnormalities during embryonic growth.

See also **General Resources** on page 917

National Associations & Support Groups

1702 AboutFace USA

PO Box 158
South Beloit, IL 61080

702-769-9264
888-486-1209
Fax: 702-341-5351
e-mail: info@aboutfaceusa.org
www.aboutfaceusa.org

Provides information, services, emotional support and educational programs for and on behalf of individuals with facial differences and their families. Working to increase understanding through public awareness and education.

3M members

Debbie Oliver, Executive Director

1703 Cleft Palate/Craniofacial Birth Defects: Cleft Palate Foundation

1504 East Franklin Street, Suite 102
Chapel Hill, NC 27514

919-933-9044
800-242-5338
Fax: 919-933-9604
e-mail: info@cleftline.org
www.cleftline.org

The Cleft Palate Foundation operates a toll-free CLEFTLINE for parents with children born with cleft lip, palate and other craniofacial birth defects. Referrals are made to cleft palate/craniofacial healthcare teams and to parent-support groups. Free information is available to parents.

Earl J Seaver PhD, President
Nancy Smythe, Executive Director

1704 Craniofacial Foundation of America
975 E 3rd Street
Chattanooga, TN 37403

423-778-9192
800-418-3223
Fax: 423-778-8172
www.erlanger.org/cranio

Organization assists families with both the physical and emotional aspects, trying to make the everyday events a little easier.

Terri Farmer, Coordinator

1705 FACES: National Association for the Craniofacially Handicapped
PO Box 11082
Chattanooga, TN 37401

423-266-1632
800-332-2373
Fax: 423-267-3124
e-mail: faces@faces-cranio.org
www.faces-cranio.org

Assists individuals with facial disfigurations and their families They maintain a registry of centers offering corrective surgery for craniofacial deformities and financial assistance to qualified applicants.

Lynne Mayfield, President

1706 Genetic Alliance
4301 Connecticut Avenue NW
Washington, DC 20008

202-966-5557
800-336-4363
Fax: 202-966-8553
e-mail: info@geneticalliance.org
www.geneticalliance.org

A coalition of voluntary genetic support groups, consumers and professionals addressing the needs of individuals and families affected by genetic disorders from a national perspective.

Sharon Terry, President/CEO

1707 March of Dimes Birth Defects Foundation
1275 Mamaroneck Avenue
White Plains, NY 10605

888-663-4637
Fax: 914-997-4763
www.marchofdimes.com

The March of Dimes Resource Center answers questions about preparing for pregnancy, pregnancy, genetic diseases, birth defects and related topics.

Dr Jennifer Howse, President

1708 Prescription Parents
45 Brentwood Circle
Needham, MA 02492

617-499-1936
www.samizdat.com/pp1.html

Organization that gives information and support to children with cleft lip and cleft palate through its educational and support materials, including its directory, newsletter and brochures.

1709 Wide Smiles
PO Box 5153
Stockton, CA 95205

209-942-2812
Fax: 209-464-1497
e-mail: josmiles@yahoo.com
www.widesmiles.org

Wide Smiles was formed to ensure that parents of cleft-affected children do not have to feel alone. We offer support, inspiration,

information and networking for families everywhere who may be dealing with the challenges associated with clefting.

Joanne Green, Founding Director

Web Sites

1710 AboutFace USA
www.aboutfaceusa.org

Provides information, services, emotional support and educational programs for and on behalf of individuals with facial differences and their families. Working to increase understanding through public awareness and education.

1711 Cleft Palate/Craniofacial Birth Defects: Cleft Palate Foundation
www.cleftline.org

The Cleft Palate Foundation operates a toll-free CLEFTLINE for parents with children born with cleft lip, palate and other craniofacial birth defects. Referrals are made to cleft palate/craniofacial healthcare teams and to parent-support groups. Free information is available to parents.

1712 Craniofacial Foundation of America
www.erlanger.org/cranio

Organization assists families with both the physical and emotional aspects, trying to make the everyday events a little easier.

1713 FACES: National Association for the Craniofacially Handicapped
www.faces-cranio.org

Assists individuals with facial disfigurations and their families They maintain a registry of centers offering corrective surgery for craniofacial deformities and financial assistance to qualified applicants.

1714 March of Dimes Birth Defects Foundation
www.marchofdimes.com

The March of Dimes Resource Center answers questions about preparing for pregnancy, pregnancy, genetic diseases, birth defects and related topics.

1715 Online Mendelian Inheritance in Man
www.ncbi.nlm.nih.gov

This database is a catalog of human genes and genetic disorders.

1716 Prescription Parents
www.samizdat.com/pp1.html

Organization that gives information and support to children with cleft lip and cleft palate through its educational and support materials, including its directory, newsletter and brochures.

1717 Wide Smiles
www.widesmiles.org

Wide Smiles was formed to ensure that parents of cleft-affected children do not have to feel alone. We offer support, inspiration, information and networking for families everywhere who may be dealing with the challenges associated with clefting.

Book Publishers

1718 Children with Facial Difference
Woodbine House
6510 Bells Mill Road
Bethesda, MD 20817

301-468-8800
800-843-7323
Fax: 301-897-5838
e-mail: info@woodbinehouse.com
www.woodbinehouse.com

The first guide for parents about their child's congenital craniofacial anomaly-a condition that affects the appearance and function of the head and face. This accessible book discusses conditions such as cleft lip, cleft palate, Teacher Collins syndrome, Crouzon syndrome, and more. Parents learn about the diagnostic process, interdisciplinary treatment approach, education, speech and language issues, and how to help their child and family adjust emotionally.

361 pages Softcover
ISBN: 0-933149-61-1

1719 Communicative Disorders Related to Cleft Lip and Palate - Fifth Edition
Pro-Ed
8700 Shoal Creek Boulevard
Austin, TX 78757

512-451-3246
800-897-3202
Fax: 512-451-8542
e-mail: info@proedinc.com
www.proedinc.com

Being successfully used to train professional graduate students of speech pathology and audiology. Explains how to conduct clinical research in the area of communicative disorders related to cleft lip and palate and related craniofacial disorders.

Newsletters

1720 AboutFace USA
AboutFace
PO Box 158
South Beloit, IL 61080

888-486-1209
Fax: 702-341-5351
e-mail: info@aboutfaceusa.org
www.aboutfaceusa.org

A free newsletter.

8 pages

Rickie Anderson, Executive Director

Pamphlets

1721 As You Get Older: Information for Teens Born with Cleft Lip and Palate
Cleft Palate Foundation
1504 East Franklin Street, Suite 102
Chapel Hill, NC 27514

919-933-9044
Fax: 919-933-9604
e-mail: info@cleftline.org
www.cleftline.org

Describes medical treatment and social skilld that may be necessary for teens born with clefts. Concludes with three essays written by teens and a list of resources for more information

2002 20 pages

1722 Cleft Lip & Palate
March of Dimes Resource Center
1275 Mamaroneck Avenue
White Plains, NY 10605

914-997-4488
888-663-4637
Fax: 914-997-4763
www.marchofdimes.com

Various pamphlets and articles.

1723 Cleft Lip and Cleft Palate: The First Four Years
Cleft Palate Foundation
1504 East Franklin Street, Suite 102
Chapel Hill, NC 27514

919-933-9044
Fax: 919-933-9604
e-mail: info@cleftline.org
www.cleftline.org

Provides a basic explanation of cleft lip and palate and an overview of the care that a baby born with a cleft requires. Presents information on feeding, hearing testing, care of the ears, speech development, dental care, and a brief discussion of what to expect at the time of surgery.

1998 24 pages

1724 Cleft Lip and Palate: The Adult Patient
Cleft Palate Foundation
1504 East Franklin Street, Suite 102
Chapel Hill, NC 27514

919-933-9044
Fax: 919-933-9604
e-mail: info@cleftline.org
www.cleftline.org

Designed to empower adults to make informed decisions about what additional treatment, if any, they want to seek out in relation to their clefts. Provides instructions for how adults can get in touch with either cleft palate/craniofacial treatment teams or parent/patient support groups in their area.

1998 31 pages

1725 Cleft Lip and Palate: The School-Aged Child
Cleft Palate Foundation
1504 East Franklin Street, Suite 102
Chapel Hill, NC 27514

919-933-9044
Fax: 919-933-9604
e-mail: info@cleftline.org
www.cleftline.org

Divided into two sections, one addressing the medical concers of a school-aged child born with a cleft and the other providing information about the school experience for these children.

1998 27 pages

1726 Feeding an Infant with a Cleft
Cleft Palate Foundation
1504 East Franklin Street, Suite 102
Chapel Hill, NC 27514

919-933-9044
Fax: 919-933-9604
e-mail: info@cleftline.org
www.cleftline.org

Provides detailed instructions for feeding a newborn with cleft lip and/or palate. Recommendations about feeding positions, timing, and supplies are offered, with drawings and ordering information for the various bottles which are manufactured or can be adapted for babies with clefts.

1999 15 pages

1727 Hemangiomas and Vascular Malformations
Cleft Palate Foundation
1504 East Franklin Street, Suite 102
Chapel Hill, NC 27514

919-933-9044
Fax: 919-933-9604
e-mail: info@cleftline.org
www.cleftline.org

Provides an overview of the various types of vascular borthmarks and the treatment options for each. Also contains an essay written by an adult patient, as well as a glossary of terms. Includes 24 before and after color photos of the various vascular birthmarks.

1999 25 pages

1728 Managing Speech Problems: Physical Treatment of Velopharyngeal Dysfunction

Cleft Palate Foundation
1504 East Franklin Street, Suite 102
Chapel Hill, NC 27514

919-933-9044
Fax: 919-933-9604
e-mail: info@cleftline.org
www.cleftline.org

Describes additional procedures that may be needed to improve speech in people with repaired cleft palate. Explains surgical procedures including palate lengthening, pharyngeal flap, sphincter pharyngoplasty, and pharyngeal wall augmentation. Non-surgical prosthetic treatments are also described.

2004 12 pages

1729 The Genetics of Cleft Lip and Palate: Information for Families

Cleft Palate Foundation
1504 East Franklin Street, Suite 102
Chapel Hill, NC 27514

919-933-9044
Fax: 919-933-9604
e-mail: info@cleftline.org
www.cleftline.org

Contains a brief overview of genetic biology and a summary of what is known about the causes of clefting. Features a graph for affected individuals, parents, and siblings, showing each group's approximate chances of having a child with cleft.

1998 7 pages

DESCRIPTION

1730 CLUBFOOT

Synonym: Talipes
Covers these related disorders: Talipes equinovarus
Involves the following Biologic System(s):
Orthopedic and Muscle Disorders

Clubfoot, also known as congenital talipe equinovarus, is a deformity in which the foot is abnormally twisted out of position at birth (congenital). There are a number of foot deformities that are sometimes loosely classified as clubfoot. These include defects in which the inner portion of the foot is raised with the sole turned inward (metatarsus varus) or the front area of the foot is raised and the heel is turned outward (talipes calcaneovalgus). However, the term "clubfoot" is most commonly used to refer to a specific deformity in which the heel is turned inward and the sole is flexed with the toes downward (plantar flexion). More specifically, in infants with this condition, the forefoot is turned upward and inward toward the body; the heel is inverted; and the arch is high due to plantar flexion. These abnormalities are thought to occur as a result of deformity of the ankle bone (talus) and dislocation of the ankle (i.e., talonavicular joint). Depending upon the severity of the deformity, the affected foot may have varying levels of stiffness and inflexibility. In addition, the foot and lower leg may be unusually small. Muscles of the foot and calf are also typically underdeveloped, which may become more apparent with advancing age.

Talipes equinovarus is approximately twice as common in males than in females. In about 50 percent of children with this condition, both feet are affected. When one foot is affected, the right side is most often involved. Talipes equinovarus, however, often occurs an an isolated condition. Such cases occur randomly for unknown reasons or may be familial. In familial cases, the condition is thought to result from the interaction of an abnormal (mutated) gene, possibly in association with the involvement of other genes or certain environmental factors (multifactorial inheritance). Although deformity of the ankle bone was considered the primary abnormality, researchers speculate that a neuromuscular abnormality may be the underlying cause of the talus deformities and associated findings.

In some cases, talipes equinovarus may also occur due to or in association with certain neuromuscular disorders (e.g., arthrogryposis multiplex congenita) or other underlying disorders or syndromes. In addition, some researchers suspect that the deformity may also result from abnormal positioning of the foot during fetal development. Talipes equinovarus may affect up to one in 1,000 newborns.

The treatment of talipes equinovarus usually begins soon after birth. Treatment measures may include repeated, gentle manipulations of the affected foot toward a more normal position and the use of taping, casts, or splints (e.g., malleable splints, serial plaster casts) to hold the foot in a corrected position; casts to maintain proper positioning (e.g., holding casts); and other orthopedic appliances and corrective shoes to assist with walking. If the use of taping, splints, or casts does not result inappropriate correction, surgical methods may be recommended. Physicians should continue to regularly monitor affected children to detect possible recurrence and to ensure ongoing improvement.

See also **General Resources** on page 917

Government Agencies

1731 National Center for Environmental Health
Division of Birth Defects & Developmental Disabled
1600 Clifton Road
Atlanta, GA 30333

404-639-3311
800-331-3435
www.cdc.gov

Strives to promote health and quality of life by preventing or controlling those diseases or deaths that result from interactions between people and their enviroment.

Julie Louise Gerberding MD MPH, Director
Lynn Austin, Chief of Staff

National Associations & Support Groups

1732 Center for Pediatric Orthopaedic Surgery
NYU Hospital for Joint Diseases
301 E 17th Street, Suite 413
New York, NY 10003

212-598-6403
Fax: 212-598-6084

A specialized sector of the Center for Children at the Hospital for Joint Diseases, offering information, consultation, and comprehensive treatment of clubfoot deformities.

Wallace B Lehman MD, Physician

1733 Genetic Alliance
4301 Connecticut Avenue NW, Suite 404
Washington, DC 20008

202-966-5557
800-336-4363
Fax: 202-966-8553
e-mail: info@geneticalliance.org
www.geneticalliance.org

A nonprofit tax exempt organization founded in 1986 as a national coalition of consumers, professionals and genetic support groups to voice the common concerns of children and adults and families living with, and at risk of, genetic conditions. The Alliance builds partnerships among consumers and professionals and the private and public sectors to promote optimum healthcare and enhanced quality of life for individuals identified with genetic conditions.

Sharon Terry, President/CEO

1734 March of Dimes Birth Defects Foundation
1275 Mamaroneck Avenue
White Plains, NY 10605

914-428-7100
888-663-4637
Fax: 914-428-8203
e-mail: resourcecenter@modimes.org
www.marchofdimes.com

Partnership of volunteers and professionals dedicated to improving the health of babies by preventing birth defects and infant mortality. Over 100 chapters are located across the country and can be located through the National Office.

Dr Jennifer Howse, President

Web Sites

1735 CLIPS: Clubfoot Information and Parental Support
ixprss.com/clubfoot

A web site dedicated to providing clubfoot information and parental support, created by a parent as a resource for information, support and understanding.

1736 Children with Talipes (Clubfoot)
www.clubfoot.co.uk

Created by a parent of a child with talipes, the web site offers a first-hand account of treatment and description of clubfoot, as well as links to other sites.

1737 Johns Hopkins Department of Orthopaedic Surgery
www.hopkinsmedicine.org/orthopedicsurgery

A web site serving as a learning resource for patients and physicians alike, offering insight into the services provided by the university's professional staff members.

1738 Orthoseek
www.orthoseek.com/articles/clubfoot.html

A source of authoritative information on pediatric orthopedics and pediatric sports medicine.

1739 ParentsPlace Clubfoot Bulletin Board
pages.ivillage.com/clubfootboard/

Web pages offering information and links to help families choose the right treatment course.

1740 TIPS: Talipes Information and Parental Support
home.vicnet.net.au/~tips/

A support group run by parents whose children have, or had, talipes, offering comprehensive information and many web links, as well as a bi-monthly newletter, stories from parents, email correspondence, and emotional support.

1741 Virtual Children's Hospital: Treatment of Congenital Clubfoot
www.vh.org/pediatric/provider/orthopaedics/clubfoot

A digital library of pediatric information committed to educating patients, healthcare providers and students for the purpose of improving patients' care, outcome and lives; uses current, authoritative, trustworthy health information created by the University of Iowa, while serving as a platform for research into the challenges facing world-wide information distribution.

1742 Wheeless' Textbook of Orthopaedics
www.wheelessonline.com

Derives from a variety of sources, including journals, articles, national meetings, lectures and other textbooks.

Pamphlets

1743 Club Foot
March of Dimes Resource Center
1275 Mamaroneck Avenue
White Plains, NY 10605

888-663-4637
Fax: 914-997-4763
www.marchofdimes.com

Provides information on Club Foot.

1744 Club Foot and Other Foot Deformities
March of Dimes Resource Center
1275 Mamaroneck Avenue
White Plains, NY 10605

888-663-4637
Fax: 914-997-4763
TTY: 914-997-4764
e-mail: resourcecenter@modimes.org
www.modimes.org

Fact Sheets: one to two page review written for the general public. Also available electronically from our website www.modimes.org. Brochures: 3 panel color brochures written for the general public.

Camps

1745 Hemlocks Easter Seals Recreation
85 Jones Street
Hebron, CT 06248

860-228-9496
800-832-4409
Fax: 860-228-2091
e-mail: info@eastersealscamphemlocks.org
www.eastersealscamphemlocks.org

Accepts campers, ages 6 and under, whose major disability is orthopedic. First preference is given to Connecticut residents. A computer camp is also available.

Carl Larson

DESCRIPTION

1746 COARCTATION OF THE AORTA

Involves the following Biologic System(s):

Cardiovascular Disorders

Coarctation of the aorta is a congenital heart defect characterized by a narrowing or constriction of the body's main artery. This artery, known as the aorta, carries blood away from the heart to nourish the tissues of the body. Most of these defects are located just below the origin of the artery that supplies blood to the left arm, (left subclavian artery). Because this constriction reduces blood flow to the lower portion of the body, affected individuals may have unusually low blood pressure and weak or absent pulses in their legs. In addition, there may be higher blood pressure and strong pulses in the arms.

The severity of associated symptoms relates to the degree of pressure changes resulting from aortic narrowing. Although some children have no symptoms, others may experience dizziness, headache, weakness, fainting, nosebleeds, cold legs, and leg pain or cramps. Some affected infants may develop heart failure within the first few days or weeks of life. In some newborns, heart failure may result in decreased blood flow and abnormally high levels of acid in the blood (metabolic acidosis), sometimes accompanied by severe diarrhea and kidney (renal) failure. This life-threatening situation requires immediate treatment. Treatment of coarctation in a newborn requires surgery. (As these infants age, the narrowing may recur [restenosis] necessitating dilation or opening of the vessel through a procedure called balloon angioplasty, during which a balloon-tipped tube [catheter] is inflated inside the aorta, thus helping to expand the narrowed area of the vessel.) Correction of coarctation of the aorta through surgery or balloon catheterization may be recommended in older children with significant impairment. Because coarctation of the aorta is very often accompanied by other heart defects, early intervention is crucial. Other cardiac anomalies often associated with this defect include bicuspid aortic valve (i.e., the heart valve between the left ventricle and the aorta is composed of only two leaflets, or cusps, instead of the normal three); abnormalities of the mitral valve (located between the left atrium and the left ventricle); and an abnormal opening in the wall between the left and right ventricles (ventricular septal defect).

The cause of coarctation of the aorta is unknown. Some researchers think that it develops in the fetus in association with certain types of cardiac abnormalities. Coarctation of the aorta is more prevalent in males than in females by a ratio of about two to one.

See also **General Resources** on page 917

See also **General Resources** on page 917

Government Agencies

1747 NIH/National Heart, Lung and Blood Institu te
National Institute of Health
31 Center Dr MSC 2486, Bldg 31, Room 5A48
Bethesda, MD 20892

301-592-8573
Fax: 240-629-3246
TTY: 240-629-3255
e-mail: NHLBIinfo@nhlbi.nih.gov
www.nhlbi.nih.gov

Primary responsibility of this organization is the scientific investigation of heart, blood vessel, lung and blood disorders. Oversees research, demonstration, prevention, education, control and training activities in these fields and emphasizes the prevention and control of heart diseases.

Elizabeth G Nabel, MD, Director
Susan Shurin, MD, Deputy Director

1748 NIH/National Institute of Child Health and Human Development
31 Center Drive, Building 31
Bethesda, MD 20892

301-496-5133
Fax: 301-496-1104
www.nichd.nih.gov

Established in 1962 by congress, today the institute conducts and supports research on topics related to the health of children, adults, families and populations. Some of these topics include: developmental disabilities, growth and development, infant death, reproductive health and birth defects.

Nancy D Wirth, Director
Lisa Kaeser, Program & Public Liaison

National Associations & Support Groups

1749 American Heart Association
7272 Greenville Avenue
Dallas, TX 75231

214-373-6300
800-242-8721
Fax: 214-706-1341
e-mail: inquire@amhrt.org
www.amhrt.org

Supports research, education and community service programs with the objective of reducing premature death and disability from cardiovascular diseases and stroke; coordinates the efforts of health professionals, and others engaged in the fight against heart and circulatory disease.

M Cass Wheeler, CEO

1750 Genetic Alliance
4301 Connecticut Avenue NW
Washington, DC 20008

202-966-5557
800-336-4363
Fax: 202-966-8553
e-mail: info@geneticalliance.org
www.geneticalliance.org

A coalition of voluntary genetic support groups, consumers and professionals addressing the needs of individuals and families affected by genetic disorders from a national perspective.

Sharon Terry, President/CEO

1751 March of Dimes Birth Defects Foundation
1275 Mamaroneck Avenue
White Plains, NY 10605

914-428-7100
888-663-4637
Fax: 914-428-8203
e-mail: resourcecenter@modimes.org
www.marchofdimes.com

Partnership of volunteers and professionals dedicates to improving the health of babies by preventing birth defects and infant mortality. Over 100 chapters are located across the country and can be located through the National Office.

Dr Jennifer Howse, President

Research Centers

1752 Children's Hospital: Academic Pediatric Surgery Department
1056 E 19th Avenue
Denver, CO 80218

303-861-8888
800-624-6553
Fax: 303-764-5997
www.thechildrenshospital.org

Strives to improve the health of children through the provision of high quality, coordinated programs of patient care, education, research and advocacy.

Web Sites

1753 Congenital Heart Information Network
www.tchin.org

An international organization that provides reliable information, support services and resources to families of children with congenital heart defects and acquired heart disease, adults with congenital heart defects, and the professionals who work with them.

1754 Southern Illinois University School of Medicine
www.siumed.edu/peds/index.htm

Mission is to meet the health care needs of children and their families in central and Southern Illinois through provision of high quality, coordinated care of children with acute and chronic conditions with inpatient, ambulatory, and community-based programs.

1755 Yale University School of Medicine
www.info.med.yale.edu/intmed/cardio/chd

A site that offers information on congential heart conditions including Coarctation of the Aorta.

Book Publishers

1756 Congenital Disorders Sourcebook
Omnigraphics
PO Box 625
Holmes, PA 19043

800-234-1340
Fax: 800-875-1340
e-mail: info@omnigraphics.com
www.omnigraphics.com

Basic consumer health information on disorders aquired during gestation, including spina bifida, hydrocephalus, cerebral palsy, heart defects, craniofacial abnormalities and fetal alcohol syndrome.

650 pages
ISBN: 0-780809-45-9

DESCRIPTION

1757 COLIC

Synonyms: Infantile colic, Three-month colic
Involves the following Biologic System(s):
Gastrointestinal Disorders, Neonatal and Infant Disorders

Colic refers to a condition in which infants experience frequent episodes of abdominal pain, accompanied by irritability and intense crying. These episodes usually begin suddenly and continue for several hours. Symptoms and physical findings of colic may also include flushing of the face, swelling of the abdomen, repeated extending or flexing of the legs, and unusually cold feet.

It is suspected that colic is intestinal in origin; however, its exact cause is not known. Contributing factors may include the excessive swallowing of air during episodes of unceasing crying, overfeeding, hunger, certain foods, intestinal allergy, and environmental stress. Attacks of colic usually commence within the first few weeks of life and occur most often in the afternoon or evening. Colic often resolves spontaneously within three or four months, without residual effects.

Infants with symptoms associated with colic should be evaluated to determine if another, perhaps more serious disorder, is causing the pain and discomfort. The treatment of colic may include soothing, comforting gestures such as holding, patting, stroking, rocking, and other repetitive movements. Some affected infants may benefit from white noise or other comforting background sounds; the application of a warm wash cloth, hot water bottle, or warm heating pad under the stomach when the child is lying prone; or a ride in the car. Some episodes of colic may resolve with the passing of gas or stool. In addition, parents and caregivers may be advised to refrain from overstimulating, overfeeding, or underfeeding babies with colic. The toll colic takes on parents can be considerable. Physicians often advise that parents or caregivers try to get enough sleep as fatigue, may sometimes add to the already stressful situation.

See also **General Resources** on page 917

National Associations & Support Groups

1758 American College of Gastroenterology
PO Box 342260
Bethesda, MD 20827

301-263-9000
www.acg.gi.org

To advance the scientific study and medical practice of diseases of the gastrointestinal tract.

1932

Jack A DiPalma, President
Amy E Foxx-Orenstein, VP

1759 Digestive Disease National Coalition
507 Capitol Court NE, Suite 200
Washington, DC 20002

202-544-7497
Fax: 202-546-7105
www.ddnc.org

Advocacy organization comprised of 22 voluntary and professional societies concerned with the many diseases of the digestive tract and liver.

Nancy Norton, Chairperson
Dr. Maurice Cerulli, President

1760 Intestinal Disease Foundation
100 W Station Square Drive
Pittsburgh, PA 15219

412-261-5888
877-587-9606
Fax: 412-471-2722
e-mail: info@intestinalfoundation.org
www.intestinalfoundation.org

Nonprofit organization whose mission is to improve the quality of life of adults and children affected by chronic digestive illness through information, guidance and support. IDF offers a quarterly newsletter, Intestinal Fortitude, educational seminars, volunteer phone network, and Pittsburgh area support groups.

1761 North American Society for Pediatric Gastroenterology/Hepatology/Nutrition
PO Box 6
Flourtown, PA 19031

215-233-0808
Fax: 215-233-3918
e-mail: naspghan@naspghan.org
www.naspghan.org

Strives to improve the care of infants, children and adolescents with digestive disorders by promoting advances in clinical care of children with chronic abdominal pain, diarrhea, constipation, vomiting, bleeding from the GI tract, inflammatory bowel disease, liver diseases, diseases of the pancreas, poor weight gain and nutritional problems.

Philip Sherman, President
Margaret K Stallings, Executive Director

Libraries & Resource Centers

1762 Family Resource Center at Lucile Packard Children's Hospital
725 Welch Road
Palo Alto, CA 94304

650-497-8102
www.lpch.org/healthLibrary

Provides hospital patients, their families and staff with access to a wide variety of information about child and maternal health and well-being. The FRC collection includes books, periodicals and pamphlets on a variety of topics from coping with chronic illness such as colic to parenting skills and child development. The Family Resource Center also maintains a large collection of recreational reading materials and video tapes.

1763 National Digestive Diseases Information Clearinghouse
2 Information Way
Bethesda, MD 20892

301-654-3810
800-891-5389
Fax: 703-738-4929
e-mail: nddic@info.niddk.nih.gov
www.digestive.niddk.nih.gov

The National Institute of Diabetes and Digestive and Kidney Diseases conducts and supports research on many of the most serious diseases affecting public health. The Institute supports much of the clinical research on the diseases of internal medicine and related subspecialty fields as well as many basic science disciplines.

Kathy Kranzfelder, Project Officer

Research Centers

1764 CNS Clinical Trials: Atlanta
6065 Roswell Road, Suite 820
Atlanta, GA 30328

404-459-6699
877-749-4419
Fax: 404-459-6524
e-mail: sm_atlanta@cnsmail.com

Katie Neri BSN RN CCRC, Director

1765 CRI Worldwide Pediatric Center for Excellence
CRI Worldwide
130 White Horse Pike
Clementon, NJ 08021

856-566-9000
Fax: 856-566-4302
e-mail: dkrefetz@cnsresearchinstitute.com
www.cnsresearchinstitute.com

Formerly called CNS Research Institute; Psychiatrists and Child Psychologists maintains a major emphasis in the area of pediatric research. Working hard with parents and their children to educate and treat the entire family.

Dr David Krefetz, Director

1766 Central DuPage Hospital Center for Digestive Disorders
25 N Winfield Road
Winfield, IL 60190

630-933-1600
Fax: 630-933-1300
www.cdh.org

Bringing together the best research about colic and weighed up the evidence about how to treat it.

Luke McGuinness, President/CEO
Dr. Kenneth Heaps, Medical Affairs VP

1767 Cincinnati Digestive Diseases Research Development Center
Cincinnati Children's Hospital Medical Center
3333 Burnet Avenue
Cincinnati, OH 45229

513-636-4200
800-344-2462
TTY: 513-636-4900
www.cincinnatichildrens.org

Promote research that will yield insights into the fundamental processes of growth and development in the digestive tract and lead to novel or improved therapies.

Mitchell Cohen, MD, Director
Jorge Bezerra, MD, Associate Director

1768 Infant Behavior, Cry and Sleep Clinic
Women & Infants Hospital of Rhode Island
50 Holden Street, 1st Floor
Providence, RI 02908

401-453-7690
Fax: 401-453-7697
e-mail: Barry_Lester@brown.edu
www.womenandinfants.com

A clinical service developed to diagnose and treat infants with crying, sleeping, feeding and associated early behavior problems by helping parents understand and manage their infant and to adjust to the disruption caused by having an infant who has behavioral problems in the first few months of life.

Barry Lester, Director

Web Sites

1769 Ask NOAH About: Stomach and Intestinal (Gastrointestinal) Disorders
noah-health.org/english/illness/gastro/gastro.html

NOAH provides access to high quality full-text consumer health information in English and Spanish that is accurate, timely, relevenat and unbiased.

Journals

1770 Journal of Pediatric Gastroenterology and Nutrition
NASPGHAN, author

Lippincott Williams & Wilkins
530 Walnut Street
Philadelphia, PA 19106

215-521-8300
Fax: 215-521-8902
www.lww.com

Publication of the North American Society for Pediatric Gastroenterolgy, Hepatology and Nutrition, which strives to improve the care of infants, children and adolescents with digestive disorders by promoting advances in clinical care of children with chronic abdominal pain, diarrhea, constipation, vomiting, bleeding from the GI tract, inflammatory bowel disease, liver diseases, diseases of the pancreas, poor weight gain and nutritional problems.

Newsletters

1771 NASPGHAN News
PO Box 6
Flourtown, PA 19031

215-233-0808
Fax: 215-233-3939
e-mail: naspghan@naspghan.org
www.naspgn.org

Publication of the North American Society for Pediatric Gastroenterolgy, Hepatology and Nutrition, which strives to improve the care of infants, children and adolescents with digestive disorders by promoting advances in clinical care of children with chronic abdominal pain, diarrhea, constipation, vomiting, bleeding from the GI tract, inflammatory bowel disease, liver diseases, diseases of the pancreas, poor weight gain and nutritional problems.

DESCRIPTION

1772 CONDUCT DISORDER

Covers these related disorders: Group conduct disorder, Solitary aggressive conduct disorder, Undifferentiated conduct disorder

Involves the following Biologic System(s):
Developmental/Behavioral/Psychiatric Disorders

Conduct disorder refers to a group of distinct behavioral abnormalities characterized by the repetition of certain types of disruptive or antisocial behaviors. Children or adolescents with conduct disorder may often lie, steal, skip school, run away from home, use drugs or alcohol, hurt animals, commit arson or vandalism, engage in physical violence, use weapons, and commit other criminal acts. Those affected with solitary aggressive conduct disorder are usually selfish, rarely get along with or relate well to others, and often lack remorse for their behavior. Children and adolescents with group conduct disorder, however, may be attached and faithful to a particular clique, gang, or other group of friends while at the same time violating the rights of or displaying antisocial behavior toward those outside of the group. In some cases, affected individuals may display behavior characteristic of both solitary aggressive and group conduct disorders and, subsequently, may be diagnosed with undifferentiated conduct disorder.

Conduct disorder may be caused by a variety of factors including genetic as well as environmental influences (e.g., childrearing, etc.). In many cases, children with this type of behavioral irregularity have parents or caregivers who display similar patterns of conduct. In addition, parents or caregivers often have inconsistent parenting skills or may be overly aggressive in punishing or disciplining. Some parents or caregivers may be unsupportive of the child, or may lack other basic skills that help the child to develop a sense of self-worth, respect for others, etc. Several factors may influence whether affected children carry these characteristic patterns of behavior into adulthood. Some factors include parental or caregiver influences, the age of onset, the severity and type of behavior, the number of different types of antisocial behaviors exhibited, and whether the episodes of disruptive behavior continue to increase.

Treatment of conduct disorder may include individual, group, and family therapy, as well as parental or caregiver management training. In some cases, children with severe conduct disorder may benefit from hospitalization for psychiatric evaluation and treatment. Medication is, in most cases, not indicated for the treatment of conduct disorder; however, it is sometimes prescribed to treat other underlying disorders (e.g, depression, attention deficit hyperactivity disorder, etc.). Other treatment is supportive.

See also **General Resources** on page 917

Government Agencies

1773 NIH/National Institute of Mental Health
6001 Executive Boulevard, Room 8184, MSC 9663
Bethesda, MD 20892

301-443-4513
866-615-6464
Fax: 301-443-4279
TTY: 301-443-8431
e-mail: nimhinfo@nih.gov
www.nimh.nih.gov

Conducts strategic planning for specific research areas as well as for the Institute as a whole.

Dr Thomas R Insel, Director

National Associations & Support Groups

1774 American Mental Health Foundation
191 Presidential Boulevard, Suite 3-W, PO Box 345
Bala Cynwyd, PA 19004
USA

Dedicated to the extensive and intensive research in the theories and techniques of treatment of emotional illness and to the implementation of reforms in the mental health system. Efforts have resulted in development of better and less expensive treatment methods. Findings are disseminated in English and other major languages.

Monroe W Spero, MD

1775 Association for Behavioral and Cognitive Therapies
305 7th Avenue, 16th Floor
New York, NY 10001

212-647-1890
Fax: 212-647-1865
e-mail: membership@abct.org
www.aabt.org

Formerly known as the Association for Advancement of Behavior Therapy; this organization is concerned with the application of behavioral and cognitive sciences to understanding human behavior, developing interventions to enhance the human condition, and promoting the appropriate utilization of these interventions.

Mary Jane Eimer, Executive Director
Lisa Yarde, Membership Services Manager

1776 Center for Mental Health Services Knowledge Exchange Network
US Department of Health and Human Services
PO Box 42557
Washington, DC 20015

800-789-2647
Fax: 240-747-5470
TDD: 866-889-2647
http://mentalhealth.samhsa.gov

Supplies the public with responses to their commonly asked questions about health issues and services.

1777 Federation of Families for Children's Mental Health
9605 Medical Center Drive, Suite 280
Rockville, MD 20850

240-403-1901
Fax: 240-403-1909
e-mail: ffcmh@ffcmh.org
www.ffcmh.org

The National family run organization is dedicated exclusively to helping children with mental health needs and their families achieve a better quality of life.

Sandra Spencer, Executive Director

1778 NADD: National Association for the Dually Diagnosed
132 Fair Street
Kingston, NY 12401

845-331-4336
800-331-5362
Fax: 845-331-4569
e-mail: info@thenadd.org
www.thenadd.org

Nonprofit organization designed to promote the interests of professional and parent development with resources for individuals who have the coexistence of mental illness and mental retardation. Provides conferences, educational services and training materials to professionals, parents, concerned citizens and service organizations.

Dr Robert Fletcher, CEO

1779 National Alliance for the Mentally Ill
2107 Wilson Blvd, Ste 300, Colonial Place Three
Arlington, VA 22201

703-524-7600
800-950-6264
Fax: 703-524-9094
TDD: 703-516-7227
e-mail: info@nami.org
www.nami.org

NAMI is a nonprofit, grassroots, self-help, support and advocacy organization of consumers, families and friends of people with severe mental illness, such as schizophrenia, bipolar disorder, major despressive disorder, obsessive compulsive disorder, anxiety disorders, autism and other severe and persistent mental illnesses that affect the brain.

Suzanne Vogel-Scibilia MD, President

1780 National Association for the Dually Diagno sed
132 Fair Street
Kingston, NY 12401

845-331-4336
800-331-5362
Fax: 845-331-4569
e-mail: thenadd@aol.com
www.thenadd.org

Nonprofit organization designed to promote interests of professional and parent development with resources for individuals who have the coexistence of mental illness and mental retardation. Provides conferences, educational services and training materials to professionals, parents, concerned citizens and service organizations.

Robert Fletcher, Executive Director

1781 National Mental Health Association
2000 N Beauregard Street, 6th Floor
Alexandria, VA 22311

703-684-7722
800-969-6642
Fax: 703-684-5968
TTY: 800-433-5959
www.nmha.org

Dedicated to promoting mental health, preventing mental disorders and achieving victory over mental illness through advocacy, education, research and service.

David L Shern PhD, President & CEO

1782 National Mental Health Consumers' Self-Help Clearinghouse
1211 Chestnut Street, Suite 1207
Philadelphia, PA 19107

215-751-1810
800-553-4539
Fax: 215-636-6312
e-mail: info@mhselfhelp.org
www.mhselfhelp.org

Offers information, support and appropriate referrals; and promotes public and professional education. Provides networking for those with special interests related to albinism. Promotes and supports research and funding that will improve diagnosis and management of albinism and hypopigmentation.

Joseph Rogers, Executive Director & Founder

State Agencies & Support Groups

1783 Center for Disabilities and Development
University of Iowa Hospitals and Clinics
100 Hawkins Drive
Iowa City, IA 52242

319-353-6900
877-686-0031
e-mail: cdd-webmaster@uiowa.edu
www.healthcare.uiowa.edu/cdd

A trusted resource for healthcare, training, research and information for people with disabilities that include: behavior disorders, brain injury, cerebral palsy, diabetes, down syndrome, learning disabilities, mental retardation, sleep disorders and spina bifida.

Elayne Sexsmith, Administrator
Amy Mikelson, Supervisor Info Resource Service

Research Centers

1784 Menninger Child & Family Program
Menninger Clinic
2801 Gessner Drive, PO Box 809045
Houston, TX 77280

713-275-5000
800-351-9058
Fax: 713-275-5107
www.menninger.edu

Menninger's research strategies are developed through the Menninger Child & Family Program. Projects are designed to develop a better understanding of the mind in order to more effectively treat mental disorders.

Peter Fonagy, Ph.D, Program Director

1785 National Technical Assistance Center for Children's Mental Health
Georgetown University
Box 571485
Washington, DC 20057

202-687-5000
Fax: 202-687-1954
TDD: 202-687-5503
e-mail: childrensmh@georgetown.edu
www.gucchd.georgetown.edu

Devoted to helping states, tribes, territories, and communities discover, apply, and sustain innovative and collaborative solutions that improve the social, emotional, and behavioral well being of children and families.

DJ Ida, Executive Director

1786 Research & Training Center for Children's Mental Health at University of South FL
Louis de la Parte Florida Mental Health Institute
13301 Bruce B. Downs Boulevard
Tampa, FL 33612

813-974-4661
Fax: 813-974-6257
e-mail: friedman@fmhi.usf.edu
www.rtckids.fmhi.usf.edu/

Working towards increasing the effectiveness of service systems by strengthening the empirical base for such systems through research and dissemination to key audiences. With its new, five-year research program, the Center expands its mission with an integrated research, training, and dissemination program targeted specifically at implementation issues for developing effective systems of care.

Robert M Friedman, Ph.D, Center Director
Krista Kutash, Ph.D, Research Deputy Director

1787 Research and Training Center on Family Support and Children's Mental Health
1600 SW 4th Avenue, Suite 900
Portland, OR 97201

503-725-4040
Fax: 503-725-4180
e-mail: flemingd@pdx.edu
www.rtc.pdx.edu

Funded to pursue an integrated set of research, training, technical assistance, and dissemination activities. The center's work will focus on two related themes; community integration for children and adolescents with emotional and behavioral disorders and their families; and strengthening family and youth participation in child and adolescent mental health services.

Donna Flemming, Information Director

1788 Technical Assistance Partnership for Child and Family Mental Health
1000 Thomas Jefferson Street NW, Suite 400
Washington, DC 20007

202-342-5600
Fax: 202-342-5007
e-mail: tapartnership@air.org
www.air.org/tapartnership

A staff of family members and professionals with extensive practice experience, grounded in an organization with vast research experience in children with serious emotional disturbance and their families.

Leigh Meredith, Research Associate
Regenia Hicks, Project Director

Audio Video

1789 Managing the Defiant Child
Courage To Change Publishing
PO Box 486
Wilkes-Barres, PA 18703

800-440-4003
Fax: 800-772-6499
www.couragetochange.com

An information-packed video brings to life a proven approach to behavior management. Shows clinicians, school practitioners, teachers, parents and students how enhanced parenting skills can dramatically improve the parent-child relationship.

Russell A Barkley, Editor

1790 Understanding and Treating the Hereditary Psychiatric Spectrum Disorders
Hope Press
PO Box 188
Duarte, CA 91009

818-303-0644
800-321-4039
Fax: 818-358-3520
hopepress.com

Learn with ten hours of audio tapes from a two day seminar given in May 1997 by David E Comings MD. Tapes cover: ADHD, Tourette syndrome, Obsessive-Compulsive Disorder, Conduct Disorder, Oppositional Defiant Disorder, Autism and other Hereditary Psychiatric Spectrum Disorders. Eight audio tapes.

David E Comings, MD, Presenter

1791 Understanding the Defiant Child
Courage To Change
PO Box 486
Wilkes-Barres, PA 18703

800-440-4003
Fax: 800-772-6499
www.couragetochange.com

Provides a vivid picture of what we know about Oppositional Defiant Disorder and presents real-life scenes of family interactions and commentary from parents. Illuminates the nature and causes of ODD, why it should be dealt with early, and what can be done. Ideal viewing for school practitioners, clinical child psychologists, counselors and parents coping with a defiant child.

Russell A Barkley, Editor

Web Sites

1792 Conductdisorders.com
www.conductdisorders.com

Site for parents, teachers, and family members who deal with a child with one of the defined behavioral disorders.

1793 Internet Mental Health
www.mentalhealth.com

Our goal is to improve understanding, diagnosis, and treatment of mental illness throughout the world.

1794 Online Mendelian Inheritance in Man
www.ncbi.nlm.nih.gov

This database is a catalog of human genes and genetic disorders.

1795 Planetpsych
www.planetpsych.com

Planetpsych is an online resource for mental health information.

Book Publishers

1796 Aggression and Violence Throughout the Life Span
Sage Publications
2455 Teller Road
Thousand Oaks, CA 91320

805-499-0721
Fax: 805-499-0871
e-mail: info@sagepub.com
www.sagepub.com

A unique life span developmental perspective on some of society's most perplexing and pernicious problems, aggressive and violent behaviors. Examines issues in the development of aggressive behaviors in young children, the progression of these behaviors to older children and adolescents and cause, effect and treatment of aggressive and violent behaviors in adults. Integrates empirical research with clinical applications.

360 pages Softcover
ISBN: 0-803945-51-5

Ray Peters, Editor
Robert J McMahon, Editor

1797 Antisocial Behavior by Young People

Cambridge University Press
32 Avenue of the Americas
New York, NY 10013

212-924-3900
Fax: 212-619-3239
www.cambridge.org

Written by a child psychiatrist, a criminologist and a social psychologist, this book is a major international review of research evidence on anti-social behavior. Covers all aspects of the field, including descriptions of different types of delinquency and time trends, the state of knowledge on the individuals, social-psychological and cultural factors involved and recent advances in prevention and intervention.

490 pages Paperback
ISBN: 0-521646-08-1

Michael Rutter, Editor
Ann Hagell, Editor

1798 Conduct Disorders in Childhood and Adolescence (Developmental Clinical)

Sage Publications
2455 Teller Road
Thousand Oaks, CA 91320

805-499-0721
800-818-7243
Fax: 805-499-0871
e-mail: info@sagepub.com
www.sagepub.com

Conduct disorder is a clinical problem among children and adolescents that includes aggressive acts, theft, vandalism, firesetting, running away, truancy, defying authority and other antisocial behaviors. This book describes the nature of conduct disorder and what is currently known from research and clinical work. Topics include psychiatric diagnosis, parent psychopathology and child-rearing processes.

192 pages Hardcover
ISBN: 0-803971-81-8

Alan E Kazdin, Editor

1799 Conduct Disorders in Children and Adolescents

American Psychiatric Publishing
1000 Wilson Boulevard, Suite 1825
Arlington, VA 22009

703-907-7322
800-368-5777
Fax: 703-907-1091
e-mail: appi@psych.org
www.appi.org

Examines the phenomenology, etiology, and diagnosis of conduct disorders, and describes therapeutic and preventive interventions. Includes the range of treatments now available, including individual, family, group, and behavior therapy; hospitalization; and residential treatment.

1995 414 pages Hardcover
ISBN: 0-880485-17-5

G Pirooz Sholevar, MD, Editor

1800 Conduct Problem/Emotional Problem Interventions: A Holistic Perspective

Slosson Educational Publications
PO Box 544
East Aurora, NY 14052

716-625-0930
888-756-7766
Fax: 800-655-3840
e-mail: slosson@slosson.com
www.slosson.com

This innovative book is broad in scope and addresses the now what sensation that many professionals get when charged with the education or treatment of individuals with conduct disorders or emotional disturbance. Distinct intervention and screening strategies and patient involvement strategies are offered in clear and practical terms.

Edward J Kelly, Editor

1801 Difficult Child

Random House
1745 Broadway
New York, NY 10019

212-782-9000
Fax: 212-782-9700
www.randomhouse.com

One of the nation's most respected experts on children and discipline; Dr. Stanley Turecki a father of a once difficult child offers compassionate and practical advice to parents of hard-to-raise children.

320 pages Paperback

Stanley Turecki, Writer

1802 Disruptive Behavior Disorders in Children and Adolescents

Robert L Hendren, DO, author

American Psychiatric Publishing
1000 Wilson Boulevard, Suite 1825
Arlington, VA 22209

703-907-7322
800-368-5777
Fax: 703-907-1091
e-mail: appi@psych.org
www.appi.org

Discusses attention deficit hyperactivity disorder, conduct disorder, substance abuse and disruptive behavior disorders. Examines the relationship between violence and mental illness in adolescence.

1999 216 pages Paperback
ISBN: 0-880489-60-7

1803 Preventing Antisocial Behavior: Interventions

Guilford Press
72 Spring Street
New York, NY 10012

212-431-9800
800-365-7006
Fax: 212-966-6708
e-mail: info@guilford.com
www.guilford.com

Establishes the crucial link between theory, measurement and intervention. Brings together a collection of studies that utilize experimental approaches for evaluating intervention programs, both the feasibility, and necessity of independent evaluation. Also shows how the information obtained in such studies can be used to test and refine prevailing theories about human behavior in general, and behavior changes in particular.

1992 391 pages
ISBN: 0-898628-82-2

Joan McCord, Editor
Richard Tremblay, Editor

1804 Skills Training for Children with Behavior Disorders
Courage To Change
PO Box 486
Wilkes-Barres, PA 18703

800-440-4003
Fax: 800-772-6499
www.couragetochange.com

Designed for use by both parents and therapists, provides background information, step-by-step instructions and many useful, reproducible worksheets. Techniques offered help children with anger management, compliance and following rules, academic success, emotional well-being and self-esteem and much more.

272 pages

Michael L Bloomquist, Editor

Pamphlets

1805 Conduct Disorder in Children and Adolescents
National Mental Health Information Center
PO Box 42557
Washington, DC 20015

800-789-2647
Fax: 240-747-5470
TDD: 866-889-2647
e-mail: ken@mentalhealth.org
www.mentalhealth.samhsa.gov

This fact sheet defines conduct disorder, identifies risk factors, discusses types of help available, and suggests what parents or other caregivers can do.

1997 2 pages

1806 Mental, Emotional, and Behavior Disorders in Children and Adolescents
National Mental Health Information
PO Box 42557
Washington, DC 20015

240-747-5484
800-789-2647
Fax: 240-747-5470
mentalhealth.samhsa.gov

This fact sheet describes mental, emotional, and behavioral problems that can occur during childhood and adolescence and discusses related treatment, support services, and research.

4 pages

1807 Treatment of Children with Mental Disorder
National Institute of Mental Health
6001 Executive Boulevard
Bethesda, MD 20892

301-443-4513
866-615-6464
Fax: 301-443-4279
TTY: 301-443-8431
e-mail: nimhinfo@nih.gov
www.nimh.nih.gov/publicat

A short booklet that contains questions and answers about therapy for children with mental disorders. Includes a chart of mental disorders and medications used.

Joan Abell, Chief IRIB
Sharon Maarsen, Technical Information Specialist

Camps

1808 Adventure Learning Center Camp Programs
Eagle Village
4507 170th Avenue
Hersey, MI 49639

231-832-7262
800-748-0061
Fax: 231-832-1468
e-mail: summercamp@eaglevillage.org
www.eaglevillage.org

Offers a variety of fun camp experiences for children, including those with emotional and/or behavioral impairments. A low staff-to-camper ratio and exciting, challenging activities make the camps rewarding experiences. As funding is available, we will offer camp scholarships to eligible participants.

Sara Kofal, Camp Director

1809 Bennington School
992 Fairview Street
Bennington, VT 800-6

802-447-1557
800-800-639
Fax: 802-447-3234

A 115 bed residential treatment center serving emotionally and behaviorally disordered adolescent male and female students. Offer a fully accredited on-grounds educational program in addition to comprehensive clinical and residential components. The beautiful rural setting provides many recreational opportunities as well as cultural experiences.

Patrick Ramsay, Admissions Director
Jeff LaBonte, Executive Director

1810 Camp Niobe
4580 S Mill Road
Dryden, MI

810-796-2480

A six week summer resident camp program for boys and girls whose learning and behavior styles have made successful participation in the traditional camp program difficult. All camp activities have a special emphasis on building self-esteem and peer relationships. Strong in waterfront, nature, campcrafts and a special arts program. 2 weeks ($560.00); 4 weeks ($1075.00); Canoe Trip ($275).

Joanne Mandel, Director

1811 Life Adventure Center
Life Adventure Center of the Bluegrass
570 Milner Road
Versailles, KY 40383

859-873-3271
Fax: 859-873-2410
www.lifeadventurecamp.org

A unique experience of discovery and development where lifelong lessons are learned. Through purposeful play, using a combination of physical and mental problem-solving exercises, participants engage in opportunities to make positive choices, gain self-confidence, improve decision making, build on group strengths and much more.

1812 Talisman Summer Camps
Talisman Schools
64 Gap Creek Road
Zirconia, NC 28790

828-669-8639
Fax: 828-669-2521
e-mail: summer@talismancamps.com
www.talismansummercamp.com/

Camps for children ages 6 to 17 and young adults 18-21 with LD, ADD and ADHD, Asperger's Syndrome, and high functioning autism. Talisman has been offering such experiences since 1980 and is ACA accredited. The unique summer camps specialize in creating camps that offer not only adventure, but learning experiences, for children and teenagers with learning disabilities, attention deficit hyperactivity disorder, Asperger's syndrome and high-functioning autism.

Linda Tatsapaugh, Director
Aaron McGinley, Base Camp Program Manager

DESCRIPTION

1813 CONGENITAL ADRENAL HYPERPLASIA

Synonyms: CAH, Androgenital syndrome, Congenital virilizing adrenal hyper, 21-hydroxylase deficiency, 11-beta-hydroxylase deficiency

Involves the following Biologic System(s):

Endocrinologic Disorders

Congenital adrenal hyperplasia (CAH) refers to a group of genetic diseases that leads to the inability of the adrenal glands to make cortisol. Cortisol is a steroid hormone needed to maintain metabolism, energy, blood pressure, and a normal responses to stress or injury. There are many different steps in the production of cortisol; each step requires an enzyme for completion and as a result, a deficiency in any enzyme along the path leads to one of the forms of CAH. The inability to make cortisol leads to symptoms from both the lack of cortisol as well as from the build-up of the cortisol precursors. In CAH, male hormones (androgens) are made in excess and this will lead to exaggerated male characteristics in these patients. Some people with CAH also have deficiency in another hormone, aldosterone. Aldosterone regulates salt (sodium)levels in the body.

Symptoms of CAH can vary in girls and boys, and also may vary according to the specific type of CAH. In girls, the excess of androgens leads to masculinization of the female external genitalia (ambiguous genitalia). Symptoms in girls with milder forms of CAH include irregular menstrual periods, excessive or male pattern hair growth, or infertility. In boys, symptoms of salt-wasting CAH include adrenal crisis which typically consists of low blood pressure and sodium abnormalities. Girls can also have salt abnormalities, but are often diagnosed before an adrenal crisis because of their ambiguous external genitalia can be seen. In boys with non-salt wasting CAH, the effect of excess androgens leads to pubertal changes earlier than expected (precocious puberty).

The treatment of CAH is replacement of cortisol with glucocorticoid medications, and if needed, replacement of aldosterone with mineralocorticoid medications. It is important to remember to give extra medication (stress dose steroids during times of stress, illness, or injury because of the body's greater demand for steroids during those times.)

See also **General Resources** on page 917

National Associations & Support Groups

1814 CARES Foundation
2414 Morris Avenue, Suite 110
Union, NJ 07083

973-912-3895
866-227-3737
Fax: 973-912-8990
e-mail: kelly@caresfoundation.org
www.caresfoundation.org

CARES Foundation is a nonprofit, educational organization. Its purpose is to educate the public and physicians about all forms of Congenital Adrenal Hyperplasia, its symptoms, diagnostic protocols, treatment, genetic frequency, the necessity for early intervention and benefits of newborn screening. It is also dedicated to providing support and information to affected individuals and their families.

Kelly R Leight, Executive Director

1815 MAGIC Foundation: Major Aspects of Growth in Children
6645 West North Avenue
Oak Park, IL 60302

708-383-0808
800-362-4423
Fax: 708-383-0899
e-mail: mary@magicfoundation.org
www.magicfoundation.org

The MAGIC Foundation is a national nonprofit organization created to provide support services for the families of children afflicted with a wide variety of chronic and/or critical disorders, syndromes, and diseases that affect a child's growth.

10,000 members

Mary Andrews, CEO
Dianne Tamburrino, Executive Director

1816 National Adrenal Diseases Foundation
505 Northern Boulevard
Great Neck, NY 11021

516-487-4992
e-mail: nadfmail@aol.com
www.medhelp.org/www/nadf

NADF is committed to bringing information regarding adrenal diseases into the public's awareness to facilitate early diagnosis and treatment.NADF sponsors support groups across the countrty allowing for an exchange of ideas and feelings by individuals who share a common illness. NADF members receive quaterly newsletters, educational materials, and access to a library of related information.

Melanie G Wong, Executive Director
Paul Margulies, MD, Medical Director

Libraries & Resource Centers

1817 University of Iowa Birth Defects and Genetic Disorders Unit
2614 JCP
Iowa City, IA 52242

319-335-9901

James M Smith, Director

Web Sites

1818 CARES Foundation
www.caresfoundation.org

Provides education to the public and physicians about all forms of Congenital Adrenal Hyerplasia — symptoms, diagnostic protocols, treatment, genetic frequency, the necessity for early intervention and benefits of newborn screening. The web site also provides support and information to affected individuals and their families.

1819 MAGIC Foundation: Major Aspects of Growth in Children
www.magicfoundation.org

Created to provide support services for the families of children afflicted with a wide variety of chronic and/or critical disorders, syndromes, and diseases that affect a child's growth.

1820 National Adrenal Diseases Foundation
www.medhelp.org/nadf/index.htm

Committed to bringing information regarding rare diseases to the publics awareness to facilitate early diagnosis and treatment.

Newsletters

1821 CARES Foundation Newsletter
2414 Morris Avenue, Suite 110
Union, NJ 07083

973-912-3895
866-227-3737
e-mail: kelly@caresfoundation.org
www.caresfoundation.org

Provides support and information to affected individuals and their families.

3x year

Kelly R Leight, Executive Director

1822 NADF News
505 Northern Boulevard
Great Neck, NY 11021

516-487-4992
e-mail: nadfmail@aol.com
www.medhelp.org/www/nadf

Features important information on adrenal disorders, support groups and the latest research.

quaterly

Melanie G Wong, Executive Director
Paul Margulies, MD, Medical Director

DESCRIPTION

1823 CONGENITAL CATARACTS

Involves the following Biologic System(s):
Genetic/Chromosomal/Syndrome/Metabolic Disorders,
Ophthalmologic Disorders

Congenital cataracts refers to a condition in which cloudiness or opacities in the lens of the eye or eyes are present at birth. These opacities may vary in severity, with some resolving spontaneously as in cataracts of prematurity. Other congenital cataracts, if left untreated, may result in loss of transparency of the lens and subsequent visual impairment. In addition, in some newborns, remnants of other eye tissues may contribute to the formation of a stationary opacity of the cornea. In most instances , this type of stationary cloudiness does not contribute to visual impairment.

Congenital cataracts may occur as the result of many different factors (multifactorial), including genetic influences, associated metabolic and chromosomal disorders, congenital infections, and toxic exposure. If inherited as an isolated event, congenital cataracts are usually transmitted as an autosomal dominant or autosomal recessive trait. Several metabolic disorders are characterized by congenital cataracts, including galactosemia, in which an enzyme deficiency results in the inability to process the simple sugar galactose; oculocerebrorenal syndrome (Lowe's syndrome), an X-linked metabolic disorder that affects many systems of the body; certain metabolic diseases known as lyosomal storage disorders; and several other diseases related to inborn errors of metabolism. Other contributing metabolic factors may include low blood levels of calcium (hypocalcemia) or glucose (hypoglycemia). In addition, cataracts are sometimes diagnosed in newborns whose mothers have diabetes mellitus. Several chromosomal disorders are also characterized by congenital opacities including Down's syndrome (trisomy 21), trisomy 13 syndrome, Turner's syndrome (45XO), and others. Congenital cataracts are sometimes the result of maternal infections that occur during pregnancy. Such infections may include German measles (rubella), syphilis, measles, influenza, certain herpes infections, and others. Additional contributing factors may include toxic influences from drug substances taken by the mother during pregnancy.

Treatment for congenital cataracts depends upon the extent of the defect and its influence on vision. To restore lost transparency of the lens resulting from cataracts, surgery may be performed in which the cataract and lens are removed. To reestablish the ability of the eye to deflect light that was lost with lens removal, special contact lenses or implants are then fitted to the eye. In some cases, additional surgery may be indicated. Because congenital opacities of the lens are so often associated with other eye irregularities (e.g., amblyopia, glaucoma, strabismus, etc.) and in order to obtain the best outcome, treatment may also be directed toward any associated abnormalities. In addition, patients are followed carefully after surgery in order to prevent, correct, or treat any possible complications.

See also **General Resources** on page 917

Government Agencies

1824 NIH/National Eye Institute
31 Center Drive MSC 2510
Bethesda, MD 20892

301-496-5248
e-mail: 2020@nei.nih.gov
www.nei.nih.gov

Conducts and supports research that helps prevent and treat eye diseases and other disorders of vision. This research leads to sight-saving treatments, reduces visual impairment and blindness, and improves the quality of life for people of all ages. NEI-supported research has advanced our knowledge of how the eye functions in health and disease.

Paul A Sieving M.D., Ph.D., Director

National Associations & Support Groups

1825 American Council of the Blind
1155 15th Street NW, Suite 720
Washington, DC 20005

202-467-5081
800-424-8666
Fax: 202-467-5085
e-mail: info@acb.org
www.acb.org

A national organization established to promote the independence, dignity and well-being of blind and visually impaired people. The Council helps to improve the lives of the blind by working to enhance civil rights, employment, rehabilitation services, safe and expanded transportation, travel and recreation, Social Security benefits, accessibility and works in coalition with other disability groups.

1826 Association for Education & Rehabilitation of the Blind & Visually Impaired
1703 N Beauregard Street, Suite 440
Alexandria, VA 22311

703-671-4500
877-492-2708
Fax: 703-671-6391
e-mail: markr@aerbvi.org
www.aerbvi.org

The Association for Education and Rehabilitation of the Blind and Visually Impaired (AER) is the only international membership organization dedicated to rendering all possible support and assistance to the professionals who work in all phases of education and rehabilitation of blind and visually impaired children and adults. Our membership is comprised of more than 4,200 professionalswho provide services to people with visual impairment.

Jim Gandorf, Executive Director
Barbara Sherr, CMP, Executive Assistant

1827 Genetic Alliance
4301 Connecticut Avenue NW
Washington, DC 20008

202-966-5557
800-336-4363
Fax: 202-966-8553
e-mail: info@geneticalliance.org
www.geneticalliance.org

A coalition of voluntary genetic support groups, consumers and professionals addressing the needs of individuals and families affected by genetic disorders from a national perspective.

Sharon Terry, President/CEO

1828 National Association for Parents of Children with Visual Impairments
PO Box 317
Watertown, MA 02471

617-972-7441
800-562-6265
Fax: 617-972-7444
e-mail: napvi@perkins.org
www.spedex.com/napvi/

Offers emotional support for parents of blind or visually impaired children. Provides information, training and assistance, and help in understanding and using available resources.

Susan LaVenture, Executive Director
Mary Zabelski, President

1829 National Association for Visually Handicapped
22 W 21st Street, 6th Floor
New York, NY 10010

212-889-3141
Fax: 212-727-2931
e-mail: navh@navh.org
www.navh.org

Serves as a clearinghouse for information about all services available to the partially-sighted from public and private sources. Conducts self-help groups. Provides information on large print books, textbooks and educational tools.

Dr Lorraine Marchi, Founder & CEO

1830 National Eye Research Foundation
910 Skokie Boulevard, Suite 207A
Northbrook, IL 60062

847-564-4652
800-621-2258
Fax: 847-564-0807
e-mail: info@nerf.org
www.nerf.org

Devoted to the enhancement of care and study of eye related diseases.

1831 Parents of Cataract Kids
179 Hunter Lane
Devon, PA 19333

215-293-1917

State Agencies & Support Groups

Alabama

1832 Alabama Institute for the Deaf & Blind
PO Box 698
Talladega, AL 35160

256-761-3200
Fax: 256-761-3344
www.nectas.unc.edu

Services include central directory, representatives of agencies, service providers, families, and coordinators of infant, toddler, and preschool special education programs.

Joseph Busta, Interagency Coordinating Council

Arizona

1833 National Association for Parents of the Visually Impaired
Po Box 317
Watertown, MA 02471

617-972-7441
800-562-6265
Fax: 617-972-7444
www.spedex.com/napvi

Mary Ellen Simmons

California

1834 Helen Keller National Center SW Region
6160 Cornerstone Court E
San Diego, CA 92121

858-623-2777
Fax: 858-642-0266
TTY: 858-646-0784
e-mail: ckirscher@cspp.edu
www.helenkeller.org

Cathy Kircher, SW Regional Representative

Ohio

1835 Region 2 of the National Association for Parents of the Visually Impaired
3910 Pocahontas Avenue
Cincinnati, OH 45227

513-561-8542

Victoria Gorman Miller

Pennsylvania

1836 East Central Region-Helen Keller National Center
4351 Garden City Drive
New Carrollton, MD 20785

301-459-5474
Fax: 301-459-5070
e-mail: hkncreg3cl@aol.com
www.helenkeller.org

South Carolina

1837 Region 4 of the National Association for Parents of the Visually Impaired
1032 Trail Road
Belton, SC 29627

864-338-9593

Washington

1838 Northwestern Region-Helen Keller National Center
2366 Eastlake Avenue E
Seattle, WA 98102

206-324-9120
e-mail: nwhknc@juno.com

Libraries & Resource Centers

Alabama

1839 Mobile Association for the Blind
2440 Gordon Smith Drive
Mobile, AL 36617

334-473-3585

Offers work adjustment training, activities of daily living, mobility, communication skills and sheltered employment for adults and children who are visually impaired.

Mahlon McCracken, Executive Director

Arizona

1840 Educational Services for the Visually Impaired
PO Box 668
Little Rock, AR 72203

501-371-5710

Offers textbooks, braille books and more to the visually impaired grades K-12 in the Arkansas area.

David Beavers, Director

Arkansas

1841 Arkansas Regional Library for the Blind and Physically Handicapped
1 Capitol Mall
Little Rock, AR 72201

501-682-1155
Fax: 501-682-1529
TDD: 501-682-1002
e-mail: nlsbooks@asl.lib.ar.us
www.asl.lib.ar.us/ASL_LBPH.htm

Public library books in recorded or braille format. Popular fiction and nonfiction books for all ages, books and players are on free loan, sent to patrons by mail and may be returned postage free. Anyone who cannot see well enough to read regular print with glasses on or who has a disability that makes it difficult to hold a book or turn the pages is eligible.

John D Hall, Director

California

1842 American Action Fund for Blind Children and Adults
18440 Oxnard Street
Tarzana, CA 91356

818-343-2022
www.actinfund.org

Offers a charitable and educational fund, braille assistive devices and a lending library for the visually impaired.

1843 Blind Children's Center
4120 Marathon Street
Los Angeles, CA 90029

323-664-2153
Fax: 323-665-3828
www.blindentr.org

Offers support and informational groups.

1844 Braille Institute Desert Center
70-251 Ramon Road
Rancho Mirage, CA 92270

760-321-2555

Dedicated to providing blind and visually impaired men, women and children with the training, programs and services they need to enjoy productive lives. Services offered include child development, youth programs, library services and adult education.

1845 Braille Institute Sight Center
741 N Vermont Avenue
Los Angeles, CA 90029

213-663-1111
e-mail: bils@brailib.org

Offers help, programs, services and information to the blind and visually impaired children and adults.

Dr. Henry Chang, Librarian

1846 Braille Institute Youth Center
3450 Cahuenga Boulevard W
Los Angeles, CA 90068

213-851-5695

Offers various youth programs and services for the blind and visually impaired youngster.

1847 New Beginnings - Blind Children's Center
4120 Marathon, Street
Los Angeles, CA 90029

323-664-2153
800-222-3566
Fax: 323-665-3828

Helps children and their families become independent by creating a climate of safety and trust. Services include an infant stimulation program, educational preschool, interdisciplinary assessment services, family services, correspondence program, toll-free national hotline and a publication and research service.

1848 San Francisco Public Library for the Blind and Print Disabled
100 Larkin Street
San Francisco, CA 94102

415-557-4293
Fax: 415-557-4375
e-mail: lbphmgr@sfpl.lib.ca.us
www.library.ca.us

Foreign-language books on cassette, children's books on cassettes and more.

Martin Maqid, Librarian

1849 Variety Audio
PO Box 5731
San Jose, CA 95150

408-277-4839

Summer reading programs, braille writer, magnifiers, closed-circuit TV, large-print photocopier, cassette books and magazines, children's books on cassette, home visits and other reference materials on blindness and other handicaps.

Louisa Griehshammer

District of Columbia

1850 Council of Families with Visual Impairment
1155 15th Street NW
Washington, DC 20005

202-467-5081

Members are sighted parents of blind or visually impaired children. Offers a forum for support and outreach, sharing of experiences in parent-child relationships, and educational and cultural information about child development. Monitors developments in technical and legislative arenas.

Nola Webb, President

Florida

1851 Florida Bureau of Braille and Talking Book Library Services
420 Platt Street
Daytona Beach, FL 32114

386-239-6000
Fax: 386-239-6069
TDD: 800-226-6079
e-mail: mike_gunde@dbs.doc.state.fl.us
www.state.fl.us/dbs/lswel.html

Discs, cassettes, closed-circuit TV, large-print photocopier, films, children's books on cassettes and more.

Michael Gunde, Librarian

1852 Talking Book Library, Jacksonville Public Library
1755 Edgewood Avenue W, Suite 1
Jacksonville, FL 32208

904-765-5588
Fax: 904-768-7404
TDD: 904-768-7822
e-mail: jerryr@coj.net
neflin.org/neflin/members/jackspub.html

Discs, cassettes and reference materials on blindness and other disabilities.

Jerry Reynolds, Librarian Senior

1853 Talking Book Service - Manatee County Central Library
6081 26th Street W
Bradenton, FL 34207

941-742-5914
Fax: 941-751-7089
TDD: 941-742-5951
e-mail: patricia.schubert@co.manatee.fl.us
www.co.manatee.fl.us

Offers children's books on disc and cassette and more reference materials for the blind and physically handicapped.

Patricia Schubert, Librarian

Georgia

1854 Albany Library for the Blind and Physical Handicapped
300 Pine Avenue
Albany, GA 31701

229-420-3220
Fax: 229-420-3240
e-mail: sinquefk@mail.dougherty.public.lib.ga.us
www.docolib.org/LBPH/index.html

Offers discs, cassettes, reference materials on blindness and other handicaps, large-print photocopiers, summer reading programs, cassette books and more.

Kathryn Sinquefield, Librarian

1855 Bainbridge Subregional Library for the Blind and Physically Handicapped
301 S Monroe Street
Bainbridge, GA 31717

912-248-2680
800-795-2680
Fax: 912-248-2670
TDD: 912-248-2665
e-mail: lbph@mail.deccatur.public.lib.ga.us
www.decatur.public.lib.ga.us/local/lbph/lbph1.htm

Discs, cassettes, summer reading programs, closed-circuit TV, magnifiers and more.

Kathy Hutchins, Librarian

1856 CEL Subregional Library for the Blind and Physically Handicapped
2708 Mechanics
Savannah, GA 31401

912-354-5864
Fax: 912-354-5534
TDD: 912-652-3635
e-mail: stokesl@cel.co.chatman.ga.us

Summer reading programs, braille writer, magnifiers, closed-circuit TV, large-print photocopier, cassette books and magazines, children's books on cassette, home visits and other reference materials on blindness and other handicaps.

Linda Stokes, Librarian

Idaho

1857 Idaho State Talking Book Library
325 W State Street
Boise, ID 83702

208-334-2117
Fax: 208-334-4016
TDD: 800-377-1363
e-mail: tblbooks@isl.state.id.us
www.lili.org/isl/tblinfo.htm

Summer reading programs, braille writer, magnifiers, closed-circuit TV, large-print photocopier, cassette books and magazines, children's books on cassette, home visits and other reference materials on blindness and other handicaps.

Sue Walker, Librarian

Illinois

1858 Chicago Library Service for the Blind
1055 W Roosevelt Road
Chicago, IL 60608

312-746-9210

Summer reading programs, braille writer, magnifiers, closed-circuit TV, large-print photocopier, cassette books and magazines, children's books on cassette, home visits and other reference materials on blindness and other handicaps.

Carol Pellish, Librarian

1859 Illinois State Library, Talkng Book and Braille Service
300 S 2nd Street
Springfield, IL 62701

217-782-9435
Fax: 217-782-8261
TDD: 800-665-5576
e-mail: sruda@ilsos.net
www.cyberdriveillinois.com/library/isl/bph/bph.html

Summer reading programs, braille writer, magnifiers, closed-circuit TV, large-print photocopier, cassette books and magazines, descriptive videos, children's books on cassette, home visits and other reference materials on blindness and other handicaps.

Sharon Ruda, Librarian

1860 Mid Illinois Talking Book System
515 York Street
Quincy, IL 62301

217-224-6619
Fax: 217-224-9818

Summer reading programs, braille writer, magnifiers, closed-circuit TV, large-print photocopier, cassette books and magazines, children's books on cassette, home visits and other reference materials on blindness and other handicaps.

1861 Mid-Illinois Talking Book Center
845 Brenkman Drive
Pekin, IL 61554

309-353-4110
Fax: 309-353-8281
e-mail: hitbc@darkstar.rsa.lib.il.us
www.mitbc.org

Summer reading programs, braille writer, magnifiers, closed-circuit TV, large-print photocopier, cassette books and magazines, children's books on cassette, home visits and other reference materials on blindness and other handicaps.

Eileen Sheppard, Librarian

1862 Talking Book Center of Northwest Illinois
PO Box 125
Coal Valley, IL 61240

309-799-3137
Fax: 309-799-7916
e-mail: kodean@libby.rbls.lib.il.us
www.rbls.lib.il.us

Subregional library provides Talking Book and Braille Book programs to eligible persons unable to use standard print materials due to visual or physical disabilities. Includes cassette books and magazines; summer reading program.

Indiana

1863 Northwest Indiana Subregional Library for Blind and Physically Handicapped
1919 W Lincoln Highway
Merrillville, IN 46410

219-769-3541
Fax: 219-769-0690

Summer reading programs, braille writer, magnifiers, closed-circuit TV, large-print photocopier, cassette books and magazines, children's books on cassette, home visits and other reference materials on blindness and other handicaps.

Renee Lewis

Iowa

1864 Iowa Library for the Blind and Physically Handicapped
Iowa Department for the Blind
524 4th Street
Des Moines, IA 50309

515-281-1333
Fax: 515-281-1378
TDD: 515-281-1355
e-mail: keninger.karen@blind.state.ia.us
www.blind.state.ia.us

Summer reading programs, magnifiers, closed-circuit TV,
large-print photocopier, children's books on cassette, children's
books in Braille and Print Braille, cassette magazines, home visits
and reference materials on blindness and other handicaps.

Karen Keninger, Program Manager/Librarian

1865 University of Iowa Birth Defects and Genetic Disorders Unit
2614 JCP
Iowa City, IA 52242

319-335-9901

James M Smith, Director

Kansas

1866 CKLS Headquarters
1409 Williams Street
Great Bend, KS 67530

316-792-2393
800-362-2642
Fax: 316-792-5495
e-mail: cenks@ink.org
www.macular.org

Summer reading programs, braille writer, magnifiers, closed-circuit
TV, large-print photocopier, cassette books and magazines, children's books on cassette, home visits and other reference materials
on blindness and other handicaps.

Jerri Robinson, Librarian

1867 Services for the Visually Disabled
629 Poyntz Avenue
Manhattan, KS 66502

785-776-4741
Fax: 785-776-1545
e-mail: marionr@manhattan.lib.ks.us

Summer reading programs, braille writer, magnifiers, closed-circuit
TV, large-print photocopier, cassette books and magazines, children's books on cassette, home visits and other reference materials
on blindness and other handicaps.

Marion Rice, Librarian

Kentucky

1868 Kentucky Library for the Blind and Physically Handicapped
PO Box 818
Frankfort, KY 40602

502-564-8300
800-372-2968
Fax: 502-564-5773
e-mail: richard.feindel@kdla.net
www.kdla.net/libserv/ktbl.htm

Large-print photocopier, cassette books and magazines, children's
books on cassette, and other reference materials on blindness and
other handicaps.

5,200 members

Richard Feindel, Librarian

Maryland

1869 Maryland State Library for the Blind and Physically Handicapped
415 Park Avenue
Baltimore, MD 21201

410-230-2424
Fax: 410-333-2095
TTY: 800-934-2541
TDD: 410-333-8679
e-mail: recept@lbta.lib.md.us
www.lbph.lib.md.us

Summer reading programs, braille writer, magnifiers, large-print
photocopier, cassette books and magazines, children's books on
cassette, and other reference materials on blindness and other
handicaps.

1870 Prince George's County Memorial Library Talking Book Center
6530 Adelphi Road
Hyattsville, MD 20782

301-779-9330

Summer reading programs, braille writer, magnifiers, closed-circuit TV, large-print photocopier, cassette books and magazines,
children's books on cassette, home visits and other reference materials on blindness and other handicaps.

Shirley Tuthill, Librarian

Massachusetts

1871 Braille and Talking Book Library Perkins School for the Blind
175 N Beacon Street
Watertown, MA 02472

617-924-3434
Fax: 617-926-2027
e-mail: perkins@bpl.org
www.perkins.org

Patricia Kirk

1872 Carroll Center for the Blind
770 Centre Street
Newton, MA 02158

617-969-6200
800-852-3131
Fax: 617-969-6204
www.carroll.org

Assists blind and visually impaired adults and adolescents to adjust
to loss of vision. The goal of this dynamic program is to help the
person become more independent, to restore self-confidence, prepare for employment and improve the quality of life. Programs of
individual counseling are offered as part of the program.

Rachel Rosenbaum, President

Michigan

1873 Downtown Detroit Subregional Library for the Blind and Handicapped
121 Gratiot Avenue
Detroit, MI 48226

313-224-0580
Fax: 313-965-1977
TDD: 313-224-0584
e-mail: deveans@cms.xx.wayne.edu
www.detroit.lib.mi.us

Summer reading programs, braille writer, magnifiers, closed-circuit TV, large-print photocopier, cassette books and magazines,
children's books on cassette, home visits and other reference materials on blindness and other handicaps.

Deborah Evans, Librarian

1874 Kent County Library for the Blind
775 Ball Avenue NE
Grand Rapids, MI 49503

616-336-3250
Fax: 616-336-3201
e-mail: kdlcm@lakeland.lib.mi.us

Summer reading programs, braille writer, magnifiers, closed-circuit TV, large-print photocopier, cassette books and magazines, children's books on cassette, home visits and other reference materials on blindness and other handicaps.

Claudya Muller, Librarian

1875 Library of Michigan Service for the Blind
PO Box 30007
Lansing, MI 48909

517-373-5614
Fax: 517-373-5865
e-mail: info@sbph.libomich.lib.mi.us

Summer reading programs, braille writer, magnifiers, closed-circuit TV, large-print photocopier, cassette books and magazines, children's books on cassette, home visits and other reference materials on blindness and other handicaps.

1876 Macomb Library for the Blind and Physically Handicapped
16480 Hall Road
Clinton Township, MI 48038

586-286-1580
Fax: 586-286-0634
TDD: 810-869-40
e-mail: macbld@libcoop.net
www.macomb.lib.mi.us/macspc/

Summer reading programs, braille writer, closed-circuit TV, cassette books and magazines, children's books on cassette, reference materials on blindness and other handicaps.

Beverlee Babcock, Librarian

1877 Mideastern Michigan Library Co-op
G-4195 W Pasadena Avenue
Flint, MI 48504

810-732-1120
Fax: 810-732-1715
e-mail: cnash@genesse.freeret.org
www.fakon.edu/gdl/talking.htm

Summer reading programs, braille writer, magnifiers, closed-circuit TV, large-print photocopier, cassette books and magazines, children's books on cassette, home visits and other reference materials on blindness and other handicaps.

Carolyn Nash, Librarian

1878 Muskegon County Library for the Blind
635 Ottawa Street
Muskegon, MI 49442

231-724-6248
Fax: 231-724-6675
TDD: 231-722-4103
www.muskcolib.org

Summer reading programs, braille typewriter, magnifiers, closed-circuit TV, large-print photocopier, cassette books and magazines, children's books on cassette, home visits and other reference materials on blindness and other handicaps, The Reading Edge, Perkins Brailler and large print books.

Linda Clapp, Librarian

1879 Upper Peninsula Library for the Blind Physically Handicapped
1615 Presque Isle Avenue
Marquette, MI 49855

906-228-7697
Fax: 906-228-5627
e-mail: uproc.lib.mi.us
www.upesc.lib.mi.us/uplbph

Summer reading programs, braille writer, magnifiers, closed-circuit TV, large-print photocopier, cassette books and magazines, chil-

dren's books on cassette, home visits and other reference materials on blindness and other handicaps.

Suzanne Dees, Librarian

1880 Washtenaw County Library
PO Box 8645
Ann Arbor, MI 48107

734-222-4357
Fax: 734-222-6715
e-mail: contact us@ewashtenaw.org
www.ewashtenaw.org

Summer reading programs, braille writer, magnifiers, closed-circuit TV, large-print photocopier, cassette books and magazines, children's books on cassette, home visits and other reference materials on blindness and other handicaps.

Margeret Wolfe, Librarian

1881 Washtenaw County Library for the Blind and Physically Disabled
PO Box 8645
Ann Arbor, MI 48107

734-971-6059
Fax: 734-971-3892
e-mail: lbpd@co.washtennaw.mi.us
www.co.washten.ml.us/depts/lib/liblbpd.h

Book lovers club.adaptive technology,cassette equipment, cassette books and magazines, described videos, low vision aids reference and referral services.

Margaret Wolfe, Coordinator

1882 Wayne County Regional Library for the Blind
30555 Michigan Avenue
Westland, MI 48186

734-727-7300
Fax: 734-727-7333
TTY: 734-727-7330
e-mail: werlbph@tln.lib.mi.us
www.wayneregional.lib.mi.us

Summer reading programs, braille writer, magnifiers, closed-circuit TV, large-print photocopier, cassette books and magazines, children's books on cassette, home visits and other reference materials on blindness and other handicaps.

Reginald Williams, Wayne County Librarian

Minnesota

1883 Minnesota Library for the Blind & Physically Handicapped
Highway 298, PO Box 68
Fairbault, MN 55021

507-333-4828
800-722-0550
Fax: 507-333-4832
e-mail: libblnd@state.mn.us

Summer reading programs, braille writer, magnifiers, closed-circuit TV, large-print photocopier, cassette, large print, braille books and magazines, children's books on cassette, and other reference materials on blindness and other handicaps.

Catherine A Durivage, Program Director

Missouri

1884 Adriene Resource Center for Blind Children
1445 Boonville Avenue
Springfield, MO 65802

417-862-2781
Fax: 417-862-7566
e-mail: blind@ag.org
www.gospelpublishing.com

Offers braille and cassette lending library, braille and cassette Sunday school materials for all ages, braille and cassette periodicals and resource assistance, and resources for blind children and children of blind parents.

Paul Weingariner, Director

1885 Assemblies of God National Center for the Blind
1445 Boonville Avenue
Springfield, MO 65802

417-862-2781
Fax: 417-862-7566
e-mail: blind@ag.org
www.gospelpublishing.com

Offers braille and cassette lending library, braille and cassette Sunday school materials for all ages, braille and cassette periodicals and resource assistance, and resources for blind children and children of blind parents.

Paul Weingariner, Director

1886 Wolfner Memorial Library for the Blind
PO Box 387
Jefferson City, MO 65102

573-751-8720
Fax: 573-526-2985
TDD: 800-347-1379
e-mail: beckles@mail.sos.state.mo.us

Summer reading programs, braille writer, magnifiers, closed-circuit TV, large-print photocopier, cassette books and magazines, children's books on cassette, home visits and other reference materials on blindness and other handicaps.

Elizabeth Eckles, Librarian

Nebraska

1887 Nebraska Library Commission Talking Book & Braille Services
1200 N Street
Lincoln, NE 68508

402-471-4038
800-742-7691
Fax: 402-471-6244
TDD: 402-471-4038
e-mail: doertli@nlc.state.ne.us
www.ncl.state.ne.us/tbbs/tbbsl/html

Free loan of books and magazines on cassette and in Braille, including children's materials, along with specially designed playback equipment. Summer reading program for children, Braille embossing, closed circuit TV, large-print copier. Reference materials on blindness and other disabilities.

David Oerti, Librarian

New Jersey

1888 New Jersey Library for the Blind and Handicapped
2300 Stuyvesant Avenue
Trenton, NJ 08618

609-292-6450
800-792-8322
Fax: 609-530-6384
TDD: 877-882-5593
e-mail: nglbh@njstatelib.org
www.mjstatelib.org

Summer reading programs, braille writer, magnifiers, closed-circuit TV, large-print, cassette braille books and magazines, children's books on cassettes in braille and other reference materials on blindness and other handicaps.

Deborah Rutledeger, Director

New Mexico

1889 New Mexico State Library for the Blind and Physically Handicapped
1209 Camino Carlos Ray
Santa Fe, NM

505-476-9700
Fax: 505-476-9701
e-mail: jbrewstr@stlib.state.nm.us
www.stlib.state.nm.us

Summer reading programs, braille writer, magnifiers, closed-circuit TV, large-print photocopier, cassette books and magazines, children's books on cassette, home visits and other reference materials on blindness and other handicaps.

Glee Wenzel, Librarian

New York

1890 Helen Keller National Center
111 Middle Neck Road
Sands Point, NY 11050

516-944-8900
Fax: 516-944-7302

Provides diagnostic, evaluation, short term comprehensive rehabilitation and personal adjustment training. A technical assistance center is offered providing assistance to public and private agencies and to parent groups who work towards community integration and the enhancement of the quality of life. A national parent network is also provided that develops and shares information about advocacy, legislation, new services and achievements.

1891 New York State Talking Book & Braille Library
Empire State Plaza, CEC
Albany, NY 12230

518-474-5801
Fax: 518-474-5786
TDD: 518-474-7121
e-mail: jane@unix2.nysed.gov
www.suffolk.lib.ny.us

Books on audio cassette, cassette players, braille books, summer reading programs, braille writer, magnifiers, closed-circuit TV, large-print photocopier, cassette books and magazines, children's books on cassette, reference materials on blindness and other handicaps.

Jane Somers, Director

North Carolina

1892 North Carolina Library for the Blind
1811 Capital Boulevard
Raleigh, NC 27635

919-733-4376
Fax: 919-733-6910
TDD: 919-733-1462
e-mail: nclbph@ncsl.der.state.nc

Summer reading programs, braille writer, magnifiers, closed-circuit TV, large-print photocopier, cassette books and magazines, children's books on cassette, home visits and other reference materials on blindness and other handicaps.

Francine Martin, Librarian

Ohio

1893 American Council of Blind Parents
34400 Cedar Road, Apartment 108
University Heights, OH 44121

800-424-8666

Members are sighted parents of blind or visually impaired children. Offers a forum for support and outreach, sharing of experiences in parent-child relationships, and educational and cultural information about child development. Monitors developments in technical and legislative arenas.

Nola Webb, President

Oregon

1894 Oregon State Library, Talking Book and Braille Services
250 Winter Street NW
Salem, OR 97310

503-378-4243
Fax: 503-588-7119
TDD: 503-378-4276
e-mail: tbabs@sparkie.osl.state.or.us

Cassette books and magazines, children's books on cassette, home visits and other reference materials on blindness and other handicaps.

Donna Bensen, Regional Librarian

Virginia

1895 Alexandria Library Talking Book Service
5005 Duke Street
Alexandria, VA 22304

703-519-5900
Fax: 703-519-5915
TDD: 703-838-4568
e-mail: emccaffr@lea.eda
www.www.alexandria.lib.va.us

Summer reading programs, braille writer, magnifiers, closed-circuit TV, large-print photocopier, cassette books and magazines, children's books on cassette, home visits and other reference materials on blindness and other handicaps.

Patricia Bates, Librarian

1896 Division for the Visually Handicapped
1920 Association Drive
Reston, VA 20191

703-620-3660

Members are teachers, college faculty members, administrators, supervisors and others concerned with the education and welfare of visually handicapped and blind children and youth. This is a division of the Council For Exceptional Children.

Dr. Kay Ferrell, President

1897 Division on Visual Impairments
Council for Exceptional Children
1110 North Glebe Road, Suite 300
Arlington, VA 22201

800-224-6830
Fax: 703-264-9494
TTY: 866-915-5000
www.ed.arizona.edu/dvi/welcome.htm; www.cec.sped.org

A division within the CEC, it handles concerns for Federal, state and local issues and policies related to education of youths, children and infants with visual impairments.

Ellyn Ross, President
Shirley J Wilson, Secretary

1898 Virginia State Library for the Visually and Physically Handicapped
1901 Roane Street
Richmond, VA 23222

804-367-0014

Summer reading programs, braille writer, magnifiers, closed-circuit TV, large-print photocopier, cassette books and magazines, children's books on cassette, home visits and other reference materials on blindness and other handicaps.

Mary Ruth Halapatz, Librarian

Washington

1899 Washington Library for the Blind and Physically Handicapped
821 Lenora Street
Seattle, WA 98129

206-386-4636
Fax: 206-386-4685
e-mail: wtbbl@spl.lib.wa.us
www.spl.lib.wa.us

Summer reading programs, braille writer, magnifiers, closed-circuit TV, large-print photocopier, cassette books and magazines, children's books on cassette, home visits and other reference materials on blindness and other handicaps.

Jan Ames, Librarian

West Virginia

1900 West Virginia School for the Blind
301 E Main Street
Romney, WV 26757

304-822-3521
Fax: 304-822-4896
e-mail: cjohn@access.mountain.net

Summer reading programs, braille writer, magnifiers, closed-circuit TV, large-print photocopier, cassette books and magazines, children's books on cassette, home visits and other reference materials on blindness and other handicaps.

Cynthia Johnson, Librarian

Research Centers

1901 American Association for Pediatric Ophthalmology and Strabismus
PO Box 193832
San Francisco, CA 94119

415-561-8505
Fax: 415-561-8531
e-mail: aapos@aao.org
www.aapos.org

Provides support and resources for Pediatric Ophthalmologists, Strabismologists, related personnel and their patients by way of its Internet Website.

Maria A Schweers, Scientific Program Coordinator
Christie L Morse, MD, President

1902 Center for the Partially Sighted
12301 Wilshire Boulevard, Suite 600
Los Angeles, CA 90025

310-458-3501
Fax: 310-458-8179
e-mail: info@low-vision.org
www.low-vision.org

Provides professional, comprehensive vision rehabilitation services to visually impaired people of all ages. For those whose sight is severely limited due to macular degeneration, diabetic retinopathy, glaucoma, retinal detachment, stroke or other conditions not correctable medically or surgically.

1903 Helen Keller National Center
111 Middle Neck Road
Sands Point, NY 11050

516-944-8900
Fax: 516-944-7302

Provides diagnostic evaluation, short term comprehensive rehabilitation and personal adjustment training. A technical assistance center is offered providing assistance to public and private agencies and to parent groups who work towards community integration and the enhancement of the quality of life. A national parent network is also provided that develops and shares information about advocacy, legislation, new services and achievements.

1904 Mobile Association for the Blind
2440 Gordon Smith Drive
Mobile, AL 36617

251-473-3585
877-292-5463
Fax: 251-470-8622
e-mail: sales@mobile.blind.com
www.mobileblind.com

Offers work adjustment training, activities of daily living, mobility, communication skills and sheltered employment for adults and children who are visually impaired.

Mahlon McCracken, Executive Director

1905 National Eye Research Foundation
910 Skokie Boulevard, Suite 207A
Northbrook, IL 60062

847-564-4652
800-621-2258
Fax: 847-564-0807
e-mail: info@nerf.org
www.nerf.org

Devoted to the enhancement of care and study of eye related diseases.

1906 New Beginnings - The Blind Children's Center
4120 Marathon Street
Los Angeles, CA 90029

213-664-2153

The purpose of the Center is to turn initial fears into hope. Helps children and their families become independent by creating a climate of safety and trust. Children learn to develop self confidence and to master a wide range of skills. Services include an infant stimulation program, educational preschool, interdisciplinary assessment services, family services, correspondence program, toll free national hotline and a publication and research service.

1907 Pediatric Ophathalmology and Adult Strabis mus Service Research
Indiana University
702 Rotary Circle
Indianapolis, IN 46202

317-274-2128
Fax: 317-274-2277
e-mail: dplager@iupui.edu
www.iupui.edu/~ophthal/

Improve techniques and treatment modalities for children with eye and vision problems, such as cataracts, glaucoma, retinopathy of prematurity, and for both children and adults with eye muscle abnormalities.

David A Plager, MD, Director

1908 Research to Prevent Blindness
645 Madison Avenue
New York, NY 10022

212-752-4333
800-621-0026
www.rpbusa.org

Provides research grants to scientists interested in eye disease and vision disorders.

Audio Video

1909 Heart to Heart
Blind Children's Center
4120 Marathon Street
Los Angeles, CA 90029

323-644-2153
Fax: 323-665-3828
www.blindcntr.org

Parents of blind and partially sighted children talk about their feelings.

Videotape

1910 Let's Eat
Blind Children's Center
4120 Marathon Street
Los Angeles, CA 90029

213-664-2153
Fax: 213-665-3828

Teaches competent feeding skills to children with visual impairments.

Videotape

1911 See What I Feel
Britannica Film Co.
345 4th Street
San Francisco, CA 94107

415-597-5555

A blind child tells her friends about her trip to the zoo. Each experience was explained as a blind child would experience it. A teacher's guide comes with this video.

Films

Web Sites

1912 American Association for Pediatric Ophthalmology and Strabismus
www.aapos.org

Provides support and resources for Pediatric Ophthalmologists, Strabismologists, related personnel and their patients by way of its Internet Website.

1913 Lighthouse International
www.lighthouse.org

The mission is to overcome vision impairment for people of all ages through worldwide leadership in rehabilitation services, education, research, prevention and advocacy.

1914 National Alliance of Blind Students
www.blindstudents.org

The leading national advocacy and consumer organization for students in high school or college who are blind or visually impaired.

1915 National Association for Visually Handicapped
www.navh.org

Helps to cope with the difficulties of vision impairment.

1916 Online Mendelian Inheritance in Man
www.ncbi.nlm.nih.gov

This database is a catalog of human genes and genetic disorders.

1917 Royal National Institute of the Blind
www.rnib.org.uk

Offering information, support and advice to people with sight problems.

Book Publishers

1918 Children with Visual Impairments: A Parents' Guide
Peytral Publications
PO Box 1162
Minnetonka, MN 55345

952-949-8707
877-739-8725
Fax: 952-906-9777
www.peytral.com

Covers visual impairments ranging from low vision to total blindness. Offers authoritative information and empathy, parental insight on diagnosis and treatment, orientation and mobility, literacy, legal issues and more. Valuable to parents, educators and support staff.

395 pages

M Cay Holbrook PhD, Editor

1919 Ophthalmic Disorders Sourcebook
Omnigraphics Editorial Office
615 Griswold
Detroit, MI 48226

313-961-1340
800-234-1340
Fax: 313-961-1383
e-mail: editorial@omnigraphics.com
www.omnigraphics.com

Basic consumer information about glaucoma, cataracts, macular degeneration, strabismus, refractive disorders and more.

1996 631 pages Hardcover
ISBN: 0-780800-81-8

Linda M Ross, Editor

Magazines

1920 Journal of Visual Impairment and Blindness

American Foundation for the Blind
11 Penn Plaza, Suite 300
New York, NY 10001

212-502-7600
Fax: 212-502-7777
e-mail: afbinfo@afb.net
www.afb.org

Published in braille, regular print and on cassette this journal contains a wide variety of subjects including rehabilitation, psychology, education, legislation, medicine, technology, employment, sensory aids and childhood development as they relate to visual impairments.

10x Year

1921 Reaching, Crawling, Walking - Let's Get Moving

Blind Children's Center
4120 Marathon Street
Los Angeles, CA 90029

323-664-2153
Fax: 323-665-3828
e-mail: info@blindchildrenscenter.org
www.blindchildrenscenter.org

Orientation and mobility for visually impaired preschool children.

24 pages

1922 Seeing Candy

National Association for Visually Handicapped
22 W 21st Street, 6th Floor
New York, NY 10010

212-889-3141
Fax: 212-727-2931
e-mail: staff@navh.org
www.navh.org

This newsletter offers short stories, news, medical updates, assistive device information, poems, resources, crossword puzzles and more for the visually impaired.

Biannually

1923 Tactic

Clovernook Home and School for the Blind
7000 Hamilton Avenue
Cincinnati, OH 45231

513-522-3860
Fax: 513-728-3950
e-mail: clovernook@aol.com

Quarterly

Newsletters

1924 Gleams

Glaucoma Research Foundation
251 Post Street, Suite 600
San Francisco, CA 94104

415-986-3162
800-826-6693
Fax: 415-986-3763
e-mail: info@glaucoma.org
www.glaucoma.org

Includes information about glaucoma, new treatments, updates on research findings, and more.

3x/year

Andrew Jackson, Communications Director

1925 National Library Service for the Blind & Physically Handicapped

Library of Congress Reference Section
1291 Taylor Street NW
Washington, DC 20542

202-707-5100
800-424-8567
Fax: 202-707-0712
TTY: 202-707-0744
TDD: 202-707-0744
e-mail: nis@loc.gov
www.loc.gov/nls

Provides information and advocacy resources for families and professionals, including listings of organizations focusing on more specific areas of concern to families and young adults who have disabilities. Administers a natural library service that provides recorded and braille reading materials to eligible children and adults who cannot read standard print.

12 pages Quarterly
ISSN: 1046-1663

Vicki Fitzpatrick, Editor

1926 Talking Book Topics

National Library Services for the Blind
1291 Taylor Street NW
Washington, DC 20542

202-707-5100
Fax: 202-707-0712
www.loc.gov/nls

Offers hundreds of listings of books, fiction and nonfiction, for adults and children on cassette. Also offers listings on foreign language books on cassette, talking magazines and reviews.

Bimonthly

Pamphlets

1927 Dancing Cheek to Cheek

Blind Children's Center
4120 Marathon Street
Los Angeles, CA 90029

213-664-2153
Fax: 213-665-3828
www.blindchildrenscenter.org

Discusses beginning social, play and language interactions.

33 pages

1928 Family Guide - Growth and Development of the Partially Seeing Child

National Association for Visually Handicapped
22 W 21st Street, 6th Floor
New York, NY 10010

212-889-3141
Fax: 212-727-2931
e-mail: staff@navh.org
www.navh.org

Offers information for parents and guidelines in raising a partially seeing child.

1929 Family Guide to Vision Care

American Optometric Association
243 N Lindbergh Boulevard
Saint Louis, MO 63141

314-991-4100
Fax: 314-991-4101
www.aoanet.org

Offers information on the early developmental years of your vision, finding a family optometrist and how to take care of your eyesight through the learning years, the working years and the mature years.

1930 Heart to Heart
Blind Children's Center
4120 Marathon Street
Los Angeles, CA 90029

213-664-2153
Fax: 213-665-3828
www.blindchildrenscenter.org

Parents of blind and partially sighted children talk about their feelings.

12 pages

1931 Learning to Play
Blind Children's Center
4120 Marathon Street
Los Angeles, CA 90029

213-664-2153
Fax: 213-665-3828
www.blindchildrenscenter.org

Discusses how to present play activities to the visually impaired preschool child.

12 pages

1932 Let's Eat
Blind Children's Center
4120 Marathon Street
Los Angeles, CA 90029

213-664-2153
Fax: 213-665-3828
www.blindchildrenscenter.org

Teaches competent feeding skills to children with visual impairments.

28 pages

1933 Move with Me
Blind Children's Center
4120 Marathon Street
Los Angeles, CA 90029

213-664-2153
Fax: 213-665-3828
www.blindchildrenscenter.org

A parent's guide to movement development for visually impaired babies.

12 pages

1934 Selecting a Program
Blind Children's Center
4120 Marathon Street
Los Angeles, CA 90029

213-664-2153
Fax: 213-665-3828
www.blindchildrenscenter.org

A guide for parents of infants and preschoolers with visual impairments.

28 pages

1935 Standing on My Own Two Feet
Blind Children's Center
4120 Marathon Street
Los Angeles, CA 90029

323-664-2153
Fax: 323-665-3828
e-mail: info@blindchildrenscenter.org
www.blindchildrenscenter.org

A step-by-step guide to designing and constructing simple, individually tailored adaptive mobility devices for preschool-age children who are visually impaired.

36 pages

1936 Talk to Me
Blind Children's Center
4120 Marathon Street
Los Angeles, CA 90029

213-664-2153
Fax: 213-665-3828
www.blindchildrenscenter.org

A language guide for parents of deaf children.

11 pages

1937 Talk to Me II
Blind Children's Center
4120 Marathon Street
Los Angeles, CA 90029

213-664-2153
Fax: 213-665-3828
www.blindchildrenscenter.org

A sequel to Talk To Me, available in English and Spanish.

15 pages

Camps

1938 Bloomfield
5300 Angeles Vista Boulevard
Los Angeles, CA 90043

323-295-4555
800-352-2290
Fax: 323-296-0424
e-mail: info@juniorblind.org
www.juniorblind.org

This camp is dedicated to serving blind and developmentally disabled children and adults.

1939 Florida School-Deaf and Blind
207 San Marco Avenue
Saint Augustine, FL 32084

800-800-344
www2.kidscamps.com

1940 National Camps for Blind Children
Christian Record
4444 S 52nd Street
Lincoln, NE 68516

402-488-0981
Fax: 402-488-7582
e-mail: info@christianrecord.org
www.christianrecord.org

Camps throughout the US and Canada are offered at no cost to the legally blind, ages 9-65. Activities include archery, beeper basketball, water sports, hiking and rock climbing and horseback riding. $35 registration fee.

Keith Elliott, Director

1941 VISIONS/Vacation Camp for the Blind
500 Greenwich Street, 3rd Floor
New York, NY 10013

212-625-1616
888-245-8333
Fax: 212-219-4078
e-mail: tmdecker@visionvcb.org
www.visionvcb.org

Family programs at Vacation Camp for the Blind in Rockland County, NY for children who are blind, severely visually impaired or multi-handicapped. Parent or guardian must attend winter weekends and summer session.

Thomas M Decker, Camp Director
Nancy D Miller, Executive Director

DESCRIPTION

1942 CONGENITAL DIAPHRAGMATIC HERNIA

Synonym: CDH

Involves the following Biologic System(s):

Gastrointestinal Disorders, Respiratory Disorders

Congenital diaphragmatic hernia (CDH) is a birth defect characterized by projection or bulging of organs of the abdomen into the chest cavity. This occurs as a result of an abnormal opening in the diaphragm, the dome-shaped muscle that separates the abdomen from the chest and plays an essential role in breathing. Approximately one in 5,000 newborns are affected by the condition. CDH is thought to result due to failed closure of a certain area of the embryonic diaphragm (i.e., the foramen of Bochdalek) during fetal development. In some cases, disrupted development in other areas of the growing fetus may also cause CDH. This birth defect may occur as an isolated condition or, in about 20 to 30 percent of patients, in association with other abnormalities or underlying malformation syndromes, such as Down syndrome (trisomy 21), trisomy 18 syndrome, or trisomy 13 syndrome. There are reports of several infants with isolated CDH in certain families (kindreds). In such cases, the condition is thought to result from abnormal changes (mutations) of different genes, possibly in association with certain environmental factors (multifactorial inheritance).

In newborns with CDH, the diaphragmatic defect may be small or can affect up to half of the diaphragm. The left side of the diaphragm is most commonly involved. The lungs may also be unusually small and underdeveloped (pulmonary hypoplasia), and abnormalities of the blood vessels supplying the lungs may also be present. In addition, the intestines may not be positioned properly (intestinal malformation). Most newborns with CDH experience increasing difficulties breathing (respiratory distress) within the first 24 hours after birth. Associated symptoms include labored breathing (dyspnea), grunting upon exhalation, drawing in of the chest wall during inhalation, and a bluish discoloration of the skin and mucous membranes (cyanosis). These findings may potentially result in life-threatening complications. In addition, in some affected newborns, air may collect in the chest cavity, causing the lung(s) to collapse (pneumothorax). Symptoms associated with CDH may not become apparent until after the first few weeks of life. These infants may experience mild respiratory symptoms or intestinal obstruction and associated vomiting (emesis).

In newborns with CDH, immediate measures may be necessary to prevent or treat potentially life-threatening complications. Surgery to repair the diaphragmatic defect is deferred until the newborn's respiratory status has been stabilized. Ongoing supportive measures may be employed before surgery, such as use of a device known as an extracorporeal membrane oxygenator (ECMO). This device supplies oxygen to the infant's blood and returns this oxygenated blood to the body. In addition, certain medications may also be used (e.g., surfactant therapy to help improve oxygenation, etc.).

See also **General Resources** on page 917

Government Agencies

1943 NIH/National Institute of Child Health and Human Development

31 Center Drive, Building 31
Bethesda, MD 20892

301-496-5133
Fax: 301-496-1104
www.nichd.nih.gov

Established in 1962 by congress, today the institute conducts and supports research on topics related to the health of children, adults, families and populations. Some of these topics include: developmental disabilities, growth and development, infant death, reproductive health and birth defects.

Nancy D Wirth, Director
Lisa Kaeser, Program & Public Liaison

National Associations & Support Groups

1944 CHERUBS: Association of Congenital Diaphragmatic Hernia Research & Advocacy

270 Coley Road
Henderson, NC 27537

252-492-6003
866-603-1944
Fax: 815-425-9155
e-mail: info@cherubs-cdh.org
www.cherubs-cdh.org

Goal is to not only help parents of children born with CDH but to lead the medical community into finding the cause and prevention of this devastating birth defect

Dawn Torrence, President/Founder

1945 Digestive Disease National Coalition

507 Capitol Court NE, Suite 200
Washington, DC 20002

202-544-7497
Fax: 202-546-7105
www.ddnc.org

Advocacy organization comprised of 22 voluntary and professional societies concerned with the many diseases of the digestive tract and liver.

Nancy Norton, Chairperson
Dr. Maurice Cerulli, President

1946 Genetic Alliance
4301 Connecticut Avenue NW
Washington, DC 20008

202-966-5557
800-336-4363
Fax: 202-966-8553
e-mail: info@geneticalliance.org
www.geneticalliance.org

A coalition of voluntary genetic support groups, consumers and professionals addressing the needs of individuals and families affected by genetic disorders from a national perspective.

Sharon Terry, President/CEO

Libraries & Resource Centers

1947 National Digestive Diseases Information Clearinghouse
2 Information Way
Bethesda, MD 20892

301-654-3810
800-891-5389
Fax: 703-738-4929
e-mail: nddic@info.niddk.nih.gov
www.digestive.niddk.nih.gov

The National Institute of Diabetes and Digestive and Kidney Diseases conducts and supports research on many of the most serious diseases affecting public health. The Institute supports much of the clinical research on the diseases of internal medicine and related subspecialty fields as well as many basic science disciplines.

Kathy Kranzfelder, Project Officer

1948 University of Iowa Birth Defects and Genetic Disorders Unit
2614 JCP
Iowa City, IA 52242

319-335-9901

James M Smith, Director

Web Sites

1949 Ask NOAH About: Stomach and Intestinal (Gastrointestinal) Disorders
noah-health.org/english/illness/gastro/gastro.html

Information on many conditions, including colic, celiac disease, ulcerative colitis, Crohn's disease, diarrhea, hernia and Hirschsprung's disease.

1950 Family Village
www.familyvillage.wisc.edu

A global community that integrates information, resources and communication opportunities on the Internet for persons with cognitive and other disabilities, for their families and for those that provide them services and support.

Book Publishers

1951 Digestive Diseases & Disorders Sourcebook
Omnigraphics Editorial Office
615 Griswold
Detroit, MI 48226

313-961-1340
800-234-1340
Fax: 313-961-1383
e-mail: editorial@omnigraphics.com
www.omnigraphics.com

Provides basic information for the layperson about common disorders of the upper and lower digestive tract. It also includes information about medications and recommendations for maintaining a healthy digestive tract. A glossary of important terms and a directory of digestive diseases organizations are also provided.

2000 335 pages Hardcover
ISBN: 0-780803-27-2

Karen Bellenir, Editor

DESCRIPTION

1952 CONGENITAL DYSPLASIA OF THE HIP

Synonyms: CDH, Congenital dislocation of the hip, DDH, Developmental dysplasia of the hip

Covers these related disorders: Teratologic congenital dysplasia of the hip, Typical congenital dysplasia of the hip (Developmental dysplasia)

Involves the following Biologic System(s):
Neonatal and Infant Disorders, Orthopedic and Muscle Disorders

Congenital dysplasia of the hip (CDH) refers to a condition present at birth or soon thereafter in which one or both hips are dislocated. This occurs when the ball-shaped head of the upper thigh bone (femur) does not fit appropriately into the hip socket of the pelvis (acetabulum). Congenital hip dysplasia may be classified as typical, which occurs shortly after birth in infants with no underlying neurologic irregularities, or teratologic, which develops before birth. The typical form of this condition is commonly referred to as developmental dysplasia of the hip.

The cause of CDH is unknown, although it is more prevalent in newborns who were surrounded by an unusually small amount of amniotic fluid during the gestational period (oligohydramnios). Those infants who present in a breech position; those with other close family members with this condition may also be at increased risk for CDH. In addition, it is more predominant in girls than it is in boys by a ratio of nine to one. Teratologic dysplasia of the hip in the developing fetus may occur as part of a pattern of abnormalities associated with certain underlying disorders affecting the neuromuscular system such as arthrogryposis multiplex congenita and myelodysplasia.

Assessment of the hips is part of the newborn physical exam. The Ortalani and Barlow maneuvers help to detect both anterior and posterior dislocations for the femoral head. Children with certain risk factors (i.e. breech delivery) should have a hip ultrasound at 3 months.

Treatment during infancy may include manipulation of the hip joint into its proper position followed by immobilization and splinting of the thigh for a period of several months. Some infants may benefit from wearing two or three diapers at a time. In some patients, delayed detection of this birth defect may necessitate the use of traction to restore the femoral head to its correct position. However, if the dislocation is not discovered until late childhood, surgery followed by fitting with a plaster cast may be necessary to correct this condition. Delayed treatment may result in chronic difficulties with walking. Untreated dysplasia of the hip may result in degenerative changes in the joint (osteoarthritis). Approximately 4 of every 1,000 infants are affected by congenital dysplasia of the hip; however, in approximately 70 percent of these children, the dislocation corrects itself.

See also **General Resources** on page 917

Government Agencies

1953 NIH/National Institute of Arthritis & Musculoskeletal & Skin Diseases
National Institutes of Health
1 AMS Circle
Bethesda, MD 20892

301-495-4484
877-226-4267
Fax: 301-718-6366
TDD: 301-565-2966
e-mail: niamsinfo@mail.nih.gov
www.niams.nih.gov

The mission of the NIAMS, a part of the NIH, is to support research into the causes, treatment and prevention of arthritis and musculoskeletal and skin diseases, the training of basic and clinical scientists to carry out this research, and the dissemination of information on research progress in these diseases.

Stephen I Katz, MD/Ph.D, Director
Steven J Hausman, Deputy Director

1954 NIH/National Institute of Child Health and Human Development
31 Center Drive, Building 31
Bethesda, MD 20892

301-496-5133
Fax: 301-496-1104
www.nichd.nih.gov

Established in 1962 by congress, today the institute conducts and supports research on topics related to the health of children, adults, families and populations. Some of these topics include: developmental disabilities, growth and development, infant death, reproductive health and birth defects.

Nancy D Wirth, Director
Lisa Kaeser, Program & Public Liaison

National Associations & Support Groups

1955 Genetic Alliance
4301 Connecticut Avenue NW
Washington, DC 20008

202-966-5557
800-336-4363
Fax: 202-966-8553
e-mail: info@geneticalliance.org
www.geneticalliance.org

A coalition of voluntary genetic support groups, consumers and professionals addressing the needs of individuals and families affected by genetic disorders from a national perspective.

Sharon Terry, President/CEO

1956 March of Dimes Birth Defects Foundation
1275 Mamaroneck Avenue
White Plains, NY 10605

914-428-7100
888-663-4637
Fax: 914-428-8203
e-mail: resourcecenter@modimes.org
www.marchofdimes.com

Partnership of volunteers and professionals dedicated to improving the health of babies by preventing birth defects and infant mortality. Over 100 chapters are located across the country and can be located through the National Office.

James E Sproull, Jr, Esq, Board-Directors Chairman
Thomas A Russo, Board-Directors Vice Chairman

1957 National Dissemination Center for Children with Disabilities
PO Box 1492
Washington, DC 20013

202-884-8200
800-695-0285
Fax: 202-884-8441
e-mail: nichcy@aed.org
www.nichcy.org

A national information and referral center that provides information on disabilities and disability-related issues for families, educators and other professionals.

Suzanne Ripley, Executive Director

Libraries & Resource Centers

1958 University of Iowa Birth Defects and Genetic Disorders Unit
2614 JCP
Iowa City, IA 52242

319-335-9901

James M Smith, Director

Web Sites

1959 Dr. Koop
www.drkoop.com/

Information on the condition, causes, symptoms, tests and treatment.

Book Publishers

1960 Let's Talk About Going to the Hospital
Rosen Publishing Group's PowerKids Press
29 E 21st Street
New York, NY 10010

212-777-3017
800-237-9932
Fax: 888-436-4643
e-mail: rosenpub@tribeca.ios.com
www.powerkidspress.com

If a child has to check into the hospital, chances are he or she is already upset about being ill. Knowing how a hospital functions and what the procedures are, such as when family members can visit, will help in what is already a stressful situation. Grades K-5.

24 pages
ISBN: 0-823950-36-0

DESCRIPTION

1961 CONGENITAL GLAUCOMA

Synonym: Infantile glaucoma

Covers these related disorders: Primary glaucoma, Secondary glaucoma

Involves the following Biologic System(s):
Ophthalmologic Disorders

Glaucoma refers to a condition in which the fluid pressure within the eyes (intraocular pressure) is abnormally elevated. This may occur as a result of the buildup of fluid (aqueous humor) due to obstruction or other problems with the eyes. Glaucoma that develops by the third year of life is referred to as congenital or infantile glaucoma, which is a very rare occurrence. Primary glaucoma refers to the condition as it relates to an irregularity in the mechanism that drains the eye. Secondary glaucoma refers to increased intraocular pressure that results from other types of irregularities that may or may not be accompanied by a drainage deficit.

Symptoms associated with congenital glaucoma may include an abnormal sensitivity to light (photophobia), involuntary, repeated squeezing and closing of the eyelids (blepharospasm), abnormal tearing, swelling and enlargement of the cornea, difficulty in seeing, and other ocular irregularities. Affected infants under three months of age are at additional risk of incurring tissue damage due to heightened sensitivity of the cornea to elevated fluid pressure within the eye. Eye irregularities may be observed by a physician upon ophthalmic examination.

Congenital glaucoma may develop subsequent to certain congenital problems such as trauma, bleeding (hemorrhage) within the eye, or tumors and inflammation. Other associated abnormalities may include the lack of transparency (opacity) of the lenses of the eye (cataracts), displacement of the lenses (ectopia lentis), partial absence of the iris (aniridia), and other abnormalities. Disorders often associated with congenital glaucoma include certain chromosomal disorders that may affect various systems of the body such as Sturge-Weber syndrome, oculocerebrorenal syndrome, neurofibromatosis, and Marfan syndrome.

Treatment for congenital glaucoma includes surgery to relieve the pressure within the eye to prevent optic nerve damage and preserve vision. In some cases, more than one surgery may be necessary and follow-up therapy may be required. Additional treatment is directed toward associated irregularities and complications.

See also **General Resources** on page 917

Government Agencies

1962 NIH/National Eye Institute
31 Center Drive MSC 2510
Bethesda, MD 20892

301-496-5248
e-mail: 2020@nei.nih.gov
www.nei.nih.gov

Conducts and supports research that helps prevent and treat eye diseases and other disorders of vision. This research leads to sight-saving treatments, reduces visual impairment and blindness, and improves the quality of life for people of all ages. NEI-supported research has advanced our knowledge of how the eye functions in health and disease.

Paul A Sieving M.D., Ph.D., Director

National Associations & Support Groups

1963 Children's Glaucoma Foundation
2 Longfellow Place, Suite 201
Boston, MA 02114

617-227-3011
Fax: 617-227-9538
e-mail: childglau@worldnet.att.net
www.childrensglaucoma.com

A nonprofit organization dedicated to supporting programs for children with glaucoma. Serves to increase awareness of the symptoms and encourage parents and doctors to screen infants and children for glaucoma.

David S Walton, MD, President

1964 Genetic Alliance
4301 Connecticut Avenue NW
Washington, DC 20008

202-966-5557
800-336-4363
Fax: 202-966-8553
e-mail: info@geneticalliance.org
www.geneticalliance.org

A coalition of voluntary genetic support groups, consumers and professionals addressing the needs of individuals and families affected by genetic disorders from a national perspective.

Sharon Terry, President/CEO

1965 Glaucoma Research Foundation
251 Post Street, Suite 600
San Francisco, CA 94102

415-986-3162
800-826-6693
Fax: 415-986-3763
www.glaucoma.org

Mission is to preserve the sight and independence of individuals with glaucoma through research and education with the ultimate goal of finding a cure.

Thomas M Brunner, President/CEO
Catalina San Agustin, Operations Director

1966 Glaucoma Support Network
Glaucoma Research Foundation
490 Post Street, Suite 1427
San Francisco, CA 94102

415-986-3162
800-826-6693
Fax: 415-986-3763
e-mail: info@glaucoma.org
www.glaucoma.org

The Glaucoma Research Foundation's mission is to preserve the sight and independence of individuals with glaucoma through research and education with the ultimate goal of finding a cure.

1967 National Association for Visually Handicapped
22 W 21st Street, 6th Floor
New York, NY 10010

212-889-3141
Fax: 212-727-2931
e-mail: navh@navh.org
www.navh.org

Serves as a clearinghouse for information about all services available to the partially-sighted from public and private sources. Conducts self-help groups. Provides information on large print books, textbooks and educational tools.

Dr Lorraine Marchi, Founder & CEO

1968 Prevent Blindness America
500 E Remington Road
Schaumburg, IL 60173

847-843-2020
800-331-2020
Fax: 847-843-8458
e-mail: info@preventblindness.org
www.preventblindness.org

A volunteer eye health and safety organization dedicated to fighting blindness and saving sight. Focused on promoting a continuum of vision care, Prevent Blindness America touches the lives of millions of people each year through public and professional education, advocacy, certified vision screening training, community and patient service programs and research.

State Agencies & Support Groups

Alabama

1969 Alabama Institute for the Deaf & Blind
PO Box 698
Talladega, AL 35160

256-761-3200
Fax: 256-761-3344
www.nectas.unc.edu

Services include central directory, representatives of agencies, service providers, families, and coordinators of infant, toddler, and preschool special education programs.

Joseph Busta, Interagency Coordinating Council

Arizona

1970 National Association for Parents of the Visually Impaired
Po Box 317
Watertown, MA 02471

617-972-7441
800-562-6265
Fax: 617-972-7444
www.spedex.com/napvi

Mary Ellen Simmons

California

1971 Helen Keller National Center SW Region
6160 Cornerstone Court E
San Diego, CA 92121

858-623-2777
Fax: 858-642-0266
TTY: 858-646-0784
e-mail: ckirscher@cspp.edu
www.helenkeller.org

Cathy Kircher, SW Regional Representative

Ohio

1972 Region 2 of the National Association for Parents of the Visually Impaired
3910 Pocahontas Avenue
Cincinnati, OH 45227

513-561-8542

Victoria Gorman Miller

Pennsylvania

1973 East Central Region-Helen Keller National Center
4351 Garden City Drive
New Carrollton, MD 20785

301-459-5474
Fax: 301-459-5070
e-mail: hkncreg3cl@aol.com
www.helenkeller.org

South Carolina

1974 Region 4 of the National Association for Parents of the Visually Impaired
1032 Trail Road
Belton, SC 29627

864-338-9593

Washington

1975 Northwestern Region-Helen Keller National Center
2366 Eastlake Avenue E
Seattle, WA 98102

206-324-9120
e-mail: nwhknc@juno.com

Libraries & Resource Centers

Alabama

1976 Mobile Association for the Blind
2440 Gordon Smith Drive
Mobile, AL 36617

334-473-3585

Offers work adjustment training, activities of daily living, mobility, communication skills and sheltered employment for adults and children who are visually impaired.

Mahlon McCracken, Executive Director

Arizona

1977 Educational Services for the Visually Impaired
PO Box 668
Little Rock, AR 72203

501-371-5710

Offers textbooks, braille books and more to the visually impaired grades K-12 in the Arkansas area.

David Beavers, Director

Arkansas

1978 Arkansas Regional Library for the Blind and Physically Handicapped
1 Capitol Mall
Little Rock, AR 72201

501-682-1155
Fax: 501-682-1529
TDD: 501-682-1002
e-mail: nlsbooks@asl.lib.ar.us
www.asl.lib.ar.us/ASL_LBPH.htm

Public library books in recorded or braille format. Popular fiction and nonfiction books for all ages, books and players are on free loan, sent to patrons by mail and may be returned postage free. Anyone who cannot see well enough to read regular print with glasses on or who has a disability that makes it difficult to hold a book or turn the pages is eligible.

John D Hall, Director

California

1979 American Action Fund for Blind Children and Adults
18440 Oxnard Street
Tarzana, CA 91356

818-343-2022
www.actinfund.org

Offers a charitable and educational fund, braille assistive devices and a lending library for the visually impaired.

1980 Blind Children's Center
4120 Marathon Street
Los Angeles, CA 90029

323-664-2153
Fax: 323-665-3828
www.blindcntr.org

Offers support and informational groups.

1981 Braille Institute Desert Center
70-251 Ramon Road
Rancho Mirage, CA 92270

760-321-2555

Dedicated to providing blind and visually impaired men, women and children with the training, programs and services they need to enjoy productive lives. Services offered include child development, youth programs, library services and adult education.

1982 Braille Institute Sight Center
741 N Vermont Avenue
Los Angeles, CA 90029

213-663-1111
e-mail: bils@brailib.org

Offers help, programs, services and information to the blind and visually impaired children and adults.

Dr. Henry Chang, Librarian

1983 Braille Institute Youth Center
3450 Cahuenga Boulevard W
Los Angeles, CA 90068

213-851-5695

Offers various youth programs and services for the blind and visually impaired youngster.

1984 New Beginnings - Blind Children's Center
4120 Marathon, Street
Los Angeles, CA 90029

323-664-2153
800-222-3566
Fax: 323-665-3828

Helps children and their families become independent by creating a climate of safety and trust. Services include an infant stimulation program, educational preschool, interdisciplinary assessment services, family services, correspondence program, toll-free national hotline and a publication and research service.

1985 San Francisco Public Library for the Blind and Print Disabled
100 Larkin Street
San Francisco, CA 94102

415-557-4293
Fax: 415-557-4375
e-mail: lbphmgr@sfpl.lib.ca.us
www.library.ca.us

Foreign-language books on cassette, children's books on cassettes and more.

Martin Maqid, Librarian

1986 Variety Audio
PO Box 5731
San Jose, CA 95150

408-277-4839

Summer reading programs, braille writer, magnifiers, closed-circuit TV, large-print photocopier, cassette books and magazines, children's books on cassette, home visits and other reference materials on blindness and other handicaps.

Louisa Griehshammer

District of Columbia

1987 Council of Families with Visual Impairment
1155 15th Street NW
Washington, DC 20005

202-467-5081

Members are sighted parents of blind or visually impaired children. Offers a forum for support and outreach, sharing of experiences in parent-child relationships, and educational and cultural information about child development. Monitors developments in technical and legislative arenas.

Nola Webb, President

Florida

1988 Florida Bureau of Braille and Talking Book Library Services
420 Platt Street
Daytona Beach, FL 32114

386-239-6000
Fax: 386-239-6069
TDD: 800-226-6079
e-mail: mike_gunde@dbs.doe.state.fl.us
www.state.fl.us/dbs/lswel.html

Discs, cassettes, closed-circuit TV, large-print photocopier, films, children's books on cassettes and more.

Michael Gunde, Librarian

1989 Talking Book Library, Jacksonville Public Library
1755 Edgewood Avenue W, Suite 1
Jacksonville, FL 32208

904-765-5588
Fax: 904-768-7404
TDD: 904-768-7822
e-mail: jerryr@coj.net
neflin.org/neflin/members/jackspub.html

Discs, cassettes and reference materials on blindness and other disabilities.

Jerry Reynolds, Librarian Senior

1990 Talking Book Service - Manatee County Central Library
6081 26th Street W
Bradenton, FL 34207

941-742-5914
Fax: 941-751-7089
TDD: 941-742-5951
e-mail: patricia.schubert@co.manatee.fl.us
www.co.manatee.fl.us

Offers children's books on disc and cassette and more reference materials for the blind and physically handicapped.

Patricia Schubert, Librarian

Georgia

1991 Albany Library for the Blind and Physical Handicapped
300 Pine Avenue
Albany, GA 31701

229-420-3220
Fax: 229-420-3240
e-mail: sinquefk@mail.dougherty.public.lib.ga.us
www.docolib.org/LBPH/index.html

Offers discs, cassettes, reference materials on blindness and other handicaps, large-print photocopiers, summer reading programs, cassette books and more.

Kathryn Sinquefield, Librarian

1992 Bainbridge Subregional Library for the Blind and Physically Handicapped
301 S Monroe Street
Bainbridge, GA 31717

912-248-2680
800-795-2680
Fax: 912-248-2670
TDD: 912-248-2665
e-mail: lbph@mail.deccatur.public.lib.ga.us
www.deccatur.public.lib.ga.us/local/lbph/lbph1.htm

Discs, cassettes, summer reading programs, closed-circuit TV, magnifiers and more.

Kathy Hutchins, Librarian

1993 CEL Subregional Library for the Blind and Physically Handicapped
2708 Mechanics
Savannah, GA 31401

912-354-5864
Fax: 912-354-5534
TDD: 912-652-3635
e-mail: stokesl@cel.co.chatman.ga.us

Summer reading programs, braille writer, magnifiers, closed-circuit TV, large-print photocopier, cassette books and magazines, children's books on cassette, home visits and other reference materials on blindness and other handicaps.

Linda Stokes, Librarian

Idaho

1994 Idaho State Talking Book Library
325 W State Street
Boise, ID 83702

208-334-2117
Fax: 208-334-4016
TDD: 800-377-1363
e-mail: tblbooks@isl.state.id.us
www.lili.org/isl/tblinfo.htm

Summer reading programs, braille writer, magnifiers, closed-circuit TV, large-print photocopier, cassette books and magazines, children's books on cassette, home visits and other reference materials on blindness and other handicaps.

Sue Walker, Librarian

Illinois

1995 Chicago Library Service for the Blind
1055 W Roosevelt Road
Chicago, IL 60608

312-746-9210

Summer reading programs, braille writer, magnifiers, closed-circuit TV, large-print photocopier, cassette books and magazines, children's books on cassette, home visits and other reference materials on blindness and other handicaps.

Carol Pellish, Librarian

1996 Illinois State Library, Talkng Book and Braille Service
300 S 2nd Street
Springfield, IL 62701

217-782-9435
Fax: 217-782-8261
TDD: 800-665-5576
e-mail: sruda@ilsos.net
www.cyberdriveillinois.com/library/isl/bph/bph.html

Summer reading programs, braille writer, magnifiers, closed-circuit TV, large-print photocopier, cassette books and magazines, descriptive videos, children's books on cassette, home visits and other reference materials on blindness and other handicaps.

Sharon Ruda, Librarian

1997 Mid Illinois Talking Book System
515 York Street
Quincy, IL 62301

217-224-6619
Fax: 217-224-9818

Summer reading programs, braille writer, magnifiers, closed-circuit TV, large-print photocopier, cassette books and magazines, children's books on cassette, home visits and other reference materials on blindness and other handicaps.

1998 Mid-Illinois Talking Book Center
845 Brenkman Drive
Pekin, IL 61554

309-353-4110
Fax: 309-353-8281
e-mail: hitbc@darkstar.rsa.lib.il.us
www.mitbc.org

Summer reading programs, braille writer, magnifiers, closed-circuit TV, large-print photocopier, cassette books and magazines, children's books on cassette, home visits and other reference materials on blindness and other handicaps.

Eileen Sheppard, Librarian

1999 Talking Book Center of Northwest Illinois
PO Box 125
Coal Valley, IL 61240

309-799-3137
Fax: 309-799-7916
e-mail: kodean@libby.rbls.lib.il.us
www.rbls.lib.il.us

Subregional library provides Talking Book and Braille Book programs to eligible persons unable to use standard print materials due to visual or physical disabilities. Includes cassette books and magazines; summer reading program.

Indiana

2000 Northwest Indiana Subregional Library for Blind and Physically Handicapped
1919 W Lincoln Highway
Merrillville, IN 46410

219-769-3541
Fax: 219-769-0690

Summer reading programs, braille writer, magnifiers, closed-circuit TV, large-print photocopier, cassette books and magazines, children's books on cassette, home visits and other reference materials on blindness and other handicaps.

Renee Lewis

Iowa

2001 Iowa Library for the Blind and Physically Handicapped
Iowa Department for the Blind
524 4th Street
Des Moines, IA 50309

515-281-1333
Fax: 515-281-1378
TDD: 515-281-1355
e-mail: keninger.karen@blind.state.ia.us
www.blind.state.ia.us

Summer reading programs, magnifiers, closed-circuit TV, large-print photocopier, children's books on cassette, children's books in Braille and Print Braille, cassette magazines, home visits and reference materials on blindness and other handicaps.

Karen Keninger, Program Manager/Librarian

2002 University of Iowa Birth Defects and Genetic Disorders Unit
2614 JCP
Iowa City, IA 52242

319-335-9901

James M Smith, Director

Kansas

2003 CKLS Headquarters
1409 Williams Street
Great Bend, KS 67530

316-792-2393
800-362-2642
Fax: 316-792-5495
e-mail: cenks@ink.org
www.macular.org

Summer reading programs, braille writer, magnifiers, closed-circuit TV, large-print photocopier, cassette books and magazines, children's books on cassette, home visits and other reference materials on blindness and other handicaps.

Jerri Robinson, Librarian

2004 Services for the Visually Disabled
629 Poyntz Avenue
Manhattan, KS 66502

785-776-4741
Fax: 785-776-1545
e-mail: marionr@manhattan.lib.ks.us

Summer reading programs, braille writer, magnifiers, closed-circuit TV, large-print photocopier, cassette books and magazines, children's books on cassette, home visits and other reference materials on blindness and other handicaps.

Marion Rice, Librarian

Kentucky

2005 Kentucky Library for the Blind and Physically Handicapped
PO Box 818
Frankfort, KY 40602

502-564-8300
800-372-2968
Fax: 502-564-5773
e-mail: richard.feindel@kdla.net
www.kdla.net/libserv/ktbl.htm

Large-print photocopier, cassette books and magazines, children's books on cassette, and other reference materials on blindness and other handicaps.

5,200 members

Richard Feindel, Librarian

Maryland

2006 Maryland State Library for the Blind and Physically Handicapped
415 Park Avenue
Baltimore, MD 21201

410-230-2424
Fax: 410-333-2095
TTY: 800-934-2541
TDD: 410-333-8679
e-mail: recept@lbta.lib.md.us
www.lbph.lib.md.us

Summer reading programs, braille writer, magnifiers, large-print photocopier, cassette books and magazines, children's books on cassette, and other reference materials on blindness and other handicaps.

2007 Prince George's County Memorial Library Talking Book Center
6530 Adelphi Road
Hyattsville, MD 20782

301-779-9330

Summer reading programs, braille writer, magnifiers, closed-circuit TV, large-print photocopier, cassette books and magazines, children's books on cassette, home visits and other reference materials on blindness and other handicaps.

Shirley Tuthill, Librarian

Massachusetts

2008 Braille and Talking Book Library Perkins School for the Blind
175 N Beacon Street
Watertown, MA 02472

617-924-3434
Fax: 617-926-2027
e-mail: perkins@bpl.org
www.perkins.org

Patricia Kirk

2009 Carroll Center for the Blind
770 Centre Street
Newton, MA 02158

617-969-6200
800-852-3131
Fax: 617-969-6204
www.carroll.org

Assists blind and visually impaired adults and adolescents to adjust to loss of vision. The goal of this dynamic program is to help the person become more independent, to restore self-confidence, prepare for employment and improve the quality of life. Programs of individual counseling are offered as part of the program.

Rachel Rosenbaum, President

Michigan

2010 Downtown Detroit Subregional Library for the Blind and Handicapped
121 Gratiot Avenue
Detroit, MI 48226

313-224-0580
Fax: 313-965-1977
TDD: 313-224-0584
e-mail: deveans@cms.xx.wayne.edu
www.detroit.lib.mi.us

Summer reading programs, braille writer, magnifiers, closed-circuit TV, large-print photocopier, cassette books and magazines, children's books on cassette, home visits and other reference materials on blindness and other handicaps.

Deborah Evans, Librarian

2011 Kent County Library for the Blind
775 Ball Avenue NE
Grand Rapids, MI 49503

616-336-3250
Fax: 616-336-3201
e-mail: kdlem@lakeland.lib.mi.us

Summer reading programs, braille writer, magnifiers, closed-circuit TV, large-print photocopier, cassette books and magazines, children's books on cassette, home visits and other reference materials on blindness and other handicaps.

Claudya Muller, Librarian

2012 Library of Michigan Service for the Blind
PO Box 30007
Lansing, MI 48909

517-373-5614
Fax: 517-373-5865
e-mail: info@sbph.libomich.lib.mi.us

Summer reading programs, braille writer, magnifiers, closed-circuit TV, large-print photocopier, cassette books and magazines, children's books on cassette, home visits and other reference materials on blindness and other handicaps.

2013 Macomb Library for the Blind and Physically Handicapped
16480 Hall Road
Clinton Township, MI 48038

586-286-1580
Fax: 586-286-0634
TDD: 810-869-40
e-mail: macbld@libcoop.net
www.macomb.lib.mi.us/macspe/

Summer reading programs, braille writer, closed-circuit TV, cassette books and magazines, children's books on cassette, reference materials on blindness and other handicaps.

Beverlee Babcock, Librarian

2014 Mideastern Michigan Library Co-op
G-4195 W Pasadena Avenue
Flint, MI 48504

810-732-1120
Fax: 810-732-1715
e-mail: cnash@genesse.freeret.org
www.fakon.edu/gdl/talking.htm

Summer reading programs, braille writer, magnifiers, closed-circuit TV, large-print photocopier, cassette books and magazines, children's books on cassette, home visits and other reference materials on blindness and other handicaps.

Carolyn Nash, Librarian

2015 Muskegon County Library for the Blind
635 Ottawa Street
Muskegon, MI 49442

231-724-6248
Fax: 231-724-6675
TDD: 231-722-4103
www.muskcolib.org

Summer reading programs, braille typewriter, magnifiers, closed-circuit TV, large-print photocopier, cassette books and magazines, children's books on cassette, home visits and other reference materials on blindness and other handicaps, The Reading Edge, Perkins Brailler and large print books.

Linda Clapp, Librarian

2016 Upper Peninsula Library for the Blind Physically Handicapped
1615 Presque Isle Avenue
Marquette, MI 49855

906-228-7697
Fax: 906-228-5627
e-mail: uproc.lib.mi.us
www.upesc.lib.mi.us/uplbph

Summer reading programs, braille writer, magnifiers, closed-circuit TV, large-print photocopier, cassette books and magazines, children's books on cassette, home visits and other reference materials on blindness and other handicaps.

Suzanne Dees, Librarian

2017 Washtenaw County Library
PO Box 8645
Ann Arbor, MI 48107

734-222-4357
Fax: 734-222-6715
e-mail: contact us@ewashtenaw.org
www.ewashtenaw.org

Summer reading programs, braille writer, magnifiers, closed-circuit TV, large-print photocopier, cassette books and magazines, children's books on cassette, home visits and other reference materials on blindness and other handicaps.

Margeret Wolfe, Librarian

2018 Washtenaw County Library for the Blind and Physically Disabled
PO Box 8645
Ann Arbor, MI 48107

734-971-6059
Fax: 734-971-3892
e-mail: lbpd@co.washtennaw.mi.us
www.co.washten.ml.us/depts/lib/liblbpd.h

Book lovers club.adaptive technology,cassette equipment, cassette books and magazines, described videos, low vision aids reference and referral services.

Margaret Wolfe, Coordinator

2019 Wayne County Regional Library for the Blind
30555 Michigan Avenue
Westland, MI 48186

734-727-7300
Fax: 734-727-7333
TTY: 734-727-7330
e-mail: werlbph@tln.lib.mi.us
www.wayneregional.lib.mi.us

Summer reading programs, braille writer, magnifiers, closed-circuit TV, large-print photocopier, cassette books and magazines, children's books on cassette, home visits and other reference materials on blindness and other handicaps.

Reginald Williams, Wayne County Librarian

Minnesota

2020 Minnesota Library for the Blind & Physically Handicapped
Highway 298, PO Box 68
Fairbault, MN 55021

507-333-4828
800-722-0550
Fax: 507-333-4832
e-mail: libblnd@state.mn.us

Summer reading programs, braille writer, magnifiers, closed-circuit TV, large-print photocopier, cassette, large print, braille books and magazines, children's books on cassette, and other reference materials on blindness and other handicaps.

Catherine A Durivage, Program Director

Missouri

2021 Adriene Resource Center for Blind Children
1445 Boonville Avenue
Springfield, MO 65802

417-862-2781
Fax: 417-862-7566
e-mail: blind@ag.org
www.gospelpublishing.com

Offers braille and cassette lending library, braille and cassette Sunday school materials for all ages, braille and cassette periodicals and resource assistance, and resources for blind children and children of blind parents.

Paul Weingariner, Director

2022 Assemblies of God National Center for the Blind
1445 Boonville Avenue
Springfield, MO 65802

417-862-2781
Fax: 417-862-7566
e-mail: blind@ag.org
www.gospelpublishing.com

Offers braille and cassette lending library, braille and cassette Sunday school materials for all ages, braille and cassette periodicals and resource assistance, and resources for blind children and children of blind parents.

Paul Weingariner, Director

2023 Wolfner Memorial Library for the Blind
PO Box 387
Jefferson City, MO 65102

573-751-8720
Fax: 573-526-2985
TDD: 800-347-1379
e-mail: beckles@mail.sos.state.mo.us

Summer reading programs, braille writer, magnifiers, closed-circuit TV, large-print photocopier, cassette books and magazines, children's books on cassette, home visits and other reference materials on blindness and other handicaps.

Elizabeth Eckles, Librarian

Nebraska

2024 Nebraska Library Commission Talking Book & Braille Services
1200 N Street
Lincoln, NE 68508

402-471-4038
800-742-7691
Fax: 402-471-6244
TDD: 402-471-4038
e-mail: doertli@nlc.state.ne.us
www.ncl.state.ne.us/tbbs/tbbsl/html

Free loan of books and magazines on cassette and in Braille, including children's materials, along with specially designed playback equipment. Summer reading program for children, Braille embossing, closed circuit TV, large-print copier. Reference materials on blindness and other disabilities.

David Oerti, Librarian

New Jersey

2025 New Jersey Library for the Blind and Handicapped
2300 Stuyvesant Avenue
Trenton, NJ 08618

609-292-6450
800-792-8322
Fax: 609-530-6384
TDD: 877-882-5593
e-mail: nglbh@njstatelib.org
www.njstatelib.org

Summer reading programs, braille writer, magnifiers, closed-circuit TV, large-print, cassette braille books and magazines, children's books on cassettes in braille and other reference materials on blindness and other handicaps.

Deborah Rutledeger, Director

New Mexico

2026 New Mexico State Library for the Blind and Physically Handicapped
1209 Camino Carlos Ray
Santa Fe, NM

505-476-9700
Fax: 505-476-9701
e-mail: jbrewstr@stlib.state.nm.us
www.stlib.state.nm.us

Summer reading programs, braille writer, magnifiers, closed-circuit TV, large-print photocopier, cassette books and magazines, children's books on cassette, home visits and other reference materials on blindness and other handicaps.

Glee Wenzel, Librarian

New York

2027 Helen Keller National Center
111 Middle Neck Road
Sands Point, NY 11050

516-944-8900
Fax: 516-944-7302

Provides diagnostic, evaluation, short term comprehensive rehabilitation and personal adjustment training. A technical assistance center is offered providing assistance to public and private agencies and to parent groups who work towards community integration and the enhancement of the quality of life. A national parent network is also provided that develops and shares information about advocacy, legislation, new services and achievements.

2028 New York State Talking Book & Braille Library
Empire State Plaza, CEC
Albany, NY 12230

518-474-5801
Fax: 518-474-5786
TDD: 518-474-7121
e-mail: jane@unix2.nysed.gov
www.suffolk.lib.ny.us

Books on audio cassette, cassette players, braille books, summer reading programs, braille writer, magnifiers, closed-circuit TV, large-print photocopier, cassette books and magazines, children's books on cassette, reference materials on blindness and other handicaps.

Jane Somers, Director

North Carolina

2029 North Carolina Library for the Blind
1811 Capital Boulevard
Raleigh, NC 27635

919-733-4376
Fax: 919-733-6910
TDD: 919-733-1462
e-mail: nclbph@ncsl.der.state.nc

Summer reading programs, braille writer, magnifiers, closed-circuit TV, large-print photocopier, cassette books and magazines, children's books on cassette, home visits and other reference materials on blindness and other handicaps.

Francine Martin, Librarian

Ohio

2030 American Council of Blind Parents
34400 Cedar Road, Apartment 108
University Heights, OH 44121

800-424-8666

Members are sighted parents of blind or visually impaired children. Offers a forum for support and outreach, sharing of experiences in parent-child relationships, and educational and cultural information about child development. Monitors developments in technical and legislative arenas.

Nola Webb, President

Oregon

2031 Oregon State Library, Talking Book and Braille Services
250 Winter Street NW
Salem, OR 97310

503-378-4243
Fax: 503-588-7119
TDD: 503-378-4276
e-mail: tbabs@sparkie.osl.state.or.us

Cassette books and magazines, children's books on cassette, home visits and other reference materials on blindness and other handicaps.

Donna Bensen, Regional Librarian

Virginia

2032 Alexandria Library Talking Book Service
5005 Duke Street
Alexandria, VA 22304

703-519-5900
Fax: 703-519-5915
TDD: 703-838-4568
e-mail: emccaffr@lea.eda
www.www.alexandria.lib.va.us

Summer reading programs, braille writer, magnifiers, closed-circuit TV, large-print photocopier, cassette books and magazines, children's books on cassette, home visits and other reference materials on blindness and other handicaps.

Patricia Bates, Librarian

2033 Division for the Visually Handicapped
1920 Association Drive
Reston, VA 20191

703-620-3660

Members are teachers, college faculty members, administrators, supervisors and others concerned with the education and welfare of visually handicapped and blind children and youth. This is a division of the Council For Exceptional Children.

Dr. Kay Ferrell, President

2034 Division on Visual Impairments
Council for Exceptional Children
1110 North Glebe Road, Suite 300
Arlington, VA 22201

800-224-6830
Fax: 703-264-9494
TTY: 866-915-5000
www.ed.arizona.edu/dvi/welcome.htm; www.cec.sped.org

A division within the CEC, it handles concerns for Federal, state and local issues and policies related to education of youths, children and infants with visual impairments.

Ellyn Ross, President
Shirley J Wilson, Secretary

2035 Virginia State Library for the Visually and Physically Handicapped
1901 Roane Street
Richmond, VA 23222

804-367-0014

Summer reading programs, braille writer, magnifiers, closed-circuit TV, large-print photocopier, cassette books and magazines, children's books on cassette, home visits and other reference materials on blindness and other handicaps.

Mary Ruth Halapatz, Librarian

Washington

2036 Washington Library for the Blind and Physically Handicapped
821 Lenora Street
Seattle, WA 98129

206-386-4636
Fax: 206-386-4685
e-mail: wtbbl@spl.lib.wa.us
www.spl.lib.wa.us

Summer reading programs, braille writer, magnifiers, closed-circuit TV, large-print photocopier, cassette books and magazines, children's books on cassette, home visits and other reference materials on blindness and other handicaps.

Jan Ames, Librarian

West Virginia

2037 West Virginia School for the Blind
301 E Main Street
Romney, WV 26757

304-822-3521
Fax: 304-822-4896
e-mail: cjohn@access.mountain.net

Summer reading programs, braille writer, magnifiers, closed-circuit TV, large-print photocopier, cassette books and magazines, children's books on cassette, home visits and other reference materials on blindness and other handicaps.

Cynthia Johnson, Librarian

Research Centers

2038 Center for the Partially Sighted
12301 Wilshire Boulevard, Suite 600
Los Angeles, CA 90025

310-458-3501
Fax: 310-458-8179
e-mail: info@low-vision.org
www.low-vision.org

Provides professional, comprehensive vision rehabilitation services to visually impaired people of all ages. For those whose sight is severely limited due to macular degeneration, diabetic retinopathy,

glaucoma, retinal detachment, stroke or other conditions not correctable medically or surgically.

2039 Florida Ophthalmic Institute
7106 NW 11th Place
Gainesville, FL 32605

352-331-2020

Nonprofit organization that understands and treats ocular diseases including glaucoma.

Norman S Levy, MD, Director

2040 Foundation for Glaucoma Research
200 Pine Street, Suite 200
San Francisco, CA 94104

415-986-3162
Fax: 415-986-3763

Clinical and laboratory studies of glaucoma.

Robert N Shaffer, MD, Chairman

2041 Glaucoma Laser Trabeculoplasty Study
Sinai Hospital of Detroit
29275 Northwestern Highway
Southfield, MI 48034

248-493-5157

Examines the effectiveness and safety of the treatments of glaucoma.

Hugh Beckman, Chairman

2042 Glaucoma Research Foundation
251 Post Street, Suite 600
San Francisco, CA 94104

415-986-3162
800-826-6693
Fax: 415-986-3763
e-mail: questions@glaucoma.org
www.glaucoma.org

Conducts patient education activities, maintains eye donor network, provides multi-disciplinary seminars and conducts collaborative studies.

Jennifer Rulon, Research/Education Specialist

2043 Helen Keller National Center
111 Middle Neck Road
Sands Point, NY 11050

516-944-8900
Fax: 516-944-7302

Provides diagnostic evaluation, short term comprehensive rehabilitation and personal adjustment training. A technical assistance center is offered providing assistance to public and private agencies and to parent groups who work towards community integration and the enhancement of the quality of life. A national parent network is also provided that develops and shares information about advocacy, legislation, new services and achievements.

2044 Mobile Association for the Blind
2440 Gordon Smith Drive
Mobile, AL 36617

251-473-3585
877-292-5463
Fax: 251-470-8622
e-mail: sales@mobile.blind.com
www.mobileblind.com

Offers work adjustment training, activities of daily living, mobility, communication skills and sheltered employment for adults and children who are visually impaired.

Mahlon McCracken, Executive Director

2045 National Eye Research Foundation
910 Skokie Boulevard, Suite 207A
Northbrook, IL 60062

847-564-4652
800-621-2258
Fax: 847-564-0807
e-mail: info@nerf.org
www.nerf.org

Devoted to the enhancement of care and study of eye related diseases.

2046 National Ophthalmic Research Institute
Retina Consultants of Southwest, Florida
6901 International Center Boulevard
Ft. Myers, FL 33912

239-938-1284
Fax: 239-938-1270
e-mail: NORI@eye.md

A physician-owned clinical research center specializing in innovative investigational treatments for ophthalmic, retinal and vitreous diseases.

Cherly Kiesel, Research Director
Eileen Knips, RN, Clinical Research Coordinator

2047 New Beginnings - The Blind Children's Center
4120 Marathon Street
Los Angeles, CA 90029

213-664-2153

The purpose of the Center is to turn initial fears into hope. Helps children and their families become independent by creating a climate of safety and trust. Children learn to develop self confidence and to master a wide range of skills. Services include an infant stimulation program, educational preschool, interdisciplinary assessment services, family services, correspondence program, toll free national hotline and a publication and research service.

2048 Research to Prevent Blindness
645 Madison Avenue
New York, NY 10022

212-752-4333
800-621-0026
www.rpbusa.org

Provides research grants to scientists interested in eye disease and vision disorders.

Audio Video

2049 Heart to Heart
Blind Children's Center
4120 Marathon Street
Los Angeles, CA 90029

323-644-2153
Fax: 323-665-3828
www.blindcntr.org

Parents of blind and partially sighted children talk about their feelings.

Videotape

2050 Let's Eat
Blind Children's Center
4120 Marathon Street
Los Angeles, CA 90029

213-664-2153
Fax: 213-665-3828

Teaches competent feeding skills to children with visual impairments.

Videotape

2051 See What I Feel
Britannica Film Co.
345 4th Street
San Francisco, CA 94107

415-597-5555

A blind child tells her friends about her trip to the zoo. Each experience was explained as a blind child would experience it. A teacher's guide comes with this video.

Films

Web Sites

2052 Glaucoma Associates
www.glaucoma.net

Developed to promote research into the basic causes of Glaucoma, develop new treatments for Glaucoma, and to develop public education into the treatment of Glaucoma.

2053 Glaucoma Research Foundation
www.glaucoma.org

Mission is to preserve the sight and independence of individuals with glaucoma through research and education with the ultimate goal of finding a cure.

2054 Lighthouse International
www.lighthouse.org

The mission is to overcome vision impairment for people of all ages through worldwide leadership in rehabilitation services, education, research, prevention and advocacy.

2055 National Alliance of Blind Students
www.blindstudents.org

The leading national advocacy and consumer organization for students in high school or college who are blind or visually impaired.

2056 National Association for Visually Handicapped
www.navh.org

Helps to cope with the difficulties of vision impairment.

2057 Online Mendelian Inheritance in Man
www.ncbi.nlm.nih.gov

This database is a catalog of human genes and genetic disorders.

2058 Royal National Institute of the Blind
www.rnib.org.uk

Offering information, support and advice to over two million people with sight problems.

Book Publishers

2059 Childhood Glaucoma: A Reference Guide for Families
Nat'l Assn for Parents of Children with Visual
PO Box 317
Watertown, MA 02272

617-972-7441
800-562-6265
Fax: 617-972-7444
www.spedex.com/napvi

Provides nontechnical information about childhood glaucoma and its treatment. The book also discusses educational issues and family concerns, gives a resource list, and includes a glossary.

1997 36 pages

Susan LaVenture, Editor/Executive Director

2060 Children with Visual Impairments: A Parents' Guide
Peytral Publications
PO Box 1162
Minnetonka, MN 55345

952-949-8707
877-739-8725
Fax: 952-906-9777
www.peytral.com

Covers visual impairments ranging from low vision to total blindness. Offers authoritative information and empathy, parental insight on diagnosis and treatment, orientation and mobility, literacy, legal issues and more. Valuable to parents, educators and support staff.

395 pages

M Cay Holbrook PhD, Editor

2061 Ophthalmic Disorders Sourcebook
Omnigraphics Editorial Office
615 Griswold
Detroit, MI 48226

610-461-3548
800-234-1340
Fax: 610-532-9001
e-mail: editorial@omnigraphics.com
omnigraphics.com

Basic Information about glaucoma, cataracts, macular degeneration, strabismus, refractive disorders, and more.

1996 631 pages
ISBN: 0-780800-81-8

Linda M Ross, Editor

Magazines

2062 Journal of Visual Impairment and Blindness
American Foundation for the Blind
11 Penn Plaza, Suite 300
New York, NY 10001

212-502-7600
Fax: 212-502-7777
e-mail: afbinfo@afb.net
www.afb.org

Published in braille, regular print and on cassette this journal contains a wide variety of subjects including rehabilitation, psychology, education, legislation, medicine, technology, employment, sensory aids and childhood development as they relate to visual impairments.

10x Year

2063 Reaching, Crawling, Walking - Let's Get Moving
Blind Children's Center
4120 Marathon Street
Los Angeles, CA 90029

323-664-2153
Fax: 323-665-3828
e-mail: info@blindchildrenscenter.org
www.blindchildrenscenter.org

Orientation and mobility for visually impaired preschool children.

24 pages

2064 Seeing Candy
National Association for Visually Handicapped
22 W 21st Street, 6th Floor
New York, NY 10010

212-889-3141
Fax: 212-727-2931
e-mail: staff@navh.org
www.navh.org

This newsletter offers short stories, news, medical updates, assistive device information, poems, resources, crossword puzzles and more for the visually impaired.

Biannually

2065 Tactic
Clovernook Home and School for the Blind
7000 Hamilton Avenue
Cincinnati, OH 45231

513-522-3860
Fax: 513-728-3950
e-mail: clovernook@aol.com

Quarterly

Newsletters

2066 National Library Service for the Blind & Physically Handicapped
Library of Congress Reference Section
1291 Taylor Street NW
Washington, DC 20542

202-707-5100
800-424-8567
Fax: 202-707-0712
TTY: 202-707-0744
TDD: 202-707-0744
e-mail: nis@loc.gov
www.loc.gov/nls

Provides information and advocacy resources for families and professionals, including listings of organizations focusing on more specific areas of concern to families and young adults who have disabilities. Administers a natural library service that provides recorded and braille reading materials to eligible children and adults who cannot read standard print.

12 pages Quarterly
ISSN: 1046-1663

Vicki Fitzpatrick, Editor

2067 Talking Book Topics
National Library Services for the Blind
1291 Taylor Street NW
Washington, DC 20542

202-707-5100
Fax: 202-707-0712
www.loc.gov/nls

Offers hundreds of listings of books, fiction and nonfiction, for adults and children on cassette. Also offers listings on foreign language books on cassette, talking magazines and reviews.

Bimonthly

Pamphlets

2068 Dancing Cheek to Cheek
Blind Children's Center
4120 Marathon Street
Los Angeles, CA 90029

213-664-2153
Fax: 213-665-3828
www.blindchildrenscenter.org

Discusses beginning social, play and language interactions.

33 pages

2069 Family Guide - Growth and Development of the Partially Seeing Child
National Association for Visually Handicapped
22 W 21st Street, 6th Floor
New York, NY 10010

212-889-3141
Fax: 212-727-2931
e-mail: staff@navh.org
www.navh.org

Offers information for parents and guidelines in raising a partially seeing child.

2070 Family Guide to Vision Care
American Optometric Association
243 N Lindbergh Boulevard
Saint Louis, MO 63141

314-991-4100
Fax: 314-991-4101
www.aoanet.org

Offers information on the early developmental years of your vision, finding a family optometrist and how to take care of your eyesight through the learning years, the working years and the mature years.

2071 Glaucoma

Foundation for Glaucoma Research
251 Post Street, Suite 600
San Francisco, CA 94104

415-986-3162
800-826-6693
Fax: 415-986-3763
www.glaucoma.org

Offers information on what glaucoma is, the causes, treatments, types of glaucoma, eye exams and prevention.

2072 Glaucoma: The Sneak Thief of Sight

National Association for Visually Handicapped
22 W 21st Street, 6th Floor
New York, NY 10010

212-889-3141
Fax: 212-727-2931
e-mail: navh@navh.org
www.navh.org

A pamphlet describing the disease, treatment and medications.

22 pages

Donna A Esposito, MD, Editor

2073 Heart to Heart

Blind Children's Center
4120 Marathon Street
Los Angeles, CA 90029

213-664-2153
Fax: 213-665-3828
www.blindchildrenscenter.org

Parents of blind and partially sighted children talk about their feelings.

12 pages

2074 Information on Glaucoma

Foundation for Glaucoma Research
200 Pine Street, Suite 200
San Francisco, CA 94104

415-986-3162
Fax: 415-986-3763
www.glaucoma.org

2075 Learning to Play

Blind Children's Center
4120 Marathon Street
Los Angeles, CA 90029

213-664-2153
Fax: 213-665-3828
www.blindchildrenscenter.org

Discusses how to present play activities to the visually impaired preschool child.

12 pages

2076 Let's Eat

Blind Children's Center
4120 Marathon Street
Los Angeles, CA 90029

213-664-2153
Fax: 213-665-3828
www.blindchildrenscenter.org

Teaches competent feeding skills to children with visual impairments.

28 pages

2077 Move with Me

Blind Children's Center
4120 Marathon Street
Los Angeles, CA 90029

213-664-2153
Fax: 213-665-3828
www.blindchildrenscenter.org

A parent's guide to movement development for visually impaired babies.

12 pages

2078 Selecting a Program

Blind Children's Center
4120 Marathon Street
Los Angeles, CA 90029

213-664-2153
Fax: 213-665-3828
www.blindchildrenscenter.org

A guide for parents of infants and preschoolers with visual impairments.

28 pages

2079 Standing on My Own Two Feet

Blind Children's Center
4120 Marathon Street
Los Angeles, CA 90029

323-664-2153
Fax: 323-665-3828
e-mail: info@blindchildrenscenter.org
www.blindchildrenscenter.org

A step-by-step guide to designing and constructing simple, individually tailored adaptive mobility devices for preschool-age children who are visually impaired.

36 pages

2080 Talk to Me

Blind Children's Center
4120 Marathon Street
Los Angeles, CA 90029

213-664-2153
Fax: 213-665-3828
www.blindchildrenscenter.org

A language guide for parents of deaf children.

11 pages

2081 Talk to Me II

Blind Children's Center
4120 Marathon Street
Los Angeles, CA 90029

213-664-2153
Fax: 213-665-3828
www.blindchildrenscenter.org

A sequel to Talk To Me, available in English and Spanish.

15 pages

Camps

2082 Bloomfield

5300 Angeles Vista Boulevard
Los Angeles, CA 90043

323-295-4555
800-352-2290
Fax: 323-296-0424
e-mail: info@juniorblind.org
www.junoirblind.org

This camp is dedicated to serving blind and developmentally disabled children and adults.

2083 Florida School-Deaf and Blind
207 San Marco Avenue
Saint Augustine, FL 32084

800-800-344
www2.kidscamps.com

2084 National Camps for Blind Children
Christian Record
4444 S 52nd Street
Lincoln, NE 68516

402-488-0981
Fax: 402-488-7582
e-mail: info@christianrecord.org
www.christianrecord.org

Camps throughout the US and Canada are offered at no cost to the legally blind, ages 9-65. Activities include archery, beeper basketball, water sports, hiking and rock climbing and horseback riding. $35 registration fee.

Keith Elliott, Director

2085 VISIONS/Vacation Camp for the Blind
500 Greenwich Street, 3rd Floor
New York, NY 10013

212-625-1616
888-245-8333
Fax: 212-219-4078
e-mail: tmdecker@visionvcb.org
www.visionvcb.org

Family programs at Vacation Camp for the Blind in Rockland County, NY for children who are blind, severely visually impaired or multi-handicapped. Parent or guardian must attend winter weekends and summer session.

Thomas M Decker, Camp Director
Nancy D Miller, Executive Director

DESCRIPTION

2086 CONJUNCTIVITIS

Synonym: Pinkeye

Covers these related disorders: Infectious conjunctivitis, Noninfectious conjunctivitis

Involves the following Biologic System(s):

Infectious Disorders, Ophthalmologic Disorders

Conjunctivitis refers to a condition characterized by acute inflammation of the delicate mucous membranes (conjunctiva) that line the inside of the eyelids and the whites of the eyes (sclerae). This condition may be caused by a virus or bacterium. Allergic reactions or exposure to certain chemicals and other environmental factors may also play a role in certain types of conjunctivitis. Neonatal conjunctivitis (also known as neonatal ophthalmia or ophthalmia neonatorum) becomes apparent during the first four weeks of life and is considered an infectious disease resulting from bacterial or viral infections carried by the mother and passed to the child during the birthing process. Bacteria responsible for neonatal conjunctivitis infections may be common disease-causing organisms (pathogens) or may include Chlamydia trachomatis, the bacteria that causes the sexually transmitted disease (STD) chlamydia or Neisseria gonorrhoeae, responsible for the STD gonorrhea. In addition, viral transmission may be caused by herpes simplex type 2 virus, which is responsible for genital herpes. In addition, bacterial contamination may occur in a hospital nursery (Pseudomonas aeruginosa) and may, in some cases, cause severe infection.

The characteristic symptoms associated with infectious neonatal conjunctivitis include redness and severe swelling of the conjunctiva, including the eyelids and whites of the eyes, and a discharge from the eyes that may or may not contain pus (purulent). Symptoms of neonatal infection resulting from transmission during the birthing process may be present at birth or may appear during the second week of life, depending on the bacterium or virus responsible. Any early conjunctival infection should be evaluated as soon as possible to determine its cause and, subsequently, the appropriate course of treatment in order to prevent complications that could potentially lead to impaired vision or blindness.

Soon after delivery, erythromycin, or tetracycline drops or ointment are routinely administered to the eyes of the newborn to prevent gonococcal (gonorrheal) conjunctivitis. The use of 1% silver nitrate drops as prophylaxis (prevention) against gonococcal ophthalmia soon after birth has reduced its incidence in the United States to less than 0.03% of infants. Although silver nitrate is effective, it also may cause a chemical conjunctival inflammation that typically resolves on its own within 48 hours. Other preventive measures are directed toward identification and treatment of pregnant women with gonococcal infection.

Treatment for bacteria-caused neonatal conjunctivitis includes the use of particular antibiotics. In addition, washing (irrigating) the eye with a solution containing salt (saline) or direct application of antibiotic ointment to the eyes is often effective in relieving itching and discomfort and clearing up the discharge. Conjunctivitis caused by viral transmission may be treated with antiviral eye drops or ointment. Sometimes the antiviral drug acyclovir may be administered to prevent viral spread.

Additional causes of conjunctivitis in children may include other viruses associated with systemic diseases such as measles, some viruses of the adenovirus family, and intestinal viruses of the enterovirus family. This type of conjunctivitis is usually characterized by a watery discharge from the eyes, is usually self-limited, and treatment is symptomatic. However, one such adenovirus may cause severe itching and burning of the eyes, sensitivity to light (photophobia), and involvement of the cornea. This type of conjunctivitis is known as keratoconjunctivitis and affects the membranes lining the eyelids as well as the corneas. This virus is transmitted by direct contact. Conjunctivitis caused by allergies is usually seasonal and is characterized by swelling, tearing, and itching. Treatment is symptomatic and may include the application of antihistamine eye drops. Certain chemicals or environmental factors may also cause noninfectious, allergic-type conjunctivitis. In addition to silver nitrate used in preventive treatment in newborns, other irritating substances may include cleaning products, different types of sprays, smoke, pollen, and other materials. Treatment is directed toward prevention and relief of symptoms.

In the United States, as mentioned, the occurrence of neonatal conjunctivitis caused by Neisseria gonorrhoeae is extremely rare, while that caused by Chlamydia trachomatis is slightly more than eight out of every 1,000 births.

See also **General Resources** on page 917

Government Agencies

2087 Centers for Disease Control
1600 Clifton Road
Atlanta, GA 30333

404-639-3311
www.cdc.gov

Mission is to promote health and quality of life by preventing and controlling disease, injury, and disability.

2088 NIH/National Eye Institute
31 Center Drive MSC 2510
Bethesda, MD 20892

301-496-5248
e-mail: 2020@nei.nih.gov
www.nei.nih.gov

Conducts and supports research that helps prevent and treat eye diseases and other disorders of vision. This research leads to sight-saving treatments, reduces visual impairment and blindness, and improves the quality of life for people of all ages. NEI-supported research has advanced our knowledge of how the eye functions in health and disease.

Paul A Sieving M.D., Ph.D., Director

2089 NIH/National Institute of Allergy and Infectious Diseases
6610 Rockledge Drive, MSC 6612
Bethesda, MD 20892

301-496-5717
Fax: 301-402-3573
TDD: 800-877-8339
www.niaid.nih.gov

Conducts and supports basic and applied research to better understand, treat, and ultimately prevent infectious, immunologic, and allergic diseases.

Anthony S Fauci MD, Director

National Associations & Support Groups

2090 American Institute for Preventive Medicine
30445 Northwestern Highway, Suite 350
Farmington Hills, MI 48334

248-539-1800
800-345-2476
Fax: 248-539-1808
e-mail: aipm@healthylife.com
www.healthylife.com

An internationally recognized authority on the development and implementation of health promotion, wellness, medical self-care, and disease management programs and publications.

Don R Powell, Ph.D, President/CEO

2091 World Health Organization
Avenue Appia 20
CH-1211 Geneva 27,
Switzerland

www.who.int

WHO is the directing and coordinating authority for health within the United Nations system.

Dr Margaret Chan, Director General

Web Sites

2092 American Academy of Family Physicians
www.aafp.org

Represents more than 94,300 family physicians, family practice residents and medical students nationwide. Its mission is to preserve and promote the science and art of family medicine and to ensure high-quality, cost effective health care for patients of all ages.

2093 Dr. Koop
www.drkoop.com

Information on the condition, causes, symptoms, tests and treatment.

2094 LSU Health Sciences Center
www.lsuhsc.edu

An online library of resources.

2095 MedicineNet.com
www.medicinenet.com

An online, healthcare media publishing company providing easy-to-read, in-depth, authoritative medical information for consumers via its user-friendly, interactive web site. MedicineNet.com has had a highly accomplished, uniquely experienced team of qualified executives in the fields of medicine, healthcare, internet tehnology, and business to bring you the most comprehensive, sought after healthcare information anywhere.

2096 Virtual Children's Hospital
www.vh.org

Mission is to educate patients, healthcare providers, and students in a free and anonymous manner, for the purpose of improving patients' care, outcome and lives.

DESCRIPTION

2097 CORNELIA DE LANGE SYNDROME

Synonyms: BDLS, Brachmann-de Lange syndrome, CdLS, De Lange syndrome

Involves the following Biologic System(s):
Genetic/Chromosomal/Syndrome/Metabolic Disorders

Cornelia de Lange syndrome is a genetic disorder characterized by growth delays before and after birth (prenatal growth retardation); delays in the acquisition of skills that require the coordination of physical and mental activities (psychomotor retardation), and mild to severe mental retardation. Characteristic physical abnormalities include delays in the maturation of bone; malformations of the head and facial (craniofacial) area that result in a distinctive facial appearance; abnormalities of the arms, legs, hands, and feet (limbs); or other abnormalities. Associated symptoms and findings may vary in range and severity from case to case.

Infants with Cornelia de Lange syndrome often have feeding difficulties (e.g., projectile vomiting, regurgitation, swallowing difficulties); fail to grow and gain weight at the expected rate (failure to thrive); and have a weak, growling cry. Affected infants usually experience breathing problems, such as episodes in which there is temporary cessation of breathing (apnea), inhalation (aspiration) of food into the air passages of the lungs, and increased susceptibility to repeated respiratory infections. Affected infants and children also typically have arched, bushy eyebrows that grow together (synophrys); unusually long, curly eyelashes; a low hair line; and generalized excessive hair growth (hirsutism). Characteristic craniofacial abnormalities may include an abnormally prominent vertical groove in the center of the upper lip (philtrum); thin, downturned lips; and a small jaw (micrognathia). In addition, in many affected children, the teeth may erupt later than expected and are widely spaced.

Many infants and children with Cornelia de Lange syndrome also have malformations of the upper limbs, such as small hands or abnormal positioning of the fifth fingers (clinodactyly) or thumbs. In rare cases, the forearms, hands, and fingers may be absent (phocomelia and oligodactyly). Many affected infants and children also may have abnormally small, short feet with webbing of the second and third toes (syndactyly).

In many cases, additional symptoms and findings are present. For example, in most affected males, the testes may fail to descend into the scrotum (cryptorchidism). Some af-fected infants may also have digestive abnormalities (e.g., gastroesophageal reflux, pyloric stenosis, bowel obstruction); heart defects (e.g., ventricular septal defects); episodes of uncontrolled electrical activity in the brain (seizures); or other physical abnormalities. In addition, many affected children experience hearing loss and speech delays and may demonstrate behavioral problems, such as self-destructive tendencies.

Treatment of infants and children with Cornelia de Lange syndrome includes symptomatic and supportive measures, such as the prescription of certain medications to help prevent or control seizures (i.e., anticonvulsants); supportive therapies to ensure the proper intake of nutrients and to helpprevent or treat respiratory problems; and surgical or other appropriate methods to treat heart or digestive defects.

In most cases, Cornelia de Lange syndrome appears to occur randomly for unknown reasons. However, in a few reported cases, autosomal dominant inheritance has been suggested. The disorder is thought to affect approximately one in 10,000 newborns.

See also **General Resources** on page 917

National Associations & Support Groups

2098 Children's Craniofacial Association
13140 Colt Road, Suite 307
Dallas, TX 75240

214-570-9099
800-535-3643
Fax: 214-570-8811
e-mail: contactCCA@ccakids.com
www.ccakids.com

A national, nonprofit organization dedicated to improving the quality of life for people with facial differences and their families. CCA's mission is to empower and give hope to facially disfigured children and their families.

Tony Davis, Chairman
Heather Lermont-Pape, Secretary

2099 Cornelia de Lange Syndrome Foundation
302 W Main Street, Suite 100
Avon, CT 06001

860-676-8166
800-223-8355
Fax: 860-676-8337
e-mail: info@cdlsusa.org
www.cdlsusa.org

Provides a host of services that attract, educate, and unite families touched by this rare birth disorder which causes individuals to develop at a slower rate, both physically and mentally.

Julie Mairanu, Executive Director
Barbara Koontz, Information Coordinator

2100 FACES: The National Craniofacial Association
PO Box 11082
Chattanooga, TN 37401

800-332-2373
e-mail: faces@faces-cranio.org
www.faces-cranio.org

Serving children and adults throughout the United States with severe craniofacial deformities resulting from birth defects, injuries or disease. There is never a charge for any service provided by the association.

2101 Genetic Alliance
4301 Connecticut Avenue NW
Washington, DC 20008

202-966-5557
800-336-4363
Fax: 202-966-8553
e-mail: info@geneticalliance.org
www.geneticalliance.org

A coalition of voluntary genetic support groups, consumers and professionals addressing the needs of individuals and families affected by genetic disorders from a national perspective.

Sharon Terry, President/CEO

2102 March of Dimes Birth Defects Foundation
1275 Mamaroneck Avenue
White Plains, NY 10605

914-428-7100
888-663-4637
Fax: 914-428-8203
e-mail: resourcecenter@modimes.org
www.marchofdimes.com

Partnership of volunteers and professionals dedicated to improving the health of babies by preventing birth defects and infant mortality. Over 100 chapters are located across the country and can be located through the National Office.

Dr Jennifer Howse, President

Web Sites

2103 Online Mendelian Inheritance in Man
www.ncbi.nlm.nih.gov

This database is a catalog of human genes and genetic disorders.

Journals

2104 Facing the Challenges
Cornelia de Lange Syndrome Foundation
302 W Main Street, Suite 100
Avon, CT 06001

860-676-8166
800-223-8355
Fax: 860-676-8337
e-mail: info@cdlusa.org
www.cdlsusa.org/publications

The purpose of this book is to provide emotional support and factual information to those facing the challenges of caring for a person with Cornelia de Lange Syndrome.

Newsletters

2105 Reaching Out
Cornelia de Lange Syndrome Foundation
302 W Main Street, Suite 100
Avon, CT 06001

860-676-8166
800-223-8355
Fax: 860-676-8337
e-mail: info@cdlusa.org
www.cdlsusa.org/publications

Up-to-date on issues relevant to the syndrome and connected to a community of families who share in the joys and sorrows of CdLS.

1977 Bi-Monthly

Sue Anthony, Editor

DESCRIPTION

2106 CRANIOSYNOSTOSIS

Synonyms: Craniostenosis, Craniostosis

Covers these related disorders: Frontal plagiocephaly, Kleeblattschadel deformity, Scaphocephaly, Trigonocephaly, Turricephaly (oxycephaly or acrocephaly)

Involves the following Biologic System(s):

Orthopedic and Muscle Disorders

Craniosynostosis is a developmental abnormality in which early closure of one or more of the fibrous joints (sutures) between bones of the skull results in deformity of the skull and an abnormally shaped head. The severity of the deformity depends upon which fibrous joint or joints close prematurely as well as the ability of other joints in the skull to expand and compensate for the other closed joint or joints. Craniosynostosis may occur as an isolated condition or in association with certain chromosomal or malformation syndromes. In most instances of isolated craniosynostosis, the condition appears to occur randomly for unknown reasons. However, there have been reports of isolated craniosynostosis in members of several multigenerational families (kindreds), indicating autosomal dominant or autosomal recessive inheritance. Many genetic malformation syndromes have been identified in the medical literature that are associated with craniosynostosis. The specific underlying cause of craniosynostosis is not fully understood. Craniosynostosis occurs in approximately one in every 1,000 to 2,000 births and is more prevalent in males than females.

In infants with craniosynostosis, because the skull is unable to enlarge in certain directions relative to the affected fibrous joint in the skull, there is compensatory growth and enlargement in other directions at the sites of open joints. This causes deformity of the skull and an abnormally shaped head. For example, in the most common form of craniosynostosis, there is premature closure of the joint between the upper sides of the skull (sagittal suture), causing the head to appear abnormally long and narrow (scaphocephaly). Affected infants also tend to have a broad forehead and a prominent back portion of the head (occiput). This condition appears to be more common in males than females.

In the form of craniosynostosis known as frontal plagiocephaly, there is early closure of a suture between the upper sides of the head and one of the bones of the forehead (e.g., coronal suture). This results in flattening of one side of the forehead, prominence of the ear, and elevation of the eyebrow and eye on the affected side. Frontal plagiocephaly appears to affect females more commonly than males.

Trigonocephaly, another form of craniosynstosis, is characterized by premature fusion of the suture between the bones forming the forehead (metopic suture). Affected infants have a keel-shaped forehead and closely spaced eyes (hypotelorism). In infants with the form of craniosynostosis known as turricephaly (also called oxycephaly or acrocephaly), premature fusion of coronal and sagittal sutures causes the head to have an abnormally long, narrow, cone-like appearance. In addition, a rare form of craniosynostosis, known as Kleeblattschadel deformity, is characterized by premature closure of multiple cranial sutures, causing the skull to appear cloverleaf-like in shape. Affected infants have a high forehead, marked protrusion of the eyes (proptosis), abnormal prominence of the lower sides of the skull (temporal bones), and other associated abnormalities. Many affected infants also experience hydrocephalus, a condition in which obstruction or impaired absorption of the fluid surrounding the brain and spinal cord (cerebrospinal fluid) causes fluid accumulation under increasing pressure within the brain, resulting in abnormal enlargement of the brain.

In infants with craniosynostosis, premature closure of one suture is rarely associated with increased pressure within the skull or associated neurologic abnormalities, such as mental retardation. In such patients, surgery may be considered for cosmetic purposes. Premature closure of two or more sutures is more likely to cause increased pressure within the skull, potentially resulting in brain damage and associated mental retardation. Additional findings associated with increased pressure may include vomiting, headaches, and swelling of the area where the optic nerve enters the eye and joins with the nerve-rich membrane at the back of the eye (papilledema). In these infants, surgery is necessary to increase the capacity of the skull in order to prevent excessive pressure within the skull. If craniosynostosis is diagnosed before three months of age, surgery may be conducted to create artificial cranial joints in the skull, allowing skull growth and preventing abnormal shaping of the head.

See also **General Resources** on page 917

National Associations & Support Groups

2107 AboutFace USA
PO Box 158
South Beloit, IL 61080

702-769-9264
888-486-1209
Fax: 702-341-5351
e-mail: info@aboutfaceusa.org
www.aboutfaceusa.org

Provides information, services, emotional support and educational programs for and on behalf of individuals with facial differences and their families. Working to increase understanding through public awareness and education.

3M members

Debbie Oliver, Executive Director

2108 Children's Craniofacial Association
13140 Coit Road, Suite 307
Dallas, TX 75240

214-570-9099
800-535-3643
Fax: 214-570-8811
e-mail: contactCCA@ccakids.com
www.ccakids.com

Devoted to the dispersion of medical knowledge of this and similar disorders, along with providing emotional support for the sufferers and their families.

Tony Davis, Chairman
Heather Lermont-Pape, Secretary

2109 Craniosynostosis and Positional Plagiocephaly Support
6905 Xandu Court
Fredericksburg, VA 22407

703-445-1078
Fax: 703-445-1078
e-mail: cappsorg@aol.com
www.cappskids.org/

Established by a mother whose child had Craniosynostosis to offer support and information to other families who had a child with Craniosynostosis.

2110 FACES: National Association for the Craniofacially Handicapped
PO Box 11082
Chattanooga, TN 37401

423-266-1632
800-332-2373
Fax: 423-267-3124
e-mail: faces@faces-cranio.org
www.faces-cranio.org

Assists individuals with facial disfigurations and their families They maintain a registry of centers offering corrective surgery for craniofacial deformities and financial assistance to qualified applicants.

2111 FACES: National Craniofacial Foundation
PO Box 11082
Chattanooga, TN 37401

800-332-2373
www.faces-cranio.org

A nonprofit organization serving children and adults throughout the United States with severe craniofacial deformities resulting from birth defects, injuries, or disease. There is never a charge for any service provided by the foundation.

2112 Forward Face
317 E 34th Street, Suite 901A
New York, NY 10016

212-684-5860
Fax: 212-684-5864
e-mail: info@forwardface.org
www.forwardface.org

Mission is to help children and their families find immediate support to manage the medical and social effects of facial differences. Working to educate, advocate and raise public awareness.

Barbara Robertson, President
Camille Walsh, Assistant to Executive Director

2113 Genetic Alliance
4301 Connecticut Avenue NW
Washington, DC 20008

202-966-5557
800-336-4363
Fax: 202-966-8553
e-mail: info@geneticalliance.org
www.geneticalliance.org

A coalition of voluntary genetic support groups, consumers and professionals addressing the needs of individuals and families affected by genetic disorders from a national perspective.

Sharon Terry, President/CEO

2114 Guardians of Hydrocephalus Research Foundation
2618 Avenue Z
Brooklyn, NY 11235

718-743-4473
800-458-8655
Fax: 718-743-1171
e-mail: ghrf2618@aol.com
www.ghrf.homestead.com

Non-profit organization made up of concerned parents and dedicated volunteers. The goal of this foundation is to wipe out this top ranking birth defect.

Kathy Soriano

2115 Hydrocephalus Parent Support Group
Exceptional Family Resource Center
9245 Sky Park Court, Suite 130
San Diego, CA 92123

619-594-7416
800-281-8252
Fax: 858-268-4275
www.efrconline.org

Determined to provide support to the parents and relatives of the children stricken with the disorder.

2116 Let's Face It
University of Michigan
1011 N University
Ann Arbor, MI 48109

360-676-7325
e-mail: letsfaceit@faceit.org
www.faceit.org

A nonprofit network for people with facial difference, their families, friends and professionals. The mission is to advance knowledge about, by, and for people with facial differences and to promote their full and equal participation in society.

Betsy Wilson, Founder/Director

2117 March of Dimes Birth Defects Foundation
1275 Mamaroneck Avenue
White Plains, NY 10605

914-428-7100
888-663-4637
Fax: 914-428-8203
e-mail: resourcecenter@modimes.org
www.marchofdimes.com

Partnership of volunteers and professionals dedicates to improving the health of babies by preventing birth defects and infant mortality. Over 100 chapters are located across the country and can be located through the National Office.

Dr Jennifer Howse, President

2118 National Foundation for Facial Reconstruction
317 E 34th Street, Room 901
New York, NY 10016

212-263-6656
Fax: 212-263-7534
e-mail: info@nffr.org
www.nffr.org

Created to address the plight of children with a facial disfigurement by supporting state-of-the-art treatment, innovative research, psychosocial support and medical training that inspires a new generation of pediatric doctors.

Whitney Burnett, Executive Director
Michele B Golombuski, Associate Executive Director

2119 National Hydrocephalus Foundation
12413 Centralia Road
Lakewood, CA 90715

562-924-6666
888-857-3434
e-mail: hydrobrat@earthlink.net
www.nhfonline.org

Nonprofit public service organization that assembles and disseminates information about Hydrocephalus. Promotes communication networks among those affected and their families, helps others gain a deeper understanding of those areas affected by Hydrocephalus, such as education, tax and estate planning, employment and family. Also promotes and supports research on the causes, treatment and prevention of Hydrocephalus.

Michael Fields, President/Treasurer
Debbie Fields, Executive Director

Libraries & Resource Centers

2120 University of Illinois at Chicago, Craniofacial Center
College of Medicine
808 S Wood Street
Chicago, IL 60680

312-996-6979
Fax: 312-413-1526

Dr. Allen Goldman, Director

Research Centers

2121 Craniofacial Center at University of Illin ois, Chicago
811 S Paulina
Chicago, IL 60612

312-996-7546
Fax: 312-413-1157
e-mail: dreisber@uic.edu
uic.edu/com/surgery/plastic/craniofacial_cntr.htm

Dr David J Reisberg, Director

Audio Video

2122 Face First
Fanlight Productions
4196 Washington Street, Suite 2
Boston, MA 02131

617-469-4999
800-937-4113
Fax: 617-469-3379
e-mail: fanlight@fanlight.com
www.fanlight.com

Profiles of several people born with facial deformities; they chronicle both physical pain and the pain of rejection, as well as the strengths that have enabled them to achieve successful adult lives.

1998 29 Minutes VHS
ISBN: 1-572952-59-8

Nicole Johnson, Publicity Coordinator

Book Publishers

2123 Congenital Disorders Sourcebook
Omnigraphics
PO Box 625
Holmes, PA 19043

800-234-1340
Fax: 800-875-1340
e-mail: info@omnigraphics.com
www.omnigraphics.com

Basic consumer health information on disorders aquired during gestation, including spina bifida, hydrocephalus, cerebral palsy, heart defects, craniofacial abnormalities and fetal alcohol syndrome.

650 pages
ISBN: 0-780809-45-9

DESCRIPTION

2124 CROHN'S DISEASE

Synonym: Regional enteritis
Involves the following Biologic System(s):
Gastrointestinal Disorders

Crohn's disease is an inflammatory bowel disease (IBD) characterized by chronic inflammation of any region of the digestive (gastrointestinal) tract from the mouth to the anus. The disease most commonly involves the lower region of the small intestine (ileum) and the major part of the large intestine (colon). Chronic inflammation of these areas causes thickening and scarring of the intestinal wall. The range and severity of Crohn's disease is extremely variable and depends on the intestinal region affected, the severity of symptoms and findings of inflammation, and associated complications. In children, Crohn's disease usually becomes apparent during the late teens; however, symptoms may begin during early childhood. In developed countries, inflammatory bowel disease, including Crohn's disease, is the most common cause of chronic intestinal inflammation during mid-childhood. Crohn's disease affects males and females in equal numbers. In the U.S., the disease affects approximately 30 to 100 per 100,000 individuals in the general population and occurs more frequently among Caucasians and African-Americans, (and is more common in Jewish individuals than in Hispanic-Americans and Asian-Americans. Although the exact cause of Crohn's disease is unknown, genetic, immune, and environmental factors are thought to play a role. Some researchers suspect that the disorder may result from an exaggerated immune response to an invading microorganism, such as a particular virus or bacterium.

In most children, Crohn's disease initially involves both the lower region of the small intestine and the major part of the large intestine (ileocolitis). However, initial inflammation may be restricted to the small intestine or the colon. The inflammatory process tends to be segmental in nature, and diseased regions of the intestine are often separated by apparently normal segments (skip lesions). Chronic inflammation causes thickening, ulceration, and scarring of affected areas of the intestinal walls and may lead to the development of abnormal channels (fistulas) between regions of the colon, the intestine and the urinary bladder, or the intestine and the surface of the skin. Additional complications may include the development of pus-filled pockets of infection (abscesses) or intestinal obstruction due to abnormal narrowing of certain intestinal regions.

Many children with Crohn's disease experience episodes of cramping; abdominal discomfort and pain; diarrhea that may contain blood; persistent spasms of the rectum (tenesmus); and a compelling urge to defecate. Additional symptoms and findings typically include fever, chills, easy fatigability, a general feeling of ill health (malaise), lack of appetite (anorexia), weight loss, and malnutrition due to impaired intestinal absorption of fats and nutrients (malabsorption). Many patients also develop deep grooves or cracks (fissures) in the mucous membranes of the anus. Some children have delayed bone maturation, retarded physical growth, or delayed sexual development as much as one to two years before the onset of other symptoms.

Many patients with Crohn's disease may also develop more generalized, systemic symptoms. These may include joint swelling and inflammation (arthritis); inflammation of the outermost layers of the eye's tough, white, outer coat (episcleritis); eruption of multiple, inflamed, reddish-purplish swellings on the legs and possibly the arms (erythema nodosum); and abnormal concentrations of mineral salts (calculi or stones) in the kidneys or the muscular sac (gall bladder) that stores and concentrates bile from the liver. Patients may also be prone to developing ankylosing spondylitis, a chronic, progressive, inflammatory disease that affects joints of the spine and results in pain, stiffness, and possible loss of spinal mobility. In addition, it is suspected that patients who have Crohn's disease for many years may have an increased risk of colon cancer as compared with the general population.

Symptoms typically flare up at irregular intervals throughout life. These episodes may be mild or severe and last for relatively short or prolonged periods. The treatment of Crohn's disease is directed at minimizing symptoms. Therapy may include the use of certain medication, such as sulfasalazine, azathioprine, or metronidazole. For example, azathioprine or metronidazole may be helpful in treating anal fistulas, and metronidazole has been beneficial in treating some patients who have not responded to other medications. Oral steroids may be added if needed. They are highly effective in reducing symptoms but should be used for short-term treatment only. Steroids should be tapered as soon as possible to reduce the risk of long-term side effects. In many children, treatment may include the administration of nutrients in liquid form (total parenteral nutrition) via a tube through the nose to the stomach (nasogastric tube). Some patients who experience severe, sudden episodes may require hospitalization to ensure proper intake of nutrients and fluids and to receive appropriate medical therapy. In addition, some patients may eventually require surgery to remove diseased portions of the intestine. However, such surgery is reserved for very specific indications, because the recurrence rate is high and the risk of needing additional surgery increases after such a procedure. Additional treatment is symptomatic and supportive.

See also **General Resources** on page 917

National Associations & Support Groups

2125 Crohn's & Colitis Foundation of America Hotline
Crohn's & Colitis Foundation of America
386 Park Avenue S, 17th Floor
New York, NY 10016

212-685-3440
800-932-2423
Fax: 212-779-4098
e-mail: info@ccfa.org
www.ccfa.org

The mission of the Crohn's & Colitis Foundation of America (CCFA), is to cure and prevent Crohn's disease and ulcerative colitis through research and to improve the quality of life of children and adults affected by these digestive diseases through education and support. Known collectively as inflammatory bowel disease (IBD), these painfaul chronic illnesses affect up to one million Americans, including approximately 100,000 children under the age of 18. CCFA was founded in 1967.

2126 Digestive Disease National Coalition
507 Capitol Court NE, Suite 200
Washington, DC 20002

202-544-7497
Fax: 202-546-7105
www.ddnc.org

Advocacy organization comprised of 22 voluntary and professional societies concerned with the many diseases of the digestive tract and liver.

Nancy Norton, Chairperson
Dr. Maurice Cerulli, President

2127 Genetic Alliance
4301 Connecticut Avenue NW
Washington, DC 20008

202-966-5557
800-336-4363
Fax: 202-966-8553
e-mail: info@geneticalliance.org
www.geneticalliance.org

A coalition of voluntary genetic support groups, consumers and professionals addressing the needs of individuals and families affected by genetic disorders from a national perspective.

Sharon Terry, President/CEO

2128 International Foundation for Bowel Dysfunction
PO Box 170864
Milwaukee, WI 53217

414-964-1799
888-964-2001
Fax: 414-964-7176
e-mail: iffgd@iffgd.org
www.iffgd.org

A nonprofit education and research organization. Our mission is to inform, assist, and support people affected by gastrointestinal disorders.

2129 International Foundation for Functional Gastrointestinal Disorders
PO Box 170864
Milwaukee, WI 53217

414-964-1799
888-964-2001
Fax: 414-964-7176
e-mail: iffgd@iffgd.org
www.iffgd.org

Nonprofit education and research organization founded in 1991. IFFGD addresses the issues surrounding life with gastrointestinal (GI) functional and mobility disorders and increases the awareness about these disorders among the general public, researchers and the clinical care community.

Nancy J Norton, Founder
William Norton, VP

2130 March of Dimes Birth Defects Foundation
1275 Mamaroneck Avenue
White Plains, NY 10605

914-428-7100
888-663-4637
Fax: 914-428-8203
e-mail: resourcecenter@modimes.org
www.marchofdimes.com

Partnership of volunteers and professionals dedicates to improving the health of babies by preventing birth defects and infant mortality. Over 100 chapters are located across the country and can be located through the National Office.

Dr Jennifer Howse, President

State Agencies & Support Groups

Alabama

2131 Alabama/Northwest Florida Chapter of Crohn 's Colitis Foundation of America
244 Goodwin Crest Drive, Suite 120
Birmingham, AL 35209

205-941-9900
800-249-1993
Fax: 205-941-1411
e-mail: ccfaal@aol.com
www.ccfa.org

Crohn's and Colitis Foundation of America is a nonprofit, voluntary health organization dedicated to improving the quality of life for persons with Crohn's disease or ulcerative colitis.

Pat Talty, Executive Director

Arizona

2132 Arizona Chapter of Crohn's & Colitis Foundation of America
8098 Via de Negocio, Suite 201
Scottsdale, AZ 85258

480-246-3676
877-259-2104
Fax: 480-246-3679
e-mail: ccfaal@aol.com
www.ccfa.org

Crohn's and Colitis Foundation of America is a nonprofit, voluntary health organization dedicated to improving the quality of life for persons with Crohn's disease or ulcerative colitis.

Bridgette Haley, Executive Director

California

2133 Greater Los Angeles/Orange County Chapter of Chron's & Colitis Foundation
1640 S Sepulveda Boulevard, Suite 214
Los Angeles, CA 90025

310-478-4500
866-831-9157
Fax: 310-478-4546
e-mail: losangeles@ccfa.org
www.ccfa.org

Crohn's and Colitis Foundation of America is a nonprofit, voluntary health organization dedicated to improving the quality of life for persons with Crohn's disease or ulcerative colitis.

Ronni Epstein, Executive Director

2134 Greater San Diego/Desert Chapter of Crohn's & Colitis Foundation of America
6920 Miramar Road, Suite 101
San Diego, CA 92109

858-547-8200
Fax: 858-547-8204
e-mail: sandiego@ccfa.org
www.ccfa.org

Crohn's and Colitis Foundation of America is a nonprofit, voluntary health organization dedicated to improving the quality of life for persons with Crohn's disease or ulcerative colitis.

Pamela Meistrell, Executive Director

2135 Northern California Chapter of Crohn's and Colitis Foundation
111 New Montgomery Street, Suite 208
San Francisco, CA 94105

415-356-2232
800-241-0758
Fax: 415-356-0880
e-mail: ncal@ccfa.org
www.ccfa.org

Supports basic and clinical scientific research to find the cause of, and cure for, Crohn's disease and ulcerative colitis; provides educational programs for patients, medical professionals and the general public; offers supportive services for patients, their families and friends including support groups, information packets, education seminars, physician referral hotline and a quarterly newsletter called Rumblings.

Tamara Block, Executive Director

Colorado

2136 Rocky Mountain Chapter of Crohn's & Colitis Foundation of America
1777 S Bellaire Street, Suite 120
Denver, CO 80222

303-639-9163
800-768-2232
Fax: 303-639-9166
e-mail: rockymountain@ccfa.org
www.ccfa.org

Crohn's and Colitis Foundation of America is a nonprofit, voluntary health organization dedicated to improving the quality of life for persons with Crohn's disease or ulcerative colitis.

Connecticut

2137 Central Connecticut Chapter of Crohn's & Colitis Foundation of America
PO Box 185431
Hamden, CT 06518

203-393-8964
Fax: 203-876-1693
e-mail: sallyconnolly@sbcglobal.net
www.ccfa.org

Crohn's and Colitis Foundation of America is a nonprofit, voluntary health organization dedicated to improving the quality of life for persons with Crohn's disease or ulcerative colitis.

2138 Fairfield/Westchester Chapter of Crohn's & Colitis Foundation of America
200 Bloomingdale Road
White Plains, NY 10605

914-328-2874
Fax: 914-328-2946
e-mail: westfield@ccfa.org
www.ccfa.org

Crohn's and Colitis Foundation of America is a nonprofit, voluntary health organization dedicated to improving the quality of life for persons with Crohn's disease or ulcerative colitis.

Ren,e Krutoff, Executive Director

2139 Northern Connecticut Affiliate Chapter of Crohn's & Colitis Foundation of America
PO Box 370614
West Hartford, CT 06137

www.ccfa.org

Crohn's and Colitis Foundation of America is a nonprofit, voluntary health organization dedicated to improving the quality of life for persons with Crohn's disease or uilcerative colitis.

Florida

2140 Florida Chapter of Crohn's & Colitis Found ation of America
21301 Powerline Road #301

Boca Raton, FL 33433

561-218-2929
877-664-2929
Fax: 561-218-2240
e-mail: florida@ccfa.org
www.ccfa.org

Crohn's and Colitis Foundation of America is a nonprofit, voluntary health organization dedicated to improving the quality of life for persons with Crohn's disease or ulcerative colitis.

Debra Farnham-Bartels, Development Manager

Georgia

2141 Georgia Chapter of Crohn's & Colitis Foundation of America
2250 N Druid Hills Road, Suite 250
Atlanta, GA 30329

404-982-0616
800-472-6795
Fax: 404-982-0656
e-mail: georgia@ccfa.org
www.ccfa.org

Crohn's and Colitis Foundation of America is a nonprofit, voluntary health organization dedicated to improving the quality of life for persons with Crohn's disease or ulcerative colitis.

Marcia Greenburg, Regional Executive Director
Karen Rittenbaum, Development Director

Illinois

2142 Crohn's & Colitis Foundation of America
2250 E Devon Avenue, Suite 244
Des Plaines, IL 60018

847-827-0404
800-886-6664
Fax: 847-827-6563
www.ccfa.org

Crohn's and Colitis Foundation of America is a nonprofit, voluntary health organizaiton dedicated to finding the cause of, and cure for Crohn's disease and ulcerative colitis. The foundation is committed to conquering these devastating diseases.

$25.00 Dues

Kathleen Durkin, Executive Director

Indiana

2143 Indiana Chapter of Crohn's & Colitis Found ation of America
8555 Cedar Place Drive, Suite 112
Indianapolis, IN 46240

317-259-8071
800-332-6029
Fax: 317-259-8091
e-mail: indiana@ccfa.org
www.ccfa.org

Provides support and education to adults, children, and families dealing with Crohn's disease and ulcerative colitis. Raises funds for research and programs. Quarterly newsletter, national magazine, award winning website. 55 chapters nationwide.

Scott Baumruck, Development Director

Iowa

2144 Iowa Chapter of Crohn's Colitis Foundation of America
PO Box 145
Cedar Falls, IA 50613

319-277-6293
Fax: 319-277-6293
e-mail: iowa@ccfa.org
www.ccfa.org

Crohn's and Colitis Foundation of America is a nonprofit, voluntary health organization dedicated to improving the quality of life for persons with Crohn's disease or ulcerative colitis.

Dan D'Alessandro, Chapter President

Kansas

2145 Mid-America Chapter of Crohn's & Colitis F oundation of America
8420 Delmar Boulevard, Suite 303
St. Louis, MO 63124

314-991-0220
800-783-8006
Fax: 314-991-8756
www.ccfa.org

Crohn's and Colitis Foundation of America is a nonprofit, voluntary health organization dedicated to improving the quality of life for persons with Crohn's disease or ulcerative colitis.

Jan Baron, Executive Director

Kentucky

2146 Kentucky Chapter of Crohn's & Colitis Foundation of America
8555 Cedar Place Lane, Suite 112
Indianapolis, IN 46240

317-259-8071
Fax: 317-259-8091
e-mail: kentucky@ccfa.org
www.ccfa.org

Crohn's and Colitis Foundation of America is a nonprofit, voluntary health organization dedicated to improving the quality of life for persons with Crohn's disease or ulcerative colitis.

Steve Picton, President

Louisiana

2147 Louisiana/Mississippi Chapter of Crohn's & Colitis Foundation of America
7611 Maple Street, Suite B
New Orleans, LA 70118

504-861-3433
Fax: 504-861-3466
e-mail: lams@ccfa.org
www.ccfa.org

Crohn's and Colitis Foundation of America is a nonprofit, voluntary health organization dedicated to improving the quality of life for persons with Crohn's disease or ulcerative colitis.

David Lee Thomas, Development Director

Maryland

2148 Maryland/South Delaware Chapter of Crohn's & Colitis Foundation of America
10400 Little Patuxent Parkway, Suite 270
Columbia, MD 21044

443-276-0861
877-807-5271
Fax: 443-276-0865
e-mail: maryland@ccfa.org
www.ccfa.org

Our mission is to fund research to find a cure for Crohn's disease and ulcerative colitis and to educate and provide support to patients and families with these diseases.

Robert J Milanchus, Regional Executive Director

Massachusetts

2149 New England Chapter of Crohn's & Colitis Foundation of America
280 Hillside Avenue
Needham, MA 02494

781-449-0324
800-314-3459
Fax: 781-449-0325
e-mail: ne@ccfa.org
www.ccfa.org

Crohn's and Colitis Foundation of America is a nonprofit, voluntary health organization dedicated to improving the quality of life for persons with Crohn's disease or ulcerative colitis.

Michelle Mosher Cibotti, Development Manager

Michigan

2150 Michigan Chapter of Crohn's & Colitis Foundation of America
31313 Northwestern Highway, Suite 209
Farmington Hills, MI 48334

248-737-0900
Fax: 248-737-0904
e-mail: miccfa@aol.com
www.ccfa.org

Crohn's and Colitis Foundation of America is a nonprofit, voluntary health organization dedicated to improving the quality of life for persons with Crohn's disease or ulcerative colitis.

Bernard L Riker, Executive Director

Minnesota

2151 Minnesota/Dakotas Chapter of Crohn's & Colitis Foundation of America
1885 University Avenue W, Suite 355
Saint Paul, MN 55104

651-917-2424
888-422-3266
Fax: 651-917-2425
e-mail: minnesota@ccfa.org
www.ccfa.org

Voluntary health organization providing education service and support to Crohn's disease and ulcerative colitis patients and the professional community.

James J Fennell, Midwest Regional Executive Director

Mississippi

2152 Louisiana/Mississippi Chapter of Crohn's & Colitis Foundation of America
7611 Maple Street
New Orleans, LA 70118

504-861-3433
Fax: 504-861-3466
e-mail: lams@ccfa.org
www.ccfa.org

Crohn's and Colitis Foundation of America is a nonprofit, voluntary health organization dedicated to improving the quality of life for persons with Crohn's disease or ulcerative colitis. Your local chapter can supply you with a list of CCFA physician members in your area.

David Lee Thomas, Development Director

Missouri

2153 Saint Louis Chapter of Crohn's & Colitis Foundation of America
8420 Delmar Boulevard, Suite 303
Saint Louis, MO 63124

314-991-0220
Fax: 314-991-8756
e-mail: missouri@ccfa.org
www.ccfa.org

Crohn's and Colitis Foundation of America is a nonprofit, voluntary health organization dedicated to improving the quality of life for persons with Crohn's disease or ulcerative colitis.

Jan Baron, Executive Director

New Jersey

2154 New Jersey Chapter of Crohn's & Colitis Foundation of America
45 Wilson Avenue
Manalapan, NJ 07726

732-786-9960
Fax: 732-786-9964
e-mail: newjersey@ccfa.org
www.ccfa.org

Crohn's and Colitis Foundation of America is a nonprofit, voluntary health organization dedicated to improving the quality of life for persons with Crohn's disease or ulcerative colitis.

Rosemarie Golombos, Executive Director

New Mexico

2155 Southwest Chapter of Crohn's & Colitis Foundation of America
8098 Via de Negocio, Suite 201
Scottsdale, AZ 85258

480-246-3676
877-259-2104
Fax: 480-246-3679
www.ccfa.org

Crohn's and Colitis Foundation of America is a nonprofit, voluntary health organization dedicated to improving the quality of life for persons with Crohn's disease or ulcerative colitis.

Bridgette Haley, Executive Director

New York

2156 Central New York Chapter of Crohn's & Colitis Foundation of America
PO Box 47
Syracuse, NY 13206

315-424-1093
e-mail: centralny@ccfa.org
www.ccfa.org

Crohn's and Colitis Foundation of America is a nonprofit, voluntary health organization dedicated to improving the quality of life for persons with Crohn's disease or ulcerative colitis. Your local chapter can supply you with a list of CCFA physician members in your area.

2157 Fairfield/Westchester Chapter of Crohn's & Colitis Foundation of America
200 Bloomingdale Road
White Plains, NY 10605

914-328-2874
Fax: 914-328-2946
e-mail: westfield@ccfa.org
www.ccfa.org

Crohn's and Colitis Foundation of America is a nonprofit, voluntary health organization dedicated to improving the quality of life for persons with Crohn's disease or ulcerative colitis. Your local chapter can supply you with a list of CCFA physician members in your area.

Ren,e Krutoff, Executive Director

2158 Greater New York Chapter of Crohn's & Colitis Foundation of America
386 Park Avenue S, 14th Floor
New York, NY 10016

212-679-1570
Fax: 212-679-3567
e-mail: newyork@ccfa.org
www.ccfa.org

Crohn's and Colitis Foundation of America is a nonprofit, voluntary health organization dedicated to improving the quality of life for persons with Crohn's disease or ulcerative colitis.

Marilyn Haggerty-Blom, Executive Director

2159 Long Island Chapter of Crohn's & Colitis Foundation of America
585 Stewart Avenue, Suite 414
Garden City, NY 11530

516-222-5530
Fax: 516-222-5535
e-mail: longisland@ccfa.org
www.ccfa.org

Crohn's and Colitis Foundation of America is a nonprofit, voluntary health organization dedicated to improving the quality of life for persons with Crohn's disease or ulcerative colitis.

2160 Rochester Chapter of Crohn's & Colitis Foundation of America
3177 Latta Road, Suite 301
Rochester, NY 14612

585-234-1214
e-mail: rochester@ccfa.org
www.ccfa.org

Crohn's and Colitis Foundation of America is a nonprofit, voluntary health organization dedicated to improving the quality of life for persons with Crohn's disease or ulcerative colitis.

2161 Upstate/Northeast New York Chapter of Crohn's & Colitis Foundation of America
4 Normanskill Boulevard
Delmar, NY 12054

518-439-0252
Fax: 518-458-7509
e-mail: upstateny@ccfa.org
www.ccfa.org

The chapter encompasses the following: Albany, Schenectady, Rensselaer, Northern Dutchess, Jefferson, Sullivan, Greene, Columbia, Schoharie, Fulton, Montgomery, Oneida, Saratoga, Ulster, Washington, Warren, Essex, Clinton, Franklin, and Herkimer counties.

Linda Winston, Chapter President

2162 Western New York Chapter of Crohn's & Colitis Foundation of America
PO Box 224
Williamsville, NY 14231

716-833-2870
e-mail: westernny@ccfa.org
www.ccfa.org

Crohn's and Colitis Foundation of America is a nonprofit, voluntary health organization dedicated to improving the quality of life for persons with Crohn's disease or ulcerative colitis. Your local chapter can supply you with a list of CCFA physician members in your area.

North Carolina

2163 Carolinas Chapter of Crohn's & Colitis Foundation of America
2901 N Davidson Street, Suite 160
Charlotte, NC 28205

704-332-1611
888-883-2232
Fax: 704-332-1612
e-mail: kking@ccfa.org
www.ccfa.org

Crohn's and Colitis Foundation of America is a nonprofit, voluntary health organization dedicated to improving the quality of life for persons with Crohn's disease or ulcerative colitis.

Kelli King, Development Director

Ohio

2164 Central Ohio Chapter of Crohn's & Colitis Foundation of America
5008 Pine Creek Drive, Suite A
Westerville, OH 43081

614-865-1933
800-625-5977
Fax: 614-865-1934
e-mail: centralohio@ccfa.org
www.ccfa.org

Crohn's and Colitis Foundation of America is a nonprofit, voluntary health organization dedicated to improving the quality of life for persons with Crohn's disease or ulcerative colitis.

Andrea Rothfelder, Executive Director

2165 Northeast Ohio Chapter of Crohn's & Colitis Foundation of America
23775 Commerce Park Road
Beachwood, OH 44122

216-831-2692
866-345-2232
Fax: 216-831-2792
e-mail: neohio@aol.com
www.ccfa.org

Crohn's and Colitis Foundation of America is a nonprofit, voluntary health organization dedicated to improving the quality of life for persons with Crohn's disease or ulcerative colitis.

Andrea Rothfelder, Executive Director
Patty Kaplan, Development Manager

2166 Southwest Ohio Chapter of Crohn's & Colitis Foundation of America
8 Triangle Park Drive, Suite 800
Cincinnati, OH 45246

513-772-3550
877-283-7513
Fax: 513-772-7599
e-mail: swohio@ccfa.org
www.ccfa.org

CCFA is the only national nonprofit organization dedicated to finding the cause of and cure for Crohn's disease and ulcerative colitis. We offer monthly connection and education groups, education symposium, one-on-one support through our Ambassador Program and for our children, a four day regional camp. CCFA offers free

Teacher's Guides, Parent's Guide and Children's Guides to Crohn's Disease and Ulcerative Colitis. This chapter also serves Greater Dayton, Northern Kentucky and SW Indiana.

Andr‚a Rothfelder, Executive Director
Jenny Sothers, Development Manager

Oklahoma

2167 Oklahoma Chapter of Crohn's & Colitis Foundation of America
4504 E 67th Street, Suite 125
Tulsa, OK 74136

918-523-8540
800-658-1533
Fax: 918-523-8560
e-mail: ccfa@aol.org
www.ccfa.org

Crohn's and Colitis Foundation of America is a nonprofit, voluntary health organization dedicated to improving the quality of life for persons with Crohn's disease or ulcerative colitis.

Judy Summers, Regional Executive Director

Pennsylvania

2168 Pennsylvania/Delaware Valley Chapter of Crohn's & Colitis Foundation of America
367 E Street Road
Trevose, PA 19053

215-396-9100
888-340-4744
Fax: 215-396-1170
e-mail: philaelphia@ccfa.org
www.ccfa.org

Crohn's and Colitis Foundation of America is a nonprofit, voluntary health organization dedicated to improving the quality of life for persons with Crohn's disease and ulcerative colitis.

Barbara Berman, Executive Director

2169 Western Pennsylvania Chapter of Crohn's & Colitis Foundation of America
580 S Aiken Avenue, Suite 202
Pittsburgh, PA 15232

412-687-9775
800-627-6467
Fax: 412-687-8544
e-mail: wpawy@ccfa.org
www.ccfa.org

National nonprofit research-oriented voluntary health organization dedicated to improving the quality of life for people with Crohn's disease and ulcerative colitis. Our mission: support basic and clinical scientific research to find a cause and cure for Crohn's disease and ulcerative colitis, provide educational programs for patients, medical professioinals, and general public, and offer supportive services for patients, their families and friends.

600 Members

Susan Kukic, Executive Director

South Carolina

2170 South Carolina Chapter of Crohn's & Colitis Foundation of America
2901 N Davidson Street, Suite 160
Charlotte, NC 28205

704-332-1611
877-632-1611
Fax: 704-332-1612
e-mail: kking@ccfa.org
www.ccfa.org

Crohn's and Colitis Foundation of America is a nonprofit, voluntary health organization dedicated to improving the quality of life for persons with Crohn's disease.

Kelli King, Development Director

Tennessee

2171 Tennessee Chapter of Crohn's & Colitis Foundation of America
2200 21st Avenue S, Suite 406
Nashville, TN 37212

615-383-0020
866-814-2232
Fax: 615-383-0889
e-mail: tennessee@ccfa.org
www.ccfa.org

Crohn's and Colitis Foundation of America is a nonprofit, voluntary health organization dedicated to improving the quality of life for persons with Crohn's disease or ulcerative colitis.

Steve Wallace, Executive Director

Texas

2172 Houston-Gulf Coast/South Texas Chapter of Crohn's & Colitis Foundation of America
5120 Woodway, Suite 8008
Houston, TX 77056

713-752-2232
800-785-2232
Fax: 713-572-2433
e-mail: infohouston@ccfa.org
www.ccfa.org

Crohn's and Colitis Foundation of America is a nonprofit, voluntary health organization dedicated to improving the quality of life for persons with Crohn's disease or ulcerative colitis.

Ann Swift, Development Manager

2173 North Texas Chapter of Crohn's & Colitis Foundation of America
12801 N Central Expressway
Dallas, TX 75234

972-386-0607
Fax: 972-386-0509
e-mail: ntexas@ccfa.org
www.ccfa.org

Crohn's and Colitis Foundation of America is a nonprofit, voluntary health organization dedicated to improving the quality of life for persons with Crohn's disease or ulcerative colitis.

Leslie Martin, Development Manager

Washington

2174 Washington State Chapter of Crohn's & Colitis Foundation of America
9 Lake Bellevue Drive, Suite 116
Bellevue, WA 98005

425-451-8455
Fax: 425-451-1708
e-mail: northwest@ccfa.org
www.ccfa.org

Crohn's and Colitis Foundation of America is a nonprofit, voluntary health organization dedicated to improving the quality of life for persons with Crohn's disease or ulcerative colitis.

Steve Wright MPA, Executive Director

Wisconsin

2175 Wisconsin Chapter of Crohn's & Colitis Foundation of America
1126 S 70th Street, Suite S210A
West Allis, WI 53214

414-475-5520
877-586-5588
Fax: 414-475-5502
e-mail: wisconsin@ccfa.org
www.ccfa.org

Crohn's and Colitis Foundation of America is a nonprofit, voluntary health organization dedicated to improving the quality of life for persons with Crohn's disease or ulcerative colitis.

Jan Lenz, Executive Director

Libraries & Resource Centers

2176 National Digestive Diseases Information Clearinghouse
2 Information Way
Bethesda, MD 20892

800-891-5389
Fax: 703-738-4929
e-mail: nddic@info.niddk.nih.gov
www.digestive.niddk.nih.gov

The National Institute of Diabetes and Digestive and Kidney Diseases conducts and supports research on many of the most serious diseases affecting public health. The Institute supports much of the clinical research on the diseases of internal medicine and related subspecialty fields as well as many basic science disciplines.

Research Centers

2177 Crohn's & Colitis Foundation of America
386 Park Avenue S, 17th Floor
New York, NY 10016

212-685-3440
800-932-2423
Fax: 212-779-4098
e-mail: info@ccfa.org
www.ccfa.org

Since 1967, CCFA has been the only national voluntary health agency dedicated to funding research to find a cure for Crohn's disease and ulcerative colitis. The Foundation provides educational and patient support services to both the lay and medical communities and plans to provide grants dedicated to pediatric research.

2178 Krancer Center for Inflammatory Bowel Disease Research
Hahnemann University
Broad & Vine Streets
Philadelphia, PA 19102

215-762-8618
Fax: 215-762-1998

Research into the causes and treatments of ulcerative colitis and Crohn's disease.

Harris Clearfield, Director

Web Sites

2179 Crohn's & Colitis Foundation of America
www.ccfa.org

Information regardin Crohn's disease and ulcerative colitis.

2180 Health Answers
www.healthanswers.com

HealthAnswers offers a breadth of services in medical education, sales force training, patient support, solutions, professional promotion and consumer solutions.

Book Publishers

2181 Crohn's Disease and Ulcerative Colitis Fact Book
Crohn's & Colitis Foundation of America
386 Park Avenue S, 17th Floor
New York, NY 10016

212-685-3440
800-932-2423
Fax: 212-779-4098
e-mail: info@ccfa.org
www.ccfa.org

Written in layman's language, this first, complete guide is helpful in understanding and coping with inflammatory bowel diseases.

2182 Digestive Diseases & Disorders Sourcebook

Omnigraphics
PO Box 625
Holmes, PA 19043

800-234-1340
Fax: 800-875-1340
e-mail: info@omnigraphics.com
omnigraphics.com

Basic consumer health information including celiac disease, Crohn's disease, diarrhea, hernias, irritable bowel syndrome and ulcers.

335 pages
ISBN: 0-780803-27-2

2183 Let's Talk About Going to the Hospital

Rosen Publishing Group's PowerKids Press
29 E 21st Street
New York, NY 10010

212-777-3017
800-237-9932
Fax: 888-436-4643
e-mail: rosenpub@tribeca.ios.com
www.powerkidspress.com

If a child has to check into the hospital, chances are he or she is already upset about being ill. Knowing how a hospital functions and what the procedures are, such as when family members can visit, will help in what is already a stressful situation. Grades K-5.

24 pages
ISBN: 0-823950-36-0

2184 Managing Your Child's Crohn's Disease or Ulcerative Colitis

Crohn's & Colitis Foundation of America
386 Park Avenue S, 17th Floor
New York, NY 10016

212-685-3440
800-932-2423
Fax: 212-779-4098
e-mail: info@ccfa.org
www.ccfa.org

This first full-length book on Crohn's disease and ulcerative colitis, specifically targeted for parents of children and teenagers, includes topics on cause and diagnosis, treatment, surgery, hospitalization, diet and nutrition, school and social issues, and resources for the patient.

$16.95 Members

2185 New People...Not Patients: a Source Book for Living with Bowel Disease

Crohn's & Colitis Foundation of America
386 Park Avenue S, 17th Floor
New York, NY 10016

212-685-3440
800-932-2423
Fax: 212-779-4098
e-mail: info@ccfa.org
www.ccfa.org

This book contains the essential information you need to help you cope with Crohn's disease and ulcerative colitis after you leave the doctor's office.

2186 Treating IBD

Crohn's & Colitis Foundation of America
386 Park Avenue S, 17th Floor
New York, NY 10016

212-685-3440
800-932-2423
e-mail: info@ccfa.org
www.ccfa.org

A patient's guide to the medical and surgical management of Inflammatory Bowel Disease, this book gives information on treating Crohn's disease and ulcerative colitis, including drug therapies, ad-

vances in nutritional care, and recently developed surgical alternatives.

2187 Understanding Crohn Disease and Ulcerative Colitis

University Press of Mississippi
3825 Ridgewood Road, Unit 9
Jackson, MS 39211

601-432-6205
800-737-7788
Fax: 601-432-6246
e-mail: press@ihl.state.ms.us
www.upress.state.ms.us

For patients and caregivers, an overview of the nature and treatments of inflammatory bowel disease.

128 pages Paperback
ISBN: 1-578062-03-9

Magazines

2188 Take Charge

Crohn's & Colitis Foundation of America
386 Park Avenue S, 17th Floor
New York, NY 10016

800-932-2423
e-mail: info@ccfa.org
www.ccfa.org

Offers the most up-to-date information on IBD research, treatment, and legislative initiatives for patients, families, and friends.

Newsletters

2189 Under the Microscope

Crohn's & Colitis Foundation of America
386 Park Avenue S, 17th Floor
New York, NY 10016

212-685-3440
800-932-2423
Fax: 212-779-4098
e-mail: info@ccfa.org
www.ccfa.org

Includes a variety of relevant information such as information on new research projects, clinical trials, conference notes, and breaking news about partnerships and grants.

Pamphlets

2190 CCFA: A Case for Support

Crohn's & Colitis Foundation of America
386 Park Avenue S, 17th Floor
New York, NY 10016

212-685-3440
800-932-2423
Fax: 212-779-4098
e-mail: info@ccfa.org
www.ccfa.org

Reviews the work of the Crohn's and Colitis Foundation of America, sponsors a nationally recognized research program, which seeks to improve treatment, and ultimately find the cure for inflammatory bowel disease.

2191 Coping with Crohn's and Colitis is Tough

Crohn's & Colitis Foundation of America
386 Park Avenue S, 17th Floor
New York, NY 10016

212-685-3440
800-932-2423
Fax: 212-779-4098
e-mail: info@ccfa.org
www.ccfa.org

Offers information on the Crohn's and Colitis Association. Also offers factual information and statistics on the diseases.

2192 Crohn's Disease, Ulcerative Colitis, and Your Child

Crohn's & Colitis Foundation of America
386 Park Avenue S, 17th Floor
New York, NY 10016

212-685-3440
800-932-2423
Fax: 212-779-4098
e-mail: info@ccfa.org
www.ccfa.org

Answers questions about IBD in children, providing information on early signs, growth and developments, treatments and special problems in school.

2193 Guide for Children and Teenagers to Crohn's Disease/Ulcerative Colitis

Crohn's & Colitis Foundation of America
386 Park Avenue S, 17th Floor
New York, NY 10016

212-685-3440
800-932-2423
Fax: 212-779-4098
e-mail: info@ccfa.org
www.ccfa.org

Offers important information on these illnesses to children and teens.

2194 Questions & Answers About Diet and Nutrition

Crohn's & Colitis Foundation of America
386 Park Avenue S, 17th Floor
New York, NY 10016

212-685-3440
800-932-2423
Fax: 212-779-4098
e-mail: info@ccfa.org
www.ccfa.org

Raises important facts about how diet and nutrition affect persons with Crohn's Disease.

2195 Questions and Answers About Complications

Crohn's & Colitis Foundation of America
386 Park Avenue S, 17th Floor
New York, NY 10016

212-685-3440
800-932-2423
Fax: 212-779-4098
e-mail: info@ccfa.org
www.ccfa.org

Medical facts and complications from surgery.

2196 Questions and Answers About Crohn's Disease & Ulcerative Colitis

Crohn's & Colitis Foundation of America
386 Park Avenue S, 17th Floor
New York, NY 10016

212-685-3440
800-932-2423
Fax: 212-779-4098
e-mail: info@ccfa.org
www.ccfa.org

Offers information on the illness and answers the most frequently asked questions about Crohn's Disease. Also includes a glossary of IBD terms.

2197 Questions and Answers About Emotional Factors In Ileitis and Colitis

Crohn's & Colitis Foundation of America
386 Park Avenue S, 17th Floor
New York, NY 10016

212-685-3440
800-932-2423
Fax: 212-779-4098
e-mail: info@ccfa.org
www.ccfa.org

Answers some of the most commonly asked questions about ileitis and colitis and the role of emotional factors in their cause and course.

2198 Teacher's Guide to Crohn's Disease & Ulcerative Colitis

Crohn's & Colitis Foundation of America
386 Park Avenue S, 17th Floor
New York, NY 10016

212-665-3440
800-932-2423
Fax: 212-779-4098
e-mail: info@ccfa.org
www.ccfa.org

DESCRIPTION

2199 CRYPTORCHIDISM

Synonyms: Cryptorchidy, Cryptorchism

Covers these related disorders: Ectopic (maldescended) testes, True undescended testes

Involves the following Biologic System(s):
Renal and Urologic Disorders

Cryptorchidism is characterized by failure of one or both testes to descend into the pouch-like structure known as the scrotum. The testes are the paired, oval-shaped glands that produce the male reproductive cells (sperm). Early during male fetal growth, the testes develop within the abdomen near the kidneys. The testes then descend into the scrotum through a tubular canal that passes through lower muscular layers of the abdominal wall (inguinal canal). In males with cryptorchidism, one or both testes fail to complete their descent into the scrotum. Undescended testes that are located along the proper path of descent are known as true undescended testes, whereas those that have completed their descent through the inguinal canal yet have become located in areas other than the scrotum are referred to as ectopic or maldescended testes.

In most cases, one testis is affected (unilateral cryptorchidism); however, both testes may fail to descend (bilateral cryptorchidism) in up to 30 percent of affected male infants. In many cases, undescended testes may move down into the scrotum before one year of age. However, testes that fail to spontaneously descend during the first year of life typically fail to develop properly, may decrease in size, and have decreased numbers of reproductive cells. Without treatment, affected males are at an increased risk of infertility; malignant tumor development in affected testes during the third or fourth decade of life; or pain, swelling, and, in some cases, localized areas of tissue loss (necrosis).

Treatment of cryptorchidism often includes early surgery to relocate undescended testes into the scrotum (i.e., orchiopexy) and to correct inguinal hernias, which typically occur in association with true undescended testes and ectopic testes. Inguinal hernias are characterized by bulging of portions of the intestine into the inguinal canal. Surgical correction of cryptorchidism is typically recommended in the first years of life to help improve proper testicular development and fertility in adulthood.

Cryptorchidism affects about three and a half percent of full-term male newborns and increases in incidence in newborns who are born before 37 weeks of pregnancy (preterm). The condition may occur as an isolated abnormality or, in some cases, due to or in association with a number of different underlying syndromes or conditions.

See also **General Resources** on page 917

Government Agencies

2200 NIH/National Institute of Child Health and Human Development
31 Center Drive, Building 31
Bethesda, MD 20892

301-496-5133
Fax: 301-496-1104
www.nichd.nih.gov

Established in 1962 by congress, today the institute conducts and supports research on topics related to the health of children, adults, families and populations. Some of these topics include: developmental disabilities, growth and development, infant death, reproductive health and birth defects.

Nancy D Wirth, Director
Lisa Kaeser, Program & Public Liaison

National Associations & Support Groups

2201 Genetic Alliance
4301 Connecticut Avenue NW, Suite 404
Washington, DC 20008

202-966-5557
800-336-4363
Fax: 202-966-8553
e-mail: info@geneticalliance.org
www.geneticalliance.org

A coalition of voluntary genetic support groups, consumers and professionals addressing the needs of individuals and families affected by genetic disorders from a national perspective.

Sharon Terry, President/CEO

2202 March of Dimes Birth Defects Foundation
1275 Mamaroneck Avenue
White Plains, NY 10605

914-428-7100
888-663-4637
Fax: 914-428-8203
e-mail: resourcecenter@modimes.org
www.marchofdimes.com

Partnership of volunteers and professionals dedicated to improving the health of babies by preventing birth defects and infant mortality. Over 100 chapters are located across the country and can be located through the National Office.

Michelle King, Director

2203 NIH/National Institute of Mental Health
6001 Executive Boulevard, Room 8184, MSC 9663
Bethesda, MD 20892

301-443-4513
866-615-6464
Fax: 301-443-4279
TTY: 301-443-8431
e-mail: nimhinfo@nih.gov
www.nimh.nih.gov

Conducts strategic planning for specific research areas as well as for the Institute as a whole.

Dr Thomas R Insel, Director

Web Sites

2204 European Society for Pediatric Urology

www.espu.org

A nonprofit society whose main purpose is to promote pediatric urology, appropriate practice, education as well as exchanges between practitioners involved in the treatment of genito urinary disorders in children.

2205 National Center for Biotechnology Information

www.ncbi.nlm.nih.gov

NCBI's mission is to develop new information technologies to aid in the understanding of fundamental molecular and genetic processes that control health and disease.

2206 Online Mendelian Inheritance in Man

www.ncbi.nlm.nih.gov

This database is a catalog of human genes and genetic disorders.

DESCRIPTION

2207 CUSHING'S SYNDROME

Synonyms: Cushing's basophilism, Hyperadrenocorticism, Pituitary basophilism

Involves the following Biologic System(s):

Endocrinologic Disorders

Cushing's syndrome refers to a condition characterized by excessive levels of the corticosteroid hormone, cortisol, in the blood. Cortisol is produced in the outer portion (cortex) of the adrenal glands in response to the secretion of adrenocorticotropic hormone (ACTH; corticotropin). ACTH stimulates the growth of the adrenal cortex and thus the production of cortisol. Cushing's syndrome may be caused by a variety of factors including tumors of the adrenal glands or the pituitary gland, tumors of certain other organs, and excessive intake of corticosteroid drugs. In the very young, Cushing's syndrome occurs in more girls than boys by a ratio of approximately three to one.

Because cortisol assists in the metabolism of fat, protein, and glucose, many characteristic symptoms and findings associated with this disorder are related to the levels and distribution of body fat. For example, children with Cushing's syndrome may be somewhat obese with very full cheeks, a reddish moonface appearance, double chin, and excessive fat deposits on the back of the neck. In addition, the adrenal glands may be stimulated to secrete excessive amounts of other hormones that are converted in the liver to testosterone and estrogen. Overproduction of these androgenic hormones may result in symptoms such as increased amounts of hair on the face and trunk (hypertrichosis), the development of acne, and deepening of the voice as well as other masculine traits. Other findings that may appear over a period of time include elevated blood pressure (hypertension), kidney (renal) stones, and increased vulnerability to infection. Children with Cushing's syndrome may also experience growth delays or may not achieve height (short stature). However, those children who develop masculinization symptoms may reach average or above average height. Older children may experience a delay in onset of puberty and develop purplish stretch marks (striae) on the abdomen, breasts, hips, and thighs. In addition, their skin may become thin and fragile, leading to easy tissue injury. Affected children may develop headaches and weakness, experience increasing difficulty with school work, or become depressed or experience other emotional disturbances.

Treatment of Cushing's syndrome is dependent upon the underlying cause. If the disease results from a benign or malignant tumor or enlargement of the adrenal gland, surgical removal of the tumor or the adrenal gland (adrenalectomy) may be advised. A tumor in the pituitary gland may either be surgically removed or treated with radiation. Subsequent management of surgical or other procedures often includes appropriate hormone replacement therapy. Cushing's syndrome associated with prolonged or excessive intake of corticosteroids may be re|versed by a monitored and gradual (tapered) withdrawal of the medication. Other treatment is symptomatic and supportive.

See also **General Resources** on page 917

National Associations & Support Groups

2208 American Association of Clinical Endocrinologists
245 Riverside Avenue, Suite 200
Jacksonville, FL 32202

904-353-7878
Fax: 904-353-8185
e-mail: info@aace.com
www.aace.com

A professional medical organization aimed at promoting the quality of clinical epidemiologic research and improving the knowledge base for the diagnosis, prognosis, prevention and treatment of health conditions through the advancement and application of innovative methods.

2209 Cushing's Support & Research Foundation
65 E India Row, Suite 22B
Boston, MA 02110

617-723-3674
Fax: 617-723-3674
e-mail: cushinfo@csrf.net
www.csrf.net

To provide information and support for Cushing's Disease and Cushing's Syndrome to patients and their families to increase awareness and to educate the public about Cushing's Disease and Cushing's Syndrome. To be a resource for information and support to healthcare professionals, to raise and distribute funds for Cushing's Disease and Cushing's Syndrome research.

Louise Pace, Founding President

2210 Human Growth Foundation
997 Glen Cove Avenue, Suite 5
Glen Head, NY 11545

800-451-6434
Fax: 516-671-4055
e-mail: hgfl@hgfound.org
www.hgfound.org

A voluntary, nonprofit organization whose mission is to help children and adults with disorders of growth and growth hormones through research, education, support and advocacy. The foundation is dedicated to helping medical science to better understand the process of growth. It is composed of concerned parents and friends of children and adults with growth problems and interested health professionals.

Patricia D Costa, Executive Director

2211 Lawson Wilkins Pediatric Endocrine Society
867 Allardice Way
Stanford, CA 94305

650-494-3133
Fax: 650-649-2615
e-mail: secretary@lwpes.org
www.lwpes.org

To promote the acquisition and dissemination of knowledge of endocrine and metabolic disorders from conception through adolescence.

Kenneth Copeland, President

2212 National Adrenal Diseases Foundation
505 Northern Boulevard
Great Neck, NY 11021

516-487-4992
e-mail: nadfmail@aol.com
www.nadf.us

A nonprofit organization dedicated to providing support, information and education to individuals having Addison's disease as well as related diseases such as Cushing's Syndrome and Congenital Adrenal Hyperplasia. Promotes early diagnosis and treatment, and sponsors support groups and offers a quarterly newsletter, educational materials and access to a library of related information.

Melanie G Wong, Executive Director

Web Sites

2213 Cushing's Support and Research Foundation
csrf.net

The mission is to provide information and support for Cushing's Disease and Cushing's Syndrome patients and their families, to increase awareness and to educate the public about Cushing's Disease and Cushing's Syndrome, to be a resource for information and support to health care professionals, to raise and distribute funds for Cushing's Disease and Cushing's Syndrome research.

Book Publishers

2214 Endocrine & Metabolic Disorders Sourcebook
Omnigraphics
PO Box 625
Holmes, PA 19043

800-234-1340
Fax: 800-875-1340
e-mail: info@omnigraphics.com
www.omnigraphics.com

Basic information for the lay person about pancreatic and insulin-related disorders such as pancreatitis, diabetes and hypoglycemia; adrenal gland disorders such as Cushing's syndrome, Addison's disease and congenital adrenal hyperplasia; pituitary gland disorders such as growth hormone deficiency, acromegaly and pituitary tumors; and thyroid disorders such as hypothyroidism, Grave's disease, Hashimoto's disease and goiter.

574 pages hardcover
ISBN: 0-780802-07-1

2215 Let's Talk About Going to the Hospital
Rosen Publishing Group's PowerKids Press
29 E 21st Street
New York, NY 10010

212-777-3017
800-237-9932
Fax: 888-436-4643
e-mail: rosenpub@tribeca.ios.com
www.powerkidspress.com

If a child has to check into the hospital, chances are he or she is already upset about being ill. Knowing how a hospital functions and what the procedures are, such as when family members can visit, will help in what is already a stressful situation. Grades K-5.

24 pages
ISBN: 0-823950-36-0

Journals

2216 Endocrine Practice
245 Riverside Avenue, Suite 200
Jacksonville, FL 32202

904-353-7878
Fax: 904-353-8185
e-mail: info@aace.com
www.aace.com

Peer-reviewed journal published six-times a year and is the official journal of the American College of Endocrinology (ACE) and the American Association of Clinical Endocrinologists (AACE).

Newsletters

2217 NADF News
National Adrenal Diseases Foundation
505 Northern Boulevard
Great Neck, NY 11021

516-487-4992
e-mail: nadfmail@aol.com
www.medhelp.org/nadf

Provides support and information to those living with adrenal diseases.

DESCRIPTION

2218 CYSTIC FIBROSIS

Synonyms: CF, Mucoviscidosis

Involves the following Biologic System(s):

Respiratory Disorders

Cystic fibrosis (CF) is an inherited multisystem disorder that results in the abnormal production of mucus by almost all exocrine glands, causing obstruction of those glands and ducts. Glands of the respiratory and reproductive systems as well as pancreatic glands and sweat glands are affected. CF is considered one of the most common autosomal recessive disorders affecting Caucasians. Cystic fibrosis occurs in approximately one in 2,500 to 3,000 Caucasian infants and about one in 17,000 African-American infants. It is considered extremely rare in other populations. The disorder results from abnormal changes (mutations) of a gene on the long arm (q) of chromosome 7 (7q31.2). More than 400 different mutations of the CF gene have been identified.

In infants, children, and adults with cystic fibrosis, mucus-secreting glands within the air passages of the lungs (bronchi) produce unusually thick secretions, clogging and obstructing the airways and promoting the growth of certain bacteria. As a result, affected individuals may experience chronic obstruction and infection of the airways. In addition, the pancreas lacks sufficient digestive enzymes to break down food materials (malabsorption). Other exocrine gland abnormalities may also be present. For example, the sweat glands produce secretions containing abnormally high levels of salt; glands of the neck of the uterus (cervix) in affected females may produce abnormally increased, thickened secretions of mucus; and certain ducts of the male reproductive system (e.g., epididymis, ductus [vas] deferens, seminal vesicles) may be absent (atretic).

During the first or second day of life, some newborns with cystic fibrosis may experience bloating of the abdomen (abdominal distension), vomiting (emesis), and abnormal blockage of the lower region of the small intestine with meconium (meconium ileus). Meconium is the thick, sticky, darkish green material that accumulates in the fetal intestines and forms a newborn's first stools. Infants with cystic fibrosis also usually fail to grow and gain weight at the expected rate (failure to thrive). Additional symptoms and findings may include abnormally decreased muscle mass; a protruding abdomen; and loose, foul-smelling stools that contain an excessive amount of fat (steatorrhea). Children with cystic fibrosis often have respiratory abnormalities including wheezing; a chronic cough that may be accompanied by gagging and vomiting; recurrent inflammation of the air passages (bronchiolitis); and an increased susceptibility to lower respiratory infections (e.g., pneumonia). Affected adolescents may experience abnormally slow growth and delayed sexual development (i.e., average delay of two years); in addition, affected males may be infertile due to lack of sperm development (azoospermia). As the disease progresses, individuals with cystic fibrosis tend to experience increasingly severe respiratory abnormalities that may result in life-threatening complications.

Cystic fibrosis may be diagnosed based upon characteristic physical findings (e.g., chronic obstructive pulmonary disease, exocrine pancreatic insufficiency), specialized laboratory tests (e.g., sweat testing), and a positive family history (including DNA analysis). The treatment of cystic fibrosis is symptomatic and supportive and includes early intervention, ongoing monitoring, preventive measures, the use of certain medications, and other specialized treatment techniques. Approaches to treatment may include physical therapy, a high protein, high calorie diet, pancreatic enzyme replacement therapy, vitamin supplementation, specialized respiratory therapy, medications to help clean mucus from the airways and prevent or treat respiratory infections (e.g., antibiotic therapy). Median survival is about 31 years of age.

See also **General Resources** on page 917

National Associations & Support Groups

2219 American Lung Association
61 Broadway, 6th Floor
New York, NY 10006

212-315-8700
800-586-4872
www.lungusa.org

The American Lung Association fights lung disease in all its forms, with special emphasis on asthma, tobacco control and environmental health. The American Lung Association is funded by contributions from the public, along with gifts and grants from corporations, foundations and government agencies. The association achieves its many successes through the work of thousands of committed volunteers and staff.

2220 Cystic Fibrosis Foundation
6931 Arlington Road
Bethesda, MD 20814

301-951-4422
800-344-4823
Fax: 301-951-6378
e-mail: info@cff.org
www.cff.org

The mission of CF Foundation is to assure the development of means to cure and control CF and to improve the quality of life for those with the disease. It funds medical research and care programs which are improving the length and quality of life for people with cystic fibrosis.

Robert J Beall PhD, President/CEO

2221 Cystic Fibrosis Research
2672 Bayshore Parkway, Suite 520
Mountain View, CA 94043

650-404-9575
Fax: 650-404-9981
e-mail: cjenkins@cfri.org
www.cfri.org

Cystic Fibrosis Research's mission is to alleviate the emotional and physical suffering associated with cystic fibrosis and to offer educational and support programs for people with CF and their families.

Carroll Jenkins, Executive Director
David Soohoo, Program Services Manager

2222 Genetic Alliance
4301 Connecticut Avenue NW
Washington, DC 20008

202-966-5557
800-336-4363
Fax: 202-966-8553
e-mail: info@geneticalliance.org
www.geneticalliance.org

A coalition of voluntary genetic support groups, consumers and professionals addressing the needs of individuals and families affected by genetic disorders from a national perspective.

Sharon Terry, President/CEO

2223 March of Dimes Birth Defects Foundation
1275 Mamaroneck Avenue
White Plains, NY 10605

914-428-7100
888-663-4637
Fax: 914-428-8203
e-mail: resourcecenter@modimes.org
www.marchofdimes.com

Partnership of volunteers and professionals dedicates to improving the health of babies by preventing birth defects and infant mortality. Over 100 chapters are located across the country and can be located through the National Office.

Dr Jennifer Howse, President

Libraries & Resource Centers

2224 National Digestive Diseases Information Clearinghouse
2 Information Way
Bethesda, MD 20892

301-654-3810
800-891-5389
Fax: 703-738-4929
e-mail: nddic@info.niddk.nih.gov
www.digestive.niddk.nih.gov

The National Institute of Diabetes and Digestive and Kidney Diseases conducts and supports research on many of the most serious diseases affecting public health. The Institute supports much of the clinical research on the diseases of internal medicine and related subspecialty fields as well as many basic science disciplines.

Kathy Kranzfelder, Project Officer

Research Centers

Alabama

2225 Gregory Fleming James Cystic Fibrosis Cent er
1530 3rd Avenue S
Birmingham, AL 35294

205-934-9640
Fax: 205-934-7593
e-mail: sorscher@uab.edu
www.cfcenter.uab.edu

Eric J Sorscher MD, Director

Arizona

2226 Cystic Fibrosis Center: Phoenix Children's Hospital
1919 E Thomas Road
Phoenix, AZ 85016

602-546-0985
www.phxchildrens.com

Wayne J Morgan MD, Director

California

2227 Brian Wesley Ray Cystic Fibrosis Center
San Bernadino County Medical Center
780 E Gilbert Street
San Bernardino, CA 92415

909-387-8111

Gerald Greene, MD

2228 Children's Hospital of Los Angeles
4650 W Sunset Boulevard
Los Angeles, CA 90027

213-660-2450
e-mail: webmaster@chla.usc.edu
www.chla.org

Monique F Margetis MD, Contact

2229 Children's Hospital of Orange County: Depa rtment of Pulmonology - Cystic Fibrosis
455 S Main Street
Orange, CA 92868

714-997-3000
e-mail: mail@choc.org
www.choc.org

2230 Children's Hospital: Pediatric Pulmonary Center
747 52nd Street
Oakland, CA 94609

510-428-3000

2231 Cystic Fibrosis Center: Cedars-Sinai Medical Center
8700 Beverly Boulevard, N Tower, Fourth Floor
Los Angeles, CA 90048

800-233-2771
Fax: 310-423-1402

2232 Cystic Fibrosis Center: University of California at San Francisco
8700 Beverly Boulevard, N Tower, Fourth Floor
San Francisco, CA 94143

800-233-2771
Fax: 310-423-1402

2233 Cystic Fibrosis Research
2672 Bayshore Parkway, Suite 520
Mountain View, CA 94043

650-404-9975
Fax: 650-404-9981
e-mail: cjenkins@cfri.org
www.cfri.org

Cystic Fibrosis Research Inc.'s mission is to alleviate the emotional and physical suffering associated with cystic fibrosis, to offer educational and support programs for people with CF and their families. Membership: $15 annual; $50 lifetime.

Carroll Jenkins, Executive Director

2234 Cystic Fibrosis and Pediatric Respiratory Diseases Center
University of California at Davis
2315 Stockton Boulevard
Sacramento, CA 95817

Fax: 916-734-0491
e-mail: children@ucdavis.edu
www.ucdmc.ucdavis.edu/children

2235 Kaiser Permanente Medical Center
Kaiser Permanente Oakland Medical Center
280 W MacArthur Boulevard
Oakland, CA 94611

410-752-1000
www.kaiserpermanente.org

2236 Memorial Miller Children's Hospital Cystic Fibrosis Center
2801 Atlantic Avenue
Long Beach, CA 90806

562-933-8521
Fax: 562-933-8539
www.memorialcare.org

2237 Pulmonary Care and Cystic Fibrosis Center
Lucille Packard Children's Hospital
770 Welch Road, Suite 350
Palo Alto, CA 94304

650-723-5191
Fax: 650-498-4209
www.lpch.org

Deals with children's breathing in all its aspects.

Richard B Boss MD, Director

2238 Stanford CF Center
Packard Children's Hospital At Stanford
730 Welch Road
Palo Alto, CA 94304

650-497-8841
e-mail: jkirby@leland.stanford.edu
cfcenter.stanford.edu

Richard Moss MD, Director

Colorado

2239 Denver Children's Hospital
1056 E 19th Avenue
Denver, CO 80218

303-837-2522
Fax: 303-837-2924

Frank J Accurso MD, Pulmonology Pediatrics

Connecticut

2240 University of Connecticut Health Center
282 Washington Street
Hartford, CT 06106

860-545-9440
Fax: 860-545-9445
e-mail: kdaigle@ccmckids.org

Karen Daigle MD, Pediatric Pulmonary Division

2241 Yale University Cystic Fibrosis Research Center
School of Medicine Department
333 Cedar Street, PO Box 208064
New Haven, CT 06520

203-785-4638
Fax: 203-688-7864
www.med.yale.edu

Respiratory Medicine in the Department of Pediatrics at Yale University and Yale-New Haven Hospital is a multi-disiplinary section that has developed considerably since the early 90's and continues to develop and refine its clinical and research activities. We have also reorganized our Cystic Fibrosis Care Center, increased the clinical research activities pertaining to the care of CF patients and organized a number of CF family group meetings to dissimenate new knowledge of care of patients.

Marie E Egan MD, Cystic Fibrosis Center

Florida

2242 CF & Pediatric Pulmonary Disease Center
University of Florida
PO Box 100225
Gainesville, FL 32610

352-392-2666
Fax: 352-392-0821

Dr Veena B Antony MD, Director Adult CF Program

2243 Cystic Fibrosis Center - All Children's Hospital
801 6th Street S
St Petersburg, FL 33701

727-898-7451
800-456-4543

2244 Miami Children's Hospital, Division of Pulmonology
3100 SW 62nd Street
Miami, FL 33155

305-666-6511

Moises Simpser MD, Director

2245 Pulmonary Wellness Program
Orlando Regional Medical Center
1414 Kuhl Avenue
Orlando, FL 32806

321-841-4194
www.arnoldpalmerhospital.org

Our staff is trained in all diagnostic tests as well as a variety of Cystic Fibrosis therapies, including therapy vest treatments. Our professionals will work with your child and your family to create a more enriched diet including vitamin and enzyme supplements to help counteract the effects of Cystic Fibrosis. We also administer antibiotics in pill form as well as intravenously and through medicated vapors.

Georgia

2246 Department of Pediatrics, Medical College of Georgia
1120 15th Street, BT-1852
Augusta, GA 30912

706-721-3466
Fax: 706-721-7311

Dr William P Kanto Jr, Chairperson Pediatrics

2247 Egleston Cystic Fibrosis Center: Departmen t of Pediatrics
Emory University
2015 Uppergate Drive
Atlanta, GA 30322

404-727-5728
Fax: 404-727-4828
www.emory.edu

Daniel Caplan MD, Director

Illinois

2248 Cystic Fibrosis Center: Children's Memoria l Hospital
Northwestern University
2300 N Children's Plaza, #43
Chicago, IL 60614

773-880-4382
e-mail: cf@childrensmemorial.org

Susanna McColley MD, Head, Pulmonary Medicine

2249 Loyola University Medical Center/ Department of Pediatrics
2160 S First Avenue
Maywood, IL 60153

888-584-7888

Youngran Chung MD FAAP, Pediatric Pulmonary

2250 Park Ridge, Cystic Fibrosis Center
Advocate Lutheran General Hospital
1775 Dempster Street
Park Ridge, IL 60068

847-723-5437

2251 Saint Francis Medical Center Specialty Clinics, CF Center
Hillcrest Medical Plaza
200 E Pennsylvania Avenue #LO1
Peoria, IL 61603

309-655-4184
www.childrenshospitalofil.org

2252 University of Chicago Children's Hospital, Department of Pediatrics
University of Chicago Hospitals and Clinics
5721 S Maryland Avenue
Chicago, IL 60637

773-702-1000
Fax: 773-702-4753
www.uchicagokidshospital.org

Provides comprehensive, innovative medical care to children of all social and economic backgrounds. Dedicated to enhancing the health and wellness through patient care, education and research into the causes and cure of childhood diseases. Immediate access to the full resources of The University of Chicago Hospitals and to faculty of the division of Biological Sciences. The hospital sees children from the Chicago area, the Midwest and around the world who have the most complex medical problems.

Maria Dowell MD, Assistant Professor of Pediatrics

Indiana

2253 Cystic Fibrosis and Chronic Pulmonary Disease Clinic
Saint Joseph's Regional Medical Center
801 E LaSalle Avenue
South Bend, IN 46617

574-239-6126
800-206-0879
Fax: 574-472-6067

2254 Riley Cystic Fibrosis Center
Riley Hospital for Children
702 Barnhill Drive
Indianapolis, IN 46202

317-274-5000

Iowa

2255 Blank Children's Hospital: Department of Pulmonology
1212 Pleasant Street, Suite 300
Des Moines, IA 50309

515-241-6548

Ricardo Flores MD, Contact

2256 University of Iowa Hospitals & Clinics
Allergy and Pulmonary Division: Cystic Fibrosis Ct
200 Hawkins Drive
Iowa City, IA 52242

319-356-8486

Miles Weinberger MD, Director

Kansas

2257 Kansas University Medical Center: Departme nt of Pulmonology
Department of Pediatrics
3901 Rainbow Boulevard
Kansas City, KS 66160

913-588-6301

2258 Via Christi Specialty Clinics: Cystic Fibr osis, Adult and Pediatrics
St Joseph Campus
3600 E Harry Street
Wichita, KS 67218

316-685-1111

Kentucky

2259 University of Kentucky: Pediatric Pulmonar y Medicine
Department of Pediatrics
740 S Limestone
Lexington, KY 40536

859-323-6211
Fax: 859-257-7706

Michael I Anstead MD, Director

Louisiana

2260 Louisiana State University Health Sciences Center
Department of Pediatrics: Critical Care/Pulmonary
200 Henry Clay Avenue
New Orleans, LA 70118

504-896-2723
Fax: 504-896-2720
e-mail: dhoppe@lsuhsc.edu

Robert Hopkins MD, Professor of Clinical Pediatrics

Maine

2261 Central Maine Medical Center
Department of Pediatrics
12 High Street, Suite 301
Lewiston, ME 04240

207-795-5730
Fax: 207-797-7241
www.cmmc.org

Focuses special attention on the services that it provides to Cystic Fibrosis patients. In microbiology, for example, the lab employs a number of techniques supporting the special needs of CF patients. The CMMC pathology departments's chemistry section provides quantitative sweat analysis for the diagnosis of patients to other laboratories in the region, thereby assisting in diagnosis.

David R Baker DO, Special Interst: Cystic Fibrosis

2262 Eastern Maine Medical Center: Cystic Fibrosis Center
489 State Street
Bangor, ME 04401

207-973-7000
www.emmc.org

2263 Pediatric Cystic Fibrosis Center
Maine Medical Center: Dept. of Resp. Care
887 Congress Street, Suite 320
Portland, ME 04102

207-828-8226
Fax: 207-775-6024
www.mmc.org

Services offered: pediatric pulmonary consultation, flexible bronchoscopy of the pediatric airway, full pediatric and infant pulmonary function testing, including exercise testing, bronchopulmonary challenge, and accredited sleep lab. Also offered, full-time inpatient consultation service for neonates through adolesence, a bimonthly Cystic Fibrosis Clinic, and a biweekly outpatient pulmonary clinic.

Maryland

2264 John Hopkins Children's Hospital
Division of Pulmonary
600 N Wolfe Street
Baltimore, MD 21287

410-955-2035
Fax: 410-955-1030
www.hopkinschildrens.org

Massachusetts

2265 Baystate Medical Center
3300 Main Street
Springfield, MA 01199

413-794-0815
Fax: 413-794-7408

Annabelle I Quizon MD, Chief, Pediatric Pulmonary

2266 Children's Hospital Boston
Pulmonary and Critical Care Unit
55 Fruit Street, Bulfinch 148
Boston, MA 02114

617-726-3735
Fax: 617-724-9948
www.mgh.harvard.edu/pulmonary

Charles A Hales MD, Chief, Pulmonary and Critical Care

2267 Massachusetts General Hospital
Pulmonary and Critical Care Unit
55 Lake Avenue N
Worcester, MA 01605

www.umass.edu/pediatrics

Brian O'Sullivan MD, Professor

2268 Tufts New England Medical Center
Division of Pulmonary, Critical Care and Sleep
750 Washington Street, NEMC #369
Boston, MA 02111

617-636-6377

Nicholas Hill MD, Chief, Division of Pulmonary

Michigan

2269 Butterworth Hospital, Cystic Fibrosis Center
426 Michigan Street NE
Grand Rapids, MI 49503

616-454-1509

John Schuen, MD, Director

2270 Children's Hospital of Michigan Cystic Fibrosis Care, Teaching & Resource
Children's Hospital of Michigan
3901 Beaubien Boulevard
Detroit, MI 48201

313-745-5437

Debbie Toder, MD, Director

2271 Cystic Fibrosis Center
Children's Hospital of Michigan
3901 Beaubien Boulevard
Detroit, MI 48201

313-745-5541
Fax: 313-993-2948
www.chmkids.org

Physicians provide consultation for the diagnoses and care of unexplained, recurrent and chronic symptoms or diseases related to the respiratory system such as cystic fibrosis (CF), asthma, bronchopulmonarydysplasia, infant apnea and sleep disorders.

Debbie Toder, MD, Director

2272 Cystic Fibrosis Center/Pediatric Pulmonary and Sleep Medicine
330 Barclay Avenue NE, Suite 200
Grand Rapids, MI 49503

616-391-2125
Fax: 616-391-2131

John Schuen, MD, Director
Susan Millard, MD, Director

2273 East Lansing Cystic Fibrosis Center
Michigan State University
401 W Greenlawn Avenue
Lansing, MI 48910

517-482-4443

Richard Honicky, MD

2274 Kalamazoo Center for Medical Studies
Michigan State University
1000 Oakland Drive
Kalamazoo, MI 49008

616-337-6430

Douglas Homnick, MD, Director

2275 University of Michigan, Cystic Fibrosis Center
1500 E Medical Center Drive
Ann Arbor, MI 48109

734-936-3236

Samya Nasrimo, Director

Minnesota

2276 Minnesota Cystic Fibrosis Center
Fairview University Medical Center
420 Delaware Street SE
Minneapolis, MN 55455

612-273-3000
Fax: 612-625-4955
www.fairview-university.fairview.org

Comprehensive and coordinated care approach that is designed to prevent and slow the rate of disease progression. Since 1961, this care approach used by the University of Minnesota physicians has led to an increase in the average age of survival for patients with Cystic Fibrosis from 2 1/2 to 39 years.

2277 University of Minnesota Cystic Fibrosis Center
University of Minnesota Hospital
420 Delaware Street SE
Minneapolis, MN 55455

612-626-5147

Warren J Warwick, Director

Mississippi

2278 University of Mississippi Medical Center
2500 N State Street
Jackson, MS 39216

601-984-5046

Suzanne Miller, MD, Director

Missouri

2279 Children's Mercy Hospital, University of Missouri
Kansas City School of Medicine
24th & Gillham Road
Kansas City, MO 64108

816-231-8895

Michael McCubbin, MD, Director

2280 Cystic Fibrosis, Pediatric Pulmonary and Pediatric Gastrointestinal Center
Cardinal Glennon Memorial Hospital for Children
1465 S Grand
Saint Louis, MO 63104

314-577-5600

Anthony J Rejent, MD, Center Director

2281 University of Missouri-Columbia Cystic Fibrosis Center
University of Missouri/Department of Child Health
One Hospital Drive
Columbia, MO 65212

573-882-6921

Peter Konig, MD, Director

2282 Washington University Cystic Fibrosis Center
Saint Louis Children's Hospital
1 Childrens Plaza
Saint Louis, MO 63110

314-721-0072

George B Mallory, MD, Director

Nebraska

2283 University of Nebraska at Omaha Pediatric Pulmonary/Cystic Fibrosis Center
600 S 42nd Street
Omaha, NE 68198

402-559-4156
Fax: 402-559-7062

John L Colombo, MD, Director

Nevada

2284 Children's Lung Specialists
2200 S Rancho Drive
Las Vegas, NV 89102

702-598-4411
Fax: 702-598-1988

Ruben Diaz, MD, Director

New Hampshire

2285 New Hampshire Cystic Fibrosis Care and Teaching Center
Dartmouth Hitchcock Medical Center
1 Medical Center Drive
Lebanon, NH 03756

603-650-6244
Fax: 603-650-8601

William Boyle Jr, MD, Director

New Jersey

2286 Monmouth Medical Center, Cystic Fibrosis & Pediatric Pulmonary Center
279 3rd Avenue
Long Branch, NJ 07740

908-222-4474
Fax: 908-222-4472

Robert Zanni, MD, Director

2287 New Jersey Medical School
185 S Orange Avenue, Room Msb-F534
Newark, NJ 07103

201-982-4815
800-482-3627
Fax: 201-982-7597

Nelson Turcios, MD, Director

New Mexico

2288 University of New Mexico School of Medicine
2211 Lomas Boulevard NE
Albuquerque, NM 87131

505-272-6633
Fax: 505-272-0329

Bennie C McWilliams, PhD, Director

New York

2289 Albany Medical College Pediatric Pulmonary & Cystic Fibrosis Center
Department of Pediatrics
47 New Scotland Avenue
Albany, NY 12208

518-262-6880
Fax: 518-262-6472

Robert Kaslovsky, MD, Director

2290 Armond V. Mascia CF Center
NY Medical College
Munger Pavillion, Room 106
Valhalla, NY 10595

914-285-7585
Fax: 914-993-4336

Allen Dozer, MD, Director

2291 CF & Pediatric Pulmonary Care Center
Mt. Sinai School of Medicine
5th Avenue at 100th Street
New York, NY 10029

212-241-7788

Richard J Bonforte, MD, Director

2292 CF, Pediatric Pulmonary & GI Center
Saint Vincent's Hospital & Medical Center of NY
36 7th Avenue
New York, NY 10011

212-604-8895

Joan DeGelie-Germana, MD, Director

2293 Children's Lung and Cystic Fibrosis Center
Children's Hospital of Buffalo
219 Bryant Street
Buffalo, NY 14222

716-878-7524
Fax: 716-888-3945

Services for infants, children and teenagers with cystic fibrosis and other chronic respiratory conditions.

Drucy Borowitz, MD, Director

2294 Long Island College Hospital
340 Henry Street
Brooklyn, NY 11201

718-780-1025
www.lich.org

Robert Giusti, MD, Director

2295 Pediatric Pulmonary Center
Babies Hospital & Columbia Presbyterian Med Center
630 W 168th Street
New York, NY 10032

212-305-5122
Fax: 212-805-6103

Lynne M Quittell, MD, Director

2296 Schneider Children's Hospital of Long Island
Albert Einstein College of Medicine

New Hyde Park, NY 14040

716-470-3250

Jack D Gorvoy, MD

2297 State University Hospital/Upstate Medical Center
750 E Adams Street
Syracuse, NY 13210

315-473-5834

Ran Anbar, MD, Director

2298 University of Rochester Medical Center
Strong Memorial Hospital/Division of Pediatrics
601 Elmwood Avenue, #667
Rochester, NY 14642

716-275-2100
ww.urmc.rochester.edu/peds/

Karen Z Voter, MD, Director

North Carolina

2299 Duke University Medical Center/ CF Center
302 Bell Bldg
Durham, NC 27710

919-684-3364
Fax: 919-681-6943

Marc Majure, MD, Director

2300 UNC CF Center
Department of Pediatrics
509 Burnett-Womack Building
Chapel Hill, NC 27599

919-966-1055

Gerald W Fernald, MD, Director

North Dakota

2301 Saint Alexius Medical Center/CF Center
311 N 9th Street
Bismarck, ND 58501

701-224-7500
Fax: 701-224-7560

Allan Stillerman, MD, Director

Ohio

2302 Case Western Reserve University Cystic Fibrosis Center
2101 Adelbert Road
Cleveland, OH 44106

216-844-3264
Fax: 216-844-5916

Pamela B Davis, MD, Director

2303 Columbus Children's Hospital, Cystic Fibrosis Center
700 Childrens Drive
Columbus, OH 43205

614-722-4766
Fax: 614-722-4755

Karen S McCoy, MD, Director

2304 Lewis H. Walker, MD, Cystic Fibrosis Center
Children's Hospital Medical Center of Akron
1 Perkins Square
Akron, OH 44308

330-543-1000
www.alchonchildrens.org

Part of the Robert T Stone Respiratory Center, one of six centers in the state of Ohio providing comprehensive care for patients who suffer from this disease. Caused by a defective gene, CF is characterized by a thick, sticky mucus in the lungs, intestines and other excretory organs that leads to severe respiratory and digestive problems.

Robert T Stone, MD, Director

2305 Pediatric Pulmonary Center
Children's Medical Center
1 Childrens Plaza
Dayton, OH 45404

513-226-8376
Fax: 937-463-5390

Michael E Steffan, MD, Director

2306 University of Cincinnati College of Medicine/Division of Pediatrics
Children's Hospital Medical Center
3333 Burnet Avenue
Cincinnati, OH 45229

513-636-4200
800-344-2462
www.chmcc.org

Robert Wilmott, MD, Director

Oklahoma

2307 University of Oklahoma Cystic Fibrosis Center
940 NW 13th Street
Oklahoma City, OK 73106

405-271-6390
Fax: 405-271-7866

John E Grunow, MD, Director

Oregon

2308 Oregon Health Sciences Unit
3181 SW Sam Jackson Park Road
Portland, OR 97201

503-494-7820

Michael A Wall, MD, Research Director

Pennsylvania

2309 CF Center at The Children's Hospital of Philadelphia
34th & Civic Center Boulevard
Philadelphia, PA 19104

215-590-3749
Fax: 215-590-4298

The CF center consists of pediatric and adult specialists who collaorate to provide multidisciplinary care for CF patients through their entire life span. The interdisiplinary health care team forms the core of our Centerand meets regularly to assess the clinical, educational and psychosocial needs of the family and to plan and evaluate the care provided. The CF center also provides educational programs for health professionals and reserch focused on improved treatments.

Thomas F Scanlin MD, Director
LeeAnn Webb CRNP, Coordinator

2310 Cystic Fibrosis Center at Polyclinic Medical Center
Polyclinic Medical Center
2601 N 3rd Street
Harrisburg, PA 17110

717-782-4105
800-334-1007
Fax: 717-782-2597

Muttiah Ganeshananthan, MD, Director

2311 Pediatric Pulmonary and Cystic Fibrosis Center
Saint Christopher's Hospital For Children
Erie Avenue at Front Street
Philadelphia, PA 19134

215-427-5183

Daniel Schidlow, MD, Director

2312 University of Pittsburgh Cystic Fibrosis Center/Children's Hospital
3705 5th Avenue
Pittsburgh, PA 15213

412-648-9670

Raymond A Frizzell, MD, Director

Rhode Island

2313 Rhode Island Hospital, Cystic Fibrosis Center
CDC-APC
593 Eddy Street
Providence, RI 02903

401-444-5685
Fax: 401-444-6115

Mary Ann Passero, MD, Director

South Carolina

2314 CF Center/Medical University of South Carolina
158 Rutledge Avenue
Charleston, SC 29425

803-792-3561
Fax: 803-792-0732

Robert Baker, MD, Director

South Dakota

2315 Sioux Valley Hospital, South Dakota Cystic Fibrosis Center
1100 S Euclid Avenue, PO Box 5039
Sioux Falls, SD 57117

605-333-1000

Rodney Parry, MD, Director

Tennessee

2316 Memphis Cystic Fibrosis Center
LeBonheur Children's Medical Center
One Children's Plaza
Memphis, TN 38103

901-572-5222
Fax: 901-572-3337

Robert Schoumacher, MD, Director

2317 Pediatric Pulmonary Medicine
S-0119 McN
Nashville, TN 37232

615-343-7617
Fax: 615-343-7727
www.vanderbiltchildrens.com

Texas

2318 CF Center, Pulmonary Section
Baylor College of Medicine/Dept. of Pediatrics
1 Baylor Plaza
Houston, TX 77030

713-798-4945

Peter W Hiatt, MD, Director

2319 Cook-Ft. Worth Medical Center, CF Center
801 7th Avenue
Fort Worth, TX 76104

817-885-4207
Fax: 817-885-1090

James C Cunningham, MD, Director

2320 Cystic Fibrosis Care, Teaching and Research Center
Children's Medical Center
1935 Motor Street
Dallas, TX 75235

214-640-2000

Claude Prestidge, MD, Director

2321 Cystic Fibrosis-Lung Disease Center Santa Rosa Children's Hospital
519 W Houston Street
San Antonio, TX

210-228-2058
Fax: 210-224-2132

2322 Tri-Services Military CF Center
Brooke Army Medical Center
3851 Roger Brooke Drive
Fort Sam Houston, TX 78234

210-916-3400
e-mail: bamac/home.hm
www.grmc.amed d.army.nil/

Stephen Inscore, LTC, MC, Director

Utah

2323 University of Utah Intermountain Cystic Fibrosis Center
50 N Medical Drive
Salt Lake City, UT 84132

801-581-7715
Fax: 801-581-2177

Dennis W Neilson, Center Co-Director

Vermont

2324 Medical Center Hospital of Vermont
Cystic Fibrosis Center
50 Timber Lane
South Burlington, VT 05403

802-862-5529
Fax: 802-864-0294

Donald Swartz, MD, Director

Virginia

2325 Cystic Fibrosis Center/University of Virginia Health System
Department of Pediatrics
PO Box 800386
Charlottesville, VA 22908

434-924-2250
Fax: 434-243-6618

Comprehensive care for children and adults with cystic fibrosis.

Deborah K Froh, MD, Director Children's Program
Mark Robbins, MD, Director Adult Program

2326 Cystic Fibrosis Program of the Medical College of Virginia
9000 Stony Point Parkway
Richmond, VA 23298

804-786-9445
Fax: 804-560-7347

David Draper, MD, Director

2327 Eastern Virginia Medical Center
Children's Hospital of The King's Daughters
601 Childrens Lane
Norfolk, VA 23507

804-668-7132
Fax: 804-668-9767

Thomas Rubio, MD, Director

Washington

2328 University of Washington CF Center
4800 Sand Point Way NE
Seattle, WA 98105

206-526-2024
Fax: 206-528-2639

Bonnie W Ramsey, MD, Director

West Virginia

2329 West Virginia University Cystic Fibrosis Center
PO Box 9214
Morgantown, WV 26506

304-293-4341
Fax: 304-293-4341

Stephen C Aronoff, MD, Director

2330 West Virginia University Mountain State Cystic Fibrosis Center
PO Box 9214
Morgantown, WV 26506

304-293-1217
800-982-8242
Fax: 304-293-1216
e-mail: kmoffett@hsc.wvu.edu

Cathryn S Moffett, MD, Director

Wisconsin

2331 Medical College of Wisconsin Cystic Fibrosis Center
Children's Hospital of Wisconsin
9000 W Wisconsin Avenue, MS #777A
Milwaukee, WI 53226

414-266-6730
Fax: 414-266-2653

Mark Splaingard, MD, Director

2332 University of Wisconsin-Madison Cystic Fibrosis/Pulmonary Center
Clinical Science Center H4/430
600 Highland Avenue
Madison, WI 53792

608-263-8555
Fax: 608-263-0440

Michael J Rock, MD, Director

Audio Video

2333 Don't Cry for Me
Fanlight Productions
4196 Washington Street
Boston, MA 02131

617-469-4999
Fax: 617-469-3379
e-mail: fanlight@tiac.net
www.fanlight.com

Profiles five exceptional young people living with cystic fibrosis. This film is not about death, but about living with the intensity created by the knowledge of a shortened life expectancy.

54 minutes
ISBN: 1-572950-95-1

2334 Embers of the Fire
Fanlight Productions
4196 Washington Street, Suite 2
Boston, MA 02131

617-469-4999
Fax: 617-469-3379
e-mail: fanlight@tiac.net
www.fanlight.com

Offers a straight-forward explanation of cystic fibrosis with a primary focus on the stories of several courageous young people with cystic fibrosis during a week at summer camp. Addresses their fears of rejection, isolation, and death while demonstrating the ways they have learned to lead fulfilling lives.

28 minutes
ISBN: 1-572950-98-6

2335 Living with Cystic Fibrosis
Aquarius Health Care Videos
5 Powderhouse Lane, PO Box 1159
Sherborn, MA 01770

508-651-2963
888-440-2963
Fax: 508-650-4216
e-mail: info@aquariusproductions.com
www.aquariusproductions.com

People diagnosed with this genetic disorder are surviving longer than ever. Many patients live well into their thirties and beyond. This film looks at the hope that current research offers to those with cystic fibrosis, their caregivers and families.

Donna Kaufman

Web Sites

2336 American Lung Association of the City of New York
www.lungusa.org

The American Lung Association fights lung disease in all its forms, with special emphasis on asthma, tobacco control and environmental health. The American Lung Association is funded by contributions from the public, along with gifts and grants from corporations, foundations and government agencies. The association achieves its many successes through the work of thousands of committed volunteers and staff.

2337 CF Index of Online Resources
vmsb.csd.mu.edu/~541lukasr/cystic.html

2338 CF Web
cf-web.mit.edu

2339 Healing Well
www.healingwell.com

An online health resource guide to medical news, chat, information and articles, newsgroups and message boards, books, disease-related web sites, medical directories, and more for patients, friends, and family coping with disabling diseases, disorders, or chronic illnesses.

2340 Onhealth
www.onhealth.com

Provides over 50 links to information on cystic fibrosis.

2341 Online Mendelian Inheritance in Man
www.ncbi.nlm.nih.gov

This database is a catalog of human genes and genetic disorders.

Book Publishers

2342 Alex: The Life of a Child Rutledge Press
Frank Deford, author

PO Box 141000
Nashville, TN 37214

Paperback
ISBN: 1-558535-52-7

2343 Cystic Fibrosis
Franklin Watts
90 Old Sherman Turnpike
Danbury, CT 06816

203-797-3500
Fax: 203-797-3197
www.grolier.com

1994 128 pages
ISBN: 0-531125-52-1

2344 Cystic Fibrosis: A Guide for Patient and Family
Raven Press
1185 Avenue of the Americas
New York, NY 10036

212-930-9500

253 pages Softcover
ISBN: 0-397516-53-3

2345 Cystic Fibrosis: The Facts
Oxford University Press
2001 Evans Road
Cary, NC 27513

212-726-6000
Fax: 919-677-1303
www.oup-usa.org

1995 128 pages Paperback
ISBN: 0-192625-43-8

2346 Give Me One Wish
Norton Publishers
500 5th Avenue
New York, NY 10110

212-354-5500
www.scholastic.com/

This book reads like a novel because it reenacts the author's daughter's bout with cystic fibrosis.

Grades 10-12

2347 Let's Talk About Going to the Hospital
Rosen Publishing Group's PowerKids Press
29 E 21st Street
New York, NY 10010

212-777-3017
800-237-9932
Fax: 888-436-4643
e-mail: rosenpub@tribeca.ios.com
www.powerkidspress.com

If a child has to check into the hospital, chances are he or she is already upset about being ill. Knowing how a hospital functions and what the procedures are, such as when family members can visit, will help in what is already a stressful situation. Grades K-5.

24 pages
ISBN: 0-823950-36-0

2348 Lung Disorders Sourcebook
Omnigraphics
615 Griswold
Detroit, MI 48226

800-234-1340
Fax: 800-875-1340
e-mail: info@omnigraphics.com
omnigraphics.com

Basic consumer health information on lung disorders including tuberculosis, asthma and cystic fibrosis.

678 pages
ISBN: 0-780803-39-6

2349 Robyn's Book: A True Diary
Scholastic
730 Broadway
New York, NY 10003

212-505-3000

This book chronicles the life of the author and her battle with cystic fibrosis.

Grades 7-12

2350 Toothpick
Holiday
40 E 49th Street
New York, NY 10017

212-688-0085

This book uses relationships between two different teenagers to parallel the life of a person with cystic fibrosis.

Grades 6-9

2351 Understanding Cystic Fibrosis
University Press of Mississippi
3825 Ridgewood Road, Unit 9
Jackson, MS 39211

601-982-6205
Fax: 601-982-6217

This book charts the progress that has been made in identifying the mutations that cause CF and understanding how these genetic errors cause a disease whose symptoms can range from mild respiratory distress to life-threatening lung infections.

128 pages Hardcover
ISBN: 0-878059-66-0

Newsletters

2352 Commitment
Cystic Fibrosis Foundation
6931 Arlington Road
Bethesda, MD 20814

301-951-4422
Fax: 301-951-6378
e-mail: info@cff.org
www.cff.org

Offers medical news, fund-raising features, public policy and news from across the nation on cystic fibrosis.

Pamphlets

2353 An Introduction to Cystic Fibrosis for Patients and Families
Cystic Fibrosis Foundation
6931 Arlington Road
Bethesda, MD 20814

301-951-4422

Offers up-dated medical information, the latest news on assistive technology and treatments, answers to some frequently asked questions on the illness and more.

94 pages

2354 Consumer Fact Sheet
Cystic Fibrosis Foundation
6931 Arlington Road
Bethesda, MD 20814

301-951-4422

Offers a brief introduction to cystic fibrosis, symptoms, causes, treatments and offers illustrations pertaining to drainage positions.

2355 Cystic Fibrosis: Guide for Parents
American Lung Association
1740 Broadway
New York, NY 10019

212-315-8700
800-586-4872
Fax: 212-765-7876
e-mail: info@lungusa.org
www.lungusa.org

Comprehensive booklet covering topics such as treatment, social aspects, inheritance, genetics and outlook for the future.

24 pages

2356 Here's Everything You'll Need to Save Money with the CFF Health Services
CFF Home Health & Pharmacy Services
6931 Arlington Road
Bethesda, MD 20814

Fax: 800-233-3504

Offers information on the Cystic Fibrosis Foundation's home health services.

2357 Here's Everything You'll Need to Start Saving Money with the CFF Pharmacy
CFF Home Health And Pharmacy Services
6931 Arlington Road
Bethesda, MD 20814

Fax: 800-233-3504

Offers information on money-saving medications and patient information for the Cystic Fibrosis Pharmacy.

2358 Home Line
Cystic Fibrosis Foundation
6931 Arlington Road
Bethesda, MD 20814

301-951-4422

This bimonthly newsletter offers information on services and programs offered by the Foundation.

Bimonhtly

2359 On the Threshold of a Cure...You Can Make the Difference!
Cystic Fibrosis Foundation
6931 Arlington Road
Bethesda, MD 20814

301-951-4422

Offers information on what Cystic Fibrosis is and what people can do to help support the foundation's research.

Camps

2360 LA Lions Camp Pelican
PO Box 171
Leesville, LA

337-239-0782
800-348-6567
Fax: 337-239-9975
e-mail: lalions@lionscamp.org
www.lionscamp.org

Provides residential camp for children with lung disorders.

Troy Ricard

DESCRIPTION

2361 CYTOMEGALOVIRUS

Synonyms: Child care virus, CMV, Cytomegalic inclusion disease

Involves the following Biologic System(s):

Infectious Disorders

Cytomegalovirus (CMV) is a member of the herpesvirus family. This very common, worldwide viral infection often causes no apparent disease; however, in some patients, CMV infection results in symptoms and physical findings that may range from mild to potentially life-threatening.

Cytomegalovirus may be transmitted from mother to child before birth through the placenta, during birth through genital tract secretions, or after birth through breast milk. CMV is present in the environment; therefore, infection may be acquired at virtually any age. Because this virus may be shed in the urine and saliva for months or years after infection, children and adults who work in child-care settings are especially vulnerable. This is such a common occurrence that CMV infection is sometimes called the child-care virus. CMV may also be excreted in feces or transmitted through blood transfusions and in transplanted organs such as the kidneys, heart, and bone marrow. In the case of transmission through donated organs, CMV symptoms may be particularly severe due to immune suppression that occurs with the use of immune-suppressive drugs used to prevent organ rejection. In this way, these individuals are less capable of mounting a defense against the virus. Other individuals with impaired immune systems, such as the elderly and those with acquired immunodeficiency syndrome (AIDS), are also at increased risk of potentially life-threatening complications.

Fetal infection is more common when the mother is infected by CMV for the first time as opposed to recurrent infection. The majority of CMV-infected infants have no symptoms at birth; however, approximately five to 10 percent may exhibit symptoms and physical findings involving different organs of the body. Symptomatic CMV infection in the newborn (congenital CMV) may include such characteristic findings as an unusually small head (microcephaly); accumulations of calcium salts in the tissues of the brain; enlargement of the liver and spleen (hepatosplenomegaly); yellowish discoloration of the skin, eyes, and mucous membranes (jaundice); purplish skin lesions; eye abnormalities (i.e., chorioretinitis); and other irregularities of the central nervous system that may result in loss of sight and hearing, paralysis, and mental retardation. Approximately 10 to 20

percent of asymptomatic newborns later develop similar difficulties associated with the central nervous system. Infants who contract CMV infection after birth may have enlargement of the liver and spleen, inflammation of the liver (hepatitis), or pneumonia. In addition, premature, low birth weight infants who acquire CMV infection through blood transfusion may develop inflammation of the lungs (pneumonitis), jaundice, enlargement of the liver and spleen, grayish skin coloring, and irregularities of the blood. CMV-infected children with AIDS or transplanted organs may develop potentially life-threatening conditions, including pneumonitis, inflammation of the retinas of the eyes (retinitis), and gastrointestinal abnormalities. Primary cytomegalovirus infections in children receiving transplants are more likely to have more severe symptoms than those of recurrent infection.

Older affected children and adults with cytomegalovirus infection may develop symptoms and physical findings similar to those of mononucleosis. These findings usually last about two to three weeks and may include fever, rash, headache, fatigue, muscle pain, and hepatosplenomegaly. In addition, mild CMV infections in many children and adults often subside with no treatment.

In some cases, preventive treatment for CMV infection includes administration of intravenous immunoglobulin. Although this therapy is not usually effective in preventing disease acquired through most types of organ transplantation, it may be beneficial to bone marrow recipients whose compromised immune systems may not be capable of preventing a primary CMV infection. Other preventive measures may include screening of blood and organ donors for cytomegalovirus. In addition, pregnant child-care workers are urged to practice good hygiene, including frequent and thorough handwashing. Certain antiviral drugs (e.g., gancyclovir) are sometimes used to treat symptoms associated with life-threatening disease. However, symptoms tend to recur after treatment is stopped and serious side effects associated with this type of treatment are common. Separate studies on vaccine development and the use of antiviral drugs in the treatment of congenital cytomegalovirus are ongoing. Other treatment is supportive.

See also **General Resources** on page 917

Government Agencies

2362 NIH/National Institute of Allergy and Infectious Diseases
6610 Rockledge Drive, MSC 6612
Bethesda, MD 20892

301-496-5717
Fax: 301-402-3573
TDD: 800-877-8339
www.niaid.nih.gov

Conducts and supports basic and applied research to better understand, treat, and ultimately prevent infectious, immunologic, and allergic diseases.

Anthony S Fauci MD, Director

2363 NIH/National Institute of Child Health and Human Development
31 Center Drive, Building 31
Bethesda, MD 20892

301-496-5133
Fax: 301-496-1104
www.nichd.nih.gov

Established in 1962 by congress, today the institute conducts and supports research on topics related to the health of children, adults, families and populations. Some of these topics include: developmental disabilities, growth and development, infant death, reproductive health and birth defects.

Nancy D Wirth, Director
Lisa Kaeser, Program & Public Liaison

National Associations & Support Groups

2364 March of Dimes Birth Defects Foundation
1275 Mamaroneck Avenue
White Plains, NY 10605

914-428-7100
888-663-4637
Fax: 914-428-8203
e-mail: resourcecenter@modimes.org
www.marchofdimes.com

Partnership of volunteers and professionals dedicates to improving the health of babies by preventing birth defects and infant mortality. Over 100 chapters are located across the country and can be located through the National Office.

Dr Jennifer Howse, President

2365 National Congenital CMV Disease Registry
Feigin Center
1102 Bates MC3-2371, Suite 1150
Houston, TX 77030

713-770-4387
Fax: 713-770-4387
e-mail: cmv@bcm.tmc.edu
www.bcm.tmc.edu

Provides copies of pertinent information pieces regarding the disorder along with support facilities.

Web Sites

2366 Kid's Health
www.kidshealth.org

Kids health is the largest and most visited site on the web providing doctor-approved health information about children from before birth through adolescence. Kids health provides families with accurate, up to date and jargon free health information they can use.

Book Publishers

2367 Let's Talk About Going to the Hospital
Rosen Publishing Group's PowerKids Press
29 E 21st Street
New York, NY 10010

212-777-3017
800-237-9932
Fax: 888-436-4643
e-mail: rosenpub@tribeca.ios.com
www.powerkidspress.com

If a child has to check into the hospital, chances are he or she is already upset about being ill. Knowing how a hospital functions and what the procedures are, such as when family members can visit, will help in what is already a stressful situation. Grades K-5.

24 pages
ISBN: 0-823950-36-0

DESCRIPTION

2368 DENTAL CONDITIONS

Covers these related disorders: Anodontia, Dental Caries, Discoloration of the Teeth, Malocclusion, Supernumerary Teeth

Involves the following Biologic System(s):

Dental Disorders

This chapter will discuss the following pediatric dental conditions: anodontia; dental caries; discoloration of the teeth; malocclusion; supernumerary teeth; teeth grinding.

Anodontia refers to a condition in which some or all of the teeth are missing as the result of a congenital defect or of damage sustained from disease. Ectodermal dysplasias are a group of congenital disorders characterized by abnormalities of the teeth, hair, nails, skin glands, the skin, nervous system, ears and eyes, and the membranes that line the anus and the mouth. Partial anodontia may also result from a common birth defect such as cleft palate, in which the roof of the mouth does not close completely. Partial anodontia is often a component of certain disorders or syndromes including pseudohypoparathyroidism, cleidocranial dysplasia, and other disorders affecting the face and skull. The absence of some teeth may result in malocclusion, or misalignment, of the upper and lower teeth.

Treatment of anodontia may include the use of full or partial dentures, other dental prosthetics (bridgework), and dental implants. These approaches may be delayed until underlying structural deficits, such as cleft palate, are surgically corrected.

Dental caries, or tooth decay, is a common condition characterized by the gradual destruction (erosion) of the enamel and, potentially, the dentin and interior pulp of a tooth. The main cause of dental caries is plaque, a sticky film consisting of food debris, saliva and mucus. Certain bacteria that reside in the mouth break down dietary carbohydrates within plaque, creating acids that gradually wear down the outer tooth surfaces. Dental caries initially appear as whitish spots. As loss of dental tissue progresses, the enamel is gradually destroyed. Without treatment, the dentin and pulp may erode, causing pain, infection, and eventual tooth loss. In affected infants or children, dental caries typically appear on the minute grooves on the grinding surfaces of the back molars, or on the contact surfaces between adjacent teeth.

Dental caries are thought to be caused more by the frequency of carbohydrate consumption than by the quantity of carbohydrates consumed. For example, baby bottle tooth decay, which becomes apparent between 1 and 2 years, is extensive decay due to sleeping with, and constant use of, bottles with milk, juice and other sugary liquids. The same amount of such liquids consumed during a single meal is much less likely to cause decay. The frequency of dental caries has decreased 35 to 50 percent during the past 20 years due to fluorinated water and toothpaste. Dental caries are treated by drilling out the decayed area and filling the cavity with a dental material. Treatment of advanced decay may include removal of the pulp (root canal), restoration (crown), or extraction of the tooth.

Permanent discoloration of the teeth is caused by the incorporation of particular substances into de veloping tooth enamel, such as taking certain antibiotic medications (e.g. tetracyclines), excessive fluoride consumption, particular pediatric conditions or disorders, or other factors. Since tetracycline medications are highly absorbed into the teeth and bones, taking such medications during the development of enamel may result in thin, deficient tooth enamel (hyypoplasia) that is permanently stained yellowish brown. The risk for this condition is from the fourth month of fetal development to 10 months for primary teeth and from four months to 16 years for secondary teeth. Risk varies with type of medication, dose, and duration of treatment. Excessive fluoride may also result in tooth discoloration known as mottling. This primarily affects children in areas with higher-than-recommended levels of fluoride in the water supply. Permanent discoloration may also result from certain vitamin deficiencies, infectious disorders, or certain pediatric conditions. The use of certain specialized dental procedures and devices may help to minimize or cover discolored teeth. Children may also experience temporary tooth staining on the surface of teeth due to certain bacteria or food dyes. These may be removed by professional tooth polishing.

Malocclusion is a dental condition in which there is improper positioning of the teeth of the upper jaw in relation to those of the lower jaw. There are three main classes of malocclusion. In proper contact of the teeth (occlusion) the front teeth of the upper jaw slightly overlap the front teeth of the lower jaw and the ridges (cusps) of the back teeth (premolars and molars) in the lower jaw interlock slightly ahead and inside the cusps of the corresponding teeth in the upper jaw. In class I malocclusion, certain upper and lower teeth do not have appropriate contact due to crowding. In class II malocclusion (retrognathism), the most common, the cusps of the back teeth in the lower jaw are positioned behind and inside the cusps of the corresponding teeth in the upper jaw. In class III malocclusion (prognathism), the cusps of the back teeth in the lower jaw are abnormally positioned in front of corresponding maxillary teeth and the front teeth of the lower jaw meet or protrude beyond the upper front teeth. Malocclusion usually occurs during childhood as the bones of the jaws grow and the teeth develop and, in most cases, is genetic. Some cases of malocclusion may result due to other dental abnormalities, such as improper development or crowding of teeth, or constant thumbsucking. Treating malocclusion may avoid strain, stiffness, or pain that may result from an abnormal bite, may improve facial appearance, and may prevent tooth decay and loss. Treatment may include a variety of measures: tooth extraction in cases of dental crowding; orthodontic appliances to correct the positioning of teeth; or, in severe cases, surgical correction of abnormal protrusion or recession of the lower jaw.

Supernumerary teeth refers to the presence of one or more teeth in excess of the normal 20 primary teeth or 32 secondary teeth. These teeth are usually abnormal in shape and size and may erupt through the gums or may remain impacted in the gums or the jaw bone. In addition, a primary or secondary tooth is typically not present to replace the supernumerary (super = "extra") tooth. In most cases, only one supernumerary tooth is present; however, instances of multiple supernumerary teeth have been reported. The presence of supernumerary teeth may cause delayed eruption, abnormal positioning, or impaction of nearby teeth. Therefore, early diagnosis is important in removal or extraction of the extra tooth, or in regular monitoring to assess the need for possible extraction. Natal teeth, which are teeth that are present at birth, may be supernumerary or primary teeth that have erupted unusually early. Natal teeth usually have little bony support or root formation and are typically loose and mobile. If natal teeth are determined to be supernumerary, they are often extracted; if they are primary teeth, attempts may be made to maintain them. Supernumerary teeth develop in different locations in the mouth, and have different names: mesiodens develop between the central front teeth in the upper jaw; paramolars form between molars in the upper jaw; disomolars, also known as retromolars, develop in the back of the third molars (widsom teeth); peridens erupt outside the dental arches, such as in the roof of the mouth. Supernumerary teeth may be the result of abnormalities during embryonic development, and may occur with other conditions, such as cleft lip and palate. There have been reports that suggest supernumerary teeth are inherited.

Teeth grinding, or bruxism, refers to compulsive, involuntary, rhythmic, and nonfunctional grinding, clenching, or gnashing of the teeth. This habitual grinding is most evident during sleep, so the individual may be oblivious to it, but family members may notice. Affected individuals may also unconsciously grind their teeth during the day as well. Daytime teeth grinding is known as bruxomania. In some, teeth grinding may be considered a habit or habit disorder, depending upon the degree of severity and the impact upon daily functioning. Bruxism most often results from unresolved or unexpressed anger, aggression, fear, frustration, resentment, or other negative emotions. Teeth grinding that occurs during sleep exerts more force than that of normal daytime chewing or grinding. For this reason, bruxism may cause muscle pain or tightness in the jaw area, headache, earache as well as irregularities in the surface contact between the upper and lower teeth. In addition, bruxism may wear down or loosen the teeth. The goals of treatment are to reduce pain, prevent permanent damage to the teeth, and reduce clenching behaviors as much as possible. Treatment for teeth grinding may include stress management and behavior therapy. Other treatment is symptomatic, and involves a dental appliance, such as a mouthguard, worn at night to help reduce associated dental injury.

See also **General Resources** on page 917

Government Agencies

2369 NIH/National Institute of Child Health and Human Development
31 Center Drive, Building 31
Bethesda, MD 20892

301-496-5133
Fax: 301-496-1104
www.nichd.nih.gov

Established in 1962 by congress, today the institute conducts and supports research on topics related to the health of children, adults, families and populations. Some of these topics include: developmental disabilities, growth and development, infant death, reproductive health and birth defects.

Nancy D Wirth, Director
Lisa Kaeser, Program & Public Liaison

2370 NIH/National Institute of Dental and Crani ofacial Research
National Institutes of Health
31 Center Drive, MSC 2290, Building 31
Bethesda, MD 20892

301-496-4261
Fax: 301-402-2185
e-mail: nidcrinfo@mail.nih.gov
www.nidcr.nih.gov

The Institute promotes the general health of the American people by improving their oral, dental and craniofacial health. The

NIDCR aims to promote health, to prevent diseases and conditions, and to develop new diagonistics and therapeutics.

Dr Lawrence A Tabak, Director
Thomas G Murphy, Acting Executive Director

National Associations & Support Groups

2371 American Academy of Pediatric Dentistry Foundation
211 E Chicago Avenue, Suite 700
Chicago, IL 60611

312-337-2169
Fax: 312-337-6329
e-mail: bwilliams@aapd.org
www.aapd.org

The AAPD is the membership organization representing the specialty of pediatric dentistry. Our members serve as primarily care providers for millions of children from infancy through adolescence, providing advanced specialty level of care for infants, children, adolescents and patients with special healthcare needs in private offices, clinics and hospital settings.

4500 members

John S Rutkauskes, Executive Director
C Scott Litch, Deputy Executive Director

2372 American Association of Orthodontics
401 N Lindbergh Boulevard
Saint Louis, MO 63141

314-993-1700
800-424-2841
Fax: 314-997-1745
e-mail: info@aaortho.org
www.aaortho.org/

A professional association of educationally qualified orthodontic specialists dedicated to advancing the art and science of orthodontics and dentofacial orthopedics, improving the health of the public by promoting quality othodontic care, and supporting the successful practice of orthodontics.

2373 American Dental Association
211 E Chicago Avenue
Chicago, IL 60611

312-440-2500
Fax: 312-440-2800
www.ada.org

Professional association of dentists committed to the public's oral health, ethics, science and professional advancement; leading a unified profession through initiatives in advocacy, education, research and the development of standards.

Dr Robert Brandjord, President

Libraries & Resource Centers

2374 University of Illinois at Chicago, Craniofacial Center
College of Medicine
808 S Wood Street
Chicago, IL 60680

312-996-6979
Fax: 312-413-1526

Dr. Allen Goldman, Director

2375 University of Mississippi Medical Center
2500 N State Street
Jackson, MS 39216

601-984-1100
e-mail: cporter@pubaffairs.umsmed.edu
www.umc.edu

The health sciences campus of the University of Mississippi. It houses schools of Medicine, Nursing, Health Related Professions and Dentistry.

Suzanne Miller, MD, Director

Audio Video

2376 Face First
Fanlight Productions
4196 Washington Street, Suite 2
Boston, MA 02131

617-469-4999
800-937-4113
Fax: 617-469-3379
e-mail: fanlight@fanlight.com
www.fanlight.com

Profiles of several people born with facial deformities; they chronicle both physical pain and the pain of rejection, as well as the strengths that have enabled them to achieve successful adult lives.

1998 29 Minutes VHS
ISBN: 1-572952-59-8

Nicole Johnson, Publicity Coordinator

Web Sites

2377 American Academy of Pediatric Dentistry Foundation
www.aapd.org

Supports and promotes education, research, service and policy development that advances the oral health of infants and children through adolescence, including those with special healthcare needs.

2378 Dental Consumer Advisory
www.toothinfo.com/

The purpose of this site is to provide uselful and pracitcal information for the public concerning issues of dental care.

2379 Dental Resources on the Web
www.dental-resources.com

Dental sites for education, practices, laboratories, office supplies, dental care and associations.

Book Publishers

2380 Understanding Dental Health
University Press of Mississippi
3825 Ridgewood Road
Jackson, MS 39211

601-432-6205
800-737-7788
Fax: 601-432-6217
e-mail: press@ihl.state.ms.us
www.upress.stat.ms.us

A user friendly manual on the basics of dental health.

128 pages Hard/Soft cover
ISBN: 1-578060-09-5

DESCRIPTION

2381 DEPRESSION

Involves the following Biologic System(s):
Developmental/Behavioral/Psychiatric Disorders

Depression refers to an emotional state characterized by exaggerated feelings of sadness, discouragement, loneliness, low self-esteem, and despair. These feelings may follow a recent loss or other tragic event. However, if feelings of depression worsen and are prolonged, or occur for no apparent reason, this may indicate a chronic (formerly called "endogenous") depressive disorder. Although clinical depression occurs more commonly among the adult population (2-3 times more common in females than in males, depression may be evident as early as infancy and is increasingly common among adolescents.

Symptoms and findings associated with depression are variable. It has a chronic course with relapses. The mood is typically depressed, irritable, and/or anxious, often accompanied by preoccupation with guilt, decreased ability to concentrate, diminished interest in usual activities (anhedonia), social withdrawal, hopelessness, and recurrent thoughts of death and suicide. Symptoms associated with depression in school-age children are similar to those seen in adults and include overwhelming feelings of sadness, crying, loss of interest in pleasurable activities, eating and sleeping irregularities, and, in some cases, suicidal thoughts (ideation). Some affected children may exhibit symptoms that belie a diagnosis of depression, such as overactivity and aggression. Adolescents with depression may have feelings of hopelessness and helplessness with no corresponding periods of happiness or well-being. However, inappropiate displays of euphoria together with such behavior as truancy, substance abuse, or other antisocial behaviors may also be symptomatic of depression. Other symptoms and findings associated with adolescent depression may include a decline in school grades, boredom, repetitive accidents, drug or alcohol abuse, absenteeism, feelings or delusions of guilt, and thoughts of suicide. Physical symptoms may sometimes include fatigue, headaches, and abdominal pain. Those who are psychotically depressed may experience delusions and hallucinations.

Depression in infants may be precipitated by such events as sudden separation from the mother or caregiver after six months of age (anaclitic depression of infancy) and may be manifested by ceaseless crying, panic, apprehension, withdrawal, and eating and sleeping disturbances. Eventually, indifference and unresponsiveness may develop and result in deficiencies in intellectual, physical, and social development. Endogenous depression may be caused by many different factors including genetic influences, hormonal disturbances, certain medications, infectious or neurologic disorders, physical conditions (i.e., stroke, etc.), certain tumors, nutritional influences, and psychosocial factors. In addition, depression may occur in association with other psychological disorders such as bipolar or other mood disorders (e.g., schizoaffective disorder).

Most persons with depression get treated as outpatients. Treatment of depression most often includes the administration of certain antidepressant medications. Most studies indicate that cognitive, interpersonal, and behavior therapy are effective, especially in combination with antidepressant medications. Electroconvulsive therapy (ECT) is effective but is usually reserved for severely depressed patients or patients who do not respond to or are not tolerant of medications. Children and adolescents with this disorder also often require individual psychotherapy and, in many cases, group and family therapy. Overall, the suicide rate is estimated at 15%. All patients with depression should be be asked gently but directly about suicidal ideas or plans. All communications about self-destruction should be taken seriously.

See also **General Resources** on page 917

See also **General Resources** on page 917

Government Agencies

2382 NIH/National Institute of Mental Health
6001 Executive Boulevard, Room 8184, MSC 9663
Bethesda, MD 20892

301-443-4513
866-615-6464
Fax: 301-443-4279
TTY: 301-443-8431
e-mail: nimhinfo@nih.gov
www.nimh.nih.gov

Conducts strategic planning for specific research areas as well as for the Institute as a whole.

Dr Thomas R Insel, Director

National Associations & Support Groups

2383 Anxiety Disorders Association of America
8730 Georgia Avenue, Suite 600
Silver Spring, MD 20910

240-485-1001
Fax: 240-485-1035
e-mail: anxdis@adaa.org
www.adaa.org

Offers help, support and information for persons with anxiety disorders, manic and depressive disorders and mental illness.

Francine Greenberg, Communications/PR Manager

2384 Depression & Related Affective Disorders Association
Meyer 3-181 600 N Wolfe Street
Baltimore, MD 21287

410-955-4647
Fax: 410-614-3241
e-mail: drada@jhmi.edu
www.drada.org

Provides education, information and support services for individuals with depression of bipolar illness, their families and mental health professionals.

2385 Depression and Bipolar Support Alliance
730 N Franklin Street, Suite 501
Chicago, IL 60610

312-642-0049
800-826-3632
Fax: 312-642-7243
www.dbsalliance.org

Patient-directed organization focusing on the most prevelant mental illnesses- depression and bipolar disorder. Fosters an understanding about the impact and management of these life-threatning illnesses by providing up-to-date, scientifically-based tools and information written in language the general public can understand.

Susan Bergeson, President

2386 Depressives Anonymous: Recovery from Depression
329 E 62nd Street
New York, NY 10021

212-689-2600

Individuals suffering from depression or anxiety. A self-help organization with meetings and sharing of experiences. Conducts research and offers classes. Disseminates information. Publications: Newsletter, three-four times a year. Brochures and pamphlets.

Dr. Helen DeRosis, Founder

2387 Federation of Families for Children's Mental Health
9605 Medical Center Drive, Suite 280
Rockville, MD 20850

240-403-1901
Fax: 240-403-1909
e-mail: ffcmh@ffcmh.org
www.ffcmh.org

The National family run organization is dedicated exclusively to helping children with mental health needs and their families achieve a better quality of life.

Sandra Spencer, Executive Director

2388 NADD: National Association for the Dually Diagnosed
132 Fair Street
Kingston, NY 12401

845-331-4336
800-331-5362
Fax: 845-331-4569
e-mail: info@thenadd.org
www.thenadd.org

Nonprofit organization designed to promote the interests of professional and parent development with resources for individuals who have the coexistence of mental illness and mental retardation. Provides conferences, educational services and training materials to professionals, parents, concerned citizens and service organizations.

Dr Robert Fletcher, CEO
Michelle Jordan, Office Manager

2389 National Alliance for Research on Schizophrenia and Affective Disorders
60 Cutter Mill Road, Suite 404
Great Neck, NY 11021

516-829-0091
800-829-8289
Fax: 516-487-6930
e-mail: info@narsad.org
www.narsad.org

Raises and distributes funds for scientific research into the causes, cures, treatments, and prevention of severe mental illness, primarily schizophrenia and affective disorders.

Stephen G Doochin, Executive Director

2390 National Alliance for the Mentally Ill
2107 Wilson Blvd, Ste 300, Colonial Place Three
Arlington, VA 22201

703-524-7600
800-950-6264
Fax: 703-524-9094
TDD: 703-516-7227
e-mail: info@nami.org
www.nami.org

NAMI is a nonprofit, grassroots, self-help, support and advocacy organization of consumers, families and friends of people with severe mental illness, such as schizophrenia, bipolar disorder, major despressive disorder, obsessive compulsive disorder, anxiety disorders, autism and other severe and persistent mental illnesses that affect the brain.

Suzanne Vogel-Scibilia MD, President

2391 National Anxiety Foundation
3135 Custer Drive
Lexington, KY 40517

859-272-7166
www.lexington-on-line.com/naf.html

Offers information and help to persons with panic disorders, manic and depressive disorders and mental illness.

Stephen Cox MD, President & Medical Director
Linda Vernon Blair, Vice President

2392 National Foundation for Depression
2 Penn Plaza, Suite 1981
New York, NY 10121

212-268-4260

Amy Russell

2393 National Foundation for Depressive Illness
PO Box 2257
New York, NY 10116

212-268-4260
800-248-4344
Fax: 800-248-4344
www.depression.org

Corrects the myths and misconceptions surrounding the illness and helps to reverse the devastating effects of depression. Informs the public, health care providers, health care professionals and corporations about depression, manic depression and provides the information about correct diagnosis and treatment and the availability of qualified doctors and support groups. Psychiatric referral service and information packets on childhood, adolescent depression.

2394 National Organization for Seasonal Affective Disorder (SAD)
19217 Orbit Drive
Gaithersburg, MD 20879

301-869-5908
800-548-3968
Fax: 301-977-2281
e-mail: info@sunbox.com
www.sunbox.com

A newly identified medical disorder characterized by winter symptoms which include fall and winter weight gain, carbohydrate cravings, oversleeping, decreased intrest in normal activities and low mood and energy.

2395 Recovery
802 N Dearborn Street
Chicago, IL 60610

312-337-5661
Fax: 312-337-5756
e-mail: spot@recovery-inc.com
recovery-inc.com

Techniques for controlling behavior, changing attitudes.

Shirley Sachs, Executive Director

State Agencies & Support Groups

2396 Depressive and Manic-Depressive Assocation of Mount Sinai
100 LaSalle Street, Suite 5A
New York, NY 10027

917-445-2399
e-mail: jgg17@columbia.edu
www.columbia.edu/~jgg17/DMDA/PAGE_1.html

The NYC Depressive and Manic-Depressive Group is a support group for persons with mood disorders, depression and bipolar disorder, as well as their family members and friends.

Research Centers

2397 National Alliance for Research on Schizophrenia & Depression
60 Cutter Mill Road, Suite 404
Great Neck, NY 11021

516-829-0091
800-829-8289
Fax: 516-487-6930
e-mail: info@narsad.org
www.narsad.org

Largest private 501 (c) (3) not for profit corporation and registered public chairty. Raises and distributes funds for scientific research into the causes, cures, treatments and prevention of brain disorders.

Stephen G Doochin, Executive Director

2398 University of Pennsylvania, Depression Research Unit
School of Medicine, Department of Psychiatry
3600 Spruce Street
Philadelphia, PA 19104

215-662-3462
Fax: 215-662-6443

Focuses on mental health and depression.

Jay D Amsterdam, MD, Director

2399 University of Texas, Mental Health Clinical Research Center
5323 Harry Hines Boulevard
Dallas, TX 75235

214-648-2951

Research activity of major and atypical depression.

A John Rush, MD, Director

2400 Yale University, Behavioral Medicine Clinic
Yale School of Medicine
333 Cedar Street
New Haven, CT 06510

203-785-4184

Focuses on mental disorders including schizophrenia and depression.

Hoyle Leigh, MD, Director

2401 Yale University, Ribicoff Research Facilities
CT Medical Health Center
34 Park Street
New Haven, CT 06511

203-764-9765
Fax: 203-688-2491

Clinical research in the areas of schizophrenia, depression and mental disorders.

George Heninger, MD, Director

Audio Video

2402 Coping with Depression
New Harbinger Publications
5674 Shattuck Avenue
Oakland, CA 94609

510-652-2002
800-748-6273
Fax: 510-652-5472
e-mail: customerservice@newharbinger.com
newharbinger.com

60 minute videotape that offers a powerful message of hope for anyone struggling with depression.

ISBN: 1-879237-62-8

2403 Cry for Help - How to Help a Friend Who is Depressed or Suicidal
Aquarius Health Care Videos
5 Powderhouse Lane, PO Box 1159
Sherborn, MA 01770

508-651-2963
888-440-2963
Fax: 508-650-4216
e-mail: info@aquariusproductions.com
www.aquariusproductions.com

Most suicidal young people don't really want to die; they just want their pain to end. Teen sucide is often preventable if young people know the signs to look for and the steps to take when they suspect a friend is suicidal. This video teaches young people to recognize the warning signs and to take specific actions to help a friend.

22 Minutes

Donna Kaufman

2404 Day for Night: Recognizing Teenage Depression
DRADA-Depression and Related Affective Disorders
600 N Wolfe Street
Baltimore, MD 21287

410-955-4647
Fax: 410-614-3241

2405 Depression and Manic Depression
Fanlight Productions
47 Halifax Street
Boston, MA 02130

617-469-4999
Fax: 617-469-3379
e-mail: fanlight@tiac.net
www.fanlight.com

This video explores the realities of depression and manic depression, as well as providing an overview of available treatments, and a listing of other resources.

28 minutes

2406 Living with Depression and Manic Depression
New Harbinger Publications
5674 Shattuck Avenue
Oakland, CA 94609

510-652-2002
800-748-6273
Fax: 510-652-5472
e-mail: customerservice@newharbinger.com
newharbinger.com

Describes a program based on years of research and hundreds of interviews with depressed persons. Warm, helpful, and engaging, this tape validates the feelings of people with depression while it encourages positive change.

ISBN: 1-879237-63-6

2407 Why Isn't My Child Happy? A Video Guide About Childhood Depression
ADD WareHouse
300 NW 70th Avenue
Plantation, FL 33317

954-792-8944
800-233-9273
Fax: 954-792-8545
addwarehouse.com

The first of its kind, this new video deals with childhood depression. Informative and frank about this common problem, this book offers helpful guidance for parents and professionals trying to better understand childhood depression. 110 minutes.

Web Sites

2408 AACAP
www.aacap.org

Assisting parents and families in understanding developmental, behavioral, emotional and mental disorders affecting children and adolescents.

2409 Dr. Ivan's Depression Central
www.psycom.net/depression.central.html

This site is the Internet's central clearinghouse for information on all types of depressive disorders and on the most effective tratments for individuals suffering from Major Depression, Manic Depression (Bipolar Disorder), Cyclothymia, Dysthymia and other mood disorders.

2410 Internet Mental Health
www.mentalhealth.com/

Our goal is to improve understanding, diagnosis, and teatment of meantal illness throughout the world.

2411 Mental Health Net
www.mentalhelp.net

We wish to provide the following: to discuss, develop and debate in an open forum the future of the mental health field in America and throughout the world. To help coordinate various components of the mental health field so as to bring about greater communication between them. To educate the public about mental health issues, to promote active collaboration between professionals in all segments of mental health development, implementation and policy.

2412 Online Mendelian Inheritance in Man
www.ncbi.nlm.nih.gov

This database is a catalog of human genes and genetic disorders.

2413 Seasonal Affective Disorder
www.alt.support.depression.seasonal

The SAD Association is a voluntary organization and registered charity which informs the public and health professions about SAD and supports and advises sufferers of the illness.

2414 Understanding and Treating Depression
www.couns.uiuc.edu/depression.htm

Offers an understanding of depression, causes, how to help yourself, things to do, what to avoid while in the depression state, and treatments of the depression.

2415 Wing of Madness: A Depression Guide
www.wingofmadness.com

Is a nonprofit organization dedicated to disseminating information about depression to consumers.

Book Publishers

2416 Anxiety & Depression In Adults & Children
Sage Publications
2455 Teller Road
Newbury Park, CA 91320

805-499-0721

1994 304 pages Softcover
ISBN: 0-803970-21-8

2417 Ask the Doctor: Depression
Andrews McMeel Publishing
PO Box 419150
Kansas City, MO 64141

816-932-6700
800-233-2336
Fax: 212-698-7336

A look at depression, its symptoms, what causes it, and what you can do about it. Learn the difference between mood problems and genuine depression, and how to read warning signs such as sleep abnormalities, nervousness, and suicidal thoughts. Information on chemicals, genetics, and medical solutions.

128 pages Softcover
ISBN: 0-836227-11-5

2418 Coping with Depression
Rosen Publishing Group
29 E 21st Street
New York, NY 10010

800-237-9932
Fax: 888-436-4643
e-mail: rosenpub@tribeca.ios.com
www.rosenpublishing.com

With an emphasis on life's myriad difficulties, the authors help teens find practical ways to cope with depression.

ISBN: 0-823919-51-0

2419 Dealing with Depression: Five Ways to Help
Haworth Press
10 Alice Street
Binghamton, NY 13904

607-722-8277
Fax: 607-722-1424

1995
ISBN: 1-560249-33-1

2420 Depression and Its Treatment
Warner Books
1271 Avenue of the Americas
New York, NY 10020

212-522-7200

A layman's guide to help one understand and cope with America's number one mental health problem.

157 pages

2421 Depression, the Mood Disease
Johns Hopkins University Press
2715 N Charles Street
Baltimore, MD 21218

410-516-6900
800-537-5487
Fax: 410-516-6998

This book explores the many faces of an illness that will affect as many as 36 million Americans at some point in their lives. Updated to reflect state-of-the-art treatment.

1993 240 pages
ISBN: 0-801851-84-X

2422 Depressive Illnesses: Treatments Bring New Hope
Superintendent of Documents
PO Box 371954
Pittsburgh, PA 15250
202-512-2250

Offers the general public an overview of the various depressive illnesses. Topics include causes, symptoms and types of depression, clinical evaluation and treatment, helpful suggestions for family and friends, and other sources of information.

28 pages

2423 Encyclopedia of Depression
Facts on File
Department M274, 11 Penn Plaza
New York, NY 10001
212-290-8090
800-322-8755
Fax: 212-678-3633

This volume defines and explains all terms and topics relating to depression.

170 pages Hardbound

2424 Essential Guide to Psychiatric Drugs
Saint Martin's Press
175 5th Avenue
New York, NY 10010
212-674-5151
800-221-7945
Fax: 212-420-9314

Basic information on 123 drugs used for depression, anxiety and bipolar illness.

2425 Everything You Need To Know About Depression
Rosen Publishing Group
29 E 21st Street
New York, NY 10010
212-777-3017
800-237-9932
Fax: 212-436-4643
e-mail: rosenpub@tribeca.ios.com

An important resource for teens who are looking for help with depression.

Grades 7-12
ISBN: 0-823926-06-0

2426 Handbook of School-Based Interventions
Courage to Change
PO Box 1268
Newburgh, NY 12551
800-440-4003
Fax: 800-772-6499

Comprehensive volume that describes interventions for virtually every major problem behavior students may exhibit from K-12. All interventions are research-based and guidance is given for practical application of the techniques. Topics range from dishonesty, academic performance, procrastination and low self-esteem to obsessive-compulsive behavior, substance abuse, AIDS and depression.

512 pages Hardcover

2427 Help Me, I'm Sad
Penguin Putnam
PO Box 999
Bergenfield, NJ 07621
800-526-0275
Fax: 800-227-9604

Helping and understanding a child with depression.

2428 Helping Your Child Cope with Depression and Suicidal Thoughts
Jossey-Bass
111 River Street
Hoboken, NJ 07030
201-748-6000
800-956-7739
Fax: 201-748-6088
www.josseybass.com

Shows parents how to learn to talk, listen, and communicate effectively with a depressed child; signs to watch for and situations which may cause a wish to commit suicide.

192 pages
ISBN: 0-787908-44-4

2429 Helping Your Depressed Child
Prima Publishing
PO Box 1260
Rocklin, CA 95677
916-624-5718

Reasurring guide to the causes and treatment of childhood and adolescent depression.

284 pages

2430 Kid Power Tactics for Dealing with Depression & Parent's Survival Guide
Childs Work/Childs Play
135 Dupont Street
Plainville, NY 11803
800-962-1141
Fax: 800-262-1886
e-mail: info@Childswork.com
Childswork.com

2 volume set was wriiten by a child who suffered from depression and his mother. Plain language and a wealth of information for children ages 8 and over, plus their parents and teachers.

2431 Mood Apart
Basic Books
10 E 53rd Street
New York, NY 10022
212-207-7057

An overview of depression and manic depression and the available treatments for them.

363 pages

2432 Overcoming Depression
Harper & Row
10 E 53rd Street
New York, NY 10022
212-207-7000

1987 318 pages Softcover

2433 Panic Disorder in the Medical Setting
Superintendent of Documents
PO Box 371954
Pittsburgh, PA 15250
202-512-2250

This book serves the primary care physicians as a helpful guide in recognizing and treating panic disorder in patients and in identifying those who need psychiatric consultation or referrals.

1993 135 pages

2434 Prozac Nation: Young & Depressed in America, A Memoir
Houghton Mifflin Company
222 Berkeley Street
Boston, MA 02116
617-351-3698
800-225-3362

Struck with depression at 11, now 27, Wurtzel chronicles her struggle with the illness. Witty, terrifying and sometimes funny, it tells the story of a young life almost destroyed by depression.

317 pages

2435 Psychotherapy of Severe and Mild Depression
Jason Aronson
400 Keystone Industrial Park
Dunmore, PA 18521

800-782-0015
Fax: 201-840-7242
www.aronson.com

464 pages Softcover
ISBN: 1-568211-46-5

2436 Report of the Secretary's Task Force on Youth Suicide
Superintendent of Documents
PO Box 371954
Pittsburgh, PA 15250

202-512-2250

A comprehensive review of information about youth suicide. The task force recommendations are presented in Volume 1.

110 pages

2437 Sad Days, Glad Days
National Alliance for the Mentally Ill
PO Box 753
Waldorf, MD 20604

703-524-7600
www.NIMF.org

Helps five to nine-year-olds understand a parent's depression.

1995

2438 Suicide, Why?
National Alliance for the Mentally Ill
PO Box 753
Waldorf, MD 20604

703-524-7600
www.NAMI.org

An authoritative book, noting that suicide is usually caused by brain disorders.

1989

2439 Surprising Truth About Depression: Medical Breakthroughs That Can Work
Zondervan
5300 Patterson SE
Grand Rapids, MI 49530

616-698-6900
Fax: 616-698-3439
www.zondervan.com

1994 224 pages Softcover
ISBN: 0-310401-01-1

2440 Treating Depressed Children
New Harbinger Publications
5674 Shattuck Avenue
Oakland, CA 94609

800-748-6273
Fax: 510-652-5472
e-mail: customerservice@newharbinger.com
www.newharbinger.com

This book explains a 12-session treatment program to help children change their negative thoughts, gain confidence and recognize their emotions. These actions are achieved with the help of cartoons and role-playing games.

160 pages Hardcover
ISBN: 1-572240-61-X

Laseu Pfaff, Publicist

2441 Treating Depression
Jossey-Bass
111 River Street
Hoboken, NJ 07030

201-748-6000
800-956-7739
Fax: 201-748-6088
www.josseybass.com

Offers guidelines and specific models for intervention in the treatment of numerous types and subtypes of depression. Also will assist you in deciding if it is appropriate to prescribe medication, if psychotherapy is the proper course of action, or if it is best to use a combination of medication and psychotherapy.

1997 223 pages
ISBN: 0-787915-85-8

2442 Understanding Depression
University Press of Mississippi
3825 Ridgewood Road
Jackson, MS 39211

601-432-6205
800-737-7788
Fax: 601-432-6217
e-mail: press@ihl.state.ms.us
www.upress.state.ms.us

A clear explanation for those who know the illness personally and for those who want to understand them.

120 pages Hardcover/Ppbck
ISBN: 1-578061-68-7

2443 Understanding Your Teenager's Depression
Berkley Books
200 Madison Avenue
New York, NY 10016

212-951-8800

1994 352 pages Softcover
ISBN: 0-399518-56-8

2444 When Nothing Matters Anymore: A Survival Guide for Depressed Teens
Free Spirit Publishing
217 5th Avenue N
Minneapolis, MN 55401

612-338-2068
800-735-7323
Fax: 612-337-5050
e-mail: help4kids@freespirit.com
freespirit.com

Written for teens with depression and those who feel despondent, dejected or alone. This powerful book offers help, hope, and potentially lifesaving facts and advice.

176 pages
ISBN: 1-575420-36-8

Penne Post, Tradesales Associate

2445 Working with Children and Adolescents in Groups
Courage to Change
PO Box 1268
Newburgh, NY 12551

800-440-4003
Fax: 800-772-6499

Step-by-step guide that discusses how to effectively treat problem behavior in children and adolescents using small groups. Based on empirical research and their own work with groups, the authors show how a variety of approaches can be effectively combined to help resolve such problem behaviors as fighting and low self-esteem.

384 pages Hard Cover

2446 Yesterday's Tomorrow
Hazelden
15251 Pleasant Valley Road
Center City, MN 55012

612-257-4010
800-328-9000
Fax: 917-339-0325
www.hazelden.org

A meditation book that shows why and how recovery works, from the author's own experiences.

432 pages Softcover
ISBN: 1-568381-60-3

Magazines

2447 New Message
Emotions Anonymous
PO Box 4245
Saint Paul, MN 55104

651-647-9712
Fax: 651-647-1593
e-mail: caisc@mtn.org
EmotionsAnonymous.org

Quarterly magazine.

Karen Mead, Executive Director

Newsletters

2448 National Foundation for Depressive Illness
PO Box 2257
New York, NY 10116

212-268-4260
800-248-4344
Fax: 212-268-4434
www.depression.org

Information on the myths and misconceptions surrounding the illness. Informs the public, health care providers, healthcare professionals and corporations about depression and manic depression, and provides the information about correct diagnosis and treatment and the availability of qualified doctors and support groups.

4 pages Quarterly

Amy C Russell, Editor

2449 Outreach
Depression and Bipolar Support Alliance
730 N Franklin Street, Suite 501
Chicago, IL 60610

800-826-3632
Fax: 312-642-7243
www.dbsalliance.org

Quarterly publication serving members and constituents of the organization. National DMDA educates patients, families, professionals, and the public concerning the nature of depressive and manic-depressive illnesses as treatable medical diseases; fosters self-help for patients and families; eliminates discrimination and stigma; improves access to care; advocates for research toward the elimination of these illnesses.

Lydia Lewis, Executive Director
Gloria Pope, External Relations Director

2450 Smooth Sailing
Depression & Related Affective Disorders Assoc.
Meyer 3-181, 600 N Wolfe Street
Baltimore, MD 21287

410-955-4647
Fax: 410-614-3241
e-mail: drada@jhmi.edu
www.drada.org

Contains a variety of information including medical, educational and first hand experiences about mood disorders. Newsletter is free with membership.

Quarterly

Pamphlets

2451 Depression Is a Treatable Illness: A Patients Guide
Department of Health & Human Services
2101 E Jefferson Street, Suite 501
Rockville, MD 20852

301-217-1245

Tells about major depressive disorder, which is only one form of depressive illness. This booklet answers important questions regarding this disorder and gives information on where to go for more help.

2452 Depression in Children and Adolescents: A Fact Sheet for Physicians
National Institute of Mental Health
6001 Executive Boulevard
Bethesda, MD 20892

301-443-4513
Fax: 301-443-4279
TTY: 301-443-8431
e-mail: nimhinfo@nih.gov
nih.gov/publicat

Discusses the scope of the problem and the screening tools used in evaluating children with depression.

8 pages

2453 Let's Talk About Depression
Superintendent of Documents
PO Box 371954
Pittsburgh, PA 15250

202-512-2250

Targeted especially for inner-city youth. The colorful design will capture attention and focus on depression in a way that young people will understand and identify with.

2454 Let's Talk Facts About Childhood Disorders
American Psychiatric Association
1400 K Street NW
Washington, DC 20005

202-682-6220

Offers information on depression and depressive disorders including the causes, symptoms, treatments, anxiety, and various other phobias.

2455 Living Without Depression & Manic Depression: A Workbook
National Alliance for the Mentally Ill
PO Box 753
Waldorf, MD 20604

703-524-7600
www.NAMI.org

Workbook offering checklists and helpful advice targeted for individuals whose depressive illness is stabilized.

1994

2456 Major Depression in Children and Adolescents
Center for Mental Health Services
PO Box 42490
Washington, DC 20015

800-789-2647
Fax: 301-984-8796
e-mail: ken@mentalhealth.org
mentalhealth.org

This fact sheet defines depression and its signs, identifies types of help available, and suggests what parents or other caregivers can do.

2 pages

2457 Now We Can Successfully Treat the Illness Called Depression

National Foundation for Depressive Illness (NAFDI)
PO Box 2257
New York, NY 10116

212-268-4260
800-248-4344
Fax: 212-268-4434
www.depression.org

Basic information on depression and manic depression, gives symptoms, encourages persons who have symptoms to seek medical treatment. Tips on managing depressive illness.

Amy C Russell, Editor

2458 Panic Disorder

National Institutes of Health
5600 Fishers Lane, Room 7C-02
Rockville, MD 20857

301-443-4707
Fax: 301-443-6000

Written for the lay public, this pamphlet contains a description of panic disorder, gives the symptoms, describes treatment methods, and encourages the person who has the symptoms to seek treatment.

2459 Plain Talk About Depression

Superintendent of Documents
PO Box 371954
Pittsburgh, PA 15250

202-512-2250

A flyer discussing types of depression, major depression; symptoms and causes.

2460 Understanding Panic Disorder

National Institutes of Health
5600 Fishers Lane, Room 7C-02
Rockville, MD 20857

301-443-4707
Fax: 301-443-6000

Offers information on what panic disorder is, symptoms, causes, treatment, medications and therapy.

2461 Useful Information on Phobias and Panic

Superintendent of Documents
PO Box 371954
Pittsburgh, PA 15250

202-512-2250

This booklet provides information on both phobias and panic. Symptoms, causes and treatments of these disorders are referred to. If you know someone who is excessively fearful, this booklet will be of great help to them in understanding their problem.

40 pages 50 copies

2462 What to Do When a Friend Is Depressed: Guide for Students

Superintendent of Documents
PO Box 371954
Pittsburgh, PA 15250

202-512-2250

Offers information on depression and its symptoms and suggests things a young person can do to guide a depressed friend in finding help.

DESCRIPTION

2463 DIABETES MELLITUS

Involves the following Biologic System(s):

Endocrinologic Disorders

Diabetes mellitis refers to an inability of the body to utilize glucose. There are two types of DM: Insulin-dependent diabetes mellitus, referred to as Type I diabetes, is a disorder in which insufficient production of insulin by the pancreas results in abnormally high levels of the sugar glucose in the blood. Insulin is a hormone that regulates and stabilizes blood glucose levels by promoting the movement of energy-rich glucose into body cells for energy production or into the liver and fat cells for storage. Type I diabetes may also cause impaired fat metabolism and long-term complications affecting certain large and small blood vessels (angiopathy), the nerve-rich membranes at the back of the eyes (retinas), skin, kidneys, nerves, or other tissues of the body. The exact cause of Type I diabetes is unknown. However, researchers speculate that certain environmental factors, such as a viral infection, may inappropriately trigger the immune system to destroy insulin-producing cells within the pancreas (beta cells), resulting in severe insulin deficiency. Genetic factors are also thought to play some role in causing a predisposition for the disorder.

Type I diabetes is the major form of diabetes affecting children. It affects 1 million patients in the United States, most often in young people, 10-14 years of age. The other major type of diabetes, Type II diabetes, may be characterized by a resistance to the effects of insulin. Although this type of diabetes may occur at any age, it most commonly becomes apparent in middle-aged or older people, but is increasingly common during childhood and adolescence. It is most common in obese patients. In some children, various forms of diabetes may occur secondary to certain genetic multisystemic disorders that affect the pancreas, such as cystic fibrosis; other endocrine disorders, such as Cushing's syndrome; the administration of particular drugs; or exposure to certain poisons.

In most children with Type I diabetes, associated symptoms and findings may appear to occur suddenly and may include excessive urine production by the kidneys, causing increased urination (polyuria) and excessive thirst (polydipsia); weight loss; and abnormally increased hunger (polyphagia). Additional abnormalities may include exhaustion, blurred vision, abnormal sensations (paresthesias) in the hands and feet, and increased irritability. Without prompt diagnosis and treatment, symptoms may rapidly progress to a metabolic condition known as ketoacidosis. Because of deficient insulin production, the body's cells begin to rely on sources of energy other than glucose, causing an excessive breakdown of fats and an abnormal accumulation of certain chemical compounds (ketones) in body tissues and fluids. Early symptoms associated with ketoacidosis may be relatively mild, including increased urination, vomiting and dehydration but, without appropriate treatment, coma and potentially life-threatening complications may occur. The treatment of ketoacidosis may include the immediate administration of intravenous fluids; replacement of electrolytes, such as sodium and potassium; initiation of intravenous insulin therapy; measures to prevent or appropriately treat increased fluid pressure within the brain; and other therapies as required.

Patients with either Type I or Type II diabetes may eventually develop certain long-term complications associated with the disease. Complications may include thickening and leaking of the walls of certain small blood vessels, narrowing of medium and large-size arteries due to plaque development (atherosclerosis), abnormally high blood pressure (hypertension), poor blood circulation, and problems affecting the eyes, kidneys, nerves, and skin. For example, kidney damage may result in impaired kidney function and kidney failure; damage to blood vessels within the nerve-rich membranes at the back of the eyes (diabetic retinopathy) may lead to visual impairment; and nerve damage may cause weakness or the loss of certain sensations, such as changes in temperature or pressure, increasing the risk of injury. In addition, impaired blood supply to certain skin areas may increase the risk of developing skin sores (ulcers). Poor wound healing and susceptibility to infected foot ulcers may lead to localized loss of tissue (necrosis), potentially requiring amputation. Diet is central to management of diabetes and must be individualized according to the patient's activity level, food preferences, and need to attain and maintain ideal weight. Regular exercise is also correlated with better glucose control. Individuals with Type I diabetes take insulin, delivered either by injection or by insulin pump. Type II diabetics can take oral blood-sugar lowering (hypoglycemic) drugs that potentiate insulin secretion. Other drugs help regulate glucose storage or release.

See also **General Resources** on page 917

National Associations & Support Groups

2464 American Association of Diabetes Educators
100 W Monroe Street, Suite 400
Chicago, IL 60603

312-424-2427
800-832-6874
www.aabenet.org

An independent, multidisciplinary organization of health professionals involved in teaching persons with diabetes. The mission is to enhance the competence of health professionals who teach persons with diabetes education and care for all those affected by diabetes.

Cheryl Hunt, RN, MSED, CDE, President

2465 American Diabetes Association
1701 North Beauregard Street
Alexandria, VA 22311

703-549-1500
800-342-2383
Fax: 703-549-6995
www.diabetes.org

The nation's leading voluntary organization concerned with diabetes and its complications. The mission of the organization is to prevent and cure diabetes and to improve the lives of persons with diabetes. Offers a network of 52 affiliates with over 55,000 volunteers, including a professional membership of more than 10,000 physicians, social workers, nutritionists, educators and nurses.

Bruce R Zimmerman, MD

2466 Juvenile Diabetes Foundation International
120 Wall Street
New York, NY 10005

212-785-9500
800-533-2873
Fax: 212-785-9595
e-mail: info@jdfcure.com
www.jdrf.org

Focuses energies on fund-raising, referrals, educational materials and information pertaining to juvenile diabetes.

Stephen H Leeper, DDS, President

2467 National Diabetes Action Network for the Blind
National Federation of the Blind
1800 Johnson Street, Suite 2
Baltimore, MD 21230

410-659-9314
Fax: 410-685-5653

Leading support and information organization of persons losing vision due to diabetes. Provides personal contact and resource information with other blind diabetics about non-visual techniques of independently managing diabetes, monitoring glucose levels, measuring insulin and other matters concerning diabetes. Publishes Voice of the Diabetic, the leading publication about diabetes and blindness.

State Agencies & Support Groups

2468 Center for Disabilities and Development
University of Iowa Hospitals and Clinics
100 Hawkins Drive
Iowa City, IA 52242

319-353-6900
877-686-0031
e-mail: cdd-webmaster@uiowa.edu
www.healthcare.uiowa.edu/cdd

A trusted resource for healthcare, training, research and information for people with disabilities that include: behavior disorders, brain injury, cerebral palsy, diabetes, down syndrome, learning disabilities, mental retardation, sleep disorders and spina bifida.

Elayne Sexsmith, Administrator
Amy Mikelson, Supervisor Info Resource Service

Libraries & Resource Centers

2469 National Diabetes Information Clearinghouse
One Information Way
Bethesda, MD 20205

301-654-3327
800-860-8747
Fax: 301-907-8906
e-mail: ndic@info.niddk.nih.gov
www.kidney.niddk.nih.gov

Offers various materials, resources, books, pamphlets and more for persons and families in the area of diabetes.

Research Centers

2470 Center for the Partially Sighted
12301 Wilshire Boulevard, Suite 600
Los Angeles, CA 90025

310-458-3501
Fax: 310-458-8179
e-mail: info@low-vision.org
www.low-vision.org

Provides professional, comprehensive vision rehabilitation services to visually impaired people of all ages. For those whose sight is severely limited due to macular degeneration, diabetic retinopathy, glaucoma, retinal detachment, stroke or other conditions not correctable medically or surgically.

Audio Video

2471 Diabetes: Not So Sweet
Fanlight Productions
47 Halifax Street
Boston, MA 02130

617-469-4999
Fax: 617-469-3379
e-mail: fanlight@fanlight.com
www.fanlight.com

Exciting new approaches to the prevention and control of diabetes, and a look at its prevalence in Native American communities in particular.

47 minutes

2472 Juvenile Diabetes
Fanlight Productions
47 Halifax Street
Boston, MA 02130

617-469-4999
Fax: 617-469-3379
e-mail: fanlight@fanlight.com
www.fanlight.com

Features a number of youngsters with diabetes, and stresses the importance of young people managing as much of their own care as possible.

28 minutes

Web Sites

2473 Mediconsult
www.mediconsult.com

We are committed to provide excellent and professional services to our business partners. Through a team approach we will develop, provide and continuously improve our knowledge and competency. We work towards the betterment of healthcare delivery systems for the community.

2474 National Diabetes Information Clearinghouse
www.kidney.niddk.nih.gov

The National Kidney and Urologic Diseases Information Clearinghouse is an information dissemination service of the National Institute of Diabetes and Digestive and Kidney Diseases.

Book Publishers

2475 Diabetes 101
Wiley
1 Wiley Drive
Somerset, NJ 08875

732-469-4400
800-225-5945
Fax: 732-302-2300
e-mail: bookinfo@wiley.com
www.wiley.com

Revised and expanded second edition. A layman's guide to everything you need to know to live healthfully with diabetes.

175 pages
ISBN: 1-565610-24-5

2476 Diabetes Dictionary
National Diabetes Information Clearinghouse
2 Information Way
Bethesda, MD 20892

301-654-3810
Fax: 301-907-8906
e-mail: nddic@info.niddk.nih.gov
www.niddk.nih.gov

Illustrated glossary of more than 300 diabetes-related terms.

2477 Diabetes Medical Nutition Therapy
American Diabetes Association
1660 Duke Street, Suite 100
Alexandria, VA 22314

800-232-3472
Fax: 703-549-6995
www.diabetes.org

A professional guide to management and nutrition education resources. Provides in-depth coverage of nutrition assessment, goal setting, intervention, and outcome evaluation. Information is provided on specific resources and case studies are cited for practical examples.

2478 Diabetes Teaching Guide for People Who Use Insulin
Joslin Diabetes Center
1 Joslin Place
Boston, MA 02215

617-732-2400

Discusses the causes of diabetes, the role of diet and exercise, meal planning and complications. Also provides information on drawing blood, mixing and injecting insulin.

2479 Endocrine & Metabolic Disorders Sourcebook
Omnigraphics
PO Box 625
Holmes, PA 19043

800-234-1340
Fax: 800-875-1340
e-mail: info@omnigraphics.com
omnigraphics.com

Basic information for the lay person about pancreatic and insulin-related disorders such as pancreatitis, diabetes and hypoglycemia; adrenal gland disorders such as Cushing's syndrome, Addison's disease and congenital adrenal hyperplasia; pituitary gland disorders such as growth hormone deficiency,

acromegaly and pituitary tumors; and thyroid disorders such as hypothyroidism, Grave's disease, Hashimoto's disease and goiter.

574 pages
ISBN: 0-780802-07-1

2480 Even Little Kids Get Diabetes
Albert Whitman & Company
6340 Oakton Street
Morton Grove, IL 60053

847-531-0033
800-255-7675
Fax: 847-531-0039
www.awhitmanco.com

A preschooler tells how when she was only two, that she was diagnosed with this common disease and describes her daily treatment and the precautions her family must observe.

ISBN: 0-807521-58-2

Joseph Boyd, President
Joe Campbell, Customer Service

2481 Everyone Likes to Eat
Wiley
1 Wiley Drive
Somerset, NJ 08875

732-469-4400
800-225-5945
Fax: 732-302-2300
e-mail: custserv@wiley.com
www.wiley.com

Revised and up-to-date second edition. How children can eat most of the foods they enjoy and still take care of their diabetes. Intended for elementary-school-age children, this guide is filled with activities, puzzles, and problem-solving exercises.

ISBN: 1-565610-26-1

2482 Grilled Cheese
American Diabetes Association
1660 Duke Street, Suite 100
Alexandria, VA 22314

800-232-3472
Fax: 703-549-6995
www.diabetes.org

Story designed to ease children's fears and frustrations of having diabetes.

2483 If Your Child Has Diabetes: An Answer Book for Parents
Putnam Publishing Group
200 Madison Avenue
New York, NY 10016

212-951-8400

Provides information and recommendations for parents of children with diabetes on subjects such as school, recreation, medical and life insurance and employment as well as general information about diabetes.

2484 In Control: Guide for Teens with Diabetes
Wiley
1 Wiley Drive
Somerset, NJ 08875

732-469-4400
800-225-5945
Fax: 732-302-2300
e-mail: custserv@wiley.com
www.wiley.com

Dispels myths and tackles the real issues that teens with diabetes face. Teaches how to care for their diabetes without letting it get in the way of their lives.

ISBN: 1-565610-61-X

2485 Kiss the Candy Days Good-Bye
Delacorte Press
1540 Broadway
New York, NY 10036

212-354-6500

This book focuses on Jimmy who is surprised to learn he has diabetes after seeming so healthy and fit. The story contains information on symptoms and the dangers of untreated diabetes.

2486 Let's Talk About Diabetes
Rosen Publishing Group's PowerKids Press
29 E 21st Street
New York, NY 10010

212-777-3017
800-237-9932
Fax: 888-436-4643
e-mail: rosenpub@tribeca.ios.com
www.powerkidspress.com

Defines diabetes and shows how a child can live a very normal life with the disease. Grades K-5.

24 pages
ISBN: 0-823951-96-0

2487 Life with Diabetes: A Series of Teaching Outlines
American Diabetes Association
1660 Duke Street, Suite 100
Alexandria, VA 22314

800-232-3472
Fax: 703-549-6995
www.diabetes.org

Presents a comprehensive curriculum for diabetes education. Each outline includes a statement of purpose, pre-requisites for attending the session, materials needed for teaching the session, recommended teaching method, a content outline, instructor notes, and evaluation and documentation plan, and suggested readings related to each topic.

2488 Raising a Child with Diabetes: A Guide for Parents
American Diabetes Association
1660 Duke Street, Suite 100
Alexandria, VA 22314

800-232-3472
Fax: 703-549-6995
www.diabetes.org

You'll learn how to help your child adjust to insulin, to allow for favorite foods, have a busy schedule and still feel healthy and strong, negotiate the twists and turns of being different, and much more.

Magazines

2489 Countdown
Juvenile Diabetes Foundation International
432 Park Avenue S
New York, NY 10016

212-889-7575
Fax: 212-532-7891

Offers the latest news and information in diabetes research and treatment to everyone from an international arena of diabetes investigators to parents of small children with diabetes, from physicians to school teachers, from pharmacists to corporate executives.

Sandy Dylak, Editor

2490 Diabetes Forecast
American Diabetes Association
166 Duke Street, Suite 100
Alexandria, VA 22314

800-232-3472
Fax: 703-549-6995
www.diabetes.org

The monthly lifestyle magazine for people with diabetes, featuring complete, in-depth coverage of all aspects of living with diabetes.

2491 Voice of the Diabetic
National Federation of the Blind
1800 Johnson Street, Suite 2
Baltimore, MD 21230

410-659-9314
Fax: 410-685-5653

The leading publication in the diabetes field. Each issue addresses the problems and concerns of diabetes, with a special emphasis for those who have lost vision due to diabetes. Available in print and on cassette.

Journals

2492 Diabetes
American Diabetes Association
166 Duke Street, Suite 100
Alexandria, VA 22314

800-232-3472
Fax: 703-549-6995
www.diabetes.org

A peer-reviewed journal focusing on laboratory research.

2493 Diabetes Care
American Diabetes Association
166 Duke Street, Suite 100
Alexandria, VA 22314

800-232-3472
Fax: 703-549-6995
www.diabetes.org

A peer-reviewed journal emphasizing reviews, documentaries and original research on topics of interest to clinicians.

2494 Diabetes Spectrum: From Research to Practice
American Diabetes Association
166 Duke Street, Suite 100
Alexandria, VA 22314

800-232-3472
Fax: 703-549-6995
www.diabetes.org

A journal translating research into practice and focusing on diabetes education and counseling.

Newsletters

2495 Clinical Diabetes
American Diabetes Association
166 Duke Street, Suite 100
Alexandria, VA 22314

800-232-3472
Fax: 703-549-6995
www.diabetes.org

A bimonthly newsletter providing practical treatment information for primary care physicians.

2496 Diabetes Advisor
American Diabetes Association
166 Duke Street, Suite 100
Alexandria, VA 22314

800-232-3472
Fax: 703-549-6995
www.diabetes.org

Offers informative articles and research in the area of diabetes for professionals and patients. Offers facts and research on diagnosis, symptoms, technology and the newest devices for persons with diabetes, as well as referral and hotline numbers.

2497 Diabetes Dateline
National Diabetes Information Clearinghouse
2 Information Way
Bethesda, MD 20892

301-654-3810
Fax: 301-907-8906
e-mail: nddic@info.niddk.nih.gov
www.niddk.nih.gov

2498 Diabetes Educator
American Association of Diabetes Educators
444 N Michigan Avenue, Suite 1240
Chicago, IL 60611

312-424-2426
800-338-3633
Fax: 312-424-2427
www.aadenet.org

Offers information to health professionals working with persons with diabetes.

James J Balija, Executive Director

2499 Kid's Corner
American Diabetes Association
166 Duke Street, Suite 100
Alexandria, VA 22314

800-232-3472
Fax: 703-549-6995
www.diabetes.org

A mini-magazine for kids that offers word searches, puzzles and jokes-plus an encouraging story in each issue about kids with diabetes.

Pamphlets

2500 Alternative Ways To Take Insulin
Information Clearinghouse
2 Information Way
Bethesda, MD 20892

301-654-3810
Fax: 301-907-8906
e-mail: nddic@info.niddk.nih.gov
www.niddk.nih.gov

2501 Children with Diabetes
2 Information Way
Bethesda, MD 20892

301-654-3810
Fax: 301-907-8906
e-mail: nddic@info.niddk.nih.gov
www.niddk.nih.gov

2502 Complementary and Alternative Therapies for Diabetes Treatment
2 Information Way
Bethesda, MD 20892

301-654-3810
Fax: 301-907-8906
e-mail: nddic@info.niddk.nih.gov
www.niddk.nih.gov

2503 Diabetes Insipidus
2 Information Way
Bethesda, MD 20892

301-654-3810
Fax: 301-907-8906
e-mail: nddic@info.niddk.nih.gov
www.niddk.nih.gov

2504 Diabetes Overview
2 Information Way
Bethesda, MD 20892

301-654-3810
Fax: 301-907-8906
e-mail: nddic@info.niddk.nih.gov
www.niddk.nih.gov

2505 Diabetes in African Americans
2 Information Way
Bethesda, MD 20892

301-654-3810
Fax: 301-907-8906
e-mail: nddic@info.niddk.nih.gov
www.niddk.nih.gov

2506 Diabetes in Hispanic Americans
2 Information Way
Bethesda, MD 20892

301-654-3810
Fax: 301-907-8906
e-mail: nddic@info.niddk.nih.gov
www.niddk.nih.gov

2507 Diabetic Neuropathy: the Nerve Damage of Diabetes
2 Information Way
Bethesda, MD 20892

301-654-3810
Fax: 301-907-8906
e-mail: nddic@info.niddk.nih.gov
www.niddk.nih.gov

2508 Diabetics Control and Complications Trial
2 Information Way
Bethesda, MD 20892

301-654-3810
Fax: 301-907-8906
e-mail: nddic@info.niddk.nih.gov
www.niddk.nih.gov

2509 Financial Help for Diabetics Care
Information Clearinghouse
2 Information Way
Bethesda, MD 20892

301-654-3810
Fax: 301-907-8906
e-mail: nddic@info.niddk.nih.gov
www.niddk.nih.gov

2510 Gastoparesis in Diabetes
Information Clearinghouse
2 Information Way
Bethesda, MD 20892

301-654-3810
Fax: 301-907-8906
e-mail: nddic@info.niddk.nih.gov
www.niddk.nih.gov

2511 Glycemic Index and Diabetes
Information Clearinghouse
2 Information Way
Bethesda, MD 20892

301-654-3810
Fax: 301-907-8906
e-mail: nddic@info.niddk.nih.gov
www.niddk.nih.gov

2512 I Have Diabetes: How Much Should I Eat?
2 Information Way
Bethesda, MD 20892

301-654-3810
Fax: 301-907-8906
e-mail: nddic@info.niddk.nih.gov
www.niddk.nih.gov

2513 I Have Diabetes: What Should I Eat?
2 Information Way
Bethesda, MD 20892

301-654-3810
Fax: 301-907-8906
e-mail: nddic@info.niddk.nih.gov
www.niddk.nih.gov

2514 I Have Diabetes: When Should I Eat?
2 Information Way
Bethesda, MD 20892

301-654-3810
Fax: 301-907-8906
e-mail: nddic@info.niddk.nih.gov
www.niddk.nih.gov

2515 Joint and Bone Conditions Related to Diabetes
Information Clearinghouse
2 Information Way
Bethesda, MD 20892

301-654-3810
Fax: 301-907-8906
e-mail: nddic@info.niddk.nih.gov
www.niddk.nih.gov

2516 Kidney Disease of Diabetes
Information Clearinghouse
1 Information Way
Bethesda, MD 20892

301-654-3820
Fax: 301-907-8906
e-mail: ndoc@info.niddk.nih.gov
www.niddk.nih.gov

2517 Looking for Diabetes Recipes and Cookbooks
2 Information Way
Bethesda, MD 20892

301-654-3810
Fax: 301-907-8906
e-mail: nddic@info.niddk.nih.gov
www.niddk.nih.gov

2518 Skin Problems and Diabetes
2 Information Way
Bethesda, MD 20892

301-654-3810
Fax: 301-907-8906
e-mail: nddic@info.niddk.nih.gov
www.niddk.nih.gov

2519 Travel and Diabetes
2 Information Way
Bethesda, MD 20892

301-654-3810
Fax: 301-907-8906
e-mail: nddic@info.niddk.nih.gov
www.niddk.nih.gov

Camps

2520 American Diabetes Association
149 Madison Avenue
New York, NY

212-725-4925
888-888-DIA
Fax: 212-725-8916
www.diabetes.org

The American Diabetes Association provides research, and provides information and advocacy for people with diabetes and their families. The Asssociation also provides seminars for health care professionals.

Lynne Perry

2521 Camp Discovery American Diabetes Association
837 S Hillside
Wichita, KS 800-3

316-684-6091
800-800-362
Fax: 316-684-5675
e-mail: lgiles@diabetes.org
www.diabetes.org

Offers young people with diabetes a week of fun at rock springs 4-H Center. Special attention to diabetes makes Camp Discovery a safe environment for active youth while providing valuable diabetes management education. Call the American Diabetes Association-Kansas area office for more information.

Lindsay Giles, District Manager

2522 Camp Joslin
1 Joslin Plaza
Boston, MA

617-735-1925
Fax: 617-732-2455
e-mail: sarah.gorman@joslin.harvard.edu
www.joslin.org

For boys, ages 7-16, with diabetes. This program offers active summer sports and activities, supplemented by medical treatment and diabetes education. Coed Winter Camp and Coed Weekend Retreats are offered during the school year. Tuition: $625/wk-scholarships available.

Michael Kasparian, Camp Director
Sarah Gorman, Camp Coordinator

2523 Camp de los Ninos - Diabetes Society
1165 Lincoln Avenue
San Jose, CA 800-9

408-287-3785
800-800-989
Fax: 408-287-2701
e-mail: camp@diabetesscv.org
www.diabetesscv.org

Since 1974, the Diabetes Society of Santa Clara Valley has sponsored Camp de los Ninos, a resident camp for children 6 through 14. This camp provides an opportunity for children with diabetes to go to camp, meet other children and gain a better understanding of their diabetes. The total experience can help campers develop more confidence in their abilities to control their diabetes effectively while enjoying the traditional camp experience.

Sharon Ogbor, Executive Director

2524 Clara Barton Camp
PO Box 356
North Oxford, MA

508-987-2056
Fax: 508-987-2002
e-mail: bcdecamp@aol.com
www.bartoncenter.org

Girls, ages 6-17, with diabetes participate in a well-rounded camp program with special education in diabetes, health and safety. Activities include swimming, boating, sports, dance, music and arts and crafts. Tuition: $1600 for 2 weeks. Two week adventure camp for high school girls offering camping, hiking, canoeing, etc. Also a minicamp (one week) for girls 6-12. Tuition $800. Day camps are offered in Worcester, Boston, and New York City.

Brooke Beverly, Resident Camp Director
Kerry Packard, Day Camp Director

2525 EDI
1460 Pepperhill Drive
Florissant, MO

Youngsters with diabetes learn how to care for themselves while participating in a wide variety of outdoor activities and trips. The camp, managed and financed by the American Diabetes Association Greater St. Louis Affiliate, offers camperships to children from the Greater St. Louis area, ages 7-16, but nonresidents may also apply. Tuition $300-500 for 2 weeks.

Fred Schaljo

2526 Florida Camp for Children and Youth
PO Box 14136
Gainesville, FL

352-334-1323

An adventure camp for children and youth with diabetes.

Rhonda Rogers

2527 Floyd Rogers
PO Box 31536
Omaha, NE

402-341-0866

A camp for diabetic children.

Sherman Poska

2528 Hickory Hill
PO Box 1942
Columbia, MO

573-698-2510

Educates diabetic children concerning diabetes and its care. In addition to daily educational sessions on some aspects of diabetes, campers participate in swimming, sailing, arts and crafts and overnight camping. Tuition: $200 for 2 weeks.

William Mees

2529 John Warvel
American Diabetes Association
7363 E 21st Street
Indianapolis, IN 800-2

317-352-9226
800-800-228
e-mail: bookorders@diabetes.org

Provides an enjoyable, safe and educational out-of-doors experience for children with insulin-dependent diabetes. A unique learning atmosphere for children to acquire new skills in caring for their disease. The camp experience instills confidence for the child's self-management of diabetes. Offers one-week sessions and can accommodate 200 campers.

Carol Helming, Executive Director

2530 Nejeda
PO Box 156
Stillwater, NJ

973-383-2611
Fax: 973-383-9891
e-mail: nejeda@nac.net

For children with diabetes, ages 5-15, provides an active and safe camping experience which enables the children to learn about and understand diabetes. Activities include boating, swimming, fishing, archery, as well as camping skills. Tuition: $850 for 2 weeks.

Cheryl Lyding, Executive Director
James Daschbach, Camp Director

2531 Sweeney
PO Box 918
Gainesville, TX

940-665-9502
Fax: 940-665-2833
e-mail: info@campsweeney.org
www.campsweeney.org

Teaches self-care and self-reliance to children with diabetes. Campers participate in such activities as swimming, fishing, horseback riding, arts and crafts while learning about diabetes and how to cope with it. Tuition: $450 for 1 week; $1,400 for 3 weeks.

Marlene E Gray, Foundation Development Director

2532 Utada Camp
American Diabetes Association
250 E 3rd Street
Salt Lake City, UT

801-363-3024
Fax: 801-363-3031
e-mail: gburns@diabetes.org
www.diabetes.org

Campers with diabetes aged 6-17.

Gayle Burns, Field Services Associate

DESCRIPTION

2533 DIGEORGE SYNDROME

Synonyms: DiGeorge sequence, Thymic agenesis immunodeficiency

Involves the following Biologic System(s):
Genetic/Chromosomal/Syndrome/Metabolic Disorders, Immunologic and Rheumatologic Disorders

DiGeorge syndrome is a disorder present at birth (congenital) that is characterized by some combination of absence (aplasia) or underdevelopment (hypoplasia) of the thymus gland and the parathyroid glands, malformations of the heart and its major blood vessels (cardiovascular abnormalities), and characteristic malformations of the head and facial (craniofacial) area. Due to absence or underdevelopment of the thymus gland, affected children may have abnormalities of the immune system, causing impaired resistance to certain infections. DiGeorge syndrome occurs as the result of abnormal development of certain embryonic structures (third and fourth pharyngeal pouches) that later develop into the thymus and parathyroid glands. In some cases, other embryonic structures that are forming during the same approximate period may also be affected, resulting in certain cardiovascular, craniofacial, or other malformations. The thymus, a lymphoid tissue organ located in the upper portion of the chest, plays an essential role in the immune system beginning at approximately the 12th week of fetal development and lasts until puberty. It serves as a source of certain white blood cells (lymphocytes) before birth and then promotes the development of certain specialized lymphocytes, known as T lymphocytes, through secretion of particular hormones (e.g., thymosin). The actions of the T lymphocytes help to defend the body against certain microorganisms (i.e., cell-mediated immunity). The parathyroid glands, which are two pairs of small glands on the sides of the thyroid gland, produce parathyroid hormone, which helps to maintain normal levels of calcium in the blood.

DiGeorge syndrome usually occurs randomly and is caused by spontaneous, minute deletions of material from the long arm of chromosome 22 (22q11.2). DiGeorge syndrome may also occur in association with certain chromosomal abnormalities (e.g., chromosome 10, monosomy 10p; chromosome 22, monosomy 22q). In addition, there have been some cases in which DiGeorge syndrome affected individuals within certain families (kindreds) yet did not appear to result from known chromosome syndromes. In some familial cases, DiGeorge syndrome may have autosomal dominant inheritance. The disorder is thought to affect approximately one in 20,000 newborns.

In infants and children with DiGeorge syndrome, associated symptoms and findings may be extremely variable. Patients who have absence or severe underdevelopment of the thymus gland are prone to frequent infections from fungi, viruses, and certain bacteria (such as Pneumocystis jiroveci, previously knowns as Pneumocystis carinii). These patients often experience chronic inflammation of the mucous membranes of the nose (rhinitis), recurrent inflammation of the lungs (pneumonia), fungal infection of the mucous membranes of the mouth (oral candidiasis), recurrent diarrhea, or systemic infections in which invading microorganisms or their toxins are present inthe blood circulation (septicemia). In some cases of serious infection, life-threatening complications may result. Infants and children with mild underdevelopment (hypoplasia) of the thymus are said to have partial DiGeorge syndrome and may have little difficulty with recurring infections. Because of absence or underdevelopment of the parathyroid glands (hypoparathyroidism), many affected infants experience certain symptoms and findings during the first days of life, including abnormally low calcium levels in the blood (hypocalcemia) and muscle twitching, tremors and cramps, (neonatal tetany) and even seizures. Such symptoms and findings can be treated with calcium supplementation and are usually temporary but may recur later in life.

Some newborns with DiGeorge syndrome may also have defects of the heart and its great arteries. Some of these may be simple defects while others may be more complex, such as interrupted aortic arch, ventricular septal defects, and tetralogy of Fallot.

Infants with DiGeorge syndrome may have an unusually narrow or blind-ending esophagus (esophageal atresia) that does not form a passageway into the stomach. In addition, affected newborns may have characteristic malformations of the head and facial (craniofacial) area, such as widely spaced eyes (ocular hypertelorism); downwardly slanting eyelid folds (palpebral fissures); a small mouth; an unusually short, vertical groove in the center of the upper lip (philtrum); and low-set, notched ears. Some patients may also have mild to moderate mental retardation.

The treatment of infants and children with DiGeorge syndrome is symptomatic and supportive. Treatment measures may include the administration of calcium in those with hypoparathyroidism and hypocalcemia, therapies to help prevent and aggressively treat infections (e.g., antiviral, antifungal, and antibiotic agents) in patients with immuno-deficiency, medical and surgical measures for cardiovascular malformations, or other measures as required. If patients with immunodeficiency require blood transfusions, donor blood must be exposed to high levels of radiation (irradiated) to kill the donor lymphocytes and thus prevent the occurrence of graft-versus-host disease, a serious disease caused by an immune response of donor cells against the recipient's tissues.

See also **General Resources** on page 917

National Associations & Support Groups

2534 22Q and You Center
34th Street and Civic Center Boulevard
Philadelphia, PA 19104

215-590-2920
Fax: 215-590-3298
e-mail: lunny@email.chop.edu
cbil.humgen.upenn.edu

Services offered by the Department of Clinical Genetics in the Children's Hospital of Philadelphia, include literature, support groups and referrals.

2535 Genetic Alliance
4301 Connecticut Avenue NW
Washington, DC 20008

202-966-5557
800-336-4363
Fax: 202-966-8553
e-mail: info@geneticalliance.org
www.geneticalliance.org

A coalition of voluntary genetic support groups, consumers and professionals addressing the needs of individuals and families affected by genetic disorders from a national perspective.

Sharon Terry, President/CEO

2536 Immune Deficiency Foundation
40 W Chesapeake Avenue, Suite 308
Towson, MD 21204

410-321-6647
800-296-4433
Fax: 410-321-9165
e-mail: IDF@primaryimmune.org
www.primaryimmune.org

The only national charitable organization aimed at fighting the primary immune deficiency diseases. The founders included parents of children with primary immune deficiency, immunologists who treat immune deficient patients and other individuals with an interest in helping others. The Foundation's main goal is to improve the care and treatment of adults and children with primary immune deficiency diseases and to promote public education and awareness about the diseases.

2537 March of Dimes Birth Defects Foundation
1275 Mamaroneck Avenue
White Plains, NY 10605

914-428-7100
888-663-4637
Fax: 914-997-4763
TDD: 914-997-4764
e-mail: askus@marchofdimes.com
www.marchofdimes.com

A national not-for-profit organization that was established in 1938. The mission of the Foundation is to improve the health of babies by preventing birth defects and infant mortality.

Dr Jennifer Howse, President

Conferences

2538 Immune Deficiency Foundation National Conference
Meetings Manager
40 W Chesapeake Avenue, Suite 308
Towson, MD 21204

410-321-6647
800-296-4433
Fax: 410-321-9165
e-mail: IDF@primaryimmune.org
www.primaryimmune.org

Annual conference hosted by an organization aimed at fighting the primary immune deficiency diseases. The founders included parents of children with primary immune deficiency, immunologists who treat immune deficient patients and other individuals with an interest in helping others. The Foundation's main goal is to improve the care and treatment of adults and children with primary immune deficiency diseases and to promote public education and awareness about the diseases.

June

Richard Barr MD, Chairman
Kathy Crews, Vice Chairman

Web Sites

2539 International Patient Organization for Primary Immunodeficiencies
ipopi.org

IPOPI is an international organization whose members are national patient organizations for the primary immunodeficiencies (PID's). It was formed to benefit and serve its members and patients with expertise and resources and influence of members in order to achieve worlwide improvement in the care and treatment of patients with PID's.

2540 Jeffrey Modell Foundation
www.jmfworld.com

The foundation is dedicated to the early and precise diagnosis, meaningful treatment, and ultimate cure of Primary Immunodeficiencies.

2541 Kansas University Medical Center
www.kumc.edu/gec/support/velo.html

Offers information for genetic professionals, information on genetic conditions and support groups, and genetic educational information.

2542 Online Mendelian Inheritance in Man
www.ncbi.nlm.nih.gov

This database is a catalog of human genes and genetic disorders.

Book Publishers

2543 Let's Talk About Going to the Hospital
Rosen Publishing Group's PowerKids Press
29 E 21st Street
New York, NY 10010

212-777-3017
800-237-9932
Fax: 888-436-4643
e-mail: rosenpub@tribeca.ios.com
www.powerkidspress.com

If a child has to check into the hospital, chances are he or she is already upset about being ill. Knowing how a hospital functions and what the procedures are, such as when family members can visit, will help in what is already a stressful situation. Grades K-5.

24 pages
ISBN: 0-823950-36-0

DESCRIPTION

2544 DOWN SYNDROME

Synonyms: Chromosome 21, trisomy 21, Trisomy 21 syndrome

Covers these related disorders: Trisomy 21 mosaicism, Trisomy 21 translocation

Involves the following Biologic System(s):
Genetic/Chromosomal/Syndrome/Metabolic Disorders

Down syndrome, also known as trisomy 21, is a chromosomal disorder that affects approximately one in 660 newborns, making it the most common genetic syndrome. Cells of the body (with the exception of reproductive cells) typically contain 23 pairs of chromosomes that are numbered from 1 to 22. The 23rd pair consists of one X chromosome from the mother and an X or Y chromosome from the father. However, in infants with Down syndrome, all or a portion of chromosome 21 is present three times rather than twice in cells of the body (trisomy). In rare cases, a certain percentage of cells contain the extra chromosome 21, whereas other cells have the normal two. This finding is known as chromosomal mosaicism.

The symptoms and physical findings associated with Down syndrome vary in range and severity and depend in part on the exact location and the percentage of body cells containing the extra chromosome 21.

Down syndrome is usually the result of errors during the division of a parent's reproductive cells. Increased maternal age (over 35) presents additional risk. The disorder may also result due to a chromosome 21 translocation that is transmitted by a parent or occurs sporadically. Translocations are chromosomal abnormalities in which pieces of two or more chromosomes break off and are rearranged, resulting in an altered set of chromosomes.

Many infants with Down syndrome have abnormally diminished muscle tone (hypotonia), a tendency to keep the mouth open, protrusion of the tongue, excessive mobility of the joints, absence of certain reflexes, and excessive skin on the back of the neck. Other abnormalities may include a small, short head, flattened facial features, upwardly slanting eyelid folds, vertical skin folds over the eyes' inner corners, a highly arched roof of the mouth, a small nose and depressed nasal bridge, and small, misshapen ears. Abnormalities of the limbs may also be present, including unusually short arms and legs; short, broad hands; improper positioning of the fifth fingers (clinodactyly); abnormal skin ridge patterns on the fingers, hands, toes, and feet (dermatoglyphics); and a wide gap between the first and second toes. Infants with Down syndrome have an increased frequency of intestinal narrowing or obstruction (atresia) at birth. Patients also tend to have relatively short stature, progressive delays in the acquisition of skills requiring the coordination of physical and mental activities (psychomotor delays), poor coordination, an awkward manner of walking (gait), and varying levels of mental retardation.

Approximately 40 percent of infants with Down syndrome have heart defects at birth (congenital heart defects). In some patients, such heart defects may require surgical repair. In addition, some individuals with Down syndrome are prone to recurrent respiratory infections and chronic inflammation of the membranes that line the eyes and eyelids (conjunctivitis) or the nasal cavity (rhinitis). Treatment of individuals with Down syndrome includes symptomatic and supportive measures, such as possible surgical correction of congenital heart defects, and special education.

See also **General Resources** on page 917

Government Agencies

2545 NIH/National Institute of Child Health and Human Development
31 Center Drive, Building 31
Bethesda, MD 20892

301-496-5133
Fax: 301-496-1104
www.nichd.nih.gov

Established in 1962 by congress, today the institute conducts and supports research on topics related to the health of children, adults, families and populations. Some of these topics include: developmental disabilities, growth and development, infant death, reproductive health and birth defects.

Nancy D Wirth, Director
Lisa Kaeser, Program & Public Liaison

National Associations & Support Groups

2546 ARC of the United States
1010 Wayne Avenue, Suite 650
Silver Spring, MD 20910

301-565-3842
Fax: 301-565-5342
e-mail: info@thearc.org
www.thearc.org

The ARC of the United States advocates for the rights and full participation of all children and adults with intellectual and developmental disabilities. Together with our network of members and affiliated chapters, we improve systems of supports and services; connect families; inspire communities an influence public policy.

Michael Coburn, Assistant Executive Director
Adam Aaronson, Public Inquiries Director

2547 Aleh Foundation
Aleh Institutions USA
5317 13th Avenue
Brooklyn, NY 10001

718-851-4597
Fax: 718-851-4597
e-mail: info@aleh.org
www.aleh.org

The Aleh Rehabilitation Center in Bnei Break has served as a residential facility to close to 200 children with multiple, physical and mental disabilities. These children and their families have benefited from our wide range of services in an atmosphere of warmth and love.

2548 Arc of Montgomery County
11600 Nebel Street
Rockville, MD 20852

301-984-5777
Fax: 301-816-2429
e-mail: info@arcmontmd.org
www.arcmontmd.org

Aims to provide support, advocacy and choices for people who have mental retardation and related developmental disabilities and their families.

Peter Holden, Executive Director
John Slavcoff, President

2549 Association for Children with Down Syndrome
4 Fern Place
Plainview, NY 11803

516-933-4700
Fax: 516-933-9524
e-mail: information@acds.org
www.acds.org

Dedicated to providing lifetime resources of exceptional quality, innovation and inclusion for individuals with Down syndrome and other developmental disabilities and their families.

Michael Smith, Executive Director
Jane Shimkin, Educational Coordinator

2550 Birth Defects Research for Children
930 Woodcock Road, Suite 224
Orlando, FL 32803

407-895-0802
e-mail: staff@birthdefects.org
www.birthdefects.org

An organization that provides parents and expectant parents with information about birth defects and support services for their children. BDRC has a parent-matching program that links families who have children with similar birth defects.

Betty Mekdeci, Executive Director

2551 Down Syndrome Guild
PO Box 821174
Dallas, TX 75382

972-422-5354
e-mail: president@downsyndromedallas.com
www.downsyndromedallas.com

Provides new baby/parent hospital visits, monthly newsletter, support and encouragement for individuals with Down Syndrome and their families. Bi-lingual group. Job coaching scholarships.

Stephanie Crow, Executive Director

2552 Genetic Alliance
4301 Connecticut Avenue NW
Washington, DC 20008

202-966-5557
800-336-4363
Fax: 202-966-8553
e-mail: info@geneticalliance.org
www.geneticalliance.org

A coalition of voluntary genetic support groups, consumers and professionals addressing the needs of individuals and families affected by genetic disorders from a national perspective.

Sharon Terry, President/CEO

2553 March of Dimes Birth Defects Foundation
1275 Mamaroneck Avenue
White Plains, NY 10605

914-428-7100
888-663-4637
Fax: 914-428-8203
e-mail: resourcecenter@modimes.org
www.marchofdimes.com

Partnership of volunteers and professionals dedicates to improving the health of babies by preventing birth defects and infant mortality. Over 100 chapters are located across the country and can be located through the National Office.

Dr Jennifer Howse, President

2554 National Association for Down Syndrome (NADS)
PO Box 206
Wilmette, IL 60091

630-325-9112
e-mail: info@nads.org
www.nads.org

Established by parents of children with Down syndrome who felt a need to create a better environment and bring about understanding and acceptance of people with Down syndrome.

2555 National Dissemination Center for Children with Disabilities
PO Box 1492
Washington, DC 20013

202-884-8200
800-695-0285
Fax: 202-884-8441
e-mail: nichcy@acd.org
www.nichcy.org

A national information and referral center that provides information on disabilities and disability-related issues for families, educators and other professionals.

Suzanne Ripley, Executive Director

2556 National Down Syndrome Congress
1370 Center Drive, Suite 102
Atlanta, GA 30338

770-604-9500
800-232-6372
Fax: 770-604-9898
e-mail: info@ndsccenter.org
www.ndsccenter.org

It is the mission of the National Down Syndrome Congress to be the national advocacy organization for Down syndrome and to provide leadership in all areas of concern related to persons with Down syndrome. In that capacity, NDSC will function as a major source of support and empowerment to persons with down syndrome and their families.

David Tolleson, Executive Director
Sue Joe, Resource Specialist

2557 National Down Syndrome Society
666 Broadway
New York, NY 10012

800-221-4602
Fax: 212-979-2873
e-mail: info@ndss.org
www.ndss.org/

Established with the goals of promoting research, education and advocacy for individuals with Down syndrome and their families. NDSS works to obtain a better understanding of Down syndrome, the potential of people with Down syndrome, to support research about the condition, and to provide information and referral services for families and professionals.

Elizabeth F Goodwin, President
Jon Colman, Chief Operating Officer

2558 National Down Syndrome Society Hotline
666 Broadway, 8th Floor
New York, NY 10012

212-460-9330
800-221-4602
Fax: 212-979-2873
e-mail: info@ndss.org
www.ndss.org

NDSS supports researchers seeking the causes of and answers to many of the medical, genetic, behavioral and learning problems associated with Down syndrome; sponsors symposia and conferences for parents and professionals; performs advocacy; provides information and referral through a toll-free number; and develops and disseminates educational materials.

Myra Madnick, Executive Director

2559 National Early Childhood Technical Assistance System
University of North Carolina, Chapel Hill
Campus Box 8040
Chapel Hill, NC 27599

919-962-2001
Fax: 919-966-7463
TDD: 919-843-3269
e-mail: nectac@unc.edu
www.unc.edu

Supports the national implementation of the early childhood provisions of the Individuals with Disabilities Education Act (IDEA). The mission is to strengthen systems at all levels to ensure that children (birth through five) with disabilities and their families receive and benefit from high quality, culturally appropriate and family centered supports and services.

Pascal Trohanis, Director
Judi Shaver, Operations Coordinator

State Agencies & Support Groups

2560 Parents of Children with Down Syndrome Arc of Montgomery County
11600 Nebel Street
Rockville, MD 20852

301-984-5777
Fax: 301-816-2429
e-mail: info@arcmontmd.org
www.arcmontmd.org

Aims to provide support, advocacy and choices for people who have mental retardation and related developmental disabilities and their families.

Peter Holden, Executive Director
John Slavcoff, President

Arizona

2561 Foundation for Children with Down Syndrome
17646 N Cave Creek Road, Suite 152
Phoenix, AZ 85032

602-493-7688
Fax: 602-265-8216
www.ffcwds.org

California

2562 Down Syndrome Association of Los Angeles
315 Arden Avenue, Suite 25
Glendale, CA 91203

818-242-7871
Fax: 818-242-7819
e-mail: info@dsala.org
www.dsala.org

Offers information on Down syndrome, counseling, resources, facts, laws and other forms of information.

Margie Thomas, Program Administrator
Thomas Von Der Ahe, Jr, President

Colorado

2563 Mile High Down Syndrome Association
1899 Gaylord Street
Littleton, CO 80162

303-797-1699
Fax: 303-336-5669
e-mail: mhdsa@aol.com
www.mhdsa.org

Serves families of children and adults with Down syndrome, and interested professionals in the Mountain States region. Provides education, resources and support in partnership with individuals, families, professionals, and the community.

Linda Barth, Executive Director
Robin Zaborek, Program/Resource Manager

Connecticut

2564 Connecticut Down Syndrome Congress
C/O: A.J. Pappanikou, University of Connecticut
263 Farmington Avenue
Farmington, CT 06030

860-563-9114
888-486-8537
e-mail: manager@ctdownsyndrome.org
www.ctdownsyndrome.org/

Established as a special interest group to advocate for persons with Down syndrome in the State of Connecticut. The mission is to advocate for the realization and enhancement of the full spectrum of human and civil rights for persons with Down syndrome, gather and disseminate accurate information regarding Down syndrome, provide support to families of children with Down syndrome, and to encourage quality services for persons with Down syndrome.

Walter Glomb, President
Karen Zbierski, Executive VP

Florida

2565 Gold Coast Down Syndrome Organization
5300 Broken Sound Boulevard NW
Boca Raton, FL 33487

561-912-1231
Fax: 561-912-1232
e-mail: gcdso@bellsouth.net
www.goldcoastdownsyndrome.org

Gold Coast Down Syndrome Organization is a private, nonprofit corporation dedicated to making the future brigher for people with Down syndrome in Palm Beach County, Florida.

Diane De Braga, Executive Director

2566 Goodwill Industries-Suncoast
10596 Gandy Boulevard
St. Petersburg, FL 33702

727-523-1512
888-279-1988
Fax: 727-563-9300
TDD: 727-579-1068
e-mail: gw.marketing@goodwill-suncoast.com
www.goodwill-suncoast.org

Nonprofit organization that helps people achieve their full potential through the dignity and power of work.The agency offers a variety of employment and training services to promote self-sufficiency, and contribute to community conservation through recycling.

Deborah Passerini, Operations VP
R Lee Waits, President/CEO

Georgia

2567 Down Syndrome Association of Atlanta
4355 J Cobb Parkway, Suite 213
Atlanta, GA 30339

404-320-3233
Fax: 770-946-9687
e-mail: contactus@atlantadsaa.org
www.atlantadsaa.org

A source of information and support to families, as well as working to promote public awareness and encouraging a better understanding of Down syndrome and individuals with Down syndrome.

Michelle Norweck, Executive Director

Hawaii

2568 Hawaii Down Syndrome Congress
419 Keoniana Street, Suite 804
Honolulu, HI 96815

808-949-1999
e-mail: Conkay@AOL.com
www.hawaiidownsyndrome.com

An organization of families and professionals concerned with all aspects of Down Syndrome. We provide outreach to parents of newborns to foster fellowship and social interaction, educational opportunities and resources, public relation activities to inform the general public about Down syndrome, monthly meetings that provide emotional and psychological support, and serve as activists and advocates on behalf of children with special needs.

Connie Smith, President

Indiana

2569 Down Syndrome Association of NWI
2927 Jewett Avenue
Highland, IN 46322

219-838-3656
Fax: 219-838-6959
e-mail: dsa@netnitco.net

Provides informational and emotional support to parents who have a child, adolescent, or adult family member with special needs. Program offers an important connection for a parent who is seeking support for a special disability issue, by matching him or her with a trained veteran parent.

2570 Down Syndrome Support Association of Southern Indiana (DSSASI)
PO Box 3262
Clarksville, IN 47131

812-948-5182

Provides informational and emotional support to parents who have a child, adolescent, or adult family member with special needs. Program offers an important connection for a parent who is seeking support for a special disability issue, by matching him or her with a trained veteran parent.

Iowa

2571 Center for Disabilities and Development
University of Iowa Hospitals and Clinics
100 Hawkins Drive
Iowa City, IA 52242

319-353-6900
877-686-0031
e-mail: cdd-webmaster@uiowa.edu
www.healthcare.uiowa.edu/cdd

A trusted resource for healthcare, training, research and information for people with disabilities that include: behavior disorders, brain injury, cerebral palsy, diabetes, down syndrome, learning disabilities, mental retardation, sleep disorders and spina bifida.

Elayne Sexsmith, Administrator
Amy Mikelson, Supervisor Info Resource Service

Massachusetts

2572 Massachusetts Down Syndrome Congress (MDSC)
PO Box 866
Melrose, MA 02176

800-664-6372
www.mdsc.org

An all-volunteer, non-profit organization made up of parents, professionals and anyone interested in gaining a better understanding of Down syndrome. The mission is to enhance on a continuous ba-

sis the lives of individuals with Down syndrome through the education and support of people with Down syndrome, their families, their friends, their teachers, and the community as a whole. To ensure individuals are valued, included, and live fulfilling lives in the community.

Suzanne Boudrot Shea, President
Jonathan Fee, Vice President

Minnesota

2573 Down Syndrome Association of Minnesota
656 Transfer Road
St. Paul, MN 55114

651-603-0720
800-511-3696
e-mail: dsamn@dsamn.com
www.dsamn.org/

A nonprofit organization composed of some 3,000 members; more than 900 people with Down syndrome, their families and friends, plus health-care, education and developmental professionals. We are the only organization in our region devoted exclusively to the needs of people with Down syndrome and their families.

Kathleen Forney, Executive Director
Connie Gunderson Warner, Program Coordinator

New Jersey

2574 Foundation for Children with Down Syndrome
355 Bennetts Mills Road
Jackson, NJ 08527

732-833-1331
www.ffcwds.org

New York

2575 Center for Family Support
333 7th Avenue, 9th Floor
New York, NY 10001

212-629-7939
Fax: 212-239-2211
www.cfsny.org

The Center for Family Support (CFS) is a not-for-profit human service agency providing support and assistance to individuals with developmental disabilities and traumatic brain injuries throughout New York City, Long Island, the lower Hudson Valley region and New Jersey.

Steven Vernickofs, Executive Director

Ohio

2576 Miami Valley Downs Syndrome Association
1133 Edwin C Moses Boulevard, Suite 190
Dayton, OH 45408

937-222-0744
Fax: 937-222-0396
www.mvdsa.org

Informational and emotional support to parents who have a child, adolescent, or adult family member with special needs.

Tennessee

2577 Down Syndrome Association of Middle Tennessee
111 N Wilson Boulevard
Nashville, TN 37205

615-386-9002
Fax: 615-386-9754
e-mail: dsamt@bellsouth.net
www.dsamt.org

A nonprofit organization that is affiliated with the National Down Syndrome Society and the National Down Syndrome Congress. DSAMT works closely with The Arc of Tennessee and other disability organizations locally and throughout the state to provide support for individuals with Down syndrome.

Sheila Moore, Executive Director

Texas

2578 Down Syndrome Guild of Dallas
701 N Central Expressway, Building I
Richardson, TX 75080

214-267-1374
e-mail: kelly@thompson-realty.com
www.downsyndromedallas.org

Aims to impact the community so that everyone will acknowledge the inherent dignity and abilities of people with Down syndrome with full participation in society.

Elizabeth Longworth, President
Kelly Drablos, Vice President

2579 Texas Association on Mental Retardation
PO Box 28076
Austin, TX 78755

512-349-7470
Fax: 512-349-2117
e-mail: pat.holder@tamr-web.com
www.tamr-web.com

An organization made up of professionals, parents, consumers and advocates. The goal is to create an accessible system of services and resources which support personal choice and promotes lives of dignity and self-determination. An Annual Convention is a forum for sharing ideas and research, offering opportunities for exchanging information, and developing an understanding for other perspectives.

Pat Holder, Executive Director
Robert Welsh, President

Research Centers

Alabama

2580 Down Syndrome Clinic, Children's Hospital of Alabama
1600 7th Avenue S
Birmingham, AL 35233

205-939-9141
Fax: 205-975-6330

Dr. Diane K Donley

California

2581 Children's Hospital & Research Center of Oakland
747 52nd Street
Oakland, CA 94609

510-428-3000
www.childrenshospitaloakland.org

Scientific research is an important part of the work that goes on at Children's Hospital & Research Center Oakland. Researchers are making significant progress in such areas as diagnosing and treating pediatric cancers, sickle cell disease, AIDS and HIV, hemophilia, cystic fibrosis, developing prenatal techniques for diagnosing mental retardation and birth defects, and improving infant nutrition.

Vipul N Mankad, MD, Senior VP/Chief Medical Officer
Nancy Shibata, RN, Nursing VP

2582 Pediatric Disabilities Clinic, Down Syndrome Clinic
University of California Medical Center
400 Parnassus, Box 0374
San Francisco, CA 94143

415-476-2841
www.ucsfhealth.org

Lucy Crain, MD

Georgia

2583 Pediatric Neurodevelopmental Center at Marcus Institute
Marcus Institute
1920 Briarcliff Road
Atlanta, GA 30329

404-419-5300
Fax: 404-419-5410
e-mail: ccoles@emory.edu
www.marcus.org

Provides an array of evaluation and treatment services for individuals from infancy through adolescence. As well as providing individual evaluations, we feature a number of unique multispecialty programs. Once a child is evaluated, the proper course of treatment and/or therapy can be determined. The evaluation may result in a recommendation for further treatment at the Marcus Institute, or may involve other programs and services in the child's community.

Howard S Schub, MD, Medical Director

Illinois

2584 Adult Down Syndrome Center of Lutheran General Hospital
1999 Dempster Street
Park Ridge, IL 60068

847-318-2303
Fax: 847-318-2377
www.advocatehealth.com/adultdown

A comprehensive medical resource providing multidisciplinary medical and psychosocial care for adults with Down syndrome, with an emphasis on health promotion.

Brian Chicoine, MD, Medical Director
Jenny Lobough-Howard, Outreach Specialist

2585 Advocate Lutheran General Children's Hospital, Pediatric Research
1775 Dempster Street
Park Ridge, IL 60068

847-723-5180
e-mail: denise.angst@advocatehealth.com
www.advocatehealth.com

An organization of physicians and health care professionals dedicated to serving the health needs of individuals, families and communities in Northern Illinois. Ongoing research on Pediatric disorders are being conducted and finding new procedures and medicines.

Nancy Keck, MD, Medical Director
Denise B Angst, DNSc, Research Director

2586 LaRabida Children's Hospital, Down Syndrome Clinic
E 65th Street and Lake Michigan
Chicago, IL 60649

773-753-8626
Fax: 773-363-7160
e-mail: info@larabida.org
www.larabida.org

Recognized as a leader in the diagnosis and treatment of children with developmental disabilities and delays. La Rabida provides comprehensive care and services for children with Down syndrome. The Down syndrome program at La Rabida is designed to provide medical and developmental evaluations and be a resource for both parents and pediatricians caring for children with this chronic condition.

Paula Kienberger Jaudes, MD, President/CEO

Indiana

2587 Ann Whitehill Down Syndrome Program
Riley Hospital for Children
702 Barnhill Drive
Indianapolis, IN 46202

317-274-4846
Fax: 317-274-4471
www.rileychildrenshospital.com

Brings together specialists from many areas to address the medical and psychosocial needs of children with Down Syndrome. A developmental pediatrician, pediatric nurse practitioner, pediatric social worker, pediatric occupational therapist, physical therapist and certified speech pathologist work closely with the primary care physician to help each child achieve his or her optimal potential. We also refer the family to local resources for therapy and developmental programs.

Marilyn Bell, MD

Iowa

2588 Center for Disabilities and Development

University of Iowa Hospitals and Clinics
100 Hawkins Drive
Iowa City, IA 52242

319-353-6900
877-686-0031
Fax: 319-356-8284
e-mail: cdd-webmaster@uiowa.edu
www.uihealthcare.com/cdd

Comprehensive health care and services to people with disabilities of all ages and their families through a combination of outpatient, inpatient, and community based programs. CDD provides information, evaluation, treatment recommendations, and training related to aging and disabilities. CDD provides both preservice and inservice training programs for service providers and others who provide services to individuals with disabilities.

Elayne Sexsmith, Assistant Administrator

Maryland

2589 Behavioral and Developmental Pediatrics Division, University of Maryland

22 S Greene Street
Baltimore, MD 21201

410-328-2214
Fax: 410-328-3981
www.umm.edu

Offers comprehensive consultation, evaluation and treatment for children, birth to age 21, with developmental and behavioral problems.

Linda Grossman, MD, Associate Professor

2590 Kennedy Krieger Institute, Down Syndrome Clinic

1750 E Fairmount Avenue
Baltimore, MD 21231

410-550-9000
Fax: 410-550-9292
e-mail: koller@kennedykrieger.org
www.kennedykrieger.org/

Develop and conduct clinical research studies into the neurobiologic basis of cognitive impairment and co-morbid psychiatric disorders in Down syndrome; to study potential therapies for safety and efficacy; and to investigate genetic and environmental factors relevant to AV Canal defect.

George Capone, MD, Director
Char Koller, Research Contact

2591 Mt. Washington Pediatric Clinic

1708 W Rogers Avenue
Baltimore, MD 21209

410-578-8600
800-999-9442
Fax: 419-466-4311
e-mail: dgreenberg@mwph.org
www.mwph.org

David A Greenberg, VP Outpatient

Massachusetts

2592 Down Syndrome Program, Children's Hospital Boston

300 Longwood Avenue
Boston, MA 02115

617-355-7971
Fax: 617-735-7429
e-mail: CROCKER_A@A1.TCH.Harvard.edu
www.childrenshospital.org/

Medical and developmental monitoring for children from birth to 3 years of age. Evaluations are provided every 4 to 6 months by an interdisciplinary team comprised of a developmental pediatrician, physical therapist, nutritionist, audiologist, speech pathologist, and social worker. Individual support is available for families, along with information, referral, and case management assistance.

Dr. Allen Crocker, Director

Minnesota

2593 Down Syndrome Clinic of Minneapolis Children's Medical Center

2525 Chicago Avenue
Minneapolis, MN 55404

612-813-7800
Fax: 612-813-6100
e-mail: dmcconn606@aol.com

Mission of the clinic is to improve the quality of life for children and adolescents with Down syndrome and to help them reach their full potentials. A multi-disciplinary team of professionals provide care to the children and adolescents who come to the clinic. Because of the full spectrum of services available, the program can provide consultation for specific medical and developmental problems, developmental assessments, management of behavioral difficulties, and family support.

Dr. Kim McConnell, Director
Mary Bergs, Social Worker

Missouri

2594 Children's Mercy Hospital, Down Syndrome Clinic

2401 Gillham Road
Kansas City, MO 64108

816-234-3000
Fax: 816-842-6107
e-mail: webmaster@cmh.edu
http://www.childrens-mercy.org/

Medical staff of nearly 600 pediatric specialists with a comprehensive range of programs and services, representing more than 40 pediatric specialities.

V Fred Burry, MD, Executive Medical Director/SVP
Barbara Mueth, Community Relations VP

2595 Down's Syndrome Medical Clinic

Washington University Medical Center
400 S Kingshighway Boulevard
Saint Louis, MO 63110

314-454-6026
www.washington.edu/medical/

Dr. Arnold Strauss

New Hampshire

2596 Medical Genetics Clinic

Dartmouth-Hitchcock Medical Center
1 Medical Center Drive
Lebanon, NH 03756

603-653-6044
Fax: 603-650-8268
www.dhmc.org

Provides specialty consultations for diagnosis and treatment of suspected inherited conditions or syndromes.

John Moeschler, MD, Program Director
Mary Beth Dinulos, MD, Medical Geneticist

New Jersey

2597 Bancroft School
110 Shore Drive
Worcester, MA 01605

508-853-7824
Fax: 508-853-2640
e-mail: bbrooks@bancroft.put.k12.ma.us
www.bancroft.put.k12.ma.us

Dr. Donald Younkin

New York

2598 Child Development Clinical Services
Westchester Institute for Human Development

Valhalla, NY 10595

914-285-8178
Fax: 914-285-1973
e-mail: KEdwards@wihd.org
www.wihd.org/childdev

Diagnostic evaluation and treatment services are provided for children with developmental concerns, communication disorders, attention deficit disorders (including ADHD) and learning disabilities, as well as cerebral palsy and other neuromotor disorders, spina bifida, mental retardation, and autism.

Mark Bertin, MD, Director
Karen Edwards, MD, Pediatrics Director

2599 Institute for Basic Research in Developmental Disabilities
1050 Forest Hill Road
Staten Island, NY 10314

718-494-0600
Fax: 718-494-0833
www.omr.state.ny.us/ws/ws_ibr_resources.jsp

Research arm of the New York State Office of Mental Retardation and Developmental Disabilities (OMRDD). IBR conducts basic and clinical research into the causes, treatment, and prevention of mental retardation and other developmental disabilities. It also provides specialized biomedical, psychological, and laboratory services to individuals with developmental disabilities and their families, and educates the public and professionals regarding the causes, diagnosis, prevention, and treatment.

W Ted Brown, MD; Ph.D, Director

North Dakota

2600 Children's Hospital Merit Care Down Syndrome Service
737 Broadway
Fargo, ND 58102

701-234-2568
Fax: 701-234-6965

Dr. Guy Carter

Ohio

2601 Down Syndrome Clinic, Department of Pediatrics
Medical College of Ohio, Health Center
Box 10008
Toledo, OH 43699

419-381-4000
www.mco.edu

Dr. Eileen Quinn

2602 Down Syndrome Clinic, Rainbow Babies and Children's Hospital
11100 Euclid Avenue
Cleveland, OH 44106

216-844-8260
Fax: 216-844-8444

Dr. Joanne Mortimer

2603 Jane and Richard Thomas Center for Down Syndrome
Cincinnati Children's Hospital Medical Center
3333 Burnet Avenue
Cincinnati, OH 45229

513-636-0520
800-344-2462
Fax: 513-559-9669
www.cincinnatichildrens.org

Conducts research and offers interdisciplinary evaluations and intervention for infants, children, adolescents and young adults with Down syndrome. By providing a range of comprehensive services within one center, families can now spend less time pursuing services through multiple agencies and professionals.

David J Schonfeld, MD, Division Head

2604 Pediatric Clinical Trials International
700 Childrens Drive
Columbus, OH 43205

614-722-2551
Fax: 614-722-2662
e-mail: Marketing@PedCTI.com
www.centerwatch.com/

Consists of inpatient and outpatient capabilities. The inpatient facility includes research beds, a psychophysiological recording and observation/recording center. The latter, located on the neuromonitoring unit, consists of a subject testing room equipped with video cameras and psychological recording systems, and the second is the monitoring room equipped with computer programming and audio-video monitoring, etc.

Milo Hilty, MD, Medical Director
John P Niles, CEO

Pennsylvania

2605 Children's Hospital of Pittsburgh General Clinical Research Center
3705 5th Avenue
Pittsburgh, PA 15213

412-692-7963
Fax: 412-692-5723
e-mail: Clined@chplink.chp.edu
www.chp.edu/research

Established to increase medical knowledge about childhood diseases and to improve the management and treatment of these diseases. Participation is of great importance and value to medical research. We have a dedicated staff of physicians, nurses and health care professionals experienced in health care delivery and research who will ensure your comfort and safety as you participate in medical studies.

Silva Arslanian, MD, Program Director
Diane E Cline, Administrative Manager

2606 Children's Seashore House
Children's Hospital in Philadelphia
3405 Civic Center Boulevard
Philadelphia, PA 19104

215-590-1734
e-mail: rac@email.chop.edu
www.chop.edu

Leading research institution quickly bringing scientific discoveries into the clinical setting and community to improve care. Some current research studies include: cognitive studies of the development of mathematical competence in normal children and in those with congenital defects, studies of language development in children with inherited syndromes, and development of novel strategies to prevent violence in the school setting.

Marc Yudkoff, MD, Division Chief
Nathan Blum, MD, Behavioral Pediatrics

2607 Down Syndrome Clinic
MS Hershey Medical Center, Division of Genetics
PO Box 850
Hershey, PA 17033

717-531-8414
www.hmc.psu.edu

Maria Mascari, PhD

2608 Dr. Gertrude A. Barber National Institute
136 E Avenue
Erie, PA 16507

814-453-7661
Fax: 814-455-1132
e-mail: BNIerie@barberinstitute.org
www.barbercenter.org/

Committed to remaining on the cutting-edge of breakthrough technologies and practices. We seek out research opportunities that will enhance our services and will provide the most current proven information to present to the public.

John Barber, President/CEO
Maureen Barber-Carey, Executive VP

2609 International Foundation for Genetic Research/Michael Fund
4371 Northern Pike
Pittsburgh, PA 15146

412-374-0111
www.michaelfund.org

Research is directed toward preventing and treating the harmful consequences of the extra chromosome in Down's Syndrome. Also; dedicated to reversing this destructive universal trend by opening up new doors of therapy in the field of mental retardation associated with chromomal disorders such as Down Syndrome and continuing the curative research program.

Randy Engel, Executive Director

Rhode Island

2610 Children's Neurodevelopment Center at Hasbro Children's Hospital
Rhode Island Hospital
593 Eddy Street
Providence, RI 02903

401-444-5685
Fax: 401-444-6115
e-mail: sigpueschel@aol.com
www.lifespan.org/hch/services/

A site for the evaluation and treatment of children with neurological, genetic, developmental, metabolic and behavioral disorders.

David Mandelbaum, MD; Ph.D, Director

Texas

2611 Down Syndrome Specialty Clinic
Children's Medical Center
1935 Motor Street
Dallas, TX 75235

214-640-2357
Fax: 214-456-2567
www.childrens.com

Comprehensive care for children with Down syndrome and their families including; medical management, genetic counseling, speech and oral motor developmental evaluation and recommendations, psychosocial support, screening and referral for behavioral or psychiatric problems, and referrals to community agencies for educational intervention or therapies.

Lewis Waber, MD; Ph.D, Clinical Medical Doctor
Joanna Spahis, RN, Clinical Nurse Specialist

2612 Santa Rosa Medical Center
PO Box 7330
San Antonio, TX 78207

210-228-2386

Dr. Robert Clayton

Washington

2613 University of Washington: Experimental Education Unit
University of Washington
Columbia Road, Gate #6
Seattle, WA 98195

206-543-2100
www.depts.washington.edu/

Provide clinical services to children and their families, and conduct interdisciplinary research.

Rick Neel, Director
Kate Ahern, Admissions Coordinator

Wisconsin

2614 Center for the Study of Bioethics
Medical College of Wisconsin
8701 Watertown Plank Road
Milwaukee, WI 53226

414-527-8191
e-mail: centerbioethics@mcw.edu
www.mcw.edu/bioethics

Center for the Study of Bioethics is a leader in the field of bioethics. The Center has conscientiously served the functions of a typical institution of higher learning; research, education, and service.

Robyn S Shapiro, Director
Kristen Tym, Assistant Director

Conferences

2615 National Down Syndrome Society Annual National Conference
666 Broadway
New York, NY 10012

212-763-4365
800-221-4602
e-mail: jfalik@ndss.org
www.ndss.org

The focus is on working together to improve the lives of individuals with Down syndrome, enabling them to enjoy the benefits of, and contribute to, their communities.

Jennifer Falik, Special Events Director

Audio Video

2616 A Different Kind of Beginning
Association for Children with Down Syndrome
2616 Martin Avenue
Bellmore, Long Island, NY 11710

516-221-4700

Demonstrates the independence and capabilities of individuals with Down syndrome as seen in various settings from early intervention programs to adult employment.

2617 A New Set of Fears, a New Set of Hopes
Meyer Children's Rehabilitation Institute
Resource Center, 444 S 44th Street
Omaha, NE 68131

402-559-7467
800-232-6372

Explores the way a family adjusts as they go through the life cycle with their child who has Down syndrome.

2618 A Special Love
Association for Children with Down Syndrome
2616 Martin Avenue
Bellmore, NY 11710

516-221-4700
Fax: 516-221-4311

A candid video of a ten-year-old brother playing with his six-year-old sister with Down Syndrome. The brother describes his perceptions of mental retardation and his feelings towards his sister.

4 minutes, b/w

DB Shalom, Editor

2619 Adaptation to the Initial Crisis
Lawren Productions
930 Pitner Avenue
Evanston, IL 60202

847-328-6700

A family learns to adapt to the birth of a child with a handicap.

2620 Congratulations? An Introduction to Down Syndrome for Parents/Family/Friends
New Challenges
96 Ogden Avenue
White Plains, NY 10605

914-287-0723

A film for parents which addresses some of the most commonly asked questions about raising a child with Down syndrome.

57 mins.

2621 Daddy's Girl
Carle Media
110 W Main Street
Urbana, IL 61801

217-384-4838

Dina Lev, a 12-year-old actress with Down syndrome, portrays Nancy, a girl trying to deal with her divorced father's inability to accept the fact that his daughter has Down syndrome.

28 mins.

Bruce Postman, Producer
Regina Conroy, Writer/Director

2622 Down Syndrome Preschool Program
Association for Children with Down Syndrome
2616 Martin Avenue
Bellmore, NY 11710

516-221-4700

A look at preschool programs for children with Down syndrome birth to five years.

2623 Down Syndrome, See the Potential
Down Syndrome Association of Charlotte
PO Box 3136
Charlotte, NC 28210

704-536-2163

Video highlighting the capability of children with Down syndrome.

2624 Down Syndrome: Parent's Perspective
Aquarius Productions
18 N Main Street
Sherborn, MA 01770

888-440-2963
Fax: 508-650-1665
e-mail: info@aquariusproductions.com
www.aquariusproductions.com

Presents a candid and positive portrayal of how a group of parents with children with Down syndrome have managed to maintain a focus on quality-of-life needs. The video does not emphasize traumatic incidents, but demonstrates in a dynamic manner how parents support each other and their expectations of professionals.

20 Minutes
ISBN: 6-304166-69-9

Elizabeth S Graham, Director
W Carl Cooley, Medical Consultant

2625 Educating Peter
State of the Art Production
2470 Fox Hill Road
State College, PA 16803

814-355-8004
800-458-3401
Fax: 814-355-2714
e-mail: sales@resistor.com
www.resistor.com

Thought-provoking film follows a child with Down syndrome through a year of inclusion in a public school in Mrs. Stallings' third grade class. The film raises many questions about inclusion by honestly presenting the reactions to, and methods of, dealing with Peter's behavior problems.

30 Minutes

Thomas C Goodwin, Producer/Director
Gerardine Wurzburg, Producer/Director

2626 Gifts of Love
National Down Syndrome Society
666 Broadway
New York, NY 10012

212-460-9330
Fax: 212-979-2873
e-mail: info@ndss.org
www.ndss.org

Four families of children with Down syndrome talk about their feelings and experiences with their children, particularly during the first six years. All the children live at home and attend programs in their communities.

25 minutes

2627 Infant Motor Development: A Look at the Phases
Therapy Skill Builders

San Antonio, TX 78283

732-441-0404

Shows normal infant motor development from birth to 12 months. Identifies components of movement and specific skills that are acquired during 4 phases of motor development: infantile, preparation, modification, and refinement. Transitional movement patterns and their relationship to skill acquisition are also described.

20 Minutes

Kerry Goudy, Producer
Joan Winger, Producer

2628 New Expectations
Altschul Group Corporation
1560 Sherman Avenue, Suite 100
Evanston, IL 60201

800-421-2363
e-mail: agcmedia@starnetinc.com

Focuses on the emotional and technical aspects of Down syndrome. Highlights four persons at various life stages from infancy to adulthood in the areas of education and employment.

2629 Opportunities to Grow
National Down Syndrome Society
666 Broadway, 8th Floor
New York, NY 10012

800-221-4602
Fax: 212-979-2873
e-mail: info@ndss.org
www.ndss.org

Sequel to Gifts of Love video shows how people with Down Syndrome, ages six to twenty-six, participate equally in all phases of community life. Vignettes of fifteen young men and women illustrate how inclusion, education, computer facilitation, socialization programs, and employment training help them to fulfill their potential.

25 Minutes

2630 Stepping Stones
AIT
PO Box A
Bloomington, IN 47402

Series of video programs on teaching basic skills to at-risk, special needs and normally developed children.

Web Sites

2631 ARC of the United States
www.thearc.org

The ARC is the national organization of and for people with mental retardation and related developmental disabilities and their families. Devoted to promoting and improving supports and services for people with mental retardation and their families. The association also fosters research and education regarding the prevention of mental retardation in infants and young children. The ARC was founded in 1950 by a small group of parents and other concerned individuals.

2632 Aleh Foundation
www.aleh.org

Aleh is a nonprofit organization that believes that every child, no matter how severe his/her disability, has potential. We are committed to providing severely disabled children through Israel with the high-level medical and rehabilitative care they need to grow beyond the boundaries of their prognoses.

2633 Association for Children with Down Syndrome
www.acds.org

Dedicated to providing lifetime resources of exceptional quality, innovation and inclusion for individuals with Down syndrome and other developmental disabilities and their families.

2634 Birth Defects Research for Children
www.birthdefects.org

An organization that provides parents and expectant parents with information about birth defects and support services for their children. BDRC has a parent-matching program that links families who have children with similar birth defects.

2635 Down Syndrome Guild
www.downsyndromedallas.com

Provides new baby/parent hospital visits, monthly newsletter, support and encouragement for individuals with Down Syndrome and their families. Bi-lingual group. Job coaching scholarships.

2636 Health Answers
www.healthanswers.com

HealthAnswers offers a breadth of services in medical education, sales force training, patient support, solutions, professional promotion and consumer solutions.

2637 National Association for Down Syndrome (NADS)
www.nads.org

Established by parents of children with Down syndrome who felt a need to create a better environment and bring about understanding and acceptance of people with Down syndrome.

2638 National Down Syndrome Congress
www.ndsccenter.org

It is the mission of the National Down Syndrome Congress to be the national advocacy organization for Down syndrome and to provide leadership in all areas of concern related to persons with Down syndrome. In that capacity, NDSC will function as a major

source of support and empowerment to persons with down syndrome and their families.

2639 National Down Syndrome Society
www.ndss.org

Our mission is to benefit people with Down Syndrome and their families through national leadership in education research and advocacy.

2640 Online Mendelian Inheritance in Man
www.ncbi.nlm.nih.gov

This database is a catalog of human genes and genetic disorders.

Book Publishers

2641 Adolescents with Down Syndrome
University of Victoria
3800 Finnerty Road
Victoria, BC, V8P
Canada

250-721-7211
www.uvic.ca

Adolescents with Down syndrome: International perspectives on research and programme development: Implications for parents, researchers, and practitioners.

165 pages
ISBN: 0-919955-16-9

Carey Denholm, Editor

2642 Babies with Down Syndrome
Woodbine House
6510 Bells Mill Road
Bethesda, MD 20817

301-897-3570
800-843-7323
Fax: 301-897-5838

Praised as the finest book ever written for new parents, this book covers everything they need to know about rearing these beautiful and special children in a loving environment.

340 pages Paperback
ISBN: 0-933149-64-6

Karen Stray-Gundersen, Editor

2643 Biomedical Concerns in Persons with Down's Syndrome
Brookes Publishing Company
PO Box 10624
Baltimore, MD 21285

410-337-9580
800-638-3775
Fax: 410-337-8539
www.brookespublishing.com

Written by leading authorities and spanning many disciplines and specialties, this comprehensive resource provides vital information on biomedical issues concerning individuals with Down's syndrome.

336 pages Hardcover
ISBN: 1-557660-89-1

Siegfried M Pueschel, Editor
Jeanette K Pueschel, Editor

2644 Cara: Growing with a Retarded Child
Temple University Press
USB Room 305, Broad & Oxford
Philadelphia, PA 19122

215-204-8787
www.temple.edu/templepress/

Despite the fact that Cara Jablow was born with Down's syndrome, formerly known as mongolism, she was reading before she was five. Her mother, a journalist, dramatically recounts Cara's development from birth to age seven, revealing how a family reacts to the news that their baby is retarded, how they now can make use of early intervention programs, and what Cara's prospects are for the future.

210 pages Paperback
ISBN: 0-877222-69-X

Martha Moraghan Jablow, Editor

2645 Communication Skills in Children with Down Syndrome: A Guide for Parents
Woodbine House
6510 Bells Mill Road
Bethesda, MD 20817

301-468-8800
800-843-7323
Fax: 301-897-5838
e-mail: info@woodbinehouse.com
www.woodbinehouse.com

Offers parents a chance to learn what to expect as communication skills progress from infancy through early teenage years. Discussions are included on speech and language therapy, hearing problems, school performance and intelligibility issues.

241 pages Paperback
ISBN: 0-933149-53-0

Libby Kumin, Editor

2646 Count Us In: Growing up with Down Syndrome
Harvest Book Company
185 Commerce Drive
Fort Washington, PA 19034

877-512-3022
www.harvestbooks.com/

Mitchell Levitz and Jason Kingsley share their innermost thoughts, feelings, hopes and dreams, their lifelong friendship and their experiences of growing up with Down Syndrome.

1994 208 pages Paperback
ISBN: 0-156226-60-X

Jason Kingsley, Editor
Mitchell Levitz, Editor

2647 Current Approaches to Down's Syndrome
Greenwood Publishing Group
88 Post Road W, Suite 5007
Westport, CT 06880

203-226-3571
www.greenwood.com

An exploration of current initiatives relating to Down syndrome in the medical, educational and social fields.

447 pages Hardcover
ISBN: 0-275902-12-9

David Lane, Editor
Brian Stratford, Editor

2648 Differences in Common: Straight Talk on Mental Retardation/Down Syndrome & Life
Woodbine House
6510 Bells Mill Road
Bethesda, MD 20817

301-468-8800
800-843-7323
Fax: 301-897-5838
e-mail: info@woodbinehouse.com
www.woodbinehouse.com

A collection of essays by the mother of an adult son who has Down syndrome. Focuses on mainstreaming, terminology, parent groups and advocacy.

231 pages Paperback
ISBN: 0-933149-40-9

Marilyn Trainer, Editor

2649 Down Sydrome: Living and Learning in the Community
Wiley & Sonecial Children
10475 Crosspoint Boulevard
Indianapolis, IN 46256
0

877-762-2974
Fax: 800-597-3299
www.wiley.com

Four parents' personal observations. Challenges of people with DS as they become integrated into community, family role, cognitive development and acquisition of language, education, health care, independent living arrangement.

1995 312 pages Hardcover
ISBN: 0-471022-01-2

Lynn Nadel, Editor
Donna Rosenthal, Editor

2650 Down Syndrome-An Update and Review for Primary Care Physician's
Dartmouth-Hitchcock Medical Center
1 Medical Center Drive
Lebanon, NH 03756

603-650-5000

An excellent medical review of Down Syndrome. Intended for physicians.

WC Cooley, Editor

2651 Down Syndrome: Birth to Adulthood: Giving Families an Edge
Love Publishing Company
9101 E Kenyon Evenue
Denver, CO 80237

303-221-7333
Fax: 303-221-7444
e-mail: lovepublishing@1pc.com
www.lovepublishing.com

Provides a collection of longitudinal perspectives on experiences of individuals with Down Syndrome, from birth to adulthood.

1995 356 pages Paperback
ISBN: 0-891082-36-0

John R Rynders, Editor

2652 Down Syndrome: Living & Learning in the Community
John Wiley & Sons
605 3rd Avenue
New York, NY 10158

212-850-6000
Fax: 212-850-6088
e-mail: info@wiley.com
www.witey.com.uk

1995 312 pages Paperback
ISBN: 0-471022-01-2

2653 Down Syndrome: The Facts
Oxford University Press
2001 Evans Road
Cary, NC 27513

212-726-6000
800-451-7556
Fax: 919-677-1303
www.oup-usa.org

A book for parents who have a child with Down Syndrome, written by a pediatrician who works with Down syndrome children.

208 pages Paperback
ISBN: 0-192626-62-0

Mark Selikowitz, Editor

2654 From 17 Months to 17 Years...A Look At Down Syndrome
Bonnie Lavender
Rural Route 1, Box 102C
Richville, NY 13681

315-287-2973

Includes profiles of six families who have children with Down syndrome. Offers photographs and accompanying text that detail each family's experiences with Down syndrome.

B Lavender, Editor
GJ Lega

2655 Let's Talk About Down Syndrome
Rosen Publishing Group's PowerKids Press
29 E 21st Street
New York, NY 10010

212-777-3017
800-237-9932
Fax: 888-436-4643
e-mail: rosenpub@tribeca.ios.com
www.rosenpublishing.com

By stressing that children with Down syndrome are wonderful, viable members of society, this book lessens the stigma attached to this rather common genetic condition.

Ages: 4-8 24 pages Library Binding
ISBN: 0-823951-97-9

Melanie Apel Gordon, Editor

2656 Medical and Surgical Care for Children with Down Syndrome
Woodbine House
6510 Bells Mill Road
Bethesda, MD 20817

301-897-3570
800-843-7323
Fax: 301-897-5838
www.woodbinehouse.com

Provides detailed and easy-to-understand information for parents on a wide range of medical conditions and treatments including: heart disease, recurrent infections, thyroid problems, eye problems, skin conditions, ear, nose and throat problems, orthopedic conditions, leukemia, facial and dental concerns and neurological problems.

395 pages Paperback
ISBN: 0-933149-54-9

Philip Matheis, MD, Editor
Don Van Dyke, MD, Editor

2657 Nursing Your Baby with Down Syndrome
Childbirth Graphics
PO Box 21207
Waco, TX 76702

254-755-6885

2658 Our Brother Has Down's Syndrome: An Introduction for Children
Annick Press
15 Patricia Avenue
Toronto, ON, M2M
Canada

416-221-4802
Fax: 416-221-8400
www.annickpress.com

Two young sisters tell about their little brother Jai, who has Down's Syndrome. The text stresses the ways in which he is like all children, although he needs extra help to walk, use a spoon, stack blocks, etc. The color photographs show an engaging little boy going about his daily activities, often with other family members.

24 pages Paperback
ISBN: 0-920303-31-5

Shelly Cairo, Editor
Jasmine Cairo, Editor

2659 Parent's Guide to Down Syndrome: Toward a Brighter Future
Brookes Publishing Company
PO Box 10624
Baltimore, MD 21285

410-337-9580
Fax: 410-337-8539
e-mail: custserv@brookespublishing.com
www.brookespublishing.com

A comprehensive reference book especially for new parents, but useful and informative to seasoned parents as well. Range of topics include a history of Down syndrome, physical characteristics, developmental expectations, early intervention, feeding the young child and the school years.

352 pages Paperback
ISBN: 1-557664-52-8

Siegfried M Pueschel, Editor

2660 Parents of Down Syndrome Children
11600 Nebel Street
Rockville, MD 20852

301-984-5792

Activities include formal and informal meetings; parent-to-parent counseling; contacting new parents of Down syndrome children to offer support and information on community resources; providing information on doctors, hospitals and professionals.

2661 Perceptual-Motor Behavior in Down Syndrome
Human Kinetics Publishing
1607 N Market Street
Champaign, IL 61825

217-351-5076
800-747-4457
Fax: 217-351-2674
www.humankinetics.com

A comprehensive collection of contemporary research and provides readers a window into the life of someone with Down Syndrome.

365 pages Hardcover
ISBN: 0-880119-75-6

Daniel J Weeks, Editor
Romeo Chua, Editor

2662 Screening for Down Syndrome
Cambridge University Press
40 W 20th Street
New York, NY 10011

212-924-3900
Fax: 212-691-3239
www.cambridge.org

Summarises the recent exciting advances in screening for Down's syndrome. It addresses important clinical questions such as; risk assessment, whom to screen, when to screen, which techniques to use and the organisation of screening programmes nationally and internationally.

1995 358 pages Hardcover
ISBN: 0-521452-71-6

J G Grudzinskas, Editor
T Chard, Editor

2663 Secret Place of the Stairs
Harper & Row
10 E 53rd Street
New York, NY 10022

212-207-7000

A story that weaves many themes, including the institutionalizing of the protagonist's sister, her parents' divorce and her own expectations.

Grades: 7-10 151 pages Hardcover
ISBN: 0-060251-42-5

Susan Sallis, Editor

2664 Shattered Dreams - Lonely Choices: Birth Parents of Babies with Disabilities

Bergin & Garvey/Greenwood Publishing
88 Post Road W, PO Box 5007
Westport, CT 06880

203-226-3571
800-225-5800
Fax: 203-222-1502
e-mail: custserv@greenwood.com
www.greenwood.com

Joanne Finnegan shares her personal experience and that of several families she interviewed who, like herself, explored options other than raising their child with a disability. Parents express with candor the overwhelming pain they felt when receiving the news, the frustration when searching for options, the no-win feeling of decision making, the resolve with a final decision, and finally, life after the decision.

208 pages Hardcover
ISBN: 0-897892-86-0

Joanne Finnegan, Editor

2665 Show Me No Mercy: Compelling Story of Remarkable Courage

Abingdon Press
201 8th Avenue South
Nashville, TN 37202

800-251-3320
www.abingdonpress.com

A father of a young adult man with Down syndrome relates the experience of his attempt to be reunited with his son after a family tragedy separates them.

144 pages Paperback
ISBN: 0-687384-35-4

Robert Perske, Editor

2666 Since Owen

Johns Hopkins University Press
2715 N Charles Street
Baltimore, MD 21218

410-516-6900
Fax: 410-516-6968
www.press.jhu.edu

A well written book displaying understanding from a veteran parent communicating with other parents of children with disabilities.

488 pages Paperback
ISBN: 0-801839-64-5

Charles R Callanan, Editor

2667 Special Kids Make Special Friends

Association for Children with Down Syndrome
4 Fern Place
Plainview, NY 11803

516-933-4700
Fax: 516-933-9524
e-mail: information@acds.org
www.acds.org

Written to assist young children, new parents, siblings, and professionals in developing a better understanding of Down syndrome. Photographs depict children in preschool, emphasizing similarities and strengths of youngsters with Down syndrome rather than their differences.

1995 Paperback
ISBN: 9-995007-64-9

Debra Shalom, Editor

2668 Teaching the Infant with Down Syndrome: Guide for Parents & Professionals

Pro-Ed
8700 Shoal Creek Boulevard
Austin, TX 78757

512-451-3246
800-897-3202
Fax: 512-451-8542
e-mail: info@proedinc.com
www.proedinc.com

A manual providing teaching ideas and activities that can be used to assist an infant's development.

268 pages Hardcover
ISBN: 0-890791-03-1

Marci J Hanson, Editor

2669 To Give An Edge: A Guide for New Parents of Children with Down's Syndrome

Colwell Systems
1031 Mendola Heights Road
St. Paul, MN 55120

651-232-7800

A guide for new parents designed to provide information about the disorder and how other parents of children with Down syndrome have coped.

Paperback
ISBN: 9-993370-55-X

JM Horrobin, Editor

2670 Understanding Down Syndrome

Brookline Books
PO Box 1047
Cambridge, MA 02238

617-868-0360
800-666-2665
Fax: 617-868-0362
e-mail: brooklinebks@delphi.com
www.brooklinebooks.com

The author provides answers and explanations to the countless questions directed to him during his twenty years' involvement with Down syndrome individuals and their families.

243 pages Paperback
ISBN: 1-571290-09-5

Cliff Cunningham, Editor

2671 Where's Chimpy?

Albert Whitman & Company
6340 Oakton Street
Morton Grove, IL 60053

847-581-0033
800-255-7675
Fax: 847-581-0039
e-mail: mail@awhitmancod.com
www.awhitmanco.com

Text and photographs show Misty, a little girl with Down syndrome and her father reviewing her day's activities in their search for her stuffed monkey.

32 pages Paperback
ISBN: 0-807589-27-6

Berniece Rabe, Editor
Diane Schmidt, Illustrator

Magazines

2672 Down Syndrome News
National Down Syndrome Congress
1370 Center Drive, Suite 102
Atlanta, GA 30338

770-604-9500
Fax: 770-604-9898
e-mail: info@ndscenter.org
www.ndscenter.org

Down Syndrome News provides advocacy news and information to parents and family members of individuals with Down syndrome and those working with them.

6x/year

2673 Down Syndrome, Papers and Abstracts for Professionals
200 Rabbit Road
Gaithersburg, MD 20878

301-963-1857

Quarterly review of research literature pertaining to Down syndrome.

Monthly

2674 Upbeat
National Down Syndrome Society
666 Broadway
New York, NY 10012

800-221-4602
Fax: 212-979-2893
e-mail: info@ndss.org
www.ndss.org

For and by people with Down syndrome that comes out three times a year.

Newsletters

2675 Communicating Together
PO Box 6395
Columbia, MD 21045

410-995-0722
Fax: 410-997-8735
www.kidsource.com

An excellent resource for parents and professionals. Each issue includes a feature article, a question and answer section and home activities.

6x/year

Dr. Libby Kumin, Editor

2676 Down Syndrome News
National Down Syndrome Congress
7000 Peachtree Dunwoody Road NE, Suite 100
Atlanta, GA 30328

770-604-9500
800-232-NDSC
e-mail: NDSC.center@aol.com
www.ndsccenter.org

Contains book reviews, articles and items of interest to those touched by Down syndrome.

10x Annually

Frank J Murphy, Executive Director

2677 Down Syndrome Today
Down Syndrome Today Publications
PO Box 212
Holtsville, NY 11742

516-654-3242

Offers information, articles, resources and materials for the parent and professional working and nurturing patients and persons with Downs syndrome.

Debra Hoeft, Publisher

2678 Down Syndrome Update
National Down Syndrome Society
666 Broadway
New York, NY 10012

800-221-4602
Fax: 212-979-2873
e-mail: info@ndss.org
www.ndss.org

Offers information on the activities of the society, new breakthroughs in medical technology, articles offering state of the art information to families and individuals with Down syndrome, and answers to questions about the illness.

12 pages Quarterly

Fran Goldstein, Editor

Pamphlets

2679 Down Syndrome
National Down Syndrome Congress
1370 Center Drive, Suite 102
Atlanta, GA 30338

770-604-9500
Fax: 770-604-9898
www.ndsccenter.org

Pertinent information ranging from education to medicine to legal or legislative issues.

2680 Heart and Down Syndrome
National Down Syndrome Society
666 Broadway
New York, NY 10012

212-460-9330
www.pcsltd.com/ndss/

1995

2681 Life Planning and Down Syndrome
National Down Syndrome Society
666 Broadway
New York, NY 10012

212-460-9330
www.pcsltd.com/ndss/

2682 Neurology of Down Syndrome
National Down Syndrome Society
666 Broadway
New York, NY 10012

212-460-9330
www.pcsltd.com/ndss/

1995

2683 New Parents
Association for Children with Down Syndrome
2616 Martin Avenue
Bellmore, NY 11710

516-221-4700
Fax: 516-221-4311

A bibliography compiled for parents who have just given birth to a child with Down syndrome.

**2684 Speech and Language Skills in Children and Adults
with Down Syndrome**
National Down Syndrome Society
666 Broadway
New York, NY 10012

212-460-9330
800-221-4602
Fax: 212-979-2873
e-mail: info@ndss.org
www.ndss.org

1995

DESCRIPTION

2685 DYSLEXIA

Involves the following Biologic System(s):

Neurologic Disorders

Dyslexia refers to a specific learning disability characterized by the impaired ability to process written symbols. Although individuals with dyslexia are able to see and recognize letters, this disorder impairs their ability to read, write, and spell. Affected individuals typically have no problems with the correct recognition of pictures and objects.

No definition of dyslexia is universally accepted, thus incidence is difficult to determine. An estimated 15% of public school children receive special education for reading problems of whom 3 to 5% are probably dyslexic. Young children with dyslexia may have difficulty remembering the correct names of letters and numbers. Articulating proper speech may be difficult. Some children of school age may reverse letters and words when writing. For example, affected children may substitute the letter p for q or the word was for saw, while transposing letters so that bets may become best. Children with dyslexia may also have difficulty reading due to an impaired ability to determine the sequence of letters within words and to distinguish right from left. The hallmark of this learning disability is the fact that, despite the difficulties associated with dyslexia, affected children are of average or above average intelligence as evidenced by I.Q. testing as well as their success in other scholastic achievements.

Early diagnosis of dyslexia is an important factor in treating this learning disability. Children nearing the end of first grade who exhibit difficulties with word skills or any children whose reading and writing ability is not commensurate with that of their other scholastic abilities may be tested for dyslexia. Although dyslexia is not related to eye defects, an ophthalmologic evaluation is beneficial in determining if ocular abnormalities may be eliminated as a cause of symptoms. Also, eye irregularities may be present in addition to dyslexia and, therefore, may be diagnosed and corrected at that time. Treatment for dyslexia is geared toward remedial teaching techniques specific to this disability.

Dyslexia is thought to be a familial disorder that may be inherited through an autosomal dominant trait. Boys are more frequently affected than girls.

See also **General Resources** on page 917

Government Agencies

2686 NIH/National Institute of Child Health and Human Development

31 Center Drive, Building 31
Bethesda, MD 20892

301-496-5133
Fax: 301-496-1104
www.nichd.nih.gov

Established in 1962 by congress, today the institute conducts and supports research on topics related to the health of children, adults, families and populations. Some of these topics include: developmental disabilities, growth and development, infant death, reproductive health and birth defects.

Nancy D Wirth, Director
Lisa Kaeser, Program & Public Liaison

National Associations & Support Groups

2687 American Speech Language Hearing Associati on (ASHA)

10801 Rockville Pike
Rockville, MD 20852

301-897-5700
800-638-8255
Fax: 301-571-0457
e-mail: productsales@asha.org
www.asha.org

The mission of the American Speech-Language-Hearing Association is to promote the interests of and provide the highest quality services for professionals in audiology, speech-language pathology, speech and hearing science, and to advocate for people with communication disabilities.

Arlene A Pietranton, Executive Director
Maureen E Thompson, Director Governance Operations

2688 Davis Dyslexia Association International

1601 Bayshore Highway, Suite 245
Burlingame, CA 94010

650-692-7141
888-999-3324
Fax: 650-692-7075
e-mail: ddai@dyslexia.com
www.dyslexia.com

Offers books, materials, workshops and certification in the Davis Dyslexia Correction method.

Ron Davis, Founder

2689 Genetic Alliance

4301 Connecticut Avenue NW
Washington, DC 20008

202-966-5557
800-336-4363
Fax: 202-966-8553
e-mail: info@geneticalliance.org
www.geneticalliance.org

A coalition of voluntary genetic support groups, consumers and professionals addressing the needs of individuals and families affected by genetic disorders from a national perspective.

Sharon Terry, President/CEO

2690 International Dyslexia Association
8600 La Salle Road, Chester Building
Baltimore, MD 21286

410-296-0232
800-222-3123
Fax: 410-321-5069
e-mail: info@interdys.org
www.interdys.org

Our mission is to pursue and provide the most comprehensive range of information and services that address the full scope of dyslexia and related difficulties in learning to read and write.

Megan P. Cohen, MPA, CAE, Executive Director
Gerri Morris, Coordinator Information/Referral

2691 Learning Disabilities Association of Ameri ca
4156 Library Road
Pittsburgh, PA 15234

412-341-1515
888-300-6710
Fax: 412-344-0224
e-mail: info@LDAAmerica.org
www.LDAAmerica.org

Helps families of the affected individual through information and referral to professionals in their area. A membership organization with affiliates in 43 states.

Sheila Buckley, Executive Director

2692 March of Dimes Birth Defects Foundation
1275 Mamaroneck Avenue
White Plains, NY 10605

914-428-7100
888-663-4637
Fax: 914-428-8203
e-mail: resourcecenter@modimes.org
www.marchofdimes.com

Partnership of volunteers and professionals dedicates to improving the health of babies by preventing birth defects and infant mortality. Over 100 chapters are located across the country and can be located through the National Office.

Dr Jennifer Howse, President

2693 National Network of Learning Disabled Adults
808 N 82nd Street, Suite F2
Scottsdale, AZ 75827

602-941-5112

Provides information and referral for LD adults involved with or in search of support groups and networking opportunities. The network publishes a quaterly newsletter.

2694 Option Institute: Son Rise Program
Autism Treatment Center of America
2080 S Undermountain Road
Sheffield, MA 01257

413-229-2100
800-714-2779
Fax: 413-229-3202
e-mail: information@son-rise.org
www.son-rise.org

Describes an effective, loving and respectful method for treating children with autism. It teaches parents and healing professionals how to set up a home based program using the child's motivation to reach their special child.

Barry Neil Kaufman, Co-Founder/Co-Creator
Samahria Lyte Kaufman, Co-Founder/Co-Creator

State Agencies & Support Groups

2695 Center for Disabilities and Development
University of Iowa Hospitals and Clinics
100 Hawkins Drive
Iowa City, IA 52242

319-353-6900
877-686-0031
e-mail: cdd-webmaster@uiowa.edu
www.healthcare.uiowa.edu/cdd

A trusted resource for healthcare, training, research and information for people with disabilities that include: behavior disorders, brain injury, cerebral palsy, diabetes, down syndrome, learning disabilities, mental retardation, sleep disorders and spina bifida.

Elayne Sexsmith, Administrator
Amy Mikelson, Supervisor Info Resource Service

Research Centers

2696 Dyslexia Research Institute
5746 Centerville Road
Tallahassee, FL 32309

850-893-2216
Fax: 850-893-2440
e-mail: dri@talstar.com
www.dyslexia-add.org

Searching for new and better methods to deal with the unique needs of Dyslexics.

Patricia K Hardman, PhD, Director
Robyn A Rennick, MS, Director

Conferences

2697 International Dyslexia Association Conference
8600 La Salle Road, Chester Building
Baltimore, MD 21286

410-296-0232
800-222-3123
Fax: 410-321-5069
e-mail: info@interdys.org
www.interdys.org

Focuses on the latest advances in dyslexia, related language difficulties and related fields. Individual sessions are geared towards educators and educational administrators, educational diagnosticians and therapists, parents, speech and language pathologists and of course, individuals with dyslexia and their families.

Megan P. Cohen, MPA, CAE, Executive Director
Noreen A. Frohme, Director Conferences

Audio Video

2698 Dyslexia
Fanlight Productions
4196 Washington Street, Suite 2
Boston, MA 02131

617-469-4999
800-937-4113
Fax: 617-469-3379
e-mail: fanlight@fanlight.com
www.fanlight.com

Looks at the experiences of people with these learning disabilities as well as the potential value to society of their alternative ways of learning. Dartmouth Hitchcock Medical Center Series, The Doctor is In...

1997 28 Minutes VHS

Nicole Johnson, Publicity Coordinator

Web Sites

2699 American Speech Language Hearing Associati on (ASHA)
www.asha.org

An organization working to promote a better quality of life for children and adults with communication disorders. Our mission is to advance knowledge about the causes and treatment of hearing, speech, and language problems.

2700 British Dyslexia Association
www.bda-dyslexia.ork.uk

The BDA offers a range of practical help for dyslexic children, dyslexic adults, parents and professionals in education.

2701 Davis Dyslexia Association
www.dyslexia.com

The goals of DDA are to increase worldwide awareness of: the perceptual gifts, talents or potentials for genius that accompany and give rise to dyslexia; effective methods for resolving the learning disability aspects of dyslexia.

2702 Davis Dyslexia Association International Dyslexia: The Gift
www.dyslexia.com

Offers information and training in methods for overcoming learning problems developed by Ron Davis, author of 'The Gift of Dyslexia,' listings of Davis Dyslexia Correction providers worldwide, a forum for networking and articles and reports on learning styles and educational approaches.

2703 International Dyslexia Association
www.interdys.org

Dyslexia is a neurological disorder that impairs reading. If undetected in children, it can create major learning problems. Contact the IDA for free information. Publications are available for a range of fees.

2704 Learning Disabilities Association of Ameri ca
www.ldaamerica.org

Helps families of the affected individual through information and referral to professionals in their area. A membership organization with affiliates in 42 states.

2705 Mental Health Net
www.mentalhelp.net

We wish to provide the following: to discuss, develop and debate in an open forum the future of the mental health field in America and throughout the world. To help coordinate various components of the mental health field so as to bring about greater communication between them.

2706 NIH/National Institute of Child Health and Human Development
www.nichd.nih.gov

Established in 1962 by congress, today the institute conducts and supports research on all stages of human dveeloptment to better understand the health of children, adults, families and communities. Topics of research include: birth defects, mental retardation, developmental disabilities, reproductive health, growth and development, and infant death.

2707 Option Institute
www.son-rise.org

Describes an effective, loving and respectful method for treating children with autism. It teaches parents and healing professionals how to set up a home based program using the child's motivation to reach their special child.

Book Publishers

2708 Let's Talk About Dyslexia

Melanie Apel Gordon, author

Rosen Publishing Group's PowerKids Press
29 E 21st Street
New York, NY 10010

212-777-3017
800-237-9932
Fax: 888-436-4643
e-mail: rosenpub@tribeca.ios.com
www.powerkidspress.com

Children will learn what dyslexia is and how to tell if they have it. This book stresses that children with dyslexia are just as smart as their classmates. Tells about Albert Einstein and other well known people who were dyslexic. Grades K-5.

24 pages
ISBN: 0-823951-99-5

2709 Misunderstood Child

Larry B Silver, MD, author

Active Parenting Publishers
1995 Vaughn Road NW, Suite 108
Kennesaw, GA 30144

770-429-0565
800-825-0060
Fax: 770-429-0334
e-mail: cservice@activeparenting.com
www.activeparenting.com

The fully revised and updated must-have resource to help you become a supportive and assertive advocate for your child. The Misunderstood Child, Fourth Edition has become the go-to reference guide for families of children with learning disorders. Item #8825.

432 pages

2710 Overcoming Dyslexia in Children, Adolescents, and Adults

Dale R Jordan, author

Pro-Ed
8700 Shoal Creek Boulevard
Austin, TX 78757

512-451-3246
800-897-3202
Fax: 800-397-7633
www.procdinc.com

The third edition summarizes what science knows today about what causes the forms of dyslexia that are related to left-brain language processing. This book also discusses in detail nonverbal types of learning disabilities (LD) and social and emotional types of LD. All forms of dyslexia are described in detail with graphic illustrations of how dyslexia impacts classroom learning, social behavior, emotional maturity and development.

432 pages Softcover
ISBN: 0-890796-42-4

2711 Straight Talk about Psychological Testing for Kids

Ellen Braaten PhD, Gretcen Felopulos PhD, author

Active Parenting Publishers
1955 Vaughn Road NW, Suite 108
Kennesaw, GA 30144

770-429-0565
800-825-0060
Fax: 770-429-0334
e-mail: cservice@activeparenting.com
www.activeparenting.com

This authoritative guide gives parents the inside scoop on how psychological testing works and how to use testing to get the best help for their children. Item #8670.

260 pages Softcover

Camps

2712 Dunnabeck at Kildonan
425 Morse Hill Road
Amenia, NY 12501

845-373-8111
Fax: 845-373-2004
www.kildonan.org

Specializes in helping intelligent children with specific reading, writing and spelling disablities. Provides Orton-Gillingham tutoring with camp activities, including swimming, sailing, waterskiing, horseback riding, ceramics, tennis and woodworking.

Ages 9-15

Ron Wilson, Headmaster
Bea Sattler, Administrative Assistant

2713 Dyslexia Centers
New Mexico State University
755 S Telshor Boulevard
Las Cruces, NM

505-524-6450

Participants must enroll at the Audiology Center for a minimum of two weeks. Children and adults who are learning disabled or speech handicapped receive speech therapy and psychotherapy in addition to tutoring, academic instruction and remedial reading.

Janice Kolosseus

2714 Marvelwood Summer
Marvelwood School
476 Skiff Mountain Road, PO Box 3001
Kent, CT 06757

860-927-0047
800-440-9107
Fax: 860-927-5325
e-mail: summerschool@marvelwood.org
www.themarvelwoodschool.com

The emphasis in this summer program is on diagnosis and remediation of individual reading, spelling, writing, mathematics and study problems. Participants are boys and girls entering grades 6-10.

Scott E Pottbecker, Head of School
Katherine Almquist, Summer Admissions

2715 Tower Program at Regis College
Regis College
235 Wellesley Street
Weston, MA

781-768-7000
www.regiscollege.edu

Helps average and above average college-bound students, ages 16-17, having a diagnosed dyslexic learning disability, to adjust to a college setting. Emphasis is on instruction and academic reinforcement, affective support, awareness of support services available on most college campuses and strategy training.

S Marilyn MacGregor

DESCRIPTION

2716 DYSTONIA

Covers these related disorders: Dopa-responsive dystonia (DRD) or Segawa syndrome, Drug-induced dystonia, Dystonia musculorum deformans (DMD) or torsion, Fecal dystonia

Involves the following Biologic System(s):
Neurologic Disorders, Orthopedic and Muscle Disorders

Dystonia is a neurologic movement disorder characterized by relatively slow, involuntary, writhing motions that may result in twisting or distorted posturing of affected muscles. The abnormal motions associated with dystonia result from unusually increased muscle rigidity due to simultaneous contractions of certain muscles termed agonists and antagonists. In unaffected individuals, when voluntary movements occur, there are usually coordinated contractions and simultaneous relaxations of several muscles. Muscles known as agonists are primarily responsible for producing a particular movement, and other muscles, called synergists, contract to assist the agonist muscles. While these muscles contract, other muscles known as antagonists normally simultaneously relax, helping to ensure smooth rather than jerky, uncoordinated motions. However, in patients with dystonia, agonist and antagonist muscles simultaneously contract, resulting in abnormally distorted movements. Depending upon the form of dystonia present, abnormal motions may vary greatly in severity and may be limited to one muscle group or may affect many muscles of the body, causing severely distorted postures and significantly interfering with activities of daily living.

Dystonias that are limited to certain specific muscle groups may be referred to as focal dystonias. Focal dystonias may be confined to muscles of the neck (cervical dystonia or spasmodic torticollis); the eyelids, causing near or complete closure of the eyelids (blepharospasm) and functional blindness; the mouth and jaw (buccomandibular dystonia); the hand (writer's cramp); or certain other areas of the body. Although such conditions are considered the most prevalent forms of dystonia, they occur much more commonly in adults than children. The main causes of dystonia during childhood include certain genetic disorders, such as dystonia musculorum deformans, dopa-responsive dystonia, Wilson disease, or Hallervorden-Spatz disease; lack of oxygen during labor, delivery, or immediately after birth (perinatal asphyxia), causing brain damage (hypoxicischemic encephalopathy); or exposure to particular medications.

The most pronounced form of dystonia is observed in a group of genetic disorders known as dystonia musculorum deformans (DMD) or torsion dystonia. One form of the disorder is thought to most commonly affect individuals of Eastern European Ashkenazi Jewish descent. Symptoms typically become apparent between the ages of six to 14 years and initially include involuntary movement or posturing of one area of the body, particularly the foot. Most patients first experience abnormal periodic bending of one foot with the toes downward (plantar flexion), potentially causing tip-toe walking. Such posturing of the foot gradually becomes constant, and muscles in other areas of the body, such as the shoulders, pelvis, and spine, begin to develop periodic, involuntary, spasmodic, twisting movements. With disease progression, spasms become frequent and, eventually, are ongoing, causing contortion and severely distorted posturing of affected muscles. Although dystonic movements may initially subside during sleep, they may eventually be present at all times, severely restricting activities of daily living and causing a high level of functional disability. Treatment may include administration of the drug trihexyphenidyl or certain other medications, such as carbamazepine, bromocriptine, levodopa, or diazepam.

Dopa-responsive dystonia (DRD), also known as Segawa syndrome, is a genetic disorder that is thought to be transmitted as an autosomal dominant trait. The disorder more commonly affects females and usually becomes apparent between four to eight years of age. Initial symptoms often include periodic, involuntary stiffening and abnormal posturing of the foot. As the disease progresses, dystonia may also eventually affect muscles of the arms, torso, and, in some patients, the neck. Within about four to five years, all areas of the body are usually affected. Some patients may also have unusually slow movements (bradykinesia) and involuntary, rhythmic movements (tremors) of certain muscles while at rest. Symptoms usually subside with sleep and gradually worsen during the day. Administration of the medication levodopa, a biological forerunner or precursor of the neurotransmitter dopamine, typically causes a dramatic improvement of symptoms.

Wilson disease is an autosomal recessive disorder in which copper metabolism causes an abnormal accumulation of copper in the liver, brain, kidneys, corneas, and other tissues of the body. The disorder is often characterized by progressive liver disease, degenerative changes of the brain, kidney failure, and the presence of characteristic grayish-green or reddish-gold rings at the outer margins of the corneas (Kayser-Fleischer rings). Neurologic symptoms, which rarely become apparent before age 10, are thought to result from progressive involvement of a region of the brain that assists in regulating muscular movements (basal ganglia). Such symptoms usually initially include progressive dystonia that is characterized by abnormalities of muscle tone, muscle stiffness and rigidity, muscle spasms, and abnormal movement patterns and fixed postures, such as a fixed smile due to drawing back of the upper lip. Patients also experience involuntary, rhythmic, quivering movements of the extremities on one side of the body (unilateral) that eventually become generalized and disabling. The treatment of patients with Wilson disease often consists of administration of penicillamine, a medication that binds with copper and enables it to be excreted from the body; supplementation of vitamin B6; and a diet that is low in copper intake (less than one mg/day).

Hallervorden-Spatz disease is a rare autosomal recessive disorder characterized by an abnormal accumulation of iron pigment in certain areas of the brain. Symptoms usually develop during childhood and may include progressive dystonia characterized by muscle stiffness, rigidity, and relatively slow, involuntary, twisting and distorted posturing of affected muscles. By adolescence, patients may have restricted movements of certain muscles due to increased muscle rigidity (spasticity); an inability to coordinate voluntary movements (ataxia); difficulty speaking (dysarthria); and progressive confusion, disorientation, and deterioration of intellectual abilities (dementia). The treatment of patients with Hallervorden-Spatz disease is symptomatic and supportive.

In some children, the administration of certain drugs may cause a sudden (acute) development of dystonia, such as certain antiseizure (anticonvulsant) medications or antipsychotic drugs (phenothiazines). In addition, particular medications may cause acute or chronic progressive dystonia, such as the antiseizure medications phenytoin or carbamazepine, or the antipsychotic drug haloperidol. Treatment may include the withdrawal of the offending drug and intravenous administration of the medication, diphenhydramine.

Depending upon its underlying cause or specific form, treatment measures for chronic dystonia may include the administration of certain medications (anticholinergic agents), such as trihexyphenidyl or ethopropazine. These drugs inhibit the transmission of particular nerve impulses to muscles.|In addition, focal dystonias such as dystonia limited to muscles of the neck (cervical dystiodic torticollis), are often treated with periodic injections of botulin (botulinum toxin) into affected muscles. Botulin is a bacterial toxin that blocks the release of a particular neurotransmitter (acetylcholine), resulting in temporary paralysis and thus relief from discomfort and disability associated with muscle rigidity.

See also **General Resources** on page 917

Government Agencies

2717 NIH/National Institute of Neurological Dis orders and Stroke (NINDS)
PO Box 5801
Bethesda, MD 20824

301-496-5751
800-352-9424
Fax: 301-496-0296
TTY: 301-468-5981
www.ninds.nih.gov

Supports and conducts research and research training on the normal structure and function of the nervous system and on the causes, prevention, diagnosis and treatment of nervous system disorders including stroke, epilepsy, multiple sclerosis, Parkinson's disease, head and spinal cord injury, Alzheimer's disease and brain tumors.

Story C Landis Ph.D., Director
Audrey S Penn M.D., Deputy Director

National Associations & Support Groups

2718 American Speech Language Hearing Associati on (ASHA)
10801 Rockville Pike
Rockville, MD 20852

301-897-5700
800-638-8255
Fax: 301-571-0457
e-mail: pr@asha.org
www.asha.org

Works to promote a better quality of life for children and adults with communication disorders. Part of their mission is to advance knowledge about the causes and treatment of hearing, speech, and language problems.

Arlene A Pietranton, Executive Director

2719 Dystonia Medical Research Foundation
One E Wacker Drive, Suite 2430
Chicago, IL 60601

312-755-0198
Fax: 312-803-0138
e-mail: dystonia@dystonia-foundation.org/
www.dystonia-foundation.org/

The mission of the Dystonia Medical Research Foundation is to advance research for more treatments and ultimately a cure; to promote awareness and education; and to support the needs and well being of affected individuals and families.

Claire A. Centralla, President
Janet Hieshetter, Executive Director

2720 Genetic Alliance
4301 Connecticut Avenue NW
Washington, DC 20008

202-966-5557
800-336-4363
Fax: 202-966-8553
e-mail: info@geneticalliance.org
www.geneticalliance.org

A coalition of voluntary genetic support groups, consumers and professionals addressing the needs of individuals and families affected by genetic disorders from a national perspective.

Sharon Terry, President/CEO

2721 March of Dimes Birth Defects Foundation
1275 Mamaroneck Avenue
White Plains, NY 10605

914-428-7100
888-663-4637
Fax: 914-428-8203
e-mail: resourcecenter@modimes.org
www.marchofdimes.com

Partnership of volunteers and professionals dedicates to improving the health of babies by preventing birth defects and infant mortality. Over 100 chapters are located across the country and can be located through the National Office.

Dr Jennifer Howse, President

2722 Muscular Dystrophy Association
3300 E Sunrise Drive
Tuscon, AZ 85718

520-529-2000
800-572-1717
Fax: 520-529-5300
e-mail: mda@mdausa.org
www.mdausa.org

Voluntary health agency aimed at conquering nucromuscular diseases that affect more than 1,000,000 Americans. The diseases in MDA's program include nine forms of muscular dystrophy, amyotrophic lateral sclerosis (Lou Gehrig's disease), spinal muscular atrophy, Charcot-Marie-Tooth disease and other neuromuscular conditions. With nearly 200 offices across the country, MDA conducts research, medical and community services, clinics, support groups, summer camp for youngsters and much more.

Bob Mackle, Director Public Information
Carol Sowell, Director Publications

2723 National Foundation for Jewish Genetic Diseases
One Gustave L Levy Place, Box 1497
New York, NY 10029

212-659-6774
Fax: 212-241-6947
www.nfjgd.org

2724 National Spasmodic Torticollis Association
9920 Talbert Avenue, Suite 233
Fountain Valley, CA 92708

714-378-7837
800-487-8385
Fax: 714-378-7830
e-mail: nstamail@aol.com
www.torticollis.org

Nonprofit organization, providing support, referrals and information for ST patients and family members.

Cheryl Lynne Sullivan, Executive Director

2725 WE MOVE (Worldwide Education and Advocacy Movement Disorders)
204 W 84th Street
New York, NY 10024

212-241-8567
800-437-6682
Fax: 212-875-8389
e-mail: wemove@wemove.org
www.wemove.org

WE MOVE provides movement disorder information and educational materials to physicians, patients, the media, and the public via its comprehensive Web sites training courses, and more. It's goal is to make early diagnosis, up-to-date treatment and patient support a reality for all people living with movement disorders.

Susan Bressman MD, President

Research Centers

2726 Benign Essential Blepharospasm Research Foundation
637 N 7th Street, Suite 102, PO Box 12468
Beaumont, TX 77726

409-832-0788
Fax: 409-832-0890
e-mail: bebrf@blapharospasm.org
www.blepharospasm.org

The purpose of BEBRF is to undertake, promote, develop and carry on the search for the cause and a cure for benign essential blepharospace and other related disorders and infirmities of the facial musculature.

Mary Lou Thompson, President
Don Peaslee, First Vice President

2727 Dystonia Medical Research Foundation
One E Wacker Drive, Suite 2430
Chicago, IL 60601

312-755-0198
Fax: 312-803-0138
e-mail: dystonia@dystonia-foundation.org
www.dystonia-foundation.org/

Dedicated to serving people with dystonia, a neurological disorder. The goals of the Foundation is to advance research into the causes of and treatments for dystonia; to build awareness of dystonia in both the medical and lay communities; and to sponsor patient and family support groups and programs.

Claire A. Centralla, President
Jane Hieshetter, Executive Director

Web Sites

2728 American Speech Language Hearing Associati on (ASHA)
www.asha.org

An organization working to promote a better quality of life for children and adults with communication disorders. Our mission is to advance knowledge about the causes and treatments of hearing, speech, and language problems.

2729 Dystonia Medical Research Foundation
www.dystonia-foundation.org

Dedicated to serving people with dystonia, a neurological disorder. The goals of the the Foundation is to advance research into the causes of and treatments for dystonia; to build awareness of dystonia in both the medical and lay communities; and to sponsor patient and family support groups and programs.

2730 MGH Neurology Web Forums
www.mgh.harvard.edu/forum

2731 Muscular Dystrophy Association
www.mdausa.org

Voluntary health agency aimed at conquering nucromuscular disease that affect more than 1,000,000 Americans.

2732 NIH/National Institute of Neurological Dis orders and Stroke (NINDS)
www.ninds.nih.gov

Supports and conducts research and research training on the normal structure and function of the nervous system and on the causes, prevention, diagnosis and treatment of nervous system disorders including stroke, epilepsy, multiple sclerosis, Parkinson's disease, head and spinal cord injury, Alzheimer's disease and brain tumors.

2733 National Spasmodic Torticollis Association
www.torticollis.org

Nonprofit organization, providing support, referrals and information for ST patients and family members.

2734 Online Mendelian Inheritance in Man
www.ncbi.nlm.nih.gov

This database is a catalog of human genes and genetic disorders.

2735 WE MOVE (Worldwide Education and Advocacy Movement Disorders)
www.wemove.org

WE MOVE provides movement disorder information and educational materials to physicians, patients, the media, and the public via its comprehensive Web sites training courses, and more. It's goal is to make early diagnosis, up-to-date treatment and patient support a reality for all people living with movement disorders.

Newsletters

2736 Benign Essential Blepharospasm Research Foundation
637 N 7th Street, Suite 102, PO Box 12468
Beaumont, TX 77726

409-832-0788
Fax: 409-832-0890
e-mail: bebrf@blepharospasm.org
www.blepharospasm.org

BEBRF Focus for 2006: Twenty-five years of hope, and progress.

12 pages Bimonthly

Mary Lou Thompson, President
Don Peaslee, First Vice President

2737 Dystonia Dialogue
Dystonia Medical Research Foundation
One E Wacker Drive, Suite 2430
Chicago, IL 60601

312-755-0198
Fax: 312-803-0138
e-mail: dystonia@dystonia-foundation.org
www.dystonia-foundation.org/

The official publication of the Dystonia Medical Research Foundation. Provides information to individuals with dystonia, their families, health care professionals, and supporters of the foundation.

Quarterly

Claire A. Centralla, President
Janet Hieshetter, Executive Director

Pamphlets

2738 Classification and Definition of Disorders Causing Hypertonia in Childhood
National Inst. of Neurological Disorders/Stroke
NIH, 31 Center Drive, MSC 2540, Bldg. 31, Rm 8A06
Bethesda, MD 20892

301-496-5751
800-352-9424
www.ninds.nih.gov

Report on an April, 2001 meeting.

2739 DMRF/NINDS Dystonia Workshop: From Gene to Function in Dystonia
National Inst. of Neurological Disorders/Stroke
PO Box 5801
Bethesda, MD 20824

301-496-5751
800-352-9424
www.ninds.nih.gov

Health Disparities: Working Group-Cognitive and Emotional Health in Minority Children Workshop.

Story C. Landis, PhD, Director
Audrey S. Penn, MD, Deputy Director

2740 Dytonias: Fact Sheet
National Inst. of Neurological Disorders/Stroke
PO Box 5801
Bethesda, MD 20824

301-496-5751
800-352-9424
www.ninds.nih.gov

Fact Sheet listing the following contents: What are the Dystonias, What are the symptoms, How are the Dystonias classified, What do scientists know about the Dystonias, When do symptoms occur, Are their any treatments, What research is being done, Where can I get more information.

Story C. Landis, PhD, President
Audrey S. Penn, MD, Deputy Director

2741 NINDS Seeks Patients with Generalized Dystonia
National Inst. of Neurological Disorders/Stroke
PO Box 5801
Bethesda, MD 20824

301-496-5751
800-352-9424
www.ninds.nih.gov

NINDS program announcements, requests for applications and clinical studies seeking patients.

Story C. Landis, PhD, Director
Audrey S. Penn, MD, Deputy Director

2742 Patients with Cervical or Focal Hand Dystonia Sought
National Inst. of Neurological Disorders/Stroke
PO Box 5801
Bethesda, MD 20824

301-496-5751
800-352-9424
e-mail: karpb@ninds.nih.gov
www.ninds.nih.gov

NINDS program announcements, requests for applications and clinical studies seeking patients.

Story C. Landis, PhD, Director
Audrey S. Penn, MD, Deputy Director

DESCRIPTION

2743 EATING DISORDERS

Synonyms: Anorexia Nervosa, Bulima Nervosa, Binge Eating Disorder, Impulsive Overeating

Involves the following Biologic System(s):
Developmental/Behavioral/Psychiatric Disorders

There are two principal eating disorders — Anorexia Nervosa and Bulimia Nervosa. Although different in the symptoms they manifest, the two disorders are quite similar in their underlying pathology: an obsessive concern with body image and body weight. Approximately 90% of patients are female, and the average age of onset is 17 years. It is commonly believed that eating disorders are, in part, culturally determined. In the Western world, particularly in the U.S., a pervasive cultural preference for slimness causes many young women to spend extraordinary amounts of time, money, and energy dieting and exercising to stay slim.

Those with eating disorders may cause grave physical damage to their bodies, so treatment first involves restoring patients to a safe and healthy body weight. Once the patient is out of physical danger, treatment is usually a long-term process that includes medication and psychotherapy. Fortunately, most people who undergo appropriate treatment do recover from eating disorders.

Anorexia nervosa is diagnosed when a person refuses to maintain a body weight at or above 85 percent of their normal weight. Patients have an intense fear of gaining weight or becoming fat, despite being underweight. They are disturbed by the way their body weight or shape is experienced, give it undue influence, and deny the seriousness of low body weight. Patients with anorexia nervosa may be severely depressed, and may experience insomnia and irritability. They also may exhibit a strong need to control their environment, and may be socially and emotionally withdrawn. In menstruating females, anorexia may create an absence of at least three consecutive menstrual cycles.

Bulima nervosa consists of recurrent episodes of binge eating — eating more food than most people would eat under similar circumstances, during which the person feels out of control over eating. This behavior is then followed by purging in order to prevent weight gain, and includes self-induced vomiting and misuse of laxatives or diuretics. Excessive fasting or exercise may be evident in both anorexia and bulimia. Self evaluation is unduly influenced by body weight and shape.

Patients with binge eating disorder may eat unusually large amounts of food or eat much more quickly than usual and until they are uncomfortable. They may eat even when they are not hungry, and often eat alone because of embarrassment over the amount of food they are eating. Binge eating disorder is associated with feelings of guilt and/or depression.

Those with bulimia nervosa are often within the normal weight range, but may have been overweight prior to developing the disorder. People with eating disorders also share many features of obsessive compulsive disorder, i.e. hoarding food and spending unusual amounts of time researching and reading about food. They may also have symptoms of mood and anxiety disorders.

Prevalence studies in adolescent females show rates of 0.5 to one percent for anorexia nervosa, and one to three percent for bulimia nervosa. Patients rarely seek treatment; family members usually are first to bring it to attention. A multidisciplinary approach to treatment is essential. Medications, especially the newest SSRIs (Selective Serotonin Reuptake Inhibitors, which were originally developed as antidepressants) have been found to be very effective in the treatment of eating disorders. They can help restore and build self-esteem, and thereby help the patient maintain a positive attitude as well as a safe and healthy body image and body weight. Because of the physical damage that eating disorders can create, nutritional counseling and monitoring is often vital to restore and maintain proper body weight. Hospitalization often is indicated in anorexia, especially if the patients is more than 20% below the expected body weight. There is a high (10%) mortality rate. Restoration of fluids and chemicals in the blood (electrolytes) is critical. Outpatient management for anorexia also includes a supervised weight-gain program. The outcome (prognosis) for patients with bulimia is better than that for patients with anorexia. They are also more likely to seek treatment. Eating disorders are extremely complex, and patients often have conflicting psychological issues that trigger the compulsion to binge, or the morbid fear of gaining weight. Psychotherapy and cognitive behavior therapy may be required for a number of years.

See also **General Resources** on page 917

Government Agencies

2744 NIH/National Institute of Mental Health Eating Disorders Program
Public Information and Communications Branch
6001 Executive Boulevard, Room 8184, MSC 9663
Bethesda, MD 20892

301-496-1891
866-615-6464
Fax: 301-443-4279
TTY: 866-415-8051
e-mail: nimhinfo@nih.gov
www.nimh.nih.gov/publicat/eatingdisorders.cfm

A nonprofit organization developed to coordinate nationwide mental health screening programs and to ensure cooperation, professionalism, and accountability in mental illness screenings.

Thomas R Insel, MD, NIMH Director
Richard Nakamura, MD, NIMH Deputy Director

National Associations & Support Groups

2745 Anorexia Nervosa & Related Eating Disorders
Box 5102
Eugene, OR 97405

541-344-1144
e-mail: jarinor@rio.com
www.anred.com

A national nonprofit organization that provides free and low-cost information about anorexia, bulimia, compulsive eating and compulsive exercising. Offers a free booklet as well as brochures, fact sheets and a monthly newsletter.

J Bradley Rubel, President

2746 Change for Good Coaching
Change for Good Coaching
3801 Connecticut Avenue NW
Washington, DC 20008

202-362-3009
Fax: 433-645-2420
e-mail: brockhansenlcsw@aol.com
www.change-for-good.org/

Change for Good Coaching provides services to individuals that are designed to: help an individual to clarify their goals; helping an individual to craft an action plan, and, support the individual in following through to their own satisfaction. Interested individuals can contact Change for Good Coaching for a free complimentary telephone coaching session.

Brock Hansen, LCSW, Director

2747 Compulsive Eaters Anonymous
5500 E Atherton Street, Suite 227-B
Long Beach, CA 90815

562-342-9344
Fax: 562-342-9346
e-mail: gso@ceahow.org
www.ceahow.org

Purpose is to stop eating compulsively and carry the message to those that still suffer.

Eric R Florida, Chairman
N Woody, President

2748 Council on Size and Weight Discrimination (CSWD)
PO Box 305
Mount Marion, NY 12456

845-679-1209
Fax: 845-679-1206
e-mail: info@cswd.org
www.cswd.org

Works to influence public policy and opinion in an effort to eliminate oppression and discrimination based on body size, shape, or weight standards. Projects include International No Diet Coalition.

Publications: Annotated Bibliography on Size Acceptance, Anti-Dieting, Eating Disorders and Related Issues, book. International No Diet Coalition Directory of Resources, books.

Miriam Berg, President
Lynn McAfee, Medical Advocacy Director

2749 Eating Disorders Group
Renfrew Center
11 East 36th Street
New York, NY 10016

800-736-3739
Fax: 212-686-1865
www.renfrew.org/

Women struggling to overcome anorexia, bulimia or other disordered eating patterns involving binge eating or restricting can benefit from these weekly groups. Led by experienced therapists, the sessions provide a safe, sympathetic atmosphere where group members explore what triggers their eating disorders as well as issues concerning body image, relationships, school, work and home.

Jane Fleming, Executive Director

2750 Food Addicts Anonymous
World Service Office
4623 Forest Hill Boulevard, #109-4
West Palm Beach, FL 33415

561-967-3871
Fax: 561-967-9815
e-mail: info@foodaddictsanonymous.org
foodaddictsanonymous.org

A 12-step fellowship of men and women who are willing to recover from the disease of food adiction. Primary purpose is to maintain abstinence from sugar, flour, and wheat. Information and referral, pen pals, online contacts, conferences. Assistance in starting groups.

Charlotte Brinkey, Program Coordinator

2751 International Association of Eating Disorders Professionals
PO Box 1295
Pekin, IL 61555

309-346-3341
800-800-8126
Fax: 390-346-2874
www.iaedp.com

The International Association of Eating Disorders Professionals provides first-quality education and high-level training standards to an international multidisciplinary group of various healthcare treatment providers and helping professions, who treat the full spectrum of eating disorder problems.

Shirley Klein, Executive Director
Emmett R Bishop, MD/CEDS, Board-Directors President

2752 Klaman Eating Disorders Center at McLean Hospital
McClean Hospital
115 Mill Street
Belmont, MA 02478

617-855-2000
800-333-0338
e-mail: mcleaninfo@mclean.harvard.edu
www.mclean.harvard.edu/patient/child/edc.php

Founded with the generous support of the Klarman Family Foundation, the Klarman Eating Disorders Center at Harvard-affiliated McLean Hospital provides state-of-the-art treatment for eating disorders in girls and young women ages 13 to 23. Housed in its own newly renovated building on the grounds of McLean, the Center provides a unique therapeutic environment that is conducive to recovery.

Esther Dechant, MD, Medical Director
Patricia Tarbox, LICSW, Program Director

2753 Largesse, The Network for Size Esteem
PO Box 9404
New Haven, CT 06534

203-787-1624
Fax: 203-787-1624
e-mail: size_esteem@yahoo.com
eskimo.com/~largesse

International clearinghouse for organizations and people concerned with weight-based bias. Acts as a support and information resource for people and groups who promote size esteem and oppose discrimination based on weight. Seeks 'the empowerment of all women, regardless of size or shape' and develops educational and support materials. Publications: The Fat Underground, book. Legal Resource Kit. Room to Grow, poetry of size. Size Esteem, periodical.

Richard K Stimson, Co-Director
Karen W Stimson, Co-Director

2754 McCallum Place
615 S New Ballas Road
Saint Louis, MO 63141

314-569-6898
Fax: 314-995-4197
www.mccallumplace.com/

McCallum Place provides comprehensive medical and psychiatric care, specialized psychotherapies and nutritional support for patients with eating disorders. Our state-of-the-art treatment and programs, which integrate the latest findings from eating disorders research with experienced clinical practice, are designed to create an environment of structure and support.

Kimberli McCallum, MD, Medical Director
Lynn Stark, Program Director

2755 National Association of Anorexia Nervosa and Associated Disorders (ANAD)
PO Box 7
Highland Park, IL 60035

847-831-3438
Fax: 847-433-4632
e-mail: anad20@aol.com
www.anad.org

Sponsors national and local programs to prevent eating disorders and assist people with eating disorders and their families. Provides a national clearinghouse of information and is a grassroots association for laypeople and professionals. It operates a national network of free support groups for people with eating disorders and their families, and provides prevention information and education to students and lecturers.

Vivian Hanson Meehan, President

2756 National Association to Advance Fat Acceptance (NAAFA)
PO Box 225100
Oakland, CA 94609

916-558-6880
800-442-1214
Fax: 415-863-8596
e-mail: naafa@naafa.org
naafa.org

Nonprofit organization dedicated to improving the quality of life for fat people. Opposes discrimination against fat people including discrimination in advertising, employment, fashion, medicine, insurance, social acceptance, the media, schooling and public accommodations. Monitors legislative activity and litigation affecting fat people. Publications: NAAFA Newsletter, bimonthly. Annual conference and symposium, always mid-August.

Maryanne Bodoky, Executive Director
Marilyn Wann, Activism Chair

2757 National Center for Overcoming Overeating
Old Chelsea Station, PO Box 1257
New York, NY 10113

212-875-0442
e-mail: webmaster@overcomingovereating.com
OvercomingOvereating.com

The National Center for Overcoming Overeating is an educational and training organization working to end body hatred and dieting. It was started in 1989 by Carol Munter and Jane Hirschmann, authors of Overcoming Overeating and When Women Stop Hating Their Bodies.

Carol Munter, Co-Founder
Jane Hirschmann, Co-Founder

2758 National Eating Disorders Association
603 Stewart Street, Suite 803
Seattle, WA 98101

206-382-3587
800-931-2237
Fax: 206-829-8501
e-mail: info@NationalEatingDisorders.org
www.NationalEatingDisorders.org

Dedicated to the elimination of eating disorders through prevention efforts, education, referral and support services, advocacy, training, and research. Offers free information and referrals as well as educational curriculum and materials for sale. We also operate a Toll-Free Information and Referral HelpLine at 800-931-2237, the first eating disorders information source of its kind in the world, linking more than 1,200 callers per month to vital information and life-saving treatment.

Tonia Brown, Program Assistant

2759 National Eating Disorders Association (NED A)
603 Stewart Street, Suite 803
Seattle, WA 98101

206-382-3587
800-931-2237
e-mail: info@NationalEatingDisorders.org
www.NationalEatingDisorders.org

The National Eating Disorders Association (NEDA) is the largest not-for-profit organization in the United States working to prevent eating disorders and provide treatment referrals to those suffering from anorexia, bulimia and binge eating disorder and those concerned with body image and weight issues. Formerly known as The American Anorexia Bulimia Association.

Tracy L Kahlo, Chief Operating Officer
Lynn S Grefe, Chief Executive Officer

2760 Overeaters Anonymous World Service Office
PO Box 44020
Rio Ranch, NM 87174

505-891-2664
Fax: 505-891-4320
e-mail: info@oa.org
www.oa.org/index.htm

For families and friends of compulsive overeaters. Provides support groups that offer opportunities for the sharing of experiences and viewpoints to offer comfort, hope and friendship. Also to grow spiritually by working with the Twelve Steps and to give understanding and encouragement to the compulsive overeater. Works in cooperation with Overeaters Anonymous. Publications: newsletter, three to four times a year. Offers periodic retreats and workshops.

Jack Finley, Chairman
Naomi Lippel, Managing Director

2761 Overeaters Anonymous, World Service Office
PO Box 44020
Rio Rancho, NM 87174

505-891-2664
Fax: 505-891-4320
e-mail: info@overeatersanonymous.org
www.overeatersanonymous.org

Overeaters Anymonous is a 12 step program dealing with food and compulsive overeating. There are no fees or dues. The only requirement for membership is the desire to stop eating compulsively. Call the World Service Office for a location near you.

2762 TOPS Club
4575 South 5th Street
Milwaukee, WI 53207

414-482-4620
800-932-8677
e-mail: topsinteractive@tops.org
www.tops.org/

Weight control self-help association using group dynamics, competition and recognition to help members lose weight. TOPS is medically oriented requiring physician-approved individual diet programs and physician-set weight goals. Publications: TOPS News, monthly, a magazine that contains member news, success stories, inspirational materials and features on diet-related subjects, chapter news, medical questions and answers. Annual International Recognition Days.

Lily Files, Chairman of the Board
Barb Cady, President/Officers

2763 We Insist on Natural Shapes (WINS)
PO Box 19938
Sacramento, CA 95819

800-600-9467
e-mail: winsnews@aol.com
winsnews.org

Nonprofit organization educates about normal, healthy shapes in recognizing that the shape of one's body is determined by one's genes. Genetic makeup determines healthy weight, whether it be thin or heavy, and a moderate amount of balanced food, with a moderate amount of exercise will allow one to achieve her/his natural, healthy shape.

June Preston, Executive Director
Mary Jane Ray, Committee Chair

State Agencies & Support Groups

Connecticut

2764 Renfrew Center of Connecticut
436 Danbury Road
Wilton, CT 06897

800-736-3739
Fax: 203-563-9936
e-mail: info@renfrewcenter.com
www.renfrewcenter.com/locations/wilton.asp

The Renfrew Center of Connecticut provides an Eating Disorders Group led by experienced therapists the sessions of which provide a safe, sympathetic atmosphere where group members explore what triggers their eating disorders as well as issues concerning body image, relationships, school, work and home. A therapeutic approach that allows women to recognize and confront negative thoughts and feelings about their bodies and to replace them with realistic and healthy views about themselves is used.

Jane Fleming, Executive Director
Gayle Brooks, Ph.D, Clinical Director

Florida

2765 Coconut Creek Eating Disorders Support Group
Renfrew Center
7700 Renfrew Lane
Coconut Creek, FL 33073

954-698-9222
800-736-3739
Fax: 954-698-9007
e-mail: info@renfrewcenter.org
www.renfrewcenter.com/locations/coconut-creek.asp

The Coconut Creek Eating Disorders Support Group at the Renfrew Center is led by experienced therapists where the sessions provide a safe, sympathetic atmosphere in which group members

explore what triggers their eating disorders as well as issues concerning body image, relationships, school, work and home.

Jane Fleming, Executive Director
Gayle Brooks, Ph.D, Clinical Director

2766 Renfrew Center of Miami
151 Majorca Avenue
Coral Gables, FL 33134

800-736-3739
Fax: 605-445-2779
e-mail: info@renfrewcenter.org
www.renfrewcenter.com/locations/coral-gables.asp

The Renfrew Center of Miami provides an Eating Disorders Group led by experienced therapists the sessions of which provide a safe, sympathetic atmosphere where group members explore what triggers their eating disorders as well as issues concerning body image, relationships, school, work and home.

Jane Fleming, Executive Director
Gayle Brooks, Ph.D, Clinical Director

2767 Renfrew Center of South Florida
7700 Renfrew Lane
Coconut, FL 33073

Fax: 954-698-9007
e-mail: info@renfrewcenter.org
www.renfrew.org

Illinois

2768 Academy for Eating Disorders (AED)
60 Revere Drive, Suite 500
Northbrook, IL 60060

847-498-4274
Fax: 847-480-9282
e-mail: info@aedweb.org
www.aedweb.org/index.cfm

The Academy for Eating Disorders is an international transdisciplinary professional organization that promotes excellence in research, treatment and prevention of eating disorders. The AED provides education, training and a forum for collaboration and professional dialogue.

Sally Finney, Executive Director
Eric Van Furth, Ph.D, President/Officers Board

Maryland

2769 Center for Eating Disorders
Saint Josephs Medical Center
7601 Osler Drive
Towson, MD 21204

410-337-1000
Fax: 410-337-1337
www.sjmcmd.org

At the Center for Eating Disorders, the staff focuses on each patient's personal needs and works with him or her to gain new confidence and coping skills. The center offers a full spectrum of services in a supportive environment.

Harry A Brandt, MD, Executive Director
Steven Crawford, MD, Associate Director

Massachusetts

2770 Anorexia/Bulimia Care
PO Box 213
Lincoln, MA 01773

781-259-9767

Sponsors support groups throughout Massachusetts for sufferers and their patients.

2771 Massachusetts Eating Disorder Association (MEDA)
92 Pearl Street
Newton, MA 02458

617-558-1881
Fax: 617-558-1771
e-mail: info@medainc.com
www.medainc.org

MEDA is a non-profit organization dedicated to the prevention and treatment of eating disorders and disordered eating. MEDA's mission is to prevent the continuing spread of eating disorders through educational awareness and early detection. MEDA serves as a support network and resource for clients, loved ones, clinicians, educators and the general public.

100+ Members

Beth Mayer, Executive Director
Aiden Winslow, Assistant Director

New Jersey

2772 Eating Disorders Association of New Jersey
10 Sation Place, Suite 15
Metuchen, NJ 08840

732-549-6886
800-522-2230
Fax: 609-688-1544
www.edanj.org/PAGE_TEMPLATE.htm

Eating Disorders Association of New Jersey is dedicated to the study, prevention and treatment of eating disorders: anorexia nervosa, bulimia nervosa and binge eating disorder. We are a non-profit organization that provides education and support services in New Jersey to individuals affected by eating disorders, including sufferers, family members, friends, educators, and therapists.

Leigh Garfield, LCSW, President
Maureen Kritzer Lange, LCSW, Support Group Coordinator

2773 New Jersey Support Groups
Anorexia/Bulimia Association of New Jersey
114 Main Street
Kingston, NJ 08528

609-252-0202

Offers various support groups across the state for anorexics and bulimics. Call for details.

2774 Renfrew Center of Northern New Jersey
174 Union Street
Ridgewood, NJ 07450

800-736-3739
Fax: 201-562-6253
e-mail: info@renfrewcenter.org
www.renfrew.org

A weekly group that helps women overcome compulsive overeating and make positive lifestyle changes. The group focuses on the needs of the participants and may include looking deeper at culture, family and self within a sympathetic and safe atmosphere.

Jane Fleming, Executive Director
Gayle Brooks, Ph.D, Clinical Director

New York

2775 Eating Disorder Council of Long Island
8214 262nd Street
Floral Park, NY 11004

718-962-2778
www.edcli.org

2776 Metro Intergroup of Overeaters Anonymous
PO Box 1235
New York, NY 10159

212-946-4599
e-mail: NYOAMetroOffiice@yahoo.com
www.oanyc.org/oanyc/

Overeaters Anonymous offers a program of recovery from compulsive overeating using the Twelve Steps and Twelve Traditions of OA. Worldwide meetings and other tools provide a fellowship of experience, strength and hope where members respect one another's anonymity. OA charges no dues or fees; it is self-supporting through member contributions.

Naomi Lippel, Managing Director
Sarah Armstrong, Associate Director

2777 National Eating Disorders Association-Long Island (NEDA-LI)
50 Charles Lindbergh Blvd
Uniondale, NY 11553

516-229-2393
www.nationaleatingdisorders.org/p.asp?WebPage_ID=717

NEDA LI is a non-profit organization devoted to prevention, education and support: prevention of eating disorders, education about eating disorders and support to sufferers of eating disorders, their families and their friends. The organization is comprised of professionals who specialize in eating disorders including psychiatrists, psychologists, social workers, counselors and nutritionists.

Sondra Kronberg, MS/RD/CDN, Executive Director
Vivian Delman, MS/RD/CDN, Board-Directors President

2778 New York City Support Group
Park West Presbyterian Church
186 W 86th Street
New York, NY 10024

212-362-4890
Fax: 212-362-5043
www.commerce.prodigybiz.com

2779 Overeaters Anonymous Support Group
Holliswood Hospital
87-37 Palermo Street
Holliswood, NY 11423

718-776-8181
800-486-3005
Fax: 718-716-8572
e-mail: HolliswoodInfo@libertymgt.com
www.holliswoodhospital.com/

The Holliswood Hospital, a 110-bed private psychiatric hospital located in a quiet residential Queens community, is a leader in providing quality, acute inpatient mental health care for adult, adolescent, geriatric and dually diagnosed patients. Services include an Overeaters Anonymous Support Group.

Susan Clayton, Suppport Group Program Coordinator
Angela Hurtado, Support Group Program Coordinator

2780 Renfrew Center of New York City
11 East 36th Street
New York, NY 10016

800-736-3739
Fax: 212-686-1865
e-mail: info@renfrewcenter.org
www.renfrewcenter.com/locations/new-york.asp

Women struggling to overcome anorexia, bulimia or other disordered eating patterns involving binge eating or restricting can benefit from these weekly groups. Led by experienced therapists, the sessions provide a safe, sympathetic atmosphere where group members explore what triggers their eating disorders as well as issues concerning body image, relationships, school, work and home.

Jane Fleming, Executive Director
Gayle Brooks, Clinical Director

2781 Westchester Center for Eating Disorders
14 Rolling Way
New Rochelle, NY 10804

914-633-7654
Fax: 914-633-7349

Program and support group for individuals struggling with eating disorders.

Ann Rothstein, LCSW, Executive Director

Oregon

2782 Rainrock Treatment Center
1863 Pioneer Parkway, Suite 304 (Mailing Only)
Springfield, OR 97477

541-896-9300
Fax: 541-896-9320
e-mail: mntc@montenido.com
www.montenido.com/rainrock/

Rainrock is a private residential treatment center designed and created by Annie Laughlin and Carolyn Costin to heal women suffering from anorexia, bulimia, and exercise addiction. RainRock, an affiliate of the Monte Nido Treatment Center in Malibu, California, opened in Summer 2006. It is located on four beautifully maintained acres along the McKenzie River just outside Eugene, Oregon with an ideal therapeutic environment for self-reflection, personal growth, and healing.

Carolyn Costin, LMFT, Founder/Executive Director
Annie Lauglin, Founder/Program Coordinator

Pennsylvania

2783 Pennsylvania Chapter of the American Anorexia Bulimia Association
4200 Monument Avenue, PO Box 1287
Philadelphia, PA 19047

215-221-1864
e-mail: mjcjbs@sosbbs.com
www.aabaphila.org/

The American Anorexia / Bulimia Association of Philadelphia (American Anorexia and Bulimia (AABAP), is non-profit, providing services and programs for anyone interested in or affected by, Anorexia, Bulimia and/or related disorders. Its purpose is to aid in the education and prevention of these life threatening disorders. AABAP is a member organization of the Eating Disorders Coalition.

Samuel A Menaged, Board-Directors President EDC

2784 Pennsylvania Educational Network for Eating Disorders (PENED)
7805 McKnight Road
Pittsburgh, PA 15237

412-366-9966
Fax: 412-487-6850
e-mail: pened1@aol.com
www.pened.org/

PENED is a non-profit organization providing educational, supportive and referral services to the general and professional public on the causes, treatment, and prevention of eating disorders and related issues.

Anita Sinicrope-Maier, MSW, Executive Director

2785 Philadelphia Support Group
34th Street & Civic Center Boulevard
Philadelphia, PA 19104

215-750-7087

2786 Renfrew Center of Bryn Mawr
735 Old Lancaster Road
Bryn Mawr, PA 19010

800-736-3739
Fax: 610-527-9361
e-mail: info@renfrewcenter.org
www.renfrewcenter.com/locations/bryn-mawr.asp

Support group for women to overcome compulsive overeating and make positive lifestyle changes. Focuses on the needs of the participants and may include looking deeper at culture, family and self within a sympathetic and safe atmosphere. Led by experienced therapists, sessions provide safe, sympathetic atmosphere where women in midlife faced with new stresses such as divorce, empty-nest syndrome, chronic illness or career changes come together to explore what triggers their eating disorders.

Jane Fleming, Executive Director
Gayle Brooks, Clinical Director

2787 Renfrew Center of Philadelphia
475 Spring Lane
Philadelphia, PA 19128

800-736-3739
Fax: 215-482-7390
e-mail: info@renfrewcenter.org
www.renfrewcenter.com/locations/location.asp?id=2

Women struggling to overcome anorexia, bulimia or other disordered eating patterns involving binge eating or restricting can benefit from this weekly group. Led by experienced therapists, the sessions provide a safe, sympathetic atmosphere where group members explore what triggers their eating disorders as well as issues concerning body image, relationships, school, work and home.

Jane Fleming, Executive Director
Gayle Brooks, Clinical Director

2788 University of Pennsylvania Weight and Education Program
3535 Market Street, Suite 3108
Philadelphia, PA 19104

215-898-7314
Fax: 215-898-2878
e-mail: weight@uphsnet.med.upenn.edu
www.med.upenn.edu/weight/

The Center for Weight and Eating Disorders was founded by Albert J. Stunkard, M.D., over 45 years ago to better understand the causes of weight and weight-related disorders. The Center continues to conduct a wide variety of studies on the causes and treatment of weight-related disorders. More recently, the Center for Weight and Eating Disorders has begun to offer professional services to the general public rather than only to participants in research studies.

Dr. Albert Stunkard, Founder
Thomas A Wadden, Ph.D, Director

Libraries & Resource Centers

2789 Association of Gastrointestinal Motility Disorders
AGMD International Corporate
12 Roberts Drive
Bedford, MA 01730

781-275-1300
Fax: 781-275-1304
e-mail: gimotility@msn.com
www.AGMD-GIMOTILITY.org

Support and education for persons affected by digestive motility disorders. Serves as educational resource and information base for medical professionals. Physician referrals, video tapes, educational materials, networking support, symposiums, and several publications.

Mary-Angela Degrazia-Ditucci, President/Founder
Thomas Abell, MD, Advisory Board Member

2790 National Eating Disorder Association of Long Island (NEDA-LI)
50 Charles Lindbergh Blvd, Suite 400
Uniondale, NY 11553

516-229-2393
www.edap.org/p.asp?WebPage_ID=717

The National Eating Disorders Association (NEDA) was formed in 2001, when Eating Disorders Awareness & Prevention (EDAP) joined forces with the American Anorexia Bulimia Association (AABA). NEDA LI is a non-profit organization devoted to prevention, education and support: prevention of eating disorders, education about eating disorders and support to sufferers of eating disorders, their families and their friends.

Vivian Delman, MS/RD/CDN, Board-Directors President
Susan Morin, NPP, Board-Directors Vice President

Research Centers

2791 Center for the Research and Treatment of Anorexia Nervosa
UCLA Neuropsychiatric Institute
760 Westwood Plaza
Los Angeles, CA 90024

310-825-9822
800-825-1192
e-mail: research.ucla@yahoo.com
www.wpic.pitt.edu/research/angenetics/contact.html

Appointed to the faculty of the department of psychiatry at the UCLA School of Medicine in 1975, Michael Strober, Ph.D., now holds the rank of full professor, and is director of the eating disorders program and the adolescent mood disorders program at the UCLA Neuropsychiatric Institute and Hospital. Dr. Strober's primary research activities center on the long-term course and outcome, psychopathology and genetics of eating disorders.

Michael Strober, Ph.D, Program Director

2792 Center for the Study of Anorexia and Bulimia
1841 Broadway @ 60th Street, 4th Floor
New York, NY 10023

212-333-3444
Fax: 212-333-5444
e-mail: Info@csabnyc.org
www.csabnyc.org/

The Center for the Study of Anorexia and Bulimia was established as a division of the Institute for Contemporary Psychotherapy in 1979 and is the oldest non-profit eating disorders clinic in New York City. Using an eclectic approach, the professional staff and affiliates are on the cutting edge of treatment in their field. The treatment staff includes social workers, psychologists, registered nurses and nutritionists, all with special training in the treatment of eating disorders.

Jill M Pollack, LCSW/BCD, Executive Director

2793 Eating Disorders Research and Treatment Program
Michael Reese Hospital and Medical Center
2929 Ellis Avenue
Chicago, IL 60616

312-791-2000
e-mail: info@michaelreesehospital.com
www.michaelreesehospital.com/Services

Michael Reese Hospital maintains a full spectrum psychiatric care for children, adolescents and adults including inpatient hospitalization for acute psychiatric cases as well as an intensive outpatient program for individuals in need of ongoing support, including that of eating disorders.

Regina Casper, Director
Enrique Beckman, MD, Chairman/CEO

2794 New York Obesity Research Center
Saint Luke's-Roosevelt Hospital
1090 Amsterdam Avenue, 14th Floor
New York, NY 10025

212-523-3622
Fax: 212-523-3571
e-mail: j9lpdylan@yahoo.com
www.nyorc.org/index.html

The mission of the New York Obesity Research Center is to help reduce the incidence of obesity and related diseases through leadership in basic research, clinical research, epidemiology and public health, patient care, and public education.

Dr. Xavier Pi-Sunyer, MD/MPH, Director
Richard Weil, M.Ed/CDE, Exercise Physiologist

Audio Video

2795 Bulimia
Baxley Media Group
510 West Main Street
Urbana, IL 61801

217-384-4838
Fax: 217-384-8280
e-mail: baxley@baxleymedia.com
www.baxleymedia.com/

Award-winning video presentation explores the causes and effects of bulimia. Addresses the fact that many high school and college women view this type of behavior as routine aspect of their everyday lives.

Videotape

Carolyn Baxley, President

2796 Eating Disorder Video
Active Parenting Publishers
1955 Vaughn Road Northwest, Suite 108
Kennesaw, GA 30144

770-429-0565
800-825-0060
Fax: 770-429-0334
e-mail: cservice@activeparenting.com
activeparenting.com

Features compelling interviews with several young people who have suffered from anorexia nervosa, bulimia and compulsive eating. Discusses the treatments, causes, and techniques for prevention with field experts.

Michael H Popkin, Ph.D, Founder/President
Harry Popkin, Secretary/Office of the President

2797 Eating Disorders
Research Press
PO Box 9177
Champaign, IL 61826

217-352-3273
Fax: 217-352-1221
e-mail: rp@researchpress.com
www.researchpress.com

This video shows young people how easily they can become victims of eating disorders such as anorexia, bulimia and compulsive overeating.

Videotape

2798 In Our Own Words
Gurze Books
5145 B Avenida Envinas, PO Box 2238
Carlsbad, CA 92008

760-434-7533
800-756-7533
Fax: 760-434-5476
e-mail: gzcatl@aol.com
gurze.com

Stunningly honest profiles offer viewers a first-hand look at what it feels like to have anorexia and bulimia, and what it takes to recover.

VHS pages 30 minutes

Lindsey Hall, Co-Director/Co-Owner
Leigh Cohn, Co-Director/Co-Owner

2799 Inside Out: Stories of Bulimia
Fanlight Productions
4196 Washington Street
Boston, MA 02131

617-469-4999
800-937-4113
Fax: 617-469-3379
e-mail: info@fanlight.com
www.fanlight.com

This documentary takes us into the lives of women and men who are struggling to cope with bulimia and its consequences on their health, on their work and play, and on their relationships. It combines interviews and observational footage of each of them, and their family members and partners, with abstract imagery and an original score evoking the feelings of compulsion, confusion, and desperation endemic to the disorder - but also of humor and the hope of recovery.

56 minutes

Ben Achtenberg, President
Sandy St. Louis, Marketing Director

2800 It Only Takes One Bite: Food Allergy and Anaphylaxis
Food Allergy Network
11781 Lee Jackson Hwy, Suite 160
Fairfax, VA 22033

800-929-4040
Fax: 703-691-2713
e-mail: faan@foodallergy.org
www.foodallergy.org/

Nonprofit organization dedicated to bringing about a clearer understanding of the issues surrounding food allergies and providing helpful resources. Explains food induced anaphylaxis and how to live with it. An excellent resource for training parents, teachers, caregivers and patients.

18 mins.

Hugh A Simpson, Medical Director
Anne Munoz Furlong, Founder/CEO

Web Sites

2801 Alt.support.eating.disord
www.alt.support.eating.disord

Information for anorexics, also a bulletin board.

2802 Anorexia Nervosa and Related Eating Disorders
www.anred.com

We are a nonprofit organization that provides information about anorexia nervosa, bulimia nervosa, binge eating disorder, and other less-well-known food and weight disorders. Our material includes self-help tips and information about recovery and prevention.

2803 Close to You
Close to You
www.eatingdisordersonline.com

Is a resource for information about Eating Disorders, Anorexia, Bulimia, Binge Eating Disorder, Compulsive Overeating, Over Exercising, and more. Also, a list of treatment options around the world, current news, and info on recovery.

2804 Eating Disorders Awareness and Prevention
www.edap.org

NEDA is dedicated to expanding public understanding of eating disorders and promoting access to quality treatment for those affected along with support for their families through education, advocacy and research.

2805 Eating Disorders Online.com: 15 Styles of Distorted Thinking
//eatingdisordersonline.com/specific/disthink.php

Reference useful for cognitive therapy.

2806 Food Allergy Network
www.foodallergy.org

Mission is to raise public awareness, to provide advocacy and education, and to advance research on behalf of all those affected by food allergies and anaphylaxis.

2807 Gurze Bookstore
www.gurze.com/titlecat.html

Specializes in information about eating disorders including anorexia nervosa, bulimia nervosa, and binge eating, plus related topics such as body image and obesity. We offer books at discounted prices, many free articles about eating disorders, newsletters, links to treatment facilities, organizations, other websites and much more.

2808 Harvard Eating Disorders Center
www.hedc.org

Advances understanding, prevention, and treatment of eating disorders through research, education, and outreach.

2809 Health Answers
www.healthanswers.com

HealthAnswers offers a breadth of services in medical education, sales force training, patient support, solutions, professional promotion and consumer solutions.

2810 Mental Help Net- Eating Disorders
www.mentalhelp.net/guide/eating.htm

We wish to provide the following: to discuss, develop and debate in an open forum the future of the mental health field in America and throughout the world. To help coordinate various components of the mental health field, so as to bring about greater communication between them and to educate the public about mental health issues.

2811 Mirror, Mirror
www.mirror-mirror.org/eatdis.htm

Helps with eating disorders, like how to get help, myths and realities, other websites, and about recovery.

2812 National Association for Anorexia Nervosa and Associated Disorders (ANAD)
www.anad.org

We provide hotline counseling, a national network of free support groups, referrals to healh care professionals, and education and prevention programs to promote self-acceptance and health lifesyles. All of our services are free of charge. ANAD also lobbies for state and national health insurance parity, undertakes and encourages advocacy campaigns to protect potential victims of eating disorders. ANAD stands with individuals and families and helps them win.

2813 National Eating Disorders Association (NED A)
www.NationalEatingDisorders.org

The mission of the National Eating Disorder Association is to eliminate eating disorders and body disatisfaction through prevention efforts, education, referral, and support services, advocacy, training, and research.

2814 Something Fishy
www.something-fishy.org

Dedicated to raising awareness, emphasizing always that Eating Disorders are NOT about food and weight, they are just the symptoms of something deeper going on, inside. We are determined to remind each and every sufferer that they are not alone, and that complete recovery is possible.

Book Publishers

2815 Anorexia Nervosa & Recovery: A Hunger for Meaning
The Haworth Press
10 Alice Street
Binghamton, NY 13904

607-771-0012
800-895-0582
e-mail: getinfo@haworthpress.com
www.haworthpress.com/

Anorexia Nervosa and Recovery lets the reader hear the personal struggles of women who have fought this powerful disease. They describe how anorexia controlled their lives and how, once they overcame their obsessions with food, weight, and thinness, they were able to lead fulfilling lives.

1993 142 pages Paperback
ISBN: 0-918393-95-7

William Cohen, President/Publisher
Al Horowitz, Chief Financial Officer

2816 Barely Any Fat Cookbook

Obesity Foundation
5600 S Quebec Street
Englewood, CO 80111

303-850-0328
e-mail: editor@obesity.org
www.obesity.org

Perfect cookbook to assist anyone in a weight reduction program.

2817 Billy's Story

Overeaters Anonymous World Service Office
PO Box 44020
Rio Rancho, NM 87174

505-891-2664
Fax: 505-891-4320
e-mail: info@oa.org
www.oa.org/

An inspirational story written for younger children suffering from eating disorders and weight problems.

Naomi Lippel, Managing Director
Sarah Armstrong, Associate Director

2818 Body Betrayed

Gurze Books
PO Box 2238
Carlsbad, CA 92018

760-433-4753
800-756-7533
Fax: 760-434-5476
e-mail: mylo@gurze.net
www.gurze.com/

A book concentrating on women, eating disorders and treatments. This widely-read, beautifully-written book covers the most important aspects of diagnosis and treatment for eating disorders. Zerbe is compassionate, knowledgeable, and a considerable poet. Particularly appropriate for parents and loved ones who want a deeper, more thorough understanding of eating disorders

447 pages Paperback
ISBN: 0-880485-22-1

Lindsey Hall, Co-Founder/Co-Director
Leigh Cohn, Co-Founder/Co-Director

2819 Bulimia Nervosa & Binge Eating: A Guide to Recovery

New York University Press
838 Broadway, Third Floor
New York, NY 10003

212-998-2575
800-996-6987
Fax: 212-995-3833
e-mail: customerservice@nyupress.org
www.nyupress.nyu.edu

Book offers guidance and advice for the understanding of the eating disorder bulimia and inspiring hope for change and regaining control of one's life.

1995 170 pages
ISBN: 0-814715-23-0

Steve Maikowski, Director
Ilene Kalish, Executive Editor

2820 Bulimia: A Guide to Recovery

Gurze Books
PO Box 2238
Carlsbad, CA 92018

760-434-7533
800-756-7533
Fax: 760-434-5476
e-mail: mylo@gurze.net
www.gurze.com

This intimate guidebook offers a complete understanding of bulimia and a plan for recovery. It includes a two-week program to stop binging, things-to-do instead of bingeing, a two week guide for support goups, specific advice for loved ones, and Eating Without Fear, Hall's story of self-cure which has inspired thousands of other bulimics.

190 pages Paperback

Lindsey Hall, Co-Founder/Co-Director
Leigh Cohn, Co-Founder/Co-Director

2821 Conversation with Anorexics: A Compassionate & Hopeful Journey

Rowman & Littlefield Publisher
4501 Forbes Blvd, Suite 200
Lanham, MD 20706

301-459-3366
Fax: 301-429-5748
e-mail: custserv@rowman.com
www.rowmanlittlefield.com/aronsonp/

Book is a collection of case studies on anorexia more aptly geared toward the professional as it does not provide guidance but more of an overview on the treatment of the eating disorder.

1994 238 pages Paperback
ISBN: 1-568212-61-5

Jonathan Sisk, Publisher
Christopher Anzalone, Washington Editor

2822 Coping with Eating Disorders

Rosen Publishing Group
29 East 21st Street
New York, NY 10010

212-777-3017
800-237-9932
Fax: 888-436-4643
e-mail: rosenpub@tribeca.ios.com
www.rosenpublishing.com/

This book offers practical suggestions on coping with eating disorders, explaining how to set positive goals, and briefly discusses where to go for additional help.

ISBN: 0-823929-74-4

Miriam Gilbert, Sales and Marketing Director

2823 Cult of Thinness

Oxford University Press
198 Madison Avenue
New York, NY 10016

212-726-6000
800-445-9714
Fax: 212-726-6453
e-mail: custserv.us@oup.com
www.oup.com/usa

Examining the testimonies of young women concerning the practice of body rituals, the author Hesse-Biber observes the extent to which these women sacrifice their bodies and minds to the pursuit of the ultra-slender ideal. Hesse-Biber provides new frameworks for envisioning femininity and personal power, overcoming body insecurity, strengthening the inner self, and changing the cultural environment itself.

1996 256 pages
ISBN: 0-195178-78-5

Joan Bossert, Psych/Behavioral Sciences Editor
Catharine Carlin, Health Psychology Editor

2824 Deadly Diet: Recovering From Anorexia and Bulimia
New Harbinger Publications
5674 Shattuck Avenue
Oakland, CA 94605

510-652-0215
800-748-6273
Fax: 510-652-5472
e-mail: customerservice@newharbinger.com
www.newharbinger.com

This book provides the reader with a great discussion of the use of cognitive-behavioral therapy in the treatment of eating disorders. The author also provides the reader with a step-by-step guide to implementing this approach in his or her own life during recovery from an eating disorder.

1993 248 pages Paperback
ISBN: 1-879237-42-3

Matthew McKay, Ph.D, Publisher
Earlita Chenault, Publicist

2825 Do I Look Fat in This?: Life Doesn't Begin Five Pounds From Now
Simon & Schuster Free Press
866 3rd Avenue
New York, NY 10022

877-989-0009
Fax: 800-943-9831
www.simonsays.com

For any woman who has bonded with a stranger by complaining about how fat she feels, here is a thoughtful and inspiring guide to breaking the cycle of body criticism and creating a powerful and healthy self-image.

2006 200 pages
ISBN: 1-416913-57-2

Jack Romanos, President/CEO
David England, SVP/Chief Financial Officer

2826 Eating Disorder Sourcebook
Gurze Books
PO Box 2238
Carlsbad, CA 92018

760-434-7533
800-756-7533
Fax: 760-434-5476
e-mail: mylo@gurze.net
www.gurze.com

An ideal book for someone with a loved one who has an eating disorder but who knows little about this subject, this new release presents a clear overview of basic issues.

222 pages Paperback

Lindsey Hall, Co-Founder/Co-Director
Leigh Cohn, Co-Founder/Co-Director

2827 Eating Disorders
Thomson Gale
PO Box 95501
Chicago, IL 60694

800-877-4253
Fax: 800-414-5043
e-mail: gale.galeord@thomson.com
www.gale.com/lucent/index.htm

This book examines how eating disorders can be identified, who is affected by them, and how they can be treated.

1991
ISBN: 1-560061-29-4

Andrew Becker, Director
John Barnes, EVP Strategic Business Development

2828 Eating Disorders & Obesity
Guilford Press
72 Spring Street
New York, NY 10012

212-431-9800
800-365-7006
Fax: 212-966-6708
e-mail: info@guilford.com
www.guilford.com

Presents and integrates virtually all that is currently known about eating disorders and obesity in one authorative, accessible, and eminently practical volume.

1995 583 pages
ISBN: 9-781572-30-6

Robert Matloff, President
Seymoure Weingarten, Editor-in-Chief

2829 Eating Disorders Resource Catalogue
Gurze Books
5145 B Avenida Encinas, PO Box 2238
Carlsbad, CA 92018

760-434-4366
800-756-7533
Fax: 760-434-5476
e-mail: mylo@gurze.net
www.gurze.com/

This catalogue of resources contains over 140 books, videos, and audiotapes, lists of national organizations and treatment facilities, and basic facts about eating disorders. It is widely distributed by individuals who are suffering, their loved-ones, the health care professionals who treat them, and educators who are working towards prevention.

24 pages Annually

Lindsey Hall, Co-Founder/Co-Director
Leigh Cohn, Co-Founder/Co-Director

2830 Eating Disorders: When Food Turns Against You
Franklin Watts c/o Grolier
90 Old Sherman Turnpike
Danbury, CT 06816

203-797-3500
Fax: 203-797-3197
www.grolier.com

Anorexia nervosa and bulimia are specifically examined, including a listing of the danger signals of each. A final chapter suggests places to secure help.

1993 96 pages
ISBN: 0-531111-75-0

Richard Robinson, President/Chairman/CEO
Mary Winston, EVP/Chief Financial Officer

2831 Encyclopedia of Obesity and Eating Disorders
Facts on File
132 West 31st Street, 17th Floor
New York, NY 10001

212-967-8800
800-322-8755
Fax: 800-678-3633
e-mail: CustServ@factsonfile.com
www.factsonfile.com/

This revised and expanded edition includes more than 450 entries, more than 140 of them new. Complete with a history of obesity and eating disorders; chronology of key events, research, and breakthroughs; tables listing key facts and statistics; and a directory of resources and Web sites, this single-volume reference is the first stop in any serious research of these troubling health afflictions.

2006 384 pages Hardcover
ISBN: 0-816061-97-1

Laurie Katz, Publicity Director
Coreena Schultz, Library Sales Director

2832 Endorphins: Eating Disorders & Other Addictive Behavior

WW Norton & Company
500 5th Avenue
New York, NY 10110

212-354-5500
Fax: 212-869-0856
www.wwnorton.com

Dr. Huebner discusses anorexia nervosa and bulimia as addictions to endorphins, and presents a treatment model involving education about the addictive process, cognitive/behavioral strategies, and psychotherapy. He then reveals the role of endorphin addiction in other compulsive behaviors such as obsessive exercise, religious fanatacism, and cult involvement.

1993 320 pages
ISBN: 0-393701-56-5

William Drake McFeely, President

2833 Etiology and Treatment of Bulimia Nervosa

Jason Aronson
230 Livingston Street
Northvale, NJ 07647

201-767-4093
www.aronson.com

352 pages Softcover
ISBN: 1-568213-39-5

2834 Fear of Being Fat

Rowman & Littlefield Publishers
4501 Forbes Blvd, Suite 200
Lanham, MD 20706

301-459-3366
Fax: 301-429-5748
www.rowmanlittlefield.com/aronsonj/

This book, which presents one psychoanalytic approach to the treatment of anorexia nervosa, has been written by a number of authors, all members of the Psychosomatic Study Group of the Psychoanalytic Association of New York. The theoretical positions and therapeutic approaches are, consequently, conclusions based on extensive clinical experience acquired over many years. Geared more for the professional.

366 pages
ISBN: 0-876688-99-7

Thomas Koerner, Ph.D, VP/Editorial Director
Wanda Mathews, Marketing Manager

2835 Food for Recovery

Crown Publishing Group/Random House
280 Park Avenue
New York, NY 10017

212-572-6117
Fax: 212-940-7868
e-mail: crownpublicity@randomhouse.com
www.randomhouse.com/

Written for those in recovery from alcohol and drug abuse and eating disorders, this is an excellent basic book on nutrition. Beasley, director of a clinic that focuses on addictive diseases and nutritional medicine, and Knightly, a faculty member of Manhattan's Natural Gourmet Cooking School, discuss nutrition basics and explain how to select wholesome, unprocessed food.

1994 374 pages
ISBN: 0-517586-94-0

Jenny Frost, President/Publisher
Tina Constable, VP/Publicity Executive Director

2836 Getting Better Bit(e) by Bit(e)

Gurze Books
5145 B Avenida Encinas, PO Box 2238
Carlsbad, CA 92008

760-434-7533
800-756-7533
Fax: 760-434-5476
e-mail: mylo@gurze.net
www.gurze.com

This practical book on recovery from bulimia and binge eating is packed with lists, exercises, case studies, discussions, insights, and specific things to do. This book also addresses the day-to-day problems faced by eating disorder sufferers and concentrates on key behavior changes necessary for progress.

143 pages Paperback

Lindsey Hall, Co-Founder/Co-Director
Leigh Cohn, Co-Founder/Co-Director

2837 Golden Cage, The Enigma of Anorexia Nervosa

Gurze Books
5145 B Avenida Encinas, PO Box 2238
Carlsbad, CA 92008

760-434-7533
800-756-7533
Fax: 760-434-5476
e-mail: mylo@gurze.net
www.gurze.com

First published more than 20 years ago, The Golden Cage is still the classic book on anorexia nervosa for patients, parents, mental health workers, and sufferers.

Lindsey Hall, Co-Founder/Co-Director
Leigh Cohn, Co-Founder/Co-Director

2838 Group Psychotherapy for Eating Disorders

American Psychiatric Press
1000 Wilson Boulevard, Suite 1825
Arlington, VA 22209

703-907-7322
800-368-5777
Fax: 703-907-1091
e-mail: appi@psych.org
www.appi.org/

The first book to fully explore the use of group therapy in the treatment of eating disorders.

353 pages Hardcover
ISBN: 0-880484-19-5

Robert E Hales, MD, Editor-in-Chief
Ron McMillen, Chief Executive Officer

2839 Helping Athletes with Eating Disorders

Gurze Books
5145 B Avenida Encinas, PO Box 2238
Carlsbad, CA 92008

760-434-7533
800-756-7533
Fax: 760-434-5476
e-mail: mylo@gurze.net
www.gurze.com/

Gives readers the information they need to identify and address major eating disorders such as: anorexia, bulimia nervosa, and eating disorders not otherwise specified.

208 pages Cloth
ISBN: 0-873223-83-7

Lindsey Hall, Co-Founder/Co-Director
Leigh Cohn, Co-Founder/Co-Director

2840 Hope and Recovery: A Mother-Daughter Story About Anorexia Nervosa & Bulimia
Franklin Watts
90 Old Sherman Turnpike
Danbury, CT 06816

800-621-1115
e-mail: custserv@scholastic.com
www.scholastic.com/aboutscholastic/

Mother and daughter tell a story of a young woman's recovery from the horror of an eating disorder. This compelling account shows how anorexia and bulimia can affect an entire family.

192 pages
ISBN: 0-531111-40-7

Richard Robinson, Chairman/President/CEO
Mary A Winston, EVP/Chief Financial Officer

2841 How to get Your Kid to Eat...
Bull Publishing
PO Box 1377
Boulder, CO 80306

800-676-2855
Fax: 303-545-6354
e-mail: bullpublishing@msn.com
www.bullpub.com

Touches on the various reasons for a child not wanting to eat, as well as continuos snacking, and not eating vegetables.

408 pages
ISBN: 0-915950-83-9

Jim Bull, Publisher

2842 Hungry Self; Women, Eating and Identity
Gurze Books
5145 B Avenida Encinas, PO Box 2238
Carlsbad, CA 92008

760-434-7533
800-756-7533
Fax: 760-434-5476
e-mail: mylo@gurze.net
www.gurze.com

The author, Chermin, looks at the association between self-identity and eating disorders, connecting the often troubled relationship between mothers and daughters.

Lindsey Hall, Co-Founder/Co-Director
Leigh Cohn, Co-Founder/Co-Director

2843 I Was a Fifteen-Year-Old Blimp
Harper & Row
10 East 53rd Street
New York, NY 10022

212-207-7000
www.harpercollins.com/

This story focuses on Gabby, a teenage girl who overhears others discuss her weight and takes radical steps to become popular.

Grades 6-9

Jane Friedman, President/CEO
Lisa Herling, SVP/Corporate Communications

2844 Insights in the Dynamic Psychotherapy of Anorexia And Bulimia
Rowman & Littlefield Publishers
4501 Forbes Blvd, Suite 200
Lanham, MD 20706

301-459-3366
Fax: 301-429-5748
www.rowmanlittlefield.com/

Discusses the eating disorders of anorexia and bulimia providing an overview of the dynamics in diagnosing the disease in addition to developmental and sociocultural issues, therapy and hospitalization.

320 pages Hardcover
ISBN: 0-876685-68-8

Shiela Burnett, Vice President/Marketing Director
Christopher Anzalone, Washington Editor/Director

2845 It's Not Your Fault
Gurze Books
5145 B Avenida Encinas, PO Box 2238
Carlsbad, CA 92008

760-434-7533
800-756-7533
Fax: 760-434-5476
e-mail: mylo@gurze.net
www.gurze.com

In this comprehensive, medically sound guide to overcoming eating disorders, Dr. Marx defines the warnings signs of eating disorders, explores causes, at-risk populations, the role of drug therapy, and advises patients and families where and how they can find help.

1991 237 pages
ISBN: 0-394574-02-8

Lindsey Hall, Co-Founder/Co-Director
Leigh Cohn, Co-Founder/Co-Director

2846 Making Peace with Food
Gurze Books
5145 B Avenida Encinas, PO Box 2238
Carlsbad, CA 92008

760-434-7533
800-756-7533
Fax: 760-434-5476
e-mail: mylo@gurze.net
www.gurze.com

This unique, full sized workbook is designed to help anyone who experienced compulsive eating, yo-yo dieting, food and body anxiety, or associated eating disorders. Filled with ideas, workbook pages, exercises, and resources, Kano's book is an excellent aid to clarifying and overcoming your personal diet/weight struggle.

1989 272 pages Paperback
ISBN: 0-060963-28-X

Lindsey Hall, Co-Founder/Co-Director
Leigh Cohn, Co-Founder/Co-Director

2847 Management of Eating Disorders and Obesity
Humana Press Scientific and Medical Publishers
999 Riverview Drive, Suite 208
Totowa, NJ 07512

973-256-1699
Fax: 973-256-8341
e-mail: humana@humanapr.com
www.humanapress.com/

Stressing human physiology, treatment, and disease prevention, the authors take advantage of the new molecular understanding of the biological regulation of energy. Updated chapters review specific evidence-based and future treatment modalities, present an objective evaluation of the treatment, and identify the positives and negatives that have been seen during clinical studies, as well as cumulative data derived from clinical practice.

2004 448 pages Hardcover
ISBN: 1-588293-41-6

Paul Dolgert, Editorial Director
Ellie Shaw, Developmental Editor

2848 Meals Without Squeals Sense
Bull Publishing
PO Box 1377
Boulder, CO 80306

800-676-2855
Fax: 303-545-6354
e-mail: bullpublishing@msn.com
www.bullpub.com

Straightforward information on childrens, growth accompanies age-specific, child-tested recipes. Explained is how common feeding problems can be solved and show ways to offer children positive experiences with food.

288 pages
ISBN: 0-923521-39-9

Jim Bull, Publisher/President

2849 My Name is Caroline
Gurze Books
5145 B Avenida Encinas, PO Box 2238
Carlsbad, CA 92008

760-434-7533
800-756-7533
Fax: 760-434-5476
e-mail: mylo@gurze.net
www.gurze.com/

A poignant tale of one woman's battle with bulimia throughout her life as a successful student, athlete, scholar and musician.

Grades 10-12

Lindsey Hall, Co-Founder/Co-Director
Leigh Cohn, Co-Founder/Co-Director

2850 Obesity: Theory and Therapy
Raven Press
1185 Avenue of the Americas
New York, NY 10036

212-930-9500

A classic reference for clinicians dealing with obesity, this volume provides the most up-to-date research, preclinical and clinical information.

1992 388 pages
ISBN: 0-881678-84-8

2851 Overeaters Anonymous
World Service Office
PO Box 44020
Rio Rancho, NM 87174

505-891-2664
Fax: 505-891-4320
e-mail: nlippel@oa.org
www.oa.org/

World Service Office offers literature, provides information or meetings world wide. Free sample of Lifeline Magazine available.

204 pages Hardcover

Naomi Lippel, Managing Director
Sarah Armstrong, Associate Director

2852 Overeaters Anonymous Lifeline Sampler
Metro Intergroup of Overeaters Anonymous
117 W 26th Street
New York, NY 10001

212-206-8621

2853 Practice Guidelines for Eating Disorders
American Psychiatric Publishing
1000 Wilson Boulevard, Suite 1825
Arlington, VA 22209

703-907-7322
800-368-5777
Fax: 703-907-1091
e-mail: appi@psych.org
www.appi.org/books.cfx

Designed for health care professionals, this guideline includes information on all aspects of anorexia nervosa and bulimia nervosa, including self-induced vomiting, use of laxatives and vigorous exercise to prevent weight gain.

38 pages Paperback
ISBN: 0-890423-00-8

Robert S Pursell, Marketing
John McDuffie, Product Information

2854 Self-Starvation: from Individual to Family Therapy in the Treatment of Anorexia Ne

rvosa, author

Rowman & Littlefield Publishers
4501 Forbes Blvd, Suite 200
Lanham, MD 20706

301-459-3366
Fax: 301-429-5748
e-mail: custserv@rowman.com
www.rowmanlittlefield.com/

Discusses the eating disorder anorexia nervosa and how it affects both the individual and family members alike, including information on possible treatment options.

1978 296 pages Hardcover
ISBN: 0-876683-10-3

Sheila Burnett, Marketing
Jack Meinhardt, Acquisitions Editor

2855 Starving to Death in a Sea of Objects
Rowman & Littlefield Publishers
4501 Forbes Blvd, Suite 200
Lanham, MD 20706

301-459-3366
Fax: 301-429-5748
e-mail: custserv@rowan.com
www.rowmanlittlefield.com

How emanciation becomes security for anorexics.

464 pages Softcover
ISBN: 0-876684-35-5

Sheila Burnett, Marketing
Jack Meinhardt, Acquisitions Editor

2856 Surviving an Eating Disorder Perspectives and Strategies
Gurze Books
5145 B Avenida Encinas, PO Box 2238
Carlsbad, CA 92008

760-434-7533
800-756-7533
Fax: 760-434-5476
e-mail: mylo@gurze.net
www.gurze.com

Parents, spouses, and friends of individuals with food problems will find practical guidelines in this book for helping themselves and their loved-ones.

222 pages Paperback

Lindsey Hall, Co-Founder/Co-Director
Leigh Cohn, Co-Founder/Co-Director

2857 Treating Bulimia: A Psychoeducational Approach
American Anorexia/Bulimia Association
4200 Monument Avenue
Philadelpha, PA 19131

215-877-2000
e-mail: jbsmje@epix.net
www.aabaphila.org/

Book discusses the eating disorder bulimia focusing on utlizing the multifaceted treatment approach through the incorporation of education, self-monitoring, goal setting, assertion training, relaxation, and cognitive restructuring.

ISBN: 0-080323-99-5

Randi E Wirth, Ph.D, Executive Director

2858 Twelve Steps of Overeaters Anonymous
Overeaters Anonymous World Service Office
PO Box 44020
Rio Rancho, NM 87174

505-891-2664
Fax: 505-891-4320
e-mail: nlippel@oa.org
www.oa.org/

The ideas expressed in the Twelve Steps, which originated in Alcoholics Anonymous, reflect practical experience and application of spiritual insights recorded by thinkers throughout the ages. Their greatest importance lies in the fact that they work! They enable compulsive overeaters and millions of other Twelve-Steppers to lead happy, productive lives. They represent the foundation upon which Overeaters Anonymous is built.

Naomi Lippel, Managing Director
Sarah Armstrong, Associate Director

2859 When Food is Love
Gurze Books
5145 B Avenida Encinas, PO Box 2238
Carlsbad, CA 92008

760-434-7533
800-756-7533
Fax: 760-434-5476
e-mail: mylo@gurze.net
www.gurze.com

Drawing on her own personal experience, Roth explores similarities between eating and loving such as fantasizing, wanting the forbidden, creating drama, control issues, and the experience of relationship.

205 pages Paperback
ISBN: 0-452268-18-4

Lindsey Hall, Co-Founder/Co-Director
Leigh Cohn, Co-Founder/Co-Director

2860 Withering Child
University of Georgia Press
330 Research Drive
Athens, GA 30602

404-542-2830
Fax: 709-369-6131
e-mail: books@ugapress.uga.edu
www.uga.edu/ugapress

Non-fiction book of a parents' struggle with their son and his diagnosis of borderline attention deficit disorder, therapy and his eventual return to school.

1993 288 pages
ISBN: 0-820315-60-5

Nicole Mitchell, Administrative Director
Lane Stewart, Development Director

Journals

2861 BASH Magazine
Bulimia Anorexia Self-Help/Behavior Adaptation
6125 Clayton Avenue, Suite 215
Saint Louis, MO 63139

314-567-4080
800-227-4785
www.caringonline.com/eatdis/treatment.htm

A journal of eating and mood disorders.

Monthly

Newsletters

2862 AABA Newsletter
American Anorexic and Bulimia Association
4200 Monument Avenue
Philadelphia, PA 19131

215-877-2000
e-mail: jbsmje@epix.net
www.aabaphila.org/

The American Anorexia Bulimia Association is a national, non-profit organization dedicated to the prevention and treatment of eating disorders. Publishes a monthly newsletter.

Randi E Wirth, Ph.D, Executive Director

2863 Eating Disorders Review
Gurze Books
5145 B Avenida Encinas, PO Box 2238
Carlsbad, CA 92008

760-434-7533
800-756-7533
Fax: 760-434-5476
e-mail: mylo@gurze.net
www.gurze.com/

Presents current clinical information for the professional treating eating disorders. Features summeries of relevant research from journals and unpublished studies, abstracts, nutritional notes, questions and answers, book reviews, and reproducible client handouts.

8 pages Bimonthly

Lindsey Hall, Co-Founder/Co-Director
Leigh Cohn, Co-Founder/Co-Director

2864 Food Allergy News
Food Allergy & Anaphylaxis Network
11781 Lee Jackson Highway, Suite 160
Fairfax, VA 22033

800-929-4040
Fax: 703-691-2713
e-mail: faan@foodallergy.org
www.foodallergy.org/

Contains tips for parents, including notices on ingredients in various foods, and recipes are published annually.

Bimonthly

Hugh A Sampson, Medical Director

2865 Working Together
Anorexia Nervosa and Associated Disorders
PO Box 7
Highland Park, IL 60035

847-831-3438
Fax: 847-433-4632
e-mail: anad20@aol.com
www.anad.org

Designed for individuals, families, group leaders and professionals concerned with eating disorders. Provides updates on treatments, resources, conferences, programs, articles by therapists, recovered victims, group members and leaders.

Quarterly

Vivian Hanson, D.Sc, Founder/President

Pamphlets

2866 About Overeaters Anonymous
Metro Intergroup of Overeaters Anonymous
117 W 26th Street
New York, NY 10001

212-206-8621

2867 An Inside View

Metro Intergroup of Overeaters Anonymous
117 W 26th Street
New York, NY 10001

212-206-8621

2868 Anonymity

Metro Intergroup of Overeaters Anonymous
117 W 26th Street
New York, NY 10001

212-206-8621

2869 Applying New Attitudes & Directions

Anorexia Nervosa and Associated Disorders
PO Box 7
Highland Park, IL 60035

847-831-3438
Fax: 847-433-4632
e-mail: anad20@aol.com
www.anad.org

Self-help booklet offering an eight-step program to recovery with suggestions, information and recovery stories.

Dawn Ries, Administrator

2870 Before You Take That First...

Metro Intergroup of Overeaters Anonymous
117 W 26th Street
New York, NY 10001

212-206-8621

2871 Body Image

ETR Associates
4 Carbonero Way
Scotts Valley, CA 95066

831-438-4060
800-321-4407
Fax: 800-435-8433
e-mail: customerservice@etr.org
www.etr.org

Discusses the difference between healthy and disorted body image; the link between poor body image and low self esteem; five point list to help people check out their own body image.

2872 Bulimia: Am I at Risk?

ETR Associates
PO Box 1830
Santa Cruz, CA 95061

831-438-4060
800-321-4407
Fax: 800-435-8433

Includes a clear overview of bulimia, symptoms to watch for, and health problems that result from this serious eating disorder.

DESCRIPTION

2873 ECTODERMAL DYSPLASIAS

Involves the following Biologic System(s):

Dental Disorders, Dermatologic Disorders

Ectodermal dysplasias are a group of inherited disorders that are apparent at birth (congenital) and are characterized by abnormalities of the teeth, hair, nails, skin glands (i.e., eccrine and sebaceous glands), the skin, nervous system, ears and eyes, or the delicate mucous membranes that line the mouth and the anus. Ectodermal dyplasia is an integral part of several different syndromes that include anhidrotic ectodermal dysplasia, hidrotic ectodermal dysplasia, and EEC (Ectrodactyly-Ectodermal Dysplasia-Clefting) syndrome.

Anhidrotic ectodermal dysplasia, also known as hypohidrotic ectodermal dyplasia or Christ-Siemens-Touraine syndrome, is usually inherited as an X-linked recessive trait that is fully expressed in boys; however, some children may inherit this disorder as an autosomal recessive trait that affects boys and girls in equal numbers. Anhidrotic ectodermal dysplasia is characterized by absent (aplastic) or underdeveloped (hypoplastic) sweat glands, dental irregularities such as absent or widely-spaced, cone-shaped teeth, and sparse hair (hypotrichosis) that is light in color. Characteristic facial features may include a large chin; thick lips; bulging forehead (frontal bossing); flat nasal bridge; prominent, low-set ears; wrinkled, dark skin around the eyes; and other facial irregularities. Other findings may include light-colored, dry, and wrinkled skin that peels easily. Occasionally, children with anhidrotic ectodermal dysplasia have certain irregularities of the eyes such as cataracts, and abnormalities of the ears that can result in hearing loss. Affected children may be at increased risk for gastrointestinal infections as well as potentially life-threatening respiratory infections. Other life-threatening findings may include abnormally elevated body temperature coupled with an inability to sweat. Treatment for this disorder is preventive, cosmetic, symptomatic, and supportive. For example, parents and caregivers are counseled to protect children from high environmental temperatures. In addition, intervention for teeth and eye irregularities may include evaluation and treatment with dental appliances (e.g., bridgework, implants) and other dental and ocular corrective measures.

Hidrotic ectodermal dysplasia, also known as Clouston's syndrome, is inherited as an autosomal dominant trait. This form of the disorder is characterized by defective or absent nails, thickening of the skin on the palms of the hands and soles of the feet (palmar/plantar hyperkeratosis), and sparse hair. Other occasional findings may include abnormally increased coloration of the skin over major joints and the development of unusually small teeth that are prone to decay. Treatment is symptomatic and supportive.

EEC syndrome is inherited as an autosomal dominant trait. Symptoms and physical findings associated with this disorder are variable and may include lightly-pigmented skin, sparse hair and eyebrows, absent eyelashes, a split or opening (cleft) in the lip and palate, defective nails, tear duct irregularities, and absence of all or part of one or more fingers or toes (ectrodactyly). Other findings may include deafness and irregularities of the teeth, eyes, and urinary tract. Treatment is symptomatic and supportive.

See also **General Resources** on page 917

Government Agencies

2874 NIH/National Institute of Arthritis and Musculoskeletal and Skin Diseases
1AMS Circle
Bethesda, MD 20892

301-402-4484
Fax: 301-718-6366
e-mail: ord@od.nih.gov
rarediseases.info.nih.gov

The mission of the National Institute of Arthritis and Musculoskeletal and Skin Diseases is to support research into the causes, treatment, and prevention of arthritis and musculoskeletal and skin diseases, the training of basic and clinical scientists to carry out this research, and the dissemination of information on research progress in these diseases.

Stephen I Katz MD PhD, Director

2875 NIH/National Institute of Dental and Crani ofacial Research
National Institutes of Health
31 Center Drive, MSC 2290, Building 31
Bethesda, MD 20892

301-496-4261
Fax: 301-402-2185
e-mail: nidcrinfo@mail.nih.gov
www.nidcr.nih.gov

Provides leadership for a national research program designed to understand, treat and prevent the infectious and inherited craniofacial-oral-dental diseases and disorders.

Dr Lawrence A Tabak, Director
Thomas G Murphy, Acting Executive Director

National Associations & Support Groups

2876 American Dental Association
211 E Chicago Avenue
Chicago, IL 60611

312-440-2500
Fax: 312-440-2800
www.ada.org

Professional association of dentists committed to the public's oral health, ethics, science and professional advancement; leading a unified profession through initiatives in advocacy, education, research and the development of standards.

Dr Robert Brandjord, President

2877 Genetic Alliance
4301 Connecticut Avenue NW
Washington, DC 20008

202-966-5557
800-336-4363
Fax: 202-966-8553
e-mail: info@geneticalliance.org
www.geneticalliance.org

A coalition of voluntary genetic support groups, consumers and professionals addressing the needs of individuals and families affected by genetic disorders from a national perspective.

Sharon Terry, President/CEO

2878 HED Hypohidrotic Ectodermal Dysplasia Foundation & Related Disorders
PO Box 9421
Hampton, VA 23670

757-826-0065
e-mail: smoody@hedfoundation.org

2879 March of Dimes Birth Defects Foundation
1275 Mamaroneck Avenue
White Plains, NY 10605

914-428-7100
888-663-4637
Fax: 914-428-8203
e-mail: resourcecenter@modimes.org
www.marchofdimes.com

Partnership of volunteers and professionals dedicates to improving the health of babies by preventing birth defects and infant mortality. Over 100 chapters are located across the country and can be located through the National Office.

Dr Jennifer Howse, President

2880 National Foundation for Ectodermal Dysplasias
410 E Main Street, PO Box 114
Mascoutah, IL 62258

618-566-2020
Fax: 618-566-4718
e-mail: info@nfed.org
www.nfed.org

Seeks to enrich the lives of individuals affected by all forms of the ectodermal dysplasia syndromes.

Mary K Richter, Founder/Executive Director

2881 Society for Pediatric Dermatology
8365 Keystone Crossing, Suite 107
Indianapolis, IN 46240

317-202-0224
Fax: 317-205-9841
e-mail: spd@hp-assoc.com
www.pedsderm.net

National organization dedicated to promote, develop and advance edcuation, research and care of skin disease in all pediatric age groups.

Kent Lindeman, Executive Director

State Agencies & Support Groups

2882 National Foundation for Ectodermal Dysplasias-Regional Office
PO Box 2069
Auburn, WA 98071

253-735-5195
Fax: 253-735-5195
TTY: 800-688-4889
e-mail: nfed3@aol.com
www.nfed.org

Disseminates information on this and related disorders for people of any age to access and use in everyday life situations.

Mary K Richter, Executive Director
Betsy Howe, Regional Rep

Libraries & Resource Centers

2883 International Center for Skeletal Dysplasia Registry
St. Joseph Hospital
7620 York Road
Townson, MD 21204

310-423-9915
Fax: 310-423-9939

Provides patient services for those with skeletal dysplasia; does s research in dwarfism.

Dr. Steven Kopitis, Director

Web Sites

2884 American Dental Association
www.ada.org

The ADA foundation enhances health by securing contributions and providing grants for sustainable programs in dental research, education, access to care and assistance for dentists and their families in need.

2885 Dental Consumer Advisory
www.toothinfo.com

Purpose is to provide useful and practical information for the public concerning issues of dental care.

2886 Dental Resources on the Web
www.dental-resources.com

Dental sites for education, practices, laboratories, office supplies, dental care and associations.

2887 Online Mendelian Inheritance in Man
www.ncbi.nlm.nih.gov

This database is a catalog of human genes and genetic disorders.

DESCRIPTION

2888 ECZEMA

Synonym: Eczematous dermatitis

Covers these related disorders: Allergic contact dermatitis, Atopic dermatitis, Dyshidrosis, Irritant contact dermatitis, Seborrheic dermatitis

Involves the following Biologic System(s):

Dermatologic Disorders

Eczema is a common inflammatory condition of the skin (dermatitis) characterized by redness, itching, blistering, and oozing of affected areas. As the condition progresses, the skin often becomes abnormally dry and may scale, crust over, thicken, or develop increased or decreased areas of coloration. There are several different types of eczema that may be caused by various internal or external factors. Children are mostly affected by certain forms of the condition, including atopic dermatitis, irritant and allergic contact dermatitis, seborrheic dermatitis, or dyshidrosis.

Approximately two to eight percent of children develop atopic dermatitis, which is the most common form of childhood eczema. Also known as infantile eczema when it occurs during childhood, this form of eczema is characterized by an excessive immune response to particular substances that the body perceives as foreign (sensitizing antigen). Such responses, known as allergic or hypersensitive reactions, occur upon exposure to previously encountered, usually environmental substances (allergens). Patients with atopic dermatitis are thought to have an inherited tendency toward allergy. This may be supported by the fact that many affected infants and children later develop additional conditions due to exposure to certain allergens, particularly inflammation of the nose's mucous membranes (allergic rhinitis) and inflammation and narrowing of the airways (asthma).

Atopic dermatitis usually begins during the first year of life, and up to 90 percent of affected patients have symptoms by five years of age. The disorder often occurs with the introduction of particular foods into a child's diet, such as wheat, cow's milk, soy, eggs, or peanuts. Although atopic dermatitis tends to subside with advancing age, the condition may recur over many years before completely disappearing. Atopic dermatitis is characterized by the development of reddish, inflamed, intensely itchy (pruritic) patches that rapidly begin to ooze and crust over. During infancy, the condition usually initially affects the skin of the cheeks and gradually extends to involve the rest of the face; the neck, abdomen, wrists, and hands; the inside of the elbows; behind the knees; or other areas. Due to intense itching, infants may rub affected areas against their crib, their clothes, or other surfaces in an attempt to obtain relief. Secondary bacterial infections may occur as the result of the repeated rubbing or scratching. Over time, skin areas may become dry and scaly and develop changes in color. In addition, the skin may thicken, accentuating skin lines and causing an unusual, "bark-like" skin appearance (lichenification).

The treatment of atopic dermatitis may include measures to eliminate or avoid certain factors that may worsen the condition, such as certain foods, extremes of humidity and temperature, detergents or soaps, or potentially abrasive textures, such as wool. Affected children should be dressed in garments with smooth textures, such as cotton; their fingernails should be kept as short as possible to discourage scratching; and excessive bathing should be avoided. Adding bath oil to bath water and applying moisturizing lotions and creams to damp skin after bathing may help to alleviate some symptoms. In addition, when inflammation is severe, the application of wet dressings may reduce inflammation and associated itching. Treatment may also include the use of topical medicated skin creams and ointments, such as corticosteroid preparations, as well as certain medications such as oral antihistamines to help reduce itching. Secondary bacterial infections are treated with appropriate antibiotics.

Contact dermatitis, another common form of eczema, is a skin inflammation that is typically confined to a particular area and may have clearly defined boundaries. This disorder is often subdivided into irritant and allergic contact dermatitis. Irritant contact dermatitis is a skin inflammation caused by repetitive or prolonged exposure to certain substances that damage the skin. Allergic contact dermatitis is a hypersensitive, inflammatory response of the skin due to exposure to a previously encountered substance (allergen).

Irritant contact dermatitis may be caused by repetitive or prolonged exposure to certain soaps or detergents, citrus juices, bubble bath, or other substances. In many infants, saliva from drooling may cause inflammation of the skin of the face and neck folds. Diaper dermatitis is another common form of irritant contact dermatitis. Affected infants may develop reddish, scaling, blistering skin inflammation and secondary bacterial infections due to prolonged contact with waste materials, diaper soaps, and topical skin lotions. The treatment of irritant contact dermatitis includes removal or avoidance of the responsible irritants and administration of topical corticosteroid creams or ointments. In addition, affected areas should be carefully, regularly washed with warm water and a mild soap. To help prevent diaper dermatitis, physicians may recommend frequent changing of diapers; gentle, thorough cleansing of genitals with warm water and mild soaps and application of mild protective topical preparations during the diaper changes; or use of disposable diapers with absorbent materials.

Allergic contact dermatitis is characterized by a hypersensitive or allergic response to previously encountered allergens. Common causes include metal compounds in jewelry; particular plants, such as poison ivy, poison oak, or poison sumac; medications in skin creams, such as certain antibiotic- or antihistamine-containing creams; shoes; or clothing. Patients may develop intensely itchy, reddish, blistering skin inflammations that may later develop scaling, cracking, (fissuring), changes in color, or an abnormal thickened, bark-like appearance. Treatment includes removal or avoidance of the allergen and application of cool compresses, corticosteroid ointments or oral medications, antihistamine medications, and antibiotic therapy for secondary bacterial infections.

Seborrheic dermatitis is a chronic inflammatory disorder of unknown cause that may occur at any age and may appear to follow the distribution of sebaceous glands in skin tissue. These relatively small glands, which open into hair follicles, produce an oily secretion known as sebum that helps to lubricate the hair and skin and protect the skin from drying. In children, the condition most commonly occurs during infancy. Affected infants may initially develop localized or widespread crusting and scaling of the scalp, known as cradle cap. In some patients, this may be the only finding of the condition. Other infants may develop reddish, greasy, scaling patches that may be localized or may spread to affect most of the body. Affected areas often include the face, behind the ears, the neck, the diaper region, or under the arms. Patients may experience associated itching, hair loss, or changes in skin color. Treatment may include the use of special antiseborrheic shampoos or the application of wet compresses or topical corticosteroid creams or ointments.

Dyshidrosis, also known as pompholyx, is another form of eczema that may occur during chi|ldhood. This is a recurrent, potentially seasonal blistering condition that affects the palms of the hands and soles of the feet. The condition is initially characterized by recurrent crops of severely itchy blisters. Affected skin areas gradually become abnormally thickened and may have areas of fissuring. Many patients also experience excessive sweating (hyperhidrosis) in affected areas and may develop secondary bacterial infections due to scratching. Because this is typically a recurrent condition, patients should take appropriate measures to protect their hands and feet from harsh soaps, chemicals, the effects of excessive sweating or adverse weather, or other potential triggering factors. Treatment may include the application of wet dressings, topical corticosteroid ointments or creams, or mild topical preparations that promote skin softening and peeling (keratolytic agents) and the administration of antibiotics to treat secondary bacterial infections.

See also **General Resources** on page 917

Government Agencies

2889 NIH/National Institute of Allergy and Infectious Diseases
6610 Rockledge Drive, MSC 6612
Bethesda, MD 20892

301-496-5717
Fax: 301-402-3573
TDD: 800-877-8339
www.niaid.nih.gov

Conducts and supports basic and applied research to better understand, treat, and ultimately prevent infectious, immunologic, and allergic diseases.

Anthony S Fauci MD, Director

2890 NIH/National Institute of Arthritis and Musculoskeletal and Skin Diseases
1AMS Circle
Bethesda, MD 20892

301-402-4484
Fax: 301-718-6366
e-mail: ord@od.nih.gov
rarediseases.info.nih.gov

The mission of the National Institute of Arthritis and Musculoskeletal and Skin Diseases is to support research into the causes, treatment, and prevention of arthritis and musculoskeletal and skin diseases, the training of basic and clinical scientists to carry out this research, and the dissemination of information on research progress in these diseases.

Stephen I Katz MD PhD, Director

National Associations & Support Groups

2891 Eczema Association for Science and Education
1211 SW Yanhill
Portland, OR 97205

503-228-4430

Offers research and information to persons with eczema and other skin disorders.

2892 National Eczema Association
4460 Redwood Highway, Suite 16-D
San Rafael, CA 94903

415-499-3474
800-818-7546
Fax: 415-472-5345
e-mail: info@nationaleczema.org
www.nationaleczema.org

Works to improve the health and the quality of life of persons living with atopic dermatitis/eczema, including those who have the disease as well as their loved ones.

2893 Society for Pediatric Dermatology
8365 Keystone Crossing, Suite 107
Indianapolis, IN 46240

317-202-0224
Fax: 317-205-9841
e-mail: spd@hp-assoc.com
www.pedsderm.net

National organization dedicated to promote, develop and advance education, research and care of skin disease in all pediatric age groups.

Kent Lindeman, Executive Director

Libraries & Resource Centers

California

2894 University of California, San Francisco Dermatology Drug Research
515 Spruce
San Francisco, CA 94143

415-476-2001
Fax: 415-476-6014
cc.ucsf.edu/people

Conducts clinical testing of new or existing pharmalogic agents used in the treatment of skin disorders.

John Koo, MD, Director

Delaware

2895 Delaware Division of Libraries for the Blind and Physically Handicapped
43 S Dupont Highway
Dover, DE 19901

302-736-4748
800-282-8676
Fax: 302-736-6787
TDD: 302-739-4748
e-mail: bedpg@lib.de.us

Braille readers receive service from Philadelphia and Pennsylvania, summer reading program, braille writer and cassettes.

Beth Landon, Librarian

Illinois

2896 Dermatology Information Network (DERMINFONET)
American Academy of Dermatology
PO Box 4014
Schaumburg, IL 60168

847-330-0230
Fax: 847-330-0050

Consists of a collection of dermatologic databases that are available to members on a subscription and/or purchase basis. These databases are designed to run on a wide variety of personal computers.

2897 National Library of Dermatologic Teaching Slides
American Academy of Dermatology
930 N Meacham Road
Shaumburg, IL 60173

847-330-0230
Fax: 847-330-0050
www.aad.org

A collection of dermatologic teaching slides offering the most comprehensive series ever assembled. Each set offers a realistic presentation of classic clinical skin conditions encountered by the dermatologist.

New York

2898 Laboratory of Dermatology Research
Memorial Sloan-Kettering Cancer Center
1275 York Avenue
New York, NY 10021

212-639-2000
Fax: 212-639-3576
www.mskcc.org

Specific studies on the identification of skin disorders and dermatology.

Biijan Safai, MD, Head

2899 Rockefeller University Laboratory for Investigative Dermatology
1230 York Avenue
New York, NY 10021

212-327-7458
Fax: 212-327-7459

Research into skin disorders and the whole specialty of dermatology in general.

D Martin Carter, MD, PhD, Head

Research Centers

2900 University of California, San Francisco Dermatology Drug Research
515 Spruce
San Francisco, CA 94143

415-476-2001
Fax: 415-221-4751

Conducts clinical testing of new or existing pharmacologic agents used in the treatment of skin disorders.

John Koo, MD, Director

Audio Video

2901 National Library of Dermatologic Teaching Slides
American Academy Of Dermatology
PO Box 94020
Palatine, IL 60094

847-330-0230
Fax: 847-330-0050

A collection of dermatologic teaching slides offering the most comprehensive series ever assembled. Each set offers a realistic presentation of classic clinical skin conditions encountered by the dermatologist.

Magazines

2902 International Journal of Dermatology
International Society of Dermatology
138 Palm Coast Parkway, NE No 333
Palm Coast, FL 32137

386-437-4405
Fax: 386-437-4427
e-mail: info@intsocdermatol.org
www.intsocderm.org

Focuses on information for dermatologists and the whole specialty of dermatology research and education.

10 times a year

2903 Journal of Dermatologic Surgery and Oncology
International Society for Dermatologic Surgery
930 N Meachan Road
Schaumburg, IL 60173

847-330-9830
Fax: 847-330-1135

Focuses on medical updates and information on dermatology.

Monthly

Newsletters

2904 Awareness
NAPVI
PO Box 317
Watertown, MA 02471

617-972-7441
800-562-6265
Fax: 617-972-7444
www.spedex.com/napvi

Newsletter offering regional news, sports and activities, conferences, camps, legislative updates, book reviews, audio reviews, professional question and answer column and more for the visually impaired and their families.

Quarterly

2905 DVH Quarterly
University of Arkansas at Little Rock
2801 S University Avenue
Little Rock, AR 72204

Fax: 501-663-3536

Offers information on upcoming events, conferences and workshops on and for visual disabilities. Book reviews, information on the newest resources and technology, educational programs, want ads and more.

Quarterly

Bob Brasher, Editor

2906 Dermatology Focus
Dermatology Foundation
1560 Sherman Avenue
Evanston, IL 60201

847-328-2256
Fax: 847-328-0509
dermatologyfoundation.org

Includes membership activities, research articles and lists recipients of foundation awards.

Quarterly

2907 Dermatology World
American Academy of Dermatology
PO Box 94020
Palatine, IL 60094

847-330-0230
Fax: 847-330-0050

Offers Academy members information outside the clinical realm. It carries news of government actions, reports of socioeconomic issues, societal trends and other events which impinge on the practice of dermatology.

Monthly

2908 Progress in Dermatology
Dermatology Foundation
1560 Sherman Avenue
Evanston, IL 60201

847-328-2256
Fax: 847-328-0509
dermatologyfoundation.org

Bulletin offering information on research reports and clinical trials.

Quarterly

Pamphlets

2909 Eczema/Atopic Dermatitis
American Academy of Dermatology
PO Box 4014
Schaumburg, IL 60168

847-240-1280
866-503-7546
Fax: 847-240-1859
e-mail: mrc@aad.org
www.aad.org

Explains how to recognize and treat dermatitis.

1995

2910 Hand Eczema
American Academy of Dermatology
PO Box 4014
Schaumburg, IL 60168

847-240-1280
866-503-7546
Fax: 847-240-1859
e-mail: mrc@aad.org
www.aad.org

Shows examples of hand rashes, explains causes, lists protective measures and treatments.

1993

DESCRIPTION

2911 EHLERS-DANLOS SYNDROME

Involves the following Biologic System(s):

Connective Tissue Disorders

Ehlers-Danlos syndrome is a group of hereditary connective tissue disorders characterized by abnormalities of collagen, the major structural protein in the body. At least 10 forms of the disorder have been identified based upon underlying biochemical and genetic abnormalities and associated symptoms and findings. Although such subtypes were previously indentified by Roman numerals (e.g., I to X), different classification systems have since been proposed. Most forms of Ehlers-Danlos syndrome are thought to have autosomal dominant inheritance. However, other subtypes have been identified that may be inherited as an autosomal recessive or an X-linked recessive trait. Although certain symptoms and findings are commonly associated with Ehlers-Danlos syndrome, other abnormalities may be variable in range and severity, depending upon the form of the disorder present.

Although infants with Ehlers-Danlos syndrome often appear normal at birth, associated symptoms and findings soon become apparent. The main symptoms associated with the disorder may include abnormally thin, elastic skin that is excessively fragile and unusually loose, flexible (hyperextensible) joints that may be prone to recurrent dislocation. Due to abnormal fragility of the skin, blood vessels, and other tissues, patients may be prone to tearing or splitting of the skin, be susceptible to easy bruising and bleeding, and tend to heal slowly. Healing of skin wounds may leave distinctive, cigarette paper-like scars, such as over the knees, shins, elbows, and forehead. In addition, due to abnormal accumulations of scar tissue, patients may develop small, rounded skin growths that resemble tumors (molluscoid pseudotumors). In some cases, small, round, hard lumps (calcified spheroids) may also develop under the skin.

Depending upon the form of the disorder present, affected children may have additional, variable symptoms, such as certain skeletal, blood vessel, or eye (ocular) abnormalities. Associated skeletal malformations may include front-to-back and sideways curvature of the spine (kyphoscoliosis); short, wide collarbones (clavicles); bowing of bones of the arms and legs; bone fragility; short stature; or other abnormalities. Fragility of certain blood vessels may lead to ballooning of the wall of the major artery in the body (aortic aneurysm) or spontaneous rupture of certain intermediate- or large-sized arteries, potentially causing life-threatening complications. In addition, in some patients, ocular abnormalities may include fragility of the front, transparent region of the eye (cornea); noninflammatory protrusion of the cornea (keratoconus); rupture of the cornea or the tough, fibrous, outer coating of the eye (sclera); or detachment of the nerve-rich membrane at the back of the eye (retina). Additional symptoms and findings may include diminished muscle tone (hypotonia); abnormal prominence of blood vessels under the skin; protrusion of one of the heart valves back into the left upper chamber (atrium) of the heart during contraction of the left lower heart chamber (mitral valve prolapse); severe inflammation of the tissues that surround and support the teeth (periodontitis), leading to premature tooth loss; rupture of the intestine; or other abnormalities.

The treatment of children with Ehlers-Danlos syndrome is symptomatic and supportive. Appropriate measures must be taken to avoid trauma and injuries, such as those that may occur in contact sports. Wearing protective clothing and padding may be beneficial. In addition, appropriate precautions must be taken during dental or surgical procedures.

See also **General Resources** on page 917

Government Agencies

2912 NIH/National Institute of Arthritis and Musculoskeletal and Skin Diseases

1AMS Circle
Bethesda, MD 20892

301-402-4484
Fax: 301-718-6366
e-mail: ord@od.nih.gov
rarediseases.info.nih.gov

The mission of the National Institute of Arthritis and Musculoskeletal and Skin Diseases is to support research into the causes, treatment, and prevention of arthritis and musculoskeletal and skin diseases, the training of basic and clinical scientists to carry out this research, and the dissemination of information on research progress in these diseases.

Stephen I Katz MD PhD, Director

National Associations & Support Groups

2913 Ehlers-Danlos National Foundation

3200 Wilshire Boulevard, Suite 1601, South Tower
Los Angeles, CA 90010

213-368-3800
Fax: 213-427-0057
e-mail: staff@ednf.org
www.ednf.org

Provides emotional support and updated information to the individuals and their families who are affected by the disease. The foundation produces educational and support pamphlets, brochures, audiovisual aids, journal article reprints, newsletter, and a referral service.

Cindy Lauren, President/CEO
Edzel Lejano, Member Services Coordinator

2914 Genetic Alliance
4301 Connecticut Avenue NW
Washington, DC 20008

202-966-5557
800-336-4363
Fax: 202-966-8553
e-mail: info@geneticalliance.org
www.geneticalliance.org

A coalition of voluntary genetic support groups, consumers and professionals addressing the needs of individuals and families affected by genetic disorders from a national perspective.

Sharon Terry, President/CEO

2915 March of Dimes Birth Defects Foundation
1275 Mamaroneck Avenue
White Plains, NY 10605

914-428-7100
888-663-4637
Fax: 914-428-8203
e-mail: resourcecenter@modimes.org
www.marchofdimes.com

Partnership of volunteers and professionals dedicates to improving the health of babies by preventing birth defects and infant mortality. Over 100 chapters are located across the country and can be located through the National Office.

Dr Jennifer Howse, President

Web Sites

2916 Wheeless' Textbook of Orthopaedics
www.wheelessonline.com

Derives from a variety of sources, including journals, articles, national meetings lectures and other textbooks.

Pamphlets

2917 Ehlers-Danlos Syndrome
Arthritis Foundation
PO Box 7669
Atlanta, GA 30357

404-872-7100
Fax: 404-872-0457

DESCRIPTION

2918 ENCEPHALOCELE

Involves the following Biologic System(s):

Neurologic Disorders

Encephalocele is an abnormality that is present at birth (congenital)and belongs to a group of birth defects known as neural tube defects. These defects develop during the early stages of pregnancy at which time a specialized layer of tissue forms and extends along the back portion of the developing embryo. As the embryo grows, this tissue, known as the neural plate, forms a groove that is bordered by folds. This groove eventually deepens and closes to form the neural tube. Later in development, the neural tube gives rise to tissue that later forms the brain and spinal cord. The neural tube is surrounded and protected by the bones of the back (vertebrae). Failure in this sequence of developmental events results in a neural tube defect.

In newborns with encephalocele, a portion of the brain protrudes through a defect in the skull. This defect may be located at the back of the head (occipital region), the forehead (frontal region), or the area of the forehead and nose (nasofrontal region). Affected children may experience visual abnormalities, mental retardation, an abnormally small head (microcephaly), and seizures. Affected newborns may also have an increase in the volume of fluid surrounding the brain (hydrocephalus), possibly resulting in increased pressure within the skull, enlargement of the head, and convulsions.

Encephalocele may occur as the result of different genetic and environmental factors (multifactorial), alone or in combination. Such factors may include vitamin deficiencies or toxic factors. Genetic transmission in some children is supported by the fact that multiple cases of this neural tube defect have been reported in some families. In addition, encephalocele may sometimes be associated with other disorders. For example, physical characteristics of Meckel-Gruber syndrome, a rare, life-threatening disorder inherited as an autosomal recessive trait, include encephalocele in the back of the head; an abnormal ridge (cleft) or opening in the lip or palate; a sloping forehead, extra fingers or toes (polydactyly); and enlarged kidneys that contain multiple cysts (polycystic kidneys).

Treatment of encephalocele may often involve a team of medical specialists working together to determine the best course of therapy or management. Such treatment may include surgery, medication, or the insertion of a tube known as a shunt into the brain. This shunt diverts fluid away from the brain into the abdominal cavity where it is harmlessly absorbed into the systemic circulation.

The risk of neural tube defects is significantly reduced when supplemental folic acid is consumed in addition to a healthful diet prior to and during the first month following conception. Women who could become pregnant, especially those at risk who may have previously delivered a child with a neural tube defect, are advised to eat foods fortified with folic acid or take a folic acid supplement in addition to eating folate-rich foods to reduce the risk of some serious birth defects.

See also **General Resources** on page 917

Government Agencies

2919 NIH/National Institute of Child Health and Human Development

31 Center Drive, Building 31
Bethesda, MD 20892

301-496-5133
Fax: 301-496-1104
www.nichd.nih.gov

Established in 1962 by congress, today the institute conducts and supports research on topics related to the health of children, adults, families and populations. Some of these topics include: developmental disabilities, growth and development, infant death, reproductive health and birth defects.

Nancy D Wirth, Director
Lisa Kaeser, Program & Public Liaison

National Associations & Support Groups

2920 AboutFace USA

PO Box 158
South Beloit, IL 61080

702-769-9264
888-486-1209
Fax: 702-341-5351
e-mail: info@aboutfaceusa.org
www.aboutfaceusa.org

Provides information, services, emotional support and educational programs for and on behalf of individuals with facial differences and their families. Working to increase understanding through public awareness and education.

3M members

Debbie Oliver, Executive Director

2921 Birth Defect Research for Children

930 Woodcock Road, Suite 225
Orlando, FL 32803

407-895-0802
Fax: 407-895-0824
e-mail: staff@birthdefects.org
www.birthdefects.org

Organization that helps families with free birth defect information, parent matching that links families of children with similar defects and research through the National Birth Defect Registry to discover the causes of birth defects. Support group information and newsletter on Internet.

Betty Mekdeci, Executive Director

2922 Children's Craniofacial Association
13140 Coit Road, Suite 307
Dallas, TX 75240

214-570-9099
800-535-3643
Fax: 214-570-8811
e-mail: contactCCA@ccakids.com
www.ccakids.com

Devoted to the dispersion of medical knowledge of this and similar disorders, along with providing emotional support for the sufferers and their families.

Jeffrey Fearon, MD, Chief Medical Advisor

2923 Fighters for Encephalocele Support Group
332 Brereton Street
Pittsburgh, PA 15219

412-261-5363

2924 Forward Face
317 E 34th Street, Suite 901A
New York, NY 10016

212-684-5860
Fax: 212-684-5864
e-mail: info@forwardface.org
www.forwardface.org

Founded in 1978 by parents of children with facial differences; helps children and their families find immediate support to manage the medical and social effects of facial differences.

Barbara Robertson, President

2925 Guardians of Hydrocephalus Research Foundation
2618 Avenue Z
Brooklyn, NY 11235

718-743-4473
800-458-8655
Fax: 718-743-1171
e-mail: ghrf2618@aol.com
http://ghrf.homestead.com/ghrf.html

Nonprofit group dedicated to research into the cause and treatment of hydrocephalus. Guardians operate a laboratory in the Department of Neurology at New York University Medical Center, in which information from clinical and research facilities is integrated to provide for better diagnosis and treatment of hydrocephalus, a frequently occuring congenital disorder that can also occur shortly after birth. Hydrocephalus accounts for a large propotion of adult patients with a diagnosis of dementia.

Kathy Soriano

2926 Hydrocephalus Association
870 Market Street, Suite 705
San Francisco, CA 94102

415-732-7040
888-598-3789
Fax: 415-732-7044
e-mail: info@hydroassoc.org
www.hydroassoc.org

A national nonprofit organization devoted exclusively to hydrocepahalus. We provide support, education and an extensive range of resources to families and professionals dealing with the complex issues of hydrocephalus, the abnormal accumulation of cerebrospinal fluid within the brain. Our resources cover all age groups, from prenatal to adults with normal pressure hydrocepahalus. Our office is staffed daily from 10 AM to 4 PM Pacific time.

Dory Kranz, Executive Director
Gina DeGennaro, Development Director

2927 Hydrocephalus Support Group
9245 Sky Park Court, Suite 130
San Diego, CA 92123

619-268-8252
Fax: 619-268-4275
e-mail: cfrc@mail.sdsu.edu

Provides education and support for hydrocephalus patients and their families. The HSG puts out a quarterly newspaper, gives parent referrals and has a library with articles and tapes about hydrocephalus.

2928 March of Dimes Birth Defects Foundation
1275 Mamaroneck Avenue
White Plains, NY 10605

914-428-7100
888-663-4637
Fax: 914-428-8203
e-mail: resourcecenter@modimes.org
www.marchofdimes.com

Partnership of volunteers and professionals dedicated to improving the health of babies by preventing birth defects and infant mortality. Over 100 chapters are located across the country and can be located through the National Office.

Dr Jennifer Howse, President

2929 National Craniofacial Foundation
PO Box 11082
Chattanooga, TN 37401

800-332-2373
e-mail: faces@faces-cranio.org
www.faces-cranio.org

Provides information to affected individuals; families of affected individuals; the public or media and professionals. We also provide peer support; professional counseling; medical referrals; referrals for non-medical services and to local chapters or groups. We offer pamphlets; fact sheets; newsletter; booklets; video's and movies.

Lynne Mayfield, Director

2930 National Hydrocephalus Foundation
12413 Centralia Road
Lakewood, CA 90715

562-402-3523
888-857-3434
Fax: 562-924-6666
e-mail: hydrobrat@earthlink.net
www.nhfonline.org

Nonprofit public service organization that assembles and disseminates information pertaining to hydrocephalus, its treatments and outcomes. Facilitates a communication network among affected families and individuals. Helps others gain a deeper understanding of those areas affected by hydrocephalus, such as education, insurance, tax and estate planning, employment and family. Promotes and supports research on the causes, treatment and prevention of hydrocephalus.

Debbie Fields, Executive Director

Web Sites

2931 Rare Genetic Diseases in Children (NYU)
www.med.nyu.edu/rgdc/homenow.htm

We target issues arising from rare genetic diseases affecting children. Also, to assist in the endeavor to bring knowledge and hope to those for whom there is, at present, so little.

Book Publishers

2932 Congenital Disorders Sourcebook
Omnigraphics
PO Box 625
Holmes, PA 19043

800-234-1340
Fax: 800-875-1340
e-mail: info@omnigraphics.com
www.omnigraphics.com

Basic consumer health information on disorders aquired during gestation, including spina bifida, hydrocephalus, cerebral palsy, heart defects, craniofacial abnormalities and fetal alcohol syndrome.

650 pages
ISBN: 0-780809-45-9

Newsletters

2933 AboutFace USA
AboutFace
PO Box 158
South Beloit, IL 61080

888-486-1209
Fax: 702-341-5351
e-mail: info@aboutfaceusa.org
www.aboutfaceusa.org

A free newsletter.

8 pages

Rickie Anderson, Executive Director

DESCRIPTION

2934 ENCOPRESIS

Involves the following Biologic System(s):

Developmental/Behavioral/Psychiatric Disorders, Gastrointestinal Disorders

Encopresis refers to the passage of feces in inappropriate or unacceptable places by children who have no detectable disorder or organic abnormality and who are past the age when toilet training is typically completed. This type of soiling may be considered primary encopresis, in which fecal incontinence persists from birth, or secondary encopresis, a regressive form of this disorder in which fecal incontinence occurs in children who were previously toilet trained. Children with this disorder may refuse to use a commode, may soil their clothing, or may defecate in secret places. Other associated findings may include chronic constipation leading to the presence of large, hardened fecal masses in the colon or rectum (fecal impaction) that, in turn, may result in an abnormally enlarged or dilated colon (megacolon). Encopresis occurs in approximately one percent of school children and is much more common in boys than it is in girls.

The causes of encopresis may sometimes be linked to anger, defiance, resistance, or fear of toilet training and, as such, may indicate the need for psychotherapeutic intervention that includes parents or caregivers, as well as the affected child. Treatment is often supportive. For example, a reward system may be established so that the child has an incentive to cooperate. In addition, the affected child may be encouraged to use the bathroom at specific times (e.g., after meals) and for specified periods of time. Parents are advised to remain nonjudgmental and nonretaliatory, so that consequences for noncompliance are minor. Additional treatment for primary encopresis may initially include the carefully monitored, short-term use of laxatives and enemas to relieve constipation and subsequent complications. Affected children may sometimes benefit from biofeedback, during which individuals learn how to control certain involuntary physiologic functions such as, in this case, the anal sphincter muscle. In addition, the careful administration of mineral oil, together with a high fiber diet, may be effective in relieving constipation and associated complications in children with secondary encopresis. Other treatment is symptomatic and supportive.

See also **General Resources** on page 917

Government Agencies

2935 NIH/National Institute of Child Health and Human Development
31 Center Drive, Building 31
Bethesda, MD 20892

301-496-5133
Fax: 301-496-1104
www.nichd.nih.gov

Established in 1962 by congress, today the institute conducts and supports research on topics related to the health of children, adults, families and populations. Some of these topics include: developmental disabilities, growth and development, infant death, reproductive health and birth defects.

Nancy D Wirth, Director
Lisa Kaeser, Program & Public Liaison

National Associations & Support Groups

2936 International Foundation for Functional Gastrointestinal Disorders
PO Box 170864
Milwaukee, WI 53217

414-964-1799
888-964-2001
Fax: 414-964-7176
e-mail: iffgd@iffgd.org
www.iffgd.org

The organization offers responses to those commonly asked questions for families and individuals whose lives have been touched with the disorder.

Nancy J Norton, Founder
William Norton, VP

2937 March of Dimes Birth Defects Foundation
1275 Mamaroneck Avenue
White Plains, NY 10605

914-428-7100
888-663-4637
Fax: 914-428-8203
e-mail: resourcecenter@modimes.org
www.marchofdimes.com

Partnership of volunteers and professionals dedicates to improving the health of babies by preventing birth defects and infant mortality. Over 100 chapters are located across the country and can be located through the National Office.

Dr Jennifer Howse, President

Web Sites

2938 Mental Help Net
mentalhelp.net

We wish to provide the following: to develop and debate in an open forum the future of the mental health field in America and throughout the world; to help coordinate various components of the mental health field, so as to bring about greater communication between them; also to educate the public about mental health issues.

Book Publishers

2939 What I Need to Know About Constipation
Nat'l Digestive Diseases Information Clearinghouse
2 Information Way
Bethesda, MD 20892

301-654-3810
Fax: 301-907-8906
e-mail: nddic@info.niddk.nih.gov
www.niddk.nih.gov

Defines constipation and includes a list of steps for prevention, as well as a list of additional resources

Pamphlets

2940 Constipation
NDDIC
2 Information Way
Bethesda, MD 20892

301-654-3810
800-891-5389
Fax: 301-907-8906
e-mail: nddic@info.niddk.nih.gov
www.niddk.nih.gov

Includes a definition of constipation and information on how it develops, how it is diagnosed, and how it can be treated. Also provides details on misconceptions about constipation.

8 pages

2941 Constipation in Children
Nat'l Digestive Diseases Information Clearinghouse
2 Information Way
Bethesda, MD 20892

301-654-3810
Fax: 301-907-8906
e-mail: nddic@info.niddk.nih.gov
www.niddk.nih.gov

2942 Fecal Incontinence
NDDIC
2 Information Way
Bethesda, MD 20892

301-654-3810
800-891-5389
Fax: 301-907-8906
e-mail: nddic@info.niddk.nih.gov
www.niddk.nih.gov

8 pages

DESCRIPTION

2943 EPIDERMOLYSIS BULLOSA

Covers these related disorders: Epidermolysis bullosa dystrophica, Epidermolysis bullosa simplex, Junctional epidermolysis bullosa

Involves the following Biologic System(s):

Dermatologic Disorders

Epidermolysis bullosa is a group of inherited diseases that are often apparent at birth (congenital) and characterized by blistering of the skin after minor injury or trauma. In addition, blistering tends to worsen in warm temperatures. These disorders vary in severity, specific features, and mode of inheritance, and are classified under one of three groupings.

Epidermolysis bullosa simplex is a relatively mild, non-scarring form of this disorder that is inherited as an autosomal dominant trait. Epidermolysis bullosa simplex is further categorized as generalized or localized. The generalized type is usually apparent at birth or soon thereafter. The blisters, also known as bullae, are usually located on areas of the body that are prone to injury such as the hands, feet, elbows, knees, etc. Blistering tendencies usually lessen with advancing age with no long-term effects or scarring. The localized form of this disorder, known as Weber-Cockayne syndrome, affects the hands and feet and may not become apparent until walking commences or, in some cases, adolescence or adulthood. Blistering may be mild, but may severely worsen with such activities as extended walking. Treatment is symptomatic and supportive and may be directed toward prevention and treatment of secondary infections.

Junctional epidermolysis bullosa is inherited as an autosomal recessive trait and is also apparent at birth or soon thereafter. Characteristic findings and symptoms associated with this|potentially life-threatening form of the disorder may include severe blistering around the mouth and on the scalp, trunk, diaper area, and legs. In addition, slow-healing lesions may develop in the mucous membranes of the respiratory, gastrointestinal, and genitourinary tracts. Affected infants are also at increased risk for infections such as septicemia, a life-threatening condition in which harmful bacteria multiply in the bloodstream. In addition, the nails may appear defective and teeth may decay easily. Other findings may include growth retardation and abnormally low levels of circulating red blood cells (anemia). Treatment for junctional epidermolysis bullosa may include the administration of antibiotics to treat infections and blood transfusions to treat anemia. In addition, nutritional supplementation may be beneficial. Other treatment is symptomatic and supportive.

Epidermolysis bullosa dystrophica may be inherited as an autosomal dominant trait, an autosomal recessive trait, or it may appear sporadically. Findings associated with autosomal dominant inheritance are less severe than those of autosomal recessive transmission. This form of epidermolysis bullosa may be further categorized as the albopapuloid Pasini variant and the Cockayne-Touraine variant. The albopapuloid Pasini variant may first appear as early as infancy or as late as adolescence and is characterized by extensive, scarring-type blistering of the skin on the joints, arms, and legs; the appearance during adolescence of flesh-colored (albopapuloid) lesions on the trunk; and involvement of certain mucuous memberanes. The Cockayne-Touraine variant of this disorder develops during infancy or early childhood and is characterized by blisters that most commonly appear on the arms and legs. Epidermolysis bullosa dystrophica that is inherited as an autosomal recessive trait is a severe form of this disorder that may be characterized at birth by extensive blistering and erosions of the body surfaces and mucous membranes. As the lesions heal, scarring may result in deformity and limited mobility. In addition, healing of the mucous membranes of the esophagus may cause narrowing of this structure, leading to difficulties in feeding and eating. Treatment may include the implementation of a special diet or use of special feeding devices necessitated by scarring or narrowing of the esophagus. Additional treatment may be directed toward the prevention or care of associated secondary infections. Other treatment is symptomatic and supportive.

See also **General Resources** on page 917

Government Agencies

2944 NIH/National Institute of Arthritis and Musculoskeletal and Skin Diseases

1AMS Circle
Bethesda, MD 20892

301-402-4484
Fax: 301-718-6366
e-mail: ord@od.nih.gov
rarediseases.info.nih.gov

The mission of the National Institute of Arthritis and Musculoskeletal and Skin Diseases is to support research into the causes, treatment, and prevention of arthritis and musculoskeletal and skin diseases, the training of basic and clinical scientists to carry out this research, and the dissemination of information on research progress in these diseases.

Stephen I Katz MD PhD, Director

National Associations & Support Groups

2945 DebRA: Dystrophic Epidermolysis Bullosa Research Association of America
5 West 36th Street, Suite 404
New York, NY 10018

212-868-1573
866-332-7276
Fax: 212-513-4099
e-mail: staff@debra.org
www.debra.org

Committed to providing referrals, patient advocacy and lobbying, offers networking services, and engages in patient and professional education.

Suzanne J Cohen, Executive Director
Abby Meadows, Development Manager

2946 Genetic Alliance
4301 Connecticut Avenue NW
Washington, DC 20008

202-966-5557
800-336-4363
Fax: 202-966-8553
e-mail: info@geneticalliance.org
www.geneticalliance.org

A coalition of voluntary genetic support groups, consumers and professionals addressing the needs of individuals and families affected by genetic disorders from a national perspective.

Sharon Terry, President/CEO

2947 March of Dimes Birth Defects Foundation
1275 Mamaroneck Avenue
White Plains, NY 10605

914-428-7100
888-663-4637
Fax: 914-428-8203
e-mail: resourcecenter@modimes.org
www.marchofdimes.com

Partnership of volunteers and professionals dedicates to improving the health of babies by preventing birth defects and infant mortality. Over 100 chapters are located across the country and can be located through the National Office.

Dr Jennifer Howse, President

2948 National Epidermolysis Bullosa Registry
Clinical Coordinating Center, Univ. of N Carolina
Chapel Hill, Department Derm., Room 137-NCMH
Chapel Hill, NC 27514

919-966-3321
Fax: 919-966-6383
www.nationaleidermolysisbullosaregistry

Web Sites

2949 EB Medical Research Foundation
www-med.stanford.edu/school/dermatology/ebmrf/

The EBMRF is a nonprofit, whose sole purpose is dedicated to the support of medical research of epidermolysis bullosa — its causes, its cure, and the development of successful treatments.

2950 Family Village
www.familyvillage.wisc.edu

A global community that integrates information, resources and communication opportunities on the Internet for persons with cognitive and other disabilities, for their families and for those that provide them services and support.

2951 Online Mendelian Inheritance in Man
www.ncbi.nlm.nih.gov

This database is a catalog of human genes and genetic disorders.

Book Publishers

2952 Epidermolysis Bullosa

Clinical, epidemiologic, and laboratory advances and the findings of the National Epidermolysis Bullosa Registry. The first comprehensive examination of EB employing a large, well-characterized research study population and using the latest epidemiological and biostatistical research principles. Includes the assessment of over 2,000 patients with EB. Topics discussed are molecular and cell biology, epidemiology, diagnosis, classification, medical and surgical treatments, and clinical outcomes.

510 pages
ISBN: 0-801860-24-5

Jo-David Fine, MD, MPH, Editor
Eugene A Bauer, MD, Editor

Newsletters

2953 DebRA Currents
DebRA
5 West 36th Street, Suite 404
New York, NY 10018

212-868-1573
866-332-7276
Fax: 212-513-4099
e-mail: staff@deba.org
www.debra.org

Suzanne J Cohen, Executive Director

DESCRIPTION

2954 ERB'S PALSY

Synonym: Erb-Duchenne paralysis

Involves the following Biologic System(s):

Neurologic Disorders

Erb's palsy is a form of paralysis in newborns resulting from injury to certain nerves (i.e., fifth and sixth cervical nerves of upper brachial plexus) that supply specific muscles of the shoulder and arm. Nerve injury may be the result of a difficult delivery (e.g., breech presentation, delivery of an unusually large newborn, etc.). During delivery, lateral traction of the head and neck may occur and lead to stretching of these nerves, potentially resulting in such injury.

Newborns with Erb's palsy typically experience swelling and inflammation of the affected nerves and paralysis of the affected shoulder and arm muscles (e.g., deltoid, biceps, brachialis). This causes the arm to hang loosely with the elbow extended and inwardly rotated. Newborns with the condition are unable to move the affected arm away from the shoulder or rotate the arm away from the body. In addition, although they may extend the forearm, affected newborns lack a startle reflex known as Moro's reflex on the affected side. Moro's reflex, which is usually present at birth, involves stretching of the arms and legs forward and out and extension of the fingers when startled. In some severe cases, paralysis and associated loss of the muscle mass (atrophy)in the shoulder area (deltoid muscle) may cause drop shoulder, which is characterized by depression of the affected shoulder below the level of the other. Some infants may experience impairment of sensation in affected areas. Movements of the hand are typically not affected.

The effectiveness of certain treatments for Erb's palsy may vary, depending upon whether affected nerves (i.e., fifth and sixth cervical nerves) were torn or injured in a manner that allows a return of function within a few months. Treatment measures may include initial immobilization of the affected arm and shoulder with braces or splints and physical therapy including range of motion exercises, massage, and active and passive corrective exercises. Such therapy may help to improve muscle function and prevent permanent bending of affected joints in a fixed posture (flexion contractures). If paralysis continues at three to six months of age, surgical measures may be considered in some cases.

See also **General Resources** on page 917

National Associations & Support Groups

2955 Brachial Plexus Injury/Erb's Palsy Support & Information Network
PO Box 533
Manasha, WI 54952

441-836-3843

Furnishes a variety of support tools including reading and audio materials.

2956 Brachial Plexus Palsy Foundation
210 Springhaven Circle
Royersford, PA 19468

610-792-0974
e-mail: contact@brachialplexuspalsyfoundation.or
www.brachialplexuspalsyfoundation.org

A non profit organizaztion designed to raise funds for activities in support of families with children who have suffered brachial plexus injuries. The Foundation also provides information about a brachial plexus injury ti better educate families who do not have the time or resources.

2957 March of Dimes Birth Defects Foundation
1275 Mamaroneck Avenue
White Plains, NY 10605

914-428-7100
888-663-4637
Fax: 914-428-8203
e-mail: resourcecenter@modimes.org
www.marchofdimes.com

Partnership of volunteers and professionals dedicates to improving the health of babies by preventing birth defects and infant mortality. Over 100 chapters are located across the country and can be located through the National Office.

Dr Jennifer Howse, President

2958 National Brachial Plexus/Erb's Palsy Association
PO Box 23
Larsen, WI 54947

920-836-9955
Fax: 920-836-9587
e-mail: erbspalsy@usa.net
www.nbpepa.org

Provides support, promotes public awareness, serves as a resource to families and professionals and provides a network of information to incearse the understanding of Brachial Pelxus injuries and to discover new and better way to treat children with the injury.

2959 United Brachial Plexus Network
1610 Kent Street
Kent, OH 44240

866-877-7004
Fax: 866-877-7004
e-mail: info@ubpn.org
www.ubpn.org

A registered non-profit organization devoted to providing information, support, and leadership for families and those concerned with brachial plexus injuries worldwide. Also provided is an online registry, various outreach and awareness programs and publications.

Nancy Birk, President

Libraries & Resource Centers

2960 National Rehabilitation Information Center
4200 Forbes Blvd, Suite 202
Lanham, MD 20706

301-459-5900
800-346-2742
Fax: 301-562-2401
TTY: 301-459-5984
e-mail: naricinfo@heitechservices.com
www.naric.com

Committed to providing direct, personal and high quality information services to anyone interested in disability and rehabilitation issues. We are committed to serving customers, researchers, family members, health professionals, educators, counselors and students throughout the country.

Mark Odum, Director

Web Sites

2961 Texas Children's Hospital
www.texaschildrenshospital.org

Is an internationally recognized full-care prediatric hospital located in the Texas Medical Center in Houston. The largest pediatric hospital in the United States, Texas Children's is nationaly ranked in the top 5 among children's hospitals.

Newsletters

2962 Outreach
United Brachial Plexus Network
1610 Kent Street
Kent, OH 44240

866-877-7004
Fax: 866-877-7004
e-mail: nancy@ubpn.org
www.ubpn.org

Brachial Plexus/Erb's Palsy newsletter.

DESCRIPTION

2963 ERYTHEMA INFECTIOSUM

Synonyms: EI, Fifth disease, Sticker's disease, Parvovirus, Slapped Cheek

Involves the following Biologic System(s):

Infectious Disorders

Erythema infectiosum, or Fifth disease, is a contagious infection caused by the human parvovirus B19. It is characterized by a three-stage rash. First, there is the sudden appearance of a red rash on the face that may look as if the cheeks had been slapped. Then the rash progresses to a reddish, raised-spot, blotchy eruption that spreads to the trunk, buttocks, arms, and legs. When it begins to fade, the rash takes on a lacy-type appearance. The rash usually subsides within five to 10 days, but may reappear within a month's time, especially after exercise, stress, skin irritation, or exposure to sunlight. Transmission of this virus is through inhalation of droplets exhaled or coughed into the air by infected individuals. The incubation period for erythema infectiosum is approximately four to 14 days.

Erythema infectiosum occurs most commonly in preschool and young school-age children. The first symptoms may be low-grade fever and headache. Once the rash appears or shortly thereafter, fever and other signs of illness may be absent. However, some older children and adults may develop mild itching (pruritus), joint pain (arthralgia), and inflammation of the joints (arthritis). In addition, under certain circumstances, exposure to human parvovirus B19 may result in more severe complications. For example, individuals with certain blood disorders such as thalessemia or sickle cell anemia may develop a temporary inability to produce red blood cells, resulting in a decrease in the body's capacity to supply oxygen to the tissues of the body (anemia). Symptoms associated with severe anemia may include weakness, discomfort, pale skin (pallor), rapid breathing (tachypnea), and rapid heartbeat (tachycardia). In addition, those who have impaired immune function may experience severe consequences upon exposure to human parvovirus B19. For example, individuals undergoing certain types of chemotherapy, those with acquired immunodeficiency syndrome (AIDS), or those with certain types of primary, inherited immune defects may experience recurrent or prolonged infections, anemia, or other blood abnormalities.

Pregnant women infected with parvovirus B19 may transmit it to their unborn children, resulting, in rare cases, in miscarriage or stillbirth; however, most of those exposed in utero are born with no apparent consequences. Other viral-exposed infants may have abnormal accumulations of fluid in the tissues or cavities of the body (hydrops). If this condition is diagnosed before birth, special blood transfusions delivered by way of the umbilical vein may be of benefit to the affected fetus. Treatment for this viral infection is symptomatic.

See also **General Resources** on page 917

Government Agencies

2964 Centers for Disease Control
1600 Clifton Road
Atlanta, GA 30333

404-639-3311
www.cdc.gov

Mission is to promote health and quality of life by preventing and controlling disease, injury, and disability.

2965 NIH/National Institute of Allergy and Infectious Diseases
6610 Rockledge Drive, MSC 6612
Bethesda, MD 20892

301-496-5717
Fax: 301-402-3573
TDD: 800-877-8339
www.niaid.nih.gov

Conducts and supports basic and applied research to better understand, treat, and ultimately prevent infectious, immunologic, and allergic diseases.

Anthony S Fauci MD, Director

National Associations & Support Groups

2966 March of Dimes Birth Defects Foundation
1275 Mamaroneck Avenue
White Plains, NY 10605

914-428-7100
888-663-4637
Fax: 914-428-8203
e-mail: resourcecenter@modimes.org
www.marchofdimes.com

Partnership of volunteers and professionals dedicates to improving the health of babies by preventing birth defects and infant mortality. Over 100 chapters are located across the country and can be located through the National Office.

Dr Jennifer Howse, President

2967 World Health Organization
Avenue Appia 20
CH-1211 Geneva 27,
Switzerland

www.who.int

WHO is the directing and coordinating authority for health within the United Nations system.

Dr Margaret Chan, Director General

Web Sites

2968 Kid's Health
kidshealth.org

Kids health is the largest and most visited site on the web providing doctor-approved health information about children from before birth through adolescence. Kids health provides families with accurate, up to date and jargon free health information they can use.

2969 Med Help International
www.medhelp.org

Is dedicated to helping patients find the highest quality medical information in the world today. We offer patients the tools necessary to make informed treatment decisions within the short time lines dedicated by their illness or disease.

2970 New York State Department of Health
www.medhelp.org/lib/fifth.htm

Information on erythema infectiosum, like how does anyone get it, what is the treatment, and what can be done to prevent this disease from occuring.

DESCRIPTION

2971 ESOPHAGEAL ATRESIA

Synonyms: Tracheo-esophageal fistula, Vacterl, Vater

Involves the following Biologic System(s):

Gastrointestinal Disorders

Esophageal atresia is a defect that is present at birth (congenital). The esophagus, which is a muscular tube, is that portion of the digestive system that connects the throat and the stomach. In infants with esophageal atresia, the channel (lumen) within the tubular esophagus fails to develop properly, resulting in an esophagus that ends in a blind pouch, failing to provide a continuous passage to the stomach. In some infants, the upper section of the esophagus may be dramatically narrowed or it may be closed at its lower end. In others, the closed-end lower portion extends upward from the stomach and there is no through connection between the two. Most affected infants also have an abnormal tube-like connection or opening between the windpipe (trachea) and either the upper or lower portion of the esophagus. This is known as a tracheoesophageal fistula. In some children, there is a double connection in which there is an abnormal passage between the trachea and part of the esophagus, as well as between the trachea and a lower region of the esophagus.

Infants with esophageal atresia cannot swallow at all and therefore salivate and regurgitate excessively. If a tracheoesophageal fistula exists between the windpipe and upper portion of the esophagus, fluid may enter the lungs, resulting in coughing, choking, a bluish discoloration (cyanosis) of the nail beds, lips, and mucous membranes, and possibly pneumonia. The presence of an abnormal passage between the trachea and the lower section of the esophagus may allow air to enter the abdomen, resulting in excessive abdominal swelling (distension) that may interfere with normal breathing. In addition, contents of the abdomen may enter the lungs and severe inflammation may occur. If esophageal atresia is present without a fistula, characteristic findings may include a boat-shaped abdomen that is devoid of air.

Treatment includes surgery to join or connect the two sections of the esophagus. This procedure is known as an esophageal anastomosis. Tracheoesophageal fistulas may be surgically corrected by ligation, a procedure in which the passageway is tied off. Before surgery, special care is taken to ensure the infants do not draw fluid (aspirate) into their lungs through the esophagus.

As many as 50 percent of infants with esophageal atresia have associated structural malformations of other organs. For example, if a tracheoesophageal fistula is present, other abnormalities of the trachea may also be apparent. In addition, approximately half of all affected infants have a complex of congenital anomalies (VACTERL syndrome) characterized by additional malformations involving the heart, skeleton, kidneys, and urinary and genital systems. Treatment for esophageal atresia includes management or correction of associated anomalies. Esophageal atresia occurs in approximately one in 3,500 births in the United States. About 33 percent of these infants are born prematurely.

See also **General Resources** on page 917

National Associations & Support Groups

2972 American College of Gastroenterology
PO Box 342260
Bethesda, MD 20827

301-263-9000
www.acg.gi.org

Founded to advance the scientific study and medical practice of diseases of the gastrointestinal (GI) tract.

Jack A DiPalma, President
Amy E Foxx-Orenstein, VP

2973 Digestive Disease National Coalition
507 Capitol Court NE, Suite 200
Washington, DC 20002

202-544-7497
Fax: 202-546-7105
www.ddnc.org

Advocacy organization comprised of 22 voluntary and professional societies concerned with the many diseases of the digestive tract and liver.

Nancy Norton, Chairperson
Dr. Maurice Cerulli, President

2974 EA/TEF Child and Family Support Connection
111 W Jackson Boulevard, Suite 1145
Chicago, IL 60604

312-987-9085
Fax: 312-987-9086
e-mail: eatef2@aol.com
www.eatef.org

2975 International Foundation for Functional Gastrointestinal Disorders
PO Box 170864
Milwaukee, WI 53217

414-964-1799
888-964-2001
Fax: 414-964-7176
e-mail: iffgd@iffgd.org
www.iffgd.org

Nonprofit education and research organization founded in 1991. IFFGD addresses the issues surrounding life with gastrointestinal (GI) functional and mobility disorders and increases the awareness about these disorders among the general public, researchers and the clinical care community.

Nancy J Norton, Founder
William Norton, VP

2976 North American Society for Pediatric Gastroenterology/Hepatology/Nutrition
PO Box 6
Flourtown, PA 19031

215-233-0808
Fax: 215-233-3918
e-mail: naspghan@naspghan.org
www.naspghan.org

Strives to improve the care of infants, children and adolescents with digestive disorders by promoting advances in clinical care of children with chronic abdominal pain, diarrhea, constipation, vomiting, bleeding from the GI tract, inflammatory bowel disease, liver diseases, diseases of the pancreas, poor weight gain and nutritional problems.

Philip Sherman, President
Margaret K Stallings, Executive Director

Libraries & Resource Centers

2977 National Digestive Diseases Information Clearinghouse
2 Information Way
Bethesda, MD 20892

301-654-3810
800-891-5389
Fax: 703-738-4929
e-mail: nddic@info.niddk.nih.gov
www.digestive.niddk.nih.gov

The National Institute of Diabetes and Digestive and Kidney Diseases conducts and supports research on many of the most serious diseases affecting public health. The Institute supports much of the clinical research on the diseases of internal medicine and related subspecialty fields as well as many basic science disciplines.

Kathy Kranzfelder, Project Officer

Web Sites

2978 National Digestive Diseases Information Clearinghouse
www.digestive.niddk.nih.gov

The National Institute of Diabetes and Digestive and Kidney Diseases conducts and supports research on many of the most serious diseases affecting public health. The Institute supports much of the clinical research on the diseases of internal medicine and related subspecialty fields as well as many basic science disciplines.

Journals

2979 Journal of Pediatric Gastroenterology and Nutrition

NASPGHAN, author

Lippincott Williams & Wilkins
530 Walnut Street
Philadelphia, PA 19106

215-521-8300
Fax: 215-521-8902
www.lww.com

Publication of the North American Society for Pediatric Gastroenterolgy, Hepatology and Nutrition, which strives to improve the care of infants, children and adolescents with digestive disorders by promoting advances in clinical care of children with chronic abdominal pain, diarrhea, constipation, vomiting, bleeding from the GI tract, inflammatory bowel disease, liver diseases, diseases of the pancreas, poor weight gain and nutritional problems.

Newsletters

2980 NASPGHAN News
PO Box 6
Flourtown, PA 19031

215-233-0808
Fax: 215-233-3939
e-mail: naspghan@naspghan.org
www.naspgn.org

Publication of the North American Society for Pediatric Gastroenterolgy, Hepatology and Nutrition, which strives to improve the care of infants, children and adolescents with digestive disorders by promoting advances in clinical care of children with chronic abdominal pain, diarrhea, constipation, vomiting, bleeding from the GI tract, inflammatory bowel disease, liver diseases, diseases of the pancreas, poor weight gain and nutritional problems.

2981 TEF/VATER International Support Network
15301 Grey Fox Road
Upper Marlboro, MD 20722

301-952-6837
Fax: 301-952-9152
e-mail: info@tefvater.org
www.tefvater.org

Provides support to children and adults born with esophageal atresia.

DESCRIPTION

See also **General Resources** on page 917

2982 EWING'S SARCOMA

Synonym: Ewing's tumor

Involves the following Biologic System(s):

Hematologic and Oncologic Disorders, Orthopedic and Muscle Disorders

Ewing's sarcoma is a malignant tumor that typically occurs in individuals under the age of 20 years. The tumor most often arises in the long bones of the shin (tibia), thigh (femur), or upper arm (humerus) or the flat bones of the pelvis, vertebrae, or chest wall. Ewing's sarcoma often invades surrounding soft tissues and tends to spread (metastasize) to other bones, the lungs, and, less frequently, to the bone marrow or other organs. In some cases, the primary tumor may develop in soft tissue. Approximately 75 percent of these tumors occur in the legs or arms as well as the bones of the shoulders.

The most common symptoms of Ewing's sarcoma include fever, as well as pain, tenderness, and swelling in the area of the tumor. Some children may also experience weight loss, low levels of circulating red blood cells (anemia), and elevated levels of circulating white blood cells (leukocytosis). In addition, the tumor may weaken the surrounding bone and thus increase vulnerability to bone fracture. The diagnosis of Ewing's tumor is established through the use of x-rays along with examination of tissue samples obtained through biopsy. In addition, other procedures such as bone scanning, computed tomography (CT), and magnetic resonance imaging (MRI) may be used to confirm the presence of lung, bone, or other metastases.

Ewing's sarcoma develops most frequently between the ages of 10 and 20 years of age and affects boys more often than girls by a ratio of two to one. These tumors rarely occur in black children. Treatment of Ewing's sarcoma may include the use of chemotherapy and radiation. Patients are also evaluated for possible surgical removal of the tumor. Other treatment is symptomatic and supportive. Outcome (prognosis) for children with Ewing's sarcoma depends on several factors that include the extent of the disease, the size and location of the tumor, presence or absence of metastases, the tumor's response to therapy, and the age and overall health of the child. Prompt medical attention and aggressive therapy are important for the best prognosis.

Government Agencies

2983 NIH/National Cancer Institute
6116 Executive Boulevard, Room 3036A
Bethesda, MD 20892

800-422-6237
www.cancer.gov

The National Cancer Institute coordinates the National Cancer Program, which conducts and supports research, training, health information dissemination, and other programs with respect to the cause, diagnosis, prevention, and treatment of cancer, rehabilitation from cancer, and the continuing care of cancer patients and the families of cancer patients.

John E Niederhuber MD, Director

National Associations & Support Groups

2984 American Cancer Society
Brain Tumor Support Group
ACS Building, 8900 Carpenter Freeway
Dallas, TX 75247

214-819-1200
800-227-2345
Fax: 214-631-3869
www.cancer.org

Attacks the support aspect of this disease from every angle including data on lowering risks to dealing with grief.

Maria Clarke, Executive Director

2985 B.A.S.E. Camp Children's Cancer Foundation
7501 Glenmoor Lane
Winter Park, FL 32792

407-673-5060
Fax: 407-673-5095
e-mail: email@basecamp.org
basecampcf.org

Provides a year round base of support for children and families facing the challenge of living with cancer, hemophilia and other blood related illnesses.

Terri Jones, Executive Director

2986 Believe In Tomorrow National Children's Foundation
6601 Fredrick Road
Baltimore, MD 21228

800-933-5470
Fax: 410-774-1984
e-mail: info@believeintomorrow.org
www.believeintomorrow.org

Provides exceptional hospital and retreat housing services to critically ill children and their families. The Foundation also provides a unique Hands On adventures program that allows children to experience unique once in a lifetime opportunities.

Brian R Morrison, Founder/ National Director

2987 Candlelighters Childhood Cancer Foundation
PO Box 498
Kensington, MD 20895

301-962-3520
800-366-2223
Fax: 310-962-3521
e-mail: staff@candlelighters.org
www.candlelighters.org

The Candlelighters Childhood Cancer Foundation National Office was founded in 1970 by concerned parents of children with cancer.

Today our membership of over 50,000 members of the national office and more than 100,000 members across the across the country, including Candlelighters affiliate groups, includes, parents of children who are being treated or have been treated for cancer.

Ruth Hoffman, Executive Director

2988 Hair Club for Kids: Hair Club for Men
270 Farmington Avenue, Suite 232
Farmington, CT 06032

860-674-0202
888-888-8986
Fax: 860-676-0805
www.hairclub.com/kids

If your child expresses an interest in wearing a wig, send pictures prior to hair loss with snippets of hair for a good match of original color and texture. The cost of the wig may be covered by insurance.

2989 Just In Time
PO Box 27693
Philadelphia, PA 19118

215-247-8777
Fax: 215-247-0956
www.softhats.com

100% cotton hat, turbans and caps designed for women with hair loss due to cancer, chemotherapy, alopecia or trichotillomania.

2990 National Childhood Cancer Foundation
4600 East West Highway, Suite 600
Bethesda, MD 20814

800-458-6223
e-mail: info@curesearch.org
www.curesearch.org

CureSearch unites the world's largest childhood cancer research organization, the Children's Oncology Group, and the National Childhood Cancer Foundation through our mission to cure childhood cancer. Research is the key to the cure.

2991 National Coalition for Cancer Survivorship
1010 Wayne Road, Suite 770
Silver Spring, MD 20910

301-650-9127
877-622-7937
Fax: 301-565-9670
e-mail: info@canceradvocacy.org
www.canceradvocacy.org

Furnishes information about legal rights and advocacy services for cancer survivors of all ages. Publications include: Health Insurance and Cancer: What You Need to Know; Working It Out: Your Employment Rights As a Cancer Survivor; and Charting the Journey: An Almanac of Practical Resources for Cancer Survivors.

Ellen Stovall, President & CEO
Michael Bergin, Chief Operating Officer

Web Sites

2992 CancerCare
www.cancercare.org

Dedicated to providing emotional support, information, and practical help to people with cancer and their loved ones. CancerCare is the oldest, largest, nonprofit agency devoted to offering professional services.

2993 Children's Cancer Web
www.cancerindex.org/ccw

An independent nonprofit site, established to provide a directory of childhood cancer resources.

2994 Ewing's Sarcoma Support Group Resources Page
www.cureourchildren.org

2995 OncoLink: The University of Pennslyvania Cancer Center Resource
www.oncolink.upenn.edu

Book Publishers

2996 Let's Talk About Going to the Hospital
Rosen Publishing Group's PowerKids Press
29 E 21st Street
New York, NY 10010

212-777-3017
800-237-9932
Fax: 888-436-4643
e-mail: rosenpub@tribeca.ios.com
www.powerkidspress.com

If a child has to check into the hospital, chances are he or she is already upset about being ill. Knowing how a hospital functions and what the procedures are, such as when family members can visit, will help in what is already a stressful situation. Grades K-5.

24 pages
ISBN: 0-823950-36-0

2997 Let's Talk About when Kids Have Cancer
Rosen Publishing Group's PowerKids Press
29 E 21st Street
New York, NY 10010

212-777-3017
800-237-9932
Fax: 888-436-4643
e-mail: customerservice@rosenpub.com
www.powerkidspress.com

In a straightforward yet comforting way, this book explains what cancer is, what kinds of treatments surround the disease and how to cope if a child or the friend of a child has cancer.

24 pages
ISBN: 0-823951-95-2

2998 Pediatric Cancer Sourcebook
Omnigraphics
PO Box 625
Holmes, PA 19043

800-234-1340
Fax: 800-875-1340
e-mail: info@omnigraphics.com
omnigraphics.com

Basic consumer health information about leukemias, brain tumors, sarcomas, lymphomas and other cancers in infants, children and adolescents.

587 pages
ISBN: 0-780802-45-4

DESCRIPTION

2999 FAMILIAL DYSAUTONOMIA

Synonyms: FD, HSAN-III, Riley-Day syndrome

Involves the following Biologic System(s):

Genetic/Chromosomal/Syndrome/Metabolic Disorders, Neurologic Disorders

Familial dysautonomia (FD) is a rare inherited disorder of that part of the nervous system responsible for regulating various essential involuntary functions (autonomic nervous system). This disorder is characterized in infants by feeding difficulties, including excessive salivation and poor swallowing and sucking reflexes. The breathing in of liquid or other substances into the lungs (aspiration) may lead to repeated episodes of bronchial pneumonia. Other associated symptoms and findings include skin blotching, sweating, fluctuating extremes in body temperature, and defective tear secretion (lacrimation). Affected children develop an reduced sensitivity to temperature and pain. This may lead to frequent injuries such as irritation of the corneas of the eyes. Corneal injury may also occur as the result of decreased tear production. In addition, slurred speech and drooling may become evident. Children with familial dysautonomia typically have weak reflex responses (hyporeflexia) and experience delays in walking accompanied by the inability to coordinate voluntary movements (motor incoordination). After three years of age, affected children often develop severe vomiting episodes (hyperemesis) that may occur three or four times an hour and, in some cases, may last for three days or more. These episodes may sometimes be accompanied by elevated blood pressure (hypertension), abdominal pain and swelling, increased irritability, or breathing difficulties (dyspnea). As children with this disorder reach adolescence, a sideward curvature of the spine (scoliosis) may become evident along with leg cramping and weakness. In addition, some children may experience a delay in the onset of puberty. Older children may develop emotional and behavioral changes, such as irritability and depression. Intolerance for anesthetics is a common finding among children with FD.

Treatment for familial dysautonomia is symptomatic and supportive. Artificial tears, drops, or ointments may be placed in the eyes to prevent injury to corneas. Certain medications known as antiemetics may be prescribed to help control episodes of vomiting. In addition, replacement fluids and electrolytes may be administered to prevent excessive fluid loss (dehydration) resulting from vomiting episodes. Other treatment may include surgery or the use of orthopedic aids to correct scoliosis.

Familial dysautonomia is inherited as an autosomal recessive trait and occurs most commonly among certain individuals of eastern European descent, particularly Ashkenazi Jews at a rate of one out of 10,000 to 20,000 births. The disease gene for this disorder is located on the long arm of chromosome 9 (9q31-33).

See also **General Resources** on page 917

National Associations & Support Groups

3000 Dysautonomia Foundation
315 West 39th Street, Suite 701
New York, NY 10018

212-279-1066
Fax: 212-279-2066
e-mail: info@familialdysautonomia.org
www.familialdysautonomiafoundation.org

Provides parents the knowledge regarding both national and international facilities that specialize in the treatment of the disorder.

David Brenner, Executive Director

3001 Familial Dysautonomia Hope Foundation
605 5th Avenue
Conover, NC 28613

828-695-1060
Fax: 828-695-1060
e-mail: info@fdhope.org
www.fdvillage.org

To find a cure and new treatment options for Familial Dysautonomia by funding relevant research programs, to provide a support network aimed at addressing the needs of patients and families and to promote Familial Dysautonomia education and awareness programs in the medical community.

3002 Genetic Alliance
4301 Connecticut Avenue NW
Washington, DC 20008

202-966-5557
800-336-4363
Fax: 202-966-8553
e-mail: info@geneticalliance.org
www.geneticalliance.org

A coalition of voluntary genetic support groups, consumers and professionals addressing the needs of individuals and families affected by genetic disorders from a national perspective.

Sharon Terry, President/CEO

3003 March of Dimes Birth Defects Foundation
1275 Mamaroneck Avenue
White Plains, NY 10605

914-428-7100
888-663-4637
Fax: 914-428-8203
e-mail: resourcecenter@modimes.org
www.marchofdimes.com

Partnership of volunteers and professionals dedicates to improving the health of babies by preventing birth defects and infant mortality. Over 100 chapters are located across the country and can be located through the National Office.

Dr Jennifer Howse, President

3004 National Foundation for Jewish Genetic Diseases
250 Park Avenue, Suite 1000
New York, NY 10017

212-371-1030
Fax: 212-319-5808
e-mail: nfjgd@aol.com
www.nfjgd.org

Provides the information regarding this and related disorders for
the people suffering from them.

Web Sites

3005 Family Village
www.familyvillage.wisc.edu

A global community that integrates information, resources and
communication opportunities on the Internet for persons with cognitive and other disabilities, for their families and for those that
provide them services and support.

3006 NYU
www.med.nyu.edu/fd/fdcenter.html

Offers information about Familial Dysautonomia.

3007 Online Mendelian Inheritance in Man
www.ncbi.nlm.nih.gov

This database is a catalog of human genes and genetic disorders.

DESCRIPTION

See also **General Resources** on page 917

3008 FETAL ALCOHOL SYNDROME

Synonyms: FAS, Fetal alcohol effect (FAE), Alcohol-related neurodevelopmental, Alcolol-related birth defects

Involves the following Biologic System(s):

Genetic/Chromosomal/Syndrome/Metabolic Disorders

Fetal alcohol syndrome, or FAS, is a condition that is present at birth and the result of persistent maternal alcohol consumption during pregnancy. This condition is characterized by various birth defects such as low birth weight, short birth length, and an unusually small head (microcephaly) that may be associated with slowed development of the brain. Infants with FAS may also have several abnormalities of the face and skull including an unusually short opening between the margins of the upper and lower eyelids (palpebral fissures), vertical folds of skin that extend from the inner corners of the upper eyelids to the sides of the nose (epicanthal folds), an abnormally small lower jaw (micrognathia), or a poorly developed upper jaw (maxillary hypoplasia). Additional unusual features may include an abnormal opening in the roof of the mouth (cleft palate), a prominent forehead (frontal bossing), a flattened nasal bridge, and a thin, smooth upper lip. Other characteristic findings may include heart defects, abnormalities of the limbs and joints (e.g., dislocated hip, etc.), and irregular skin crease patterns on the palms of the hands. Within the first day of life, affected newborns may also exhibit characteristic symptoms of alcohol withdrawal such as tremor, increased irritability, muscle spasms, vomiting, or other problems. The development of the brain may also be impaired resulting in moderate to severe mental retardation. Approximately 20 percent of newborns with fetal alcohol syndrome risk life-threatening symptoms and complications within the first few weeks of life.

Alcohol consumption during pregnancy affects the growth and development of the fetus within the uterus and may result not only in birth defects but, in some cases, miscarriage or stillbirth. Although it is believed that fetal alcohol syndrome results from persistent moderate or heavy drinking, no safe levels of alcohol intake during pregnancy have been established; therefore, pregnant women are counseled to avoid alcohol consumption. It has, however, been determined that the more alcohol consumed, the greater the chances of giving birth to children with associated abnormalities. Therefore, treatment is directed toward identification, counseling, and education of women at risk. Other treatment is symptomatic and supportive.

Government Agencies

3009 NIH/National Institute of Child Health and Human Development
31 Center Drive, Building 31
Bethesda, MD 20892

301-496-5133
Fax: 301-496-1104
www.nichd.nih.gov

Established in 1962 by congress, today the institute conducts and supports research on topics related to the health of children, adults, families and populations. Some of these topics include: developmental disabilities, growth and development, infant death, reproductive health and birth defects.

Nancy D Wirth, Director
Lisa Kaeser, Program & Public Liaison

3010 NIH/National Institute of Mental Health
6001 Executive Boulevard, Room 8184, MSC 9663
Bethesda, MD 20892

301-443-4513
866-615-6464
Fax: 301-443-4279
TTY: 301-443-8431
e-mail: nimhinfo@nih.gov
www.nimh.nih.gov

Conducts strategic planning for specific research areas as well as for the Institute as a whole.

Dr Thomas R Insel, Director

3011 NIH/National Institute on Alcohol Abuse an d Alcoholism
5635 Fishers Lane, MSC 9304
Bethesda, MD 20892

301-443-3885
877-266-4267
Fax: 301-443-7043
www.niaaa.nih.gov

Established in 1970, NIAAA conducts research focused on improving the treatment and prevention of alcoholism and alcohol-related problems to reduce the enormous health, social, and econmic consequences of this disease.

Dr Ting-Kai Li, Director

National Associations & Support Groups

3012 ARC of the United States
1010 Wayne Avenue, Suite 650
Silver Spring, MD 20910

301-565-3842
Fax: 301-565-5342
e-mail: info@thearc.org
www.thearc.org

The ARC is the national organization of and for people with mental retardation and related developmental disabilities and their families. Devoted to promoting and improving supports and services for people with mental retardation and their families. The association also fosters research and education regarding the prevention of mental retardation in infants and young children. The ARC was founded in 1950 by a small group of parents and other concerned individuals.

Sue Swenson, Executive Director
Adam Aaronson, Public Inquiries Director

3013 Family Empowerment Network: Supporting Families Affected by FAS/FAE
777 South Mills Street
Madison, WI 53703

608-262-6590
800-462-5254
Fax: 608-263-5813
e-mail: fen@fammed.wisc.edu
www.fammed.wisc.edu/fen/index.html

Provides education, resources and referrals to families affected by Fetal Alcohol Synadrome (FAS/FAE) and other professionals involved with them.

Georgiana Wilton, PhD, Director
Patricia Cameron, BS/FAS, Family Advocacy Specialist

3014 Fetal Alcohol Education Program
7 Kent Street
Brookline, MA 02146

617-739-1424
Fax: 617-566-4019

Works to educate the professional and community on the affects of alcohol consumption during pregnancy.

3015 Fetal Alcohol Syndrome Family Resource Institute
PO Box 2525
Lynwood, WA 98036

253-531-2878
800-999-3429
Fax: 253-531-2668
e-mail: vicky@fetalalcoholsyndrome.org
www.fetalalcoholsyndrome.org

Provides information packets, a statewide hotline for information, crisis and referral and a newsletter. Parents are available to give talks throughout the United States and Canada.

3016 March of Dimes Birth Defects Foundation
1275 Mamaroneck Avenue
White Plains, NY 10605

914-428-7100
888-663-4637
Fax: 914-428-8203
e-mail: resourcecenter@modimes.org
www.marchofdimes.com

Partnership of volunteers and professionals dedicates to improving the health of babies by preventing birth defects and infant mortality. Over 100 chapters are located across the country and can be located through the National Office.

Dr Jennifer Howse, President

3017 National Mental Health Association
2000 N Beauregard Street, 6th Floor
Alexandria, VA 22311

703-684-7722
800-969-6642
Fax: 703-684-5968
TTY: 800-433-5959
www.nmha.org

Addresses all aspects of mental health and mental illness. NMHA with over 340 affiliates works to improve the mental health of all Americans.

David L Shern PhD, President & CEO

3018 National Mental Health Consumers' Self-Help Clearinghouse
1211 Chestnut Street, Suite 1207
Philadelphia, PA 19107

215-751-1810
800-553-4539
Fax: 215-636-6312
e-mail: info@mhselfhelp.org
www.mhselfhelp.org

Offers information, support and appropriate referrals; and promotes public and professional education. Provides networking for those with special interests related to albinism. Promotes and supports research and funding that will improve diagnosis and management of albinism and hypopigmentation.

Joseph Rogers, Executive Director & Founder

3019 National Organization on Fetal Alcohol Syndrome
216 G Street NE
Washington, DC 20002

202-785-4585
800-666-6327
Fax: 202-466-6456
www.nofas.org

Dedicated to eliminating birth defects caused by alcohol consumption during pregnancy and to improving the quality of life for those affected individuals and families.

Tom Donaldson, President
Kathleen Tavenner Mitchell, MHS/LCADC, VP/National Spokesperson

3020 National Resource Center for Prevention of Perinatal Abuse of Alcohol
CSAP Division of Communications Programs
5600 Fishers Lane, Building 2
Rockville, MD 20857

301-443-9936

Offers information and resources to pregnant women on substance abuse, alcoholism and drugs pertaining to their unborn child's health.

Book Publishers

3021 Alcohol, Tobacco and Other Drugs May Harm the Unborn
National Clearinghouse for Alcohol and Drug Info.
PO Box 2345
Rockville, MD 20847

800-729-6686

Presents the most recent findings of basic research and clinical studies conducted on the effects of alcohol, drugs and tobacco on the unborn.

3022 Congenital Disorders Sourcebook
Omnigraphics
PO Box 625
Holmes, PA 19043

800-234-1340
Fax: 800-875-1340
e-mail: info@omnigraphics.com
www.omnigraphics.com

Basic consumer health information on disorders aquired during gestation, including spina bifida, hydrocephalus, cerebral palsy, heart defects, craniofacial abnormalities and fetal alcohol syndrome.

650 pages
ISBN: 0-780809-45-9

3023 Drugs and Pregnancy: It's Not Worth The Risk
American Council On Drug Education
204 Monroe Street, Suite 110
Rockville, MD 20850

800-488-3784

A scientific monograph for health care providers which teaches them to identify alcohol and drug problems in their patients.

48 pages

3024 Pregnancy and Exposure to Alcohol and Other Drug Use
National Clearinghouse for Alcohol and Drug Info.
PO Box 2345
Rockville, MD 20849

800-729-6686
www.health.org

This report is for health care professionals presenting state-of-the-art information about preventing alcohol use among women of childbearing age.

3025 Prevention Resource Guide: Pregnant, Postpartum Women and Their Infants
National Clearinghouse for Alcohol and Drug Info.
PO Box 2345
Rockville, MD 20849

800-729-6686
www.health.org

This resource guide targets health care providers, prevention program planners and counselors of pregnant and postpartum women between the ages of 15 and 44.

30 pages

Pamphlets

3026 Alcohol and Pregnancy
March of Dimes Resource Center
1275 Mamaroneck Avenue
White Plains, NY 10605

888-663-4637
Fax: 914-997-4763
e-mail: contactus@marchofdimes.com
www.marchofdimes.com

Discusses the dangers of drinking alcohol during pregnancy and brestfeeding; also gives tips and referrals to help pregnant women stop drinking alcohol.

3027 Drinking During Pregnancy
March of Dimes Resource Center
1275 Mamaroneck Avenue
White Plains, NY 10605

888-663-4637
Fax: 914-997-4763
www.marchofdimes.com

3028 Effects of Alcohol on Pregnancy National Clearinghouse for Alcohol Information
PO Box 2345
Rockville, MD 20847

301-468-2600

Free publications are available that discuss the effects of alcohol on pregnancy: Fetal Alcohol Syndrome; and The Fact Is Alcohol and Other Drugs Can Harm an Unborn Baby.

3029 Fetal Alcohol Syndrome
Hazelden
15251 Pleasant Valley Road
Center City, MN 55012

612-257-4010
800-328-9000
Fax: 612-257-1331
www.hazelden.org

A source of information about the effects of drinking while pregnant.

3030 Fight Drug Abuse at Home, Work, School and in the Community
American Council for Drug Education
204 Monroe Street, Suite 110
Rockville, MD 20850

800-488-3784

A catalog of print and video materials pertaining to substance abuse, alcoholism and drugs.

3031 How to Take Care of Your Baby Before Birth
National Clearinghouse for Alcohol and Drug Info.
PO Box 2345
Rockville, MD 20849

800-729-6686
www.health.org

A low-literacy brochure aimed at pregnant women that describes what they should and should not do during pregnancy.

DESCRIPTION

3032 FETAL RETINOID SYNDROME

Covers these related disorders: Etretinate embryopathy, Isotretinoin embryopathy, Retinol embryopathy
Involves the following Biologic System(s):
Neonatal and Infant Disorders

Fetal retinoid syndrome is a characteristic pattern of birth defects caused by exposure to vitamin A (retinol) or its derivatives during early pregnancy. The term retinoid refers to retinol or any natural or artificially created derivative of vitamin A. In newborns with fetal retinoid syndrome, characteristic symptoms and findings include small, low-set ears or complete absence of the outer ears and external ear canals (microtia); an abnormally small head (microcephaly); enlargement of the cavities (ventricles) within the brain; and underdevelopment (hypoplasia) of the thymus, a small gland in the upper portion of the chest that functions as an essential part of the immune system during infancy and childhood.

Several studies have reported fetal retinoid syndrome in newborns as a result of maternal use of vitamin A derivatives such as isotretinoin during early pregnancy. In addition, an increasing number of studies reveal the occurrence of such birth defects due to maternal use of other vitamin A derivatives, particularly the medication etretinate, or large doses of vitamin A (e.g., greater than 15,000 units daily) during early embryonic development. Although the frequency of fetal retinoid syndrome is unknown, reported cases represent only a small percentage of actual occurrences of the syndrome. Moreover, there is ongoing concern that increasing use of high dose vitamin A preparations and of vitamin A derivatives to treat certain common skin conditions, such as cystic acne or psoriasis, may result in additional cases of fetal retinoid syndrome. The most well known retinoid is isotretinoin. Because it can cause severe birth defects, including mental retardation and physical malformations, a woman must not become pregnant while taking it. If a woman of childbearing age requests isotretinoin, her doctor will ask her to sign a detailed consent form before presribing it. If a woman accidentally becomes pregnant while taking the medication, she should immediately consult her doctor. Dosage levels and the stage of embryonic development during which retinoid exposure occurs are thought to be the major factors influencing the occurrence of fetal retinoid syndrome. The period of greatest risk may occur between approximately two to five weeks after conception. The specific underlying abnormality that causes fetal retinoid syndrome is not known.

Studies indicate that retinoid exposure may cause disrupted development in the embryonic region that later becomes the brain and spinal cord (neural crest). The role that genetic influences or other environmental factors may have in contributing to fetal retinoid syndrome is unknown.

Although the symptoms and findings associated with fetal retinoid syndrome vary somewhat from case to case, affected newborns typically have a characteristic pattern of malformations. Affected newborns may have abnormalities of the head and face, including premature closure of the fibrous joint between the bones forming the forehead (metopic craniosynostosis); downslanting eyelid folds (palpebral fissures); widely spaced eyes (ocular hypertelorism) that may be abnormally small (microphthalmia); a short or broad nose; a small jaw (micrognathia); or incomplete closure of the roof of the mouth (cleft palate) and a groove in the upper lip (cleft lip). Abnormalities of the brain and spinal cord (central nervous system) are also common and include obstruction of the flow of cerebrospinal fluid around the brain, causing the fluid to accumulate under increasing pressure within the cavities of the brain (hydrocephalus); loss of vision; or other abnormalities (e.g., holoprosencephaly [failure of the forebrain (prosencephalon) to grow as two separate hemispheres in the first few weeks of fetal life], posterior fossa cyst). Additional neurologic problems may include paralysis of the nerves that supply muscles responsible for eye movements (oculomotor paralysis) or weakness or paralysis of the nerve that supplies the forehead, scalp, eyelids, cheeks, jaws, and muscles of facial expression (facial nerve palsy).

Newborns with fetal retinoid syndrome may also have clouding of the lenses of the eyes (congenital cataracts); malformations of the heart and its major blood vessels (e.g., ventricular septal defects, hypoplastic aortic arch, transposition of the great arteries); underdevelopment (hypoplasia) of the kidneys and tubes (ureters) that carry urine from the kidneys into the bladder; and ab normalities of the liver. Many affected newborns may also have malformations of the arms, legs, hands, and feet, such as webbing or fusion of the fingers and toes (syndactyly); malformations of the bone on the thumb side of the forearm (radial defects); a defect in which the foot is twisted out of shape or position (clubfoot or talipes); or fusion of the lower legs and absence of the feet (sirenomelia). In some patients, life-threatening complications may occur soon after birth. Treatment of newborns with fetal retinoid syndrome includes symptomatic and supportive measures.

See also **General Resources** on page 917

Government Agencies

3033 NIH/National Institute of Child Health and Human Development
31 Center Drive, Building 31
Bethesda, MD 20892

301-496-5133
Fax: 301-496-1104
www.nichd.nih.gov

Established in 1962 by congress, today the institute conducts and supports research on topics related to the health of children, adults, families and populations. Some of these topics include: developmental disabilities, growth and development, infant death, reproductive health and birth defects.

Nancy D Wirth, Director
Lisa Kaeser, Program & Public Liaison

National Associations & Support Groups

3034 Association of Children's Prosthetic/ Orthotic Clinics
6300 N River Road, Suite 727
Rosemont, IL 60018

847-698-1637
Fax: 847-823-0536
e-mail: raymond@aaos.org
www.acpoc.org

The Association of Children's Prosthetic Clinics is an association of professionals who are involved in clinics providing prosthetic-orthotic care for children with limb loss or orthopaedic disabilities.

Melody Raymond, Contact

3035 March of Dimes Birth Defects Foundation
1275 Mamaroneck Avenue
White Plains, NY 10605

914-428-7100
888-663-4637
Fax: 914-428-8203
e-mail: resourcecenter@modimes.org
www.marchofdimes.com

Partnership of volunteers and professionals dedicated to improving the health of babies by preventing birth defects and infant mortality. Over 100 chapters are located across the country and can be located through the National Office.

Dr Jennifer Howse, President

3036 National Rehabilitation Information Center
4200 Forbes Blvd, Suite 202
Lanham, MD 20706

301-459-5984
800-364-2742
Fax: 301-459-4263
e-mail: naricinfo@heitechservices.com
www.naric.com

NARIC is a library and information center focusing in disability and rehabilitation research. Information specialists provide quick information and referrals free of charge. Other sevices include customized searches of REHABDATA, the premier database of disability and rehabilitation literature.

Mark Odum, Director

Web Sites

3037 Association of Children's Prosthetic/ Orthotic Clinics
www.acpoc.org

An association of professionals who are involved in clinics which provide prosthetic-orthotic care for children with limb loss or orthopaedic disabilities.

3038 March of Dimes Birth Defects Foundation
www.marchofdimes.com

Partnership of volunteers and professionals dedicated to improving the health of babies by preventing birth defects and infant mortality. Over 100 chapters are located across the country and can be located through the National Office.

3039 National Rehabilitation Information Center
www.naric.com/naric

NARIC is a library and information center focusing in disability and rehabilitation research. Information specialists provide quick information and referrals free of charge. Other sevices include customized searches of REHABDATA, the premier database of disability and rehabilitation literature.

DESCRIPTION

3040 FRAGILE X SYNDROME

Synonyms: Marker X Syndrome, Martin-Bell Syndrome
Involves the following Biologic System(s):
Genetic/Chromosomal/Syndrome/Metabolic Disorders

Fragile X Syndrome, a disorder that results from an inherited defect of the X chromosome, is the most common cause of mental retardation in males. The disorder is thought to affect approximately one in 2,000 to 4,000 males and to be slightly less frequent in females. Although symptoms may be variable, the most common feature associated with fragile X syndrome is mental retardation.

Most males with fragile X syndrome have mild to profound mental retardation (e.g., an intelligence quotient or I.Q. ranging from approximately 30 to 55.) However, some may have an I.Q. that is considered borderline normal. Affected males with mild mental retardation may have a distinctive speech pattern characterized by rapid speech with a variable rhythm (cluttering). Those with more severe retardation typically communicate in bursts of repetitive speech. Affected males with severe or profound mental retardation may lack the ability to speak. In addition, most males with fragile X syndrome may have poor eye contact or experience emotional difficulties. Some may have poor concentration associated with hyperactivity or engage in autistic-like behaviors, such as hand biting or hand flapping.

In many cases, affected males may also have physical abnormalities. For example, many males with fragile X syndrome may have unusually large testes (macroorchidism), a finding that is most apparent after puberty; however, testicular function is normal. Affected males may also typically have characteristic facial features, such as a large head (macrocephaly) and forehead, a relatively long face and prominent jaw, thick lips, and prominent ears. Other findings may include crowding of the teeth, excessive flexibility of the finger joints, or flat feet (pes planus). In addition, approximately 50 percent of affected females have varying degrees of mental retardation or learning difficulties. In some cases, females with fragile X syndrome may also have physical abnormalities, such as irregular teeth or unusually flexible finger joints. The treatment of children with fragile X syndrome includes symptomatic and supportive measures, such as special education, speech therapy, and, in some cases, multidisciplinary techniques such as behavioral therapies to help manage hyperactivity or autistic-like behaviors.

Individuals with fragile X syndrome inherit a fragile area or site on the long arm (q) of the X chromosome (Xq27.3). Chromosomal analysis reveals that the genetic material on the end of this arm appears to be broken off. In reality, this genetic material is actually dangling from the end of the long arm. The diseased gene within this area is known as the FRAXA gene. This region (locus) of the X chromosome contains abnormally long repeats (e.g., over 200 repeats) of coded DNA instructions (CGG trinucleotide repeat expansion). Males have only one X chromosome; therefore, if they inherit a fragile X locus containing more than 200 CGG repeats, they generally express the symptoms associated with this syndrome and are typically more severely affected than females. However, because females have two X chromosomes, certain disease traits may be masked by the presence of a normal gene on the other X chromosome, resulting in lower frequency and decreased severity of the disease among females.

See also **General Resources** on page 917

Government Agencies

3041 NIH/National Institute of Child Health and Human Development
31 Center Drive, Building 31
Bethesda, MD 20892

301-496-5133
Fax: 301-496-1104
www.nichd.nih.gov

Established in 1962 by congress, today the institute conducts and supports research on topics related to the health of children, adults, families and populations. Some of these topics include: developmental disabilities, growth and development, infant death, reproductive health and birth defects.

Nancy D Wirth, Director
Lisa Kaeser, Program & Public Liaison

National Associations & Support Groups

3042 ARC of the United States
1010 Wayne Avenue, Suite 650
Silver Spring, MD 20910

301-565-3842
Fax: 301-565-5342
e-mail: info@thearc.org
www.thearc.org

The ARC is the national organization of and for people with mental retardation and related developmental disabilities and their families. Devoted to promoting and improving supports and services for people with mental retardation and their families. The association also fosters research and education regarding the prevention of mental retardation in infants and young children. The ARC was founded in 1950 by a small group of parents and other concerned individuals.

Sue Swenson, Executive Director
Adam Aaronson, Public Inquiries Director

3043 FRAXA Research Foundation
45 Pleasant Street
Newburyport, MA 01950

978-462-1866
Fax: 978-463-9985
e-mail: info@fraxa.org
www.fraxa.org

FRAXA supports research on fragile X syndrome, a genetic disorder which is the most common inherited cause of mental retardation.

2,500 members

Katherine Clapp, Co-Founder/President
Megan Massey, RN, Vice President

3044 Genetic Alliance
4301 Connecticut Avenue NW
Washington, DC 20008

202-966-5557
800-336-4363
Fax: 202-966-8553
e-mail: info@geneticalliance.org
www.geneticalliance.org

A coalition of voluntary genetic support groups, consumers and professionals addressing the needs of individuals and families affected by genetic disorders from a national perspective.

Sharon Terry, President/CEO

3045 National Fragile X Foundation
PO Box 190488
San Francisco, CA 94119

925-938-9300
800-688-8765
Fax: 925-938-9315
e-mail: NATLFX@FragileX.org
www.fragilex.org

Provides a wide variety data for people suffering from the disorder to access at any time with ease.

Jeffrey S. Cohen, President
Randi J. Hagerman, MD, Medical Chair

State Agencies & Support Groups

California

3046 Fragile X Association of Southern California
PO Box 6924
Burbank, CA 91510

818-754-4227
Fax: 310-276-9251
e-mail: info@fraxsocal.org
www.fraxsocal.org

Promotes awareness of Fragile X syndrome with special emphasis on educators and health professionals; provides a forum for families of children with fragile X to meet and share their ideas, concerns and problems; and supports scientific research on fragile X syndrome.

Naomi Star, President
Diane Bateman, Vice President

3047 Fragile X Center of San Diego
PO Box 19551
San Diego, CA 92119

619-697-6468
Fax: 619-697-6468
e-mail: info@fragilesandiego.org
www.fragilexsandiego.org

Provides information for families and professionals. Activities include: family support, improving awareness of fragile X syndrome, increasing the identification for affected families, promoting research into fragile X syndrome.

Cindy de Gruchy, MPA, President

Ohio

3048 Fragile X Alliance of Ohio
6790 Ridgecliff Drive
Solon, OH 44139

440-519-1517
Fax: 440-519-1518
e-mail: fraxohio@adelphia.org
www.fragilexohio.org

Promotes awareness of Fragile X syndrome with special emphasis on educators and health professionals; provides a forum for families of children with fragile X to meet and share their ideas, concerns and problems; and supports scientific research on fragile X syndrome.

Leslie A. Bagdasarian, President

Web Sites

3049 ARC of the United States
www.thearc.org

The ARC is the national organization of and for people with mental retardation and related developmental disabilities and their families. Devoted to promoting and improving supports and services for people with mental retardation and their families. The association also fosters research and education regarding the prevention of mental retardation in infants and young children.

3050 American College of Medical Genetics
www.acmg.net

Offers information about fragile X syndrome.

3051 FRAXA Research Foundation
www.fraxa.org

FRAXA supports research on fragile X syndrome, a genetic disorder which is the most common inherited cause of mental retardation.

3052 National Fragile X Foundation
www.fragilex.org

Provides a wide variety data for people suffering from the disorder to acces at any time with ease.

Book Publishers

3053 Children With Fragile X Syndrome

Jayne Dixon Weber, author

Peytral Publications
PO Box 1162
Minnetonka, MN 55345

952-949-8707
877-739-8725
Fax: 952-906-9777
www.peytral.com

A complete, sensitive infroduction to Fragile X Syndrome, covering diagnosis, parental emotions, therapies and medications, early intervention, education, daily care, legal rights and more. Item #WP-307X.

472 pages

3054 Children with Fragile X Syndrome
Peytral Publications
PO Box 1162
Minnetonka, MN 55345

952-949-8707
877-739-8725
Fax: 952-906-9777
www.peytral.com

Provides a complete, sensitive introduction to fragile X syndrome, an inherited, genetic condition. Covers diagnosis, parental emotions, therapies and medications, early intervention, education, daily care, legal rights and advocacy.

472 pages

3055 Educating Boys with Fragile X Syndrome

Gail Spiridigliozzi, PhD, author

FRAA Research Foundation
45 Pleasant Street
Newburyport, MA 01950

978-462-1866
Fax: 978-463-9985
e-mail: info@fraxa.org
www.fraxa.org

Guide for parents, teachers and therapist to give specific strategies for education.

20 pages

3056 Fragile X - A to Z: Guide for Families by Families

Sally Nantais, Mary Beth Langan, Wendy Dillworth, author

FRAA Research Foundation
45 Pleasant Street
Newburyport, MA 01950

978-462-1866
Fax: 978-463-9985
e-mail: info@fraxa.org
www.fraxa.org

Intended to help families cope with many daily challenges of living with a child or adult who has fragile X syndrome.

100 pages

3057 My Brother has Fragile X

Charles Stieger, author

FRAA Research Foundation
45 Pleasant Street
Newburyport, MA 01950

978-462-1866
Fax: 978-463-9985
e-mail: info@fraxa.org
www.fraxa.org

Suitable for young children and for reading in an elementary school classroom to educate children about what it's like to have fragile X.

23 pages

Newsletters

3058 FRAXA Research Foundation Newsletter

45 Pleasant Street
Newburyport, MA 01950

978-462-1866
Fax: 978-463-9985
e-mail: info@fraxa.org
www.fraxa.org

FRAXA supports research on fragile X syndrome, a genetic disorder which is the most common inherited cause of mental retardation.

Quarterly

Katherine Clapp, Co-Founder/President
Megan Massey, RN, Vice President

Pamphlets

3059 A Fragile X Planation

L Elbaum, author

Health Resources and Services Administration
PO Box 2910
Merrifield, VA 22116

703-356-1964
888-275-4772
Fax: 703-821-2098
TTY: 877-489-4772
TDD: 877-489-4772
www.ask.hrsa.gov

An explanation of fragile X syndrome intended to be used, in conjunction with genetic counseling, as an aid for family members who are considering molecular testing for the fragile X syndrome.

8 pages Booklet

3060 Fragile X Planation

National Maternal and Child Health Clearinghouse
2070 Chain Bridge Road
Vienna, VA 22182

703-356-1964
Fax: 703-821-2098

An explanation of fagile X syndrome intended to be used, in conjunction with genetic counseling, as an aid for family members who are considering molecular testing for the fragile X syndrome.

DESCRIPTION

3061 GALACTOSEMIA

Covers these related disorders: Classic galactosemia, Galactokinase deficiency, Deficiency of uridyl diphosphogalactose-4-epimerase

Involves the following Biologic System(s):
Gastrointestinal Disorders,
Genetic/Chromosomal/Syndrome/Metabolic Disorders

Galactosemia is a genetic disorder transmitted as an autosomal recessive trait and characterized by the inability of the body to process or metabolize galactose, a simple sugar found in milk and milk products, certain fruits and vegetables, and seaweed. This inborn error of metabolism occurs as the result of a deficiency of one of three different enzymes and is thus divided into three distinct galactosemic disorders.

Classic galactosemia results from a deficiency of galactose-1-phosphate uridyl transferase, an enzyme that breaks down galactose-1-phosphate, a component of the milk sugar lactose. Galactose-1-phosphate begins to accumulate in the tissues of the body and may lead to damage of the functional tissues in the brain, liver, and kidneys. Symptoms may include a yellowish discoloration of the skin, eyes, and mucous membranes (jaundice); opacity of the lenses of the eyes (cataracts); vomiting; convulsions; increased irritability; sluggishness; difficulty in feeding; and failure to gain weight. Characteristic findings may include enlargement of the liver and spleen (hepatosplenomegaly), low blood sugar (hypoglycemia), the presence of amino acids in the urine (aminoaciduria), an abnormal accumulation of fluid in the abdomen (ascites), the formation of scar tissue in the liver (cirrhosis), and mental retardation. Treatment is directed toward the elimination of galactose from the diet to prevent the appearance of or progressive worsening of cirrhosis, mental retardation, cataracts, and other findings associated with galactosemia. In addition, a pregnant woman who has galactosemia or is aware that she carries the gene for this disorder should eliminate galactose-containing foods from her diet in order to prevent galactose from crossing the placental barrier, possibly resulting in injury to the fetus. Although strict dietary regulation may prevent many of the severe complications of classic galactosemia, some affected children and adults may experience delays in growth and development, speech irregularities, and difficulties with motor function. Approximately one of every 60,000 newborns is affected with classic galactosemia.

Galactokinase deficiency results from the absence of or decreased levels of galactokinase, an enzyme that is responsible for assisting in the first step of the chemical reaction that allows utilization of galactose. This deficiency results in findings associated with galactosemia, the presence of increased levels of galactose in the blood and urine, and the formation of cataracts. Treatment includes the institution of a galactose-free diet. Approximately one in 40,000 newborns is affected with galactosemia resulting from galactokinase deficiency.

Galactose epimerase deficiency, a very rare form of galactosemia, results from defective uridyl diphosphogalactose-4-epimerase (UDP glucose-4-epimerase), another enzyme that assists in the metabolism of galactose. This deficiency may be present in a benign form in which the deficiency is limited to the blood cells, usually resulting in no symptoms or long-term effects. However, in those with more widespread epimerase deficiency, symptoms, findings, and treatment may be similar to those of classic galactosemia.

See also General Resources on page 917

National Associations & Support Groups

3062 American Liver Foundation
75 Maiden Lane, Suite 603
New York, NY 10038

212-668-1000
800-465-4837
Fax: 212-483-8179
e-mail: info@liverfoundation.org
www.liverfoundation.org

Nonprofit, national voluntary health organization dedicated to the prevention, treatment and cure of hepatitis and other liver diseases through research, education, and advocacy on behalf of those affected by or at risk of liver disease.

Alan P Brownstein, President/CEO
James L Boyer MD, Chair

3063 Genetic Alliance
4301 Connecticut Avenue NW
Washington, DC 20008

202-966-5557
800-336-4363
Fax: 202-966-8553
e-mail: info@geneticalliance.org
www.geneticalliance.org

A coalition of voluntary genetic support groups, consumers and professionals addressing the needs of individuals and families affected by genetic disorders from a national perspective.

Sharon Terry, President/CEO

3064 March of Dimes Birth Defects Foundation
1275 Mamaroneck Avenue
White Plains, NY 10605

914-428-7100
888-663-4637
Fax: 914-428-8203
e-mail: resourcecenter@modimes.org
www.marchofdimes.com

Partnership of volunteers and professionals dedicates to improving the health of babies by preventing birth defects and infant mortality. Over 100 chapters are located across the country and can be located through the National Office.

Dr Jennifer Howse, President

3065 Parents of Galactosemic Children
1519 Magnolia Bluff Drive
Gautier, MS 39553

228-497-5886
e-mail: president@galactosemia.org
www.galactosemia.org

National nonprofit, volunteer organization whose misssion is to provide information, support and networking opportunities to families affected by galactosemia.

Michelle Fowler, President & Treasurer
Nishkala Rao, Secretary

Libraries & Resource Centers

3066 National Digestive Diseases Information Clearinghouse
2 Information Way
Bethesda, MD 20892

301-654-3810
800-891-5389
Fax: 703-738-4929
e-mail: nddic@info.niddk.nih.gov
www.digestive.niddk.nih.gov

The National Institute of Diabetes and Digestive and Kidney Diseases conducts and supports research on many of the most serious diseases affecting public health. The Institute supports much of the clinical research on the diseases of internal medicine and related subspecialty fields as well as many basic science disciplines.

Kathy Kranzfelder, Project Officer

Web Sites

3067 American Liver Foundation
www.liverfoundation.org

Nonprofit, national voluntary health organization dedicated to the prevention, treatment, and cure of hepatitis and other liver diseases through research, education and advocacy on behalf of those affected by or at risk of liver disease.

3068 Disability Information and Resource Center
www.dircsa.org.au/pub/docs/galac.txt

DIRC provides a professional and friendly information and referral service to the people of South Australia.

3069 Galactosemia Resources and Information
www.galactosemia.com

Information about galactosemia.

3070 Online Mendelian Inheritance in Man
www.ncbi.nlm.nih.gov

This database is a catalog of human genes and genetic disorders.

3071 Parents of Galactosemic Children
www.galactosemia.org

National nonprofit, volunteer organization whose mission is to provide information, support and networking opportunities to families affected by galactosemia.

3072 Rare Genetic Diseases in Children (NYU)
www.med.nyu.edu/rgdc/homenow.htm

We target issues arising from rare genetic diseases affecting children. Also, to assist in the endeavor to bring knowledge and hope to those for whom there is, at present, so little.

3073 Save Babies Through Screening Foundation
www.savebabies.org

Is a national, nonprofit, public charity run by volunteers. Its mission is to improve the lives of babies by working to prevent disabilities and early death resulting from disorders detectable through newborn screening.

DESCRIPTION

3074 GAUCHER'S DISEASE

Synonyms: Gaucher disease, Glucosylceramide lipidosis, Glucosyl cerebroside lipidosis

Covers these related disorders: Chronic Gaucher's disease (Adult or Classic Gaucher's disease), Infantile Gaucher's disease, Juvenile Gaucher's disease

Involves the following Biologic System(s): Genetic/Chromosomal/Syndrome/Metabolic Disorders

Gaucher's disease is an inherited metabolic disorder characterized by a deficiency of the enzyme glucocerebrosidase (glucosylceramidase), which assists in the metabolism of certain fats (lipidosis). This deficiency results in the accumulation of certain fatty substances (glucocerebroside or glucosylceramide) throughout the body. Although uncommon, Gaucher's disease is the lipidosis seen most often by physicians. Gaucher's disease is subdivided into three main types. The first, known as chronic, adult, or classic Gaucher's disease, may develop at any age from birth to 80 years old. This form of the disease is common among eastern European Jews, with an incidence rate of as many as one in 500 births. Findings associated with chronic Gaucher's disease include enlargement of the spleen (splenomegaly) or liver (hepatomegaly), or both (hepatosplenomegaly); a decrease in levels of hemoglobin in the blood (anemia); decreased numbers of circulating white blood cells (leukopenia); and abnormally low levels of circulating platelets (thrombocytopenia), which may lead to easy bruising or bleeding. Symptoms may include a brownish-pigmented skin; yellow spots in the eyes resulting from accumulation of fatty substances; and bone pain resulting from accumulations in the bone marrow. Treatment for chronic Gaucher's disease includes enzyme replacement therapy.

Infantile Gaucher's disease, a life-threatening form of this disorder, affects the central nervous system of the newborn. Symptoms and findings may include enlargement of the spleen, crossed eyes (strabismus); muscle spasms in the jaw (trismus or lockjaw); seizures; backward bending of the head; or a rigid, arched back. Additional abnormalities of the central nervous system may become apparent.

Juvenile Gaucher's disease may appear at any time during childhood. Characteristic findings may include enlargement of the liver and spleen (hepatosplenomegaly), bone abnormalities resulting in pain and swelling of the joints, anemia, and abnormally low levels of circulating white blood cells and platelets. Affected children may be pale, weak, and particularly susceptible to bleeding and recurring infection. Symptoms related to nervous system involvement include lack of motor coordination and loss of balance, inflammation of the nerves in the arms and legs accompanied by abnormal sensations and discomfort, muscle spasms, paralysis of the nerves of the eye (ophthalmoplegia), and impairment of mental function.

Enzyme replacement therapy is usually not effective in the treatment of the infantile and juvenile forms of Gaucher's disease. Alternative treatment may include removal of the spleen (splenectomy). Other treatment is symptomatic and supportive.

Gaucher's disease is inherited as an autosomal recessive trait. The gene responsible for the regulation of the enzyme glucocerebrosidase is located on the long arm of chromosome 1 (1q21-q31).

See also **General Resources** on page 917

National Associations & Support Groups

3075 ARC of the United States
1010 Wayne Avenue, Suite 650
Silver Spring, MD 20910

301-565-3842
Fax: 301-565-5342
e-mail: info@thearc.org
www.thearc.org

The ARC is the national organization of and for people with mental retardation and related developmental disabilities and their families. Devoted to promoting and improving supports and services for people with mental retardation and their families. The association also fosters research and education regarding the prevention of mental retardation in infants and young children. The ARC was founded in 1950 by a small group of parents and other concerned individuals.

Sue Swenson, Executive Director
Adam Aaronson, Public Inquiries Director

3076 National Foundation for Jewish Genetic Diseases
250 Park Avenue, Suite 1000
New York, NY 10017

212-371-1030

Provides the information regarding this and related disorders for the people suffering from them.

3077 National Gaucher Foundation
11140 Rockville Place, Suite 350
Rockville, MD 20852

301-816-1515
800-428-2437
Fax: 301-816-1516
e-mail: ngf@gaucherdisease.org
www.gaucherdisease.org

A nonprofit organization whose primary objective is to assist in perfecting a treatment program and discovering a cure for Gaucher disease. The Foundation supports medical research and clinical programs which enhance the current understanding of Gaucher disease.

Robin A. Ely, MD, President
Rhonda P. Buyers, Executive Director

3078 National Lipid Diseases
1201 Corbin Street
Elizabeth, NJ 07201

908-527-8000
800-527-8005
Fax: 908-527-8004

Focuses on the facilities that specialize on the disease and helping people choose the one that is right for them.

3079 National Tay-Sachs and Allied Diseases Association
2001 Beacon Street, Suite 204
Boston, MA 02135

617-277-4463
800-906-8723
Fax: 617-277-0134
e-mail: info@ntsad.org
www.ntsad.org

Dedicated to the treatment and prevention of Tay-Sachs and related diseases, and to provide information and support services to individuals, and families affected by these diseases, through education, research, genetic screening, family services and advocacy.

Diana Pangonis, Interim Executive Director

Audio Video

3080 Pain & Hope
National Gaucher Foundation
5410 Edson Lane, Suite 260
Rockville, MD 20852

301-816-1515
800-428-2437
Fax: 301-816-1516
e-mail: ngf@gaucherdisease.org
www.gaucherdisease.org

A patient and family perspective on Gaucher Disease.

Web Sites

3081 ARC of the United States
www.thearc.org

The ARC is the national organization of and for people with mental retardation and related developmental disabilities and their families. Devoted to promoting and improving supports and services for people with mental retardation and their families.

3082 Children's Gaucher Research Fund
www.childrensgaucher.org

We are a nonprofit organization, that raises funds to coordinate and support research to find a cure for type 2 and type 3 Gaucher disease.

3083 Gaucher Registry
www.gaucherregistry.com

Our goal is to significantly contribute to the medical understanding of Gaucher disease and to improve the quality of care for Gaucher patients worldwide through active publication of Registry findings and disease management approaches.

3084 Health Answers
www.healthanswers.com

HealthAnswers offers a breadth of services in medical education, sales force training, patient support, solutions, professional promotion and consumer solutions.

3085 National Gaucher Foundation
www.gaucherdisease.org

The mission of the NGF is to find a cure for Gaucher Disease by funding vital research programs, to meet the ever-increasing needs

of patients and families, as well as to promote community/physician awareness and educational programs.

3086 Rare Genetic Diseases in Children (NYU)
www.med.nyu.edu/rgdc/homenow.htm

We target issues arising from rare genetic diseases affecting children. Also, to assist in the endeavor to bring knowledge and hope to those for whom there is, at present, so little.

Newsletters

3087 Gaucher Disease Newsletter
National Gaucher Foundation
11140 Rockville Pike
Rockville, MD 20852

301-816-1515
800-427-2437
Fax: 301-816-1516
e-mail: ngf@gaucherdisease.org
www.gaucherdisease.org

Offers information on the latest research, treatments and technology for persons affected by Gaucher Disease. Also includes legislative and medical information.

Quarterly

Robin A. Ely, MD, President
Rhonda P. Buyers, Executive Director

Pamphlets

3088 Gaucher Disease Fact Sheet
National Gaucher Foundation
11140 Rockville Pike
Rockville, MD 20852

301-816-1515
800-428-2437
Fax: 301-816-1516
e-mail: ngf@gaucherdisease.org
www.gaucherdisease.org

Offers information on what Gaucher Disease is, the symptoms, risks, treatments and the workings of the National Gaucher Foundation.

Robin A. Ely, MD, President
Rhonda P. Buyers, Executive Director

3089 Living with Gaucher Disease
National Gaucher Foundation
11140 Rockville Pike
Rockville, MD 20852

301-816-1515
800-427-2437
Fax: 301-816-1516
e-mail: ngf@gaucherdisease.org
www.gaucherdisease.org

A guide for parents, families and relatives that teach them how to deal with and cope with a diagnosis of Gaucher Disease.

24 pages

Robin A. Ely, MD, President
Rhonda P. Buyers, Executive Director

DESCRIPTION

3090 GROWTH HORMONE DEFICIENCY

Synonym: GH deficiency

Involves the following Biologic System(s):

Endocrinologic Disorders

Growth hormone deficiency is a condition characterized by deficient production or impaired response to growth hormone, resulting in growth impairment and short stature with normal proportions (pituitary dwarfism). Growth hormone, also known as GH, stimulates body growth and development by promoting the production of protein in cells, releasing energy from the breakdown of fats, and performing other vital functions. GH is secreted by the pituitary gland. Also known as the master gland, the pituitary gland is connected to a region of the brain known as the hypothalamus by a stalk of nerve fibers (pituitary stalk). The hypothalamus controls the functioning of the pituitary gland through direct nerve stimulation as well as through the actions of certain nerve cells that secrete hormones (hormone-releasing and hormone-inhibiting factors) into the bloodstream for transport directly to the pituitary gland. The region of the pituitary gland known as the anterior pituitary gland secretes GH in response to a particular hormone-releasing factor (growth hormone releasing factor) from the hypothalamus. Depending upon the underlying cause of GH deficiency, some patients may also have deficiencies of additional hormones that are produced by the anterior pituitary gland, such as thyroid-stimulating hormone (TSH), which stimulates the production of thyroid hormones, or adrenocorticotropic hormone (ACTH), which promotes the growth and production of hormones by cells in the outer region (cortex) of the adrenal gland. Inadequate functioning of the pituitary gland is known as hypopituitarism.

Growth hormone deficiency may be due to many different causes, including absence, underdevelopment, or malformation of the pituitary gland or hypothalamus at birth; tumors of the anterior pituitary gland, pituitary stalk, or hypothalamus, particularly pituitary tumors known as craniopharyngiomas; or radiation therapy for the treatment of certain malignancies in the brain or skull region. GH deficiency may also result from trauma affecting the pituitary gland or hypothalamus, such as injury during delivery or lack of oxygen to the brain (anoxia). In addition, the condition may occur in association with certain chromosomal or genetic syndromes or may appear to occur randomly for unknown reasons (idiopathic hypopituitarism). There are also genetic forms of hypopituitarism that may be limited to GH deficiency or may be characterized by additional anterior pituitary hormone deficiencies.

There are several genetic subtypes of isolated growth hormone deficiency (IGHD), including those that may be inherited as an autosomal recessive, autosomal dominant, or X-linked trait. Patients with autosomal recessive IGHD may have complete deletions of a particular gene, known as the GH1 gene, which is located on the long arm of chromosome 17 (17q22-24). This form of the disorder is typically characterized by marked growth delays after birth and severe short stature. Other patients with autosomal recessive IGHD have various abnormal changes (mutations) of the GH1 gene, causing variable degrees of growth failure and short stature. Some patients with autosomal dominant IGHD may also have mutations of the GH1 gene. The disease gene responsible for X-linked IGHD has not yet been located. Another genetic form of hypopituitarism, known as Laron syndrome, is thought to result from an impaired response to growth hormone and is characterized by abnormally increased levels of circulating GH.

Most children with GH deficiency appear to be of normal weight and length at birth. By the first year of life, children with severe GH deficiency or Laron syndrome may be significantly shorter than would be expected (e.g., more than four standard deviations below the mean) for their age and sex. Patients with less severe GH deficiency experience regular growth spurts that alternate with periods during which no growth occurs. Patients may continue to experience growth beyond the age when most individuals attain their adult height. This is due to abnormal delays in the fusion of the growing ends (epiphyseal plates) and the shafts of the long bones. If children with GH deficiency do not receive treatment, their adult height may range from four to 12 standard deviations below the mean.

Children with GH deficiency typically have normally proportioned arms and legs; however, they may have relatively small hands and feet. Many also have a characteristic facial appearance, including a short, broad face and relatively round head; and undeveloped upper and lower jaw; a small, saddle-shaped nose with a depressed nasal bridge; a small neck; delayed eruption and crowding of the teeth; and fine, sparse scalp hair. Due to abnormal smallness of the voice box (larynx), many patients have a high-pitched voice. Other findings may include underdeveloped genitals, delayed or absent sexual development, and abnormally low blood sugar (hypoglycemia).

Children with GH deficiency due to tumors of the pituitary gland or hypothalamus may develop additional symptoms, depending upon the location, nature, and growth of the tumor. In some patients, invasion and destruction of the pituitary gland cause degeneration (atrophy) of the thyroid gland, sex glands (gonads), and outer regions of the adrenal glands (adrenal cortex). Associated findings may include absence of sweating, weight loss, abnormal sensitivity to cold, delayed or absent sexual maturation, lack of response to certain stimuli (torpor), or other abnormalities. Tumor growth may also cause total growth failure, abnormally increased urination (polyuria), vomiting, headaches, visual disturbances, episodes of abnormally increased electrical activity in the brain (seizures), and other abnormalities.

The treatment of GH deficiency varies and depends on the underlying cause and nature of the condition. If the condition results due to tumor growth, treatment measures may include surgery, radiation therapy, or other appropriate measures to remove the tumor. Pituitary function should be carefully evaluated after such measures to determine any necessary therapies for pituitary abnormalities. The treatment of children with IGHD includes early replacement therapy with synthetic growth hormone that is continued until there is no longer a response. The maximum response usually occurs during the first year of therapy with slower subsequent growth. Because such therapy may cause abnormally decreased activity of the thyroid gland (hypothyroidism), thyroid function should be regularly evaluated. Children who have deficiencies of other anterior pituitary hormones in association with GH deficiency may receive additional hormone replacement therapies as required. Additional treatment is symptomatic and supportive. Some athletes abuse growth hormone because they believe it will increase their muscle growth and strength while decreasing their body fat. Use of growth hormone without medical need over a long period can cause an increase in fat levels in the blood, diabetes, and an increase in heart size that may result in heart failure. Human growth hormone has also been touted as being able to reverse or slow the effects of aging. However, there is little or no evidence of a positive effect on the processes of aging.

See also **General Resources** on page 917

Government Agencies

3091 NIH/National Institute of Child Health and Human Development
31 Center Drive, Building 31
Bethesda, MD 20892

301-496-5133
Fax: 301-496-1104
www.nichd.nih.gov

Established in 1962 by congress, today the institute conducts and supports research on topics related to the health of children, adults, families and populations. Some of these topics include: developmental disabilities, growth and development, infant death, reproductive health and birth defects.

Nancy D Wirth, Director
Lisa Kaeser, Program & Public Liaison

National Associations & Support Groups

3092 Dwarf Athletic Association of America
418 Willow Way
Lewisville, TX 75077

972-317-8299
Fax: 972-966-0184
e-mail: daaa@flash.net
www.daaa.org

The DAAA mission is to encourage people with dwarfism to participate in sports regardless of their level of skills. We promote and provide quality amateur level athletic opportunities for dwarf athletics in the US.

Jimmy Loyless, President
Gerry Graff, Vice President

3093 Genetic Alliance
4301 Connecticut Avenue NW
Washington, DC 20008

202-966-5557
800-336-4363
Fax: 202-966-8553
e-mail: info@geneticalliance.org
www.geneticalliance.org

A coalition of voluntary genetic support groups, consumers and professionals addressing the needs of individuals and families affected by genetic disorders from a national perspective.

Sharon Terry, President/CEO

3094 Human Growth Foundation
997 Glen Cove Avenue, Suite 5
Glen Head, NY 11545

516-671-4041
800-451-6434
Fax: 516-671-4055
e-mail: hgfl@hgfound.org
www.hgfound.org

A nonprofit, national organization committed to expanding and accelerating research into growth and growth disorders, provides education and support to those affected by growth disorders and their families, and fosters the exchange of information with the medical community.

Patricia D Costa, Executive Director

3095 Lawson Wilkins Pediatric Endocrine Society
867 Allardice Way
Stanford, CA 94305

650-302-0940
Fax: 650-494-3133
e-mail: secretary@lwpes.org
www.lwpes.org

To promote the acquisition and dissemination of knowledge of endocrine and metabolic disorders from conception through adolescence.

Kenneth Copeland, President
Ronald Rosenfield, President-Elect

3096 Little People of America

5289 NE Elam Young Parkway, Suite F-100
Hillsboro, OR 97124

503-846-1562
888-572-2001
Fax: 503-846-1590
e-mail: info@lpaonline.org
www.lpaonline.org

A nonprofit organization that provides support and information to people of short stature and their families.

Lois Gerage-Lamb, President
Bill Bradford, VP Programs

3097 MAGIC Foundation: Major Aspects of Growth in Children

6645 W North Avenue
Oak Park, IL 60302

708-383-0808
800-362-4423
Fax: 708-383-0899
e-mail: mary@magicfoundation.org
www.magicfoundation.org

A national nonprofit organization providing support and education regarding growth disorders in children and related adult disorders. Provides educational information, networking, a national conference, a kids' program and an extensive medical library.

Mary Andrews, CEO
Dianne Tamburrino, Executive Director

3098 March of Dimes Birth Defects Foundation

1275 Mamaroneck Avenue
White Plains, NY 10605

914-428-7100
888-663-4637
Fax: 914-428-8203
e-mail: resourcecenter@modimes.org
www.marchofdimes.com

A unique partnership of volunteers and professionals that provides leadership in the treatment and prevention of birth defects and prematurity. It is funded by voluntary contributions from individuals and a variety of organizations.

Dr Jennifer Howse, President

State Agencies & Support Groups

Colorado

3099 Little People of America - Front Range Chapter

7117 E Euclid Drive
Englewood, CO 80111

303-740-8555

Informational and emotional support to parents who have a child, adolescent, or adult family member with special needs.

Research Centers

3100 Case Western Research University, Bolton Brush Growth Study Center

2123 Abington Road
Cleveland, OH 44106

216-368-6715
Fax: 216-368-3204
e-mail: mgh4@cwru.edu
www.dental.cwru.edu/bolton-brush

Investigations and research into the growth and development of the human body.

B Holly Broadbent Jr, DDS, Director

3101 International Center for Skeletal Dysplasia

Saint Joseph Hospital, 7620 York Road
Towson, MD 21204

301-337-1250

3102 Jackson Laboratory

600 Main Streeet
Bar Harbor, ME 04609

207-288-6000
800-474-9880
Fax: 207-288-6150
www.jax.org

Studies focusing on growth disorders and human genetics.

Richard Woychik, PhD, Director

3103 New Jersey Institute of Technology Center for Biomedical Engineering

323 Martin Luther King Jr Boulevard
Fenster Hall, Sixth Floor, University Heights
Newark, NJ 07102

973-596-5268
Fax: 973-596-5222
www.njit.edu

Offers research into facial and bone disorders.

Richard Foulds, Director, Masters Program
Judith D. Redling, Coordinator, Undergraduate Program

3104 University of Colorado, R.F. Stolinsky Research Laboratories

4200 E 9th Street, Box C233
Denver, CO 80262

303-315-8017

Focuses on genetic disorders and growth diseases.

Stephen Goodman, MD, Director

3105 W.M. Krogman Center for Research In Child Growth and Development

University of Pennsylvania
3451 Walnut Street
Philadelphia, PA 19104

215-898-1470

Focuses research and studies on growth disorders and birth defects.

Solomon Katz, MA, PhD, Director

Web Sites

3106 Alliance of Genetic Support Groups

www.geneticalliance.org

Is an international coalition comprised of millions of individuals with genetic conditions and more than 600 advocacy, research and health care orgainizations that represent their interests. As a broad-based coalition of key stakeholders, the Alliance builds partnerships to promote healthy lives for all those living with genetic condtions.

3107 Dwarf Athletic Association of America

www.daaa.org

The DAAA mission is to encourage people with dwarfism to participate in sports regardless of their level of skills. We promote and provide quality amateur level athletic opportunities for dwarf athletiecs in the US.

3108 Health Answers

www.healthanswers.com

HealthAnswers offers a breadth of services in medical education, sales force training, patient support solutions, professional promotion and consumer solutions.

3109 Human Growth Foundation
www.hgfound.org

Information regarding disorders related to growth or growth hormone.

3110 OHSU Homepage Search
www.ohsu.edu

Educates health and high-technology professionals, scienists and enviromental engineers, and it undertakes the indispendible functions of patient care, community service and biomedical research.

3111 Online Mendelian Inheritance in Man
www.ncbi.nlm.nih.gov

This database is a catalog of human genes and genetic disorders.

3112 Society for Endocrinology
www.endocrinology.org

Aims to advance education and research in endocrinology for the public benefit.

Book Publishers

3113 Endocrine & Metabolic Disorders Sourcebook
Linda M. Shin, author

Omnigraphics
PO Box 625
Holmes, PA 19043

610-461-3548
800-234-1340
Fax: 800-875-1340
e-mail: info@omnigraphics.com
omnigraphics.com

Basic information for the lay person about pancreatic and insulin-related disorders such as pancreatitis, diabetes and hypoglycemia; adrenal gland disorders such as Cushing's syndrome, Addison's disease and congenital adrenal hyperplasia; pituitary gland disorders such as growth hormone deficiency, acromegaly and pituitary tumors; and thyroid disorders such as hypothyroidism, Grave's disease, Hashimoto's disease and goiter.

574 pages Hardcover
ISBN: 0-780802-07-1

3114 Growing Children: A Parent's Guide
Human Growth Foundation
977 Glen Cove Avenue, Suite 5
Glen Head, NY 11545

516-671-4041
800-451-6434
Fax: 516-671-4055
e-mail: hgfl@hgfound.org
www.hgfound.org

Offers parents information on the normal pattern of their child's growth, growth charts, recognition of growth problems, evaluation of growth problems and resources for more information. Available to members.

Frank Diamond, MD, President
Emily Germain-Lee, MD, Vice President

3115 Short Mort Meets a Big Bully
Assosiation for the Care of Children's Health
7910 Woodmont Avenue
Bethesda, MD 20814

301-654-6549
Fax: 301-986-4553

This fictional story helps children and families address issues surrounding short stature. It offers helpful strategies for dealing with self-esteem issues, peers, and siblings. The book, illustrated dramatically with full-color pictures, is intended for children 8 to 11 years of age, but it can be read with younger children.

1997

3116 Short and OK

Patricia Rieser, Heino FL Mayer-Bahlbug, author

Human Growth Foundation
977 Glen Cove Avenue, Suite 5
Glen Head, NY 11545

516-671-4041
800-451-6434

This is a guide for parents of short children offering information on behavior issues, medical issues and psychological warning signs.

54 pages

3117 Two Very Little Sisters
Clarion Books/Houghton Mifflin Company
215 Park Avenue S
New York, NY 10003

www.hougtonmifflinbooks.com

This story is based on the lives of two real Little People. Small in height but large in will, these sisters enjoyed a happy New England childhood and later had very successful careers in the Ringling Brothers Circus.

32 pages Grades K-3
ISBN: 0-395609-27-5

Newsletters

3118 MAGIC Foundation: Major Aspects of Growth in Children
6645 W North Avenue
Oak Park, IL 60302

708-383-0808
800-362-4423
Fax: 708-383-0899
TTY: 123-019-99
e-mail: mary@magicfoundation.org
www.magicfoundation.org

A national nonprofit organization providing support and education regarding growth disorders in children and related adult disorders. Provides educational information, networking, a national conference, a kids' program and an extensive medical library.

36 pages Quarterly

Mary Andrews, CEO
Dianne Tamburrino, Executive Director

3119 Orphan Disease Update
National Organization for Rare Disorders
55 Kenosia Avenue, PO Box 1968
Danbry, CT 06813

203-744-0100
800-999-6673
Fax: 203-798-2291
e-mail: orphan@rarediseases.org
www.rarediseases.org

It provides updates on research, advocacy, and special events, as well as advice and sources of help for caregivers, Web sites of interest, current clinical trials, and funding opportunities.

16 pages 3/year

Carolyn Asbury, PhD, Chair
Sami I. Said, MD, Chair Medical Advisory Committee

Pamphlets

3120 Dental Problems with Growth Hormone Deficiency
Human Growth Foundation
997 Glen Cove Avenue, Suite 5
Glen Head, NY 11545

516-671-4041
800-451-6434
Fax: 516-671-4055
e-mail: hgfl@hgfound.org
www.hgfound.org

Growth hormone has a strong effect on bone growth, including the bones of the upper and lower jaws.

3121 Growth Hormone Deficiency
Human Growth Foundation
997 Glen Cove Avenue, Suite 5
Glen Head, NY 11545

516-671-4041
800-451-6434
Fax: 516-671-4055
e-mail: hgfl@hgfound.org
www.hgfound.org

Causes and control of growth hormone deficiency.

3122 Growth Hormone Testing
Human Growth Foundation
997 Glen Cove Avenue, Suite 5
Glen Head, NY 11545

516-671-4041
800-454-6434
Fax: 516-671-4055
e-mail: hgfl@hgfound.org
www.hgfound.org

Describes how growth hormone testing is used, when growth hormone test is ordered, and what growth hormone test results might mean.

3123 Intrauterine Growth Retardation
Human Growth Foundation
977 Glen Cove Avenue, Suite 5
Glen Head, NY 11545

516-671-4041
800-451-6434
Fax: 516-761-4055
e-mail: hglf@hgfound.org
hgfound.org

Offers information on how to understand this growth disorder and how to cope with it.

3124 Most Frequently Asked Questions with Growth Hormone Deficiency
Human Growth Foundation
977 Glen Cove Avenue, Suite 5
Glen Head, NY 11545

516-671-4041
800-451-6434
Fax: 516-671-4055
e-mail: hgfl@hgfound.org
www.hgfound.org

Discusses the consequences of growth hormone deficiency in chidlren and adults.

3125 Psychosocial Issues of Growth Delayed Children
Human Growth Foundation
7777 Leesburg Pike, Suite 202S
Falls Church, VA 22043

703-883-1773
800-451-6434

DESCRIPTION

3126 GUILLAIN-BARRE SYNDROME

Synonyms: Acute ascending polyneuritis, Acute febrile polyneuritis, Acute idiopathic polyneuritis, Acute postinfectious polyneuropathy, GBS, Landry's paralysis

Involves the following Biologic System(s):

Neurologic Disorders

Guillain-Barre syndrome (GBS) (pronounced gE-Ian-ba-rA) is a progressive neurologic disorder that affects many nerves (polyneuropathy) and is characterized by unusual sensations (paresthesias) in the arms, legs, or both. GBS generally causes progressive muscle weakness over days and, in some cases, paralysis accompanied by lack of muscle tone. Guillain-Barre syndrome is thought to be an autoimmune disorder and may occur as a reaction to a previous viral infection, immunization, or bacterial infection (e.g., Lyme disease). Autoimmune disorders involve the body's inappropriate immune response to its own healthy tissues.e symptoms of GBS typically begin approximately one to three weeks following the triggering event.

Symptoms associated with Guillain-Barre syndrome range from mild to severe and may include numbness, tingling, muscle weakness, and sometimes paralysis that begins in the legs and then usually spreads upward toward the trunk, arms, muscles of the chest, and sometimes the face (ascending paralysis). Affected children may become irritable and unable or unwilling to walk. As weakness spreads to the chest and facial areas, muscles required for speech, breathing, and eating may become affected. In addition, if the nerves of the autonomic nervous system which control vital involuntary functions are affected, individuals with GBS may develop fluctuations in blood pressure and heart rate as well as other heart irregularities. A rare form of Guillain-Barreyndrome called the Miller-Fisher syndrome is characterized by paralysis of the nerves and muscles of the eyes (ophthalmoplegia), an absence of normal reflexes (areflexia), and an inability to coordinate voluntary movement (ataxia).

Most children with Guillain-Barre syndrome recover completely within two to three weeks. Some may experience ongoing muscular weakness. In addition, in rare cases, affected individuals may experience prolonged or recurring episodes of GBS that may last for months or years. These uncommon manifestations are referred to as chronic unremitting polyradiculoneuropathy and chronic relapsing polyradiculoneuropathy.

Guillain-Barre syndrome may be diagnosed through specialized tests of the fluid that surrounds the brain and spinal cord (cerebrospinal fluid) and other clinical findings. Early diagnosis and hospitalization allow for observation and monitoring of affected individuals. If the progression of muscle weakness or paralysis is very slow and limited, treatment may include observation and supportive care until recovery is complete. If, however, paralysis progresses to involve breathing and swallowing, appropriate support is necessary. Other treatment may include plasma exchange (plasmapheresis), a procedure during which blood is withdrawn and the liquid portion (plasma) removed in order to filter out harmful substances. A plasma substitute is then mixed with the blood, and the reconstituted blood is then returned to the body. Alternative treatment may include the intravenous administration of immunoglobulin (IVIG). In some cases, certain immunosuppressive drugs or corticosteroids may be effective. Physical therapy may aid in the maintenance of joint and muscle function. Other treatment is symptomatic and supportive.

See also **General Resources** on page 917

National Associations & Support Groups

3127 American Autoimmune Related Diseases Association
22100 Gratiot Avenue
E Detroit, MI 48021

586-776-3900
www.aarda.org

The American Autoimmune Related Diseases Association is dedicated to the eradication of autoimmune diseases and the alleviation of suffering and the socioeconomic impact of autoimmunity through fostering and facilitating collabration in the areas of education, public awareness, research,and patient in an effective, ethical and efficient manner.

Virginia Ladd, Director

3128 GBS/CIDP Foundation International
Holly Bldg, 104 1/2 Forrest Avenue
Narberth, PA 19072

610-667-0131
Fax: 610-667-7036
e-mail: info@gbsfi.com
www.gbsfi.com

Provides emotional support and assistance to people affected by this rare disease. Arranges personal visits to affected individuals in hospitals and rehabilitation centers. Fosters research into the cause, treatment, and other aspects of the disorder and directs affected individuals with long-term disabilities to resources for vocational, financial, and other aspects of the disorder.

Sara Voorhees, PMP, President
Estelle L. Benson, Executive Director

Web Sites

3129 GBS Support Group of the UK
www.gbs.org.uk/

Objectives are to: provide emotional support to patients, families and friends; provide, when possible, personal visits by former patients to those currently in hospitals and rehabilitation centres and those recovering; supply a comprehensive short guide for patients, relatives and friends, and other literature, so that patients and their families can learn what to expect during the illness; and to educate the public and medical community about the Support Group.

Book Publishers

3130 Immune System Disorders Sourcebook

Joyce Brennfleck Shannon, author

Omnigraphics
PO Box 625
Holmes, PA 19043

610-461-3548
800-234-1340
Fax: 800-875-1340
e-mail: info@omnigraphics.com
www.omnigraphics.com

Basic information about lupus, multiple sclerosis, guillain-barre syndrome and more.

671 pages Hardcover
ISBN: 0-780807-48-0

Pamphlets

3131 Fact Sheet: Guillain-Barre Syndrome

National Inst. of Neurological Disorders/Stroke
PO Box 5801
Bethesda, MD 20824

301-496-5751
800-352-9424

Information about Guillain-Barren Syndrome, what causes Guillain-Barren Syndrome, how is it diagnosed and treated, etc. Also available in Spanish.

DESCRIPTION

3132 HIV INFECTION

Synonyms: Fetal AIDS, Acquired Immune Deficiency Syndrome

Involves the following Biologic System(s):
Immunologic and Rheumatologic Disorders, Infectious Disorders

HIV Infection destroys the body's ability to fight infections, resulting in Acquired Immune Deficiency, or AIDS. T-cells, which are responsible for responding to infections, are destroyed by the virus. The process is slow and silent, which means that HIV can be contracted unwittingly years before any symptoms appear. As the T-cells are destroyed, organisms that are usually defeated by a normal immune system, infect the body. Patients suffer from one infection after another. HIV is usually spread from an infected person to a non-infected person by unprotected sexual intercourse, or by sharing needles. Most young children with AIDS contract the disease through in utero transmission; however, infants may occasionally acquire the infection through mother's milk. In addition, children with hemophilia and others who may have received transfusions of blood or blood products before HIV blood-screening became standard in 1985 may have become infected by contaminated blood.

Some children with HIV infection develop symptoms in the first or second year of life, while the majority may not show signs of infection for several years. AIDS is diagnosed in about 50 percent of HIV-infected children by three years of age. Early signs may include chronic or recurrent fevers and diarrhea, rashes, swollen lymph glands (lymphadenopathy), enlarged liver and spleen (hepatosplenomegaly), and delays in growth and nervous system development. Some infants and young children are anemic, experience weight and appetite loss, decreased energy, and irregularities of the heart and kidneys. Early symptoms may include chronic or recurrent bacterial infections and uncommon viral, fungal, and other types of infections caused by microorganisms that do not ordinarily cause disease or infections. As the immune system continues to weaken, children may develop lung inflammations and potentially life-threatening pneumocystis pneumonia. Children with AIDS are also at increased risk for certain types of malignant diseases such as non-Hodgkin's lymphoma.

Most infants born to mothers with HIV show antibodies in their blood for approximately 12 to 14 months. In infants who are not infected with the virus, these passive antibodies disappear. For this reason, standardized HIV testing is not conclusive in children younger than 18 months. However, HIV infection in these children may often be detected through the use of virus cultures and a specialized DNA-copying technique called polymerase chain reaction or PCR.

Prevention of HIV and subsequent AIDS infection in infants may be directed toward counseling of at-risk women of child-bearing age who may be advised to avoid becoming pregnant. The strictly prescribed administration of the drug AZT during the last six months of pregnancy, as well as during labor and delivery, has been shown to greatly improve the chances of an HIV-infected mother delivering an infant who is not infected with HIV. In fact, congenitally acquired HIV has been reduced dramatically in recent years. Delivery by Cesarean section may also reduce risk of transmission to the newborn. In addition, mothers with HIV should refrain from breast-feeding their infants, as there is some evidence of HIV transmission from mother to child in women who may have contracted the virus after pregnancy.

Infants and children with HIV may be treated with antibiotics to prevent pneumocystis pneumonia. Intravenous gamma globulin therapy may be used to maintain or increase the ability of the immune system to fight the effects of secondary infections. In addition, certain steroidal drugs may be administered to treat lymphoid interstitial pneumonitis, while AZT, alone or in combination, is often used to treat children and has been found to be particularly effective against neurologic irregularities. Additional therapies are also being tested in children. Other treatment is symptomatic and supportive.

See also **General Resources** on page 917

Government Agencies

3133 Centers for Disease Control
1600 Clifton Road
Atlanta, GA 30333

404-639-3311
www.cdc.gov

Mission is to promote health and quality of life by preventing and controlling disease, injury, and disability.

3134 NIH/National Institute of Allergy and Infectious Diseases
6610 Rockledge Drive, MSC 6612
Bethesda, MD 20892

301-496-5717
Fax: 301-402-3573
TDD: 800-877-8339
www.niaid.nih.gov

Conducts and supports basic and applied research to better understand, treat, and ultimately prevent infectious, immunologic, and allergic diseases.

Anthony S Fauci MD, Director

National Associations & Support Groups

3135 American Social Health Association
PO Box 13827
Research Triangle Park, NC 27709

919-361-8400
800-783-9877
Fax: 919-361-8425
www.ashastd.org

Dedicated to improving the health of individuals, families, and communities with a focus on preventing sexually transmitted diseases and their harmful consequences.

Lynn Barclay, President/CEO
Deborah Arrindell, VP Health Policy

3136 Elizabeth Glazer Pediatric AIDS Foundation
2950 31st Street, Suite 125
Santa Monica, CA 90405

310-314-1459
800-499-4673
Fax: 310-314-1469
e-mail: info@pedsaids.org
www.pedsaids.org

A national nonprofit organization dealing with medical problems unique to children infected with HIV/AIDS. The foundation is focused specifically on creating a future that will offer hope, finding effective therapies and issues of pregnancy and HIV. The foundation encourages students to enter the world of pediatric AIDS through a student intern program and more.

Pamela Barnes, President/CEO
Trish Carlin, Vice President Programs

3137 Foundation for Children with AIDS
1800 Columbus Avenue
Roxbury, MA 02119

617-442-7442
Fax: 617-442-1705

A national, nonprofit organization founded to improve the quality of life for drug-affected and HIV-infected children and their families. The foundation raises funds for family and community-based services for children and their families affected by HIV infection and drug exposure. Offers Project STAR which is a child and family care program offering therapeutic child care, early intervention, transportation, counseling and case management services.

Geneva Woodruff, PhD, Executive Director

3138 Immune Deficiency Foundation
Immune Deficiency Foundation
40 W Chesapeake Avenue, Suite 308
Towson, MD 21204

410-321-6647
800-296-4433
Fax: 410-321-9165
e-mail: idf@primaryimmune.org
www.primaryimmune.org

The only national charitable organization aimed at fighting the primary immune deficiency diseases. The founders included parents of children with primary immune deficiency, immunologists who treat immune deficient patients and other individuals with an interest in helping others. The Foundation's main goal is to improve the care and treatment of adults and children with primary immune deficiency diseases and to promote public education and awareness about the diseases.

Marcia Boyle, Founder/Chairman/President
Katherine Antilla, Vice Chair

3139 National AIDS Hotline
American Social Association
PO Box 13827
Research Triangle Park, NC 27709

919-361-8400
800-342-2437
Fax: 919-361-8425
TDD: 800-243-7889
www.ashastd.org

Information and advocacy resources for families and professionals. Includes listings of organizations providing general information and organizations focusing on more specific areas of concern to families and young adults who have disabilities.

Lynn Barclay, President/CEO
Deborah Arrindell, VP Health Policy

3140 National Abandoned Infants Assistance Resource Center
University of California, Berkeley
1950 Addison Street, Suite 104, #7402
Berkeley, CA 94720

510-643-8390
Fax: 510-643-7019
e-mail: aia@berkeley.edu
www.aia.berkeley.edu

The Center's vision is to enhance the quality of social and health services delivered to drug and HIV-affected children and their families. Its strategy is to provide state-of-the-art training, technical assistance, research, and information to professionals who serve these families. Services include a national newsletter, telephone seminars, conferences, monographs, guides and reports.

Jeanne Pietrzak, Director
Neil Gilbert PhD, Principal Investigator

3141 National Association of People with AIDS
8041 Colesville Road, Suite 750
Silver Spring, MD 20910

240-247-0880
Fax: 240-247-0574
e-mail: info@napwa.org
www.napwa.org

Advocates on behalf of all people with HIV and AIDS in order to end the pandemic and the human suffering caused by HIV/AIDS.

Frank Oldham, Jr, Executive Director
Vanessa Johnson, Deputy Executive Director

3142 Support for Children with AIDS
1222 T Street NW, Grandma's House
Washington, DC 20009

202-234-4128
Fax: 202-234-8145
e-mail: terrific03@aol.com
www.grandmashouse-terrific.org

A support organization that provides service, care, and preventive education for children and adults with AIDS. It provides housing for children with AIDS (e.g. Grandma's House® in Washington, DC).

Susan McCarley, Vice President

3143 World Health Organization
Avenue Appia 20
CH-1211 Geneva 27,
Switzerland

www.who.int

WHO is the directing and coordinating authority for health within the United Nations system.

Dr Margaret Chan, Director General

Research Centers

3144 American Foundation for AIDS Research
120 Wall Street, 13th Floor
New York, NY 10005

212-806-1600
800-392-6327
Fax: 212-806-1601
www.amfar.org

Dedicated to the support of HIV/AIDS research, HIV prevention, treatment education, and the advocacy of sound AIDS related public policy.

Jerome J. Radwin, Chief Executive Officer
Deborah C. Hernan, VP Public Information

3145 Children's Clinical Research Center
New York Hospital, Cornell Medical Center
525 E 68th Street, Box 149
New York, NY 10021

212-746-4745
Fax: 212-746-8922
www.ccrc.med.cornell.edu

Offers research into the study of pediatric AIDS and other disorders.

Julianne Imperato-McGinley, MD, Program Director
Patricia Giardina, MD, Associate Program Director

3146 Developmental Medicine Center
Children's Hospital
300 Longwood Avenue
Boston, MA 02115

617-355-6000
Fax: 617-735-7429
TTY: 617-355-0443
e-mail: webteam@tch.harvard.edu
www.childrenshospital.org

The Developmental Medicine Center (DMC) at Children's Hospital Boston provides developmental evaluation and treatment services for children aged birth to adolescence with a wide range of developmental, behavioral and learning difficulties. The Center was founded for the purpose of enhancing the coordination of services for children and families with special needs.,

Leonard A. Rappaport MD, MS, Program Director

3147 National Training Center for Professional AIDS Education
1800 Columbus Avenue
Roxbury, MA 02119

617-442-7442
Fax: 617-442-1705

Program training teachers, health care providers and other professionals who serve HIV-infected children and their families. Offers education, site workshops, technical assistance, regional conferences, printed materials and publication of articles in the media and professional journals. Training is designed for providers and administrators of early childhood/intervention programs, public school, preschool and special education programs.

Geneva Woodruff, PhD, Executive Director

Conferences

3148 Immune Deficiency Foundation National Conference
40 West Chesapeake Avenue, Suite 308
Towson, MD 21204

410-321-6647
800-296-4433
Fax: 410-321-9165
e-mail: idf@primaryimmune.org
www.primaryimmune.org

Annual conference hosted by an organization aimed at fighting the primary immune deficiency diseases. The founders included par-

ents of children with primary immune deficiency, immunologists who treat immune deficient patients and other individuals with an interest in helping others. The Foundation's main goal is to improve the care and treatment of adults and children with primary immune deficiency diseases and to promote public education and awareness about the diseases.

June

Marcia Boyle, Founder/Chairman/President
Katherine Antilla, Vice Chair

Audio Video

3149 Families And Health: a Child's Voice
Aquarius Health Care Videos
18 North Main Street
Sherborn, MA 01770

508-650-1616
888-440-2963
Fax: 508-650-1665
e-mail: info@aquariusproductions.com
www.aquariusproductions.com

A moving documentary about children communicating their concerns over a family health condition - be it their own, a sibling or parent. These children talk openly about conditions such as HIV, diabetes, asthma and cancer and how they affect them at home, the hospital and school.

22 minutes

Donna Kaufman

3150 Kid Called Troy
Fanlight Productions
4196 Washington Street
Boston, MA 02131

617-469-4999
800-937-4113
Fax: 617-524-8838
e-mail: orders@fanlight.com
www.fanlight.com

Troy, a seven-year-old from Australia, has lived with the HIV virus his entire life. Narrated by Troy's father, this film shows how Troy manages to remain happy and engaged and also offers a portrait of parental love and dedication.

54 minutes
ISBN: 1-572952-21-0

Ben Achtenberg, President
Sandy St. Louis, Distribution Director

3151 Pediatric AIDS: A Time of Crisis
Association for the Care of Children's Health
8701 Hartsdale Avenue
Bethesda, MD 20817

301-493-5113

Families caring for children who are HIV positive speak about the kinds of services and programs they need to meet the needs of these children in the hospital, at home and in the community.

24 minutes

Web Sites

3152 AEGIS
www.aegis.com/
Web based reference for HIV/AIDS-related information.

3153 AIDS Knowledge Base
hivinsite.ucsf.edu/InSite
A comprehensive, on-line textbook of HIV disease from the University of California San Francisco and San Francisco Hospital.

3154 American Social Health Association

www.ashastd.org

Dedicated to improving the health of individuals, families, and communities with a focus on preventing sexually transmitted diseases and their harmful consequences.

3155 Children with AIDS Project

www.aidskids.org/

The mission is to transform the silence that surrounds HIV infected, children and AIDS orphans into an audible sound. This sound must be amplified until the needs are met for all children in the nation and globally affected by the AIDS epidemic.

3156 Elizabeth Glazer Pediatric AIDS Foundation

www.pedaids.org/

The foundation created a future of hope for children and families worldwide by eradicating pediatric AIDS, providing care and treatment to people with HIV/AIDS, and accelerating the discovery of new treatments for other serious and life-threatening pediatric illnesses.

3157 Food and Drug Administration

www.fda.gov

The FDA is responsible for protecting the public health by assuring the safety, efficacy, and security of human and veterinary drugs, biological products, medical devices, our nation's food supply, cosmetics, and products that emit radiation. The FDA is also responsible for advancing the public health by helping to speed innovations that make medicines and foods more effective, safer, and more affordable and helping the public get accurate, science-based information they need to improve health.

3158 Immune Deficiency Foundation

www.primaryimmune.org

The only national charitable organization aimed at fighting the primary immune deficiency diseases. The founders included parents of children with primary immune deficiency, immunologists who treat immune deficient patients and other individuals with an interest in helping others.

3159 National Association of People with AIDS

www.napwa.org

Advocates on behalf of all people with HIV and AIDS in order to end the pandemic and the human suffering caused by HIV/AIDS.

3160 National Pediatric & Family HIV Resource Center

www.womenchildrenhiv.org

The goal of this site is to contribute to an improvement in the scale and quality of international HIV/AIDS prevention care and treatment programs for women and children by increasing access to authoritative HIV/AIDS information.

3161 National Pediatric AIDS Network

www.npan.org/

Is a nonprofit organization, that works collaboratively with a number of other HIV/AIDS information providers.

3162 Parents Helping Parents

www.php.com

Mission is to help children with special needs receive the resources, love, hope, respect, health care, education, and other services they need to reach their full potential by providing them with strong families, dedicated professionals, and responsive systems to serve them.

3163 Pediatric AIDS Clinical Trials Group

pactg.s-3.com

Goals are: to optimize strategies to maintain or improve mother to infant transmission at less than 2% without long termn toxicity to exposed infants or treated pregnant women in the United States; and to enable more than 90% of children perinatally infected with HIV to achieve normal growth and development, and more than 20 years survival in the United States.

3164 Sunshine for HIV Kids

www.sunshinesite.com

Is a nonprofit tax exempt organization that identifies and raises funds for charities who directly deliver care to children afficted with HIV/AIDS and their familes.

3165 Wayne State University

www.research.wayne.edu

Advances in therapy to prevent HIV transmission from mothers to infants have brought hope to thousands, but transmission of HIV continues to increase in developing countries. We must identify effective intervention strategies usable by all nations if we are to reduce the incidence of mother to infant HIV transmission worldwide.

Book Publishers

3166 AIDS Awareness Library

Anna Forbes, MSS, author

Rosen Publishing Group
29 E 21st Street
New York, NY 10010

212-777-3017
800-237-9932
Fax: 888-436-4643
e-mail: info@rosenpub.com
www.rosenpublishing.com

This series of eight 24-page books for grades K-5, speaks to children in nonthreatening langauge that provides vital information without graphic detail. This series is meant to be a gentle introduction to this frightening epidemic. Titles in series: Heroes Against AIDS, Kids with AIDS, Living in a World with AIDS, Myths and Facts About AIDS, What is AIDS?, What You Can Do About AIDS, When Someone You Know Has AIDS, Where Did AIDS Come From?.

24 pages
ISBN: 0-823974-06-5

3167 AIDS and the Education of Our Children

Consumer Information Center
US Department of Education
Pueblo, CO 81009

719-948-3334
888-878-3256
www.pueblo.gsa.gov

A guide for parents and teachers offering helpful information on the topic of AIDS education.

28 pages

3168 Alex, the Kid with AIDS

Albert Whitman & Company
6340 Oakton Street
Morton Grove, IL 60053

847-581-0033
800-225-7675
Fax: 847-581-0039
e-mail: mail@awhitmanco.com
www.awhitmanco.com

A boy with AIDS decides he doesn't want to use his illness to get special consideration in school and makes a friend in the process. With a compassionate but humorous touch, the author shows how a very real child reacts to a terrible disease and how others react to him.

32 pages Grades 2-5
ISBN: 0-807502-45-6

Joseph Boyd, President
Joe Campbell, Customer Service

3169 Be a Friend-Children Who Live with AIDS Speak

Compassion Books
477 Hannah Branch Road
Burnsville, NC 28714

828-675-5909
Fax: 828-675-5909

Through writings and drawings children living with HIV infection and AIDS candidly share their feelings, hopes, and fears.

Softcover

3170 Community Service Delivery for Children with HIV Infection and Families

South Shore Mental Health Center
500 Victory Road
Quincy, MA 02171

617-847-1950
800-852-2844
TTY: 617-847-1922
www.ssmh.org

A manual providing guidelines for developing community-based, family-centered services for children with HIV infection and their families. Describes how services can be planned and delivered using guiding principles and practices of transagency case management.

3171 Heroes Against AIDS

Anna Forbes, MSS, author

Rosen Publishing Group
29 E 21st Street
New York, NY 10010

212-777-3017
800-237-9932
Fax: 888-436-4643
e-mail: info@rosenpub.com
www.rosenpublishing.com

Ryan White and Magic Johnson are just two of the heroes in this book who demonstrate through their courage and kindness their strength in adversity.

K-5 24 pages
ISBN: 0-823923-71-1

3172 How Can I Tell You? Secrecy with Children When a Family Member Has AIDS

Association for the Care of Children's Health
8701 Hartsdale Avenue
Bethesda, MD 20817

301-493-5113

Assists families and professionals as they explore issues surrounding the disclosure of an HIV diagnosis to children.

84 pages

3173 Kids with AIDS

Anna Forbes, MSS, author

Rosen Publishing Group
29 E 21st Street
New York, NY 10010

212-777-3017
800-237-9932
Fax: 888-436-4643
e-mail: info@rosenpub.com
www.rosenpublishing.com

This book is written so as not to scare kids but teach compassion for their peers who might have AIDS. It stresses the importance of eliminating blame from this disease.

K-5 24 pages
ISBN: 0-823923-72-X

3174 Let's Talk About Going to the Hospital

Rosen Publishing Group's PowerKids Press
29 E 21st Street
New York, NY 10010

212-777-3017
800-237-9932
Fax: 888-436-4643
e-mail: rosenpub@tribeca.ios.com
www.powerkidspress.com

If a child has to check into the hospital, chances are he or she is already upset about being ill. Knowing how a hospital functions and what the procedures are, such as when family members can visit, will help in what is already a stressful situation. Grades K-5.

24 pages
ISBN: 0-823950-36-0

3175 Living in a World with AIDS

Anna Forbes, MSS, author

Rosen Publishing Group
29 E 21st Street
New York, NY 10010

212-777-3017
800-237-9932
Fax: 888-436-4643
e-mail: info@rosenpub.com
www.rosenpublishing.com

AIDS is a reality. Kids hear about it on TV, at school, and on the streets. This introductory volume reassures kids about their basic safety and provides gentle preventative advice that is age appropriate.

K-5 24 pages
ISBN: 0-823923-67-3

3176 Myths and Facts About AIDS

Rosen Publishing Group's PowerKids Press
29 E 21st Street
New York, NY 10010

212-777-3017
800-237-9932
Fax: 888-436-4643
e-mail: rosenpub@tribeca.ios.com
www.powerkidspress.com

In a simple and reassuring manner, the author demystifies this disease and puts to rest many misconceptions. Grades K-5.

K-5 24 pages
ISBN: 0-823923-66-5

3177 What Is AIDS?

Rosen Publishing Group's PowerKids Press
29 E 21st Street
New York, NY 10010

212-777-3017
800-237-9932
Fax: 888-436-4643
e-mail: rosenpub@tribeca.ios.com
www.powerkidspress.com

Accessible scientific look at AIDS puts it in the context of other diseases, teaching about the human organism in an age-appropriate manner. Grades K-5.

K-5 24 pages
ISBN: 0-823923-68-1

3178 What You Can Do About AIDS

Anna Forbes, MSS, author

Rosen Publishing Group
29 E 21st Street
New York, NY 10010

212-777-3017
800-237-9932
Fax: 888-436-4643
e-mail: info@rosenpub.com
www.rosenpublishing.com

It's never too early to teach kids about social responsibility. This book emphasizes community participation.

K-5 24 pages
ISBN: 0-823923-70-3

3179 When Someone You Know Has AIDS

Anna Forbes, MSS, author

Rosen Publishing Group
29 E 21st Street
New York, NY 10010

212-777-3017
800-237-9932
Fax: 888-436-4643
e-mail: info@rosenpub.com
www.rosenpublishing.com

This unique volume helps kids who might know someone with AIDS to approach that person with love and compassion as one would any sick person.

K-5 24 pages
ISBN: 0-823923-69-X

3180 Where Did AIDS Come From?

Anna Forbes, MSS, author

Rosen Publishing Group
29 E 21st Street
New York, NY 10010

212-777-3017
800-237-9932
Fax: 888-436-4643
e-mail: info@rosenpub.com
www.rosenpublishing.com

AIDS is frightening, especially to young children who sense the secrecy around it. This is a gentle introduction to the topic. It treats AIDS like any other epidemic.

K-5 24 pages
ISBN: 0-823923-65-7

3181 You and HIV: A Day At a Time

Association for the Care of Children's Health
8701 Hartsdale Avenue
Bethesda, MD 20817

301-493-5113

This is a well-written book for teenagers that covers HIV. Although the text is for young people, it can be used very effectively by students, social workers, teachers, health administrators, policy makers and anyone else who is interested in children and AIDS. The illustrations may be somewhat crude, but they are very effective in illustrating what is being discussed. This is a very good book that is recommended for school and public libraries.

258 pages

Newsletters

3182 Children with AIDS

Foundation for Children with AIDS
1800 Columbus Avenue
Roxbury, MA 02119

617-442-7442
Fax: 617-442-1705

Offers information on AIDS/HIV and hemophilia disorders affecting children. Gives housing information, medical research, projects, and publications for children and their families.

Bimonthly

3183 Just Kids

3 Corners
5th Avenue
New York, NY 10014

212-634-4879

Covers medical and social issues faced by HIV-positive children, teens and their parents.

Annual

Pamphlets

3184 Children with AIDS: Guidelines for Parents and Caregivers

AIDS Task Force of Central New York
627 W Genesee Street
Syracuse, NY 13204

315-415-2430

Offers general information on AIDS, diet and feeding, household chores, and coping with the illness.

3185 Hope for Children with AIDS

Elizabeth Glazer Pediatric AIDS Foundation
1140 Connecticut Avenue NW, Suite 200
Washington, DC 20036

202-296-9165
888-499-4693
Fax: 202-296-9185
www.pedaids.org

The Elizabeth Glaser Pediatric AIDS Foundation creates a future of hope for children and families worldwide by eradicating pediatric AIDS, providing care and treatment to people with HIV/AIDS, and accelerating the discovery of new treatments for other serious and life-threatening pediatric illnesses. In working toward our mission the foundation is committed to ensuring that the vast majority of every dollar raised goes directly into our research education and outreach program.

Camps

3186 Camp Heartland

1845 N Farwell Avenue, Suite 310
Milwaukee, WI 53202

414-272-1118
800-724-4673
Fax: 414-272-9916
e-mail: helpkids@campheartland.org
www.campheartland.org

Set up to provide children impacted by HIV/AIDS with the best week of their lives. Provides children forever affected by the isolation and tragedy of the disease the opportunity to experience - sometimes for the first time - the pure joys of being a kid.

Neil Willenson, Founder/CEO
Jeffrey Maiken, President

3187 Hole in the Wall Gang Camp
565 Ashford Center Road
Ashford, CT

860-429-3444
Fax: 860-429-7295
e-mail: ashford@holeinthewallgang.org
www.holeinthewallgang.org

Nonprofit organization that provides a recreational camp experience for children ages 7-15 with cancer, genetic blood diseases and HIV/AIDS.

Matthew Cook, Camp Director
James Canton, Executive Director

DESCRIPTION

3188 HEAD INJURIES

Synonyms: Closed head injury, Concussion, Traumatic brain injury

Involves the following Biologic System(s):

Neurologic Disorders

Head injuries describe trauma to the head that results in damage to the scalp, skull, or brain and associated membranes, nerves, or blood vessels. Every year in the United States, approximately 100,000 children require hospitalization because of head injuries. Many of these injuries are the result of motor vehicle and bicycle accidents. The risk of sustaining head or brain injury during a vehicular or bicycle accident is reduced by the proper use of restraint systems such as approved car seats, seat belts, or helmets. There are different types of head injuries, some of which are minor and, after healing, of no further significance; however, certain injuries that impact upon the brain may have severe complications and be potentially life-threatening. These include skull fractures, concussions, brain contusions and lacerations, and bleeding in the brain (e.g., subdural or epidural hematomas). Brain injury may result in mild, moderate, or severe functional disabilities, depending upon the particular area of brain tissue that is damaged or destroyed. Disabilities may affect physical, emotional, or intellectual development and include impairment in the comprehension or production of speech and language (aphasia); the inability to remember or perform certain familiar tasks requiring sequential movements (apraxia); the failure to remember past events or experiences (amnesia); the lack of ability to recognize familiar persons or objects (agnosia); and the development of episodes of uncontrolled electrical activity in the brain (posttraumatic epilepsy), usually within two years of the initial head injury.

In children with skull fractures or an open-head injury, there is an actual break in the skull bone (cranium). Many skull fractures do not interfere with normal brain function and will heal with no complications. However, in some patients, fractures may damage blood vessels or the membranes surrounding the brain (meninges), resulting in leakage of the fluid that surrounds the brain and spinal cord (cerebrospinal fluid). The break in the skull may also serve as an entry point for bacteria that may subsequently cause serious infection. A thorough evaluation is necessary to determine the extent of the injury. Surgical intervention may sometimes be necessary.

Concussions are closed-head injuries that occur as a result of a jarring of the brain within the skull. Symptoms and findings associated with this type of injury in children may include a temporary loss of consciousness, lack of muscle tone, poor or absent reflexes (areflexia), dilated pupils, blurred vision, irritability, or restlessness. These signs of concussion may be followed by rapid heartbeat (tachycardia), vomiting, listlessness, drowsiness, apathy, a pale skin color, or confusion. Treatment for concussion always involves observation. Although most children recover completely, hospitalization may be required for those whose level of consciousness continues to drop or those who appear listless, drowsy, or confused. Those who vomit excessively or experience seizures or other neurological symptoms may also require hospitalization.

Other closed-head injuries may include contusions, characterized by bruises on the brain; lacerations, characterized by tears in the brain tissue; subdural hematomas, characterized by accumulations of blood under the outermost membrane layer surrounding the brain (dura mater); and epidural hematomas, characterized by blood between the dura mater and the skull. Hematomas may result from ruptures or lacerations in certain blood vessels. Contusions and hematomas may cause the brain to swell with an accompanying buildup of fluid (edema). Increasing pressure within the skull may result in brain damage. Symptoms and findings may include headache; seizures; altered levels of consciousness sometimes leading to coma; loss of strength; numbness; paralysis; confusion; amnesia; or life-threatening complications such as respiratory distress and heart irregularities. Treatment is aimed at the maintenance of respiratory and cardiovascular function in order to prevent further injury. If necessary, the upper spine (cervical spine) is stabilized. The monitoring and management of brain swelling and fluid accumulation may include the careful administration of intravenous fluids and medications, bed elevation, and the use of supplemental oxygen. In addition, surgical intervention may be required to relieve intracranial pressure, remove blood clots, or control bleeding around the brain. Further treatment may include medication for the control of seizures. Recovery from major head or brain trauma may be a very slow, progressive process and, as such, may require the assistance of a team of specialists who will work with the family or caregivers of the child to coordinate symptomatic and supportive care.

See also **General Resources** on page 917

Government Agencies

3189 NIH/National Institute of Neurological Dis orders and Stroke (NINDS)
PO Box 5801
Bethesda, MD 20824

301-496-5751
800-352-9424
Fax: 301-496-0296
TTY: 301-468-5981
www.ninds.nih.gov

The mission of NINDS is to reduce the burden of neurological disease, a burden borne by every age group, by every segment of society, by people all over the world.

Story C Landis PhD, Director
Audrey S Penn MD, Deputy Director

National Associations & Support Groups

3190 Acoustic Neuroma Association
600 Peachtree Parkway, Suite 108
Cumming, GA 30041

770-205-8211
877-200-8211
Fax: 770-205-0239
e-mail: info@anausa.org
www.anausa.org

The Acoustic Neuroma Association provides information and support to patients who have been diagnosed with or experienced an acoustic neuroma or other benign problem affecting the cranial nerves. The ANA is an incorporated, nonprofit organization, and is supported by contributions from its members. The association also furnishes information on patient rehabilitation to physicians and health care personnel, promotes research on acoustic neuroma, and educates the public.

3191 Brain Injury Association of America Helpli ne
8201 Greensboro Drive, Suite 611
McLean, VA 22102

703-761-0750
800-444-6443
Fax: 703-761-0755
e-mail: familyhelpline@biausa.org
www.biausa.org

The mission of the Brain Injury Association is to create a better future through brain injury prevention, research, education and advocacy. This national number can link people to local BIA affiliates.

Susan H Connors, President/CEO
Mary S Reitter, CAE, Executive VP/COO

3192 Brain Injury Association of America Nation al Office
8201 Greensboro Drive, Suite 611
McLean, VA 22102

703-761-0750
800-444-6443
Fax: 703-761-0755
e-mail: info@biausa.org
www.biausa.org

Our mission is to create a better future through brain injury prevention, research, education and advocacy.

Susan H Connors, President/CEO
Mary S Reitter, CAE, Executive VP/COO

3193 Brain Injury Association of Michigan
8619 W Grand River, Suite I
Brighton, MI 48116

810-229-5880
800-772-4323
Fax: 810-229-8947
e-mail: info@biami.org
www.biami.org

Information center for persons with brain injury, their families, and concerned professionals.

Michael Dabbs, President
Carolyn Laughton, Director Administration

3194 Brain Trauma Foundation
708 Third Avenue
New York, NY 10017

212-772-0608
Fax: 212-772-0357
e-mail: info@braintrauma.org
www.braintrauma.org

The Brain Trauma Foundation mission is to improve the outcome of Traumatic Brain Injury (TBI) patients nationwide.

Jamshid Ghajar, MD/PhD, President
Pamela Drexel, Executive Director

3195 Coma Recovery Association
8300 Republic Airport, Suite 106
Farmingdale, NY 11735

763-756-1826
Fax: 631-756-1827
e-mail: office@comarecovery.org
www.comarecovery.org

Our purpose is to help families of coma and head injury survivors by providing information and referrals, enabling them to make informed choices regarding treatment, rehabilitation and socialization alternatives as well as support from others who struggle with similar concerns.

3196 Head Injury Hotline
212 Pioneer Building
Seattle, WA 98104

206-621-8558
Fax: 206-329-4355
e-mail: brain@headinjury.com
www.headinjury.com

Sponsors public information seminars designed to bring together survivors of head injuries, their families and professionals for networking and information sharing, as well as operating a national helpline for people suffering from a head injury.

Constance Miller, MA, Founder

3197 Perspectives Network
PO Box 121012
W Melbourne, GA 30028

770-844-6898
800-685-6302
Fax: 770-844-6898
e-mail: TPN@tbi.org
www.tbi.org

Primary focus is positive communication between persons with brain injury, family members, caregivers and friends of persons with brain injury, the many professionals who treat persons with brain injury and community members in order to create positive changes and enhance public awareness and knowledge of acquired and traumatic brain injury.

State Agencies & Support Groups

Alabama

3198 Alabama Head Injury Foundation
3100 Lorna Road, Suite 226
Hoover, AL 35216

205-823-3818
800-433-8002
Fax: 205-823-4544
e-mail: ahif1@aol.com
www.ahif.org

Our mission is to improve the quality of life for survivors of traumatic brain injury and for their families and to increase public awareness of (TBI).

Tom Novack, President
Charles D Priest, Executive Director

3199 Brain Injury Association of Alabama
3100 Lorna Road, Suite 226
Hoover, AL 35216

205-823-3818
800-433-8002
Fax: 205-823-4544
e-mail: Ahif@aol.com
www.ahif.org

The purpose is to increase public awareness of Traumatic Brain Injury (TBI) and to stimulate the development of supportive services. Today AHIF is amoung the largest state brain injury associations in the nation with model programs and statewide services.

Mary Watkins, President
Tom Novack, VP

Alaska

3200 Brain Injury Association of Alaska
313 Cindy Circle
Kenai, AK 99611

907-283-5711
888-945-4323
www.alaska.net/~drussell/bia-ak/

Debi Russell, Contact Person

3201 Brain Injury Association of Alaska - Helpline
1251 Muldoon Road
Anchorage, AK 99504

907-338-9800
www.alaska.net/~drussell/bia-ak/

Debi Russell, Contact Person

Arizona

3202 Brain Injury Association of Arizona
4250 E Camelback Road, Suite K-280
Phoenix, AZ 85018

602-508-8024
888-305-0073
Fax: 602-508-8285
e-mail: info@biaaz.org
www.biaaz.org

A non-profit membership organiation of people with brain injuries, their families, friends and service providers working together since 1983 to provide information and referrels, education, advocacy and support for those affected by brain injury.

Theresa Armstrong, MA, President
Mattie Smith, Executive Director

Arkansas

3203 Brain Injury Association of Arkansas
PO Box 26236
Little Rock, AR 72221

501-374-3585
800-325-2443
Fax: 501-918-6595
e-mail: info@brainassociation.org
www.brainassociation.org

Creating a better future through brain injury prevention, research, education and advocacy.

Dianne Gutierrez, President

California

3204 California Brain Injury Association
2658 Mt Vernon Avenue
Bakersfield, CA 93306

661-872-4903
888-662-4222
Fax: 661-873-2508
e-mail: calbiainfo@yahoo.com
www.calbia.org

Our mission is to serve and empower the community of many thousands of persons living in California with brain injuries and to enable them to live with dignity and to access all therapy, hospitalization, long term care, and all possible means for recovery and rehabilitation and to support their families.

Paula Daoutis, Contact

3205 Jodi House
1235 C Veronica Springs Road
Santa Barbara, CA 83105

805-563-2882
Fax: 805-593-3982
e-mail: info@jodihouse.org

The mission of Jodi House is to create a nurturing place of order, caring, acceptance and motivation for people with acquired brain injury,and to provide opportunities for each person to discover new paths to regain responsible independence and effective interdependence to the best of our ability, in order to achieve worthwhile purposes in our community.

Jim Cook, President
Andrew Chung, VP

Colorado

3206 Brain Injury Association of Colorado
4200 W Conejos Place, # 524
Denver, CO 80204

303-355-9969
800-955-2443
Fax: 303-355-9968
e-mail: informationreferralbiacolorado.org
www.biacolorado.org

The Brain Injury Association of Colorado began in April 1980. BIAC was formed by a group of family members and professionals in Denver and Colorado Springs who were concerned with the lack of support services for survivors and family members affected by head injury.The mission is to improve the quality of life for survivors of brain injury and their families, and to support programs that prevent brain injury.

Daniel Sloane, Esq, President
Peggy Spaulding, Executive Director

Connecticut

3207 Brain Injury Association of Connecticut
333 East River Drive, Suite 106
East Hartford, CT 06108

860-721-8111
800-278-8242
Fax: 860-721-9008
e-mail: general@biact.org
www.biact.org

Supports persons with brain injuries and their families by promoting services to facilitate full inclusion within their local community, and to increase awareness and understanding of brain injury and its prevention through community education.

500 Members

Charles Lyons, President Board of Directors
Julie Peters, Program Director

3208 TBI Support Group for Families & Survivors
Gaylord Hospital Conference Room
Wallingford, CT 06492

203-284-2800
TDD: 203-284-2700

Our mission is to preserve and enhance a person's health and function. We offer people a comprehensive continuum of care ranging from our Medically Complex Program and inpatient rehabilitation programs to outpatient services and sleep services.

Delaware

3209 Brain Injury Association of Delaware
32 West Loockerman Street, Suite 103
Dover, DE 19904

302-346-2083
800-411-0505
Fax: 302-678-3183
e-mail: biadresources@cavtel.net
www.biausa.org/delaware/bia.htm

A nonprofit organization whose mission is to advocate for and with people who survive traumatic brain injury; to secure and develop community-bases services for survivors and their families; to support research leading to better outcomes that enhance the lives of those who sustain brain injuries; and to promote prevention of brain injury through awareness, education and legislation.

John Goodier, President

District of Columbia

3210 Brain Injury Association of Washington DC
2100 Mayflower Drive
Lake Ridge, VA 22192

202-877-1464
Fax: 202-291-5366
e-mail: FamilyHelpline@biausa.org

Provide support to survivors of brain injury and their families, education to those who are being effected by brain injury, including the general public, and advocacy, to give the many suffering from this silent epidemic a public voice.

Karen Tyner, Contact Person

Florida

3211 Brain Injury Association of Florida
N Broward Medical Center, 201 E Sample Road
Pompano Beach, FL 33064

954-786-2400
800-992-3442
Fax: 954-786-2437
e-mail: info@biaf.org
www.biaf.org

A non profit organization founded in 1985, with the mission to improve the quality of life for persons with brain injury and their families by creating a better future through brain injury prevention, research, education, suport services and advocacy.

Mark Todd, PhD, President
Elynor Kazuk, Executive Director

3212 Family/Community Support Group of the Brain Injury Association of Florida
North Broward Medical Center
201 E Sample Road
Pompano Beach, FL 33064

954-786-2400
800-992-3442
www.biaf.org

Helping individuals with traumatic brain injuries and their families find practical solutions to the difficult problems faced when living with the long-term consequences of a traumatic brain injury (TBI).

3213 Goodwill Industries-Suncoast: Choices for Work Program
Goodwill Industries-Suncoast
10596 Gandy Boulevard
St. Petersburg, FL 33702

727-577-6411
888-297-1988
Fax: 727-579-0850
www.goodwill-suncoast.org

Provides short-term, light-duty work options for individuals recovering from on-the-job injuries. Participants are sponsored by a referring insurance company. This service is available in Hillsborough, Pinellas, Pasco and Polk counties through Suncoast Business Solutions.

Deborah A Passerini, Operations VP
R Lee Waits, President/CEO

3214 Pensacola Brain Injury
TBI/ABI Support Group
2001 N East Street
Pensacola, FL 32507

850-455-4117
Fax: 850-455-8474
e-mail: iccpots@people.com
pcolatbisupport.homestead.com/tbiinde

Survivors and caregivers oriented association. Publishes monthly magazine.

Georgia

3215 Brain Injury Resource Foundation
1841 Montreal Road, Suite 220
Tucker, GA 30084

678-937-1555
888-334-2424
Fax: 678-937-1557
e-mail: info@birf.info
www.birf.info/index.shtml

A nonprofit charitable orginazation working together with families and professionals since 1982 to provide education, advocacy and support for those effected by brain injury. Our mission is to empower individuals with brain injury by making available resources that may improve the quality of their lives.

Karen Parsley, Executive Director

Hawaii

3216 Brain Injury Association of Hawaii
2201 Waimano Home Road, Hale E
Pearl City, HI 96826

808-454-0699
Fax: 808-454-1975
e-mail: biahi@verizon.net
www.biausa.org/Hawaii

Dedicated to improving the quality of life of persons with brain injury and the families of such persons in Hawaii and other areas of the Pacific Basin. The goals of BIA-HI include promoting the rights of individuals experiencing disability caused by brain injury, io increase public awareness of brain injury, and to provide education for individuals who have sustained a brain injury and their families.

Mary Isley-Wilson, President
Angie Enoka, VP

3217 Pacific Head Injury Association
1775 S Beretania Street, Room 203
Honolulu, HI 96826

808-941-0372
www.waikiki-gallery.com/tbi.ht

Lyna Burnian

3218 Special Education Center of Hawaii
708 Palekaua Street
Honolulu, HI 96816

808-734-0233
Fax: 808-734-0391
e-mail: info@secoh.org
www.secoh.org

Committed to providing individual and family supports that promote successful community living in the lifestyle of choice. Services and supports are provided to people with developmental disabilities, or acquired disabilities due to aging or head injury. Services include day care, respite care, and supported employment.

Idaho

3219 Brain Injury Association of Idaho
PO Box 414
Boise, ID 83701

208-342-0999
888-374-3447
Fax: 208-333-0026
e-mail: info@biad.org
www.biad.org

A non-profit organization helping persons with brain injuryand their familiy members.

Michelle Featherson, President

Illinois

3220 Brain Injury Association of Illinois
PO Box 64420
Chicago, IL 60664

312-726-5699
800-699-6443
Fax: 312-630-4011
e-mail: info@biail.org
www.biail.org

A not-for-profit statewide membership organization comprised of people with brain injuries, family members, friends and professionals, with the mission to create a better future through brain injury awareness, prevention, education and advocacy.

Ginny Lazzara, President
Philicia Deckard, Executive Director

Indiana

3221 Brain Injury Association of Indiana
9531 Valparaiso Court, Suite A
Indianapolis, IN 46268

317-356-7722
Fax: 317-808-7770
e-mail: info@biai.org
www.biausa.org/Indiana

A nonprofit service organization comprised of people with brain injury, their families, and concerned stakeholders who are dedicated to creating a better future by reducing the incidence and effects of brain injury through public and professional education, advocacy, support, and by facilitating inter-agency commitment and collaboration.

J Michael Antrim, Esq, Chairman

Iowa

3222 Brain Injury Association of Iowa
2101 Kimball Avenue, LL7
Waterloo, IA 50702

319-272-2312
800-475-4442
Fax: 319-272-2109
e-mail: biaa@cedarnet.org
www.biausa.org/Iowa

Founded in 1980, exists to support, assist, and advocate for persons with acquired brain damage and for their families; advocates for and with people with brain injury and family members by responding to their challenges and representing their concerns through legislative efforts and active support of programs created for their needs.

Julie Dixon, President

3223 Center for Disabilities and Development
University of Iowa Hospitals and Clinics
100 Hawkins Drive
Iowa City, IA 52242

319-353-6900
877-686-0031
e-mail: cdd-webmaster@uiowa.edu
www.healthcare.uiowa.edu/cdd

A trusted resource for healthcare, training, research and information for people with disabilities that include: behavior disorders, brain injury, cerebral palsy, diabetes, down syndrome, learning disabilities, mental retardation, sleep disorders and spina bifida.

Elayne Sexsmith, Administrator
Amy Mikelson, Supervisor Info Resource Service

Kansas

3224 Brain Injury Association of Kansas & Greater Kansas City
PO Box 413072
Kansas City, MO 64105

816-842-8607
800-783-1356
Fax: 816-842-1531
e-mail: Lliggett@biaks.org
www.biaks.org

Offers support services to individuals and their families in the greater Kansas City area and throughout the state of Kansas who are recovering from traumatic brain injury.

Leigh Liggett, Executive Director
Dave Banks, Baord President

Kentucky

3225 Brain Injury Association of Kentucky
7410 New LaGrange Road, Suite 100
Louisville, KY 40222

816-842-8607
800-592-1117
Fax: 502-426-2993
e-mail: dir@braincenter.org
www.biak.us

Serves those affected by brain injury through advocacy, education, injury prevention, research, service and support.

Debbie Nelson, President
Melinda Mast, Executive Director

Louisiana

3226 Brain Injury Association of Louisiana
PO Box 57527
Ne Orleans, LA 70157

504-619-9989
800-500-2026
www.biala.org

A non-profit organization that serves the needs of persons with brain injury, their families, and care providers. The focus is to create a better future for individuals who have survived brain injury through brain injury prevention awareness, promotion of research, public education, and advocacy.

William E Moak, President/Executive Director

Maine

3227 Brain Injury Association of Maine
325 Main Street
Waterville, ME 04901

207-861-9900
800-275-1233
Fax: 207-861-4617
e-mail: info@biame.org
www.biame.org

A nonprofit organization that looks to create a better future for the people of Maine, through brain injury awareness, prevention, education and advocacy.

Bev Bryant, President
John Bott, Executive Director

Maryland

3228 Brain Injury Association of Maryland
2200 Kernan Drive
Baltimore, MD 21207

> 410-448-2924
> 800-221-6443
> Fax: 410-448-3541
> e-mail: info@biamd.org
> www.biamd.org

Our mission is to create a better future through brain injury prevention, research, education and advocacy.

Patricia Janus, President
Diane Triplett, Executive Director

Massachusetts

3229 Brain Injury Association of Massachusetts
30 Lyman Street
Westborough, MA 01581

> 508-475-0032
> 800-242-0030
> Fax: 508-475-0400
> e-mail: biama@biama.org
> www.biama.org

Our mission is to serve as an information and resource center for persons with brain injury, their families and friends, and providers and professionals in the field of brain injury treatment and rehabilitation.

Gregory L Zagloba, President
Arlene Korab, Executive Director

3230 VALT Support Group (Vital Active Life After Trauma)
53 Linden Street
Brookline, MA 02149

> 617-277-6327

Michigan

3231 Brain Injury Association of Michigan
8619 W Grand River, Suite 1
Brighton, MI 48116

> 810-229-5880
> 800-772-4323
> Fax: 810-229-8947
> e-mail: info@biami.org
> www.biami.org

A nonprofit organization that brings together people with brain injury, their families, friends, and concerned professionals to improve the quality of life that people experience after brain injury.

William Buccalo, Chair
Michael F Dabbs, President

3232 Rehabilitation Institute of Michigan
261 Mack Avenue
Detroit, MI 48201

> 313-745-1203
> Fax: 313-745-9863
> www.rimrehab.org

Providing quality patient care, academic excellence and cutting-edge research in physical medicine and rehabilitation.

Terry Reiley, President

Minnesota

3233 Brain Injury Association of Minnesota
34 13th Avenue NE, Suite B001
Minneapolis, MN 55413

> 612-378-2742
> 800-669-6442
> Fax: 612-378-2789
> e-mail: info@braininjurymn.org
> www.braininjurymn.org

The only non-profit organization in the state devoted solely to serving the needs of the 100,000 Minnesotans who live with a disabil-

ity due to brain injury. Providing hope, help and a voice for brain injured persons for over 20 years.

quaterly 20-24 pages

Russ Philstrom, Chair
Ardis Sandstrom, Executive Director

Mississippi

3234 Brain Injury Association of Mississippi
PO Box 55912
Jackson, MS 39296

> 601-981-1021
> 800-641-6442
> Fax: 601-981-1039
> e-mail: biaofms@aol.com
> www.members.aol.com/biaofms/index.htm

Enhances the quality of life for Traumatic Brain Injury survivors and their families, and to develop and support programs that prevent brain injury.

Howard Katz, PhD, Chair/President
Paul Gospodarski, EdD, Executive Director

Missouri

3235 Brain Injury Association of Missouri
10270 Page Avenue, Suite 100
Saint Louis, MO 63132

> 314-426-4024
> 800-377-6442
> Fax: 314-426-3290
> e-mail: info@biamo.org
> www.biamo.org

Founded in 1982, a community based organization serving persons with brain injury, their families, caregivers, physicians, therapists, case managers, and others throught the state of Missouri.

Terri Price, PhD, President
Scott Gee, Executive Director

Montana

3236 Brain Injury Association of Montana
1280 S 3rd West, Suite 4
Missoula, MT 59801

> 406-541-6442
> 800-241-6442
> Fax: 604-541-4360
> e-mail: biam@biamt.org
> www.biamt.org

To create a better future through brain injury prevention, research, education and advocacy.

Luke Foust, President
Stacy Rye, Executive Director

Nebraska

3237 Brain Injury Association of Nebraska
1108 Avenue H, PO Box 124
Gothenburg, NE 69158

> 308-537-7875
> 800-444-6443
> Fax: 308-537-7663
> e-mail: FamilyHelpline@biausa.org
> www.biausa.org/Nebraska/bia

Genenne Didier, President

Nevada

3238 Brain Injury Association of Northern Nevada
PO Box 2789
Gardnerville, NV 89410

> 702-782-8336

Carol Swan, Contact Person

3239 Brain Injury Association of Southern Nevada
2820 W Charleston Boulevard, Suite D37
Las Vegas, NV 89102

702-259-1903

Francis Laura, Contact Person
Robert Hogan

New Hampshire

3240 Brain Injury Association of New Hampshire
109 N State Street, Suite 2
Concord, NH 03301

603-225-8400
800-773-8400
Fax: 603-228-6749
e-mail: mail@bianh.org
www.bianh.org

Founded in 1983, a private, non-profit family and consumer run organization representing over 5000 New Hamphire residents with acquired brain disorders and stroke.

Carolyn Ramsay, President
Steven Wade, Executive Director

New Jersey

3241 Brain Injury Association of New Jersey
1090 King George Post Road, Suite 708
Edison, NJ 08837

732-738-1002
800-669-4323
Fax: 732-738-1132
e-mail: info@bianj.org
www.bianj.org

A nonprofit organization that brings together people with brain injury, their families and friends, and concerned allied health professionals to improve the quality of life people experience after brain injury.

Glenn Mccreesh, President
Barbara Geiger-Parker, Executive Director

New Mexico

3242 Brain Injury Association of New Mexico
121 Cardenas NE
Albuquerque, NM 87108

505-292-7414
888-292-7415
Fax: 505-271-8983
e-mail: info@braininjurynm.com
www.braininjurynm.org

Actively supports progressive public policy for persons with traumatic brain injury on both state and federal levels.

John Tiwald, Board President
Clara Holguin, Executive Director

New York

3243 Brain Injury Association of New York
10 Colvin Avenue
Albany, NY 12206

518-459-7911
800-228-8201
Fax: 518-482-5285
e-mail: info@bianys.org
www.bianys.org

Not-for-profit dedicated to improving the lives of persons, and their families, who have sustained traumatic brain injury. A clearinghouse providing information resources and referral, statewide support groups, and family support services coordinators, as well as educational programs to increase public and professional awarenesss.

Judith Avner, Executive Director
Michael Kaplen, Esq, President

3244 Brain Injury Association of New York State
10 Colvin Avenue
Albany, NY 12206

518-459-7911
800-228-8201
Fax: 518-482-5285
e-mail: info@bianys.org
www.bianys.org

A statewide non-profit membership organization that advocates on behalf of individuals with brain injury and their families, and promotes prevention. Established in 1982, provides education, advocacy, and community support services that lead to improved outcomes for children and adults with brain injuries and their families.

Michael Kaplen, Esq, President
Judy Avner, Executive Director

3245 Hy Feinstein Clubhouse
Long Island Head Injury Association
65 Austin Boulevard
Commack, NY 11725

631-543-2245
Fax: 631-543-2261
e-mail: club@lihia.org
lihia.org/club.htm

A non-profit organization whose primary mission is to provide a place for people with head injuries to participate in meaningful work; to have the opportunity to meet and build friendships; and ulimately seek employment within the community.

3246 Mount Sinai Traumatic Brain Injury
Mt Sinai Medical Center
1 Gustav L Levy Place, Dept. of Rehab Medicine
New York, NY 10029

212-241-7917
www.mssm.edu/rehab

Specializing not only in helping patients regain mastery over their physical environment, but also in addressing the cognitive and emotional aftermaths, including anxiety and depression, which are frequently triggered by such injuries. The program contains different treatment levels to address the very specific needs of this population.

Steven Flanagan, MD, Director

North Carolina

3247 Brain Injury Association of North Carolina
PO Box 748
Raleigh, NC 27601

919-833-9634
800-377-1464
Fax: 919-833-5415
e-mail: Sandra.farmer@bianc.net
www.bianc.net

Founded in 1982 by families and concerned professionals. The Association is an affiliate of the Brain Injury Association of America. Today, the Association has Family and Community Support Centers in Raleigh, Greenville, and Charlotte and 29 local chapters and support groups across the state.

Marylin Lash, President
Sandra Farmer, Executive Director

North Dakota

3248 Brain Injury Association of North Dakota
Open Door Center
2111 Main Avenue E
West Fargo, ND 58078

701-845-1124
Fax: 701-845-1175

Mary Simonson, President

Ohio

3249 Brain Injury Association of Ohio
1335 Dublin Road, Suite 271D
Columbus, OH 43215

614-481-7100
866-664-6242
Fax: 614-481-7103
e-mail: help@biaoh.org
www.biaoh.org

A statewide advocacy and education organization incorporated in 1982 to improve services and supports to Ohioans with brain injury and their families, and to promote prevention.

Jon Fishpaw, President
Suzanne Minnich, Executive Director

3250 Ohio Brain Injury Association
1335 Dublin Road, Suite 217D
Columbus, OH 43215

614-481-7100
800-686-956
Fax: 614-481-7103
e-mail: help@biaoh.org
www.biaoh.org

State-wide advocacy and education organization affiliated with the National Brain Injury Association serving Ohioans with brain injury and their families through assistance in locating services, supports, educational materials, conferences, prevention initiatives and legislative advocacy. Membership fee is $50.00 for professionals

400 members

Suzanne Minnich, Executive Director/Helpline Staff

Oklahoma

3251 Brain Injury Association of Oklahoma
PO Box 88
Hillsdale, OK 73743

580-233-4363
800-765-6809
Fax: 580-233-4546
e-mail: information@braininjuryoklahoma.org
www.braininjuryoklahoma.org

Tracy Grammer, President

Oregon

3252 Brain Injury Association of Oregon
2145 NW Overton Street
Portland, OR 97210

503-413-7707
800-544-5243
Fax: 503-413-6849
e-mail: biaor@biaoregon.org
www.biaoregon.org

To improve the quality of life of persons with brain injury and their families; and to prevent brain injury.

Wayne Eklund, President
Sherry Stock, Executive Director

3253 Oregon Brain Injury Resource Network
345 N Monmouth Avenue
Monmouth, OR 97361

503-413-7707
877-872-7246
e-mail: tbi@wou.edu
www.tr.wou.edu/tbi/

Aims to improve access to information and services for individuals with brain injuries, their families, and the professionals who serve them. The Resource Network houses information on all aspects of brain injury, from the point of initial injury throughout the life span of the individual.

Pennsylvania

3254 Brain Injury Association of Pennsylvania
2400 Park Drive
Harrisburg, PA 17110

717-657-3601
800-383-8889
e-mail: info@biapa.org
www.biapa.org

To prevent brain injury and improve the quality of life for people who have experienced brain injury and their family members through support, education, advocacy, and research.

Drew Nagele, President

3255 Pittsburgh Area Brain Injury Alliance
630 Bascom Avenue
Pittsburgh, PA 15212

412-481-0443
e-mail: jp@pabia.org
www.pabia.org

Dedicated to the people recovering from Brain Injury and who live with the consequences of Traumatic Brain Injury. The purpose is to provide a forum for peer-to-peer support and to assist in the development of peer-to-peer support groups in Western Pennsylvania.

Ed Crinnion, President

Rhode Island

3256 Brain Injury Association of Rhode Island
935 Park Avenue, Suite 8
Cranston, RI 02910

401-461-6599
Fax: 401-461-6561
e-mail: braininjuryctr@biaofri.org
biaofri.org

To improve the quality of life for people with brain injuries and their families, and to develop and support programs that prevent brain injuries.

Paula O'Connor, President
Sharon Brinkworth, Executive Director

South Carolina

3257 Brain Injury Alliance of South Carolina
920 St. Andrews Road
Columbia, SC 29210

803-731-9823
800-290-6461
Fax: 803-731-0589
e-mail: scbraininjury@bellsouth.net
www.biausa.org/SC/

Mission is to create a better future through brain injury prevention, research, education and advocacy.

Philip Clarkson, President
Robert E Brabham, PhD, Executive Director

3258 Brain Injury Association of South Carolina
920 St Andrews Road
Columbia, SC 29210

803-731-9823
800-290-6461
Fax: 803-731-0589
e-mail: scbraininjury@bellsouth.net
www.biausa.org/SC/

To create a better future through brain injury prevention, education, and advocacy.

Philip Clarkson, President
Joyce Davis, Executive Director

3259 South Carolina Brain Injury Task Force Affiliated with National Brain Injury
1030 St Andrews Road
Columbia, SC 29210

803-731-0588
800-290-6461
Fax: 803-731-0589
e-mail: scbraininjury@mindspring.com

Robert Bramble, MD, Executive Director

Tennessee

3260 Brain Injury Association of Tennessee
151 Athens Way, Suite 100
Nashville, TN 37228

615-248-5878
877-757-2428
Fax: 615-248-5879
e-mail: biaoftn@yahoo.com
www.biaoftn.org

The mission is to improve the quality of life for persons with brain injuries and their families and to reduce the incidence of brain injury.

Cheryl Spencer, President
Stephanie Pruitt, Executive Director

Texas

3261 Brain Injury Association of Texas
316 W 12th Street, Suite 405
Austin, TX 78701

512-326-1212
800-392-0040
Fax: 512-478-3370
e-mail: info@biatx.org
www.biatx.org

A non-profit public service organization, strives to meet the urgent need to develop programs for public awareness and education, to support research and rehabilitation and to provide family guidance.

Dr Margaret Struchen, President

Utah

3262 Brain Injury Association of Utah
1800 SW Temple, Suite 203
Salt Lake City, UT 84115

801-484-2240
800-281-8442
Fax: 801-484-5932
e-mail: biau@sisna.com
www.biau.org

Created in 1984, the only non-profit organization dedicated exclusively to education and support for the issues of prevention and recovery of brain injury in the state of Utah. The mission of the Brain Injury Association of Utah is to create a better future through brain injury prevention, research, education and advocacy.

Jeffrey Eisenberg, President
Ron Roskos

Vermont

3263 Brain Injury Association of Vermont
PO Box 226
Shelburne, VT 05482

802-985-8440
877-856-1772
e-mail: biavtinfo@adelphia.net
www.biavt.org

To create a better future through brain injury, prevention, research, education, and advocacy.

Bob Luce, President

Virginia

3264 Brain Injury Association of Virginia
3212 Cutshaw Avenue, Suite 315
Richmond, VA 23230

804-355-5748
800-334-8443
Fax: 804-355-6381
e-mail: infoa@biav.net
www.biav.net

Nonprofit organization Creating a better future through brain injury education, awareness, advocacy, and support.

Irv Cantor, President
Anne McDonnell, Executive Director

Washington

3265 Brain Injury Association of Washington
800 Jefferson Street, Suite 600
Seattle, WA 98104

206-388-0900
800-523-5438
Fax: 206-388-0901
e-mail: biawa@biawa.org
www.biawa.org

The mission, which begins with prevention, is to provide support to survivors of brain injury and their families, education to those who are being effected by brain injury, including the general public, and advocacy, to give the many suffering from this silent epidemic a public voice.

Richard Adler, President
Gene van den Bosch, Executive Director

3266 Head Injury Hotline
Brain Injury Resource Center
212 Pioneer Building
Seattle, WA 98104

206-621-8558
Fax: 206-624-4961
e-mail: brain@headinjury.com
www.headinjury.com

Disseminates head injury information and provides referrals to facilitate adjustment to life following head injury. Organizes seminars for professionals, head injury survivors, and their families. Our intention is to help you avoid much of the greif and loss of brain injury, and perhaps to inspire you to get involved.

Constance Miller, Founder

West Virginia

3267 Brain Injury Association of West Virginia
PO Box 574
Institute, WV 25112

304-766-2564
800-356-6443
Fax: 304-766-4940
e-mail: biawv@aol.com
www.biausa.org/WVirginia/

A nonprofit agency dedicated to providing support, advocacy, education and training on behalf of survivors of brain injuries, their families and those who provide services or care for them.

Michael W Davis, President

Wisconsin

3268 Brain Injury Association of Wisconsin
N 35 W21100 Capitol Drive, Suite 5
Pewaukee, WI 53072

262-790-9660
800-882-9282
Fax: 262-790-9678
e-mail: biaw@execpc.com
www.biaw.org

Established in 1980 by a group of individuals with brain injury, their families, friends, and professionals. BIAW is a chartered member affiliate of the national Brain Injury Association, Inc.

BIAW provides services in these 5 core areas: information and resources, education, prevention, advocacy, and support services

Jeff Cameron, President
Patricia David, Operations Director

Wyoming

3269 Brain Injury Association of Wyoming
111 W 2nd Street, Suite 106
Casper, WY 82601

307-473-1767
800-643-6457
Fax: 307-237-5222
e-mail: biaw@tricsp.com
www.biausa.org/Wyoming

The mission is to create a better future through brain injury prevention, research, education, and advocacy.

Dr Larry Plemmons, President
Dorothy Cronin, Executive Director

Libraries & Resource Centers

3270 Brain Injury Association of Michigan
8619 W Grand River, Suite I
Brighton, MI 48116

810-229-5880
800-772-4323
Fax: 810-229-8947
e-mail: info@biami.org
www.biami.org

A resource and information center addressing the needs of persons with brain injury, their families, and concerned professionals. Resources include written materials, and videos on various topics regarding the understanding and rehabilitation of brain injury.

Michael F Dabbs, President
Cheryl Burda, Program/Services Director

Illinois

3271 University of Illinois at Chicago, Craniofacial Center
College of Medicine
808 S Wood Street
Chicago, IL 60680

312-996-6979
Fax: 312-413-1526

Dr. Allen Goldman, Director

Research Centers

3272 Brain Injury Research Center of the Institute for Rehabilitation & Research
1333 Moursund Avenue
Houston, TX 77030

713-799-5000
e-mail: tirrreferrals@tirr.tmc.edu
www.tirr.org/research

Brings together world-renowned researchers to study the many complicated facets of recovery from brain injury. BIRC has been able to leverage resources from the US Department of Education's National Institute for Rehabilitation and Research (NIDRR) and from NIH to conduct its research in a manner that facilitates the greatest progress in identifying effective treatments.

William Donovan, MD, EVP Medical Affairs
Gerard Francisco, MD, Brain Injury Program Physician

3273 Brain Research Institute
Brain Research Institute UCLA
Box 951761
Los Angeles, CA 90095

310-825-5061
Fax: 310-206-5855
e-mail: lmaninger@mednet.ucla.edu
www.bri.ucla.edu

An organization research unit within the School of Medicine at the University of California , Los Angeles.

Christopher Evans, PhD, Director
Bernard W Balleine, PhD, Associate Director for Research

3274 Dana Alliance for Brain Initiatives
745 5th Avenue, Suite 900
New York, NY 10151

212-223-4040
Fax: 212-317-8721
e-mail: dabiinfo@dana.org
www.dana.org/brainweb

A nonprofit organization of more than 250 pre-eminent scientists dedicated to advancing education about the progress and promise of brain research.

Edward F Rover, President

3275 Rehabilitation Research and Training Center on Traumatic Brain Injury
Mt. Sinai School of Medicine, Dept. Rehabilitation
1 Gustave L Levy Place, Box 1240
New York, NY 10029

212-659-9372
Fax: 212-348-5901
e-mail: wayne.gordon@mssm.edu
www.mssm.edu/tbicentral/rrtc

Research to improve mood in people with TBI; analyze the content and quality of recently published post-TBI intervention studies; development of new measures of rehabilitation outcomes that incorporates both objective and subjective perspectives on participation in home and community activities; and a capacity building program to better educate professionals in identifying, assessing and providing appropriate interventions, treatments and accommodations for people with TBI.

Wayne A Gordon, PhD, Project Director
Allen Hafina, Research Associate

California

3276 Brain Imaging Center at the University of California, Irvine
University of California, Irvine

Irvine, CA 92697

949-824-8040
Fax: 949-824-7873
e-mail: bic@msx.hsis.uci.edu
www.bic.uci.edu

Performs clinical assessment of regional brainmetabolism for Parkinson's disease, epilepsy, brain tumor evaluation, Alzheimer'sdisease, and head injury. Other neuropsychiatric illnesses that are assessed with PETscans at UCI include stroke, psychotic disorders, and movement disorders.

Steven G Potkin, MD, Director
Jill Upton, Research Coordinator

3277 Brain and Spinal Injury Center (BASIC) Research at University of California
UCSF Department of Neurological
500 Parnassus Avenue, M779
San Francisco, CA 94143

415-476-4590
Fax: 415-476-9687
www.neurosurgery.medschool.ucsf.edu

Established to promote collaborative basic, translational, and clinical studies on injuries to the brain and spinal cord. BASIC is a joint effort between the Departments of Neurological Surgery and Neurology. Both departments bring their particular areas of expertise to a multidisciplinary effort centered on translational research.

Linda Noble-Haeusslein, PhD, Co-Director
Geoffrey T Manley, MD; PhD, Co-Director

3278 Southern California Neuropsychiatric Institute
6794 La Jolla Boulevard
La Jolla, CA 92037

619-454-2102
Fax: 619-454-2104

Sydney Walker III, MD, Director

Louisiana

3279 Tulane University, US-Japan Biomedical Research Laboratories
Herbert Research Center
3705 Main Street
Belle Chasse, LA 70037

504-394-7199
Fax: 504-394-7169
e-mail: arimura@tulane.edu
www.omi.tulane.edu/labs/usjamed

Focuses research efforts on neuroendocrinology and neurosciences.

Massachusetts

3280 Harold Goodglass Aphasia Research Center
150 S Huntington Avenue (12A)
Boston, MA 02130

617-232-9500
Fax: 617-522-4786
e-mail: aphasia@bu.edu
www.bu.edu/aphasia

Research done into cognitive and language impairment following brain damage and closely related topics.

Harold Goodglass, MD, Director

Michigan

3281 Bioengineering Center of Wayne State University
Wayne State University
818 W Hancock
Detroit, MI 48202

313-577-1347
Fax: 313-577-8333
e-mail: king@rrb.eng.wayne.edu
www.ttb.cng.wayne.edu

A leading laboratory doing research work in the areas of impact trauma, low back pain and orthopedic biomechanics. Current projects in impact trauma include research on side impact, rear end collisions, head injury and lower extremity injuries.

Albert I King, Director

3282 Rehabilitation Institute of Michigan
Detroit Medical Center/Wayne State University
261 Mack Avenue
Detroit, MI 48201

313-745-1203
Fax: 313-745-9863
www.rimrehab.org

Our dedicated group of board certified physicians are committed to improving the lives of their patients by providing quality, compassionate medical care and contributing to the science of rehabilitation medicine.

Terry Reiley, MBA/CHE, President

New York

3283 Brady Institute for Traumatic Brain Injury
Jamaica Hospital Medical Center
8900 Van Wyck Expressway
Jamaica, NY 11418

718-206-6000
e-mail: hr@jhmc.org
www.jamaicahospital.org

Provides general medical, pediatric,and psychiatric emergency services, ambulatory care, on and off campus ambulatory surgery, a broad spectrum of diagnostic and treatment services, and home health services.

3284 Stroke Rehabilitation & Traumatic Brain Injury Research
Ruft Institute at NYU Medical Center
400 E 34th Street
New York, NY 10016

212-263-5870
Fax: 212-263-8510
e-mail: yehuda.ben-yishay@med.nyu.edu
www.med.nyu.edu/rusk/research

Ways of improving problem-solving behavior in individual with acquired brain damage are being investigated and instruments measuring problem solving in interpersonal situations are being developed.

Mathew Lee, Medical Director

Ohio

3285 Ohio State University Laboratory of Psychobiology
225 Psychology Bldg., 1835 Neil Avenue
Columbus, OH 43210

614-292-8185
Fax: 614-292-4537
www.psy.ohio-state.edu

Studies done on recovery of function after brain damage.

Pennsylvania

3286 Institutes for Achievement of Human Potential
8801 Stenton Avenue
Wyndmoor, PA 19038

215-233-2050
800-344-8322
Fax: 215-233-9312
e-mail: institutes@iahp.org
www.iahp.org

A teaching institute that focuses on home-based neurological training for brain-injured children. Commited to the significant increases of the ability of all children to perform in the physical, intellectual and social realms. Our work has led to powerful insights about the brain and, especially, about its development in the neonate and very young children. We have developed exciting concepts and practices applied by parents at home, to mulitply the intelligence of tiny children.

500 members

Janet Duman, Director
Glenn Doman, Founder

3287 Thomas Jefferson University Brain Injury Rehabilitation Program
Thomas Jefferson University Hospital
111 South 11th Street
Philadelphia, PA 19107

215-587-3398
www.jeffersonhospital.org/rehab/

Provides coordinated, multidisciplinary acute medical and surgical care for all levels of brain injury. The program delivers care for the acute phases of injury at Jefferson and shifts follow-up care to Magee Rehabilitation Hospital.

Daniel Weinstein, MD, Medical Director

Tennessee

3288 University of Memphis Neuropsychology Lab

Department of Psychology
202 Psychology Building, Room 126
Memphis, TN 38152

901-678-2147
Fax: 901-678-2579
www.psyc.memphis.edu/psc

Evaluation and development of assessment and treatment procedures for neurologically impaired persons.

Dr. Charles Long, Director

Texas

3289 Institute for Rehabilitation and Research

1333 Moursund Avenue
Houston, TX 77030

713-799-5000
800-477-3422
e-mail: tirrreferrals@tirr.tmc.edu
www.tirr.org

Our mission is to create partnerships, exceed expectations, excel in care, optimize resources, provide value, research for breakthroughs, serve the community, share knowledge and unleash human potential.

L Don Lehmkuhl, PhD, Director

Virginia

3290 Virginia Commonwealth University Department of Neurosurgery Research

PO Box 980631
Richmond, VA 23298

804-828-9165
Fax: 804-828-0374
www.neurosurgery.vcu.edu

Studies include work on cerebral blood flow, subarachnoid hemorrhage, vasospasm, ischemia, metabolism, cerebral edema, elevated intracranial pressure, trauma, secondary neural insults, CNS tumor biology, clinical trials for new brain tumor therapies, spinal biomechanics, computer imaging on the CNS and immunology of the nervous system.

M.R. Bullock, MD, Research Director

Audio Video

3291 Face First

Fanlight Productions
4196 Washington Street, Suite 2
Boston, MA 02131

617-469-4999
800-937-4113
Fax: 617-469-3379
e-mail: fanlight@fanlight.com
www.fanlight.com

Profiles of several people born with facial deformities; they chronicle both physical pain and the pain of rejection, as well as the strengths that have enabled them to achieve successful adult lives.

1998 29 Minutes VHS
ISBN: 1-572952-59-8

Nicole Johnson, Publicity Coordinator

3292 Surviving Coma: the Journey Back

Brain Injury Association of Mississippi
2727 Old Canton Road
Jackson, MS 39296

601-981-1021
Fax: 601-981-1039
e-mail: biaofms@aol.com

A realistic presentation about coma survival and the problems encountered during the long journey through rehabilitation.

19 Minutes

Paul Gospodarski, Ed.D, Executive Director

Web Sites

3293 Brain Injury Association

www.biausa.org

Founded in 1980, the leading national organization serving and representing individuals, families and professionals who are touched by a life-altering, often devastating, traumatic brain injury (TBI).

3294 Brain Research Institute (BRI) School of Medicine University of California LA

www.bri.ucla.edu

BRI's mission is to increase understanding of how the brain works, how it dvelops, and how it responds to experience, injury and disease, and to help make UCLA the preeminent center for translating basic knowledge into medical interventions and new technologies.

3295 Centre for Neuro Skills

www.neuroskills.com

The TBI Resource Guide is the internet's central source of information, services, and products relating to traumatic brain injury, brain injury recovery, and post-acute rehabilitation.

3296 Dana Alliance for Brain Initiatives

www.dana.org/brainweb

Is a nonprofit organization of more then 200 neuroscientists, formed to help provide information about the personal and public benefits of brain research. Today one out of five Americans suffers from a brain-related disease or disorder, ranging from cocain addiction to learning diabilities from Alzheimer's disease to spinal cord injuries.

3297 Family Caregiver Alliance

www.caregiver.org

The FCA is a public voice for caregivers. Our pioneering programs, information, education, services, research, and advocacy, support and sustain the important work of families nationwide caring for loved ones with chronic, disabling health conditions.

3298 NIH/National Institute of Neurological Dis orders and Stroke (NINDS)

www.ninds.nih.gov

The mission of NINDS is to reduce the burden of neurological disease, a burden borne by every age group, by every segment of society, by people all over the world.

3299 Northeast Rehabilitation Health Network

www.northeastrehab.com

We provide services within a continuum of care to individuals and families whos lives have been impcated by illness or injury in order to restore stability and maximize their potential for independence, functional abilites, and quality of life. In addition, we provide services that encourage well being. Our customers include: patients, families, physicians, referrers, payers, employees and the community.

3300 Perspectives Network

www.tbi.org

It's primary focus is positive communications between persons with brain injury, family members, caregivers, friends of persons with brain injury, those many professionals who treat persons with brain injury and community members in order to create positive changes and enhance public awareness and knowledge of acquired, traumatic brain injury.

3301 Traumatic Brain Injury Model Systems Natio nal Data and Statistical Center

www.tbindc.org

The TBIMS program seeks to improve the lives of persons who experience traumatic brain injury, their families and their communities by creating and disseminating new knowledge about the course, treatment and outcomes relating to their condtion.

Book Publishers

3302 Children With Traumatic Brain Injury: A Pa rents Guide

Lisa Schoenbrodt, EdD, author

Peytral Publications
P.O. Box 1162
Minnetonka, MN 55345

952-949-8707
877-739-8725
Fax: 952-906-9777
www.peytral.com

Informative handbook for parents of children and teens; covers medical, educational, legal, family life, daily care, emotional issues and more.

482 pages

3303 Children with Traumatic Brain Injury

Peytral Publications
PO Box 1162
Minnetonka, MN 55345

952-949-8707
877-739-8725
Fax: 952-949-8707
www.peytral.com

Comprehensive, must-have reference that provides parent with the support and information needed to help their child recover from a closed-head injury. Written by a team of medical specialists, therapists, educators and an attorney this publications covers medical concerns, rehabilitation, treatment, adjustment, effects on learning, thinking, language behavior and more.

482 pages

Lisa Schoenbrodt, EdD, Editor

3304 Cognitive Effects of Early Brain Injury

John's Hopkins University Press
2715 N Charles Street
Baltimore, MD 21218

410-516-6900
Fax: 410-516-6998
www.press.jhu.edu

This book offers a detailed overview of the effects of genetic, prenatal, and perinatal brain disorders on cognitive development and learning in children. Summarizing the available data as well as presenting previously unpublished research, the book provides clinicians with practical information that will aid their diagnostic and therapeutic work with children who have sustained early brain injury.

1994 336 pages Hardcover
ISBN: 0-801848-56-3

3305 Cognitive Rehabilitation for Persons with Traumatic Brain Injury

Paul H Brookes Publishing/Brookes
PO Box 10624
Baltimore, MD 21285

410-337-9580
800-638-3775
Fax: 410-337-8539
e-mail: custserv@brookespublishing.com
www.brookespublishing.com

Virtually all persons with brain injury retain ability to learn. Cognitive rehab is a set of stategies to improve problems. Reports on theory, practices, research, consequences of brain trauma and assessment & intervention. Case studies.

1991 299 pages Hardcover
ISBN: 1-557660-71-9

Jeffrey S Kreutzer, Editor
Paul H Wehman, Editor

3306 Communication Following Traumatic Brain Injury

Pro-Ed
8700 Shoal Creek Boulevard
Austin, TX 78757

512-451-3246
800-897-3202
Fax: 512-451-8542
e-mail: feedback@proedinc.com
www.proedinc.com

For graduates and professionals, this text takes a holistic approach toward treating the client with traumatic brain injury.

1990 439 pages Paperback
ISBN: 0-316092-51-7

3307 From the Ashes

Brain Injury Resource Center
212 Pioneer Building
Seattle, WA 98104

206-621-8558
e-mail: brain@headinjury.com
www.headinjury.com/ashesord.htm

An enduring resource for survivors, families and the professionals serving them.

1987 108 pages
ISBN: 0-963659-40-5

Constance Miller, Editor
Kay Campbell, Editor

3308 Handbook of Head Truma: Acute Care to Recovery

Springer Publishing Company
11 W 42nd Street, 15th Floor
New York, NY 10036

877-687-7476
e-mail: contactus@springerpub.com
www.springerpub.com

Providing a thorough collection of information regarding clinical aspects of head injury from acute care to recovery, this treatise interrelates a variety of neural specialties and broadens the rehabilitation process to include the family

1992 472 pages
ISBN: 0-306439-47-6

Charles Long, Editor
Leslie Ross, Editor

3309 Head Injury in Children and Adolescents: A Resource and Review for School

John Wiley & Sons
10475 Crosspoint Boulevard
Indianapolis, IN 46256

877-762-2974
Fax: 800-597-3299
e-mail: consumers@wiley.com
www.wiley.com

Complex nature of traumatic brain injury and its implications are examined carefully from medical, neuropsychological, rehabilitative and educational perspectives. Contents are arranged in a spiraling manner to provide the reader with a progressive and practical appreciation of traumatic brain injury and its neurobehavioral effects.

260 pages Hardcover
ISBN: 0-884220-98-2

Vivian Begali, Editor

3310 Head Trauma Sourcebook
Omnigraphics
PO Box 625
Holmes, PA 19043

800-234-1340
Fax: 800-875-1340
e-mail: info@omnigraphics.com
omnigraphics.com

Basic consumer information for the layperson about open-head and closed-head injuries, treatment advances, recovery and rehabilitation.

414 pages
ISBN: 0-780802-08-X

Karen Bellenir, Editor

3311 Let's Talk About Going to the Hospital
Rosen Publishing Group's PowerKids Press
29 E 21st Street
New York, NY 10010

212-777-3017
800-237-9932
Fax: 888-436-4643
e-mail: rosenpub@tribeca.ios.com
www.powerkidspress.com

If a child has to check into the hospital, chances are he or she is already upset about being ill. Knowing how a hospital functions and what the procedures are, such as when family members can visit, will help in what is already a stressful situation. Grades K-5.

24 pages
ISBN: 0-823950-36-0

3312 What To Do About Your Brain Injured Child
National Book Network
8801 Stenton Avenue
Wyndmoor, PA 19038

215-233-2050
800-344-8322
Fax: 215-233-3940
e-mail: institutes@iahp.org
www.iahp.org

The author reveals life saving techniques to measure mobility, language, and manual, visual, auditory and tactile development.

318 pages
ISBN: 1-591170-23-0

Glen Doman, Editor

Magazines

3313 Brain Injury Source
Brain Injury Association of America
8201 Greensboro Drive, Suite 611
McLean, VA 22102

703-761-0750
Fax: 703-761-0755
e-mail: Publications@biausa.org
www.biausa.org

Written for and by professionals in the field. Blends professionally written articles on information and research in brain injury with a user friendly format that incorporates graphics and charts to effectively deliver the messages. Full color.

50+ pages Quarterly

Susan H Connors, President/CEO
Pat Britz, Information Director

Journals

3314 Journal of Head Trauma Rehabilitation
Aspen Publishers
7201 McKinney Circle
Frederick, MD 21704

800-234-1660
Fax: 800-901-9075
www.aspenpublishers.com

A leading, peer-reviewed resource that provides up-to-date information on the clinical management and rehabilitation of persons with traumatic brain injuries. The journal is comprised of feature articles, brief reports, pharmacological updates, legislative and public policy updates, columns on ethics, book reviews, abstracts of selected literature, and more.

Mitchell Rosenthal, MD, Editor

Newsletters

3315 American Brain Tumor Association Message Line
2720 River Road
Des Plaines, IL 60018

847-827-9910
800-886-2282
Fax: 847-827-9918
e-mail: abta@aol.com
www.abta.org

Offers association news, events, fundraising and convention news, as well as medical and legislative updates for patients and their families.

Quarterly

3316 Headlines
Brain Injury Association of Minnesota
34 13th Avenue NE
Minneapolis, MN 55414

612-378-2742
800-669-6442
Fax: 612-378-2789
e-mail: info@braininjurymn.org
www.braininjurymn.org

Published for the families and professionals who are involved with brain injuries. We also have an e-mail newsletter that reaches several hundred.

Quarterly

Ardis Sandstrom, Executive Director
Brad Donaldson, Associate Director of Operations

3317 Heads Up Ohio
Brain Injury Association of Ohio
1335 Dublin Road, Suite 217D
Columbus, OH 43215

614-481-7100
800-686-9563
Fax: 614-481-7103
e-mail: help@biaoh.org
www.biaoh.org

Reports on the members' achievements, public policy affecting the disability community and information and opportunities about services, supports and/or training.

16 pages Quarterly

Suzanne Minnich, Editor

3318 Headway

Brain Injury Association of Virginia
3212 Cutshaw Avenue, Suite 315
Richmond, VA 23230

804-355-5748
800-334-8443
Fax: 804-355-6381
e-mail: biav@visi.net
www.nvbia.org

Information and resources for individuals with brain injury, their family members and professionals dealing with brain injury.

16 pages Quarterly

Michelle Ward, Editor
Stephen Smith, President

3319 TBI Challenge

Brain Injury Association of America
8201 Greensboro Drive, Suite 611
McLean, VA 22102

703-761-0750
Fax: 703-761-0755
e-mail: familyhelpline@biausa.org
www.biausa.org

Exclusively for and about persons with brain injury. Provides information to individuals with brain injury and their families. Professionals will benefit from the perspectives provided in Kid's Corner, Relatively Speaking, Ask the Lawyer, Information and Resources and Ask the Doctor.

Quarterly

Susan H Connors, President/CEO
Pat Britz, Information Director

3320 The Headliner

Brain Injury Association of Oregon
2145 NW Overton Street
Portland, OR 97210

503-413-7707
800-544-5243
Fax: 503-413-6849
e-mail: biaor@biaoregon.org
www.biaoregon.org

To improve the quality of life of persons with brain injury and their families; and to prevent brain injury.

16 pages Quarterly

Sherry Stock, Executive Director

Pamphlets

3321 Brain Injury Glossary

HDI Publishers
2407 Waugh Drive, PO Box 131401
Houston, TX 77219

713-526-6900
800-321-7037
Fax: 713-526-7787
www.braininjurybooks.com

Contains special sections on terms relating to insurance, definitions relating to The Americans with Disabilities Act and descriptions of commonly prescribed medications. The Brain Injury Glossary is a must for all persons working or involved in brain injury rehabilitation.

1993 46 pages

L Don Lehmkuhl, Editor

3322 Brain Injury Update

HDI Publishers
2407 Waugh Drive, PO Box 131401
Houston, TX 77219

713-526-6900
800-321-7037
Fax: 713-526-7787
www.braininjurybooks.com

Monthly digest of news and information from the brain injury research and rehabilitation fields. Expanded summaries of journal articles, research papers, news releases and government reports are provided in a concise, time saving format. Brain Injury Update also provides information on grant opportunities, pharmacological intervention, calls for papers, people in the news, listings of upcoming conferences and symposia, legal and legislative developments and advances in prevention.

1991 Annual

Dr. Linda Thoi, Editor-in-Chief
Nathan D Zasler, MD, Contributing Editor

3323 Clinical Trials in Head Injury

National Inst. of Neurological Disorders/Stroke
31 Center Drive, MSC 2540, Building 31, Room 8A06
Bethesda, MD 20892

301-496-5751
800-352-9424

3324 Shaken Baby Syndrome

National Inst. of Neurological Disorders/Stroke
PO Box 5801
Bethesda, MD 20892

301-496-5751
800-352-9424

Camps

3325 Association for Neurologically Impaired Brain Injured Children

212-12 26th Avenue
Bayside, NY

718-423-9550
Fax: 718-423-9838
e-mail: info@anibic.org

ANIBIc is a voluntary, multi-service organization that is dedicated to serving individuals with severe learning disabilities, neurological impairments and other developmental disabilities. Services include: residential, vocational, family support services, recreation (children and adults), respite (adult), summer day camp, counseling, and tramatic brain injury services (adults).

Jeanne Parisi, Executive Director
Lisa Eisenberg, Director Family Support Services

3326 Bancroft NeuroHealth

Hopkins Lane
Haddonfield, NJ 800-7

856-429-0010
800-800-774
Fax: 856-429-4755
www.bancroftneurohealth.org

The Bancroft Institution is a nonprofit organization which provides professional training; disseminates information and best practices in the fields of developmental disabilities and brain injury.

George Niemann, PhD, Chief Executive
Joseph Hess Jr, President

3327 Camp Barefoot

Brain Injury Association of Michigan
8619 W Grand River, Suite I
Brighton, MI 48116

810-229-5880
800-772-4323
Fax: 810-229-8947
e-mail: info@biami.org
www.biami.org

Primary goal of our recreational programming is to give people who have experienced a brain injury a normal camping experience. Dedicated to providing quality summer camping experiences for people who sustained a brain injury. Over six days, Camp Barefoot provides structured, enriching personal and recreational experiences for people with brain injury.

Cheryl Burda, Programs/Services Director
Katie Walsh, Program Coordinator

3328 Camp Hickory Wood

Traumatic Brain Injury Program
425 5th Avenue N, Cordell Hull Building
Nashville, TN 37243

800-882-0611
www2.state.tn.us/health/TBI

Each year the TBI Program in collaboration with Easter Seals Tennessee Inc. sponsors a weekend and a weeklong camp for adult and youth survivors of brain injury. These camps focus on providing a unique social and recreational opportunity to persons with brain injury. Nestled between the banks of Old Hickory Lake and surrounded by protective woods, camp offers great outdoor fun.

3329 Oklahoma Brain Injury Camp

Oklahoma Brain Injury Association
PO Box 88
Hillsdale, OK 73743

405-364-8118
e-mail: information@braininjuryoklahoma.org
www.braininjuryoklahoma.org

An annual camp for brain injury survivors sponsored by the Brain Injury Association of Oklahoma. Great fun had by all with music, games, crafts, a hayride, cookout, bingo, fishing, and paddle boat rides.

Cathe Fox, Camp Director

DESCRIPTION

3330 HEARING IMPAIRMENT/DEAFNESS

Covers these related disorders: Conductive deafness or hearing loss, Mixed hearing loss, Sensorineural deafness or hearing loss

Involves the following Biologic System(s):

Neurologic Disorders

Hearing impairment may be defined as a loss of the ability to hear that is sufficient enough to impede the ability to communicate. Deafness refers to severe or profound hearing loss. Hearing loss or deafness may occur as the result of hereditary factors or birth defects. Hearing loss may also be acquired and occur after birth (e.g., from disease or physical damage to the hearing mechanism). However, genetic factors are thought to be responsible for moderate to severe hearing loss in about half of affected children. Hearing loss may be further categorized into three types: conductive, sensorineural, or mixed.

Conductive hearing loss occurs as a result of the faulty transmission of sound through the external or middle ear to the inner ear. This transmission problem may be due to infections of the middle ear (otitis media), damage to the eardrum or bones of the middle ear, the absence or the narrowing of the ear canal, impacted earwax (cerumen), foreign bodies in the ear canal, or other physical causes. In addition, conductive hearing loss is sometimes inherited as a feature of certain syndromes such as Klippel-Feil syndrome, Crouzon syndrome, osteogenesis imperfecta, and others. In children with sensorineural hearing loss, sounds are conducted to the inner ear through the external and middle ear, but are not transmitted from there to the brain. This occurs as the result of a defect in the structure of the inner ear or problems with the nerve that conveys impulses from the inner ear to the brain (auditory nerve; acoustic nerve; eighth cranial nerve). Sensorineural hearing loss that results from defects of inner ear structures is considered sensory and include the absence or underdevelopment of the snail shell-type tubular structure of the inner ear (cochlea); damage to hair cells or other inner ear structures from prolonged exposure to loud noise, certain drugs, viral infections or other diseases; and other irregularities. Sensorineural hearing loss that results from damage to the auditory nerve pathway is considered neural and may be due to brain lesions or tumors; childhood disorders such as German measles, mumps, inner ear infections, etc.; certain hereditary disorders (e.g., Waardenburg syndrome, Usher syndrome, etc.); diseases that affect the myelin sheath, which is the fatty, protective, insulating covering on certain nerve fibers (demyelinating diseases); or seizures. Mixed hearing loss refers to a combination of both conductive and sensorineural hearing loss.

Early screening for hearing loss is important in order to provide early intervention that will allow the best outcome for educational and social development. Treatment may require the cooperation of parents, caregivers, pediatricians, speech and language pathologists, and specialists in hearing loss (aud|iologists) who assess the extent of hearing loss through the use of specialized tests. Infant screening by specialists may include tests that gauge behavioral responses to noise through observation, , such as a startle response to a sudden hand clap. Other tests may electronically assess hearing loss (audiometry); measure the head-turning response of an infant or toddler using animated aids in conjunction with sounds emitted through a loudspeaker (visual reinforcement audiometry or VRA); measure the lowest intensity at which certain words are heard or understood (speech recognition threshold or SRT); measure the ability of the middle ear to impede or resist sound energy (tympanometry); differentiate between sensory and neural hearing loss (auditory brain stem response); measure the integrity of the cochlea (otoacoustic emissions or OAEs); or other specialized tests. Treatment for conductive hearing loss may include the removal of fluid, earwax, or foreign bodies through drainage or other means. Surgical intervention may be indicated for the correction of structural abnormalities. Children as well as infants with hearing loss may benefit from the use of certain types of hearing aids; however, repeat testing is necessary to provide more exact hearing aid specification. In addition, cochlear implants are now available to children with severe or profound hearing loss. Other treatment is directed toward the teaching of communication skills such as lip-reading, sign language, and speech. Cooperation and support of family, me|dical specialists, and educators is important in determining the best approach for the education and social development of the individual child.

See also **General Resources** on page 917

Government Agencies

3331 Deafness and Communicative Disorders Branch
Department of Education
400 Maryland Avenue SW
Washington, DC 20202

202-205-5465
Fax: 202-205-9772
TTY: 202-205-8352
cd.gov

Promotes improved and expanded rehabilitation services for deaf and hard-of-hearing people and individuals with speech or language impairments.

Victor Galloway, EdD, Branch Chief

National Associations & Support Groups

3332 Academy of Rehabilitative Audiology
PO Box 952
DeSoto, TX 55426

952-920-0484
Fax: 952-920-6098
e-mail: ara@audrehab.org
www.audrehab.org

The primary purpose of ARA is to promote excellence in hearing care through the provision of comprehensive rehabilitative and habilitative services.

350 Members

Perry C Hanavan, President
Kemberly Peters, Secretary

3333 Alexander Graham Bell Association for the Deaf and Hearing Impaired
Alexander Graham Bell Association for the Deaf
3417 Volta Place NW
Washington, DC 20007

202-337-5220
800-432-7543
Fax: 202-337-8314
TTY: 202-337-5221
e-mail: info@agbell.org
www.agbell.org

The Alexander Graham Bell Association for the Deaf and Hard of Hearing (AG bell) is a lifelong resource,support network and advocate for listening,learning,talking and living independently with hearing loss. Through publications, advocacy,training,scholarships and financial aid,AG Bell promotes the use of spoken language and hearing technology.

Wendy Will, Executive Assistant

3334 American Academy of Audiology
11730 Plaza America Drive, Suite 300
Reston, VA 20190

703-790-8466
800-222-2336
Fax: 703-790-8631
e-mail: info@audiology.org
www.audiology.org

A professional organization dedicated to providing high quality and balanced hearing care to the public. Provides professional development, education and research and provides increased public awareness of hearing disorders and audiologic services.

Laura Fleming Doyle, CAE, Executive Director
Cheryl Kreider Carey, Deputy Executive Director

3335 American Association of the Deaf-Blind
8630 Fenton Street, Suite 121
Silver Spring, MD 20910

301-495-4403
Fax: 301-495-4404
TTY: 301-495-4402
e-mail: ADDB-Info@aadb.org
www.aadb.org

The American Association of the Deaf-Blind is a national consumer organization of, by, and for people with both vision and hearing losses. AADB is a non-profit organization governed by by-laws and a board of directors, the majority of whom are deaf-blind. Its mission is to enable deaf-blind persons to achieve their maximum potential through increased independence, productivity and integration into the community.

600 Members

Arthur Roehrig, President
Marilyn Fernandez, Secretary

3336 American Deafness and Rehabilitation Assoc iation (ADARA)
PO Box 251554
Little Rock, AR 72225

501-868-8850
Fax: 501-868-8812

A network of professionals who serve people who are deaf or hard of hearing

3337 American Hearing Research Foundation
8 S Michigan Avenue, Suite 814
Chicago, IL 60603

312-726-9670
Fax: 312-726-9695
e-mail: ahrf@american-hearing.org
www.american-hearing.org

As a not-profit organization, a major source of our income is through donations. We have received generous contributions from individuals, corporations, and institutions, and continue to rely on these donations to found future research.

William L. Lederer, Executive Director
Lorraine L. Koch, Assistant Director

3338 American Society for Deaf Children
3820 Hartzdale Drive
Camp Hill, PA 17011

717-703-0073
866-895-4206
Fax: 717-909-5599
e-mail: asdc@deafchildren.org
www.deafchildren.org

A nonprofit parent-helping-parent organization promoting a positive attitude toward signing and deaf culture. Also provides support, encouragement, and current information about deafness to families with deaf and hard-of-hearing children.

Roger Williams, Co-President
Sherry Williams, Co-President

3339 American Speech Language Hearing Associati on (ASHA)
10801 Rockville Pike
Rockville, MD 20852

301-897-5700
800-638-8255
Fax: 301-571-0457
TTY: 301-897-0157
e-mail: actioncenter@asha.org
www.asha.org

ASHA is the professional, scientific and credentialling association for more than 123,000 members and affiliates who are speech-language pathologists, audiologists, and speech, language, and hearing scientists. Their mission is to promote the interests of and provide the highest quality services for proesstionals, and to advocate for people with communication disabilities.

Arlene A Pietranton, Executive Director

3340 Auditory - Verbal International
2121 Eisenhower Avenue, Suite 402
Alexandria, VA 22314

703-739-1049
Fax: 703-739-0395
TTY: 703-739-0874
e-mail: audiverb@aol.com

Provides the choice of listening and speaking as the way of life for children and adults who are deaf or hard of hearing. Through the use of assistive technology such as digital hearing aids or cochlear implants and auditory-verbal therapy, many deaf and hard of hearing children can learn to listen and speak.

900 members

Sara Lake, Executive Director/CEO
Steven Rech JD, President

3341 BEGINNINGS for Parents of Hearing Impaired Children
PO Box 17646
Raleigh, NC 27619

919-850-2746
800-541-4327
Fax: 919-850-2804
TTY: 919-850-2746
e-mail: raleigh@ncbegin.org
www.ncbegin.com

BEGINNINGS provides emotional support and access to information to information as a central resource for families with deaf or hard of hearing children, age birth through 21. These services are also available to deaf parents who have hearing children. Their mission is to help parents to be informed, empowered and supported as they make decisions about their child. In addition, they are committed to providing technical assistance to professionals who work with these families.

Joni Y Alberg, Executive Director
Christene A Tashjian, Assistant Executive Director

3342 Better Hearing Institute
515 King Street, Suite 420
Alexandria, VA 22314

703-684-3391
800-327-9355
Fax: 703-684-6048
TTY: 703-642-0580
e-mail: mail@betterhearing.org
www.betterhearing.org

A nonprofit educational organization that implements national public information programs on hearing loss and available medical, surgical, hearing aid, and rehabilitation assistance for millions with uncorrected hearing problems. Its award-winning series of television, radio, and print media public service messages include many celebrities who overcame hearing loss. BHI maintains a toll-free Hotline HelpLine telephone service that provides information on hearing loss and hearing help to callers.

Sergei Kochkin, PhD, Executive Director
Sasha Ward, Administrative Director

3343 Center for Early Intervention of Deafness (CEID)
1035 Grayson Street
Berkeley, CA 94710

510-848-4800
Fax: 510-848-4801
TDD: 510-527-5196
e-mail: ceid@ceid.org
www.ceid.org

A non-profit organization dedicated to providing a program of intensive and comprehensive early intervention services to young children up to five years old who have hearing losses or severe speech/language delays and their families. CEID uses 'Total Communication', which includes the simultaneous use of spoken English, audition, and literal representation of sign language (SEE signing), in a play based curriculum incorporting thematic active learning strategies and total family involvement.

Jill Ellis, MEd, Executive Director
Cindy Dickeson, Program Manager

3344 Children's Legal Advocacy Program (CLA)
Alexander Graham Bell Association for the Deaf
3417 Volta Place NW
Washington, DC 20007

202-337-5220
800-432-7543
Fax: 202-337-8314
TTY: 202-337-5221
e-mail: ghanna@agbell.org
www.agbell.org

Supports families of children who are deaf or hard of hearing by providing legal representation and technical assistance to families who need help obtaining appropriate services in their communities.

3345 Cochlear Implant Assocciation
5335 Wisconsin Avenue NW, Suite 440
Washington, DC 20015

202-895-2781
Fax: 202-895-2782
e-mail: C_I_A_I_info@cici.org
www.cici.org

A non-profit organization dedicated to educating and supporting cochlear implant recipients and their familiies; advocating and promoting cochlear implants.

John McCelland, President
Lorie Singer, VP

3346 Council on Education of the Deaf
California State University, Deaf Study Department
405 White Hall College of Education
Kent, OH 44242

330-672-0735
Fax: 330-672-2498
TTY: 330-672-2396
e-mail: mhoverst@kent.edu
www.monster.educ.kent.edu/deaf

Offers information and referral services to the hearing impaired.

Lawrence R Fleischer, EdD, President

3347 Deaf REACH
3512 12th Street NE
Washington, DC 20017

202-832-6681
Fax: 202-832-8454
TTY: 202-832-6681
www.deaf-reach.org

Nonprofit organization: our mission is to maximize the self-sufficiency of deaf adults needing special services by providing referral, education, advocacy, counseling, and housing.

Rudy Gawlik, President
Peter Goodman, VP

3348 Dial-a-Hearing Screening Test
300 S Chester Road
Swathmore, PA 19018

610-544-7700
800-222-3277
Fax: 610-543-2802
e-mail: dahst@aol.com
www.dialatest.com

National telephone hearing screening test service. Consumers receive a copy of their hearing screening test results and referral to a hearing health care center in the Dial A Hearing Screening Test network. Flexible participation plans for hearing health care providers.

George Biddle, President
James Biddle, Vice President

3349 EAR Foundation
PO Box 330867
Nashville, TN 37203

615-627-2724
800-545-4327
Fax: 615-627-2728
TDD: 615-627-2724
e-mail: info@earfoundation.org
www.earfoundation.org

The EAR foundation has three basic purposes: to provide the general public support services promoting the integration of the hearing and balance impaired into mainstream society; to provide practicing ear specialists continuing medical education courses and related programs specifically regarding rehabilitation and hearing preservation; and to educate young people and adults about hearing preservation and early detection of hearing loss, enabling them to prevent hearing and balance disorders.

Michael E Glasscock, III, MD, Founder and President
Steve Masic, Chair

3350 Genetic Center
800 Florida Avenue NE, HMB
Washington, DC 20002

202-651-5385
800-451-8834
Fax: 202-651-5521
TDD: 202-651-5258
e-mail: david.snyder@gallaudet.edu

Professional genetic services are available for deaf and hard-of-hearing individuals and couples who wish to better understand the cause and future implications of their deafness; parents of deaf and hard-of-hearing children who want information about the cause of their children's hearing loss and the potential for having other chidren with hearing loss; and individuals with a history of hearing loss in their family who have questions about the effects on future generations

3351 Hands Organization
2501 W 103rd Street
Chicago, IL 60655

773-239-6632

Advocacy for the deaf and hard-of-hearing; information and referrals, educational events, sign language summer youth camps and newsletters.

Kate Kubey, Contact

3352 Hear Now
9745 E Hampden Avenue, Suite 300
Denver, CO 80231

303-695-7797
800-648-4327
Fax: 303-695-7789
TTY: 800-648-4327
e-mail: 76350.650@compuserve.com

Committed to making technology accessible to deaf and hard-of-hearing individuals throughout the United States. Also raises funds to provide hearing aids, cochlear implants and related services to children and adults who have hearing losses but do not have financial resources to purchase their own devices.

Bernice Dinner, MA, CCC, President/Founder
Elaine Hansen

3353 Hearing Impairments Better Hearing Institute
PO Box 1840
Washington, DC 20013

800-327-9355
Fax: 703-750-9302
TTY: 800-EAR-WELL

To educate the public and medical profession about hearing loss, its treatment and prevention.

3354 HearingPlanet
100 Westwood Place, Suite 300
Brentwood, TN 37027

615-248-5910
800-432-7669
Fax: 615-248-5903
www.hearingplanet.com

A hearing specialist is ready to answer questions about hearing aids, hearing loss and treatments.

3355 Hearts and Homes For Youth
1320 Fenwick Lane, Suite 800
Silver Spring, MD 20910

301-589-8444
Fax: 301-495-0923
e-mail: sponlts@juno.com
www.hh4y.org

Helps troubled children and youth who are abused, neglected or runaways, become independent, productive adults. To fulfill this mission, HHY provides a broad spectrum of educational, residential, independent living and mental health programs to a culturally diverse client population.

Shirley Carozza, Chiar
Hilda Douglas, Secretary

3356 House Ear Institute
2100 W 3rd Street
Los Angeles, CA 90057

213-483-4431
Fax: 213-483-8789
TDD: 800-388-8612
e-mail: info@hei.org
www.hei.org

A non-profit organization dedicated to advancing hearing science through research and education to improve the quality of life. HEI scientists explore the developing ear, hearing loss and ear disease at the cell and molecular level, as well as the complex relationship between the ear and the brain. They are also working to improve hearing aids and auditory implants, diagnostics, clinical treatments and intervention methods. HEI employs more than 180 staff members within 22 departments.

John W House, MD, President
James D Boswell, CEO

3357 International Hearing Society
16880 Middlebelt Road, Suite 4
Livonia, MI 48154

734-522-7200
800-521-5247
Fax: 734-522-0200
e-mail: chelms@ihsinfo.org
www.ihsinfo.org

IHS is the professional association that represents Hearing Instrument Speicalists worldwide. IHS members are engaged in the practice of testing human hearing and selecting, fitting and dispensing hearing instruments. The Society continues to recognize the need for promoting and maintaining the highest possible standards for its members in the best interest of the hearing impaired it serves.

3000 members

Cindy Helms, Exeuctive Director
Felicia Anderson, Manager Marketing/Communications

3358 International Kaf/Tek
330 N Wabash Avenue, Suite 2300
Chicago, IL 60611

312-840-8422
Fax: 312-840-8432
TTY: 508-620-1777

International electronic mail service dedicated to communities that are deaf or hard-of-hearing. The service is used by individuals, organizations, agencies, schools, colleges and universities, service providers, and professionals in the field of deafness.

Brenda Monene, RN, MeD, President

3359 International Organization for the Education of the Hearing Impaired
Alexander Graham Bell Association for the Deaf
3417 Volta Place NW
Washington, DC 20007

202-337-5220
800-432-7543
Fax: 202-337-8314
TTY: 202-337-5220
e-mail: agbell2@aol.com
www.agbell.org

IOEHI promotes excellence in education for children and adults who are deaf or hard-of-hearing, encourages scientific study of the educational and communicative processes and stimulates the exchange of information among educators through seminars.

Elizabeth Wilkes, PhD, Chairperson
Elizabeth Quigley

3360 John Tracy Clinic
806 W Adams Boulevard
Los Angeles, CA 90007

213-748-5481
800-522-4582
Fax: 213-749-1651
TTY: 213-747-2924
e-mail: canguita@jtc.org
www.johntracyclinic.org

A private, non-profit education center whose mission is to offer hope, guidance and encouragement to families of infants and pre-school children with hearing loss by providing free, parent-centered services worldwide. The center has over 60 years of expertise in the spoken language option.

Barbara Hecht, PhD, President
Kevin Matthew, VP Finance and Administration

3361 National Association for Hearing and Speech Action
American Speech Language Hearing Association
10801 Rockville Pike
Rockville, MD 20852

301-897-5700
Fax: 301-571-0457
TDD: 301-897-0157
e-mail: actioncenter@asha.org

Provides general information on speech, language and hearing disorders to members and the public. Provides referrals to speech/language pathologists and audiologists.

77,346 members

3362 National Association of the Deaf
8630 Fention Street, Suite 820
Silver Spring, MD 20910

301-587-1789
Fax: 301-587-1791
TTY: 301-587-1788
e-mail: nadinfo@nad.org
www.nad.org

NAD was established in 1880 in Cincinnati, Ohio. Its mission is to promote, protect, and preserve the rights and quality of life of deaf and hard of hearing individuals in the United States of America.

Nancy J Bloch, CEO
Anita B Farb, Director Outreach/Communications

3363 National Captioning Institute
1900 Gallows Road, Suite 3000
Vienna, VA 22182

703-917-7600
Fax: 703-917-9853
TTY: 703-917-7600
e-mail: mail@ncicap.org
www.ncicap.org

NCI was established in 1979 as a non-profit corporation with the mission of ensuring that deaf and hard of hearing people, as well as others who can benefit from the same service, have access to television's entertainment and news through the technology of closed captioning. NCI employs almost 200 individuals.

Gene Chao, CEO
Jack Gates, President

3364 National Center for Voice and Speech
University of Iowa
677 Phillips Hall
Iowa City, IA 52242

319-335-2238
Fax: 319-335-8851
e-mail: ASL-Program@uiowa.edu
www.uiowa.ude

This is a consortium of the following institutions focusing on voice and speech disorders: University of Iowa, Denver Center for Performing Arts, University of Wisconsin-Madison, University of Utah. NCVS trains scientists interested in careers in voice and speech research, provides continuing education for professionals, and conducts research on voice and speech production.

Ingo Titze, PhD, Director
Cynthia Kintigh, MA

3365 National Cued Speech Association
23970 Hermitage Road
Cleveland, OH 44122

216-292-6213
800-459-3529
TTY: 216-292-6213
e-mail: cuedspdisc@aol.com
www.cuedspeech.org

A non-profit membership organization founded in 1982 to promote and support the effective use of Cued Speech. They raise awareness of Cued Speeck and its applications, provide educational services, assist local affiliate chapters, establish standards for Cued Speech and certify Cued Speech instructors and transliterators. Their mission and goals are to promote and support the effectuve use of Cued Speech for communication, language acquistion and literacy.

Sarina Roffe, President
Carolyn Ostrander, VP

3366 National Family Association for Deaf-Blind
141 Middle Neck Road
Sands Point, NY 11050

800-255-0411
Fax: 516-883-9060
TTY: 516-944-8637
e-mail: nfadb@aol.com
www.nfadb.org

A nonprofit, volunteer based, family association that believes individuals who are deaf-blind are valued members of society and are entitled to the same opportunity and choices as other members of the community

Lynda Syler, President
Pearl Veesart, VP

3367 National Information Center on Deafness
Gallaudet Univ. Press c/o Chicago Distrib. Center
800 Florida Avenue NE
Washington, DC 20002

202-651-5300
800-621-2736
Fax: 202-651-5477
TTY: 888-630-9347
e-mail: infotech.services@galludet.edu
www.gallaudet.edu

Provides information or referrals on questions about deafness, including general information, education, research, legislation, assistive devices and more. Offers a bibliography of readings available on 30 topics relating to deafness.

Loraine DiPietro, Director

3368 National Information Clearinghouse on Children Who Are Deaf-Blind
Teaching Research
345 N Monmouth Avenue
Monmouth, OR 97361

503-838-8391
800-438-9376
Fax: 503-838-8150
TTY: 800-854-7013
e-mail: dblink@tr.wou.edu
www.tr.wou/dblink

Collects, organizes and disseminates information related to children and youth who are deaf-blind and connects consumers of deaf-blind information to sources of information about deaf-blindness, assistive technology and deaf-blind people.

John Reiman, PhD, Director

3369 National Organization for the Advancement of the Deaf
Lamar University Station
PO Box 10078
Beaumont, TX 77710

409-880-8230
Fax: 409-880-2265
e-mail: intladm@hal.lumar.edu

Dedicated to facilitating communication on issues related to the deaf and providing technical assistance for professionals and parents working with deaf and hard-of-hearing children, adolescents, and adults.

Michael Bienenstock, President

3370 National Rehabilitation Information Center
4200 Forbes Blvd, Suite 202
Lanham, MD 20706

301-459-5900
800-346-2742
Fax: 301-459-4263
TTY: 301-459-5984
e-mail: naricinfo@heitchservices.com
www.naric.com

Its mission is to generate, disseminate and promote new knowledge to improve the options available to disabled persons. The ultimate goal is to allow these individuals to perform their regular activities in the community and to bolster society's ability to provide full opportunities and appropriate supports for its disabled citizens.

Mark Odum, Director

3371 National Technical Institute for the Deaf
Rochester Institute of Technology
52 Lomb Memorial Drive
Rochester, NY 14623

585-475-6400
Fax: 585-475-5978
TTY: 585-475-6400
e-mail: ntidmc@rit.edu
www.rit.edu

Technical college for students who are deaf or hard of hearing. Its mission is to provide these students with outstanding state-of-the-art technical and professional programs, complemented by a strong liberal arts and sciences curriculum, that prepare them to live and work in the mainstream of a rapidly changing global community and enhances their lifelong learning.

Alan Hurwitz, Vice President/Dean

3372 SEE Center for the Advancement of Deaf Chi ldren
PO Box 1181
Los Alamitos, CA 90720

562-430-1467
Fax: 562-795-6614
TTY: 562-430-1467
e-mail: seecenter@seecenter.org
www.seecenter.org

Established in 1984 as a nonprofit organization to work with parents and educators of hearing impared children. Their goals are to promote early identification and intervention; to promote development of improved English skills; to promote development and understanding of principles of Signing Exact English and its uses; to promote information to parents on deafness and related topics; and to foster the positive development of self concept in the deaf child.

Esther Zawolkow, Director

3373 Self Help for Hard of Hearing People Hearing Loss Association of America
7910 Woodmont Avenue, Suite 1200
Bethesda, MD 20814

301-657-2248
Fax: 301-913-9413
TTY: 301-657-2248
e-mail: info@hearingloss.org
www.shhh.org

The HLAA exists to open the world of communication for people with hearing loss through information, education, advocacy and support. They believe people with hearing loss can help themselves and one another to participate fully and successfully in society. HLAA promotes self-confidence; empowers individuals with skills to improve their lives; and provides an opportunity for affiliation among people with hearing loss and their friends, families, and professionals.

Anne T Pope, President
Victor M Matsui, Vice President

3374 Signing Exact English Center Advancement of Deaf Children
PO Box 1181
Los Alamitos, CA 90720

562-430-1467
Fax: 562-795-6614
e-mail: seecenter@seecenter.org
seecenter.org

Information and referral center for parents and educators of hearing impaired children. Conducts workshops on the use of Signing Exact English, educational interpreting, education-related communication topics. Sign skill evaluations for teachers/teachers aids, educational interpreters also available.

Esther Zawolkow, Director

3375 Telecommunications for the Deaf
8630 Fenton Street, Suite 604
Silver Spring, MD 20910

301-589-3786
Fax: 301-589-3797
TTY: 301-589-3006
e-mail: info@tdi-online.org
www.tdi-online.org

An active national advocacy organization focusing its energies and resources to address equal access issues in telecommunications and media for four constituences in deafness and hearing loss, specifically people who are deaf, hard-of-hearing, late-deafened, or deaf-blind.

Claude Stout, Executive Director
Scott Recht, Business Manager

3376 Tripod
1727 W Burbank Boulevard
Burbank, CA 91506

800-972-2080
Fax: 818-972-2090
TTY: 818-972-2080
e-mail: info@tripod.org
www.tripod.org

In partnership with the Burbank Unified School District, provides a co-enrollment educational program for deaf and hard-of-hearing children and support services for their families. The program begins with a parent-infant/toddlergroup and continues through the 12th grade. Additionally, TRIPOD Captioned Films, a public service of the TRIPOD Model School program, distributes first-run open feature films to deaf and hard-of-hearing movie going audiences nationwide.

Christopher Opie, Executive Director

3377 USA Deaf Sports Federation
102 N Krohn Place
Sioux Falls, SD 57103

605-367-5760
800-393-8710
Fax: 605-367-5958
TTY: 605-367-5761
e-mail: homeoffice@usadsf.org
www.usadsf.org

Information on adaptive sports and recreation activities for people of many abilities. Including local chapters, referrals, fun and social interaction and support groups.

Bobbie Beth Scoggins, President

State Agencies & Support Groups

3378 Communication Matters Association
PO Box 898
Freeeport, IL 61032

815-232-7963
TDD: 815-832-7963
e-mail: hearno@aeroinc.net

Not-for-profit organization dedicated to assisting families when hearing loss is identified. Provides family support, community awareness, educational advocacy, communication training, including basic sign language instruction and lending library/demonstration center full of books, videos, games and technology for deaf needs. Affiliated with Illinois Families for Hands and Voices.

Cathleen Varner, Director/Educator

Alabama

3379 Alabama Institute for the Deaf & Blind
PO Box 698
Talladega, AL 35160

256-761-3200
Fax: 256-761-3344
www.nectas.unc.edu

Services include central directory, representatives of agencies, service providers, families, and coordinators of infant, toddler, and preschool special education programs.

Joseph Busta, Interagency Coordinating Council

Libraries & Resource Centers

Alabama

3380 University of Alabama Speech and Hearing Center
Deparment of Communicative Disorders
Box 870242
Tuscaloosa, AL 35487

205-348-7131
Fax: 205-348-5936
e-mail: gculton@ed.ua.edu
http://universityrelations.ua.edu

Enhancing the educational mission of the Department, the Speech and Hearing Center is further dedicated to reducing the impact of communicative disorders affecting diverse populations across a life-span.

Gerald Chulton, MD, Director

California

3381 Hear Center
301 E Del Mar Boulevard
Pasadena, CA 91101

626-796-2016
Fax: 626-796-2320
e-mail: auditory@hearcenter.org
www.hearcenter.org

The Hear Center's mission is to help individuals with hearing loss or speech and language impairments integrate into the mainstream of the community by providing them with the means for developing auditory and oral communication skills.

Josephine Wilson, Executive Director

District of Columbia

3382 Center for Auditory and Speech Sciences-Gallaudet University
800 Florida Avenue NE
Washington, DC 20002

202-651-5000
Fax: 202-651-5295
www.gallaudet.edu

The Hearing and Speech Center provides comprehensive speech, language, and audiology services to Gallaudet students, faculty, staff and to clients in the Washington, D.C. area. These services include hearing and hearing aid evaluations, hearing aid dispensing, assistive devices evaluations, speech-language evaluations and therapy, communication therapy, and speech reading classes.

I King Jordon, President
Jane K Fernandes, Provost

3383 District of Columbia Public Library/ Librarian for the Deaf Community
901 G Street NW, Room 215
Washington, DC 20001

202-727-2145
Fax: 202-727-1129
e-mail: lbphb_2000@yahoo.com
www.dclibrary.org

Offers reference services through TDD, portable TDD for public use at pay phones, signers for library programs, sign language classes, information about deafness, print and nonprint materials for persons who are deaf.

3384 Laurent Clerc National Deaf Education Center-Gallaudet Universty
800 Florida Avenue NE
Washington, DC 20002

202-651-5300
Fax: 202-651-5477
TTY: 202-651-5300
www.gallaudet.edu

Gallaudet University's Laurent Clerc National Deaf Education Center provides deaf and hard of hearing children through the Model Secondary School for the Deaf and the Kendall Demonstration Elementary School and also collects, evaluates and disseminates best practices in deaf education.

I King Jordan, President
Katherine Jankowski, Dean

3385 Volta Bureau Library
Alexander Graham Bell Association for the Deaf
3417 Volta Place NW
Washington, DC 20007

202-337-5220
866-337-5220
Fax: 202-337-8314
TTY: 202-337-5221
e-mail: agbell2@aol.com
www.agbell.org

Contains one of the world's largest historical collections of publications, documents and information on deafness. In addition to the main collection, which includes books, periodicals and indexed clipping files dating from the turn of the century, the library also houses a significant archival collection dealing with the history of deafness since the 16th century. Membership dues for professionals are $50.00.

4500 members

Rebecca Parlakian, Director Member Services

Illinois

3386 Loyola University of Children, Parmly Hearing Institute
6525 N Sheridan Road
Chicago, IL 60626

773-508-2766
Fax: 773-508-2719
e-mail: ssheft@luc.edu

The Parmly Hearing Institute is part of Loyola University Chicago.

Stanley Edward Sheft PhD, Director

Maine

3387 University of Maine, Conley Speech and Hearing Center
5724 Dunn Hall, Room 336
Orono, ME 04469

207-581-2006

The Madelyn E and Albert D Conley Speech, Language and Hearing Center is a center for clinical education and research as well as a facility for comprehensive state-of-the-art speech, language and hearing services. Both the Audiology Clinic and the Speech-Language Clinic provide services for individuals across the lifespan. The Speech-Language Clinic includes a Diagnostic Clinic, a Family-Based Treatment Clinic, and a Stuttering Clinic.

Susan K Riley MS, Clinic Director

Massachusetts

3388 Eaton-Peabody Laboratory of Auditory Physiology
Massachusetts Eye & Ear Institute
243 Charles Street
Boston, MA 02114

617-573-7900
Fax: 617-720-4408
TDD: 617-523-5498
www.meei.harvard.edu

A consortium between the Massachusetts Eye and Ear Infirmary, the Harvard Medical School, the Research Laboratory of Electronics at Massachusetts Institute of Technology, and the Massachusetts General Hospital. Research interests span the auditory system from peripheral to central, from normal to abnormal function, from neurophysiology to behavior, and from the molecular and genetic bases of deafness, to its treatment via hearing aids and cochlear implants.

Nelson YS Kiang, PhD, Director

Nebraska

3389 University of Nebraska, Lincoln Barkley Memorial Center
Barkley Center 301
Lincoln, NE 68583

402-472-2145
Fax: 402-472-7697
www.unl.edu.barkley/index.shtml

The University of Nebraska-Lincoln Barkley Memorial Center and Boys Town National Research Hospital have joined forces to offer an exciting future in the audiology profession.

John E Bernthal, Director

New Jersey

3390 Princeton University, Cutaneous Communication Laboratory
Psychology Department, Green Hall

Princeton, NJ 08544

609-258-4442
Fax: 609-258-1113
e-mail: psych@princeton.edu

Dr. Roger Cholewiak

New York

3391 Wallace Memorial Library
Rochester Institute of Technology
90 Lomb Memorial Drive
Rochester, NY 14623

585-475-2562
http://library.rit.edu/collections/wallace.html

A multimedia resource center with a collection of more than 750,000 items. Resource materials include more than 350,000 books; 2900 print journals subscriptions; 380,000 microforms; 3,100 audio cassettes and recordings; 6,700 film and video titles. They have an extensive web-based online collection which features over 150 research databases, 7,000+ eBooks, 16,000 electronic journal subscriptions and thousands of digital images in various collections.

Melanie Norton, Reference Librarian

Oregon

3392 Regional Resource Center on Deafness
Western Oregon State College
345 N Monmouth Avenue
Monmouth, OR 97361

503-838-8444
877-877-1593
Fax: 503-838-8228
e-mail: education@wou.edu

Prepares professionals in the Northwest to be qualified to serve the unique communication, rehabilitation, and educational needs of deaf and hard of hearing individuals. The Center offers graduate and undergraduate degree programs for professionals entering fields that serve people who are deaf or hard of hearing, continuing education opportunities for currently practicing professionals, and consultation and community service activities designed to enhance the quality of life for all affected.

John Freeburg, Director
Hilda Rosselli PhD, Dean

South Carolina

3393 Described and Captioned Media Program
National Association of the Deaf
1447 E Main Street
Spartanburg, SC 29307

864-585-1778
800-237-6213
Fax: 864-585-2611
TTY: 864-585-2617
e-mail: info@cfv.org
www.dcmp.org

Renamed the Described and Captioned Media Program, CMP continues to provide all persons who are deaf or hard of hearing awareness of and equal access to communication and learning through the use of captioned educational media and supportive collateral materials. They also act as a captioning information and training center. Their ultimate goal is to permit media to be an integral part in the lifelong learning process for all stakeholders in the deaf and hard of hearing community.

Bill Stark, Project Director

Virginia

3394 University of Virginia Communication Disorders Program
PO Box 400260
Charlottesville, VA 22904

434-924-3334
Fax: 434-924-0747

Richard Talbott, MD, Director

Research Centers

Alabama

3395 Civitan International Research Center
CIRC 329, 1719 6th Avenue S
Birmingham, AL 35294

205-934-8900
800-822-2472
Fax: 205-975-6330
e-mail: info@uab.edu
www.uab.edu

An interdisciplinary center dedicated to improving lives through brain research and the prevention and treatment of developmental disabilities. Among the many program areas are mental retardation, autism spectrum disorders, treating brain tumors, neonaltal scizures, constraint therapy, Rett syndrome, Alexander's Disease, Kernicterus and many more.

Harald Sontheimer, Director
Alan Percy, Medical Director

Arkansas

3396 Arkansas Rehabilitation Research and Training Center for Deaf Persons
University of Arkansas
4601 W Markham Street
Little Rock, AR 72205

501-686-9691
Fax: 501-686-9698
TTY: 501-686-9698

The center focuses on issues affecting the employability of deaf and hard-of-hearing rehabilitation clients.

Douglas Watson, PhD, Director

Massachusetts

3397 National Temporal Bone, Hearing and Balance Pathology Resource Registry
Massachusetts Eye & Ear Infirmary
243 Charles Street
Boston, MA 02114

800-822-1327
Fax: 617-573-3838
TTY: 888-561-3277
e-mail: tbregistry@meei.harvard.edu
www.tbregistry.org

The Registry, established by the National Institute on Deafness and Other Communication Disorders, maintains a database of human temporal bone collections, responds to inquiries from the public and researchers interested in temporal bone donation or research, disseminates information about temporal bone collection and its importance, implements professional educational activities in the field of temporal bone and auditory brain cell stem study and implements a national acquistion network.

Julie Rose, Coordinator

Michigan

3398 University of Michigan, Kresge Hearing Research Institute
1301 E Ann Street, Room 5032
Ann Arbor, MI 48109

734-763-9600
Fax: 734-764-0014
TTY: 734-764-8110

Research programs include multi-disciplinary projects in behavior, morphology, physiology, molecular biology and genetics, bioengineering, pharmacology and biochemistry. They include: the genetics of hearing and deafness, mechanisms of auditory processing, molecular otology, cochlear prosthesis and tissue bioengineering, and training.

Jochen Schacht PhD, Scientific Director
Diana Gilham, Finance

Missouri

3399 Central Institute for the Deaf
4560 Clayton Avenue
Saint Louis, MO 63110

314-977-0000
888-444-4565
Fax: 314-977-0223
TTY: 314-997-0001
TDD: 314-977-0037
e-mail: rfeder@cid.wustl.edu
www.cid.wustl.edu

Central Institute for the Deaf is a private, nonprofit institute composed of research laboratories in which scientists study the normal

aspects as well as the disorders of hearing, language, and speech; a school for children who have hearing impairments; speech, language, and hearing clinics; and professionals with hearing impairment, and communication sciences.

Robin M Feder, Executive Director

Nebraska

3400 Lied Learning and Technology Center for Childhood Deafness and Vision Disorders
Boys Town National Research Hospital
14100 Crawford Street
Boys Town, NE 68010

402-498-1300
800-448-3000
Fax: 402-498-1348
TTY: 402-498-6543
e-mail: hotline@girlsandboystown.org
www.boystown.org/chlc

A not-for-profit corporation closely affiliated with the Boys Town National Research Hospital. The center houses Model Childhood Education Classrooms, a Cochlear Implant Clinic and Research Center, Educational Media Production Studios, Distance Learning and Family Outreach Center, Hearing and Vision Laboratories, Bio-informatics and Computer Center and a Communication Technology Development Center.

Patrick E Brookhouser MD, President

New York

3401 Montifiore Medical Center
3415 Bainbridge Avenue, at Gunhill Road
Bronx, NY 10467

718-920-2484
Fax: 718-405-9014
e-mail: ruben@aecom.vu.edu
www.montefiore.org

Provides diagnosis, treatment and research of diseases of the ear, nose and throat.

3402 New York Foundation for Otologic Research
920 Park Avenue
New York, NY 10021

212-980-3100

Unsolved hearing problems and deafness research.

Alan Austin Scheer, MD, Director

3403 State University College at Plattsburgh Auditory Research Laboratory
101 Broad Street
Plattsburgh, NY 12901

518-564-2040
888-673-0012
Fax: 518-564-2045
e-mail: hamernrp@plattsburgh.edu
www.plattsburgh.edu

The Auditory Research Laboratory (ARL) is home to several laboratories, including acoustics lab, anatomy lab, auditory evoked potential lab, and otoacoustic emissions lab. Facilities include: acoustics and vibrations laboratory, otoacoustic emmissions laboratory, middle ear analysis laboratory, auditory evoked potential laboratory, and cochlear anatomy laborator.

Roger Hamernik, MD, Director

3404 Syracuse University, Institute for Sensory Research
Merrill Lane
Syracuse, NY 13244

315-443-4164
Fax: 315-443-1184
e-mail: robert-smith@isr5yr.edu
www.isr.syr.edu

Research center dedicated to the discovery and application of knowledge of the sensory systems. Integration of engineering, life, and physical sciences, combining rigorous experimental methodology with mathematical analysis is stressed.

Robert Smith, MD, Director

Oregon

3405 Oregon Health Sciences University Research Center
3181 SW Sam Jackson Park Road
Portland, OR 97201

503-494-8311
Fax: 503-494-5656
e-mail: contact@ohsuhealth.com
www.ohsuhealth.com

OSHU blends education, research, patient care and community outreach into one shared mission: to improve the well-being of people in Oregon and beyond. They incorporate the latest medical research, technology and innovation.

Pennsylvania

3406 Temple University, Section of Auditory Research
SW Corner Broad and Tioga Streets, 1st Floor
Philadelphia, PA 19140

215-707-3663
Fax: 215-707-7523
e-mail: anita@ent.temple.edu
www.temple.edu

The Auditory Research Section includes the Garfied Auditory Research Laboratory, the Hearing Science Research Program and the Electrophysiology Progject.

Anita Cilea, Departmental Administrator
Kate Haney, Financial Administrator

Tennessee

3407 Bill Wilkerson Center
1215 21st Avenue South
Nashville, TN 37212

615-936-5000
Fax: 615-936-5013
e-mail: kate.carney@vanderbilt.edu
www.mc.vanderbilt.edu

The Vanderbilt Bill Wilkerson Center for Otolaryngology and Communication Sciences is dedicated to serving persons with diseases of the ear, nose, throat, head and neck, and hearing, speech, language and related disorders.

Robert H Ossoff DMD MD, Director
Fred H Bess PhD, Associate Director

Texas

3408 Houston Ear Research Foundation
7737 SW Freeway, Suite 630
Houston, TX 77074

713-771-9966
800-843-0808
Fax: 713-771-0546
TTY: 800-843-0807
e-mail: jangil@hern.org

The Foundation was incorporated in August, 1983 as a center to provide excellence in service dedicated to the cochlear implant.

Jan Gilden, Executive Director

Audio Video

3409 50th Anniversary Collection
Harris Communications
15155 Technology Drive
Eden Prairie, MN 55344

952-906-1180
800-825-6758
Fax: 952-906-1099
TTY: 952-906-1198
e-mail: info@harriscomm.com
www.harriscomm.com

Stories: A picture for Harold's Room; Corduroy; Danny and the Dinosaur; Harry the Dirty Dog; Click, clack moo, Cows that type. DVD-R, voiced; signed in ASL, no captions.

3410 A Few Errands
Modern Sign Press
10443 Los Alamitos Boulevard, PO Box 1181
Los Alamitos, CA 90720

562-596-8548
800-572-7332
Fax: 562-795-6614
TTY: 562-493-4168
e-mail: modsigns@modernsignspress.com
www.modernsignspress.com

Basic level videotape of signed story for Expressive and Receptive practice. Story is repeated three times for ease of use. Watch how the visual features are incorporated. Turn the sound off for receptive practice. Written script and tape use suggestions included.
VHS

3411 A Lesson With Heart
American Sign Language Productions
15155 Technology Drive
Eden Prairie, MN 55344

952-906-1180
800-767-4461
Fax: 952-906-1099
TTY: 952-906-1198
e-mail: ASLProductions@harriscomm.com
www.americansignlanguageproductions.com

A skilled 4th grade teacher presents a lesson on Anatomy including the respiratory system, digestive system, and the heart that will increase your familiarity with this vocabulary and content. Improve your interpreting skills for this subject matter and grade level by accepting this assignment. You won't be alone...we provide two interpreters to demonstrate it for your. 55 minutes. DVD - $59.95; VHS - 49.95

3412 A Mother's Persepctive on the IEP Process
American Sign Language Productions
15155 Technology Drive
Eden Prairie, MN 55344

952-906-1180
800-767-4461
Fax: 952-906-1099
TTY: 952-906-1198
e-mail: ASLProductions@harriscomm.com
www.americansignlanguageproductions.com

Maxine Camvel is a parent of a Deaf daughter wanting to make it easier for other parents. She gives valuable insight into how to advocate for your children by maximizing parent input to the Individualized Education Plan (IEP) process. This program also provides an opportunity to interpret vocabulary and emotional content commonly expressed by parents. Your two team interpreters demonstrate how to interpret this sample. 1 hour. DVD - $59.95; VHS - $49.95

3413 ABC Stories

Sign Media
4020 Blackburn Lane
Burtonsville, MD 20866

800-475-4756
Fax: 301-421-0270
www.signmedia.com

You will marvel at the skill of these Deaf performers as they use every letter of the manual alphabet, in sequence, to tell a story. To capture the creativity and genius of the stories, the videotape uses slow motion and graphic displays. VHS, 1 hour.

3414 ABCs of AVT: Analyzing Auditory-Verbal Therapy

Alexander Graham Bell Association for the Deaf
3417 Volta Place NW
Washington, DC 20007

202-337-5220
800-432-7543
Fax: 202-337-8314
TTY: 202-337-5221
e-mail: info@agbell.org
www.agbell.org

An Educational Tool for Professionals. Developed for use in university classrooms and training environments; provides an overview of Auditory-Verbal techniques and guidance on appropriate intervention for children experiencing difficulties with language development.

2005 104 pages 46 Minute video

Warren Estabrooks MEd, Author
Rhonda Schwartz MA, Co-Author

3415 ASL Stories: Christmas Stories

Harris Communications
15155 Technology Drive
Eden Prairie, MN 55344

952-906-1180
800-825-6758
Fax: 952-906-1099
TTY: 952-906-1198
e-mail: info@harriscomm.com
www.harriscomm.com

This video is one in a collection of videotapes featuring classic fairy tales signed by Deaf storytellers, and is a wonderful way to get into the spirit of Christmas. This video also makes a welcome gift. Stories include: The Night Before Christmas, A Christmas Carol, The First Christmas Tree, The Birth of Christ, In the Great Walled City, and The Little Match Girl. For ages 10 and over. VHS: 80 minutes; signed in ASL; no captions; voice over.

3416 ASL Stories: Fairy Tales I

Harris Communications
15155 Technology Drive
Eden Prairie, MN 55344

952-906-1180
800-825-6758
Fax: 952-906-1099
TTY: 952-906-1198
e-mail: info@harriscomm.com
www.harriscomm.com

This video is one of a collection of videotapes featuring classic fairy tales signed by Deaf storytellers. Stories include Rapunzel, Snow White and Rose Red, The Frog Prince, Hansel and Gretel, and The Brave Little Tailor. For ages 10 and over. VHS: 114 minutes; signed in ASL; no captions; voice-over.

3417 ASL Stories: Fairy Tales II

Harris Communications
15155 Technology Drive
Eden Prairie, MN 55344

952-906-1180
800-825-6758
Fax: 952-906-1099
TTY: 952-906-1198
e-mail: info@harriscomm.com
www.harriscomm.com

This video is one of a collection of videotapes featuring classic fairy tales signed by Deaf storytellers. Stories include Sleeping Beauty, The Golden Goose, Little Red Riding Hood, The Princess and the Pea, and The Tinder Box. For ages 10 and over. VHS: 83 minutes; signed in ASL; no captions; voice-over.

3418 Acoustics, Audition and Speech Reception

Daniel Lind OC, PhD, author

Alexander Graham Bell Association for the Deaf
3417 Volta Place NW
Washington, DC 20007

202-337-5220
202-337-8314
TTY: 202-337-5221
e-mail: info@agbell.org
www.agbell.org

This videotape of four professionals provides viewers with an overview of the properties of speech and the ways children can get the most from their hearing aids or cochlear implants. The tape is a practical how-to guide in which team members demonstrate how speech sounds are created in the vocal tract, how distance affects the intensity of spoken language and how patterns are distorted by profound hearing loss.

3419 American Sign Language Handshape Dictionar y DVD

Gallaudet University Press
800 Florida Avenue NE
Washington, DC 20002

202-651-5448
Fax: 202-651-5489
TTY: 202-651-5448
e-mail: gupress@gallaudet.edu
http://gupress.gallaudet.edu

A perfect complement to the dictionary, this new DVD features a diverse cast of native signers forming more than 1,400 ASL signs organized by 40 basic handshapes, with a complete list of English glosses and synonyms for each sign.

Richard Tennant, Co-Producer
Marianne Gluszak Brown, Co-Producer

3420 American Sign Language Phrase Series

Sign Media
4020 Blackburn Lane
Burtonsville, MD 20866

800-475-4756
Fax: 301-421-0270
www.signmedia.com

It's easy to learn ASL with these videos where you learn actual ASL phrases. You can begin conversing in ASL even before you master the grammar. Each videotape is keyed to the text and contains phrases, expressions, sentences, and questions that come up in everyday conversation. Over 200 sentences or phrases organized by commonly occurring themes are included on each videotape. Perfect for beginning signers. Three tape set, each tape one hour.

3421 American Sign Language Video Series
DeBee Communications/TJ Publishers
2544 Tarpley Road, Suite 108
Carrollton, TX 75006

972-416-0800
800-999-1168
Fax: 972-416-0944
TTY: 972-416-0933
e-mail: customerservice@tjpublishers.com
www.tjpublishers.com

Learning ASL with the Deaf Robinson family. The family acts out scenes that occur in everyday life in this videotape series. Each situation is reviewed in an ASL classroom with a deaf teacher. This series also includes sections on Deaf culture and grammar, rounding off a complete and effective instructional tool. Work Day-VHS-90 minutes, School Day-VHS-90 minutes, Shopping-VHS-90 minutes, Softball Game-VHS-90 minutes. $39.95 each

3422 American Sign Language: Green Books Text a nd Tapes
Sign Media
4020 Blackburn Lane
Burtonsville, MD 20866

800-475-4756
Fax: 301-421-0270
www.signmedia.com

The classic ASL series. This unique set of texts, written by Dennis Cokely and Charlotte Baker-Shenk, is complimented by videotapes. The videotapes explain difficult concepts and offer practice situations to improve your sign language skills. The series may be ordered as a complete set of books and tapes, a complete set of tapes only, individual books and tapes, or a specific tape and book combination set. VHS.

3423 Ancient Greece
American Sign Language Productions
15155 Technology Drive
Eden Prairie, MN 55344

952-906-1180
800-767-4461
Fax: 952-906-1099
TTY: 952-906-1198
e-mail: ASLProductions@harriscomm.com
www.americansignlanguageproductions.com

We often think about interpreting for Deaf children, but often need to understand the speech and thought patterns of their hearing classmates. Krisjana is a hearing child presenting a report on Ancient Greece. A great way to practice with vocabulary from the classroom before you have to sit in the hot seat. Is it all Greek to you? No need to worry. Two interpreters will show you how. 30 minutes. DVD - $59.95; VHS - $49.95

3424 Animals, Insects, School, Colors Spanish/E nglish Videos
Modern Signs Press
10443 Los Alamitos Boulevard, PO Box 1181
Los Alamitos, CA 90720

562-596-8548
800-572-7332
Fax: 562-795-6614
TTY: 562-493-4168
e-mail: modsigns@modernsignspress.com
www.modernsignspress.com

Entertaining sign language instructional videos in Spanish and English. Great tool to help bridge the gap between Spanish, English and Sign Language. The videos have a split screen - Connie and Merced teach you the sign and say the word in both Spanish and English. Vocabulary words are used in sentences to reinforce the signs. There are graphics showing the vocabulary they are reviewing. 10 titles available, either alone or in a complete package.

3425 Art Show
Modern Sign Press
10443 Los Alamitos Boulevard, PO Box 1181
Los Alamitos, CA 90720

562-596-8548
800-572-7332
Fax: 562-795-6614
TTY: 562-493-4168
e-mail: modsigns@modernsignpress.com
www.modernsignspress.com

Basic level videotape of signed story for Expressive and Receptive practice. Story is repeated three times for ease of use. Watch how the visual features are incorporated. Turn the sound off for receptive practice. Written script and tape use suggestions included. VHS

3426 Baby See 'n Sign
Harris Communications
15155 Technology Drive
Eden Prairie, MN 55344

952-906-1180
800-825-6758
Fax: 952-906-1099
TTY: 952-906-1198
e-mail: info@harriscomm.com
www.harriscomm.com

Features American Sign Language signs and real-life images in full color. They may be used as an educational tool for effectively promoting communication with people who are autistic, have Down Syndrome, or are ESL. For parents who have decided to sign to their children, this is a great video. Over 60 basic American Sign Language signs and real-life images are presented in full-color, making it enjoyable for parents and children to watch. A parental question and answer guide is included.

6 months + DVD 45 minutes

3427 Baby See 'n Sign II
Harris Communications
15155 Technology Drive
Eden Prairie, MN 55344

952-906-1180
800-825-6758
Fax: 952-906-1099
TTY: 952-906-1198
e-mail: info@harriscomm.com
www.harriscomm.com

This DVD shows over 100 real-life images that relate to your child's daily life, including animals, foods, toys and activities. Volume II has beginning abstract concepts and continues with object-word association. It is never too late to begin signing. Ages 6 months and up. DVD: 50 minutes.

3428 Baby Signing Time
Harris Communications
15155 Technology Drive
Eden Prairie, MN 55344

952-906-1180
800-825-6758
Fax: 952-906-1099
TTY: 952-906-1198
e-mail: info@harriscomm.com
www.harriscomm.com

Designed specifically for babies 3-36 months old, the DVD combines sign-along songs, playful animation and the positive reinforcement of signing babies - who are all ages 2 and under - to teach you and your baby to sign the easy way. Baby Signing Time sets your baby's day to music as you learn sign and sogns for everyday events in baby's life - eating, family, pets and more.

3429 Baby Signing Time DVD 2

Harris Communications
15155 Technology Drive
Eden Prairie, MN 55344

952-906-1180
800-825-6758
Fax: 952-906-1099
TTY: 952-906-1198
e-mail: info@harriscomm.com
www.harriscomm.com

This video sets your baby's day to music as you learn signs and sogns for everyday events in baby's life - eating, family, pets and more. Designed specifically for babies 3-36 months old, this DVD combines sign-along songs, playful animation and the positive re-inforcement of signing babies - who are all ages 2 and under - to teach you and your baby to sign the easy way.

3430 Bachelor Father

Modern Sign Press
10443 Los Alamitos Boulevard, PO Box 1181
Los Alamitos, CA 90720

562-596-8548
800-572-7332
Fax: 562-795-6614
TTY: 562-493-4168
e-mail: modsigns@modernsignspress.com
www.modernsignspress.com

Basic level videotape of signed story for Expressive and Receptive practice. Story is repeated three times for ease of use. Watch how the visual features are incorporated. Turn the sound off for recep-tive practice. Written script and tape use suggestions included. VHS

3431 Basic Course in American Sign Language Videotape Package

TJ Publishers
2544 Tarpley Road, Suite 108
Carrollton, TX 75006

800-999-1168
Fax: 972-416-0944
TTY: 972-416-0933
e-mail: customerservice@tjpublishers.com
www.tjpublishers.com

This videotape features four Deaf models signing each vocabulary word contained in all 22 lessons of the text plus the alphabet and numbers. The tape has captions and voice which can be turned off to sharpen visual acuity. It is ideal for classroom reinforcement and independent home study. Available on VHS or DVD.

Video

Angela K Thames, President

3432 Beginning Level Curriculum Tapes Complete Set

Modern Signs Press
PO Box 1181
Los Alamitos, CA 90720

562-596-8548
800-572-7332
Fax: 562-795-6614
TTY: 562-493-4168
e-mail: modsigns@modernsignspress.com
www.modernsignspress.com

A good way to learn the beginning lessons of Signing Exact Eng-lish with Dr. Gerilee Gustason, co-author of SEE. The full set of tapes introduce more than 700 words and signs. There are 14 les-sons with approximately 50 vocabulary items and practice sen-tences in each lesson. Words and sentences are presented twice allowing time for observation and ability to imitate presenter. Words are also shown in text form for both the individual vocabu-lary words and sentences to help with clarity.

VHS and DVD

3433 Beginning Reading and Sign Language Video

TJ Publishers
2544 Tarpley Road, Suite 108
Carrollton, TX 75006

972-416-0800
800-999-1168
Fax: 972-416-0944
TTY: 972-416-0933
e-mail: customerservice@tjpublsihers.com
www.tjpublishers.com

Great for kids from 2 to 12, this video picture book feature Deaf actress Susan Bressler signing over a hundred words at the zoos, at home and around the community. Don't tell your kids that learning Sign language improves reading, motor skills and visual perception and increases language acquisition abilities. English captions give reading practice, too. Great for hearing and Deaf children. VHS 30 minutes.

Video
ISBN: 0-932314-00-7

Angela K Thames, President

3434 Blue's Clues: All Kinds of Signs

Harris Communications
15155 Technology Drive
Eden Prairie, MN 55344

952-906-1180
800-825-6758
Fax: 952-906-1099
TTY: 952-906-1198
e-mail: info@harriscomm.com
www.harriscomm.com

Preschoolers play along with Steve and Blue with the two episodes in this video. The video uses different kinds of signs - from direc-tional signs to American Sign Language - to figure out where Blue wants to eat in Where does Blue want to have her snack?, and where she would like to go in Where does Blue want to go? Guest appearance by Marlee Matline. Approximately 50 minutes. Closed captioned. VHS.

3435 Bold as Brianna

American Sign Language Productions
15155 Technology Drive
Eden Prairie, MN 55344

952-906-1180
800-767-4461
Fax: 952-906-1099
TTY: 952-906-1198
e-mail: ASLProductions@harriscomm.com
www.americanlanguageproductions.com

Elementary: 7-Year-Old Deaf Child. A Confident, articulate seven-year-old willing and able to give you an eye-full. Precious and precocious, Briana will entertain you as you improve your re-ceptivity and sign-to-voice interpreting skills. Two certified inter-preters provide interpretations for your to compare and contrast to each other and your own work. 33 minutes. DVD - $59.95; VHS - $49.95

3436 Building Cue Reading

Melanie Metzger, PhD and Earl Fleetwood, MA, author

Alexander Graham Bell Association for the Deaf
3417 Volta Place NW
Washington, DC 20007

202-337-5220
202-337-8314
TTY: 203-337-5221
e-mail: info@agbell.org
www.agbell.org

Designed for hearing individuals who already cue expressively, this two videotape set offers lessons to develop receptive Cued English skills. The videos comprise 15 lessons with drills and prac-tice exercises.

3437 Communication Rules for Hard-of-Hearing People

Self Help for Hard-of-Hearing People
7910 Woodmont Avenue, Suite 1200
Bethesda, MD 20814

301-657-2248
Fax: 301-913-9413
TTY: 301-657-2249
e-mail: national@shhh.org
www.shhh.org

For use with manual (listed separately).

1987 Open-captioned

3438 Deaf Children Signers

Harris Communications
15155 Technology Drive
Eden Prairie, MN 55344

952-906-1180
800-825-6758
Fax: 952-906-1099
TTY: 952-906-1198
e-mail: info@harriscomm.com
www.harriscomm.com

This five-part collection of children signers is great for children, teachers, parents and interpreters. Available in VHS and DVD

Bill Williams, National Sales Manager

3439 Delightful as Derek

American Sign Language Productions
15155 Technology Drive
Eden Prarie, MN 55344

952-906-1180
800-767-4461
Fax: 952-906-1099
TTY: 952-906-1198
e-mail: ASLProductions@harriscomm.com
www.americansignlanguageproductions.com

Join Derek, a bright and linguistically advanced 10-year-old, as he shares his passion for creative projects and home schooling. His use of ASL will delight and assist you to enhance you own signing and voicing skills. Benefit from two certified interpreters demonstrating how to interpret for Derek. 40 minutes. DVD - $59.95; VHS - $49.95

3440 Discovering Cued Speech

Pamela H. Beck, author

Alexander Graham Bell Association for the Deaf
3417 Volta Place NW
Washington, DC 20007

202-337-5220
202-337-8314
TTY: 203-337-5221
e-mail: info@agbell.org
www.agbell.org

Two-volume video and personal workbook are used in conjunction to make the learning and practice of Cued Speech interesting and effective. A Quick Review at the beginning of each workbook lesson lists the specific goals of that lesson. Participants will read through the lesson in the workbook, use the video instruction to learn, return to the workbook to practice, then return to the video as needed.

78 pages VHS 2:52 min

3441 Economic Glitch

Modern Sign Press
10443 Los Alamitos Boulevard, PO Box 1181
Los Alamitos, CA 90720

562-596-8548
800-572-7332
Fax: 562-795-6614
TTY: 562-493-4168
e-mail: modsigns@modernsignspress.com
www.modernsignspress.com

Basic level videotape of signed story for Expressive and Receptive practice. Story is repeated three times for ease of use. Watch how the visual features are incorporated. Turn the sound off for receptive practice. Written script and tape use suggestions included.
VHS

3442 Family Traditions

Modern Sign Press
10443 Los Alamitos Boulevard, PO Box 1181
Los Alamitos, CA 90720

562-596-8548
800-572-7332
Fax: 562-795-6614
TTY: 562-493-4168
e-mail: modsigns@modernsignspress.com
www.modernsignspress.com

Basic level videotape of signed story for Expressive and Receptive practice. Story is repeated three times for ease of use. Watch how the visual features are incorporated. Turn the sound off for receptive practice. Written script and tape use suggestions included.
VHS

3443 Fantastic Videos: Colonial Times, Chocolat e, and Cars

Gallaudet University Press
800 Florida Avenue NE
Washington, DC 20002

202-651-5488
Fax: 202-651-5489
e-mail: gupress@gallaudet.edu
http://gupress.gallaudet.edu

Young viewers visit Colonial Williamsburg in Virginia to see various crafts. Other parts show chocolate being made, and films of old cars. VHS, color, voice-over, captions.

VHS 28 minutes
ISBN: 1-563680-06-8

3444 Fantastic Videos: Dogs at Work and Play

Gallaudet University Press
800 Florida Avenue NE
Washington, DC 20002

202-651-5488
Fax: 202-651-5489
e-mail: gupress@gallaudet.edu
http://gupress.gallaudet.edu

See how dogs are trained, including Fantastic's own hearing-ear dog, police dogs, plus puppies and dogs in space? VHS, color, voice-over, captions.

VHS 28 minutes
ISBN: 1-563680-03-3

3445 Fantastic Videos: Exciting People, Places and Things!

Gallaudet University Press
800 Florida Avenue NE
Washington, DC 20002

202-651-5488
Fax: 202-651-5489
e-mail: gupress@gallaudet.edu
http://gupress.gallaudet.edu

In this program, Rita Corey welcomes young viewers for a trip to a crayon factory, a jump rope tournament, and mime by actor Bernard Bragg. VHS, color, voice-over captions.

VHS 28 minutes
ISBN: 1-563680-01-7

3446 Fantastic Videos: From Post Offices to Dai ry Goats!

Gallaudet University Press
800 Florida Avenue NE
Washington, DC 20002

202-651-5488
Fax: 202-651-5489
e-mail: gupress@gallaudet.edu
http://gupress.gallaudet.edu

In this program, children follow the route of a letter from mailbox through the post office to its final destination. Also, they visit dairy goats and other animals. VHS, color, voice-over, captions

VHS 28 minutes
ISBN: 1-563680-05-X

3447 Fantastic Videos: Imagination, Actors, and 'Deaf Way!'
Gallaudet University Press
800 Florida Avenue NE
Washington, DC 20002

> 202-651-5488
> Fax: 202-651-5489
> e-mail: gupress@gallaudet.edu
> http://gupress.gallaudet.edu

Deaf clowns, mimes and actors display the wonders of imaginagion, along with performances at the international cultural celebration 'Deaf Way.' VHS, color, voice-over, captions.

VHS 28 minutes
ISBN: 1-563680-04-1

3448 Fantastic Videos: Roller Coasters, Maps, a nd Ice Cream!
Gallaudet University Press
800 Florida Avenue NE
Washington, DC 20002

> 202-651-5488
> Fax: 202-651-5489
> e-mail: gupress@gallaudet.edu
> http://gupress.gallaudet.edu

Mike Montangino leads the way on rides at Kings Dominion, and also to see how maps are drawn and how ice cream is made. VHS, color, voice-over, captions.

VHS 28 minutes
ISBN: 1-563680-07-6

3449 Fantastic Videos: Skiing, Factories, and R ace Horses
Gallaudet University Press
800 Florida Avenue NE
Washington, DC 20002

> 202-651-5488
> Fax: 202-651-5489
> e-mail: gupress@gallaudet.edu
> http://gupress.gallaudet.edu

Snow Skiing starts this program, which continues in a factory where 'who-knows-what' is made. Also, young viewers learn about horse care, and also the making of Oreos. VHS, color, voice-over, captions.

VHS 28 minutes
ISBN: 1-563680-08-4

3450 Fantastic Videos: The Wonderful Worlds of Sports and Travel
Gallaudet University Press
800 Florida Avenue NE
Washington, DC 20002

> 202-651-5488
> Fax: 202-651-5489
> e-mail: gupress@gallaudet.edu
> http://gupress.gallaudet.edu

In this program, young viewers ride on a train, watch deaf athletes compete, and see actor Bernard Bragg perform The Lion and the Mouse. VHS, color, voice-over, captions.

VHS 28 minutes
ISBN: 1-563680-02-5

3451 Fingerspelling: Expressive and Receptive Fluency
DawnSign Press
6130 Nancy Ridge Drive
San Diego, CA 92121

> 858-625-0600
> Fax: 858-625-2336
> e-mail: info@dawnsign.com
> www.dawnsign.com

This videotape makes the elements of fingerspelling understandable to ASL students. Based on her highly successful and popular workshopes, Joyce Lindene Groode presents a variety of strategies for building and improving the skills for producing fingerspelled words. VHS.

120 minutes
ISBN: 0-915035-13-8

Joyce Linden Groode

3452 Four for You! Fables and Fairy Tales Serie s
Sign Media
4020 Blackburn Lane
Burtonsville, MD 20866

> 800-475-4756
> Fax: 301-421-0270
> www.signmedia.com

Aesop's fables and classic fairy tales performed in ASL. Stars four Sign Language performers and storytellers. Each volume contains four Aesop's fables and two classic fairy tales. The fables are presented twice - first as a straightforward rendition of the story: the second as a dramatized version using minimal sets and props. Voice-over is provided. Activity Packets include printed text of each story in the volume, crossword puzzles, word find challenges, secret message decoding and more.

5 tapes/packets

3453 From Mime to Sign
TJ Publishers
2544 Tarpley Road, Suite 108
Carrollton, TX 75006

> 972-416-0800
> 800-999-1168
> Fax: 972-416-0944
> TTY: 972-416-0933
> e-mail: customerservice@tjpublishers.com
> www.tjpublishers.com

More than 1,000 photographs illustrate how natural gestures, mime and facial expressions used every day can become the basis for learning sign language. Three videotapes accompany and enhance the text, demonstrating techniques chapter by chapter. Learn to synthesize gesture, mime, facial expression and American Sign Language to truly open the door to visual thinking. VHS or DVD.

1989

Gilbert G Eastman

3454 Generating Business
Modern Sign Press
10443 Los Alamitos Boulevard, PO Box 1181
Los Alamitos, CA 90720

> 562-596-8548
> 800-572-7332
> Fax: 562-795-6614
> TTY: 562-493-4168
> e-mail: modsigns@modernsignpress.com
> www.modernsignspress.com

Basic level videotape of signed story for Expressive and Receptive practice. Story is repeated three times for ease of use. Watch how the visual features are incorporated. Turn the sound off for receptive practice. Written script and tape use suggestions included. VHS

3455 Getting In Touch - Communicating with a Ch ild Who is Deaf-Blind
Research Press
PO Box 9177 Dept 26W
Champaign, IL 61826

> 217-352-3273
> 800-519-2707
> Fax: 217-352-1221
> e-mail: rp@researchpress.com
> www.researchpress.com

Shows how to create an individualized communications system based on the abilites and needs of the child. It stresses using verbal communication and sign language when possible and encouraging children to use whatever residual hearing and or sight they may have.

Video 19 min

3456 Getting Ready for the Big Date
Modern Sign Press
10443 Los Alamitos Boulevard, PO Box 1181
Los Alamitos, CA 90720

562-596-8548
800-572-7332
Fax: 562-795-6614
TTY: 562-493-4168
e-mail: modsigns@modernsignspress.com
www.modernsignspress.com

Basic level videotape of signed story for Expressive and Receptive practice. Story is repeated three times for ease of use. Watch how the visual features are incorporated. Turn the sound off for receptive practice. Written script and tape use suggestions included. VHS

3457 Getting Through Audiotape
Self Help for Hard-of-Hearing People
7910 Woodmont Avenue, Suite 1200
Bethesda, MD 20814

301-657-2248
Fax: 301-913-9413
TTY: 301-657-2249
e-mail: national@shhh.org
www.shhh.org

Simulates hearing loss for better understanding of communication difficulties. The tape features a hearing test.

Audiotape

3458 Ghost Investigation
Modern Sign Press
10443 Los Alamitos Boulevard, PO Box 1181
Los Alamitos, CA 90720

562-596-8548
800-572-7332
Fax: 562-795-6614
TTY: 562-493-4168
e-mail: modsigns@modernsignspress.com
www.modernsignspress.com

Basic level videotape of signed story for Expressive and Receptive practice. Story is repeated three times for ease of use. Watch how the visual features are incorporated. Turn the sound off for receptive practice. Written script and tape use suggestions included. VHS

3459 Governor's Campaign
Modern Sign Press
10443 Los Alamitos Boulevard, PO Box 1181
Los Alamitos, CA 90720

562-596-8548
800-572-7332
Fax: 562-795-6614
TTY: 562-493-4168
e-mail: modsigns@modernsignspress.com
www.modernsignspress.com

Basic level videotape of signed story for Expressive and Receptive practice. Story is repeated three times for ease of use. Watch how the visual features are incorporated. Turn the sound off for receptive practice. Written script and tape use suggestions included. VHS

3460 Graduate School
Modern Sign Press
10443 Los Alamitos Boulevard, PO Box 1181
Los Alamitos, CA 90720

562-596-8548
800-572-7332
Fax: 562-795-6614
TTY: 562-493-4168
e-mail: modsigns@modernsignspress.com
www.modernsignspress.com

Basic level videotape of signed story for Expressive and Receptive practice. Story is repeated three times for ease of use. Watch how the visual features are incorporated. Turn the sound off for receptive practice. Written script and tape use suggestions included. VHS

3461 High Five! Fables and Fairy Tales
Sign Media
4020 Blackburn Lane
Burtonsville, MD 20866

800-475-4756
Fax: 301-421-0270
www.signmedia.com

The cast of Four for You retuns with the addition of one new member for even more enjoyment. The same format is used here. Each tape includes five fables and two fairy tales. As an added bonus, two fables and one fairy tale are told twice. The first version is the traditional story, the second is how Deaf people would tell each tale. Each tape has a translated voice-over. Set of five 90 minute tapes.

3462 House Guests
Modern Sign Press
10443 Los Alamitos Boulevard, PO Box 1181
Los Alamitos, CA 90720

562-596-8548
800-572-7332
Fax: 562-795-6614
TTY: 562-493-4168
e-mail: modsigns@modernsignspress.com
www.modernsignspress.com

Basic level videotape of signed story for Expressive and Receptive practice. Story is repeated three times for ease of use. Watch how the visual features are incorporated. Turn the sound off for receptive practice. Written script and tape use suggestions included. VHS

3463 Hungry Caterpillar and Goodnight Moon
Modern Signs Press
10443 Los Alamitos Boulevard, PO Box 1181
Los Alamitos, CA 90720

562-596-8548
800-572-7332
Fax: 562-795-6614
TTY: 562-493-4168
e-mail: modsigns@modernsignspress.com
www.modernsignspress.com

Two favorite stories beautifully animated and signed using Signing Exact English. VHS

3464 I Can Hear
Alexander Graham Bell Association for the Deaf
3417 Volta Place NW
Washington, DC 20007

202-337-5220
800-432-7543
Fax: 202-337-8314
TTY: 202-337-5220
e-mail: agbell2@aol.com
www.agbell.org

This inspirational video describes the auditory-verbal approach for developing speech and language for hearing impaired children and adults.

1992 23 minutes

3465 I Can Hear-II

Alexander Graham Bell Association for the Deaf
3417 Volta Place NW
Washington, DC 20007

202-337-5220
800-432-7543
Fax: 202-337-8314
TTY: 202-337-5220
e-mail: agbell2@aol.com
www.agbell.org

An exciting videotape that gives more examples of auditory-verbal therapy and a variety of kids who have been taught to speak using this method.

1996 19 Minute video

3466 I Remember it Well

Modern Sign Press
10443 Los Alamitos Boulevard, PO Box 1181
Los Alamitos, CA 90720

562-596-8548
800-572-7332
Fax: 562-795-6614
TTY: 562-493-4168
e-mail: modsigns@modernsignspress.com
www.modernsignspress.com

Basic level videotape of signed story for Expressive and Receptive practice. Story is repeated three times for ease of use. Watch how the visual features are incorporated. Turn the sound off for receptive practice. Written script and tape use suggestions included. VHS

3467 Joy of Signing

Gallaudet Univ. Press c/o Chicago Distrib. Center
11030 S Langley Avenue
Chicago, IL 60628

202-651-5000
800-621-2736
Fax: 800-621-8476
TTY: 888-630-9347
www.gallaudet.edu/~gupress

Three tapes full of useful information to help increase skill and comfort with sign.

1 Videotape

3468 Kudos to Kuualoha

American Sign Language Productions
15155 Technology Drive
Eden Prairie, MN 55344

952-906-1180
800-767-4461
Fax: 952-906-1099
TTY: 952-906-1198
e-mail: ASLProductions@harriscomm.com
www.americansignlanguageproductions.com

From Hawaii, Kuuolaha, a beautiful, doe eyed child provides commentary on a number of subjects, along with the opportunity to practice reading a child's signs. Prepares you for interpreting in the middle school environment. Two certified interpreters demonstrate for you to compare, contrast and incorporate what you learn to your own skills. 30 minutes. DVD - $59.95; VHS - $49.95

3469 Language Says it All - 3 Part Video Set

Aquarius Health Care Videos
18 N Main Street
Sherborn, MA 01770

508-650-1616
888-440-2963
Fax: 508-650-1665
e-mail: info@aquariusproductions.com
www.aquariusproductions.com

We meet four families in which parent and siblings have learned to fulfill their deaf child's need for language. We learn from parents who candidly express the fears and uncertainties. Deaf educator, Cynthia Lebuffe, clearly explains the special challenge of bringing up a deaf child in a hearing family. Part 2 is an inspirational music video about Jacob Shamburg, a football player who is deaf. Part 3 reminds us of how important story time is to parents and their hearing impaired children.

Closed captions

Leslie Kussmann, President/Producer

3470 Learning to Communicate: The First Three Years Videotape

Alexander Graham Bell Association for the Deaf
3417 Volta Place NW
Washington, DC 20007

202-337-5220
800-432-7543
Fax: 202-337-8314
TTY: 202-337-5220
e-mail: agbell2@aol.com
www.agbell.org

This video shows normal communication development in young children under three years-of-age. It discusses factors which can affect speech and language development, including anatomy and environment. Closed-captioned.

11 Minutes

3471 Let's Eat

Modern Sign Press
10443 Los Alamitos Boulevard, PO Box 1181
Los Alamitos, CA 90720

562-596-8548
800-572-7332
Fax: 562-795-6614
TTY: 562-493-4168
e-mail: modsigns@modernsignspress.com
www.modernsignspress.com

Basic level videotape of signed story for Expressive and Receptive practice. Story is repeated three times for ease of use. Watch how the visual features are incorporated. Turn the sound off for receptive practice. Written script and tape use suggestions included. VHS

3472 Life in the Country

Modern Sign Press
10443 Los Alamitos Boulevard, PO Box 1181
Los Alamitos, CA 90720

562-596-8548
800-572-7332
Fax: 562-795-6614
TTY: 562-493-4168
e-mail: modsigns@modernsignspress.com
www.modernsignspress.com

Basic level videotape of signed story for Expressive and Receptive practice. Story is repeated three times for ease of use. Watch how the visual features are incorporated. Turn the sound off for receptive practice. Written script and tape use suggestions included. VHS

3473 Lipreading Made Easy
Alexander Graham Bell Association for the Deaf
3417 Volta Place NW
Washington, DC 20007

202-337-5220
800-432-7543
Fax: 202-337-8314
TTY: 202-337-5220
e-mail: agbell2@aol.com
www.agbell.org

Program gives you the much-needed practice-at-home material and provides the basic building blocks of lipreading. Video teaches you to see the sounds that make up the English conversation.

Video & Book

3474 Listen Learn and Talk
Alexander Graham Bell Association for the Deaf
3417 Volta Place NW
Washington, DC 20007

202-337-5220
202-337-8314
TTY: 203-337-5221
e-mail: info@agbell.org
www.agbell.org

Three-volume videotape and guidebook set provides general guiding theory, support materials and age-appropriate strategies for parents, families, and early interventionists who practice listening skills with young children. Videos are age specific and include the following developmental categories: 0-15 months, 16-30 months, and 31 months to school age. Softcover, spiral binding manual and three tape VHS set, 1:20 minutes.

3475 Listen to This, Volume One

Warren Eastabrooks, Karen MacIver Lux, Lisa Katz, author

Alexander Graham Bell Association for the Deaf
3417 Volta Place NW
Washington, DC 20007

202-337-5220
202-337-8314
TTY: 203-337-5221
e-mail: info@agbell.org
www.agbell.org

An Auditory-Verbal Therapy Videotape and Guidebook for Professionals and Parents designed for professionals in the fields of Auditory-Verbal therapy, auditory learning and professional education who want to enhance their service delivery of Auditory-Verbal therapy and auditory based learning and for parents of children who are participating in Auditory-Verbal therapy. Workbook - 76 pp., VHS - 47:14 minutes.

3476 Listen to This, Volume Two

Warren Eastabrooks, Karen MacIver Lux, Lisa Katz, author

Alexander Graham Bell Association for the Deaf
3417 Volta Place NW
Washington, DC 20007

202-337-5220
202-337-8314
TTY: 203-337-5221
e-mail: info@agbell.org
www.agbell.org

For health professional and parents of children with hearing loss, this interactive training resource builds upon the Auditory-Verbal therapy skills introduced in Volume 1 and chronicles the journey of Annie, a young girl who lost her hearing as an infant to meningitis. The DVD and step-by-step guidebook models more advance Auditory-Verbal therapy techniques and strategies and features the parent-professional partnership critical to guiding children with hearing loss along the path to listening.

DVD

3477 Literacy, Classroom Amplification and the Brain DVD

Carol Flexer, PhD, author

Alexander Graham Bell Association for the Deaf
3417 Volta Place NW
Washington, DC 20007

202-337-5220
202-337-8314
TTY: 203-337-5221
e-mail: info@agbell.org
www.agbell.org

This intermediate level program focuses on the essential components for enhancing classrooms to optimize the listening environment for school-age children. This video will provide educational information about sound field technology and how to create a favorable listening environment for enhanced development of learning, language and literacy.

DVD

3478 Literacy, Classroom Amplification and the Brain

Carol Flexer, PhD, author

Alexander Graham Bell Association for the Deaf
3417 Volta Place NW
Washington, DC 20007

202-337-5220
202-337-8314
TTY: 203-337-5221
e-mail: info@agbell.org
www.agbell.org

This intermediate level program focuses on the essential components for enhancing classrooms to optimize the listening environment for school-age children. This video will provide educational information about sound field technology and how to create a favorable listening environment for enhanced development of learning, language and literacy.

VHS

3479 Lydia's Lessons
American Sign Language Productions
15155 Technology Drive
Eden Prairie, MN 55344

952-906-1180
800-767-4461
Fax: 952-906-1099
TTY: 952-906-1198
e-mail: ASLProductions@harriscomm.com
www.americansignlanguageproductions.com

Lydia shares her school and camp experiences along with a rare opportunity to practice receptive skills and interpreting with a 12-year-old client. Here's your stress-free chance to hone your skills for middle school interpreting. Remember, you have two team interpreters to demonstrate how to interpret for Lydia. 40 minutes. DVD - $59.95; VHS - $49.95

3480 Mercer Mayer Frog Stories
Harris Communications
15155 Technology Drive
Eden Prairie, MN 55344

952-906-1180
800-825-6758
Fax: 952-906-1099
TTY: 952-906-1198
e-mail: info@harriscomm.com
www.harriscomm.com

Three classic Mercer Mayer stories on DVD-R; voiced; signed in ASL; no captions. Features: A Boy, a Dog and a Frog; Frog on His Own; and Frog, Where are You?

3481 My Baby Can Talk: First Signs
Harris Communications
15155 Technology Drive
Eden Prairie, MN 55344

952-906-1180
800-825-6758
Fax: 952-906-1099
TTY: 952-906-1198
e-mail: info@harriscomm.com
www.harriscomm.com

This is the only baby sign language video that features a young baby signing all the words presented and is considered engaging for young babies. Brightly colored toys, beautiful live footage, engaging images and a young baby signing captivate your baby and as a result your baby learns to sign. This DVD was specifically developed to respect the developmental stage, attention span and intellect of babies from 10 to 24 months. Teaches elementary signs based upon ASL. Ages 10 months and up.

2004 DVD 45 minutes

3482 My Surprise
Modern Sign Press
10443 Los Alamitos Boulevard, PO Box 1181
Los Alamitos, CA 90720

562-596-8548
800-572-7332
Fax: 562-795-6614
TTY: 562-493-4168
e-mail: modsigns@modernsignspress.com
www.modernsignspress.com

Basic level videotape of signed story for Expressive and Receptive practice. Story is repeated three times for ease of use. Watch how the visual features are incorporated. Turn the sound off for receptive practice. Written script and tape use suggestions included. VHS

3483 New Neighbors
Modern Sign Press
10443 Los Alamitos Boulevard, PO Box 1181
Los Alamitos, CA 90720

562-596-8548
800-572-7332
Fax: 562-795-6614
TTY: 562-493-4168
e-mail: modsigns@modernsignspress.com
www.modernsignspress.com

Basic level videotape of signed story for Expressive and Receptive practice. Story is repeated three times for ease of use. Watch how the visual features are incorporated. Turn the sound off for receptive practice. Written script and tape use suggestions included. VHS

3484 Number Signs for Everyone: Numbering in American Sign Language
DawnSign Press
6130 Nancy Ridge Drive
San Diegoe, CA 92121

858-625-0600
Fax: 858-625-2336
e-mail: info@dawnsign.com
www.dawnsign.com

Presenter Cinnie MacDougall shows you all the different rules and handshapes for clearly and accurately communicating numbers within ASL sentences in proper context. VHS.

90 minutes
ISBN: 0-915035-32-4

Cinnie MacDougall, Presenter

3485 Opinion Section
Modern Sign Press
10443 Los Alamitos Boulevard, PO Box 1181
Los Alamitos, CA 90720

562-596-8548
800-572-7332
Fax: 562-795-6614
TTY: 562-493-4168
e-mail: modsigns@modernsignspress.com
www.modernsignspress.com

Basic level videotape of signed story for Expressive and Receptive practice. Story is repeated three times for ease of use. Watch how the visual features are incorporated. Turn the sound off for receptive practice. Written script and tape use suggestions included. VHS

3486 Parent Sign Series
Sign Media
4020 Blackburn Lane
Burtonsville, MD 20866

900-475-4756
Fax: 301-421-0270
www.signmedia.com

Learn sign language within the situations that you face everyday. Rather than wasting time learning vocabulary that doesn't fit your needs, learn the signs that help you communicate quickly with your deaf child. Each tape shows conversations and interactions within a family followed by review sentences and vocabulary items. Perfect for parents to use at home or for sign language programs that offer instruction to parents and beginning signers. Comes in ten one-hour tapes.

VHS

3487 Rainbow's End
Sign Media
4020 Blackburn Lane
Burtonsville, MD 20866

800-475-4756
Fax: 301-421-0270
www.signmedia.com

It's like Sesame Street but with Deaf characters who use ASL. Designed to enhance the self-image of Deaf children, these five videotapes teach while they entertain. They encourage and lead children to acquisition of English language and reading skills. The Pot of Gold Resource Workbook contains activities and exercises and is fully reproducible. Set includes five 30 minute tapes and workbook.

3488 Rather Strange Stories
Modern Sign Press
10443 Los Alamitos Boulevard, PO Box 1181
Los Alamitos, CA 90720

562-596-8548
800-572-7332
Fax: 562-795-6614
TTY: 562-493-4168
e-mail: modsigns@modernsignspress.com
www.modernsignspress.com

Created to provide practice in word groups at the intermediate level in Signing Exact English. The word groups were established by topic, and the stories created to use all the words in a given group in the shortest story possible...which is why they are Rather Strange Stories at time. 14 titles: Math/Science, Words Around the House, Prepositions, Words for People, Education/English, Body & Health, Nature, Picnic, Playacting, Sports, Grand Ball, Rabbit/Beaver, Transportation and Religion.

$15 each tape

3489 Russian Soldier
Modern Sign Press
10443 Los Alamitos Boulevard, PO Box 1181
Los Alamitos, CA 90720

562-596-8548
800-572-7332
Fax: 562-795-6614
TTY: 562-493-4168
e-mail: modsigns@modernsignspress.com
www.modernsignspress.com

Basic level videotape of signed story for Expressive and Receptive practice. Story is repeated three times for ease of use. Watch how the visual features are incorporated. Turn the sound off for receptive practice. Written script and tape use suggestions included. VHS

3490 Science, Math
Modern Sign Press
10443 Los Alamitos Boulevard, PO Box 1181
Los Alamitos, CA 90720

562-596-8548
800-572-7332
Fax: 562-795-6614
TTY: 562-493-4168
e-mail: modsigns@modernsignspress.com
www.modernsignspress.com

Basic level videotape of signed story for Expressive and Receptive practice. Story is repeated three times for ease of use. Watch how the visual features are incorporated. Turn the sound off for receptive practice. Written script and tape use suggestions included. VHS

3491 Sign Songs: Fun Songs to Sign and Sing
Aylmer Press/TJ Publishers
2544 Tarpley Road, Suite 108
Carrollton, TX 75006

972-416-0800
800-999-1168
Fax: 972-416-0944
TTY: 972-416-0933
e-mail: customerservice@tjpublishers.com
www.tjpublishers.com

Features performers John Kinstler, formerly with the National Theatre of the Deaf, signing along to the lyrics of the eleven kids' songs written and performed by guitarist/singer Ken Lonnquist. Songs include 'Alligator Rag,' 'One Speed Bike,' 'Nattie of the Jungle' plus eight more delightful and fun songs. Lyrics included. VHS.

29 minutes
ISBN: 0-932314-45-7

3492 Sign With Your Baby-Complete Learning Kit
Modern Sign Press
10443 Los Alamitos Boulevard, PO Box 1181
Los Alamitos, CA 90720

562-596-8548
800-572-7332
Fax: 562-795-6614
TTY: 562-493-4168
e-mail: modsigns@modernsignspress.com
www.modernsignspress.com

Includes video, book and quick reference guide. The video makes learning easy with instruction, demonstrations and tips from the author and Speech-Language Pathologist. Interviews with parents and grandparents who share their experiences and footage of signing babies offers inspirational vision of the power of the system. The book is filled with anecdotes, practical guidelines and humor and offers an effective way to teach parents and infants how to communicate through sign.

VHS and DVD

Joseph Garcia, Author
Alice Stroutsos, Speech-Language Pathologist

3493 Signing Naturally
TJ Publishers
2544 Tarpley Road, Suite 108
Carrollton, TX 75006

972-416-0800
800-999-1168
Fax: 972-416-0944
TTY: 972-416-0933
e-mail: customerservice@tjpublishers.com
www.tjpublishers.com

This series is based on the functional-notional approach to teaching sign language developed at Vista Community College at Berkeley. Signing Naturally organizes language lessons around everyday interaction. Exercises in the student workbooks coincide with exercises on the videotapes. VHS and DVD

Cheri Smith, Producer
Ella Mae Lentz, Producer

3494 Sleeping Beauty
Gallaudet University Press
800 Florida Avenue NE
Washington, DC 20002

202-651-5488
Fax: 202-651-5489
e-mail: gupress@gallaudet.edu
http://gupress.gallaudet.edu

The Sleeping Beauty videotape features the full story in ASL and includes vocabulary and sentence structure focusing on adjectives, with a voice-over throughout. Color, 30 minutes

VHS
ISBN: 0-930323-98-X

3495 Sound & Fury
Aquarius Health Care Videos
18 N Main Street, PO Box 1159
Sherborn, MA 01770

508-650-1616
888-440-2963
Fax: 508-650-1665
e-mail: info@aquariusproductions.com
www.aquariusproductions.com

This film takes viewers inside the seldom seen world of the deaf to witness a painful family struggle over a controversial medical technology called the cochlear implant. Illuminates the ongoing struggle for identity among deaf people today. Available in VHS and DVD

55 Minutes

Leslie Kussman, President/Producer

3496 Sound and Fury: Six Years Later
Aquarius Health Care Media
18 North Main Street, PO Box 1159
Sherborn, MA 01770

888-440-2963
Fax: 508-650-1665
e-mail: orders@aquariusproductions.com
www.aquariousproductions.com

In 2000, the first Sound & Fury captured audiences around the world and an Academy Award nomination through the riveting story of the Artinian family of Long Island. This sequel gives a new look at the family as it follows them in the next six years of their life. An excellent film for anyone dealing with issues of hearing loss. A must for both professionals and families to see. 2006 - 29 minutes, DVD

3497 Stories About Growing Up
Harris Communciations
15155 Technology Drive
Eden Prairie, MN 55344

952-906-1180
800-825-6758
Fax: 952-906-1099
TTY: 952-906-1198
e-mail: info@harriscomm.com
www.harriscomm.com

DVD-R - voiced; signed in ASL; no captions. Three Scholastic stories: Leo the Late Bloomer by Robert Kraus (One day, in his own good time, Leo shows everyone how glorious it is to finally bloom); A Weekend with Wendell by Kevin Henkes (Three cheers for compromise as quiet-as-a-mouse Sophie learns to assert herself with big-mouthed Wendell), and Joey Runs Away by Jack Kent (Joey looks for another home when he doesn't like cleaning his room).

3498 Teaching Strategies for the Development of Auditory Verbal Communication
Alexander Graham Bell Association for the Deaf
3417 Volta Place NW
Washington, DC 20007

202-337-5220
800-432-7543
Fax: 202-337-8314
TTY: 202-337-5220
e-mail: agbell2@aol.com
www.agbell.org

This educational series of five-hour videotapes demonstrates teaching strategies for developing auditory-verbal communication in young children with severe to profound hearing loss.

Set of 5

3499 The Big Test
Modern Sign Press
10443 Los Alamitos Boulevard, PO Box 1181
Los Alamitos, CA 90720

562-596-8548
800-572-7332
Fax: 562-795-6614
TTY: 562-493-4168
e-mail: modsigns@modernsignspress.com
www.modernsignspress.com

Basic level videotape of signed story for Expressive and Receptive practice. Story is repeated three times for ease of use. Watch how the visual features are incorporated. Turn the sound off for receptive practice. Written script and tape use suggestions included.
VHS

3500 The Driving Test
Modern Sign Press
10443 Los Alamitos Boulevard, PO Box 1181
Los Alamitos, CA 90720

562-596-8548
800-572-7332
Fax: 562-795-6614
TTY: 562-493-4168
e-mail: modsigns@modernsignspress.com
www.modernsignspress.com

Basic level videotape of signed story for Expressive and Receptive practice. Story is repeated three times for ease of use. Watch how the visual features are incorporated. Turn the sound off for receptive practice. Written script and tape use suggestions included.
VHS

3501 The Gossip
Modern Sign Press
10443 Los Alamitos Boulevard, PO Box 1181
Los Alamitos, CA 90720

562-596-8548
800-572-7332
Fax: 562-795-6614
TTY: 562-493-4168
e-mail: modsigns@modernsignspress.com
www.modernsignspress.com

Basic level videotape of signed story for Expressive and Receptive practice. Story is repeated three times for ease of use. Watch how the visual features are incorporated. Turn the sound off for receptive practice. Written script and tape use suggestions included.
VHS

3502 The Grocer and the Cook
Modern Sign Press
10443 Los Alamitos Boulevard, PO Box 1181
Los Alamitos, CA 90720

562-596-8548
800-572-7332
Fax: 562-795-6614
TTY: 562-493-4168
e-mail: modsigns@modernsignspress.com
www.modernsignspress.com

Basic level videotape of signed story for Expressive and Receptive practice. Story is repeated three times for ease of use. Watch how the visual features are incorporated. Turn the sound off for receptive practice. Written script and tape use suggestions included.
VHS

3503 The Memo
Modern Sign Press
10443 Los Alamitos Boulevard, PO Box 1181
Los Alamitos, CA 90720

562-596-8548
800-572-7332
Fax: 562-795-6614
TTY: 562-493-4168
e-mail: modsigns@modernsignspress.com
www.modernsignspress.com

Basic level videotape of signed story for Expressive and Receptive practice. Story is repeated three times for ease of use. Watch how the visual features are incorporated. Turn the sound off for receptive practice. Written script and tape use suggestions included.
VHS

3504 The Pet Show
Modern Sign Press
10443 Los Alamitos Boulevard, PO Box 1181
Los Alamitos, CA 90720

562-596-8548
800-572-7332
Fax: 562-795-6614
TTY: 562-493-4168
e-mail: modsigns@modernsignspress.com
www.modernsignspress.com

Basic level videotape of signed story for Expressive and Receptive practice. Story is repeated three times for ease of use. Watch how the visual features are incorporated. Turn the sound off for receptive practice. Written script and tape use suggestions included.
VHS

3505 The Race
Modern Sign Press
10443 Los Alamitos Boulevard, PO Box 1181
Los Alamitos, CA 90720

562-596-8548
800-572-7332
Fax: 562-795-6614
TTY: 562-493-4168
e-mail: modsigns@modernsignspress.com
www.modernsignspress.com

Basic level videotape of signed story for Expressive and Receptive practice. Story is repeated three times for ease of use. Watch how the visual features are incorporated. Turn the sound off for receptive practice. Written script and tape use suggestions included. VHS

3506 The Snowman
HEAR-MORE
42 Executive Boulevard
Farmingdale, NY 11735

800-881-4327
Fax: 631-752-0689
TTY: 800-281-4327
www.hearmore.com

This delightful animation weaves a spell of magic enchantment as a young boy's snowman comes to life and escorts him on a fantasy dream visit to the North Pole.

3507 The Treasure Chest

Drs Michelle Anthony and Reyna Lindert, author

HEAR-MORE
42 Executive Boulevard
Farmingdale, NY 11735

800-881-4327
Fax: 631-752-0689
TTY: 800-281-4327
www.hearmore.com

Children of all ages will be delighted by this magical journey of discovery. Join us as we lead you and your child to a treasure trove of toys, plays, songs, and signs. The visually engaging images in the video present families with endless opportunities to make meaningful connections with their little ones. Designed for children aged 0-36 months. Running time is approximately 30 minutes. Includes more than 35 ASL signs.

DVD

3508 The World According to Pat: Reflections of Residential School Days
TJ Publishers
2544 Tarpley Road, Suite 108
Carrollton, TX 75006

972-416-0800
800-999-1168
Fax: 972-416-0944
TTY: 972-416-0933
e-mail: customerservice@tjpublishers.com
www.tjpublishers.com

Pat Graybill's one-man show offers humerous and touching insights into life in a residential school dormitory. Includes appearances by others who provide their own recollections of residential school days. VHS

90 minutes

3509 University Professor
Modern Sign Press
10443 Los Alamitos Boulevard, PO Box 1181
Los Alamitos, CA 90720

562-596-8548
800-572-7332
Fax: 562-795-6614
TTY: 562-493-4168
e-mail: modsigns@modernsignspress.com
www.modernsignspress.com

Basic level videotape of signed story for Expressive and Receptive practice. Story is repeated three times for ease of use. Watch how the visual features are incorporated. Turn the sound off for receptive practice. Written script and tape use suggestions included. VHS

3510 Videos on Hearing-Impaired Children TRIPOD Grapevine
2901 N Keystone Street
Burbank, CA 91504

800-352-8888
TDD: 800-287-4763

TRIPOD Grapevine will loan to parents upon request two excellent videos (open captioned) for families with hearing-impaired children. 'Language Says It All' focuses on the importance of establishing clear communication in the home. Parents talk about concerns for their children. 'Once Upon a Time' reminds us how important story time is to parents and their hearing-impaired child. Parents describe the ways in which they learned to share a rich story heritage with their children.

3511 Why We Can Hear And Speak
Alexander Graham Bell Association for the Deaf
3417 Volta Place NW
Washington, DC 20007

202-337-5220
202-337-8314
TTY: 203-337-5221
e-mail: info@agbell.org
www.agbell.org

This documentary was developed to show the children of Natural Communication, Inc. at different stages of language development. Each vignette inclueds an introductory biography that briefly describes the child's diagnosis, current age, therapy history and amplification technology. The principles of Auditory-Verbal philosophy are described throughout the tape. All children featured use the Auditory-Verbal approach.

VHS 23 minutes

Computer Software

3512 ASL Clip and Create Version 3
HEAR-MORE
42 Executive Boulevard
Farmingdale, NY 11735

800-881-4327
Fax: 631-752-0689
TTY: 800-281-3555
www.hearmore.com

Design learning materials, posters, cards, labels, postcards, and banners using over 3,500 American Sign Language pictures. Four sign-skill enhancing games. Six different templates to customize. Custom design & printing capabilities. Suggestions for learning activities and games. Minimum requirements: Windows 98 SE, Pentium II or equivalent, 64 Mb memory.

3513 ASL Songs for Kids
HEAR-MORE
42 Executive Bouldevard
Farmingdale, NY 11735

800-881-4327
Fax: 631-752-0689
TTY: 800-281-3555
www.hearmore.com

This CD-Rom presents six songs typically learned by young children-sung and signed. The CD contains two short songs-Twinkle, Twinkle Little Star & Happy Birthday, and four songs that have multiple verses-The Ants Go Marching, Old McDonald, The Wheels on the Bus and The Green Grass Grows All Around. ÆAs the songs are sung, Paws the dog sings, and graphics convey the lyrics, as well as information about the notes and volume. The songs can be viewed with signs in English word order or in ASL.

3514 ASL Tales and Games for Kids

HEAR-MORE
42 Executive Boulevard
Farmingdale, NY 11735

800-881-4327
Fax: 631-752-0689
TTY: 800-281-3555
www.hearmore.com

This CD series follows Paws, the signing dog, and his friends as they explore their neighborhood. This program contains 3 community-focused stories and 10 games. The neighborhood children are deaf or hard of hearing and represent different ethnic groups. Minimum system requirements: Windows (95,98,NT,ME,2000), 166 MHz Pentium, 4x CD-ROM Drive

3515 ASL Tales and Games for Kids 2

HEAR-MORE
42 Executive Bouldevard
Farmingdale, NY 11735

800-881-4327
Fax: 631-752-0689
TTY: 800-281-3555
www.hearmore.com

In this CD-ROM, Biscuit Boulevard focuses on events that take place on one street in Pawstown, Biscuit Boulevard. The stories are original and written to promote good English literacy, while simultaneously teaching important aspects of ASL. Each story can be viewed continuously, without the child needing to manipulate the mouse, or the child can control the story himself.

3516 ASL Tales and Songs for Kids CD-1

Harris Communications
15155 Technology Drive
Eden Prairie, MN 55344

952-906-1180
800-825-6758
Fax: 952-906-1099
TTY: 952-906-1198
e-mail: info@harriscomm.com
www.harriscomm.com

In 'Woof, Woof Way' Paws the Dog helps children build their skills with colorful graphics. Paws, the signing dog, and the Pawstown neighborhood kids on adventures in their own community. System requirements: Windows 95, 98, NT, ME, 2000; Pentium 166MHz; 4X or more CD-ROM drive; works with most popular monochrome and color printers supported by Windows.

CD-ROM

3517 ASL Tales and Songs for Kids CD-2

Harris Communications
15155 Technology Drive
Eden Prairie, MN 55344

952-906-1180
800-825-6758
Fax: 952-906-1099
TTY: 952-906-1198
e-mail: info@harriscomm.com
www.harriscomm.com

Paws, the signing dog, and the Pawstown neighborhood kids on adventures in their own community. In CD-2, 'Biscuit Boulevard,' Paws the Dog helps children build their skills with colorful graphics. System requirements: Windows 95, 98, NT, ME, 2000; Pentium 166MHz; 4X or more CD-ROM drive; works with most popular monochrome and color printers supported by Windows.

CD-ROM

3518 American Sign Language V2.0

HEAR-MORE
42 Executive Boulevard
Farmingdale, NY 11735

800-881-4327
Fax: 631-752-0689
TTY: 800-281-3555
www.hearmore.com

This updated version comes as a 5 CD-ROM set. Customize signing pace with the speed control feature. Takes you from beginner to advanced intermediate levels. Set includes SigningAvatar, HyperSign Jr, Ready! Set! Sign! Starter version, ASL Condensed Dictionary, and ASL introduction which aids children in developing essential analytical skills. System requirements: 500 MHz or faster, Windows 98/ME/XP, 128 MB RAM, 100 MB hard drive.

3519 American Sign Language Vocabulary

HEAR-MORE
42 Executive Boulevard
Farmingdale, NY 11735

800-881-4327
Fax: 631-752-0689
TTY: 800-281-3555
www.hearmore.com

PC requirements: Pentium 120 MHz or faster, Win 95, 98, NT4, 2000, 64 MB RAM, active movie 1.0 or higher, DirectShow 6.0 recommended, Active X Network libraries. Macintosh Requirements: PowerPC or later, 120 MHz or faster, MacOS 7+, 64 MB RAM, Quicktime 3 or higher, Quicktime mpeg extension v1.1.1 or higher.

3520 Baby's First Book of Signs: An ASL Word Bo ok (Volume 1-3)

HEAR-MORE
42 Executive Bouldevard
Farmingdale, NY 11735

800-881-4327
Fax: 631-752-0689
TTY: 800-281-3555
www.hearmore.com

Three sweet little electronic books depict the signs for basic words. Signs are shown in video and pictures. English equivalents, as well as concept graphics, are included. Easy to use-just click to turn each page. Volume 1 includes: Animals, Clothes, Colors, Food and Toys. Volume 2 includes: Actions, Descriptions, Feelings, When and Where. Volume 3 includes: Alphabet, Numbers, Home, Outside and People. CD-ROM

3521 Baby's First Book of Signs: Volumes I-III

Harris Communications
15155 Technology Drive
Eden Prairie, MN 55344

952-906-1180
800-825-6758
Fax: 952-906-1099
TTY: 952-906-1198
e-mail: info@harriscomm.com
www.harriscomm.com

An ASL Word Book with Video and Audio Clips. Each CD-ROM contains an electronic flip book for basic words in video and pictures. English equivalents (in print and audio), as well as concept graphics, are included. In these three CD-ROMs, you can learn 390 words in sign language. Minimum PC requirements: Windows 98, ME, 2000, XP; 64 MB RAM, 800x600 pixels screen area; Pentium II Æ300 MHz; 16-bit color display; CD-ROM drive.

3522 Cochlear Impant Auditory Training Guide

David Sindrey, Cert. AVT, author

Alexander Graham Bell Association for the Deaf
3417 Volta Place NW
Washington, DC 20007

202-337-5220
202-337-8314
TTY: 203-337-5221
e-mail: info@agbell.org
www.agbell.org

This second edition comes with games pieces, peg boards, and two print CDs. The manual presents easy to follow hierarchy and the CDs include a placement test, lesson plan forms, acoustic screens, and hundreds of discrimination cards and activities for single word, multiple element and broader language listening at all levels. The Wordplay product Vattier Boards has now been incorporated into this package.

3523 Elf on a Shelf for Minimal Pairs: Giant CD Print Program

David Sindrey, Cert. AVT, author

Alexander Graham Bell Association for the Deaf
3417 Volta Place NW
Washington, DC 20007

202-337-5220
202-337-8314
TTY: 203-337-5221
e-mail: info@agbell.org
www.agbell.org

Print more than 1100 English words. This program organizes effective word-pair practice into the following formats: Lotto games, Dixie Cup games, Matrix games, Fiv. Operates on any PC or MAC system.

3524 Fingerspelling & Numbers Software

Sign Enhancers
10568 SE Washington Street
Portland, OR 97216

800-767-4461
Fax: 503-304-1063
TTY: 888-283-5097
e-mail: HeyYou@SignEnhancers.com
www.signenhancers.com

Fingerspelling practice partner that allows you to control the speed and vocabulary level. Requires Windows 3.1 or greater.

Software

Michele Paoletti-Schelp, President/CEO
Johann Paoletti-Schelp, COO

3525 Foundation In Speech Perception Computer Program

Alexander Graham Bell Association for the Deaf
3417 Volta Place NW
Washington, DC 20007

202-337-5220
800-432-7543
Fax: 202-337-8314
TTY: 202-337-5220
e-mail: agbell2@aol.com
www.agbell.org

This computerized auditory training program for children, ages three and up, fosters learning and literacy by developing skills in speech perception, speech production, vocabulary, reading, writing, and computer skills in children with a variety of hearing impairments, this software progresses at the child's pace and allows unlimited exploration opportunities. Each module varies the amount of visual support that a child can use.

3526 Hear & Listen! Talk & Sing!

Warren Estabrooks MEd, Lois Birkenshaw-Fleming BA, author

Alexander Graham Bell Association for the Deaf
3417 Volta Place NW
Washington, DC 20007

202-337-5220
202-337-8314
TTY: 203-337-5221
e-mail: info@agbell.org
www.agbell.org

This music book and CD integrates songs with speech sounds to enable young children with hearing loss to develop melodic, natural-sounding voices and enhance linguistic skills. Songs include sounds that are acoustically relevant to children with severe or profound hearing loss ages 18 months to 7 years. Songs are grouped in categories such as animals, weather and holidays and vary in difficulty.

3527 Hearing is Believing, Volume One

Dimity Dornan, BA, author

Alexander Graham Bell Association for the Deaf
3417 Volta Place NW
Washington, DC 20007

202-337-5220
Fax: 202-337-8314
TTY: 202-337-5221
e-mail: info@agbell.org
www.agbell.org

The first volume of the Hearing is Believing distance education series on CD-ROM offers self-directed learning through four hours of lectures on the following Auditory-Verbal topics: Current Auditory-Verbal PRactice and Research, Auditory Learning, Listening for Older Children, Integration into the Mainstream School. Includes lectures within the framework of the Auditory-Verbal Curriculum, accompanying PowerPoint slides, video excerpts of Auditory-Verbal therapy sessions and transcripts.

3528 Hearing is Believing, Volume Three

Dimity Dornan, BA, author

Alexander Graham Bell Association for the Deaf
3417 Volta Place NW
Washington, DC 20007

202-337-5220
Fax: 202-337-8314
TTY: 202-337-5221
e-mail: info@agbell.org
www.agbell.org

This third volume in the Hearing is Believing series provides four hours of self-directed learning on the following Auditory-Verbal topics: Teaching Spoken Language, Speech Development, Working with Parents and Infants. Includes lectures within the framework of the Auditory-Verbal curriculum, accompanying PowerPoint slides, video excerpts of Audio-Verbal therapy sessions and transcripts. A note-taking feature allows you to jot down ideas and questions as you learn.

3529 Hearing is Believing, Volume Two

Judith A Marlow, PhD, author

Alexander Graham Bell Association for the Deaf
3417 Volta Place NW
Washington, DC 20007

202-337-5220
Fax: 202-337-8314
TTY: 202-337-5221
e-mail: info@agbell.org
www.agbell.org

This interactive CD-ROM, the second volume in the Hearing is Believing distance eduction series includes two hours of lectures on early detection and intervention: The Rationale for Early Detection and Current Status, Achieving Timely Evaluation and Intervention, Shifting Paradigms. Includes lectures within the framework of the Auditory-Verbal curriculum, accompanying PowerPoint slides, video excerpts of Auditory-Verbal therapy sessions and transcripts.

3530 Holidays CD-ROM

Harris Communications
15155 Technology Drive
Eden Prairie, MN 55344

952-906-1180
800-825-6758
Fax: 952-906-1099
TTY: 952-906-1198
e-mail: info@harriscomm.com
www.harriscomm.com

This electronic book teaches 303 basic signs for 13 holidays: New Year, Valentine's Day, Patriotic Days, St. Patrick's Day, Easter, Graduation, Jewish Holidays, Parents' Days, Halloween, Christmas, Birthdays, Weddings and Thanksgiving. Minimum PC requirements: Windows 98, ME, 2000, XP; Pentium II 300MHz; 64 MB RAM; 16-bit color display; 800x600 pixels screen area; CD-ROM drive.

3531 Holidays: An ASL Word Book

HEAR-MORE
42 Executive Bouldevard
Farmingdale, NY 11735

800-881-4327
Fax: 631-752-0689
TTY: 800-281-3555
www.hearmore.com

This electronic book teaches all of the basic signs for 13 holidays. Signs are shown in video and pictures. English equivalents, as well as concept graphics, are included. Holidays covered include: New Year, Valentine's Day, Patriotic Days, St. Patrick's Day, Easter, Christmas, Jewish Holidays, Thanksgiving, Graduation, Weddings/Anniversaries, Hallowwen, Birthday, and Parents' Days. Easy to use-just click to turn each page. Windows 98/ME/2000/XP, Pentium 2 300 MHz, 64 MB Ram, CD drive

3532 I Cue, U Cue

HEAR-MORE
42 Executive Bouldevard
Farmingdale, NY 11735

800-881-4327
Fax: 631-752-0689
TTY: 800-281-3555
www.hearmore.com

This software provides information about Cued Speech. Cued Speech combines hand-shapes and placements with mouth movements to represent the consonants and vowels of a language. The complete American English system is taught through 14 classes, with an additional class providing extra practice. Includes guide. Windows 98SE, ME, 2000, XP; CD-ROM drive, 16X; Pentium III, 600 MHz or eqivalent; 190 MD hard drive space.

3533 Illustrated Dictionary - 3D ASL

HEAR-MORE
42 Executive Boulevard
Farmingdale, NY 11735

800-881-4327
Fax: 631-752-0689
TTY: 800-281-3555
www.hearmore.com

This CD-ROM Dictionary is designed for everyone who wants to learn American Sign Language. Choose one of nine characters with different personalities and ethnic backgrounds. Characters fidget while waiting and show emotions, like impatience or happiness. Every word in the dictionary is represented by a picture, used in a sentence and signed by your selected character. System require-

ments: 300 MHz PC, Windows 98/ME/NT/2000/XP, Internet Explorer 4+, CD-ROM, 1024X768 monitor, 100MB hard drive space

3534 Johnny Rock's Christmas

HEAR-MORE
42 Executive Boulevard
Farmingdale, NY 11735

800-881-4327
Fax: 631-752-0689
TTY: 800-281-3555
www.hearmore.com

This software is specially designed to enhance vocabulary development for deaf and hard of hearing students and elementary aged students with similar language needs. Teachers and Parents will love it as much as the kids will. Delightful graphics. Easy installation. Non-auditory. On-line technical support. Two 3.5 diskettes. Runs on Windows/Win95/Win98.

3535 Ling Series

Daniel Ling, PhD, author

Alexander Graham Bell Association for the Deaf
3417 Volta Place NW
Washington, DC 20007

202-337-5220
Fax: 202-337-8314
TTY: 202-337-5221
e-mail: info@agbell.org
www.agbell.org

Learn at your own pace with this CD-ROM distance education program featuring lectures from the University of Ottawa seminar in Auditory-Verbal practices. Topics include: Assessment of Spoken Language, Phonological Processes, Remediation of Deviant Speech. The CD includes the lecture, accompanying PowerPoint slides, clips of Ling's students, full lecture transcripts and a note-taking feature that allows you to jot down ideas and questions as you learn.

3536 Marvin Teaches Fingerspelling

HEAR-MORE
42 Executive Boulevard
Farmingdale, NY 11735

800-881-4327
Fax: 631-752-0689
TTY: 800-281-3555
www.hearmore.com

This CD is the coolest way yet to improve your receptive fingerspelling skills. Beginners can learn to recognize the different handshapes that make up the letters of the alphabet. Signers of every ability level can practice reading many fingerspelled words at speeds varying from novice to expert. Minimum system requirements: Pentium I, Windows 95, CD drive.

3537 MyTTY Phone Messenger Software for Windows

HEAR-MORE
42 Executive Bouldevard
Farmingdale, NY 11735

800-881-4327
Fax: 631-752-0689
TTY: 800-281-3555
www.hearmore.com

myTTY Phone Messenger is out-dialing software. It allows you to send pre-recorded TTY text and/or voice message to each telephone number on a customizable list. It can be used for such purposes as emergency, informational, meeting, and advertising notifications. Requires Windows 2000 or XP; 32 MB memory, Pentium Processor or compatible, CD-Rom dirve; TAPI-complieant voice modem.

3538 MyTTY for Windows 95, 98, ME, 2000, XP
HEAR-MORE
42 Executive Boulevard
Farmingdale, NY 11735

800-881-4327
Fax: 631-752-0689
TTY: 800-281-3555
www.hearmore.com

Now you can use your PC as a TTY too. myTTY is a computer program that runs under the Microsoft Windows operating system. If the computer is equipped with a voice modem, myTTY will make the computer perform like a TTY. The program allows your computer to communicate with any Baudot TTY over a telephone line. Requirements: Windows 98, SE or later (XP compatible) with Internet Explorer 4.0 or later, a Pentium processor or equivalent, CD drive, TAP compliant modem and 32 MB of memory.

3539 Paws Sign Stories
Harris Communications
15155 Technology Drive
Eden Prairie, MN 55344

952-906-1180
800-825-6758
Fax: 952-906-1099
TTY: 952-906-1198
e-mail: info@harriscomm.com
www.harriscomm.com

An educational and entertaining program designed for deaf and hard of hearing children who want to learn American Sign Language. Includes 5 stories and 15 games. Click on individual words or whole sentences to have them signs and voiced. Includes video clips of a person dressed as Paws, using ASL so all information is accessible to deaf and hard of hearing children. Ages 3-7.

CD-ROM

3540 Ready! Set! Sign!
HEAR-MORE
42 Executive Boulevard
Farmingdale, NY 11735

800-881-4327
Fax: 631-752-0689
TTY: 800-281-3555
www.hearmore.com

Begin with 100 signs you already know. Then continue learning over 1,000 more using video clips, photos, animations and graphics as visual aids for learning and remembering signs. Afterwards study the topics that interest you: fingerspelling, numbers, grammar concepts, and more. Learn the vocabulary you want, when you want it. Test your current sign language knowledge by reading over 1,750 signed practice sentences, phrases, words and numbers. View one or more of twenty-three Cultural Moments.

3541 School Days
Harris Communications
15155 Technology Drive
Eden Prairie, MN 55344

952-906-1180
800-825-6758
Fax: 952-906-1099
TTY: 952-906-1198
e-mail: info@harriscomm.com
www.harriscomm.com

An ASL Word Book with Video and Audio Clips. Prepare your child for school with this fun electronic book of 76 basic school vocabulary words. Each page shows the sign in both video and a picture. English equivalents in print and audio, plus concept graphics are included. Minimum system requirements: Windows 98, ME, 2000, XP; Pentium II 300MHz; 64MB RAM; 16-bit color display; 800x600 pixels screen area; CD-ROM drive.

CD-ROM

3542 School Days: An ASL Word Book
HEAR-MORE
42 Executive Boulevard
Farmingdale, NY 11735

800-881-4327
Fax: 631-752-0689
TTY: 800-281-3555
www.hearmore.com

Prepare your child for school with this fun little electronic book of basic school signs. Each page shows the sign in both video and a picture. English equivalents (in print and audio), as well as concept graphics, are included. 76 signs in all. Easy to use-just click to turn each page. Minimum system requirements: Windows 98/ME/2000/XP, Pentium 2 300 MHz, 64 MB Ram, 16-bit color display, 800x600 pixels screen area, CD drive.

3543 Sign Fine - Vacations
HEAR-MORE
42 Executive Bouldevard
Farmingdale, NY 11735

800-881-4327
Fax: 631-752-0689
TTY: 800-281-3555
www.hearmore.com

Join Paws, the signing dog, as he goes to 14 different travel destinations. Just click on any of the items in the picture to see a video of Paws signing the vocabulary word and an English word equivalent. This CD-Rom software for Windows has over 550 American Sign Language videos that illustrate signs and three fun games to play. Requires Windows 98, ME, 200, XP, Pentium III, 600 MHZ or equivalent, CD-Rom drive and 90 MB of hard drive space.

3544 Simser Series
Judith Simser, author

Alexander Graham Bell Association for the Deaf
3417 Volta Place NW
Washington, DC 20007

202-337-5220
Fax: 202-337-8314
TTY: 202-337-5221
e-mail: info@agbell.org
www.agbell.org

Enhance your knowledge with this interactive CD-ROM distance education program featuring lectures from the University of Ottawa seminar in Auditory-Verbal practices. Topics include: Auditory-Verbal Techniques and Hierarchies, Ongoing Assessment, The Why and How of Toys and Games, Goals for the Cochlear Implant User. The CD includes the lectures, accompanying PowerPoint slides, demonstrations of an Auditory-Verbal therapy session, audio clips of students, and full lecture transcripts.

3545 Smile
Enid G Wolf-Schein, EdD, CCC-SLP, author

Alexander Graham Bell Association for the Deaf
3417 Volta Place NW
Washington, DC 20007

202-337-5220
202-337-8314
TTY: 203-337-5221
e-mail: info@agbell.org
www.agbell.org

SMILE is a multisensory program that teaches speech, reading, and writing to children with severe language and communication delays, including those with hearing loss, dyslexia, or autism. Unique in its engaging yet simple focus, SMILE uses expressive and receptive modalities to improve the reading skills of target and general populations. Softcover manual 138 pp. CD and five-Teacher's Guide set.

3546 Snap! Kids American Sign Language
HEAR-MORE
42 Executive Boulevard
Farmingdale, NY 11735

800-881-4327
Fax: 631-752-0689
TTY: 800-281-3555
www.hearmore.com

This CD-ROM focuses on ASL basics. Especially for young readers, this disc is full of interactive games and animated vocabulary allowing kids to master new signs while having fun. 26 vocabulary 'books' covering subjects from Action words to Animals; Transportation to Telling Time. Instructional Demos featuring Live-action video signing. ASL Games including Tic Tac Toe and Multiple Choice. System Requirements: Processor 386 DX/33 MHz or faster, Win 3.1, 8 MB RAM, 6 MB HD, 2X CD-ROM, Sound card

3547 Software to Go
Gallaudet Univ. Press c/o Chicago Distrib. Center
11030 S Langley Avenue
Chicago, IL 60628

202-651-5000
800-621-2736
Fax: 800-621-8476
TTY: 888-630-9347
www.gallaudet.edu/~gupress

Lists and describes commercial software that may be borrowed by educators of hearing impaired students.

100 pages

3548 Songs for Listening! Songs for Life!
Warren Estabrooks MEd, Lois Birkenshaw-Fleming BA, author

Alexander Graham Bell Association for the Deaf
3417 Volta Place NW
Washington, DC 20007

202-337-5220
202-337-8314
TTY: 203-337-5221
e-mail: info@agbell.org
www.agbell.org

A song book/CD set and therapy guide. Designed to teach children with hearing loss how to listen and talk through the use of singing and music. It includes early intervention activities as well as resources for parents and professionals who work to develop audition and spoken language in children with hearing loss and/or other communicative disorders. This publication incorporates current language-learning therapy, is presented in an easy-to-read format, and includes technical references.

3549 The Ultimate ASL Dictionary
HEAR-MORE
42 Executive Boulevard
Farmingdale, NY 11735

800-881-4327
Fax: 631-752-0689
TTY: 800-281-3555
www.hearmore.com

Over 2400 signs included. Identify words through ASL or English, Words and definitions in video clips, graphics, text and audio, variations of English words that relate to a single sign, spell-check and parameter check.

3550 Troll In A Bowl: Games and Card Print Factory

David Sindrey, Cert. AVT, author

Alexander Graham Bell Association for the Deaf
3417 Volta Place NW
Washington, DC 20007

202-337-5220
202-337-8314
TTY: 203-337-5221
e-mail: info@agbell.org
www.agbell.org

Features over 2000 articulation, minimal pair, and vocabulary cards organized by a Speech-Language Pathologist. Operates on any PC or MAC system. Includes 54 page soft-cover spiral-binding workbook, game piece and CD

Book Publishers

3551 50 Frequently Asked Questions About Auditory-Verbal Therapy
Warren Estabrooks, MEd, author

Alexander Graham Bell Association for the Deaf
3417 Volta Place NW
Washington, DC 20007

202-337-5220
Fax: 202-337-8314
TTY: 202-337-5221
e-mail: info@agbell.org
www.agbell.org

A prolific collection of responses to most frequently asked questions about auditory-verbal therapy and its application for children who are deaf and hard of hearing. Parents, professionals and everyone concerned with deafness will welcome the guidance, encouragement and knowledge found within this collaboration of professionals who have joined both hearts and minds to provide an extraordinary, informative and invaluable worldwide resource.

213 pages Softcover

3552 A Basic Course in American Sign Lanuage, Second Edition
Tom Humphries, Carol Padden, Terrenc J O'Rourke, author

TJ Publishers
2544 Tarpley Road, Suite 108
Carrollton, TX 75006

972-416-0800
800-999-1168
Fax: 972-416-0944
TTY: 972-416-0933
e-mail: customerservice@tjpublishers.com
www.tjpublishers.com

Features a new introduction, which includes a section on Deaf Culture and Community, expanded dialogue introductions that incorporate cultural information, revised grammar notes and an updated bibliography.

288 pages Spiral bound
ISBN: 0-932666-42-6

3553 A Basic Vocabulary: American Sign Language for Parents and Children

Terrence J O'Rourke, author

TJ Publishers
2544 Tarpley Road, Suite 108
Carrollton, TX 75006

972-416-0800
800-999-1168
Fax: 972-416-0944
TTY: 972-416-0933
e-mail: customerservice@tjpublishers.com
www.tjpublishers.com

Carefully selected words and signs include those families use every day. Alphabetically organized vocabulary incorporates developmental lists helpful to both Deaf and hearing children and over 1000 clear sign language illustrations.

240 pages Softcover
ISBN: 0-932666-00-0

3554 A Book of Colors: Baby's First Sign Book

Kim Votry and Curt Waller, author

Gallaudet University Press
800 Florida Avenue NE
Washington, DC 20002

202-651-5488
Fax: 202-651-5489
e-mail: gupress@gallaudet.edu
http://gupress.gallaudet.edu

Depicts the charming character with the favorite hat signing all of the primary and secondary colors - red, yellow, blue, orange green and purple - in interesting settings. The other pages display a wide variety of appealing colors, too, including pink, white, black, gray, brown, and tan, topped off with a richly rendered illustration of a rainbow.

16 pages Board book
ISBN: 1-563681-47-1

3555 A Season of Change

Lois L Hodge, author

Gallaudet University Press
800 Florida Avenue NE
Washington, DC 20002

202-651-5488
Fax: 202-651-5489
e-mail: gupress@gallaudet.edu
http://gupress.gallaudet.edu

Okay, so she can't hear as well as other people, but do they believe she can't think as well? Everyone, it seems, in 13-going-on-14-year-old Biney Richmond's life treats her as though she should be wrapped in cotton and set on a shelf. Her parents act as though she can't do things for herself. The only one who seems to have any confidence in her is her best friend, Pat. When Pat's older brother, Gene-who secretly wants to date Biney-gets in trouble, Biney proves to everyone how grown up she is.

108 pages Softcover
ISBN: 0-930323-27-0

3556 ABC's of Finger Spelling

Modern Signs Press
PO Box 1181
Los Alamitos, CA 90720

562-596-8548
800-572-7332
Fax: 562-795-6614
TTY: 310-493-4168
e-mail: modsigns@modernsignspress.com
www.modernsignspress.com

Helps teach upper and lower case letters of the alphabet. Includes printed letters and easy-to-follow drawings of the hand shapes.

1984 60 pages paperback

3557 ABCs of AVT: Analyzing Auditory-Verbal The rapy

Warren Estabrooks, MEd and Rhonda Schwartz, MA, author

Alexander Graham Bell Association for the Deaf
3417 Volta Place NW
Washington, DC 20007

202-337-5220
Fax: 202-337-8314
TTY: 202-337-5221
e-mail: info@agbell.org
www.agbell.org

Provides an overview of Auditory-Verbal techniques and guidance on appropriate intervention for children experiencing difficulties with language development. Task analysis exercises outlined in the manual and demonstrated in the video, which contains excerpts of therapy sessions and longitudinal studies, are designed to help students and professionals of all levels of experience hone their clinical skills. Softcover/Spiral binding/manual and VHS set/Open-Captioned 46:04

104 pages Softcover

3558 APT/HI: Auditory Perception Test for the Hearing Impaired

Alexander Graham Bell Association for the Deaf
3417 Volta Place NW
Washington, DC 20007

202-337-5220
800-432-7543
Fax: 202-337-8314
TTY: 202-337-5220
e-mail: agbell2@aol.com
www.agbell.org

This test, modeled on children with hearing losses, allows speech therapists and audiologists to assess functional use of residual hearing. The test identifies auditory processing and auditory training, prioritizes speech targets and auditory functioning, and assesses amplification.

1994 25-Tests

3559 ASL Babies: First Signs

Tina Jo Breindel and Michael Carter, author

Harris Communications
15155 Technology Drive
Eden Prairie, MN 55344

952-906-1180
800-825-6758
Fax: 952-906-1099
TTY: 952-906-1198
e-mail: info@harriscomm.com
www.harriscomm.com

A toddler signs 14 words that first appear in a child's vocabulary: airplane, baby, bath, bed, dad, help, hot, hurt, mom, more, please, thank you, tired and toilet.

16 pages Board book

3560 ASL Babies: Let's Eat

Tina Jo Breindel and Michael Carter, author

Harris Communications
15155 Technology Drive
Eden Prairie, MN 55344

952-906-1180
800-825-6758
Fax: 952-906-1099
TTY: 952-906-1198
e-mail: info@harriscomm.com
www.harriscomm.com

Food-related vocabulary words in English and American Sign Language are beautifully illustrated in this board book.

16 pages Board book

3561 AUSPLAN Auditory Speech and Language

Adeline McClatchie, LCST and MaryKay Therres, MS, author

Alexander Graham Bell Association for the Deaf
3417 Volta Place NW
Washington, DC 20007

202-337-5220
Fax: 202-337-8314
TTY: 202-337-5221
e-mail: info@agbell.org
www.agbell.org

AuSpLan is a communication therapy manual for children using choclear implants or hearing aids. It addresses auditory, speech/articulation, and language skills of children between the ages of 18 months and 5 years.

212 pages Softcover

3562 Academic Acceptance of ASL

Gallaudet Univ. Press c/o Chicago Distrib. Center
11030 S Langley Avenue
Chicago, IL 60628

202-651-5000
800-621-2736
Fax: 800-621-8476
TTY: 888-630-9347
www.gallaudet.edu/~gupress

This monograph presents a dozen articles that demonstrate clearly and convincingly that the study of ASL affords the same educational values and the same intellectual rewards as the study of any other foreign language.

196 pages

3563 Access for All: Integrating Deaf, Hard-of- Hearing and Hearing Preschoolers

Gallaudet Univ. Press c/o Chicago Distrib. Center
11030 S Langley Avenue
Chicago, IL 60628

202-651-5000
800-621-2736
Fax: 800-621-8476
TTY: 888-630-9347
www.gallaudet.edu/~gupress

Describes a model program for integrating the deaf and hard-of-hearing in early education.

69 pages Book & Video

3564 Advocacy Handbook

Alexander Graham Bell Association for the Deaf
3417 Volta Place NW
Washington, DC 20007

202-337-5220
800-432-7543
Fax: 202-337-8314
TTY: 202-337-5220
e-mail: agbell2@aol.com
www.agbell.org

A comprehensive guide including sections on effective advocacy, parent concerns, special education and IEPs, adolescence, the Americans with Disabilities Act, inclusion, technology and taxes.

1995 150 pages

3565 Advocacy for Deaf Children

Charles C Thomas Publishing
2600 S 1st Street
Springfield, IL 62794

217-789-8980
800-258-8980
Fax: 217-789-9130
www.ccthomas.com

Professional text on attitudes toward the deaf children in America.

114 pages

3566 Alandra's Lilacs

Tressa Bowers, author

Gallaudet University Press
800 Florida Avenue NE
Washington, DC 20002

202-651-5488
Fax: 202-651-5489
e-mail: gupress@gallaudet.edu
http://gupress.gallaudet.edu

When, in 1968, 19-year-old Tressa Bowers took her baby daughter to an expert on deaf children, he pronounced that Alandra was 'stone deaf,' she most likely would never be able to talk, and she probably would not get much of an education because of her communication limitations. Tressa refused to accept this stark assessment of Alandra's prospects. Instead, she began the arduous process of starting her daughter's education.

158 pages Softcover
ISBN: 1-563680-82-3

3567 All of Us Together

Jeri Banks, author

Gallaudet University Press
800 Florida Avenue NE
Washington, DC 20002

202-651-5488
Fax: 202-651-5489
e-mail: gupress@gallaudet.edu
http://gupress.gallaudet.edu

John H. Kinzie Elementary School, in Chicago, for decades was the pride of its neighborhood until changing demographics, racial conflict, and desegregation mandates threatened its existance. Then, its new principal, James Burke, welcomed 15 classes of deaf and hard of hearing children. This is the story of the Kinzie School from 1982, when hearing and nonhearing populations were kept in separate parts of the school, to the present in which all students intermingle freely and achieve together.

212 pages Hardcover
ISBN: 1-563680-28-9

3568 Alone in the Mainstream: A Deaf Women Reme mbers Public School

Gina A Oliva, author

Gallaudet University Press
800 Florida Avenue NE
Washington, DC 20002

202-651-5488
Fax: 202-651-5489
e-mail: gupress@gallaudet.edu
http://gupress.gallaudet.edu

When Gina Oliva first went to school in 1955, she didn't know that she was 'different.' If the kindergarten teacher played a tune on the piano to signal the next exercise, Olivia didn't react because she couldn't hear the music. So began her journey as a 'solitary,' her term for being the only deaf child in the entire school. Gina felt alone because she couldn't communicate easily with her class-mates, but also because none of them had a hearing loss like hers.

224 pages Softcover
ISBN: 1-563683-00-8

3569 Alphabet of Animal Signs
HEAR-MORE
42 Executive Boulevard
Farmingdale, NY 11735

800-881-4327
Fax: 631-752-0689
TTY: 800-281-4327
www.hearmore.com

This book includes animal illustrations and associated signs for each letter of the alphabet.

3570 American Deaf Culture: An Anthology
Sign Media
4020 Blackburn Lane
Burtonsville, MD 20866

301-421-0268
800-475-4756
Fax: 301-421-0270
TDD: 301-421-4460
e-mail: signmedia@aol.com
www.signmedia.com

Features deaf and hearing authors offering their experience and perspectives on cultural values, ASL, social interaction in the deaf community, education, folklore and more.

202 pages Paperback
ISBN: 0-932130-09-7

Barbara Olmert, Director Marketing

3571 American Sign Language Dictionary Third Ed ition

Martin L A Stemberg, author

TJ Publishers
2544 Tarpley Road, Suite 108
Carrollton, TX 75006

972-416-0800
800-999-1168
Fax: 972-416-0944
TTY: 972-416-0933
e-mail: customerservice@tjpublishers.com
www.tjpublishers.com

Completely updated and revised, this easy to use abridged version of the American Sign Language: A Comprehensive Dictionary has more than 500 new signs and 1500 new illustrations. It contains more than 5000 of the most widely used words, phrases, and idi-oms, accompanied by 8000 easy-to-follow illustrations of the hand, arm and facial movements that express each one.

772 pages Softcover
ISBN: 0-062736-34-5

3572 American Sign Language: A Student Text; Units 10-18
Sign Media
4020 Blackburn Lane
Burtonsville, MD 20866

800-475-4756
Fax: 301-421-0270
www.signmedia.com

These texts were designed to help students acquire conversational abilities in American Sign Language. Each unit targets a specific grammatical feature of ASL and presents a dialogue focusing on that grammatical feature. Dialogues are presented three times - the first is a shot of both conversational participants, the second and third presentations each focus on one of the participants. Following the dialogues are anecdotes, stories and poems.

ISBN: 0-930323-87-4

3573 American Sign Language: A Student Text; Units 1-9
Sign Media
4020 Blackburn Lane
Burtonsville, MD 20866

800-475-4756
Fax: 301-421-0270
www.signmedia.com

These texts were designed to help students acquire conversational abilities in American Sign Language. Each unit targets a specific grammatical feature of ASL and presents a dialogue focusing on that grammatical feature. Dialogues are presented three times - the first is a shot of both conversational participants, the second and third presentations each focus on one of the participants. Following the dialogues are anecdotes, stories and poems.

ISBN: 0-930323-86-6

3574 American Sign Language: A Student Text; Un its 19-27
Sign Media
4020 Blackburn Lane
Burtonsville, MD 20866

800-475-4756
Fax: 301-421-0270
www.signmedia.com

These texts were designed to help students acquire conversational abilities in American Sign Language. Each unit targets a specific grammatical feature of ASL and presents a dialogue focusing on that grammatical feature. Dialogues are presented three times - the first is a shot of both conversational participants, the second and third presentations each focus on one of the participants. Following the dialogues are anecdotes, stories and poems.

ISBN: 0-930323-88-2

3575 American Sign Language: Beginning Course - Teacher's Manual
National Association of the Deaf
814 Thayer Avenue
Silver Spring, MD 20910

301-587-1788
Fax: 301-587-1791
TTY: 301-587-1789
e-mail: nadinfo@nad.org
www.nad.org

Provides a quick reference to the vocabulary and grammar in the student text, with lists of props and pictures needed for each les-son, and stories and dialogues for classroom instruction.

Deborah L Jacobs

3576 Amplification for Children with Auditory Deficits
Alexander Graham Bell Association for the Deaf
3417 Volta Place NW
Washington, DC 20007

202-337-5220
800-432-7543
Fax: 202-337-8314
TTY: 202-337-5220
e-mail: agbell2@aol.com
www.agbell.org

This text offers an overview of the field of pediatric amplification and is a valuable addition to any audiologist's reference collection. Based on papers presented at the International Symposium on Amplification for children with Auditory Defects, this volume of work represents years of study related to amplification devices and the various issues facing the children who wear them.

1996 578 pages

3577 Animal Signs: A First Book of Sign Languag e
Debbie Slier, author

Gallaudet University Press
800 Florida Avenue NE
Washington, DC 20002

202-651-5488
Fax: 202-651-5489
e-mail: gupress@gallaudet.edu
http://gupress.gallaudet.edu

Charming, full-color photographs of basic animals plus illustrations of their corresponding signs offer children ages 1 to 4 a fun way to learn their first signs and vocabulary words.

16 pages Board Book
ISBN: 1-563680-49-1

3578 Approaching Equality
TJ Publishers
2544 Tarpley Road, Suite 108
Carrollton, TX 75006

972-416-0800
800-999-1168
Fax: 972-416-0944
TTY: 972-416-0933
e-mail: customerservice@tjpublishers.com
www.tjpublsihers.com

Public education laws guarantee special education programs for all Deaf children, but many find the special education system confusing, or are unsure of their rights under the current law. Those with an interest in education, advocacy and the Deaf community will find this review of dramatic developments in the education of Deaf children, youth and adults most informative. Written by the former chair of the Commission on the Education of the Deaf.

1991 112 pages Softcover
ISBN: 0-932666-39-6

Frank Bowe, Author

3579 Assessment and Management of Mainstreamed Hearing-Impaired Children
Pro-Ed
8700 Shoal Creek Boulevard
Austin, TX 78757

512-451-3246
800-897-3202
Fax: 512-451-8542
e-mail: info@proedinc.com
www.proedinc.com

Covers the development of appropriate programming for children with hearing impairments (primarily oral/aural).

415 pages Hardcover
ISBN: 0-890794-58-8

3580 Auditory Training
Alexander Graham Bell Association for the Deaf
3417 Volta Place NW
Washington, DC 20007

202-337-5220
800-432-7543
Fax: 202-337-8314
TTY: 202-337-5220
e-mail: agbell2@aol.com
www.agbell.org

Experience with hearing-impaired children to develop a practical hearing guide for teachers and parents of hearing-impaired children.

1982 197 pages

3581 Auditory-Verbal Therapy and Practice
Alexander Graham Bell Association for the Deaf
3417 Volta Place NW
Washington, DC 20007

202-337-5220
800-432-7543
Fax: 202-337-8314
TTY: 202-337-5221
e-mail: info@agbell.org
www.agbell.org

A comprehensive book introducing auditory-verbal therapy and its impact on children with hearing impairments and their families.

Warren Estabrooks MEd, Editor

3582 Aural Habilitation
Alexander Graham Bell Association for the Deaf
3417 Volta Place NW
Washington, DC 20007

202-337-5220
800-432-7543
Fax: 202-337-8314
TTY: 202-337-5220
e-mail: agbell2@aol.com
www.agbell.org

This classic text for professionals, educators and parents teaches how to assess and plan individualized educational programs for young children with hearing impairments.

1986 64 pages paperback
ISBN: 0-890790-82-5

3583 Baby Sign Language Basics
Monta Z Briant, author

Harris Communications
15155 Technology Drive
Eden Prairie, MN 55344

952-906-1180
800-825-6758
Fax: 952-906-1099
TTY: 952-906-1198
e-mail: info@harriscomm.com
www.harriscomm.com

This is the perfect book for new parents - now, they can understand what their baby is trying to tell them. This books makes learning fun and easy, and it is small enough to take anywhere. It includes 60 baby-friendly American Sign Language signs like bird, happy, baby, and mommy, just to name a few. There are also baby-specific signing techniques, black and white photographs, songs and games.

329 pages Softcover

3584 Baby's First Signs

Kim Voltry and Curt Waller, author

Gallaudet University Press
800 Florida Avenue NE
Washington, DC 20002

202-651-5488
Fax: 202-651-5489
e-mail: gupress@gallaudet.edu
http://gupress.gallaudet.edu

A durable board book, lavishly colored in bright reds, blues, greens, and yellows sure to please your child's eye. Each page features an illustration of a toddler signing a word as well as demonstrating what the sign is about. For example, on the baby page, a toddler makes the sign for baby by mimicking the cradling of a child in his arms while also smiling at his baby sister sitting beside him. The illustrations include both a diagram box that depicts how to perform the sign and English word.

16 pages Board Book
ISBN: 1-563681-14-5

3585 Basic Course in Manual Communication

National Association of the Deaf
814 Thayer Avenue
Silver Spring, MD 20910

301-587-1788
Fax: 301-587-1791
TTY: 301-587-1789
e-mail: nadinfo@nad.org
www.nad.org

Over 700 signs are grouped according to shape, location, and movement. Also includes dialogues for practice.

Deborah L Jacobs

3586 Basic Vocabulary and Language Thesaurus for Hearing-Impaired Children

Alexander Graham Bell Association for the Deaf
3417 Volta Place NW
Washington, DC 20007

202-337-5220
800-432-7543
Fax: 202-337-8314
TTY: 202-337-5220
e-mail: agbell2@aol.com
www.agbell.org

This simple thesaurus lists spontaneous vocabulary used by normally hearing children and lets patients and teachers check so that children with hearing losses have mastered these words.

1977 76 pages

3587 Be Careful

HEAR-MORE
42 Executive Boulevard
Farmingdale, NY 11735

800-881-4327
Fax: 631-752-0689
TTY: 800-281-4327
www.hearmore.com

A What-Will-Happen-Next Book of Safety, a book of cautions. It shows the child, in an amusing and dramatic manner, just what can happen to a careless or thoughtless child. Read the story aloud and sign to the child while looking at the pictures together. Let the child see your lips when you read and sign.

3588 Be Happy Not Sad

Modern Signs Press
PO Box 1181
Los Alamitos, CA 90720

562-596-8548
800-572-7332
Fax: 562-795-6614
TTY: 310-493-4168
e-mail: modsigns@modersignspress.com
www.modernsignspress.com

These books help children understand hard to explain emotions through signing. Includes Be Happy Not Sad coloring workbook.

1988 2 Book Set
ISBN: 0-916708-19-5

3589 Belonging

Virginia M Scott, author

Gallaudet University Press
800 Florida Avenue NE
Washington, DC 20002

202-651-5488
Fax: 202-651-5489
e-mail: gupress@gallaudet.edu
http://gupress.gallaudet.edu

Gustie is 15 when she contracts meningitis during which she loses the small amount of residual hearing she had seemed to retain, Gustie tires to pick up the pieces of her life. Her parents are unrealistic and over protective; her best friend rejects her; her teachers run the gamut from being convinced Gustie cannot function in the mainstream to being supportive...through a new boyfriend who has a deaf brother and sister-in-law, and through visits with an understanding special education teacher

176 pages Softcover
ISBN: 0-903233-35-5

3590 Blueprint for Developing Conversational Competence

Alexander Graham Bell Association for the Deaf
3417 Volta Place NW
Washington, DC 20007

202-337-5220
800-432-7543
Fax: 202-337-8314
TTY: 202-337-5220
e-mail: agbell2@aol.com
www.agbell.org

A book that develops conversational skills in children with hearing impairments.

1988 175 pages

3591 Book of Name Signs

Gallaudet Univ. Press c/o Chicago Distrib. Center
11030 S Langley Avenue
Chicago, IL 60628

202-651-5000
800-621-2736
Fax: 800-621-8476
TTY: 888-630-9347
www.gallaudet.edu/~gupress

This text discusses the rules for ASL name sign formulation and their appropriate uses and presents a list of over 400 name signs.

112 pages

3592 CHATS: The Miami Cochlear Implant, Auditory & Tactile Skills Curriculum

Alexander Graham Bell Association for the Deaf
3417 Volta Place NW
Washington, DC 20007

202-337-5220
800-432-7543
Fax: 202-337-8314
TTY: 202-337-5220
e-mail: agbell2@aol.com
www.agbell.org

A comprehensive curriculum for educators and clinicians providing educational tools and techniques to maximize the potential of children with hearing impairments who wear sensory aids.

1994 327 pages

3593 Can't Your Child Hear?

Gallaudet Univ. Press c/o Chicago Distrib. Center
11030 S Langley Avenue
Chicago, IL 60628

202-651-5000
800-621-2736
Fax: 800-621-8476
TTY: 888-630-9347
www.gallaudet.edu/~gupress

Is deafness a difference to be accepted or a defect to be corrected? This comprehensive reference will help parents, as well as educators and other professionals, recognize their options in understanding and handling a child who is deaf.

340 pages Softcover

3594 Carolina Picture Vocabulary Test for Deaf and Hearing Impaired Children

Pro-Ed
8700 Shoal Creek Boulevard
Austin, TX 78757

512-451-3246
800-897-3202
Fax: 512-451-8542
e-mail: info@proedinc.com
www.proedinc.com

The CPVT is a norm-referenced, validated, individually administered, receptive sign vocabulary test for children between the ages of four and 11 1/2 who are deaf or hearing impaired.

Thomas Layton, Co-Author
David Holmes, Co-Author

3595 Challenge of Educating Together

Charles C Thomas Publishing
2600 S 1st Street
Springfield, IL 62704

217-789-8980
800-258-8980
Fax: 217-789-9130
e-mail: books@ccthomas.com
www.ccthomas.com

This book is for those who have this challenge of education; the author believes that deaf and hearing youth can be educated together and without outrageously expensive devices and programs.

198 pages $28.95 paper
ISBN: 0-398056-65-X

3596 Children with Hearing Difficulties

Scholars International Corporation
2630 W Barry Avenue
Chicago, IL 60618

410-337-3775
800-638-3775
Fax: 410-337-8539
e-mail: scholars@ameritech.net

Based on ten years of research into hearing and hearing-impaired children, this book looks at the impact of deafness on all aspects of the development and education of young children.

192 pages Softcover
ISBN: 0-304317-24-1

David Wood, Co-Author
Alec Webster, Co-Author

3597 Choices In Deafness: A Parent's Guide to Communication Options

Alexander Graham Bell Association for the Deaf
3417 Volta Place NW
Washington, DC 20007

202-337-5220
800-432-7543
Fax: 202-337-8314
TTY: 202-337-5220
e-mail: agbell2@aol.com
www.agbell.org

Serving as an invaluable guide to the world of deaf education, this expanded edition covers a wide variety of communication options for children with hearing impairments. Provides medical, audiological, and educational information and numerous case studies.

1996 304 pages

3598 Chris Gets Ear Tubes

Gallaudet University Press
800 Florida Avenue NE
Washington, DC 20002

202-651-5488
800-621-2736
Fax: 202-651-5489
TTY: 202-651-5488
e-mail: gupress@gallaudet.edu
http://gupress.gallaudet.edu

A helpful book for parents and children to share concerning ear tubes and hospitals.

48 pages paperback
ISBN: 0-930323-36-x

3599 Chris Gets Ear Tubes: Spanish Edition

Betty Pace, author

Gallaudet University Press
800 Florida Avenue NE
Washington, DC 20002

202-651-5488
Fax: 202-651-5489
e-mail: gupress@gallaudet.edu
http://gupress.gallaudet.edu

Chris Get Ear Tubes describes what happens, before, during, and after the surgery in a language a child understands. It takes away the child's natural fear of the unknown. Also available in English

48 pages Softcover
ISBN: 1-563680-93-9

3600 Classroom GOALS

Jill B Firszt, MA and Ruth M Reeder, MA, author

Alexander Graham Bell Association for the Deaf
3417 Volta Place NW
Washington, DC 20007

202-337-5220
Fax: 202-337-8314
TTY: 202-337-5221
e-mail: info@agbell.org
www.agbell.org

Classroom GOALS was designed to help teachers incorporate auditory goals into academic lessons after those specific goals have been identified. Objectives accommodate students with hearing loss regardless of the degree of loss, sensory devise, grade level, mode of communication or school placement.

199 pages Softcover

3601 Classroom Notetaker

Jimmie Joan Wilson, author

Alexander Graham Bell Association for the Deaf
3417 Volta Place NW
Washington, DC 20007

202-337-5220
Fax: 202-337-8314
TTY: 202-337-5221
e-mail: info@agbell.org
www.agbell.org

How to organize a program serving students with hearing impairments. Designed to help teachers incorporate auditory goals into academic lessons, after those specific goals have been identified. Objectives accommodate students with hearing loss regardless of the degree of loss, sensory device, grade level, mode of communication or school placement. This guide describes practical ways for teachers to create situations during academic instruction that encourage the use of residual hearing.

127 pages Softcover

3602 Cochlear Implant Auditory Training Guidebook

Alexander Graham Bell Association for the Deaf
3417 Volta Place NW
Washington, DC 20007

202-337-5220
800-432-7543
Fax: 202-337-8314
TTY: 202-337-5221
e-mail: publications@agbell.org
www.agbell.org

Designed for parents and professionals working with children ages four and up who have cochlear implants. It includes an easy to follow hierarchy for listening goals and a quick placement test to help you find where to start. Comes with CD

236 pages

David Sindrey

3603 Cochlear Implantation for Infants and Children

Alexander Graham Bell Association for the Deaf
3417 Volta Place NW
Washington, DC 20007

202-337-5220
800-432-7543
Fax: 202-337-8314
TTY: 202-337-5220
e-mail: agbell2@aol.com
www.agbell.org

This comprehensive text presents the surgical, medical, audiological speech and language, and habilitation aspects of cochlear implants in infants and children.

1997 263 pages

3604 Cochlear Implants for Kids

Warren Estabrooks, MEd, author

Alexander Graham Bell Association for the Deaf
3417 Volta Place NW
Washington, DC 20007

202-337-5220
Fax: 202-337-8314
TTY: 202-337-5221
e-mail: info@agbell.org
www.agbell.org

Written to educate parents and the professional community about cochlear implants for the pediatric population. Sections include: History and ethical issues, Surgery and programming, Habilitation, Family stories from around the world. Its accessible language and photography make this text a perfect resource for anyone interested

in therapy for pre and post cochlear implantation and in the entire family experience.

404 pages Softcover

3605 Cochlear Implants in Children

John B Christiansen and Irene W Leigh, author

Alexander Graham Bell Association for the Deaf
3417 Volta Place NW
Washington, DC 20007

202-337-5220
Fax: 202-337-8314
TTY: 202-337-5221
e-mail: info@agbell.org
www.agbell.org

Based on a survey of 439 parents of children who have cochlear implants, this book addresses every facet of the controversy over early implantation.

360 pages Hardcover

3606 Cochlear Implants in Children: Ethics and Choices

John B Christiansen and Irene W Leigh, author

Gallaudet University Press
800 Florida Avenue NE
Washington, DC 20002

202-651-5488
Fax: 202-651-5489
e-mail: gupress@gallaudet.edu
http://gupress.gallaudet.edu

Addresses every facet of the ongoing controversy about implanting cochlear hearing devices in children as young as 12 months old and in some cases, younger. The authors analyzed the sensitive issues connected witht he procedure by reviewing 439 responses to a survey of parents with children who have cochlear implants. They followed up with interviews of the parents of children who have had a year's experience using the implants, and also the children themselves.

340 pages Hardcover
ISBN: 1-563681-16-1

3607 Cognition, Eduction, and Deafness: Directi ons for Research and Instruction

David S Martin, Editor, author

Gallaudet University Press
800 Florida Avenue NE
Washington, DC 20002

202-651-5488
Fax: 202-651-5489
e-mail: gupress@gallaudet.edu
http://gupress.gallaudet.edu

This book integrates the work of 54 contributors to the 1984 symposium on cognition, education and deafness. It focuses on cognition and deaf students' growth and development, problem-solving strategies, thinking processes, language development, reading methodology, measurement of potential, and intervention programs. A synthesis of these discoveries establishes directions for new research and outlines implications for all professionals working with hearing-impaired learners.

248 pages Softcover
ISBN: 1-563681-49-8

3608 Colors

HEAR-MORE
42 Executive Boulevard
Farmingdale, NY 11735

800-881-4327
Fax: 631-752-0689
TTY: 800-281-4327
www.hearmore.com

The Early Sign Language Series: A fascinating and enjoyable way for children and adults to learn sign language. Colors presents the early concepts of color recognition. It fosters both receptive and expressive language through signs and pictures, and it is perfect for young children whether hearing impaired, hearing, pre-verbal or verbal. Reviews ten colors in bright cheery illustrations.

3609 Come Sign With Us: Sign Language Activitie s for Children

David S Martin, Editor, author

Gallaudet University Press
800 Florida Avenue NE
Washington, DC 20002

202-651-5488
Fax: 202-651-5489
e-mail: gupress@gallaudet.edu
http://gupress.gallaudet.edu

Completely revised, this book now offers more follow-up activities, including many in context, to teach children sign language. The second edition of this fun, fully illustrated activities manual features more than 300 line drawings of both adults and children signing familiar words, phrases, and sentences using American Sign Language signs in English word order. Twenty lively lessons each introduce ten selected target vocabulary words in a format familiar and exciting to children.

160 pages Softcover
ISBN: 1-563680-51-3

3610 Come Sign with Us Sign Language Activities for Children

Gallaudet University Press
800 Florida Avenue NE
Washington, DC 20002

202-651-5488
800-621-2736
Fax: 202-651-5489
TTY: 202-651-5488
e-mail: gupress@gallaudet.edu
http://gupress.gallaudet.edu

Revised version, offering more follow-up activities, including many in context, to teach children sign language. Features more than 300 line drawings of both adults and children signing familiar words, phrases, and sentences using ASL. Shows how to form each sign exactly and also presents the origins of ASL, facts about deafness, and the deaf community.

2002 160 pages Softcover
ISBN: 1-563680-51-3

3611 Communication Training for Hearing Impaired Children and Teenagers

Alexander Graham Bell Association for the Deaf
3417 Volta Place NW
Washington, DC 20007

202-337-5220
866-337-5220
Fax: 202-337-8314
TTY: 202-337-5221
e-mail: agbell112@aol.com
www.agbell.org

Program combines speech, reading, listening, and repair strategy training using speech materials that are meaningful to children and teenagers. The training activities are simple to present and do not require advance preparation.

1997 265 pages

3612 Cosmo Gets An Ear

Gary Clementine, author

Modern Signs Press
10443 Los Alamitos Boulevard, PO Box 1181
Los Alamitos, CA 90720

562-596-8548
800-572-7332
Fax: 562-795-6614
TTY: 562-493-4168
e-mail: modsigns@modernsignspress.com
www.modernsignspress.com

Welcome to the world of 'Cosmo'. Once you get past the normal turmoil of his impossible room, you find a boy who needs to have the TV loud and his mother shouting at him to respond. Cosmo has a hearing problem. This story was written by a man who is hearing impaired and regretfully did not use an aid until much later in life. It is colorfully and humorously illustrated by an artist who captures the exuberance and fears of the youngster. An excellent way to help others understand what it is like.

48 pages

3613 Cued Speech Resource Book

Orin Cornett and Mary Elsie Daisey, author

Alexander Graham Bell Association for the Deaf
3417 Volta Place NW
Washington, DC 20007

202-337-5220
Fax: 202-337-8314
TTY: 202-337-5221
e-mail: info@agbell.org
www.agbell.org

A fact book for parents and professionals who want to use this system of hand cues with speech to help children affected by hearing loss or auditory neuropathy learn spoken languages. Explains Cued Speech and how to use it and includes personal accounts, practice materials, and guidance. Second edition revisions describe legal rights and the mechanics of cueing. This classic text explains: Initiating communication, Language development, Reading, Speech Production, Multiple Disabilities and more.

832 pages Hardcover

3614 Cued Speech Resource Guide for Parents of Deaf Children

Alexander Graham Bell Association for the Deaf
3417 Volta Place NW
Washington, DC 20007

202-337-5220
800-432-7543
Fax: 202-337-8314
TTY: 202-337-5220
e-mail: agbell2@aol.com
www.agbell.org

A comprehensive book describing Cued Speech, getting started, your child's rights in and out of school, and families expectations with special attention on siblings and peer relationships.

1992 832 pages Hardcover

3615 Curriculum Guide: Hearing-Impaired Children, Birth to Three Years

Alexander Graham Bell Association for the Deaf
3417 Volta Place NW
Washington, DC 20007

202-337-5220
800-432-7543
Fax: 202-337-8314
TTY: 202-337-5220
e-mail: agbell2@aol.com
www.agbell.org

An invaluable book providing guidelines for professionals in the organization and administration of an auditory-oral infant/preschool program for children with hearing impairments stressing an equal partnership between parents and the team of teachers.

1977 291 pages

3616 Dad and Me in the Morning

Patricia Lakin and Robert G steele, author

Harris Communications
15155 Technology Drive
Eden Prairie, MN 55344

952-906-1180
800-825-6758
Fax: 952-906-1099
TTY: 952-906-1198
e-mail: info@harriscomm.com
www.harriscomm.com

Warm and fuzzy and beautifully illustrated! This delightful book will provide enjoyable reading and superb pictures for a cozy, shared reading adventure for parent and a hard of hearing child.

3617 Deaf Children in China

Alison Callaway, author

Gallaudet University Press
800 Florida Avenue NE
Washington, DC 20002

202-651-5488
Fax: 202-651-5489
e-mail: gupress@gallaudet.edu
http://gupress.gallaudet.edu

Provides a striking profile of the views and attitudes of well-educated Chinese parents with preschool-age deaf children. The author's inclusion of a survey of 122 English mothers of deaf children reveals the differences between Western and Chinese parents, who rely upon grandparents to help them and who frequently search for medical cures. She also discovered that many issues cross cultures and contexts, especially the problems of achieving early diagnosis and intervention for all deaf children

256 pages Hardcover
ISBN: 1-563680-85-8

3618 Deaf Children in Public Schools: Placement , Context, and Consequences

Claire L Ramsey, author

Gallaudet University Press
800 Florida Avenue NE
Washington, DC 20002

202-651-5488
Fax: 202-651-5489
e-mail: gupress@gallaudet.edu
http://gupress.gallaudet.edu

Assesses the progress of three second-grade deaf students to demonstrate the importance of placement, context, and language in their development. The autor points out that these deaf children were placed in two different environments, with the general population of hearing students, and separately with other deaf and hard of hearing children. The answers found in this cohesive book offer educators and parents a remarkable stage for assessing and enhancing the education context for deaf children.

142 pages Hardcover
ISBN: 1-563680-62-9

3619 Deaf Children, Their Families, and Professionals: Dismantling Barriers

David Fulton Publishers
2 Barbon Close, Great Ormond Street
London, WC1N

171-405-5606
Fax: 171-831-4840

Concerns about the growing need among parents of deaf children and professionals (including student practitioners) who work with them for clear illustrations of what deaf children and their families have to say for themselves about their experiences.

1995 176 pages Softcover
ISBN: 1-853463-29-9

3620 Deaf Daughter, Hearing Fahter

Richard Medugno, author

Gallaudet University Press
800 Florida Avenue NE
Washington, DC 20002

202-651-5488
Fax: 202-651-5489
e-mail: gupress@gallaudet.edu
http://gupress.gallaudet.edu

A father shares practical information on many of the common challenges faced by hearing parents. e provides a list of games that hearing and deaf children can play together, a consideration for many families. His enthusiasm for all possibilities, from exploring the potential of video phones to helping stage CSD musicals, reveals his abiding devotion to Miranda. This has enabled her to feel proud, confident and happy in her pursuits. Medugno realizes that the rewards of having a deaf daughter

184 pages Softcover
ISBN: 1-563681-77-X

3621 Deaf Side Story: Deaf Sharks, Hearing Jets , and a Classic American Musical

Mark Rigney, author

Gallaudet University Press
800 Florida Avenue NE
Washington, DC 20002

202-651-5488
Fax: 202-651-5489
e-mail: gupress@gallaudet.edu
http://gupress.gallaudet.edu

The 1957 classic American Musical West Side Story has been staged by many community and school theater groups. At a small school in Jacksonville, IL, the new drama head, determined to add an extra element to the usual demands of putting on a show by having deaf students perform half of the parts. The author portrays the progress of the production, including the frustrations and triumphs of the leads, the campus and community politics, and the clashes between the deaf cast members and hearing.

232 pages Softcover
ISBN: 1-563681-45-5

3622 Deaf Students Can Be Great Readers

Modern Signs Press
10443 Los Alamitos Boulevard, PO Box 1181
Los Alamitos, CA 90720

562-596-8548
800-572-7332
Fax: 562-795-6614
TTY: 562-493-4168
e-mail: modsigns@modernsignspress.com
www.modernsignspress.com

Detailed analytical review of a case study of one deaf child. Also, information about the place on phonological awareness in developing reading capability. Includes a comprehensive annotated bibliography related to education of deaf and hard of hearing children.

3623 Directory of Auditory-Oral Programs

Alexander Graham Bell Association for the Deaf
3417 Volta Place NW
Washington, DC 20007

202-337-5220
800-432-7543
Fax: 202-337-8314
TTY: 202-337-5220
e-mail: agbell2@aol.com
www.agbell.org

This directory lists auditory-oral programs in public and private schools, auditory-oral programs in speech and hearing centers, and therapists who offer private tutoring and auditory-oral therapy.

1995 204 pages

3624 Discovering Sign Language

Gallaudet Univ. Press c/o Chicago Distrib. Center
11030 S Langley Avenue
Chicago, IL 60628

202-651-5000
800-621-2736
Fax: 800-621-8476
TTY: 888-630-9347
www.gallaudet.edu/~gupress

Fascinating book explaining different kinds of hearing losses and the significance of when the loss occurred.

104 pages Softcover

3625 Ear Gear: A Student Workbook on Hearing and Hearing Aids

Gallaudet Univ. Press c/o Chicago Distrib. Center
11030 S Langley Avenue
Chicago, IL 60628

202-651-5000
800-621-2736
Fax: 800-621-8476
TTY: 888-630-9347
www.gallaudet.edu/~gupress

Attractive workbook designed to teach elementary-age children about hearing loss and the use of hearing aids.

75 pages

3626 Educating Deaf Students: Global Perspectiv es

Des Power and Greg Leigh, Editors, author

Gallaudet University Press
800 Florida Avenue NE
Washington, DC 20002

202-651-5488
Fax: 202-651-5489
e-mail: gupress@gallaudet.edu
http://gupress.gallaudet.edu

The 19 chapters of this book present a select cross-section of the issues addressed at the 19th International Congress of Education of the Deaf. Divided into four distinct parts - Contemporary Issus for all Learners, The Eary Years, The School Years, and Contemporary Issues in Postsecondary Education - the themes considered here span the entire student age range. Authored by 27 different researchers and practitioners from six different countries.

248 pages Hardcover
ISBN: 1-563683-08-3

3627 Education of the Hearing Impaired Child

A book of information about educational programs and devices used in teaching the hearing impaired child.

180 pages Softcover

3628 Educational Audiology for the Limited- Hearing Infant and Preschooler

Alexander Graham Bell Publishing
3417 Volta Place NW
Washington, DC 20007

202-337-5220
866-337-5220
Fax: 202-337-8314
TTY: 202-337-5221
e-mail: agbell2@aol.com
www.agbell.org

The third edition of this popular book focuses on current concepts and practices in audio-logic screening, evaluation and the role of parents.

1997 390 pages

3629 Educational Audiology for the Limited-Hear ing Infant and Preschooler

Charles C Thomas Publishers
2600 South First Street
Springfield, IL 62704

217-789-8980
800-258-8980
e-mail: books@ccthomas.com
www.ccthomas.com

The third edition of this book brings up to date the material that so many readers found helpful in the previous editions. The entire text has been rewritten and reorganized with revised chapters focusing on current concepts and practices in audiologic screening and evaluation, development of language, the role of parents, parent education, mainstreaming of the limited-hearing child, and program modifications for the severely learning disabled child. Includes 18 tables.

430 pages Softcover

3630 Educational Interpreting: How It Can Succe ed

Elizabeth A Winston, Editor, author

Gallaudet University Press
800 Florida Avenue NE
Washington, DC 20002

202-651-5488
Fax: 202-651-5489
e-mail: gupress@gallaudet.edu
http://gupress.gallaudet.edu

This book explores the current state of educational interpreting and how it is failing deaf students. The contributors, all experts in their field, include former educational interpreters, teachers of deaf students, interpreter trainers, and deaf recipients of interpreted educations. It presents the salient issues in three distinct sections. Part 1 focuses on deaf students. Part 2 raises the questions about the support and training intrepreters receive. Part 3 presents possible suggestions.

224 pages Hardcover
ISBN: 1-563683-09-1

3631 Educational and Development Aspects of Deafness

Gallaudet University Press
800 Florida Avenue NE
Washington, DC 20002

202-651-5488
Fax: 202-651-5489
TTY: 202-651-5488
e-mail: gupress@gallaudet.edu
http://gupress.gallaudet.edu

Book detailing the ongoing revolution in the education of deaf children.

415 pages

Donald F Moores, Editor
Kathryn P Meadow-Orlans, Editor

3632 Educational and Developmental Aspects of D eafness

Donald Moores and Kathryn Meadow-Orlans, Editors, author

Gallaudet University Press
800 Florida Avenue NE
Washington, DC 20002

202-651-5488
Fax: 202-651-5489
e-mail: gupress@gallaudet.edu
http://gupress.gallaudet.edu

Details the ongoing revolution in the eduction of deaf children. More than 20 researchers contributed their discoveries in anthropology, education, linguistics, psychology, sociology, and other major disciplines, with special concentration upon the education of deaf children. Divided into two parts on education at home and in school, this book documents breakthroughs such as the public's interest in sign language, the increasing availability of interpreters, and other positive trends.

451 pages Hardcover
ISBN: 0-930323-52-1

3633 Effectiveness of Cochlear Implants and Tactile Aids for Deaf Children

Alexander Graham Bell Association for the Deaf
3417 Volta Place NW
Washington, DC 20007

> 202-337-5220
> 800-432-7543
> Fax: 202-337-8314
> TTY: 202-337-5220
> e-mail: agbell2@aol.com
> www.agbell.org

This monograph presents a fascinating study to evaluate differences in the rate of change in speech perception, speech production and spoken language skills among children using the Nucleus 22-channel cochlear implant, tactile aids and conventional hearing aids. This monograph also offers teaching strategies in perception, lipreading, and spoken language.

1994 232 pages Softcover

3634 FM Auditory Trainers: A Winning Choice for Students, Teachers and Parents

Alexander Graham Bell Association for the Deaf
3417 Volta Place NW
Washington, DC 20007

> 202-337-5220
> 800-432-7543
> Fax: 202-337-8314
> TTY: 202-337-5220
> e-mail: agbell2@aol.com
> www.agbell.org

Written for teachers, parents, and professionals, this booklet describes how FM technology is used at school and at home. Programming guidelines, general component care, and troubleshooting hints are examined.

1991 67 pages

3635 Facilitating Hearing and Listening in Young Children

Alexander Graham Bell Association for the Deaf
3417 Volta Place NW
Washington, DC 20007

> 202-337-5220
> 800-432-7543
> Fax: 202-337-8314
> TTY: 202-337-5220
> e-mail: agbell2@aol.com
> www.agbell.org

Emphasizes the need to create an auditory world for children, as their auditory brain centers continue to develop the neurological and experiential foundations for literacy and learning. Information provided is: the structure and function of the ear, types and degrees of hearing loss, behavioral and objective measurement of hearing, technological management of hearing, and facilitation of listening skills.

1999 312 pages

3636 Families and Their Hearing-Impaired Children

Alexander Graham Bell Association for the Deaf
3417 Volta Place NW
Washington, DC 20007

> 202-337-5220
> 800-432-7543
> Fax: 202-337-8314
> TTY: 202-337-5220
> e-mail: agbell2@aol.com
> www.agbell.org

Looks at specific family issues that have not had much play in the literature to date. Discussions include a range of family members, problems, solutions and more.

150 pages

3637 Finger Alphabet

Gallaudet Univ. Press c/o Chicago Distrib. Center
800 Florida Avenue NE
Washington, DC 20002

> 202-651-5000
> 800-621-2736
> Fax: 800-621-8476
> TTY: 202-651-5000
> www.gallaudet.edu/~gupress

Includes activities for improving fingerspelling.

1992 30 pages paperback
ISBN: 0-931993-46-6

3638 Fire Fighter Brown

HEAR-MORE
42 Executive Boulevard
Farmingdale, NY 11735

> 800-881-4327
> Fax: 631-752-0689
> TTY: 800-281-4327
> www.hearmore.com

The Fire Fighter Brown book tells about the Fire Fighter Brown's work, the clothes he wears, and the equipment he uses in rescuing a little boy from a burning building. Use the signs when reading the book to your child, and let the child see your lips as you read and sign. This will help your child learn to associate the signs with sounds and lip shapes.

3639 First Signs at Home

HEAR-MORE
42 Executive Boulevard
Farmingdale, NY 11735

> 800-881-4327
> Fax: 631-752-0689
> TTY: 800-281-4327
> www.hearmore.com

The Early Sign Language Series: A fascinating and enjoyable way for children and adults to learn sign language. First Signs present some of the very first words for parents and children.

3640 First Signs at Play

HEAR-MORE
42 Executive Boulevard
Farmingdale, NY 11735

> 800-881-4327
> Fax: 631-752-0689
> TTY: 800-281-4327
> www.hearmore.com

The Early Sign Language Series: A fascinating and enjoyable way for children and adults to learn sign language. First Signs present some of the very first words for parents and children.

3641 Foundations of Spoken Language for Hearing -Impaired Children

Daniel Ling, PhD, author

Alexander Graham Bell Association for the Deaf
3417 Volta Place NW
Washington, DC 20007

> 202-337-5220
> Fax: 202-337-8314
> TTY: 202-337-5221
> e-mail: info@agbell.org
> www.agbell.org

Emphasizes the perception of speech through residual hearing, either through the use of modern hearing aids or cochlear implants.

A feature of the book is the presentation of the aspects of speech that appear in the octave bands centered on frequencies depicted in audiograms. This konowledge, in conjunction with the Six-Sound Test, allows teachers and clinicians to determine whether the frequency response charachteristics of hearing aids are adjusted to provide optimal levels of hearing.

447 pages Softcover

3642 Free Hand: Enfranchising the Education of Deaf Children

TJ Publishers
2544 Tarpley Raod, Suite 108
Carrollton, TX 75006

972-416-0800
800-999-1186
Fax: 972-416-0944
TTY: 972-416-0933
e-mail: customerservice@tjpublishers.com
www.tjpublishers.com

Based on the proceedings of a 1990 symposium on the educational uses of ASL, A Free Hand presents papers by prominent educators, researchers and linguists in the changing role of American Sign Language in the classroom.

1992 204 pages Softcover
ISBN: 0-932666-40-X

Angela K Thames, President
Jerald Murphy, Vice President

3643 From Gesture to Language in Hearing and De af Children

Virginia Volterra and Carol J Ertling, Editors, author

Gallaudet University Press
800 Florida Avenue NE
Washington, DC 20002

202-651-5488
Fax: 202-651-5489
e-mail: gupress@gallaudet.edu
http://gupress.gallaudet.edu

In 21 essays on communicative gesturing in the first two years of life, this collection demonstrates the importance of gesture in a child's transition to a linguistic system. Introductions preceding each section emphasize the parallels between the findings in these studies and the general body of scholarship devoted to the process of spoken language acquisition. Scholars contributing to this volume include Ursula Bellugi, Judy Snitzer Reilly, Susan Goldwin-Meadow, Andrew Lock, and many others.

358 pages Softcover
ISBN: 1-563680-78-5

3644 Functional Signs: New Approach from Simple to Complex

Pro-Ed
8700 Shoal Creek Boulevard
Austin, TX 78757

512-451-3246
800-897-3202
Fax: 800-397-7633
e-mail: feedback@proedinc.com
www.proedinc.com

A unique dictionary of 330 American Sign Language signs for persons with disabilities. Each of the signs has been analyzed for a percentage of understandability.

1984

3645 Genetics, Disability and Deafness

John Vickrey Van Cleve, Editory, author

Gallaudet University Press
800 Florida Avenue NE
Washington, DC 20002

202-651-5488
Fax: 202-651-5489
e-mail: gupress@gallaudet.edu
http://gupress.gallaudet.edu

This volume brings together 13 essays from science, history, and the humanities, history and the present, to show the many ways that disability, deafness and the new genetetics interact and what that interaction means for society. Prize-winning author Louis Menand begins this volume by expressing the position shared by most authors in this wide-ranging forum—the belief in the value of human diversity and skepticism of actions that could eliminate it through modification of the human genome.

240 pages Hardcover
ISBN: 1-563683-07-5

3646 Go Togethers

HEAR-MORE
42 Executive Boulevard
Farmingdale, NY 11735

800-881-4327
Fax: 631-752-0689
TTY: 800-281-4327
www.hearmore.com

The Early Sign Language Series: A fascinating and enjoyable way for children and adults to learn sign language. Go-Togethers presents early objects and concepts that are complimentary. It fosters both receptive and expressive language through signs and pictures, and it is perfect for young children whether hearing impaired, hearing, pre-verbal or verbal. Learn 10 go-together items (20 in total).

3647 Goldilocks and the Three Bears Told in Sig ned English

Harry Bornstein and Karen L Saulnier, author

Gallaudet University Press
800 Florida Avenue NE
Washington, DC 20002

202-651-5488
Fax: 202-651-5489
e-mail: gupress@gallaudet.edu
http://gupress.gallaudet.edu

Offers children ages 3-8 all of the fun their parents had when they first read about the little girl with the golden curls who turned the Bears' house upside down. In this exciting new edition, children can learn new words and the matching signs, which will help them to remember both.

48 pages
ISBN: 1-563680-57-2

3648 Grandfather Moose!

Harley Hamilton, author

Modern Signs Press
10443 Los Alamitos Boulevard, PO Box 1181
Los Alamitos, CA 90720

562-596-8548
800-572-7332
Fax: 562-795-6614
TTY: 562-493-4168
e-mail: modsigns@modernsignspress.com
www.modernsignspress.com

Move over 'Mother Goose'...here comes 'Grandfather Moose'! Exciting and beautifully illustrated book of rhythms, games, and chants in sign language. Hearing children enjoy the sound of rhyming words. Deaf and hard of hearing children will delight in the rythmic quality of these signing tales. Rhymes are made up of words whose signs have similar hand shapes. Games and chants provide group sign language activities for home and school.

32 pages

3649 Growing Together: Information for Parents of Deaf & Hard of Hearing Children
Gallaudet Univ. Press c/o Chicago Distrib. Center
11030 S Langley Avenue
Chicago, IL 60628

> 202-651-5000
> 800-621-2736
> Fax: 800-621-8476
> TTY: 888-630-9347
> www.gallaudet.edu/~gupress

This publication answers questions often asked by parents of children with a hearing loss.

92 pages

3650 Hearing Aid Handbook: User's Guide for Children
Alexander Graham Bell Association for the Deaf
3417 Volta Place NW
Washington, DC 20007

> 202-337-5220
> 800-432-7543
> Fax: 202-337-8314
> TTY: 202-337-5220
> e-mail: agbell2@aol.com
> www.agbell.org

Explains exactly how to conduct the initial visit, fit ear molds, learn and maintain hearing aids and adjust amplification.

1990 36 pages Softcover

3651 Hearing Care for Children
Alexander Graham Bell Association for the Deaf
3417 Volta Place NW
Washington, DC 20007

> 202-337-5220
> 800-432-7543
> Fax: 202-337-8314
> TTY: 202-337-5220
> e-mail: agbell2@aol.com
> www.agbell.org

This professional text for audiologists provides a comprehensive overview of childhood hearing loss and rehabilitation options. Among the topics covered are the causes and effects of childhood hearing loss, the identification and evaluation of such hearing loss, counseling options for affected children and their families, amplification and auditory stimulation, and intervention and education options for children with hearing losses.

1996 372 pages Hardcover
ISBN: 0-131247-02-6

Mark Ross, Editor

3652 Hearing Impairments in Young Children
Alexander Graham Bell Association for the Deaf
3417 Volta Place NW
Washington, DC 20007

> 202-337-5220
> 800-432-7543
> Fax: 202-337-8314
> TTY: 202-337-5220
> e-mail: agbell2@aol.com
> www.agbell.org

A useful text that helps educators and professionals effectively manage early intervention programs for children with hearing impairments from birth to five years-of-age and their families.

1988 239 pages

3653 Hearing Loss
Franklin Watts c/o Grolier
90 Old Sherman Turnpike
Danbury, CT 06816

> 203-797-3500
> 800-272-2665
> Fax: 203-797-3197
> www.grolier.com

Offers a concise explanation of how and why hearing losses occur, how the ear works and how to protect your hearing.

1991 144 pages hardcover
ISBN: 0-531125-19-0

3654 Hearing-Impaired Child
Alexander Graham Bell Association for the Deaf
3417 Volta Place NW
Washington, DC 20007

> 202-337-5220
> 800-432-7543
> Fax: 202-337-8314
> TTY: 202-337-5220
> e-mail: agbell2@aol.com
> www.agbell.org

This indispensable book provides speech-language pathologists and audiologists with essential information to help diagnose and treat children with all degrees of hearing loss.

1992 183 pages
ISBN: 1-563720-13-2

3655 Hearing-Impaired Children and Youth with Developmental Disabilities
Gallaudet Univ. Press c/o Chicago Distrib. Center
11030 S Langley Avenue
Chicago, IL 60628

> 202-651-5000
> 800-621-2736
> Fax: 800-621-8476
> TTY: 888-630-9347
> www.gallaudet.edu/~gupress

The insights of 24 experts help clarify relationships between hearing impairment and developmental difficulties and propose interdisciplinary cooperation as an approach to the problems created.

394 pages

3656 Hearing-Impaired Children in the Mainstream
Alexander Graham Bell Association for the Deaf
3417 Volta Place NW
Washington, DC 20007

> 202-337-5220
> 800-432-7543
> Fax: 202-337-8314
> TTY: 202-337-5220
> e-mail: agbell2@aol.com
> www.agbell.org

This comprehensive book advises educators to integrate students with hearing impairments into regular classrooms and covers many areas that will help students to become appropriately mainstreamed from elementary school to the college level.

1990 336 pages

Mark Ross, Editor

3657 How Children Learn Language

James McLean, PhD And Lee Snyder-McLean, PhD, author

Alexander Graham Bell Association for the Deaf
3417 Volta Place NW
Washington, DC 20007

202-337-5220
Fax: 202-337-8314
TTY: 202-337-5221
e-mail: info@agbell.org
www.agbell.org

This introductory text guides professionals in nonlanguage fields and students in education/special education courses through the miracle of typical child's language development.

227 pages Softcover

3658 Hug Just Isn't Enough

Gallaudet University Press
11030 S Langley Avenue
Chicago, IL 60628

202-651-5000
800-621-2736
Fax: 800-621-8476
TTY: 888-630-9347
www.gallaudet.edu/~gupress

Photos of deaf children and excerpts from interviews with parents of deaf youngsters.

1985
ISBN: 0-913586-27-

3659 I Can Sign my ABCs

Susan Gibbons Chaplin, author

Harris Communications
15155 Technology Drive
Eden Prairie, MN 55344

952-906-1180
800-825-6758
Fax: 952-906-1099
TTY: 952-906-1198
e-mail: info@harriscomm.com
www.harriscomm.com

In this full-color picture book, each letter's manual alphabet handshape is followed by the picture, name, and sign of an object beginning with that letter. Ideal for teaching children the English and the American Manual alphabets.

52 pages Hardcover

3660 I Can't Hear You in the Dark: How to Learn and Teach Lipreading

Betty Woerner Carter, author

Charles C Thomas Publishers
2600 South First Street
Springfield, IL 62704

217-789-8980
800-258-8980
e-mail: books@ccthomas.com
www.ccthomas.com

'I can't hear you in the dark, but I can lipread you in the light.' Lipreading is one of the ways that hearing-impaired people can communicate and strengthen relationships with others. Written for the beginning lipreader and the experienced, this book shows how lipreading can be taught by supplying ready-to-use lessons.

226 pages Softcover
ISBN: 0-393067-89-9

3661 I Heard That! A Developmental Sequence of Listening Activities for the Young Child

Alexander Graham Bell Association for the Deaf
3417 Volta Place NW
Washington, DC 20007

202-337-5220
800-432-7543
Fax: 202-337-8314
TTY: 202-337-5220
e-mail: agbell2@aol.com
www.agbell.org

This handbook provides a practical framework for teachers, clinicians, and parents by setting objectives and designing activities to develop listening skills in children with hearing losses. Includes auditory communication, listening skill development, auditory learning objectives, and experience charts.

1978 360 pages

3662 I Love You Story

Walter Paul Kelly, author

Harris Communications
15155 Technology Drive
Eden Prairie, MN 55344

952-906-1180
800-825-6758
Fax: 952-906-1099
TTY: 952-906-1198
e-mail: info@harriscomm.com
www.harriscomm.com

A black and white illustrated story on how love and eventually the ILY handsign in American Sign Language got started.

Hardcover

3663 I'M Deaf and It's Okay

Lorraine Aseltine, Evelyn Mueller, Nancy Tate, author

Harris Communications
15155 Technology Drive
Eden Prairie, MN 55344

952-906-1180
800-825-6758
Fax: 952-906-1099
TTY: 952-906-1198
e-mail: info@harriscomm.com
www.harriscomm.com

A young boy explains how lonely and frustrated he feels because he can't hear. He dislikes the hearing aids he wears and is angered because he will never be rid of them. His feelings begin to change when he is befriended by a teenage boy who also wears hearing aids. This book is well-illustrated with sensitive line drawings done by Helen Cogancherry.

36 pages Hardcover

3664 I.D.E.A. Advocacy for Children Who Are Deaf or Hard-of-Hearing

Alexander Graham Bell Association for the Deaf
3417 Volta Place NW
Washington, DC 20007

202-337-5220
800-432-7543
Fax: 202-337-8314
TTY: 202-337-5220
e-mail: agbell2@aol.com
www.agbell.org

This book offers up-to-date information about the 1997 Individuals with Disabilities Education Act which affects children who are deaf or hard of hearing.

1997 126 pages

3665 In Our House

Carolyn Norris, author

Modern Signs Press
10443 Los Alamitos Boulevard, PO Box 1181
Los Alamitos, CA 90720

562-596-8548
800-572-7332
Fax: 562-795-6614
TTY: 562-493-4168
e-mail: modsigns@modernsignspress.com
www.modernsignspress.com

This colorful picture book tells the story of Joy and Jason helping Mom and Dad around the house. Demonstrates cooking, cleaning, gardening, etc. Has a 140 word vocabulary listed in an alphabetical glossary and the manual alphabet.

3666 In Silence: Growing Up Hearing in a Deaf World

Ruth Sidransky, author

Gallaudet University Press
800 Florida Avenue NE
Washington, DC 20002

202-651-5488
Fax: 202-651-5489
e-mail: gupress@gallaudet.edu
http://gupress.gallaudet.edu

This is an account of growing up as the hearing daughter of deaf Jewish parents in the Bronx and Brooklyn during the 1930s and 1940s. It reveals the challenges deaf people faced during the Depression and afterward. The author portrays her family with deep affection and honesty, and her frank account provides a living narrative of the Deaf experience in pre- and post-World War II America.

352 pages Softcover
ISBN: 1-563682-87-7

3667 Inclusion?

Gallaudet Univ. Press c/o Chicago Distrib. Center
11030 S Langley Avenue
Chicago, IL 60628

202-651-5000
800-621-2736
Fax: 800-621-8476
TTY: 888-630-9347
www.gallaudet.edu/~gupress

This book defines quality education for deaf and hard of hearing students.

213 pages

3668 Infants and Toddlers with Hearing Loss: Family Centered Assessment/Intervention

Alexander Graham Bell Association for the Deaf
3417 Volta Place NW
Washington, DC 20007

202-337-5220
800-432-7543
Fax: 202-337-8314
TTY: 202-337-5220
e-mail: agbell2@aol.com
www.agbell.org

A scholarly title for early intervention professionals examining clinical, legislative, and philosophical issues affecting the delivery of early intervention services to hearing impaired and hard-of-hearing children.

1994 360 pages
ISBN: 0-912752-28-9

3669 Inner Lives of Deaf Children: Interviews and Analysis

Martha Sheridan, author

Gallaudet University Press
800 Florida Avenue NE
Washington, DC 20002

202-651-5488
Fax: 202-651-5489
e-mail: gupress@gallaudet.edu
http://gupress.gallaudet.edu

Conducting interviews with seven deaf children between the ages of 7 and 10, the author offers a fresh look at the private thoughts and feels of deaf children. 'What does it mean to be a child who is deaf or hard of hearing?' Sheridan asks in the beginning of her study. She turns to Danny, Angie, Joe, Alex, Lisa, Mary and Pat for the answer. Footnotes, bibliography, index.

256 pages Softcover
ISBN: 1-563682-89-3

3670 International Directory of Periodicals Related to Deafness

Gallaudet Univ. Press c/o Chicago Distrib. Center
11030 S Langley Avenue
Chicago, IL 60628

202-651-5000
800-621-2736
Fax: 800-621-8476
TTY: 888-630-9347
www.gallaudet.edu/~gupress

Offers information on more than 500 magazines and journals related to deafness.

150 pages

3671 Joy of Listening: An Auditory Training Program

Alexander Graham Bell Association for the Deaf
3417 Volta Place NW
Washington, DC 20007

202-337-5220
800-432-7543
Fax: 202-337-8314
TTY: 202-337-5220
e-mail: agbell2@aol.com
www.agbell.org

This manual contains lessons to improve listening skills, auditory discrimination, attention span, memory, and sequencing in children with hearing losses. The lessons can be used when working with children alone, or in small groups.

1978 148 pages paperback
ISBN: 0-882001-19-1

3672 Joy of Signing

National Association of the Deaf
814 Thayer Avenue
Silver Spring, MD 20910

301-587-1788
Fax: 301-587-1791
TTY: 301-587-1789
e-mail: nadinfo@nad.org
www.nad.org

Illustrated sign language text with descriptions of the origin of selected signs and examples of how each is used. Second edition.

1987 hardcover

Deborah L Jacobs

3673 Kaleidoscope of Deaf America

Harris Communications
15159 Technology Drive
Eden Prairie, MN 55344

612-906-1180
800-825-6758
Fax: 612-902-1099
e-mail: mail@harriscomm.com
www.harriscomm.com

Puts you in touch with trends, events and thinking that is shaping the future of deaf Americans.

79 pages paperback

3674 Keys to Raising a Deaf Child

Barron's Education Series
250 Wireless Boulevard
Hauppauge, NY 11788

800-645-3476
Fax: 631-434-3723
e-mail: info@barronseduc.com
www.barronseduc.com

Two educators offer positive advice and encouragement on helping children adapt to deafness. They show how problems related to deafness can be overcome so that the child interacts as a social and intellectual equal with children who can hear. The authors recommend bimodal communication, having the child, parents, and other non-deaf family members combine sign language and speech as a first step in normal communication.

208 pages Paperback
ISBN: 0-764107-23-2

3675 Kid-Friendly Parenting with Deaf and Hard of Hearing Children

Gallaudet University Press
800 Florida Avenue NE
Washington, DC 20002

202-651-5488
Fax: 202-651-5489
TTY: 202-651-5488
e-mail: gupress@gallaudet.edu
http://gupress.gallaudet.edu

A step-by-step guide offering parents hundreds of ideas and play activities for children ages three to 12.

320 pages

3676 King Midas

Robert Newby, author

Gallaudet University Press
800 Florida Avenue NE
Washington, DC 20002

202-651-5488
Fax: 202-651-5489
e-mail: gupress@gallaudet.edu
http://gupress.gallaudet.edu

Now the tale of King Midas and his golden touch is retold with full-color illustrations, and key sentences shown in American Sign Language. The line drawings of the story teller (who appears in both the book and videotape) recreate 44 sentences, making this ideal for helping both hearing and deaf children to learn reading skills. The videotape shows the entire classic story performed in ASL by the storyteller accompanied by a voiceover. A perfect complement to the book. VHS, color, 30 minutes.

VHS-$39.95 72 pages Hardcover book
ISBN: 0-930323-75-0

3677 Language Learning Practices with Deaf Children, Third Edition

Pro-Ed
8700 Shoal Creek Boulevard
Austin, TX 78757

512-451-3246
800-897-3202
Fax: 512-451-8542
e-mail: info@proedinc.com
www.proedinc.com

Provides future and practicing teachers of deaf children with basic theoretical and research knowledge as well as specific principles and practices for fostering the development of language and reading. In this third edition, the authors have added a section on language assessment address high-stakes or large-scale testing and a new chapter on special programs, including ASL-English programs for children from multicultural homes and technology for language learning.

3678 Language-Children Living with Deafness

Gareth Stevens
1555 N River Center Drive
Milwaukee, WI 53212

414-225-0333
800-341-3569
Fax: 414-336-0156

Did you know you can't whisper in sign language? To share a secret, you have to be sure that no one else can see what you're signing. Linda is nearly deaf, and some of her friends at school can't hear at all. Read about how they speak to each other with their hands, in sign language. Learn what special dangers deaf children face. Find out how you can play and talk with children who are deaf.

ISBN: 1-555329-16-0

3679 Learning Ladder: Assessing and Teaching T ext Comprehension

Elisabeth H Wiig, PhD and Carolyn C Wilson, MS, author

Alexander Graham Bell Association for the Deaf
3417 Volta Place NW
Washington, DC 20007

202-337-5220
Fax: 202-337-8314
TTY: 202-337-5221
e-mail: info@agbell.org
www.agbell.org

A general education program developed for students, aged 7 to 12 years, with reading comprehension difficulties. Major sections of the text include two components: assessment and interventions. The assessment component describes typical home and school social interactions. The intervention component introduces intervention options including grade-level activities, resources, and graphic organizers. The intervention component also responds to the Least Restrictive Environment provision of IDEA.

269 pages Softcover/CD

3680 Learning to See: American Sign Language as a Second Language

Gallaudet University Press
800 Florida Avenue NE
Washington, DC 20002

202-651-5488
Fax: 202-651-5489
TTY: 202-561-5488
e-mail: gupress@gallaudet.edu
http://gupress.gallaudet.edu

Provides a comprehensive introduction to the history and structure of ASL to the deaf community.

160 pages
ISBN: 1-563680-59-9

3681 Least Restrictive Environment: The Paradox of Inclusion

National Association of the Deaf
814 Thayer Avenue
Silver Spring, MD 20910

301-587-1788
Fax: 301-587-1791
TTY: 301-587-1789
e-mail: nadinfo@nad.org
www.nad.org

Analyzes relevant federal law and the inclusion reform movement, and discusses the premise that forcing one generic placement on all children will be more problematic.

1994 304 pages

Deborah L Jacobs

3682 Legal Rights for the Deaf and Hard of Hearing

Hearing Loss Association of America
7910 Woodmont Avenue, Suite 1200
Bethesda, MD 20814

301-657-2248
Fax: 301-913-9413
TTY: 301-657-2249
e-mail: bookstore@hearingloss.org
www.hearingloss.org

A comprehensive analysis of recent laws passed to protect the rights of and guarantee equal access for people with hearing loss. In this revised, fifth edition, the book explains in layman's terminology how legislation affects individuals with disabilities in everyday life.

Softcover

3683 Legal Rights: The Guide for Deaf and Hard of Hearing People - Fifth Edition

Gallaudet University Press
800 Florida Avenue NE
Washington, DC 20002

202-651-5488
Fax: 202-651-5489
TTY: 202-651-5488
e-mail: gupress@gallaudet.edu
http://gupress.gallaudet.edu

Includes updated interpretations of legislation affecting hearing-impaired people, including chapters dealing with the ADA.

3684 Let's Learn About Deafness

Gallaudet Univ. Press c/o Chicago Distrib. Center
800 Florida Avenue NE
Washington, DC 20002

202-651-5000
800-621-2736
Fax: 800-621-8476
TTY: 888-630-9347
www.gallaudet.edu/~gupress

Hands-on school classroom activities for the deaf student.

1988 82 pages spiralbound

3685 Listen Little Star

Dimity Dornan, BA, author

Alexander Graham Bell Association for the Deaf
3417 Volta Place NW
Washington, DC 20007

202-337-5220
Fax: 202-337-8314
TTY: 202-337-5221
e-mail: info@agbell.org
www.agbell.org

Maximize your child's auditory potential with this series of parent-child activities designed to help your baby develop listening and speaking skills using techniques based on the Auditory-Verbal approach. Designed to take approximately four-to-six months to complete. Includes:12 parent-child activities that build auditory skills, a caregiver workbook to guide you through each exercise, a note-taking section to document your child's progress, a reminder checklist, and a plush toy star.

3686 Listen with the Heart: Relationships and Hearing Loss

Michael Harvey, author

Hearing Loss Association of America
7910 Woodmont Avenue, Suite 1200
Bethesda, MD 20814

301-657-2248
Fax: 301-913-9413
TTY: 301-657-2249
e-mail: bookstore@hearingloss.org
www.hearingloss.org

True stories of how parents, children and spouses are transformed by helping each other heal and grow. Unique insights into the consequences of this challenge for individuals and their loved ones. Told with a deep human wisdom and touch of humor, these accounts are a genuine look at the opportunities life gives us to listen with the heart.

3687 Listening and Talking

Alexander Graham Bell Association for the Deaf
3417 Volta Place NW
Washington, DC 20007

202-337-5220
800-432-7543
Fax: 202-337-8314
TTY: 202-337-5220
e-mail: agbell2@aol.com
www.agbell.org

This research-based text for professionals promotes communication by developing language, audition, and speech in early intervention programs for young children with hearing loss.

1992 191 pages Softcover

3688 Listening to Learn: A Handbook for Parents with Hearing-Impaired Children

Alexander Graham Bell Association for the Deaf
3417 Volta Place NW
Washington, DC 20007

202-337-5220
800-432-7543
Fax: 202-337-8314
TTY: 202-337-5220
e-mail: agbell2@aol.com
www.agbell.org

Developed by teachers, this handbook provides parents with the essential steps necessary to develop effective spoken communication with their children.

1990 98 pages

3689 Literacy and Your Deaf Child: What Every Parent Should Know

David A Steward and Bryan R Clarke, author

Gallaudet University Press
800 Florida Avenue NE
Washington, DC 20002

202-651-5488
Fax: 202-651-5489
e-mail: gupress@gallaudet.edu
http://gupress.gallaudet.edu

This book begins by introducing some common concepts, among them the importance of parental involvement in a deaf child's education. It outlines how children acquire language and describes the auditory and visual links to literacy. With this information, parents can make informed decisions regarding hearing aids, cochlear implants, speechreading, and sign communication all of which can have a marked influence on their child's language development.

240 pages Softcover
ISBN: 1-563681-36-6

3690 Little Read Riding Hood: Told in Signed En lish

Harry Bornstein and Karen Luczak Saulnier, author

Gallaudet University Press
800 Florida Avenue NE
Washington, DC 20002

202-651-5488
Fax: 202-651-5489
e-mail: gupress@gallaudet.edu
http://gupress.gallaudet.edu

Now one of the most beloved of all folktales, Little Red Riding Hood in a new Signed Enlish edition illustrated in full color. It presents a vivacious version of this favorite story that will intrigue and delight children. Along with the story illustrations, line drawings showing the characters and a narrator signing the story in Signed English, a system that uses American Sign Language in English grammatical order.

48 pages Hardcover
ISBN: 0-930323-63-7

3691 Living with Deafness

Franklin Watts c/o Grolier
90 Old Sherman Turnpike
Danbury, CT 06816

203-797-3500
800-272-2665
Fax: 203-797-3197
www.grolier.com

Shows how deaf persons can overcome their disability and live happy, productive lives.

0989 32 pages hardcover
ISBN: 0-531108-42-2

3692 Living with Hearing Loss

Marcia B Dugan, author

Gallaudet University Press
800 Florida Avenue NE
Washington, DC 20002

202-651-5488
Fax: 202-651-5489
TTY: 888-630-9347
e-mail: gupress@gallaudet.edu
gupress.gallaudet.edu

192 pages
ISBN: 1-563681-34-0

3693 Mainstreaming Deaf and Hard of Hearing Students

Gallaudet Univ. Press c/o Chicago Distrib. Center
11030 S Langley Avenue
Chicago, IL 60628

202-651-5000
800-621-2736
Fax: 800-621-8476
TTY: 888-630-9347
www.gallaudet.edu/~gupress

Booklet presenting mainstreaming as one educational option.

40 pages

3694 Mandy

Barbara D Booth, author

Harris Communications
15155 Technology Drive
Eden Prairie, MN 55344

952-906-1180
800-825-6758
Fax: 952-906-1099
TTY: 952-906-1198
e-mail: info@harriscomm.com
www.harriscomm.com

Mandy is a young deaf girl who goes searching in the woods for her grandmother's silver pin as a thunderstorm approaches. She will touch readers with her peceptions of the world and her wonder of what sound is.

32 pages Hardcover

3695 Medical Sign Language: Easily Understood D efinitions of Commonly Used Medical Term

W Joseph Garcia, author

Charles C Thomas Publishers
2600 South First Street
Springfield, IL 62704

217-789-8980
800-258-8980
e-mail: books@ccthomas.com
www.ccthomas.com

In this glossary, a multitude of medical and dental terms are accurately defined and precisely translated, through description and illustration, into American Sign Language. The book easily lends itself to use at both ends of the chain of communication that links health care professionals with their deaf patients. Includes bibliography. Comes in both hardcover and softcover

726 pages

3696 Messy Monsters Jungle Joggers and Bubble B aths

Nehama Pluznik and Rochelle Sobel, author

Alexander Graham Bell Association for the Deaf
3417 Volta Place NW
Washington, DC 20007

202-337-5220
Fax: 202-337-8314
TTY: 202-337-5221
e-mail: info@agbell.org
www.agbell.org

An illustrated book of poetry for children with hearing loss. Poems are organized according to the accepted group of speechreading phonemes which are classified by their appearance on the lips. Each poem emphasizes a particular phoneme which appears in the initial, medial, or final position of the word. Four worksheets accompany each poem: About the poem, Tell me more, Speech practice, and Language activities.

97 pages Softcover

3697 My First Book of Sign

TJ Publishers
817 Silver Spring Avenue, Suite 206
Silver Spring, MD 20910

301-585-4440
800-999-1168
Fax: 301-585-5930
TTY: 301-585-4440
TDD: 301-585-4441
e-mail: TJPubinc@aol.com

Full-color book gives alphabetically grouped signs for 150 words most frequently used by young children.

1990 80 pages Hardcover
ISBN: 0-903023-20-3

3698 Negotiating the Special Education Maze

Alexander Graham Bell Association for the Deaf
3417 Volta Place NW
Washington, DC 20007

202-337-5220
800-432-7543
Fax: 202-337-8314
TTY: 202-337-5220
e-mail: agbell2@aol.com
www.agbell.org

This guidebook, written primarily for parents, teachers, and school administrators, provides easy to understand information about developing an effective educational program for children with special needs.

1997 446 pages hardcover

3699 None So Deaf - Student Text

National Association of the Deaf
814 Thayer Avenue
Silver Spring, MD 20910

301-587-1788
Fax: 301-587-1791
TTY: 301-587-1789
e-mail: nadinfo@nad.org
www.nad.org

A student history of the education of deaf people and the development of sign language. Stories about deaf children illustrate the struggle toward equal recognition and the right to education, and modern systems of communication.

Deborah L Jacobs

3700 Nursery Rhymes from Mother Goose: Told in Signed English

Harry Bornstein and Karen L Saulnier, author

Gallaudet University Press
800 Florida Avenue NE
Washington, DC 20002

202-651-5488
Fax: 202-651-5489
e-mail: gupress@gallaudet.edu
http://gupress.gallaudet.edu

More than a dozen favorite nursery rhymes are presented in this unique edition of Mother Goose. All of the rhymes are illustrated with full-color paintings accompanied by more than 389 drawings showing the verses in Signed English. Young readers, both hearing and deaf, will learn the special charm of rhyme while also discovering new vocabulary and new ways to experience English through signing. As they learn and memorize their favorite verses, children will also strengthen their language skills.

64 pages Hardcover
ISBN: 0-930323-99-8

3701 Operation SHHH

Self Help for Hard-of-Hearing People
7910 Woodmont Avenue, Suite 1200
Bethesda, MD 20814

301-657-2248
Fax: 301-913-9413
TTY: 301-657-2249
e-mail: national@shhh.org
www.shhh.org

Features SHHHerman, the lion who does not roar. This program is designed for elementary school children. Includes video, posters, brochures and more.

3702 Opposites

HEAR-MORE
42 Executive Boulevard
Farmingdale, NY 11735

800-881-4327
Fax: 631-752-0689
TTY: 800-281-4327
www.hearmore.com

The Early Sign Language Series: A fascinating and enjoyable way for children and adults to learn sign language. Opposites presents the early concepts of opposite relationships. It fosters both receptive and expressive language through signs and pictures, and it is perfect for young children whether hearing impaired, hearing, pre-verbal or verbal. Reviews 10 opposite items (20 in total).

3703 Out for a Walk: Baby's First Sign Book

Kim Votry and Curt Waller, author

Gallaudet University Press
800 Florida Avenue NE
Washington, DC 20002

202-651-5488
Fax: 202-651-5489
e-mail: gupress@gallaudet.edu
http://gupress.gallaudet.edu

Offers toddlers their first look at signs for the world around them. As they follow our distinctively hatted youngster on a stroll, they encounter familiar animals and insect, among them a dog, cat, butterfly, and squirrel, and learn which ones can be pets. They'll enjoy imaginative images of senses, too - sight, smell, hearing, taste, and touch.

16 pages Board Book
ISBN: 1-563681-46-3

3704 Parent's Guide to Chochlear Implants

Patricia M Chute and Mary Ellen Nevins, author

Gallaudet University Press
800 Florida Avenue NE
Washington, DC 20002

202-651-5488
Fax: 202-651-5489
e-mail: gupress@gallaudet.edu
http://gupress.gallaudet.edu

Now, parents of deaf children have at hand a complete guide to the process of cochlear implantation. It explains in a friendly easy-to-follow style each stage of the process. Parents will discover how to have their child evaluated to determine his or her suitability for an implant. They'll learn about implant device options, how to choose an implant center, and every detail of the surgical procedure. The initial 'switch-on' is described along with counseling about device maintainance.

208 pages Softcover
ISBN: 1-563681-29-3

3705 Parents and Teachers: Partners in Language Development

Alexander Graham Bell Association for the Deaf
3417 Volta Place NW
Washington, DC 20007

202-337-5220
800-432-7543
Fax: 202-337-8314
TTY: 202-337-5220
e-mail: agbell2@aol.com
www.agbell.org

Outlines the essential role of the teacher and parent in the development of language in the school-aged child with hearing impairment.

1990 386 pages

3706 Parents and Their Deaf Children: The Early Years
Gallaudet University Press
800 Florida Avenue NE
Washington, DC 20002

202-651-5488
Fax: 202-651-5489
e-mail: gupress@gallaudet.edu
http://gupress.gallaudet.edu

This book stems from a nationwide survey of parents with 6-7 year old deaf or hard of hearing children, followed up by interviews with 80 parents. The authors not only discuss the parents' communication choices for their children, but also provide how parents' experiences differ, especially for those whose children are hard of hearing, have additional conditions, or have cochlear implants. One chapter is devoted to minority cultures. Includes tables, figures, references and index.

272 pages Hardcover
ISBN: 1-563681-37-4

Kathryn P Meadow-Orlans, Co-Author
Donna M Mertens, Co-Author

3707 Parents' Guide to Speech and Deafness
Alexander Graham Bell Association for the Deaf
3417 Volta Place NW
Washington, DC 20007

202-337-5220
800-432-7543
Fax: 202-337-8314
TTY: 202-337-5220
e-mail: agbell2@aol.com
www.agbell.org

A guide to help parents play an active role in the speech development of children with hearing impairment.

1984 paperback
ISBN: 0-882001-55-8

3708 Patrick Gets Hearing Aids
Alexander Graham Bell Association for the Deaf
3417 Volta Place NW
Washington, DC 20007

202-337-5220
800-432-7543
Fax: 202-337-8314
TTY: 202-337-5220
e-mail: agbell2@aol.com
www.agbell.org

A children's book where Patrick the rabbit finds himself out of touch because he has a hearing loss. Also available in Spanish.

1994 44 pages spanish avail.

3709 Pediatric Audiology 0 to 5 Years
Alexander Graham Bell Association for the Deaf
3417 Volta Place NW
Washington, DC 20007

202-337-5220
800-432-7543
Fax: 202-337-8314
TTY: 202-337-5220
e-mail: agbell2@aol.com
www.agbell.org

A professional title that examines childhood hearing impairments and the impact of hearing loss on speech and language.

1993 446 pages
ISBN: 1-897635-25-7

3710 Police Officer Jones
HEAR-MORE
42 Executive Boulevard
Farmingdale, NY 11735

800-881-4327
Fax: 631-752-0689
TTY: 800-281-4327
www.hearmore.com

This beginning book describes a police officer and his exciting job. Use the signs when reading the book to your child and speak when you sign so the child will learn to associate the sign with sound and lip shape.

3711 Raising Your Hearing-Impaired Child
Alexander Graham Bell Association for the Deaf
3417 Volta Place NW
Washington, DC 20007

202-337-5220
800-432-7543
Fax: 202-337-8314
TTY: 202-337-5220
e-mail: agbell2@aol.com
www.agbell.org

This practical book is written by the mother of two children with hearing impairments offering support, information, and practical suggestions for parents who discover their child has a hearing problem.

1982 256 pages paperback
ISBN: 0-882001-50-7

3712 Reading Between the Lips
Alexander Graham Bell Association for the Deaf
3417 Volta Place NW
Washington, DC 20007

202-337-5220
800-432-7543
Fax: 202-337-8314
TTY: 202-337-5220
e-mail: agbell2@aol.com
www.agbell.org

In a frank and witty celebration of the advantages and pitfalls of speaking and lipreading, the author shows that total deafness is not an impenetrable barrier but one to get over or around.

1995 363 pages hardcover

3713 Religious Signing: A Comprehensive Guide f or All Faiths

Elaine Costello, author

TJ Publishers
2544 Tarpley Road, Suite 108
Carrollton, TX 75006

972-416-0800
800-999-1168
Fax: 972-416-0944
TTY: 972-416-0933
e-mail: customerservice@tjpublishers.com
www.tjpublishers.com

Contains over 500 religious signs and their meanings for all denominations. Clearly demonstrated and defined through illustrations that show movement of hands, body and face. Includes a special section on favorite verses, prayers and blessings.

219 pages Softcover
ISBN: 0-553342-44-4

3714 Rhode Island Test of Language Structure RITLS
Pro Ed
8700 Shoal Creed Boulevard
Austin, TX 78757

512-451-3246
800-897-3202
Fax: 800-397-7633
e-mail: info@proedinc.com
www.proedinc.com

The Rhode Island Test of Language Structure (RITLS) provides a measure of English language development and assessment data. It is designed primarily for use with children who are hearing impaired, but also useful in other areas where level of language development is of concern, including mental retardation, learning disability, and bilingual programs. The RITLS focuses on syntax, unlike other tests compared with other reading, language, intelligence, and achievement tests frequently used.

1983

3715 Rural Habilitation
Alexander Graham Bell Association for the Deaf
3417 Volta Place NW
Washington, DC 20007

202-337-5220
800-432-7543
Fax: 202-337-8314
TTY: 202-337-5220
e-mail: agbell2@aol.com
www.agbell.org

Provides essential information in the planning of individual educational programs for hearing-impaired children from early infancy to emphasize the optimal use of residual hearing, the assessment of each child for placement in the least restrictive educational setting and more.

336 pages

3716 Schedules of Development for Hearing Impaired Infants and Their Parents
Alexander Graham Bell Association for the Deaf
3417 Volta Place NW
Washington, DC 20007

202-337-5220
Fax: 202-337-8314
TTY: 202-337-5221
e-mail: publications@agbell.org
www.agbell.org

Written for parents and teachers, this assessment record of verbal learning will help to evaluate each child's language development.

1977 14 pages

Agnes Ling Philips PhD, Author

3717 Science Curriculum: Clarke Curriculum Series
Alexander Graham Bell Association for the Deaf
3417 Volta Place NW
Washington, DC 20007

202-337-5220
800-432-7543
Fax: 202-337-8314
TTY: 202-337-5220
e-mail: agbell2@aol.com
www.agbell.org

This comprehensive science curriculum for young students with hearing losses teaches classroom units about the process of science, technology, and society. Teaches science through language activities, central science concepts, scientific processes, objectives, resources, and related children's literature.

1994 455 pages

3718 Screening Children for Auditory Function
Alexander Graham Bell Association for the Deaf
3417 Volta Place NW
Washington, DC 20007

202-337-5220
800-432-7543
Fax: 202-337-8314
TTY: 202-337-5220
e-mail: agbell2@aol.com
www.agbell.org

This current source of information on early recognition of children with hearing impairments from infancy to school-age is based on papers by 58 distinguished authors.

1992 560 pages Hardcover
ISBN: 0-963143-90-5

3719 Screening for Hearing Loss and Otitis Medi a in Children

Jackson Roush PhD, author

Alexander Graham Bell Association for the Deaf
3417 Volta Place NW
Washington, DC 20007

202-337-5220
Fax: 202-337-8314
TTY: 202-337-5221
e-mail: info@agbell.org
www.agbell.org

Provides a concise yet comprehensive guide to hearing and middle ear screening in children. From acoustic emissions and automated ABR in newborns to hearing screening of school-age children.

245 pages Softcover

3720 Secret Signing: A Sign Language Activity Book
Gallaudet Univ. Press c/o Chicago Distrib. Center
11030 S Langley Avenue
Chicago, IL 60628

202-651-5000
800-621-2736
Fax: 800-621-8476
TTY: 888-630-9347
www.gallaudet.edu/~gupress

Children will enjoy this activity book with signs.

64 pages Level K-1

3721 Sign Language Coloring Books
Gallaudet Univ. Press c/o Chicago Distrib. Center
800 Florida Avenue NE
Washington, DC 20002

202-651-5000
800-621-2736
Fax: 800-621-8476
TTY: 202-651-5000
www.gallaudet.edu/~gupress

A mischievous mouse and a spinning top, a doll on the sofa, a hobo clown with his friend the elephant: these coloring books are a FUNtastic way for children to learn to sign, fingerspell, read and write.

paperback
ISBN: 0-915035-52-9

3722 Sign Language Talk
Franklin Watts c/o Grolier
90 Old Sherman Tpke
Danbury, CT 06816

203-797-3500
800-621-1115
Fax: 203-797-3197
www.grolier.com

Using 300 easy-to-follow illustrations, this book introduces the structure of sign language, shows how sentences are formed and how signed conversations differ from spoken ones.

1989 96 pages hardcover
ISBN: 0-531105-97-0

3723 Sign Language for Babies

Walter Paul Kelly, author

Harris Communications
15155 Technology Drive
Eden Prairie, MN 55344

952-906-1180
800-825-6758
Fax: 952-906-1099
TTY: 952-906-1198
e-mail: info@harriscomm.com
www.harriscomm.com

A black and white illustrated story on how love and eventually the ILY handsign in American Sign Language got started.

Hardcover

3724 Sign Numbers

Nancy Bartusch, author

Modern Signs Press
10443 Los Alamitos Boulevard, PO Box 1181
Los Alamitos, CA 90720

562-596-8548
800-572-7332
Fax: 562-795-6614
TTY: 562-493-4168
e-mail: modsigns@modernsignspress.com
www.modernsignspress.com

Mandy helps Handy teach manual and written numbers. Includes printed numbers and easy-to-follow drawings of the number hand shapes. Also shows words and signs for the objects counted in a picture on each page. Black and white drawings make this a coloring book, too.

60 pages

3725 Sign With Kids Supplement

Modern Signs Press
10443 Los Alamitos Boulevard, PO Box 1181
Los Alamitos, CA 90720

562-596-8548
800-572-7332
Fax: 562-795-6614
TTY: 562-493-4168
e-mail: modsigns@modernsignspress.com
www.modernsignspress.com

The supplement contains easy to use illustrations for all the signs in every lesson of Sign With Kids. Both volumes together provide a comprehensive program for teaching sign language to hearing kids.

3726 Sign with Me Books

Gallaudet University Press
800 Florida Avenue NE
Washington, DC 20002

202-651-5000
800-621-2736
Fax: 800-621-8476
TTY: 202-651-5000
www.gallaudet.edu/~gupress

Bold, colorful pictures and accurate diagrams make it fun to learn everyday signs. Titles in this series include ABC Sign With Me; Colors Sign With Me; and 1,2,3 Sign With Me.

1987 paperback

3727 Sign-Me-Fine

Gallaudet University Press
800 Florida Avenue NE
Washington, DC 20002

202-651-5488
Fax: 202-651-4589
TTY: 202-651-5488
e-mail: gupress@gallaudet.edu
http://gupress.gallaudet.edu

Written for young adults, this book introduces American Sign Language and how it differs from English.

1997 120 pages paperback
ISBN: 0-930323-76-9

3728 Signed English Starter

Harris Communications
15159 Technology Drive
Eden Prairie, MN 55344

612-906-1180
800-825-6758
Fax: 612-902-1099
TTY: 800-825-9187
e-mail: mail@harriscomm.com
www.harriscomm.com

The first book to use when learning Signed English.

1984 208 pages softcover

3729 Signing Exact English Using Affixes

Modern Signs Press
10443 Los Alamitos Boulevard, PO Box 1181
Los Alamitos, CA 90720

562-596-8548
800-572-7332
Fax: 562-795-6614
TTY: 562-493-4168
e-mail: modsigns@modernsignspress.com
www.modernsignspress.com

A catalog of signed vocabulary extended by prefixes, suffixes, contractions and tenses.

3730 Signing Family: What Every Parent Should K now About Sign Communication

David A Stewart and Barbara Leutke-Stahlman, author

Gallaudet University Press
800 Florida Avenue NE
Washington, DC 20002

202-651-5488
Fax: 202-651-5489
e-mail: gupress@gallaudet.edu
http://gupress.gallaudet.edu

Parents of deaf children concerned with finding the best means of communication for their family will welcome the straightforward, reader-friendly information in this book. In a style both positive and pragmatic, the authors employ common-sense reasoning to establish the importance of teach deaf children language fundamentals as early as possible. This essential book for parents continues by explaining why the visual-gestural nature of signing is generally the best langue mode for deaf children

192 pages Softcover
ISBN: 1-563680-69-6

3731 Signing Fun: American Sign Language Vocabu lary, Phrases, Games and Activities

Penny Warner and Paula Gray, author

Gallaudet University Press
800 Florida Avenue NE
Washington, DC 20002

202-651-5488
Fax: 202-651-5489
e-mail: gupress@gallaudet.edu
http://gupress.gallaudet.edu

For young adults age 11 and up. Signing is visual, easy to learn, and fun to use. Offers 441 useful signs on a variety of favorite topics: activities, animals, fashion, food, holidays, home, outdoors, parties, people, places, play, emotions, school, shopping, travel, plus extra fun signs for especially popular words. Each chapter includes practice sentences using everyday phrases to help new signers learn in a fun way. Provides dozens of entertaining games and activities.

192 pages Softcover
ISBN: 1-563629-23-6

3732 Signing Illustrated

Gallaudet University Press
800 Florida Avenue NE
Washington, DC 20002

202-651-5000
800-621-2736
Fax: 800-621-8476
TTY: 888-630-9347
www.gallaudet.edu/~gupress

A guide presenting illustrations of over 1,350 signs. Features key elements of the most popular sign language systems.

1994 288 pages paperback
ISBN: 0-399521-34-8

3733 Signing for Kids

Gallaudet University Press
800 Florida Avenue NE
Washington, DC 20002

202-651-5000
800-621-2736
Fax: 800-621-8476
TTY: 202-651-5000
www.gallaudet.edu/~gupress

Contains 17 chapters dealing with special areas of interest to children, like pets, family, friends and people.

1991 142 pages paperback
ISBN: 0-399516-72-7

3734 Signing: How to Speak With Your Hands, Sec ond Edition

Elaine Costello, author

TJ Publishers
2544 Tarpley Road, Suite 108
Carrollton, TX 75006

972-416-0800
800-999-1168
Fax: 972-416-0944
TTY: 972-416-0933
e-mail: customerservice@tjpublishers.com
www.tjpublishers.com

This book presents more than 1300 signs and their descriptions. Linguistic principles are described at the beginning of each chapter giving insight into the rules which govern American Sign Language.

248 pages Softcover
ISBN: 0-553375-39-3

3735 Signs for Me

Ben Bahan and Joe Dannis, author

Harris Communications
15155 Technology Drive
Eden Prairie, MN 55344

952-906-1180
800-825-6758
Fax: 952-906-1099
TTY: 952-906-1198
e-mail: info@harriscomm.com
www.harriscomm.com

Ideal for youngsters and other sign language beginners, a unique illustrated approach to presenting basic vocabulary. While the book

provides a multidimentional sign vocabulary for pre-school and elementary school children, its appealing format makes it suitable for signers of all ages.

111 pages Softcover

3736 Signs for Me: Basic Sign Vocabulary for Ch ildren, Parents and Teachers

Ben Bahan and Joe Dannis, author

TJ Publishers
2544 Tarpley Road, Suite 108
Carrollton, TX 75006

972-416-0800
800-999-1168
Fax: 972-416-0944
TTY: 972-416-0933
e-mail: customerservice@tjpublishers.com
www.tjpublishers.com

Sign language vocabulary for preschool and elementary school children introduces household items, animals, family members, actions, emotions, safety concerns and other concepts. Over 300 vocabulary words, pictures and sign illustrations.

112 pages Softcover
ISBN: 0-915035-27-8

3737 Signs of Sharing: An Elementary Sign Language and Deaf Awareness Curriculum

Charles C Thomas Publisher
2600 S 1st Street
Springfield, IL 62704

217-789-8980
800-258-8980
Fax: 217-789-9130
e-mail: books@ccthomas.com
www.ccthomas.com

A unique set of materials that provides educators whose responsibilities include the integration of hearing-impaired children, with a multifaceted tool to teach sign language and deaf awareness.

1993 380 pages
ISBN: 0-398058-51-2

Sue F V Rakow, Co-Author
Carol B Carpenter, Co-Author

3738 Silent Garden

Paul W Ogden, author

Gallaudet University Press
800 Florida Avenue NE
Washington, DC 20002

202-651-5488
Fax: 202-651-5489
e-mail: gupress@gallaudet.edu
http://gupress.gallaudet.edu

This completely rewritten edition presents parents of deaf children with more crucial information enhanced by the advances made in the general understanding of what it means to be deaf and the greater possibilities afforded deaf children today. Provides parents with a firm foundation for making the difficult decisions necessary to begin their child on the road to realizing his or her full potential.

304 pages Softcover
ISBN: 1-563680-58-0

3739 Silent Garden: Raising Your Deaf Child

Alexander Graham Bell Association for the Deaf
3417 Volta Place NW
Washington, DC 20007

202-337-5220
800-432-7543
Fax: 202-337-8314
TTY: 202-337-5220
e-mail: agbell2@aol.com
www.agbell.org

This book provides parents of deaf children with crucial information on the possibilities afforded their children. Ogden, deaf since birth and a professor of deaf studies, offers parents the foundation for making the difficult decisions necessary to start their children on the road to realizing their full potential.

1996 313 pages

3740 Silent Observer

Christy MacKinnon, author

Gallaudet University Press
800 Florida Avenue NE
Washington, DC 20002

202-651-5488
Fax: 202-651-5489
e-mail: gupress@gallaudet.edu
http://gupress.gallaudet.edu

An affectionage, poignant memoir of childhood as seen through the eyes of a vivacious young girl. Teachers, parents, and children will share in their enjoyment of this beautiful, sensitive story of a harder but wonderful time that has passed.

48 pages Hardcover
ISBN: 1-563680-22-X

3741 Simple Signs

Cindy Wheeler, author

Harris Communications
15155 Technology Drive
Eden Prairie, MN 55344

952-906-1180
800-825-6758
Fax: 952-906-1099
TTY: 952-906-1198
e-mail: info@harriscomm.com
www.harriscomm.com

Children have a lot to say, whether through gestures, movement, pictures or words. American Sign Language incorporates all these natural skills. With pictures, clear diagrams, and hints, learn from these 28 signs. Ages 3-6 years.

30 pages Softcover

3742 Six-Sound Song

Warren Estabrooks MEd, author

Alexander Graham Bell Association for the Deaf
3417 Volta Place NW
Washington, DC 20007

202-337-5220
Fax: 202-337-8314
TTY: 202-337-5221
e-mail: info@agbell.org
www.agbell.org

Based on the Six-Sound Tests developed by the late Daniel Ling, PhD. Used for both individual and group therapy sessions in auditory and oral environments. Children will enjoy the illustrations created by seven-year-old Hunter Jackson who received his cochlear implant while the Auditory-Verbal Centre of the Learning to Listen Foundation. Hardcover Book and CD set

3743 Songs in Sign

S Harold Collins, author

TJ Publishers
2544 Tarpley Road, Suite 108
Carrollton, TX 75006

972-416-0800
800-999-1168
Fax: 972-416-0944
TTY: 972-416-0933
e-mail: customerservice@tjpublishers.com
www.tjpublishers.com

Presents six songs in Signed English. The easy-to-follow illustrations enable you to sign: Twinkle, Twinkle Litt Star; The Mullberry Bush; Row, Row, Row Your Boat; If You're Happy; Bingo and The Muffin Man.

16 pages Softcover
ISBN: 0-931993-71-7

3744 Speak to Me (Second Edition)

Marcia Calhoun Forecki, author

Gallaudet University Press
800 Florida Avenue NE
Washington, DC 20002

202-651-5488
Fax: 202-651-5489
e-mail: gupress@gallaudet.edu
http://gupress.gallaudet.edu

An engrossing, personal account of life with Charlie, an adorable, active, deaf seven-year-old. The story of an ordinary person confronted with an overwhelming reality - the fact that her son is deaf. Forecki's struggle as a single parent to care for her child, to find the right schools, and to establish communication with her son will strike a familiar chord in all hearing parents of deaf children. All readers will be touched by the mixture of pathos and humor in this account.

154 pages Softcover
ISBN: 0-930323-68-8

3745 Speech and Deafness

Alexander Graham Bell Association for the Deaf
3417 Volta Place NW
Washington, DC 20007

202-337-5220
800-432-7543
Fax: 202-337-8314
TTY: 202-337-5220
e-mail: agbell2@aol.com
www.agbell.org

Practical examination of the major current methodologies of teaching of the deaf. There are more down-to-earth recommendations for selecting and assessing the appropriate approach for each child.

1983 304 pages paperback
ISBN: 0-882000-70-5

3746 Speech and the Hearing Impaired Child (Second Edition)

Daniel Ling, PhD, author

Alexander Graham Bell Association for the Deaf
3417 Volta Place NW
Washington, DC 20007

202-337-5220
Fax: 202-337-8314
TTY: 202-337-5221
e-mail: info@agbell.org
www.agbell.org

An extension of the original text published by the late Daniel Ling in 1976. It looks much more closely at the development of speech in the context of spoken language. It incorporates informal strategies for promoting spoken language development that are appropriate for use with modern technology such as digital hearing aids and cochlear implants. Considerable emphasis is placed on the ongoing evaluation of speech in the context of spoken language.

440 pages Softcover

3747 Speechreading: A Way to Improve Understanding
Gallaudet University Press
800 Florida Avenue NE
Washington, DC 20002

202-651-5488
Fax: 202-651-5489
TTY: 202-651-5488
e-mail: gupress@gallaudet.edu
http://gupress.gallaudet.edu

This useful guide for teachers and therapists approaches speechreading instruction with the help of context cues.

160 pages

3748 Sport Signs
Modern Signs Press
PO Box 1181
Los Alamitos, CA 90720

562-596-8548
800-572-7332
Fax: 562-795-6614
TTY: 310-493-4168
e-mail: modsigns@modernsignspress.com

Objects and actions are depicted with illustrations, and manual signs are shown with the printed words.

1985 paperback
ISBN: 0-317427-69-7

3749 Student Study Guide to A Basic Course in A merican Sign Language
Frances DeCapite, author

TJ Publishers
2544 Tarpley Road, Suite 108
Carrollton, TX 75006

972-416-0800
800-999-1168
Fax: 972-416-0944
TTY: 972-416-0933
e-mail: customerservice@tjpublishers.com
www.tjpublishers.com

Designed to supplement the text of A Basic Course in American Sign Language, the guide provides a wide array of supplemental practice materials for student and teacher. Exercises and practice sentences allow students to practice receptive and expressive skills.

197 pages Spiral bound
ISBN: 0-932666-33-7

3750 Supporting Young Adults Who Are Deaf-Blind in Their Communities
National Association of the Deaf
814 Thayer Avenue
Silver Spring, MD 20910

301-587-1789
Fax: 301-587-1791
TTY: 301-587-1789
e-mail: nadinfo@nad.org
www.nad.org

Provides specific strategies to help individuals who are deaf-blind to achieve greater integration into the community.

1995 384 pages
Deborah L Jacobs

3751 Talking Finger Series - At Grandma's House
Modern Signs Press
10443 Los Alamitos Boulevard, PO Box 1181
Los Alamitos, CA 90720

562-596-8548
800-572-7332
Fax: 562-795-6614
TTY: 562-493-4168
e-mail: modsigns@modernsignspress.com
www.modernsignspress.com

Pictures, signs and printed words tell the tale of April, a cuddly little rabbit who loves to play with her beloved Grandma. Uses 27-word vocabulary, includes manual alphabet and glossary of signs.

3752 Talking Finger Series - Little Green Monst er
Modern Signs Press
10443 Los Alamitos Boulevard, PO Box 1181
Los Alamitos, CA 90720

562-596-8548
800-572-7332
Fax: 562-795-6614
TTY: 562-493-4168
e-mail: modsigns@modernsignspress.com
www.modernsignspress.com

This storybook features Becky and Barry, two playful little bears who keep you in suspense. The 45-word vocabulary in signs and printed words introduces concept of directionality (here, there, behind, etc.). Includes manual alphabet and glossary of signs.

36 pages

3753 Teach Your Tot to Sign
Stacy A Thompson and Valerie Nelson-Metlay, author

Gallaudet University Press
800 Florida Avenue NE
Washington, DC 20002

202-651-5488
Fax: 202-651-5489
e-mail: gupress@gallaudet.edu
http://gupress.gallaudet.edu

This book provides parents and teachers the opportunity to teach more than 500 basic American Sign Language signs to their infants, toddlers, and young children. It features fundamental signs of great appeal to young children and concise instructions on how to sign, including the critical importance of facial expression. Anticipates all of the common desires and interests of young children - food, pets, planes, trains, cars and boats, games, holidays, vegetables, family - nearly everything.

232 pages Softcover
ISBN: 1-563683-11-3

3754 Teaching Reading to Deaf Children
Alexander Graham Bell Association for the Deaf
3417 Volta Place NW
Washington, DC 20007

202-337-5220
800-432-7543
Fax: 202-337-8314
TTY: 202-337-5220
e-mail: agbell2@aol.com
www.agbell.org

Developed by Lexington School for the Deaf, this practical hand book for educators and parents presents a step-by-step program to guide children's reading growth.

1978 221 pages paperback

3755 Test of Early Reading Ability, Deaf or Hard-of-Hearing
Pro-Ed
8700 Shoal Creek Boulevard
Austin, TX 78757

512-451-3246
800-897-3202
Fax: 512-451-8542
e-mail: info@proedinc.com
www.proedinc.com

This is the only individually administered test of reading designed for children with moderate to profound sensory hearing loss (i.e. ranging from 41 to beyond 91 decibels, corrected). Ages: 3 through 13. Testing time: 20 to 30 minutes

3756 The Development of Deaf Children: Academic Achievement Levels and Social Processes

Kerstin Heiling, author

Gallaudet University Press
800 Florida Avenue NE
Washington, DC 20002

202-651-5488
Fax: 202-651-5489
e-mail: gupress@gallaudet.edu
http://gupress.gallaudet.edu

This revealing volume presents the research from a videotape study of the behavior of 20 deaf children for 14 years, and a comprehensive test at age 15 to assess their development.

280 pages Hardcover
ISBN: 3-927731-58-7

3757 The Handbook of Pediatric Audiology

Sanford E Gerber, Editor, author

Gallaudet University Press
800 Florida Avenue NE
Washington, DC 20002

202-651-5488
Fax: 202-651-5489
e-mail: gupress@gallaudet.edu
http://gupress.gallaudet.edu

Presents 14 comprehensive chapters written by expert in each discipline. Clinicians and students now can refer to specific subjects in pediatric audiology for treating children from infancy through their elementary school years. Contributors include: Yash Pal Kapur, Franklin A. Katz, Robert J. Ruben, Allen O. Diefendorf, Judith S. Gravel, Jane R. Madell, Shlomo Silman, Carol A. Silverman, Herbert Jay Gold, and Maurice Mendel. Tables, figures, references, bibliography, author and subject index

478 pages Softcover
ISBN: 1-563680-99-7

3758 The Hearing Aid Handbook: Clinician's Guid e to Client Orientation

Donna S Wayner, author

Gallaudet University Press
800 Florida Avenue NE
Washington, DC 20002

202-651-5488
Fax: 202-651-5489
e-mail: gupress@gallaudet.edu
http://gupress.gallaudet.edu

This handbook consists of three volumes for audiologists and other clinicians to help clients learn to use hearing aids. Planned for three classes, the guide explains exactly how to conduct the initial visit, fit ear molds, clean and maintain hearing aids and adjust amplification. Clinicians will also learn to encourage the use of visual cues, speechreading, and contextual clues to ensure a high rate of success for their clients. Users Guides feature information and worksheets.

172 pages Softcover
ISBN: 0-930323-56-4

3759 The Joy of Signing Second Edition

Lottie L Riekehof, author

TJ Publishers
2544 Tarpley Road, Suite 108
Carrollton, TX 75006

972-416-0800
800-999-1168
Fax: 972-416-0944
TTY: 972-416-0933
e-mail: customerservice@tjpublishers.com
www.tjpublishers.com

This popular dictionary of approximately 1500 known signs makes them easier to remember. Sentences present signs in proper context. Appendix gives information about the most effective way to add signs to spoken English.

352 pages Hardcover
ISBN: 0-882435-20-5

3760 The Listener

Warren Estabrooks, MEd, author

Alexander Graham Bell Association for the Deaf
3417 Volta Place NW
Washington, DC 20007

202-337-5220
Fax: 202-337-8314
TTY: 202-337-5221
e-mail: info@agbell.org
www.agbell.org

Subject material is centered around listening, speech, language, spoken communication, and cognitive, social and psychological development of children who are deaf or hard of hearing and their families. Articles address: Making sense of complex skills lesson planning, Morphosyntax: evidence-based AVT, Your young child's newly diagnosed hearing loss: knowing how to cope, What is Auditory-Verbal Therapy?, Teachers' perceptions of the integration of children with hearing loss.

64 pages Softcover

3761 The Night Before Christmas told in Signed english

Adapted By Harry Bornstein and Karen L Saulnier, author

Gallaudet University Press
800 Florida Avenue NE
Washington, DC 20002

202-651-5488
Fax: 202-651-5489
e-mail: gupress@gallaudet.edu
http://gupress.gallaudet.edu

Now this wonderful, seasonal poem can be enjoyed in a new way by both hearing and deaf children. Accompanying the complete verses and full-color illustrations, line drawings show this holiday favorite in Signed English, the system that uses American Sign Language signs in English word order. Uses both rhyme and signing to help children practice their vocabulary and learn English grammar. Entertains at the same time that it teaches.

64 pages Hardcover
ISBN: 1-563680-20-3

Clement C Moore, Original Author

3762 The Rising of Lotus Flowers: Self-Educatin g Deaf Children in Thai Boarding Schools

Charles B Reilly and Nipapon Reilly, author

Gallaudet University Press
800 Florida Avenue NE
Washington, DC 20002

202-651-5488
Fax: 202-651-5489
e-mail: gupress@gallaudet.edu
http://gupress.gallaudet.edu

In developed nations around the world, residential schools for deaf students are giving way to the trend of inclusion in regular classrooms. Nonetheless, deaf education continues to lag as students struggle to communicate. In the Bua School in Thialand, however, 400 residential deaf students ranging in age from 6 to 19 have met with great success in teaching each other Thai Sign Language and a world of knowledge once thought to be lost to them.

272 pages Hardcover
ISBN: 1-563682-75-3

3763 The Young Deaf Child

David Luterman, PhD, author

Alexander Graham Bell Association for the Deaf
3417 Volta Place NW
Washington, DC 20007

202-337-5220
Fax: 202-337-8314
TTY: 202-337-5221
e-mail: info@agbell.org
www.agbell.org

A valuable resource for audiologists, early interventionists and special educators who provide diagnostic or therapeutic services to parents of newborns and children with hearing loss. Discusses the history of deaf education in the United States and offers valuable information on the pros and cons of screening, elements essential to effective programming and therapy, a model for intervention centered on the parent-child connection, assistive hearing technologies and counseling techniques.

3764 There's a Hearing Impaired Child in my Class

Gallaudet Univ. Press c/o Chicago Distrib. Center
800 Florida Avenue NE
Washington, DC 20002

202-651-5000
800-621-2736
Fax: 800-621-8476
TTY: 202-651-5000
www.gallaudet.edu/~gupress

This complete package provides basic facts about deafness, practical strategies for teaching hearing impaired children, and the question-and-answer information for all students.

44 pages

3765 Today's Hearing Impaired Child: Into The Mainstream of Education

Alexander Graham Bell Association for the Deaf
3417 Volta Place NW
Washington, DC 20007

202-337-5220
800-432-7543
Fax: 202-337-8314
TTY: 202-337-5220
e-mail: agbell2@aol.com
www.agbell.org

A practical guide to the educational rights of hearing-impaired children under the law, guidelines for mainstreaming, educational assessment, special instructions for the regular classroom teacher, suggestions for developing and enhancing reading skills necessary for successful mainstreaming and an overview of hearing impairment for the regular classroom teacher.

1981 240 pages paperback
ISBN: 0-882001-43-4

3766 Un Curso Basico de Lenguaje Americano de S enas

TJ Publishers
2544 Tarpley Road, Suite 108
Carrollton, TX 75006

972-416-0800
800-999-1168
Fax: 972-416-0944
TTY: 972-416-0933
e-mail: customerservice@tjpublishers.com
www.tjpublishers.com

Features English and Spanish translations side by side. It is designed for teachers, parents and students working with Deaf Hispanic American children and adults learning English and American Sign Language.

356 pages Spiral bound
ISBN: 0-932666-35-3

3767 Very Special Friend

Gallaudet University Press
800 Florida Avenue NE
Washington, DC 20002

202-651-5000
800-621-2736
Fax: 800-621-8476
TTY: 202-651-5000
www.gallaudet.edu/~gupress

Six-year-old Frannie finds a very special friend who talks in sign language. She learns to sign and the two become best friends.

1992 32 pages Hardcover
ISBN: 1-878363-24-7

3768 We Can

Alexander Graham Bell Association for the Deaf
3417 Volta Place NW
Washington, DC 20007

202-337-5220
800-432-7543
Fax: 202-337-8314
TTY: 202-337-5220
e-mail: agbell2@aol.com
www.agbell.org

Hearing-impaired children need hearing-impaired role models. Written at a 4th-grade level, the books can also be used in the classroom for career education, as well as for reading and language instruction.

1980 88 pages hardcover
ISBN: 0-882001-35-3

3769 We Can Hear and Speak

Alexander Graham Bell Association for the Deaf
3417 Volta Place NW
Washington, DC 20007

202-337-5220
Fax: 202-337-8314
TTY: 202-337-5221
e-mail: info@agbell.org
www.agbell.org

Written by parents for families of children who are deaf or hard-of-hearing, this work describes auditory-verbal terminology and approaches and contains personal narratives written by parents and their children who are deaf or hard-of-hearing.

1998 184 pages Softcover

Carol Flexer PhD, Contributor
Catherine Richards, Contributor

3770 When Your Child is Deaf: A Guide for Parents

Alexander Graham Bell Association for the Deaf
3417 Volta Place NW
Washington, DC 20007

202-337-5220
800-432-7543
Fax: 202-337-8314
TTY: 202-337-5220
e-mail: agbell2@aol.com
www.agbell.org

This book gives encouragement and advice to parents on their essential roles in teaching speech to their child.

1991 182 pages

3771 Winnie-the-Pooh's ABCs

HEAR-MORE
42 Executive Boulevard
Farmingdale, NY 11735

800-881-4327
Fax: 631-752-0689
TTY: 800-281-4327
www.hearmore.com

In this special edition of Winnie-the-Pooh's ABC, both hearing and deaf children are introduced to the written and ASL alphabets, Hundred Acre Wood-Style. Inspired by A.A. Milne

32 pages

3772 Word Signs: A First Book of Sign Language

Debbie Slier, author

Gallaudet University Press
800 Florida Avenue NE
Washington, DC 20002

202-651-5488
Fax: 202-651-5489
e-mail: gupress@gallaudet.edu
http://gupress.gallaudet.edu

Charming, full-cover photographs of basic animals plus illustrations of their corresponding signs offer children ages 1 to 4 a fun way to learn their first signs and vocabulary words.

164 pages Board book
ISBN: 1-563680-48-3

3773 Written-Language Assessment and Intervention: Links To Literacy

Alexander Graham Bell Association for the Deaf
3417 Volta Place NW
Washington, DC 20007

202-337-5220
800-432-7543
Fax: 202-337-8314
TTY: 202-337-5220
e-mail: agbell2@aol.com
www.agbell.org

Assessment is an important part of a written-language program because it helps to identify students' strengths and weaknesses, determine instructional objectives, monitor students' progress, and provide feedback to students on their performance.

1996 215 pages

3774 You Make the Difference In Helping Your Child Learn

Alexander Graham Bell Association for the Deaf
3417 Volta Place NW
Washington, DC 20007

202-337-5220
800-432-7543
Fax: 202-337-8314
TTY: 202-337-5220
e-mail: agbell2@aol.com
www.agbell.org

This simple, attractive book will help parents and children connect in ways that foster children's self-esteem and language learning. Full of clear cartoons, these easily understood messages are uncomplicated and perfect for parents of all children, especially those whose language and social skills are delayed or at risk.

1995 90 pages paperback
ISBN: 0-921145-06-3

3775 You and Your Deaf Child

Gallaudet University Press
800 Florida Avenue NE
Washington, DC 20002

202-651-5488
Fax: 202-651-5489
TTY: 202-651-5489
e-mail: gupress@gallaudet.edu
http://gupress.gallaudet.edu

This guide for parents explores how families interact to deal with the special impact of a child who is hearing impaired.

1997 224 pages softcover
ISBN: 0-563680-60-2

3776 You and Your Deaf Child: A Self-Help Guide for Parents of Deaf and Hard of Hearing

John W Adams, author

Gallaudet University Press
800 Florida Avenue NE
Washington, DC 20002

202-651-5488
Fax: 202-651-5489
e-mail: gupress@gallaudet.edu
http://gupress.gallaudet.edu

A guide for parents of deaf or hard of hearing children that explores how parents and their children interact. It examines the special impact of having a deaf child in the family. Eleven chapters focus on such topics as feelings about hearing loss, the importance of communication in the family, and effective behavior management. Many chapters contain practice activities and check their grasp of the material.

224 pages Softcover
ISBN: 1-563680-60-2

3777 You and Your Hearing Impaired Child: A Self-Instructional Parents Guide

TJ Publishers
817 Silver Spring Avenue, Suite 206
Silver Spring, MD 20910

301-585-4440
800-999-1168
Fax: 301-585-5930
TTY: 301-585-4440
TDD: 301-585-4441
e-mail: TJPubinc@aol.com

Designed specifically for parents who have children newly diagnosed as hearing impaired. Provides vital information on hearing impairment, setting limits, behavior management, nonverbal behavior and much more.

1988 142 pages Softcover
ISBN: 0-930323-40-8

3778 Young Deaf Child

Alexander Graham Bell Association for the Deaf
3417 Volta Place NW
Washington, DC 20007

202-337-5220
Fax: 202-337-8314
TTY: 202-337-5221
e-mail: info@agbell.org
www.agbell.org

With a foreward by Mark Ross, Ph.D., this book is based on experience by the three authors and outlines the best approach for the child, early intervention, maximization of technology and strong family involvment.

1999 235 pages

David Luterman PhD, Author

Magazines

3779 Auditory - Verbal International

2121 Eisenhower Avenue, Suite 402
Alexandria, VA 22314

703-739-1049
Fax: 703-739-0395
TTY: 703-739-0874
e-mail: audiverb@aol.com

Magazine of the organization dedicated to helping children who have hearing losses learn to listen and speak. Promotes the Auditory-Verbal Therapy approach, which is based on the belief that the overwhelming majority of these children can hear and talk by using their residual hearing and hearing aids. Membership dues for

Canada are $55, International, $60, US, $50, and students are charged $30.

Quarterly

Sara Lake, Executive Director/CEO
Mary Benson, Executive Assistant

3780 Deaf American Monograph Series
National Association of the Deaf
814 Thayer Avenue
Silver Spring, MD 20910

301-587-1788
Fax: 301-587-1791
TTY: 301-587-1789
e-mail: nadinfo@nad.org
www.nad.org

Each monograph in the series contains more than 30 articles on a single theme. Past themes have included communication issues, perspectives on deafness, viewpoints on deafness, and deafness — the next twenty years.

Annual

Mervin D Garretson, Editor
Deborah L Jacobs

3781 Deaf Life
c/o MSM Productions, LTD
PO Box 23380
Rochester, NY 14692

716-442-6370
Fax: 716-442-6371
TTY: 716-442-6370
e-mail: deaflife@deaflife.com
www.deaflife.com

This magazine focuses on profiles, news, controversial issues, cultural topics and more relating to the deaf community, first published in 1988.

64 pages Monthly
ISSN: 0898-719x

Matthew Moore, Publisher

3782 Deaf USA
Eye Festival Communications
6917B Woodley Avenue
Van Nuys, CA 91406

Fax: 818-902-9840

Provides news coverage on all activities and issues of interest to deaf and hard-of-hearing readers as well as professionals and associates within this specialized market.

Monthly

David Rosenbaum, Editor

3783 Hearing Health
PO Box 2663
Corpus Christi, TX 78403

361-776-7240
Fax: 361-776-3278
www.hearinghealthmag.com

A publication for deaf and hard-of-hearing people, as well as hearing health care professionals, libraries, agencies, schools and organizations.

Bimonthly

Paula Bartone-Bonillas, Editor

3784 Perspectives in Education and Deafness
Gallaudet University Press
11030 S Langley Avenue
Chicago, IL 60628

202-651-5000
800-621-2736
Fax: 800-621-8476
TTY: 888-630-9347
www.gallaudet.edu/~gupress

A practical, reader-friendly magazine, offering help and advice in and beyond the classroom, tuned to the needs of today's students, teachers and families.

5 times a year

Mary Abrams Perica, Editor

3785 Volta Voices
Alexander Graham Bell Association for the Deaf
3417 Volta Place NW
Washington, DC 20007

202-337-5220
800-432-7543
Fax: 202-337-8314
TTY: 202-337-5220
e-mail: agbell2@aol.com
www.agbell.org

A magazine highlighting inspirational stories from parents of children who are deaf, legislative news, technology update, and stories pertaining to speech, speech-reading, and the use of residual hearing.

Bimonthly

Brooke Rigler, Editor

Journals

3786 American Annals of the Deaf
Convention of American Instructors of the Deaf
800 Florida Avenue NE, Fowler Hall 409
Washington, DC 20002

202-651-5340
Fax: 202-651-5708
www.gallaudet.edu:80/~penmpaad/index.htm

Scholarly journal at the forefront of research related to the education of deaf people. Annual reference Issue identifies programs and services for deaf people nationwide.

5 times a year

Donald F Moores, Editor
Mary Ellen Carew, Managing Editor

3787 Journal of Speech, Language, and Hearing R esearch
American Speech Language Hearing Association
10801 Rockville Pike
Rockville, MD 20852

301-897-5700
888-498-6699
e-mail: subscriptions@asha.org
www.asha.org

Basic and applied research in communication processes, both normal and disordered.

Bi-monthly

Katherine Verdolini, Editor, Speech
Alan G Kamhi, Editor, Language

3788 Language, Speech, and Hearing in Schools
American Speech Language Hearing Association
10801 Rockville Pike
Rockville, MD 20852

301-897-5700
888-498-6699
e-mail: subscriptions@asha.org
www.asha.org

Focuses on research for speech-language pathologists and audiologists in the school setting.

Quarterly

Brian Goldstein, Editor

3789 SHHH Journal
Self Help for Hard-of-Hearing People
7910 Woodmont Avenue, Suite 1200
Bethesda, MD 20814

301-657-2248
Fax: 301-913-9413
TTY: 301-657-2249

An educational journal about hearing loss for hard-of-hearing people.

Bimonthly

Barbara G Harris, Editor

Newsletters

3790 Endeavor
American Society for Deaf Children
PO Box 3355
Gettysburg, PA 17325

717-334-7922
800-942-2732
Fax: 717-334-8808

Newsletter for parents of deaf children.

Quarterly

Barbara Aschembrenner, Editor

3791 Gallaudet Today
Gallaudet University Press
11030 S Langley Avenue
Chicago, IL 60628

202-651-5000
800-621-2736
Fax: 800-621-8476
TTY: 888-630-9347
www.gallaudet.edu/~gupress

A university alumni publication with both general and special issues on deafness-related topics.

44 pages Quarterly

Roz Prickett, Publications Manager

3792 Hear
Deafness Research Foundation
15 W 39th Street
New York, NY 10018

212-768-1181

Offers information on the Foundation's activities and events, technical updates on assistive devices, legislative and medical information on the latest breakthroughs and laws for the hearing impaired, book reviews and resources.

Monte H Jacoby, Executive Director

3793 National Association of the Deaf
814 Thayer Avenue, Suite 250
Silver Spring, MD 20910

301-587-1788
Fax: 301-587-1791
TTY: 301-587-1789
e-mail: nadinfo@nad.org
www.nad.org

Information on the nation's largest constituency organization safeguarding the accessibility and civil rights of 28 million deaf and hard of hearing Americans in education, employment, health care and telecommunications. Focus on advocacy, captioned media, deafness-related information/publications, legal assistance and more.

32-40 pages 11 times a year

Deborah L Jacobs

3794 Newsletter of American Hearing Research
American Hearing Research Foundation
55 E Washington Street, 2022
Chicago, IL 60602

312-726-9670

Concerned with hearing research and education.

William Lederer, Editor

3795 Newsline
Sertoma Foundation
1912 E Meyer Boulevard
Kansas City, MO 64132

816-333-8300

Reports on activities of the Sertoma Foundation in the field of speech and hearing impairments.

3796 Signs for Me: Basic Sign Vocabulary for Children, Parents, & Teachers
TJ Publishers
817 Silver Spring Avenue, Suite 206
Silver Spring, MD 20910

301-585-4440
800-999-1168
Fax: 301-585-5930
TTY: 301-585-4440
TDD: 301-585-4441
e-mail: TJPubinc@aol.com

Sign language vocabulary for preschool and elementary school children introduces household items, animals, family members, actions, emotions, safety concerns and other concepts.

112 pages Softcover

3797 Speech and Deafness Newsletter
Hearing, Speech
1620 18th Avenue
Seattle, WA 98122

206-323-5770

Agency newsletter for membership and community.

8 pages

Patty Tumberg, Editor

3798 Volta Review
Alexander Graham Bell Association for the Deaf
3417 Volta Place NW
Washington, DC 20007

202-337-5220
800-432-7543
Fax: 202-337-8314
TTY: 202-337-5220
e-mail: agbell2@aol.com
www.agbell.org

Offers the latest theory, research, current perspectives and practical guidance from noted specialists in education, audiology, speech and language sciences and psychology. Each issue contains a Special Focus-a group of chapters exploring a specific topic in detail.

Quarterly

Pamphlets

3799 25 Ways to Promote Spoken Language in Your Child with a Hearing Loss

Alexander Graham Bell Association for the Deaf
3417 Volta Place NW
Washington, DC 20007

202-337-5220
800-432-7543
Fax: 202-337-8314
TTY: 202-337-5220
e-mail: agbell2@aol.com
www.agbell.org

This pamphlet teaches twenty-five golden rules about preparing your child to listen and to speak.

1995 62 pages

3800 Between Two Worlds of Hearing and Not Hearing

Self Help for Hard-of-Hearing People
7910 Woodmont Avenue, Suite 1200
Bethesda, MD 20814

301-657-2248
Fax: 301-913-9413
TTY: 301-657-2249
e-mail: national@shhh.org
www.shhh.org

3801 Books for Parents of Deaf and Hard-of- Hearing Children

National Information Center on Deafness
800 Florida Avenue NE
Washington, DC 20002

202-651-5051
Fax: 202-651-5054
TTY: 202-651-5052

Identifies books written for parents and everday experiences of deaf and hard-of-hearing children.

3802 Can Your Baby Hear?

Alexander Graham Bell Association for the Deaf
3417 Volta Place NW
Washington, DC 20007

202-337-5220
800-432-7543
Fax: 202-337-8314
TTY: 202-337-5220
e-mail: agbell2@aol.com
www.agbell.org

This simple card for parents lists risk indicators and warning signs of hearing loss in babies.

3803 Care of the Ears and Hearing for Health

American Hearing Research Foundation
55 E Washington Street
Chicago, IL 60602

312-726-9670

Offers information on ear infections relating to chronic progressive deafness.

3804 Child's Perspective

Self Help for Hard-of-Hearing People
7910 Woodmont Avenue, Suite 1200
Bethesda, MD 20814

301-657-2248
Fax: 301-913-9413
TTY: 301-657-2249
e-mail: national@shhh.org
www.shhh.org

3805 Commonly-Asked Questions About Children with Minimal Hearing Loss in the Class

Self Help for Hard-of-Hearing People
7910 Woodmont Avenue, Suite 1200
Bethesda, MD 20814

301-657-2248
Fax: 301-913-9413
TTY: 301-657-2249
e-mail: national@shhh.org
www.shhh.org

3806 Communicating with People who Have a Hearing Loss

Alexander Graham Bell Association for the Deaf
3417 Volta Place NW
Washington, DC 20007

202-337-5220
800-432-7543
Fax: 202-337-8314
TTY: 202-337-5220
e-mail: agbell2@aol.com
www.agbell.org

This brochure describes ways to communicate more effectively with people who have hearing losses.

1994

3807 Deafness: A Fact Sheet

National Information Center On Deafness
800 Florida Avenue NE
Washington, DC 20002

202-651-5051
Fax: 202-651-5054
TTY: 202-651-5052

3808 Developing Cognition in Young Children Who are Deaf

Hope
55 E 100 N
Logan, UT 84321

435-752-9533
Fax: 435-752-9533

Presents interesting, updated information on the importance of early cognition development in young children who are deaf. Contains many ideas for ways to promote early thinking skills, especially those that promote and enhance early communication and language development.

3809 Educating Deaf Children: An Introduction

National Information Center on Deafness
800 Florida Avenue NE
Washington, DC 20002

202-651-5051
Fax: 202-651-5054
TTY: 202-651-5052

Describes the different settings in which deaf children are currently educated.

3810 Educational Perspective

Self Help for Hard-of-Hearing People
7910 Woodmont Avenue, Suite 1200
Bethesda, MD 20814

301-657-2248
Fax: 301-913-9413
TTY: 301-657-2249
e-mail: national@shhh.org
www.shhh.org

3811 Getting Beyond Hearing Loss: A Guide for Families

Self Help for Hard-of-Hearing People
7910 Woodmont Avenue, Suite 1200
Bethesda, MD 20814

301-657-2248
Fax: 301-913-9413
TTY: 301-657-2249
e-mail: national@shhh.org
www.shhh.org

3812 Hearing Alert Informational Brochures
Alexander Graham Bell Association for the Deaf
3417 Volta Place NW
Washington, DC 20007

202-337-5220
800-432-7543
Fax: 202-337-8314
TTY: 202-337-5220
e-mail: agbell2@aol.com
www.agbell.org

These brochures encourage early detection of hearing loss in young children; for medical facilities, speech and hearing clinics, and schools.

3813 Helping Your Hard-of-Hearing Child Succeed
Alexander Graham Bell Association for the Deaf
3417 Volta Place NW
Washington, DC 20007

202-337-5220
800-432-7543
Fax: 202-337-8314
TTY: 202-337-5220
e-mail: agbell2@aol.com
www.agbell.org

Offers information on how to help children succeed in school with speech and language development.

3814 How Does Your Child Hear and Talk?
American Speech Language Hearing Association
10801 Rockville Pike
Rockville, MD 20852

301-897-5700
800-638-8255
Fax: 301-571-0457
www.asha.org

Offers a chart to parents on children's growth pertaining to their hearing and speech.

3815 Leading National Publications of and for Deaf People
National Information Center On Deafness
800 Florida Avenue NE
Washington, DC 20002

202-651-5051
Fax: 202-651-5054
TTY: 202-651-5052

Identifies publications with national circulations to deaf audiences.

3816 Listen - Hear for Parents of Hearing Impaired Children
Alexander Graham Bell Association for the Deaf
3417 Volta Place NW
Washington, DC 20007

202-337-5220
800-432-7543
Fax: 202-337-8314
TTY: 202-337-5220
e-mail: agbell2@aol.com
www.agbell.org

Offers information that parents of deaf and hard-of-hearing children need to be aware of. Also includes information on hearing aids, hearing loss and the association in general.

3817 National Information Center on Deafness Brochure
National Information Center on Deafness
800 Florida Avenue NE
Washington, DC 20002

202-651-5051
Fax: 202-651-5054
TTY: 202-651-5052

A description of services offered by NICD.

3818 Parent Packets
Alexander Graham Bell Association for the Deaf
3417 Volta Place NW
Washington, DC 20007

202-337-5220
800-432-7543
Fax: 202-337-8314
TTY: 202-337-5220
e-mail: agbell2@aol.com
www.agbell.org

These educational packets for parents are specifically designed to address important age-related topics about your child with a hearing impairment.

Packet

3819 Parents' Perspective
Self Help for Hard-of-Hearing People
7910 Woodmont Avenue, Suite 1200
Bethesda, MD 20814

301-657-2248
Fax: 301-913-9413
TTY: 301-657-2249
e-mail: national@shhh.org
www.shhh.org

3820 Personal Quest for Educational Excellence for a Hard of Hearing Child
Self Help for Hard-of-Hearing People
7910 Woodmont Avenue, Suite 1200
Bethesda, MD 20814

301-657-2248
Fax: 301-913-9413
TTY: 301-657-2249
e-mail: national@shhh.org
www.shhh.org

3821 Perspectives Folio: Parent-Child
Gallaudet University Press
11030 S Langley Avenue
Chicago, IL 60628

202-651-5000
800-621-2736
Fax: 800-621-8476
TTY: 888-630-9347
www.gallaudet.edu/~gupress

Seven articles emphasizing family communication while providing important information for parents about deafness and the deaf culture.

29 pages

3822 Publications From the National Information Center on Deafness
National Information Center on Deafness
800 Florida Avenue NE
Washington, DC 20002

202-651-5051
Fax: 202-651-5054
TTY: 202-651-5052

Order form and explanations of NICD publications.

3823 Questions and Answers on Hearing Loss
Self Help for Hard-of-Hearing People
7910 Woodmont Avenue, Suite 1200
Bethesda, MD 20814

301-657-2248
Fax: 301-913-9413
TTY: 301-657-2249
e-mail: national@shhh.org
www.shhh.org

3824 Signs for Me: Basic Sign Vocabulary for Children, Parents, & Teachers
DawnSignPress
6130 Nancy Ridge Drive
San Diego, CA 92121

858-625-0600
800-549-5350
Fax: 858-625-2336
e-mail: info@dawnsign.com
www.dawnsign.com

ASL/English vocabulary primer. Young readers will associate a sign and picture with the English form of a word. Introduces more than 300 primary words arranged in thematic groupings. Captures students' interest through clearly illustrated signs and actions; includes an illustrated look at the English word for effective bilingual learning.

128 pages paperback
ISBN: 0-915035-27-8

Ben Bahan, Co-Author
Joe Dannis, Co-Author

3825 Situation is Serious But Not Hopeless: The Psychological Benefits of Hearing Loss
Self Help for Hard-of-Hearing People
7910 Woodmont Avenue, Suite 1200
Bethesda, MD 20814

301-657-2248
Fax: 301-913-9413
TTY: 301-657-2249
e-mail: national@shhh.org
www.shhh.org

3826 So You Have Had An Ear Operation...What Next?
American Hearing Research Foundation
55 E Washington Street
Chicago, IL 60602

312-726-9670

Offers information on ear infections and surgery.

3827 Speechreading: Methods and Materials
Self Help for Hard-of-Hearing People
7910 Woodmont Avenue, Suite 1200
Bethesda, MD 20814

301-657-2248
Fax: 301-913-9413
TTY: 301-657-2249
e-mail: national@shhh.org
www.shhh.org

3828 Statewide Services for Deaf and Hard of Hearing People
National Information Center on Deafness
800 Florida Avenue NE
Washington, DC 20002

202-651-5051
Fax: 202-651-5054
TTY: 202-651-5052

A resource list of states that have established commissions and other offices to serve deaf people.

3829 World of Sound
International Hearing Society
16880 Middlebelt Road, Suite 4
Livonia, MI 48154

734-522-7200
Fax: 734-522-0200
www.hearingihs.org

The purpose of this booklet is to provide basic information for those with questions about hearing loss, hearing aids and hearing instrument specialists.

Camps

3830 Central Michigan University Summer Clinics
444 Moore
Mount Pleasant, MI

517-774-3803

Designed for children, ages 6 and up, with speech, language and hearing disorders who can benefit from intensive clinical work. A wide range of recreational and social activities form part of the clinical program and promote the social use of skills learned in class.

3831 Children's Beach House
100 W 10th Street
Wilmington, DE

302-655-4288
Fax: 302-655-4216
e-mail: childrens.beach.house@dol.net
www.cbhinc.org

Summer camp for children from Delaware of normal mental level, with speech, language and hearing disorders are accepted, ages 6-13. Activities include aquatics, art, music, nature and dramatics. Speech and language therapy are provided. Also school-year environmental education for Delaware students of all exceptionalities.

Diane B O'Hara, Summer Program Director

3832 Emanuel-Day
Emanuel-Day and Resident
331 Marlay Road
Dayton, OH

Camp for hearing impaired and normal hearing youth.

Nan Crawford, Camp Director

3833 Florida School-Deaf and Blind
207 San Marco Avenue
Saint Augustine, FL 32084

800-800-344
www2.kidscamps.com

3834 Isola Bella
American School for the Deaf
139 N Main Street
W Hartford, CT

860-527-2681

Hearing-impaired children, ages 6-19, blend educational instruction in communications with recreational activities. Qualified deaf and hearing staff members with experience in education, child care and counseling are employed at the camp. Tuition: $165-178 week.

3835 Junior National Association of the Deaf & Youth Leadership Camp
National Association of the Deaf
814 Thayer Avenue
Silver Spring, MD 20910

301-587-1788
Fax: 301-587-1791
TTY: 301-587-1789
e-mail: nadinfo@nad.org
www.nad.org

Deborah L Jacobs

3836 Lions Camp for the Deaf
7202 Buchanan Street
Landover Hills, MD

301-577-8057

This recreational camp for deaf children offers a complete waterfront program including swimming, canoeing and fishing, for ages 6-14.

Rev. Edward Helm, Executive Director

3837 Meadowood Springs Speech and Hearing Camp
PO Box 1025
Pendleton, OR

541-276-2752
Fax: 541-276-7227
e-mail: meadowoodcamp@uci.ne
www.meadowoodsprings.org

On 143 acres in the Blue Mountains of Eastern Oregon, this camp is designed to help young people who have diagnosed clinical disorders of speech, hearing or language. A full range of activities in recreational and clinical areas is available. For cabin reservations 541-566-2191.

Rosemarie Atfield, Executive Director
Marie Story, Camp Manager

3838 Program for Children and Youth Who are Deaf or Hard of Hearing
One Commerce Plaza
Albany, NY

518-474-5652
e-mail: dsteele@mail.nysed.gov
www.nysed.gov

Dirothy Steel, Coordinator Deaf Services

3839 University of Iowa - Wendell Johnson Speech and Hearing Clinic
Wendell Johnson Speech And Hearing Center
Iowa City, IA 52242

319-335-1845
Fax: 319-335-8851

The clinic offers assessment and remediation for disordered communication in adults and children. The clinic also offers an Intensive Summer Residential Clinic for school age children needing intervention services because of speech, language, hearing and/or reading problems.

Richard Hurtig, Professor/Chair
Ann L Michael, Clinic Director

3840 Youth Leadership Camp
National Association of the Deaf
814 Thayer Avenue
Silver Spring, MD

301-587-5940

Sponsored by the National Association of the Deaf, this camp emphasizes leadership training for deaf teenagers and young adults. In addition to many recreational activities and sports, there are academic offerings and camp projects.

DESCRIPTION

3841 HEMANGIOMAS AND LYMPHANGIOMAS

Covers these related disorders: Capillary hemangiomas, Cavernous hemangiomas, Cystic hygromas, Disseminated hemangiomatosis, Mixed hemangiomas, Port-wine stains (or salmon patches), Kasabach-merritt syndrome

Involves the following Biologic System(s):

Dermatologic Disorders

Hemangiomas are the most common benign tumors in infants. In addition, during childhood, lymphangiomas, also known as lymphatic malformations, are the second most common benign tumor affecting vessels of the body. Hemangiomas consist of an abnormal distribution of relatively small blood vessels (e.g., capillaries) due to malformation of developing fetal tissue from which the vessels arise. Lymphangiomas consist of masses of abnormally enlarged (dilated), newly formed lymph vessels, which are the channels that transport lymphatic fluid throughout the body. Lymph, a thin bodily fluid that consists of proteins, fats, and certain white blood cells (lymphocytes), accumulates in spaces between tissue cells and flows back into the bloodstream via lymph vessels.

Hemangiomas usually affect blood vessels of the skin (cutaneous hemangiomas). They most commonly develop in the head and neck regions and are rarely fully formed at birth. These tumors, which occur more frequently in females than males, are usually single growths that occur randomly for unknown reasons. However, some multigenerational families (kindreds) have been reported in which several individuals developed isolated hemangiomas. In such cases, the condition may be transmitted as an autosomal dominant trait. In addition, in rare cases, certain forms of hemangiomas may occur in association with particular underlying syndromes.

Cutaneous hemangiomas may be superficial (capillary hemangiomas), deep (cavernous hemangiomas), or both (mixed hemangiomas). Capillary hemangiomas are considered the most common type of hemangioma, affecting approximately 60 percent of patients. These hemangiomas include port-wine stains (a form of nevus flammeus) and strawberry hemangiomas (strawberry nevi). Port-wine stains are present at birth (congenital) and are typically permanent defects. These lesions consist of mature, abnormally widened capillaries; are flat (macular) with sharply defined borders; and are usually reddish purple in color. They may vary greatly in size and typically develop on the head, face, and neck areas. As patients reach adulthood, port-wine stains may darken and form elevated (papular) areas that may occasionally bleed. Port-wine stains must be differentiated from salmon patches, which are flat, salmon-colored lesions that are typically present during infancy on certain facial areas, such as over the eyelids, on the middle of the forehead, or between the eyes. Salmon patches typically fade completely over time. Port-wine stains may be an isolated condition or may occur in association with several rare underlying syndromes (e.g., Klippel-Trenaunay-Weber syndrome, Sturge-Weber syndrome, etc.). Treatment may include a variety of measures, such as laser therapy, destruction of affected tissue through the use of extreme cold (cryosurgery), surgical removal (excision), transplantation of skin tissues (grafting), or masking with cosmetics.

Strawberry hemangiomas are dull or bright red and elevated, have clearly defined borders, and consist of immature capillaries. The lesions, which may develop as single or multiple growths, may affect any area of the body; however, they are most common on the scalp, face, chest, or back. Strawberry hemangiomas usually appear within approximately two months after birth. In most patients, the hemangiomas initially grow rapidly, cease such growth (stationary phase), and then gradually begin to regress in size (involution). After the lesions have reduced in size, approximately 10 percent of patients have residual discoloration or puckering of affected skin. In rare cases, complications associated with strawberry hemangiomas may include infection; destruction of the skin's surface, resulting in open sores and inflammation (ulceration); bleeding (hemorrhaging); or extensive growth that interferes with necessary functions, such as breathing difficulties due to tumor growth affecting the airways. Because most strawberry hemangiomas spontaneously regress, treatment typically consists of careful, ongoing observation. However, if hemangiomas rapidly grow, potentially causing tissue destruction, removal, using elastic bandages or other measures, may be recommended in selected patients. If there is rapid growth that may ultimately cause life-threatening complications, treatment may include the administration of corticosteroids by injection or| mouth or therapy with an artificial (synthetic) form of interferon (interferon alpha-2a). Interferons are natural proteins that are produced by the body's immune system in response to certain invading viruses or other stimuli. In the most severe cases, radiation therapy may be necessary. Other treatment is symptomatic and supportive.

Cavernous hemangiomas may be firm or form cysts. The

skin overlying such hemangiomas is often bluish in color. However, if physicians suspect that underlying structures may be affected, specialized imaging techniques, such as CT scanning or ultrasonography, are conducted to detect and characterize such involvement. Rarely, some patients develop multiple hemangiomas. In such cases, affected children may have numerous small, red or purplish, raised hemangiomas on the skin. In addition, internal hemangiomas may be present involving certain organs, particularly the liver, lungs, brain and spinal cord, and organs of the gastrointestinal tract. In such cases, affected children are said to have disseminated hemangiomatosis.

Life-threatening complications may potentially arise due to hemorrhage, tissue compression (e.g., neural tissue compression), obstruction of the airways, or an inability of the heart to effectively pump blood to the lungs and throughout the body (heart failure). In some cases, multiple internal and cutaneous hemangiomas occur in association with certain rare, underlying syndromes (e.g., macrocephaly with pseudopapilledema).

Lymphangiomas may be localized or widely distributed growths that, in some cases, may have hemangioma-like components. In almost all affected children, lymphangiomas are apparent by approximately age three. Lymphangiomas most commonly develop in the neck and facial regions, in the chest area (thorax), or under the arms (axillae). For example, some affected children may have an abnormal cystic growth consisting of dilated lymph vessels beneath the skin in the neck area (cystic hygroma). Lymphangiomas, such as cystic hygroma, may occur as isolated findings or in association with certain underlying syndromes (e.g., Noonan syndrome). Unlike hemangiomas, lymphangiomas rarely spontaneously regress. In some patients, they may expand in size and may obstruct the gastrointestinal tract or the airways, potentially causing life-threatening complications without appropriate treatment. Because most lymphangiomas are relatively widely distributed (diffuse), treatment often includes removal of the growths in several stages (staged surgical resection). Additional treatment includes symptomatic and supportive measures.

See also **General Resources** on page 917

Government Agencies

3842 NIH/National Institute of Arthritis and Mu sculoskeletal and Skin Diseases
1AMS Circle
Bethesda, MD 20892

301-402-4484
Fax: 301-718-6366
e-mail: ord@od.nih.gov
rarediseases.info.nih.gov

The mission of the National Institute of Arthritis and Musculoskeletal and Skin Diseases is to support research into the causes, treatment, and prevention of arthritis and musculoskeletal and skin diseases, the training of basic and clinical scientists to carry out this research, and the dissemination of information on research progress in these diseases.

Stephen I Katz MD PhD, Director

National Associations & Support Groups

3843 American Academy of Dermatology (AAD)
PO Box 4014
Schaumburg, IL 60618

847-240-1280
866-503-7546
Fax: 847-240-1859
e-mail: MRC@aad.org
www.aad.org

To promote and advance the art of medicine and surgery of the skin; promote the highest possible standards in clinical practice , education and research in dermatology and related disciplines.

Stephen P Stone MD, President
William P Coleman III, MD, VP

3844 American Skin Association
346 Park Avenue S, 4th Floor
New York, NY 10010

212-889-4858
800-499-7546
Fax: 212-889-4959
e-mail: AmericanSkin@compuserve.com
www.americanskin.org

The American Skin Association is the only volunteer led health organization dedicated through research, education and advocacy to saving lives and alleviating human suffering caused by the full spectrum of skin disorders.

Howard P Milstein, Chairman
George W Hambrick, Jr, President/Founder

3845 Hemangioma Support System
C/O Cynthia Schumerth
1484 Sand Acres Drive
Depere, WI 54115

920-336-9399

Provides parent-to-parent support for families with children affected by hemangiomas.

1990

3846 National Congenital Port Wine Stain Foundation
123 E 63rd Street
New York, NY 10021

516-867-5137
Fax: 516-869-1278

3847 Society for Pediatric Dermatology
8365 Keystone Crossing, Suite 107
Indianapolis, IN 46240

317-202-0224
Fax: 317-205-9841
e-mail: spd@hp-assoc.com
www.pedsderm.net

National organization dedicated to promote, develop and advance education, research and care of skin disease in all pediatric age groups.

Kent Lindeman, Executive Director

3848 Vascular Birthmarks Foundation
PO Box 106
Latham, NY 12110

518-782-9637
877-823-4646
e-mail: HVBF@aol.com
www.birthmark.org

A not for profit organization that provides support and informational resources for individuals affected by hemangiomas, port wine stains, and other vascular birthmarks and tumors.

Linda Rozell Shannon, Founder
Dr. Milton Waner, MD, Medical Chairman

Libraries & Resource Centers

3849 Children's Center for Cancer and Blood Disorders
University of South Carolina School of Medicine
5 Richland Memorial Park
Columbia, SC 29203

803-777-7000

Joint clinical and basic research of juvenile cancer and blood disorders.

Dr. Robert S Ettinger, Director

Web Sites

3850 Vascular Anomalies Center
www.hemangioma.org/

Provide the most up-to-date information to parents and patients as well as give the resources to help understand vascular anomaly.

Book Publishers

3851 Sturge-Weber Syndrome: A Resource Guide for a Reason, a Season and a Lifetime
Sturge-Weber Foundation
PO Box 418
Mt. Freedom, NJ 07970

973-895-4445
800-627-5482
Fax: 973-895-4846
e-mail: swf@sturge-weber.com
www.sturge-weber.com

Covers most of the issues and concerns of parents and individuals with SWS, PWS and KT in short essays and chapters that provide practical and helpful advice

95 pages Paperback
ISBN: 0-967048-40-0

Carol Buck, Patient/Family Services Director
Lauris Partizian, Information Services Manager

DESCRIPTION

3852 HEMOLYTIC DISEASE OF THE NEWBORN

Synonyms: Erythroblastosis fetalis, Erythroblastosis neonatorum

Involves the following Biologic System(s):

Hematologic and Oncologic Disorders, Neonatal and Infant Disorders

Hemolytic disease of the newborn, also known as erythroblastosis neonatorum or erythroblastosis fetalis, is characterized by destruction of a newborn's red blood cells by antibodies that crossed the placenta from the mother's bloodstream during pregnancy. Antibodies are produced by certain white blood cells in response to foreign proteins (antigens) that are present in some cells and invading microorganisms. In hemolytic disease of the newborn the mother's immune system treats the baby's blood cells as foreign and makes antibodies against them. In most cases, the condition occurs when a developing fetus has Rh-positive blood (i.e., inherited from the father), but the mother has Rh-negative blood.

In approximately 85 percent of individuals, red blood cells contain an antigen called the Rh factor. Those with this antigen are said to have Rh-positive blood, whereas those without the antigen have Rh-negative blood. The blood plasma does not naturally contain antibodies to inactivate or destroy the Rh antigen (anti-Rh antibodies). However, if a fetus has Rh-positive blood and the mother is Rh negative, the presence of the Rh factor in the fetus' red blood cells causes the mother's body to produce anti-Rh antibodies. If the woman becomes pregnant again and the developing fetus has Rh-positive blood, the mother's antibodies may react with the fetus' Rh-positive cells, resulting in hemolysis (breakdown of red blood cells). In many cases, mothers who are known to have Rh-negative blood may be treated with a protein to help prevent them from producing anti-Rh antibodies (e.g., injection of human anti-D globulin), thereby lowering the risk of erythroblastosis fetalis during future pregnancies.

In infants affected by hemolytic disease of the newborn, associated symptoms and findings may vary. These may range from a mild breakdown of red blood cells to severely low levels of circulating red blood cells (anemia); paleness of the skin (pallor); tiny reddish, purplish spots on the skin (petechiae) due to abnormal bleeding under the skin's surface; enlargement of the liver and spleen (hepatosplenomegaly); or development of abnormal yellowish coloring of the mucous membranes, whites of the eyes, and skin (jaundice). In extremely severe cases, affected newborns may experience low levels of oxygen supply (hypoxia), difficulty breathing (respiratory distress), heart (cardiac) failure, severe abnormal accumulations of fluid in body tissues and cavities (hydrops), and potentially life-threatening complications. Depending upon the severity of the condition, treatment may include transfusions (e.g., partial or full exchange transfusions with Rh-negative blood) and supportive measures, such as ventilation assistance.

Hemolytic disease of the newborn may also result due to other blood type incompatibilities, primarily if the mother is type O and the developing fetus is type A or B. However, the condition develops in only about 10 percent of such cases of ABO incompatibility. In addition, the condition is typically less severe than that associated with Rh incompatibility. In cases of ABO blood type incompatibility, the development of jaundice approximately a day after birth may be the only associated symptom.

See also **General Resources** on page 917

Government Agencies

3853 NIH/National Heart, Lung and Blood Institute
National Institute of Health
31 Center Dr MSC 2486, Bldg 31, Room 5A48
Bethesda, MD 20892

301-592-8573
Fax: 240-629-3246
TTY: 240-629-3255
e-mail: NHLBIinfo@nhlbi.nih.gov
www.nhlbi.nih.gov

Primary responsibility of this organization is the scientific investigation of heart, blood vessel, lung and blood disorders. Oversees research, demonstration, prevention, education, control and training activities in these fields and emphasizes the prevention and control of heart diseases.

Elizabeth G Nabel, MD, Director
Susan Shurin, MD, Deputy Director

3854 NIH/National Institute of Child Health and Human Development
31 Center Drive, Building 31
Bethesda, MD 20892

301-496-5133
Fax: 301-496-1104
www.nichd.nih.gov

Established in 1962 by congress, today the institute conducts and supports research on topics related to the health of children, adults, families and populations. Some of these topics include: developmental disabilities, growth and development, infant death, reproductive health and birth defects.

Nancy D Wirth, Director
Lisa Kaeser, Program & Public Liaison

National Associations & Support Groups

3855 American Autoimmune Related Diseases Association
22100 Gratiot Avenue
E Detroit, MI 48021

586-776-3900
www.aarda.org

Dedicated to the eradication of autoimmune diseases and the alleviation of suffering and the socio-economic impact of autoimmunity through fostering and facilitating collaboration in the areas of education, public awareness, research and patient services in an effective, ethical and efficient manner.

Virginia Ladd, Director

Web Sites

3856 NIH/National Institutes of Health/Office o f Rare Diseases
rarediseases.info.nih.gov/

Provides information about ORD-sponsored scientific activites, and ORD cosponsored genetic and rare disease information center, and a portal to databases that provide information on major topics of interest in rare disease research.

3857 Online Mendelian Inheritance in Man
www.ncbi.nlm.nih.gov

This database is a catalog of human genes and genetic disorders.

DESCRIPTION

3858 HEMOPHILIA

Synonyms: AHF, Antihemophilic factor deficiency, Classic hemophilia, Factor VIII deficiency, Hemophilia A
Covers these related disorders: Hemophilia A, Hemophilia B (Christmas disease; Factor IX deficiency), Von Willebrand's disease (Factor VIIIR deficiency)
Involves the following Biologic System(s):
Hematologic and Oncologic Disorders

The term hemophilia refers to a group of bleeding disorders including hemophilia A, hemophilia B, and von Willebrand's disease. Each of these diseases is characterized by the deficiency of a specific blood-clotting protein (factor). Hemophilia A, the most common form of the disease, affects approximately 80 percent of people with hemophilia and is caused by a deficiency of factor VIII. Hemophilia B, accounting for approximately 12 to 15 percent of all cases, results from a deficiency in clotting factor IX. In both forms of hemophilia, the severity of the disease and associated symptoms depend upon the level of coagulating activity of the individual clotting factors; the lower the activity of these factors, the more severe the disease. The most common symptoms, usually appearing at about 18 months when the child becomes more physically active, include easy bruising and bleeding into the joints (hemarthrosis) and muscles. Pain and swelling in the ankles, knees, and elbows may follow and eventually lead to degenerative changes and limited range of motion. Bleeding episodes may occur after injury, trauma, minor surgery, and, in some cases, for no apparent reason (spontaneously). Von Willebrand's disease involves a deficiency of factor VIIIR and is characterized by easy bruising, nose bleeds and bleeding into the gastrointestinal tract. In affected females, excessive uterine bleeding may occur during menstruation or childbirth. In some patients, blood may be present in the urine (hematuria). Unlike hemophilia A or B, bleeding into the joints is rare and the disorder seems to improve with advancing age.

Treatment of hemophilia A and B includes transfusions of appropriate clotting factor when a bleeding episode occurs. These concentrates may also be regularly self-administered to prevent bleeds. Other preventive measures may include the administration of certain clot-aiding drugs before surgery, the avoidance of certain drugs that may exacerbate bleeding problems, and avoidance of participation in contact sports or other similar activities that could provoke a bleeding episode. The treatment of von Willebrand's disease may include the infusion of DDAVP or VW protein prior to surgery or childbirth.

Hemophilia A and hemophilia B are transmitted as x-linked recessive traits and affect males almost exclusively. Approximately 10 males out of every 100,000 are born with hemophilia A, while the rate of occurrence of hemophilia B is about two males out of every 100,000. For the most part, von Willebrand's disease is inherited as an autosomal dominant disorder. In rare instances, the disease may be inherited as a recessive gene. Children with hemophilia who may have received transfusions of blood or blood products before HIV blood-screening became standard in 1985 may have unwittingly become infected by receiving contaminated blood.

See also **General Resources** on page 917

See also **General Resources** on page 917

National Associations & Support Groups

3859 American Red Cross Blood Services
4333 Arlington Boulevard
Arlington, VA 22203

703-527-3010
Fax: 703-527-2705
e-mail: LKeefe@arlingtonredcross.org
www.arlingtonredcross.org

Distributes a wide variety of plasma therapeutics to benefit people with hemophilia A and B, immune disorders and hypoalbuminemia.

Sandra L Mertz, Product Manager

3860 Baxter Healthcare Hyland Division
550 N Brand Boulevard
Glendale, CA 91203

818-956-3200
Fax: 818-507-5596
www.baxter.com/

Government affairs office that monitors and selectively lobbies on issues relating to Medicare, Medicaid, orphan drugs and other subjects relating to hemophilia.

Pam Koo, Programs Manager

3861 Children's Blood Foundation
333 E 38th Street, Suite 830
New York, NY 10016

212-297-4336
Fax: 212-297-4340
e-mail: info@childrensblooddoundation.org
www.childrensbloodfoundation.org

The foundation's major emphasis is on blood diseases affecting children: leukemia, thalassemia, hemophilia, sickle cell anemia, platelet disorders, retinoblastoma and AIDS.

John Calicchio, Chairman

3862 Hemophilia Health Services
6820 Charlotte Pike
Nashville, TN 37209

615-352-2500
800-800-6606
Fax: 615-352-2588
e-mail: info@HemophiliaHealth.com
www.hemophiliahealth.com

Specializes in providing pharmaceuticals, therapeutic supplies and disease management services for people with hemophilia and related bleeding disorders.

Kyle J Callahan, President

3863 National Hemophilia Foundation
116 W 23rd Street, 11th Floor
New York, NY 10001

212-328-3700
800-424-2634
Fax: 212-328-3777
e-mail: handi@hemophilia.org
www.hemophilia.org

Offers various information, articles, resources, books and more for the hemophilia and HIV/AIDS community.

Howard Balsam, CPA, COO
Marie Cramer, Human Resources Director

State Agencies & Support Groups

3864 Missouri Gateway Hemophilia Association
462 N Taylor Avenue, Suite 101
St. Louis, MO 63180

314-531-8300
877-623-8300
Fax: 314-531-8301
e-mail: hemophilia@sbcglobal.net
www.gatewayhemophilia.org

A nonprofit community based organization dedicated to the support of families affected by hemophilia and other cogenital blood coagulation disorders.

Danielle R Burton, Administrator
Dirk Stueber, President

Alabama

3865 Alabama Chapter of the National Hemophilia Foundation
802 Midland Avenue
Muscle Shoals, AL 35661

205-381-5925
Fax: 205-943-8360

Arkansas

3866 Hemophilia Center of Arkansas
Arkansas Children's Hospital
800 Marshall Street
Little Rock, AR 72202

501-364-1100
TDD: 501-364-1184
www.archildrens.org

Patients with coagulation disorders can be diagnosed and evaluated by a group of physicians, physical therapists, dentists, psychologists and geneticists to provide education, prevention and continuity of care. The Hemophilia Center of Arkansas offers the latest diagnosis, prevention and treatment modalities for children and adults.

David Becton, MD, Medical Director

California

3867 Central California Chapter of the National Hemophilia Foundation
PO Box 163689
Sacramento, CA 95821

916-448-0370
Fax: 916-489-1569
e-mail: hubbert@newfactor.com
www.hemophilia.org

An organization devoted to improving the quality of life for persons affected with bleeding disorders and their complications. This is accomplished through outreach development, educational pro-

grams, informational literature, support services and patient referrals.

Sean Hubbert, President

3868 Hemophilia Association of San Diego County
3570 Camino Del Rio N, Suite 108
San Diego, CA 92108

619-325-3570
Fax: 619-325-4350
e-mail: info@hasdc.org
www.hasdc.org

An organization devoted to improving the quality of life for persons affected with bleeding disorders and their complications. This is accomplished through outreach development, educational programs, informational literature, support services and patient referrals.

Barbara Castle, DDS, Executive Director
Antonio Pasucci, President

3869 Hemophilia Foundation of Northern California
7700 Edgewater Drive, Suite 818
Oakland, CA 94621

510-568-6243
888-749-4362
Fax: 510-568-6111
e-mail: execadmin@hfnconline.org
www.hfnconline.org

An organization devoted to improving the quality of life for persons affected with bleeding disorders and their complications. This is accomplished through outreach development, educational programs, informational literature, support services and patient referrals.

Diana Vergil-Bolling, President
Robin Bratton-Bias, Associate Administrator

3870 Hemophilia Foundation of Southern California
33 S Catalina Drive, Suite 102
Pasenda, CA 91106

626-793-6192
800-371-4123
Fax: 626-796-5605
e-mail: hfsc@hemosocal.org
www.hemosocal.org

An organization devoted to improving the quality of life for persons affected with bleeding disorders and their complications. This is accomplished through outreach development, educational programs, informational literature, support services and patient referrals.

Linda Corrente, Executive Director
Reina Castaneda, Program Coordinator

Colorado

3871 Hemophilia Society of Colorado
655 Broadway, Suite 575
Denver, CO 80203

303-629-6990
888-687-2568
Fax: 303-629-7035
e-mail: hsc@cohemo.org
www.cohemo.org

An organization devoted to improving the quality of life for persons affected with bleeding disorders and their complications. This is accomplished through outreach development, educational programs, informational literature, support services and patient referrals.

Larry Hoyle, Chapter Administrator
Daniel Reilly, President

Florida

3872 Florida Hemophilia Association
18801 Old Cutler Road, Suite 501
Palmetto Bay, FL 33157

888-880-8330
e-mail: info@floridahemophilia.org
www.floridahemophilia.org

An organization devoted to improving the quality of life for persons affected with bleeding disorders and their complications. This is accomplished through outreach development, educational programs, informational literature, support services and patient referrals.

Debbie Adamkin, Executive Director
Linda Thompson, President

3873 Hemophilia Foundation of Greater Florida
1350 N Orange Avenue, Suite 227
Winter Park, FL 32789

800-293-6527
e-mail: Hemofoundation@earthlink.net
www.hemophiliaflorida.org

An organization devoted to improving the quality of life for persons affected with bleeding disorders and their complications. This is accomplished through outreach development, educational programs, informational literature, support services and patient referrals.

Fran Haynes, Executive Director
Ron Sachs, President

Georgia

3874 Hemophilia Foundation of Georgia
8800 Roswell Road, Suite 170
Atlanta, GA 30350

770-518-8272
800-866-4366
Fax: 770-518-3310
e-mail: mail@hog.org
www.hog.org

An organization devoted to improving the quality of life for persons affected with bleeding disorders and their complications. This is accomplished through outreach development, educational programs, informational literature, support services and patient referrals.

Patricia Dominicti, CEO
Eugene F Sandor, CGO

Hawaii

3875 Hemophilia Foundation of Hawaii
1164 Bishop Street, Suite 1501
Honolulu, HI 96813

281-379-4600
Fax: 281-379-1450
e-mail: hemophiliafoundation@hawaii.rr.com
www.bleedingdisorders.org

An organization devoted to improving the quality of life for persons affected with bleeding disorders and their complications. This is accomplished through outreach development, educational programs, informational literature, support services and patient referrals.

Rita Gonzales, President

Idaho

3876 Hemophilia Foundation of Idaho
PO Box 7622
Boise, ID 83707

208-344-4476
e-mail: hfi@velocitus.net

An organization devoted to improving the quality of life for persons affected with bleeding disorders and their complications. This is accomplished through outreach development, educational pro-

grams, informational literature, support services and patient referrals.

Jeanette Angel, President

Illinois

3877 Hemophilia Foundation of Illinois
332 S Michigan Avenue, Suite 1135
Chicago, IL 60604

312-427-1495
Fax: 312-427-1602
e-mail: info@hemophiliaillinois.org
www.hemophiliaillinois.org

An organization devoted to improving the quality of life for persons affected with bleeding disorders and their complications. This is accomplished through outreach development, educational programs, informational literature, support services and patient referrals.

Robert Robinson, Executive Director
Mike Toohey, President-Elect

Indiana

3878 Hemophilia Foundation of Indiana
4905 E 56th Street
Indianapolis, IN 46220

317-396-0065
800-241-2873
Fax: 317-396-0318
e-mail: mrice@hemophiliaofindiana.org
www.hemophiliaofindiand.org

An organization devoted to improving the quality of life for persons affected with bleeding disorders and their complications. This is accomplished through outreach development, educational programs, informational literature, support services and patient referrals.

Michelle Rice, Executive Director
John Spickelmier, Marketing Director

Kentucky

3879 Kentucky Hemophilia Foundation
1850 Taylor Avenue, Suite 2
Louisville, KY 40213

502-456-3233
800-582-2873
Fax: 502-456-3234
e-mail: info@kyhemo.org
www.kyhemo.org

An organization devoted to improving the quality of life for persons affected with bleeding disorders and their complications. This is accomplished through outreach development, educational programs, informational literature, support services and patient referrals.

Ursela M Lacer, Executive Director

Louisiana

3880 Louisiana Hemophilia Foundation
3636 S Sherwood Forest Boulevard, Suite 450
Baton Rouge, LA 70816

225-291-1675
Fax: 225-291-1679
e-mail: lahemophilia@etigers.net
www.louisianahemophilia.org

An organization devoted to improving the quality of life for persons affected with bleeding disorders and their complications. This is accomplished through outreach development, educational programs, informational literature, support services and patient referrals.

Lori Keels, Executive Director
Tres Major, President

Maryland

3881 Hemophilia Foundation of Maryland
8043 Kimberly Road
Baltimore, MD 21222

410-288-3955
800-964-3131
Fax: 410-285-3271
www.hfmonline.org

An organization devoted to improving the quality of life for persons affected with bleeding disorders and their complications. This is accomplished through outreach development, educational programs, informational literature, support services and patient referrals.

Kathy Robinette-Stoneberg, President

Massachusetts

3882 Massachusetts, New England Hemophilia Association
347 Washington Street, Suite 402
Dedham, MA 02026

781-326-7645
Fax: 781-329-5122
e-mail: neha@theworld.com
www.newenglandhemophilia.org

An organization devoted to improving the quality of life for persons affected with bleeding disorders and their complications. This is accomplished through outreach development, educational programs, informational literature, support services and patient referrals.

Mary Hagerty, RN, Executive Director
Patrick Mancini, President

Michigan

3883 Hemophilia Foundation of Michigan
1921 W Michigan Avenue
Ypsilanti, MI 48197

734-544-0015
800-482-3041
Fax: 734-544-0095
e-mail: harner@hfmich.org
www.hfmich.orgm

An organization devoted to improving the quality of life for persons affected with bleeding disorders and their complications. This is accomplished through outreach development, educational programs, informational literature, support services and patient referrals.

Ivan C Harner, Executive Director
Lauren Shellenberger, President

Minnesota

3884 Hemophilia Foundation of Minnesota and the Dakotas
750 S Plaza Drive, Suite 207
Mendota Heights, MN 55120

651-406-8655
800-994-4363
Fax: 651-406-8656
e-mail: hemophiliafoundation@visi.com
www.hfmd.org

An organization devoted to improving the quality of life for persons affected with bleeding disorders and their complications. This is accomplished through outreach development, educational programs, informational literature, support services and patient referrals.

James Paist, Executive Director
Aaron Reeves, President

Mississippi

3885 Mississippi Hemophilia Foundation
36 Avery Circle, PO Box 13608
Jackson, MS 39326

601-957-2706
e-mail: patty8501@aol.com

An organization devoted to improving the quality of life for persons affected with bleeding disorders and their complications. This is accomplished through outreach development, educational programs, informational literature, support services and patient referrals.

Mike May, President
Patty Lyons, Treasurer

Missouri

3886 Gateway Hemophilia Association of Missouri
462 N Taylor Street, Suite 107
St. Louis, MO 63108

314-729-0233
866-729-0233
Fax: 314-729-7033
e-mail: hemophilia@sbcglobal.net
www.gatewayhemophilia.org

An organization devoted to improving the quality of life for persons affected with bleeding disorders and their complications. This is accomplished through outreach development, educational programs, informational literature, support services and patient referrals.

Kitty Darden, President

Nebraska

3887 Nebraska Chapter of the National Hemophilia Foundation
215 Centennial Mail South, Suite 205
Lincoln, NE 68508

402-742-5663
Fax: 402-742-5677
e-mail: office@nebraskanhf.org
www.nebraskanhf.org

An organization devoted to improving the quality of life for persons affected with bleeding disorders and their complications. This is accomplished through outreach development, educational programs, informational literature, support services and patient referrals.

Carl Clark, President

New York

3888 Bleeding Disorders Association of Northeas tern New York
61 Main Street, PO Box 3707
Albany, NY 12203

518-782-9787
Fax: 518-356-5612
e-mail: bdaneny@bdaneny.org
www.bdaneny.org

Formerly known as the Upper Hudson Valley Chapter of the National Hemophilia Foundation. The Association endeavors to meet the diverse needs of a geographically dispersed community through a variety of programs, including; emergency financial support, scholarships, Camp High Hopes, Double Hole in the Woods Ranch, HIV/AIDS education, outreach and support, and recreational community activities.

Deborah Huskie, Co-Executive Director
Kevin Pelletier, Co-Executive Director

3889 Hemophilia Center of Western New York
426 Grider Street
Buffalo, NY 14215

716-896-2470
800-669-2299
Fax: 716-898-5537
www.hemophiliawny.com

A nonprofit, licensed diagnostic and treatment center. It offers a variety of services for persons with hemophilia and other herditary blood disorders ensuring that the patient is cared for at all times whether at the hospital, at home, at the center at school or on the job.

Rosemary P Holmberg, Executive Director
Thomas H Long, President

3890 Mary M Gooley Hemophilia Center of the National Hemophilia Foundation
1415 Portland Avenue, Suite 425
Rochester, NY 14621

585-922-5700
Fax: 585-922-5775
e-mail: Robert.Fox@viahealth.org
www.hemocenter.org

Specialized diagnostic testing, expert medical evaluation and diagnosis, personal counseling and support groups, home care treatment training, routine and urgent care, education of school and daycare personnel, research to advance knowledge, improve treatment and enhance quality of life for patients and families.

Robert W Fox, President/CEO
Vicky Orto, RN, Chairperson

North Carolina

3891 Hemophila Foundation of North Carolina
42 Dorado Drive
High Point, NC 27265

336-289-4446
880-990-5557
Fax: 336-725-4873
e-mail: rbrummett@triad.rr.com

An organization devoted to improving the quality of life for persons affected with bleeding disorders and their complications. This is accomplished through outreach development, educational programs, informational literature, support services and patient referrals.

Randall Brummett, President
Tyrone Cowans, Office Manager

Ohio

3892 Central Ohio Chapter of the National Hemophilia Foundation
PO Box 345
Worthington, OH 43085

614-457-0027
800-847-0345
e-mail: steje08@aol.com

An organization devoted to improving the quality of life for persons affected with bleeding disorders and their complications. This is accomplished through outreach development, educational programs, informational literature, support services and patient referrals.

Kathy Stewart, Co-President

3893 Northern Ohio Chapter of the National Hemophilia Foundation
One Independence Place
4807 Rockside Road, Suite 380
Cleveland, OH 44131

216-834-0051
800-554-4366
Fax: 216-834-0055
e-mail: lynnecapretto@nohf.org
www.nohf.org

The mission is to enhance the quality of life for people with genetic bleeding disorders and their families, through advocacy, education, research and other constituency services.

Lynne Capretto, Executive Director
Donald Whiteaker, President

3894 Northwest Ohio Hemophilia Foundation
PO Box 12606
Toledo, OH 43606

419-291-5882
Fax: 419-479-3269
e-mail: carla@nwohemophilia.org
www.nwohemophilia.org

A volunteer nonprofit organization that serves the bleeding disorders community in Northwest Ohio.

Carla Wells, Executive Director
Scott Newsom, President

3895 Southwestern Ohio Chapter of the National Hemophilia Foundation
82 Elva Court, Suite B
Dayton, OH 45377

937-415-0644
Fax: 937-415-0604
e-mail: SWOF@aol.com

Serving people with hemophilia and blood clotting disorders in an 11 county area. Dedicated to offering people and their families; educational opportunities about the physical, psychological and social aspects of these disorders. Workshops and seminars are regularly offered to address these issues. Offers support groups, volunteer services, telephone and walk-in education, information, counseling and referrals.

Dena M Shephard, President

3896 Tri-State Bleeding Disorders Chapter of the National Hemophilia Foundation
635 W 7th Street, Suite 407
Cincinnati, OH 45203

513-961-4366
Fax: 513-961-1740
e-mail: hemophilia@fuse.net
www.tristatebleedingdisorderfoundation.org

Formerly known as the Greater Cincinnati/Northern Kentucky Chapter of the National Hemophilia Foundation. An organization devoted to improve the quality of life for persons affected with bleeding disorders and their complications. This is accomplished through outreach development, educational programs, informational literature, support services and patient referrals.

Lisa Raterman, Executive Director
Gary Dillhoff, President

Oklahoma

3897 Oklahoma Chapter of the National Hemophilia Foundation
1407 W Blake
El Reno, OK 73036

405-844-5850
800-735-3855
e-mail: ohf@dmgp.com

An organization devoted to improving the quality of life for persons affected with bleeding disorders and their complications. This is accomplished through outreach development, educational programs, informational literature, support services and patient referrals.

Tom Ayers, President
Kerri Crabtree, Vice President

Oregon

3898 Hemophilia Foundation of Oregon
5319 SW Westgate Drive, Suite 126
Portland, OR 97221

503-297-7207
Fax: 503-297-0127
e-mail: hfo@easystreet.com
www.hfo.info

An organization devoted to improving the quality of life for persons affected with bleeding disorders and their complications. This is accomplished through outreach development, educational programs, informational literature, support services and patient referrals.

Linda Charles, President
Dave Worthington, Vice President

Pennsylvania

3899 Delaware Valley Chapter of the National Hemophilia Foundation
222 S Easton Road, Suite 122
Glenside, PA 19038

215-885-6500
Fax: 215-885-6074
e-mail: hemophilia@navpoint.com
www.hemophiliasupport.org

An organization devoted to improving the quality of life for persons affected with bleeding disorders and their complications. This is accomplished through outreach development, educational programs, informational literature, support services and patient referrals.

Ann E Rogers, Executive Director
Clifford B Cohn, President

3900 Western Pennsylvania Chapter of The National Hemophilia Foundation
532 S Aiken Avenue, Suite 102
Pittsburgh, PA 15232

412-683-2231
Fax: 412-683-2568
e-mail: wpcnhf@earthlink.net

Brings together and serves as a focal point for those segments of the community most concerned with hemophilia. They include medical and social service providers, people with hemophilia and their families, educators and the general public. This chapter combines service, education and advocacy programs.

Kerry Fatula, Executive Director
Ida McFarren, President

Rhode Island

3901 Rhode Island Hemophilia Foundation
160 Plainfield Street, Suite 2
Providence, RI 02909

401-944-6950
Fax: 401-944-4161

Lidia A Grande, Executive Director
Emili Vaziri, President

South Carolina

3902 Hemophilia Association of South Carolina
PO Box 2386
Irmo, SC 29063

888-829-4849
Fax: 888-829-4849
e-mail: factoreight@aol.com

An organization devoted to improving the quality of life for persons affected with bleeding disorders and their complications. This is accomplished through outreach development, educational programs, informational literature, support services and patient referrals.

Mark Eichelberger, President
Brandy Stewart, Vice President

Tennessee

3903 Tennesse Hemophilia & Bleeding Disorders Foundation
203 Jefferson Street
Smyrna, TN 37167

615-220-4868
Fax: 615-220-4889
e-mail: mail@thbdf.org
www.thbdf.org

Offers a hemophilia clinic, social workers and consultants, a state hemophilia program, blood donor programs, counseling programs, genetic counseling, literature and resources, summer camp, grants and more for the hemophilia and HIV/AIDS community.

Warren Cranford, Executive Director
Cathy Baggett, Program Services Coordinator

Texas

3904 Lone Star Chapter of the National Hemophilia Foundation
17414 Fairgrove Park Drive
Houston, TX 77095

281-861-6644
Fax: 281-861-6644
e-mail: Director@LoneStarHemophilia.org
www.lonestarhemophilia.org

An organization devoted to improving the quality of life for persons affected with bleeding disorders and their complications. This is accomplished through outreach development, educational programs, informational literature, support services and patient referrals.

Debbie de la Riva, Executive Director
Joe Rodriguez, President

3905 Texas Central Chapter of the National Hemophilia Foundation
3530 Forest Lane, Suite 311
Dallas, TX 75234

214-351-4595
Fax: 214-654-9954
e-mail: mail@texcen.org
www.texcen.org

A group of volunteers seeking solutions to the various aspects of the hemophilia problem. Supports blood drives, sponsors a summer camp for hemophiliac children, conducts educational member meetings, arranges for genetic counseling and sponsors group support meetings.

Michael Farnell, President
Tara Benker, Administrative Director

Utah

3906 Utah Chapter of the National Hemophilia Foundation
880 E 3375 South
Salt Lake City, UT 84106

801-484-0325
Fax: 801-484-4177
e-mail: smuir@hemophiliautah.org
www.hemophiliautah.org

Offers educational information, pamphlets, fundraising events and more for persons and families affected by hemophilia.

Scott Muir, Executive Director
Reg Ecker, President

Virginia

3907 Hemophilia Association of the Capital Area
10560 Main Street, Suite 604
Fairfax, VA 22030

703-352-7182
Fax: 703-352-2145
e-mail: info@hacacares.org
www.hacacares.org

A nonprofit organization serving persons with bleeding disorders and their families in northern Virginia, Washington, DC and Montgomery and Prince George's Counties in Maryland. The mission is to improve the quality of life for persons with hemophilia and Von Willebrand's disease and their families, to educate, to act as an advocate, to provide member services and to raise money to fulfill all these purposes.

Sandi Qualley, Executive Director
Keith Bushey, President

3908 United Virginia Chapter of the National Hemophilia Foundation
1505 Leewal Court
Chesterfield, VA 23832

804-740-8643
800-266-8438
Fax: 804-740-8643
e-mail: vahemophiliaed@verizon.net
www.vahemophilia.org

An organization devoted to improving the qualit of life for persons affected with bleeding disorders and their complications. This is accomplished through outreach development, educational programs, informational literature, support servcies and patient referrals.

Kelly Waters, Executive Director
Kevin Waters, President

Washington

3909 Bleeding Disorders Foundation of Washington
9659 Firdale Avenue
Edmunds, WA 98205

206-652-5789
Fax: 206-652-5790
e-mail: regina@bdfwa.org
www.bdfwa.org

An organization devoted to improving the quality of life for persons affected with bleeding disorders and their complications. This is accomplished through outreach development, educational programs, informational literature, support services and patient referrals.

Regina Timmons, Executive Director
Reid Morgan, President

3910 Hemophilia Foundation of Washington
PO Box 4565
West Richland, WA 99353

509-967-0203
e-mail: iebd4u@verizon.net

The Foundation's mission is to provide a conduit for education and information, advocate for excellent medical care, and support affected individuals and their families via peer outreach programs and special events

Jill McCary, President
Debbie Campeau, Executive Director

West Virginia

3911 West Virginia Chapter
RR 2 Box 231
Milton, WV 25541

304-743-3966

Wisconsin

3912 Great Lakes Hemophilia Foundation
638 N 18th Street, Suite 108
Milwaukee, WI 53233

414-257-0200
888-797-4543
Fax: 414-257-1225
e-mail: glfh@execp.com
www.glfh.org

The only Wisconsin organization that addresses the physical, emotional, social and financial needs of individuals affected by hemophilia. This chapter supports high-quality, cost-effective programs for patient care, education, research and public awareness.

Kathleen Roach, Executive Director
Brian Andrew, President

Libraries & Resource Centers

Alabama

3913 Alabama Department of Rehabilitation Services
2129 E South Boulevard, PO Box 11586
Mongomery, AL 36111

334-281-8780
800-846-3697
Fax: 334-613-3553
e-mail: cboswell@rehab.state.al.us
www.rehab.state.al.us

Mission is to enable children and adolescents with special health needs and adults with hemophilia to achieve their maximum potential within a community-based, family-centered, comprehensive, culturally sensitive and coordinated system of services.

Cary Boswell, Ed.D, Director

Florida

3914 University of Florida Hemophilia Treatment Center
University of Florida
2000 SW Archer Road, PO Box 100296
Gainesville, FL 32610

352-392-5633
e-mail: mehtaps@peds.ufl.edu

Paulette Mehta, MD

Indiana

3915 Riley Hemophilia and Thrombophilia Center
702 Barnhill Drive, ROC 4270
Indianapolis, IN 46202

317-274-2153
800-769-2848
Fax: 317-278-3751
e-mail: anholcom@iupui.edu
www.rileypeds.org

We strive to improve the health and health care of children by developing and applying best scientific evidence and methods in health services research and informatics.

Richard Schreiner, MD, Chairman of Pediatrics
Anna Holcomb, Executive Director

Wisconsin

3916 Hemophilia Outreach Center
1794 E Allouez Avenue
Green Bay, WI 54311

920-965-0606
Fax: 920-965-0607
e-mail: katiedirector@hemophiliaoutreach.org
www.hemophiliaoutreach.org

A comprehensive treatment center serving individuals and families with bleeding disorders. A facility maintained and administered through the collaboration of lay people, professionals, medical providers, consumers and families. Offering a variety of programs and services in a family-oriented, safe environment directed toward a holistic approach to wellness and to living a full life, including coordinating comprehensive care, consumer advocacy and financial and emotional support.

Katie Kralovetz, Director

Research Centers

3917 Albany New York Regional Comprehensive Hemophilia Treatment Center
Albany Medical College
47 New Scotland Avenue A-52
Albany, NY 12208

518-262-5827
800-773-7080
Fax: 518-262-6320
e-mail: ALBANYHTC@mail.amc.edu
www.amc.edu/patient/services/hemophilia

Providing comprehensive health care for patients with mild to severe hemophilia A, hemophilia B, von Willebrand's disease and thrombophilia in the Albany, New York region.

Barbara Leckerling, Administrator
Joanne Porter, MD, Director

3918 Albert Einstein Medical Center Hemophilia Program
5501 Old Ypnk Road
Philadelphia, PA 19141

215-456-6140
Fax: 757-953-3331
www.einstein.edu

Our principal purpose is the provision of compassionate, high-quality healthcare in order to elevate the heath status of the greater Philadelphia region.

Mehdi K Kajani, MD

3919 American Red Cross Hemophilia Center
PO Box 5905
Madison, WI 53705

608-233-9300

Diane Nugent, MD

3920 Blood Research Institute of Saint Michael's Medical Center
Cathedral Healthcare System
111 Central Avenue
Newark, NJ 07102

973-877-5340
Fax: 973-877-5466
www.cathedralhealth.org

Dedicated to research and the treatment of blood-related disorders and cancers, the Blood Research Institute is a multi-disciplinary unit of the hematology/oncology departments.

Yale S Arkel, MD

3921 Boston Hemophilia Center
Children's Hospital Boston
300 Longwood Avenue
Boston, MA 02115

617-355-6101
Fax: 617-730-0641
www.childrenshosptial.org

A federally funded hemophilia treatment center, the program offers comprehensive care to people with hemophilia and their families. Services range from medical treatment, counseling and support to discounts on clotting-factor replacement and other products that people with hemophilia require.

Jocelyn Bessette, PNP

3922 Bowman Grey School of Medicine-Hemophilia Diagnostic Center
Wake Forest University
Department of Pediatrics
Winston Salem, NC 27157

919-716-4324
Fax: 910-716-7100

Christine A Johnson, MD

3923 Cardeza Foundation Hemophilia Center
Thomas Jefferson University Hospital
705 Curtis Building, 1015 Walnut Street
Philadelphia, PA 19107

215-955-8435
www.jeffersonhospital.org/hematology

Devoted to research into the causes of a wide v ariety of diseases of the blood and to the diagnosis and care of patients with blood and lymphatic diseases. Our members have competence in all areas of hematology, with particularly well recognized depth and experience in diseases affecting blood platelets, hemorrhagic (bleeding) and thrombotic (clotting) disorders, hematologic malignancies (leukemia, lymphoma and multiple myeloma) and other bone marrow disorders.

Jamie Siegel, MD, Director

3924 Center for Cancer and Blood Disorders at Children's Medical Center in Dallas
1935 Motor Street
Dallas, TX 75235

214-456-2382
Fax: 214-456-6133
e-mail: CCBDinfo@childrens.com
www.childrens.com/ccbd

Comprehensive diagnostic and treatment program for patients with disorders of blood coagulation which results in increased risk of bleeding or clotting.

George Buchanan, MD, Director

3925 Children's Center for Cancer and Blood Disorders of Palmetto Health Richland
7 Richland Medical Park Drive
Columbia, SC 29203

803-434-3533
800-775-2287
Fax: 803-434-4598
www.palmettohealth.org

Diagnosis and treatment of cancer and blood disorders. The staff includes a nurse practitioner and a patient and family educator who provide complex nursing management, treatment and navigation through the healthcare system. The multidisciplinary team also includes skilled social workers, therapists, nutritionists and child-life specialists, all of whom play an active role in each child's care.

Cary K Smith, President
Beth Blackmon, Public Relations Director

3926 Children's Hospital of Philadelphia Hemophilia Program
34th Street & Civic Center Boulevard
Philadelphia, PA 19104

215-590-1000
Fax: 215-426-5480
www.chop.edu

Provides multidisciplinary comprehensive care for children and adolescents with inherited bleeding disorders. Services include diagnosis, acute and chronic medical management of hemophilia and its complications, genetic counseling, physical therapy, HIV care and counseling and coordination with other services.

Catherine S Manno, MD, Program Director
Regina B Bulter, RN, Program Nurse Coordinator

3927 Comprehensive Bleeding Disorder Center
Children's Hospital of Illinois
530 NE Glen Oak Avenue
Peoria, IL 61637

309-692-4533
Fax: 309-692-4533
e-mail: CBDC@hemophilia-ctr-peoria.com
www.childrenshospitalofil.org/programs/

Provides and facilitates state-of-the-art treatment for children and adults with hemophilia and related bleeding and thrombatic disorders. The staff includes a board-certified physician in pediatrics and pediatric hematology/oncology, nurses, social worker, rural outreach coordinator, reimbursement specialist/patient advocate, physical therapist and dentist.

Paul Kramer, Executive Director
Sara Dill, Administration Director

3928 Comprehensive Hemophilia Diagnostic and Treatment Center
University of North Carolina at Chapel Hill
433 Clinical Science S Building
Chapel Hill, NC 27599

919-966-4736
Fax: 919-962-8224

Joseph Eron, MD, Director

3929 Comprehensive Pediatric Hemophilia Treatment Center
University of Miami
1601 NW 12th Avenue
Miami, FL 33136

305-585-5635
www.pediatrics.med.miami.edu

Provided excellent medical and psychological care and emotional support for patients with bleeding disorders and their families since 1987. The HTC participates in national and regional research protocols dealing with various aspects of coagulation disorders. Orthopaedic and physical therapy are also offered at the monthly comprehensive clinic.

Maria Santaella, RN, Director
Steve E Lipshultz, MD, Chairman

3930 East Tennessee Comprehensive Hemophilia Center
University of Tennessee Medical Center
1924 Alcoa Highway 4 NW, Suite 180, Building E
Knoxville, TN 37920

865-454-9170
Fax: 865-544-9876
www.utmedicalcenter.org/hemophilia_services

Provides multidisciplinary comprehensive care to persons with bleeding disorders, including information, education and counseling to families affected by these disorders. The center's professional staff and consultants serve patients with hereditary bleeding disorders in Knoxville and surrounding counties.

Cheryl Zimmerman, RN, Director

3931 Eastern Michigan Hemophilia Center
Hurley Medical Center
1 Hurley Plaza
Flint, MI 48503

800-257-9432
Fax: 810-237-6750
www.hfmich.org/medical_resources

Provide and coordinate a broad range of treatment and prevention services provided by physicians who specialize in hematology and other relevant specialties such as orthopedics, social work, psychologists, nurses with extensive training and experience with hemophilia, genetic counselors, dentists, dental hygienists, and dieticians.

Ivan Harner, Regional Director

3932 Federal Hemophilia Treatment Center Program of Los Angeles
Children's Hospital of LA
4650 Sunset Boulevard
Los Angeles, CA 90027

323-669-4141
Fax: 323-660-7128
www.childrenshospitalla.org

Provides continuing and comprehensive care to children and young adults with inherited bleeding disorders (in particular, hemophilia). The hemophilia treatment program is a federally funded resource which focuses on multidisciplinary management of bleeding disorders and collaborates with other programs in the United States to provide comprehensive care and teaching for patients and health care providers.

Wing-Yen Wong, MD, Director
Robert Miller, Coordinator

3933 Federal Hemophilia Treatment Center of Hawaii
Kapiolani Medical Center for Women and Children
1319 Punchou Street Pau
Honolulu, HI 96817

808-983-8551
Fax: 808-983-8005
www.kapiolani.org

Part of a nation-wide network established to promote comprehensive hemophilia care and to prevent hemophilia complications.

Desiree Medeiros, MD, Director
Dee Ann Omatsu, RN, Coordinator

3934 First Regional Hemophilia Center
James H Quillen College of Medicine
400 N State of Franklin Road, 1st Floor
Johnson City, TN 37604

423-433-6200
Fax: 423-433-6220

Helping patients and families to manage every aspect of living with hemophilia, from providing information about the latest medical developments to organizing support groups for parents and teens.

Sheri Miller, RN

3935 Gundersen Clinic Comprehensive Hemophilia Treatment Center
Gundersen Clinic
1836 S Avenue
LaCrosse, WI 54601

608-782-7300
800-362-9567
Fax: 608-791-6692

Susan Bock, RN

3936 Hemophilia Center of Arkansas
Arkansas Children's Hospital
800 Marshall Street
Little Rock, AR 72202

501-364-3569
Fax: 501-364-4332
www.archildrens.org/

Patients with coagulation disorders can be diagnosed and evaluated by a group of physicians, physical therapists, dentists, psychologists and geneticists to provide education, prevention and continuity of care. The Hemophilia Center of Arkansas offers the latest diagnosis, prevention and treatment modalities for children and adults.

Nikki Shock

3937 Hemophilia Center of Central Pennsylvania
MS Hershey Medical Center
500 University Drive, PO Box 852
Hershey, PA 17033

717-531-7468
Fax: 717-531-5461

M Elaine Eyster, MD

3938 Hemophilia Center of West Virginia
University Health Sciences Center
Medical Center Drive, Room 4098
Morgantown, WV 26506

304-293-4967
Fax: 304-293-3793

John S Rogers II, MD

3939 Hemophilia Center of Western New York
462 Grider Street
Buffalo, NY 14215

716-896-2470
Fax: 716-898-5537
e-mail: hemoctr@pce.net
www.wnyhemophilia.com

The center provides a variety of services to the hemophilia and HIV/AIDS community. Included among these services are diagnostics, registration, outpatient treatment, home care programs, home visits, school visits, dental services and counseling services. Offers an adult unit and a pediatric unit.

Rosemary Holmberg, Executive Director
Thomas Long, President

3940 Hemophilia Center of Western Pennsylvania
3636 Boulevard of the Allies
Pittsburgh, PA 15213

412-622-7280
Fax: 412-683-4029

Comprehensive care to all individuals who are diagnosed with Hemophilia residing in Western Pennsylvania.

Toni Gorence, Coordinator

3941 Hemophilia Center of the New England Medical Center
UMass Memorial Medical Center; Memorial Campus
119 Belmont Street
Worcester, MA 01605

508-334-1000
www.umassmemorial.org

Family-oriented, state-of-the-art medical and psychosocial services, education and research. Provides diagnostic and treatment services for individuals with bleeding disorders using a community-based, family centered and culturally sensitive approach. A hematologist is available 24 hours a day.

Doreen Brettler, MD, Director
Ann Forsberg, Program Administrator

3942 Hemophilia Clinic - Childrens' Rehabilitation Service
1870 Pleasant Avenue
Mobile, AL 36617

334-472-1035
800-879-8163

Nancy Woodall, RN

3943 Hemophilia Program at Children's National Medical Center
Hematology/Oncology Department
111 Michigan Avenue NW
Washington, DC 20010

202-884-2800
www.cnmc.org/dcchildrens

Children's Hemophilia Program offers high quality, comprehensive care for children with hemophilia and thrombophilia. Children's is the only program in the Metropolitan DC are that is supported by the National Institutes of Health. Nearly 150 patients are treated here annually.

Anne Angiolillo, MD, Director

3944 Hemophilia Treatment Center at Munson Medical Center
1105 6th Street
Traverse City, MI 49684

231-935-7227
Fax: 231-935-6582
www.munsonhealthcare.org

A program which cares for patients with all types of bleeding disorders from 26 northern Michigan counties. Provides specialty treatment to patients with hemophilia with the goal of minimizing complications from bleeding episodes.

David Rushlow, Program Coordinator

3945 Hemophilia Treatment Center at the University of Iowa
UI Health Care Department of Pediatrics
200 Hawkins Drive
Iowa City, IA 52242

319-356-4277
Fax: 319-356-7659
e-mail: melinda-schultz@uiowa.edu
www.uihealthcare.com

Committed to provide the best care for individuals with bleeding disorders. To accomplish this mission we offer state of the art comprehensive clinical care, education to patients and their families and accessibility to clinical research projects that are oriented to improve the lives of people with these type of disorders.

Jorge Di Paola, MD, Director
Donald E McFarlane, MD, Co-Director

3946 Hemophilia Treatment Center of Tidewater Virginia
Division of Pediatric Hematology
800 W Olney Road
Norfolk, VA 23507

757-628-7000

Eric J Werner, MD

3947 Hemophilia and Coagulation Programs
Norris Cotton Cancer Center
1 Medical Center Drive
Lebanon, NH 03756

603-650-5486
Fax: 603-650-7791
www.cancer.dartmouth.edu/services/hemophilia

Provides complete clinical and laboratory diagnostic facilities for evaluation and treatment of patients with cogenital bleeding disorders and disorders of thrombosis and hemostasis.

Cornelius J Cornell, Jr.; MD, Program Director

3948 Hemophilia and Thrombosis Center at the University of Minnesota Medical Center
420 Delaware Street SE, Room B-549
Minneapolis, MN 55455

612-626-6455
800-688-5252
Fax: 612-625-4955
e-mail: htc@fairview.org
www.university.fairview.org

Offers a wide range of services for patients with inherited bleeding and clotting disorders. We care for patients of all ages using a team approach. Hematologists and nurse clinicians are involved and provide services including diagnostic evaluations, treatment, education, research and care coordination.

Mark Reding, MD, Co-Director
Margaret Heisel Kurth, MD, Co-Director

3949 Hemophilia and Thrombosis Center of Nevada
2020 W Palomino Lane, Suite 110
Las Vegas, NV 89106

702-385-2702
Fax: 702-322-0158
www.htcnevada.org

Offers diagnosis and management for persons with inherited or acquired bleeding disorders including hemophilia, von Willebrand's Disease, and platelet disorders. Comprehensive care is administered using a team approach with input from social services, physical therapy, orthopedic specialists, dentist, nursing, laboratory support, and medical services.

Rinah Shopnick, MD, Medical Director/Division Chief

3950 Hemophilia and Thrombosis Center: Division of Blood Disease Center
Cincinnati Children's Hospital Medical Center
3333 Burnet Avenue
Cincinnati, OH 45229

513-636-8790
800-344-2462
Fax: 246-636-4900
e-mail: blood@cchmc.org
www.cincinnatichildrens.org

Aim is to improve the lives of children and adolescents with hemophilia and thrombophilia. This is achieved by offering compassionate, state-of-the-art clinical care to patients and their families, advancing our understanding of the disorder through research and educating future health care providers and leaders in the field.

Karen Kalinyak, MD, Director
Vinod V Balasa, Thrombosis Director

3951 Huntington Area Hemophilia Association
Marshall University School of Medicine
1600 Medical Center Drive
Huntington, WV 25703

304-691-1700
Fax: 304-691-1726

Cynthia E Gonzales, MD

3952 Huntington Hospital Hemophilia Center
10 Congress Street, #340
Pasadena, CA 91105

626-397-3737

Laurence J Logan, MD

3953 Indiana Hemophilia and Thrombosis Center
8402 Harcourt Road, Suite 420
Indianapolis, IN 46260

317-871-0000
888-256-8837
Fax: 317-871-0010
e-mail: info@ihtc.org
www.ihtc.org

Multidisciplinary evaluation and treatment facility serving the people of Indiana who have bleeding disorders or thrombotic disease (known collectively as disorders of coagulation). The center aids local medical providers in the care of individuals of all ages with blood disorders and their families.

Amy Shapiro, MD, Medical Director

3954 Kalamazoo Comprehensive Hemophilia Treatment Center
Michigan State University
1000 Oakland Drive
Kalamazoo, MI 49008

616-341-7966
www.kcms.msu.edu

Offers diagnosis, management, and genetic counseling for these patients, as well.

Charles Zeller, MD, Program Director

3955 Louisiana Comprehensive Hemophilia Care Center
Tulane University School of Medicine
1430 Tulane Avenue
New Orleans, LA 70112

504-588-5433
Fax: 504-988-6808
www1.omi.tulane.edu/

Provides diagnostic, evaluation and treatment services for individuals with hemophilia, von Willebrand disease and other coagulopathies throughout Louisiana and the Mississippi gulf coast. The Center provides comprehensive medical and psychosocial evaluations through a multi-disciplinary team of adult and pediatric hematologists, orthopedists, nurses, social workers, physical therapists and dentists.

3956 Maine Hemophilia and Thrombosis Center
Maine Medical Center
22 Bramhall Street
Portland, ME 04102

207-885-7683
Fax: 207-885-7687
www.mmc.org

Offers a wide range of services for patients with inherited bleeding and clotting disorders. We care for patients of all ages using a team approach. Hematologists and nurse clinicians are involved and provide services including diagnostic evaluations, treatment, education, research and care coordination. Also, a full-time social worker provides psychosocial assessment, counseling and resource information.

Glen Roy, RN, Contact

3957 Mayo Comprehensive Hemophilia Center
200 1st Street SW
Rochester, MN 55905

507-284-2511
Fax: 507-284-0161
www.mayoclinic.org

Specializes in treating people with hemophilia and other bleeding disorders. The Center provides evaluation and care to approximately 200 patients per year. It also assists in the management and

care of another 100 patients annually who come to Mayo Clinic for initial evaluation or consultation.

Denis Cortese, MD, CEO

3958 Miami Comprehensive Hemophilia Center
University of Miami, Department of Pediatrics
PO Box 016960
Miami, FL 33101

305-585-5635
Fax: 305-325-8387
www.pediatrics.med.miami.edu

The Comprehensive Pediatric Hemophilia Treatment Center has provided excellent medical and psychological care and emotional support for patients with bleeding disorders and their families since 1987. HTC participates in national and regional research protocols dealing with various aspects of coagulation disorders. The major goal of the HTC medical team is to improve the quality of life for patients and their families coping with the stress and discomfort of living with a chronic illness.

Joanna Davis, MD, Medical Director

3959 Michigan State University Comprehensive Center for Bleeding Disorders
138 Service Road, Suite A-225
East Lansing, MI 48824

517-353-9385
800-759-5595
Fax: 517-353-9421
www.healthteam.msu.edu/

Offering education and information to individuals and families affected by blood clots and blood clotting disorders, and to assist with research efforts relating to all aspects of thrombosis and thrombophilia.

John Penner, MD, Director
Roshni Kulkarni, MD, Coordinator

3960 Mobile Hemophilia Clinic
Children's Rehabilitation Service
1870 Pleasant Avenue
Mobile, AL 36617

334-472-1035

3961 National Hemophilia Foundation
116 W 32nd Street 11th Floor
New York, NY 10001

212-328-3700
800-424-2634
Fax: 212-328-3777
e-mail: HANDI@hemophilia.org
www.hemophilia.org

Dedicated to finding the cures for inherited bleeding disorders and to preventing and treating the complications of these disorders through education, advocacy, and research.

3962 Nebraska Regional Hemophilia Center
Nebraska Medical Center
987430 Nebraska Medical Center, Kiewit Tower
Omaha, NE 68198

402-559-3656
Fax: 402-552-2410
e-mail: nmamdani@nebraskamed.com
www.unmc.edu/

Medical and educational support for those dealing with hemophilia, and their families.

Nizar Mamdani, Executive Director

3963 North Dakota Comprehensive Hemophilia and Thrombosis Treatment Center
Roger Maris Cancer Center/MeritCare Health System
820 4th Street N
Fargo, ND 58122

701-234-7544
800-437-4010
Fax: 701-234-7577
www.meritcare.com/specialties/more/hemophilia

Provides comprehensive care for people who have hemophilia, von Willebrand's disease and many other types of bleeding and clotting disorders. Using a team approach, professionals work together to provide evaluations, recommendations, treatment plans and follow-up care. They also offer a variety of services including assistance with clotting factors and home therapy.

Dr. Nathan Kobrinsky, MD, Director

3964 Northwest Ohio Hemophilia Treatment Center
Toledo Childrens Hospital
2142 N Cove Boulevard
Toledo, OH 43606

419-291-8580
Fax: 419-479-3258
www.toledochildrens.org

A full range of inpatient and outpatient services is provided for children and adolescents with blood conditions and cancer. The patient care program also offers support for the psychosocial needs of patients and their families.

Ann Gilbert, RN, Director

3965 Oklahoma Hemophilia Foundation
1407 W Blake
El Reno, OK 73036

405-262-8909
800-735-3855
e-mail: bettyjolo@att.net

Betty Lockler, President
Karen Duncan, VP

3966 Orthopaedic Hospital's Hemophilia Treatment Center
2400 S Flower Street
Los Angeles, CA 90007

213-742-1000
e-mail: info@orthohospital.org
www.orthohospital.org

Objective of the Center is the diagnosis and optimal management of bleeding disorders and their complications. Disorders treated include hemophilia A and B, von Willebrand's disease, and other inborn deficiencies of plasma clotting factors and platelets. Adolescents and adults who have acquired blood-borne infections, including chronic hepatitis and HIV infection, through prior treatment with blood products, are also treated at the Center.

Laurence Logan, MD, Director
Carol K Kasper, MD, Emeritus Director

3967 Pediatric Hemophilia Program of Pennsylvania
Children's Hospital of Pittsburgh
3705 Fifth Avenue
Pittsburgh, PA 15213

412-692-5055
www.chp.edu

Provides high quality, comprehensive care for children with hemophilia and thrombophilia through research and clinical programs.

Margaret Ragni, MD, Director
Kim Ritchey, MD, Pediatric Program Director

3968 Phoenix Center for Cancer and Blood Disorders
Phoenix Children's Hospital
1919 E Thomas Road
Phoenix, AZ 85016

602-546-1000
www.phoenixchildrens.com

Largest program of its kind in Arizona and is making significant difference in the quality of life for pediatric and adult hemophilia patients. It is one of only two federally funded hemophilia treatment programs in the state. The Center treats children with sickle cell disease, hemophilia and other hematologic disorders, and it is a designated center for the treatment and study of Gaucher's disease, an inherited metabolic disorder that can cause multiple medical problems.

Thomas J Diederich, Human Resources VP
Deborah Wesley, Patient Care/Chief Nursing VP

3969 Puget Sound Blood Center
921 Terry Avenue
Seattle, WA 98104

206-292-6500
e-mail: HumanResources@psbc.org
www.psbc.org

Puget provides all the blood and tissue services that people in our region need. It is this longstanding pledge to the community that has guided the Blood Center to more than sixty years of unparalleled success and to a leadership position in healthcare. In addition, our work in medical research is advancing medical care and making cures possible for patients around the world.

Jose Lopez, MD, Executive VP

3970 Regional Hemophilia Program
Children's Hospital of Michigan
3901 Beaubien Street
Detroit, MI 48201

313-745-5437
888-362-2500
www.chmkids.org/

Clinical evaluations and recommendations by a team of experts, home treatment, training and educational programs, HIV/AIDS counceling and management, carrier detection and genetic counceling. Clinical trials provide our patients with the latest treatment modalities and in-depth surveillance of complications.

Lynne Thomas Gordon, COO
Herman Gray, MD, President

3971 Research at BloodCenter of Wisconsin
8739 W Watertown Plank Road
Wauwatosa, WI 53226

414-257-2424
Fax: 414-937-6580
e-mail: jeanne.mccabe@bcw.edu
www.bcw.edu

Through basic, clinical and applied research programs, the center's scientists are enable to continue discoveries that enables to extend continuum of care.

Jeanne McCabe, Research Administration Director

3972 Rhode Island Hemostasis and Thrombosis Center
Rhode Island Hospital
593 Eddy Street
Providence, RI 02903

401-444-8250
Fax: 401-444-6104
www.lifespan.org/rih/services/blood

Formerly known as the Rhode Island Hemophilia Treatment Center, we have expanded our services to offer to persons with clotting disorders the same cutting edge, comprehensive program that has been extremely successful for our bleeding disorders community.

Sandra Meech, MD, Program Director
Coleen Foley, RN, Program Coordinator

3973 SUNY Upstate Medical University Research Development
750 E Adams Street
Syracuse, NY 13210

315-464-4317
Fax: 315-464-4318
www.upstate.edu/research

In collaboration with Upstate faculty, the Center conducts research and executes data analyses designed to guide the improvement of patient care and associated patient outcomes.

John Lucas, Ph.D, Research VP

3974 South Dakota Center For Bleeding Disorders

Sioux Valley Hospital
1305 W 18th Street
Sioux Falls, SD 57117

605-333-1000
e-mail: info@siouxvalley.org
www.siouxvalley.org

Provides comprehensive care based on family centered/community based health care. Hemophilia specialists are available 24 hours a day.

3975 South Texas Comprehensive Hemophilia and Thrombophilia Treatment Center

University of Texas Medicine
7703 Floyd Curl Drive
San Antonio, TX 78207

210-567-5200
Fax: 210-567-6921
e-mail: NAVAE@UTHSCSA.EDU
www.pediatrics.uthscsa.edu

A federally funded program focusing on the evaluation, treatment, and prevention of complications from Hemophilia, Von Willebrand's disease, thrombophilia, and menorrhagia in adolescents and women.

Donna Doulton, RN, Project Coordinator
Marcia Grayson, Senior Research Associate

3976 Spectrum Health Research

DeVos Hospital/Spectrum Health
100 Michigan Street NE
Grand Rapids, MI 49503

616-391-3050
e-mail: research.department@spectrum-health.org
www.devoschildrens.org

Formerly known as the Cook Institute for Research and the Cook Research Department. The Spectrum Health research department has a reputation for selectively participating in clinical research that brings cutting-edge treatments to the people of West Michigan. Many of the diseases under study currently have limited or no treatment options.

Robert Connors, MD, President
Dominic Sanflippo, MD, Executive Medical Director

3977 Steele Children's Research Center

University of Arizona Health Sciences Center
1501 N Campbell Avenue, Suite 3301
Tucson, AZ 85724

520-626-7051
Fax: 520-626-7176
www.steelecenter.arizona.edu

One of the eight centers of excellence at The University of Arizona College of Medicine. Internationally known physicians and scientists, who also are professors in the UA Department of Pediatrics, work together to research causes and develop cures for childhood illnesses and diseases. Our goal is to advance medical knowledge to help improve the health of Arizona's children and children throughout the world.

Fayez Ghishan, MD, Director

3978 Ted R. Montoya Hemophilia Program

University of New Mexico Health Sciences Center
MSC09 5300
Albuquerque, NM 87131

505-272-5551
Fax: 505-272-6845
www.hsc.unm.edu

Division program provides comprehensive care to the individual (child and adult) with hemophilia and other hereditary bleeding disorders.

Richard Heideman, MD, Division Chief
Jami Frost, MD, Clinical Director

3979 UCD Hemophilia Treatment Center

2315 Stockton Boulevard
Sacramento, CA 95817

916-734-2011
www.ucdmc.ucdavis.edu

Offers a variety of medical, educational and social services to people with hemophilia or other inherited bleeding disorders and their families across Northern California.

Jonathan M Ducore, MD, Co-Director

3980 UCSD Hemophilia Treatment Center

200 W Arbor Drive
San Diego, CA 92103

619-543-6222
Fax: 619-325-4350
e-mail: caglass@ucsd.edu
www.ucsd.edu

Part of the federal network of over 140+ specialty centers for bleeding disorder diagnosis and management. These two HTCs are funded, in part, by grants from the Maternal and Child Health Bureau and Centers for Disease Control and Prevention. The purpose of the grants is to support a multidisciplinary team which can provide comprehensive care and conduct research to prevent hemophilia complications.

Amy Lovejoy, MD, Director
Catherine Glass, RN, Nurse Coordinator

3981 UT Southwestern Medical Center at Dallas: Hematology-Oncology Research

5323 Harry Hines Boulevard
Dallas, TX 75390

214-648-0455
Fax: 214-648-2119
www.utsouthwestern.edu

Basic science research is enhanced by the world class investigative environment at UT Southwestern that includes 4 Nobel Prize winners and other internationally known scientists with whom hematology-oncology faculty regular collaborate. Cutting edge clinical research in hemophilia/thrombophilia and ITP are also major commitments.

George R Buchanan, MD, Director

3982 United Health Services Blood Disorder Center

Wilson Regional Medical Center
33-57 Harrison Street
Johnson City, NY 13790

607-763-6436
Fax: 607-763-5514
www.uhs.net/

Provides comprehensive care for those with blood disorders from diagnosis to treatment to home care and support services. Physicians, nurse specialists, dentists, orthopedists, physical therapists, and social workers treat people diagnosed with hemophilia and vWD at a dedicated site at Wilson Memorial Regional Medical Center. They also assist family physicians throughout the region in caring for persons with blood disorders.

Matthew J Salanger, President/CEO

3983 University Treatment Center of University Hospitals of Cleveland

11100 Euclid Avenue
Cleveland, OH 44106

216-844-3345
Fax: 216-844-5431
www.uhhospitals.org

Susan B Shurin, MD

3984 University of Cincinnati Adult Hemophilia Program
Division of Hematology & Oncology
3125 Eden Avenue, Vontz Center
Cincinnati, OH 45219

513-558-4233
Fax: 513-558-6703
e-mail: palascje@ucmail.uc.edu
www.intmed.uc.edu/divisions

Patient care, teaching, and research in the area of hematology/oncology. Rapidly growing in all research, clinical, and educational components. The division participates in investigator-initiated protocols, pharmaceutical or industry-sponsored studies, as well as cooperative groups, such as the Southwest Oncology Group and Radiotherapy Oncology Group.

Joseph Palascak, MD, Director
Albert Muhleman, MD, Division Director

3985 University of Michigan Adult Hemophilia and Cougulation Disorders Program
1500 E Medical Center Drive, Floor B1
Ann Arbor, MI 48109

734-936-6393
Fax: 734-936-5953
www2.med.umich.edu/healthcenters

Provides comprehensive, coordinated assessments and management services for individuals with blood disorders. Disorders may include disorders of blood coagulation (abnormal bleeding and clotting), hematology, hematopoietic malignancies, coagulation disorders, Von Willebrand's disease, lupus anticoagulant and thrombosis, and hemophilia.

Paula L Bockenstedt, MD, Director

3986 University of Tennessee Hemophilia Clinic
UT Health Science Center
920 Madison Avenue, Suite 300
Memphis, TN 38103

901-448-6454
Fax: 901-448-7929
www.utmem.edu

Diagnosis, evaluation, management, and treatment. The Hemophilia Center uses a comprehensive model to deliver effective care coordinated in the community. Emphasis is on educating providers, educators, patients, and their families for successful management. The center also manages a hemophilia factor concentrate program.

Marion Dugdale, MD, Director

3987 University of Texas Department of Hematology Research
University of Texas Medical School at Houston
6431 Fannin, 5th Floor
Houston, TX 77030

713-500-6800
Fax: 713-500-6810
www.uth.tmc.edu

Major research activities include a multidisciplinary center for vascular and thrombosis research and diversified hematologic and oncologic research projects covering a wide scope of disciplines from molecular biology to clinical trials.

Kenneth Wu, MD; PhD, Administration Director
Rebecca Davis, Research Staff

3988 University of Virginia Hemophilia Treatment Center
Kluge Children's Rehabilitation Center
2270 Ivy Road
Charlottesville, VA 22903

804-924-5161

Julie A Kopco, RN

3989 Vanderbilt Hemostasis-Thrombosis Clinic
Vanderbilt University Medical Center
2220 Pierce Avenue, 5th Floor, Suite A
Nashville, TN 37232

615-936-1765
Fax: 615-936-1767
e-mail: VHTCClinic@vanderbilt.edu
www.vanderbiltchildrens.com

Comprehensive health promotion; preventive medical and dental services; diagnostic testing; genetic testing and counseling; individual case management; specific and prompt treatments as needed; education and training; options for home treatment; and referrals, when necessary.

Anderson B Collier III, MD, Director
Mary G Hudson, RN, Nursing Coordinator

3990 Vermont Regional Hemophilia Center
Vermont Department of Health
108 Cherry Street
Burlington, VT 05402

802-656-2296
Fax: 802-863-7635

Miriam Husted, RN

3991 West Central Ohio Hemophilia Center
Children's Medical Center of Dayton
1 Childrens Plaza
Dayton, OH 45404

937-641-3111
Fax: 937-463-5878
www.childrensdayton.org

The center provides complete care for individuals and families with hemophilia and related bleeding disorders. Some of the services offered include a comprehensive clinic, emergency treatment network, consultations, diagnostic coagulation laboratory, home infusion programs, HIV/AIDS education and counseling and more.

James French III, MD, Medical Director

3992 Yale Pediatric Hematology/Oncology Research Center
Yale School of Medicine
PO Box 208064
New Haven, CT 06520

203-785-4640
Fax: 203-737-2228
e-mail: diana.beardsley@yale.edu
www.yalepediatrics.org

Oriented toward improving the lives of children with blood disorders and childhood cancer, while working toward future improved treatments and outcomes.

Diana S Beardsley, MD; PhD, Research Director

3993 Youngstown Hemophilia Center
Western Reserve Care System South Medical Center
500 Gypsey Lane
Youngstown, OH 44502

330-740-4176
Fax: 330-740-6559

Lawrence M Pass, MD

Audio Video

3994 Song of Superman
National Hemophilia Foundation
116 W 32nd Street
New York, NY 10001

212-328-3700
Fax: 212-328-3777
e-mail: handi@hemophilia.org
www.hemophilia.org

Designed to help young people with bleeding disorders come to terms with their HIV status, sexuality, and living with HIV. The video explores issues of disclosure in relationships and safer sex through dramatic scenes and frank testimonials by young people living with hemophilia and/or HIV. The companion workbook contains group exercises that follow each of the main topics of the video and serve as a bridge to discussion.

1993 33 Mins

Web Sites

3995 American Red Cross Blood Services
www.crossnet.org

Distributes a wide variety of plasma therapeutics to benefit people with hemophilia A and B, immune disorders and hypoalbuminemia.

3996 Health Answers
www.healthanswers.com

HealthAnswers offers a breadth of services in medical education, sales force training, patient support solutions, professional promotion and customer solutions.

3997 National Hemophilia Foundation
www.hemophilia.org

Devoted to improving the quality of life for persons affected with bleeding disorders. This is accomplished through outreach development, educational programs, information literature, support services and patient referrals.

3998 Online Mendelian Inheritance in Man
www.ncbi.nlm.nih.gov

This database is a catalog of human genes and genetic disorders.

Book Publishers

3999 Adventures of Maxx
Nova Factor
1620 Century Centery Parkway, Suite 109
Memphis, TN 38137

901-385-3600
800-235-8498
Fax: 901-385-3778

An activity book for children with hemophilia, this publication is intended to be both educational and entertaining.

1991 15 pages

4000 Children's Hemophilia Book
Porton Products Limited
30401 Agoura Road
Agoura Hills, CA 91301

818-879-2200

Coloring book that discusses what hemophilia is, bleeding episodes and treatment from a child's point of view.

1990 25 pages

4001 Federal Medicaid Drug Program
1730 E Street NW
Washington, DC 20006

202-628-9292

Discusses changes in government reimbursement and its effect on plasma derived products distributed by the American Red Cross. Includes law information, individual state billing procedures and Medicaid program coverage for the hemophilia community.

4002 Genetics Coloring Book
Medical College of Virginia
Box 98033, MCV Station.
Richmond, VA 23298

804-828-9632
Fax: 804-828-3760
e-mail: bodurtha@gems.vcu.edu
www.medschool.vcu.edu/

Adventures of Gene coloring book for children ages 5-9. Two coloring books, one dealing with cystic fibrosis and one with hemophilia.

1994-1995 Comic/Coloring

4003 Guide to Insurance Coverage for People With Hemophilia
Armour Pharmaceutical Company
500 Arcola Road
Collegeville, PA 19426

215-454-3720

An educational guide designed to assist with health insurance concerns.

4004 Harold Talks About How He Inherited Hemophilia
Hemophilia Foundation
982 Eastern Parkway
Louisville, KY 40217

502-634-8161
800-582-2873
Fax: 502-634-9995
e-mail: info@kyhemo.org
www.kyhemo.org

Children's brochure explaining hemophilia causes, symptoms and living a regular life.

4005 Harold's Secret: A Boy with Hemophilia
Bayer
400 Morgan Lane
West Haven, CT 06516

203-937-2765

A comic book for youngsters pertaining to children with hemophilia and understanding of the illness among school friends.

16 pages

4006 Hemophilia Camp Directory
National Hemophilia Foundation
116 W 32nd Street
New York, NY 10001

212-328-3700
Fax: 212-328-3777
e-mail: handi@hemophilia.org
www.hemophilia.org

Lists camps in the United States for children with hemophilia and other coagulation disorders.

16 pages

4007 Hemophilia Diseases and People
Enslow Publishers
40 Industrial Road
Berkeley Heights, NJ 07922

908-771-9400
800-398-2504
Fax: 908-771-0925
e-mail: CustomerService@enslow.com
www.enslow.com

An excellent resource for basic research for personal or academic use. The disease is carefully described, with effective black-and-white graphics, charts, and photos, showing blood biology and the circulatory system and the various levels of severity (depending on what clotting factors the individual is missing).

Ages: 9-12 128 pages Library Binding
ISBN: 0-766016-84-6

Edward Willet, Editor

4008 Hemophilia Handbook
Hemophilia of Georgia
8800 Roswell Road, Suite 170
Atlanta, GA 30350

770-518-8272
Fax: 770-518-3310
e-mail: mail@hog.org
www.hog.org

A comprehensive, easy-to-read resource for people with hemophilia and their families. The fourth edition of this handbook, contains up-to-date information on all important topics.

1988 348 pages

4009 Hemophilia Nursing Handbook

National Hemophilia Foundation
116 W 32nd Street
New York, NY 10001

212-328-3700
Fax: 212-328-3777
www.hemophilia.org

A revision and expansion of the 1995 Hemophilia Nursing Handbook. Now incorporating von Willebrand disease and other bleeding disorders. It is intended to provide comprehensive information as well as practical ideas to assist nurses at all levels in caring for patients with bleeding disorders. The guide is designed to be both an introduction to nurses new to coagulation and a resource for more experienced nurses.

1995 Members: $20

4010 Let's Talk About Going to the Hospital

Rosen Publishing Group's PowerKids Press
29 E 21st Street
New York, NY 10010

212-777-3017
800-237-9932
Fax: 888-436-4643
e-mail: rosenpub@tribeca.ios.com
www.powerkidspress.com

If a child has to check into the hospital, chances are he or she is already upset about being ill. Knowing how a hospital functions and what the procedures are, such as when family members can visit, will help in what is already a stressful situation. Grades K-5.

24 pages
ISBN: 0-823950-36-0

4011 Passport: Global Treatment Centre Directory

World Federation of Hemophilia
1425 Rene Levesque Boulevard W, Suite 1010
Montreal, Quebec, H3G
Canada

514-875-7944
Fax: 514-875-8916
e-mail: wfh@wfh.org
www.wfh.org

Lists over 900 hemophilia treatment centres and national hemophilia organizations in more than 100 countries, including contact names, telephone and fax numbers, as well as e-mail and web site addresses. It is very useful for people with hemophilia who are travelling to other countries and as a directory of hemophilia treaters around the world.

1990 188 pages Members: $6

4012 Procedure Coding for Hemophilia Treatment

Armour Pharmaceutical Company
500 Arcola Road
Collegeville, PA 19426

215-454-3720

Educational guide designed to facilitate the appropriate use of CPT codes for the hemophilia community.

4013 Understanding Hemophilia: A Young Person's Guide

Armour Pharmaceuticals Company
500 Arcola Road
Collegeville, PA 19426

This publication is designed for young persons with hemophilia. Presented in very basic and accessible language, this text with colored illustrations points out what hemophilia is, how to cope and more.

1988 91 pages

Magazines

4014 Bloodstone Magazine

Hemophilia Health Services
6820 Charlotte Pike
Nashville, TN 37209

800-800-6606
e-mail: info@hemophiliahealth.com
www.hemophiliahealth.com

A premier magazine of the bleeding disorders community. Features of community news, The Adventures of Welligan Hugsley, ProToCall, and human interest stories. A must read for anyone interested in the latest hemophilia related information.

Quarterly

Kyle J Callahan, Publisher/President
Lydia Dixon Harden, Editor-in-Chief

4015 HEMALOG

Materia Medica
208 E 51st Street, Box 234
New York, NY 10022

212-725-5151
Fax: 212-725-2794
e-mail: mmca@earthlink.net
www.mmca.com

The purpose of Hemalog is to serve as a national forum for the hemophilia community, providing current news, information, opinion, and contact with others in the community. The material contained in this journal reflects the experience and opinion of a wide range of people connected with hemophilia, and encourages story and art contributions.

Quarterly

Barbara Robin Slonevsky, Publisher
Janet Spencer-King

4016 HemAware

National Hemophilia Foundation
116 W 32nd Street, 11th Floor
New York, NY 10001

212-328-3700
Fax: 212-328-3777
e-mail: handi@hemophilia.org
www.hemophilia.org

Packed with medical updates, analysis, professional news, and practical health information for people living with a bleeding disorder and for their care providers. This magazine showcases how custom publishing can deepen relationships within a community by providing useful information in a compelling format.

Bi-Monthly

4017 Human Factor

Hemophilia Health Services
6820 Charlotte Pike
Nashville, TN 37209

800-800-6606
e-mail: info@hemophiliahealth.com
www.accredahealth.net

This journal is provided as a free service for the purpose of informing, educating and empowering the hemophilia community.

Quarterly

Newsletters

4018 Artery
Hemophilia Foundation of Michigan
1921 W Michigan Avenue
Ypsilanti, MI 48197

734-544-0015
800-482-3041
Fax: 734-544-0095
www.hfmich.orgs

Features articles on people in the bleeding disorders community, information and reviews on programs and services, memorials and donors.

Quarterly

Susan Lerch, Editor

4019 Big Red Factor
National Hemophilia Foundation of Nebraska
215 Centennial Mall South, Suite 426

402-742-5663
Fax: 402-742-5677
e-mail: office@nebraskanhf.org
www.nebraskanhf.org

Chapter newsletter offering legislative and medical updates, technology, resources, assistive devices and more for persons affected by hemophilia and other blood disorders.

Loren Ortman, President

4020 Bloodlines
Hemophilia Association of San Diego County
3570 Camoni Del Rio N, Suite 108
San Diego, CA 92108

619-325-3570
Fax: 619-325-4350
e-mail: info@hasdc.org
www.hasdc.org

Updates membership on the newest techniques and technologies on the treatment of hemophilia.

Quarterly

Teresa Ramirez, Executive Director

4021 COTT Canary Bulletin
Committee of Ten Thousand
236 Massachusetts Avenue NE, Suite 609
Washington, DC 20002

202-543-0988
800-488-2688
Fax: 202-543-6720
e-mail: cott-dc@earthlink.net
www.cott1.org

Tracks safety issues in our Nation's blood supply. It provides regular reporting, information and viewpoints from the grass roots end user communities.

Quarterly

Greg Haas, Editor

4022 Common Factor
Committee of Ten Thousand
500 Belmont Street, Suite 300
Brockton, MA 02301

508-587-2512

Offers information and medical updates on research and organizations, fund-raising events and resources pertaining to blood disorders, hemophilia, HIV and AIDS.

Quarterly

Greg Haas, Editor

4023 Community Alert
National Hemophilia Foundation
116 W 32nd Street
New York, NY 10001

888-463-6643
800-424-2634
Fax: 212-328-3777
www.infonhf.org

Features advocacy updates and medical news for the entire bleeding disorders community.

8 pages Monthly

Christopher Rael, Editor

4024 Concentrate
Hemophilia of North Carolina
2 Centerview Drive
Greensboro, NC 27407

919-852-4788

Offers information on summer camps, resources, book reviews, parent information and articles pertaining to hemophilia.

Monthly

4025 Factor Nine News
Coalition for Hemophilia B
712 5th Avenue, 43rd Floor
New York, NY 10019

212-554-6823
Fax: 212-554-6900
e-mail: info@coalitionforhemophiliab.org
www.coalitionforhemophiliab.org

Offers information on FDA approvals, annual meetings and the latest in technology and information regarding hemophilia.

Quaterly

Kimberly Phelan, Executive Director

4026 Headline News
Great Lakes Hemophilia Foundation
638 N 18th Street, PO Box 704
Milwaukee, WI 53201

414-257-0200
Fax: 414-257-1225
e-mail: info@glhf.org
www.glhf.org

Provides information on research, new treatments and support groups.

Kathleen Boach, Executive Director

4027 Hemophilia Headlines
Hemophilia Foundation of Oregon
5319 SW Westgate Drive, Suite 126
Portland, OR 97204

503-297-7207
Fax: 503-297-0127
e-mail: hfo@easystreet.com
www.hfo.info

Contains local, national and international news regarding bleeding disorders. It educates its readers with legislative and medical updates, as well as a current events calendar.

Quarterly

Jamie Dessellier, Editor
Dave Worthington, Vice President

4028 Infusions
Northern California Chapter of the NHF
7700 Edgewater Drive, Suite 710
Oakland, CA 94621

650-568-6243
888-749-4362
Fax: 510-568-6111

Informs members of medical, dental and orthopedic treatment advances and the latest research in the field. Helps to keep people with hemophilia and their families aware of relevant local and national meetings and includes important updates regarding research and treatment.

Bimonthly

4029 Initiatives

Philanthropic Initiative
160 Federal Street, 8th Floor
Boston, MA 02110
60

617-338-2590
Fax: 617-338-2591
www.tpi.org

Aimed at keeping patients and other interested individuals informed on important economic trends, legislation and medical issues.

Quarterly

Jane Maddox, Senior Editor
Joe Breiteneicher, President/CEO

4030 Linking Factor

Utah Hemophilia Foundation
880 E 3375 South
Salt Lake City, UT 84106

801-484-0325
877-463-6893
e-mail: info@hemophiliautah.org
www.hemophiliautah.org

Features news pertinent to the bleeding disorders community.

Quarterly

Charles Hand, Executive Director
Linda Aagard

4031 NEHA News

New England Hemophilia Association
347 Washington Street
Dedham, MA 02026

781-326-7645
800-228-6342
Fax: 781-329-5122
e-mail: info@newenglandhemophilia.org
www.newenglandhemophilia.org

Keeps the bleeding disorders community connected and informed about NEHA's programs and events as well as relevant local and national issues affecting our community.

Quarterly

Cathy Cornell, Executive Director

4032 Newsline Eight & Nine

National Hemophilia Foundation, Florida Chapter
2176 Bent Oak Drive
Apopka, FL 32712

407-880-8330
Fax: 407-886-7649

State association news and information.

Quarterly

4033 Ways & Means

Quantum Health Resources
790 The City Drive S
Orange, CA 92868

714-750-1610

Features pertinent health care information for hemophilia patients and their families.

Quarterly

Lynne Brightman

Pamphlets

4034 Anyone Can Have a Bleeding Problem

Hemophilia Foundation of Michigan
411 Huronview Boulevard
Ann Arbor, MI 48103

734-761-2535

Offers information on hemophilia and von Willebrand's Disease, how persons can get it, prevention and causes of the illnesses.

4035 Article Reprint Exchange

HANDI - The National Hemophilia Foundation
116 W 32nd Street
New York, NY 10001

212-219-8180
Fax: 212-328-3777

Offers various reprinted articles concerning hemophilia and the newest medical technology.

4036 Avoiding Indecision and Hesitation with Hemophilia-Related Emergencies

American Health Consultants
3525 Piedmont Road, Building 6, Suite 400
Atlanta, GA 30305

404-262-7436

Provides detailed information necessary for physicians, and ED staff to deal effectively and expeditiously with hemophilia emergencies.

12 pages

4037 Caring For Your Child With Hemophilia

National Hemophilia Foundation
116 W 32nd Street, 11th Floor
New York, NY 10001

212-328-3700
Fax: 212-328-3777
www.hemophilia.org

Provides parents of children newly diagnosed with hemophilia answers to their basic questions. Many aspects are covered such as inheritance, current treatments, as well as sports, and insurance issues. The symptoms of different types of bleeding episodes are discussed explaining the severity of particular injuries. Provided are tips for babies including immunization, nutrition, and dental care. Also discussed are the social and emotional issues children with hemophilia experience.

2001 33 pages Free to Members

4038 Child With A Bleeding Disorder Guidelines For Finding Childcare

National Hemophilia Foundation
116 W 32nd Street, 11th Floor
New York, NY 10001

212-328-3700
Fax: 212-328-3777
e-mail: handi@hemophilia.org
www.hemophilia.org/resources

Provides a helpful guide for parents of children with bleeding disorders as they make choices about in-home care, cooperative childcare, center-based childcare and choosing a daycare center. Also included is a checklist of provider services and helpful hints for babysitters and other family caretakers.

8 pages Free to Members

4039 Child With A Bleeding Disorder: First Aid For School Personnel

National Hemophilia Foundation
116 W 32nd Street, 11th Floor
New York, NY 10001

212-328-3700
Fax: 212-328-3799
e-mail: handi@hemophilia.org
www.hemophilia.org

Aimed at school nurses and teachers who have a student with a bleeding disorder. Descriptions of typical injuries and other incidences when bleeding occurs are discussed with proper steps that need to be followed as well as standard precautions and medications.

4040 Clotting Agents Are Lifesavers

Hemophilia Foundation of Michigan
411 Huronview Boulevard
Ann Arbor, MI 48103

734-761-2535

Offers information on what hemophilia is, treatments, occurences, heredity, von Willebrand's disease, patient services and direct services for hemophiliacs and HIV/AIDS patients.

4041 Comprehensive Services for Persons With Hemophilia

Hemophilia Foundation of Minnesota/Dakotas
2304 Park Avenue
Minneapolis, MN 55404

612-871-3340
Fax: 612-871-1359

Offers information on what hemophilia is and information and resources for persons with hemophilia and other bleeding disorders.

4042 Countdown to a Cure

National Hemophilia Foundation-Louisiana Chapter
3636 S Sherwood Forest Boulevard
Baton Rouge, LA 70816

225-291-1675
Fax: 225-291-1679
e-mail: info@cyberview.net
www.cyberview.net/~lhf/

Offers information on chapter resources and services for hemophiliacs and their families.

4043 Fight Hemophilia with Facts Not Fiction

Great Lakes Hemophilia Foundation
8739 W Watertown Plank Road
Wauwatosa, WI 53226

414-257-0200
Fax: 414-257-1225

Offers information on what hemophilia is, research information and treatments.

4044 Hemophilia and Mild Hemophilia What To Expect

American Home Federation
PO Box 985
Enfield, CT 06083

800-243-4621
Fax: 860-763-7022
e-mail: info@ahfinfo@.com
www.ahfinfo.com

Written in clear and easy to understand language, to provide information to those living with bleeding disorders, those who serve our children in school, and those who provide our medical care. A child or adult with mild hemophilia can live a healthy and long life. Physical activity is good and will help build strong muscles. Children and adults with mild hemophilia can do most things others can do.

1991 13 pages

4045 Hemophilia, Sports, and Exercise

National Hemophilia Foundation
116 W 32nd Street, 11th Floor
New York, NY 10001

212-328-3700
Fax: 212-328-3777
e-mail: handi@hemophilia.org
www.hemophilia.org/resources/handi_pubs.htm

This fully revised guide presents valuable information for the person with a bleeding disorder or his/her parents considering participation in sports activities. Topics covered include conditioning, stretching and flexibility, strength, weight training, prophylaxis, and physical activities for infants, toddlers, preschoolers, and school-age children.

1996 30 pages Free to Members

4046 Hemophilia: Current Medical Management

National Hemophilia Foundation
116 W 32nd Street, 11th Floor
New York, NY 10001

212-328-3700
Fax: 212-328-3777
e-mail: handi@hemophilia.org
www.hemophilia.org

Provides an overview of all aspects of hemophilia treatment, including prophylaxis, home therapy, inhibitors, orthopedic solutions, surgery, and dental care.

1994 30 pages

Jonathan C Goldsmith, Author

4047 How to Control Bleeds: Inspired by Vince, an 8-year-old Boy with Hemophilia

Bayer
400 Morgan Lane
West Haven, CT 06516

203-937-2765

An educational comic book story by Vince about hemophilia and treatment for bleeds.

26 pages

4048 Inheritance of Hemophilia

National Hemophilia Foundation
116 W 32nd Street, 11th Floor
New York, NY 10001

212-328-3700
Fax: 212-328-3777
e-mail: handi@hemophilia.org
www.hemophilia.org

Booklet provides a sophisticated explanation of the genetic transmission of hemophilia. It also describes tests used to find out if the hemophilia gene is present, particularly in women who may carry the gene but show no signs of excessive bleeding. Reproductive choices for men and women with the hemophilia gene are reviewed.

1998 15 pages

4049 Living with HIV: Talking With Your Child

National Hemophilia Foundation
116 W 32nd Street, 11th Floor
New York, NY 10001

212-328-3700
Fax: 212-328-3777
e-mail: handi@hemophilia.org
www.hemophilia.org

A pamphlet directed at caregivers of young children living with hemophilia and HIV disease.

1990 8 pages

4050 What Is Hemophilia?
American Federation Home (AFH)
PO Box 985
Enfield, CT 06083

800-243-4621
Fax: 860-763-7022
e-mail: info@ahfinfo.com
www.ahfinfo.com

Offers information on what hemophilia is, common factors in hemophilia, the cost and treatments offered to hemophiliacs and more.

4051 What You Should Know About Bleeding Disorders
National Hemophilia Foundation
116 W 32nd Street, 11th Floor
New York, NY 10001

212-328-3700
800-424-2634
Fax: 212-328-3777
e-mail: info@hemophilia.org
www.hemophilia.org

Explains hemophilia, von Willebrand disease, blood safety issues, joint problems, HIV infection, hepatitis, special bleeding problems in women, prophylaxis, recombinant therapy, the cost of care, comprehensive care and other issues of concern to the bleeding disorders community.

1997 23 pages

4052 What You Should Know About Hemophilia
National Hemophilia Foundation
116 W 32nd Street, 11th Floor
New York, NY 10001

888-463-6643
Fax: 212-328-3777
www.infonhf.org

Defines hemophilia, explains its effects, and provides a historical overview of treatment and treatment complications.

1991 13 pages

Camps

4053 Hole in the Wall Gang Camp
565 Ashford Center Road
Ashford, CT

860-429-3444
Fax: 860-429-7295
e-mail: ashford@holeinthewallgang.org
www.holeinthewallgang.org

Nonprofit organization that provides a recreational camp experience for children ages 7-15 with cancer, genetic blood diseases and HIV/AIDS.

Matthew Cook, Camp Director
James Canton, Executive Director

4054 NHF Camp Directory
National Hemophilia Foundation
116 W 32nd Street, 11th Floor
New York, NY 10001

212-328-3700
Fax: 212-328-3777
e-mail: handi@hemophilia.org
www.hemophilia.org

A comprehensive national directory of camps for the bleeding disorders community collaboratively produced by NHF. Lists camps in the United States for children with hemophilia and other coagulation disorders. Now available on web site.

16 pages

Renee LaBrew, Camp Directory Coordinator

DESCRIPTION

4055 HEPATITIS

Covers these related disorders: Hepatitis A, Hepatitis B, Hepatitis C, Hepatitis D, Hepatitis E

Involves the following Biologic System(s):

Gastrointestinal Disorders, Infectious Disorders

Hepatitis refers to an inflammatory condition of the liver that may result from viral, bacterial, or parasitic infection; certain blood disorders; or exposure to certain drugs, toxins, or alcohol. However, viral infection is most frequently the cause of hepatitis. Liver inflammation may develop in association with certain viral infections such as German measles (rubella), chickenpox (varicella), or HIV. In addition, there are at least five infectious agents known as hepatotropic viruses that specifically target the liver.

Hepatitis A virus is thought to be the most common cause of hepatitis in children, with an extremely high prevalence rate in underdeveloped countries. In addition, approximately 30 percent of adults in the United States show evidence of a previous infection with hepatitis A. This form of hepatitis is usually spread by fecal-oral contamination through drinking water, food, or direct contact. Children under five years of age often have no symptoms, but still acquire immunity to future hepatitis A infection. When symptoms become evident in children, they are often mild and may include fever, weakness, general discomfort (malaise), loss of appetite (anorexia), nausea and vomiting, diarrhea, and abdominal distress. Occasionally, some children develop a very slight yellowing of the eyes (scleral icterus), skin, and mucous membranes (jaundice). Hepatitis A is an acute, self-limited form of this disease, with a return to general health typically within one month, although relapses may occur. Life-threatening complications associated with this type of hepatitis are extremely rare. Prevention of hepatitis A transmission is directed toward the teaching of good hygiene (e.g., frequent hand washing) in hospitals, child-care facilities, etc. In addition, the administration of recently developed vaccines or immunoglobulin is recommended for children and adults who plan to travel to countries with a high incidence of hepatitis A. Young children are at risk for becoming carriers of this disease while older travelers may be at risk for more significant disease involvement. Early administration of immunoglobulin is also recommended for children and adults who may have been exposed to the virus. Other treatment is symptomatic and supportive.

Hepatitis B infection in children and adolescents may be transmitted through intravenous injection of blood, blood products, or drugs; sharing of needles or razors; ear piercing with contaminated equipment; and other carrier-contact modes of transmission. For example, the hepatitis B virus may be spread by apparently healthy people who are chronic carriers. Symptoms usually develop six to seven weeks after exposure, persist for six to eight weeks, and are similar to those of hepatitis A, but are often more severe. Additional manifestations may include tenderness and enlargement of the liver (hepatomegaly), enlargement of the spleen (splenomegaly), swollen lymph glands (lymphadenopathy), accumulation of fluid within the abdomen (ascites), skin lesions, or joint pain (arthralgia). Newborns of infected mothers are at high risk for infection during delivery, possibly through infected amniotic fluid, blood, or fecal material. Although infected newborns usually do not manifest symptoms, if left untreated, most develop a chronic form of hepatitis that may result in potentially life-threatening liver disease during adulthood. Prevention of hepatitis B infection in newborns is first directed toward testing for infection in pregnant women. If a mother is positive for infection, her newborn is given a hepatitis B immune globulin injection within the first day of life, followed by immunization with hepatitis B vaccine. Immunizations are also recommended to anyone who may have been exposed to hepatitis B. Treatment is symptomatic and supportive.

Hepatitis C may be transmitted among the general population through intravenous drug use, transfusions of blood or blood products, sexual contact, and other, unknown causes. Although transmission from an infected mother to her infant is possible, it is rare except in instances where the mother also has HIV or other contributing factors. The onset of disease is approximately seven to nine weeks after exposure and symptoms are similar to those of other types of viral hepatitis. Hepatitis C is the most likely of all the hepatotropic viruses to cause chronic hepatitis, a condition associated with prolonged inflammation of the liver that persists for six months or longer. Complications may also include cirrhosis and cancer of the liver, and rarely fulminant (very severe) hepatitis. Because infection with the hepatitis C virus may occur more than once in the same person, a preventive vaccine is not effective. Treatment is symptomatic and supportive.

The hepatitis D virus cannot replicate itself without the help of the hepatitis B virus; therefore, hepatitis D only occurs in people with prior or simultaneous infection with hepatitis B. The most common mode of transmission in the

United States is through intimate contact and needle sharing; therefore, this form of hepatitis is relatively rare in children in this country. Symptoms and findings may be similar to but more severe than those of hepatitis B infection. There is no vaccine for hepatitis D; therefore, prevention is directed toward prevention of hepatitis B infection. Treatment is symptomatic and supportive.

Hepatitis E is the cause of epidemic-associated infection and is spread by fecal-oral transmission, usually through contaminated water or food. The symptoms and findings of this form of disease are similar to but more severe than those associated with hepatitis A. However, this acute, self-limited infection may pose a life-threatening risk to pregnant women. Hepatitis E is extremely rare in the United States, thus far occurring only in people who have traveled to or emigrated from indigenous countries. No vaccine is available. Treatment is symptomatic and supportive. There are some reports about the use of interferon, either alone or in combination with ribavirin, another antiviral drug, in the treatment of children with Hepatitis C. However, only a partial antiviral response response occurred.

See also **General Resources** on page 917

Government Agencies

4056 NIH/National Institute of Allergy and Infectious Diseases
6610 Rockledge Drive, MSC 6612
Bethesda, MD 20892

301-496-5717
Fax: 301-402-3573
TDD: 800-877-8339
www.niaid.nih.gov

Conducts and supports basic and applied research to better understand, treat, and ultimately prevent infectious, immunologic, and allergic diseases.

Anthony S Fauci MD, Director

National Associations & Support Groups

4057 American Liver Foundation
75 Maiden Lane, Suite 603
New York, NY 10038

212-668-1000
800-465-4837
Fax: 212-483-8179
e-mail: info@liverfoundation.org
www.liverfoundation.org

Nonprofit, national voluntary health organization dedicated to the prevention, treatment and cure of hepatitis and other liver diseases through research, education, and advocacy on behalf of those affected by or at risk of liver disease.

Alan P Brownstein, President/CEO
James L Boyer, MD, Chair

4058 Hepatitis B Coalition
1573 Selby Avenue, Suite 234
Saint Paul, MN 55104

612-647-9009
Fax: 612-647-9131
e-mail: admin@immunize.org
www.immunize.org

Works to prevent transmission of hepatitis B in high risk groups, to achieve vaccination of all infants, children and adolescents and to promote education and treatment for hepatitis B carrier.

Deborah L. Wexler, MD, Founder/Executive Director
Becky Payne, Assistant to Director

4059 Hepatitis B Foundation
3805 Old Easton Road
Doylestown, PA 18902

215-489-4900
Fax: 215-489-4313
e-mail: info@hepb.org
www.hepb.org

Dedicated to finding a cure and improving the quality of life for those affected by hepatitis B worldwide. Our commitment includes funding focused research, promoting disease awareness, supporting immunization and treatment initatives and serving as the primary source of information for patients and their families, the medical and scientific community, and the general public.

Timothy Block, PhD, President

4060 Hepatitis Education Project
4603 Aurora Avenue N
Seattle, WA 98103

206-732-0311
Fax: 206-732-0312
e-mail: hep@scn.org
www.scn.org/health/hepatitis

The mission of the Hepatitis Education Project is to help raise awareness amoung patients, medical personnel and the public of the facts concerning hepatitis patients and the resources available to help those who live with the disease.

Steve Graham, President
E Russell Alexander, MD, Vice President

4061 Hepatitis International Foundation
504 Blick Drive
Silver Spring, MD 20904

301-622-4200
800-891-0707
Fax: 301-622-4702
e-mail: hfi@intac.com
www.hepfi.org

Our mission is to teach the public and hepatitis patients how to prevent, diagnose and treat viral hepatitus; prevent viral hepatitis by promoting liver wellness and healthful lifestyles; serve as advocates for hepatitis patients and the related medical community worldwide; support research into prevention, treatment and cures for viral hepatitis.

Thelma King Theil, Chairman/CEO
Karen Wirth, MBA, Vice Chairwoman

4062 March of Dimes Birth Defects Foundation
1275 Mamaroneck Avenue
White Plains, NY 10605

914-428-7100
888-663-4637
Fax: 914-428-8203
e-mail: resourcecenter@modimes.org
www.marchofdimes.com

Partnership of volunteers and professionals dedicates to improving the health of babies by preventing birth defects and infant mortality. Over 100 chapters are located across the country and can be located through the National Office.

Dr Jennifer Howse, President

4063 National Headquarters Hepatitis C Foundation
1502 Russett Drive
Warminster, PA 18974

215-672-2606
Fax: 215-672-1518
e-mail: hepatitis_c_foundation@msn.com

4064 World Health Organization
Avenue Appia 20
CH-1211 Geneva 27,
Switzerland

www.who.int

WHO is the directing and coordinating authority for health within the United Nations system.

Dr Margaret Chan, Director General

Web Sites

4065 American Liver Foundation

Nonprofit, national voluntary health organization dedicated to the prevention, treatment and cure of hepatitis and other liver diseases through research, education, and advocacy on behalf of those affected by or at risk of liver disease.

4066 Centers for Disease Control
www.cdc.gov

Mission is to promote health and quality of life by preventing and controlling disease, injury and disability.

4067 Hepatitis B Coalition
www.immunize.org

Works to prevent transmission of hepatitis B in high risk groups, to achieve vaccination of all infants, children and adolescents and to promote education and treatment for hepatitis B carrier.

4068 Hepatitis B Foundation
www.hepb.org

Dedicated to finding a cure and improving the quality of life for those affected by hepatitis B worldwide. Our commitment includes funding focused research, promoting disease awareness, supporting immunization and treatment initatives and serving as the primary source of information for patients and their families, the medical and scientific community, and the general public.

4069 Hepatitis Education Project
www.scn.org/health/hepatitis

The mission of the Hepatitis Education Project is to help raise awareness among patients, medical personnel and the public of the facts concerning hepatitis patients and the resources available to help those who live with the disease.

4070 Hepatitis International Foundation
www.hepfi.org

Our mission is to teach the public and hepatitis patients how to prevent, diagnose and treat viral hepatitus; prevent viral hepatitis by promoting liver wellness and healthful lifestyles; serve as advocates for hepatitis patients and the related medical community worldwide; support research into prevention, treatment and cures for viral hepatitis.

4071 Hepatitis United
www.hepu.org/

Book Publishers

4072 Hepatitis B Prevention: A Resource Guide
National Digestive Diseases Info. Clearinghouse
2 Information Way
Bethesda, MD 20892

800-891-5389
Fax: 703-735-4929
e-mail: nddic@info.niddk.nih.gov
www.digestive.niddk.nih.gov

Designed to assist health care and other professionals who work in planning or administering hepatitis B prevention programs.

252 pages

Kathy Kranzfelder, Director

4073 Hepatitis C: An Information Resource
American Liver Foundation
75 Maiden Lane, Suite 603
New York, NY 10038

212-668-1000
800-223-0179
Fax: 212-483-8179
e-mail: info@liverfoundation.org
www.liverfoundation.org

Explains viral hepatitis, transmission, symptoms, testing and acute chronic hepatitis.

Alan P Brownstein, President/CEO
Paul D Berk, Chair

4074 Let's Talk About Going to the Hospital
Rosen Publishing Group's PowerKids Press
29 E 21st Street
New York, NY 10010

212-777-3017
800-237-9932
Fax: 888-436-4643
e-mail: rosenpub@tribeca.ios.com
www.powerkidspress.com

If a child has to check into the hospital, chances are he or she is already upset about being ill. Knowing how a hospital functions and what the procedures are, such as when family members can visit, will help in what is already a stressful situation. Grades K-5.

24 pages
ISBN: 0-823950-36-0

4075 Liver Disease in Children
Lippincott Williams & Wilkins
530 Walnut Street
Philadelphia, PA 19106

215-521-8300
Fax: 215-521-8902
www.lww.com

A difinitive book on pediatric liver disease, providing extensive, well-edited information that is not easily accessible or available in other textbooks.

2000 1008 pages
ISBN: 1-556443-77-2

4076 Liver Disorders in Childhood
Butterworth-Helnemann
223 Wildwood Avenue
Woburn, MA 01801

617-928-2500
800-366-2665

1994 432 pages
ISBN: 0-750610-39-5

4077 War Against Hepatitis B
University of Pennsylvania Press
418 Service Drive
Philadelphia, PA 19104

215-898-6261

It provides a unique look at the inner working of the International Task Force on hepatitis B Immunization which had long been dedicated to the fighting the hepatitis pandemic.

1995 248 pages
ISBN: 0-812232-67-4

Newsletters

4078 American Liver Foundation
75 Maiden Lane, Suite 603
New York, NY 10038

212-668-1000
800-465-4837
Fax: 212-483-8179
e-mail: info@liverfoundation.org
www.liverfoundation.org

Newsletter of the preeminent voluntary organization dedicated to promoting liver wellness and eradicating liver disease.

Quarterly

Alan P Brownstein, President/CEO
James L Boyer, MD, Chair

4079 Hepatitis B Coalition News
Hepatitis B Coalition
1573 Selby Avenue, Suite 234
Saint Paul, MN 55104

612-647-9009
Fax: 651-647-9131
e-mail: admin@immunize.org
www.immunizize.org

Newsletter with brochures, articles, videotapes, audio-cassette tapes and manuals for different ethnic populations.

24 pages

Deborah L. Wexler, MD, Founder/Executive Director
Becky Payne, Assistant to Director

Pamphlets

4080 Chronic Viral Hepatitis Backgrounder
Centers for Disease Control
1600 Clifton Road NE
Atlanta, GA 30333

404-639-3311
800-311-3435
e-mail: cdcinfo@cdc.gov
www.cdc.gov

Offers information and statistics on viral hepatitis.

Julie Louise Gerberding MD, MPH, Director
Mitch Cohen MD, Director Infectious Disease

4081 Hepatitis
National Institute of Allergy & Infectious Disease
National Institutes of Health
Bethesda, MD 20892

301-496-4000
Fax: 301-402-3573
TDD: 800-877-8339
www.3.niaid.nih.gov

A pamphlet discussing the cause, symptoms, transmission, diagnosis, tests, prevention and the latest research on hepatitis.

Anthony S. Fauci MD, Director

4082 Hepatitis B: Your Child at Risk
American Liver Foundation
1425 Pompton Avenue
Cedar Grove, NJ 07009

973-857-2626
800-223-0179

4083 Hepatitis Fact Sheet
Centers for Disease Control
1600 Clifton Road NE
Atlanta, GA 30333

404-639-3311
800-311-3435
e-mail: cdcinfo@cdc.gov
www.cdc.gov

Offers information on the causes, symptoms, prevention and treatments for hepatitis.

Julie Louis Gerberding MD, MPH, Director
Mitch Cohen MD, Director Infectious Disease

4084 How Many Times a Day Do You Risk Being Infected with Hepatitis B?
American Liver Foundation
75 Maiden Lane, Suite 603
New York, NY 10038

212-668-1000
800-465-4837
Fax: 212-483-8179
e-mail: info@liverfoundation.org
www.liverfoundation.org

A flyer emphasizing the importance of vaccination against hepatitis B.

Frederick G. Thompson, President/CEO
Gerald Jeglinski, COO/CFO

4085 Q and A: Hepatitis B Prevention
SmithKline Beecham Pharmaceuticals
1 Franklin Plaza, 200 N 16th Street
Philadelphia, PA 19010

215-751-4000
Fax: 215-751-3400
www.gsk.com

Informational booklet written for healthcare personnel by the manufacturer of Engerix-B vaccine, reviews hepatitis B prevention.

Jean-Pierre Garnier PhD, Chief Executive Officer

4086 Viral Hepatitis: Everybody's Problem?
American Liver Foundation
75 Maiden Lane, Suite 603
New York, NY 10038

212-668-1000
800-465-4837
Fax: 212-483-8179
e-mail: info@liverfoundation.org
www.liverfoundation.org

Covering a broad range of topics including: a definition of the disease, descriptions of types of infections, transmission, symptoms, treatment options and prevention.

Frederick G. Thompson, President/CEO
Gerald Jeglinski, COO/CFO

4087 What Health Care Workers Should Know About Hepatitis B
Channing L Bete Company
One Community Place
South Deerfield, MA 01373

800-477-4776
Fax: 800-499-6464
e-mail: custsvcs@channing-bete.com
www.channing-bete.com

Presents information in easy-to-read, simple English for health care
workers about hepatitis B.

16 pages

Mike Bete, President/CEO

DESCRIPTION

4088 HEREDITARY FRUCTOSE INTOLERANCE
Synonym: Deficiency of phosphofructaldolase
Involves the following Biologic System(s):
Genetic/Chromosomal/Syndrome/Metabolic Disorders

Hereditary fructose intolerance is a metabolic disorder characterized by a deficiency of the enzyme phosphofructaldolase (fructose-1,6-bisphosphate aldolase), resulting in the body's inability to process or metabolize fructose, a simple sugar (monosaccharide). Fructose is found in honey, certain sweet fruits, baby food and baby formula sweeteners. In combination with more complex sugars (disaccharides and polysaccharides), it is converted in the liver into glucose and is either distributed immediately for use as energy or converted into glycogen and stored in the liver, muscle, or fat for later energy use. The deficiency of the enzyme phosphofructaldolase results in the accumulation in the body of fructose-1-phosphate, a compound in the chain of fructose metabolism. This accumulation inhibits glucose production as well as the glycogen processing into energy-producing glucose.

Ingestion of fructose by affected infants may result in extremely low blood sugar (hypoglycemia), yellowing of the skin, eyes, and mucous membranes (jaundice), enlargement of the liver (hepatomegaly), bleeding from within the digestive tract, kidney involvement (i.e., proximal tubular dysfunction), vomiting, sluggishness, sweating, tremors, irritability, and seizures. Affected children have an aversion to sweets and fruits and typically do not have dental cavities (caries). However, physical findings and symptoms may be variable in their severity and manifestation.

Treatment for hereditary fructose intolerance includes total elimination of fructose from the diet. Vigilance is extremely important in that fructose is present in many foods and medicines as an additive. Other treatment may include administration of supplemental glucose to counteract the effects of hypoglycemia.

Hereditary fructose intolerance is transmitted as an autosomal recessive trait. The defective gene for this disorder is located on the long arm of chromosome 9 (9q22). Approximately one of every 40,000 is affected with this disorder.

See also **General Resources** on page 917

National Associations & Support Groups

4089 American College of Gastroenterology
PO Box 342260
Bethesda, MD 20827

301-263-9000
www.acg.gi.org

Founded to advance the scientific study and medical practice of diseases of the gastrointestinal (GI) tract.

Jack A DiPalma, President
Amy E Foxx-Orenstein, VP

4090 Genetic Alliance
4301 Connecticut Avenue NW
Washington, DC 20008

202-966-5557
800-336-4363
Fax: 202-966-8553
e-mail: info@geneticalliance.org
www.geneticalliance.org

A coalition of voluntary genetic support groups, consumers and professionals addressing the needs of individuals and families affected by genetic disorders from a national perspective.

Sharon Terry, President/CEO

4091 March of Dimes Birth Defects Foundation
1275 Mamaroneck Avenue
White Plains, NY 10605

914-428-7100
888-663-4637
Fax: 914-428-8203
e-mail: resourcecenter@modimes.org
www.marchofdimes.com

Partnership of volunteers and professionals dedicates to improving the health of babies by preventing birth defects and infant mortality. Over 100 chapters are located across the country and can be located through the National Office.

Dr Jennifer Howse, President

4092 North American Society for Pediatric Gastroenterology/Hepatology/Nutrition
PO Box 6
Flourtown, PA 19031

215-233-0808
Fax: 215-233-3918
e-mail: naspghan@naspghan.org
www.naspghan.org

Strives to improve the care of infants, children and adolescents with digestive disorders by promoting advances in clinical care of children with chronic abdominal pain, diarrhea, constipation, vomiting, bleeding from the GI tract, inflammatory bowel disease, liver diseases, diseases of the pancreas, poor weight gain and nutritional problems.

Philip Sherman, President
Margaret K Stalling, Executive Director

Libraries & Resource Centers

4093 National Digestive Diseases Information Clearinghouse
2 Information Way
Bethesda, MD 20892

301-654-3810
800-891-5389
Fax: 703-738-4929
e-mail: nddic@info.niddk.nih.gov
www.digestive.niddk.nih.gov

The National Institute of Diabetes and Digestive and Kidney Diseases conducts and supports research on many of the most serious diseases affecting public health. The Institute supports much of the clinical research on the diseases of internal medicine and related subspecialty fields as well as many basic science disciplines.

Kathy Kranzfelder, Project Officer

Web Sites

4094 American College of Gastroenterology
www.acg.gi.org

Founded to advance the scientific study and medical practice of diseases of the gastrointestinal (GI) tract.

4095 National Digestive Diseases Information Clearinghouse
www.digestive.niddk.nih.gov

The National Institute of Diabetes and Digestive and Kidney Diseases conducts and supports research on many of the most serious diseases affecting public health. The Institute supports much of the clinical research on the diseases of internal medicine and related subspecialty fields as well as many basic science disciplines.

4096 North American Society for Pediatric Gastroenterology/Hepatology/Nutrition
www.naspghan.org

Strives to improve the care of infants, children and adolescents with digestive disorders by promoting advances in clinical care of children with chronic abdominal pain, diarrhea, constipation, vomiting, bleeding from the GI tract, inflammatory bowel disease, liver diseases, diseases of the pancreas, poor weight gain and nutritional problems.

4097 Online Mendelian Inheritance in Man
www.ncbi.nlm.nih.gov

This database is a catalog of human genes and genetic disorders.

4098 Rare Genetic Diseases in Children (NYU)
www.med.nyu.edu/rgdc/homenow.htm

We target issues arising from rare genetic diseases affecting children. Also, to assist in the endeavor to bring knowledge and hope to those for whom there is, at present, so little.

Journals

4099 Journal of Pediatric Gastroenterology and Nutrition

NASPGHAN, author

Lippincott Williams & Wilkins
530 Walnut Street
Philadelphia, PA 19106

215-521-8300
Fax: 215-521-8902
www.lww.com

Publication of the North American Society for Pediatric Gastroenterolgy, Hepatology and Nutrition, which strives to improve the care of infants, children and adolescents with digestive disorders by promoting advances in clinical care of children with chronic abdominal pain, diarrhea, constipation, vomiting, bleeding from the GI tract, inflammatory bowel disease, liver diseases, diseases of the pancreas, poor weight gain and nutritional problems.

Newsletters

4100 NASPGHAN News
PO Box 6
Flourtown, PA 19031

215-233-0808
Fax: 215-233-3939
e-mail: naspghan@naspghan.org
www.naspgn.org

Publication of the North American Society for Pediatric Gastroenterolgy, Hepatology and Nutrition, which strives to improve the care of infants, children and adolescents with digestive disorders by promoting advances in clinical care of children with chronic abdominal pain, diarrhea, constipation, vomiting, bleeding from the GI tract, inflammatory bowel disease, liver diseases, diseases of the pancreas, poor weight gain and nutritional problems.

DESCRIPTION

4101 HERPES SIMPLEX

Covers these related disorders: Herpes simplex virus type 1 (HSV-1), Herpes simplex virus type 2 (HSV-2)

Involves the following Biologic System(s):

Infectious Disorders

Herpes simplex refers to a contagious infection caused by the herpes simplex virus. This infection is characterized by the formation of small, sometimes painful, fluid-filled, blister-like lesions (vesicles) on the skin and various mucous membranes. There are two strains of herpes simplex virus: type 1 (HSV-1) and type 2 (HSV-2). More than 85% of the U.S. population has evidence of infection with HSV-1, while 25% is infected with HSV-2. Although there is some overlap, HSV-1 is usually responsible for lesions of the lips such as cold sores (herpes labialis), the mouth (herpetic gingivostomatitis), and the eyes (e.g., corneal lesions, conjunctivitis, etc.). HSV-2 usually produces genital herpes and herpes associated with infections of the newborn that occur before or during birth (congenital herpes). HSV-1 is transmitted by direct contact through the saliva, while HSV-2 is generally transmitted through direct sexual contact. In addition, HSV-2 may be acquired by the fetus of an infected mother through the placenta or by direct contact during the birthing process.

Symptoms and findings associated with an initial or primary infection with herpes simplex virus usually appear in one to two weeks after contact and may range from no significant illness to the appearance of flu-like symptoms, sometimes in conjunction with blister-like lesions that usually scab and heal in a week to 10 days. Initial infection has a higher rate and longer duration of symptoms. Lesions associated with the first outbreak can be exceedingly painful. Newborns, malnourished infants, and individuals with compromised immune function may develop severe infection involving the entire body (systemic infection). After the primary infection, HSV becomes inactive but travels through the nerves that gave sensation to the affected area. Once it enters the roots of these nerves, it remains there for life. Recurrent episodes may be triggered by such factors as sun exposure, fever, physical and emotional stress, suppression of the immune system, the ingestion of certain medications or specific foods, and other factors. Such episodes may begin with mild irritation, itching, burning, tingling, or sometimes severe pain in the affected area followed a few hours or days later by the formation vesicles that often merge to form one large lesion. Associated symptoms and findings may include itching or discomfort in the affected area, fever, and swollen lymph nodes in the neck. The lesions sometimes become infected, especially in children. Typically, however, the lesions ulcerate and form a yellowish crust within a few days, with healing completed in about three weeks.

Symptoms associated with primary oral herpes infection (herpetic gingivostomatitis) usually appear suddenly and include pain, fever, excessive salivation, bad breath, and difficulty eating. Lesions may appear anywhere in the mouth, although the tongue and inside the cheeks are most frequently involved. In addition, the gums are usually inflamed and nearby lymph nodes may become enlarged. Primary episodes typically persist for about five to nine days. Lesions associated with recurrent oral herpes infection are often accompanied by itching, pain, or tingling that usually subsides within a week. Recurrent cold sore lesions sometimes precede oral herpes infections. Eye lesions may result from both primary and recurrent infections and include inflammation of the delicate mucous membranes that line the inside of the eyelids and the whites of the eyes (conjunctivitis) or inflammation and dryness involving the corneas as well as the conjunctiva.

Genital herpes most often affects adolescents and adults and is usually caused by HSV-2; however, approximately 10 to 25 percent of primary genital herpes infection results from HSV-1 through such factors as oral-genital transmission. This type of infection may be characterized by fever, painful urination, and swollen glands in the genital area. Females may develop herpetic lesions on the cervix and, less commonly, in the vagina and on the external genitalia while males typically develop lesions on the penis. Many patients exhibit few or no symptoms during asecondary episodes. However, infected individuals may unknowingly transmit the virus during this time through sexual activity or from a mother to her newborn.

Additional findings and complications associated with herpes simplex include a condition called herpetic whitlow, which is an infection of the finger resulting from transmission of HSV through a skin break. Whitlow is characterized by painful blistering and swelling at the fingertip. Eczema herpeticum is a severe condition in which patients with certain preexisting inflammatory skin conditions are infected with HSV and develop widespread blistering. Potentially life-threatening associated findings include high fever; excessive fluid loss (dehydration); decreases in the levels of essential elements known as electrolytes in the fluid portion of the blood (e.g., calcium, potassium, and sodium); spread of HSV to the brain and other organs; and bacterial infection. In addition, patients with suppressed immune systems are at risk for potentially life-threatening complications resulting from spread of disease to the liver, lungs, central nervous system, and other organs.

Treatment for herpes simplex is dependent upon the site affected as well as the severity and type of infection. For example, keeping affected areas dry is an important aspect of treatment as moisture tends to promote bacterial infection. Therefore, mild infections such as those associated with herpes of the lip may be treated by cleansing of the affected area with soap and water followed by careful drying of the lesion. Secondary bacterial infections may be treated with antibiotics. In addition, antiviral drugs such as acyclovir are often effective in treating various types of infection as well as preventing recurrences if administered during high-risk periods. Adolescents and young adults should receive counseling or training in order to reduce the risk of transmission. Other treatment is symptomatic and supportive. Patients with frequent outbreaks may benefit from suppressive therapy.

See also **General Resources** on page 917

Government Agencies

4102 Centers for Disease Control
1600 Clifton Road
Atlanta, GA 30333

404-639-3311
www.cdc.gov

Mission is to promote health and quality of life by preventing and controlling disease, injury, and disability.

4103 NIH/National Institute of Allergy and Infectious Diseases
6610 Rockledge Drive, MSC 6612
Bethesda, MD 20892

301-496-5717
Fax: 301-402-3573
TDD: 800-877-8339
www.niaid.nih.gov

Conducts and supports basic and applied research to better understand, treat, and ultimately prevent infectious, immunologic, and allergic diseases.

Anthony S Fauci MD, Director

National Associations & Support Groups

4104 American Social Health Association
PO Box 13827
Research Triangle Park, NC 27709

919-361-8400
800-783-9877
Fax: 919-361-8425
www.ashastd.org

The American Social Health Association is dedicated to improving the health of individuals, families and communities, with a focus

on preventing sexually transmitted diseases and their harmful consequences

Lynn Barclay, President/CEO
Deborah Arrindell, VP Health Policy

4105 March of Dimes Birth Defects Foundation
1275 Mamaroneck Avenue
White Plains, NY 10605

914-428-7100
888-663-4637
Fax: 914-428-8203
e-mail: resourcecenter@modimes.org
www.marchofdimes.com

Partnership of volunteers and professionals dedicates to improving the health of babies by preventing birth defects and infant mortality. Over 100 chapters are located across the country and can be located through the National Office.

Dr Jennifer Howse, President

4106 World Health Organization
Avenue Appia 20
CH-1211 Geneva 27,
Switzerland

www.who.int

WHO is the directing and coordinating authority for health within the United Nations system.

Dr Margaret Chan, Director General

Libraries & Resource Centers

4107 Herpes Resource Center
American Social Health Association
PO Box 13827
Research Triangle Park, NC 27709

919-361-8488
800-230-6039
www.ashastd.org

Focuses on increasing education, public awareness, and support to anyone concerned about herpes.

Lynn Barclay, President/CEO
Deborah Arrindell, VP Health Policy

Web Sites

4108 American Social Health Association
www.ashastd.org

ASHA is dedicated to improving the health of individuals, families, and communities, with a focus on preventing sexually transmitted diseases and their harmful consequences.

4109 Child Health Research Project
www.childhealthresearch.org

To help achieve USAID's strategic objectives to reduce childhood mortality and morbidity, the Child Health Research Project (CHR) conducts applied research in: diarrheal and respiratory diseases, infectious diseases, neonatal health, and malnutrition.

4110 Health Research Project (HaRP)
www.harpnet.org

A program by USAID, the project strives to improve the health status of infants, children, mothers and families through the development and research of new tools, technologies, policies and approaches.

4111 HerpeSite
www.herpesite.org

Information outlining aspects and issues relating to herpes simplex virus (HSV).

4112 Herpes.com

www.herpes.com/

Purpose of this website is to fill the desperate need for herpes education, make it easier to manage herpes, inform people of ways to limit herpes reacurrences, to inform people of the beneficial products for herpes sufferers, to show the relationship between good health and herpes, to provide an opportunity for herpes sufferers to share their personal experiences and to provide communication via our live chat.

4113 International Herpes Management Forum

www.ihmf.org/

Established to improve the awareness and understanding of herpes virus, and the counselling and management of people with these infections.

4114 Slack

www.slackinc.com

Is a leading provider of healthcare information, educational programs, and meeting and exhibit management services worldwide.

4115 Virtual Pediatric Hospital

www.virtualpediatrichospital.org

A digital library of pediatric information including resources for patients and health care professionals.

Book Publishers

4116 Understanding Herpes

Lawrence R. Stanberry MD, PhD, author

University Press of Mississippi
3825 Ridgewood Road
Jackson, MS 39211

601-432-6205
800-737-7788
Fax: 601-432-6217
e-mail: press@ihl.state.ms.us
www.upress.state.ms.us

A most informative overview of herpes written for the general reader.

120 pages Hardcover/Ppbck
ISBN: 1-578060-40-0

DESCRIPTION

4117 HIRSCHSPRUNG DISEASE

Synonyms: Aganglionic megacolon, Congenital aganglionic megacolon

Involves the following Biologic System(s):
Gastrointestinal Disorders

Hirschsprung disease is a gastrointestinal disorder that is usually apparent within the first few days after birth. However, in some affected infants, symptoms may not become apparent until the first weeks of life. Hirschsprung disease is characterized by absence of groups of certain nerve cell bodies (ganglia) in the smooth muscle wall of the large intestine. In most affected infants, the affected segment begins at the ring-shaped involuntary muscle of the anus (internal anal sphincter) and extends to the lowest region of the colon (sigmoid colon). However, in other cases, this segment may extend to involve the entire colon.

In infants with Hirschsprung disease, absence of these nerve groups results in impairment or absence of rhythmic contractions that propel food through the digestive system (peristalsis). Due to impaired peristalsis, most affected newborns have inadequate or delayed passage of meconium, the thick, sticky, darkish green material that accumulates in the fetal intestines and forms a newborn's first stools. Although some affected newborns may pass meconium normally, they may subsequently experience chronic constipation. In infants with Hirschsprung disease, failure to properly pass stools results in widening of the colon (megacolon) above the affected segment and severe abdominal bloating (abdominal distension). Additional symptoms and findings may include episodes of diarrhea, nausea and vomiting, dehydration, loss of appetite (anorexia) and malnutrition, failure to grow and gain weight at the expected rate (failure to thrive), listlessness (lethargy), and other abnormalities. In addition, widening of the colon may result in deterioration of the colon's mucous membranes (mucosal barrier), potentially allowing increased reproduction of certain bacteria and associated inflammation of the colon (i.e., enterocolitis). In severe cases, severe diarrhea and potentially life-threatening complications may result.

In infants with Hirschsprung disease, treatment includes surgical removal of the affected area of the colon and rejoining of healthy areas of the colon and rectum. In some patients, before surgical correction, a temporary colostomy may be required. Colostomy is a procedure in which the lower end of the healthy region of the colon is connected to a surgically created opening in the abdominal wall.

Hirschsprung disease affects approximately one in 5,000 newborns and is considered the most common cause of lower intestinal obstruction in infants during the first month of life. The condition is about four times as common in males as females. Hirschsprung disease may occur in association with other disorders or conditions that are apparent at birth (congenital disorders) or as an isolated finding for unknown reasons (sporadic occurrence). In addition, there have been many reports of Hirschsprung disease in infants within certain families (kindreds). Researchers suggest that sporadic and familial cases may result from abnormal changes or mutations of one of several different genes expressed either alone or together (polygenic). Depending upon the specific disease gene or genes, the condition may have autosomal dominant, autosomal recessive, or polygenic inheritance.

See also **General Resources** on page 917

National Associations & Support Groups

4118 American Hirschprung Disease Association
22 1/2 Spruce Street
Brattleboro, VT 05301

802-257-0603

4119 American Pseudo-Obstruction and Hirschsprung's Disease Society
158 Pleasant Street
North Andover, MA 01845

978-685-4477
Fax: 978-685-4488

Promotes public awareness of gastrointestinal motility disorders, in particular intestinal pseudo-obstruction and Hirschsprung's disease; provides education and support to individuals and families of children who have been diagnosed with these disorders through parent-to-parent contact, publications, and educational symposia; and encourages and supports medical research in the area of gastrointestinal motility disorders.

4120 Genetic Alliance
4301 Connecticut Avenue NW
Washington, DC 20008

202-966-5557
800-336-4363
Fax: 202-966-8553
e-mail: info@geneticalliance.org
www.geneticalliance.org

A coalition of voluntary genetic support groups, consumers and professionals addressing the needs of individuals and families affected by genetic disorders from a national perspective.

Sharon Terry, President/CEO

4121 Hirschsprung Disease-American Pseudo Obstruction/Hirschsprung Disease Society
158 Pleasant Street
North Andover, MA 01845

508-685-4477
Fax: 508-685-4488
e-mail: aphs@mail.tiac.net

4122 Intestinal Pseudoobstruction (IP) Support Network
34929 Elm
Wayne, MI 48184

313-729-7912

Offers peer support, matching individuals/families. Educational materials include Membership directory.

Colleen Kidder, Contact

4123 March of Dimes Birth Defects Foundation
1275 Mamaroneck Avenue
White Plains, NY 10605

914-428-7100
888-663-4637
Fax: 914-428-8203
e-mail: resourcecenter@modimes.org
www.marchofdimes.com

Partnership of volunteers and professionals dedicates to improving the health of babies by preventing birth defects and infant mortality. Over 100 chapters are located across the country and can be located through the National Office.

Dr Jennifer Howse, President

4124 Pull-Thru Network
2312 Savoy Street
Hoover, AL 35226

205-978-2930
e-mail: info@pullthrough.org
www.pullthrough.org

A chapter of the United Ostomy Association dedicated to the support and information needs of the families of children born with imperforate anus, cloaca, cloaca exstrophy, bladder exstrophy, VATER Syndrome, Hirschsprung's Disease and other related birth anomalies.

Bonnie McElroy, President

4125 Support for Parents of Ostomy Children
Division of United Ostomy Association
19772 MacArthur Boulevard, Suite 200
Irvine, CA 92612

800-826-0826
www.uoaa.org

4126 United Ostomy Association
19772 MacArthur Boulevard, Suite 200
Irvine, CA 92612

949-660-8624
800-826-0826
Fax: 949-660-9262
e-mail: info@uoaa.org
www.uoaa.org

An association of affiliated, non-profit, support groups committed to improving the quality of life of people who have, or will have, an intestinal or urinary diversion.

Ken Aukett, President

Libraries & Resource Centers

4127 National Digestive Diseases Information Clearinghouse
2 Information Way
Bethesda, MD 20892

301-654-3810
800-891-5389
Fax: 703-738-4929
e-mail: nddic@info.niddk.nih.gov
www.digestive.niddk.nih.gov

The National Institute of Diabetes and Digestive and Kidney Diseases conducts and supports research on many of the most serious diseases affecting public health. The Institute supports much of the clinical research on the diseases of internal medicine and related subspecialty fields as well as many basic science disciplines.

Kathy Kranzfelder, Project Officer

Web Sites

4128 Ask NOAH About: Stomach and Intestinal (Gastrointestinal) Disorders
noah-health.org/english/illness/gastro/gastro.html

Information on many conditions, including colic, celiac disease, ulcerative colitis, Crohn's disease, diarrhea, hernia and Hirschsprung's disease.

4129 NIH News Advisory
www.nih.gov/news/pr

The National Institute of Health is the steward of medical and behavioral research for the nation.

4130 Online Mendelian Inheritance in Man
www.ncbi.nlm.nih.gov

This database is a catalog of human genes and genetic disorders.

4131 Pull-Thru Network
www.pullthrough.org

A chapter of the United Ostomy Association dedicated to the support and information needs of the families of children born with imperforate anus, cloaca, cloaca exstrophy, bladder exstrophy, VATER Syndrome, Hirschsprung's Disease and other related birth anomalies.

4132 United Ostomy Association
www.uoaa.org

An association of affiliated, non-profit, support groups committed to improving the quality of life of people who have, or will have, an intestinal or urinary diversion.

Book Publishers

4133 Online Pediatric Surgery Handbook
PO Box 10426, Caparra Heights Station
San Juan, PR 00922

787-786-3496
Fax: 787-720-6103
e-mail: titolugo@coqul.net
home.coqui.net/titolugo/handbook.htm#IIIF

An online handbook about many different diseases and disabilities.

Newsletters

4134 Pediatric Surgery Update
PO Box 10426, Caparra Heights Station
San Juan, PR 00922

787-786-3496
Fax: 787-720-6103
e-mail: titolugo@coqul.net
home.coqui.net/titolugo/handbook.htm#IIIF

Periodical electronic newsletter of interest to Primary Physicians, Pediatricians, Surgeons, Residents, Medical Students, Nurses and Health-related professionals dealing with evidence-based medicine and reviews in the practice of pediatric surgery.

Humberto Lugo-Vicente MD, FACS, Editor-in-Chief

4135 Pull-Thru Network News
2312 Savoy Street
Hoover, AL 35226

205-978-2930
e-mail: info@pullthrough.org
www.pullthrough.org

Provides emotional support and information to patients and families of children who have had or will have pull-through surgery to correct an imperforate anus or associated malformation, Hirschsprung's disease, or other fecal incontinence problems; sponsors online discussion groups.

Pamphlets

4136 Hirschsprung Disease
Nat'l Digestive Diseases Information Clearinghouse
2 Information Way
Bethesda, MD 20892

301-654-3810
800-891-5389
Fax: 703-738-4929
e-mail: nddic@info.niddk.nih.gov
www.digestive.niddk.nih.gov

Defines and explains the causes, symptoms, and treatment of
Hirschsprung's Disease. Includes a glossary of terms associated
with the condition.

DESCRIPTION

4137 HISTIOCYTOSIS

Synonyms: Class I histiocytosis, Langerhans cell histiocytosis, LCH

Involves the following Biologic System(s):
Hematologic and Oncologic Disorders

Histiocytosis X, also known as Langerhans cell histiocytosis, LCH, or Class I histiocytosis, refers to a group of three similar disorders called eosinophilic granuloma, Hand-Schuller-Christian disease, and Letterer-Siwe disease. These disorders are all characterized by the excessive production and accumulation of certain types of tissue cells known as histiocytes, resulting in benign growth or scar formation. Characteristic findings and symptoms are variable and depend upon the organ or organ system affected; however, approximately 80 percent of individuals with LCH have skeletal involvement. Associated bone lesions may appear in isolation or in many parts of the body. These lesions occur most often in the skull, although their appearance in other areas of the skeleton is not uncommon. Some individuals may experience complications resulting from bone involvement. For example, involvement of a certain bone near the ear (mastoid) may result in chronic ear infections and persistent drainage. Involvement of certain weight-bearing bones may result in fractures.

Letterer-Siwe disease occurs during early childhood, usually before three years of age. This disease is characterized by skin eruptions, enlargement of the liver and spleen (hepatosplenomegaly) and certain lymph nodes (lymphadenopathy), and abnormally low levels of circulating red blood cells resulting in anemia. In addition, some children may experience involvement of the lungs, sometimes resulting in lung collapse (pneumothorax). Hand-Schuller-Christian disease often appears during early childhood and is characterized by bulging of the eyeballs (exophthalmos); excessive urinary excretion (polyuria), a decrease in body fluid volume (dehydration), and excessive thirst (polydipsia); elevated cholesterol levels (hypercholesterolemia); and involvement of soft tissues and bone. Eosinophilic granulomas most often occur during the second to fourth decade of life; however, they may develop during childhood, especially between the ages of five to 10 years. Benign growths may develop in the skull, jaw, and the long bones of the arms and legs, sometimes resulting in pain and fractures. In addition, lung involvement may result in respiratory symptoms such as coughing and shortness of breath, fever, and lung collapse.

Other findings and symptoms sometimes associated with Class I histiocytoses may include growth retardation, thyroid deficiency, and other abnormalities resulting from disruption in pituitary gland function or involvement of another gland in the brain known as the hypothalamus; difficulty walking and other neurologic symptoms resulting from involvement of the central nervous system; and additional irregularities of the blood resulting from involvement of the bone marrow.

Although the exact cause of each of the disorders that comprise Class I histiocytoses is unknown, it is believed that Letterer-Siwe disease may be inherited as an autosomal recessive trait and that the diseases develop as a result of disturbanc|es within the immune system. Treatment for LCH depends upon the extent and severity of involvement. For example, if only one organ or organ system (e.g., skeletal or skin, etc.) is affected, the disease is often self-limited; therefore, treatment may be directed toward control and resolution of specific lesions through low-dose radiation therapy or removal by means of a scraping procedure (curettage). If more than one system of the body is affected, treatment may involve a chemotherapy regimen that includes the use of one or two specific drugs (i.e., etoposide and vinblastine). More resistant disease may necessitate the use of other immunosuppressive drugs, bone marrow transplantation, or experimental treatments. Other treatment is symptomatic and supportive.

See also **General Resources** on page 917

Government Agencies

4138 NIH/National Cancer Institute
6116 Executive Boulevard, Room 3036A
Bethesda, MD 20892

800-422-6237
www.cancer.gov

The National Cancer Institute coordinates the National Cancer Program, which conducts and supports research, training, health information dissemination, and other programs with respect to the cause, diagnosis, prevention, and treatment of cancer, rehabilitation from cancer, and the continuing care of cancer patients and the families of cancer patients.

John E Niederhuber MD, Director

National Associations & Support Groups

4139 Genetic Alliance
4301 Connecticut Avenue NW
Washington, DC 20008

202-966-5557
800-336-4363
Fax: 202-966-8553
e-mail: info@geneticalliance.org
www.geneticalliance.org

A coalition of voluntary genetic support groups, consumers and professionals addressing the needs of individuals and families affected by genetic disorders from a national perspective.

Sharon Terry, President/CEO

4140 Histiocytosis Association of America
332 North Broadway
Pitman, NJ 08071

856-589-6606
800-548-2758
Fax: 856-589-6614
e-mail: association@histio.org
www.histio.org

Committed to the promotion of scientific research into the Histiocytoses and the development of improved control and management of these diseases. Provides solutions for some of the problems specific to patients suffering from this disease and offers support to such patients and their families. Promotes public education and produces educational materials.

Jeffrey M. Toughill, President
Beth Anne Miller, COO/Director Development

4141 March of Dimes Birth Defects Foundation
1275 Mamaroneck Avenue
White Plains, NY 10605

914-428-7100
888-663-4637
Fax: 914-428-8203
e-mail: resourcecenter@modimes.org
www.marchofdimes.com

Partnership of volunteers and professionals dedicates to improving the health of babies by preventing birth defects and infant mortality. Over 100 chapters are located across the country and can be located through the National Office.

Dr Jennifer Howse, President

Web Sites

4142 National Histicytosis Organizations
www.histio.org/

Is an international partnership of patients, families, physicians and friends. Is is a nonprofit organization whose goals are to promote scientific research into the hitiocytoses, seeking to develop better means of control and management of the disease and ultimatley seeking to develop scientific means to prevent and cure them and to provide solutions to some of the problems which are specific to patients suffering from this disease and to offer support to such patients and their families.

4143 Online Mendelian Inheritance in Man
www.ncbi.nlm.nih.gov

This database is a catalog of human genes and genetic disorders.

4144 Texas Children's Cancer Center
www.txcc.org

Offers innovative therapies for all forms of childhood cancer and blood disorders. The Cancer Center is working to improve the outcome for all patients afflicted with these diseases and to develop and perfect new treatment approaches that are born from only the most extraordinary scientific insights.

Book Publishers

4145 Let's Talk About Going to the Hospital
Rosen Publishing Group's PowerKids Press
29 E 21st Street
New York, NY 10010

212-777-3017
800-237-9932
Fax: 888-436-4643
e-mail: rosenpub@tribeca.ios.com
www.powerkidspress.com

If a child has to check into the hospital, chances are he or she is already upset about being ill. Knowing how a hospital functions and what the procedures are, such as when family members can visit, will help in what is already a stressful situation. Grades K-5.

24 pages
ISBN: 0-823950-36-0

DESCRIPTION

4146 HODGKIN'S DISEASE

Synonym: Hodgkin's lymphoma

Covers these related disorders: Hodgkin's disease—lymphocyte depletion type, Hodgkin's disease—lymphocyte predominance type, Hodgkin's disease—mixed cellularity type, Hodgkin's disease—nodular sclerosing type

Involves the following Biologic System(s):
Hematologic and Oncologic Disorders

Hodgkin's disease is a malignant disorder (cancer) characterized by painless, progressive enlargement of the lymph nodes, spleen, and other lymphoid tissues (lymphoma). The lymphatic system includes a network of vessels that collect a fluid known as lymph from different areas of the body and drain this fluid into the bloodstream. As lymph moves through the lymphatic system, it is filtered by a network of lymph nodes, which are small structures located along the course of the lymphatic vessels. Most lymph nodes that can be felt (palpable) are located in the neck, mouth, and groin and under the arms (axillae). Lymph nodes store certain white blood cells and are thought to play a role in producing antibodies, thus functioning as part of the body's immune system.

Malignancies of lymph tissue, known as lymphomas, are the third most common form of cancer affecting children in the United States. Approximately 13 per one million children are affected by lymphoma in the U.S. each year. There are two main categories of lymphoma, including Hodgkin's disease and non-Hodgkin's lymphoma. Although Hodgkin's disease may affect individuals of any age, it usually occurs between the ages of 15 and 35 or after age 50. In children, the disease is most common during late childhood or early adolescence and rarely affects those younger than five years of age. About 6,000 to 7,000 cases of the disease occur in the U.S. annually. Epstein-Barr virus, a member of the herpesvirus family that causes mononucleosis 35-50 percent of the time, may play some role in the disease. In addition, some familial cases have been reported, suggesting possible genetic mechanisms.

Hodgkin's disease is characterized by the presence of relatively large, abnormal white blood cells that have more than one nucleus and a distinctive appearance under a microscope. These cancerous cells, known as Reed-Sternberg cells, may be seen during the microscopic examination of small tissue samples removed from affected lymph nodes or other lymphoid tissues. Hodgkin's disease is categorized

into four main subtypes based upon the number and relative proportion of such cells as well as the proportions of certain other white blood cells (e.g., plasma cells, eosinophils, macrophages, etc.). The frequency of the different subtypes varies with age. For example, nodular sclerosing type is the most common form of the disease and affects approximately 50 percent of children and up to 70 percent of adolescents with Hodgkin's disease. Another subtype, known as the mixed cellularity type, affects about 40 to 50 percent of patients, and the lymphocyte predominance type of the disease primarily occurs in males and younger patients. The fourth subtype, called lymphocyte depletion type, is the rarest and most aggressive form of the disorder and occurs in fewer than 10 percent of patients.

Hodgkin's disease usually originates in the lymphatic vessels. As the disease progresses, the malignancy may spread from lymph nodes and infiltrate certain organs, particularly the spleen, lungs, liver, and bone marrow. Most patients initially experience painless swelling of lymph nodes in the neck or, in some cases, under the arm or in the groin area. Some may gradually develop generalized symptoms including fever, night sweats, fatigue, listlessness (lethargy), generalized itching (pruritus), loss of appetite (anorexia), and weight loss. Involvement of other organs or tissues may cause varying symptoms. For example, if the lungs are affected, patients may experience coughing and shortness of breath (dyspnea). Advanced involvement of the bone marrow may result in abnormally low levels of circulating red blood cells (anemia), platelets (thrombocytopenia), or certain white blood cells (neutropenia). Advanced disease may cause progressive impairment of the body's immune system, resulting in an increased susceptibility to certain infections. In patients with severe disease progression, infection with certain microorganisms that typically cause no or only minor symptoms in healthy individuals may result in severe or potentially life-threatening complications.

Treatment of patients with the disease varies, depending on the stage of the disease and other factors. For patients in early stages who have localized disease and have obtained full growth, radiation therapy alone may be effective; the 10-year survival rate exceeds 80 percent. However, up to 15 percent of such patients may experience recurrences, requiring therapy with certain anticancer drugs (combination chemotherapy). However, combination therapy cures more than 50 percent of patients, even those with advanced-stage disease. Combination chemotherapy may include the drugs doxorubicin (Adriamycin), bleomycin, vinblastine, and dacarbazine (known as ABVD) or a combination of mechlorethamine, vincristine (Oncovin), procarbazine, and prednisone (called MOPP). Physicians who specialize in the treatment of childhood cancers (pediatric oncologists) often select alternating therapy with MOPP and ABVD in combination with low-dose radiation therapy due to this treatment's high success and a reduction in certain long-term effects potentially associated with treatment for Hodgkin's disease. For example, such combination chemotherapy/radiation therapy may help reduce the risk of potential growth defects in affected children, damage to heart and lung tissue, infertility, or the development of certain secondary malignancies later in life, such as acute myeloid leukemia (AML) or certain solid tumors. Patients should receive ongoing monitoring throughout life to ensure prompt detection and treatment of possible recurrences or secondary malignancies.

See also **General Resources** on page 917

See also **General Resources** on page 917

Government Agencies

4147 NIH/National Cancer Institute
6116 Executive Boulevard, Room 3036A
Bethesda, MD 20892

800-422-6237
www.cancer.gov

The National Cancer Institute coordinates the National Cancer Program, which conducts and supports research, training, health information dissemination, and other programs with respect to the cause, diagnosis, prevention, and treatment of cancer, rehabilitation from cancer, and the continuing care of cancer patients and the families of cancer patients.

John E Niederhuber MD, Director

National Associations & Support Groups

4148 Candlelighters Childhood Cancer Foundation
PO Box 498
Kensington, MD 20895

301-962-3520
800-366-2223
Fax: 310-962-3521
e-mail: staff@candlelighters.org
www.candlelighters.org

The Candlelighters Childhood Cancer Foundation National Office was founded in 1970 by concerned parents of children with cancer. Today our membership of over 50,000 members of the national office and more than 100,000 members across the across the country, including Candlelighters affiliate groups, includes, parents of children who are being treated or have been treated for cancer.

Ruth Hoffman, Executive Director

4149 Leukemia & Lymphoma Society
1311 Mamaroneck Avenue, Suite 310
White Plains, NY 10605

914-949-5213
Fax: 914-949-6691
www.lls.org

Largest voluntary health organization dedicated to funding blood cancer research, education and patient services.

Dwayne Howell PhD, President & CEO
Larry Hausner, Chief Operating Officer

4150 Lymphoma Research Foundation of America California Office
8800 Venice Boulevard, Suite 207
Los Angeles, CA 90034

310-204-7040
800-500-9976
Fax: 310-204-7043
e-mail: LRF@lymphoma.org
www.lymphoma.org

National nonprofit organization dedicated to eradicating lymphoma and serving those touched by this disease. LRF funds research to develop safer, more effective treatments and ultimately, a cure for lymphoma. LRF delivers a comprehensive slate of educational and support programs, services, and publications for lymphoma patients and their loved ones.

Errol M. Cook, President
Evelyn Lipori, VP/Secretary

4151 Lymphoma Research Foundation of America - New York Office
111 Broadway 19th Floor
New York, NY 10006

212-349-2910
800-235-6848
Fax: 212-349-2886
e-mail: LRF@lymphoma.org
www.lymphoma.org

National nonprofit organization dedicated to eradicating lymphoma and serving those touched by this disease. LRF funds research to develop safer, more effective treatments and ultimately, a cure for lymphoma. LRF delivers a comprehensive slate of educational and support programs, services, and publications for lymphoma patients and their loved ones.

Errol M. Cook, President
Evelyn Lipori, VP/Secretary

4152 National Childhood Cancer Foundation
4600 East West Highway, Suite 600
Bethesda, MD 20814

800-458-6223
e-mail: info@curesearch.org
www.curesearch.org

CureSearch unites the world's largest childhood cancer research organization, the Children's Oncology Group, and the National Childhood Cancer Foundation through our mission to cure childhood cancer. Research is the key to the cure.

4153 National Foundation for Cancer Research
4600 East West Highway, Suite 525
Bethesda, MD 20814

301-654-1250
Fax: 301-654-5824
e-mail: info@nfcr.org
www.nfcr.org

The National Foundation for Cancer Research (NFCR) was founded in 1973 to support cancer research and public education relating to the prevention, early diagnosis, better treatments and ultimately, a cure for cancer. NFCR promotes and facilitates collaboration among scientists to accelerate the pace of discovery from bench to bedside.

Web Sites

4154 Children's Cancer Web
www.cancerindex.org/ccw

An independent nonprofit site, established to provide a directory of childhood cancer resources.

Book Publishers

4155 Let's Talk About Going to the Hospital
Rosen Publishing Group's PowerKids Press
29 E 21st Street
New York, NY 10010

213-777-3017
800-237-9932
Fax: 888-436-4643
e-mail: rosenpub@tribeca.ios.com
www.powerkidspress.com

If a child has to check into the hospital, chances are he or she is already upset about being ill. Knowing how a hospital functions and what the procedures are, such as when family members can visit, will help in what is already a stressful situation. Grades K-5.

24 pages
ISBN: 0-823950-36-0

4156 Let's Talk About when Kids Have Cancer
Rosen Publishing Group's PowerKids Press
29 E 21st Street
New York, NY 10010

212-777-3017
800-237-9932
Fax: 888-436-4643
e-mail: customerservice@rosenpub.com
www.powerkidspress.com

In a straightforward yet comforting way, this book explains what cancer is, what kinds of treatments surround the disease and how to cope if a child has cancer.

24 pages
ISBN: 0-823951-95-2

4157 Living with Childhood Cancer: A Practical Guide to Help Families Cope

Leigh A. Woznick, Carol D. Goodheart EdD, author

American Psychological Association
750 1st Street
Washington, DC 20002

202-336-5500
800-374-2721
Fax: 202-336-6123
www.apa.org

This book offers information for families faced with the shattering experience of having a child with cancer.

2001 359 pages Hardcover
ISBN: 1-557988-72-2

4158 Surviving Childhood Cancer: A Guide for Families
New Harbinger Publications
5674 Shattuck Avenue
Oakland, CA 94609

510-652-0215
800-748-6273
Fax: 510-652-5472
e-mail: customerservice@newharbinger.com
newharbinger.com

Cancer in a child is an overwhelming experience for a family. This book explains common medical procedures and offers readers practical advice about how to cope with emotions and stress during this time.

1998 232 pages
ISBN: 1-572241-02-0

4159 You and Your Cancer: A Child's Guide
BC Decker
PO Box 785
Lewiston, NY 14092

905-522-7017
800-568-7281
Fax: 905-522-7839
e-mail: customercare@bcdecker.com
www.bcdecker.com

Covers the different kinds of cancer, hospital stays, treatment, feelings, school, getting help, why some kids die, and recovery.

56 pages
ISBN: 1-550091-47-6

Pamphlets

4160 Hodgkin's Disease and Non-Hodgkin's Lymphomas
Leukemia and Lymphoma Society
1311 Mamaroneck Avenue
White Plains, NY 10605

914-949-5213
800-955-4572
Fax: 914-949-6691
www.leukemia-lymphoma.org

Explanation of the disease, its symptoms, diagnosis, prognosis and treatment, psychological responses to a confirmed diagnosis and current research.

36 pages

DESCRIPTION

4161 HOMOCYSTINURIA

Covers these related disorders: Homocystinuria Type I (Classic homocystinuria), Homocystinuria Type II, Homocystinuria Type III

Involves the following Biologic System(s):
Genetic/Chromosomal/Syndrome/Metabolic Disorders

Homocystinuria is a metabolic disorder characterized by an inborn error in the metabolism of the amino acid methionine. There are three types of homocystinuria, each resulting from a deficiency or defect of a specific enzyme or compound that is essential in the processing of methionine.

Homocystinuria Type I (Classic homocystinuria) is caused by a deficiency of the enzyme cystathionine synthase. Although symptoms and physical findings are not apparent at birth, early symptoms may include delays in development and failure to thrive. Characteristic findings, which are often not apparent until after the age of three years, may include eye abnormalities such as dislocation of the lens of the eyes (ectopia lentis), followed by nearsightedness (myopia) and tremors of the iris (iridodonesis). Other physical findings may include skeletal abnormalities such as osteoporosis, sideways curvature of the spine (scoliosis), either a sunken or prominent chest (pectus deformity), and a condition known as genu valgum in which the legs curve inward causing the knees to touch (knock-knee) and the space between the feet to increase. Affected children often have a fair complexion, blue eyes, sparse blonde hair, and a characteristic flushed face (malar flush). In addition, there is a tendency to develop blood clots (thromboemboli) in the veins and arteries. These clots may occur at any time, and if they lodge in the brain can result in paralysis and seizures heart problems and high blood pressure may also occur. Laboratory findings may include elevated levels of both methionine and the sulfur compound homocystine in body fluids. Mental retardation is apparent in approximately 65 percent of affected people. It is estimated that about 50 percent of patients experience some form of psychiatric disorder.

Treatment for classic homocystinuria includes aggressive vitamin B6 supplementation. In addition, restriction of foods that contain methionine is recommended in conjunction with supplementation of cysteine, also a sulfur-containing amino acid. In some affected individuals who do not respond to vitamin B6 treatment, administration of betaine may be effective. Classic homocystinuria is inherited as an autosomal recessive trait and occurs in approximately one in 200,000 live births. The gene for cystathionine synthase is located on the long arm of chromosome 21 (21q22.3).

Homocystinuria Type II is transmitted as an autosomal recessive trait and results from a defect in the formation of methylcobalamin. Characteristic symptoms and findings depend on the particular underlying defect. Some children with homocystinuria type II may also have a condition called methylmalonic aciduria characterized by excessive methylmalonic acid in the urine. Symptoms usually develop in the early months of life and may include difficulty in feeding, listlessness, vomiting, diminished muscle tone (hypotonia), and delays in development. Treatment for this form of homo stinuria includes vitamin B12 supplementation (cobalamin).

Homocystinuria Type III, a very rare form of the disorder, results from a deficiency of the enzyme methylenetetrahydrofolate reductase (MTHFR), also essential to the maintenance of methionine. Symptoms and physical findings are extremely variable and depend upon the extent of the deficiency. Complete absence of this enzyme may result in life-threatening episodes of respiratory distress as well as seizure-like muscle contractions (myoclonus). A partial enzyme deficiency may cause convulsions, an abnormally small head (microcephaly), mental retardation, and muscular irregularities. Occasional findings may include psychiatric disturbances, abnormalities of certain blood vessels, and inflammation or degenerative changes of specific nerves. In addition, blood clot activity may be apparent in some affected individuals.

Treatment for homocystinuria type III may include supplementation with folic acid, vitamin B6 (pyridoxine), vitamin B12, methionine, and betaine (also known as trimethylglycine). Early intervention with betaine has a particularly effective outcome. Homocystinuria Type III is transmitted as an autosomal recessive trait. The gene for methylenetetrahydrofolate reductase is located on the short arm of chromosome 1 (1p36.3).

See also **General Resources** on page 917

National Associations & Support Groups

4162 ARC of the United States
1010 Wayne Avenue, Suite 650
Silver Spring, MD 20910

301-565-3842
Fax: 301-565-5342
e-mail: info@thearc.org
www.thearc.org

The ARC is the national organization of and for people with mental retardation and related developmental disabilities and their families. Devoted to promoting and improving supports and services for people with mental retardation and their families. The association also fosters research and education regarding the prevention of mental retardation in infants and young children. The ARC was founded in 1950 by a small group of parents and other concerned individuals.

Sue Swenson, Executive Director
Adam Aaronson, Public Inquiries Director

4163 Genetic Alliance
4301 Connecticut Avenue NW
Washington, DC 20008

202-966-5557
800-336-4363
Fax: 202-966-8553
e-mail: info@geneticalliance.org
www.geneticalliance.org

A nonprofit tax exempt organization founded in 1986 as a national coalition of consumers, professionals and genetic support groups to voice the common concerns of children and adults and families living with, and at risk of, genetic conditions. The Alliance builds partnerships among consumers and professionals and the private and public sectors to promote optimum healthcare and enhanced quality of life for individuals identified with genetic conditions.

Sharon Terry, President/CEO

4164 March of Dimes Birth Defects Foundation
1275 Mamaroneck Avenue
White Plains, NY 10605

914-428-7100
888-663-4637
Fax: 914-428-8203
e-mail: resourcecenter@modimes.org
www.marchofdimes.com

Partnership of volunteers and professionals dedicated to improving the health of babies by preventing birth defects and infant mortality. Over 100 chapters are located across the country and can be located through the National Office.

Dr Jennifer Howse, President

Web Sites

4165 ARC of the United States
www.thearc.org

The ARC is the national organization of and for people with mental retardation and related developmental disabilities and their families. Devoted to promoting and improving supports and services for people with mental retardation and their families. The association also fosters research and education regarding the prevention of mental retardation in infants and young children. The ARC was founded in 1950 by a small group of parents and other concerned individuals.

4166 CLIMB: Children Living with Inherited Metabolic Disorders
www.climb.org.uk/

Official website for the organization, committed to fighting metabolic diseases through research, awareness and support, providing advice, information and support on all metabolic diseases to children, young adults, families, carers and professionals. Includes links to other sites.

4167 Genetic Alliance
www.geneticalliance.org

A nonprofit tax exempt organization founded in 1986 as a national coalition of consumers, professionals and genetic support groups to voice the common concerns of children and adults and families living with, and at risk of, genetic conditions. The Alliance builds partnerships among consumers and professionals and the private and public sectors to promote optimum healthcare and enhanced quality of life for individuals identified with genetic conditions.

4168 March of Dimes Birth Defects Foundation
www.marchofdimes.com

Partnership of volunteers and professionals dedicated to improving the health of babies by preventing birth defects and infant mortality. Over 100 chapters are located across the country and can be located through the National Office.

4169 Maryland Department of Health
www.dhmh.state.md.us/cpha

Our mission is to protect, promote and improve the health and well being of all Maryland citizens in a fiscally responsible way.

4170 National Center for Biotechnology Information
www.ncbi.nlm.nih.gov/

A national resource for biology information, the center creates public databases, conducts research in computational biology, develops software tools for analyzing genome data, and disseminated biomedical information, all for the better understanding of molecular processes affecting human health and disease.

4171 Online Mendelian Inheritance in Man
www.ncbi.nlm.nih.gov

This database is a catalog of human genes and genetic disorders.

4172 Rare Genetic Diseases in Children (NYU)
www.med.nyu.edu/rgdc/homenow.htm

We target issues arising from rare genetic diseases affecting children. Also, to assist in the endeavor to bring knowledge and hope to those for whom there is, at present, so little.

4173 Save Babies Through Screening Foundation
www.savebabies.org

Is a national nonprofit public charity run by volunteers. Its mission is to improve the lives of babies by working to prevent disabilities and early death resulting from disorders detectable through newborn screening.

DESCRIPTION

4174 HYDROCEPHALUS

Synonym: Hydrocephaly

Covers these related disorders: Acute hydrocephalus, Occult tension hydrocephalus, Overt tension hydrocephalus, Communicating hydrocephalus, Non-communicating hydrocephalus, Obstructive hydrocephalus, Non-obstructive hydrocephalus

Involves the following Biologic System(s):
Neurologic Disorders

Hydrocephalus is a general term used to describe a group of conditions characterized by the accumulation of cerebrospinal fluid (CSF) around the brain. This fluid, which acts as a protective shock absorber for the brain and spinal cord, flows through the four cavities in the brain (ventricles); through the cavity containing the spinal fluid (spinal canal); and between layers of the membrane that surrounds the brain and spinal cord (subarachnoid space). Obstructed flow or impaired absorption of the CSF results in increasing fluid pressure within the brain. Hydrocephalus is thought to affect approximately one in 500 to 1,500 births. The condition may occur as a result of certain malformations that are present at birth, such as Arnold-Chiari malformation or Dandy-Walker syndrome, certain infectious diseases, head injuries, bleeding within the brain, or certain tumors.

Symptoms associated with hydrocephalus may vary, depending upon the nature of the underlying abnormality, the age of onset, and the rate and duration of increasing pressure within the brain. Hydrocephalus may be apparent at birth (congenital) or develop during the first few months or years of life. Because the fibrous joints of the skull (fontanels) have not fused or completely closed, rapid enlargement of the head may occur. The forehead appears abnormally prominent; the skin over the skull is thin with obvious scalp veins; and the face may appear relatively small. Additional symptoms and findings many include difficulties feeding, irritability, sluggishness, lack of interest in surroundings, lack of normal reflex responses, and downward turning of the eyes. Progression of the condition without treatment may result in extreme drowsiness, episodes of uncontrolled electrical disturbances in the brain (seizures), and potentially life-threatening complications.

In other children, hydrocephalus becomes apparent after the bones of the skull are fused (i.e., after two years of age). Some children may have no apparent symptoms, whereas others may have mild, intermittent, or progressive symptoms. These symptoms may include headaches, easy distractibility, poor memory, and progressively impaired walking and balance. Others may experience an acute form of hydrocephalus in which there is rapidly increasing intracranial pressure, causing severe headache, vomiting, visual disturbances, increasing drowsiness over the period of minutes or hours, potential coma, and possibly life-threatening complications.

Treatment of infants and children with hydrocephalus depends upon the underlying cause of the condition. Therapeutic measures may include use of certain medications, such as acetazolamide and furosemide, which are diuretics ("water pills") that help to reduce the build up of cerebrospinal fluid. Other treatment options may include surgical removal of any obstruction or surgical implantation of a specialized device known as a shunt. Shunts allow excess fluid to drain away from the brain to another part of the body for absorption into the bloodstream. After treatment, many affected children may continue to have associated impairment, such as intellectual deficits, impaired memory, and visual abnormalities. Physicians may regularly monitor affected children and suggest a variety of multidisciplinary measures.

See also **General Resources** on page 917

National Associations & Support Groups

4175 Association of Hydrocephalus Education Advocacy & Discussion (AHEAD)
1730 Autumn Leaf Lane
Huntingdon Valley, PA 19006

215-355-4728

Organized by young adults with hydrocephalus for the purpose of providing telephone support nationwide.

Lane Borden, NE Regional Contact

4176 Birth Defect Research for Children
930 Woodcock Road, Suite 225
Orlando, FL 32803

407-895-0802
Fax: 407-895-0824
e-mail: staff@birthdefects.org
www.birthdefects.org

Organization that helps families with free birth defect information, parent matching that links families of children with similar defects and research through the National Birth Defect Registry to discover the causes of birth defects. Support group information and newsletter on Internet.

Betty Mekdeci, Executive Director

4177 Cerebrospinal Fluid Shunt Systems for the Management of Hydrocephalus
Hydrocephalus Association
870 Market Street, Suite 225
San Fransisco, CA 94102

415-732-7040
888-598-3789
Fax: 415-732-7044
e-mail: info@hydroassoc.org
www.hydroassoc.org

The nations's largest and most repected nonprofit organization devoted exclusively to hydrocepalus. Our office is staffed daily from 10 AM to 4 PM Pacific time. We invite your inquiries.Our mission is to provide support, education and advocacy for individuals, families and professionals.

Russell G. Fudge, President
Dory Kranz, Executive Director

4178 Genetic Alliance
4301 Connecticut Avenue NW
Washington, DC 20008

202-966-5557
800-336-4363
Fax: 202-966-8553
e-mail: info@geneticalliance.org
www.geneticalliance.org

A coalition of voluntary genetic support groups, consumers and professionals addressing the needs of individuals and families affected by genetic disorders from a national perspective.

Sharon Terry, President/CEO

4179 Guardians of Hydrocephalus Research Foundation
2618 Avenue Z
Brooklyn, NY 11235

718-743-4473
800-458-8655
Fax: 718-743-1171
e-mail: GHRF2618@aol.com
www.health.gov

Nonprofit group dedicated to research into the cause and treatment of hydrocephalus. Guardians operate a laboratory in the Department of Neurology at New York University Medical Center, in which information from clinical and research facilities is integrated to provide for better diagnosis and treatment of hydrocephalus, a frequently occuring congenital disorder that can also occur shortly after birth. Hydrocephalus accounts for a large portion of adult patients with a diagnosis of dementia.

Michael Fischette, Founder
Katherine Soriano, National Vice President

4180 Hydrocephalus Association
Hydrocephalus Association
870 Market Street
San Francisco, CA 94102

415-732-7040
888-598-3789
Fax: 415-732-7044
e-mail: info@hydroassoc.org
www.hydroassoc.org

This is the nation's largest and most respected nonprofit organization devoted exclusively to hydrocephalus. We provide support, education and an extensive range of resources to families and professionals dealing with the complex issues of hydrocephalus, the abnormal accumulation of cerebrospinal fluid within the brain. Our resources cover all ages, from prenatal to adult normal pressure hydrocephalus. Our office is staffed daily, we invite your inquiries.

Russell G. Fudge, President
Dory Kranz, Executive Director

4181 Hydrocephalus Foundation
910 Rear Broadway
Saugus, MA 07906

781-942-1161
Fax: 781-231-5250
e-mail: hyfll@nestcape.net
www.hydrocephalus.org

Foundation established to help assist patients and their families during the transition from their diagnosis to a resumption of their normal lifestyles. The primary focus is to contribute emotional support to patients of hydrocephalus and their families.

Greg A. Tocco MIR, Founder/Executive Director

4182 Hydrocephalus Parent Support Group
9425 Sky Park Court, Suite 130
San Diego, CA 92123

619-268-8252
Fax: 619-268-4275
e-mail: cfrc@mail.sdsu.edu

Provides support, information and educatoin for families of children with disabilities and the professionals who assist them.

4183 March of Dimes Birth Defects Foundation
1275 Mamaroneck Avenue
White Plains, NY 10605

914-428-7100
888-663-4637
Fax: 914-428-8203
e-mail: resourcecenter@modimes.org
www.marchofdimes.com

Partnership of volunteers and professionals dedicates to improving the health of babies by preventing birth defects and infant mortality. Over 100 chapters are located across the country and can be located through the National Office.

Dr Jennifer Howse, President

4184 National Foundation for Facial Reconstruction
317 E 34th Street, Room 901
New York, NY 10016

212-263-6656
Fax: 212-263-7534
e-mail: info@nffr.org
www.nffr.org

To enable patients with facial deformities lead productive and fulfilling lives. The NFFR lends its support to the mulidisciplinary craniofacial team at the Institute of Reconstructive Plastic Surgery at NYU Medical Center. An assembly of world-renowned surgeons, mental health professionals, research specialists and staff, give their time and expertise, using the latest techniques.

1951

Whitney Burnett, Executive Director
Michele Golombuski MS, Associate Executive Director

4185 National Hydrocephalus Foundation
12413 Centrailia Road
Lakewood, CA 90715

562-924-6666
888-857-3434
e-mail: hydrobrat@earthlink.net
nhfonline.org

The Foundation is a national organization whose purpose is to provide information and education, along with peer support newsletter quarterly. Group meeting quarterly in Long Beach, CA.

Jim Mazzetti, Founder
Michael Fields, President/Treasurer

State Agencies & Support Groups

Arizona

4186 Injury Prevention Center
Phoenix Children's Hospital
1919 E Thomas Road
Phoenix, AZ 85016

602-546-1000
e-mail: nquay@phxchildrens.com
www.phoenixchildrens.com

Their mission is to promote family-directed care through education and support of children and families with hydrocephalus. Biannual newsletter published, yearly educational conference.

Robert L. Meyer, President/CEO
Sally Moffat, Director Community Outreach

California

4187 Hydrocephalus Parent Support Group
9245 Sky Park Court, Suite 130
San Diego, CA 92123

619-268-8252

Determined to provide support to the parent and relatives of the children stricken with the disorder.

4188 Hydrocephalus Support Group of Southern California
412 N Coast Highway, Suite 131
Laguna Beach, CA 92651

949-551-6865
Fax: 949-497-5518
e-mail: HydroBrat@earthlink.net

This group was formed as a group of concerned families and patients with hydrocephalus to share information and experiences in dealing with this disease, locally and nationwide.

Debbi Fields, Contact

4189 Sacramento Area Hydrocephalus Group
7588 Sylvan Creek Court
Citrus Heights, CA 95610

916-721-9986

The group is divided into age groups for support.
Janet Kirkman

Florida

4190 Hydrocephalus Family Support Group of Central Florida
22 Lake Beauty Drive, Suite 204
Orlando, FL 32806

407-649-7686
Fax: 407-649-7692
e-mail: mrssm1000@aol.com

Their mission is to nurture understanding and increase awareness of hydrocephalus in their community.

Kay Taylor, RN, Pediatric Neurosurgery

Massachusetts

4191 Hydrocephalus Support Group
55 Lake Avenue N
Wooster, MA 01655

617-856-3403

The group in Wooster provides support and education to families in central Massachusetts and southern New Hampshire.

Dorothy Hutchins, Co-Facilitator
Kathleen Davidson

Michigan

4192 Hydrocephalus Support Group
Children's Hospital of Michigan
3901 Beaubien
Detroit, MI 48201

313-833-4490
Fax: 313-993-8744

Provides information to connect parents who have children with hydrocephalus in a mutual support group.

Mary Smellie-Decker RN, MSN, Clinical Nurse Specialist

4193 SW Michican Spina Bifida & Hydrocephalus Association
PO Box 212
Mattawan, MI 49071

269-385-3959
Fax: 269-342-9765

Provides support, education, and advocacy for families with spina bifida and/or hydrocephalus.

Richard Benthin, President

Missouri

4194 Hydrocephalus Support Group
PO Box 4236
Chesterfield, MO 63006

636-532-8228
Fax: 314-251-5871
e-mail: hydrodb@earthlink.com

Nonprofit organization providing education and support to individuals with hydrocephalus and their families.

Debby Buffa, Founder/Chairman

New Jersey

4195 Hydrocephalus Group - Children's Hospital of New Jersey
Children's Hospital of New Jersey
201 Lyons Avenue at Osborne Terrace
Newark, NJ 07112

973-926-7000
Fax: 973-325-2078
e-mail: info@sbhcs.com
www.sbhcs.com

Serves parents of infants and children in the local community and around the state.

Timothy S Yeh MD, FAAP, FAACM, Physician-in-Chief

4196 Hydrocephalus Parents Support Group
329 W Frech Avenue
Manville, NJ 08835

908-722-4691

The group provides support for parents of children with hydrocephalus.

Andrea Liptak, Founder

New York

4197 New York University Medical Center Auxilary of Tisch Hospital
530 1st Avenue
New York, NY 10016

212-263-5040
www.nyukidshealth.org

Conducts national symposiums on hydrocephalus.

Doris Balmer Farrelly, Co-President Auxiliary Medical Ctr

North Carolina

4198 Lipomyelomeningocele Family Support
415 Webster Street
Cary, NC 27511

919-844-2043
Fax: 919-844-2044
e-mail: bborchert@mindspring.com
www.lfsn.org

Providing support services to families and individuals affected by Occult Spinal Dysraphisms.

Bonnie Borchert, Director

Ohio

4199 Cleveland Clinic
9500 Euclid Avenue
Cleveland, OH 44195

216-445-3495
Fax: 216-444-9050
www.clevelandclinic.com

Provides education about hydrocephalus using speakers and parent-to-parent information.

Hilary Rossen LISW, Contact

Oregon

4200 Hydrocephalus Group of Portland
PO Box 2425
Gearhart, OR 97138

503-861-1713
Fax: 503-738-8247
e-mail: cdmorrow@pacifier.com

Education, advocation and research for children and families with hydrocephalus.

Debbie Morrow, Co-President
Cheryl Goeken, President

Pennsylvania

4201 Hydrocephalus Association of Philadelphia
PO Box 2099
Boothwyn, PA 19061

610-497-0375

The Association provides support, information, advocacy and telephone support to families in Pennsylvania, New Jersey, and Delaware.

Rita McAdams, Contact

Rhode Island

4202 Hydrocephalus Association of Rhode Island
PO Box 343
Valley Falls, RI 02864

401-723-6065

The mission of this Association is to provide information, support and advocacy for individuals with hydrocephalus and for friends and family members.

Gabriella Halmi, Director

Texas

4203 Hydrocephalus Association of N Texas
PO Box 670552
Dallas, TX 75367

214-528-2877
Fax: 214-528-8097

The mission is to provide information and support to parents of children with hydrocephalus in the state of Texas and neighboring states.

Jana Dransfield, Director

Washington

4204 Hydrocephalus Support Group of Seattle
2001 Eastlake Avenue E, Suite 1
Seattle, WA 98102

206-324-4084
e-mail: hydropr61@hotmail.com

The group of Seattle provides support to individuals with hydrocephalus.

Kim Anderson, Director

Wisconsin

4205 Fox Valley Hydrocephalus Support Group
W5929 Highway KK
Appleton, WI 54915

920-739-1751

The group provides referrals for parents and information to the community and throughout Wisconsin.

Donna Uitenbroek, Director

Research Centers

4206 New York University Medical Center Auxillary of Tisch Hospital
530 1st Avenue
New York, NY 10016

212-263-5040
www.nyukidshealth.org

Conducts national symposiums on hydrocephalus.

Doris Balmer Farrelly, Co-President Auxillary Medical Ctr

4207 Seeking Techniques Advancing Research in Shunts (STARS)
165 South Opdyke Road, Suite 105
Auburn Hills, MI 48326

313-384-3232
www.star-kids.org

Offers support to patients with hydrocephalus and their families.

Judy Brady, President

Audio Video

4208 Hydrocephalus, a Neglected Disease
Guardians of Hydrocephalus Research Foundation
2618 Avenue Z
Brooklyn, NY 11235

718-748-4473
Fax: 718-743-1171
e-mail: ghrf2618@aol.com
www.ghrf.homestead.com/ghrf

Information on Hydrocephalus.

Michael Fischette, Founder
Katherine Soriano, National Vice President

Web Sites

4209 Beth Israel Medical Center-Hydrocephalus
www.bimc.edu

Is a full tertiary teaching hospital that was originally dedicated to serving a vulnerable population in that community.

4210 Birth Defect Research for Children
www.birthdefects.org

Organization that helps families with free birth defect information, parent matching that links families of children with similar defects and research through the National Birth Defect Registry to discover the causes of birth defects. Support group information and newsletter on Internet.

4211 Guardians of Hydrocephalus Research Foundation
www.health.gov

Nonprofit group dedicated to research into the cause and treatment of hydrocephalus. Guardians operate a laboratory in the Department of Neurology at New York University Medical Center, in which information from clinical and research facilities is integrated to provide for better diagnosis and treatment of hydrocephalus, a frequently occuring congenital disorder that can also occur shortly after birth. Hydrocephalus accounts for a large portion of adult patients with a diagnosis of dementia.

4212 HYCEPH-L
www.geocities.com/HotSprings/Villa/2020/

The purpose of the list is to share information and support in dealing with hydrocephalus.

4213 Hydrocephalus Association
www.hydroassoc.org

Our mission is to provide support, education and advocacy for individuals families and professionals.

4214 Hydrocephalus Facts & Links
omega.nova.org/~twinkee/HydroLinks.htm

Offers information about hydrocephalus.

4215 Hydrocephalus Index
www.bgsm.edu/bgsm/surg-sci/ns/hyceph

Provides links about hydrocephalus.

4216 Hydrocephalus Links
www.ufbi.ufl.edu/~joneslab/hclinks.htm

Offers links about hydrocephalus such as centers, and associations.

4217 Hydrohaven Chat Room
www.geocities.com/HotSprings/Villa/2020/hydrohav

Hydrocephalus support group for patients, family and friends.

4218 National Hydrocephalus Foundation
nhfonline.org

The Foundation is a national organization whose purpose is to provide information and education, along with peer support newsletter quarterly. Group meeting quarterly in Long Beach, CA.

4219 Online Mendelian Inheritance in Man
www.ncbi.nlm.nih.gov

This database is a catalog of human genes and genetic disorders.

4220 Pediatric Neurosurgery-Hydrocephalus
cpmcnet.columbia.edu/dept/nsg/PNS/Hydroc

This site is dedicated to providing families regarding various aspects of the field of pediatric neurosurgery.

4221 Rare Genetic Diseases in Children (NYU)
www.med.nyu.edu/rgdc/homenow.htm

We target issues arising from rare genetic diseases affecting children. Also, to assist in the endeavor to bring knowledge and hope to those for whom there is, at present, so little.

Book Publishers

4222 A Guide to Hydrocephalus
Spina Bifida Association of America
4590 MacArthur Boulevard NW, Suite 250
Washington, DC 20007

202-944-3285
800-621-3141
Fax: 202-944-3295
e-mail: sbaa@sbaa.org
www.sbaa.org

Information to help you understand the circumstances that surround you and make the job of advocacy an easier one.

4223 Congenital Disorders Sourcebook
Omnigraphics
PO Box 625
Holmes, PA 19043

800-234-1340
Fax: 800-875-1340
e-mail: info@omnigraphics.com
www.omnigraphics.com

Basic consumer health information on disorders aquired during gestation, including spina bifida, hydrocephalus, cerebral palsy, heart defects, craniofacial abnormalities and fetal alcohol syndrome.

650 pages
ISBN: 0-780809-45-9

4224 Hydrocephalus: A Guide for Patients, Families, and Friends

Chuck Toporek, Kellie Robinson, author

O'Reilly & Associates
1005 Gravenstein Highway N
Sebastopol, CA 95472

707-827-7000
800-998-9938
Fax: 707-829-0104
e-mail: patientguides@oreilly.com
www.patientcenters.com

This book educates families so they can select a skilled neurosurgeon, understand treatments, participate in care and know what symptoms need attention, keep records needed for follow-up treatments and make wise lifestyle choices.

1999 377 pages Softcover
ISBN: 1-565924-10-X

4225 Loving Ben

Elizabeth Laird, author

Delacorte
1540 Broadway
New York, NY 10036

212-354-6500

This is a moving story of a sister who cares for her baby brother and tries to help him learn despite his birth defects and deteriorating health.

Grade 5-9 Hardcover
ISBN: 0-385298-10-2

4226 Spina Bifida Association of America Insights into Spina Bifida
Spina Bifida Association of America
4590 MacArthur Boulevard NW, Suite 250
Washington, DC 20007

202-944-3285
800-621-3141
Fax: 202-944-3295
e-mail: sbaa@sbaa.org
www.sbaa.org

News on medical, legislative and education topics relevant to individuals with spina bifida

Bimonthly

Marybeth Leamyini, Communications Director

Newsletters

4227 G. Advocacy
Genetic Alliance
4301 Connecticut Avenue NW, Suite 404
Washington, DC 20008

202-966-5557
800-336-4363
Fax: 202-966-8553
e-mail: info@geneticalliance.org
www.geneticalliance.org

Our e-newsletter features news about upcoming events, spotlights member organizations, and keeps you informed about legislation before Congress. We welcome your feedback on articles and suggestions on future topics.

Sharon F. Terry MA, President/CEO
Lisa Wise MA, Vice President

4228 Hydrocephalus Association Newsletter
Hydrocephalus Association
870 Market Street Suite 705
San Francisco, CA 94102

415-732-7040
888-598-3789
Fax: 415-732-7044
e-mail: info@hydroassoc.org
www.hydroassoc.org

Offers information on association news, conference articles, meetings, support and educational groups.

12 pages Quarterly

Russell G. Fudge, President
Dory Kranz, Executive Director

4229 Hydrocephalus Parents Support Group Newsletter
1325 Louis Street
Manville, NJ 08835

908-722-4691

The group provides support for parents of children with hydrocephalus.

Andrea Liptak, Founder

4230 Hydrocephalus Support Group Newsletter
PO Box 4236
Chesterfield, MO 63006

314-532-8228
Fax: 314-995-4108
e-mail: hydro@inlink.com

This group provides information, education and support to anyone dealing with hydrocephalus.

quaterly

Debby Buffa, Founder/Chairman

4231 LINK
Hydrocephalus Association
870 Market Street, Suite 705
San Francisco, CA 94102

415-732-7040
888-598-3789
Fax: 415-732-7044
e-mail: info@hydroassoc.org
www.hydroassoc.org

Provides members with direct access to other families and individuals coping with the complexities of hydrocephalus with the goal being to develop a nationwide network of individuals supporting one another, sharing information and strategies which enable them to become educated and empowered advocates.

12 pages Quarterly

Russell G. Fudge, President
Dory Kranz, Executive Director

4232 National Hydrocephalus Foundation Newsletter
12413 Centrailia Road
Lakewood, CA 90715

562-924-6666
888-598-3434
Fax: 415-732-7044
e-mail: hydrobrat@earthlink.net
www.nhfonline.org

The Foundation is a national organization whose purpose is to provide information and education, along with peer support newsletter quarterly. Group meeting quarterly in Long Beach, CA.

12-15 pages Quarterly

Michael Fields, President/Treasurer
Debbi Fields, Executive Director

4233 Update
Spina Bifida and Hydrocephalus Association/Canada
977-167 Lombard Avenue
Winnipeg,
Canada

204-925-3650
800-565-9488
Fax: 204-925-3654
e-mail: spinab@mts.net
www.sbhac.ca

Newsletter dedicated to improving the quality of life of individuals with spina bifida and/or hydrocephalus and their families.

4 pages Quarterly

Lorelei Fletcher, President
Gene Layton, Vice President

Pamphlets

4234 About Hydrocephalus - Book for Families
Hydrocephalus Association
870 Market Street, Suite 705
San Francisco, CA 94102

415-732-7040
888-598-3789
Fax: 415-732-7044
e-mail: info@hydroassoc.org
www.hydroassoc.org

Booklet in either English or Spanish, detailing all aspects of hydrocephalus from diagnosis and treatment to complications and follow-up care.

36 pages Paperback

Russell G. Fudge, President
Dory Kranz, Executive Director

4235 Cephalic Disorders Fact Sheet
National Inst. of Neurological Disorders/Stroke
PO Box 5801
Bethesda, MD 20824

301-496-5751
800-352-9424
www.ninds.nih.gov

Fact sheet indexing the following: What are Cephalic Disorders?, What are the Different Kinds of Cephalic Disorders?, What are Other Less Common Cephalics?, What Research is Being Done?, Where Can I Get More Information?.

Story C. Landis PhD, Director
Audrey S. Penn MD, Deputy Director

4236 Cerebrospinal Fluid Shunt Systems for the Management of Hydrocephalus
Hydrocephalus Association
870 Market Street, Suite 705
San Francisco, CA 94102

415-732-7040
888-598-3789
Fax: 415-732-7044
e-mail: info@hydroassoc.org
www.hydroassoc.org

Our resources cover hydrocephalus in all age groups from prenatal diagnosis to adult normal pressure hydrocephalus. Our office is staffed daily from 10 AM to 4 PM Pacific time. We invite your inquiries.

Russell G. Fudge, President
Dory Kranz, Executive Director

4237 Directory of Pediatric Neurosurgeons
Hydrocephalus Association
870 Market Street, Suite 705
San Francisco, CA 94102

415-732-7040
888-598-3789
Fax: 415-732-7044
e-mail: info@hydroassoc.org
www.hydroassoc.org

Names and addresses of more than 200 neurosurgeons who specialize in pediatrics, listed alphabetically and geographically.

Russell G. Fudge, President
Dory Kranz, Executive Director

4238 Durable Power of Attorney for Health Care Decisions
Hydrocephalus Association
870 Market Street, Suite 705
San Francisco, CA 94102

415-732-7040
888-598-3789
Fax: 415-732-7044
e-mail: info@hydroassoc.org
www.hydroassoc.org

Provided by The Hydrocephalus Association. Our resources cover hydrocephalus in all age groups from prenatal diagnosis to adult normal pressure hydrocepahlus. Our office is staffed daily from 10 AM to 4 PM Pacific time. We invite your inquiries.

Russell G. Fudge, President
Dory Kranz, Executive Director

4239 Endoscopic Third Ventriculoscopy
Hydrocephalus Association
870 Market Street, Suite 705
San Francisco, CA 94102

415-732-7040
888-598-3789
Fax: 415-732-7044
e-mail: info@hydroassoc.org
www.hydroassoc.org

Provided by the Hydrocephalus Association. Our resources cover all age groups from prenatal diagnosis through normal pressure hydrocephalus in older adults. Our office is staffed daily from 10 AM to 4 PM Pacific time. We invite your inquiries.

Russell G. Fudge, President
Dory Kranz, Executive Director

4240 Eye Problems Associated with Hydrocephalus in Children
Hydrocephalus Association
870 Market Street, Suite 705
San Francisco, CA 94102

415-732-7040
888-598-3789
Fax: 415-732-7044
e-mail: info@hydroassoc.org
www.hydroassoc.org

Provided by the Hydrocephalus Association. Our resources cover all age groups from prenatal diagnosis to normal pressure hydrocephalus in older adults. Our office is staffed daily from 10 AM to 4 PM Pacific time. We invite your inquiries.

Russell G. Fudge, President
Dory Kranz, Executive Directory

4241 Fact Sheet: Hydrocephalus
Hydrocephalus Association
870 Market Street, Suite 705
San Francisco, CA 94102

415-732-7040
888-598-3789
Fax: 415-732-7044
e-mail: info@hydroassoc.org
www.hydroassoc.org

Also available in Spanish, provided by the Hydrocephalus Association. Our resources cover all age groups from prenatal diagnosis to normal pressure hydrocephalus in older adults. Our office is staffed daily from 10 AM to 4 PM Pacific time. We invite your inquiries.

Russell G. Fudge, President
Dory Kranz, Executive Director

4242 Fact Sheet: Syringomyelia
National Inst. of Neurological Disorders/Stroke
6001 Executive Boulevard, Suite 3309
Bethesda, MD 20892

301-496-5751
800-352-9424

Provided by the Hydrocephalus Association. Our resources cover all age groups, from prenatal diagnosis to normal pressure hydrocephalus in older adults. We welcome your inquiries.

Story C. Landis PhD, Director
Audrey S. Penn MD, Deputy Director

4243 Headaches and Hydrocephalus
Hydrocephalus Association
870 Market Street, Suite 705
San Francisco, CA 94102

415-732-7040
888-598-3789
Fax: 415-732-7044
e-mail: info@hydroassoc.org
www.hydroassoc.org

Causes and tips for headache relief unique to hydrocephalus.

Russell G. Fudge, President
Dory Kranz, Executive Director

4244 Hospitalization Tips
Hydrocephalus Association
870 Market Street, Suite 705
San Francisco, CA 94102

415-732-7040
888-598-3789
Fax: 415-732-7044
e-mail: info@hydroassoc.org
www.hydroassoc.org

Provided by the Hydrocephalus Association. Our resources cover all age groups, from prenatal diagnosis, to normal pressure hydrocephalus in older adults. Our office is staffed daily from 10 AM to 4 PM, Pacific time. We welcome your inquiries.

1997

Russell G. Fudge, Director
Dory Kranz, Deputy Director

4245 How to be an Assertive Member of the Treatment Team
Hydrocephalus Association
870 Market Street, Suite 705
San Francisco, CA 94102

415-732-7040
888-598-3789
Fax: 415-732-7044
e-mail: info@hydroassoc.org
www.hydroassoc.org

Hydrocephalus information to ask involved treatment questions.

Russell G. Fudge, President
Dory Kranz, Executive Director

4246 How to be an Assertive Parent on the Treatment Team
Hydrocephalus Association
870 Market Street, Suite 705
San Francisco, CA 94102

415-732-7040
888-598-3789
Fax: 415-732-7044
e-mail: info@hydroassoc.org
www.hydroassoc.org

4247 Hydrocephalus
Hydrocephalus Association
870 Market Street, Suite 705
San Francisco, CA 94102

415-732-7040
888-598-3789
Fax: 415-732-7044
e-mail: info@hydroassoc.org
www.hydroassoc.org

4248 Hydrocephalus Association Survey Results/ FDA Presentation on Shunt Technology
Hydrocephalus Association
870 Market Street, Suite 705
San Francisco, CA 94102

415-732-7040
888-598-3789
Fax: 415-732-7044
e-mail: info@hydroassoc.org
www.hydroassoc.org

4249 Hydrocephalus: Fact Sheet
National Inst. of Neurological Disorders/Stroke
PO Box 5801
Bethesda, MD 20824

301-496-5751
800-352-9424
www.ninds.nih.gov

Our fact sheet covers all age groups, from prenatal diagnosis to normal pressure hydrocephalus in older adults. Also available in Spanish.

Story C. Landis PhD, Director
Audrey S. Penn MD, Deputy Director

4250 ID Card for Third Ventriculostomy Patients
Hydrocephalus Association
870 Market Street, Suite 705
San Francisco, CA 94102

415-732-7040
Fax: 415-732-7044
e-mail: hydroassoc@aol.com
www.hydroassoc.org

Patients with hydrocephalus managed by an ETV may request a free patient ID card from the Hydrocephaus Association. This card idenifies them as patients with hydrocephalus being managed by this procedure.

Russell G. Fudge, President
Dory Kranz, Executive Director

4251 Individualized Education Program (IEP) - Communication Skills for Parents
Hydrocephalus Association
870 Market Street, Suite 705
San Francisco, CA 94102

415-732-7040
888-598-3789
Fax: 415-732-7044
e-mail: info@hydroassoc.org
www.hydroassoc.org

Is a written education plan that describes the special education and related services a student will receive.

Russell G. Fudge, President
Dory Kranz, Executive Director

4252 LINK Directory Information
Hydrocephalus Association
870 Market Street, Suite 705
San Francisco, CA 94102

415-732-7040
888-598-3789
Fax: 415-732-7044
e-mail: info@hydroassoc.org
www.hydroassoc.org

A nationwide network of individuals listed in Directory format giving members direct access to others in similar circumstances.

Russell G. Fudge, President
Dory Kranz, Executive Director

4253 Learning Disabilities in Children with Hydrocephalus
Hydrocephalus Association
870 Market Street, Suite 705
San Francisco, CA 94102

415-732-7040
888-598-3789
Fax: 415-732-7044
e-mail: info@hydroassoc.org
www.hydroassoc.org

Also available in Spanish and English. Our offices are staffed daily from 10 AM to 4 PM, Pacific time. We welcome your inquiries.

Russell G. Fudge, President
Dory Kranz, Executive Director

4254 National Directory of Hydrocephalus Support Groups
Hydrocephalus Association
870 Market Street, Suite 705
San Francisco, CA 94102

415-732-7040
888-598-3789
Fax: 415-732-7044
e-mail: info@hydroassoc.org
www.hydroassoc.org

The Directory lists information on 16 hydrocephalus groups nationwide.

Russell G. Fudge, President
Dory Kranz, Executive Director

4255 Nonverbal Learning Disorder Syndrome
Hydrocephalus Association
870 Market Street, Suite 705
San Francisco, CA 94102

415-732-7040
888-598-3789
Fax: 415-732-7044
e-mail: info@hydroassoc.org
www.hydroassoc.org

Is a specific type of learning disability that affect's children's academic progress as well as their social and emotional development. This specific type of learning disability has been identified in some children with Hydrocephalus.

Russell G. Fudge, President
Dory Kranz, Executive Director

4256 Prenatal Hydrocephalus-Book for Parents
Hydrocephalus Association
870 Market Street, Suite 705
San Fransisco, CA 94102

415-732-7040
888-598-3789
Fax: 415-732-7044
e-mail: info@hydroassoc.org
www.hydroassoc.org

Provides information about the diagnosis of prenatal-onset hydrocephalus.

16 pages

Russell G. Fudge, President
Dory Kranz, Executive Director

4257 Preparing Your Child for Surgery
Hydrocephalus Association
870 Market Street, Suite 705
San Francisco, CA 94102

415-732-7040
888-598-3789
Fax: 415-732-7044
e-mail: info@hydroassoc.org
www.hydroassoc.org

Provided by The Hydrocephalus Association the nation's largest and most respected nonprofit organization devoted exclusively to hydrocephalus. Our offices are staffed daily from 10 AM to 4 PM, Pacific time. We welcome your inquiries.

4258 Primary Care Needs of Children with Hydrocephalus

Hydrocephalus Association
870 Market Street, Suite 705
San Francisco, CA 94102

415-732-7040
888-598-3789
Fax: 415-732-7044
e-mail: info@hydroassoc.org
www.hydroassoc.org

Our office is staffed daily from 10 AM to 4 PM Pacific time. We welcome your inquiries.

28 pages

Russell G. Fudge, President
Dory Kranz, Executive Director

4259 Resource Guide

Hydrocephalus Association
870 Market Street, Suite 705
San Francisco, CA 94102

415-732-7040
888-598-3789
Fax: 415-732-7044
e-mail: info@hydroassoc.org
www.hydroassoc.org

A comprehensive listing of 450 articles on all aspects of hydrocephalus. Articles may be ordered from the Association for a small fee.

Russell G. Fudge, President
Dory Kranz, Executive Director

4260 Social Skills Development in Children with Hydrocephalus

Hydrocephalus Association
870 Market Street, Suite 705
San Francisco, CA 94102

415-732-7040
Fax: 415-732-7044
e-mail: info@hydroassoc.org
www.hydroassoc.org

Russell G. Fudge, President
Dory Kranz, Executive Director

4261 Survival Skills for the Family Unit

Hydrocephalus Association
870 Market Street, Suite 705
San Francisco, CA 94102

415-732-7040
888-598-3789
Fax: 415-732-7044
e-mail: info@hydroassoc.org
www.hydroassoc.org

Our resources cover hydrocepahlus in all age groups from prenatal diagnosis through normal pressure hydrocephalus in older adults.

Russell G. Fudge, President
Dory Kranz, Executive Director

4262 Understanding Your Child's Education Needs /Individualized Education Program Packet

Hydrocephalus Association
870 Market Street, Suite 705
San Francisco, CA 94102

415-732-7040
888-598-3789
Fax: 415-732-7044
e-mail: info@hydroassoc.org
www.hydroassoc.org

From the Hydrocephalus Association the nations largest nonprofit group devoted exclusively to this disorder. Our offices are staffed

daily from 10 AM to 4 PM, Pacific time. We welcome your inquiries.

Russell G. Fudge, President
Dory Kranz, Executive Director

DESCRIPTION

4263 HYPERTROPHIC CARDIOMYOPATHY
Involves the following Biologic System(s):
Cardiovascular Disorders

Hypertrophic cardiomyopathy is a genetic disease that occurs because of mutations in the contraction mechanisms in the muscles of the heart. Because of this genetic abnormality, the heart muscle fibers are arranged in a disorganized fashion. This leads to enlargement of the left ventricular muscle (hypertrophy). This hypertrophic muscle may lead to variable amounts of obstruction of blood flow out of the heart into the general circulation and a spectrum of clinical manifestations. There have been several genes that have been found to be abnormal in patients with hypertrophic cardiomyopathy. Depending on the different genetic abnormality there may be different clinical findings ranging from no symptomatology to severe disease.

Hypertrophic cardiomyopathy is most commonly inherited in an autosomal dominant pattern, meaning that a child inherits a copy of the gene from one of his or her parents.aAs a result, the majority of children and adolescents who are diagnosed with the disease have a parent who also suffers from the entity. Sporadic cases are also well documented where neither parent has the disease but the child has the disease. It is presumed that in these cases, there has been a spontaneous mutation in the gene in the earliest stages of embryonic development.

Hypertrophic cardiomyopathy may become clinically evident at any time during the first two decades of life, though typically it is not diagnosed until the adolescent years. It is important to note that the hypertrophic changes that are the hallmark of the disease may not develop until as late as the teens or early twenties. As a result, in families where a parent has the disease, children should undergo repeated interval examination by a pediatric cardiologist through their adolescence.

The diagnosis is hypertrophic cardiomyopathy relies heavily on good history taking from the primary care provider. There are several important questions to ask in order to assess for risk. A family history should be taken, asking about unexplained deaths, family members with frequent episodes of fainting, or cardiac arrhythmia (abnormal heart rhythm). Patients should be questioned about episodes of shortness of breath (dyspnea) and chest pain. Any recent change in exercise tolerance should be evaluated closely. Additionally, a known history of family members with doc-umented hypertrophic cardiomyopathy should raise the concern of disease in other family members.

There are many patients with hypertrophic cardiomyopathy who are largely asymptomatic. When patients are symptomatic they usually exhibit a slow decline in function. Often, patients may not experience symptoms until they exert themselves. Symptoms may consist of shortness of breath with exertion or when lying down, chest pain, fainting (syncope) or lightheadedness, palpitations (racing heart), and fatigue. Although it is agreed that the thickened left ventricular muscle may cause some obstruction to blood flow out of the aora (the main blood vessel leading from the left side of the heart to the general circulation), this is not the only mechanism causing symptoms. In fact, there are some patients with a great deal of obstruction who have minimal symptoms, while other patients with minimal obstruction may have severe symptoms. Patients may also experience some of the above symptoms from decreased functioning of the heart muscle itself, or arrhythmia.

Hypertrophic cardiomyopathy is the most common cause of sudden death in young athletes who die during sports; clearly those individuals with HCM should be restricted from participating in sports.

The physical exam of patients with hypertrophic cardiomyopathy may be normal if there is no significant obstruction to blood flow. In some patients, findings may include a fourth heart sound or a systolic murmur heard best at the left lower sternal border. This murmur is often heard more easily during maneuvers that increase the amount of resistance in the body's tissues from muscular contraction, for example, when patients stand up after a sitting or squatting position, or when patients bear down (Valsalva maneuver). Additional findings may include increased carotid pulses, increased force of the heart beat felt near the left lower sternum or axilla (parasternal lift).

Patients with suspected hypertrophic cardiomyopathy should be referred to a pediatric cardiologist for further testing, which may consist of an echocardiogram (ultrasound imaging of the heart), electrocardiogram and perhaps an exercise stress test.

Treatment options are varied. Medical management may be difficult and surgical or catheter interventions may be recommended to decrease the amount of obstructing tissue in the heart. Mainstays of medical treatment include calcium channel blockers, beta blockers, and anti-arrhythmics. Most recently, the use of implantable defribrillators (small pacemaker-like devices that correct severe heart arrhythmias) have become common. It is critical that patients with confirmed hypertrophic cardiomyopathy be restricted from playing competitive sports. Additionally, patients should receive prophylactic antibiotics for prevention of endocarditis before dental or invasive procedures.

See also **General Resources** on page 917

See also **General Resources** on page 917

National Associations & Support Groups

4264 American Heart Association
7272 Greenville Avenue
Dallas, TX 75231

214-373-6300
800-242-8721
Fax: 214-706-1341
e-mail: inquire@amhrt.org
www.amhrt.org

Supports research, education and community service programs with the objective of reducing premature death and disability from cardiovascular diseases and stroke; coordinates the efforts of health professionals, and others engaged in the fight against heart and circulatory disease.

M Cass Wheeler, CEO

4265 Hypertrophic Cardiomyopathy Association
328 Green Pond Road, PO Box 306
Hibernia, NJ 07842

973-983-7429
Fax: 973-983-7870
e-mail: support@4hcm.us
www.4hcm.org/WCMS/

A not-for-profit organization that provides information, support and advocacy to patients, their families and medical providers.

Lisa Salberg, Founder & President

4266 March of Dimes Birth Defects Foundation
1275 Mamaroneck Avenue
White Plains, NY 10605

914-428-7100
888-663-4637
Fax: 914-428-8203
e-mail: resourcecenter@modimes.org
www.marchofdimes.com

Partnership of volunteers and professionals dedicated to improving the health of babies by preventing birth defects and infant mortality. Over 100 chapters are located across the country and can be located through the National Office.

Dr Jennifer Howse, President

Research Centers

4267 Hypertrophic Cardiomyopathy Program at St. Luke's-Roosevelt Hospital Center
University Medical Practice Associates
425 W 59th Street, Suite 8A
New York, NY 10019

212-523-7372
Fax: 212-523-7765
www.hcmny.org

We offer comprehensive diagnostic evaluation, a range of treatments and screening for relatives of affected patients.

Mark V Sherrid MD FACC FASE, Director

Web Sites

4268 American Heart Association
www.amhrt.org

Supports research, education and community service programs with the objective of reducing premature death and disability from cardiovascular diseases and stroke; coordinates the efforts of health professionals, and others engaged in the fight against heart and circulatory disease.

4269 Hypertrophic Cardiomyopathy Association
www.4hcm.org/WCMS/

A not-for-profit organization that provides information, support and advocacy to patients, their families and medical providers.

4270 Hypertrophic Cardiomyopathy: Heart Center Online for Patients
www.heartcenteronline.com

The mission of the HeartCenterOnline is to give our premier cardiovascular patients, their families and other site visiors with the tools they need to better understand the complex nature of heart-related conditions, treatments and preventive care, and to provide services and applications that deliver value to cardiovascular practices.

4271 Implantable Defibrillators in Preventing Sudden Death
www.findarticles.com

Article from American Family Physician magazine. Search by article name.

4272 MEDLINEplus
www.nlm.nih.gov/medlineplus/ency/article/000192.htm

MedlinePlus has extensive information from the National Institutes of Health and other trusted sources on over 650 diseases and conditions. There are also lists of hospitals and physicians, a medical encyclopedia and a medical dictionary, health information in Spanish, extensive information on perscription and nonperscription drugs, health information from the media and links to thousands of clinical trials.

4273 March of Dimes Birth Defects Foundation
www.marchofdimes.com

Partnership of volunteers and professionals dedicated to improving the health of babies by preventing birth defects and infant mortality. Over 100 chapters are located across the country and can be located through the National Office.

4274 Sudden Death of Young Athletes Can Be Prevented (Hypertrophic Cardiomyopathy)
www.findarticles.com

Article from USA Today. Search by article name.

Book Publishers

4275 Let's Talk About Going to the Hospital
Rosen Publishing Group's PowerKids Press
29 E 21st Street
New York, NY 10010

212-777-3017
800-237-9932
Fax: 888-436-4643
e-mail: rosenpub@tribeca.ios.com
www.powerkidspress.com

If a child has to check into the hospital, chances are he or she is already upset about being ill. Knowing how a hospital functions and what the procedures are, such as when family members can visit, will help in what is already a stressful situation. Grades K-5.

24 pages
ISBN: 0-823950-36-0

Newsletters

4276 HCMA - Heart Link Online
Hypertrophic Cardiomyopathy Association
328 Green Pond Road, PO Box 306
Hibernia, NJ 07842

973-983-7429
Fax: 973-983-7870
e-mail: support@4hcm.us
www.4hcm.org/WCMS/

A newsletter that provides information, support and advocacy to
patients, their families and medical providers.

DESCRIPTION

4277 HYPOPLASTIC LEFT HEART SYNDROME

Synonym: HLHS

Involves the following Biologic System(s):

Cardiovascular Disorders

Hypoplastic Left Heart Syndrome, also referred to as HLHS, is a severe and complex form of congenital heart disease, wherein the entire left side of the heart is underdeveloped and unable to pump blood to the body. Classically, this involves underdevelopment (hypoplasia) of the: 1). mitral valve, which connects the left atrium to the left ventricle, 2). left ventricle, which is the pumping chamber that delivers oxygenated blood to the body and 3). aortic valve and aorta, the valve and blood vessel, respectively, which carry oxygenated blood from the left ventricle to the organs and the tissues of the body.

Hypoplastic Left Heart Syndrome is the 4th most common congenital heart disorder diagnosed in the first year of life and almost always in the first few days of life. Typically, infants with HLHS are full term and tend to have normal birth weights and few non-cardiac defects. In those born with the disorder, males out number female. The cause of this HLHS remains unclear, but like many of the congenital heart diseases, it likely develops in most pregnancies early in the first trimester and may very well have a genetic component.

Because of the underdevelopment of the left side of the heart, infants born with Hypoplastic Left Heart Syndrome become gravely ill soon after birth. In the fetus, a specialized blood vessel, known as the ductus arteriosus, connects the aorta and the pulmonary artery. In normal fetal heart structure, the ductus arteriosus allows the deoxy genated (blue) blood pumped by the right ventricle to the pulmonary artery to avoid going to the lungs (which in the fetus are non-functioning and filled with fluid), delivering it to the placenta for oxygenation. After birth the lungs are inflated with air and the ductus arteriosus, which is no longer necessary, begins to undergo a natural closure process. In the infant with Hypoplastic Left Heart Syndrome, the ductus arteriosus is the only source of blood flow into the aorta, as the left heart is unable to pump adequate (if any) blood forward and, therefore, crucial to the survival of the infant; without it, inadequate blood flow to the organs and tissues leads to shock. Prior to the advent of specialized medications, such as prostaglandins, that prevent the closing process of the ductus arteriosus, patients with Hypoplastic Left Heart Syndrome would not be able to survive when the ductus underwent its natural closure.

Over the last two decades, congenital heart surgery techniques have been developed to surgically alter the path of blood leaving the right heart. Surgery for Hypoplastic Left Heart Syndrome typically involves three separate operations, the first being the most difficult and complicated, occurring in the first week or two of life. The second operation usually occurs between 4 and 6 months of life and the third may be undertaken between 18 and 36 months. Alternatively, some pediatric cardiac centers have promoted heart transplant for the patient with Hypoplastic Left Heart Syndrome. Children with Hypoplastic Left Heart Syndrome require lifelong follow-up by a cardiologist for repeated checks of how their heart is working. Virtually all the children will require heart medicines. They also risk infection on the heart's valves (endocarditis) and will need antibiotics, such as amoxicillin, before dental work and certain surgeries to help prevent endocarditis.

See also **General Resources** on page 917

National Associations & Support Groups

4278 Cincinnati Children's Hospital Medical Center
3333 Burnet Avenue
Cincinnati, OH 45229

513-636-4200
800-344-2462
TTY: 513-636-4900
www.cincinnatichildrens.org

Cincinnati Children's Heart Center is dedicated to serving the cardiac care needs of patients, fetus through young adult, and their families in a convenient, compassionate and high quality manner. The Heart Center is committed to providing research and teaching programs in an enviroment characterized by intergrity, innovation, excellence, and respect.

Lee A Carter, Chairman
James M Anderson, President & CEO

4279 Congenital Heart Information Network
600 North 3rd Street, First Floor
Philadelphia, PA 19123

215-627-4034
Fax: 215-627-4036
e-mail: mb@tchin.org
http://tchin.org

An international organization that provides reliable information, support services and resources to families of children with congenital heart defects and acquired heart disease, adults with congenital heart defects, and the professionals who work with them.

Mano Barmash, President

State Agencies & Support Groups

Arizona

4280 Arizona HeartLight
University Medical Center
1501 N Campbell Avenue, PO Box 245073
Tucson, AZ 85724
520-250-6252

Katie Desiato, Contact

4281 HeartLight
1501 N Campbell Avenue, PO Box 245073
Tucson, AZ 85724
520-250-6252

Katie Desiato, Contact

Colorado

4282 Cardiac Kids/Association of Volunteers
1056 E 19th Avenue, PO Box 465
Denver, CO 80218
303-861-6607
e-mail: abbbybee@msn.com

Florida

4283 Pediatric Heart Foundation
PO Box 540354
Lake Worth, FL 33454
561-738-4554
e-mail: phfheart@aol.com

Laurie Bernat, Contact

Georgia

4284 Heart to Heart
6322 Millbrance Road
Columbus, GA 31907
706-563-3112

Hawaii

4285 Kardiac Kids
C/O Kapi'olani Medical Center for Women & Children
1319 Punahou Street
Honolulu, HI 96826
808-983-8166

Lisa Rohr RN, Contact

Illinois

4286 Chilren's Heart Services
PO Box 8275
Bartlett, IL 60103
630-415-0282
e-mail: CHILDHRTSVC@aol.com

4287 Heart of the Matter
20128 Westport Drive
Frankfort, IL 60423
815-469-9146
e-mail: CT875@aol.com

Indiana

4288 Our Hearts
1738 N Shortridge Road
Indianapolis, IN 46219
317-322-1017
e-mail: ourhearts@iquest.net

Massachusetts

4289 Heart to Heart Fund
750 Washington Street, Suite 313
Boston, MA 02111
617-636-8101
e-mail: info@heart2heartfund.org

Michigan

4290 Families at Heart
100 Michigan Ave, MC117
Grand Rapids, MI 49503
616-391-8707

Gwen Fosse, Contact

Minnesota

4291 Parents For Heart of Minnesota
Attention: 32-P190
2525 Chicgo Avenue S
Minneapolis, MN 55404

Celeste Gebauer, Contact

Missouri

4292 Heart to Heart - St. Louis
St Louis Children's Hospital
One Children's Place
St Louis, MO 63110
314-577-5600

Elaine Wear, Contact
Nan Winters, Contact

New Hampshire

4293 Families with Heart
824 High Street
Candia, NH 03034
603-483-3025

Laura Briggs, Contact

4294 New Hampshire Families with Heart
824 High Street
Candia, NH 03034
603-483-3025

Laura Briggs, Contact

New Jersey

4295 Young Hearts
791 Fredrick Court
Wyckoff, NJ 07481
201-848-9608

Barbara Mcfadden, Contact

New York

4296 Big Hearts for Little Hearts
34 Sintsink Drive West
Port Washington, NY 11050
516-883-4080

Ruth Maszrik, Contact

4297 Cardiac Kids
PO Box 154
Fishkill, NY 12524
845-896-7321

Cindy-Jean Dennis, Contact

4298 Helping Hearts
601 Elmwood Avenue, PO Box 631
Rochester, NY 14642
716-275-6108
e-mail: info@helpinghearts.org

North Carolina

4299 Bless Their Hearts
PO Box 1072
Waxhaw, NC 28173
336-838-8298

Sara Szekely, Contact

Ohio

4300 Healing Hearts
1 Perkins Square
Akron, OH 44308

330-543-4325
866-230-3463
e-mail: flemings249@aol.com

Provides participants with an opportunity to share their emotions and concerns.

Katie Fleming, Contact

Pennsylvania

4301 Fontan Friends
482 Reginald Lane
Collegeville, PA 19426

610-831-9878

Barbara Lewis, Contact

South Dakota

4302 Thumpers
HC 58, Box 26
Fairburn, SD 57738

605-255-4377
e-mail: clsogge@cs.com

Tammy Sogge, Contact

Tennessee

4303 Tennessee Saving Little Hearts
2629 Barineau Lane
Knoxville, TN 37920

865-748-4650
e-mail: info@savinglittlehearts.com

Provides emotional assistance, educational information, and fun experiences for children that will help them build friendship and confidence.

Karen Coulter, President
Brad Coulter, Vice President

Texas

4304 Heart to Heart
PO Box 595
Colleyville, TX 70634

888-475-2787

Sally Pearson, Contact

4305 Jacob's Heart
3622 Indian Forest
Spring, TX 77373

281-250-1635
e-mail: TGart65885@aol.com

Jamie Garter, Contact

4306 Texas Heart to Heart
PO Box 595
Colleyville, TX 76034

888-475-2787
www.heart-to-heart-tx.org

Offering hope, education, and support to families.

Sally Pearson, Contact

Vermont

4307 Heart to Heart
60 Maple Ridge Road
Underhill, VT 05489

802-899-3798
e-mail: LamaDiaz@aol.com

Julianne Nickerson, Contact

Virginia

4308 Precious Hearts
144 Locust Avenue
Winchester, VA 22601

540-678-0654
e-mail: hurlbutK@aol.com

Washington

4309 Heart to Heart
2700 Northup Way
Bellevue, WA 98004

425-827-4600

Josephine Young MD, Contact

Wisconsin

4310 Kids With Heart
1578 Careful Drive
Green Bay, WI 54304

920-498-0058

4311 Left Hearts
250 N 6th Street
DePere, WI 54115

920-403-1154

Dyan Larmay, Contact

Web Sites

4312 Children's Heart Society
www.childrensheart.org

Reliable information and resources to families of children with congenital heart defects and acquired heart disease.

4313 Cincinnati Children's Hospital Medical Center
www.cincinnatichildrens.org

Cincinnati Children's Hospital is dedicated to serving the cardiac care needs of patiens, fetus through young adult, and is committed to providing research and teaching programs.

4314 Congenital Heart Information Network
http://tchin.org

Provides reliable information, support services and resources to families of children with congenital heart defects and acquired heart disease.

4315 Yale University School of Medicine
www.info.med.yale.edu/intmed/cardio/chd

Information on congential heart conditions, including Hypoplastic Left Heart Syndrome symptoms, treatments and support.

Book Publishers

4316 Hypoplastic Left Heart Syndrome
Kluwer Academic Publishers
233 Spring Street 7th Floor
New York, NY 10013

212-620-8000

With a focus on the advancement of surgical treatment of hypoplastic left heart syndrome, there are 23 contributions that collectively summarize the experience of their institution treating over 1000 infants with the disease. Discussions of anatomy, diagnosis, management, and long-term follow-up are included

2002 425 pages hardcover
ISBN: 1-402073-19-7

4317 Miracle of the Heart: True Story of One Little Girl's Gift of Life
America House Book Publishers
PO Box 151
Frederick, MD 21705

301-695-1707

2002 153 pages paperback
ISBN: 1-591294-24-x

4318 Parent's Guide to Children's Congenital Heart Defects
Random House
280 Park Avenue (11-3)
New York, NY 10017

800-733-3000
Fax: 212-940-7381
www.randomhouse.com/crown/

A practical and useful resource for families coping with a child who has CHD. An easy to read book uses personal stories and a question and answer format on a wide range of medical and daily living issues.

ISBN: 0-609807-75-7

4319 Young People and Chronic Illness: True Stories, Help and Hope
Congenital Heart Information Network
600 North 3rd Street, First Floor
New York, NY 19123

215-627-4034
Fax: 215-627-4036
http://tchin.org

Presents inspirational chapters based upon interviews of young people growing up with various chronic illnesses, including a chapter on Congenital Heart Disease.

ISBN: 1-575420-41-4

Newsletters

4320 Congenital Heart Information Network Newsletter
1561 Clark Drive
Yardley, PA 19067

215-493-3068
e-mail: mb@tchin.org
www.tchin.org

Features photos from events, informational articles, and news from members, support groups and organizations throughout the world.
semi-annual

Pamphlets

4321 Congenital Heart Information Network
600 North 3rd Street, First Floor
Philadelphia, PA 19123

215-627-4034
Fax: 215-627-4036
http://tchin.org

Four color brochure includes information about the programs and services offered.

DESCRIPTION

4322 HYPOTHYROIDISM

Covers these related disorders: Acquired hypothyroidism, Congenital hypothyroidism, Hoishimoto's disease
Involves the following Biologic System(s):
Endocrinologic Disorders

Hypothyroidism is a condition characterized by decreased activity of the thyroid gland, an endocrine gland that consists of two lobes on either side of the windpipe (trachea). Certain specialized cells within the thyroid gland secrete the thyroid hormones thyroxine (T-4) and triiodothyronine (T-3), which assist in regulating the rate of metabolism. Metabolism refers to the chemical activities within cells that release energy from nutrients or consume energy to create certain substances. The thyroid hormones also play a vital role in the normal mental and physical development and growth of infants and children. Other specialized cells in the thyroid gland secrete the hormone calcitonin, which helps to regulate concentrations of calcium in the body by inhibiting the loss of bone.

Hypothyroidism may result from an underlying defect that is present at birth (congenital). In children with congenital hypothyroidism, associated symptoms may begin at birth or be delayed until later during childhood, depending upon the nature of the underlying abnormality. Congenital hypothyroidism may result from several underlying causes, such as abnormal development (dysplasia) or absence (aplasia) of the thyroid gland; abnormalities in the production of certain hormones due to particular biochemical defects; or fetal exposure to particular medications or therapies (e.g., radioiodine therapy) during pregnancy. In children with malformation of the thyroid gland or abnormalities in hormonal production, the condition may appear to occur randomly for unknown reasons (sporadically) or may be familial. Congenital hypothyroidism affects approximately one in 4,000 infants worldwide and is about twice as common in females as in males.

Hypothyroidism may also occur later during childhood (acquired hypothyroidism) due to an autoimmune disorder in which the immune system develops antibodies against cells of the thyroid gland (Hashimoto's disease) or in association with other underlying disorders (e.g., nephropathic cystinosis, histiocytosis). Acquired hypothyroidism may also develop due to the use of particular medications or surgical removal of all or a portion of the thyroid gland as a treatment for certain diseases or conditions (e.g., thyroid cancer, thyrotoxicosis).

In newborns and infants with congenital hypothyroidism, associated symptoms may vary in range, severity, and rate of progression, depending upon the degree of thyroid hormone deficiency. Some patients may have an abnormally enlarged thyroid gland (goiter), causing swelling in front of the neck. In addition, early symptoms may include yellowish discoloration of the skin, mucous membranes, and whites of the eyes (jaundice); sluggishness; and feeding difficulties, including choking episodes during nursing. Many patients also have a large abdomen; a weakening of the abdominal wall muscles through which an abdominal organ or fatty tissue may protrude (umbilical hernia); constipation; widely open soft spots (fontanels) under the front and back of the scalp; and respiratory difficulties, including episodes in which there is a temporary cessation of spontaneous breathing (apnea). Some patients may have progressive retardation of mental and physical development that becomes increasingly severe without early diagnosis and prompt treatment. Patients may experience delays in obtaining certain developmental milestones, such as sitting up and standing; may not learn to speak; and may be increasingly lethargic. Additional physical findings associated with severe hypothyroidism include delayed skeletal maturation; a short, thick neck; short fingers and broad hands; a thick, protruding tongue; delayed eruption of the teeth (dentition); dry, scaly skin; coarse, scanty hair; and an abnormal, progressive accumulation of fluid within body tissues and associated swelling, particularly in the genital area, eyelids, and backs of the hands (myxedema).

The symptoms and findings associated with acquired hypothyroidism may also vary, depending upon the underlying cause, the age at onset, and the degree of thyroid hormone deficiency. Children with acquired hypothyroidism may experience an abnormally decreased rate of growth, decreased energy, puffiness of the skin (myxedematous changes), constipation, cold intolerance, headaches, visual problems, or other abnormalities.

In the United States, thyroid hormone levels in the blood are routinely tested in all newborns shortly after birth. Early diagnosis and prompt treatment of congenital hypothyroidism are essential for normal brain development during infancy. Such treatment includes thyroid hormone replacement therapy (e.g., sodium-L-thyroxine by mouth). The treatment of children with acquired hypothyroidism also includes thyroid hormone replacement therapy. Additional treatment is symptomatic and supportive.

See also **General Resources** on page 917

National Associations & Support Groups

4323 American Association of Clinical Endocrinologists
1000 Riverside Avenue, Suite 205
Jacksonville, FL 32204

904-353-7878
Fax: 904-353-8185
e-mail: info@aace.com
www.aace.com

A professional medical organization devoted to the enhancement of the practice of clinical endocrinology.

4324 Genetic Alliance
4301 Connecticut Avenue NW
Washington, DC 20008

202-966-5557
800-336-4363
Fax: 202-966-8553
e-mail: info@geneticalliance.org
www.geneticalliance.org

A coalition of voluntary genetic support groups, consumers and professionals addressing the needs of individuals and families affected by genetic disorders from a national perspective.

Sharon Terry, President/CEO

4325 Lawson Wilkins Pediatric Endocrine Society
867 Allardice Way
Stanford, CA 94305

650-302-0940
Fax: 650-494-3133
e-mail: secretary@lwpes.org
www.lwpes.org

To promote the acquisition and dissemination of knowledge of endocrine and metabolic disorders from conception through adolescence.

Raymond L Hintz, Secretary

4326 March of Dimes Birth Defects Foundation
1275 Mamaroneck Avenue
White Plains, NY 10605

914-428-7100
888-663-4637
Fax: 914-428-8203
e-mail: resourcecenter@modimes.org
www.marchofdimes.com

Partnership of volunteers and professionals dedicates to improving the health of babies by preventing birth defects and infant mortality. Over 100 chapters are located across the country and can be located through the National Office.

Dr Jennifer Howse, President

4327 Thyroid Foundation of America
One Longefellow Place, Suite 1518
Boston, MA 02114

617-534-1500
800-832-8321
Fax: 617-534-1515
e-mail: info@allthyroid.org
www.allthyroid.org

TFA's mission is to become the best at providing credible, unbiased information on thyroid topics using electronic, print, and voice technology for benefit of patients with thyroid disorders, their families and the general public. It is also to ensure timely diagnosis, appropriate treatment, and ongoing support for all individuals with thyroid disease.

4328 Thyroid Society for Education and Research
7515 S Main Street, Suite 545
Houston, TX 77030

713-799-9909
800-849-7643
Fax: 713-799-9919
e-mail: help@the-thyroid-society.org
www.the-thyroid-society.org

A nonprofit organization whose mission is to pursue the prevention, treatment and cure of thyroid disease.

Libraries & Resource Centers

4329 National Digestive Diseases Information Clearinghouse
2 Information Way
Bethesda, MD 20892

301-654-3810
800-891-5389
Fax: 703-738-4929
e-mail: nddic@info.niddk.nih.gov
www.digestive.niddk.nih.gov

The National Institute of Diabetes and Digestive and Kidney Diseases conducts and supports research on many of the most serious diseases affecting public health. The Institute supports much of the clinical research on the diseases of internal medicine and related subspecialty fields as well as many basic science disciplines.

Kathy Kranzfelder, Project Officer

Web Sites

4330 American Association of Clinical Endocrinologists
www.aace.com

The American Association of Clinical Endocrinologists is a professional medical organization devoted to the enhancement of the practice of clinical endocrinology.

4331 Online Mendelian Inheritance in Man
www.ncbi.nlm.nih.gov/entrez/query.fcgi?db=OMIM

Is an online database catalog of human genes and genetic disorders. The database contains textual information and references. It also contains copious links to MEDLINE and sequence records in the Entrenz System, and links to additional related resources at NCBI and elsewhere.

4332 Thyroid Federation International
www.thyroid-fed.org/

The Thyroid Federation International aims to work for the benefit of those affected by thyroid disorders throughout the world. Its objectives are to encourage and assist the formation of patient oriented thyroid organizations, to work closely with the medical professions to promote awareness and understanding of thyroid disorders and their complications, to provide through member organizations, information and moral support to those affected by thyroid disorders and to promote education.

Book Publishers

4333 Endocrine & Metabolic Disorders Sourcebook
Omnigraphics
PO Box 625
Holmes, PA 19043

800-234-1340
Fax: 800-875-1340
e-mail: info@omnigraphics.com
omnigraphics.com

Basic information for the lay person about pancreatic and insulin-related disorders such as pancreatitis, diabetes and hypoglycemia; adrenal gland disorders such as Cushing's syndrome, Addison's disease and congenital adrenal hyperplasia; pituitary gland disorders such as growth hormone deficiency, acromegaly and pituitary tumors; and thyroid disorders such as hypothyroidism, Grave's disease, Hashimoto's disease and goiter.

574 pages
ISBN: 0-780802-07-1

Journals

4334 Journal of Clinical Endocrinology
1000 Riverside Avenue, Suite 205
Jacksonville, FL 32204

904-353-7878
Fax: 904-353-8185
www.aace.com

Original research and articles, visual vignettes and other clinical information spanning the science of endocrinology.

Pamphlets

4335 Congenital & Acquired Hypothyroidism
Human Growth Foundation
7777 Leesburg Pike, Suite 202S
Falls Church, VA 22043

703-883-1773
800-451-6434
Fax: 703-883-1776
e-mail: hgfound@erols.com
www.genetic.org/hgf

DESCRIPTION

4336 ICHTHYOSIS

Covers these related disorders: Collodion baby, Congenital ichthyosiform erythroderma, Epidermolytic hyperkeratosis, Harlequin fetus, Ichthyosis vulgaris, X-linked ichthyosis

Involves the following Biologic System(s):
Dermatologic Disorders

Ichthyosis, literally meaning "fish skin," is a group of disorders characterized by abnormal thickening, dryness, and scaling of the skin due to abnormalities in the production of keratin, a protein that is the primary component of the skin, hair, and nails. Most forms of ichthyosis are genetic disorders that are usually apparent at birth (congenital) or during the first months of life. The genes that cause some congenital forms of ichthyosis have been mapped to particular chromosomes. Ichthyosis may also be due to other underlying genetic syndromes or may be an acquired condition due to certain nutritional deficiencies, the administration of particular drugs, or certain conditions, such as abnormally decreased activity of the thyroid gland (hypothyroidism) or Hodgkin's disease, a malignancy of the lymphatic system.

One congenital form of ichthyosis is known as harlequin fetus and may result from several different genetic abnormalities, most of which are thought to be transmitted as an autosomal recessive trait. Affected newborns may be covered with thickened, ridged, armor-like plates that confine the fingers and toes, restrict movements of the joints, and flatten the nose and ears. Additional features may include eyelids that are turned outward (ectropion), causing eyes to be indistinct; gaping lips; and absent hair and nails. Newborns with the condition may experience difficulties breathing, be susceptible to repeated skin infections, and develop life-threatening complications during the first days or weeks of life.

Another congenital form of ichthyosis, known as collodion baby, may also result from many different genetic abnormalities. Affected newborns are covered by a thick membrane that resembles an oiled parchment (collodion membrane), causing flattening of the nose and ears, abnormalities of the eyelids (ectropion), gaping of the lips, or other abnormalities. The membrane begins to crack as patients breathe and is gradually shed in large sheets. This condition is usually an early manifestation of specific genetic forms of ichthyosis (e.g., lamellar ichthyosis or congenital ichthyosiform erythroderma). Patients may develop potentially life-threatening symptoms due to skin infection, inflammation of the lungs (pneumonia), excessive loss of bodily fluids (dehydration), or other abnormalities.

Congenital ichthyosiform erythroderma is an autosomal recessive disorder that typically becomes apparent shortly after birth and may often present as collodion baby, the name given to a baby who is born encased in a skin that resembles a yellow, tight and shiny film or dried collodion (sausage skin) This form of ichthyosis is characterized by abnormal redness of the skin (erythroderma); generalized, fine, white scaling of the skin; and potentially severe itching (pruritus). Many children also have abnormally thickened skin (hyperkeratosis) on the palms of the hands and soles of the feet as well as around the knees, ankles, and elbo. Additional findings may include unusually sparse hair and abnormalities of the nails. Another form of the disorder, known as lamellar ichthyosis or nonbullous congenital ichthyosiform erythroderma, is usually inherited as an autosomal recessive trait. This form of ichthyosis becomes apparent shortly after birth and may also present as a collodion baby. After the collodion membrane is shed, the skin becomes covered with relatively large, coarse scales. Scaling often affects all surfaces of the body and may be associated with pruritus. Patients may also have thickened skin on the palms and soles, usually small ears, ectropion, and abnormally sparse, fine hair.

Another form of the disorder, known as X-linked ichthyosis, is often apparent at birth or during early infancy. Although males are primarily affected, some females who carry a single copy of the disease gene may also experience some symptoms. Patients develop prominent darkened scales on the scalp, ears, neck, arms and legs, torso, or other areas. Scaling may gradually worsen in severity and progress to affect other areas of the skin. By late childhood or adolescence, many patients develop clouding of the corneas (corneal opacities) that does not interfere with vision.

The most common form of the disorder is ichthyosis vulgaris, also known as ichthyosis simplex, an autosomal dominant disorder that affects about one in 250 to 300 children. Symptoms, which typically become apparent by the age of six months, may include slight roughness and scaling of the skin, particularly of the back and the legs. Scaling may worsen upon exposure to cold temperatures and may subside during warm months of the year. There may also be overgrowth of hair follicles (keratosis pilaris), particularly those of the thighs and upper arms, as well as abnormal thickening of the skin of the palms and soles. The condition may gradually improve or subside with age.

Another form of ichthyosis, known as epidermolytic hyperkeratosis or bullous congenital ichthyosiform erythroderma, may occur randomly for unknown reasons or be inherited as an autosomal dominant trait. This form of ichthyosis typically becomes apparent shortly after birth and is characterized by erythroderma, hyperkeratosis in certain areas, and small, rough, wart-like scales over body surfaces. Skin overgrowth may be most apparent on the neck and hips, under the arms, or at the elbows or knees and may affect the skin of the palms and soles. Recurrent blistering (bullae) may also develop, particularly on the lower legs, knees, or elbows.

The methods used to treat ichthyosis depend upon the specific disorder type as well as the severity and extent of associated symptoms. In severe neonatal forms, such as collodion baby and harlequin fetus, supportive measures may include administration of fluids to prevent dehydration; use of specialized support equipment such as an incubator that provides a heated, appropriately moisturized (hum idified) environment; and use of measures to help prevent or aggressively treat infections. Treatment may also include the administration of certain vitamin A derivatives (retinoids) or emulsifying ointments or lubricants. Bathing with oils may help to moisten the skin, and the application of certain emulsifying ointments and lubricants that soften the skin may alleviate dryness and scaling. In addition, applying topical agents that promote skin softening and peeling (keratolytic agents) may facilitate the removal of scales. In some patients, the use of air conditioning in warmer months and exposure to a high-humidity environment during the colder months may also be beneficial. Additional treatment is symptomatic and supportive.

See also **General Resources** on page 917

Government Agencies

4337 NIH/National Institute of Allergy and Infectious Diseases
6610 Rockledge Drive, MSC 6612
Bethesda, MD 20892

301-496-5717
Fax: 301-402-3573
TDD: 800-877-8339
www.niaid.nih.gov

Conducts and supports basic and applied research to better understand, treat, and ultimately prevent infectious, immunologic, and allergic diseases.

Anthony S Fauci MD, Director

4338 NIH/National Institute of Arthritis and Mu sculoskeletal and Skin Diseases
1AMS Circle
Bethesda, MD 20892

301-402-4484
Fax: 301-718-6366
e-mail: ord@od.nih.gov
rarediseases.info.nih.gov

The mission of the National Institute of Arthritis and Musculoskeletal and Skin Diseases is to support research into the causes, treatment, and prevention of arthritis and musculoskeletal and skin diseases, the training of basic and clinical scientists to carry out this research, and the dissemination of information on research progress in these diseases.

Stephen I Katz MD PhD, Director

4339 NIH/National Institute of Child Health and Human Development
31 Center Drive, Building 31
Bethesda, MD 20892

301-496-5133
Fax: 301-496-1104
www.nichd.nih.gov

Established in 1962 by congress, today the institute conducts and supports research on topics related to the health of children, adults, families and populations. Some of these topics include: developmental disabilities, growth and development, infant death, reproductive health and birth defects.

Nancy D Wirth, Director
Lisa Kaeser, Program & Public Liaison

National Associations & Support Groups

4340 FIRST: Foundation for Ichthyosis and Related Skin Types
1364 Welsh Road G2
North Wales, PA 19454

215-619-0670
800-545-3286
Fax: 215-619-0780
e-mail: info@scalyskin.org
www.scalyskin.org

Dedicated to helping individuals and families affected by the inherited skin diseases collectively called the Ichthyoses. Provides support, information, education, and advocacy for individuals and families affected by ichthyosis.

Jean Pickford, Executive Director

4341 Genetic Alliance
4301 Connecticut Avenue NW
Washington, DC 20008

202-966-5557
800-336-4363
Fax: 202-966-8553
e-mail: info@geneticalliance.org
www.geneticalliance.org

A coalition of voluntary genetic support groups, consumers and professionals addressing the needs of individuals and families affected by genetic disorders from a national perspective.

Sharon Terry, President/CEO

4342 March of Dimes Birth Defects Foundation
1275 Mamaroneck Avenue
White Plains, NY 10605

914-428-7100
888-663-4637
Fax: 914-428-8203
e-mail: resourcecenter@modimes.org
www.marchofdimes.com

Partnership of volunteers and professionals dedicates to improving the health of babies by preventing birth defects and infant mortality. Over 100 chapters are located across the country and can be located through the National Office.

Dr Jennifer Howse, President

4343 National Registry for Ichthyosis and Related Disorders
University of Washington, Dermatology Department
Box 356524, 1959 NE Pacific Street
Seattle, WA 98195

800-595-1265
Fax: 206-543-2489
e-mail: info@skinregistry.org
www.skinregistry.org

Identifies individuals in the USA who have an inherited disorder of keratinization; confirms the diagnosis by strict clinical, histiopathic and biological criteria, and by using molecular resources to assist in diagnosis, assistance with research, and a means of empowerment for affected individuals and their families.

Philip Fleckman, MD, Principal Investigator
Kim Pinetta, Registery Secretary

4344 Society for Pediatric Dermatology
8365 Keystone Crossing, Suite 107
Indianapolis, IN 46240

317-202-0224
Fax: 317-205-9841
e-mail: spd@hp-assoc.com
www.pedsderm.net

National organization dedicated to promote, develop and advance education, research and care of skin disease in all pediatric age groups.

Patricia Fraser, Administrator
Carol Caldwell, Office Secretary

Web Sites

4345 Family Village
www.familyvillage.wisc.edu

A global community that integrates information, resources and communication opportunities on the Internet for persons with cognitive and other disabilities, for their families and for those that provide them services and support.

4346 Ichthyosis Information
www.ichthyosis.com/

This website is to furnish users with general information.

Pamphlets

4347 Ichthyosis: An Overview
FIRST: Foundation for Ichthyosis and Related Skin
1364 Welsh Road G2
North Wales, PA 19454

215-619-0670
800-545-3286
Fax: 215-619-0780
e-mail: info@scalyskin.org
www.scalyskin.org

Descriptions of the primary types of ichthyosis and frequently asked questions. Available in Spanish.

18 pages

Jean Pickford, Executive Director

4348 Ichthyosis: The Genetics of Its Inheritance
FIRST: Foundation for Ichthyosis and Related Skin
1364 Welsh Road G2
North Wales, PA 19454

215-619-0670
800-545-3286
Fax: 215-619-0780
e-mail: info@scalyskin.org
www.scalyskin.org

A description of the genetic inheritance patterns for the different forms of ichthyosis: autosomal dominant, autosomal recessive and X-linked recessive. With illustrations.

23 pages

Jean Pickford, Executive Director

DESCRIPTION

4349 INTRAVENTRICULAR HEMORRHAGE

Synonyms: IVH, germinal matrix hemorrhage, GMH, Periventricular hemorrhage, PVH

Involves the following Biologic System(s):

Neonatal and Infant Disorders, Neurologic Disorders

Intraventricular Hemorrhage (IVH) is a disease of premature infants in which there is bleeding inside or around the ventricles, the spaces in the brain that contain the cerebrospinal fluid (CSF). Bleeding in the brain can put pressure on the nerve cells and damage them. Severe damage to cells can lead to brain injury. Intraventricular hemorrhage is most common in premature babies, especially very low birthweight babies. The younger the gestational age, the higher the incidence of IVH. It is not clear why IVH occurs. Bleeding can occur because blood vessels in a premature baby's brain are very fragile and immature and easily rupture. The risk of rupture is greatest in the first 4-5 days after birth. Abrupt changes in cerebral blood flow are thought to be one of the causes of IVH. Symptoms of IVH include apnea (stopped breathing), bradycardia (slow heart rate), pale or blue coloring (cyanosis), weak suck, high-pitched cry, and seizures.

IVH is diagnosed by cranial ultrasound and graded I through IV (IV being most severe). Infants with IVH are at higher risk for neurological disease including seizures, developmental delay, and hydrocephalus. Infants with IVH also have a higher incidence of death. With higher grades of IVH, the risk of future morbidity and mortality increases.

The treatment of IVH is supportive care. The best prevention of IVH is to prevent premature birth. When this is unavoidable, the use of anti-inflammatory medication (indomethacin) in the first 48 hours of life has been shown to decrease the incidence of IVH.

See also **General Resources** on page 917

National Associations & Support Groups

4350 Children's Hospital at Montefiore
3415 Bainbridge Avenue
Bronx, NY 10467

718-741-2426
Fax: 718-741-2460
e-mail: montekids@montefiore.org
www.montekids.org

The Children's Hospital at Montefiore is one of the most technologically advanced hospitals for children in the world. Staffed by the nationally renowned faclty of the Albert Einstein College of Medicine, our pediatric specialists and caregivers are ranked amoung the best in the nation.

4351 Children's Hospital of New York Presbyterian
3959 Broadway (165th Street and Broadway)
New York, NY 10032

212-305-5437
www.childrensnyp.org

Provides a comprehensive continuum of accessible, high-quality, family-centered children's services. Improves the health status of children in our community and maintain a world class academic center for children's health care services, teaching and research.

Cynthia N Sparer, Executive Director

4352 IVH Parents
PO Box 56-1111
Miami, FL 33256

305-232-0381
Fax: 305-232-9890
e-mail: mailto:72167.633@compuserve.com
www.familyvillage.wisc.edu

Support group for parents of children suffering from intaventricular hemorrhage.

4353 Lucile Packard Children's Hospital
725 Welch Road
Palo Alto, CA 94304

650-497-8000
800-690-2282
www.lpch.org/index.html

Devoted entirely to the care of babies, children, adolescents and expectant mothers. To best serve our communitites we advocate on behalf of the children and expectant mothers, advance family centered care, foster innovation, and educate health care providers and leaders.

Christopher Dawes, CEO

Web Sites

4354 Children's Hospital at Montefiore
www.montekids.org

Web site of one of the most technologically advanced hospitals with highly ranked pediatric specialists and caregivers.

4355 Children's Hospital of New York Presbyterian
www.childrensnyp.org

Provides comprehensive information for children with serious disearse, associated with Children's Hospital of New York Presbyterian.

4356 IVH Parents
www.familyvillage.wisc.edu

Provides support for parents of children with intaventricular hemorrhage.

4357 Yale University School of Medicine
www.info.med.yale.edu/intmed/cardio/chd

Information on heart conditions, including Intraventricular Hemorrhage — symptoms, treatments and support.

DESCRIPTION

4358 JUVENILE RHEUMATOID ARTHRITIS

Synonym: JRA

Covers these related disorders: Pauciarticular juvenile arthritis, Systemic-onset juvenile arthritis (Still's disease), Type I polyarticular juvenile arthritis, Type II polyarticular juvenile arthritis

Involves the following Biologic System(s):
Immunologic and Rheumatologic Disorders

Juvenile rheumatoid arthritis (JRA) is a group of disorders of childhood characterized by inflammation (arthritis), tenderness, pain, and swelling of one or more joints, potentially causing impaired development, limited movements, and permanent bending or extension of affected joints in various fixed postures (contractures). The symptoms and findings associated with JRA occur as the result of inflammation of the synovial membrane of affected joints (synovitis). Synovial membranes are connective tissue membranes that line the spaces between joints and bones and secrete a thick fluid to lubricate the joints. Although the cause of JRA is unknown, researchers speculate that the disorder may be the result of infection by an unidentified microorganism, an excessive immune response to a substance that the body perceives as foreign (hypersensitivity response), or abnormal immune responses against the body's own cells or tissues (autoimmune response). Certain antibodies often present in the blood of adults with rheumatoid arthritis (e.g., rheumatoid factors) are only rarely present in children with JRA. In such cases, researchers indicate that affected children may have some genetic predisposition for certain forms of JRA. Approximately 250,000 children are thought to be affected by JRA in the United States. Females are more commonly affected than males.

There are three major categories of JRA: polyarticular (30 percent), pauciarticular (50 percent), and systemic-onset juvenile arthritis (20 percent). Polyarticular juvenile arthritis typically involves several joints. Associated symptoms and findings include inflammation, swelling, abnormal warmth, tenderness, and pain of affected joints. This form of JRA often affects joints of the elbows, wrists, fingers, knees, feet, and ankles. In addition, patients may have involvement of joints of the jaw (temporomandibular joints), causing limited opening of the mouth; the neck (cervical spine), resulting in neck pain and stiffness; and the hips, causing pain, stiffness, and limited movements. Normal growth may be delayed during periods of active disease, causing such abnormalities as unusually short fingers, small feet, or underdevelopment of the jaw (micrognathia). Some children with polyarticular juvenile arthritis may also experience more generalized symptoms, such as low-grade fever, lack of appetite (anorexia), increased irritability, a mild decrease in the level of circulating red blood cells (anemia), swelling of certain lymph nodes (lymphadenopathy), or mild enlargement of the liver and spleen (hepatosplenomegaly).

Pauciarticular juvenile arthritis is characterized by involvement of larger joints, usually four or fewer for six consecutive weeks. Type I pauciarticular juvenile arthritis primarily affects females andhas an early onset. Affected joints typically include the elbows, knees, and ankles. In addition, other joints may sometimes be affected, such as those of a single finger or toe, the wrists, the neck, or the jaw. Patients are also at risk (girls more than boys) for chronic inflammation of the colored region of the eye (iris) and its muscle (iridocyclitis). One or both eyes may be affected. Some patients may experience associated redness, sensitivity to light (photophobia), pain, or decreased clearness of vision (visual acuity). Without appropriate treatment, visual impairment or, in severe cases, blindness may result. Boys are at higher risk of arthritis of the spine. Symptoms may include a general feeling of ill health (malaise), low-grade fever, mild hepatosplenomegaly, and mild anemia. Type II pauciarticular juvenile arthritisis most common in males older than age eight. Affected joints usually include those of the hips, knees, toes, and heels. In some patients, joints of the elbows, fingers, wrists, or jaw may also be affected. In patients with this form of JRA, associated foot and hip pain may sometimes be disabling. In addition, chronic, progressive, inflammatory disease of joints of the spine (spondyloarthropathy) may develop. Symptoms may include pain, stiffness, and loss of mobility of joints of the upper and lower back (ankylosing spondylitis). In addition, some affected children may experience sudden (acute) episodes of iridocyclitis.

Systemic-onset juvenile arthritis appears to affect females and males equally. This form of JRA usually begins with generalized symptoms, such as a high, intermittent fever that rapidly returns to normal; a characteristic rash; anemia; hepatosplenomegaly; lymphadenopathy; mild liver dysfunction (hepatitis); and, in about one third of patients, inflammation of the membranous sac surrounding the heart (pericarditis) or the membrane lining the lungs and chest cavity (pleuritis). The fever associated with systemic JRA tends to rise in the evenings, although it may also be elevated in the mornings, and is often associated with shaking chills. During fever episodes, a temporary, salmon-colored rash often appears on the trunk or arms or legs (extremities), although it may appear anywhere on the body. Such a rash may also temporarily appear in association with heat exposure or stress. In patients with systemic disease, joint inflammation, swelling, stiffness, and pain may occur at disease onset or months later. Joint involvement is usually similar to that seen in patients with polyarticular juvenile arthritis. Systemic symptoms and findings typically have a self-limited course that lasts for several months. However, such findings may recur in some patients.

In approximately 75 percent of affected children, symptoms associated with JRA completely disappear with little loss of function or deformity. However, other patients, particula|rly those with multiple joint involvement or rheumatoid factor, may experience repeated or chronic joint inflammation and permanent stiffness, limited movement, and deformity of certain affected joints. In addition, some patients with pauciarticular juvenile arthritis may later experience additionaljoint involvement (polyarthritis) or ongoing symptoms due to progressive, inflammatory disease of joints of the spine (spondyloarthropathy).

Children with JRA should receive regular eye (e.g., slit-lamp) examinations to ensure early detection and treatment of iridocyclitis. Treatment of iridocyclitis includes the use of corticosteroid eyedrops and drugs that widen (dilate) the pupil. Joint inflammation, pain, and stiffness may be alleviated with aspirin, nonsteroidal anti-inflammatory drugs (NSAIDs), medications such as methotrexate or hydroxychloroquine, or, in extremely severe cases, corticosteroids administered by mouth (orally). Due to the potential association of aspirin and the occurrence of Reye's syndrome, NSAIDs (e.g., tolmetin, naproxen, etc.) are currently being prescribed more frequently than aspirin as a treatment for JRA. Children with JRA who do not respond to NSAIDs therapy may be treated with low-dose methotrexate. If JRA is severe and systemic or, in patients in whom iridocyclitis is uncontrolled by corticosteroid eyedrops, oral corticosteroid therapy may be prescribed. However, oral corticosteroid therapy is usually avoided in children, if possible, since such therapy may slow the growth rate and is associated with other negative side effects. Children who don't respond well to methotrexate can be offered similar medications, sometimes referred to as disease-modifying antirheumatic drugs (DMARDs). Agents being tried in therapy of JRA include sulfasalazine, intravenous immunoglobulin, and cyclosporine. Splints may be used during the day to help rest inflamed joints and at night to minimize the risk of contracture development and associated deformity. Special exercises may also be recom-

mended to help reduce possible muscle wasting and contractures. In some patients, surgery may be required to help correct contractures. Children should also be monitored for growth abnormalities, nutritional deficiencies, and school/social impairment.

See also **General Resources** on page 917

Government Agencies

4359 NIH/National Institute of Arthritis & Musculoskeletal & Skin Diseases
National Institutes of Health
1 AMS Circle
Bethesda, MD 20892

301-495-4484
877-226-4267
Fax: 301-718-6366
TDD: 301-565-2966
e-mail: niamsinfo@mail.nih.gov
www.niams.nih.gov

The mission of the NIAMS, a part of the NIH, is to support research into the causes, treatment, and prevention of arthritis and musculoskeletal and skin diseases, the training of basic and clinical scientists to carry out this research, and the dissemination of information on research progress in these diseases.

Lillian Hatch, Librarian

4360 NIH/National Institute of Arthritis and Mu sculoskeletal and Skin Diseases
1AMS Circle
Bethesda, MD 20892

301-402-4484
Fax: 301-718-6366
e-mail: ord@od.nih.gov
rarediseases.info.nih.gov

The mission of the National Institute of Arthritis and Musculoskeletal and Skin Diseases is to support research into the causes, treatment, and prevention of arthritis and musculoskeletal and skin diseases, the training of basic and clinical scientists to carry out this research, and the dissemination of information on research progress in these diseases.

Stephen I Katz MD PhD, Director

National Associations & Support Groups

4361 American Juvenile Arthritis Organization
1330 West Peachtree Street Suite 100
Atlanta, GA 30309

404-872-7100
800-283-7800
Fax: 404-872-9559
e-mail: info.ga@arthritis.org
www.arthritis.org

Devoted to serving the special needs of children, teens, and young adults with childhood rheumatic diseases and their families. Offers both support and information through national and local programs that serve the needs of families, friends and health professionals. Serves as a clearinghouse of information, sponsors an annual national conference, monitors and promotes legislation, sponsors research, and offers training to both parents and health professionals.

Sage Rhodes, President
Sharon Davenport

4362 Arthritis Foundation
PO Box 7669
Atlanta, GA 30357

404-872-7100
800-568-4045
Fax: 404-872-0457
www.arthritis.org

The only nonprofit organization that supports the more than 100 types of arthritis and related conditions with advocacy, programs, services and research.

John H Klippel MD, President & CEO

4363 Genetic Alliance
4301 Connecticut Avenue NW
Washington, DC 20008

202-966-5557
800-336-4363
Fax: 202-966-8553
e-mail: info@geneticalliance.org
www.geneticalliance.org

A coalition of voluntary genetic support groups, consumers and professionals addressing the needs of individuals and families affected by genetic disorders from a national perspective.

Sharon Terry, President/CEO

4364 Kids on the Block Arthritis Programs
Arthritis Foundation
9385-C Gerwig Lane
Columbia, MD 21046

800-368-5437
Fax: 404-872-0457
e-mail: kob@kotb.com
www.kotb.com/kob2.htg/arth.htm

State and local programs that use puppetry to help children understand what it is like for children and adults who have arthritis.

Research Centers

4365 Pediatric Rheumatoid Clinic
Duke Medical Center
Box 3212
Durham, NC 27710

919-684-6575

Clinical and laboratory pediatric rheumatoid studies.

Dr. Deborah Kredich, Chairman
Stacy Ardman

Web Sites

4366 Online Mendelian Inheritance in Man
www.ncbi.nlm.nih.gov

This database is a catalog of human genes and genetic disorders.

Book Publishers

4367 Arthritis
Franklin Watts
90 Old Sherman Turnpike
Danbury, CT 06816

203-797-3500
800-621-1115
Fax: 203-797-3197
www.grolier.com

This book offers a clear explanation of the various forms and effects of the disease of arthritis and what treatments are available.

96 pages Grades 7-12
ISBN: 0-531108-01-5

4368 Arthritis Sourcebook
Omnigraphics
PO Box 625
Holmes, PA 19043

800-234-1340
Fax: 800-875-1340
e-mail: info@omnigraphics.com
omnigraphics.com

Basic consumer health information on specific forms of arthritis and related disorders.

550 pages Hardcover
ISBN: 0-780802-01-2

4369 Educational Rights for Children With Arthritis: Parents Manual
AJAO
PO Box 7669
Atlanta, GA 30357

404-872-7100
Fax: 404-872-9559
e-mail: help@arthritis.org
www.arthritis.org

A self-instructional manual helping parents to identify and obtain school services needed by their child with arthritis. Covers laws and special services, explores strategies for working with school personnel and stresses good communication and advocacy techniques.

4370 JRA and Me
American Juvenile Arthritis Organization
PO Box 19000
Atlanta, GA 30326

800-283-7800

A workbook for school-aged children who have juvenile arthritis. This book offers a variety of educational games, puzzles and worksheets to teach children about their illness and how to take care of themselves.

57 pages

4371 Living with Arthritis
Franklin Watts
90 Old Sherman Turnpike
Danbury, CT 06816

203-797-3500
800-621-1115
Fax: 203-797-3197
www.grolier.com

Shows how people with arthritis can overcome their pain and lead productive, full lives.

32 pages Grades 5-7

4372 Understanding Juvenile Rheumatoid Arthritis
American Juvenile Arthritis Organization
PO Box 7669
Atlanta, GA 30357

404-872-7100
800-568-4045

A manual for health professionals to use in teaching children with JRA and their families about disease management and self-care.

372 pages

4373 We Can: Guide for Parents of Children with Arthritis
American Juvinile Arthritis Association
P.O. Box 7669
Atlanta, GA 30357

404-872-7100
800-568-4045
Fax: 404-872-9559
e-mail: help@arthritis.org
www.arthritis.org

Offers parents tips for daily living and practical points for helping their child toward independent adulthood.

Katie Bitner, AJAO Assistant

4374 Yard Sale Coloring Book
American Juvenile Arthritis Organization
PO Box 19000
Atlanta, GA 30326

800-283-7800

A coloring/activity book based on a Kids on the Block script, written for third and fourth grade students. It can be used with Kids on the Block performances, as a stand-alone piece or with a free lesson plan packet.

Newsletters

4375 AJAO Newsletter
American Juvenile Arthritis Organization
P.O. Box 7669
Atlanta, GA 30357

404-872-7100
800-568-4045
Fax: 404-872-9559
e-mail: kgatmail@arthritis.org
www.arthritis.org

This reliable and comprehensive newsletter for families coping with childhood arthritis and related conditions contains the latest research findings, responsible advice from pediatric specialists, practical methods to help improve quality of life, and informative updates about medications and how they affect children. Articles are written in clear understandable language. Timely medical insights and life enhancing information that provides solutions to everyday problems.

Quarterly

Beth Blaney, Editor

Pamphlets

4376 Arthritis Information: Children
Arthritis Foundation
PO Box 7669
Atlanta, GA 30357

404-872-7100
800-283-7800
Fax: 404-872-0457
www.arthritis.org

4377 Arthritis in Children and La Artritis Infantojuvenil
American Juvenile Arthritis Organization
PO Box 7669
Atlanta, GA 30357

404-872-7100
800-568-4045

A medical information booklet about juvenile rheumatoid arthritis. This booklet is written for parents or other adults and includes details about different forms of JRA, medications, therapies and coping issues.

4378 Arthritis in Children: Resources for Children, Parents and Teachers
National Arthritis and Skin Diseases Clearinghouse
9000 Rockville Pike
Bethesda, MD 20892

301-495-4484

A resource offering information on juvenile arthritis, causes, treatments and prevention.

38 pages

4379 Rheumatoid Arthritis
NAMSIC, National Institutes of Health
1 AMS Circle
Bethesda, MD 20892

301-495-4484
Fax: 301-587-4352
TTY: 301-565-2966
www.nih.gov/niams/

Offers an introduction and definition of rheumatoid arthritis, treatments, causes, objectives, daily living, resources and medical information.

4380 When Your Student Has Arthritis: Guide for Teachers
Arthritis Foundation
PO Box 7669
Atlanta, GA 30357

404-872-7100
800-283-7800
Fax: 404-872-0457
www.arthritis.org

A medical information booklet written for teachers or other adults who have arthritis. The booklet describes different forms of juvenile arthritis, how arthritis might affect the child at school, and how to help the child work around these problems.

DESCRIPTION

4381 KAWASAKI DISEASE

Synonyms: MLNS, Mucocutaneous lymph node syndrome

Involves the following Biologic System(s):

Cardiovascular Disorders, Immunologic and
Rheumatologic Disorders

Kawasaki disease is a syndrome of unknown origin that primarily affects infants and young children. The disease was initially observed in Japanese children after World War II. Kawasaki disease is becoming increasingly frequent in the United States, has been reported worldwide, and is currently considered the leading cause of acquired heart disease in children in the U.S. Although Kawasaki disease has been reported in people in all racial groups, individuals of Japanese descent appear to be most commonly affected. The disease may occur commonly in a random or an isolated manner (sporadic form) or, rarely, may suddenly affect large numbers of individuals (epidemic form). Although the cause of Kawasaki disease is unknown, researchers suspect that toxic substances produced by certain bacteria (e.g., staphylococcal toxins) may play some role. There is no evidence of transmission of the disease from one affected individual to another (person-to-person transmission).

Kawasaki disease most commonly affects children who are five years of age or younger. Affected children typically develop a sudden, sustained, high fever that is often greater than 104 degrees and unresponsive to therapy with fever-reducing (antipyretic) medications. Most patients also have inflammation of the whites of both eyes and the lining inside the eyelids (bilateral conjunctivitis), causing redness but no associated discharge; dry, red (erythematous), cracked (fissured) lips; a strawberry-red tongue; and swelling of one or several lymph nodes, particularly those of the neck (cervical lymphadenopathy). Patients also typically develop a reddish skin rash that may consist of flat, discolored spots and small, raised areas (maculopapular) or appear similar to that seen in measles (morbilliform). The trunk, the hands and feet, and the face may be affected. Patients usually experience subsequent swelling and associated pain of the hands and feet. By approximately the second to third week, affected skin may begin to peel (desquamate) from the palms of the hands, the soles of the feet, and the tips of the fingers and toes. Such peeling may also involve other affected areas, such as the trunk. In addition, children with Kawasaki disease are usually irritable and may develop joint swelling and pain (arthritis), abdominal pain, diarrhea, vomiting, coughing, inflammation of the gall bladder, or enlargement of the liver and spleen (hepatosplenomegaly). Additional symptoms and findings may include inflammation of certain muscles (myositis), nasal discharge of a thin fluid (rhinorrhea), episodes of increased electrical activity in the brain (seizures), mild inflammation of the protective membrane surrounding the brain (aseptic meningitis), or other abnormalities.

The most serious complication potentially associated with Kawasaki disease is involvement of the heart. Within the first few weeks after disease onset, approximately 25 percent of untreated patients develop inflammation of arteries that carry blood to the heart muscle (coronary arteritis) and associated widening or bulging (aneurysms) of the walls of these arteries. In rare cases, affected children, particularly those under the age of one year, may experience few early symptoms associated with the disease, yet later develop coronary arteritis. Patients with cardiac involvement may develop inflammation of heart muscle (myocarditis); deficient blood supply to heart muscle (myocardial ischemia), resulting in localized loss of tissue (infarction); and inflammation of the membranous sac surrounding the heart (pericarditis). Additional findings may include inflammation of the membrane lining the internal surfaces of the cavities of the heart (endocarditis), an inability of the heart to sufficiently pump blood to the lungs and the rest of the body (heart failure), or abnormalities of the rhythm or rate of the heartbeat (arrythmias). In some cases, without appropriate treatment, patients with severe cardiac involvement may experience potentially life-threatening complications.

All patients with diagnosed or suspected Kawasaki disease should undergo specialized diagnostic tests, such as chest x-rays, electrocardiograms, and echocardiograms. Additional testing (e.g., two-dimensional echocardiogram) may also be conducted during the first two weeks of disease. The treatment of children with Kawasaki disease should include intravenous (IV) infusion with a preparation of antibodies (immunoglobulins) obtained from plasma, the liquid portion of the blood (intravenous gammaglobulin), and therapy with high-dose aspirin (salicylate therapy). Early (within 10 days of fever onset) intravenous gammaglobulin therapy helps to alleviate fever and other associated symptoms; in addition, controlled studies have demonstrated that such therapy decreases heart involvement to some patients. Once the fever has subsided, patients may receive therapy with lower doses of aspirin. Such therapy typically continues until coronary arteritis resolves. In the rare patient with large or multiple coronary artery aneurysms, treatment may include therapy with anticlotting medications, such as warfarin or heparin. Other treatment is symptomatic and supportive. All children diagnosed with Kawasaki disease receive outpatient follow-up with a pediatric cardiologist.

See also **General Resources** on page 917

Government Agencies

4382 Centers for Disease Control
1600 Clifton Road
Atlanta, GA 30333

404-639-3311
www.cdc.gov

Mission is to promote health and quality of life by preventing and controlling disease, injury, and disability.

4383 NIH/National Heart, Lung and Blood Institu te
National Institute of Health
31 Center Dr MSC 2486, Bldg 31, Room 5A48
Bethesda, MD 20892

301-592-8573
Fax: 240-629-3246
TTY: 240-629-3255
e-mail: NHLBlinfo@nhlbi.nih.gov
www.nhlbi.nih.gov

Primary responsibility of this organization is the scientific investigation of heart, blood vessel, lung and blood disorders. Oversees research, demonstration, prevention, education, control and training activities in these fields and emphasizes the prevention and control of heart diseases.

Elizabeth G Nabel, MD, Director
Susan Shurin, MD, Deputy Director

4384 NIH/National Institute of Allergy and Infectious Diseases
6610 Rockledge Drive, MSC 6612
Bethesda, MD 20892

301-496-5717
Fax: 301-402-3573
TDD: 800-877-8339
www.niaid.nih.gov

Conducts and supports basic and applied research to better understand, treat, and ultimately prevent infectious, immunologic, and allergic diseases.

Anthony S Fauci MD, Director

4385 NIH/National Institute of Child Health and Human Development
31 Center Drive, Building 31
Bethesda, MD 20892

301-496-5133
Fax: 301-496-1104
www.nichd.nih.gov

Established in 1962 by congress, today the institute conducts and supports research on topics related to the health of children, adults, families and populations. Some of these topics include: developmental disabilities, growth and development, infant death, reproductive health and birth defects.

Nancy D Wirth, Director
Lisa Kaeser, Program & Public Liaison

National Associations & Support Groups

4386 Kawasaki Disease Foundation
PO Box 45
Boxford, MA 01921

978-356-2070
Fax: 978-356-2079
e-mail: info@kdfoundation.org

Raising awareness among the medical community, childcare providers, and the general public is critical to early diagnosis and treatment. Facilitating support among families is essential to helping families cope with this uncommon illness and the potentially devastating effects of heart damage. Increasing funding for research is necessary to advance diagnostic guidelines, enhance the existing treatment, improve short-term and long-term follow-up care and find a cause.

Gregory Chin, President
Anthony Olaes, VP

4387 Kawasaki Families' Network
46-111 Nahewai Place
Kaneohe, HI 96744

808-525-8053
Fax: 808-525-8055
e-mail: kawasaki@compuserve.com
ourworld.compuserve.com/homepage/kawasaki

A network that works to share information on research, to share information and support through occasional mailings, and to provide links to medical literature.

DESCRIPTION

4388 KELOIDS

Synonym: Cheloids

Involves the following Biologic System(s):

Dermatologic Disorders

Keloids are firm, nodule-like overgrowths of scar tissue that occur at the sites of surgery, injury, or trauma to the skin. These overgrowths result from the formation, during the healing process, of excessive amounts of the fibrous protein collagen, which is a major structural component of connective tissue. Doctors do not understand exactly why keloids form in certain people or situations and not in others. Changes in the signals sent out by cells that control growth and proliferation may be related to the process of keloid formation, but these changes have not yet been scientifically proven. Keloids may be itchy and are usually pink in color, shiny, smooth, irregularly shaped, firm, and rubbery. Some keloids may be tender or painful. Although keloids may appear on the face, neck, earlobes, legs, or other areas, they most often occur over the breastbone (sternum) and the shoulders.

Keloid development may sometimes result following surgery, body piercing, and other types of trauma to the skin such as burns or scalds. In addition, keloids may develop in association with severe acne and occasionally with certain connective tissue disorders such as Ehlers-Danlos syndrome or skin disorders such as Touraine-Solente-Gole syndrome. In some cases, keloid development may be inherited as an autosomal recessive or autosomal dominant trait. In addition, keloids are more common in black individuals.

Without treatment, keloids tend to flatten out and become less obvious within a period of months or years. However, monthly injections of certain corticosteroid drugs directly into the lesions (intralesional) may successfully decrease their size and reduce itching, but treatment should be initiated early in their development. Treatment of large keloids may include surgical removal followed by corticosteroid injections into the lesions. Surgery alone most often results in a recurrence of the keloid. Other treatment may include laser therapy that reduces the redness of the keloid; freezing keloids (cryotherapy) may also flatten them. The direct application of silicone patches or sheeting may promote shrinkage.

See also **General Resources** on page 917

Government Agencies

4389 NIH/National Institute of Arthritis and Musculoskeletal and Skin Diseases
1AMS Circle
Bethesda, MD 20892

301-402-4484
Fax: 301-718-6366
e-mail: ord@od.nih.gov
rarediseases.info.nih.gov

The mission of the National Institute of Arthritis and Musculoskeletal and Skin Diseases is to support research into the causes, treatment, and prevention of arthritis and musculoskeletal and skin diseases, the training of basic and clinical scientists to carry out this research, and the dissemination of information on research progress in these diseases.

Stephen I Katz MD PhD, Director

National Associations & Support Groups

4390 American Academy of Dermatology (AAD)
PO Box 4014
Schaumburg, IL 60168

847-240-1280
866-503-7546
Fax: 847-240-1859
e-mail: MRC@aad.org
www.aad.org

Committed to the highest quality standards in continuing medical education. Developed a platform to promote and advance the science and art of medicine and surgery related to the skin; promotes the highest possible standards in clinical practice, education and research in dermatology and related disciplines; and supports and enhances patient care and promotes the public interest relating to dermatology.

Stephen P Stone MD, President
William P Coleman III, MD, VP

4391 American Osteopathic College of Dermatology
1501 E Illinois Street, PO Box 7525
Kirksville, MO 63501

660-665-2184
800-449-2623
Fax: 660-627-2623
e-mail: info@aocd.org
www.aocd.org

Strives to improve the standards of the practice of dermatology, to stimulate the study and extend knowledge in the field of dermatology, and to promote a more general understanding of the nature and scope of services rendered by osteopathic dermatologists to other divisions of practice, hospitals, clinics and the public.

Rebecca A Mansfield, Executive Director

4392 American Skin Association
346 Park Avenue South, 4th Floor
New York, NY 10010

212-889-4858
800-499-7546
Fax: 212-889-4959
e-mail: AmericanSkin@compuserve.com
www.americanskin.org

The American Skin Association is the only volunteer led health organization dedicated through research, education and advocacy to saving lives and alleviating human suffering caused by the full spectrum of skin disorders.

Howard P Milstein, Chairman
George W Hambrick, Jr, President/Founder

4393 Society for Pediatric Dermatology
8365 Keystone Crossing, Suite 107
Indianapolis, IN 46240

317-202-0224
Fax: 317-205-9841
e-mail: spd@hp-assoc.com
www.pedsderm.net

A national organization specifically dedicated to the field of pediatric dermatology, with the objective of promoting, developing, and advancing education, research and care of skin disease in all pediatric age groups. The organization holds meetings twice a year to educate physicians about advances in pediatric dermatology, help them support children with dermatological diseases and improve the care of these children.

Kent Lindeman, Executive Director

DESCRIPTION

4394 KERNICTERUS

Synonym: Bilirubin encephalopathy
Involves the following Biologic System(s):
Neonatal and Infant Disorders

Kernicterus refers to a rare neurologic condition in which excessive amounts of bilirubin accumulate in the brain of affected newborns, resulting in damage to the central nervous system. Bilirubin, a reddish-yellow pigment present in bile, is derived from the breakdown of the protein in red blood cells that carries oxygen (hemoglobin). Premature infants and newborns with certain congenital disorders (e.g., erythroblastosis fetalis and Crigler-Najjar syndrome) are at risk for this life-threatening condition. In premature infants, the processes needed for bilirubin excretion may not be fully developed. Factors that put extra strain on this immature metabolic process may result in increased levels of bilirubin in the blood (hyperbilirubinemia). If these levels become excessive and are left untreated, bilirubin may be deposited in the brain. For example, in infants with erythroblastosis fetalis, antibodies from the mother's blood cross the placental barrier and destroy red blood cells of the fetus, resulting in release of excessive amounts of bilirubin. In some cases, bilirubin builds up faster than the liver is able to eliminate it, resulting in hyperbilirubinemia. Signs of this condition include a yellowing of the eyes, skin, and mucous membranes (jaundice).

Crigler-Najjar syndrome results from the deficiency of an enzyme that is required to convert bilirubin to a form that may be excreted from the body, thus causing hyperbilirubinemia. Other conditions or disorders that cause hyperbilirubinemia place the newborn, especially those who are born prematurely, at risk for kernicterus.

Symptoms of kernicterus usually become apparent within the first week of life. However, hyperbilirubinemia that occurs anytime within the first month of life may result in kernicterus. Symptoms and characteristic findings may include difficulty in feeding; vomiting; lethargy; and lack of a normal response to sudden, loud noises (Moro or startle reflex). Further signs of this condition may include breathing difficulties; severe muscle spasms resulting in a backward arching of the back and neck (opisthotonos); twitching of the arms, legs, and face; a high-pitched cry; and convulsions. In some affected infants, severe involvement of the central nervous system may cause life-threatening complications. In others, findings associated with permanent disability may be observed periodically until the third year of life when the complete neurologic picture emerges. Symptoms may include involuntary spasms of the muscles, hearing loss, eye movement irregularities, deficiencies in motor development, difficulties in speech, seizures, and mental retardation. Some infants who experience only slight kernicterus may experience mild irregularities in neuromuscular coordination, moderate deafness, and slight retardation.

Treatment of kernicterus is directed toward prevention involving the correction of hyperbilirubinemia and jaundice before kernicterus can develop. Treatment may include phototherapy in which, under careful monitoring, the infant's skin is exposed to high-intensity fluorescent light. Although phototherapy is often effective in reducing levels of bilirubin, the underlying cause of hyperbilirubinemia and jaundice must be identified and treated as well. Some infants, especially those at higher risk for kernicterus, may be effectively treated with exchange blood transfusions in which small amounts of the infant's circulating blood are repeatedly withdrawn and replaced with equal amounts of whole blood from a donor until about 80 percent of the newborn's blood has been replaced. Other treatment is symptomatic and supportive.

See also **General Resources** on page 917

Government Agencies

4395 NIH/National Institute of Child Health and Human Development
31 Center Drive, Building 31
Bethesda, MD 20892

301-496-5133
Fax: 301-496-1104
www.nichd.nih.gov

Established in 1962 by congress, today the institute conducts and supports research on topics related to the health of children, adults, families and populations. Some of these topics include: developmental disabilities, growth and development, infant death, reproductive health and birth defects.

Nancy D Wirth, Director
Lisa Kaeser, Program & Public Liaison

National Associations & Support Groups

4396 American Liver Foundation
75 Maiden Lane, Suite 603
New York, NY 10038

212-668-1000
800-465-4837
Fax: 212-483-8179
e-mail: info@liverfoundation.org
www.liverfoundation.org

Nonprofit, national voluntary organization dedicated to the prevention, treatment, and cure of hepatitis and other liver diseases through research, education and advocacy on behalf of those affected by or at risk of liver disease.

Alan P Brownstein, President/CEO
James L Boyer, MD, Chair

4397 Genetic Alliance
4301 Connecticut Avenue NW
Washington, DC 20008

202-966-5557
800-336-4363
Fax: 202-966-8553
e-mail: info@geneticalliance.org
www.geneticalliance.org

A coalition of voluntary genetic support groups, consumers and professionals addressing the needs of individuals and families affected by genetic disorders from a national perspective.

Sharon Terry, President/CEO

4398 March of Dimes Birth Defects Foundation
1275 Mamaroneck Avenue
White Plains, NY 10605

914-428-7100
888-663-4637
Fax: 914-428-8203
e-mail: resourcecenter@modimes.org
www.marchofdimes.com

Partnership of volunteers and professionals dedicates to improving the health of babies by preventing birth defects and infant mortality. Over 100 chapters are located across the country and can be located through the National Office.

Dr Jennifer Howse, President

4399 United Liver Foundation
5777 W Century Boulevard
Los Angeles, CA 90045

310-670-4624
Fax: 310-670-4672
e-mail: pbrady@liver411.com
www.liver411.com

A national organization that promotes research and cures for hepatitis and other liver diseases.

Pam Brady, Contact Person
Donna Gracon, Chapter Director

Libraries & Resource Centers

4400 National Digestive Diseases Information Clearinghouse
2 Information Way
Bethesda, MD 20892

301-654-3810
800-891-5389
Fax: 703-738-4929
e-mail: nddic@info.niddk.nih.gov
www.digestive.niddk.nih.gov

The National Institute of Diabetes and Digestive and Kidney Diseases conducts and supports research on many of the most serious diseases affecting public health. The Institute supports much of the clinical research on the diseases of internal medicine and related subspecialty fields as well as many basic science disciplines.

Kathy Kranzfelder, Project Officer

Web Sites

4401 Online Mendelian Inheritance in Man
www.ncbi.nlm.nih.gov

This database is a catalog of human genes and genetic disorders.

4402 Parents of Infants and Children with Kernicterus
www.pickonline.org

Provides information and support to families of children with kernicterus.

4403 Rare Genetic Diseases in Children (NYU)
www.med.nyu.edu/rgdc/homenow.htm

We target issues arising from rare genetic diseases affecting children. Also, to assist in the endeavor to bring knowledge and hope to those for whom there is, at present, so little.

4404 Save Babies Through Screening Foundation
www.savebabies.org

Is a national nonprofit public charity run by volunteers. Its mission is to improve the lives of babies by working to prevent disabilities and early death resulting from disorders detectable through newborn screening.

DESCRIPTION

4405 KLINEFELTER SYNDROME

Synonyms: Chromosome XXY, XXY syndrome

Covers these related disorders: 45,X/46,XY/47,XXY mosaicism, 46,XY/47,XXY mosaicism, 46,XY/48,XXYY mosaicism, 46,XX/47,XXY mosaicism, 48,XXXY, 49,XXXYY

Involves the following Biologic System(s):

Genetic/Chromosomal/Syndrome/Metabolic Disorders

Klinefelter syndrome is a chromosomal disorder that appears to affect approximately one in 1,000 males. Males usually have one X and one Y chromosome; however, those with Klinefelter syndrome have an extra X chromosome in cells of the body. In some patients, only a certain percentage of cells contain the XXY chromosomal abnormality. This finding is known as chromosomal mosaicism. Other cells may have the normal XY chromosomal pair or other sex chromosome abnormalities (e.g., XX, XXYY, etc.). Some males may have Klinefelter variants in which some or all cells contain more than two X chromosomes.

Because only a few or subtle symptoms may be associated with Klinefelter syndrome, the disorder is rarely diagnosed before puberty. Males with the disorder may have extremely variable I.Q.s (intelligence quotients), ranging from well above to far below average; however, most affected males have an I.Q. within average limits (mean of 85 to 90). Some children with Klinefelter syndrome may have learning problems, such as difficulties with verbal expression, reading, and spelling, potentially requiring special assistance or full-time special education classes. Children with the disorder also tend to have behavioral problems, such as immaturity, excessive shyness, anxiety, poor judgment, aggressive activity, and poor social skills. Such behavioral difficulties tend to begin when affected children begin school.

Many children with Klinefelter syndrome have slim, tall stature; long legs; and small testes and a relatively small penis (hypogenitalism). As affected males enter puberty, they may experience partial, inadequate development of secondary sexual characteristics (impaired virilization). For example, facial hair tends to be unusually sparse, the testes remain unusually small, and, in many cases, there is abnormal enlargement of the breasts (gynecomastia). In addition, many affected males experience inadequate production of the male hormone testosterone and deficient production of male reproductive cells (azoospermia), resulting in infertility. In males with deficient testosterone production, treatment may include testosterone replacement therapy beginning at approximately 11 to 12 years of age. In most cases, Klinefelter syndrome results from errors during the division of a parent's reproductive cells (meiosis). In rare cases, the disorder may result from errors during cellular division after fertilization (mitosis).

In males with XY/XXY mosaicism (i.e., a percentage of cells containing the normal XY chromosomal pair), the range and severity of associated symptoms and findings may be less severe, and there may be an increased likelihood of fertility and improved psychosocial adjustment. Affected males with Klinefelter variants (i.e., in which cells contain more than two X chromosomes) may have more severe symptoms and findings, such as a greater risk of mental retardation and impaired virilization and fertility as well as additional physical abnormalities, including malformations of the head and facial (craniofacial) areas and other skeletal abnormalities.

See also **General Resources** on page 917

Government Agencies

4406 NIH/National Institute of Child Health and Human Development

31 Center Drive, Building 31
Bethesda, MD 20892

301-496-5133
Fax: 301-496-1104
www.nichd.nih.gov

Established in 1962 by congress, today the institute conducts and supports research on topics related to the health of children, adults, families and populations. Some of these topics include: developmental disabilities, growth and development, infant death, reproductive health and birth defects.

Nancy D Wirth, Director
Lisa Kaeser, Program & Public Liaison

National Associations & Support Groups

4407 49 XXY Syndrome Association

10001 NE 74th Street
Vancouver, WA 98662

360-892-7547
e-mail: kimbj@juno.com

4408 A&K Associates

PO Box 119
Roseville, CA 95678

916-773-2999
888-999-9428
e-mail: pediatric-info@genetic.org
www.genetic.org/ks

Nonprofit organization that provides information about Klinefelter syndrome, common characteristics, and treatment. Information on current research projects and other resources.

Melissa Aylstock, Executive Director

4409 Genetic Alliance
4301 Connecticut Avenue NW
Washington, DC 20008

202-966-5557
800-336-4363
Fax: 202-966-8553
e-mail: info@geneticalliance.org
www.geneticalliance.org

A coalition of voluntary genetic support groups, consumers and professionals addressing the needs of individuals and families affected by genetic disorders from a national perspective.

Sharon Terry, President/CEO

4410 Klinefelter Syndrome and Associates
11 Keats Court
Coto de Caza, CA 92679

916-773-2999
888-999-9428
Fax: 949-858-3443
e-mail: khenry@genetic.org
genetic.org

Nonprofit organization.

4411 Klinefelter's Syndrome Association
N5879 30th Street
Pine River, WI 54965

920-987-5782

4412 Support and Educational Exchange for Klinefelter Syndrome
1417 25th Avenue, Drive W
Bradenton, FL 34205

813-750-8044

Web Sites

4413 Klinefelter Syndrome Support Group
www.klinefeltersyndrome.org/

An online support group which offers information about the group, organizations, online pharmacies, other web sites, and current research studies.

4414 NIH/National Institute of Mental Health
www.nimh.nih.gov

The mission is to reduce the burden of mental illness and behavioral disorders through research on mind, brain, and behavior. This public health mandate demands that we harness powerful scientific tools to achieve better understanding, treatment, and eventually prevention of these disabling conditions that affect millions of Americans.

Newsletters

4415 Even Exchange Newsletter
KS&A
11 Keats Court
Coto de Caza, CA 96279

916-773-2999
888-999-9428
e-mail: pediatric-info@genetic.org
www.genetic.org

Information on support groups, meetings, research being conducted, book and product reviews, and ask the doctor column.

3 times a year

Melissa Aylstock, Executive Director

4416 Klinefelter Syndrome Newsletter
PO Box 119
Roseville, CA 95678

916-773-2999
888-999-9428
Fax: 916-773-1449
e-mail: ksinfo@genetic.org
www.genetic.org/ks/index/shtml

News on Klinefelter syndrome, education and support. You'll find a wealth of information on this very common, but underdiagnosed condition.

DESCRIPTION

4417 KLIPPEL-FEIL SYNDROME

Synonym: KFS

Covers these related disorders: Klippel-Feil syndrome Type I, Klippel-Feil syndrome Type II, Klippel-Feil syndrome Type III

Involves the following Biologic System(s):
Genetic/Chromosomal/Syndrome/Metabolic Disorders

Klippel-Feil syndrome (KFS) is a congenital malformation characterized by the fusion of two or more vertebrae, especially in the neck or cervical region (congenital synostosis) or by the absence of one or more cervical vertebrae. Klippel-Feil syndrome Type I involves extensive fusion of several cervical vertebrae and thoracic vertebrae located in the upper back. Type II involves fusion of a limited number of incompletely developed vertebrae (hemivertebrae) and vertebrae, fusion of the uppermost cervical vertebra with the bone at the back of the skull (occipital bone), and other irregularities. Klippel-Feil syndrome Type III is characterized by fusion of the cervical, lower thoracic, or lumbar vertebrae. Physical findings associated with Klippel-Feil syndrome may include a short neck with limited range of motion, a low hairline, and irregularities of the urinary tract and reproductive, cardiovascular, pulmonary, and nervous systems. Additional abnormalities may include curvatures of the spine (scoliosis or kyphosis), an inclination of the neck to one side (torticollis), webbing of the neck (pterygium colli) and fingers (syndactyly), and other irregularities of the bones and muscles.

Treatment of Klippel-Feil syndrome may be directed toward the particular physical findings and symptoms associated with this disorder. Such treatment may include measures to correct or halt the progression of various spinal irregularities and to correct other abnormalities as warranted. Other treatment is supportive.

In some children, Klippel-Feil syndrome is transmitted as an autosomal dominant trait, while transmission by autosomal recessive inheritance is possible in others. In addition, some affected children have no recognizable pattern of genetic transmission.

See also General Resources on page 917

Government Agencies

4418 NIH/National Institute of Arthritis & Musculoskeletal & Skin Diseases

National Institutes of Health
1 AMS Circle
Bethesda, MD 20892

301-495-4484
877-226-4267
Fax: 301-718-6366
TDD: 301-565-2966
e-mail: niamsinfo@mail.nih.gov
www.niams.nih.gov

The mission of the NIAMS, a part of the NIH, is to support research into the causes, treatment, and prevention of arthritis and musculoskeletal and skin diseases, the training of basic and clinical scientists to carry out this research, and the dissemination of information on research progress in these diseases.

Stephen I Katz MD PhD, Director

4419 NIH/National Institute of Child Health and Human Development

31 Center Drive, Building 31
Bethesda, MD 20892

301-496-5133
Fax: 301-496-1104
www.nichd.nih.gov

Established in 1962 by congress, today the institute conducts and supports research on topics related to the health of children, adults, families and populations. Some of these topics include: developmental disabilities, growth and development, infant death, reproductive health and birth defects.

Nancy D Wirth, Director
Lisa Kaeser, Program & Public Liaison

4420 NIH/Osteoporosis and Related Bone Diseases National Resource Center

2 AMS Circle
Bethesda, MD 20892

202-223-0344
800-624-2663
Fax: 202-293-2356
TTY: 202-466-4315
e-mail: NIAMSBoneinfo@mail.nih.gov
www.niams.nih.gov/bone/

Distributes information to health professionals, and the public on osteoporosis, Paget's disease of bone, osteogenesis imperfecta, and other metabolic bone diseases. Includes prevention, early detection, and treatment of these diseases.

Stephen I Katz MD, PhD, Director

National Associations & Support Groups

4421 Klippel-Feil Syndrome Support Group

311 Bracken Avenue
Pittsburgh, PA 15227

412-884-2969

Describes congenital fusion of at least two of the seven vertebrae in the cervical-spine. In addition there may be fusion or anomalies of vertebrae in the thoracic or lumbar-spine.

4422 March of Dimes Birth Defects Foundation
1275 Mamaroneck Avenue
White Plains, NY 10605

914-428-7100
888-663-4637
Fax: 914-428-8203
e-mail: resourcecenter@modimes.org
www.marchofdimes.com

Partnership of volunteers and professionals dedicates to improving the health of babies by preventing birth defects and infant mortality. Over 100 chapters are located across the country and can be located through the National Office.

Dr Jennifer Howse, President

Web Sites

4423 Online Mendelian Inheritance in Man
www.ncbi.nlm.nih.gov

This database is a catalog of human genes and genetic disorders.

4424 Rare Genetic Diseases in Children (NYU)
www.med.nyu.edu/rgdc/homenow.htm

We target issues arising from rare genetic diseases affecting children. Also, to assist in the endeavor to bring knowledge and hope to those for whom there is, at present, so little.

4425 Wheeless' Textbook of Orthopaedics
www.wheelessonline.com

Derives from a variety of sources, including journals, articles, national meetings lectures and other textbooks.

DESCRIPTION

4426 LEAD POISONING

Involves the following Biologic System(s):

Developmental/Behavioral/Psychiatric Disorders,
Neurologic Disorders

Children and adults exposed to lead chronically over time can develop toxic levels in their blood. Traditionally, the lead level that raises concern is 10mcg/dl or above. Lead is much more harmful to children than adults because it can affect children's developing nerves and brains. The younger the child, the more harmful lead can be. Unborn children are the most vulnerable. However, many children with these levels may be asymptomatic. There are a number of sources for lead exposure. Although paint is a common source of lead, other products that may contain lead include ceramics, crystal, gasoline, batteries, and cosmetics. In the United States, the primary sources for lead exposure include household plumbing, paint made prior to 1977, and gasoline with tetraethyl lead as an additive. Although there has been a growing movement in the US to restrict the use of lead in these products, its prior use in many products continues to pose a hazard to the general population, especially young children. Lead may be inadvertently ingested, inhaled, or absorbed through the skin. One of the most common ways small children become exposed to lead is through the ingestion of fine dust from lead based paints, by licking their hands that are coated with lead dust, or by inhaling lead dust that is then swallowed. Lead makes things taste sweet, so children are attracted to the taste of lead paint chips and especially to lead dust. Lead that enters the body gets absorbed into the blood stream. It is then deposited in soft tissue and organs, or excreted through the kidney. Most of the lead that remains in the body, though, is deposited in bones. Lead toxicity primarily involves the central nervous system and the gastrointestinal system. Although many children with lead ingestion will have asymptomatic disease, they may show increased behavioral problems, poor school performance, decreased height, and decreased cognitive function. Children with more severe lead exposure may complain of anorexia, nausea, vomiting, abdominal pain and constipation. These symptons have been reported at lead levels as low as 20 mcg/dl but more commonly seen at lead levels greater than 50 mcg/dl. Neurological symptoms may include ataxia (staggering gait), seizures, coma, and encephalopathy. Screening for lead exposure should be performed in all children under 5. A thorough history should be taken, focusing on age of the patient's home, behavioral changes, exposure to battery factories or ceramics, recent home renovations (in homes

pre-1978), and history of lead poisoning in a sibling. The frequency of the blood test screening will increase based on the patient's environmental exposure. A lead level of 10 mcg/dl or greater is considered a significant exposure and warrants further evaluation. An assessment of the home should be undertaken and the patient should have repeat blood lead levels tested no later than 3 months of age. The American Academy of Pediatrics recommends repeating a lead level by 3 months. Lead exposure may in some cases also be confirmed by x-ray, studies in the abdomen and in bones (lead lines). Therapy for lead exposure/toxicity generally focuses on removing the lead from the patient's environment, diminishing hand to mouth behaviors, improving nutrition in exposed patients and removing the lead from the patient's body. Homes may be cleaned properly by professionals and old paint must be removed from environment or sealed in a fashion that will eliminate the family's exposure to paint dust and chips. Some children will need to be moved to a lead-free safehouse while this is occurring. Frequent washing of hands and toys will cut down on exposure from hand to mouth behavior exhibited by young children. Lead levels greater than 44mcg/dl are considered significant enough to warrant chelation therapy and levels greater than 70 mcg/dl should prompt referral for chelation and hospitalization. Chelation therapy involves giving patients chelating, or binding, agents which bind to the lead and make it easier to excrete from the body. This type of therapy should begin only after the source of lead in the environment has been eliminated.

See also **General Resources** on page 917

National Associations & Support Groups

4427 National Lead Information Center
8601 Georgia Avenue Suite 503
Silver Spring, MD 20910

> 800-424-5323
> Fax: 301-585-7976
> e-mail: hotline.lead@epa.gov

Offers support and referrals for patients and their families. Provides testing kits, evaluation techniques, and resource materials, including publications and tapes.

State Agencies & Support Groups

4428 Connecticut Lead Poisoning Prevention Program
410 Capitol Avenue, Ms#51LED P.O. Box 340308
Hartford, CT 06134

> 860-509-7299
> Fax: 860-509-7295

Workshops and literature on how to diagnose and prevent lead poisoning.

Audio Video

4429 Lead Poisoning
Fanlight Productions
47 Halifax Street
Boston, MA 02130

617-469-4999
Fax: 617-469-3379
e-mail: fanlight@fanlight.com
www.fanlight.com

The disastrous effects of environmental lead on both children and adults. Dartmouth Hitchcock Medical Center Series, The Doctor is In...

28 minutes

Web Sites

4430 Consumer Product Safety Commission Hotline
www.cpsc.gov

CPSC is an Independent Federal Regulatory Agency that works to save lives and keep families safe by reducing the risk of injuries and deaths associated with consumer products.

4431 National Conference of State Legislatures
www.ncsl.org

The National Conference of State Legislatures is a bipartisan organization that serves the legislators and staffs of the nation's 50 states, its commonwealths and territories. NCSL provides research, technical assistance and opportunities for policymakers to exchange ideas on the most pressing state issues. NCSL is an effective and respected advocate for the interests of state governments before Congress and federal agencies.

4432 Safe Drinking Water Hotline
www.epa.org/safewater/

Together with the states, tribes, and its many partners, protects public health by ensuring safe drinking water and protecting ground water. Along with EPS's ten regional drinking water programs, oversees implementation of the SAFE DRINKING WATER ACT, which is the national law safeguarding tap water in America.

DESCRIPTION

4433 LEARNING DISABILITY/READING DYSLEXIA

Synonyms: Learning Disorders, LDD

Covers these related disorders: Dyscalculia, Dyslexia, Dysgraphia **Involves the following Biologic System(s):** Developmental/Behavioral/Psychiatric Disorders

Learning Disability (LD) is a general term that refers to a group of disorders characterized by problems with learning, processing, or expressing information. When LD involves speech and language, it can affect how a person hears words (receptive language disorder), how they put thoughts into words (expressive language disorder), or how words are put together when spoken (articulation disorder).

LD can also affect academic skills. Dyscalculia is a learning disability characterized by difficulty in using mathematical symbols and understanding mathematical concepts. Dysgraphia is the difficulty in the physical process of writing letters and words. A person with dyspraxia can understand sentences in a normal way, but has difficulty putting words together into a coherent sentence. Dyslexia is characterized by the impairment in the ability to process written symbols.

Young children with dyslexia may have difficulty remembering the correct names of letters and numbers. Some school aged children may reverse letters and words when writing. For example, affected children may substitute the letter P for Q, reverse the word WAS to become SAW, or transpose letters so that BETS becomes BEST. Children with dyslexia may also have difficulty reading due to an impaired ability to determine the sequence of letters within words and to distinguish right from left. The hallmark of this learning disability is the fact that despite their difficulties, affected children are of average or above average intelligence by IQ testing and scholastic achievement.

Although learning disabilities occur in very young children, the disorders are usually not recognized until the child reaches school age. Early diagnosis of LD is an important factor in treatment. Children nearing the end of first grade who exhibit difficulties with word skills, or any children whose reading, writing, or mathematical skills are not commensurate with that of their other scholastic abilities should be tested for LD. Although LD is not related to eye defects, an ophthalmologic evaluation is beneficial in eliminating vision problems as a cause for symptoms. Treatment for LD is geared towards remedial teaching techniques specific to the disability.

LD is thought to be a familial disorder and may be inherited in an autosomal dominant fashion.

See also **General Resources** on page 917

National Associations & Support Groups

4434 AVKO Dyslexia Research Foundation
3084 W Willard Road Suite W
Clio, MI 48420

810-686-9283
866-285-6612
Fax: 810-686-1101
e-mail: DonMcCabe@avko.org
www.avko.org

Nonprofit organization founded to help determine what dyslexia is, why traditional methods of teaching and writing fail and help most dyslexics learn to read and write.

1974

Don McCabe, Research Director

4435 American Speech Language Hearing Associati on (ASHA)
10801 Rockville Pike
Rockville, MD 20852

800-638-8255
Fax: 240-333-4705
e-mail: actioncenter@asha.org
www.asha.org

A certifying body of 123,000 professionals providing speech, language and hearing services to the public. It is an accrediting agency for college and university graduate school programs in speech-language pathology and audiology.

Arlene A Pietranton, Executive Director

4436 Council for Learning Disabilities
11184 Antioch Road Box 405
Overland Park, KS 66210

913-491-1011
Fax: 913-491-1012
www.cldinternational.org

An international organization that promotes effective teaching and research. CDL is composed of professionals who represent diverse disciplines and who are committed to enhancing the education and life span development of individuals with learning disabilities.

4437 Dislexia Research Institute
5746 Centerville Road
Tallahassee, FL 32309

850-893-2216
Fax: 850-893-2440
e-mail: dri@dyslexia-add.org
www,dyslexia-add.org

Addresses academic, social and self-concept issues for dyslexic and ADD children and adults. College prep courses, study skills, advocacy, diagnostic testing, seminars, teachers training, day school, tutoring and an adult literacy and life skills programs are available using an accredited MSLE approach.

Patricia K Hardman Phd, Director
Robyn A Rennick MS, Assistant Director

4438 Division for Learning Disabilities
1110 N Glebe Road Suite 300
Arlington, VA 22201

703-620-3660
888-232-7733
Fax: 703-264-9494
TTY: 703-264-9446
www.teachingld.org

The Division for Learning Disabilities is a national professional organization consisting of teacher, higher education professionals, administrators, and parents. The major purpose of DLD is to promote the education and general welfare of persons with learning disabilities, provide a forum for discussion of issues facing the field of learning disabilities, and to encourage interaction amoung the many groups whose research and service efforts impact persons with learning disabilities.

Ed Ellis, President
John Willis Lloyd, Vice President

4439 Federation for Children with Special Needs
1135 Tremont Street
Boston, MA 02120

617-236-7210
800-331-0688
Fax: 617-572-2094
e-mail: fcsninfo@fcsn.org
www.fcsn.org

The mission of the Federation for Children with Special Needs provides information, support, and assistance to parents of children with disabilities, and encouraging full participation in community life by all people, especially those with isabilities.

Sonya Andrade, Executive Assistant
Robin Foley, Director

4440 International Dyslexia Association
40 York Road 4th Floor
Baltimore, MD 21204

410-296-0232
800-223-3123
Fax: 410-321-5069
e-mail: MBIDA4@hotmail.com
www.interdys.org

Nonprofit, scientific and educational organization dedicated to the study and treatment of dyslexia. Focus in educating parents, teachers and professionals in the field of dyslexia in effective teaching methodologies. Programs and services include: information and referral; public awareness; medical and educational research; governmental affairs; conferences and publications.

Cathy Rosemond, President

4441 Learning Disabilities Association of Ameri ca
4156 Library Road
Pittsburgh, PA 15234

412-341-1515
888-300-6710
Fax: 412-344-0224
e-mail: info@LDAAmerica.org
www.LDAAmerica.org

Helps families of the affected individual through information and referral to professionals in their area. A membership organization with affiliates in 43 states.

Sheila Buckley, Executive Director

4442 National Center For Learning Disabilities With Disabilities
381 Park Avenue S Suite 1401
New York, NY 10016

212-545-7510
888-575-7373
Fax: 212-545-9665
www.ncld.org

The mission is to increase opportunities for all individuals with learning disabilities to achieve their potential.NCLD accomplishes this mission by increasing public awareness and understanding of learning disabilities, conducting educational programs and services that promote research-based knowledge, and providing national leadership in shaping public policy.

Frederic M Poses, Chairman
James H Wendorf, Executive Director

4443 National Dissemination Center for Children with Disabilities
PO Box 1492
Washington, DC 20013

202-884-8200
800-695-0285
Fax: 202-884-8441
e-mail: nichcy@aed.org
www.nichcy.org

Provides parents with information about special education and the rights children and youth with disabilities have under the law. NICHY can also provide parents and others with a State Resource Sheet, useful for identifying resources within their state. This sheet includes, names, addresses and phone numbers of state agencies disability organizations, and parent groups serving individuals with disabilities and their families. A variety of other publications are available upon request.

Suzanne Ripley, Executive Director

4444 Parents Helping Parents: Family Resources for Children with Special Needs
3041 Olcott Street
Santa Clara, CA 95054

408-727-5775
Fax: 408-727-0182
e-mail: info@php.com
www.php.com

Helping children with special needs receive the resources, love, hope, respect, health care, education and other services they need to achive their full potential by providing them with strong families and dedicated professional to serve them.

Libraries & Resource Centers

4445 Berkshire Center
18 Park Street #160
Lee, MA 01238

413-243-2576

A postsecondary program for young adults with learning disabilities ages eighteen-twenty-six. Half the students attend Berkshire Community College part-time while others go directly into the working world. Services include vocational/adacademic preparation, tutoring, college liason, life skills instruction, driver's education, money management, psychotherapy, and more. The program is year-round with an average stay of two years.

4446 University of Kansas Center for Research on Learning
3061 Dole Center
Lawrence, KS 66045

785-864-4780
Fax: 785-864-5728
www.ku-crl.org

A research center working to improve learning and performance of adolescants and adults considered to be at risk for failure in today's schools, work places, and communities. Develops products and procedures that can be used to more effectively teach these individuals. Provides support and research-validated instructional materials to an international training network that promotes system change in our schools and institutions. Newsletter for teachers containing tips and advice used in class.

Don Deshler, Director
Jean Schumaker, Associate Director

Audio Video

4447 How to Help Your Child Succeed in School

Sandra Rief, author

Peytral Publications
PO Box 1162
Minnetonka, MN 55345

952-949-8707
877-739-8725
Fax: 952-906-9777
www.peytral.com

Essential information needed by parents and educators. Topics include developiong reading, writing and math skills, building organization and study skills, surviving daily homework assignments and coping with learning disabilities.

56 minutes

4448 LOVAAS Learning Videotapes

8700 Shoal Creek Boulevard
Austin, TX 78757

512-451-3246
800-897-3202
Fax: 800-397-7633
e-mail: info@predinc.com
www.proedinc.com

Five videotapes which present valuable information on the content and execution of learning strategies for children with developmental disabilities: Getting Ready to Learn, Early Language, Basic Self-Help Skills, Advanced Language, and Expanding Your Child's World. You can purchase the complete set for $777.00 or separately.

Video

Web Sites

4449 Children's Hospital of New York Presbyterian
www.childrensnyp.org

A high quality, world class center that improves the health status of children.

4450 Division for Learning Disabilities
www.teachingld.org

Promotes the education and general welfare of persons with learning disabilities.

4451 Learning Disabilities Association of Ameri ca
www.ldanatl.org

Helps families of the affected individual through information and referral to professionals in their area. A membership organization with affiliates in 43 states.

4452 National Dissemination Center for Children with Disabilities
www.nichcy.com

Provides parents with information about special education and the rights children and youth have under law. It also provides parents with a resource sheet of organizations in their state.

4453 The Parent Educational Advocacy Training C enter
www.peatc.org

Provides general research about special education and learning disabilities.

Book Publishers

4454 Learning Disabilities and Challenging Beha viors

Nancy Mather PhD, Sam Goldstein PhD, author

Brooks Publishings
PO Box 10624
Baltimore, MD 21285

410-337-9850
800-638-3775
Fax: 410-337-8539
e-mail: custserv@brookspublishing.com
www.brookspublishing.com

A working manual for educators and others who teach children with learning disabilities. Helps readers to understand how specific developmental, behaviour, and academic problems influence school success.

416 pages

Magazines

4455 Get Ready to Read!
National Center for Learning Disabilities
381 Park Avenue S
New York, NY 10016

212-545-7510
888-575-7373
Fax: 212-545-9665
e-mail: hlp@ncld.org
www.ncld.org

Quartely

Amber Eden, Assistant Director Online Comm.
Hal Stucker, Managing Editor

4456 LD Advocate
National Center for Learning Disabilities
381 Park Avenue S
New York, NY 10016

212-545-7510
888-575-7373
Fax: 212-545-9665
e-mail: hlp@ncld.org
www.ncld.org

Quartely

Amber Eden, Assistant Director Online Comm.
Hal Stucker, Managing Editor

4457 LD News
National Center for Learning Disabilities
381 Park Avenue S
New York, NY 10016

212-545-7510
888-575-7373
Fax: 212-545-9665
e-mail: hlp@ncld.org
www.ncld.org

Quartely

Amber Eden, Assistant Director Online Comm.
Hal Stucker, Managing Editor

4458 Our World
National Center for Learning Disabilities
381 Park Avenue S
New York, NY 10016

212-545-7510
888-575-7373
Fax: 212-545-9665
e-mail: hlp@ncld.org
www.ncld.org

Quartely

Amber Eden, Assistant Director Online Comm.
Hal Stucker, Managing Editor

Newsletters

4459 International Dyslexia Association Quarterly Newsletter: Perspective
IDA
40 York Road 4th Floor
Baltimore, MD 21204

> 410-296-0232
> 800-223-3123
> Fax: 410-321-5069
> e-mail: MBIDA4@hotmail.com
> www.interdys.org

Nonprofit, scientific and educational organization dedicated to the study and treatment of dyslexia. Focus in educating parents, teachers and professionals in the field of dyslexia in effective teaching methodologies. Programs and services include: information and referral; public awareness; medical and educational research; governmental affairs; conferences and publications.

50-56 pages

Cathy Rosemond, President

Pamphlets

4460 Learning Problems or Learning Disabilities
Consumer Information Center
Department 509B
Pueblo, CO 81009

Free government publication that explains the differences between learning problems and disabilities. It contains a chart that shows language and reasoning skills to watch for at different ages.

Camps

4461 Beech Brook
3737 Lander Road
Cleveland, OH

> 216-831-2255
> Fax: 216-831-0436

A year-round residential and day treatment center, accepts summer residents when there are openings in the regular enrollment. The program is designed for emotionally disturbed, learning disabled and autistic children, providing therapeutically oriented teaching and programming techniques in a camp setting.

Don Harris, Director

4462 Big Crystal Camp
8533 Williams Road
DeWitt, MI

> 517-669-9367

One week residential camp sponsored by Lansing Area Chapter of Michigan Association for Children with Learning Disabilities.

Florence Curtis

4463 Camp Buckskin
8700 W 36th Street Suite 6w
Saint Louis Park, MN 55426

> 952-930-3544
> Fax: 952-938-6996
> e-mail: buckskin@spacestar.net
> www.campbuckskin.com

LD and ADD/ADHD youth have often experienced frustration and a lack of success. Buckskin assists these individuals to realize and develop the potentials and abilities which they possess. Teaches a combination of academic and camp activities, so the campers experience success in many areas. By necessity fairly structured, the 1:3 staff ratio ensures the program is individualized to meet each camper's needs. Parents report that their children benefit from the experience in many ways.

Thomas R Bauer, CCD, Camp Director

4464 Camp Nuhop
404 Hillcrest Drive
Ashland, OH

> 419-289-2227
> Fax: 419-289-2227
> e-mail: cnuhop@bright.net
> www.campnuhop.org

A summer residential program for any youngster from 6 to 18 with a learning disability, behavior disorder or Attention Deficit Disorder. Sixty two campers and 35 staff members live on site in groups of 7 campers to every 3 counselors. Activities focus on positive self-concept and behaviors and teach children to learn how to find their strengths, abilities and talents from a positive, yet realistic viewpoint.

Jerry Dunlap, Director

4465 Dallas Academy
950 Tiffany Way
Dallas, TX

> 214-324-1481
> Fax: 214-327-8537
> e-mail: mail@dallas-academy.com
> www.dallas-academy.com

7-week summer session for students who are having difficulty in regular school classes.

Jim Richardson, Director

4466 Developmental Center
6710 86th Avenue N
Pinellas Park, FL

Specifically designed for the learning disabled child and other children with difficulties in concentration, strategy, social skills, impulsivity, distractibility and study strategies. Programs offered include: attention training, visual-motor remediation, socialization skills training, relaxation training, horseback riding and more. The day camp meets weekdays from 9-3 for 3,4 or 5 week sessions.

Dr. Eric Larson

4467 Eagle Hill School - Summer Program
242 Old Petersham Road
Hardwick, MA 01037

> 413-477-6000
> Fax: 413-477-6837
> e-mail: admission@eaglehillschool.com
> www.ehs1.org

For the child, age 9-19, with a specific learning disability or Attention Deficit Disorder, this summer program offers a structured curriculum designed to build a basic foundation of academic competence. Extracurricular and outdoor activities complement the educational program.

Erin E Wynne, Dean of Admission

4468 Groves Learning Center
3200 Highway 100 S
Saint Louis Park, MN

A nonprofit day school in Minnesota designed especially for children with learning differences. The Center has a full day academic program from September through June, as well as an 8 week summer program. Groves also offers community services such as: psychoeducational testing for children and adults, consulting services, workshops on learning disabilities and other special learning needs, and afternoon/evening tutorial services for children and adults.

Sue Kirchhoff, Head of School

4469 Hill School of Fort Worth
4817 Odessa Avenue
Fort Worth, TX

817-923-9482
Fax: 817-923-4894
e-mail: admission@hillschool.org
www.hillschool.org

Provides an alternative learning environment for students having average or above-average intelligence with learning differences. Hill school is an established leader in North Texas with a 25 year history of effectively serving LD children. Beginning in 1961 as a tutorial service, Hill became a formal school in 1973. Our mission is to help those who learn differently develop skills and strategies to succeed. We do this by developing academic/study skills, and self-discipline.

Lucille H Helton, Principal
Cathy Allen, Admissions Director

4470 Lab School of Washington
4759 Reservoir Road NW
Washington, DC 20007

202-965-6600
Fax: 202-965-5106
www.labschool.org

The Lab School six week summer session includes individualized reading, spelling, writing, study skills, and math programs. A multisensory approach addresses the needs of bright learning disabled children. Related services such as speech/language therapy and occupational therapy are integrated into the curriculum. Elementary/Intermediate; Junior High/High School.

Sally Smith, Founder
Susan Ferley, Admissions Director

4471 Maplebrook School
5142 Route 22
Amenia, NY

845-373-8191
Fax: 845-373-7029
e-mail: mbsecho@aol.com

A coeducational boarding school for students with learning differences and ADD. A New York State registered high school servicing ages 11-18. Post secondary options offered to 18-21.

Donna M Konkolios, Head of School
Jennifer Scully, Director Admissions

4472 Oakland School & Camp
Boyd Tavern
Keswick, VA 22947

434-293-9059
Fax: 434-296-8930
e-mail: oaklanschool@earthlink.net
www.oaklandschool.net

A highly individualized program stresses improving reading ability. Subjects taught are reading, English composition, math and word analysis. Recreational activities include horseback riding, sports, swimming, tennis, crafts, archery and camping. For girls and boys, ages 8-14.

Joanne Dondero, President
Carol Smieciuch, Director

4473 Phelps School
583 Sugartown Road
Malvern, PA 19355

610-644-1754
Fax: 610-644-6679
e-mail: admis@thephelpsschool.org
www.thephelpsschool.org

Phelps School is dedicated to a personalized education for the boy who seeks success academically, personally, and socially. This philosophy is accentuated by the disciplined atmosphere, small classes, and daily tutorial support. The idea which inspired Norman T. Phelps, Sr. to begin a school dedicated to the individual boy has never been more relevant that it is today. The model of educating boys according to thier interests and abilities is designed to generate success & improve self-esteem.

Michael Reaerdon, Director of Admission
Emily Shaker, Admissions Representative

4474 Round Lake Camp
21 Plymouth Street
Fairfield, NJ

973-575-3333
Fax: 973-575-4188
e-mail: rlc@njycamps.org
www.njycamps.org

For ages 7-18, this camp provides individualized academics in reading, language development and math for children with mild learning disabilities, Round Lake also offers therapeutic recreation and Jewish cultural values to its participants.

Sheira Director, Asst. Director

DESCRIPTION

4475 LEGG-CALVE-PERTHES DISEASE

Synonyms: LCPD, Perthes disease, Avasular necrosis of femoral head

Involves the following Biologic System(s):
Orthopedic and Muscle Disorders

Legg-Calve-Perthes disease (LCPD) belongs to a group of disorders in which abnormalities of the growth centers of certain bones result in degeneration and gradual regeneration of the affected bone. This group of disorders is known as the osteochondroses. LCPD affects the growing end of the head of the thigh bone (femoral capital epiphysis). In most affected children, the thigh bone (femur) on one side of the body is affected (unilateral); however, in approximately 20 percent of patients, the disorder may eventually involve the other femur (bilateral). The age of onset and the severity and duration of the disease are variable. Legg-Calve-Perthes disease typically becomes apparent between the ages of two to 12 years, with the average age of onset approximately seven years of age. Males are affected four to five times as often as females; however, females may tend to have more severe symptoms. LCPD is thought to affect approximately one in 1,000 to 5,000 children.

Degeneration of the head of the femur is thought to occur due to insufficient blood supply (ischemia) to this area of bone, resulting in the localized loss of bone and cartilage as well as the loss of bone mass. The onset of symptoms associated with LCPD is typically slow and progressive. Many affected children initially experience muscle spasms, a limp, or mild or periodic pain that may affect the thigh, hip, knee, or groin area. As the disorder progresses, additional symptoms and findings often include delayed maturation of the thigh bone (delayed bone age); mild restriction of movements of the affected hip; potential degeneration of the front thigh muscles; abnormal positioning of the hip and thigh toward the body (internal rotation); and, in some patients, mild short stature. LCPD is considered a self-limiting disorder because, even without medical intervention, new blood supplies are eventually spontaneously reestablished (revascularization) to the femoral head, causing the formation of new bone tissue in the affected area. This may occur approximately two to four years after the onset of symptoms. In some affected children, new bony growth may be misshapen, potentially causing the affected leg to be relatively shorter than the unaffected leg, an associated limp, and an increased risk for degenerative changes of the hips, resulting in swelling, pain or tenderness, and stiffness (osteoarthritis).

Because Legg-Calve-Perthes disease is a self-limiting disorder, treatment usually is directed toward preventing deformity of the femoral head and secondary osteoarthritis. Such measures may include ongoing clinical assessment and specialized x-ray tests to monitor the progress of the disease; bed rest or special stretching exercises; the use of braces or casts; or surgery.

There is no specific cause known for LCPD and, in most cases, it is though to occur randomly for unknown reasons. However, there are some risk factors including possible links to children who are small for their age and are extremely active. Interestingly, exposure to secondhand smoke is correlated with LCPD. There have also been reports of several affected individuals within certain families (kindreds) that suggest autosomal dominant inheritance. Some reseachers suspect that LCPD may be caused by the interaction of several different genes, possibly in association with the involvement of certain environmental factors (multifactorial disorder). Although Legg-Calvé-Perthes disease cannot be prevented, much has been accomplished toward minimizing its effects.

See also **General Resources** on page 917

Government Agencies

4476 NIH/National Institute of Arthritis & Musculoskeletal & Skin Diseases
National Institutes of Health
1 AMS Circle
Bethesda, MD 20892

301-495-4484
877-226-4267
Fax: 301-718-6366
TDD: 301-565-2966
e-mail: niamsinfo@mail.nih.gov
www.niams.nih.gov

The mission of the NIAMS, a part of the NIH, is to support research into the causes, treatment, and prevention of athritis and musculoskeletal and skin diseases, the training of basic and clinical scientists to carry out this research, and the dissemination of information on research progress in these diseases.

Lillian Hatch, Librarian

4477 NIH/National Institute of Arthritis and Mu oskeletal and Skin Diseases
1AMS Circle
Bethesda, MD 20892

301-402-4484
Fax: 301-718-6366
e-mail: ord@od.nih.gov
rarediseases.info.nih.gov

The mission of the National Institute of Arthritis and Musculoskeletal and Skin Diseases is to support research into the causes, treatment, and prevention of arthritis and musculoskeletal and skin diseases, the training of basic and clinical scientists to carry out this research, and the dissemination of information on research progress in these diseases.

Stephen I Katz MD PhD, Director

4478 NIH/National Institute of Child Health and Human Development
31 Center Drive, Building 31
Bethesda, MD 20892

301-496-5133
Fax: 301-496-1104
www.nichd.nih.gov

Established in 1962 by congress, today the institute conducts and supports research on topics related to the health of children, adults, families and populations. Some of these topics include: developmental disabilities, growth and development, infant death, reproductive health and birth defects.

Nancy D Wirth, Director
Lisa Kaeser, Program & Public Liaison

National Associations & Support Groups

4479 March of Dimes Birth Defects Foundation
1275 Mamaroneck Avenue
White Plains, NY 10605

914-428-7100
888-663-4637
Fax: 914-428-8203
e-mail: resourcecenter@modimes.org
www.marchofdimes.com

Partnership of volunteers and professionals dedicates to improving the health of babies by preventing birth defects and infant mortality. Over 100 chapters are located across the country and can be located through the National Office.

Dr Jennifer Howse, President

4480 National Information Center on Deafness
Gallaudet Univ. Press c/o Chicago Distrib. Center
800 Florida Avenue NE
Washington, DC 20002

202-651-5300
800-621-2736
Fax: 202-651-5477
TTY: 888-630-9347
e-mail: infotech.services@galludet.edu
www.gallaudet.edu

Provides information or referrals on questions about deafness, including general information, education, research, legislation, assistive devices and more. Offers a bibliography of readings available on 30 topics relating to deafness.

Loraine DiPietro, Director

Web Sites

4481 Articles on Legg-Calve-Perthes
www.orthoseek.com/articles/perthes.html

A source of authoritative information on pediatric orthopedics and pediatric information regarding your child's orthopedic condition or sports injury, and you can find useful articles that you can reproduce for yourself or others.

4482 Online Support Group
www.maxpages.com/lpsupportgroup

Provides support groups for families with children diagnosed with Legg-Perthes disease.

4483 Wheeless' Textbook of Orthopaedics
www.wheelessonline.com

Derives from a variety of sources, including journals, articles, national meetings lectures and other textbooks.

DESCRIPTION

4484 LEUKODYSTROPHIES

Covers these related disorders: Adrenoleukodystrophy, ALD, Adrenomyeloneuropathy, Krabbe disease, Methachromatic leukodystrophy, Pelizaeus-Merzbacher disease

Involves the following Biologic System(s):
Genetic/Chromosomal/Syndrome/Metabolic Disorders

The leukodystrophies are a group of inherited neurodegenerative diseases that affect the white (leuko) matter of the brain and are characterized by the destruction of the fatty, protective covering around the nerve fibers (myelin sheaths). The symptoms of some forms of these diseases become obvious during childhood. These diseases include adrenoleukodystrophy (ALD), adrenomyeloneuropathy, Krabbe disease, metachromatic leukodystrophy, and Pelizaeus-Merzbacher disease.

Classic adrenoleukodystrophy, or ALD, is a metabolic disorder transmitted as an X-linked recessive trait that is fully expressed in boys. This type of adrenoleukodystrophy becomes apparent between the ages of five and 15 years and is characterized by behavioral disturbances, mental deterioration, seizures, lack of coordination, and motor weakness or partial paralysis with increased muscle tone in the arms and legs accompanied by exaggerated reflex responses (spasticity). In addition, boys with ALD may have difficulty with swallowing, language development, and speech. Vision may be impaired. Other findings include insufficient adrenal gland function characterized by a darkening or tanning of the skin. Experimental treatments include bone marrow transplantation and dietary considerations. Other treatment is symptomatic and supportive. The gene for classic ALD is located on the long arm of the X chromosome (Xq28). Adrenomyeloneuropathy is considered a milder, adult form of adrenoleukodystrophy, although its onset may occur as early as late adolescence.

Neonatal adrenoleukodystrophy is inherited as an autosomal recessive trait and is characterized by seizures, severe delays in skills that involve the coordination of mental and muscular activities (psychomotor coordination), and insufficiency of the adrenal glands. Treatment is symptomatic and supportive.

Krabbe disease, sometimes called globoid cell leukodystrophy, is a rare neurodegenerative disorder that is inherited as an autosomal recessive trait. This life-threatening, progressive disease results from a deficiency of the enzyme galactocerebrosidase and is characterized during early infancy by irritability, vomiting, extremely high fevers, difficulty feeding, and failure to thrive. Seizures may develop followed by muscular rigidity, convulsions, paralysis, , loss of vision and hearing, mental deterioration, or other irregularities. Krabbe disease may sometimes have a later onset with symptoms and findings developing during childhood or adolescence. Treatment is symptomatic and supportive. The gene for Krabbe disease is located on the long arm of chromosome 14 (14q21-q31).

Metachromatic leukodystrophy (MLD) is inherited in an autosomal recessive pattern and occurs as the result of a deficiency of the enzyme sulfatase A. Late infantile MLD usually occurs in the first or second year of life and is characterized by progressive irregularities in the manner of walking (gait), frequent falling, developmental delays, seizures, diminished muscle tone in the arms and legs, and diminished deep tendon reflexes. As the disease progresses, children may be unable to stand and signs of intellectual degeneration become apparent. Additional findings include impaired speech and deteriorating visual activity or blindness. Approximately one year after symptom onset, most children are unable to sit without support and may experience swallowing and eating difficulties. Life-threatening complications such as pneumonia may develop. Juvenile MLD occurs from the ages of four to 12 years and is characterized by behavioral and intellectual deterioration followed by walking and speech difficulties, urinary incontinence, lack of coordination, impaired muscle tone, and convulsions. This form of MLD has a slower progression than that of late infantile MLD. One variant of juvenile MLD results from a deficiency of a protein that aids in the activation of cerebroside sulfatase. The gene for metachromatic leukodystrophy is located on the long arm of chromosome 22 (22q13.31-qter).

Pelizaeus-Merzbacher disease is inherited as an X-linked recessive trait. This disorder occurs during infancy or early childhood and progresses slowly into adolescence or adulthood. This life-threatening form of leukodystrophy is characterized in infancy by head-nodding and eye irregularities such as involuntary, rhythmic movement of the eyes (nystagmus). Boys with this disorder experience developmental delays followed by tremors; well-coordinated but involuntary jerky, writhing movements; a mask-like, frozen expression (parkinsonian facies); difficulty with speech; and deterioration of mental function. Treatment is symptomatic and supportive. The gene for Pelizaeus-Merzbacher disease is located on the long arm of the X chromosome (Xq22).

Bone marrow transplantation is showing promise for a few of the leukodystrophies.

See also **General Resources** on page 917

National Associations & Support Groups

4485 Genetic Alliance
4301 Connecticut Avenue NW
Washington, DC 20008

202-966-5557
800-336-4363
Fax: 202-966-8553
e-mail: info@geneticalliance.org
www.geneticalliance.org

A coalition of voluntary genetic support groups, consumers and professionals addressing the needs of individuals and families affected by genetic disorders from a national perspective.

Sharon Terry, President/CEO

4486 March of Dimes Birth Defects Foundation
1275 Mamaroneck Avenue
White Plains, NY 10605

914-428-7100
888-663-4637
Fax: 914-428-8203
e-mail: resourcecenter@modimes.org
www.marchofdimes.com

Partnership of volunteers and professionals dedicates to improving the health of babies by preventing birth defects and infant mortality. Over 100 chapters are located across the country and can be located through the National Office.

Dr Jennifer Howse, President

4487 National Tay-Sachs and Allied Diseases Association
2001 Beacon Street, Suite 204
Boston, MA 02135

617-277-4463
800-906-8723
Fax: 617-277-0134
e-mail: info@ntsad.org
www.ntsad.org

Dedicated to the treatment and prevention of Tay-Sachs and related diseases, and to provide information and support services to individuals and families affected by these diseases through education, research, genetic screening, family services and advocacy.

Johna Crowlwy, President
Risa Ansen, Vice President

4488 Neuropathy Association
60 E 42nd Street, Suite 942
New York, NY 10165

212-692-0662
e-mail: info@neuropathy.org
www.neuropathy.org

A public, nonprofit organization which was established by people with neuropathy and their families or friends to help those who suffer from disorders that affect the peripheral nerves.

4489 United Leukodystrophy Foundation
2304 Highland Drive
Sycamore, IL 60178

815-895-3211
800-728-5483
Fax: 815-895-2432
e-mail: office@ulf.org
www.ulf.org/

Organization that aids those with leukodystrophy and those who care for them.

Paula Brazeal, President
Tim Conway, Spokesperson

Web Sites

4490 Medical College of Wisconsin
www.mcw.edu/display/router.asp?docid=208

4491 NYU
www.med.nyu/edu/neurology/subspecialties/neurogeneti

4492 Neuropathy Association
www.neuropathy.org/

Supports research into the causes and treatment of perpipheral neuropathies, provides support through education and sharing information and experiences related to pripheral neuropathy, increases the public awareness pf the nature and extent of peripheral neuropathy and the need for early intervenion and research. We encourage pharmaceutical and biotechnology companies to develop new therapies and devices for treatment of neuropathy.

4493 Online Mendelian Inheritance in Man
www.ncbi.nlm.nih.gov

This database is a catalog of human genes and genetic disorders.

4494 Virtual Pediatric Hospital
www.virtualpediatrichospital.org

A digital library of pediatric information including resources for patients and health care professionals.

Book Publishers

4495 Let's Talk About Going to the Hospital
Rosen Publishing Group's PowerKids Press
29 E 21st Street
New York, NY 10010

212-777-3017
800-237-9932
Fax: 888-436-4643
e-mail: rosenpub@tribeca.ios.com
www.powerkidspress.com

If a child has to check into the hospital, chances are he or she is already upset about being ill. Knowing how a hospital functions and what the procedures are, such as when family members can visit, will help in what is already a stressful situation. Grades K-5.

24 pages
ISBN: 0-823950-36-0

DESCRIPTION

4496 LISSENCEPHALY

Synonym: Agyria

Covers these related disorders: Isolated lissencephaly sequence, Miller-Dieker lissencephaly syndrome, Norman-Roberts lissencephaly syndrome, Walker-Warburg syndrome, X-linked lissencephaly

Involves the following Biologic System(s):

Neurologic Disorders

Lissencephaly is a developmental abnormality in which the brain has a relatively smooth surface due to incomplete formation of the folds or convolutions (gyri) of the surface of the brain (cerebral cortex). In most patients, the folds are not fully developed or are absent. Although lissencephaly was once thought to be a rare malformation, this developmental abnormality is now considered more common. This is largely due to an increase in the number of diagnosed cases resulting from the use of advanced imaging techniques.

Lissencephaly has multiple causes and may occur as an isolated finding or in association with several underlying syndromes. Affected newborns typically have a small head (microcephaly), episodes of uncontrolled electrical disturbances within the brain (seizures), and mental retardation. When an underlying syndrome is present, patients may have additional physical abnormalities. In some patients, life-threatening complications may develop during infancy or childhood. Isolated lissencephaly, which is an autosomal dominant trait, results due to changes (mutations) of a gene known as the LIS 1 gene. The gene is located on the short arm (p) of chromosome 17 (17p13.3). In addition, there are reports of numerous cases of lissencephaly in a multigenerational family due to mutations of a gene on the long arm (q) of chromosome X (Xq22.3-q23). In affected males, associated findings may include seizures that are resistant to treatment (intractable), growth failure, mental retardation, absence of the thick band of nerve fibers that connect the two cerebral hemispheres (agenesis of the corpus callosum), an abnormally small penis (microphallus), and life-threatening complications shortly after birth. In affected females who inherit a single copy of the disease gene (heterozygotes), associated abnormalities, which are milder than those in affected males, include an unusual band of brain tissue under the cerebral cortex (subcortical heterotopia) and mild mental retardation and seizures.

Lissencephaly may also occur in association with several syndromes. For example, Miller-Dieker lissencephaly syndrome is thought to result from deletions of several genes located on the short arm (p) of chromosome 17. This syndrome, which is an autosomal dominant trait, is associated with lissencephaly, profound mental retardation, seizures, agenesis of the corpus callosum, poor feeding, and failure to grow and gain weight at the expected rate (failure to thrive). Malformations of the head and face may include a small head, a prominent forehead and back portion of the head, a short nose with upturned nostrils (anteverted nares), a small jaw (micrognathia), and a prominent upper lip. In Norman-Roberts lissencephaly syndrome, an autosomal recessive trait, affected infants have profound mental retardation and seizures, severe growth deficiency after birth, abnormally increased muscle tone (hypertonia), and exaggerated reflexes (hyperreflexia). Abnormalities of the head and face may include a low, sloping forehead and prominent back portion of the head, widely set eyes (ocular hypertelorism), and a broad nasal bridge. In Walker-Warburg syndrome, also an autosomal recessive disorder, affected infants have lissencephaly associated with seizures and an abnormally small head. Malformations of the eyes may include atypical development of the nerve-rich membrane at the back of the eyes (retinal dysplasia), abnormally small eyes (microphthalmia), and clouding of the lenses (cataracts) and corneas (corneal opacities). In addition, some affected infants may experience restriction of the flow of fluid surrounding the brain and spinal cord (hydrocephalus) and abnormal widening of the cavities of the brain. The treatment of lissencephaly includes symptomatic and supportive measures.

See also **General Resources** on page 917

Government Agencies

4497 NIH/National Institute of Child Health and Human Development
31 Center Drive, Building 31
Bethesda, MD 20892

301-496-5133
Fax: 301-496-1104
www.nichd.nih.gov

Established in 1962 by congress, today the institute conducts and supports research on topics related to the health of children, adults, families and populations. Some of these topics include: developmental disabilities, growth and development, infant death, reproductive health and birth defects.

Nancy D Wirth, Director
Lisa Kaeser, Program & Public Liaison

National Associations & Support Groups

4498 AboutFace USA
PO Box 158
South Beloit, IL 61080

702-769-9264
888-486-1209
Fax: 702-341-5351
e-mail: info@aboutfaceusa.org
www.aboutfaceusa.org

To provide information, services, emotional support and educational programs for and on behalf of individuals with facial difference and their families. Working to increase understanding through public awareness and education.

David Reisberg,DDS, President
Christina Corsiqla, Vice President

4499 Birth Defect Research for Children
930 Woodcock Road, Suite 225
Orlando, FL 32803

407-895-0802
Fax: 407-895-0824
e-mail: staff@birthdefects.org
www.birthdefects.org

Organization that helps families with free birth defect information, parent matching that links families of children with similar defects and research through the National Birth Defect Registry to discover the causes of birth defects. Support group information and newsletter on Internet.

James Murphy, Associate Professor
JD Sherman, Adjunct Professor

4500 Children's Craniofacial Association
13140 Coit Road, Suite 307
Dallas, TX 75240

214-570-9099
800-535-3643
Fax: 214-570-8811
e-mail: contactCCA@ccakids.com
www.ccakids.com

Devoted to the dispersion of medical knowledge of this and similar disorders, along with providing emotional support for the sufferers and their families.

Rose Seitz, Chiar
Tony Davis DMD, Vice-Chair

4501 FACES: National Association for the Craniofacially Handicapped
PO Box 11082
Chattanooga, TN 37401

423-266-1632
800-332-2373
Fax: 423-267-3124
e-mail: faces@faces-cranio.org
www.faces-cranio.org

Assists individuals with facial disfigurations and their families They maintain a registry of centers offering corrective surgery for craniofacial deformities and financial assistance to qualified applicants.

4502 Fighters for Encephaly Support Group
332 Brereton Street
Pittsburgh, PA 15219

412-687-6437
Fax: 412-331-4365

4503 Forward Face: The Charity for Children with Craniofacial Conditions
Institute of Reconstructive Plastic Surgery
317 E 34th Street, Suite 901A
New York, NY 10016

212-684-5860
Fax: 212-684-5864
e-mail: info@forwardface.org
www.forwardface.org

Provision of data and emotional assistance to both sufferers and medical professionals.

Barbara Robertson, President
Susan Friedman, Vice President

4504 Lissencephaly Network
10408 Bitterroot Court
Fort Wayne, IN 46804

260-432-4310
Fax: 260-432-4310
e-mail: lissencephalyone@aol.com
www.lissencephaly.org

Lissencephaly is a genetic disorder that can be inherited from the parents or can occur during cell division. This web site is provided for the parents, siblings, physicians and therapists of children born with lissencephaly (smooth brain), and other neuronal migration disorders.

William Dobyns MD, Medical Director

4505 March of Dimes Birth Defects Foundation
1275 Mamaroneck Avenue
White Plains, NY 10605

914-428-7100
888-663-4637
Fax: 914-428-8203
e-mail: resourcecenter@modimes.org
www.marchofdimes.com

Partnership of volunteers and professionals dedicates to improving the health of babies by preventing birth defects and infant mortality. Over 100 chapters are located across the country and can be located through the National Office.

Dr Jennifer Howse, President

4506 National Craniofacial Foundation
3100 Carlisle Street
Dallas, TX 75204

800-535-3643

4507 National Dissemination Center for Children with Disabilities
PO Box 1492
Washington, DC 20013

202-884-8200
800-695-0285
Fax: 202-884-8441
e-mail: nichcy@aed.org
www.nichcy.org

A national information and referral center that provides information on disabilities and disability-related issues for families, educators and other professionals.

Suzanne Ripley, Executive Director

4508 National Hydrocephalus Foundation
12413 Centrailia Road
Lakewood, CA 90715

562-924-6666
888-857-3434
e-mail: debbifields@nhfonline.org
www.nhfonline.org

Promotes information and educational assistance. Establishes and facilitates a communication network and works to increase public awareness. Quarterly newsletter included with annual membership fee of $30.00.

Debbie Fields, Executive Director
Michael Fields, President/Treasurer

4509 Society for the Rehabilitation of the Facially Disfigured Inc.
317 East 34th Street Room 901
New York, NY 10016

212-263-6656
Fax: 212-263-7534
e-mail: info@nffr.org
www.niff.org

4510 World Craniofacial Foundation
P.O. Box 515838
Dallas, TX 75251

972-566-6669
800-533-3315
Fax: 972-566-3850
e-mail: worldcf@worldnet.att.net
www.worldcf.org

The World Craniofacial Foundation is a nonprofit corporation, dedicated to helping children obtain the life-changing craniofacial surgery they deserve.

Douglas Canfield, Founder And President
Chris Fashek, Vice Chairman

Web Sites

4511 Independent Holoprosencephaly Support Site
hpe.home.att.net

This site is home to an online support group for parents of children with HPE, or anyone who cares for a child with HPE.

4512 Online Mendelian Inheritance in Man
www.ncbi.nlm.nih.gov

This database is a catalog of human genes and genetic disorders.

4513 Rare Genetic Diseases in Children (NYU)
www.med.nyu.edu/pediatrics/comprehensive.html

We target issues arising from rare genetic diseases affecting children. Also, to assist in the endeavor to bring knowledge and hope to those for whom there is, at present, so little.

Book Publishers

4514 Congenital Disorders Sourcebook 2nd Edit.
Omnigraphics
PO Box 625
Holmes, PA 19043

800-234-1340
Fax: 800-875-1340
e-mail: info@omnigraphics.com
www.omnigraphics.com

Basic consumer health information on disorders aquired during gestation, including spina bifida, hydrocephalus, cerebral palsy, heart defects, craniofacial abnormalities and fetal alcohol syndrome.

647 pages
ISBN: 0-780809-45-1

Peter Ruffner, Publisher
Frederick Ruffner, Jr. Chairman

4515 Let's Talk About Going to the Hospital
Rosen Publishing Group's PowerKids Press
29 E 21st Street
New York, NY 10010

212-777-3017
800-237-9932
Fax: 888-436-4643
e-mail: rosenpub@tribeca.ios.com
www.powerkidspress.com

If a child has to check into the hospital, chances are he or she is already upset about being ill. Knowing how a hospital functions and what the procedures are, such as when family members can visit, will help in what is already a stressful situation. Grades K-5.

24 pages
ISBN: 0-823950-36-0

Roger Rosen, President

DESCRIPTION

4516 LYME DISEASE

Synonym: Deer tick disease

Covers these related disorders: Bell's palsy

Involves the following Biologic System(s):

Infectious Disorders

Lyme disease is a bacterial (Borrelia burgdorferi) infection that is transmitted by being bitten by the nymph stage of the deer tick Ixodides. It is not contagious, that is, it is not spread by contact with people or animals with Lyme disease. Lyme disease has been found in the Northeast from Maine to Virginia, the upper Midwest and on the West Coast. The most common first sign of Lyme disease is a rash at the site of the tick bite. It is a red circular rash, often with an area of central clearing (target lesion) and is called erythema migrans.

Lyme disease has three stages, early localized, early disseminated and late disease. Early localized disease is marked by the typical rash and may also include flu-like symptoms. It occurs between 7 and 10 days after the tick bite. The most common symptom of early disseminated disease is multiple erythema migrans, but patients can develop cranial nerve palsies (including Bell's palsy), meningitis, or carditis leading to heartblock on seen on an electrocardiogram (ECG). Systemic symptoms can include muscle and joint aches, fatigue and headaches. Symptoms of early disseminated disease develop from days to weeks in the untreated patient. Late Lyme disease happens weeks to months after the tick bite and is marked by arthritis of one or more large joints.

Diagnosis of Lyme disease is primarily made based on history and physical findings. Serologic testing (i.e. blood test) can be useful for diagnosis in some cases, but interpreting the immunologic tests can be difficult and it is important to utilize a high quality lab for testing. The serologic testing can not be used to assess treatment success.

Antibiotics are used to treat all stages of Lyme disease. The stage and specific symptoms determine how long treatment needs to be and whether or not the therapy can be oral or intravenous. Doxycycline is the drug of choice in patients with erythema migrans or a suspicion of Lyme disease based on clinical findings. There is no evidence supporting chronic or multiple courses of antibiotics for Lyme disease. Patients who continue to have symptoms more than six months after treatment should be evaluated for other inflammatory diseases. Prevention is important. Tick bites can be prevented by taking precautions when spending time outdoors, for instance, wearing loose fitting long sleeves and long pants; applying tick repellant; and decreasing environmental contacts with deer. A thorough search for ticks after outdoor exposure is essential. The LYMErix vaccine is no longer being manufactured, owing to its pain and at times debilitatin side effects.

See also **General Resources** on page 917

National Associations & Support Groups

4517 American Lyme Disease Foundation
P.O. Box 466
Lyme, CT 06371

914-277-6970
800-876-5963
Fax: 914-277-6974
e-mail: inquire@aldf.com
www.aldf.com

Supports research and plays a key role in providing reliable and scientifically accurate information to the public, health care provider, and government agencies about tick-borne diseases and their potentially serious effects on our health and quality of life.

Jeffrey Black, Directore Director
David Nichols, Jr., Director

4518 Lyme Disease Association
PO Box 1438
Jackson, NJ 08527

888-366-6611
e-mail: lymeliter@aol.com
www.lymediseasassociation.org

An organization which recently expanded its focus nationally, dedicated to Lyme disease education, prevention, and raising research dollars. In its search for a cure for chronic Lyme, the LDA has already funded dozens of research projects coast to coast.

Patricia Smith, President
Pam Lampe, Vice President

4519 Lyme Disease Foundation
Po Box 332
Tolland, CT 06084

860-870-0070
800-866-5963
Fax: 860-870-0080
e-mail: info@lyme.org
www.lyme.org

Nonprofit orginazation dedicated to finding solutions for tick-borne disorders. Offers support to the public and medical communities.

John F Anderson, Director
Nicole Augenti, Director

Web Sites

4520 American Lyme Disease Foundation
www.aldf.com

Provides reliable and scientifically accurate information to the public about tick borne diseases and their potentially serious effects on our life.

4521 Lyme Disease Association
www.lymedieaseassociation.org

Dedicated to lyme disease educatin, prevention, and raising money for research.

4522 Lyme Disease Foundation
www.lyme.org

Nonprofit organization that works to find solutions for tick borne disorders.

Book Publishers

4523 Aspects of Lyme Borreliosis
Springer-Verlag
11 West 42nd Street 15th Floor
New York, NY 10036

212-460-1500
877-687-7476
Fax: 201-348-4505
e-mail: contactus@springerpub.com
www.springerpub.com

1992 384 pages hardcover
ISBN: 0-387556-28-1

Ted Nardin, CEO

4524 Ecology and Enviromental Management of Lyme Disease
Rutgers University Press
100 Joyce Kilmer Avenue
Piscataway, NJ 08854

732-445-7762
800-446-9323
Fax: 732-445-7039
e-mail: bksales@rci.rutgers.edu

1993 hardcover
ISBN: 0-813519-28-4

Marlie Wasserman, Director
Christina Brianik, Assistant to the Director

4525 Let's Talk About Having Lyme Disease
Rosen Publishing Group
29 E 21st Street
New York, NY 10010

800-237-9932
Fax: 888-436-4643
e-mail: customerservice@rosenpub.com

Discusses what Lyme disease is, how one gets it, and what to do about it.

2003 24 pages hardcover
ISBN: 0-823950-29-8

Roger Rosen, President

4526 Lyme Disease
Enslow Publishers
Box 398 40 Industrial Road,
Berkeley Heights, NJ 07922

908-771-9400
800-398-2504
Fax: 908-771-0925
e-mail: customerService@enslow.com

Outlines Lyme Disease, from its discovery to current trends. The transmission of the disease from the deer tick, and its course of infection in the body are clearly discribed. Methods for protection from the disease are mixed with real life stories of patients who have contracted Lyme disease. The symptoms, diagnosis, treatment, and prevention are also covered.

104 pages hardcover
ISBN: 0-766010-52-x

Mark Enslow ., President
Brian Enslow, Vice President/Publisher

4527 Lyme Disease (Deadly Diseases and Epidemics)
Chelsea House Publishing
2080 Cabot Boulevard W, Suite 201
Langhorne, PA 19047

800-848-2665
Fax: 877-780-7300

110 pages

Journals

4528 Journal of Spirochetal and Tick-borne Diseases
1 Financial Plaza
Hartford, CT 06103

860-525-2000
Fax: 860-525-8425
e-mail: lymefnd@aol.com
www.jstd.org

Reviews all aspects of spirochetal or tick-borne disorders. Clinical topics may involve all medical disciplines, nursing, and pharmacy, as well as the social, ethnical and biological features of such disorders.

Quaterly

Ronald Schell PHD, Editor In Chief
Willy Burgdorfer PHD, Deputy Editor

Newsletters

4529 Journal of the American Medical Association
PO Box 10946
Chicago, IL 60610

312-670-7827
800-262-2350
jama.ama-assn.org

To promote the science and art of medicine and the betterment of the public health.

DESCRIPTION

4530 MACROCEPHALY

Synonyms: Macrocephalia, Megalocephaly

Covers these related disorders: Benign familial macrocephaly, Megalencephaly

Involves the following Biologic System(s): Neurologic Disorders

Macrocephaly (macro = long; cephaly = head) is a term that is used to describe an isolated or primary condition in which an infant's or a child's head circumference is more than two standard deviations above the mean for age and sex. As a rule of thumb, a newborn's head is usually about 2 centimeters larger than the chest size. Between 6 months and 2 years, both measurements are about equal. After 2 years, the chest size becomes larger than the head.

Primary macrocephaly may be apparent at birth or during early infancy. In some affected infants and children, overgrowth of the brain results in varying degrees of mental retardation. Associated symptoms and findings may include episodes of uncontrolled electrical disturbances in the brain (seizures); unusually large or small stature; and motor abnormalities ranging from diminished muscle tone (hypotonia) to muscle rigidity and associated restrictions of movement (spasticity). Patients with overgrowth of the brain (megalencephaly) have normally sized or slightly enlarged cavities of the brain (ventricles) and no evidence of underlying conditions, such as certain metabolic disorders (metabolic megalencephaly). Although infants and children with macrocephaly may have abnormal delays in the acquisition of skills requiring the coordination of physical and mental activities (psychomotor delays), they do not experience regression of such skills, a finding that is typically associated with infantile metabolic megalencephaly or certain other underlying conditions.

Some infants and children with primary macrocephaly experience no associated mental retardation or other neurologic deficits. Several such cases have been reported in individuals within certain multigenerational families. This form of benign or nonsyndromic macrocephaly, known as benign familial macrocephaly, is thought to have autosomal dominant inheritance.

Although infants with primary macrocephaly experience increasing head size, they typically do not have symptoms and findings associated with increased cerebrospinal fluid (CSF) pressure within the brain (intracranial pressure). This is in contrast to hydrocephalus, a condition in which the brain swells due to an abnormal accumulation of CSF under increasing pressure within the brain's ventricles. However, some infants with primary macrocephaly may have a slight separation of the fibrous joints (cranial sutures) between certain bones in the skull.

Although the specific underlying cause of primary macrocephaly is not understood, overgrowth of the brain is due to the presence of abnormally large or an unusually increased number of brain cells. The outer region of the brain (cerebral cortex) appears normal in some cases; however, others have structural abnormalities.

As mentioned above, overgrowth of the brain may occur as a secondary finding associated with certain progressive infantile metabolic diseases, such as Tay-Sachs disease, or other underlying geneticdisorders, such as neurofibromatosis. The condition may also occur as a result of certain structural abnormalities of the brain, such as absence of the band of nerve fibers that joins the two cerebral hemispheres (agenesis of corpus callosum), or due to a localized accumulation of blood between the outer and middle layers of the membrane that surrounds and protects the brain and spinal cord (subdural hematoma). Infants and children with macrocephaly who experience psychomotor regression should receive thorough clinical, neurologic, metabolic, and other appropriate evaluations to rule out or confirm the presence of certain underlying disorders or conditions.

The treatment of infants and children with isolated or primary macrocephaly includes symptomatic and supportive measures. These may include the prescription of certain medications to help treat or control seizures (e.g., anticonvulsants) and physical therapy, special education, and other multidisciplinary measures to ensure that patients with motor impairments and mental retardation reach their potential. In infants and children with secondary macrocephaly, treatment includes appropriate therapies for any diagnosed, underlying causes of the condition.

See also **General Resources** on page 917

Government Agencies

4531 NIH/National Institute of Child Health and Human Development
31 Center Drive, Building 31
Bethesda, MD 20892

301-496-5133
Fax: 301-496-1104
www.nichd.nih.gov

Established in 1962 by congress, today the institute conducts and supports research on topics related to the health of children, adults, families and populations. Some of these topics include: developmental disabilities, growth and development, infant death, reproductive health and birth defects.

Nancy D Wirth, Director
Lisa Kaeser, Program & Public Liaison

National Associations & Support Groups

4532 ARC of the United States
1010 Wayne Avenue, Suite 650
Silver Spring, MD 20910

301-565-3842
Fax: 301-565-5342
e-mail: info@thearc.org
www.thearc.org

The ARC is the national organization of and for people with mental retardation and related developmental disabilities and their families. Devoted to promoting and improving supports and services for people with mental retardation and their families. The association also fosters research and education regarding the prevention of mental retardation in infants and young children. The ARC was founded in 1950 by a small group of parents and other concerned individuals.

Sue Swenson, Executive Director
Adam Aaronson, Public Inquiries Director

4533 Birth Defect Research for Children
930 Woodcock Road, Suite 225
Orlando, FL 32803

407-895-0802
Fax: 407-895-0824
e-mail: staff@birthdefects.org
www.birthdefects.org

National clearinghouse that provides services to parents and professionals caring for children with disabilities. Services include data on over 300 categories of birth defects and developmental disabilities, search for links between birth defects and the mother's/father's exposure to drugs or environmental agents. Matching families of children with similar birth defects for mutual sharing and support, diagnosis and treatment. Support group information. Newsletter on Internet.

James Murphy PHD, Associate Professor
Jd Sherman MD, Adjunct Professor

4534 Genetic Alliance
4301 Connecticut Avenue NW
Washington, DC 20008

202-966-5557
800-336-4363
Fax: 202-966-8553
e-mail: info@geneticalliance.org
www.geneticalliance.org

A coalition of voluntary genetic support groups, consumers and professionals addressing the needs of individuals and families affected by genetic disorders from a national perspective.

Sharon Terry, President/CEO

4535 National Dissemination Center for Children with Disabilities
PO Box 1492
Washington, DC 20013

202-884-8200
800-695-0285
Fax: 202-884-8441
e-mail: nichcy@acd.org
www.nichcy.org

A national information and referral center that provides information on disabilities and disability-related issues for families, educators and other professionals.

Suzanne Ripley, Executive Director

Web Sites

4536 Online Mendelian Inheritance in Man
www.ncbi.nlm.nih.gov

This database is a catalog of human genes and genetic disorders.

DESCRIPTION

4537 MAPLE SYRUP URINE DISEASE

Synonyms: Branched chain ketoaciduria, MSUD

Covers these related disorders: Classic MSUD, Mild (intermediate) MSUD, Intermittent MSUD, Thiamine-responsive MSUD

Involves the following Biologic System(s):
Genetic/Chromosomal/Syndrome/Metabolic Disorders

Maple syrup urine disease (MSUD) is a metabolic disorder characterized by the deficiency of certain enzymes of the branched-chain alpha-ketoacid dehydrogenase complex that break down (catabolize) three essential organic compounds. These compounds are known as amino acids and are the building blocks of protein. These amino acids include leucine, isoleucine, and valine. A deficiency of any enzyme within this complex results in the symptoms of MSUD and leads to encephalopathy, a condition characterized by altered brain function. There are four basic types of maple syrup urine disease.

Classic MSUD, the most severe form of this disorder, becomes apparent within the first week of life and is recognizable by a characteristic maple syrup odor of the urine and on the body. Symptoms and physical findings associated with this life-threatening form of MSUD include listlessness, drowsiness, exaggerated muscular tension (hypertonicity) and rigidity with periods of loss of muscle tone (flaccidity), severe muscle spasms resulting in a backward arching of the back and neck (opisthotonus), convulsions, and coma. Additional findings include low blood sugar (hypoglycemia) and higher-than-normal acidic levels in the blood as well as abnormally low bicarbonate levels (metabolic acidosis). In addition, severe life-threatening complications may occur following infection, surgery, or other stressful events. Such complications include an excessive accumulation of fluid around the brain (cerebral edema) and acidosis accompanied by excessive levels of certain organic compounds in the tissues and body fluids (ketosis). Many affected children experience neurologic and mental deficiencies.

Treatment for classic MSUD includes the removal of leucine, isoleucine, valine, and certain other related elements from the blood by a procedure known as peritoneal dialysis. Subsequent therapy includes a diet low in leucine, isoleucine, and valine.

Intermittent MSUD develops suddenly in children who had previously exhibited no signs of the disease. Though this form of the disease is intermittent, the characteristic findings, symptoms, severity of complications, and treatment are similar to those of classic MSUD. In addition, children with this form of the disorder may exhibit more activity of certain enzymes than those with the classic form.

Mild or intermediate MSUD is a less severe form of this disorder that usually affects children after the first month of life. Affected infants may be mildly retarded and usually emit the characteristic maple syrup odor in their urine, sweat, and earwax (cerumen).

Characteristic findings and symptoms associated with thiamine-responsive MSUD are similar to those of intermittent or intermediate disease. The distinguishing feature is that treatment with high doses of vitamin B1 (thiamine) often results in a favorable response. Early diagnosis and dietary intervention prevent complications and may allow for normal intellectual development. Consequently, MSUD has been added to many newborn screening programs, and preliminary results indicate that asymptomatic newborns with MSUD have a better outcome compared with infants who are diagnosed after they become symptomatic.

Maple syrup urine disease is inherited as an autosomal recessive trait. Approximately one in 200,000 people in the United States is affected by this disorder.

See also **General Resources** on page 917

National Associations & Support Groups

4538 ARC of the United States
1010 Wayne Avenue, Suite 650
Silver Spring, MD 20910

301-565-3842
Fax: 301-565-5342
e-mail: info@thearc.org
www.thearc.org

The ARC is the national organization of and for people with mental retardation and related developmental disabilities and their families. Devoted to promoting and improving supports and services for people with mental retardation and their families. The association also fosters research and education regarding the prevention of mental retardation in infants and young children. The ARC was founded in 1950 by a small group of parents and other concerned individuals.

Sue Swenson, Executive Director
Adam Aaronson, Public Inquiries Director

4539 Association for Neuro-Metabolic Disorders
5223 Brookfield Lane
Sylvania, OH 43506

419-885-1497
e-mail: volk4olks@aol.com

Nonprofit organization that serves as an advocate organization for families of patients with the following neuro-metabolic disorders: phenylketonuria, maple syrup urine disease, galactosemia, and biotinidase deficiency. Provides educational information for parents and children; provides networking information on support groups for new parents; supports scientific research into the treatments of these four neuro-metabolic disorders.

Cheryl Volk, Contact Person

4540 Genetic Alliance
4301 Connecticut Avenue NW
Washington, DC 20008

202-966-5557
800-336-4363
Fax: 202-966-8553
e-mail: info@geneticalliance.org
www.geneticalliance.org

A coalition of voluntary genetic support groups, consumers and professionals addressing the needs of individuals and families affected by genetic disorders from a national perspective.

Sharon Terry, President/CEO

4541 MSUD:(Maple Syrup Urine Disease) Family Support Group
82 Ravine Road
Powell, OH 43065

740-548-4475
e-mail: dbulcehr@aol.com
www.msud-support.org

MSUD is a nonprofit (501)(c)(3) organization for parents of children with MSUD, adults with MSUD, health-care professionals and others interested in MSUD. Dedicated to providing opportunities for support and personal contact for those with MSUD and their families, distributing information and raising public awareness of MSUD, strengthening the liaison between families and professionals and encouraging newborn screening programs and research for MSUD.

Sandy Bulcher, Director
Kay Larsen, General Information

4542 March of Dimes Birth Defects Foundation
1275 Mamaroneck Avenue
White Plains, NY 10605

914-428-7100
888-663-4637
Fax: 914-428-8203
e-mail: resourcecenter@modimes.org
www.marchofdimes.com

Partnership of volunteers and professionals dedicates to improving the health of babies by preventing birth defects and infant mortality. Over 100 chapters are located across the country and can be located through the National Office.

Dr Jennifer Howse, President

Libraries & Resource Centers

4543 National Digestive Diseases Information Clearinghouse
2 Information Way
Bethesda, MD 20892

301-654-3810
800-891-5389
Fax: 703-738-4929
e-mail: nddic@info.niddk.nih.gov
www.digestive.niddk.nih.gov

The National Institute of Diabetes and Digestive and Kidney Diseases conducts and supports research on many of the most serious diseases affecting public health. The Institute supports much of the clinical research on the diseases of internal medicine and related subspecialty fields as well as many basic science disciplines.

Kathy Kranzfelder, Project Officer

Web Sites

4544 Family Village
www.familyvillage.wisc.edu

A global community that integrates information, resources and communication opportunities on the Internet for persons with cognitive and other disabilities, for their families and for those that provide them services and support.

Book Publishers

4545 Let's Talk About Going to the Hospital
Rosen Publishing Group's PowerKids Press
29 E 21st Street
New York, NY 10010

212-777-3017
800-237-9932
Fax: 888-436-4643
e-mail: rosenpub@tribeca.ios.com
www.powerkidspress.com

If a child has to check into the hospital, chances are he or she is already upset about being ill. Knowing how a hospital functions and what the procedures are, such as when family members can visit, will help in what is already a stressful situation. Grades K-5.

24 pages
ISBN: 0-823950-36-0

Roger Rosen, Publisher

Newsletters

4546 MSUD Newsletter
MSUD Family Support Group
82 Ravine Road
Powell, OH 43065

740-548-4475
www.msud-support.org

Provides the latest information on the treatment of the disorder, reports on the latest research, current diet information, family news and related topics.

16 pages

Sandy Bulcher, Director
K R Dollins, Editor

DESCRIPTION

4547 MARFAN SYNDROME

Synonym: MFS

Covers these related disorders: Neonatal or infantile Marfan syndrome

Involves the following Biologic System(s):
Cardiovascular Disorders,
Genetic/Chromosomal/Syndrome/Metabolic Disorders,
Orthopedic and Muscle Disorders

Marfan syndrome is a connective tissue disorder that may result in heart (cardiac), blood vessel, skeletal, and eye (ocular) abnormalities. Children with Marfan syndrome tend to be unusually tall and slim; in some cases, this may be apparent at birth. Many affected infants also have deficiency of the layer of fat under the skin and abnormally diminished muscle tone (hypotonia) that may contribute to motor delays. In addition, in some infants with Marfan syndrome, several additional characteristic symptoms and findings may be apparent during later childhood. Neonatal or infantile Marfan syndrome is characterized by abnormal flexions (contractures), dislocations, and limited ranges of movement; an abnormally long head and face (dolichocephaly); a highly arched roof of the mouth (palate); unusually large corneas of the eyes (megalocornea); abnormal quivering movements of the colored portions of the eyes (irides); and heart defects (e.g., aortic root dilatation, mitral valve prolapse).

Older children with Marfan syndrome also tend to have an unusually long, narrow face as well as a narrow, highly arched palate and abnormal crowding of the teeth. Affected children and adults also have unusually long, thin arms and legs; a wide arm span; and long, thin fingers (arachnodactyly) with abnormally increased extension (hyperflexibility). Additional skeletal abnormalities are often present, such as unusually thin, fragile ribs; abnormal protrusion or depression of the breastbone (pectus carinatum or excavatum); and, in older children and adolescents, progressive abnormal sideways curvature (scoliosis) or front-to-back curvature (kyphosis) of the spine.

In many cases, affected children also have additional ocular abnormalities, such as dislocation (subluxation) of the lenses of the eyes (ectopia lentis); abnormal bluish coloration of the tough, outer membrane of the eyes; and severe nearsightedness (myopia). In addition, in some cases, the nerve-rich membrane at the back of the eyes (retina) may become detached.

Most individuals with Marfan syndrome also experience abnormalities of the heart and certain blood vessels (cardiovascular defects) that may be life-threatening. These may include progressive widening of the major artery of the body (aorta), causing leakage of blood through the valve between the left ventricle and the aorta (aortic regurgitation). In addition, the valve between the left ventricle and the left upper chamber (atrium) of the heart may bulge backward (prolapse) into the atrium, causing leakage of blood into the atrium.

The treatment of Marfan syndrome is directed toward preventing potential complications associated with progression of the disease. Affected children should receive regular evaluations to detect ocular defects, abnormal spinal curvatures, or cardiovascular defects. Treatment includes symptomatic and supportive measures, such as orthopedic techniques to help prevent or treat scoliosis or kyphosis; therapy with certain medications (beta-adrenergic blocking agents, e.g., propranolol) that may help to prevent or reduce the progression of certain cardiovascular abnormalities (e.g., aortic dilatation and associated complications); or surgical correction of cardiovascular defects as required. At one time, affected individuals were provided with antibiotic medications before dental visits and surgical procedures to reduce the incidence of endocarditis (an infection of the heart wall or heart valvle when bacteria enter the bloodstream). The American Heart Association no longer recommends taking routine antibiotics before certain dental procedures except for people at highest risk for bad outcomes if they develop endocarditis. Individuals with Marfan syndrome do not fall into this high-risk category.

Marfan syndrome results from abnormal changes (mutations) in a gene (fibrillin gene) located on the long arm of chromosome 15 (15q21.1). Such mutations may occur spontaneously (sporadically) for unknown reasons or may be inherited as an autosomal dominant trait. In individuals with the disease gene, the range and severity of associated symptoms and findings may vary from case to case (variable expressivity). Marfan syndrome is thought to affect about one in| 10,000 individuals.

See also **General Resources** on page 917

Government Agencies

4548 NIH/National Institute of Arthritis and Mu sculoskeletal and Skin Diseases
1AMS Circle
Bethesda, MD 20892

301-402-4484
Fax: 301-718-6366
e-mail: ord@od.nih.gov
rarediseases.info.nih.gov

The mission of the National Institute of Arthritis and Musculoskeletal and Skin Diseases is to support research into the causes, treatment, and prevention of arthritis and musculoskeletal and skin diseases, the training of basic and clinical scientists to carry out this research, and the dissemination of information on research progress in these diseases.

Stephen I Katz MD PhD, Director

National Associations & Support Groups

4549 Genetic Alliance
4301 Connecticut Avenue NW
Washington, DC 20008

202-966-5557
800-336-4363
Fax: 202-966-8553
e-mail: info@geneticalliance.org
www.geneticalliance.org

A coalition of voluntary genetic support groups, consumers and professionals addressing the needs of individuals and families affected by genetic disorders from a national perspective.

Sharon Terry, President/CEO

4550 March of Dimes Birth Defects Foundation
1275 Mamaroneck Avenue
White Plains, NY 10605

914-428-7100
888-663-4637
Fax: 914-428-8203
e-mail: resourcecenter@modimes.org
www.marchofdimes.com

Partnership of volunteers and professionals dedicates to improving the health of babies by preventing birth defects and infant mortality. Over 100 chapters are located across the country and can be located through the National Office.

Dr Jennifer Howse, President

4551 National Marfan Foundation
22 Manhasset Avenue
Port Washington, NY 11050

516-883-8712
800-862-7326
Fax: 516-883-8040
e-mail: staff@marfan.org
www.marfan.org

A nonprofit voluntary health organization dedicated to saving lives and improving the quality of life for individuals and families affected by the Marfan Syndrome and related disorders.

Carolyn Levering, President/CEO
Judy Gibaldi, Senior Vice-President

Web Sites

4552 National Marfan Foundation
www.marfan.org

A nonprofit voluntary health organization dedicated to saving lives and improving the quality of life for individuals and families affected by the Marfan Syndrome and related disorders.

4553 Usenet Newsgroup
Alt.Support.Marfan

4554 Wheeless' Textbook of Orthopaedics
www.wheelessonline.com

Derives from a variety of sources, including journals, articles, national meetings lectures and other textbooks.

Book Publishers

4555 Let's Talk About Going to the Hospital
Rosen Publishing Group's PowerKids Press
29 E 21st Street
New York, NY 10010

212-777-3017
800-237-9932
Fax: 888-436-4643
e-mail: rosenpub@tribeca.ios.com
www.powerkidspress.com

If a child has to check into the hospital, chances are he or she is already upset about being ill. Knowing how a hospital functions and what the procedures are, such as when family members can visit, will help in what is already a stressful situation. Grades K-5.

24 pages
ISBN: 0-823950-36-0

Roger Rosen, Publisher

Pamphlets

4556 Marfan Syndrome
March of Dimes Resource Center
1275 Mamaroneck Avenue
White Plains, NY 10605

914-997-4488
888-663-4637
Fax: 914-997-4537
e-mail: askus@marchofdimes.com
www.marchofdimes.com

DESCRIPTION

4557 MCCUNE-ALBRIGHT SYNDROME

Synonyms: Albright syndrome, MAS, PFD, POFD, Polyostotic fibrous dysplasia, Precocious puberty with polyostotic

Involves the following Biologic System(s):

Endocrinologic Disorders, Genetic/Chromosomal/Syndrome/Metabolic Disorders

McCune-Albright syndrome is a genetic disorder characterized by multiple areas of abnormal, fiber-like tissue growths (bone lesions) that replace normal bone tissue (polyostotic fibrous dysplasia); irregular, patchy areas of light brown pigmentation on the skin (cafe-au-lait spots); and abnormalities of certain hormone-producing glands that assist in regulating the body's growth, controlling the rate of metabolism, and promoting the development of secondary sexual characteristics. Although bone lesions are most common in the pelvis and the long bones of the arms and legs, other bones may be affected, including the ribs, skull and facial bones, and bones of the spinal column (vertebrae). These bone lesions may cause abnormal thickness and deformity of affected bones, susceptibility to fractures, and bone pain. In addition, lesions may cause corresponding bones to develop unevenly. For example, one leg may appear unusually short, or one side of the face may appear different from the other (facial asymmetry). Bone lesions of the skull and face may eventually result in hearing loss and visual impairment.

Many girls with McCune-Albright syndrome undergo early development of secondary sexual characteristics (precocious puberty), including early breast development and onset of menstrual cycles (menstruation). Some boys with the disorder may also experience precocious puberty, including genital development and unusually accelerated growth. In many patients, additionalendocrine abnormalities may be present. For example, some affected children may produce excessive amounts of the hormone cortisol, resulting in Cushing's syndrome. This disorder is characterized by excessive weight gain in the chest and abdominal area; a moon-shaped, rounded face; abnormal pads of fat in certain areas of the body; high blood pressure (hypertension); weakening of bones, causing increased susceptibility to fractures; thin, and fragile skin.

Some children with McCune-Albright syndrome may also produce excessive amounts of thyroid hormones (hyperthyroidism), potentially leading to heart palpitations, anxiety, heat intolerance, excessive sweating, muscle weakness, or weight loss. In addition, some affected children may be prone to developing tumors of the pituitary gland, resulting in increased secretion of growth hormone, which stimulates body growth and development. Affected children may experience enlargement of bones and soft tissues of the hands, feet, and face (acromegaly); lengthening and coarsening of the face; and enlargement of certain organs (e.g., heart). In some patients, excessive growth during childhood (gigantism) and tall stature may occur.

McCune-Albright syndrome may be obvious at birth because of unusual skin pigmentation. Alternatively, it may not be apparent until late infancy or early childhood when precocious puberty or bone lesions become apparent. The disorder is caused by spontaneous (sporadic) changes (mutations) of a gene known as the GNAS1 gene. The disease gene is located on the long arm (q) of chromosome 20 (20q13.2). Because the gene mutation is present in only some cells of the body (mosaicism), symptoms and findings may vary among affected individuals, depending upon the specific body cells affected. Treatment of McCune-Albright syndrome includes symptomatic and supportive measures. These may include drug therapy to help prevent or treat precocious puberty, surgical removal of pituitary tumors or the thyroid gland, and appropriate treatment of bone lesions and associated abnormalities.

See also **General Resources** on page 917

Government Agencies

4558 NIH/National Institute of Arthritis and Musculoskeletal and Skin Diseases
1AMS Circle
Bethesda, MD 20892

301-402-4484
Fax: 301-718-6366
e-mail: ord@od.nih.gov
rarediseases.info.nih.gov

The mission of the National Institute of Arthritis and Musculoskeletal and Skin Diseases is to support research into the causes, treatment, and prevention of arthritis and musculoskeletal and skin diseases, the training of basic and clinical scientists to carry out this research, and the dissemination of information on research progress in these diseases.

Stephen I Katz MD PhD, Director

4559 NIH/National Institute of Child Health and Human Development
31 Center Drive, Building 31
Bethesda, MD 20892

301-496-5133
Fax: 301-496-1104
www.nichd.nih.gov

Established in 1962 by congress, today the institute conducts and supports research on topics related to the health of children, adults, families and populations. Some of these topics include: developmental disabilities, growth and development, infant death, reproductive health and birth defects.

Nancy D Wirth, Director
Lisa Kaeser, Program & Public Liaison

National Associations & Support Groups

4560 Genetic Alliance
4301 Connecticut Avenue NW
Washington, DC 20008

202-966-5557
800-336-4363
Fax: 202-966-8553
e-mail: info@geneticalliance.org
www.geneticalliance.org

A coalition of voluntary genetic support groups, consumers and professionals addressing the needs of individuals and families affected by genetic disorders from a national perspective.

Sharon Terry, President/CEO

4561 International Skeletal Dysplasia Registry
Medical Genetics Institute
8635 West Third Street, Suite 665
Los Angeles, CA 90048

310-423-9915
800-233-2771
Fax: 310-423-0462
e-mail: maryann.priore@cshs.org
www.cedars-sinai.edu/3805.html

The International Skeletal Dysplasia Registry at Cedars-Sinai Medical Center is a referral center for research into the diagnosis; management and etiology of the skeletal dysplasias.

MaryAnn Priore, Program Coordinator
David L Rimoin MD, Director

4562 MAGIC Foundation: Major Aspects of Growth in Children
6645 W North Avenue
Oak Park, IL 60302

708-383-0808
800-362-4423
Fax: 708-383-0899
e-mail: mary@magicfoundation.org
www.magicfoundation.org

A national nonprofit organization providing support and education regarding growth disorders in children and related adult disorders. Provides educational information, networking, a national conference, a kids' program and an extensive medical library.

10,000 members

Dianne Tamburrino, Executive Director
Pam Pentaris, Administrative Assistant

4563 March of Dimes Birth Defects Foundation
1275 Mamaroneck Avenue
White Plains, NY 10605

914-428-7100
888-663-4637
Fax: 914-428-8203
e-mail: resourcecenter@modimes.org
www.marchofdimes.com

Partnership of volunteers and professionals dedicates to improving the health of babies by preventing birth defects and infant mortality. Over 100 chapters are located across the country and can be located through the National Office.

Dr Jennifer Howse, President

Web Sites

4564 Human Growth Foundation
www.hgfound.org

Helps children and adults with growth or growth hormone related disorders through research, education, support and advocacy.

4565 University Alabama Birmingham
www.uab.edu/pedradpath/albright.html

Book Publishers

4566 Let's Talk About Going to the Hospital
Rosen Publishing Group's PowerKids Press
29 E 21st Street
New York, NY 10010

212-777-3017
800-237-9932
Fax: 888-436-4643
e-mail: rosenpub@tribeca.ios.com
www.powerkidspress.com

If a child has to check into the hospital, chances are he or she is already upset about being ill. Knowing how a hospital functions and what the procedures are, such as when family members can visit, will help in what is already a stressful situation. Grades K-5.

24 pages
ISBN: 0-823950-36-0

Roger Rosen, Publisher

DESCRIPTION

4567 MENINGITIS

Covers these related disorders: Bacterial meningitis, Chronic meningitis, Neonatal meningitis, Viral meningitis

Involves the following Biologic System(s):

Infectious Disorders, Neurologic Disorders

Meningitis is characterized by inflammation of the protective membranes that surround the brain and spinal cord (meninges). The condition is usually caused by infection with microorganisms, such as certain bacteria (bacterial meningitis) or viruses (viral meningitis). Prompt lumbar puncture (also called a spinal tap)is a test to evaluate the fluid that surrounds the brain and spinal cord (cerebrospinal fluid [CSF]). Repeat lumbar puncture and analysis of the CSF are curcial to assess respons to treatment. Meningitis primarily affects infants and young children.

Meningitis that occurs within the first month of life, known as neonatal meningitis, may cause a different pattern of symptoms than that seen in older infants and children. The condition affects approximately 0.2 to 0.4 in every 1,000 newborns, and the frequency increases among infants who are born before 37 weeks of pregnancy (premature infants). In newborns, meningitis may be caused by infection with certain bacteria, viruses, protozoa, or fungi. These invading microorganisms usually reach the protective membranes of the brain and spinal cord by circulating through the bloodstream (sepsis). Rarely, neonatal meningitis may be due to local infection. Affected newborns may initially experience generalized symptoms, including fever, abnormal yellowish discoloration of the skin and mucous membranes (jaundice), and breathing difficulties. Neurologic symptoms may or may not occur. When present, such symptoms typicallyinclude listlessness (lethargy), drowsiness, and episodes of abnormally increased electrical activity in the brain (seizures). In addition, pus-filled pockets of infection (abscesses) may develop in the brain, causing increased fluid pressure| in the brain, bulging of the soft spots where bones of the skull have not fully fused (fontanels), enlargement of the head (hydrocephalus), and vomiting. In some cases, life-threatening complications may result.

The treatment of newborns with neonatal meningitis includes the immediate administration of appropriate intravenous medications. Because certain bacteria are the most common causes of meningitis, such therapy may initially include a number of different antibiotics. Once the specific bacterium or other microorganism is identified, different drugs may be substituted to most effectively treat the infec-tion. Additional treatment is symptomatic and supportive.

Bacterial meningitis is a serious condition that most commonly affects children between the ages of one month to five years. Although older children and adults are rarely affected, small epidemics may periodically occur in environments where many people have close contact, such as in certain school settings, dormitories, or military camps. In children aged approximately two months to 12 years, bacterial meningitis is most commonly caused by two types of bacteria: i.e., Neisseria meningitidis, or Streptococcus pneumoniae. These microorganisms are spread by the inhalation of airborne droplets that contain the bacteria or through contact with infected respiratory secretions. Meningitis that results from the bacterium Neisseria meningitidis in the bloodstream (meningococcal sepsis) may cause a sudden onset of rapidly progressive symptoms that may lead to life-threatening complications within 24 hours. The bacteria Streptococcus pneumoniae less commonly causes rapidly progressive illness; instead, such bacteria usually initially cause several days of upper respiratory or digestive symptoms. General symptoms associated with bacterial meningitis may include fever, lack of appetite (anorexia), joint and muscle aches, or small areas of abnormal bleeding within skin layers, causing the appearance of small purplish spots on the skin (petechia). Inflammation of the meninges may cause stiffness of the neck and back pain; however, such symptoms are less common in children younger than 18 months of age. Patients may also experience increased fluid pressure in the brain, vomiting, severe headache, paralysis of nerves controlling certain eye and facial movements, and, in young children, abnormal bulging of the fontanels. Additional symptoms may include breathing difficulties, seizures, and abnormal sensitivity to light (photophobia). Without prompt treatment, patients may become irritable, confused, and increasingly drowsy; become unaware of their surroundings (stupor); progress to a coma; and develop potentially life-threatening complications.

Prompt diagnosis and immediate treatment of bacterial meningitis is essential to help prevent brain damage and potentially life-threatening complications. Treatment requires immediate therapy with intravenous antibiotics and appropriate measures to treat increased fluid pressure in the brain. A number of different antibiotics may initially be administered, based on the different bacteria that are most likely responsible for the condition. Once the specific bacterium is identified, different drugs may be substituted as required to most effectively treat the infection. Additional treatment of children with bacterial meningitis is symptomatic and supportive. Preventive antibiotic therapy may be recommended for individuals who have had close contact with patients diagnosed with bacterial meningitis. In addition, routine childhood immunization with the Haemophilus influenzae type b (Hib) vaccine now plays an essential role in preventing what used to be one of the most common causes of childhood bacterial meningitis.

Viral meningitis is a more common condition that occurs as the result of infection with a virus. This condition typically causes milder symptoms than those associated with bacterial meningitis. Patients often develop mild flu-like symptoms, including fever, headache, a general feeling of ill health (malaise), abdominal pain, nausea, and stiffness of the neck and back. Symptoms generally subside within one to two weeks. Treatment is usually symptomatic and supportive.However, in some more severe cases, antiviral medications may be prescribed.

Some patients may develop symptoms that last for a month or longer. This condition, known as chronic meningitis, may occur secondary to certain infections. In addition, chronic meningitis may be due to noninfectious causes, such as certain disorders that may affect the brain, such as sarcoidosis or multiple sclerosis; administration of particular medications, such as certain anticancer drugs; or other factors. Individuals with impaired immune systems may be more susceptible to chronic meningitis. Patients generally develop associated symptoms over a few weeks. Such symptoms may include fever, headache, a stiff neck, back pain, confusion, nausea, and vomiting. The treatment of chronic meningitis is based on the underlying cause of the condition.

Government Agencies

4568 Centers for Disease Control
1600 Clifton Road
Atlanta, GA 30333

404-639-3311
www.cdc.gov

Mission is to promote health and quality of life by preventing and controlling disease, injury, and disability.

4569 NIH/National Institute of Allergy and Infectious Diseases
6610 Rockledge Drive, MSC 6612
Bethesda, MD 20892

301-496-5717
Fax: 301-402-3573
TDD: 800-877-8339
www.niaid.nih.gov

Conducts and supports basic and applied research to better understand, treat, and ultimately prevent infectious, immunologic, and allergic diseases.

Anthony S Fauci MD, Director

See also **General Resources** on page 917

National Associations & Support Groups

4570 March of Dimes Birth Defects Foundation
1275 Mamaroneck Avenue
White Plains, NY 10605

914-428-7100
888-663-4637
Fax: 914-428-8203
e-mail: resourcecenter@modimes.org
www.marchofdimes.com

Partnership of volunteers and professionals dedicates to improving the health of babies by preventing birth defects and infant mortality. Over 100 chapters are located across the country and can be located through the National Office.

Dr Jennifer Howse, President

4571 Meningitis Foundation of America
6610 N Shadeland Avenue, Suite 220
Indianapolis, IN 46220

317-595-6395
800-668-1129
Fax: 317-595-6370
e-mail: support@musa.org
www.musa.org

Goals and objectives are: help support sufferers of Spinal Meningitis and their families; provide information to educate the public and medical professionals about meningitis so that its early diagnosis and treatment will save lives; and support development of vaccines and other preventions.

Jamie Callahan, General Manager
Scott Lawson, Development Director

Web Sites

4572 MGH Neurology Web Forums
www.mgh.harvard.edu/forum

4573 Maryland Department of Health
www.dhml.state.md.us

4574 Meningitis Foundation of America
www.musa.org

Help support sufferers of meningitis and their families and the development of vaccines and other means of treating and/or preventing meningitis.

4575 World Health Organization
www.who.int/topics/meningitis/en

WHO's objective, as set out in its Constitution, is the attainment by all peoples of the highest possible level of health.

Book Publishers

4576 Let's Talk About Going to the Hospital
Rosen Publishing Group's PowerKids Press
29 E 21st Street
New York, NY 10010

212-777-3017
800-237-9932
Fax: 888-436-4643
e-mail: rosenpub@tribeca.ios.com
www.powerkidspress.com

If a child has to check into the hospital, chances are he or she is already upset about being ill. Knowing how a hospital functions and what the procedures are, such as when family members can visit, will help in what is already a stressful situation. Grades K-5.

24 pages
ISBN: 0-823950-36-0

Roger Rosen, Editor

DESCRIPTION

4577 MENTAL RETARDATION

Synonym: Mental deficiency
Involves the following Biologic System(s):
Developmental/Behavioral/Psychiatric Disorders,
Neurologic Disorders

Mental retardation is characterized by impaired or below average intellectual functioning that results in deficits in learning ability and adaptive behaviors. The disorder is thought to affect approximately three percent of the general population. About 80 to 90 percent of patients have mild mental retardation, whereas 10 to 20 percent are affected by moderate to profound degrees of impairment.

The causes of mental retardation may be biological as well as psychosocial or sociocultural in nature. In other words, the disorder may be due to a combination of several factors and influenced both by biological abnormalities of the brain as well as the nature of a child's life experiences, such as those resulting from parent-child interactions and overall family dynamics. Biological causes of mental retardation may include fetal exposure to certain drugs, maternal infections, or radiation therapy; premature birth; or certain underlying disorders, such as inborn errors of metabolism, chromosomal abnormalities including Down syndrome and fragile X syndrome, or other genetic disorders. Mental retardation may also result from head injuries or low levels of oxygen to the brain during delivery, childhood exposure to lead, or certain infections during infancy or early childhood, such as inflammation of the protective membranes surround|ing the brain and spinal cord (meningitis). Some underlying causes may be correctable before mental retardation occurs, such as phenylketonuria (PKU), which is a metabolic disorder, or hypothyroidism, a condition characterized by decreased activity of the thyroid gland. Additional contributing factors may include malnutrition; dysfunctional interactions between caregivers and infants; or other psychosocial or sociocultural factors. In many children with mental retardation, the specific causes remain unknown. The condition may occur as the result of the interactions of several genes (polygenic inheritance), possibly in association with certain environmental influences (multifactorial).

During normal development, infants and children acquire mental, physical, and behavioral skills in certain stages known as developmental milestones. Although the particular rate of development is variable, most children acquire such skills at certain ages. However, infants and children with mental retardation typically experience delays in achieving certain developmental milestones. For example, with severe levels of mental retardation, patients may initially have delays in the acquisition of certain motor skills. With more moderate levels of retardation, children may achieve early motor milestones yet be delayed in acquiring certain skills that require the coordination of physical and mental abilities (psychomotor delays), such as delayed speech and language skills. In children with mild or borderline impairment, below average intellectual functioning may not be suspected until the early school years. Varying degrees of mental retardation are based upon the different levels of support that may be required for daily functioning as well as intelligence quotient (I.Q.), which is a standardized, age-related measure of intelligence. Mental retardation may be defined as having an I.Q. below 70 and is often subdivided into mild, moderate, severe, and profound mental retardation. Most individuals in the general population have an I.Q. between 80 and 120.

Children with what is known as borderline intellectual functioning have very mild intellectual deficits (e.g., I.Q. between 70 to 85) and minor impairments in adaptive behaviors. These behaviors include certain adaptive skills, such as social, self-care, communication, and vocational skills. Patients with mild retardation (I.Q. between 50 and 70) may develop academic skills up to the sixth grade level. In addition, with appropriate support, they may achieve social skills that enable them to function relatively independently during adulthood. Patients with moderate impairment (I.Q. between 35 and 50) may learn to communicate and tend to have only fair motor development. Although these patients rarely develop academic skills up to the second grade level, they may benefit from vocational training and achieve limited independence with appropriate supervision. Children with severe mental retardation (I.Q. between 20 and 35) typically have poor motor development and little speech or communication skills. With appropriate education and support, they may develop speech by late adolescence. In addition, with close supervision, they may learn basic hygienic skills and simple tasks by adulthood. Although children with profound impairment (I.Q. under 20) may learn some basic hygienic skills, they typically have limited psychomotor development and require close, ongoing supervision.

In infants with suspected mental retardation, a number of specialized laboratory tests may be conducted to rule out certain underlying disorders, such as fragile X syndrome or other chromosomal or genetic syndromes. The management of mental retardation is individualized for each child and may include therapeutic and special educational services as well as special social support and counseling services. Early diagnosis and the prompt development of an individualized, comprehensive intervention program is essential in helping affected children reach their potential. Prenatal screening for genetic defects, and genetic counseling for families at risk for known heritable disorders can decrease the incidence of genetically caused mental retardation. Primary care pediatricians lay an important role in consulting with specialists and other health care providers as required and developing an appropriate intervention program. As patients with mild to moderate impairment reach adolescence, specialized services may include a focus on vocational training and community living.

See also General Resources on page 917

National Associations & Support Groups

4578 ARC of the United States
1010 Wayne Avenue, Suite 650
Silver Spring, MD 20910

301-565-3842
800-433-5255
Fax: 301-565-5342
e-mail: info@thearc.org
www.thearc.org

The ARC is the national organization of and for people with mental retardation and related developmental disabilities and their families. Devoted to promoting and improving supports and services for people with mental retardation and their families. The association also fosters research and education regarding the prevention of mental retardation in infants and young children. The ARC was founded in 1950 by a small group of parents and other concerned individuals.

Sue Swenson, Executive Director
Adam Aaronson, Public Inquiries Director

4579 American Mental Health Foundation
191 Presidential Boulevard, Suite 3W, PO Box 345
Bala Cynwyd, PA 19004
USA

Dedicated to the extensive and intensive research in the theories and techniques of treatment of emotional illness and to the implementation of reforms in the mental health system. Efforts have resulted in development of better and less expensive treatment methods. Findings are disseminated in English and other major languages.

Monroe W Spero, MD

4580 Bethpage Mission
4980 W 118th Street, Suite A
Omaha, NE 68137

402-896-3884
800-628-7070
Fax: 402-896-1511
e-mail: psanchez@bethpage.org
www.bethpage.org

4581 Bethphage
2245 Midway Road, #300
Carrolton, TX 75006

972-866-9989
800-628-7070
Fax: 972-991-0834
e-mail: hbranicki@bethphage.org
www.bethphage.org

Bethphage is an affiliate of the Evangelical Lutheran Church in America, serves and advocates for people with disabilities so that they may achieve their full potential. Bethphage provides living and vocational services to individuals with developmental disabilities, including group homes, supervised apartment living and job skills training.

4582 NADD: National Association for the Dually Diagnosed
132 Fair Street
Kingston, NY 12401

845-331-4336
800-331-5362
Fax: 845-331-4569
e-mail: info@thenadd.org
www.thenadd.org

Nonprofit organization designed to promote the interests of professional and parent development with resources for individuals who have the coexistence of mental illness and mental retardation. Provides conferences, educational services and training materials to professionals, parents, concerned citizens and service organizations. Formerly known as the National Association for the Dually Diagnosed.

Dr Robert Fletcher, CEO
Michelle Jordan, Office Manager

4583 People First International
PO Box 12642
Salem, OR 97309

503-362-0336
Fax: 503-585-0287
e-mail: people1@people1.org
www.people1.org

Developmentally disabled people joining together to learn how to speak for themselves. Offers support, information, assistance and advocacy.

4584 Voice of the Retarded
5005 Newport Drive, Suite 108
Rolling Meadows, IL 60008

847-253-6020
Fax: 847-253-6054
e-mail: vor@compuserve.com
www.vor.net

Voice of the Retarded supports a full range of choices for individuals with mental retardation and their families and guardians. VOR is a national, nonprofit organization that advocates for a full continuum of quality care for persons with mental retardation.

Mary McTernan, President
Robin Sims, First Vice President

State Agencies & Support Groups

4585 Center for Disabilities and Development
University of Iowa Hospitals and Clinics
100 Hawkins Drive
Iowa City, IA 52242

319-353-6900
877-686-0031
e-mail: cdd-webmaster@uiowa.edu
www.healthcare.uiowa.edu/cdd

A trusted resource for healthcare, training, research and information for people with disabilities that include: behavior disorders, brain injury, cerebral palsy, diabetes, down syndrome, learning disabilities, mental retardation, sleep disorders and spina bifida.

Elayne Sexsmith, Administrator
Amy Mikelson, Supervisor Info Resource Service

4586 Center for Family Support
333 7th Avenue, 9th Floor
New York, NY 10001

212-629-7939
Fax: 212-239-2211
www.cfsny.org

The Center for Family Support (CFS) is a not-for-profit human service agency providing support and assistance to individuals with developmental disabilities and traumatic brain injuries throughout New York City, Long Island, the lower Hudson Valley region and New Jersey.

Steven Vernickofs, Executive Director

Web Sites

4587 American Association on Intellectual and D evelopmental Disabilities
www.aamr.org

AAMR promotes progressive policies, sound research, effective practices, and universal human rights for people with intellectual disabilites.

Hank Bersani PhD, President
Doreen Croser, Executive Director

Book Publishers

4588 Art Projects for the Mentally Retarded Child
Ellen J Sussman, author

Charles C Thomas Publishing
2600 South First Street
Springfield, IL 62704

217-789-8980
800-258-8980
Fax: 217-789-9130
e-mail: books@ccthomas.com
www.ccthomas.com

108 pages Softcover
ISBN: 0-398035-35-8

Charles Thomas, Publisher

4589 Children with Mental Retardation
Woodbine House
6510 Bells Mill Road
Bethesda, MD 20817

301-468-8800
800-843-7323
Fax: 301-897-5838
e-mail: info@woodbinehouse.com
www.woodbinehouse.com

A book for parents of children with mild to moderate mental retardation, whether or not they have a diagnosed syndrome or condition. It provides a complete and compassionate introduction to their child's medical, therapeutic, and educational needs, and discusses the emotional impact on the family. New parents can rely on Children with Mental Retardation to provide the solid foundation and confidence they need to help their child reach his or her highest potential.

437 pages Softcover
ISBN: 0-933149-39-5

4590 Music Curriculum Guidelines for Moderately Retarded Adolescents
Charles C Thomas Publishing
2600 S 1st Street
Springfield, IL 62704

217-789-8980
800-258-8980
Fax: 217-789-9130
e-mail: books@ccthomas.com
www.ccthomas.com

122 pages Spiral-Paper
ISBN: 0-398047-57-X

Charles Thomas, Publisher

4591 Retarded Isn't Stupid, Mom!
Sandra Z Kaufman, author

Brookes Publishing
PO Box 10624
Baltimore, MD 21285

410-337-9580
800-638-3775
Fax: 410-337-8539
e-mail: custserv@brookespublishing.com
www.brookespublishing.com

This book goes through the triumphs and sorrows of one young woman and her family and the emotions and events encountered as her daughter moves toward adulthood.

272 pages Softcover
ISBN: 1-557663-78-5

Paul Brooks, President
Melissa Behm, Executive Vice President

Magazines

4592 American Journal on Mental Retardation
AAMR
444 N Capitol Street NW, Suite 846
Washington, DC 20001

202-387-1968
800-424-3688
Fax: 202-387-2193
e-mail: maclean@uwyo.edu
www.aamr.allenpress.com/aamronline/?request=index.ht

AAMR promotes progressive policies, sound research, effective practices, and universal human rights for people with intellectual and developmental disabilities.

Doreen Croser, Executive Director
Paul Aitken, Director, Finance & Administration

4593 Mental Retardation
AAMR
444 N Capitol Street NW, Suite 846
Washington, DC 20001

202-387-1968
800-424-3688
Fax: 202-387-2193
e-mail: staylo01@mailbox.syr.edu
www.aamr.org

Provides information on the latest program advances, current research, and information on products and services in the developmental disabilities field.

Bimonthly

Steven J Taylor, Editor

Newsletters

4594 Association for the Help of Retarded Children
83 Maiden Lane
New York, NY 10038

212-780-2500
Fax: 212-777-5893
e-mail: ahrcnyc@dti.net
www.ahrcnyc.org

Developmentally disabled children and adults, their families, and interested individuals. Provides support services, training programs, clinics, schools and residential facilities to the developmentally disabled. Publications: The Chronicle, quarterly newsletter.

Biannually

Shirley Berenstein, Director

4595 NADD Bulletin
132 Fair Street
Kingston, NY 12401

845-331-4336
800-331-5362
Fax: 845-331-4569
e-mail: info@thenadd.org
www.thenadd.org

Official publication of the National Association for the Dually Diagnosed. It features articles that address clinical, programmatic, research or family oriented issues concerning mental health aspects in persons with disabilities.

20 pages Bimonthly

Donna Nagy Ph.D, President
Chrissoula Stavrakaki, Vice President

Camps

4596 Council for Extended Care of Mentally Retarded Citizens
1600 S Hanley Road
Saint Louis, MO

314-781-4950
Fax: 314-781-3850
e-mail: cecmrc@aol.com

Services are provided to adults and children with developmental disabilities. Supported living arrangements are located in St. Louis city and St. Charles County. Group home and camp services are located in Dittmer, MO. Travel program also available.

Cynthia Compton, Executive Director
Marge Lindhorst, Supported Living Director

4597 Ken-Crest Camp
1 Plymouth Meeting
Plymouth Meeting, PA

610-825-9360
Fax: 610-825-4127

Located on a 152-acre site in Pennsylvania, Ken-Crest provides traditional camping experiences to mentally retarded children, ages 7 and up. Among activities are swimming, biking, arts and crafts, music, and nature study.

William Nolan, Director

4598 Lions Den Outdoor Learning Center
1816 Lackland Hill Parkway
Saint Louis, MO

Varied programs for mentally retarded children, ages 6 and up, includes daily living, socialization and language skills. Sports, tent camping, crafts, and nature study are also offered. Sliding scale tuition for 2 weeks.

Cris Rodriguez

4599 New Jersey Camp Jaycee
P.O. Box 7730
North Brunswick, NJ 08902

732-246-2525
Fax: 732-214-1834
e-mail: infor@campjaycee.org
www.campjaycee.org

This camp is for children and adults with mental retardation and is sponsored jointly by the New Jersey Jaycees and the ARC of New Jersey. Activities at the 185-acre Pocono Mountain camp include arts and crafts, games and sports, music, nature, swimming, boating, horseback riding and self-help skills.

Jim Worrall, Executive Director

4600 Raven Rock Lutheran Camp
17912 Harbaugh Valley Road
Sabillasville, MD

717-794-2667

Christ-centered program for youth and mentally retarded adults.

Lee Sodowsky

DESCRIPTION

4601 MICROCEPHALY

Synonyms: Microcephalia, Microcephalism, Microencephaly **Involves the following Biologic System(s):**

Neurologic Disorders

Microcephaly is a developmental abnormality in which an infant's or child's head circumference is smaller than would be expected for his or her age and sex (i.e., two or three standard deviations below the mean). In most affected infants and children, underdevelopment of the brain (microencephaly) may result in varying degrees of mental retardation. Microcephaly is considered a relatively common condition, particularly among individuals affected by mental retardation.

In some affected infants and children, microcephaly occurs as an isolated genetic condition. Familial cases of isolated microcephaly have been reported that appear to have autosomal recessive or dominant inheritance. Autosomal recessive microcephaly is characterized by a narrow, sloping forehead; a flat back portion of the head (occiput); varying levels of mental retardation (although severe retardation is most common); and, in some cases, episodes of uncontrolled electrical disturbances in the brain (seizures). Autosomal dominant microcephaly may be characterized by mild slanting of the forehead, upslanting eyelid folds (palpebral fissures), prominent ears, short stature, and borderline or mild mental retardation. In others, the condition occurs in association with certain underlying genetic disorders, such as Cornelia de Lange syndrome. It may also be part of chromosomal malformation syndromes, such as trisomy 13 and trisomy 18 syndromes.

Microcephaly may also occur secondary to particular environmental factors, such as exposure before birth to radiation, certain chemical agents (e.g., alcohol), or certain maternal infections (e.g., rubella). In addition, the condition may result from particular conditions (e.g., meningitis, hyperthermia, etc.) during periods of rapid brain development after birth, particularly during the first two years of life.

When infants and children have a very small head circumference, the underlying abnormality may have begun during early embryonic or fetal development. Although the exact cause is not understood, the condition is thought to result from abnormal development of the outer region of the brain (cerebral cortex).

When infants or children are diagnosed with microcephaly, physicians typically take thorough family histories to determine whether other family members are affected or other disorders or syndromes may be present that are associated with microcephaly. The head circumference is measured periodically for a direct comparison to measurements at birth. Head circumference measurements may also be taken of both parents and any siblings. Additional testing may be undertaken to rule out potential underlying disorders or associated conditions. These tests may include advanced imaging techniques (e.g., CT scanning, MRI) of the brain, chromosomal testing (karyotyping), or certain laboratory tests to detect antibodies against certain infectious agents (e.g., rubella titers) in the child's and mother's bloodstream. Treatment of infants and children with microcephaly includes symptomatic and supportive measures, such as the prescription of certain medications to help treat or control seizures (e.g., anticonvulsants) and special education and other multidisciplinary measures to help ensure that affected children with mental retardation reach their potential. Prenatal screening for genetic defects, and genetic counseling for families at risk for known heritable disorders can decrease the incidence of genetically caused mental retardation. Primary care pediatricians lay an important role in consulting with specialists.

See also **General Resources** on page 917

Government Agencies

4602 ARC of the United States
Po Box 3006
Rockville, MD 20847

888-320-6942
800-370-2943
Fax: 301-984-1473
e-mail: nichdinformationresourcecenter@mail.nih
www.nichd.nih.gov

The ARC is the national organization of and for people with mental retardation and related developmental disabilities and their families. Devoted to promoting and improving supports and services for people with mental retardation and their families. The association also fosters research and education regarding the prevention of mental retardation in infants and young children. The ARC was founded in 1950 by a small group of parents and other concerned individuals.

Sue Swenson, Executive Director
Adam Aaronson, Public Inquiries Director

4603 NIH/National Institute of Child Health and Human Development
National Institues of Health
31 Center Drive
Bethesda, MD 20892

301-496-5133
Fax: 301-496-1104
www.nichd.nih.gov

Established in 1962 by congress, today the institute conducts and supports research on topics related to the health of children, adults, families and populations. These topics include: developmental disabilities, mental retardation, growth and development, infant death, reproductive health, and rehabilitation.

Nancy D Wirth, Director
Lisa Kaeser, Program & Public Liaison

National Associations & Support Groups

4604 Birth Defect Research for Children
930 Woodcock Road, Suite 225
Orlando, FL 32803

407-895-0802
Fax: 407-895-0824
e-mail: staff@birthdefects.org
www.birthdefects.org

Organization that helps families with free birth defect information, parent matching that links families of children with similar birth defects and research through the National Birth Defect Registry. Support group information and newsletter on Internet.

Betty Mekdeci, Executive Director

4605 Genetic Alliance
4301 Connecticut Avenue NW
Washington, DC 20008

202-966-5557
800-336-4363
Fax: 202-966-8553
e-mail: info@geneticalliance.org
www.geneticalliance.org

A coalition of voluntary genetic support groups, consumers and professionals addressing the needs of individuals and families affected by genetic disorders from a national perspective.

Sharon Terry, President/CEO

4606 March of Dimes Birth Defects Foundation
1275 Mamaroneck Avenue
White Plains, NY 10605

914-997-4488
888-663-4637
Fax: 914-428-8203
e-mail: resourcecenter@modimes.org
www.marchofdimes.com

Partnership of volunteers and professionals dedicated to improving the health of babies by preventing birth defects and infant mortality. Over 100 chapters are located across the country and can be located through the national office.

Dr Jennifer Howse, President

4607 National Dissemination Center for Children with Disabilities
PO Box 1492
Washington, DC 20013

202-884-8200
800-695-0285
Fax: 202-884-8441
e-mail: nichcy@aed.org
www.nichcy.org

A national information and referral center that provides information on disabilities and disability-related issues for families, educators and other professionals.

Suzanne Ripley, Executive Director

Web Sites

4608 Online Mendelian Inheritance in Man
www.ncbi.nlm.nih.gov

This database is a catalog of human genes and genetic disorders.

DESCRIPTION

4609 MICRODONTIA

Synonym: Microdontism

Involves the following Biologic System(s):

Dental Disorders

Microdontia is a term that refers to a developmental dental irregularity in which one or more teeth are abnormally small. This tooth abnormality often occurs in association with certain disorders, conditions, and syndromes and usually affects a single tooth or specific groups of teeth, namely the second or lateral incisors and the molars of the upper jaw. However, in rare instances, microdontia occurs in association with certain other disorders and may affect all or most of the teeth. These other disorders may include pituitary dwarfism, Down's syndrome, and certain forms of congenital heart disease.

Children with certain abnormalities of the face or skull (craniofacial defects) may often exhibit some form of microdontia. These disorders include Turner syndrome, a chromosomal disorder affecting females and characterized by various symptoms including a narrow palate and a small jaw (micrognathia); Crouzon's disease, an autosomal dominant disorder characterized by underdevelopment of the upper jaw and protrusion of the lower jaw (prognathism), a beaked nose, and other symptoms; and cleft lip, a congenital defect in which there is a split or fissure (cleft) in the upper lip. Microdontia is also manifested in several other disorders (e.g., focal dermal hypoplasia, progeria, oculomandibulodyscephaly, oculo-auriculo-vertebral anomaly, and others). Small teeth with a characteristic cone shape are often present in conjunction with missing teeth (anodontia) in certain syndromes known as ectodermal dysplasias, in which there is abnormal development of embryonic tissues that give rise to tooth enamel, hair, nails, skin glands, the outermost layer of the skin (epidermis), the nervous system, the ears and eyes, and mucous membranes of the anus and mouth. Other syndromes that involve microdontia include Williams syndrome, in which the second primary molar of the upper jaw is abnormally small. Aglossia-adactylia syndrome is characterized by partial or total absence of the tongue and missing or abnormally small incisors in the lower jaw.

Microdontia is thought to be genetically transmitted and results from an unknown factor or factors that affect the normal development of the main component of teeth (dentin) and their outermost covering (enamel). This condition is slightly more prevalent in females than males. Treatment may include oral surgery, orthodontic procedures, tooth restoration, and the use of implants or other dental appliances.

See also **General Resources** on page 917

Government Agencies

4610 NIH/National Institute of Child Health and Human Development

31 Center Drive, Building 31
Bethesda, MD 20892

301-496-5133
Fax: 301-496-1104
www.nichd.nih.gov

Established in 1962 by congress, today the institute conducts and supports research on topics related to the health of children, adults, families and populations. Some of these topics include: developmental disabilities, growth and development, infant death, reproductive health and birth defects.

Nancy D Wirth, Director
Lisa Kaeser, Program & Public Liaison

4611 NIH/National Institute of Dental and Crani ofacial Research

National Institutes of Health
31 Center Drive, MSC 2290, Building 31
Bethesda, MD 20892

301-496-3571
Fax: 301-402-2185
e-mail: nidcrinfo@mail.nih.gov
www.nidcr.nih.gov

Provides leadership for a national research program designed to understand, treat and prevent the infectious and inherited craniofacial-oral-dental diseases and disorders.

Dr Lawrence A Tabak, Director
Thomas G Murphy, Acting Executive Director

National Associations & Support Groups

4612 American Dental Association

211 E Chicago Avenue
Chicago, IL 60611

312-440-2500
Fax: 312-440-2800
www.ada.org

Professional association of dentists committed to the public's oral health, ethics, science and professional advancement; leading a unified profession through initiatives in advocacy, education, research and the development of standards.

Dr Robert Brandjord, President

Web Sites

4613 American Dental Association

www.ada.org

Professional association of dentists committed to the public's oral health, ethics, science and professional advancement; leading a unified profession through initiatives in advocacy, education, research and the development of standards.

4614 Dental Consumer Advisory

toothinfo.com/

Purpose is to provide useful and practical information for the public concerning issues of dental care.

4615 Dental Resources on the Web

dental-resources.com/

Dental sites for education, practices, laboratories, office supplies,
dental care and associations.

DESCRIPTION

4616 MIGRAINE HEADACHES

Covers these related disorders: Common migraine (Migraine without aura), Classic migraine (Migraine with aura)

Involves the following Biologic System(s):
Developmental/Behavioral/Psychiatric Disorders

The term migraine refers to a headache that is recurring and accompanied by three or more symptoms or findings that include the presence of certain visual, motor, or other sensations (aura or prodrome) preceding onset; head throbbing; pain on one side of the head (unilateral); nausea; vomiting; and abdominal pain. Additional associated findings include cessation of pain following sleep and a history of migraines in other family members. Migraines are the most common type of recurrent headaches that occur among children. In children younger than 10 years of age, boys are slightly more apt to develop migraines, while adolescent girls and adult females are more prone to migraines than are adolescent boys or adult men. Migraines may be caused by several different factors, alone or in combination. Such factors include genetic influences; stress-related factors; certain foods such as chocolate, citrus fruit, cheese, monosodium glutamate, etc.; red wine; stimuli such as bright lights, loud noises, etc.; medications such as birth control pills; menstruation; and other factors. Pain associated with migraines results from the narrowing and subsequent widening of the arteries that lead to the brain. This action triggers the pain receptors in that region, thus producing the characteristic pain of migraine headaches. More recent theories relate to the role played by the nervous system in the development of migraine headaches. It has been found that nerve cells in blood vessels of the migraine patient release a compound called "substance P." Substance P triggers pain and its release into the arteries is associated with the dilation of blood vessels and the release of histamine and other allergic compounds.

Migraine without aura (formerly called common migraine), is the type of migraine most likely to occur in children. Common migraine is characterized by a pounding or throbbing pain in the front or side(s) of the head. This headache may or may not be one-sided, may persist from one to 24 hours, and is usually accompanied by nausea, vomiting, and abdominal pain. Other associated symptoms may include fever, an unusual sensitivity to light (photophobia), numbness or tingling of the hands and feet, and dizziness or lightheadedness.

Migraine with aura (formerly called classic migraine), is characterized by similar symptoms and findings to those associated with common migraine; however, classic migraine is always preceded by an aura that occurs from 10 to 30 minutes before onset of the headache. This phenomenon may be characterized by visual, motor, or other sensations such as the appearance of shimmering or flashing lights (photopsia) as well as distorted images, loss of vision in part of the visual field (blind spot or scotoma), dizziness, tingling or weakness in an arm or leg, prickling or burning sensation around the mouth, and other irregularities.

In addition to the two primary types of migraine headaches, some children may develop unusual migraine headaches, called migraine variants, that may be characterized by vomiting that recurs at irregular intervals, sudden attacks of dizziness, and confusion. Children with this type of migraine, especially infants, may experience monthly episodes of severe vomiting resulting in excessive fluid loss (dehydration); the loss of essential compounds, known as electrolytes, in the fluid portion of the blood (i.e., sodium, calcium, and potassium); and associated fever, abdominal pain, and diarrhea. Children with migraine variants may at times appear disoriented, hyperactive, and nonresponsive. Other types of migraine include complicated migraine and cluster headaches. Complicated migraines refer to migraine headaches accompanied by neurologic findings that persist beyond the headache and may be further categorized as basilar migraine, ophthalmoplegic migraine, and hemiplegic migraine. These types of headaches may sometimes indicate the presence of an underlying lesion. Basilar migraine is characterized by problems with equilibrium, double or blurred vision, loss of vision in part of the visual field, lack of muscular coordination (ataxia), seizures, or other irregularities. Ophthalmoplegic migraine, which is characterized by paralysis of the eye muscles on the same side as the migraine, does not commonly occur in children. Amaurosis fugax, a variant of complicated migraine, is characterized by reversible blindness or partial blindness in one eye. Hemiplegic migraine is characterized by numbness and muscular weakness or paralysis affecting only one side of the body. It is rare for children to experience more than one hemiplegic migraine episode. Cluster headaches do not commonly occur in children.

Treatment for migraine headaches may first be directed toward prevention by identifying and removing or avoiding stimulating influences such as certain foods, medications, or underlying stress factors. Many children may benefit from simply resting in a quiet, darkened room. Treatment for pain and vomiting associated with migraine headaches may include administration of pain relievers such as acetaminophen or ibuprofen along with drugs to reduce vomiting (antiemetics). These drugs are often administered rectally in suppository form. In more severe episodes, older children and adolescents may require the administration of a preparation called ergotamine, which is most effective if taken during the early stages of the migraine episode. Ergotamine should not be administered to children with hemiplegic migraines. Some children and adolescents may benefit from behavior management therapy. Other treatment is symptomatic and supportive.

See also **General Resources** on page 917

Government Agencies

4617 NIH/National Eye Institute
31 Center Drive MSC 2510
Bethesda, MD 20892

301-496-5248
e-mail: 2020@nei.nih.gov
www.nei.nih.gov

Conducts and supports research that helps prevent and treat eye diseases and other disorders of vision. This research leads to sight-saving treatments, reduces visual impairment and blindness, and improves the quality of life for people of all ages. NEI-supported research has advanced our knowledge of how the eye functions in health and disease.

Paul A Sieving M.D., Ph.D., Director

National Associations & Support Groups

4618 American Academy of Neurology
1080 Montreal Avenue
Saint Paul, MN 55116

651-695-2717
800-879-1960
Fax: 651-695-2791
e-mail: memberservices@aan.com
www.aan.com

Medical society established to advance the art and science of neurology, and therby promote the best possible care for patients with neurological disordes by: ensuring appropriate access to neurological care, supporting and advocating for an environment which ensures ethical, high quality neurological care and supporting clinical and basic research in the neurosciences and reltated fields.

19,000 members

Stephen M Sergay, President
Robert C Griggs, President Elect

4619 American Headache Society
19 Mantua Road
Mount Royal, NJ 08061

856-423-0258
Fax: 856-423-0082
e-mail: achehq@talley.com
www.achenet.org

A professional society of health care providers dedicated to the study and treatment of headache and face pain. It was founded in 1959 and sponsors the American Council for Headache Education (ACHE), which will soon become a committee of the AHS.

Linda McGillicuddy, Executive Director
Gretchen Tietjen, MD, Chair

4620 Migraine Awareness Group: National Understanding for Migraineurs (MAGNUM)
113 South St Asaph Street, Suite 100
Alexandria, VA 22314

703-349-1929
Fax: 703-739-2432
e-mail: comments@migraines.org
www.migraines.org

Works to bring public awareness, utilizing the electronic, print, and artistic mediums, to the fact that Migraine is a true, biologic disease. Advocates on behalf of Migraine head pain sufferers worldwide.

Michael John Coleman, Founder/Executive Director
Terri Miller-Burchfield, Executive VP

4621 National Headache Foundation
820 N Orleans, Ste 217
Chicago, IL 60610

312-274-2650
888-643-5552
Fax: 312-640-9049
e-mail: info@headaches.org
www.headaches.org

Nonprofit organization dedicated to the education of headache sufferers and health care professionals about the causes and treatment of headaches.

Arthur H. Elkind MD, President
Roger K. Cadynd MD, Vice President

Research Centers

4622 Kennedy Krieger Institute
Pediatric Headache Program
707 N Broadway
Baltimore, MD 21205

443-923-9200
e-mail: malin@kennedykrieger.org
www.kennedykrieger.org/kki_cp.jsp?pid=4781

The Pediatric Headache Program was started in 2005 in order to facilitate the diagnosis, treatment and management of children and adolescents who suffer from persistent headaches, including migraine, tension and chronic daily.

Michael Malin, Program Clinical Coordinator
Terri Holbrook, Neurology/Nursing Staff Coordinator

Web Sites

4623 American Academy of Neurology
www.aan.com

Medical society established to advance the art and science of neurology, and therby promote the best possible care for patients with neurological disordes by: ensuring appropriate access to neurological care, supporting and advocating for an environment which ensures ethical, high quality neurological care and supporting clinical and basic research in the neurosciences and reltated fields.

4624 Migraine Awareness Group: A National Understanding for Migraineurs
www.migraines.org

Brings public awareness to the fact that Migraine is a true, biological neurological disease using the electronic, print and artistic mediums of expression.

4625 National Headache Foundation
www.headaches.org

A nonprofit organization dedicated to educating headache sufferers and healthcare professionals about headache causes and treatments.

Book Publishers

4626 Freedom From Headaches

Joel Saper, author

Simon & Schuster
100 Front Street
Riverside, NJ 08075

212-698-7000
800-223-2336
Fax: 212-698-7099
www.simonsays.com

236 pages paperback
ISBN: 0-671254-04-9

4627 Handbook of Headache

Lippincott Williams & Wilkins
351 W Camden Street
Baltimore, MD 21201

410-528-4000
800-638-3030
www.lww.com

2004 400 pages softbound
ISBN: 0-781752-23-0

4628 Handbook of Headache Disorders

Essential Medical Information Systems
PO Box 1607
Durant, OK 74702

580-924-0643
Fax: 580-924-9414

1993 Paperback
ISBN: 0-929240-62-6

4629 Headache Book: Prevention & Treatment for All Types of Headaches

Frank B. Minirth, author

Thomas Nelson Publishers
1 Gateway Plaza
Port Chester, NY 10573

914-937-8400

1994
ISBN: 0-785282-56-4

4630 Management of Headache & Headache Medications

Lawrence D. Robbins, author

Spring-Verlag
175 5th Avenue
New York, NY 10010

212-460-1500

1994 294 pages
ISBN: 0-387989-44-7

4631 Migraine and Other Headaches: Vascular Mechanisms

Raven Press
1185 Avenue of the Americas
New York, NY 10036

212-930-9500
www.raven.com

Leading international experts present new concepts on the mechanisms of migraine and other vascular headaches and detail the latest strategies for diagnosis and treatment of migraine with and without aura, tension-type headaches, cluster headaches and other vascular disorders.

368 pages
ISBN: 0-881677-95-7

4632 Overcoming Headaches & Migraines

Longmeadow Press
PO Box 10218
Stamford, CT 06904

203-352-2110

1993 128 pages Paperback
ISBN: 0-681417-92-7

4633 Treating the Headache Patient

Roger K. Cady, author

Marcell Dekker, Inc.
270 Madison Avenue
New York, NY 10016

212-696-9000
Fax: 800-228-1160

1994 366 pages
ISBN: 0-824791-09-6

4634 Wolff's Headaches & Other Head Pain

Stephen D. Silberstein, author

Oxford University Press
198 Madison Avenue
New York, NY 10016

212-726-6000
800-445-9714
Fax: 919-677-1303
e-mail: custserv.us@oup.com
www.us.oup.com/us

1993
ISBN: 0-195082-50-8

Newsletters

4635 Headache

American Council for Headache Education
19 Mantua Road
Mount Royal, NJ 08061

856-423-0258
Fax: 856-423-0082
e-mail: achehq@talley.com
www.achenet.org

Provides valuable and current information on new treatments, as well as time-proven headache management strategies. All articles are written or reviewed by headache experts from the American Headache Society (AHS). Recent issues have included articles by headache experts on drug and nondrug treatment options and information on new treatments and research is regularly included.

12 pages Quarterly

4636 NHF Head Lines

National Headache Foundation
820 N Orleans, Suite 217
Chicago, IL 60610

312-274-3650
888-643-5552
e-mail: info@headches.org
www.headaches.org

Offers the latest information on headaches, causes and treatments. Contains news on drugs and medical forums, in-depth discussions of headaches and preventions and a question and answer section in which physicians respond to reader inquiries and support group information.

Bimonthly

Suzanne Simons, Executive Director

Pamphlets

4637 52 Proven Stress Reducers
National Headache Foundation
820 N Orleans, Suite 217
Chicago, IL 60610

888-643-5552
Fax: 773-525-7357
www.headaches.org

Arthur H. Elkind, President
Roger K. Kady, Vice President

4638 About Headaches
National Headache Foundation
820 N Orleans, Suite 217
Chicago, IL 60610

888-643-5552
Fax: 312-640-9049
www.headaches.org

Contains an in-depth look at headaches, tips on when to seek medical advice, methods of treatment and more.

16 pages

Arthur H. Elkind MD, President
Roger C. Cady MD, Vice President

4639 Analgesic Rebound Headaches-Fact Sheet
National Headache Foundation
820 N Orleans, Suite 217
Chicago, IL 60610

888-643-5552
Fax: 312-640-9049
e-mail: info@headaches.org
www.headaches.org

Offers information on analgesic agents or drugs used to control pain including migraine and other types of headaches.

Arthur H. Elkind MD, President
Roger K. Cady MD, Vice President

4640 Cluster Headache-Fact Sheet
National Headache Foundation
820 N Orleans, Suite 217
Chicago, IL 60610

888-643-5552
Fax: 312-640-9049
e-mail: info@headaches.org
www.headaches.org

Offers information on cluster headaches and the treatment available for them.

Arthur H. Elkind MD, President
Roger K. Cady Md, Vice President

4641 Diet and Headache-Fact Sheet
National Headache Foundation
820 N Orleans, Suite 217
Chicago, IL 60610

888-643-5552
Fax: 312-640-9049
e-mail: info@headaches.org
www.headaches.org

Offers information on what foods should be avoided, and what foods trigger headaches in all migraine sufferers.

Arthur H. Elkind MD, President
Roger K. Cady MD, Vice President

4642 Headache Facts-What Everyone Should Know
American Council for Headache Education
19 Mantua Road
Mount Royal, NJ 08061

856-423-0258
Fax: 856-423-0082
e-mail: achehq@talley.com
www.achenet.org

Andrew Hershey, Chair Of Special Interest Sections
Barry Baumel, Chair Of Funding Committee

4643 Headache Handbook
National Headache Foundation
820 N Orleans, Suite 217
Chicago, IL 60610

888-643-5552
Fax: 312-640-9049
e-mail: info@headaches.org
www.headaches.org

Gives information and coauses on five common types of headaches as well as treatments available.

8 pages

Arthur H. Elkind MD, President
Roger K. Cady MD, Vice President

4644 Headache Q & A
National Headache Foundation
820 N Orleans, Suite 217
Chicago, IL 60610

888-643-5552
Fax: 312-640-9049
e-mail: info@headaches.org
www.headaches.org

Handy, fact-filled card contains the most frequently asked questions and answers concerning headache triggers and treatments.

Arthur H. Elkind MD, President
Roger K. Cady MD, Vice President

4645 Headache in Children-Fact Sheet
National Headache Foundation
820 N Orleans, Suite 217
Chicago, IL 60610

888-643-5552
Fax: 312-640-9049
e-mail: info@headaches.org
www.headaches.org

Offers information on vascular headaches, tension-type headaches, traction and inflammatory headaches and treatment.

Arthur H. Elkind MD, President
Roger K. Cady MD, Vice President

4646 How to Talk to Your Doctor About Headaches
National Headache Foundation
820 N Orleans, Suite 217
Chicago, IL 60610

888-643-5552
Fax: 312-640-9049
e-mail: info@headaches.com
www.headaches.org

Learn how to keep a headache diary to pinpoint symptoms and effective diagnosis.

Arthur H. Elkind MD, President
Roger K. Cady MD, Vice President

4647 Impact of Migraine-A Disabling and Costly Condition
American Council for Headache Education
19 Mantua Road
Mount Royal, NJ 08061

856-423-0258
Fax: 856-423-0082
e-mail: achehq@talley.com
www.achenet.org

Andrew Hershey, Chair Of Specil Interest Sections
Barry Baumel, Chair Of Funding Committee

4648 Migraine and Coexisting Conditions-Other Illnesses That May Affect Migraine
American Council for Headache Education
19 Mantua Road
Mount Royal, NJ 08061

856-423-0258
Fax: 856-423-0082
e-mail: achehq@talley.com
www.achenet.org

Andrew Hershey, Chair Of Special Interest Sections
Barry Baumel, Chair Of Funding Committee

4649 Migraine-Fact Sheet
National Headache Foundation
820 N Orleans, Suite 217
Chicago, IL 60610

888-643-5552
Fax: 312-640-9049
e-mail: info@headaches.org
www.headaches.org

Offers information on migraines and treatments.

Arthur H. Elkind MD, President
Roger K. Cady MD, Vice President

4650 Tap the Best Resource
National Headache Foundation
820 N Orleans, Suite 217
Chicago, IL 60610

888-643-5552
Fax: 312-640-9049
e-mail: info@headaches.org
www.headaches.org

Informational brochure offering facts and statistics on headaches. Everything from muscle contraction, vascular headaches, sinus headaches, TMJ, and much more.

Arthur H. Elkind MD, President
Roger K. Cady MD, Vice President

4651 What's the Best Medicine for My Headaches?
American Council for Headache Education
19 Mantua Road
Mount Royal, NJ 08061

856-423-0258
Fax: 856-423-0082
e-mail: achehq@talley.com
www.achenet.org

Andrew Hershey, Chair Of Special Interest Sections
Barry Baumel, Chair Of Funding Committee

4652 When Are Opioid (Narcotic) Drugs Appropriate for Headache?
American Council for Headache Education
19 Mantua Road
Mount Royal, NJ 08061

856-423-0258
Fax: 856-423-0082
e-mail: achehq@talley.com
www.achenet.org

4653 Women and Headache
American Council for Headache Education
19 Mantua Road
Mount Royal, NJ 08061

856-423-0258
Fax: 856-423-0082
e-mail: achehq@talley.com
www.achenet.org

DESCRIPTION

4654 MILK PROTEIN ALLERGY/LACTOSE INTOLERANCE

Involves the following Biologic System(s):

Gastrointestinal Disorders

Milk protein allergy is an allergic reaction to the proteins found in cow's milk and is the most common food allergy in children. Cow's milk is a large source of nutrition for infants and children. Infant formulas are primarily composed of cow's milk proteins, and milk products are often a major source of calories, protein, vitamins, and minerals in a child's diet. Cow's milk contains proteins, sugars (carbohydrates), as well as fats. Breastmilk can also contain these proteins from the mother's diet. There are several distinct diseases entities that would fall under the category of milk allergy or intolerance.

Most infants show symptoms of cow's milk protein allergy within the first three to six months of exposure. The immune system of the infant recognizes the milk protein as foreign and reacts by making immune proteins (antibodies also known as immunoglobulins) to defend the body against the foreign protein. Milk protein allergy can be either an immediate-onset or delayed-onset allergic reaction. Immediate-onset reactions can manifest acutely with gastrointestinal (diarrhea, vomiting, abdominal pain), respiratory (asthma, wheezing), or dermatologic (eczema, hives) symptoms. Delayed-onset reactions usually manifest with chronic diarrhea that may be bloody (hematochezia). More severe disease leads to small bowel damage and poor weight gain (failure to thrive).

The diagnosis of milk protein allergy can be made by history and physical exam. Stool, blood, skin and/or milk challenge tests may also be used to aid in diagnosis. Milk protein allergy is reported in up to 4% of infants, and usually resolves by age three. Until that time, infants on formula are fed special formulas (hydrolysate formula) and breastfeeding mothers should avoid milk and milk products. Infants with cow's milk protein allergy have a higher chance of having soy milk protein allergy and therefore soy formulas are not recommended. As children get older, milk is slowly reintroduced. Fortunately, most babies outgrow their milk allergies by their second or third year.

Lactose intolerance is not an allergic reaction, but an inability to digest the primary sugar found in milk (lactose). In the small intestine there is an enzyme (lactase) that breaks lactose down into smaller sugars to be used by the body.

Symptoms of lactose intolerance include abdominal cramping, bloating, diarrhea, and flatulence. There are large racial differences in the incidence of lactose intolerance; persons of Asian and African descent have a higher incidence in comparison to Caucasians.

Symptoms of lactose intolerance can occur any time after age 5 because lactase enzyme activity peaks in infancy and early childhood. One exception is congenital lactase deficiency. In this genetic disorder, infants are born without the enzyme lactase and symptoms, such as abdominal bloating and diarrhea, occur in the first week of life.

The treatment for lactose intolerance is avoidance of milk or lactase enzyme supplementation (available in pill form or added to milk products).

See also **General Resources** on page 917

National Associations & Support Groups

4655 International Foundation for Functional Gastrointestinal Disorders (IFFGD)
PO Box 170864
Milwaukee, WI 53217

414-964-1799
888-964-2001
Fax: 414-964-7176
e-mail: iffgd@iffgd.org
www.iffgd.org

A nonprofit education and research organization founded in 1991. IFFGD addresses the issues surrounding life with gastrointestinal functional and motility disorders and increases the awareness about these disorders among the general public, researchers, and the clinical care community.

Nancy J Norton, Founder
William Norton, VP

4656 North American Society for Pediatric Gastroenterology/Hepatology/Nutrition
PO Box 6
Flourtown, PA 19031

215-233-0808
Fax: 215-233-3918
e-mail: naspghan@naspghan.org
www.naspghan.org

Strives to improve the care of infants, children and adolescents with digestive disorders by promoting advances in clinical care of children with chronic abdominal pain, diarrhea, constipation, vomiting, bleeding from the GI tract, inflammatory bowel disease, liver diseases, diseases of the pancreas, poor weight gain and nutritional problems.

Margaret K Stallings, Executive Director
Sandy Fasoldngs, Associate Director

4657 Parents of Galactosemic Children
P.O. Box 2401
Mandeville, LA 70470

228-497-5886
866-900-7421
e-mail: president@galactosemia.org
www.galactosemia.org

A nonprofit national organization founded in 1985 by a small group of mothers in New York. It offers support and educational information to galactosemic families and facilitates communication between them and professionals.

Michelle Fowler, President & Treasurer
Nishkala Rao, Secretary

Web Sites

4658 Galactosemia Resources and Information
www.galactosemia.com

A repository for information about galactosemia and a jumping-off point to other places on the web.

4659 International Foundation for Functional Gastrointestinal Disorders (IFFGD)
www.iffgd.org

4660 NASPGHAN
www.naspghan.org

Offering information on pediatric gastroenterology, hepatology and nutrition.

4661 Parents of Galactosemic Children
www.galactosemia.org

Offering support and educational information to galactosemic families and interested professionals.

Book Publishers

4662 Infant Formulas for Allergic Infants and Dietetic Concerns for Toddlers
American Allergy Association
PO Box 7273
Menlo Park, CA 94026

650-322-1663

Offers information on reliable food labels, evaluations of infant formulas, FDA labeling requirements under the new law and more.

4663 Raising Your Child Without Milk: Reassuring Advice and Recipes For Parent
Simon & Simon
100 Front Street
Riverside, NJ 08075

530-889-4000
800-488-4308
Fax: 800-943-9831
e-mail: info@simonsays.com
www.simonsays.com

This book offers parents of milk-allergic or lactose intolerant children and the most up-to-date medical and nutritional information. It contains 125 dairy free recipes, and answers questions sent in from parents across the country.

384 pages Paperback

Jack Romanos, President/CEO
David England, VP/CFO

4664 Why Does Milk Bother Me?
NDDIC
2 Information Way
Bethesda, MD 20892

800-891-5389
Fax: 703-738-4929
e-mail: nddic@info.niddk.nih.gov
www.niddk.nih.gov

Defines lactose intolerance and provides information on symptoms, diagnosis and treatment.

16 pages

Journals

4665 Managing Food Allergy and Intolerance
Janice Vickerstaff Joneja, PhD, author

J A Hall Publications
2401-9304 Salish Court
Burnaby, BC
Canada

604-738-9688
888-993-6133
Fax: 604-738-9425
e-mail: info@hallpublications.com
www.hallpublications.com

This is a fully-referenced, extensively researched and indexed manual for health care professionals counseling those with food allergy or intolerance.

581 pages
ISBN: 0-968209-80-7

Newsletters

4666 NASPGHAN News
PO Box 6
Flourtown, PA 19031

215-233-0808
Fax: 215-233-3939
e-mail: naspghan@naspghan.org
www.naspgn.org

Publication of the North American Society for Pediatric Gastroenterolgy, Hepatology and Nutrition, which strives to improve the care of infants, children and adolescents with digestive disorders by promoting advances in clinical care of children with chronic abdominal pain, diarrhea, constipation, vomiting, bleeding from the GI tract, inflammatory bowel disease, liver diseases, diseases of the pancreas, poor weight gain and nutritional problems.

Pamphlets

4667 Lactose Intolerance
NDDIC
2 Information Way
Bethesda, MD 20892

800-891-5389
Fax: 703-738-4929
e-mail: nddic@info.niddk.nih.gov
www.niddk.nih.gov

8 pages

DESCRIPTION

4668 MUCOLIPIDOSES

Synonym: ML

Involves the following Biologic System(s):

Genetic/Chromosomal/Syndrome/Metabolic Disorders

The mucolipidoses (ML) are inborn errors of metabolism that belong to a group of diseases known as lysosomal storage disorders. Lysosomes are the major digestive structures within cells. Certain proteins known as enzymes break down or digest nutrients, such as particular fats or carbohydrates. The mucolipidoses are characterized by a deficiency or the abnormal functioning of certain lysosomal enzymes, causing the abnormal accumulation of complex carbohydrates (glycosaminoglycans) and fats (lipids) in cells within particular tissues. Such tissues may include those of the brain and spinal cord (central nervous system), skeleton, joints, heart, liver, spleen, or eyes. The mucolipidoses are thought to be inherited as an autosomal recessive trait.

Specific names as well as Roman numerals are used to classify the different forms of ML. Different types of mucolipidosis include I-Cell disease (ML II), pseudo-Hurler polydystrophy (ML III), and Berman syndrome (ML IV). Some forms of ML are further divided into different subtypes, such as sialidosis (ML I) types I and II, based on age of onset, associated symptoms, or other factors.

In children with mucolipidosis, associated symptoms and findings may be variable, depending upon the specific form of ML that is present. However, certain abnormalities occur in association with most forms of ML. Such findings include mild to severe coarsening of facial features, characteristic skeletal abnormalities (known as dysostosismultiplex), changes of the joints, and varying levels of mental retardation. In children with ML, skeletal malformations may include short stature; abnormal front-to-back or sideways curvature of the spine (kyphosis or scoliosis) or both; improper development of the hips (hip dysplasia); abnormally short neck; or premature fusion of the fibrous joints (sutures) between certain bones of the skull. Many affected children may develop joint stiffness and abnormal bending of certain joints in a fixed position (contractures). In addition, in some patients, neuromuscular abnormalities may be present, such as unusually decreased muscle tone (hypotonia) followed by abnormally exaggerated reflexes (hyperreflexia); shock-like contractions of certain muscles or muscle groups (myoclonus); or involuntary, rapid or writhing movements of the arms and legs (choreoathetoid movements).

Some forms of ML may also be associated with distinctive eye abnormalities, such as clouding of the corneas (corneal opacities), the development of abnormal red circular areas of the middle layer of the eyes (cherry-red spots), or other defects, causing visual impairment. Additional physical abnormalities associated with ML may include bulging of part of the intestine through a weak area in the abdominal wall (hernias), enlargement of the liver or spleen, enlargement of the heart or other heart defects, or increased susceptibility to repeated respiratory infections. Some children with these disorders may also experience delays in the acquisition of skills that require the coordination of physical and mental activities (psychomotor retardation) and may develop progressively severe mental retardation. Other patients may experience mild, nonprogressive mental retardation. Some of the mucolipidoses may result in potentially life-threatening complications during childhood, adolescence, or young adulthood.

The treatment of children with mucolipidosis is symptomatic and supportive. Such measures may include therapies to help prevent or aggressively treat respiratory infections; surgical correction of joint contractures, heart abnormalities, hernias, or other defects; physical therapy; special education; or other measures as required.

See also **General Resources** on page 917

National Associations & Support Groups

4669 March of Dimes Birth Defects Foundation
1275 Mamaroneck Avenue
White Plains, NY 10605

914-428-7100
888-663-4637
Fax: 914-428-8203
e-mail: resourcecenter@modimes.org
www.marchofdimes.com

Partnership of volunteers and professionals dedicates to improving the health of babies by preventing birth defects and infant mortality. Over 100 chapters are located across the country and can be located through the National Office.

Dr Jennifer Howse, President

4670 Mucolipidosis IV Foundation
719 E 17th Street
Brooklyn, NY 11230

718-434-5064
www.ml4.org

Funds three major institutions comprised of the best genetic scientists recognized worldwide.

Randy Yudenfreind, President

4671 National MPS Society
PO Box 736
Bangor, ME 04402

207-947-1445
Fax: 207-990-3074
e-mail: info@mpssociety.org
www.mpssociety.org

Organization that serves as a support group for those affected by mucopolysaccharidoses and related disorders. Raises funds to promote research and increases awareness of the disorder.

Barbara A Wedehase, Executive Director

Web Sites

4672 Healthfinder
www.healthfinder.gov

Links to carefully selected information and Web sites from over 1,500 health-related organizations.

4673 Mucolipidosis IV Foundation
www.ml4.org

Funds three major institutions comprised of the best genetic scientists recognized worldwide.

4674 National MPS Society
www.mpssociety.org

Shares information on the care and management of the children with Mucopolysaccharide diseases. The conference also brings in Medical Researchers reporting on advances in research related to these diseases.

4675 Online Mendelian Inheritance in Man
www.ncbi.nlm.nih.gov

This database is a catalog of human genes and genetic disorders.

Book Publishers

4676 Let's Talk About Going to the Hospital
Rosen Publishing Group's PowerKids Press
29 E 21st Street
New York, NY 10010

212-777-3017
800-237-9932
Fax: 888-436-4643
e-mail: rosenpub@tribeca.ios.com
www.powerkidspress.com

If a child has to check into the hospital, chances are he or she is already upset about being ill. Knowing how a hospital functions and what the procedures are, such as when family members can visit, will help in what is already a stressful situation. Grades K-5.

24 pages
ISBN: 0-823950-36-0

DESCRIPTION

4677 MUCOPOLYSACCHARIDOSES

Synonym: MPS

Involves the following Biologic System(s):

Genetic/Chromosomal/Syndrome/Metabolic Disorders

The mucopolysaccharidoses (MPS) are hereditary metabolic disorders that belong to a group of diseases known as lysosomal storage disorders. Lysosomes are the major digestive units within cells. Enzymes within lysosomes break down nutrients, such as certain fats and carbohydrates. The mucopolysaccharidoses are characterized by deficiency of certain lysosomal enzymes, causing the abnormal accumulation of complex carbohydrates in cells within particular tissues of the body. Affected tissues and organs typically include the skeleton, joints, brain and spinal cord (central nervous system), heart, liver, spleen, and eyes. The genes that encode most of these enzymes have been mapped to particular chromosomes. All of the mucopolysaccharidoses are inherited as an autosomal recessive trait, with the exception of Hunter syndrome, which has X-linked recessive inheritance. Collectively, these disorders are thought to affect approximately one in 10,000 newborns.

The various forms of MPS are typically designated by a Roman numeral and a specific name, such as Hunter syndrome (MPS II) or Sanfilippo syndrome (MPS III). In addition, some forms of MPS are divided into different subtypes, such as Hurler syndrome (MPS I H) and Hurler-Scheie syndrome (MPS I H/S), based on different changes (mutations) of the disease gene, age of onset, clinical course, or other factors. The range and severity of associated symptoms and findings may vary, depending upon the specific form of MPS that is present. However, certain findings are common to most forms of MPS, such as characteristic skeletal abnormalities (known as dysostosis multiplex), changes of the joints, growth delays, a characteristic facial appearance, and progressive mental retardation. For example, beginning in the first year of life or during later childhood, many patients develop progressively coarse facial features. Many children with MPS also experience delays in the acquisition of skills requiring the coordination of physical and mental activities (psychomotor retardation), a gradual loss of previously acquired skills (developmental regression), and progressively severe mental retardation. However, in a few forms of MPS, children may have average intelligence.

Many children with MPS also have short stature; sideways or front-to-back curvature of the spine (scoliosis or kyphosis) or both; other bone abnormalities; joint stiffness; and abnormal bending of certain joints in a fixed position (contractures). Other common findings include clouding of the corneas of the eyes and associated visual impairment, abnormal bulging of part of the intestine through a weak area in the abdominal wall (hernias), and enlargement of the liver and spleen (hepatosplenomegaly). Some patients also have associated abnormalities of the heart and its major blood vessels (cardiovascular defects), such as narrowing of the arteries supplying the heart; improper closure of one of the heart valves, allowing blood to leak back into the left upper chamber of the heart (mitral insufficiency); or other cardiac defects. Many of these disorders may result in potentially life-threatening complications during childhood or adolescence.

The treatment of children with MPS includes symptomatic and supportive measures, such as surgical correction of hernias, cardiovascular defects, joint contractures, or other abnormalities as required; physical therapy; or special education. In patients with some forms of MPS, enzyme replacement therapy has been shown to provide some temporary benefit. In addition, bone marrow transplantation may be effective in some patients with certain forms of mucopolysaccharidosis (e.g., Hurler syndrome).

See also **General Resources** on page 917

National Associations & Support Groups

4678 Association for Neuro-Metabolic Disorders
5223 Brookfield Lane
Sylvania, OH 43560

419-885-1497
e-mail: volk4olks@aol.com

Nonprofit organization that serves as an advocate organization for families of patients with the following neuro-metabolic disorders: phenylketonuria, maple syrup urine disease, galactosemia, and biotinidase deficiency. Provides educational information for parents and children; provides networking information on support groups for new parents; supports scientific research into the treatments of these four neuro-metabolic disorders.

Cheryl Volk, Parent Representative

4679 March of Dimes Birth Defects Foundation
1275 Mamaroneck Avenue
White Plains, NY 10605

914-428-7100
888-663-4637
Fax: 914-428-8203
e-mail: resourcecenter@modimes.org
www.marchofdimes.com

Partnership of volunteers and professionals dedicates to improving the health of babies by preventing birth defects and infant mortality. Over 100 chapters are located across the country and can be located through the National Office.

Dr Jennifer Howse, President

4680 National MPS Society
PO Box 736
Bangor, ME 04402

207-947-1445
Fax: 207-990-3074
e-mail: laurie@mpssociety.org
www.mpssociety.org

Organization that serves as a support group for those affected by mucopolysaccharidoses and related disorders. Raises funds to promote research and increases awareness of the disorder.

Barbara A Wdehase, Executive Director

Web Sites

4681 Canadian Society for Mucopolysaccharide & Related Diseases
Po Box 30034 RPO Parkgate
North Vancouver, BC v7h2y
canada

604-924-5130
800-667-1846
Fax: 604-924-5131
www.mpssociety.ca

Provides information and support to affected individuals and their families.

Kristen Harkins, Executive Director
Judy Byrne, Chairperson

4682 CliniWeb
www.ohsu.edu/cliniweb/C17/C17.300.550.htm

Is one of the original catalogs of health and bimedical information on the web.

4683 Healthfinder
www.healthfinder.gov

Links to carefully selected information and Web sites from over 1,500 health-related organizations.

4684 Mucopolysaccharidoes & Related Diseases
www.mpssociety.ca/

Provides information and support to affected individuals and their families.

4685 National MPS Society
www.mpssociety.org

Shares information on the care and management of the children with Mucopolysaccharide diseases. The conference also brings in Medical Researchers reporting on advances in research related to these diseases.

4686 Online Mendelian Inheritance in Man
www.ncbi.nlm.nih.gov

This database is a catalog of human genes and genetic disorders.

4687 Society for Mucopolysaccharide Diseases
www.mpssociety.co.uk

A voluntary support group that represents from throughout the UK over 1200 children and adults suffering from mucopolysaccharide and related diseases, their families, caregivers and professionals. It is a registered charity entirely supported by voluntary donations and fundraising. It is managed by the members themselves.

Book Publishers

4688 Let's Talk About Going to the Hospital
Rosen Publishing Group's PowerKids Press
29 E 21st Street
New York, NY 10010

212-777-3017
800-237-9932
Fax: 888-436-4643
e-mail: rosenpub@tribeca.ios.com
www.powerkidspress.com

If a child has to check into the hospital, chances are he or she is already upset about being ill. Knowing how a hospital functions and what the procedures are, such as when family members can visit, will help in what is already a stressful situation. Grades K-5.

24 pages
ISBN: 0-823950-36-0

DESCRIPTION

4689 MUSCULAR DYSTROPHIES

Synonyms: Duchenne muscular dystrophy, Becker muscular dystrophy, Landouzy-Dejerine disease

Involves the following Biologic System(s):

Neurologic Disorders, Orthopedic and Muscle Disorders

Muscular dystrophies are a group of inherited neuromuscular disorders characterized by the progressive weakness and degeneration of muscles without accompanying nerve tissue involvement. Each of these disorders is different from the others with respect to its age of onset, clinical manifestations, severity, course, and underlying genetic defect.

Duchenne muscular dystrophy, the most common of these disorders, is transmitted as an X-linked recessive trait and, as such, is fully expressed in boys; however, on rare occasions, girls who are carriers of the disease gene may exhibit mild symptoms. The incidence rate for this disorder is about one out of every 3,600 newborn boys. Although some affected infants may exhibit signs of diminished muscle tone such as poor head control, most boys do not develop symptoms until three to seven years of age. Early symptoms may include weakness in the pelvic girdle area that may be manifested by an unusual method of moving from the supine position to the standing position (Gowers' sign). In addition, boys with this disorder may develop a waddling manner of walking (Trendelenburg gait), be prone to stumbling and falling, or having difficulty climbing stairs and standing up from a sitting position. As the disease progresses, muscles around the joints may contract resulting in the inability to fully extend the knees and elbows. In addition, the spine may develop a side-to-side curve (scoliosis) and muscles, especially of the calves, become bulky due to the enlargement (hypertrophy) of the muscle fibers, the infiltration of fat into the muscles, and the increase of connective tissue protein (collagen) in the muscles. Other findings include involvement of the heart muscle (cardiomyopathy) and intellectual impairment ranging from learning disabilities to mental retardation. Most boys with Duchenne muscular dystrophy are able to walk until the age of 10 or 12 years, at which time they may be confined to a wheelchair. Life-threatening complications such as pneumonia, respiratory failure, and congestive heart failure often occur during late adolescence or early adulthood. This disorder is believed to result from the deficiency of the essential muscle protein dystrophin. The gene for Duchenne muscular dystrophy is located on the short arm of the X chromosome (Xp21).

Duchenne muscular dystrophy is initially diagnosed through evaluation of physical findings and through tests that show increased blood levels of the enzyme creatinine kinase. Additional diagnostic screening may include the use of an electrical muscle function test called electromyography or EMG. Confirmation, however, must be determined through microscopic examination of a muscle tissue sample (biopsy). Treatment is symptomatic and supportive. For example, nutritional vigilance and immunizations against flu and other childhood diseases may help to avoid or postpone complications. The administration of digitalis medications may help to alleviate certain heart-related complications. Some children may benefit from physical therapy, exercise, or surgical intervention to aid in walking.

Becker muscular dystrophy results in symptoms similar to those of Duchenne muscular dystrophy; however, these symptoms are usually less severe, do not appear until about the age of 10 years, and follow a long course. Patients usually remain ambulatory, and most survive into their 30s and 40s. The gene for Becker muscular dystrophy is also located on the short arm of the X chromosome (Xp21); however, the essential muscle protein dystrophin is defective and dysfunctional rather than deficient.

Less common forms of muscular dystrophy include facioscapulohumeral muscular dystrophy (Landouzy-Dejerine disease), limb-girdle muscular dystrophy, and others. Facioscapulohumeral muscular dystrophy, which is an autosomal dominant disorder occurring in both males and females, is characterized by facial and shoulder muscle weakness and sometimes weakness in the lower legs. This is a relatively mild disease that usually occurs between seven years of age and early or mid-adulthood. The gene for this disorder is located on the long arm of chromosome 4 (4q35). Limb-girdle muscular dystrophy is usually transmitted as an autosomal recessive trait, although autosomal dominant inheritance has also been documented. This disorder usually occurs in late childhood or early adulthood and is characterized by the progressive weakness and degeneration of the muscles of the hips and shoulders. Treatment for these types of muscular dystrophy is symptomatic and supportive.

See also **General Resources** on page 917

National Associations & Support Groups

4690 Duchenne Parent Project Muscular Dystrophy
1012 N University Boulevard
Middletown, OH 45042

513-424-0696
800-714-5437
Fax: 513-425-9907
e-mail: pat@parentprojectmd.org
www.parentprojectmd.org

Parent Project Muscular Dystrophy is a not-for-profit organization founded in 1994 by parents of children with Duchenne and Becker muscular dystrophy. Today, the focus is on areas such as; seeking to ensure that all families, caregivers, health care professionals and others have access to state-of-the-art information about treatment and care options for children with Duchenne and Becker MD, and to ensure that the voices of people with and affected by Duchenne and Becker are heard.

Pat Furlong, Founding President/CEO
Kimberly Galbraith, Executive VP

4691 Facioscapulohumeral Dystrophy Society
3 Westwood Road
Lexington, MA 02420

781-860-0501
Fax: 781-860-0599
e-mail: solvefshd@fshsociety.org
www.fshsociety.org

Daniel Paul Perez, President/CEO
Carol A Perez, Executive Director

4692 Muscular Dystrophy Association
3300 E Sunrise Drive
Tucson, AZ 85718

520-529-2000
800-344-4863
Fax: 520-529-5300
e-mail: mda@mdausa.org
www.mdausa.org

Voluntary health agency aimed at conquering nueromuscular diseases that affect more than 1,000,000 Americans. The diseases in MDA's program include nine forms of muscular dystrophy, amyotrophic lateral sclerosis (Lou Gehrig's disease), spinal muscular atrophy, Charcot-Marie-Tooth disease, and other neuromuscular conditions. With over 200 offices across the country, MDA conducts research, medical and community services, clinics, support groups, summer camps for youngsters and much more.

Gerald C Weinberg, President/CEO
Bob Mackle, Director Public Information

4693 Muscular Dystrophy Family Foundation
3951 N Meridian Street, Suite 100
Indianapolis, IN 46208

317-923-6333
800-544-1213
Fax: 317-923-6334
e-mail: mdff@mdff.org
www.mdff.org

Provides adaptive equipment and emotional support to individuals and families affected by one of the over forty neuromuscular diseases. Established in 1958, some of the euipment provided includes: hospital beds, wheelchairs, ramps, communication devices, and lifts.

Fred Shirley, President
Hazel M Walker, Vice President

4694 Parent to Parent Support for Muscular Dystrophy
Haiser Permanente Hospital
2025 Morse Avenue, Conference Room 3
Sacremento, CA 95825

916-863-8936
e-mail: darkrose@2xtreme.net
www.kaiserpermanente.org

A nonprofit organization whose goal is to provide compassionate support for families living with Muscular Dystrophy.

Craig Strunk, Contact
Marilyn Strunk

4695 Reflex Sympathetic Dystrophy Syndrome Association
PO Box 502
Milford, CT 06460

203-877-3790
877-662-7737
Fax: 203-882-8362
e-mail: info@rsds.org
www.rsds.org

The Reflex Sympathetic Dystrophy Syndrome Association was founded in 1984 to promote public and professional awareness of Reflex Sympathetic Dystrophy Syndrome, also known as Complex Regional Pain Syndrome. Educates those afflicted with this syndrome, their family, friends, insurance and healthcare providers, on the disabling pain the syndrome causes.

James E Tyrrell Jr. Esquire, Chairman of the Board
Paul R. Charlesworth, President

Research Centers

Minnesota

4696 Mayo Clinic and Foundation
200 First Street S.W.
Rochester, MN 55905

507-284-2511
800-323-2688
Fax: 507-284-0161
www.mayo.edu

Neuromuscular clinical research center with a primary research interest in neuropathies.

Denis Cortese M.D., CEO

New York

4697 Columbia Presbyterian Medical Center
Neurology Institute of NY/Research Center
710 W 168th Street
New York, NY 10032

212-305-2700
e-mail: alscenter@columbia.edu
www.nyp.org

Neuromuscular clinical research center.

Marc C Patterson
D Suzi Windemuth, Administrator/Executive Director

4698 Columbia University Clinical Research Center for Muscular Dystrophy
College of Physicians & Surgeons
630 W 168th Street
New York, NY 10032

212-305-1319
Fax: 212-305-3986

Salvatore DiMauro, Co-Director

4699 NYU Rusk Institute
Jerry Lewis Neuromuscular Disease Center
400 E 34th Street,
New York, NY 10016

212-263-6350
Fax: 212-263-5499
www.med.nyu.edu/rusk/services/outpatient/

Focuses on Muscular Dystrophy and related bone disorders.

Jeffrey Cohen MD, Director
Marilyn Shoo, Pediatrics Director

Ohio

4700 Parent Project for Muscular Dystrophy Research
1012 N University Boulevard
Middletown, OH 45042

513-424-0696
800-714-5437
Fax: 513-425-9907
www.parentprojectmd.org

Organization of families around the world who have children diagnosed with DMD/BMD. The goal is to invest significant amounts of money raised into medical research with clinical application.

Pat Furlong, Founding President & CEO
Kimberly Galberaith, Executive Vice President

Pennsylvania

4701 Penn Neurological Institute
Hospital of the University of Pennsylvania
3400 Spruce Street, 2nd Fl
Philadelphia, PA 19104

800-789-7366
http://pennhealth.com/neuro

Research program centering its efforts on finding better ways to prevent and treat neuromuscular disorders.

Mark J Brown MD, Director Neuromuscular Diseases

Texas

4702 Baylor College of Medicine
Neuromuscular Disease Research
6501 Fannin Street, NB302
Houston, TX 77030

713-798-5971
e-mail: neurons@bcm.tmc.edu
www.bcm.edu/neurology/research/

Offers research into biochemistry, molecular genetics and neuromuscular disorders.

Dennis Landis M.D., Professor And Chair
Michael Vincent Abene M.D., Assistant Professor

Utah

4703 University of Utah
Eccles Institute of Human Genetics
15 N 2030 E, Room 2100
Salt Lake City, UT 84112

801-581-4422
www.genetics.utah.edu

John F Atkins PhD, Research Professor
Mario R. Capecchi Ph.D, Distinguished Professor & Co-Chair

Audio Video

4704 Muscular Dystrophy
Films for Humanities/Films Media Group
PO Box 2053
Princeton, NJ 08543

800-257-5126
Fax: 609-671-0266
e-mail: custserv@filsmediagroup.comm
www.films.com

Muscular Dystrophy attacks muscles, so that people lose the ability to walk, talk, and in some cases, to breath. About two thirds of those affected are children, but symptoms can appear any time between birth and adolescence. This video looks at how people deal with a disease that has no cure. A young boy, a six year old girl, and a young mother are managing their disease and show us the medical interventions used to help them live more fully.

1990 VHS/DVD
ISBN: 1-421336-46-4

Web Sites

4705 Muscular Dystrophy Association
www.mda.org; www.mdausa.org

Information regarding muscular dystrophy.

4706 Muscular Dystrophy Family Foundation
www.mdff.org

Provides adaptive equipment and emotional support to individuals and families affected by one of the over forty neuromuscular diseases. Established in 1958, some of the euipment provided includes: hospital beds, wheelchairs, ramps, communication devices, and lifts.

4707 Parent Project Muscular Dystrophy
www.parentprojectmd.org

The Parent Project Muscular Dystrophy moblizes people in the United States and worldwide in collaborative effort to enable people with Duchenne and becker muscular dystrophy to survive, thrive and fully participate within their families and communities into adulthood and beyond.

Book Publishers

4708 Clinician's View of Neuromuscular Diseases

Micheal H. Brooke, author

Williams & Wilkins
351 W Camden Street
Baltimore, MD 21201

410-528-4000
800-638-3030

Second edition.

1986 388 pages
ISBN: 0-683010-64-6

4709 Journey of Love: Parent's Guide to Duchenne Muscular Dystrophy
Muscular Dystrophy Association
3300 E Sunrise Drive
Tucson, AZ 85718

520-529-2000
800-572-1717
Fax: 520-529-5300
e-mail: publications@mdausa.org
www.mdausa.org/publications/journey/

Complete guide for parents with children diagnosed with DMD. Information includes explanation of the disease, treatments, research, services provided by MDA, guides to finding assistance and more. Available in paperback and online.

170 pages

Carol Sowell, Director Publications

4710 Let's Talk About Going to the Hospital
Rosen Publishing Group's PowerKids Press
29 E 21st Street
New York, NY 10010

212-777-3017
800-237-9932
Fax: 888-436-4643
e-mail: rosenpub@tribeca.ios.com
www.powerkidspress.com

If a child has to check into the hospital, chances are he or she is already upset about being ill. Knowing how a hospital functions and what the procedures are, such as when family members can visit, will help in what is already a stressful situation. Grades K-5.

24 pages
ISBN: 0-823950-36-0

4711 Muscular Dystrophy
Franklin Watts
90 Old Sherman Turnpike
Danbury, CT 06816

203-797-3500
Fax: 203-797-3197
www.grolier.com

Discusses the nature of muscular dystrophy, causes, treatments and the latest research into treatments and cures.

112 pages Grades 7-12
ISBN: 0-531125-40-8

4712 Muscular Dystrophy (A Venture Book)
James A. Corrick, author

Franklin Watts
90 Old Sherman Turnpike
Danbury, CT 06816

203-797-3500
Fax: 203-797-3197
www.grolier.com

1992 96 pages
ISBN: 0-531125-40-8

4713 Muscular Dystrophy and Allied Diseases: Im pacts on Patients, Family, and Staff
Leon I Charash, author

Center for Thanatology Research & Education
391 Atlantic Avenue
Brooklyn, NY 11217

718-858-3026
Fax: 718-852-1846
e-mail: thanatology@pipeline.com
www.thanatology.org

An Internet best-seller, it covers Duchenne Muscular Dystrophy, psychosocial aspects, anticipatory grief of parents, education issues, etc.

1988 90 pages Paper
ISBN: 0-930194-38-1

4714 Muscular Dystrophy and Other Neuromuscular Diseases
Haworth Press
10 Alice Street
Binghamton, NY 13904

800-429-6784
e-mail: getinfo@haworthpress.com
www.haworthpress.com

A thoughtful book from professionals who assist persons afflicted with neuromuscular disorders to help them and their families adapt to lifestyle changes accompanying the onset of these disorders.

1991 250 pages Hardcover
ISBN: 1-560240-77-6

4715 My Life-Melinda's Story
Melinda Lawrence, author

Children's Hospice International
901 N Pitt Street, Suite 230
Alexandria, VA 22314

703-684-0330
800-242-4453
Fax: 703-684-0226
www.chionline.org/publications

Written by Melinda, a child with Muscular Dystrophy. This heartwarming story teaches children and their families how to cope with the illness.

ISBN: 0-317618-38-5

4716 Physical Medicine and Rehab Advances in The Rehab of Neuromuscular Diseases
W. M. Fowler, author

Hanley & Belfus
210 S 13th Street
Philadelphia, PA 19107

212-546-4995
www.hanleyandbelfus.com

167 pages Vol. 2, Num. 4
ISBN: 0-932883-70-2

4717 Precious Time: Children Living with Muscular Dystrophy
Thomas Bergman, author

Gareth Stevens Publishing
330 W Olive Street, Suite 100
Milwaukee, WI 53212

414-332-3520
800-542-2595
Fax: 414-332-3567
www.garethstevens.com

A leading publisher of educational books and high-quality fiction for children ages 4-16.

ISBN: 0-836815-97-1

4718 Realities in Coping with Progressive Neuromuscular Diseases
Charles C. Thomas
PO Box 15715
Philadelphia, PA 19103

215-561-2786
Fax: 215-561-0191
e-mail: mailbox@charlespresspub.com
www.charlespresspub.com

248 pages Hardcover
ISBN: 0-914783-20-3

4719 Travis:I Got Lots of Neat Stuff-Children L iving with Muscular Dystrophy
Kathy L Gordon, author

Muscular Dystrophy Association
3300 E Sunrise Drive
Tucson, AZ 85718

800-572-1717
www.mda.org/publications/travis/

Online

Magazines

4720 Quest Magazine
Muscular Dystrophy Association
3300 E Sunrise Drive
Tucson, AZ 85718

520-529-2000
800-344-4863
Fax: 520-529-5300
e-mail: publications@mdausa.org
www.mdausa.org

A national magazine that goes out to everyone registered with MDA, MDA clinics, reseacgers and subscribers. It presents news related to muscular dystrophy and other neuromuscular diseases including research, personal profiles, fund raising activities, and patient services.

125,000 circ Bimonthly

Bob Mackle, Director Public Information

Carol Sowell, Director Publications

Pamphlets

4721 101 Hints to Help-with-Ease for Patients w ith Neuromuscular Disease

Irwin M Siegel MD, author

Muscular Dystrophy Association
3300 E Sunrise Drive
Tucson, AZ 85718

520-529-2000
800-572-1717
Fax: 520-529-5300
e-mail: publications@mdausa.org
www.mdausa.org/publications/disbroch.html

A do-it-yourself guide to living with NMD's. Also available in Spanish and online.

30 pages Paperback

Carol Sowell, Director Publications

4722 Breathe Easy-Respiratory Care in Neuromusc ular Disorders

Muscular Dystrophy Association
3300 E Sunrise Drive
Tucson, AZ 85718

520-529-2000
800-572-1717
Fax: 520-529-5300
e-mail: publications@mdausa.org
www.mdausa.org

A guide to respiratory care for children with muscular dystrophy. Also available in Spanish and online.

Carol Sowell, Director Publications

4723 Conference on the Cause and Treatment of Facioscapulohumeral Muscular Dystrophy

National Inst. of Neurological Disorders/Stroke
31 Center Drive, MSC 2540, Building 31, Room 8A06
Bethesda, MD 20892

301-496-5751
800-352-9424

4724 Congressional Testimony on Muscular Dystrophy

National Inst. of Neurological Disorders/Stroke
31 Center Drive, MSC 2540, Building 31, Room 8A06
Bethesda, MD 20892

301-496-5751
800-352-9424
www.ninds.nig/gov

Testimony by Dr. Audrey Penn, Acting Director, NINDS, from February, 2001.

4725 Everybody's Different, Nobody's Perfect

Muscular Dystrophy Association
3300 E Sunrise Drive
Tucson, AZ 85718

520-529-2000
800-572-1717
Fax: 520-529-5300
www.mdausa.org/publications/nobody/

Explains how muscular dystrophy affects children and describes how people are different from each other in many ways. Emphasizing fun, friendship, and caring, this booklet is ideal for heightening awareness and encouraging understanding of persons with disabilities.

11 pages

Carol Sowell, Director Publications

4726 Facts About Duchenne and Becker Muscular Dystrophies

Muscular Dystrophy Association
3300 E Sunrise Drive
Tucson, AZ 85718

520-529-2000
800-572-1717
Fax: 520-529-5300
e-mail: publications@mdausa.org
www.mdausa.org

Describes in layman's terms Duchenne and Becker Muscular Dystrophies and addresses the most currently asked questions about these diseases, research, inheritance and treatments. Also available in Spanish or online.

23 pages

Carol Sowell, Director Publications

4727 Facts About Facioscapulohumeral Muscular Dystrophy

Muscular Dystrophy Association
3300 E Sunrise Drive
Tucson, AZ 85718

520-529-2000
800-572-1717
Fax: 520-529-5300
e-mail: publications@mdausa.org
www.mdausa.org/publications/

Explains facioscapulohumeral muscular dystrophy in layman's terms and answers commonly asked questions. Also available in Spanish.

20 pages Paperback

Carol Sowell, Director Publications

4728 Facts About Inflammatory Myopathies-DM, PM and IBM

Muscular Dystrophy Association
3300 E Sunrise Drive
Tucson, AZ 85718

520-529-2000
800-572-1717
Fax: 520-529-5300
e-mail: publications@mdausa.org
www.mdausa.org

Outlines these forms of inflammatory myopathy. Current approaches to treatment and MDA's efforts in continued research are described. Also available in Spanish.

Carol Sowell, Director Publications

4729 Facts About Limb-Girdle Muscular Dystrophy

Muscular Dystrophy Association
3300 E Sunrise Drive
Tucson, AZ 85718

520-529-2000
800-572-1717
Fax: 520-529-5300
e-mail: publications@mdausa.org
www.mdausa.org/publications

Overview of the various forms of LGMD encompassed by MDA's program. Addresses commonly asked questions and highlights MDA's research efforts aimed at finding the causes of and effective treatments for these disorders. Also available in Spanish.

19 pages

Carol Sowell, Director Publications

4730 Facts About Metabolic Diseases of Muscle

Muscular Dystrophy Association
3300 E Sunrise Drive
Tucson, AZ 85718

520-529-2000
800-572-1717
Fax: 520-529-5300
www.mda.org/publications/disbroch.html

Provides an overview of the 10 heritable metabolic diseases of muscle encompassed by MDA's program. Addresses commonly asked questions and highlights MDA's research efforts aimed at finding the causes of and effective treatments for these disorders.

Carol Sowell, Director Publications

4731 Facts About Mitochondrial Myopathies
Muscular Dystrophy Association
3300 E Sunrise Drive
Tucson, AZ 85718

520-529-2000
800-572-1717
Fax: 520-529-5300
e-mail: publications@mdausa.org
www.mdausa.org

Explains Mitochondrial myopathies in layman's terms and answers the most frequently asked questions about this disease. Also available in Spanish.

24 pages

Carol Sowell, Director Publications

4732 Facts About Muscular Dystrophy
Muscular Dystrophy Association
3300 E Sunrise Drive
Tucson, AZ 85718

520-529-2000
800-572-1717
Fax: 520-529-5300
www.mda.org/publications/fa-md-help.html

Answers many questions commonly asked about the forty-plus forms of the disease encompassed by MDA's program.

Carol Sowell, Director Publications

4733 Facts About Myasthenia Gravis
Muscular Dystrophy Association
3300 E Sunrise Drive
Tucson, AZ 85718

520-529-2000
800-572-1717
Fax: 520-529-5300
e-mail: publications@mdausa.org
www.mdausa.org/publications/fa-mg.html

Explains myasthenia gravis and Lambert-Eaton syndrome in layman's terms and answers the most frequently asked questions about these diseases. Also available in Spanish.

19 pages

Carol Sowell, Director Publications

4734 Facts About Myopathies
Muscular Dystrophy Association
3300 E Sunrise Drive
Tucson, AZ 85718

520-529-2000
800-572-1717
Fax: 520-529-5300
www.mdausa.org/publications/fa-myop.html

Describes the six inheritable myopathies encompassed by MDA's program, as well as current methods for diagnosing and managing these disorders.

Carol Sowell, Director Publications

4735 Facts About Myotonic Muscular Dystrophy
Muscular Dystrophy Association
3300 E Sunrise Drive
Tucson, AZ 85718

520-529-2000
800-572-1717
Fax: 520-529-5300
e-mail: publications@mdausa.org
www.mdausa.org

Basic knowledge about Myotonic Muscular Dystrophy, precautions, treatments, research and answers to most commonly asked questions. Also available in Spanish.

23 pages

Carol Sowell, Director Publications

4736 Facts About Plasmapheresis
Muscular Dystrophy Association
3300 E Sunrise Drive
Tucson, AZ 85718

520-529-2000
800-572-1717
Fax: 520-529-5300
e-mail: publications@mdausa.org
www.mdausa.org

Describes plasmapheresis, a plasma exchange procedure often utilized as a treatment for autoimmune diseases such as myasthenia gravis and Lambert-Eaton syndrome. Available in paperback or online.

Carol Sowell, Director Publications

4737 Facts About Rare Muscular Dystrophies
Muscular Dystrophy Association
3300 E Sunrise Drive
Tucson, AZ 85718

520-529-2000
800-572-1717
Fax: 520-529-5300
e-mail: publications@mdausa.org
www.mdausa.org

This brochure gives basic facts about four forms of muscular dystrophy (congenital, distal, Emery-Dreifuss and oculopharyngeal) and addresses commonly asked questions. Also available in Spanish.

28 pages

Carol Sowell, Director Publications

4738 Genetics and Neuromuscular Diseases
Muscular Dystrophy Association
3300 E Sunrise Drive
Tucson, AZ 85718

520-529-2000
800-572-1717
Fax: 520-529-5300
e-mail: publications@mdausa.org
www.mdausa.org

An up-to-date review of genetics information relating to neuromatic diseases, specifically describing what a genetic disorder is, genetic testing and counseling and inheritance patterns. Also available in Spanish and online.

19 pages

4739 Hey! I'm Here, Too!
Irwin M Siegel MD, author

Muscular Dystrophy Association
3300 E Sunrise Drive
Tucson, AZ 85718

520-529-2000
800-572-1717
Fax: 520-529-5300
www.mdausa.org/publications/hey/

Help for siblings of boys with Duchenne muscular dystrophy. Explores how they feel about themselves, their brothers, and their families. Also provides specific answers to some questions that siblings may wonder about. Has the option for an introduction for parents or for children.

Carol Sowell, Director Publications

4740 Learning to Live with Neuromuscular Disease: A Message To Parents
Muscular Dystrophy Association
3300 E Sunrise Drive
Tucson, AZ 85718

520-529-2000
800-572-1717
Fax: 520-529-5300
www.mdausa.org/publications/learning/

Intended to help parents and families cope with the knowledge that their child has a neuromuscular disease and with the impact the disease will have on everyday life.

Carol Sowell, Director Publications

4741 MDA Fact Sheet
Muscular Dystrophy Association
3300 E Sunrise Drive
Tucson, AZ 85718

520-529-2000
800-572-1717
Fax: 520-529-5300
www.mda.org/publications/

Outlines the history of MDA, the diseases included in MDA's program, and the services available through the Association.

4742 MDA Services for the Individual, Family and Community
Muscular Dystrophy Association
3300 E Sunrise Drive
Tucson, AZ 85718

520-529-2000
800-572-1717
Fax: 520-529-5300
www.mdausa.org/publications/mdasvcs/

Contains a list of the diseases covered by MDA as well as eligibility criteria for MDA's services program, a list of MDA-sponsored clinics nationwide, and the services available through these clinics.

4743 MDA Summer Camp
Muscular Dystrophy Association
3300 E Sunrise Drive
Tucson, AZ 85718

520-529-2000
800-572-1717
Fax: 520-529-5300
www.mdausa.org/clinics/camp.html

Highlights the activities of MDA summer camps for youngsters diagnosed with one of the more than 40 diseases in MDA's program. Shares camper and volunteer reactions. Also available in Spanish and online.

Carol Sowell, Director Publications

4744 Teacher's Guide to Neuromuscular Disease
Muscular Dystrophy Association
3300 E Sunrise Drive
Tucson, AZ 85718

520-529-2000
800-572-1717
Fax: 520-529-5300
www.mda.org/publications/tchrdmd/

A source of guidance and information to educators detailing neuromuscular disease, how it affects school participation, and ways that teachers can help meet the academic and social needs of students affected by the disorder.

4745 Workshop on Therapeutic Approaches for Duchenne Muscular Dystrophy
National Inst. of Neurological Disorders/Stroke
PO Box 5801
Bethesda, MD 20824

301-496-5751
800-352-9424
www.ninds.nih.gov/news_and_events/proceedings/

Camps

4746 MDA Summer Camp
Muscular Dystrophy Association
3300 E Sunrise Drive
Tucson, AZ 85718

520-529-2000
800-572-1717
Fax: 520-529-5300
e-mail: hjette@mdausa.org
www.mdausa.org/clinics/camp.html

Laura Cooke, Program Director

4747 Summer Camp for Children with Muscular Dystrophy
400 Vestavia Parkways
Birmingham, AL

205-823-8191

DESCRIPTION

4748 NARCOLEPSY

Synonyms: Gelineau's syndrome, Hypnolepsy, Paroxysmal sleep

Involves the following Biologic System(s):

Neurologic Disorders

Narcolepsy refers to a sleep disorder characterized by profound drowsiness during the day and sudden daytime attacks of sleep that may last from a few seconds to one or more hours. These episodes are sometimes accompanied by sudden loss of muscle tone (hypotonia) in response to emotional stimuli such as anger, fear, joy, or surprise (cataplexy). During a cataplectic episode, the patient remains conscious but is not able to speak or move. Some patients experience sleep paralysis and are unable to move at the onset of sleep or immediately upon waking.

Hypnagogic hallucinations are disquieting occurrences that take place at onset of sleep or, less commonly, upon awakening. During these hallucinations, patients may see or hear things that are not grounded in reality. In most cases, narcolepsy begins during adolescence or early adulthood and persists throughout the life of the affected individual. Sleep attacks associated with narcolepsy may occur at any time and may take place many times during the day; however, most individuals may be easily awakened.

Very few people with narcolepsy exhibit all the symptoms associated with this disorder and, occasionally, children and adults who do not have this disorder may experience similar signs and symptoms. For this reason, diagnosis of narcolepsy may necessitate confirmation by a sleep study which uses a procedure called electroencephalography (EEG), during which electrical brain-wave activity is recorded. An EEG may demonstrate an abnormal sleep pattern in which rapid eye movement or REM-type sleep occurs at the onset of sleep. There are no pathologic changes that occur in the brain. In individuals who do not have narcolepsy, REM sleep or periods of deep sleep normally follow nonrapid eye movement sleep (NREM). The cause of narcolepsy is unknown, but researchers think that, in some cases, it may be related to genetic influences as evidenced by the tendency of this disorder to occur within families. Approximately 200,000 people in the United States are affected by narcolepsy.

Treatment for narcolepsy may include regular napping and the administration of stimulant medications to control attacks of drowsiness and sleep, while antidepressant medications may help control episodes of cataplexy. Because this disorder may increase the risk of accidents, appropriate care and caution is advised in the performance of certain tasks or jobs. Other treatment is symptomatic and supportive.

See also **General Resources** on page 917

Government Agencies

4749 NIH/National Institute of Neurological Dis orders and Stroke (NINDS)
PO Box 5801
Bethesda, MD 20824

301-496-5751
800-352-9424
Fax: 301-496-0296
TTY: 301-468-5981
www.ninds.nih.gov

Works to reduce the burden of neurological disease by conducting, fostering, coordinating and guiding research on the causes, prevention, diagnosis and treatment of neurological disorders and stroke, while supporting basic research in related scientific areas.

Story C Landis Ph.D., Director
Audrey S Penn M.D., Deputy Director

National Associations & Support Groups

4750 American Academy of Sleep Medicine
1 Westbrook Corporate Center, Suite 920
Westchester, IL 60154

708-492-0930
Fax: 708-492-0943
e-mail: inquiries@aasmnet.org
www.aasmnet.org

Provides full diagnostic and treatment services to improve the quality of care for patients with all types of sleep disorders.

Michael H. Silber MBChB, President
Alejando D. Chediak, MD, President-Elect

4751 Association of Professional Sleep Societies
One Westbrook Corporate Center, Suite 920
Westchester, IL 60154

708-492-0930
Fax: 708-273-9354
e-mail: jmarkkanen@aasmnet.org
www.apss.org

A joint venture of the AASM and the Sleep Research Society. It works to facilitate the research and development of sleep disorders medically by encouraging exchange of information among members.

Jennifer Markkanen, Assistant Executive Director

4752 Florida Narcolepsy Association
2631 59th Street, PO Box 15352
Sarasota, FL 34277

941-355-5359
e-mail: sleepymc@yahoo.com
www.flnarcolepsy.org

The Association is a collective of people that helps or comforts others afflicted with Narcolepsy; as well as their families, doctors and friends.

Marion L Cikovic, Vice President

4753 Genetic Alliance
4301 Connecticut Avenue NW
Washington, DC 20008

202-966-5557
800-336-4363
Fax: 202-966-8553
e-mail: info@geneticalliance.org
www.geneticalliance.org

A coalition of voluntary genetic support groups, consumers and professionals addressing the needs of individuals and families affected by genetic disorders from a national perspective.

Sharon Terry, President/CEO

4754 NIH/National Institute of Neurological Dis orders and Stroke (NINDS)
PO Box 5801
Bethesda, MD 20824

301-496-9746
800-352-9424
Fax: 301-496-0296
TTY: 301-468-5981
www.ninds.nih.gov

Information and advocacy resources for families and professionals. Includes listings of organizations providing general tips and organizations focusing on more specific areas of concern to families and young adults who have disabilities.

Story C Landis Ph.D., Director
Walter J Koroshetz, Deputy Director

4755 Narcolepsy Institute
Montefiore Medical Center
111 E 210th Street
Bronx, NY 10467

718-920-6799
Fax: 718-654-9580
e-mail: mgoswami@narcolepsyinstitute.org
www.NarcolepsyInstitute.org

The Narcolepsy Institute, at Montefiore Medical Center, provides support services to individuals who have narcolepsy and their families in New York City. Free services are provided for people who narcolepsy qualifies as a developmental disability. The Institute provides screening, counseling, case management, crisis intervention, and advocacy for affected individuals and their families.

Dr Meeta Goswami, Phd, Director

4756 Narcolepsy Network
79 Main Street
North Kingstown, RI 02852

401-667-2523
888-292-6522
Fax: 401-633-6567
e-mail: narnet@narcolepsynetwork.org
www.narcolepsynetwok.org

Nonprofit organization that serves as a resource center, to assist support groups, to educate the public, to facilitate early diagnosis, to protect the rights of those with narcolepsy, and to encourage on-going scientific research in sleep medicine.

Dr Eveline Honig, Executive Director
Joyce Scannell, Office Assistant

4757 Narcolepsy and Cataplexy Foundation of America
445 E 68th Street, Suite 12L
New York, NY 10021

212-570-5506

Organization that provides information on narcolepsy and cataplexy. Also provides referrals, research and educational materials.

Helen Demitroff, Co-Founder & President

4758 National Narcolepsy Registry
1522 K Street NW, Suite 500
Washington, DC 20005

202-347-3471
Fax: 202-347-3472
e-mail: nsf@sleepfoundation.org
www.sleepfoundation.org

Organization that provides information to researchers that will further research, diagnosis and treatment of the disorder.

Richard Gelula, Board of Directors
Inne Barber, Board of Directors

4759 National Sleep Foundation
1522 K Street NW, Suite 500
Washington, DC 20005

202-347-3471
Fax: 202-347-3472
e-mail: nsf@sleepfoundation.org
www.sleepfoundation.org

Works to improve the quality of life for millions of Americans who suffer from sleep disorders, and to prevent the catastrophic accidents that are related to poor or disordered sleep through research, education and the dissemination of information towards the cause of the Narcolepsy Project. Seeks patients to aid new research project targeting the cause of the disorder.

Richard Gelula, CEO
Inne Barber, Board of Directors

State Agencies & Support Groups

Arizona

4760 Arizona Sleep Disorders Center
College of Medicine, Room 7303
Tucson, AZ 85724

520-626-6112
Fax: 520-626-4884

Stuart F Quan, Director

California

4761 Loma Linda University Sleep Disorders Cent er
11360 Mountain View Avenue, Hartford Bldg, Suite D
Loma Linda, CA 92354

909-558-6344
Fax: 909-558-6343
www.llu.edu/llumc/sleep/

Ralph Downwy III, PHD, Director
Philip M. Gold, Medical Director

4762 Stanford University Center for Narcolepsy
701B Welch Road, Room 143
Palo Alto, CA 94304

650-725-6517
Fax: 650-725-4913
e-mail: vdiaz1@stanford.edu
med.stanford.edu/school/psychiatry/narcolepsy/

Dr Emmanuel Mignot, Director

Connecticut

4763 Gaylord Hospital Sleep Medicine
Gaylord Farm Road, PO Box 400
Wallingford, CT 06492

203-284-2800
866-429-5673
Fax: 203-284-2700
TDD: 203-284-2700
e-mail: lcrispino@gaylord.org
www.gaylord.org

District of Columbia

4764 Georgetown University Sleep Disorders Center
3800 Reservoir Road NW
Washington, DC 20007

202-444-3610
Fax: 202-444-2920
e-mail: pmc2@gunet.georgetown.edu

Anne O'Donnell, Medical Director

Indiana

4765 Methodist Hospital Sleep Disorders Center
Rehab Centers
303 East 89th Street
Merrillville, IN 46410

219-736-4074
Fax: 219-736-4074

4766 MidWest Medical Center - Sleep Disorders Center
3232 N Meridian Street
Indianapolis, IN 46208

317-927-2100

Kenneth Wiesert, MD

4767 Sleep Disorder Center, St Elizabeth Medica l Center
1501 Hartford Street, PO Box 7501
Lafayette, IN 47903

766-423-6518
800-371-6011
Fax: 765-423-6525
www.glhsi.org

Dr Shahid M Ahsan, Medical Director

4768 Sleep Disorders Center-Good Samaritan Hospital
520 S 7th Street
Vincenne, IN 47591

812-885-3988
812-885-3660
e-mail: gsh@gshvin.org
www.gshvin.org/goodsamaritan/

4769 Sleep/Wake Disorders Center-Community Heal th Network
1500 N Ritter Avenue, Suite 451
Indianapolis, IN 46219

317-355-4275
Fax: 317-351-2785
e-mail: sleepcenter@ecommunity.com
www.ecommunity.com/sleep/

Marvin E Vollmer, MD, Co-Director

Maryland

4770 Johns Hopkins University Sleep Disorders Center
Francis Scott Key Medical Center
301 Bayview Boulevard
Baltimore, MD 21224

410-550-0571
Fax: 410-550-3374
e-mail: nschube1@jhmi.edu

Alan Schwartz, MD, Medical Director

Massachusetts

4771 Sleep Disorders Unit, Beth Israel Hospital
330 Brookline Avenue
Boston, MA 02215

617-667-3237
Fax: 617-975-5506
e-mail: patsite@bidmc.harvard.edu
www.bidmc.harvard.edu/sites/bidmc/home.asp

Jean K Matheson, MD

Michigan

4772 Center for Sleep Science at University of Michigan
University of Michigan Health System
2799 West Grand Boulevard Cfp3
Detroit, MI 48202

313-916-5176
Fax: 313-916-5150
e-mail: dhudgel1@hfhs.org
www.med.umich.edu/umsleepscience/

The center's main goal is to advance knowledge and understanding in these three areas: the physiology of normal sleep; the diagnosis of sleep disorders; and the treatment of sleep problems.

Ronald D Chervin MD, Director
Barbara T Felts MD, Pediatrics

Minnesota

4773 Center for Sleep Diagnostics
1455 St. Frances Ave.
Shakopee, MN 55379

952-403-3000
e-mail: askstfrancis@allina.com
www.stfrancis-shakopee.com/index.htm

Is dedicated to providing information, education, and support for all your sleep needs. Our goal is to be the center of sleep information and discussion on the internet.

Michael Biber, MD, Director

New Hampshire

4774 Dartmouth-Hitchcock Sleep Disorders Center
Dartmouth Medical Center
One Medical Center Drive
Lebanon, NH 03756

603-650-5000
Fax: 603-650-7820
www.dhmc.org

Michael Sateia, MD, Director
Glen Greenough MD, Fellowship Director

4775 Sleep/Wake Disorders Center, Hampstead Hospital
East Road
Hampstead, NH 03841

603-329-5311
Fax: 603-329-4746
www.hampsteadhospital.com

Kenneth M. Brown MD, Medical Director
Emad Milad MD, Child/Adolescent Psychiatrist

New Jersey

4776 Newark Sleep Disorders Center
Newark Beth Israel Medical Center
201 Lyons Avenue
Newark, NJ 07112

973-926-6668
Fax: 973-926-6672
e-mail: mkaretzky@sbhcs.com
www.njsleephelp.com

Dr Monroe S Karetzky, Director

New York

4777 Capital Regional Sleep-Wake Disorders Center
Saint Peter's Hospital & Albany Medical Center
Pine West Plaza #1
Albany, NY 12205

518-464-9999
Fax: 518-464-9650
e-mail: bwenzel@stpetershealthcare.org
www.stpetershealthcare.org

Aaron Sher, MD, Medical Director

4778 Center for Sleep Medicine of the Mount Sinai Medical Center
Box 1232, One Gustave L Levy Place
New York, NY 10029

212-241-5098
Fax: 212-987-5584
www.mountsinai.org

Gabriele Barthlen, MD
Carol Rosenbaum, MD

4779 Columbia Presbyterian Medical Center Sleep Disorders Center
161 Fort Washington Avenue
New York, NY 10032

212-305-1860
Fax: 212-305-5496
www.cpmcnet.columbai.edu/dept/sleep

Neil B Kavey, MD

4780 Saint Joseph's Hospital Health Center Sleep Laboratory
945 East Genesee Street Suite 300
Syracuse, NY 13210

315-475-3379
888-785-6371
www.sjhsyr.org/sjhhc/stj_patient_3.asp?id=269

Theodore M Pasinski, President

4781 Sleep Center, Community General Hospital
Broad Road
Syracuse, NY 13215

315-492-5877
www.chg.org/sleep.html

Robert Westlake, MD

4782 Sleep Disorders Center of Rochester, St. Mary's Hospital
2110 South Clinton Avenue
Rochester, NY 14618

585-442-4141
Fax: 585-442-6259
www.unityhealth.org

Robert H. Israel,MD
Margarita D. Zhavoronkova, MD

4783 Sleep Disorders Center of Western New York Millard Fillmore Hospital
3 Gates Circle
Buffalo, NY 14209

716-887-5337
Fax: 716-887-5332
e-mail: drifkin@kaleidahealth.org
www.kaleidahealth.org

Daniel Rifkin MD, Medical Director

4784 Sleep Disorders Center, University Hospital
MR 120A
Stony Brook, NY 11794

631-444-6654
Fax: 631-444-8821
e-mail: russell.rozensky@stonybrook.edu
www.hsc.stonybrook.edu/shtm/rcsleep

Wallace Mendelson, MD

4785 Sleep-Wake Disorders Center, Montefiore Sleep Disorders Center
111 E 210th Street
Bronx, NY 10583

718-920-4841
Fax: 718-798-4352
e-mail: thorpy@aecom.yu.edu
www.cloud9.net/~thorpy/mmc

Center that provides diagnostic and treatment services for children with sleep disorders, such as sleep apnea, narcolepsy, insomnia, daytime sleepiness, sleepwalking, or night terrors.

Michael J Thorpy, MD, Medical Director
Karen Balaban-Gil, MD

4786 Sleep-Wake Disorders Center, New York Presbyterian Hospital
Cornell Medical Center
21 Bloomingdale Road
White Plains, NY 10605

914-997-5751
800-694-7533
Fax: 914-682-6911
e-mail: mmoline@med.cornell.edu
www.cornellphysicians.com/sleepWake/

Provides outpatient diagnostic evaluation and treatment for adults and children with problems associated with sleeping and waking. More common pediatric sleep problems include complaints of difficulty falling asleep and staying asleep, snoring, sleep apnea, sleepwalking, sleep terrors, nightmares, excessive diffculty waking up, bedwetting, and narcolepsy. Many can be successfully treated in one or several visits although some may require an overnight or daytime sleep study.

Margaret Moline, PHD, Director

4787 Winthrop-University Hospital Sleep Disorders Center
222 Station Plaza North Suite 400
Mineola, NY 11501

516-663-3907
Fax: 516-663-4788
e-mail: mweinstein@winthrop
www.winthrop.org/departments/specialtycenters/?id=31

Michael D. Weinstein, MD, Medical Director

Ohio

4788 Bethesda Oak Hospital, Sleep Disorders Center
10475 Montgomery Rd. Ste 1-D
Cincinnati, OH 45242

513-745-1690
Fax: 513-745-1691
e-mail: michael_fletcher@trihealth.com

Milton Kramer, MD

4789 Center for Sleep & Wake Disorders, Miami Valley Hospital
Thirty Apple Sreet
Dayton, OH 45409

937-208-2515
Fax: 937-208-5685
e-mail: khuban@wor.rr.com
www.miamivalleyhospital.com/0406-sleep.htm

Mohammed M. Dallel, MD, Director

4790 Cleveland Clinic Foundation, Sleep Disorders Center
11203 Stokes Blvd
Cleveland, OH 44106

216-444-2200
Fax: 216-445-6205
e-mail: foldvan@ccf.org
www.clevelandclinic.org/neurology

Nancy Foldvary-Schaefer, DO, Medical Director

4791 Kettering Medical Center, Sleep Disorders Center
3535 Southern Boulevard
Kettering, OH 45429

937-723-5835
www.kmcnetwork.org/sleep/gv

Michael J. Valle, D.O. FACN, Medical Director

4792 NW Ohio Sleep Disorders Center
Toledo Hospital
2121 Hughes Drive Harris-McIntosh Tower 2nd Floor
Toledo, OH 43606

419-291-3879
Fax: 419-479-6954
e-mail: pam.lang@promedica.org

Frank O Horton, III, MD, Director

4793 Ohio Sleep Medicine Institute
4975 Bradenton Avenue
Dublin, OH 43017

614-766-0773
Fax: 614-766-2599
e-mail: betty@sleepmedicine.com
www.sleepmedicine.com

Helmut S. Schmidt, MD, Medical Director

4794 Ohio State University Hospitals, Sleep Disorders Center
410 W 10th Avenue
Columbus, OH 43210

614-257-2500
Fax: 614-257-2551
www.medicalcenter.osu.edu/index.cfm

Gregory Landholt, Director

4795 Saint Vincent Medical Center, Sleep Disorders Center
3829 Woodley Road Suite 1
Toledo, OH 43606

419-250-5702
Fax: 419-251-0574

Joseph Schaffer, PhD, Director

Pennsylvania

4796 Community Medical Center, Sleep Disorders Clinic
1800 Mulberry Street
Scranton, PA 18510

570-969-8931
www.cmchealthsys.org/sleep.html

John Goodnow, Director

4797 Crozer-Chester Medical Center
Sleep Disorders Center
Department of Neurology
Upland-Chester, PA 19013

610-447-2689

Calvin Stafford, MD, Director

4798 Geisinger Wyoming Valley Medical Center, Sleep Disorders Center
620 Baltimore Drive
Wilkes-Barre, PA 18711

570-820-6066
Fax: 570-826-7650
e-mail: lvender@geisinger.edu
www.geisinger.org

John W. McBurney, MD, Medical Director

4799 Lankenau Hospital, Sleep Disorders Center
100 Lancaster Avenue
Wynnewood, PA 19096

610-645-3400
Fax: 610-645-2291
e-mail: pressmanm@mlhs.org
www.mlhs.org

Donald D. Peterson, MD, Director

4800 Medical College of Pennsylvania, Sleep Disorders Center
3300 Henry Avenue
Philadelphia, PA 19129

215-842-6990

June M Fry, MD, PhD, Director

4801 Mercy Hospital of Johnstown, Sleep Disorders Center
1020 Franklin Street
Johnstown, PA 15905

814-533-1661

Richard Parcinski, Director

4802 Penn Center for Sleep Disorders, Hospital of the University of Pennsylvania
3400 Spruce Street, 11 Gates
Philadelphia, PA 19104

215-590-3703
Fax: 215-590-2632

Joanne Getsy, MD, Director

4803 Presbyterian-University Hospital, Pulmonary Sleep Evaluation Center
DeSoto at O'Hara Street
Pittsburgh, PA 15213

412-647-3475

Mark Sanders, MD, Director

4804 Thomas Jefferson University Sleep Disorders Center
Jefferson Medical College
1025 Walnut Street
Philadelphia, PA 19107

215-955-6980
Fax: 215-923-8219

Karl Doghramji, MD, Director

4805 Western Psychiatric Institute & Clinic, Sleep Evaluation Center
3811 O'Hara Street
Pittsburgh, PA 15213

412-624-2100
Fax: 412-246-5300

Charles F Reynolds, III, MD, Director

Rhode Island

4806 Sleep Disorders Center of Lifespan Hospitals
Rhode Island Hospital
593 Eddy Street Apc 701
Providence, RI 02903

401-431-5420
Fax: 404-431-5429
e-mail: millman@lifespan.org
www.lifespan.org/services/sleep/

Dr Judith Owens, Pediatrics Director
Dr Richard Millman, Center Director

Texas

4807 Sleep Disorders Center for Children
Children's Medical Center of Dallas
1935 Motor Street
Dallas, TX 75235

214-456-2793
Fax: 214-456-8740
e-mail: larry.brewer@childrens.com
www.childrens.com

Dr S K Naqvi, Medical Director
Dr John Herman PhD, Contact for Children

4808 Sleep Medicine Associates of Texas
5477 Glen Lakes Drive, Suite 100
Dallas, TX 75231

214-750-7776
Fax: 214-750-4621
www.sleepmed.com

Philip M Becker MD, President

4809 University of Texas Sleep/Wake Disorders Center
Southwestern Medical Center
5323 Harry Hines Boulevard
Dallas, TX 75235

214-648-3111
Fax: 214-648-3112

Studies sleep/wake disorders including insomnia, apnea and narcolepsy.

Howard Roffwrag, MD, Director

Research Centers

Illinois

4810 Center for Narcolepsy Research at the University of Illinois at Chicago
College of Nursing M/C 802
845 S Damen Avenue
Chicago, IL 60612

312-996-5176
Fax: 312-996-7008
e-mail: fmeyer@uic.edu
www.uic.edu/nursing/cnshr/index.html

David W. Carley, PhD, Director
James Herdegen, MD, Associate Professor

Iowa

4811 Mercy Sleep Laboratory
Mercy Medical Center
1111 6th Avenue
Des Moines, IA 50314

515-643-6374
Fax: 515-643-8905
e-mail: cmann@mercydesmoines.org
www.mercydesmoines.org

Sleep is an integral part of life, but it's not always a welcome or peaceful close to a busy day. Some people suffer almost unbearable torture as they toss and turn. Others find sleepiness an uncontrollable intruder. It's been estimated that 30 to 40 percent of the population suffers from a sleeping problem at some time in their lives. Mercy's Sleep Center helps patients with sleep problems.

Donald L. Burrows, MD, Medical Director

Maine

4812 Sleep Laboratory, Maine Medical Center
930 Congress Street
Portland, ME 04102

207-662-4535
Fax: 207-662-6005

George E Bokinsky, Jr, Medical Director

Maryland

4813 University of Maryland Medical Center
Pediatric Sleep Disorders Center
22 S Greene Street
Baltimore, MD 21201

410-328-8667
800-492-5538
TDD: 401-328-9600
www.umm.edu/pediatrics/sleep_disorders.htm

Carol J Blaisdell MD, Director

Ohio

4814 Tri-State Sleep Disorders Center Center for Research in Sleep Disorders
1275 E Kemper Road
Cincinnati, OH 45246

513-671-3101
800-838-4322
Fax: 513-671-4159
e-mail: web@tristatesleep.com
www.tristatesleep.com

Provides diagnostics and treatment services to thousands of people in Cincinnati and throughout the country at our state-of-the-art sleep clinic through cutting edge research efforts.

Dr Martin Scharf, Director
Dr. David Berkowitz

Texas

4815 Baylor Sleep Wellness Center
Baylor Clinic
6620 Main Street
Houston, TX 77030

713-798-2500
800-229-5671
www.bcm.edu/baylorclinic

A comprehensive program with a multidisciplinary approach to sleep disorders.

Sr Shyam Subramanian, Director
Dr Mary Rose, Clinical Psychologist

4816 University of Texas Medical Branch at Galveston, Clinical Research Center
301 University Boulevard
Galveston, TX 77555

409-772-1011
800-228-1841
Fax: 409-772-6216
e-mail: public.affairs@utmb.edu

Research focusing on sleep disorders including apnea and narcolepsy.

Charles A Stuart, Program Director

Audio Video

4817 Narcolepsy
Fanlight Productions
4196 Washington Street, Suite 2
Boston, MA 02131

617-469-4999
800-937-4113
Fax: 617-469-3379
e-mail: info@fanlight.com
www.fanlight.com

Presents the experiences of three individuals whose lives and relationships have been disrupted by narcolepsy, while offering solid, comprehensive scientific information about the disorder.

2000 25 Minutes VHS
ISBN: 1-572953-23-2

Ben Achtenberg, President
Anthony Sweeney, Marketing Director

4818 Narcolepsy: A Guide for Understanding, Dia gnosing & Treating Narcolepsy
National Sleep Foundation
1522 K Street NW, Suite 500
Washington, DC 20005

202-347-3471
www.sleepfoundation.org

A comprehensive PowerPoint™, 114 slide presentation to educate health care providers about narcolepsy.

4819 Narcolepsy: Evaluation and Treatment
American Academy of Sleep Medicine
1 Westbrook Corporate Center, Suite 920
Westchester, IL 60154

708-492-0930
Fax: 708-492-0943
www.aasmnet.org

A 97 slide presentation designed as a foundation for a teaching curriculum on the recognition and treatment of narcolepsy.

Web Sites

4820 Narcolepsy
www.narcolepsy.org

Narcolepsy Internet jumpstation.

4821 Online Mendelian Inheritance in Man
www.ncbi.nlm.nih.gov

This database is a catalog of human genes and genetic disorders.

4822 Sleep Disorders
http://talhost.net/sleep/narcolepsy.htm

Descriptions of certain sleep disorders and useful links.

4823 Talk About Sleep
www.talkaboutsleep.com

Sleep disorder information and resources.

Book Publishers

4824 Narcolepsy Primer
Montefiore Medical Center
111 E 210th Street
Bronx, NY 10467

718-920-6054
e-mail: info@montefiore.org

A guide for physicians, patients and their families on the affects, causes and prevention of narcolepsy.

4825 Psychosocial Aspects of Narcolepsy

Meeta Goswami, author

Haworth Press
10 Alice Street
Binghamton, NY 13904

800-234-1340
Fax: 800-875-1340
e-mail: info@omnigraphics.com
www.omnigraphics.com

Addresses the diagnosis, treatment and management of narcolepsy with particular emphasis on psychological and social aspects of care.

567 pages Hardcover
ISBN: 1-560242-22-1

4826 Sleep Disorders Sourcebook
Omnigraphics
PO Box 625
Holmes, PA 19043

800-234-1340
Fax: 800-875-1340
e-mail: info@omnigraphics.com
omnigraphics.com

Basic consumer health information about sleep and its disorders, including narcolepsy, insomnia, sleepwalking, sleep apnea, and restless leg syndrome.

567 pages 2nd edition
ISBN: 0-780807-43-0

4827 Sleep Disorders and Psychiatry

Daniel J Buysse MD, author

American Psychiatric Publishing
1000 Wilson Boulevard, Ste 1825
Arlington, VA 22209

703-907-7322
800-368-5777
Fax: 703-907-1091
e-mail: appi@psych.org
www.appi.org

Summarizes the major categories of sleep disorders including parasomnias and narcolepsy.

2005 256 pages Paperback
ISBN: 1-585622-29-0

Newsletters

4828 Eye Opener
American Narcolepsy Association
Po Box 26230
San Francisco, CA 94126

800-222-6085
Fax: 415-788-4795

Offers information on sleep disorders including a question and answer column for persons suffering from disorders.

Pamphlets

4829 Living with Narcolepsy
National Sleep Foundation
1522 K Street NW, Suite 500
Washington, DC 20005

202-347-3471
Fax: 202-347-3472
e-mail: nsf@sleepfoundation.org
www.sleepfoundation.org

For people with narcolepsy and their families; defines and describes narcolepsy, as well as the effects on education, social and family life.

packet of 25

4830 Narcolepsy
American Academy of Sleep Medicine
1 Westbrook Corporate Center, Suite 920
Westchester, IL 60154

708-492-0930
Fax: 708-482-0943
www.aasmnet.org

Describes the causes, symptoms and treatments of a disorder characterized by excessive sleepiness.

Lot of 50

Jerome Barrett, Executive Director

4831 When You Can't Sleep
Narcolepsy Network
10921 Reed Hartman Highway, Suite 119
Cincinnati, OH 45242

513-891-3522
Fax: 513-891-3836
e-mail: narnet@narcolepsynetwork.org
www.narcolepsynetwork.org

A primer on sleep basics, including getting enough sleep, why sleep is important, and sleep stealers. Plus a sleep quotient quiz.

DESCRIPTION

4832 NEONATAL HERPES SIMPLEX

Synonym: Congenital herpes

Involves the following Biologic System(s):

Infectious Disorders, Neonatal and Infant Disorders

Neonatal herpes simplex refers to an infection of the newborn caused by the herpes simplex virus (HSV) that is transmitted before birth from mother to fetus through the placenta, or more commonly, during birth as the baby passes through the birth canal. There are two strains of herpes simplex virus known as HSV-1 and HSV-2. Herpes simplex virus type 1 commonly causes infections of the skin and mucous membranes of the lips, mouth, and eyes, while type 2 typically causes genital herpes as well as approximately 75 percent of all neonatal herpes simplex infections.

Herpes simplex may be categorized as an initial (primary) infection or a recurrent infection. After an initial infection, the virus becomes inactive or latent; however, the virus may be reactivated by many different factors including stress, sun exposure, suppression of the immune system, and certain foods or drugs. Mothers with a primary genital herpes simplex virus infection have an approximately 45 percent chance of transmitting HSV-2 to their infants, while risk of transmission from a recurrent infection is less than five percent. In addition, newborns are at risk for HSV-1 transmission through such direct contact as kissing near the eyes or mouth by someone with a cold sore.

Symptoms of HSV infection transmitted through contact with infectious secretions during the birthing process may occur anywhere from one to four weeks after birth and may sometimes commence with the appearance of small, fluid-filled blisters (vesicles) on the skin or inflammation of the front part of the eyeball (cornea) and the delicate mucous membranes (conjunctiva) that line the inside of the eyelids and the whites of the eyes (keratoconjunctivitis). Other findings may include fever, drowsiness, loss of muscle tone, irritability, seizures, and inflammation of the liver (hepatitis) and brain (encephalitis), as well as other severe irregularities. If left untreated, HSV infection may cause potentially life-threatening complications. Some infants may have no skin involvement but manifest such symptoms as fluctuating temperature, listlessness, poor sucking, chills, shaking, nausea, vomiting, and diarrhea.

Transmission of the herpes simplex virus through the placenta is a rare but potentially life-threatening occurrence.

This type of infection usually affects the skin, eyes, and central nervous system and is characterized by blister-type rashes and scarring, abnormally small eyes (microphthalmia) and other eye abnormalities, an abnormally small head (microcephaly), and brain and spinal cord irregularities. Some infants may also have hepatitis or lung involvement.

Prevention of neonatal herpes simplex infection may include delivery by Cesarean section, especially if the mother has a primary genital herpes infection. Treatment is directed toward early diagnosis and intervention. Such therapy may include the intravenous administration of antiviral drugs such as acyclovir in conjunction with regular testing to preclude possible associated toxic side effects related to kidney dysfunction. Eye involvement may indicate the application of antiviral ointments or drops directly into the eyes. Other treatment is symptomatic and supportive.

See also **General Resources** on page 917

Government Agencies

4833 NIH/National Institute of Allergy and Infectious Diseases

6610 Rockledge Drive, MSC 6612
Bethesda, MD 20892

301-496-5717
Fax: 301-402-3573
TDD: 800-877-8339
www.niaid.nih.gov

Conducts and supports basic and applied research to better understand, treat, and ultimately prevent infectious, immunologic, and allergic diseases.

Anthony S Fauci MD, Director

National Associations & Support Groups

4834 American Social Health Association

PO Box 13827
Research Triangle Park, NC 27709

919-361-8400
800-227-8922
Fax: 919-361-8425
e-mail: info@ashastd.org
www.ashastd.org

The American Social Health Association is dedicated to improving the health of individuals, families, and communities, with a focus on preventing sexually transmitted diseases and their harmful consequences.

Lynn Barclay, President/CEO

4835 National Health Information Center

PO Box 1133
Washington, DC 20013

301-565-4137
800-336-4797
Fax: 301-984-4256
e-mail: info@nhif.org
www.nhic.org

The National Health Information Center can put you in touch with organizations that can answer your health-related questions. The National Health Information Center can provide you with names and addresses of appropriate organizations.

Libraries & Resource Centers

4836 Herpes Resource Center
American Social Health Association
PO Box 13827
Research Triangle Park, NC 27709

919-361-8488
800-227-8922
www.ahsastd.org/herpes/herpes_overview.cfm

Web Sites

4837 American Social Health Association
www.ashastd.org

Dedicated to improving the health of individuals, families, and communities, with a focus on preventing sexually transmitted diseases and their harmful consequences.

4838 Child Health Research Project
www.childhealthresearch.org

To help achieve USAID's strategic objectives to reduce childhood mortality and morbidity, the Child Health Research Project (CHR) conducts applied research in: diarrheal and respiratory diseases, infectious diseases, neonatal health, and malnutrition.

4839 Health Research Project (HaRP)
www.harpnet.org

A program by USAID, the project strives to improve the health status of infants, children, mothers and families through the development and research of new tools, technologies, policies and approaches.

4840 HerpeSite
www.herpesite.org

Provides online personal empowerment and support; a compendium of information outlining aspects and issues relating to Herpes Simplex Virus.

4841 Herpes.com
www.herpes.com

Purpose of this website is to fill the desperate need for herpes education, make it easier to manage herpes, inform people of ways to limit herpes reoccurrences, to inform people of the beneficial products for herpes sufferers, to show the relationship between good health and herpes, to provide an opportunity for herpes sufferers to share their personal experiences and to provide communication via our live chat.

4842 Infectious Diseases in Children
http://idinchildren.com

A leading provider of healthcare information, educational programs, and meeting and exhibit management services worldwide.

4843 International Herpes Alliance
www.herpesalliance.org

4844 Virtual Pediatric Hospital
www.virtualpediatrichospital.org

A digital library of pediatric informaion dedicated to helping patients find the highest quality medical information in the world today. Offers patients the tools necessary to make informed treatment decisions within the short time lines dictated by their illness or disease.

Book Publishers

4845 Understanding Herpes

Dr Lawrence R Stanberg, author

University Press of Mississippi
3825 Ridgewood Road
Jackson, MS 39211

601-432-6205
800-737-7788
Fax: 601-432-6217
e-mail: press@ihl.state.ms.us
www.upress.state.ms.us

A most informative overview of herpes written for the general reader.

120 pages Cloth
ISBN: 1-578060-40-0

Seetha Srinivasan, Director
Cynthia Foster, Administrative Assistant

DESCRIPTION

4846 NEONATAL JAUNDICE

Synonym: Icterus neonatorum

Involves the following Biologic System(s):

Neonatal and Infant Disorders

Neonatal jaundice refers to a condition of the newborn in which high blood levels of the reddish-orange bile pigment bilirubin cause a yellowing of the skin, eyes, and mucous membranes. Bilirubin is derived from the breakdown of the protein, hemoglobin, in red blood cells. Neonatal jaundice may be the result of many different factors including metabolic disturbances or deficiencies; certain genetic disorders; conditions associated with an increased rate of red blood cell destruction (hemolysis); conditions that affect liver function; and certain types of infections.

Blood levels of bilirubin may be somewhat elevated after the first day of life, usually peak by the fourth day, and fall to normal levels by the end of the first week. This temporary rise, frequently accompanied by jaundice, results from the increased destruction of fetal red blood cells and the inability of a still-developing metabolic mechanism to efficiently eliminate bile from the body. In addition, an enzyme present in the intestines of newborns may convert bilirubin to a form that allows it to be reabsorbed into the blood, resulting in even higher bilirubin blood levels. Premature infants are particularly at risk for jaundice. If no other underlying cause is responsible, jaundice typically resolves spontaneously along with bilirubin level stabilization.

The appearance of jaundice in a newborn is carefully evaluated for underlying causes. Factors that may indicate the presence of an underlying disorder may include jaundice within the first 24 hours of life; a higher and faster-than-expected rise in bilirubin levels; birth defects, especially those that affect the liver such as biliary atresia; a family history of diseases that cause the early destruction of red blood cells such as hemolytic disease of the newborn; or rare disorders associated with hyperbilirubinemia (e.g., Crigler-Najjar syndrome, transient familial neonatal hyperbilirubinemia, etc.). Other suspect findings may include an enlarged liver (hepatomegaly), enlarged spleen (splenomegaly), lethargy, unusual paleness, difficulty in feeding, vomiting, or excessive weight loss.

Treatment of neonatal jaundice depends upon the underlying cause. Some infants with jaundice associated with breast-feeding may benefit from phototherapy. During this treatment, which is carefully monitored, the infant's bare skin is exposed to high intensity fluorescent lights that speed up the excretion and elimination of bilirubin in the skin. Other treatment is symptomatic and supportive.

See also **General Resources** on page 917

Government Agencies

4847 NIH/National Institute of Child Health and Human Development

31 Center Drive, Building 31
Bethesda, MD 20892

301-496-5133
Fax: 301-496-1104
www.nichd.nih.gov

Established in 1962 by congress, today the institute conducts and supports research on topics related to the health of children, adults, families and populations. Some of these topics include: developmental disabilities, growth and development, infant death, reproductive health and birth defects.

Nancy D Wirth, Director
Lisa Kaeser, Program & Public Liaison

National Associations & Support Groups

4848 American College of Gastroenterology

PO Box 342260
Bethesda, MD 20827

301-263-9000
Fax: 301-263-9025
www.acg.gi.org

Founded to advance the scientific study and medical practice of diseases of the gastrointestinal (GI) tract.

Jack A DiPalma, President
Amy E Foxx-Orenstein, VP

4849 American Liver Foundation

75 Maiden Lane, Suite 603
New York, NY 10038

212-668-1000
800-465-4837
Fax: 212-483-8179
e-mail: info@liverfoundation.org
www.liverfoundation.org

Nonprofit, national, voluntary health organization dedicated to the prevention, treatment and cure of hepatitis and other liver diseases through research, education, and advocacy on behalf of those affected by or at risk of liver disease.

Frederick G Thompson, President/CEO
Marie P Bresnahan, VP Programs

4850 Digestive Disease National Coalition

507 Capitol Court NE, Suite 200
Washington, DC 20002

202-544-7497
Fax: 202-546-7105
www.ddnc.org

Advocacy organization comprised of 22 voluntary and professional societies concerned with the many diseases of the digestive tract and liver.

Nancy Norton, Chairperson
Dr. Maurice Cerulli, President

4851 Greater Los Angeles Chapter
American Liver Foundation
5777 W Century Boulevard, Ste 865
Los Angeles, CA 90045

310-670-4624
Fax: 310-670-4672
e-mail: cshort@liverfoundation.org
www.liverfoundation.org/greaterla

A national organization that promotes research and cures for hepatitis and other liver diseases.

Cynthia Short, Executive Director

4852 International Foundation for Functional Gastrointestinal Disorders
PO Box 170864
Milwaukee, WI 53217

414-964-1799
888-964-2001
Fax: 414-964-7176
e-mail: iffgd@iffgd.org
www.iffgd.org

Nonprofit education and research organization founded in 1991. IFFGD addresses the issues surrounding life with gastrointestinal (GI) functional and mobility disorders and increases the awareness about these disorders among the general public, researchers and the clinical care community.

Nancy J Norton, Founder
William Norton, VP

4853 March of Dimes Birth Defects Foundation
1275 Mamaroneck Avenue
White Plains, NY 10605

914-428-7100
888-663-4637
Fax: 914-428-8203
e-mail: resourcecenter@modimes.org
www.marchofdimes.com

Partnership of volunteers and professionals dedicates to improving the health of babies by preventing birth defects and infant mortality. Over 100 chapters are located across the country and can be located through the National Office.

Dr Jennifer Howse, President

4854 North American Society for Pediatric Gastroenterology/Hepatology/Nutrition
PO Box 6
Flourtown, PA 19031

215-233-0808
Fax: 215-233-3918
e-mail: naspghan@naspghan.org
www.naspghan.org

Strives to improve the care of infants, children and adolescents with digestive disorders by promoting advances in clinical care of children with chronic abdominal pain, diarrhea, constipation, vomiting, bleeding from the GI tract, inflammatory bowel disease, liver diseases, diseases of the pancreas, poor weight gain and nutritional problems.

Philip Sherman, President
Margaret K Stallings, Executive Director

Libraries & Resource Centers

4855 National Digestive Diseases Information Clearinghouse
2 Information Way
Bethesda, MD 20892

301-654-3810
800-891-5389
Fax: 703-738-4929
e-mail: nddic@info.niddk.nih.gov
www.digestive.niddk.nih.gov

The National Institute of Diabetes and Digestive and Kidney Diseases conducts and supports research on many of the most serious diseases affecting public health. The Institute supports much of the clinical research on the diseases of internal medicine and related subspecialty fields as well as many basic science disciplines.

Kathy Kranzfelder, Project Officer

Web Sites

4856 American Liver Foundation
www.liverfoundation.org

Nonprofit, national, voluntary health organization dedicated to the prevention, treatment and cure of hepatitis and other liver diseases through research, education, and advocacy on behalf of those affected by or at risk of liver disease.

4857 Cliniweb

One of the original sites for health and bimedical information on the web.

4858 Liver 411
www.liver411.com

4859 National Digestive Diseases Information Clearinghouse
www.digestive.niddk.nih.gov

The National Institute of Diabetes and Digestive and Kidney Diseases conducts and supports research on many of the most serious diseases affecting public health. The Institute supports much of the clinical research on the diseases of internal medicine and related subspecialty fields as well as many basic science disciplines.

4860 Online Mendelian Inheritance in Man
www.ncbi.nlm.nih.gov

This database is a catalog of human genes and genetic disorders.

Journals

4861 Journal of Pediatric Gastroenterology and Nutrition

NASPGHAN, author

Lippincott Williams & Wilkins
530 Walnut Street
Philadelphia, PA 19106

215-521-8300
Fax: 215-521-8902
www.lww.com

Publication of the North American Society for Pediatric Gastroenterolgy, Hepatology and Nutrition, which strives to improve the care of infants, children and adolescents with digestive disorders by promoting advances in clinical care of children with chronic abdominal pain, diarrhea, constipation, vomiting, bleeding from the GI tract, inflammatory bowel disease, liver diseases, diseases of the pancreas, poor weight gain and nutritional problems.

Newsletters

4862 NASPGHAN News
PO Box 6
Flourtown, PA 19031

215-233-0808
Fax: 215-233-3939
e-mail: naspghan@naspghan.org
www.naspgn.org

Publication of the North American Society for Pediatric Gastroenterolgy, Hepatology and Nutrition, which strives to improve the care of infants, children and adolescents with digestive disorders by promoting advances in clinical care of children with chronic abdominal pain, diarrhea, constipation, vomiting, bleeding from the GI tract, inflammatory bowel disease, liver diseases, diseases of the pancreas, poor weight gain and nutritional problems.

DESCRIPTION

4863 NEPHROTIC SYNDROME

Synonyms: Minimal change nephrotic syndrome, MCNS

Covers these related disorders: Infantile nephrotic syndrome, Primary nephrotic syndrome, Secondary nephrotic syndrome

Involves the following Biologic System(s):
Renal and Urologic Disorders

Nephrotic syndrome is characterized by an abnormality of the kidney that allows proteins to leak out of the blood and into the urine. The loss of these proteins leads to proteinuria (protein in the urine), edema (swelling) of the body, hypoproteinemia (low blood levels of protein), hyperlipidemia (high fat levels in the blood) and lipiduria (fat in the urine). Clinical examination of a patient with nephrotic syndrome will reveal swelling of the eyelids and skin around the eyes (periorbital edema), swelling of the extremities, especially feet and lower legs, and fluid in the abdomen (ascites). Laboratory examination will show large amounts of urinary protein, low serum albumin and high cholesterol.

There are three categories of nephrotic syndrome: infantile; primary; and secondary:

Infantile nephrotic syndrome is usually the result of an inherited form and symptoms occur in the first few months of life. Secondary nephrotic syndrome is nephrotic syndrome associated with another disease process. These can include infection, connective tissue disorders such as lupus erythematosus, allergen exposure and medications.

Primary nephrotic syndrome results from disease in the kidney alone. The most common form is minimal change nephrotic syndrome (MCNS), or minimal change disease. It is called minimal change because little change is seen in the kidneys when a biopsy of the kidney is examined. Minimal change nephrotic syndrome almost always responds to steroids. Although relapses are not uncommon the long-term prognosis is excellent. Other causes of primary nephrotic syndrome, such as focal segmental glomerulosclerosis, mesangial proliferative glomeruloephritis, and membranous nephropathy, may or may not improve with the steroids and generally have a worse prognosis than MCNS. These patients can be treated with immunosuppressive therapy but may progress to end-stage renal disease requiring dialysis or kidney transplant.

Children with nephrotic syndrome are at risk for several complications. These include increased risk of infection, blood clots and cardiovascular disease. Dietary management includes restriction of sodium and fluid intake. Excessive sunlight should be avoided, because sensitivity to light (photosensitivity) is common.

See also **General Resources** on page 917

National Associations & Support Groups

4864 American Kidney Fund
6110 Executive Boulevard, Suite 1010
Rockville, MD 20852

301-984-6657
800-638-8299
Fax: 301-881-3311
e-mail: helpline@kidneyfund.org
www.akfinc.org

The American Kidney Fund is the nation's leading voluntary health organization serving people with and at risk for kidney disease through direct financial assistance, comprehensive education, clinical research and community service programs.

LaVarne A Burton, CEO
Tamara Ruggiero, Director Communications

4865 National Kidney Foundation
30 E 33rd Street
New York, NY 10016

212-889-2210
800-622-9010
Fax: 212-689-9261
e-mail: info@kidney.org
www.kidney.org

A major voluntary health organization, seeking to prevent kidney and urinary tract diseases, improve the health and well-being of individuals and families affected by these diseases, and increases the availability of all organs for transplant.

John Davis, CEO
Joseph A Vassalotti MD, Chief Medical Officer

4866 NephCure Foundation
15 Waterloo Avenue, Suite 200
Berwyn, PA 19312

610-540-0186
866-637-4287
Fax: 610-540-0190
e-mail: info@nephcure.org
www.nephcure.org

The only organization solely committed to seeking a cause and cure for two potentially devastating kidney conditions, Nephrotic Syndrome and Focal Segmental Glomerulosclerosis (FSGS). NephCure is made up of patients, their families and friends, researchers, physicians and other healthcare professionals joining forces to create awareness and generate funding for research.

Henry Brehm, Executive Director
Kerri Kennedy, Director Development

Web Sites

4867 American Kidney Fund
www.akfinc.org

Providing information for people with and at risk for kidney disease such as Nephrotic Syndrome.

4868 National Kidney Foundation

www.kidney.org

A site that offers information to prevent kidney and urinary tract diseases, improve the health and well-being of individuals and families affected by these diseases, and increases the availability of all organs for transplant.

4869 NephCure Foundation

www.nephcure.org

Information pertaining to seeking a cause and cure for two potentially devastating kidney conditions, Nephrotic Syndrome and Focal Segmental Glomerulosclerosis.

Book Publishers

4870 The Official Parent's Sourcebook on Childhood Nephrotic Syndrome

James N. Parker, author

Icon Group International
7404 Trade Street
San Diego, CA 92121

Fax: 858-635-9414
e-mail: orders@icongroupbooks.com
www.icongrouponline.com

A comprehensive manual for anyone interested in self-directed research on childhood Nephrotic Syndrome. Fully referenced with ample internet listings and glossary.

2002 136 pages Paperback
ISBN: 0-597832-16-1

Newsletters

4871 NephCure Now

NephCure Foundation
15 Waterloo Avenue, Suite 200
Berwyn, PA 19312

610-540-0186
Fax: 610-540-0190
e-mail: info@nephcure.org
www.nephcure.org/news_nephnow.html

The NephCure Foundation's newsletter that contains news and information on a variety of topics including the latest research updates, NephCure events and fundraisers and much more.

Henry Brehm, Executive Director
Miriam Wagner Long, Marketing

4872 Renalink

National Kidney Foundation
30 E 33rd Street
New York, NY 10016

212-889-2210
800-622-9010
Fax: 212-689-9261
e-mail: renalink@kidney.org
www.kidney.org/professionals/journals/login.cfm

Renalink is the joint newsletter of the Council of Nephrology Nurses and Technicians, the Council of Nephrology Social Work and the Council of Renal Nutrition of the National Kidney Foundation. Renalink includes news for each Council, information vital to the renal care team and ideas that should lead to further collaboration among allied health professionals in the renal field.

Quarterly

Pamphlets

4873 Childhood Nephrotic Syndrome

Information Clearinghouse
2 Information Way
Bethesda, MD 20892

301-654-3810
Fax: 301-907-8906
e-mail: nddic@info.niddk.nih.gov
www.niddk.nih.gov

4874 Children and Kidney Disease

American Kidney Fund
6110 Executive Boulevard, #1010
Rockville, MD 20852

301-881-3052
800-638-8299
Fax: 301-881-0898
www.kidney.org

4875 Financial Assistance and Insurance for People with Kidney Disease

Information Clearinghouse
2 Information Way
Bethesda, MD 20892

301-654-3810
Fax: 301-907-8906
e-mail: nddic@info.niddk.nih.gov
www.niddk.nih.gov

4876 Kidney Disease and African Americans

Information Clearinghouse
2 Information Way
Bethesda, MD 20892

301-654-3810
Fax: 301-907-8906
e-mail: nddic@info.niddk.nih.gov
www.niddk.nih.gov

4877 Kidney Disease of Diabetes

Information Clearinghouse
1 Information Way
Bethesda, MD 20892

301-654-3820
Fax: 301-907-8906
e-mail: ndoc@info.niddk.nih.gov
www.niddk.nih.gov

DESCRIPTION

4878 NEUROFIBROMATOSIS

Synonym: NF

Covers these related disorders: Neurofibromatosis type I (von Recklinghausen disease) (NF1), Neurofibromatosis type II (NF2)

Involves the following Biologic System(s):
Dermatologic Disorders, Orthopedic and Muscle Disorders

The term neurofibromatosis is often used to refer to neurofibromatosis I (NF1), an autosomal dominant disorder that affects approximately one in 3,500 to 4,000 individuals. Neurofibromatosis type I, also known as von Recklinghausen disease, is characterized by the appearance of pale tan or light brown discolorations (macules) on the skin (cafe-au-lait spots) and multiple benign, fibrous tumors of nerves and skin (neurofibromas). A second, distinctive form of neurofibromatosis (NF), known as neurofibromatosis type II (NF2), accounts for about 10 percent of all cases of NF. Neurofibromatosis type II, also an autosomal dominant disorder, is characterized by the development of benign tumors on both acoustic nerves (bilateral acoustic neuromas), resulting in progressive hearing impairment.

In most children with neurofibromatosis type I, skin discoloration may develop by the age of one year. Such skin lesions typically increase in number and size over time, and most affected individuals have six or more spots measuring 1.5 centimeters or more in diameter after the onset of puberty. Although these cafe-au-lait spots are often distributed in various areas of the body, they are most commonly present on the trunk. In addition, after three years of age, areas of freckling, particularly under the arms (axillary) and in the groin (inguinal) area, may also be present.

In approximately 95 percent of children with NF1 over six years of age, two or more benign, tumor-like nodules, known as Lisch nodules, are present on the pigmented areas of the eyes. Benign, fibrous tumors of the skin (cutaneous neurofibromas) tend to develop during the second decade of life, typically appearing as small, soft, raised, and slightly purplish discolorations of the overlying skin. These tumors, which rarely develop before six years of age, may increase in number and size during puberty. In addition, large benign tumors composed of bundles of nerves (plexiform neurofibromas) may be apparent at birth or during early childhood. Approximately two to four percent of individuals with NF1 may develop malignant tumors (e.g., neurofibrosarcomas). Physical findings that may be associated with malignant transformation include increasing tumor size, associated pain, or various neurologic symptoms due to tumor growth. Approximately 15 percent of affected individuals may also develop tumors of the optic nerve (optic glioma), which is the cranial nerve that carries visual impulses from the back of the eye (retina) to the brain. These tumors are usually considered relatively benign and may cause no associated symptoms (asymptomatic). However, in some cases, depending upon their specific location, growth, and nature, such tumors may affect vision. In these patients, associated findings may include visual impairment; degenerat|ion (atrophy) of the optic nerve; abnormal deviation of the eye (strabismus); or involuntary, rhythmic eye movements (nystagmus). In addition, some affected individuals may have an increased risk of developing tumors of the brain and spinal cord (e.g., astrocytomas, meningiomas, neurilemmomas, etc.).

Some individuals with NF1 may also experience associated skeletal abnormalities, such as bowing of the lower legs; improper development of a bone at the base of the skull (sphenoid wing dysplasia), potentially causing pronounced bulging of the eyes (exophthalmos); and progressive sideways curvature of the spine (scoliosis). Additional abnormalities may be present, such as mild short stature, abnormal largeness of the head (macrocephaly), and episodes of uncontrolled electrical activity in the brain (seizures). In addition, many affected children may have learning disabilities and speech abnormalities. Neurofibromatosis type I is caused by abnormal changes (mutations) of a gene located on the long arm of chromosome 17 (17q11.2). In approximately 50 percent of patients, the disease gene is inherited an an autosomal dominant trait; the remaining cases result from new (sporadic) mutations of the gene that occur for unknown reasons.

Neurofibromatosis type II (NF2) is also characterized by bilateral acoustic neuromas that are responsible for carrying sound impulses from the inner ear to the brain. Symptoms may become apparent during childhood or the second or third decades of life. These may include a facial numbness or weakness, headache, dizziness, unsteadiness, and progressive hearing loss. Individuals with NF2 may also develop clouding of the lenses of the eyes (i.e., posterior subcapsular opacities), have an increased risk of developing tumors of the brain and spinal cord (e.g., gliomas, meningiomas, schwannomas, etc.), or experience progressive visual impairment. NF2 is caused by a disease gene located on the long arm of chromosome 22 (22q12.2). R
The treatment of neurofibromatosis is directed toward

ensuring early detection and prompt, appropriate management of potentially associated findings or complications. Affected individuals are typically regularly monitored with complete neurologic evaluations (e.g., including visual and auditory screening) and thorough examinations to detect potential complications associated with NF. In most cases, symptoms of NF1 are mild, and patients live normal and productive lives. In some cases, however, NF1 can be severely debilitating. In some cases of NF2, the damage to nearby vital structures, such as other cranial nerves, can be life-threatening. Some tumors may be surgically removed or treated using other appropriate methods (e.g., radiation or chemotherapy for certain malignancies). Other treatment is symptomatic and supportive.

See also **General Resources** on page 917

National Associations & Support Groups

4879 Children's Tumor Foundation
95 Pine Street, 16th Floor
New York, NY 10005

> 212-344-6633
> 800-323-7938
> Fax: 212-747-0004
> e-mail: info@ctf.org
> www.ctf.org

A nonprofit, medical foundation dedicated to improving the health and well-being of individuals and families affected by neurofibromatosis through: support and accessible information; research support; assistance in developing clinical centers; and expanding public awareness.

John Risner, President
Catherine Silberstein, Volunteer Training/Development Dir

4880 Genetic Alliance
4301 Connecticut Avenue NW
Washington, DC 20008

> 202-966-5557
> 800-336-4363
> Fax: 202-966-8553
> e-mail: info@geneticalliance.org
> www.geneticalliance.org

A coalition of voluntary genetic support groups, consumers and professionals addressing the needs of individuals and families affected by genetic disorders from a national perspective.

Sharon Terry, President/CEO

4881 March of Dimes Birth Defects Foundation
1275 Mamaroneck Avenue
White Plains, NY 10605

> 914-428-7100
> 888-663-4637
> Fax: 914-428-8203
> e-mail: resourcecenter@modimes.org
> www.marchofdimes.com

Partnership of volunteers and professionals dedicates to improving the health of babies by preventing birth defects and infant mortality. Over 100 chapters are located across the country and can be located through the National Office.

Dr Jennifer Howse, President

4882 National Brain Tumor Foundation
22 Battery Street, Suite 612
San Francisco, CA 94111

> 415-834-9970
> 800-934-2873
> e-mail: nbtf@braintumor.org
> www.braintumor.org

NBTF is a national nonprofit health organization dedicated to providing information and support for brain tumor patients, family members, and healthcare professionals, while supporting innovative research into better treatment options and a cure for brain tumors.

Walter S. Newman, Chair Emeritus, Co-Founder
Allison Jones Thomson, Chair, Business And Marketing

4883 Neurofibromatosis Support & Information Gr oup
Parents Helping Parents
3041 Olcott Street
Santa Clarka, CA 95054

> 408-727-5775
> Fax: 408-727-0182
> e-mail: info@php.com
> www.php.com

Helping children with special needs receive the resources, love, hope, respect, health care, education and other services they need to achieve their full potential by providing them with strong families and dedicated professionals to serve them.

Alexandra Cramer, Receptionist/Admin. Assistant
Carlos A. Gallegos, Kids on the Block Coordinator

4884 Neurofibromatosis, Inc
PO Box 18246
Minneapolis, MN 55418

> 301-918-4600
> 800-942-6825
> Fax: 301-918-0009
> www.nfinc.org

An organization of independent state and regional chapters that provides support and services to familes coping with neurofibromatosis. Works closely with clinical and research professionals who specialize in the treatment of NF. Has a newsletter and other printed materials.

Miguel Lessing, President

State Agencies & Support Groups

Arizona

4885 Neurofibromatosis, Inc - Arizona Chapter
PO Box 2718
Chandler, AZ 85244

> 480-945-9650
> e-mail: nfaz1@cox.net
> www.nfinc.org

Arkansas

4886 Children's Tumor Foundation-Arkansas Chapt er
1005 Flamingo Road
Rogers, AR 72756

> 479-619-4137
> e-mail: paws4mc@cox.net
> www.ctf.org/arkansas/

Julie Jarrett, Contact

4887 Children's Tumor Foundation-Arkansas Infor mation & Support
139 Rainbow Lane
Bigelow, AR 72016

> 501-759-2710
> e-mail: lesleyo@arbbs.net
> www.ctf.org

Lesley Oslica

California

4888 Neurofibromatosis, Inc - California Chapte r
PO Box 1234
Vacaville, CA 95696

707-469-0467
e-mail: info@nfcalifornia.org
www.nfinc.org

Colorado

4889 Children's Tumor Foundation - Colorado Cha pter
70 N Ranch Road
Littleton, CO 80127

303-734-9942
e-mail: ilaskey@peakpeak.com
www.ctf.org

Mark Ebel, Chapter President

Florida

4890 Children's Tumor Foundation - Florida Chap ter
6147 Donegal Drive
Orlando, FL 32819

407-909-1946
800-540-5721
e-mail: hehrli@aol.com
www.ctf.org/florida/

Hannah Erli, Chapter President
Sue Bresnahan, Office Contact

Georgia

4891 Children's Tumor Foundation - Georgia
5 Ardmore Circle
Cartersville, GA 30120

678-428-9711
e-mail: ctfgeorgia@bellsouth.net
www.ctf.org/georgia/

Randy Watkins

Hawaii

4892 NNFF Hawaii Chapter
852 Kaahue Street
Honolulu, HI 96825

808-395-4505
e-mail: pdorinson@nf.org
www.nf.org

Ruth Watanabe, Chapter President

Idaho

4893 NNFF Idaho Chapter
4419 E Linden Street
Caldwell, ID 83605

208-459-6022

Suzy Crici, Chapter President

Illinois

4894 Children's Tumor Foundation - Illinois
5604 West Henderson 3 West
Chicago, IL 60634

773-286-2802
e-mail: debbie.callahan@att.net
www.ctf.org/illinois/

2500 members

Debbie Callahan, Vice President

4895 Children's Tumor Foundation - Illinois Cha pter
PO Box 213
Emden, IL 62635

217-732-8568
Fax: 217-732-8568
e-mail: beachph@cs.com
www.ctf.org/illinois/

Paul Beach, Chapter President

4896 Neurofibromatosis, Inc - Illinois/Midwest
PO Box 1923
Lombard, IL 60148

630-932-8111
800-322-6363
Fax: 630-932-8119
e-mail: ilnfinc@sbcglobal.net
www.nfinc.org

Indiana

4897 Children's Tumor Foundation - Indiana Affi liate
863 West Roache Street
Indiannapolis, IN 46208

317-924-4725
e-mail: kym1577@sbcglobal.net
www.ctf.org

Kim Bebley, Affiliate Representative

Iowa

4898 Children's Tumor Foundation - Iowa Chapter
321 Glenview Drive
Des Moines, IA 50312

515-277-8494
Fax: 515-277-1526
e-mail: Drev@aol.com

Sheila Drevyanko, Chapter President

Kansas

4899 Neurofibromatosis, Inc - Kansas & Central Plains
PO Box 1792
Hutchinson, KS 67504

316-669-8453
800-942-6825
e-mail: nprieb@southwind.net
www.nfinc.org

Nancy Prieb, President

Kentucky

4900 NNFF of Kentucky
5482 B Jamison Street
Fort Knox, KY 40121

502-943-0861
e-mail: rrogers@bbtel.com

Lisa Rogers, Chapter President

Maryland

4901 Neurofibromatosis, Inc - MidAtlantic
8855 Annapolis Road, Suite 110
Lanham, MD 20706

301-577-8984
Fax: 301-918-0009
e-mail: NFMidAtlantic@aol.com
www.nfinc.org

Massachusetts

4902 Children's Tumor Foundation - Northern New England
275 Grove Street Suite 200-4
Newton, MA 02466

508-879-5638
888-585-5316
Fax: 617-663-4801
e-mail: seburne@ctf.org
www.ctf.org

Samantha Eburne, Vp, NE Development

4903 NNFF Massachusetts Chapter
31 Springhill Avenue
Marlborough, MA 01752

508-624-4533
888-585-5316
Fax: 508-624-7553

Nancy Brown, Chapter President

4904 Neurofibromatosis, Inc - New England/North east
9 Bedford Street
Burlington, MA 01803

781-272-9936
e-mail: info@nfincne.org
www.nfinc.org

Michigan

4905 Children's Tumor Foundation - Michigan Cha pter
6069 Brynthrop
Shelby Township, MI 48316

586-731-7811
e-mail: hawkeyenf@wideopenwest.com
www.ctf.org/michigan/

Peter Dingeman, Chapter President
Wendy Schaffer, Treasurer

4906 NF Support Group of West Michigan Spectrum Health-East Campus
Neurofibromatosis
240 Hillview Avenue NE
Grand Rapids, MI 49506

616-451-3699
www.nfinc.org/local.html

4907 NNFF Michigan Chapter - Ann Arbor
3212 Tiger Lily Ridge
Ann Arbor, MI 48103

734-662-0568

Cindy Pfiefle, Chapter Co-President

Minnesota

4908 Neurofibromatosis - Minnesota
Po Box 18246
Minneapolis, MN 55418

651-225-1720
e-mail: NFIncMN@aol.com
www.nfinc.org

Mississippi

4909 Neurofibromatosis - Mississippi
2643 Highway 80 E
Brandon, MS 39402

601-825-0433
e-mail: Bbboptical@aol.com
www.nfinc.org

Missouri

4910 Children's Tumor Foundation - Missouri Cha pter
Thompson Coburn LLP
One US Bank Plaza
St Louis, MO 63101

314-552-6139
Fax: 314-552-7139
e-mail: dcox@thompsoncoburn.com
www.ctf.org/missouri/

Dan Cox, Chapter President
Sue Slocomb, Treasurer

Nevada

4911 Children's Tumor Foundation - Nevada
8065 White Falls Drive
Reno, NV 89506

775-972-1882
Fax: 775-972-1885
e-mail: daverenorice@yahoo.com
www.ctf.org

David Rice

New Hampshire

4912 NNFF of Northern New England
3 Friar Tuck
Nashua, NH 03062

603-882-5405

New Jersey

4913 NNFF of New Jersey
271 B Reichelt Road
New Milford, NJ 07646

201-265-3296
800-323-7938
Fax: 201-265-3296
e-mail: DonnaNF@aol.com
www.nf.org

Donna Oettinger, VP

New York

4914 NNFF of New York/New Jersey
95 Pine Street, 16th Floor
New York, NY 10005

212-344-6633
Fax: 212-747-0004

Thomas Livingston, Chapter President

Ohio

4915 Children's Tumor Foundation - Ohio
523 W Main Street
Crestline, OH 44827

419-683-6158
e-mail: atadda1313@aol.com
www.ctf.org

Amy Tadda, Representative

4916 NNFF of Ohio
1377 Collinsdale
Cincinnati, OH 45230

513-231-2240

Jenny Ely, Chapter President

Oklahoma

4917 NNFF of Oklahoma
16 7th NW
Ardmore, OK 73401

580-223-3513
e-mail: rhedr35594@aol.com

Richard Hedrick, President

Oregon

4918 Children's Tumor Foundation - Oregon Support Group
18989 NE Marine Drive, Slip #65
Portland, OR 97230

503-674-9255
Fax: 503-674-9256
e-mail: walktours1@aol.com
www.ctf.org

Jean Fitzgerald, Facilitator

4919 Legacy Good Samaritan Hospital & Medical Center
Neurofibromatosis Support Group
1015 NW 22nd Avenue, N-300
Portland, OR 97210

503-413-7711
e-mail: mflorian@lhs.org

Marty Florian, Coordinator

Rhode Island

4920 NNFF of Rhode Island - Coventry
52 Stone Street
Coventry, RI 02816

401-823-4421

Diane Sisson, Chapter Co-President

4921 NNFF of Rhode Island - Warwick
43 Ithaca Street
Warwick, RI 02886

401-732-6094

Deb Thornlimb, Chapter Co-President

South Carolina

4922 Children's Tumor Foundation - South Carolina Chapter
111 Oakview Drive
Darlington, SC 29532

843-393-9672
Fax: 843-393-9673
e-mail: pmchrisley@aol.com
www.ctf.org

Pat Chrisley

South Dakota

4923 NNFF of South Dakota - Northern Plains
6008 Tecumseh Court
Sioux Falls, SD 57106

605-362-7279
e-mail: dakotanf@aol.com

Bobbie Milton, Chapter President

Tennessee

4924 Children's Tumor Foundation - Tennessee Affiliate
7029 Terry Drive
Knoxville, TN 37924

865-633-5858
Fax: 865-633-5859

Gracie Greenway, Affiliate Representative

4925 NNFF Tennessee Chapter
1006 Valencia Court
Ashland City, TN 37015

615-792-9821
Fax: 615-792-8980
e-mail: tess22@earthlink.net

Terrisa Decker, Co-President

Texas

4926 Neurofibromatosis Texas Foundation
4514 Travis Street, Suite 313
Dallas, TX 75205

214-528-5557
e-mail: texsnf@aol.com

Utah

4927 Children's Tumor Foundation - Utah Chapter
2647 S 1175 West
Syracuse, UT 84075

801-277-4041
Fax: 801-277-4042
e-mail: tick2100@comcast.net
www.ctf.org/utah/

Kathy Gift
Steve Gift

4928 NNFF of Utah
6179 S Impressions Drive
Kearns, UT 84118

801-968-3664
Fax: 801-968-0981
www.ctf.org

Jennifer Newman, Chapter President

Virginia

4929 Children's Tumor Foundation - MidAtlantic Region Chapter
11135 Rich Meadow Drive
Great Falls, VA 22066

703-444-1624
e-mail: bentleyaw@aol.com
www.ctf.org

Anne Bentley

Washington

4930 Children's Tumor Foundation - Washington Chapter
20427 NE 41st Sreet
Sammamish, WA 98074

425-868-9358
e-mail: ctfwa@yahoo.com
www.ctf.org/washington/

Provides information, support services and referrals for patients
and families afffected by neurfibromatosis, while supporting medical research toward effective treatments and a cure.

Amy Barley

4931 NNFF Washington State Chapter
6628 212th Street SW, Suite 100
Lynnwood, WA 98036

425-672-9610
Fax: 425-672-9518

Roseanne McKeown, Chapter President

West Virginia

4932 NNFF West Virginia Chapter
4505 Butler Street
Parkersburg, WV 26104

304-428-4184

Wendy Robinson, President

4933 Neurofibromatosis - West Virginia
PO Box 297
Woodville, WV 25572

304-524-7812
www.nfinc.org

Wisconsin

4934 Children's Tumor Foundation - Wisconsin Chapter
6562 W Glenbrook Road
Brown Deer, WI 53223

414-362-0211
Fax: 414-362-0212
e-mail: epankownf@aol.com
www.ctf.org

Elaine Pankow, President

4935 Neurofibromatosis - Wisconsin
2637 S Fulton Avenue
Bay View, WI 53207

414-461-9641
e-mail: mflamingo@usa.net
www.nfinc.org

Wyoming

4936 NNFF Wyoming Chapter
110 Reed Street
Rock Springs, WY 82901

307-382-5893
e-mail: moadams@wyoming.com

Molly Adams, Chapter President

4937 NNFF of Wyoming
307 S 5th Avenue
Casper, WY 82604

307-473-7723
e-mail: ngood13@juno.com

Norma Good, Chapter President

Research Centers

Florida

4938 Neurofibromatosis Center at North Broward Medical Center
201 E Sample Road
Deerfield Beach, FL 33064

954-941-8300
www.browardhealth.org

Oklahoma

4939 Neuroscience Institute at Mercy Hospital
4300 W Memorial Road
Oklahoma City, OK 73120

405-755-1515
Fax: 405-752-3977

Gary Brown PhD, Contact

Pennsylvania

4940 NF Clinic - University of Pittsburgh Child ren's Hospital
3705 Fifth Avenue
Pittsburgh, PA 15213

412-692-5520
Fax: 412-692-6787

Gulay Alpers MD, Contact

Web Sites

4941 Children's Tumor Foundation
www.ctf.org

A nonprofit medical foundation dedicated to improving the health and well being of individuals and families affected by NF.

4942 Neurofibromatosis, Inc
www.nfinc.org

An organization made up of independent state and regional chapters, providing support and services to NF families. In addition to assisting individuals and families, NF, Inc. works closely with clinical and research professionals who specialize in the treatment of NF.

4943 Online Mendelian Inheritance in Man
www.ncbi.nlm.nih.gov

This database is a catalog of human genes and genetic disorders.

Book Publishers

4944 Let's Talk About Going to the Hospital
Rosen Publishing Group's PowerKids Press
29 E 21st Street
New York, NY 10010

212-777-3017
800-237-9932
Fax: 888-436-4643
e-mail: rosenpub@tribeca.ios.com
www.powerkidspress.com

If a child has to check into the hospital, chances are he or she is already upset about being ill. Knowing how a hospital functions and what the procedures are, such as when family members can visit, will help in what is already a stressful situation. Grades K-5.

24 pages
ISBN: 0-823950-36-0

4945 Neurofibromatosis: A Handbook for Patients , Families and Health Care Professionals

Dr Bruce R Korf; Dr Allan E Rubenstein, author

Children's Tumor Foundation
95 Pine Street, 16th Floor
New York, NY 10005

212-344-6633
800-323-7938
www.ctf.org/patientinfo/

2005-2nd Ed 264 pages Hardbound

4946 Who Says It Has to Be Fair

Theda Schott, author

PublishAmerica
PO Box 151
Frederick, MD 21705

301-695-1707
www.nfinc.org; www.publishamerica.com

A mother's story about raising a child with neurofibromatosis.

2006 184 pages Paperback
ISBN: 1-424118-09-3

Newsletters

4947 Neurofibromatosis Ink
Neurofibromatosis, Inc
PO Box 18246
Minneapolis, MN 55418

301-918-4600
800-942-6825
Fax: 301-918-0009
e-mail: NFInfo@nfinc.org
www.nfinc.org

Miguel Lessing, President

4948 Neurofibromatosis News
Children's Tumor Foundation
95 Pine Street, 16th Floor
New York, NY 10005

212-344-6633
800-323-7938
Fax: 212-747-0004
www.ctf.org

Offers information on the newest advances in neurofibromatosis, related events and foundation activities.

Quarterly

Susan Blalock, Editor

Pamphlets

4949 Achieving in Spite of...A Booklet on Learn ing Disabilities

Children's Tumor Foundation
95 Pine Street, 16th Floor
New York, NY 10005

212-344-6633
800-323-7938
Fax: 212-747-0004
www.ctf.org

Designed for use by parents, teachers and health professionals- information on learning disabilities and what to do about them.

34 pages

4950 Child with Neurofibromatosis Type 1

Children's Tumor Foundation
95 Pine Street, 16th Floor
New York, NY 10005

212-344-6633
800-323-7938
Fax: 212-747-0004
www.ctf.org

Offers information on the prognosis, management, complications, genetic implications, and sources of support for children with neurofibromatosis 1. It attempts to put mild or early forms of the disorder into perspective.

4951 Facing Neurofibromatosis: A Guide for Teen s

Children's Tumor Foundation
95 Pine Street, 16th Floor
New York, NY 10005

212-344-6633
800-323-7938
Fax: 212-747-0004
e-mail: info@ctf.org
www.ctf.org

Offers information for teenagers on how to face neurofibromatosis on a daily basis.

4952 Neurofibromatosis Type 1: A Guide for Educ ators

Children's Tumor Foundation
95 Pine Street, 16th Floor
New York, NY 10005

212-344-6633
800-323-7938
Fax: 212-747-0004
e-mail: info@ctf.org
www.ctf.org/patientinfo/

Offers concise and practical information as well as recommendations about the cognitive, physical and behavioral manifestations of the disorder.

12 pages

4953 Neurofibromatosis Type 2: Information for Patients and Families

Children's Tumor Foundation
95 Pine Street, 16th Floor
New York, NY 10005

212-344-6633
800-323-7938
Fax: 212-747-0004
e-mail: info@ctf.org
www.ctf.org/patientinfo/

Offers extensive information on what NF2 is and answers the most asked about questions regarding the illness.

4954 Neurofibromatosis: Information for Patient s and Families

Children's Tumor Foundation
95 Pine Street, 16th Floor
New York, NY 10005

212-344-6633
800-323-7938
Fax: 212-747-0004
e-mail: info@ctf.org
www.ctf.org/patientinfo/

A pamphlet offering information for patients and families; designed to answer questions.

4955 Neurofibromatosis: Questions and Answers

Children's Tumor Foundation
95 Pine Street, 16th Floor
New York, NY 10005

212-344-6633
803-237-938
Fax: 212-747-0004
www.ctf.org

Information about neurofibromatosis.

Camps

4956 Camp New Friends

Neurofibromatosis, Inc
PO Box 18246
Minneapolis, MN 55418

301-918-4600
800-942-6825
Fax: 301-918-0009
e-mail: NFMidAtlantic@aol.com
www.nfinc.org

A summer camp for those affected with NF1 or NF2, between the ages of 7 and 15. Those aged 18 and over may apply as counselors or counselors-in-training. The camp is held in collaboration with Children's National Medical Center.

Sandy Cushner-Weinstein, Contact

4957 International NF Summer Camp

Children's Tumor Foundation
95 Pine Street, 16th Floor
New York, NY 10005

212-344-6633
800-323-7938
Fax: 212-747-0004
e-mail: info@ctf.org
www.ctf.org

DESCRIPTION

4958 NEUROBLASTOMA

Synonym: NB

Involves the following Biologic System(s):
Hematologic and Oncologic Disorders

Neuroblastomas are malignant tumors that account for approximately eight to 10 percent of childhood cancers. They are the most common solid tumors that develop outside the skull in children. About 500 to 600 new cases are reported each year in the United States, with males affected slightly more frequently than females. In approximately 90 percent of affected infants and children, neuroblastoma is diagnosed before age five. Neuroblastoma sometimes occurs in members of certain families (kindreds), although the specific underlying cause is unknown.

Neuroblastomas may originate in any part of the sympathetic nervous system but most commonly develop in the inner region of the adrenal gland (adrenal medulla). In other patients, neuroblastomas may arise in the chest. The sympathetic nervous system controls certain involuntary activities during times of stress, such as raising blood pressure and increasing the heart rate. The adrenal glands, two relatively small organs that curve over the top of each kidney, secrete certain hormones directly into the bloodstream.

A neuroblastoma often invades surrounding tissues and spreads to small, node-like structures located along the course of the lymphatic vessels (lymph nodes). The tumor may then spread to other parts of the body (metastasize), particularly the liver, skeleton, and bone marrow. Rarely, neuroblastomas spread to the lungs or the brain. Associated symptoms and findings are highly variable and depend upon the specific location of the tumor and the extent to which it may have spread. Many infants and children may have a hard, solid, painless lump or mass in the neck or a large mass that may be felt in the abdomen or on the back. Patients often have a general feeling of ill health (malaise) and appear pale (pallor). Those with skeletal involvement typically experience tumor-associated bone pain. In addition, because the bone marrow is a blood-producing tissue, tumor infiltration of the bone marrow may result in abnormally decreased levels of the different blood cells, including circulating red blood cells (anemia), platelets (thrombocytopenia), and certain white blood cells, (neutropenia). Due to low levels of platelets, patients may experience abnormal bleeding and easy bruising. Decreased levels of white blood cells may cause an increased susceptibility to certain infections.

Depending upon the location and potential spread of the tumor, additional symptoms and findings may occur. If a neuroblastoma spreads to the bony cavities surrounding the eyes, associated symptoms may include abnormal protrusion of the eyes (proptosis) and the appearance of bluish-purple patches (ecchymosis) around the eyes. Tumor development near the spinal cord may result in weakness or paralysis of the legs (paresis). In addition, involvement of the liver typically causes abnormal liver enlargement (hepatomegaly). Tumor growth within the adrenal glands may cause excessive secretion of the hormones epinephrine and norepinephrine, resulting in increased irritability, high blood pressure (hypertension), increased heart rate (tachycardia), flushing of the skin, severe diarrhea, and other symptoms.

Some patients may also develop Horner's syndrome, which is characterized by ptosis, absence of sweating (anhidrosis), and narrowing of the pupil of the eye (miosis). Skin abnormalities may also be present, including firm, bluish nodules under the skin or skin lesions on the scalp. Approximately four percent of patients experience a sudden onset of neuromuscular symptoms due to abnormal functioning of the cerebellum (acute cerebellar encephalopathy). The cerebellum is a region of the brain that plays an essential role in maintaining normal postures, sustaining balance, and producing coordinated movements. Neuroblastoma symptoms may include an impaired ability to coordinate voluntary movements (cerebellar ataxia); random, rapid, uncontrolled eye movements (opsoclonus); and shock-like contractions of certain muscles or muscle groups (myoclonic jerks).

In infants and children with neuroblastoma, treatment may depend upon the location of the tumor, whether it has spread, the patient's age, or other factors. If the tumor is contained and has not spread, treatment may consist of surgical removal of the tumor. When the tumor may not be removed surgically or has spread to other parts of the body, treatment measures may include the use of certain drugs (chemotherapy) or radiation therapy. Additional treatments for advanced disease may be considered.

See also **General Resources** on page 917

Government Agencies

4959 NIH/National Cancer Institute
6116 Executive Boulevard, Room 3036A
Bethesda, MD 20892

800-422-6237
www.cancer.gov

The National Cancer Institute coordinates the National Cancer Program, which conducts and supports research, training, health information dissemination, and other programs with respect to the cause, diagnosis, prevention, and treatment of cancer, rehabilitation from cancer, and the continuing care of cancer patients and the families of cancer patients.

John E Niederhuber MD, Director

National Associations & Support Groups

4960 Candlelighters Childhood Cancer Foundation
PO Box 498
Kensington, MD 20895

301-962-3520
800-366-2223
Fax: 310-962-3521
e-mail: staff@candlelighters.org
www.candlelighters.org

The Candlelighters Childhood Cancer Foundation National Office was founded in 1970 by concerned parents of children with cancer. Today our membership of over 50,000 members of the national office and more than 100,000 members across the across the country, including Candlelighters affiliate groups, includes, parents of children who are being treated or have been treated for cancer.

Ruth Hoffman, Executive Director

4961 Children's Wish Foundation International
8615 Roswell Road
Atlanta, GA 30350

770-393-9474
800-323-9474
Fax: 770-393-0683
e-mail: wish@childrenswish.org
www.childrenswish.org

Children's Wish Foundation International is dedicated to bringing joy and hope to seeiously ill children and their families world wide by involving the public in putting children first with opportunities to experience the enhanced value and quality of life through the magic of a fulfilled wish.

Arthur Stein, President/CEO
Linda Dozoretz, Founder/Executive Director

4962 Genetic Alliance
4301 Connecticut Avenue NW
Washington, DC 20008

202-966-5557
800-336-4363
Fax: 202-966-8553
e-mail: info@geneticalliance.org
www.geneticalliance.org

A coalition of voluntary genetic support groups, consumers and professionals addressing the needs of individuals and families affected by genetic disorders from a national perspective.

Sharon Terry, President/CEO

4963 Neuroblastoma Children's Cancer Society
PO Box 957672
Hoffman Estates, IL 60195

847-605-1245
800-532-5162
Fax: 847-605-0705
e-mail: info@neuroblastomacancer.org
www.neuroblastomacancer.org

The Neuroblastoma Children's Cancer Society is a group made up of volunteers, many of whom have children or relatives who are victims or survivors of this disease. The organization is an advocate for the children who suffer from neuroblastoma and is dedicated to serving as a support center for their families.

Research Centers

4964 Children's Cancer Research Institute
University of Texas Health Science Ctr
8403 Floyd Curl Drive
San Antonio, TX 78229

210-562-9000
Fax: 210-562-9014
e-mail: chessher@uthscsa.edu
ccri.uthscsa.edu

It is the mission of the institute to advance scientific knowledge relevant to childhood cancer and to accelerate the translation of knowledge into therapies.

Sharon Murphy MD, Director
Bill Chessher, Administrator

Web Sites

4965 CancerCare
www.cancercare.org

A national nonprofit organization dedicated to providing free, professional support services to those affected by cancer.

4966 Children's Cancer Web
www.cancerindex.org/ccw

An independent nonprofit site, established to provide a directory of childhood cancer resources.

4967 Online Mendelian Inheritance in Man
www.ncbi.nlm.nih.gov

This database is a catalog of human genes and genetic disorders.

Book Publishers

4968 Let's Talk About Going to the Hospital
Rosen Publishing Group's PowerKids Press
29 E 21st Street
New York, NY 10010

212-777-3017
800-237-9932
Fax: 888-436-4643
e-mail: rosenpub@tribeca.ios.com
www.powerkidspress.com

If a child has to check into the hospital, chances are he or she is already upset about being ill. Knowing how a hospital functions and what the procedures are, such as when family members can visit, will help in what is already a stressful situation. Grades K-5.

24 pages
ISBN: 0-823950-36-0

4969 Let's Talk About When Kids Have Cancer

Melanie Apel Gordon, author

Rosen Publishing Group's PowerKids Press
29 E 21st Street
New York, NY 10010

212-777-3017
800-237-9932
Fax: 888-436-4643
e-mail: customerservice@rosenpub.com
www.powerkidspress.com

In a straightforward yet comforting way, this book explains what cancer is, what kinds of treatments surround the disease and how to cope if a child or the friend of a child has cancer.

24 pages Papperback
ISBN: 0-823951-95-2

4970 Pediatric Cancer Sourcebook

Edward J. Prucha, author

Omnigraphics
PO Box 625
Holmes, PA 19043

800-234-1340
Fax: 800-875-1340
e-mail: info@omnigraphics.com
www.omnigraphics.com

Basic consumer health information about leukemias, brain tumors, sarcomas, lymphomas and other cancers in infants, children and adolescents.

1999 587 pages
ISBN: 0-780802-45-4

4971 Resource Survival Handbook

Neuroblastoma Children's Cancer Society
PO Box 957672
Hoffman Estates, IL 60195

847-605-1245
800-532-5162
Fax: 847-605-0705
www.neuroblastomacancer.org/content/handbook.htm

An accumulation of resource information of facts about neuroblastoma and related treatments, national and local resources for families and patients, health claim forms, pamphlets, and other relevant forms.

Online

4972 Surviving Childhood Cancer: A Guide for Families

Margot Joan Fromer, author

New Harbinger Publications
5674 Shattuck Avenue
Oakland, CA 94609

510-652-0215
800-748-6273
Fax: 510-652-5472
e-mail: customerservice@newharbinger.com
www.newharbinger.com

Cancer in a child is an overwhelming experience for a family. This book explains common medical procedures and offers readers practical advice about how to cope with emotions and stress during this time.

232 pages Paperback
ISBN: 1-572241-02-0

Journals

4973 Candlelighters Childhood Cancer Foundation

PO Box 498
Kensington, MD 20895

301-962-3520
800-366-2223
Fax: 310-962-3521
e-mail: staff@candlelighters.org
www.candlelighters.org

Provides the latest information on CCCF programs and childhood cancer.

Quarterly

Ruth Hoffman, Executive Director

DESCRIPTION

4974 NEUTROPENIA

Covers these related disorders: Chronic neutropenia, Transient neutropenia

Involves the following Biologic System(s):
Hematologic and Oncologic Disorders

Neutropenia is a blood condition characterized by decreased numbers of circulating white blood cells known as neutrophils. These white blood cells play an essential role in fighting bacterial infections by detecting, engulfing, and digesting invading bacteria (phagocytosis). Neutrophils mature in the bone marrow and are then released into the bloodstream, where they may circulate for approximately six to eight hours. When responding to invading microorganisms or inflammation, neutrophils may leave the blood circulation, move into affected tissues, and digest microbes or other invaders as required.

Neutropenia is specifically defined as the presence of fewer than 1,500 neutrophils per microliter of blood. The condition may result from deficient production of neutrophils by the bone marrow or abnormally increased loss of neutrophils from the blood circulation. Depending upon the nature of the condition, its underlying cause, and other factors, neutropenia may occur for only days or weeks (transient neutropenia) or be present for months or a patient's lifetime (chronic neutropenia). In addition, the findings potentially associated with neutropenia are extremely variable and may include no apparent symptoms (asymptomatic), mild infections of the mucous membranes and the skin, or, in severe cases, potentially life-threatening complications.

In children, transient neutropenia may be caused by certain viral or bacterial infections; a deficiency of folic acid or vitamin B12; or the administration of certain medications, such as a class of antipsychotic drugs (phenothiazines), penicillin preparations, nonsteroidal anti-inflammatory agents, or anticancer drugs that may suppress bone marrow production. Chronic neutropenia also has several different causes and occurs in many different forms. Benign chronic neutropenia is a condition of childhood in which patients have chronically low levels of circulating neutrophils in the blood. This may result in increased susceptibility to recurrent infections of the skin, the mouth, or other areas. The condition typically resolves on its own by age four. Patients with immune deficiency disorders that are present at birth (primary inherited immunodeficiencies) or acquired (such as acquired immune deficiency syndrome, AIDS) often develop chronic neutropenia during infancy or early childhood. These children often fail to grow and gain weight at the expected rate (failure to thrive) and may experience recurrent bacterial infections, enlargement of the liver and spleen (hepatosplenomegaly), and potentially life-threatening complications.

Other uncommon forms of childhood neutropenia include cyclic neutropenia and Kostmann's disease. In patients with cyclic neutropenia, neutropenia recurs in regular cycles (e.g., every 18 to 21 days). When circulating neutrophils are abnormally decreased, these patients may experience fever, a general feeling of ill health (malaise), and susceptibility to mouth ulcers and infections of the skin, mucous membranes, and tissues that surround and support the teeth. Cyclic neutropenia typically becomes apparent during childhood and often runs in certain families. Kostmann's disease, also known as genetic infantile agranulocytosis, is a rare, autosomal recessive disorder characterized by persistent, extremely low levels of circulating neutrophils (fewer than 200 per microliter), frequent bacterial infections, and potentially life-threatening complications by approximately age three.

Neutropenia may also occur as a component of certain genetic, multisystemic diseases, such as Shwachman syndrome and metaphyseal chondrodysplasia, or in association with certain cancers, including leukemia and lymphoma.

The treatment of children with neutropenia depends upon the condition's severity and its underlying cause. In those with mild neutropenia, treatment may not be required. If a particular medication is responsible for the condition, such drug therapy is discontinued if possible. In patients with chronic neutropenia, physicians may recommend steps to help prevent bacterial infection and institute immediate antibiotic therapy should infections occur. In severe cases of bacterial infection, hospitalization may be required. In addition, in some patients with severe neutropenia, therapies may be administered to help stimulate the bone marrow's production of neutrophils (granulocyte colony-stimulating factor [G-CSF]). In some cases, bone marrow transplantation is an option, a procedure in which healthy bone marrow is given to replace defective bone marrow.

See also **General Resources** on page 917

Government Agencies

4975 NIH/National Heart, Lung and Blood Institu te
National Institute of Health
31 Center Dr MSC 2486, Bldg 31, Room 5A48
Bethesda, MD 20892

301-592-8573
Fax: 240-629-3246
TTY: 240-629-3255
e-mail: NHLBIinfo@nhlbi.nih.gov
www.nhlbi.nih.gov

Primary responsibility of this organization is the scientific investigation of heart, blood vessel, lung and blood disorders. Oversees research, demonstration, prevention, education, control and training activities in these fields and emphasizes the prevention and control of heart diseases.

Elizabeth G Nabel, MD, Director
Susan Shurin, MD, Deputy Director

4976 NIH/National Institute of Child Health and Human Development
31 Center Drive, Building 31
Bethesda, MD 20892

301-496-5133
Fax: 301-496-1104
www.nichd.nih.gov

Established in 1962 by congress, today the institute conducts and supports research on topics related to the health of children, adults, families and populations. Some of these topics include: developmental disabilities, growth and development, infant death, reproductive health and birth defects.

Nancy D Wirth, Director
Lisa Kaeser, Program & Public Liaison

National Associations & Support Groups

4977 American Autoimmune Related Diseases Association
22100 Gratiot Avenue
E Detroit, MI 48021

586-776-3900
www.aarda.org

Dedicated to the eradication of autoimmune diseases and the alleviation of suffering and the socio-economic impact of autoimmunity through fostering and facilitating collaboration in the areas of education, public awareness, research and patient services in an effective, ethical and efficient manner.

Virginia Ladd, Director

4978 Genetic Alliance
4301 Connecticut Avenue NW
Washington, DC 20008

202-966-5557
800-336-4363
Fax: 202-966-8553
e-mail: info@geneticalliance.org
www.geneticalliance.org

A coalition of voluntary genetic support groups, consumers and professionals addressing the needs of individuals and families affected by genetic disorders from a national perspective.

Sharon Terry, President/CEO

4979 March of Dimes Birth Defects Foundation
1275 Mamaroneck Avenue
White Plains, NY 10605

914-428-7100
888-663-4637
Fax: 914-428-8203
e-mail: resourcecenter@modimes.org
www.marchofdimes.com

Partnership of volunteers and professionals dedicates to improving the health of babies by preventing birth defects and infant mortality. Over 100 chapters are located across the country and can be located through the National Office.

Dr Jennifer Howse, President

4980 National Neutropenia Network

Brighton, MI

e-mail: leereeves99@comcast.net
www.neutropenia.org

Supports general and clinical research and provides information to the families, the medical community and the general public. Also committed to helping affected families and individuals work with hospitals, physicians, nurses, and other health care professionals.

Lee Reeves, President
Lucy Lyman, Board Member

4981 Severe Chronic Neutropenia International Registry (SCNIR)
Plaza 600 Bldg, 600 Stewart Street, Suite 1503
Seattle, WA 98101

206-543-9749
800-726-4463
Fax: 206-543-3668
e-mail: registry@u.washington.edu
www.depts.washington.edu/registry

The SCNIR was established in the United States, Australia, Canada, and the European Community. The SCNIR is directed by a scientific advisory board of physicians from around the world who care for SCN patients. Our mission is to established a world-wide database of treatment and disease-related outcomes for persons diagnosed with SCN. Collection of this information will lead to improved medical care and is used for research to determine the causes of neutropenia.

Audrey Anna Bolyard, Clinical Manager

Web Sites

4982 Online Mendelian Inheritance in Man
www.ncbi.nlm.nih.gov

This database is a catalog of human genes and genetic disorders.

Book Publishers

4983 Let's Talk About Going to the Hospital
Rosen Publishing Group's PowerKids Press
29 E 21st Street
New York, NY 10010

212-777-3017
800-237-9932
Fax: 888-436-4643
e-mail: rosenpub@tribeca.ios.com
www.powerkidspress.com

If a child has to check into the hospital, chances are he or she is already upset about being ill. Knowing how a hospital functions and what the procedures are, such as when family members can visit, will help in what is already a stressful situation. Grades K-5.

24 pages
ISBN: 0-823950-36-0

DESCRIPTION

4984 NIGHTMARES

Involves the following Biologic System(s):

Developmental/Behavioral/Psychiatric Disorders

Nightmares are a type of sleep disturbance that occurs during the rapid eye movement (REM) phase of sleep, or deep sleep stage. Vivid, disturbing dreams often evoke feelings of extreme and inescapable fear, terror, anxiety, and distress. Nightmares are often so intense that they awaken the sleeping individual, who is then usually able to recall all or most details of the dream.

Nightmares are quite common in children, particularly in the eight to 10 year old age group. Girls are more prone to this type of sleep disturbance than boys. Precipitating factors vary and may include breathing irregularities caused by the common cold or other illnesses; violent movies or television programs, especially in younger children; separation anxiety; and other traumatic experiences or events. In addition, children with certain types of psychological disturbances (e.g., affective, mood, or anxiety disorders) may experience repeated episodes of nightmares.

It is common for most children to experience occasional nightmares and, until the anxiety or fear of the experience passes, understanding and comfort by parents or caregivers is usually helpful. However, children who experience frequent nightmares may require a careful evaluation to determine if these episodes are a manifestation of an underlying psychologic disorder or other irregularity. If this is the case, treatment may be directed toward the underlying condition. Other treatment is supportive. For example, parents and caregivers are encouraged to be reassuring, understanding, and firm but nonthreatening. Reading or other quiet or soothing activities or rituals before bedtime may also be beneficial. In addition, night lights or other reasonable accommodations may be provided to reassure or comfort affected children.

See also **General Resources** on page 917

Government Agencies

4985 Center for Mental Health Services Knowledge Exchange Program

US Department of Health and Human Services
PO Box 42557
Washington, DC 20015

800-789-2647
Fax: 240-221-4295
TDD: 866-889-2647
http://mentalhealth.samhsa.gov

Supplies the public with responses to their commonly asked questions about mental health issues and services.

Kathryn Power, M.Ed., Director
Edward B. Searle M.B.A., Deputy Director

4986 NIH/National Institute of Mental Health

6001 Executive Boulevard, Room 8184, MSC 9663
Bethesda, MD 20892

301-443-4513
866-615-6464
Fax: 301-443-4279
TTY: 301-443-8431
e-mail: nimhinfo@nih.gov
www.nimh.nih.gov

Conducts strategic planning for specific research areas as well as for the Institute as a whole.

Dr Thomas R Insel, Director

National Associations & Support Groups

4987 American Academy of Sleep Medicine

1 Westbrook Corporate Center, Suite 920
Westchester, IL 60154

708-492-0930
Fax: 708-492-0943
www.aasmnet.org

National not-for-profit professional membership organization dedicated to the advancement of sleep medicine. The Academy's mission is to assure quality care for patients with sleep disorders, promote the advancement of sleep research and provide public and professional education. The AASM delivers programs, information and services to and through its members and advocates sleep medicine supportive policies in the medical community and the public sector.

Jerome Barrett, Executive Director
Jennifer Markkanen, Assistant Executive Director

4988 American Mental Health Foundation

1049 5th Avenue
New York, NY 10028
USA

212-639-1561
Fax: 212-737-9027

Dedicated to the extensive and intensive research in the theories and techniques of treatment of emotional illness and to the implementation of reforms in the mental health system. Efforts have resulted in development of better and less expensive treatment methods. Findings are disseminated in English and other major languages.

Monroe W Spero, MD

4989 Christian Horizons

PO Box 3381
Grand Rapids, MI 49501

616-956-7063
Fax: 616-956-7064
e-mail: info@christianhorizonsinc.org
www.christianhorizonsinc.org

To share Christ's love as we equip and support Adults with developmental disabilities.

4990 Federation of Families for Children's Mental Health
9605 Medical Center Drive, Suite 280
Rockville, MD 20850

240-403-1901
Fax: 240-403-1909
e-mail: ffcmh@ffcmh.org
www.ffcmh.org

The National family run organization is dedicated exclusively to helping children with mental health needs and their families achieve a better quality of life.

Sandra Spencer, Executive Director

4991 NADD: National Association for the Dually Diagnosed
132 Fair Street
Kingston, NY 12401

845-331-4336
800-331-5362
Fax: 845-331-4569
e-mail: info@thenadd.org
www.thenadd.org

Nonprofit organization designed to promote the interests of professional and parent development with resources for individuals who have the coexistence of mental illness and mental retardation. Provides conferences, educational services and training materials to professionals, parents, concerned citizens and service organizations.

Dr Robert Fletcher, CEO

4992 National Alliance for the Mentally Ill
2107 Wilson Blvd, Ste 300, Colonial Place Three
Arlington, VA 22201

703-524-7600
800-950-6264
Fax: 703-524-9094
TDD: 703-516-7227
e-mail: info@nami.org
www.nami.org

NAMI is a nonprofit, grassroots, self-help, support and advocacy organization of consumers, families and friends of people with severe mental illness, such as schizophrenia, bipolar disorder, major despressive disorder, obsessive compulsive disorder, anxiety disorders, autism and other severe and persistent mental illnesses that affect the brain.

Suzanne Vogel-Scibilia MD, President

4993 National Mental Health Association
2000 N Beauregard Street, 6th Floor
Alexandria, VA 22311

703-684-7722
800-969-6642
Fax: 703-684-5968
TTY: 800-433-5959
www.nmha.org

Addresses all aspects of mental health and mental illness. NMHA with over 340 affiliates works to improve the mental health of all Americans.

David L Shern PhD, President & CEO

4994 National Mental Health Consumers' Self-Help Clearinghouse
1211 Chestnut Street, Suite 1207
Philadelphia, PA 19107

215-751-1810
800-553-4539
Fax: 215-636-6312
e-mail: info@mhselfhelp.org
www.mhselfhelp.org

Offers information, support and appropriate referrals; and promotes public and professional education. Provides networking for those with special interests related to albinism. Promotes and supports research and funding that will improve diagnosis and management of albinism and hypopigmentation.

Joseph Rogers, Executive Director & Founder

4995 National Sleep Foundation
1522 K Street NW, Suite 500
Washington, DC 20005

202-347-3471
Fax: 202-347-3472
e-mail: nsf@sleepfoundation.org
www.sleepfoundation.org

An independent, nonprofit organization dedicated to improving public health and safety by achieving public understanding of sleep and sleep disorders, and by supporting public education, sleep-related research, and advocacy. Actively collaborates with sleep centers, support groups for patients with sleep disorders and safety organizations.

Richard Gelula, CEO

State Agencies & Support Groups

4996 Center for Family Support
333 7th Avenue, 9th Floor
New York, NY 10001

212-629-7939
Fax: 212-239-2211
www.cfsny.org

The Center for Family (CFS) is a not-for-profit human service agency providing support and assistance to individuals with developmental disabilities and traumatic brain injuries throughout New York City, Long Island, the lower Hudson Valley region and New Jersey.

Steven Vernickoff, Executive Director

Libraries & Resource Centers

4997 American Academy of Somnology
PO Box 27077
Las Vegas, NV 89126

702-371-0947
e-mail: somnology@aol.com
www.hopperinstitute.com/aas_intro.html

Covers about 75 physicians, dentists, nurses, psychologists, technicians, and students and sponsoring organizations, including associations, institutions, and corporations, with a special interest in sleep.

Web Sites

4998 CyberPsych
www.cyberpsych.org

CyberPsych presents information about psychoanalysis, psychotherapy, and special topics such as anxiety disorder, the problematic use of alcohol, homophobia, and the traumatic effects of racism. CyberPsych is a nonprofit network which offers free web hosting and technical support for internet communication, to non profit groups and individuals.

4999 Planetpsych
www.planetpsych.com

Planetpsych is an online resource for mental health information.

5000 Psych Central
www.psychcentral.com

Offers free informational and educational articles and resources on psychology, support and mental health online.

5001 Sleep Disorders
http://talhost.net/sleep/parasomnia.htm

For those who have sleep disorders and have a problem sleeping.

5002 Sleepdisorders.com

www.sleepdisorders.com

Updated monthly and organized by sleep disorders with quality links.

Book Publishers

5003 Concise Guide to Evaluation and Management of Sleep Disorders

American Psychiatric Publishing
1000 Wilson Boulevard, Suite 1825
Arlington, VA 22209

703-907-7322
800-368-5777
Fax: 703-907-1091
e-mail: appi@psych.org
www.appi.org

Overview of sleep disorders medicine, sleep physiology and pathology, insomnia complaints, excessive sleepiness disorders, parasomnias, medical and psychiatric disorders and sleep, medications with sedative-hypnotic properties, special problems and populations.

2002 296 pages Paper 3rd Ed
ISBN: 1-585620-45-6

5004 Depression and Sleep

American Psychiatric Press
1400 K Street, NW
Washington, DC 20005

202-682-6262
800-368-5777
Fax: 202-789-2648
e-mail: order@appi.com
www.appi.com

Contents include normal sleep, neurochemistry of sleep, sleep in depression, neurochemistry of depression, antidepressent drugs and sleep, and clinical management of sleep disorders in depression.

1996 64 pages

5005 Sleep Disorders Diagnosis and Treatment: Current Clinical Practice Series

Humana Press
999 Riverview Drive Suite 208
Totowa, NJ 07512

973-256-1699
Fax: 973-256-8341
e-mail: humana@humanapr.com
www.appi.com

1998 250 pages
ISBN: 0-896035-27-1

5006 Sleep Disorders and Psychiatry

Daniel J Buysse MD, author

American Psychiatric Publishing
1000 Wilson Boulevard, Ste 1825
Arlington, VA 22209

703-907-7322
800-368-5777
Fax: 703-907-1091
e-mail: appi@psych.org
www.appi.org

Summarizes the major categories of sleep disorders including parasomnias and narcolepsy.

2005 256 pages Paperback
ISBN: 1-585622-29-0

5007 Snoring From A to Zzzz

Spencer Press
2525 NW Lovejoy Street, Suite 402
Portland, OR 97210

503-223-4959
Fax: 503-223-1608
e-mail: dereklipman@aol.com

Covers organizations, associations, support groups, and manufacturers of sleep-related medical products relevant to sleep disorders. Discussess every aspect of snoring abd sleep apnea from causes to cures.

256 pages Paperback
ISBN: 0-965070-81-6

Derek Lipman MD, Author/Editor

DESCRIPTION

5008 NIGHT TERRORS

Synonyms: Pavor nocturnus, Sleep-terror disorder

Involves the following Biologic System(s):

Developmental/Behavioral/Psychiatric Disorders

Night terrors is a sleep disorder characterized by episodes of sudden awakening from sleep in an extremely anxious or terrified state. This sleep disturbance occurs in from two to five children out of every hundred, and, in most cases, begins during the fourth to seventh year of life. Sleep-terror disorder more commonly affects boys than girls and often disappears before the onset of adolescence.

Episodes of night terrors usually take place during the third or fourth stage of the nonrapid eye movement or NREM phase of sleep. Each stage of NREM sleep is a successively deeper sleep leading up to rapid eye movement sleep or a deep REM during which dreams may occur. Typically, affected children awaken abruptly and may be screaming and extremely frightened. They may be in a semiconscious state and unaware of or unable to recognize people or surroundings. These children are generally inconsolable and may exhibit such physical symptoms as sweating; widening (dilation) of the pupils; elevated heart rate (tachycardia); abnormally deep, rapid breathing (hyperventilation); and violent thrashing. In about a third of patients, sleepwalking (somnambulism) may also occur. Children are usually able to fall back to sleep within minutes of these short-lived episodes and have no memory of the event when they awaken.

Night terrors are most often confused with nightmares, but unlike night terrors, a child having a nightmare is usually easily woken up and comforted. Sleep disorders such as night terrors often result from childhood fears or anxieties. For example, some young children may be apprehensive about going to bed because this actually represents a temporary separation from their parents (separation anxiety). In addition, any issues affecting the family or child (e.g., separation, divorce, death, school performance, social interactions, etc.) may translate into disturbances in normal sleep patterns. Other contributing factors may include the presence of a fever,depression, or other emotional disorders.

Although the administration of certain antianxiety and antidepressant drugs may, in some cases, be of benefit, treatment of night terrors is mainly supportive. If the precipitating cause can be determined, steps may then be taken to alleviate the fear or anxiety. In any case, parents or caregivers are encouraged to be supportive and firm, but nonjudgmental. Excitement before bedtime is discouraged; however, reading or other quiet, pleasurable activities may be beneficial.

See also **General Resources** on page 917

Government Agencies

5009 Center for Mental Health Services Knowledge Exchange Program
US Department of Health and Human Services
PO Box 42557
Washington, DC 20015

800-789-2647
Fax: 240-747-5470
TDD: 866-889-2647
http://mentalhealth.samhsa.gov

Supplies the public with responses to their commonly asked questions about mental health issues and services.

5010 NIH/National Institute of Mental Health
6001 Executive Boulevard, Room 8184, MSC 9663
Bethesda, MD 20892

301-443-4513
866-615-6464
Fax: 301-443-4279
TTY: 301-443-8431
e-mail: nimhinfo@nih.gov
www.nimh.nih.gov

Conducts strategic planning for specific research areas as well as for the Institute as a whole.

Dr Thomas R Insel, Director

National Associations & Support Groups

5011 American Academy of Sleep Medicine
1 Westbrook Corporate Center, Suite 920
Westchester, IL 60154

708-492-0930
Fax: 708-492-0943
www.aasmnet.org

National not-for-profit professional membership organization dedicated to the advancement of sleep medicine. The Academy's mission is to assure quality care for patients with sleep disorders, promote the advancement of sleep research and provide public and professional education. The AASM delivers programs, information and services to and through its members and advocates sleep medicine supportive policies in the medical community and the public sector.

Michael H. Silber MBChb, President
Clete A. Kushida MD PhD, Rpsgt, Secretary/Treasurer

5012 American Mental Health Foundation
1049 5th Avenue
New York, NY 10028
USA

212-639-1561
Fax: 212-737-9027

Dedicated to the extensive and intensive research in the theories and techniques of treatment of emotional illness and to the implementation of reforms in the mental health system. Efforts have resulted in development of better and less expensive treatment methods. Findings are disseminated in English and other major languages.

Monroe W Spero, MD

5013 Christian Horizons
PO Box 3381
Grand Rapids, MI 49501

616-956-7063
Fax: 616-956-7063
e-mail: info@christianhorizonsinc.org
www.christianhorizonsinc.org

Devoted to assisting individuals, with developmental disabilities, on a day-to-day basis.

5014 Federation of Families for Children's Mental Health
9605 Medical Center Drive, Suite 280
Rockville, MD 20850

240-403-1901
Fax: 240-403-1909
e-mail: ffcmh@ffcmh.org
www.ffcmh.org

The National family run organization is dedicated exclusively to helping children with mental health needs and their families achieve a better quality of life.

Sandra Spencer, Executive Director

5015 NADD: National Association for the Dually Diagnosed
132 Fair Street
Kingston, NY 12401

845-331-4336
800-331-5362
Fax: 845-331-4569
e-mail: info@thenadd.org
www.thenadd.org

Nonprofit organization designed to promote the interests of professional and parent development with resources for individuals who have the coexistence of mental illness and mental retardation. Provides conferences, educational services and training materials to professionals, parents, concerned citizens and service organizations.

Dr Robert Fletcher, CEO

5016 National Mental Health Consumers' Self-Help Clearinghouse
1211 Chestnut Street, Suite 1207
Philadelphia, PA 19107

215-751-1810
800-553-4539
Fax: 215-636-6312
e-mail: info@mhselfhelp.org
www.mhselfhelp.org

Offers information, support and appropriate referrals; and promotes public and professional education. Provides networking for those with special interests related to albinism. Promotes and supports research and funding that will improve diagnosis and management of albinism and hypopigmentation.

Joseph Rogers, Executive Director & Founder

5017 National Sleep Foundation
1522 K Street NW, Suite 500
Washington, DC 20005

202-347-3471
Fax: 202-347-3472
e-mail: nsf@sleepfoundation.org
www.sleepfoundation.org

An independent, nonprofit organization dedicated to improving public health and safety by achieving public understanding of sleep and sleep disorders, and by supporting public education, sleep-related research, and advocacy. Actively collaborates with sleep centers, support groups for patients with sleep disorders and safety organizations.

Richard Gelula, CEO

State Agencies & Support Groups

5018 Center for Disabilities and Development
University of Iowa Hospitals and Clinics
100 Hawkins Drive
Iowa City, IA 52242

319-353-6900
877-686-0031
e-mail: cdd-webmaster@uiowa.edu
www.uihealthcare.com

A trusted resource for healthcare, training, research and information for people with disabilities that include: behavior disorders, brain injury, cerebral palsy, diabetes, down syndrome, learning disabilities, mental retardation, sleep disorders and spina bifida.

Elayne Sexsmith, Administrator
Amy Mikelson, Supervisor Info Resource Service

5019 Center for Family Support
333 7th Avenue, 9th Floor
New York, NY 10001

212-629-7939
Fax: 212-239-2211
www.cfsny.org

The Center for Family (CFS) is a not-for-profit human service agency providing support and assistance to individuals with developmental disabilities and traumatic brain injuries throughout New York City, Long Island, the lower Hudson Valley region and New Jersey.

Steven Vernickofs, Executive Director

Libraries & Resource Centers

5020 American Academy of Somnology
PO Box 27077
Las Vegas, NV 89126

702-371-0947
e-mail: somnology@aol.com
www.hopperinstitute.com/aas_intro.html

Covers about 75 physicians, dentists, nurses, psychologists, technicians, and students and sponsoring organizations, including associations, institutions, and corporations, with a special interest in sleep.

Research Centers

5021 UC Berkeley School of Social Welfare
Mental Health & Social Welfare Research Group
303 Haviland Hall
Berkeley, CA 94720

510-642-3949
e-mail: spsegal@berkeley.edu
socialwelfare.berkeley.edu/mhswrg/mhswrg.html

Steven P Segal, Director

Web Sites

5022 About.com on Sleep Disorders
www.sleepdisorders.about.com

Well-organized information including new developments and a chat room.

5023 CyberPsych
www.cyberpsych.org

Presents information about psychoanalysis, psychtherapy and special topics such as anxiety disorder, the problamatic use of alcohol, homophobia, and the traumatic effects of racism.

5024 Planetpsych
www.planetpsych.com

Online resource for mental health information.

5025 Psych Central
www.psychcentral.com

Offers free informational and educational articles and resources on psychology, support and mental health online.

5026 Sleep Disorders
http://talhost.net/sleep/parasomnia.htm

For those who have sleep disorders and have a problem sleeping.

5027 Sleepdisorders.com
www.sleepdisorders.com

Updated monthly and organized by sleep disorders with quality links.

Book Publishers

5028 Concise Guide to Evaluation and Management of Sleep Disorders
American Psychiatric Publishing
1000 Wilson Boulevard, Suite 1825
Arlington, VA 22209

703-907-7322
800-368-5777
Fax: 703-907-1091
e-mail: appi@psych.org
www.appi.org

Overview of sleep disorders medicine, sleep physiology and pathology, insomnia complaints, excessive sleepiness disorders, parasomnias, medical and psychiatric disorders and sleep, medications with sedative-hypnotic properties, special problems and populations.

2002 296 pages Paper 3rd Ed
ISBN: 1-585620-45-6

5029 Depression and Sleep
American Psychiatric Press
1400 K Street NW
Washington, DC 20005

202-682-6262
800-368-5777
Fax: 202-789-2648
e-mail: order@appi.com
www.appi.com

Contents include normal sleep, neurochemistry of sleep, sleep in depression, neurochemistry of depression, antidepressent drugs and sleep, and clinical management of sleep disorders in depression.

1996 64 pages

5030 Principles and Practice of Sleep Medicine
Elsevier Health Sciences Division
1600 John F Kennedy Blvd, Suite 1800
Philadelphia, PA 19103

215-239-3900
800-545-2522
Fax: 215-239-3990
www.us.elsevierhealth.com

Covers the recent advances in basic sciences as well as sleep pathology in adults. Encompasses developments in this rapidly advancing field and also includes topics related to psychiatry, circadian rhythms, cardiovascualr diseases and sleep apnea diagnosis and treatment. Hardcover.

2005 1552 pages 4th Edition
ISBN: 0-721607-97-7

5031 Sleep Disorders Diagnosis and Treatment: Current Clinical Practice Series
American Psyciatric Publishing Group
1400 K Street NW
Washington, DC 20005

202-682-6262
800-368-5777
Fax: 202-789-2648
e-mail: order@appi.com
www.appi.com

1998 250 pages

5032 Sleep Disorders and Psychiatry
Daniel J Buysse MD, author

American Psychiatric Publishing
1000 Wilson Boulevard, Ste 1825
Arlington, VA 22209

703-907-7322
800-368-5777
Fax: 703-907-1091
e-mail: appi@psych.org
www.appi.org

Summarizes the major categories of sleep disorders including parasomnias and narcolepsy.

2005 256 pages Paperback
ISBN: 1-585622-29-0

5033 Snoring From A to Zzzz
Spencer Press
2525 NW Lovejoy Street, Suite 402
Portland, OR 97210

503-223-4959
Fax: 503-223-1608
e-mail: dereklipman@aol.com

Covers organizations, associations, support groups, and manufacturers of sleep-related medical products relevant to sleep disorders. Discussess every aspect of snoring abd sleep apnea from causes to cures.

256 pages Paperback
ISBN: 0-965070-81-6

Derek S Lipman, MD, Author/Editor

5034 Snoring From A to Zzzz: Proven Cures for the Night's Worst Nuisance
2525 NW Lovejoy Street, Suite 402
Portland, OR 97210

503-223-4959
Fax: 503-223-1608
e-mail: dereklipman@aol.com
www.foxcontent.com/snoring/htm

This book by a medical expert contains every aspect of snoring and sleep apnea from causes to cures. The latest edition includes an expanded section on sleep disordered breathing in children, a subject of great interest in the pediatric world.

Softcover

Derek S Lipman, MD, Author/Editor

DESCRIPTION

5035 NOCTURNAL ENURESIS

Synonym: Bed-wetting

Involves the following Biologic System(s):

Developmental/Behavioral/Psychiatric Disorders, Renal and Urologic Disorders

Nocturnal enuresis or bed-wetting refers to the discharge of urine during the night by children who have achieved urinary control during other periods of the day. It affects an estimated 5 to 7 million children in the United States. This type of bed-wetting is considered primary enuresis if nightly urinary incontinence has persisted since birth. Nocturnal enuresis that occurs in children who were previously continent during the night for a period of one year or more is considered secondary enuresis, a regressive form of this abnormality. Bed-wetting is a very common problem that occurs more often in boys than in girls and tends to run in families. In most cases, enuresis resolves spontaneously. The causes of nocturnal enuresis are varied and may include delayed maturation of certain functions of the nervous system that regulate bladder control, psychological influences, spinal abnormalities (e.g., spina bifida), structural abnormalities or defects, underlying disease (e.g., diabetes mellitus), urinary tract infection, or other physical causes. Secondary enuresis may be precipitated by stressful or traumatic events such as the birth of another child, death, divorce, or other situations that impact on the normal day-to-day routine.

Children with enuresis may undergo evaluation in order to determine if the condition is caused by neurological or physical problems. If this is the case, treatment is geared toward the underlying problem. Other treatment may include such supportive measures as establishing a reward system to give the child incentive to cooperate, charting the child's progress in order to offer positive reinforcement, limiting liquid intake before bedtime, having the child urinate directly before going to bed, and having affected older children take part in laundering soiled clothing and remaking the bed. Parents and caregivers are typically counseled to remain supportive and nonjudgmental. Additional treatment may include behavioral therapy and other counseling that involves both the parents or caregivers and the affected child. Bed-wetting alarms that detect small amounts of urine and certain types of medication (e.g., imipramine and desmopressin acetate nasal spray) may also be used to control enuresis. Imipramine is an antidepressant drug that is usually effective within two weeks; however, relapses are common after the drug is gradually stopped and, therefore, a longer course of administration may become necessary. Desmopressin acetate nasal spray reduces urine output in approximately 70 percent of affected children; however, its beneficial effect is temporary. Other treatment is supportive.

See also **General Resources** on page 917

Government Agencies

5036 NIH/National Institute of Mental Health
6001 Executive Boulevard, Room 8184, MSC 9663
Bethesda, MD 20892

301-443-4513
866-615-6464
Fax: 301-443-4279
TTY: 301-443-8431
e-mail: nimhinfo@nih.gov
www.nimh.nih.gov

Conducts strategic planning for specific research areas as well as for the Institute as a whole.

Dr Thomas R Insel, Director

5037 National Kidney and Urologic Diseases Information Clearinghouse
3 Information Way
Bethesda, MD 20892

800-891-5390
Fax: 703-738-4929
e-mail: nkudic@info.niddk.nih.gov
www.2.niddk.nih.gov

To increase knowledge and understanding about diseases of the kidneys and urologic system among people with these conditions and their families, health care professionals and the general public.

Josie Briggs MD, Director

National Associations & Support Groups

5038 American Urological Association Foundation
1000 Corporate Boulevard, Suite 410
Linthicum, MD 21090

410-689-3700
866-746-4282
Fax: 410-689-3800
e-mail: auafoundation@auafoundation.org
www.auafoundation.org

Partners with physicians, researchers, healthcare professionals, patients, families, caregivers and the public to support, promote research, and patient/public education and advocacy in improving the prevention, detection, treatment and cure of urologic diseases.

Lawrence S Ross, President
Robert C. Flannigan MD, Secretary

5039 Association for the Bladder Exstrophy Community
3075 First Street
La Salle, MI 48145

734-243-9912
866-300-2222
Fax: 734-243-9912
e-mail: admin@bladderexstrophy.com
www.bladderexstrophy.com

The ABC is an international support network of individuals with bladder exstrophy (includes classic exstrophy, cloacal exstrophy, and epispadias), local parent-exstrophy support groups, and health care providers working with patients and families living with bladder exstrophy.

Cindy Buckly, Executive Director
Barbara Ward, President, Webmaster & Int. Liaison

5040 Federation of Families for Children's Mental Health
9605 Medical Center Drive, Suite 280
Rockville, MD 20850

240-403-1901
Fax: 240-403-1909
e-mail: ffcmh@ffcmh.org
www.ffcmh.org

The National family run organization is dedicated exclusively to helping children with mental health needs and their families achieve a better quality of life.

Sandra Spencer, Executive Director

5041 National Mental Health Association
2000 N Beauregard Street, 6th Floor
Alexandria, VA 22311

703-684-7722
800-969-6642
Fax: 703-684-5968
TTY: 800-433-5959
www.nmha.org

Addresses all aspects of mental health and mental illness. NMHA with over 340 affiliates works to improve the mental health of all Americans.

David L Shern PhD, President & CEO

5042 National Mental Health Consumers' Self-Help Clearinghouse
1211 Chestnut Street, Suite 1207
Philadelphia, PA 19107

215-751-1810
800-553-4539
Fax: 215-636-6312
e-mail: info@mhselfhelp.org
www.mhselfhelp.org

Offers information, support and appropriate referrals; and promotes public and professional education. Provides networking for those with special interests related to albinism. Promotes and supports research and funding that will improve diagnosis and management of albinism and hypopigmentation.

Joseph Rogers, Executive Director & Founder

5043 National Sleep Foundation
1522 K Street NW, Suite 500
Washington, DC 20005

202-347-3471
Fax: 202-347-3472
e-mail: nsf@sleepfoundation.org
www.sleepfoundation.org

Works to improve the quality of life for millions of Americans who suffer from sleep disorders, and to prevent the catastrophic accidents that are related to poor or disordered sleep through research, education and the dissemination of information towards the cause of the Narcolepsy Project. Seeks patients to aid new research project targeting the cause of the disorder.

Richard Gelula, CEO

Web Sites

5044 American Urological Association Foundation
www.urologyhealth.org

Provides information on enuresis as well as other pediatric disorders related to the kidneys and bladder.

5045 Bedwetting Online
www.bedwetting.ferring.ca

Helps parents and children deal with Nocturnal Enuresis.

5046 Child Development Institute
childdevelopmentinfo.com/disorders/bedwetting.shtml

Child development and parent information for learning, health and safety, as well as child disorders.

5047 Dr. Koop
www.drkoop.com/ency/93/003144.html

Information on the condition, causes, symptoms, tests and treatment.

5048 National Kidney Foundation
www.kidney.org/patients/bw/index.cfm

Information for parents, kids and teens, and medical professionals on bed-wetting.

DESCRIPTION

5049 NON-HODGKIN'S LYMPHOMA

Synonym: NHL

Covers these related disorders: Non-Hodgkin's lymphoma, large cell type, Non-Hodgkin's lymphoma, lymphoblastic type, Non-Hodgkin's lymphoma, small noncleaved cell(SNC)

Involves the following Biologic System(s):
Hematologic and Oncologic Disorders

Non-Hodgkin's lymphoma is a group of diseases characterized by malignant tumors of lymphoid tissue (lymphoma). These cancerous tumors usually develop due to uncontrolled growth of certain white blood cells (B and T lymphocytes) that are components of the lymphatic and immune systems. The lymphatic system includes a network of vessels that collect lymphatic fluid (lymph) from the different areas of the body and drain this fluid into the bloodstream. As lymph moves through the lymphatic system, it is filtered by a network of lymph nodes, which are relatively small structures located along the course of the lymphatic vessels. Lymph nodes store certain white blood cells (lymphocytes) and are thought to play a role in producing antibodies, thus functioning as part of the body's immune system. Some of the white blood cells known as T lymphocytes (i.e., helper cells) assist in the recognition of foreign proteins and help to activate other T lymphocytes (killer cells), which bind to cells invaded by viruses or other microorganisms and destroy them (cell-mediated immunity). The white blood cells known as B lymphocytes produce antibodies, which recognize and help to neutralize or destroy invading microorganisms (humoral-mediated immunity).

Malignancies of lymph tissue, known as lymphomas, are the third most common form of childhood cancer in the United States, affecting about 13 per one million children annually. There are two major categories of lymphoma, including non-Hodgkin's lymphoma (NHL) and Hodgkin's disease. Although NHL most often affects individuals over age 50, these malignancies may develop in children, particularly those with impaired immune systems. These include patients with acquired immune deficiency syndrome (AIDS) or certain genetic immunodeficiency disorders that are present at birth (primary immunodeficiencies), such as Wiskott-Aldrich syndrome, X-linked lymphoproliferative syndrome, or ataxia-telangiectasia. About 50,000 patients are diagnosed with NHL in the U.S. each year. Although the cause of the disease is unknown, researchers suggest that immune mechanisms play an important role.

A common feature of the various non-Hodgkin's lymphomas is the absence of a particular cancerous cell type that is seen in patients with Hodgkin's disease. These cancerous cells, known as Reed-Sternberg cells, are relatively large, abnormal white blood cells that have more than one nucleus (multinucleated) and a distinctive appearance under a microscope. Children with NHL typically have highly malignant forms of lymphoma that rapidly infiltrate entire, affected lymph nodes (diffuse, high-grade tumors). There are several classification systems used to categorize the different forms of non-Hodgkin's lymphoma. However, the high-grade lymphoid tumors typically seen in children with the disease are often classified based upon their cellular structure and composition, including the type of white blood cells from which the tumor cells are derived (e.g., B or T lymphocytes). Primary, high-grade subtypes of NHL include small noncleaved cell (SNCC) NHL, including Burkitt's and non-Burkitt subtypes; large cell NHL; and lymphoblastic NHL.

In children with NHL, initial symptoms and findings vary and depend upon the specific location and extent of the disease. Most forms of NHL arise from lymph nodes in the head and neck region, the space in the chest cavity between the lungs (mediastinum), or the abdomen. Rarely, NHL may develop in other lymph nodes or affect the skin, bone, thyroid gland, or other areas. There is a close association between specific NHL subtypes and initial disease sites. For example, SNCC NHL usually initially develops in the head and neck or abdominal region. Lymphoblastic NHL tends to arise in the head and neck region or in the front of the chest cavity between the lungs (anterior mediastinum). Large cell NHL may develop in any area of the body.

Depending on disease location, associated findings often include painless swelling of lymph nodes in the neck, the groin area, or deep within the abdominal or chest region. Tumor development in the area of the mediastinum may result in abnormal accumulations of fluid between layers of the membrane lining the lungs and the chest cavity (pleural effusion), difficulties breathing, and abnormal swelling of tissues of the face, neck, and arms. Involvement of the tonsils may cause difficulty in swallowing. Children with abdominal involvement typically experience nausea, vomiting, lack of appetite (anorexia), abdominal pain and swelling (distension), severe constipation, or other digestive symptoms. In those with NHL that affects the skin, associated findings include dark, thickened, itchy patches of skin. Tumor infiltration of the bone marrow may result in abnormally low levels of circulating red blood cells (anemia) or platelets (thrombocytopenia). In advanced cases, involvement of the brain may cause increased fluid pressure around the brain, severe headache, paralysis of certain nerve pairs arising from the brain (cranial nerve palsies), or other findings. In addition, advancing disease may cause progressive impairment of the body's immune system, leading to potentially severe or life-threatening complications due to certain infections.

NHL is classified into different stages, based upon the number and location of lymphatic tumors or affected node-like areas (nodules), the degree that the disease may have spread , and other factors. The treatment of children with NHL varies, depending on the stage of the disease and other factors. Therapy with certain anticancer drugs (combination chemotherapy), such as CHOP, a regimen containing cyclophosphamide, doxorubicin hydrochloride, vincristine (also called Oncovin, and prednisilone, is effective for many children. Radiation therapy is not used as a primary treatment in most children with NHL. New treatment, known as immunotherapy, uses an ant ibody that is designed specifically against cancer cells. In individuals with advanced disease, treatment may include measures to prevent brain involvement and potentially associated neurologic symptoms. Bone marrow transplantation has been shown to be an effective treatment for some children with NHL who experience replapse or have advanced disease that is unresponsive to combination chemotherapy.

See also **General Resources** on page 917

See also **General Resources** on page 917

Government Agencies

5050 NIH/National Cancer Institute
6116 Executive Boulevard, Room 3036A
Bethesda, MD 20892

800-422-6237
www.cancer.gov

The National Cancer Institute coordinates the National Cancer Program, which conducts and supports research, training, health information dissemination, and other programs with respect to the cause, diagnosis, prevention, and treatment of cancer, rehabilitation from cancer, and the continuing care of cancer patients and the families of cancer patients.

John E Niederhuber MD, Director

National Associations & Support Groups

5051 Candlelighters Childhood Cancer Foundation
PO Box 498
Kensington, MD 20895

301-962-3520
800-366-2223
Fax: 310-962-3521
e-mail: staff@candlelighters.org
www.candlelighters.org

The Candlelighters Childhood Cancer Foundation National Office was founded in 1970 by concerned parents of children with cancer. Today our membership of over 50,000 members of the national office and more than 100,000 members across the across the country, including Candlelighters affiliate groups, includes, parents of children who are being treated or have been treated for cancer.

Ruth Hoffman, Executive Director

5052 Leukemia & Lymphoma Society
1311 Mamaroneck Avenue, Suite 310
White Plains, NY 10605

914-949-5213
Fax: 914-949-6691
www.leukemia-lymphoma.org

Large voluntary health organization dedicated to funding blood cancer research, education and patient services.

Dwayne Howell, President & CEO
Larry Hausner, Chief Operating Officer

5053 Lymphoma Research Foundation
111 Broadway, 19th Floor
New York, NY 10006

800-235-6848
www.lymphoma.org

Voluntary lymphoma-focused voluntary health organization devoted to funding lymphoma research and providing critical information on the disease.

Errol M Cook, President
Evelyn Lipori, VP/Secretary

5054 National Childhood Cancer Foundation
4600 East West Highway, Suite 600
Bethesda, MD 20814

800-458-6223
e-mail: info@curesearch.org
www.curesearch.org

CureSearch unites the world's largest childhood cancer research organization, the Children's Oncology Group, and the National Childhood Cancer Foundation through our mission to cure childhood cancer. Research is the key to the cure.

5055 Wellness Community
2716 Ocean Park Boulevard, #1040
Santa Monica, CA 90405

310-314-2555
Fax: 310-314-7586
e-mail: info@twc-wla.org
www.twc-wla.org

Helps people with cancer and their loved ones enhance their health and well-being by providing a professional program of emotional support, education and hope.

Janet Galea, Executive Director
Bonnie Schuman, Communications & Media Relations

Web Sites

5056 CancerCare
www.cancercare.org

A national nonprofit organization dedicated to providing free, professional support services to those affected by cancer.

5057 Children's Cancer Web
www.cancerindex.org/ccw

An independent nonprofit site, established to provide a directory of childhood cancer resources.

5058 Leukemia and Lymphoma Society of America
www.leukemia.org

Is the largest voluntary health organization dedicated to funding blood cancer research, education and patient services. The mission is to cure leukemia, lymphoma, Hodgkin's disease and myeloma, and to improve the quality of life of patients and their families.

5059 Lymphoma Innovations
www.lymphomainnovations.com

Targeted information for people with Non Hodgkins Lymphoma.

Book Publishers

5060 Let's Talk About Going to the Hospital
Rosen Publishing Group's PowerKids Press
29 E 21st Street
New York, NY 10010

212-777-3017
800-237-9932
Fax: 888-436-4643
e-mail: rosenpub@tribeca.ios.com
www.powerkidspress.com

If a child has to check into the hospital, chances are he or she is already upset about being ill. Knowing how a hospital functions and what the procedures are, such as when family members can visit, will help in what is already a stressful situation. Grades K-5.

24 pages
ISBN: 0-823950-36-0

5061 Let's Talk About When Kids Have Cancer

Melanie Apel Gordon, author

Rosen Publishing Group's PowerKids Press
29 E 21st Street
New York, NY 10010

212-777-3017
800-237-9932
Fax: 888-436-4643
e-mail: customerservice@rosenpub.com
www.powerkidspress.com

In a straightforward yet comforting way, this book explains what cancer is, what kinds of treatments surround the disease and how to cope if a child or the friend of a child has cancer.

24 pages Paperback
ISBN: 0-823951-95-2

5062 Pediatric Cancer Sourcebook
Omnigraphics
PO Box 625
Holmes, PA 19043

800-234-1340
Fax: 800-875-1340
e-mail: info@omnigraphics.com
www.omnigraphics.com

Basic consumer health information about leukemias, brain tumors, sarcomas, lymphomas and other cancers in infants, children and adolescents.

1999 587 pages
ISBN: 0-780802-45-4

5063 Surviving Childhood Cancer: A Guide for Families
New Harbinger Publications
5674 Shattuck Avenue
Oakland, CA 94609

510-652-0215
800-748-6273
Fax: 510-652-5472
e-mail: customerservice@newharbinger.com
www.newharbinger.com

Cancer in a child is an overwhelming experience for a family. This book explains common medical procedures and offers readers practical advice about how to cope with emotions and stress during this time.

232 pages Paperback
ISBN: 1-572241-02-0

DESCRIPTION

5064 NOONAN SYNDROME

Synonyms: Female Pseudo-Turner syndrome, Male Turner syndrome, NS

Involves the following Biologic System(s):

Cardiovascular Disorders,

Genetic/Chromosomal/Syndrome/Metabolic Disorders

Noonan syndrome is a genetic disorder that is usually apparent at birth (congenital). The symptoms and findings associated with the disorder may be extremely variable, differing in range and severity from case to case. However, children with Noonan syndrome often have short stature, webbing of the neck (pterygium colli), and characteristic abnormalities of the head and facial (craniofacial) area, such as downwardly slanting eyelid folds (palpebral fissures), drooping of the upper eyelids (ptosis), a small jaw (micrognathia), and prominent, low-set ears that are rotated toward the back of the head. In addition, in many affected males, the testes fail to descend into the scrotum (cryptorchidism) before birth or during the first year of life. Therefore, in some cases, the male reproductive cells (sperm) may fail to develop appropriately within the testes, potentially causing infertility. Many children with Noonan syndrome also have distinctive skeletal malformations, such as abnormal depression of the lower portion of the breastbone (pectus excavatum) and protrusion of the upper portion of the breastbone (pectus carinatum); outward deviation of the elbows upon extension (cubitus valgus); sideways curvature of the spine (scoliosis); or front-to-back curvature of the spine (kyphosis). Affected children may also have structural heart abnormalities that are present at birth (congenital heart defects), particularly obstruction of the normal blood flow from the lower right pumping chamber (ventricle) of the heart to the lungs (pulmonary valvular stenosis). During infancy, there may also be an abnormal accumulation of lymph fluid in and associated swelling of body tissues (lymphedema) due to lymphatic system malformations. Additional symptoms and findings may include deficient functioning of certain blood cells known as platelets that play an essential role in preventing or stopping bleeding, abnormally low levels of circulating platelets (thrombocytopenia), or blood clotting (coagulation factor) deficiencies, potentially causing abnormal bleeding and susceptibility to bruising. In some cases, affected children may also have mental retardation or experience delays in acquiring certain skills that require the coordination of physical and mental activities (psychomotor retardation). The treatment of children with Noonan syndrome includes symptomatic and supportive measures, such as certain medications or surgical intervention for those with congenital heart defects; surgery to move undescended testes into the scrotum (orchiopexy) in males with cryptorchidism; possible hormone replacement therapy (i.e., human growth hormone therapy); appropriate preventive or supportive measures for those with platelet dysfunction, thrombocytopenia, coagulation deficiences, or lymphedema; special education; and other treatment measures as required.

In most cases, Noonan syndrome appears to occur randomly (sporadically) due to spontaneous genetic changes (mutations). In other cases, the disorder may be inherited as an autosomal dominant trait. A gene responsible for Noonan syndrome has been located on the long arm (q) of chromosome 12 (12q24). Most estimates in the literature indicate that the disorder may affect approximately one in 1,000 to 2,500 newborns. However, due to the wide variablity of associated symptoms and findings, it may be difficult to determine the true frequency of Noonan syndrome in the general population. Genetic counseling is recommended if there is a family history of Noonan syndrome.

See also **General Resources** on page 917

See also **General Resources** on page 917

National Associations & Support Groups

5065 Genetic Alliance
4301 Connecticut Avenue NW
Washington, DC 20008

202-966-5557
800-336-4363
Fax: 202-966-8553
e-mail: info@geneticalliance.org
www.geneticalliance.org

A coalition of voluntary genetic support groups, consumers and professionals addressing the needs of individuals and families affected by genetic disorders from a national perspective.

Sharon Terry, President/CEO

5066 Human Growth Foundation
997 Glen Cove Avenue, Suite 5
Glen Head, NY 11545

516-671-4041
800-451-6434
Fax: 516-671-4055
e-mail: hgfl@hgfound.org
www.hgfound.org

Nonprofit organization devoted to research and advocacy regarding people with growth and growth hormone disorders.

Patricia D Costa, Executive Director

5067 MAGIC Foundation: Major Aspects of Growth in Children
6645 W North Avenue
Oak Park, IL 60302

708-383-0808
800-362-4423
Fax: 708-383-0899
e-mail: mary@magicfoundation.org
www.magicfoundation.org

A national nonprofit organization providing support and education regarding growth disorders in children and related adult disorders. Provides educational information, networking, a national conference, a kids' program and an extensive medical library.

Mary Andrews, CEO
Dianne Tamburrino, Executive Director

5068 March of Dimes Birth Defects Foundation
1275 Mamaroneck Avenue
White Plains, NY 10605

914-428-7100
888-663-4637
Fax: 914-428-8203
e-mail: resourcecenter@modimes.org
www.marchofdimes.com

Partnership of volunteers and professionals dedicates to improving the health of babies by preventing birth defects and infant mortality. Over 100 chapters are located across the country and can be located through the National Office.

Dr Jennifer Howse, President

5069 Noonan Syndrome Support Group
PO Box 145
Upperco, MD 21155

410-374-5245
888-686-2224
e-mail: info@noonansyndrome.org
www.noonansnydrome.org

Sharing of information and encouragement among individuals who have been affected by the syndrome. The organization offers forums where physicians and other professionals can provide information on living with the daily challenges. Offers an online newsletter.

Wanda Robinson, President
Dave Robinson, VP

Web Sites

5070 Family Village
www.familyvillage.wisc.edu

A global community that integrates information, resources and communication opportunities on the Internet for persons with cognitive and other disabilities, for their families and for those that provide them services and support.

5071 Online Mendelian Inheritance in Man
www.ncbi.nlm.nih.gov

This database is a catalog of human genes and genetic disorders.

Book Publishers

5072 Let's Talk About Going to the Hospital
Rosen Publishing Group's PowerKids Press
29 E 21st Street
New York, NY 10010

212-777-3017
800-237-9932
Fax: 888-436-4643
e-mail: rosenpub@tribeca.ios.com
www.powerkidspress.com

If a child has to check into the hospital, chances are he or she is already upset about being ill. Knowing how a hospital functions and what the procedures are, such as when family members can visit, will help in what is already a stressful situation. Grades K-5.

24 pages
ISBN: 0-823950-36-0

Newsletters

5073 Noonan Connection
Noonan Syndrome Support Group
PO Box 145
Upperco, MD 21155

410-374-5245
888-686-2224
e-mail: info@noonansyndrome.org
www.noonansnydrome.org

Provides basic information on Noonan syndrome and related current news and events.

DESCRIPTION

5074 NYSTAGMUS

Covers these related disorders: Jerky nystagmus, Pendular nystagmus

Involves the following Biologic System(s):
Neurologic Disorders, Ophthalmologic Disorders

Nystagmus is a condition characterized by involuntary, rhythmic movements of the eyes. These movements may be vertical, horizontal, circular, or a mixture of two varieties (mixed). Nystagmus may be present at birth (congenital) or develop later in life (acquired). There are two general categories or types of nystagmus: jerky nystagmus and pendular nystagmus.

Jerky nystagmus is the most common form of the condition. It is characterized by relatively slow movements of the eyes in one direction followed by rapid, corrective movements or jerks in the opposite direction. In many patients with jerky nystagmus, head movements accompany the eye movements. These unusual head movements are thought to represent so-called compensatory posturing, that is, turning of the head to bring the eyes to a position in which the nystagmus lessens and vision is best (null positioning) In pendular nystagmus, movements of the eyes are approximately equal in rate in both directions. The different forms of nystagmus result due to abnormalities in certain mechanisms that regulate the movements and positioning of the eyes. These include conjugate gaze, fixation, and vestibular mechanisms. Conjugate gaze is the normal movement of both eyes in the same direction to bring objects into view. Fixation describes the direction of the gaze so that visual images fall on a certain area of the retina, which is the nerve-rich membrane at the back of the eye (fovea centralis). The vestibular mechanism is the balancing mechanism of the inner ear.

In some affected individuals, pendular or jerky nystagmus is present at birth or develops during early infancy or childhood. Pendular nystagmus often occurs in association with eye and visual defects (e.g., congenital glaucoma, congenital cataract, albinism, etc.). In other patients, pendular nystagmus may be an isolated finding that occurs in the absence of such conditions. Jerky nystagmus is usually unassociated with other eye or visual defects, and its cause is unknown. Familial cases of isolated pendular or jerky nystagmus are reported in which the condition appears to be transmitted as an autosomal dominant, autosomal recessive, or X-linked trait.

A specific, acquired form of pendular nystagmus, known as spasmus nutans, may also affect some infants or children. This condition typically develops at approximately four months to two years of age. In spasmus nutans, nystagmus is accompanied by head nodding and, in some children, abnormal tightness or contractions of the neck muscles, resulting in twisting of the neck and abnormal positioning of the head (torticollis). In most children with spasmus nutans, pendular nystagmus is limited to or more pronounced in one eye. Symptoms usually spontaneously resolve within months or a few years.

Some infants or children may also have a form of nystagmus in which there is repetitive jerking of the eyes toward each other or backward into the eye sockets (convergent nystagmus). This form of nystagmus often occurs with impaired vertical gaze in association with certain underlying syndromes (e.g., Parinaud syndrome, sylvian aqueduct syndrome, etc.).

The development of persistent nystagmus later in life may occur in association with certain disorders of the nervous system (e.g., brain tumors, multiple sclerosis) or disorders affecting the balancing (vestibular) mechanism of the inner ear (labyrinthine-vestibular disease). Individuals with acquired nystagmus should receive immediate, thorough evaluations to diagnose the underlying cause and ensure prompt, appropriate treatment. Medications can cause nystagmus. Causes include excessive drinking of alcohol or use of medications such as those given for seizure control.

In infants and children with nystagmus, diagnostic evaluations typically include the use of a specialized imaging technique (electronystagmography) that records eye movements and helps to determine or confirm the type of nystagmus present. Treatment of patients with nystagmus includes appropriate therapies for any diagnosed, underlying causes of the condition. Other treatment includes symptomatic and supportive measures.

See also **General Resources** on page 917

Government Agencies

5075 NIH/National Eye Institute
31 Center Drive MSC 2510
Bethesda, MD 20892

301-496-5248
e-mail: 2020@nei.nih.gov
www.nei.nih.gov

Conducts and supports research that helps prevent and treat eye diseases and other disorders of vision. This research leads to sight-saving treatments, reduces visual impairment and blindness, and improves the quality of life for people of all ages. NEI-supported research has advanced our knowledge of how the eye functions in health and disease.

Paul A Sieving M.D., Ph.D., Director

National Associations & Support Groups

5076 American Nystagmus Network
303-D Beltline Place, Suite 321
Decatur, AL 35603

www.nystagmus.org

A nonprofit organization founded in 1999 to serve the needs and interests of those affected by nystagmus, and to provide information to health care providers, educators and researchers.

Jeff Lowry, President
Laura Weigand, VP

5077 Genetic Alliance
4301 Connecticut Avenue NW
Washington, DC 20008

202-966-5557
800-336-4363
Fax: 202-966-8553
e-mail: info@geneticalliance.org
www.geneticalliance.org

A coalition of voluntary genetic support groups, consumers and professionals addressing the needs of individuals and families affected by genetic disorders from a national perspective.

Sharon Terry, President/CEO

5078 March of Dimes Birth Defects Foundation
1275 Mamaroneck Avenue
White Plains, NY 10605

914-428-7100
888-663-4637
Fax: 914-428-8203
e-mail: resourcecenter@modimes.org
www.marchofdimes.com

Partnership of volunteers and professionals dedicates to improving the health of babies by preventing birth defects and infant mortality. Over 100 chapters are located across the country and can be located through the National Office.

Dr Jennifer Howse, President

5079 National Association for Visually Handicapped
22 W 21st Street, 6th Floor
New York, NY 10010

212-889-3141
Fax: 212-727-2931
e-mail: navh@navh.org
www.navh.org

Serves as a clearinghouse for information about all services available to the partially-sighted from public and private sources. Conducts self-help groups. Provides information on large print books, textbooks and educational tools.

Dr Lorraine Marchi, Founder & CEO

5080 National Eye Research Foundation
910 Skokie Boulevard, Suite 207A
Northbrook, IL 60062

847-564-4652
800-621-2258
Fax: 847-564-0807
e-mail: info@nerf.org
www.nerf.org

Devoted to the enhancement of care and study of eye related diseases.

State Agencies & Support Groups

Alabama

5081 Alabama Institute for the Deaf & Blind
PO Box 698
Talladega, AL 35160

256-761-3200
Fax: 256-761-3344
www.nectas.unc.edu

Services include central directory, representatives of agencies, service providers, families, and coordinators of infant, toddler, and preschool special education programs.

Joseph Busta, Interagency Coordinating Council

Arizona

5082 National Association for Parents of the Visually Impaired
Po Box 317
Watertown, MA 02471

617-972-7441
800-562-6265
Fax: 617-972-7444
www.spedex.com/napvi

Mary Ellen Simmons

California

5083 Helen Keller National Center SW Region
6160 Cornerstone Court E
San Diego, CA 92121

858-623-2777
Fax: 858-642-0266
TTY: 858-646-0784
e-mail: ckirscher@cspp.edu
www.helenkeller.org

Cathy Kircher, SW Regional Representative

Ohio

5084 Region 2 of the National Association for Parents of the Visually Impaired
3910 Pocahontas Avenue
Cincinnati, OH 45227

513-561-8542

Victoria Gorman Miller

Pennsylvania

5085 East Central Region-Helen Keller National Center
4351 Garden City Drive
New Carrollton, MD 20785

301-459-5474
Fax: 301-459-5070
e-mail: hkncreg3cl@aol.com
www.helenkeller.org

South Carolina

5086 Region 4 of the National Association for Parents of the Visually Impaired
1032 Trail Road
Belton, SC 29627

864-338-9593

Washington

5087 Northwestern Region-Helen Keller National Center
2366 Eastlake Avenue E
Seattle, WA 98102

206-324-9120
e-mail: nwhknc@juno.com

Libraries & Resource Centers

Alabama

5088 Mobile Association for the Blind
2440 Gordon Smith Drive
Mobile, AL 36617

334-473-3585

Offers work adjustment training, activities of daily living, mobility, communication skills and sheltered employment for adults and children who are visually impaired.

Mahlon McCracken, Executive Director

Arizona

5089 Educational Services for the Visually Impaired
PO Box 668
Little Rock, AR 72203

501-371-5710

Offers textbooks, braille books and more to the visually impaired grades K-12 in the Arkansas area.

David Beavers, Director

Arkansas

5090 Arkansas Regional Library for the Blind and Physically Handicapped
1 Capitol Mall
Little Rock, AR 72201

501-682-1155
Fax: 501-682-1529
TDD: 501-682-1002
e-mail: nlsbooks@asl.lib.ar.us
www.asl.lib.ar.us/ASL_LBPH.htm

Public library books in recorded or braille format. Popular fiction and nonfiction books for all ages, books and players are on free loan, sent to patrons by mail and may be returned postage free. Anyone who cannot see well enough to read regular print with glasses on or who has a disability that makes it difficult to hold a book or turn the pages is eligible.

John D Hall, Director

California

5091 American Action Fund for Blind Children and Adults
18440 Oxnard Street
Tarzana, CA 91356

818-343-2022
www.actinfund.org

Offers a charitable and educational fund, braille assistive devices and a lending library for the visually impaired.

5092 Blind Children's Center
4120 Marathon Street
Los Angeles, CA 90029

323-664-2153
Fax: 323-665-3828
www.blindentr.org

Offers support and informational groups.

5093 Braille Institute Desert Center
70-251 Ramon Road
Rancho Mirage, CA 92270

760-321-2555

Dedicated to providing blind and visually impaired men, women and children with the training, programs and services they need to enjoy productive lives. Services offered include child development, youth programs, library services and adult education.

5094 Braille Institute Sight Center
741 N Vermont Avenue
Los Angeles, CA 90029

213-663-1111
e-mail: bils@brailib.org

Offers help, programs, services and information to the blind and visually impaired children and adults.

Dr. Henry Chang, Librarian

5095 Braille Institute Youth Center
3450 Cahuenga Boulevard W
Los Angeles, CA 90068

213-851-5695

Offers various youth programs and services for the blind and visually impaired youngster.

5096 New Beginnings - Blind Children's Center
4120 Marathon, Street
Los Angeles, CA 90029

323-664-2153
800-222-3566
Fax: 323-665-3828

Helps children and their families become independent by creating a climate of safety and trust. Services include an infant stimulation program, educational preschool, interdisciplinary assessment services, family services, correspondence program, toll-free national hotline and a publication and research service.

5097 San Francisco Public Library for the Blind and Print Disabled
100 Larkin Street
San Francisco, CA 94102

415-557-4293
Fax: 415-557-4375
e-mail: lbphmgr@sfpl.lib.ca.us
www.library.ca.us

Foreign-language books on cassette, children's books on cassettes and more.

Martin Maqid, Librarian

5098 Variety Audio
PO Box 5731
San Jose, CA 95150

408-277-4839

Summer reading programs, braille writer, magnifiers, closed-circuit TV, large-print photocopier, cassette books and magazines, children's books on cassette, home visits and other reference materials on blindness and other handicaps.

Louisa Griehshammer

District of Columbia

5099 Council of Families with Visual Impairment
1155 15th Street NW
Washington, DC 20005

202-467-5081

Members are sighted parents of blind or visually impaired children. Offers a forum for support and outreach, sharing of experiences in parent-child relationships, and educational and cultural information about child development. Monitors developments in technical and legislative arenas.

Nola Webb, President

Florida

5100 Florida Bureau of Braille and Talking Book Library Services
420 Platt Street
Daytona Beach, FL 32114

386-239-6000
Fax: 386-239-6069
TDD: 800-226-6079
e-mail: mike_gunde@dbs.doe.state.fl.us
www.state.fl.us/dbs/lswel.html

Discs, cassettes, closed-circuit TV, large-print photocopier, films, children's books on cassettes and more.

Michael Gunde, Librarian

5101 Talking Book Library, Jacksonville Public Library
1755 Edgewood Avenue W, Suite 1
Jacksonville, FL 32208

904-765-5588
Fax: 904-768-7404
TDD: 904-768-7822
e-mail: jerryr@coj.net
neflin.org/neflin/members/jackspub.html

Discs, cassettes and reference materials on blindness and other disabilities.

Jerry Reynolds, Librarian Senior

5102 Talking Book Service - Manatee County Central Library
6081 26th Street W
Bradenton, FL 34207

941-742-5914
Fax: 941-751-7089
TDD: 941-742-5951
e-mail: patricia.schubert@co.manatee.fl.us
www.co.manatee.fl.us

Offers children's books on disc and cassette and more reference materials for the blind and physically handicapped.

Patricia Schubert, Librarian

Georgia

5103 Albany Library for the Blind and Physical Handicapped
300 Pine Avenue
Albany, GA 31701

229-420-3220
Fax: 229-420-3240
e-mail: sinquefk@mail.dougherty.public.lib.ga.us
www.docolib.org/LBPH/index.html

Offers discs, cassettes, reference materials on blindness and other handicaps, large-print photocopiers, summer reading programs, cassette books and more.

Kathryn Sinquefield, Librarian

5104 Bainbridge Subregional Library for the Blind and Physically Handicapped
301 S Monroe Street
Bainbridge, GA 31717

912-248-2680
800-795-2680
Fax: 912-248-2670
TDD: 912-248-2665
e-mail: lbph@mail.deccatur.public.lib.ga.us
www.decatur.public.lib.ga.us/local/lbph/lbph1.htm

Discs, cassettes, summer reading programs, closed-circuit TV, magnifiers and more.

Kathy Hutchins, Librarian

5105 CEL Subregional Library for the Blind and Physically Handicapped
2708 Mechanics
Savannah, GA 31401

912-354-5864
Fax: 912-354-5534
TDD: 912-652-3635
e-mail: stokesl@cel.co.chatman.ga.us

Summer reading programs, braille writer, magnifiers, closed-circuit TV, large-print photocopier, cassette books and magazines, children's books on cassette, home visits and other reference materials on blindness and other handicaps.

Linda Stokes, Librarian

Idaho

5106 Idaho State Talking Book Library
325 W State Street
Boise, ID 83702

208-334-2117
Fax: 208-334-4016
TDD: 800-377-1363
e-mail: tblbooks@isl.state.id.us
www.lili.org/isl/tblinfo.htm

Summer reading programs, braille writer, magnifiers, closed-circuit TV, large-print photocopier, cassette books and magazines, children's books on cassette, home visits and other reference materials on blindness and other handicaps.

Sue Walker, Librarian

Illinois

5107 Chicago Library Service for the Blind
1055 W Roosevelt Road
Chicago, IL 60608

312-746-9210

Summer reading programs, braille writer, magnifiers, closed-circuit TV, large-print photocopier, cassette books and magazines, children's books on cassette, home visits and other reference materials on blindness and other handicaps.

Carol Pellish, Librarian

5108 Illinois State Library, Talkng Book and Braille Service
300 S 2nd Street
Springfield, IL 62701

217-782-9435
Fax: 217-782-8261
TDD: 800-665-5576
e-mail: sruda@ilsos.net
www.cyberdriveillinois.com/library/isl/bph/bph.html

Summer reading programs, braille writer, magnifiers, closed-circuit TV, large-print photocopier, cassette books and magazines, descriptive videos, children's books on cassette, home visits and other reference materials on blindness and other handicaps.

Sharon Ruda, Librarian

5109 Mid Illinois Talking Book System
515 York Street
Quincy, IL 62301

217-224-6619
Fax: 217-224-9818

Summer reading programs, braille writer, magnifiers, closed-circuit TV, large-print photocopier, cassette books and magazines, children's books on cassette, home visits and other reference materials on blindness and other handicaps.

5110 Mid-Illinois Talking Book Center
845 Brenkman Drive
Pekin, IL 61554

309-353-4110
Fax: 309-353-8281
e-mail: hitbc@darkstar.rsa.lib.il.us
www.mitbc.org

Summer reading programs, braille writer, magnifiers, closed-circuit TV, large-print photocopier, cassette books and magazines, children's books on cassette, home visits and other reference materials on blindness and other handicaps.

Eileen Sheppard, Librarian

5111 Talking Book Center of Northwest Illinois
PO Box 125
Coal Valley, IL 61240

309-799-3137
Fax: 309-799-7916
e-mail: kodean@libby.rbls.lib.il.us
www.rbls.lib.il.us

Subregional library provides Talking Book and Braille Book programs to eligible persons unable to use standard print materials due to visual or physical disabilities. Includes cassette books and magazines; summer reading program.

Indiana

5112 Northwest Indiana Subregional Library for Blind and Physically Handicapped
1919 W Lincoln Highway
Merrillville, IN 46410

219-769-3541
Fax: 219-769-0690

Summer reading programs, braille writer, magnifiers, closed-circuit TV, large-print photocopier, cassette books and magazines, children's books on cassette, home visits and other reference materials on blindness and other handicaps.

Renee Lewis

Iowa

5113 Iowa Library for the Blind and Physically Handicapped
Iowa Department for the Blind
524 4th Street
Des Moines, IA 50309

515-281-1333
Fax: 515-281-1378
TDD: 515-281-1355
e-mail: keninger.karen@blind.state.ia.us
www.blind.state.ia.us

Summer reading programs, magnifiers, closed-circuit TV, large-print photocopier, children's books on cassette, children's books in Braille and Print Braille, cassette magazines, home visits and reference materials on blindness and other handicaps.

Karen Keninger, Program Manager/Librarian

Kansas

5114 CKLS Headquarters
1409 Williams Street
Great Bend, KS 67530

316-792-2393
800-362-2642
Fax: 316-792-5495
e-mail: cenks@ink.org
www.macular.org

Summer reading programs, braille writer, magnifiers, closed-circuit TV, large-print photocopier, cassette books and magazines, children's books on cassette, home visits and other reference materials on blindness and other handicaps.

Jerri Robinson, Librarian

5115 Services for the Visually Disabled
629 Poyntz Avenue
Manhattan, KS 66502

785-776-4741
Fax: 785-776-1545
e-mail: marionr@manhattan.lib.ks.us

Summer reading programs, braille writer, magnifiers, closed-circuit TV, large-print photocopier, cassette books and magazines, children's books on cassette, home visits and other reference materials on blindness and other handicaps.

Marion Rice, Librarian

Kentucky

5116 Kentucky Library for the Blind and Physically Handicapped
PO Box 818
Frankfort, KY 40602

502-564-8300
800-372-2968
Fax: 502-564-5773
e-mail: richard.feindel@kdla.net
www.kdla.net/libserv/ktbl.htm

Large-print photocopier, cassette books and magazines, children's books on cassette, and other reference materials on blindness and other handicaps.

5,200 members

Richard Feindel, Librarian

Maryland

5117 Maryland State Library for the Blind and Physically Handicapped
415 Park Avenue
Baltimore, MD 21201

410-230-2424
Fax: 410-333-2095
TTY: 800-934-2541
TDD: 410-333-8679
e-mail: recept@lbta.lib.md.us
www.lbph.lib.md.us

Summer reading programs, braille writer, magnifiers, large-print photocopier, cassette books and magazines, children's books on cassette, and other reference materials on blindness and other handicaps.

5118 Prince George's County Memorial Library Talking Book Center
6530 Adelphi Road
Hyattsville, MD 20782

301-779-9330

Summer reading programs, braille writer, magnifiers, closed-circuit TV, large-print photocopier, cassette books and magazines, children's books on cassette, home visits and other reference materials on blindness and other handicaps.

Shirley Tuthill, Librarian

Massachusetts

5119 Braille and Talking Book Library Perkins School for the Blind
175 N Beacon Street
Watertown, MA 02472

617-924-3434
Fax: 617-926-2027
e-mail: perkins@bpl.org
www.perkins.org

Patricia Kirk

5120 Carroll Center for the Blind
770 Centre Street
Newton, MA 02158

617-969-6200
800-852-3131
Fax: 617-969-6204
www.carroll.org

Assists blind and visually impaired adults and adolescents to adjust to loss of vision. The goal of this dynamic program is to help the person become more independent, to restore self-confidence, prepare for employment and improve the quality of life. Programs of individual counseling are offered as part of the program.

Rachel Rosenbaum, President

Michigan

5121 Downtown Detroit Subregional Library for the Blind and Handicapped
121 Gratiot Avenue
Detroit, MI 48226

313-224-0580
Fax: 313-965-1977
TDD: 313-224-0584
e-mail: deveans@cms.xx.wayne.edu
www.detroit.lib.mi.us

Summer reading programs, braille writer, magnifiers, closed-circuit TV, large-print photocopier, cassette books and magazines, children's books on cassette, home visits and other reference materials on blindness and other handicaps.

Deborah Evans, Librarian

5122 Kent County Library for the Blind
775 Ball Avenue NE
Grand Rapids, MI 49503

616-336-3250
Fax: 616-336-3201
e-mail: kdlem@lakeland.lib.mi.us

Summer reading programs, braille writer, magnifiers, closed-circuit TV, large-print photocopier, cassette books and magazines, children's books on cassette, home visits and other reference materials on blindness and other handicaps.

Claudya Muller, Librarian

5123 Library of Michigan Service for the Blind
PO Box 30007
Lansing, MI 48909

517-373-5614
Fax: 517-373-5865
e-mail: info@sbph.libomich.lib.mi.us

Summer reading programs, braille writer, magnifiers, closed-circuit TV, large-print photocopier, cassette books and magazines, children's books on cassette, home visits and other reference materials on blindness and other handicaps.

5124 Macomb Library for the Blind and Physically Handicapped
16480 Hall Road
Clinton Township, MI 48038

586-286-1580
Fax: 586-286-0634
TDD: 810-869-40
e-mail: macbld@libcoop.net
www.macomb.lib.mi.us/macspe/

Summer reading programs, braille writer, closed-circuit TV, cassette books and magazines, children's books on cassette, reference materials on blindness and other handicaps.

Beverlee Babcock, Librarian

5125 Mideastern Michigan Library Co-op
G-4195 W Pasadena Avenue
Flint, MI 48504

810-732-1120
Fax: 810-732-1715
e-mail: cnash@genesse.freeret.org
www.fakon.edu/gdl/talking.htm

Summer reading programs, braille writer, magnifiers, closed-circuit TV, large-print photocopier, cassette books and magazines, children's books on cassette, home visits and other reference materials on blindness and other handicaps.

Carolyn Nash, Librarian

5126 Muskegon County Library for the Blind
635 Ottawa Street
Muskegon, MI 49442

231-724-6248
Fax: 231-724-6675
TDD: 231-722-4103
www.muskcolib.org

Summer reading programs, braille typewriter, magnifiers, closed-circuit TV, large-print photocopier, cassette books and magazines, children's books on cassette, home visits and other reference materials on blindness and other handicaps, The Reading Edge, Perkins Brailler and large print books.

Linda Clapp, Librarian

5127 Upper Peninsula Library for the Blind Physically Handicapped
1615 Presque Isle Avenue
Marquette, MI 49855

906-228-7697
Fax: 906-228-5627
e-mail: uproc.lib.mi.us
www.upesc.lib.mi.us/uplbph

Summer reading programs, braille writer, magnifiers, closed-circuit TV, large-print photocopier, cassette books and magazines, children's books on cassette, home visits and other reference materials on blindness and other handicaps.

Suzanne Dees, Librarian

5128 Washtenaw County Library
PO Box 8645
Ann Arbor, MI 48107

734-222-4357
Fax: 734-222-6715
e-mail: contact us@ewashtenaw.org
www.ewashtenaw.org

Summer reading programs, braille writer, magnifiers, closed-circuit TV, large-print photocopier, cassette books and magazines, children's books on cassette, home visits and other reference materials on blindness and other handicaps.

Margeret Wolfe, Librarian

5129 Washtenaw County Library for the Blind and Physically Disabled
PO Box 8645
Ann Arbor, MI 48107

734-971-6059
Fax: 734-971-3892
e-mail: lbpd@co.washtennaw.mi.us
www.co.washten.ml.us/depts/lib/liblbpd.h

Book lovers club.adaptive technology,cassette equipment, cassette books and magazines, described videos, low vision aids reference and referral services.

Margaret Wolfe, Coordinator

5130 Wayne County Regional Library for the Blind
30555 Michigan Avenue
Westland, MI 48186

734-727-7300
Fax: 734-727-7333
TTY: 734-727-7330
e-mail: werlbph@tln.lib.mi.us
www.wayneregional.lib.mi.us

Summer reading programs, braille writer, magnifiers, closed-circuit TV, large-print photocopier, cassette books and magazines, children's books on cassette, home visits and other reference materials on blindness and other handicaps.

Reginald Williams, Wayne County Librarian

Minnesota

5131 Minnesota Library for the Blind & Physically Handicapped
Highway 298, PO Box 68
Fairbault, MN 55021

507-333-4828
800-722-0550
Fax: 507-333-4832
e-mail: libblnd@state.mn.us

Summer reading programs, braille writer, magnifiers, closed-circuit TV, large-print photocopier, cassette, large print, braille books and magazines, children's books on cassette, and other reference materials on blindness and other handicaps.

Catherine A Durivage, Program Director

Missouri

5132 Adriene Resource Center for Blind Children
1445 Boonville Avenue
Springfield, MO 65802

417-862-2781
Fax: 417-862-7566
e-mail: blind@ag.org
www.gospelpublishing.com

Offers braille and cassette lending library, braille and cassette Sunday school materials for all ages, braille and cassette periodicals and resource assistance, and resources for blind children and children of blind parents.

Paul Weingariner, Director

5133 Assemblies of God National Center for the Blind
1445 Boonville Avenue
Springfield, MO 65802

417-862-2781
Fax: 417-862-7566
e-mail: blind@ag.org
www.gospelpublishing.com

Offers braille and cassette lending library, braille and cassette Sunday school materials for all ages, braille and cassette periodicals and resource assistance, and resources for blind children and children of blind parents.

Paul Weingariner, Director

5134 Wolfner Memorial Library for the Blind
PO Box 387
Jefferson City, MO 65102

573-751-8720
Fax: 573-526-2985
TDD: 800-347-1379
e-mail: beckles@mail.sos.state.mo.us

Summer reading programs, braille writer, magnifiers, closed-circuit TV, large-print photocopier, cassette books and magazines, children's books on cassette, home visits and other reference materials on blindness and other handicaps.

Elizabeth Eckles, Librarian

Nebraska

5135 Nebraska Library Commission Talking Book & Braille Services
1200 N Street
Lincoln, NE 68508

402-471-4038
800-742-7691
Fax: 402-471-6244
TDD: 402-471-4038
e-mail: doertli@nlc.state.ne.us
www.ncl.state.ne.us/tbbs/tbbsl/html

Free loan of books and magazines on cassette and in Braille, including children's materials, along with specially designed playback equipment. Summer reading program for children, Braille embossing, closed circuit TV, large-print copier. Reference materials on blindness and other disabilities.

David Oerti, Librarian

New Jersey

5136 New Jersey Library for the Blind and Handicapped
2300 Stuyvesant Avenue
Trenton, NJ 08618

609-292-6450
800-792-8322
Fax: 609-530-6384
TDD: 877-882-5593
e-mail: nglbh@njstatelib.org
www.njstatelib.org

Summer reading programs, braille writer, magnifiers, closed-circuit TV, large-print, cassette braille books and magazines, children's books on cassettes in braille and other reference materials on blindness and other handicaps.

Deborah Rutledeger, Director

New Mexico

5137 New Mexico State Library for the Blind and Physically Handicapped
1209 Camino Carlos Ray
Santa Fe, NM

505-476-9700
Fax: 505-476-9701
e-mail: jbrewstr@stlib.state.nm.us
www.stlib.state.nm.us

Summer reading programs, braille writer, magnifiers, closed-circuit TV, large-print photocopier, cassette books and magazines, children's books on cassette, home visits and other reference materials on blindness and other handicaps.

Glee Wenzel, Librarian

New York

5138 Helen Keller National Center
111 Middle Neck Road
Sands Point, NY 11050

516-944-8900
Fax: 516-944-7302

Provides diagnostic, evaluation, short term comprehensive rehabilitation and personal adjustment training. A technical assistance center is offered providing assistance to public and private agencies and to parent groups who work towards community integration and the enhancement of the quality of life. A national parent network is also provided that develops and shares information about advocacy, legislation, new services and achievements.

5139 New York State Talking Book & Braille Library
Empire State Plaza, CEC
Albany, NY 12230

518-474-5801
Fax: 518-474-5786
TDD: 518-474-7121
e-mail: jane@unix2.nysed.gov
www.suffolk.lib.ny.us

Books on audio cassette, cassette players, braille books, summer reading programs, braille writer, magnifiers, closed-circuit TV, large-print photocopier, cassette books and magazines, children's books on cassette, reference materials on blindness and other handicaps.

Jane Somers, Director

North Carolina

5140 North Carolina Library for the Blind
1811 Capital Boulevard
Raleigh, NC 27635

919-733-4376
Fax: 919-733-6910
TDD: 919-733-1462
e-mail: nclbph@ncsl.der.state.nc

Summer reading programs, braille writer, magnifiers, closed-circuit TV, large-print photocopier, cassette books and magazines, children's books on cassette, home visits and other reference materials on blindness and other handicaps.

Francine Martin, Librarian

Ohio

5141 American Council of Blind Parents
34400 Cedar Road, Apartment 108
University Heights, OH 44121

800-424-8666

Members are sighted parents of blind or visually impaired children. Offers a forum for support and outreach, sharing of experiences in parent-child relationships, and educational and cultural information about child development. Monitors developments in technical and legislative arenas.

Nola Webb, President

Oregon

5142 Oregon State Library, Talking Book and Braille Services
250 Winter Street NW
Salem, OR 97310

503-378-4243
Fax: 503-588-7119
TDD: 503-378-4276
e-mail: tbabs@sparkie.osl.state.or.us

Cassette books and magazines, children's books on cassette, home visits and other reference materials on blindness and other handicaps.

Donna Bensen, Regional Librarian

Virginia

5143 Alexandria Library Talking Book Service
5005 Duke Street
Alexandria, VA 22304

703-519-5900
Fax: 703-519-5915
TDD: 703-838-4568
e-mail: emccaffr@lea.eda
www.www.alexandria.lib.va.us

Summer reading programs, braille writer, magnifiers, closed-circuit TV, large-print photocopier, cassette books and magazines, children's books on cassette, home visits and other reference materials on blindness and other handicaps.

Patricia Bates, Librarian

5144 Division for the Visually Handicapped
1920 Association Drive
Reston, VA 20191

703-620-3660

Members are teachers, college faculty members, administrators, supervisors and others concerned with the education and welfare of visually handicapped and blind children and youth. This is a division of the Council For Exceptional Children.

Dr. Kay Ferrell, President

5145 Division on Visual Impairments
Council for Exceptional Children
1110 North Glebe Road, Suite 300
Arlington, VA 22201

800-224-6830
Fax: 703-264-9494
TTY: 866-915-5000
www.ed.arizona.edu/dvi/welcome.htm; www.cec.sped.org

A division within the CEC, it handles concerns for Federal, state and local issues and policies related to education of youths, children and infants with visual impairments.

Ellyn Ross, President
Shirley J Wilson, Secretary

5146 Virginia State Library for the Visually and Physically Handicapped
1901 Roane Street
Richmond, VA 23222

804-367-0014

Summer reading programs, braille writer, magnifiers, closed-circuit TV, large-print photocopier, cassette books and magazines, children's books on cassette, home visits and other reference materials on blindness and other handicaps.

Mary Ruth Halapatz, Librarian

Washington

5147 Washington Library for the Blind and Physically Handicapped
821 Lenora Street
Seattle, WA 98129

206-386-4636
Fax: 206-386-4685
e-mail: wtbbl@spl.lib.wa.us
www.spl.lib.wa.us

Summer reading programs, braille writer, magnifiers, closed-circuit TV, large-print photocopier, cassette books and magazines, children's books on cassette, home visits and other reference materials on blindness and other handicaps.

Jan Ames, Librarian

West Virginia

5148 West Virginia School for the Blind
301 E Main Street
Romney, WV 26757

304-822-3521
Fax: 304-822-4896
e-mail: cjohn@access.mountain.net

Summer reading programs, braille writer, magnifiers, closed-circuit TV, large-print photocopier, cassette books and magazines, children's books on cassette, home visits and other reference materials on blindness and other handicaps.

Cynthia Johnson, Librarian

Research Centers

5149 Center for the Partially Sighted
12301 Wilshire Boulevard, Suite 600
Los Angeles, CA 90025

310-458-3501
Fax: 310-458-8179
e-mail: info@low-vision.org
www.low-vision.org

Provides professional, comprehensive vision rehabilitation services to visually impaired people of all ages. For those whose sight is severely limited due to macular degeneration, diabetic retinopathy, glaucoma, retinal detachment, stroke or other conditions not correctable medically or surgically.

5150 Helen Keller National Center
111 Middle Neck Road
Sands Point, NY 11050

516-944-8900
Fax: 516-944-7302

Provides diagnostic evaluation, short term comprehensive rehabilitation and personal adjustment training. A technical assistance center is offered providing assistance to public and private agencies and to parent groups who work towards community integration and the enhancement of the quality of life. A national parent network is also provided that develops and shares information about advocacy, legislation, new services and achievements.

5151 Mobile Association for the Blind
2440 Gordon Smith Drive
Mobile, AL 36617

251-473-3585
877-292-5463
Fax: 251-470-8622
e-mail: sales@mobile.blind.com
www.mobileblind.com

Offers work adjustment training, activities of daily living, mobility, communication skills and sheltered employment for adults and children who are visually impaired.

Mahlon McCracken, Executive Director

5152 National Eye Research Foundation
910 Skokie Boulevard, Suite 207A
Northbrook, IL 60062

847-564-4652
800-621-2258
Fax: 847-564-0807
e-mail: info@nerf.org
www.nerf.org

Devoted to the enhancement of care and study of eye related diseases.

5153 New Beginnings - The Blind Children's Center
4120 Marathon Street
Los Angeles, CA 90029

213-664-2153

The purpose of the Center is to turn initial fears into hope. Helps children and their families become independent by creating a climate of safety and trust. Children learn to develop self confidence and to master a wide range of skills. Services include an infant stimulation program, educational preschool, interdisciplinary assessment services, family services, correspondence program, toll free national hotline and a publication and research service.

5154 Research to Prevent Blindness
645 Madison Avenue
New York, NY 10022

212-752-4333
800-621-0026
www.rpbusa.org

Provides research grants to scientists interested in eye disease and vision disorders.

Audio Video

5155 Heart to Heart
Blind Children's Center
4120 Marathon Street
Los Angeles, CA 90029

323-644-2153
Fax: 323-665-3828
www.blindcntr.org

Parents of blind and partially sighted children talk about their feelings.

Videotape

5156 Let's Eat
Blind Children's Center
4120 Marathon Street
Los Angeles, CA 90029

213-664-2153
Fax: 213-665-3828

Teaches competent feeding skills to children with visual impairments.

Videotape

5157 See What I Feel
Britannica Film Co.
345 4th Street
San Francisco, CA 94107

415-597-5555

A blind child tells her friends about her trip to the zoo. Each experience was explained as a blind child would experience it. A teacher's guide comes with this video.

Films

Web Sites

5158 American Nystagmus Network
www.nystagmus.org

Is a nonprofit organization established to serve the needs and interests of those affected by Nystagmus.

5159 Lighthouse International
www.lighthouse.org

The mission is to overcome vision impairment for people of all ages through worldwide leadership in rehabilitation services, education, research, prevention and advocacy.

5160 National Alliance of Blind Students
www.blindstudents.org

The leading national advocacy and consumer organization for students in high school or college who are blind or visually impaired.

5161 National Association for Visually Handicapped
www.navh.org

Serves as a clearing house for information about all services available to the partially-sighted from public and private sources. Conducts self help groups. Provides information on large print books, textbooks, and educational tools.

5162 Nystagmus Network
www.nystagmusnet.org

A UK-based self-help group set up to provide support for adults and children with nystagmus, their parents and teachers and foster research into the condition.

5163 Online Mendelian Inheritance in Man
www.ncbi.nlm.nih.gov

This database is a catalog of human genes and genetic disorders.

5164 Royal National Institute of the Blind
www.rnib.org.uk

A leading UK charity offering information, support and advice to over two million people with sight problems.

Magazines

5165 Journal of Visual Impairment and Blindness
American Foundation for the Blind
11 Penn Plaza, Suite 300
New York, NY 10001

212-502-7600
Fax: 212-502-7777
e-mail: afbinfo@afb.net
www.afb.org

Published in braille, regular print and on cassette this journal contains a wide variety of subjects including rehabilitation, psychology, education, legislation, medicine, technology, employment, sensory aids and childhood development as they relate to visual impairments.

10x Year

5166 Reaching, Crawling, Walking - Let's Get Moving
Blind Children's Center
4120 Marathon Street
Los Angeles, CA 90029

323-664-2153
Fax: 323-665-3828
e-mail: info@blindchildrenscenter.org
www.blindchildrenscenter.org

Orientation and mobility for visually impaired preschool children.

24 pages

5167 Seeing Candy
National Association for Visually Handicapped
22 W 21st Street, 6th Floor
New York, NY 10010

212-889-3141
Fax: 212-727-2931
e-mail: staff@navh.org
www.navh.org

This newsletter offers short stories, news, medical updates, assistive device information, poems, resources, crossword puzzles and more for the visually impaired.

Biannually

5168 Tactic
Clovernook Home and School for the Blind
7000 Hamilton Avenue
Cincinnati, OH 45231

513-522-3860
Fax: 513-728-3950
e-mail: clovernook@aol.com

Quarterly

Newsletters

5169 National Library Service for the Blind & Physically Handicapped
Library of Congress Reference Section
1291 Taylor Street NW
Washington, DC 20542

202-707-5100
800-424-8567
Fax: 202-707-0712
TTY: 202-707-0744
TDD: 202-707-0744
e-mail: nis@loc.gov
www.loc.gov/nls

Provides information and advocacy resources for families and professionals, including listings of organizations focusing on more specific areas of concern to families and young adults who have disabilities. Administers a natural library service that provides recorded and braille reading materials to eligible children and adults who cannot read standard print.

12 pages Quarterly
ISSN: 1046-1663

Vicki Fitzpatrick, Editor

5170 Talking Book Topics
National Library Services for the Blind
1291 Taylor Street NW
Washington, DC 20542

202-707-5100
Fax: 202-707-0712
www.loc.gov/nls

Offers hundreds of listings of books, fiction and nonfiction, for adults and children on cassette. Also offers listings on foreign language books on cassette, talking magazines and reviews.

Bimonthly

Pamphlets

5171 Dancing Cheek to Cheek
Blind Children's Center
4120 Marathon Street
Los Angeles, CA 90029

213-664-2153
Fax: 213-665-3828
www.blindchildrenscenter.org

Discusses beginning social, play and language interactions.

33 pages

5172 Family Guide - Growth and Development of the Partially Seeing Child
National Association for Visually Handicapped
22 W 21st Street, 6th Floor
New York, NY 10010

212-889-3141
Fax: 212-727-2931
e-mail: staff@navh.org
www.navh.org

Offers information for parents and guidelines in raising a partially seeing child.

5173 Family Guide to Vision Care
American Optometric Association
243 N Lindbergh Boulevard
Saint Louis, MO 63141

314-991-4100
Fax: 314-991-4101
www.aoanet.org

Offers information on the early developmental years of your vision, finding a family optometrist and how to take care of your eyesight through the learning years, the working years and the mature years.

5174 Heart to Heart
Blind Children's Center
4120 Marathon Street
Los Angeles, CA 90029

213-664-2153
Fax: 213-665-3828
www.blindchildrenscenter.org

Parents of blind and partially sighted children talk about their feelings.

12 pages

5175 Learning to Play
Blind Children's Center
4120 Marathon Street
Los Angeles, CA 90029

213-664-2153
Fax: 213-665-3828
www.blindchildrenscenter.org

Discusses how to present play activities to the visually impaired preschool child.

12 pages

5176 Let's Eat
Blind Children's Center
4120 Marathon Street
Los Angeles, CA 90029

213-664-2153
Fax: 213-665-3828
www.blindchildrenscenter.org

Teaches competent feeding skills to children with visual impairments.

28 pages

5177 Move with Me
Blind Children's Center
4120 Marathon Street
Los Angeles, CA 90029

213-664-2153
Fax: 213-665-3828
www.blindchildrenscenter.org

A parent's guide to movement development for visually impaired babies.

12 pages

5178 Selecting a Program
Blind Children's Center
4120 Marathon Street
Los Angeles, CA 90029

213-664-2153
Fax: 213-665-3828
www.blindchildrenscenter.org

A guide for parents of infants and preschoolers with visual impairments.

28 pages

5179 Standing on My Own Two Feet
Blind Children's Center
4120 Marathon Street
Los Angeles, CA 90029

323-664-2153
Fax: 323-665-3828
e-mail: info@blindchildrenscenter.org
www.blindchildrenscenter.org

A step-by-step guide to designing and constructing simple, individually tailored adaptive mobility devices for preschool-age children who are visually impaired.

36 pages

5180 Talk to Me
Blind Children's Center
4120 Marathon Street
Los Angeles, CA 90029

213-664-2153
Fax: 213-665-3828
www.blindchildrenscenter.org

A language guide for parents of deaf children.

11 pages

5181 Talk to Me II
Blind Children's Center
4120 Marathon Street
Los Angeles, CA 90029

213-664-2153
Fax: 213-665-3828
www.blindchildrenscenter.org

A sequel to Talk To Me, available in English and Spanish.

15 pages

Camps

5182 Bloomfield
5300 Angeles Vista Boulevard
Los Angeles, CA 90043

323-295-4555
800-352-2290
Fax: 323-296-0424
e-mail: info@juniorblind.org
www.junoirblind.org

This camp is dedicated to serving blind and developmentally disabled children and adults.

5183 Florida School-Deaf and Blind
207 San Marco Avenue
Saint Augustine, FL 32084

800-800-344
www2.kidscamps.com

5184 National Camps for Blind Children
Christian Record
4444 S 52nd Street
Lincoln, NE 68516

402-488-0981
Fax: 402-488-7582
e-mail: info@christianrecord.org
www.christianrecord.org

Camps throughout the US and Canada are offered at no cost to the legally blind, ages 9-65. Activities include archery, beeper basketball, water sports, hiking and rock climbing and horseback riding. $35 registration fee.

Keith Elliott, Director

5185 VISIONS/Vacation Camp for the Blind
500 Greenwich Street, 3rd Floor
New York, NY 10013

212-625-1616
888-245-8333
Fax: 212-219-4078
e-mail: tmdecker@visionvcb.org
www.visionvcb.org

Family programs at Vacation Camp for the Blind in Rockland County, NY for children who are blind, severely visually impaired or multi-handicapped. Parent or guardian must attend winter weekends and summer session.

Thomas M Decker, Camp Director
Nancy D Miller, Executive Director

DESCRIPTION

5186 OBESITY

Involves the following Biologic System(s):
Developmental/Behavioral/Psychiatric Disorders,
Endocrinologic Disorders

Obesity refers to a condition in which there is an excessive accumulation of fat in subcutaneous (below the skin) and other tissues of the body. Being obese and being overweight are not necessarily synonymous, as people who are overweight may have an increased body size as a result of increased muscle or skeletal tissue mass. Obesity in children may develop at any age, but peak development periods occur during the first 12 months of life, between the ages of five and six years, and during the adolescent years. The obesity epidemic is especially evident in industrialized nations where many people live sedentary lives and eat more convenience foods, which are typically high in calories and low in nutritional value, and is becoming an epidemic in the western hemisphere. Obesity may result from an increase in the actual number of fat cells or from an increase in the size of the individual fat cells. Researchers believe that fat cells increase in number in proportion to caloric intake increase and that this increase is particularly evident in the first 12 months of life. As children grow, increases in fat cell populations continue at a slower rate. Because the number of fat cells cannot be decreased, except surgically, later weight loss must result from the reduction of fat in individual cells.

Obesity usually results when caloric intake exceeds the energy demands of the body, thus increasing the storage of body fat. Fat accumulation is usually a progressive process, resulting from repeated episodes of food intake exceeding the body's demand for energy (calories). Many factors may influence appetite or obesity. Such factors may include environmental influences; psychologic disturbances that may be induced by stress or emotional upset or trauma; brain lesions that may involve certain areas of the brain such as the hypothalamus or the pituitary gland (both essential to hormone production); an overabundance of insulin in the body (hyperinsulinism); and genetic influences. In addition, in rare instances, obesity may be a feature of certain genetic disorders.

Complications of childhood obesity may include respiratory difficulties such as shortness of breath and increased cardiovascular risk factors such as high blood pressure, elevated total cholesterol levels as well as increased bad or LDL cholesterol and decreased good or HDL cholesterol, and increased levels of fatty acid and glycerol compounds (triglycerides). In addition, childhood obesity may be associated with a resistance to the hormone insulin that aids in the metabolism of glucose, fats, carbohydrates, and proteins. This resistance may lead to excessive levels of circulating insulin in the body (hyperinsulinism); however, the body is not able to appropriately use insulin and Type 2 Diabetes Mellitus results. The symptoms associated with insulin resistance may include hunger, weight loss, sweating, and tremor.

The diagnosis of obesity in children and adolescents is usually determined through the use of certain screening methods such as measurement of the body mass index (BMI) as well as the triceps skinfold thickness. In addition, special consideration may be given to certain criteria in determining differential diagnosis and possible treatment. These criteria may include elevated blood pressure; high total cholesterol levels; regular and consecutive increases in annual body mass index screenings; psychologic or emotional weight concerns; and a family history of heart disease, elevated cholesterol levels, and diabetes.

Patterns of behavior that may lead to obesity may be established as early as infancy. For example, if parents or caregivers persistently use a bottle to pacify a crying baby, the baby may learn that food is equivalent to relief of stress. Treatment for childhood and adolescent obesity should include the cooperation and support of the entire family and may be directed toward psychologic considerations, as well as proper exercise and nutrition to avoid complications. Treatment for psychologic and emotional needs may include behavior modification, as well as individual and family counseling.

See also **General Resources** on page 917

National Associations & Support Groups

5187 CHEF - Comprehensive Health Education Foun dation
22419 Pacific Highway S
Seattle, WA 98198

206-824-2907
800-323-2433
TTY: 800-833-6388
e-mail: info@chef.org
www.chef.org

Addresses issues that are pertinent to the health and well-being of today's society. A leader in prevention education, provider of skills and information and resources.

Sue Anderson, Children/Families Program Director
Larry Clark, President/CEO

5188 Compulsive Eaters Anonymous
5500 E Atherton Street, Suite 227-B
Long Beach, CA 90815

562-342-9344
Fax: 562-342-9346
e-mail: gso@ceahow.org
www.ceahow.org

A twelve-step program, with the primary purpose of, to stop eating compulsively.

Eric R Florida, Chairman
N Woody, President

5189 National Eating Disorders Association (NED A)
603 Stewart Street, Suite 803
Seattle, WA 98101

206-382-3587
800-931-2237
e-mail: info@NationalEatingDisorders.org
www.NationalEatingDisorders.org

Formed in 2001 when Eating Disorders Awareness & Prevention (EDAP) and the American Anorexia Bulimia Association (AABA) joined forces. It works to eliminate eating disorders through prevention efforts, education, referral and support services, advocacy, training, and research.

Tracy L Kahlo, Chief Operating Officer
Lynn S Grefe, Chief Executive Officer

Libraries & Resource Centers

5190 National Digestive Diseases Information Clearinghouse
2 Information Way
Bethesda, MD 20892

301-654-3810
800-891-5389
Fax: 703-738-4929
e-mail: nddic@info.niddk.nih.gov
www.digestive.niddk.nih.gov

The National Institute of Diabetes and Digestive and Kidney Diseases conducts and supports research on many of the most serious diseases affecting public health. The Institute supports much of the clinical research on the diseases of internal medicine and related subspecialty fields as well as many basic science disciplines.

Kathy Kranzfelder, Project Officer

Research Centers

5191 New York Obesity Research Center
Saint Luke's-Roosevelt Hospital Center
1090 Amsterdam Avenue, 14th Floor
New York, NY 10025

212-523-4196
Fax: 212-523-3416
www.nyorc.org

Dr F Xavier Pi-Sunyer, Director
Janine L Pangburn, Research Manager

5192 University of Chicago-Department of Psychi atry
5841 S Maryland Avenue
Chicago, IL 60637

312-702-3858
www.psychiatry.uchicago.edu

Christianne Montgomery, Research Administrator

Audio Video

5193 Eating Disorders
Research Press
PO Box 9177
Champaign, IL 61826

217-352-3273
Fax: 217-352-1221
e-mail: rp@researchpress.com
www.researchpress.com

This video shows young people how easily they can become victims of eating disorders such as anorexia, bulimia and compulsive overeating.

Videotape

5194 Our Overweight Kids
Aquarius Health Care Videos
18 N Main Street
Sherborn, MA 01770

508-650-1616
888-440-2963
Fax: 508-650-1665
e-mail: aquarius@aquariusproductions.com
www.aquariusproductions.com

With more kids being diagnosed as obese, it's important for the entire family to eat healthy meals and stay active. Take a trip to the supermarket with one mom as she tries to make healthy but fun food choices. A nutritionist and pediatrician offer important strategies for promoting a healthy diet.

1997 28 minutes VHS
ISBN: 1-581401-93-0

Leslie Kussmann, President

5195 Reality Matters - Obesity & Nutrition
Active Parenting Publishers
1955 Vaughn Road NW, Suite 108
Kennesaw, GA 30144

770-429-0565
800-825-0060
Fax: 770-429-0334
e-mail: cservice@activeparenting.com
www.activeparenting.com

For ages 11-18, it explores America's culture of obesity and its contributing factors, along with ways to help children make healthy choices.

DVD/VHS 24 minutes

Michael H Popkin PhD, Founder/President
Harry Popkin, Secretary

5196 Teaching Children to Prevent Heart Disease
Aquarius Health Care Videos
18 N Main Street
Sherborn, MA 01770

508-650-1616
888-440-2963
Fax: 508-650-1665
e-mail: aquarius@aquariusproductions.com
www.aquariusproductions.com

Breaks down difficult concepts into stories, games, lessons, and song enables children to absorb this important, life affirming action. Closed captioned.

1996 30 Minutes VHS

Leslie Kussmann, President

Web Sites

5197 American Anorexia Bulimia Association of P hiladelphia
www.aabaphila.org

Support for sufferers friends and family.

5198 Eating Disorders Awareness and Prevention

www.edap.org

NEDA is dedicated to expanding public understanding of eating disorders and promoting access to quality treatment for those affected along with support for their families through education, advocacy and research.

5199 Gurze Books

www.gurze.com

Specializes in information about eating disorders including anorexia nervosa, bulimia nervosa, and binge eating, plus related topics such as body image and obesity. Books are offered at discounted prices, many free articles about eating disorders, newsletters, links to treatment facilities, organizations, other websites and much more.

5200 National Eating Disorders Association (NED A)

www.NationalEatingDisorders.org

The mission of the National Eating Disorders Organization is to eliminate eating disorders and body disatisfaction through prevention efforts, education, referral, and support services, advocacy, training, and research.

5201 Obesity Online

www.obesity-online.com/

Is a multi-disciplinary forum for research and treatment of massive obesity, including plastics, psychiatry, endocrinology nutrition, nursing, dietetics and allied health.

Book Publishers

5202 Eating Disorders & Obesity

Guilford Press
72 Spring Street
New York, NY 10012

212-431-9800
Fax: 212-966-6708
e-mail: info@guilford.com
www.guilford.com

Presents and integrates virtually all that is currently known about eating disorders and obesity in one authorative, accessible, and eminently practical volume.

2005 633 pages 2nd Edition
ISBN: 1-593852-36-3

5203 Eating Disorders Resource Catalogue

Gurze Books
PO Box 2238
Carlsbad, CA 92018

760-434-7533
800-756-7533
Fax: 760-434-5476
e-mail: mylo@gurze.net
www.gurze.com

This catalogue of resources contains over 160 books and videos, audiotapes, lists of national organizations and treatment facilities, and basic facts about eating disorders. It is widely distributed by individuals who are suffering, their loved-ones, the health care professionals who treat them, and educators who are working towards prevention.

40 pages Annual/Free

5204 Emotional Eating: A Practical Guide to Taking Control

Free Press
866 3rd Avenue
New York, NY 10022

Fax: 800-943-9831
www.simonsays.com

1003 200 pages
ISBN: 0-029002-15-0

5205 Endorphins: Eating Disorders & Other Addictive Behavior

WW Norton & Company
500 5th Avenue
New York, NY 10110

212-354-5500
Fax: 800-458-6515
www.wwnorton.com

1993 320 pages
ISBN: 0-393701-56-5

5206 Feed Your Kids Well: How to Help You Child Lose Weight and Get Healthy

Fred Pescatore MD, author

Wiley Publishing, Inc
10475 Crosspoint Boulevard
Indianapolis, IN 46256

317-572-3000
877-762-2974
Fax: 800-597-3299
e-mail: consumer@wiley.com
www.wiley.com

Aimed toward parents, this book offers advice and tips to help their children lose excess weight. It also examines the popular fat-free diet fads and advises diets containing the small amounts of fat that are crucial to human growth.

1999 304 pages Paperback
ISBN: 0-471349-63-1

5207 Let's Talk About Being Overweight

Melanie Apel Gordon, author

Rosen Publishing Group's PowerKids Press
29 E 21st Street
New York, NY 10010

212-777-3017
800-237-9932
Fax: 888-436-4643
e-mail: rosenpub@tribeca.ios.com
www.powerkidspress.com

Reminds kids that everyone's body is different and assures them that it is okay. Readers will also learn that they will feel better if they eat right and get regular exercise. Grades K-5.

2000 24 pages
ISBN: 0-823954-13-7

5208 Making Peace with Food

Susan Kano, author

Gurze Books
PO Box 2238
Carlsbad, CA 92018

760-434-7533
800-756-7533
Fax: 760-434-5476
e-mail: mylo@gurze.net
www.gurze.com

This unique, full sized workbook is designed to help anyone who experienced compulsive eating, yo-yo dieting, food and body anxiety, or associated eating disorders. Filled with ideas, workbook pages, exercises, and resources, Kano's book is an excellent aid to clarifying and overcoming your personal diet/weight struggle.

1989 224 pages Paperback
ISBN: 0-060963-28-0

5209 Obesity Sourcebook
Omnigraphics
PO Box 625
Holmes, PA 19043

800-234-1340
Fax: 800-875-1340
e-mail: info@omnigraphics.com
www.omnigraphics.com

Basic consumer health information about diseases and other problems associated with obesity, including risk factors, prevention and management.

2001 376 pages
ISBN: 0-780803-33-7

5210 Obesity: Theory and Therapy
Raven Press
1185 Avenue of the Americas
New York, NY 10036

212-930-9500

A classic reference for clinicians dealing with obesity, this volume provides the most up-to-date research, preclinical and clinical information.

500 pages
ISBN: 0-881678-84-8

5211 Overeaters Anonymous
World Service Office
117 W 26th Street
New York, NY 10001

505-891-2664
Fax: 505-891-4320
www.overeatersanonymous.org

World Service Office offers literature and provides information on meetings world wide.

204 pages Hardcover

5212 Overeaters Anonymous Lifeline Sampler
World Service Office
6075 Zenith Court NE, PO Box 44020
Rio Rancho, NM 87144

505-891-2664
Fax: 505-891-4320
e-mail: info@overeatersanonymous.org
www.overeatersanonymous.org

A selection of articles from Lifeline magazine. Issues and topics include: relationships in recovery, food and weight, relapse, spiritual insights, abstinent living and traditions and steps.

448 pages

5213 Twelve Steps and Twelve Traditions of Over eaters Anonymous
World Service Office
6075 Zenith Court NE, PO Box 44020
Rio Rancho, NM 87144

505-891-2664
Fax: 505-891-4320
e-mail: info@overeatersanonymous.org
www.overeatersanonymous.org

Provides a detailed exploration of how the 12 traditions help members recover and how the Fellowship functions as a whole.

240 pages Softcover

5214 Understanding Childhood Obesity
J Clinton Smith MD, author

University Press of Mississippi
3825 Ridgewood Road
Jackson, MS 39211

601-432-6205
800-737-7788
Fax: 601-432-6217
e-mail: press@ihl.state.ms.us
www.upress.state.ms.us

A clear explanation of causes, diagnosis, and treatment of childhood obesity. A comprehensive guide that covers nearly every field of obesity research.

120 pages Paper
ISBN: 1-578061-34-2

5215 When Food is Love
Geneen Roth, author

Gurze Books
PO Box 2238
Carlsbad, CA 92018

760-434-7533
800-756-7533
Fax: 760-434-5467
e-mail: mylo@gurze.net
www.gurze.com

Drawing on her own personal experience, Roth explores similarities between eating and loving such as fantasizing, wanting the forbidden, creating drama, control issues, and the experience of relationship.

1991 205 pages Paperback
ISBN: 0-452268-18-4

Journals

5216 BASH Magazine
Bulimia Anorexia Self-Help/Behavior Adaptation
6125 Clayton Avenue, Suite 215
Saint Louis, MO 63139

314-567-4080

A journal of eating and mood disorders.

Monthly

Pamphlets

5217 About Overeaters Anonymous
Metro Intergroup of Overeaters Anonymous
117 W 26th Street
New York, NY 10001

212-206-8621

5218 Media-Smart Youth: Eat, Think, and Be Acti ve Fact Sheet
Natl Institute of Child Health & Human Development
31 Center Drive, Building 31
Bethesda, MD 20814

301-496-5133
www.nichd.nih.gov

Free government information on an interactive after-school education program that helps young people between the ages of 11 and 13 understand how physical activity and nutrition can influence their health.

2005 2 pages

DESCRIPTION

5219 OBSESSIVE-COMPULSIVE DISORDER

Synonyms: Obsessive-compulsive neurosis, OCD
Involves the following Biologic System(s):
Developmental/Behavioral/Psychiatric Disorders

Obsessive-compulsive disorder (OCD) is characterized by the performance of repetitive actions, rituals, or compulsions in response to recurrent, persistent thoughts or obsessions. These actions and thoughts may cause significant anxiety and interfere with personal, social, or occupational functioning. OCD may affect approximately two to three percent of the general population worldwide. In most cases, the onset of OCD is gradual and typically becomes apparent during adolescence or early adulthood. However, onset of the disorder during childhood is not rare. Males and females are thought to be affected equally.

Many children have minor compulsions that result in little or no distress, such as avoiding cracks while walking on the sidewalk. Most such compulsions typically subside later in life. However, some rituals may continue through adulthood, such as repeatedly checking that the stove is turned off. Children who develop obsessive-compulsive disorder may initially have repetitive, persistent thoughts that constantly invade their consciousness. They may conduct a repetitive action or a series of actions during certain situations, particularly during times of stress, such as preparing to go to school. Performing compulsive actions or rituals may temporarily relieve a feeling of anxiety, whereas resisting such compulsions may serve to increase their tension. Obsessions may consist of certain ideas, phrases, or strong images; impulses to perform objectionable acts; or impulses to perform objectionable acts; or impulses to repeatedly analyze certain acts before carrying them out. Some obsessions may concern bodily secretions or wastes or a need for routine or sameness. Compulsions often include repetitive hand washing, touching certain objects in a particular sequence, or checking and rechecking door locks. Attempts may be made to involve parents or other family members in the performance of certain compulsive actions or rituals. Children with OCD are usually aware of the irrationality of their obsessive thoughts and compulsive behaviors but are unable to control them. The symptoms associated with OCD often periodically decrease or increase in intensity over time. However, in some patients, a progressive worsening of the condition may result in gradual deterioration of personal and social functioning. First-line treatment of OCD may include antidepressant medications, such as fluoxetine, fluvoxamine, or clomipramine. Behavioral therapy, including gradually increased exposure to situations that typically trigger compulsive behaviors, may be helpful. Relaxation therapy has also demonstrated some benefit.

OCD may occur as an isolated condition or in association with other underlying disorders or conditions, such as Tourette syndrome, epilepsy, or anorexia nervosa. Although the exact cause of obsessive-compulsive disorder is not known, studies suggest that the disorder may result from biochemical abnormalities affecting particular areas of the brain. There are also reports of multiple cases of isolated OCD in a| multigenerational family (kindred), suggesting autosomal dominant inheritance in these patients. In addition, the occurrence of OCD in several kindreds affected by Tourette syndrome also indicates that changes (mutations) of certain genes may result in or contribute to OCD.

See also **General Resources** on page 917

Government Agencies

5220 Center for Mental Health Services Knowledge Exchange Network

US Department of Health and Human Services
PO Box 42557
Washington, DC 20015

800-789-2647
Fax: 240-747-5470
TDD: 866-889-2647
http://mentalhealth.samhsa.gov

Supplies the public with responses to their commonly asked questions about mental health issues and services.

5221 NIH/National Institute of Mental Health

6001 Executive Boulevard, Room 8184, MSC 9663
Bethesda, MD 20892

301-443-4513
866-615-6464
Fax: 301-443-4279
TTY: 301-443-8431
e-mail: nimhinfo@nih.gov
www.nimh.nih.gov

Conducts strategic planning for specific research areas as well as for the Institute as a whole.

Dr Thomas R Insel, Director

National Associations & Support Groups

5222 Awareness Foundation for OCD and Related D isorders

564 Cuesta Drive
Aptos, CA 95003

831-684-9684
e-mail: jamescallner@sbcglobal.net
www.ocdawareness.com

Combines the expertise and experience of dynamic workshop speakers with the emotional impact of film to increase professional, educational, and public understanding of OCD and related disorders. Speakers are available for consulting and workshops in school functions, for parents and students, and family and support groups.

James Callner MA, Founder/President

5223 Federation of Families for Children's Mental Health
9605 Medical Center Drive, Suite 280
Rockville, MD 20850

240-403-1901
Fax: 240-403-1909
e-mail: ffcmh@ffcmh.org
www.ffcmh.org

The National family run organization is dedicated exclusively to helping children with mental health needs and their families achieve a better quality of life.

Sandra Spencer, Executive Director

5224 Genetic Alliance
4301 Connecticut Avenue NW
Washington, DC 20008

202-966-5557
800-336-4363
Fax: 202-966-8553
e-mail: info@geneticalliance.org
www.geneticalliance.org

A coalition of voluntary genetic support groups, consumers and professionals addressing the needs of individuals and families affected by genetic disorders from a national perspective.

Sharon Terry, President/CEO

5225 NADD: National Association for the Dually Diagnosed
132 Fair Street
Kingston, NY 12401

845-331-4336
800-331-5362
Fax: 845-331-4569
e-mail: info@thenadd.org
www.thenadd.org

Nonprofit organization designed to promote the interests of professional and parent development with resources for individuals who have the coexistence of mental illness and mental retardation. Provides conferences, educational services and training materials to professionals, parents, concerned citizens and service organizations.

Dr Robert Fletcher, CEO

5226 National Alliance for the Mentally Ill
2107 Wilson Blvd, Ste 300, Colonial Place Three
Arlington, VA 22201

703-524-7600
800-950-6264
Fax: 703-524-9094
TDD: 703-516-7227
e-mail: info@nami.org
www.nami.org

NAMI is a nonprofit, grassroots, self-help, support and advocacy organization of consumers, families and friends of people with severe mental illness, such as schizophrenia, bipolar disorder, major despressive disorder, obsessive compulsive disorder, anxiety disorders, autism and other severe and persistent mental illnesses that affect the brain.

Suzanne Vogel-Scibilia MD, President

5227 National Anxiety Foundation
3135 Custer Drive
Lexington, KY 40517

859-272-7166
www.lexington-on-line.com/naf.html

A volunteer nonprofit organization. Its goal is to educate the public and health professionals about anxiety and anxiety disorders (such as panic disorder and obsessive-compulsive disorder) through printed materials and electronic media.

Stephen Cox MD, President & Medical Director
Linda Vernon Blair, Vice President

5228 National Mental Health Association
2000 N Beauregard Street, 6th Floor
Alexandria, VA 22311

703-684-7722
800-969-6642
Fax: 703-684-5968
TTY: 800-433-5959
www.nmha.org

Addresses all aspects of mental health and mental illness. NMHA with over 340 affiliates works to improve the mental health of all Americans.

David L Shern PhD, President & CEO

5229 National Mental Health Consumers' Self-Help Clearinghouse
1211 Chestnut Street, Suite 1207
Philadelphia, PA 19107

215-751-1810
800-553-4539
Fax: 215-636-6312
e-mail: info@mhselfhelp.org
www.mhselfhelp.org

A consumer run national technical assistance center serving the mental health consumer movement. We help connect individuals to self-help and advocacy resources, and we offer expertise to self-help groups, and other peer-run services for mental health consumers. Offers a newsletter.

Joseph Rogers, Executive Director
Daniele Sadres, Project Coordinator

5230 Obsessive Compulsive Anonymous
PO Box 215
New Hyde Park, NY 11040

516-739-0662
e-mail: west24th@aol.com
members.aol.com/west24th/

A fellowship of individuals dedicated to sharing their experience, strength and hope with one another to enable them to solve their common problems and help others recover from OCD. The Twelve Steps are adapted for OCA, to help obtain relief from obsessions and compulsions. Consisting of approximately 1,000 members and 50 chapters, OCA is not allied with any sect, denomination or organization.

5231 Obsessive Compulsive Foundation
676 State Street
New Haven, CT 06511

203-401-2070
Fax: 203-401-2076
e-mail: info@ocfoundation.org
www.ocfoundation.org

Provides vital support to educate the public and professional communities about OCD and related disorders, provides assistance to individuals with OCD and related disorders, their families and friends. The foundation also funds research into the causes and effective treatments of OCD and related disorders.

Joy Kant, President
Patricia Perkins, Executive Director

5232 Suncoast Residential Training Center/Developmental Services Program
Goodwill Industries-Suncoast
10596 Gandy Boulevard
Saint Petersburg, FL 33702

727-523-1512
888-279-1988
Fax: 727-563-9300
TTY: 727-579-1068
www.goodwill-suncoast.org

A large group home which serves individuals diagnosed as mentally retarded with a secondary diagnosis of psychiatric difficulties as evidenced by problem behavior. Providing residential, behavioral and instructional support and services that will promote the development of adaptive, socially appropriate behavior, each individual is assessed to determine socialization, basic academics and recreation. The primary intervention strategy is applied behavior analysis.

Martin Gladysz, Chairman
R Lee Waits, President & CEO

State Agencies & Support Groups

5233 Center for Family Support
333 7th Avenue, 9th Floor
New York, NY 10001

212-629-7939
Fax: 212-239-2211
www.cfsny.org

The Center for Family (CFS) is a not-for-profit human service agency providing support and assistance to individuals with developmental disabilities and traumatic brain injuries throughout New York City, Long Island, the lower Hudson Valley region and New Jersey.

Steven Vernickofs, Executive Director

Illinois

5234 Obsessive Compulsive Foundation of Metropo litan Chicago
2300 Lincoln Park West
Chicago, IL 60614

773-880-1635
Fax: 773-880-1966
e-mail: info@ocfchicago.org
www.ocfchicago.org

Serves adults and children with OCD, their families, and the mental health professionals who treat them. The only Chicago area organization dedicated to OCD.

Ellen Sawyer, Executive Director

Libraries & Resource Centers

5235 Obsessive Compulsive Information Center
Madison Institute of Medicine
7617 Mineral Point Road, Suite 300
Madison, WI 53717

608-827-2470
Fax: 608-827-2479
e-mail: mim@miminc.org
www.miminc.org

This is a resource for OCD and related disorders, such as trichotillomania, body dysmorphic disorder and hypochondriasis. Currently the center has over 22,000 references on file. Quick reference questions can be answered on the phone. In addition, referrals to specialists and support groups are available, as well as patient information booklets on topics related to many psychiatric disorders and their treatments.

James W Jefferson, MD, Co-Director
John H Greist, MD, Co-Director

Research Centers

5236 Lithium Information Center
Madison Institute of Medicine
7617 Mineral Point Road, Suite 300
Madison, WI 53717

608-827-2470
Fax: 608-827-2479
e-mail: mim@miminc.org
www.miminc.org

This is a resource for lithium treated disorders, and other medical and biological applications of lithium. Currently the Center has more than 32,000 references on file. Information is readily available on all aspects of the biomedical uses of lithium including his-

tory, pharmacokinetics, administration and dosage, monitoring procedures, side effects, interactions with other drugs, environmental exposure and nonphychiatric uses.

Margaret Baudhuin, MLS

5237 National Alliance for Research on Schizophrenia and Depression
60 Cutter Mill Road, Suite 404
Great Neck, NY 11021

516-829-0091
800-829-8289
Fax: 516-487-6930
e-mail: info@narsad.org
www.narsad.org

NARSAD raises and distributes funds for scientific research into the causes, cures, treatments, and prevention of severe mental illnesses, primarily schizophrenia.

Stephen G Doochin, Executive Director

Audio Video

5238 Hope and Solutions for OCD
ADD WareHouse
300 NW 70th Avenue, Suite 102
Plantation, FL 33317

954-792-8100
800-233-9273
Fax: 954-792-8545
e-mail: sales@addwarehouse.com
www.addwarehouse.com

A video series about obsessive compulsive disorder with some straight forward solutions and advice for individuals with OCD, their families, doctors, and school personnel. Viewers will learn what OCD is and how to treat it. Discusses how OCD can affect students in school and the impact on the family life.

85 Minutes
ISBN: 1-886941-37-8

5239 Hope and Solutions for Obsessive Compulsive Disorder, Part III
Awareness Foundation for OCD and Related Disorders
564 Cuesta Drive
Aptos, CA 95003

831-684-9684
e-mail: jamescallner@sbcglobal.net
www.ocdawareness.com

An educational psychologist offers educators effective classroom strategies that school personnel may implement with students who have obsessive compulsive disorder and addresses federal law as it pertains to students with disabilities.

5240 It's Not Me...It's My OCD: A Look at Behav ioral Therapy
Aquarius Health Care Videos
18 N Main Street
Sherborn, MA 01770

508-650-1616
888-440-2963
Fax: 508-650-1665
e-mail: info@aquariusproductions.com
www.aquariusproductions.com

1997 28 Minutes
ISBN: 1-581403-38-0

5241 Touching Tree

Awareness Films, author

Pyramid Media
PO Box 1048
Santa Monica, CA 90406

310-828-7577
800-421-2304
Fax: 310-453-9083
e-mail: info@pyramidmedia.com
www.pyramidmedia.com

Chronicles of a young boy trapped in the pain of OCD; how he faces his fears and begins the slow recovery with professional help. A film ideal for teaching the need for sensitivity when dealing with special children and their differences.

38 Minutes

Web Sites

5242 Anxiety Disorders Association of America
www.adaa.org

The only national nonprofit membership organization dedicated to informing the public healthcare professionals and legislators that anxiety disorders are real, serious and treatable. The ADAA promotes the early diagnosis, treatment and cure of anxiety disorders, and is committed to improving the lives of the people who suffer from them.

5243 CyberPsych
www.cyberpsych.org

CyberPsych presents information about psychoanalysis, psychotherapy, and special topics such as anxiety disorder, the problematic use of alcohol, homophobia, and the traumatic effects of racism. CyberPsych is a nonprofit network which offers free web hosting and technical support for internet communication, to nonprofit groups and individuals.

5244 Guidelines for Families Coping with OCD
www.ocdhope.com/gdlines.htm

Offers 19 guidelines for families coping with OCD.

5245 NIH/National Institute of Health
www.nih.gov

The National Institutes of Health is the stweard of medical and behavioral research for the Nation.

5246 National Anxiety Foundation
www.lexington-on-line.com/naf.html

Nonprofit organization that provides education to the public and professionals about anxiety through printed and electronic media.

5247 National Mental Health Consumers' Self-Help Clearinghouse
www.mhselfhelp.org

A consumer run national technical assistance center serving the mental health consumer movement. We help connect individuals to self-help and advocacy resources, and we offer expertise to self-help groups, and other peer-run services for mental health consumers.

5248 Obsessive Compulsive Disorder (OCD)
www.nimh.nih.gov/healthinformation/ocdmenu.cfm

Discusses the diagnosis of obsessive-compulsive disorder, its prevalence among both children and adults. Descibes types of treatment including pharmacotherapy. Gives sources of information for both the individual who has OCD and the family.

5249 Obsessive Compulsive Foundation
www.ocfoundation.org

An international nonprofit organization composed of people with obsessive compulsive disorder and related disorders, their families, friends, professionals, and other concerned individuals.

5250 Planetpsych
www.planetpsych.com

Planetpsych is an online resource for mental health information.

5251 Psych Central
www.psychcentral.com

Offers free informational and educational articles and resources on psychology, support and mental health online.

Book Publishers

5252 Boy Who Couldn't Stop Washing: The Experience and Treatment of OCD

Judith L Rapoport, author

Penguin Group
375 Hudson Street
New York, NY 10014

212-366-2952
us.penguingroup.com

A comprehensive treatment of obsessive-compulsive disorder that summarizes evidence that the disorder is neurobiological. It also describes the effect of medication combined with behavioral therapy.

1991 304 pages Paperback
ISBN: 0-451172-02-0

5253 Brain Lock: Free Yourself from Obsessive Compulsive Behavior

Jeffrey M Schwartz, author

Harper Collins
10 E 53rd Street
New York, NY 10022

212-207-7000
800-242-7737
Fax: 800-822-4090
www.harpercollins.com

A simple four-step method for overcoming OCD that is so effective, it's now used in academic treatment centers throughout the world. Proven by brain-imaging tests to actually alter the brain's chemistry, this method doesn't rely on psychopharmaceuticals but cognitive self-therapy and behavior modification to develop new patterns of response. Offers real-life stories of actual patients.

1997 256 pages Paperback
ISBN: 0-060987-11-1

5254 Brief Strategic Solution-Oriented Therapy of Phobic and Obsessive Disorders

Giorgio Nardone, author

Jason Aronson Publishers
4501 Forbes Boulevard, Suite 200
Lanham, MD 20706

301-459-3366
800-462-6420
Fax: 301-429-5748
www.aronson.com

1996 188 pages Cloth
ISBN: 1-568218-04-4

5255 Childhood Obsessive Compulsive Disorder

Greta Francis, author

Sage Publications
2455 Teller Road
Thousand Oaks, CA 91320

805-499-9774
800-818-7243
Fax: 805-499-0871
e-mail: info@sagepub.com
www.sagepub.com

1996 120 pages
ISBN: 0-803959-22-2

5256 Freeing Your Child from Obsessive-Compulsi ve Disorder

Tamar E Chansky PhD, author

Crown Publishing Group/Random House
280 Park Avenue
New York, NY 10017

212-940-7381
800-733-3000
www.randomhouse.com/crown/

ISBN: 0-812931-17-4

5257 It's Nobody's Fault-New Hope and Help for Difficult Children and Their Parents
ADD WareHouse
300 NW 70th Avenue, Suite 102
Plantation, FL 33317

954-792-8100
800-233-9273
Fax: 954-792-8545
www.addwarehouse.com

This book explains that neither the parents nor children are causes of mental disorders and related problems.

1997 320 pages Paperback
ISBN: 0-812929-21-7

5258 OCD in Children and Adolescents: A Cognitive-Behavioral Treatment Manual
Guilford Publications
72 Spring Street
New York, NY 10012

212-431-9800
800-365-7006
Fax: 212-966-6708
e-mail: info@guilford.com
www.guilford.com

Written for clinicians, the book includes tips for parents, and treatment guidelines. The cognitive-behavioral approach to OCD has been problematic for many to understand because patients with symptoms of increased anxiety are told that their treatment initially involves further increases in their anxiety levels. The authors provide this in a modified and developmentally appropriate approach.

1998 298 pages
ISBN: 1-572302-42-6

5259 Obsessive Compulsive Disorder in Children and Adolescents: A Guide
Madison Institute of Medicine
7617 Mineral Point Road, Suite 300
Madison, WI 53717

608-827-2470
Fax: 608-827-2479
e-mail: mim@miminc.org
www.miminc.org

The guide is a comprehensive introduction to obsessive-compulsive disorder for parents who are learning about the illness. Discusses treating symptoms by a combination of behavorial therapy

and medication and describes various drugs that can be used with children and adolescents in terms of their effects on brain functioning, symptom control, and side effects. The book is attuned to the difficulties families of OCD children face.

66 pages

5260 Obsessive Compulsive Disorder: Helping Children and Adolescents

Mitzi Waltz, author

O'Reilly Media
1005 Gravenstein Highway N
Sebastopol, CA 95472

707-827-7000
800-998-9938
Fax: 707-829-0104
www.oreilly.com

This book helps parents secure an accurate and complete diagnosis, and live with OCD children using effective parenting techniques. Offers support systems, medical interventions and explores therapeutic and other interventions, such as cognitive therapy; helps to secure care with an existing health plan even with no coverage of mental disorders, navigate the special education system and find resources.

2000 404 pages
ISBN: 1-565927-58-3

5261 Obsessive-Compulsive Disorder in Children and Adolescents
American Psychiatric Publishing
1000 Wilson Boulevard, Suite 1825
Arlington, VA 22209

703-907-7322
800-368-5777
Fax: 703-907-1091
e-mail: appi@psych.org
www.appi.org

Examines the early development of obsessive-compulsive disorder and describes effective treatments.

1989 368 pages Hardcover
ISBN: 0-880482-82-0

5262 School Personnel: A Critical Link in the Identification and Management of OCD

Gail B Adams, author

Obsessive Compulsive Foundation
676 State Street
New Haven, CT 06511

203-401-2070
Fax: 203-401-2076
www.ocfoundation.org

Recognizing OCD in the school setting, current treatments, the role of school personnel in identification, assessment, and educational interventions are thoroughly covered in this brief, but informative booklet especially targeted to educators and guidance counselors.

2003 32 pages Booklet

5263 Teaching the Tiger
Hope Press
PO Box 188
Duarte, CA 91009

800-321-4039
Fax: 626-358-3520
www.hopepress.com

Innovative methods of teaching children with ADD, Tourette Syndrome and Obsessive-Compulsive Disorders.

ISBN: 1-878267-34-5

Newsletters

5264 Key Update

National Mental Health Consumer's Self-Help Clrhs.
1211 Chestnut Street, Suite 1207
Philadelphia, PA 19107

215-751-1810
800-553-4539
Fax: 215-636-6312
e-mail: info@mhselfhelp.org
www.mhselfhelp.org

A monthly e-newsletter that provides timely news and notes on important mental health issues, details on upcoming events, and recent publications on policy issues. Topics addressed in the newsletter include self-advocacy, self-care, community integration, human rights and mental health treatments and services.

Monthly

5265 OCD Newsletter

Obsessive Compulsive Foundation
PO Box 9573
New Haven, CT 06535

203-401-2070
Fax: 203-401-2076
e-mail: info@ocfoundation.org
www.ocfoundation.org

For sufferers of obsessive-compulsive disorder and their families and friends.

16-20 pages 6 times/yr

Patricia B Perkins, Executive Director/Editor

Pamphlets

5266 Children and Adolescents

Madison Institute of Medicine
7617 Mineral Point Road, Suite 300
Madison, WI 53717

608-827-2470
Fax: 608-827-2479
e-mail: mim@miminc.org
www.miminc.org

Literature packet: diagnosis, treatment and other information on OCD in young children and adolescents.

5267 Obsessive Compulsive Disorder General Pack et

Madison Institute of Medicine
7617 Mineral Point Road, Suite 300
Madison, WI 53717

608-827-2470
Fax: 608-827-2479
e-mail: mim@miminc.org
www.miminc.org

Literature packet: overview of OCD, including information on prevalence, diagnosis and treatment.

5268 Obsessive-Compulsive Disorder, A Real Illn ess

National Institute of Mental Health
Public Info, 6001 Executive Blvd, Rm 8184
Bethesda, MD 20892

301-443-4513
866-615-6464
Fax: 301-443-4279
TTY: 301-443-8431
e-mail: nimhinfo@nih.gov
www.nimh.nih.gov

Easy-to read booklet on OCD, explaining what it is, when it starts, how long it lasts and how to get help. The booklet also includes a self-test.

DESCRIPTION

5269 OMPHALOCELE

Involves the following Biologic System(s):

Gastrointestinal Disorders, Neonatal and Infant Disorders

An omphalocele is a birth defect characterized by bulging or protrusion of a portion of the intestines through an abnormal opening in the abdominal wall near the navel, the region where the umbilical cord meets the abdomen during fetal growth and development. The bulging area of the intestines is covered by a thin, membrane-like sac consisting of part of the amnion and peritoneum. The amnion is the inner layer of membrane that forms the amniotic sac, the fluid-filled sac within which a fetus grows and develops. The peritoneum is the thin membrane that lines the abdominal cavity and covers the internal abdominal organs.

Depending upon the size of the abdominal wall defect in an affected newborn, varying amounts of intestine or, in severe cases, other abdominal organs, may protrude through the navel. Associated complications may include rupture of the protruding, membranous sac, damage to body tissues due to drying, or onset of infection. Because these complications may be life-threatening, an omphalocele is usually surgically repaired immediately after birth.

An omphalocele is thought to affect approximately one in 4,000 newborns. Prenatal ultrasounds often identify infants with an omphalocele before birth. Otherwise, physical examination of the infant is sufficient to diagnose this condition. In many infants, omphaloceles occur in association with other birth defects, such as abnormalities of the urinary and reproductive systems, central nervous system, or cardiovascular system. This condition may also occur in association with certain rare malformation syndromes that are apparent at birth. These include Beckwith-Wiedemann syndrome, also known as exomphalos-macroglossia-gigantism, and Shprintzen omphalocele syndrome, also called pharynx and larynx hypoplasia with omphalocele.

In other cases, omphaloceles may occur as isolated findings for unknown reasons. Omphaloceles are repaired with surgery, although not always immediately; complete recovery is expected. There have been reports of multiple cases of isolated omphaloceles within certain families (kindreds). In these families, the condition may be caused by abnormal changes (mutations) in a gene or genes that may be inherited as an autosomal recessive or X-linked trait. It is also possible that the interaction of several different genes in association with certain environmental factors (multifactorial inheritance) may play a role in the development of some omphaloceles.

See also **General Resources** on page 917

Government Agencies

5270 Division of Birth Defects & Developmental Disabilities
1600 Clifton Road
Atlanta, GA 30333

404-639-3311
800-311-3435
Fax: 404-639-3534
www.cdc.gov

Information and advocacy resources for families and professionals dealing with children with birth defects and developmental disabilities.

National Associations & Support Groups

5271 American College of Gastroenterology
PO Box 342260
Bethesda, MD 20827

301-263-9000
www.acg.gi.org

Founded to advance the scientific study and medical practice of diseases of the gastrointestinal (GI) tract.

Jack A DiPalma, President
Amy E Foxx-Orenstein, VP

5272 March of Dimes Birth Defects Foundation
1275 Mamaroneck Avenue
White Plains, NY 10605

914-428-7100
888-663-4637
Fax: 914-428-8203
e-mail: resourcecenter@modimes.org
www.marchofdimes.com

Partnership of volunteers and professionals dedicated to improving the health of babies by preventing birth defects and infant mortality. Over 100 chapters are located across the country and can be located through the National Office.

Dr Jennifer Howse, President

5273 North American Society for Pediatric Gastroenterology/Hepatology/Nutrition
PO Box 6
Flourtown, PA 19031

215-233-0808
Fax: 215-233-3918
e-mail: naspghan@naspghan.org
www.naspghan.org

Strives to improve the care of infants, children and adolescents with digestive disorders by promoting advances in clinical care of children with chronic abdominal pain, diarrhea, constipation, vomiting, bleeding from the GI tract, inflammatory bowel disease, liver diseases, diseases of the pancreas, poor weight gain and nutritional problems.

Philip Sherman, President
Margaret K Stallings, Executive Director

Libraries & Resource Centers

5274 National Digestive Diseases Information Clearinghouse
2 Information Way
Bethesda, MD 20892

301-654-3810
800-891-5389
Fax: 703-738-4929
e-mail: nddic@info.niddk.nih.gov
www.digestive.niddk.nih.gov

The National Institute of Diabetes and Digestive and Kidney Diseases conducts and supports research on many of the most serious diseases affecting public health. The Institute supports much of the clinical research on the diseases of internal medicine and related subspecialty fields as well as many basic science disciplines.

Kathy Kranzfelder, Project Officer

Web Sites

5275 Mothers of Omphaloceles
www.omphalocele.com

Support and Webring.

5276 National Digestive Diseases Information Clearinghouse
www.digestive.niddk.nih.gov

The National Institute of Diabetes and Digestive and Kidney Diseases conducts and supports research on many of the most serious diseases affecting public health. The Institute supports much of the clinical research on the diseases of internal medicine and related subspecialty fields as well as many basic science disciplines.

5277 Online Mendelian Inheritance in Man
www.ncbi.nlm.nih.gov

This database is a catalog of human genes and genetic disorders.

5278 Pediatric Surgery Update
home.coqui.net/titolugo/PSU11.htm#1152

An online handbook about many differnt diseases and disablilies.

Journals

5279 Journal of Pediatric Gastroenterology and Nutrition

NASPGHAN, author

Lippincott Williams & Wilkins
530 Walnut Street
Philadelphia, PA 19106

215-521-8300
Fax: 215-521-8902
www.lww.com

Publication of the North American Society for Pediatric Gastroenterolgy, Hepatology and Nutrition, which strives to improve the care of infants, children and adolescents with digestive disorders by promoting advances in clinical care of children with chronic abdominal pain, diarrhea, constipation, vomiting, bleeding from the GI tract, inflammatory bowel disease, liver diseases, diseases of the pancreas, poor weight gain and nutritional problems.

Newsletters

5280 NASPGHAN News
PO Box 6
Flourtown, PA 19031

215-233-0808
Fax: 215-233-3939
e-mail: naspghan@naspghan.org
www.naspgn.org

Publication of the North American Society for Pediatric Gastroenterolgy, Hepatology and Nutrition, which strives to im-

prove the care of infants, children and adolescents with digestive disorders by promoting advances in clinical care of children with chronic abdominal pain, diarrhea, constipation, vomiting, bleeding from the GI tract, inflammatory bowel disease, liver diseases, diseases of the pancreas, poor weight gain and nutritional problems.

DESCRIPTION

5281 OPPOSITIONAL DEFIANT DISORDER

Synonym: ODD

Involves the following Biologic System(s):

Developmental/Behavioral/Psychiatric Disorders

Oppositional Defiant Disorder (ODD) is a disruptive behavioral disorder along with conduct disorder. It is marked by an ongoing pattern of negativistic, argumentative, and hostile behaviors when interacting with some or all authority figures. The symptoms are usually seen in multiple settings, but may be more noticeable at home or at school. Five to fifteen percent of all school-age children have ODD. This disorder is usually apparent before age eight. Although it is more common in boys in the pre-pubertal years, the sex ratio evens out post puberty. The causes of ODD are unknown, but many parents report that their child with ODD was more rigid and demanding than the child's siblings from an early age. Biological and environmental factors may have a role. ODD can also be a precursor to conduct disorder later in life. Children with ODD also have a higher risk of other conditions, including ADHD (attention deficit hyperactivity disorder), anxiety and depression.

ODD is diagnosed by the presence of at least six months of hostile, negative and defiant behavior that is more frequent and intense than expected for a child's age. The behavior must cause significant functional impairment, either socially, academically or occupationally. ODD can not be diagnosed in patients who are actively psychotic or who meet criteria for conduct disorder or antisocial personality disorder.

Treatment for ODD centers upon evaluating the child's physical and psychosocial environment, ruling out or treating co-morbid conditions and assisting parents in anticipating and modifying behavior. Problems in the family or environment that may be driving the behaviors also need to be addressed. Many children with ODD will respond to the positive parenting techniques. A child with ODD can be very difficult for parents who need support and understanding. Older school age children and adolescents with ODD are more likely to benefit from an intensive intervention program.

See also **General Resources** on page 917

National Associations & Support Groups

5282 American Academy of Child and Adolescent Psychiatry
3615 Wisconsin Avenue NW
Washington, DC 20016

202-966-7300
Fax: 202-966-2891
www.aacap.org

The AACAP (American Academy of Child and Adolescent Psychiatry) is the leading national professional medical association dedicated to treating and improving the quality of life for children, adolescents, and families affected by these disorders. The AACAP is a 501 (c)(3) nonprofit organization established in 1953.

Thomas F Anders, MD, President

Audio Video

5283 Explosive Child

Ross W Greene PhD, author

HarperCollins Publishers
1350 Avenue of the Americas
New York, NY 10019

212-261-6500
800-242-7737
www.harpercollins.com

A new approach for understanding and parenting easily frustrated, cronically inflexible children. Dr Greene offers help for you and your child. Now updated with new practical information, The Explosive Child lays out a sensitive, practical approach to helping your child at home and school.

1999 Audio Cassette
ISBN: 0-694521-90-6

Web Sites

5284 American Academy of Child and Adolescent Psychiatry
www.aacap.org

Information on treating and improving the quality of life for children, adolescents, and families affected by such disorders as Oppositional Defiant.

Book Publishers

5285 Defiant Children

Russell A Barkley, author

Guilford Press
72 Spring Street
New York, NY 10012

212-431-9800
800-365-7006
Fax: 212-966-6708
e-mail: info@guilford.com
www.guilford.com

A clear and effective manual includes a thorough clinical guide to Dr. Barkley's 10-session parent training program, an assessment section that incorporates DSM-IV diagnostic criteria, and reproducible materials reinforcing each step of the program.

1997 264 pages 2nd Edition
ISBN: 1-572301-23-6

5286 Disruptive Behavior Disorders in Children and Adolescents

Robert L Hendren, DO, author

American Psychiatric Publishing
1000 Wilson Boulevard, Suite 1825
Arlington, VA 22209

703-907-7322
800-368-5777
Fax: 703-907-1091
e-mail: appi@psych.org
www.appi.org

Comprehensively reviews current research and clinical observations on this timely topic. The authors look at three subtypes of attention-deficit/hyperactivity disorder (ADHD), conduct disorder, and oppositional defiant disorder, all of which are common among youths and often share similar symptoms of impulse control problems.

1999 216 pages Paperback
ISBN: 0-880489-60-7

5287 Explosive Child

Ross W Greene PhD, author

HarperCollins Publishers
1350 Avenue of the Americas
New York, NY 10019

212-261-6500
800-242-7737
www.harpercollins.com

A new approach for understanding and parenting easily frustrated, cronically inflexible children. Dr Greene offers help for you and your child. Now updated with new practical information, The Explosive Child lays out a sensitive, practical approach to helping your child at home and school.

2005 334 pages Paperbcak
ISBN: 0-060931-02-7

5288 New Strong-Willed Child

James C Dobson, author

Tyndale House Publishers
351 Executive Drive
Carol Stream, IL 60188

800-323-9400
Fax: 800-684-0247
www.tyndale.com

A complete update of The Strong-Willed Child for a new generation of parents and teachers. It offers practical advice on raising difficult-to-handle children and incorporates the latest research.

2004 270 pages Hardcover
ISBN: 0-842336-22-2

Magazines

5289 EHealth

UAB Health System
619 19th Street South
Birmingham, AL 35249

205-934-9999
800-822-8816
Fax: 205-934-9991
www.health.uab.edu

A health and fitness publication packed with all the latest news and health tips from the UAB Health System.

Quarterly

Journals

5290 Official Journal of the American Academy of Child and Adolescent Psychiatry

Lippincott Williams & Wilkins
351 West Camden Street
Baltimore, MD 21201

410-528-4200
800-638-3030
Fax: 410-528-8557
www.jaacap.com

The journal is recognized as THE major journal focusing exclusively on today's psychiatric research and treatment of the child and adolescent.

12x a year

Mina K Dulcan MD, Editor
Sara Tiner, Editorial Coordinator

Newsletters

5291 AACAP News

American Academy of Child & Adolescent Psychiatry
3615 Wisconsin Avenue NW
Washington, DC 20016

202-966-7300
Fax: 202-966-2891
www.aacap.org

Official membership publication; provides the latest information on issues that directly affect child and adolescent psychiatrists.

6400 48 pages Bi-monthly

5292 DevelopMentor

American Academy of Child & Adolescent Psychiatry
3615 Wisconsin Avenue NW
Washington, DC 20016

202-966-7300
Fax: 202-966-2891
www.aacap.org

Introduces medical students and residens to the clinical, academic, and research opportunities in child and adolescent psychiatry. Ideal for training directors.

Semi-annual

DESCRIPTION

5293 OSTEOGENESIS IMPERFECTA

Synonyms: Brittle bone disease, OI

Covers these related disorders: Osteogenesis imperfecta Type I (OI Type I), Osteogenesis imperfecta Type II (OI Type II), Osteogenesis imperfecta Type III (OI Type III), Osteogenesis imperfecta Type IV (OI Type IV)

Involves the following Biologic System(s): Genetic/Chromosomal/Syndrome/Metabolic Disorders, Orthopedic and Muscle Disorders

Osteogenesis imperfecta (OI) is an inherited collagen disorder characterized by abnormally brittle, fragile bones that are prone to fracture. Collagen is a protein that forms connective tissue such as bone. This disorder is subdivided into Types I, II, III, and IV. Symptoms of this disorder are widely variable and may include a deep blue appearance of the whites of the eyes (sclerae), loose joints, multiple fractures that may result in stunted or abnormal growth, and deafness resulting from irregular development of the bones in the inner ears (otosclerosis).

Osteogenesis imperfecta Type I is the least severe and most common form of OI. It occurs in approximately one in every 30,000 live births. Common characteristics associated with Type I include bowing of the lower limbs, knock knees (genu valgum), flat feet, short stature, and irregularities of the teeth. As affected children reach adolescence, the frequency of bone fractures may be dramatically reduced. OI Type I is inherited as an autosomal dominant trait.

OI Type II is incompatible with life and is characterized by low birth weight; crumpled bones; and other skeletal abnormalities of the limbs, ribs, and face. As many as 50 percent of Type II births are stillborn, while defects in the rib cage cause death in the others soon after birth. Approximately one in 60,000 infants is affected with OI Type II. This form of the disorder is inherited as an autosomal recessive trait, an autosomal dominant trait, or represents a new spontaneous genetic mutation.

Osteogenesis imperfecta Type III is a progressive form of this disorder characterized in the newborn by multiple fractures and severely fragile bones, progressing to deformity of the skeleton and skull. Although many children reach adolescence, adulthood is rarely attained. Type III is inherited as an autosomal recessive trait or occurs as a result of a new mutation.

OI Type IV is characterized by bone mass reduction (osteoporosis) resulting in fragile bones; however, other symptoms typical of Type I may be absent or less severe. Bone fractures may be present at birth or at any time up to adulthood. Although most individuals will be short of stature, other symptoms of this disorder often improve during early puberty. Osteogenesis Type IV is inherited as an autosomal dominant trait.

Treatment for osteogenesis Types I, III, and IV may include immediate orthopedic intervention for management of bone fractures and deformity correction or surgical intervention as necessary.

See also **General Resources** on page 917

Government Agencies

5294 NIH/National Institute of Child Health and Human Development
National Institutes of Health
Building 31, Room 2A32
Bethesda, MD 20892

> 301-496-5133
> Fax: 301-496-7107
> www.nichd.nih.gov

Supports several basic and clinical research projects on osteogenesis imperfecta.

Nancy D Wirth, Director
Lisa Kaeser, Program & Public Liaison

5295 NIH/Osteoporosis and Related Bone Diseases National Resource Center
2 AMS Circle
Bethesda, MD 20892

> 202-223-0344
> 800-624-2663
> Fax: 202-293-2356
> TTY: 202-466-4315
> e-mail: NIAMSBoneinfo@mail.nih.gov
> www.niams.nih.gov/bone/

Provides patients, health professionals and the public with an important link to resources and information on osteoporosis and other metabolic bone diseases.

Stephen I Katz MD, PhD, Director

National Associations & Support Groups

5296 Genetic Alliance
4301 Connecticut Avenue NW
Washington, DC 20008

> 202-966-5557
> 800-336-4363
> Fax: 202-966-8553
> e-mail: info@geneticalliance.org
> www.geneticalliance.org

A coalition of voluntary genetic support groups, consumers and professionals addressing the needs of individuals and families affected by genetic disorders from a national perspective.

Sharon Terry, President/CEO

5297 Little People of America
5289 NE Elam Young Parkway, Suite F-100
Hillsboro, OR 97124

603-846-1562
888-572-2001
Fax: 503-846-1590
e-mail: info@lpaonline.org
www.lpaonline.org

A nonprofit organization that provides support and information to people of short stature and their families.

Lois Gerage-Lamb, President
Bill Bradford, VP Programs

5298 March of Dimes Birth Defects Foundation
1275 Mamaroneck Avenue
White Plains, NY 10605

914-428-7100
888-663-4637
Fax: 914-428-8203
e-mail: resourcecenter@modimes.org
www.marchofdimes.com

Partnership of volunteers and professionals dedicates to improving the health of babies by preventing birth defects and infant mortality. Over 100 chapters are located across the country and can be located through the National Office.

Dr Jennifer Howse, President

5299 National Dissemination Center for Children with Disabilities
PO Box 1492
Washington, DC 20013

202-884-8200
800-695-0285
Fax: 202-884-8441
e-mail: nichcy@aed.org
www.nichcy.org

A national information and referral center for families, educators and other professionals on: disabilities in children and youth; programs and services; IDEA, the nation's special education law; and research-based information on effective practices.

Suzanne Ripley, Executive Director

5300 Osteogenesis Imperfecta Foundation
804 W Diamond Avenue
Gaithersburg, MD 20878

301-947-0083
800-981-2663
Fax: 301-947-0456
e-mail: bonelink@oif.org
www.oif.org

This foundation serves the needs of people affected by osteogenesis imperfecta, a brittle bone disorder. Offers information, resources, support and a biannual conference.

Heller An Shapiro, Executive Director
Mary Beth Huber, Information/Resource Director

Libraries & Resource Centers

5301 NIH/Osteoporosis and Related Bone Diseases National Resource Center
2 AMS Circle
Bethesda, MD 20892

202-223-0344
800-624-2663
Fax: 202-293-2356
TTY: 202-466-4315
e-mail: NIAMSBoneinfo@mail.nih.gov
www.niams.nih.gov/bone/

Devoted to the dissemination of knowledge regarding the disease along with several helpful medias to explore.

Stephen I Katz MD, PhD, Director

Audio Video

5302 Plan for Success: Educator's Guide to Students with Osteogenesis Imperfecta
Osteogenesis Imperfecta Foundation
804 W Diamond Avenue, Suite 210
Gaithersburg, MD 20878

301-947-0083
800-981-2663
Fax: 301-947-0456
e-mail: bonelink@oif.org
www.oif.org

Information for parents and educators on planning steps that will help children with osteogenesis imperfecta to fully particapate in school activities.

15 minutes

Heller An Shapiro, Executive Director
Mary Beth Huber, Information/Resource Director

5303 You Are Not Alone
Osteogenesis Imperfecta Foundation
804 W Diamond Avenue, Suite 210
Gaithersburg, MD 20878

301-947-0083
Fax: 301-947-0456
e-mail: bonelink@oif.org
www.oif.org

Explores the emotional turmoil of dealing with the diagnosis of OI and offers practical and uplifting solutions for caring for infants with Type II to severe Type III OI. Also valuable for new families with the more mild forms of OI. Available open captioned or with Spanish subtitles (specify if needed). Add $5.00 per video for Canadian orders and $11.00 per video for overseas orders.

Web Sites

5304 Online Mendelian Inheritance in Man
www.ncbi.nlm.nih.gov

This database is a catalog of human genes and genetic disorders.

5305 Osteogenesis Imperfecta Foundation
www.oif.org

Is the only voluntary national health organization dedicated to helping people cope with the problems associated with osteogenesis imperfecta. The foundations mission is to improve the quality of life for individuals affected by OI through research to find treatments and a cure, education, awareness, and mutual support.

5306 Osteoporosis and Related Bone Diseases - National Resource Center
www.niams.nih.gov/bone/

The National Resource Center is dedicated to increasing the awareness, knowledge and understanding of physicians, health professionals, patients, underserves and at-risk populations and the general public about the prevention, early detection and treatment of osteoperosis and related bone diseases.

5307 Shriner's Hospital Research Study Report
www.shrinershq.org

Provides patients, health professionals, and the public with an important link to resources and information on metabolic bone disease, including osteoporosis, Paget's disease of the bone, osteogenesis imperfecta, and hyperparathyroidism. It is dedicated to increasing the underserved and at-risk populations and the general public about the prevention, early detection and treatment of osteoporosis and related bone disease.

5308 Wheeless' Textbook of Orthopaedics
www.wheelessonline.com

Derives from a variety of sources, including journals, articles, national meetings lectures and other textbooks.

Book Publishers

5309 Children with Osteogenesis Imperfecta: Str ategies to Enhance Performance
Osteogenesis Imperfecta Foundation
804 W Diamond Avenue
Gaithersburg, MD 20878

301-947-0083
Fax: 301-947-0456
e-mail: BoneLink@oif.org
www.oif.org

A guide to fitness and exercise for children and teens who have OI. It focuses on practical strategies designed to maximize mobility and function, and prevent some of the complications related to immobility.

2005 270 pages Paperback
ISBN: 0-964218-95-0

Heller An Shapiro, Executive Director
Mary Beth Huber, Information/Resource Director

5310 Growing Up with OI: Guide for Children
Osteogenesis Imperfecta Foundation
804 W Diamond Avenue, Suite 210
Gaithersburg, MD 20878

301-947-0083
800-981-2663
Fax: 301-947-0456
e-mail: bonelink@oif.org
www.oif.org

Tips and experiences from families of people who have osteogenesis imperfecta.

2001 122 pages Paperback
ISBN: 0-964218-92-5

Heller An Shapiro, Executive Director
Mary Beth Huber, Information/Resource Director

5311 Growing Up with OI: Guide for Families and Caregivers
Osteogenesis Imperfecta Foundation
804 W Diamond Avenue, Suite 210
Gaithersburg, MD 20878

301-947-0083
800-981-2663
Fax: 301-947-0456
e-mail: bonelink@oif.org
www.oif.org

Tips and experiences from families of people who have Osteogenesis Imperfecta.

2001 295 pages Paperback
ISBN: 0-964218-91-7

Heller An Shapiro, Executive Director
Mary Beth Huber, Information/Resource Director

5312 Jason's First Day!
Osteogenesis Imperfecta Foundation
804 W Diamond Avenue
Gaithersburg, MD 20878

301-947-0083
Fax: 301-947-0456
e-mail: BoneLink@oif.org
www.oif.org

This picture book tells the story of the first day of school for a child with OI. It can be read to preschool, kindergarten and first grade children. The book includes a teacher's guide and resources for educators to make the transition to school easier for children with OI or other mobility impairing disabilities.

2004 43 pages Paperback
ISBN: 0-964218-94-1

Heller An Shapiro, Executive Director
Mary Beth Huber, Information/Resource Director

5313 Let's Talk About Going to the Hospital
Rosen Publishing Group's PowerKids Press
29 E 21st Street
New York, NY 10010

212-777-3017
800-237-9932
Fax: 888-436-4643
e-mail: rosenpub@tribeca.ios.com
www.powerkidspress.com

If a child has to check into the hospital, chances are he or she is already upset about being ill. Knowing how a hospital functions and what the procedures are, such as when family members can visit, will help in what is already a stressful situation. Grades K-5.

24 pages
ISBN: 0-823950-36-0

5314 Managing Osteogenesis Imperfecta: a Medical Manual
Osteogenesis Imperfecta Foundation
804 W Diamond Avenue, Suite 210
Gaithersburg, MD 20878

301-947-0083
800-981-2663
Fax: 301-947-0456
e-mail: bonelink@oif.org
www.oif.org

The manual is designed for physicians, physical and occupational therapists, orthopedic technologists, early intervention providers and others who come in contact with persons with OI. It covers a broad range of topics including genetics, diagnosis, pregnancy, arthritis, and osteoperosis.

1997

Heller An Shapiro, Executive Director
Mary Beth Huber, Information/Resource Director

5315 Osteogenesis Imperfecta: A Guide for Nurse s
Osteogenesis Imperfecta Foundation
804 W Diamond Avenue
Gaithersburg, MD 20878

301-947-0083
Fax: 301-947-0456
e-mail: BoneLink@oif.org
www.oif.org

A comprehensive guide to assist nursing professionals as they come into contact with people who have OI of all ages. Topics include diagnosis, family education, standard treatments, emergencies and medical procedures. It is intended for nursing professionals, nursing students and familes.

2003 64 pages Paperback

Heller An Shapiro, Executive Director
Mary Beth Huber, Information/Resource Director

Newsletters

5316 Breakthrough
Osteogenesis Imperfecta Foundation
804 W Diamond Avenue
Gaithersburg, MD 20878

301-947-0083
Fax: 301-947-0456
e-mail: bonelink@oif.org
www.oif.org

Newsletter of the Osteogenesis Imperfecta Foundation that provides information on current research and OIF fundraising activities as well as support features. Free within the United States.

24 pages Quarterly

Heller An Shapiro, Executive Director
Mary Beth Huber, Information/Resource Director

Pamphlets

5317 Caring for Infants and Children with Osteogenesis Imperfecta

Osteogenesis Imperfecta Foundation
804 W Diamond Avenue
Gaithersburg, MD 20878

301-947-0083
Fax: 301-947-0456
e-mail: BoneLink@oif.org
www.oif.org

Presents information on caring for a babies and toddlers with OI. Available in Spanish.

17 pages

5318 Osteogenesis Imperfecta: A Guide for Medical Professionals, Ind. & Families

Osteogenesis Imperfecta Foundation
804 W Diamond Avenue
Gaithersburg, MD 20878

301-947-0083
Fax: 301-947-0456
e-mail: BoneLink@oif.org
www.oif.org

Briefly describes osteogenesis imperfecta, its diagnosis and treatment.

10 pages Paperback

5319 Therapeutic Strategies for OI: A Guide for Physical and Occupational Therapists

Osteogenesis Imperfecta Foundation
804 W Diamond Avenue
Gaithersburg, MD 20878

301-947-0083
Fax: 301-947-0456
e-mail: BoneLink@oif.org
www.oif.org

It covers the role of physical and occupational therapy in managing OI. Topics include safe handling of children and adults with OI and strategies for safe, successful therapy.

14 pages Paperback

Heller An Shapiro, Executive Director
Mary Beth Huber, Information/Resource Director

5320 We're Growing Stronger

Osteogenesis Imperfecta Foundation
804 W Diamond Avenue
Gaithersburg, MD 20878

301-947-0083
Fax: 301-947-0456
www.oif.org

Briefly describes osteogenesis imperfecta and introduces the Osteogenesis Imperfecta Foundation, Inc.

DESCRIPTION

5321 OTITIS MEDIA

Synonym: Tympanitis

Covers these related disorders: Acute otitis media, Chronic otitis media, Secretory otitis media

Involves the following Biologic System(s): Infectious Disorders

Otitis media refers to an infection or inflammation of the middle ear, which is an irregularly-shaped cavity that lies in the temporal bone on each side of the skull. This type of inflammation is one of the most common disorders of childhood, especially in children from the ages of six months to three years.

Acute otitis media usually occurs in conjunction with or as a complication of upper respiratory tract infections such as those caused by the common cold. Infections of the respiratory tract commonly involve the eustachian tube that extends from the rear of the nasal area to the middle ear and, in infants and young children, is narrow, short, and positioned somewhat horizontally, thus making these young patients more susceptible to the backward flow of infectious secretions into the middle ear and subsequent infection. In addition, adenoids that are swollen or enlarged from upper respiratory tract infection may block the eustachian tube, thus impairing its ability to drain pus-filled secretions resulting in an accumulation of these infection-causing substances in the middle ear.

Symptoms associated with acute otitis media often develop within a few days of the onset of a respiratory tract infection and include sudden and severe ear pain (otalgia), ringing in the ears (tinnitus), fever, temporary hearing loss, and discomfort. Infants and young children may be irritable, nauseated, and may vomit and have diarrhea. The eardrum (tympanic membrane) may rupture, thus releasing fluid, which leads to relief of pain. In the absence of further complications, the eardrum may heal within a short period of time. The development of symptoms such as dizziness, headache, sudden and significant hearing loss or deafness, chills, and fever may suggest the presence of severe complications including inflammation of the membranes surrounding the brain and spinal cord (meningitis), infection of the inner ear canals (labyrinthitis) or the mastoid bone behind the ear (mastoiditis). Treatment for acute otitis media is dependent upon the causative agent. For example, if the infection is bacterial, antibiotics may be administered. Some children may require surgical intervention through the use of a procedure called myringotomy during which an incision is made in the eardrum to relieve pressure and allow the release of pus and other secretions or through tympanocentesis, a procedure during which the eardrum is surgically punctured to release fluid. Other treatment is symptomatic and supportive. For example, pain relief may be accomplished through the use of analgesic medications.

Some children may develop secretory otitis media (otitis media with effusion), which is a condition that occurs subsequent to eustachian tube blockage or successful resolution of acute otitis media and is characterized by the escape of thin (serous), thick (mucoid), or pus-like fluid from the ear. Associated symptoms may include dizziness and a ringing or buzzing (tinnitus) in the ears. Although this condition may sometimes resolve spontaneously, treatment is often indicated in some infants and children to prevent possible hearing loss and subsequent difficulties in speech and language development. In addition, surgical incision of the eardrum along with insertion of tubes into the eardrum may allow for drainage of fluid. Children who do not respond to these medications and procedures may benefit from the removal of their adenoids (adenoidectomy). Other treatment is symptomatic and supportive.

Chronic otitis media is a persistent infection of the middle ear that is caused by perforation of the eardrum resulting from acute otitis media, eustachian tube blockage, or various injuries. Drainage of pus-filled fluid may occur subsequent to upper respiratory tract infections or after swimming or bathing. Chronic flare-ups may result in the development of relatively small growths (polyps) in the ear and in damage to the small bones (ossicles) of the middle ear, resulting in the impaired ability to conduct sound and subsequent conductive hearing loss. If the perforation is located on the perimeter of the eardrum, complications may include facial paralysis, inflammations involving other ear structures and the brain, and the formation of skinlike growths (cholesteatomas) that may damage or destroy adjacent bones. Treatment may include cleansing of the ear in conjunction with the installation of a hydrocortisone/acetic acid solution, the administration of antibiotics, and surgical removal of cholesteatomas. Surgical intervention may also be indicated to restore the mechanism of the middle ear by establishing the continuity of the small bones and repairing the eardrum through a procedure called tympanoplasty. Other treatment is symptomatic and supportive.

See also **General Resources** on page 917

Government Agencies

5322 Centers for Disease Control
1600 Clifton Road
Atlanta, GA 30333

404-639-3311
www.cdc.gov

Mission is to promote health and quality of life by preventing and controlling disease, injury, and disability.

5323 NIH/National Institute of Allergy and Infectious Diseases
6610 Rockledge Drive, MSC 6612
Bethesda, MD 20892

301-496-5717
Fax: 301-402-3573
TDD: 800-877-8339
www.niaid.nih.gov

Conducts and supports basic and applied research to better understand, treat, and ultimately prevent infectious, immunologic, and allergic diseases.

Anthony S Fauci MD, Director

National Associations & Support Groups

5324 American Academy of Audiology
11730 Plaza America Drive, Suite 300
Reston, VA 20190

703-790-8466
800-222-2336
Fax: 703-790-8631
e-mail: info@audiology.org
www.audiology.org

A professional organization dedicated to providing high quality and balanced hearing care to the public. Provides professional development, education and research and provides increased public awareness of hearing disorders and audiologic services.
ISSN: 1050-0545

Laura Fleming Doyle, CAE, Executive Director
Sydney Hawthorne Davis, Director Communications

5325 American Hearing Research Foundation
8 S Michigan Avenue, Suite 814
Chicago, IL 60603

312-726-9670
Fax: 312-726-9695
e-mail: ahrf@american-hearing.org
www.american-hearing.org

Funds medical research and education into the causes, prevention, and cures of hearing losses, and balance disorders. Also keeps physicians and the public informed of the latest developments in hearing research and education.

Bill Lederer, Executive Director
Lorraine Koch, Assistant Director

5326 March of Dimes Birth Defects Foundation
1275 Mamaroneck Avenue
White Plains, NY 10605

914-428-7100
888-663-4637
Fax: 914-428-8203
e-mail: resourcecenter@modimes.org
www.marchofdimes.com

Partnership of volunteers and professionals dedicates to improving the health of babies by preventing birth defects and infant mortality. Over 100 chapters are located across the country and can be located through the National Office.

Dr Jennifer Howse, President

5327 World Health Organization
Avenue Appia 20
CH-1211 Geneva 27,
Switzerland

www.who.int

WHO is the directing and coordinating authority for health within the United Nations system.

Dr Margaret Chan, Director General

Web Sites

5328 Baylor College of Medicine-Pathology & Pat hogenesis of Otitis Media
www.bcm.edu/oto/grand/42194.html

5329 Group Health Cooperative
www.bcm.tmc.edu/oto/grand/42194.html

5330 Indiana State University School of Medicin e
web.indstate.edu/theme/micro/otitis/otitis.htm

Provides a presentation of the disease including signs, symptoms and illustrations.

5331 PDR.net
www.pdr.net

Offers integrated medical information and education tools. Updated frequently, this site contains the drug information resources needed daily by its prescriber user base arranged together in one site for convenience and ease-of-use.

5332 University of Texas Medical Branch
www.utmb.edu/oto/

Book Publishers

5333 Hearing Care for Children
AGB Association for the Deaf and Hard of Hearing
3417 Volta Place NW
Washington, DC 20007

202-337-5220
800-432-7543
Fax: 202-337-8314
TTY: 202-337-5221
e-mail: publications@agbell.org
www.agbell.org

This professional text for audiologists provides a comprehensive overview of childhood hearing loss and rehabilitation options. Among the topics covered are the causes and effects of childhood hearing loss, the identification and evaluation of such hearing loss, counseling options for affected children and their families, amplification and auditory stimulation, and intervention and education options for children with hearing losses.

1996 372 pages Hardcover

Mark Ross, Editor

5334 Hearing Impairments in Young Children
AGB Association for the Deaf and Hard of Hearing
3417 Volta Place NW
Washington, DC 20007

202-337-5220
800-432-7543
Fax: 202-337-8314
TTY: 202-337-5221
e-mail: publications@agbell.org
www.agbell.org

A useful text that helps educators and professionals effectively manage early intervention programs for children with hearing impairments from birth to five years of age and their families.

1988 239 pages Hardcover
ISBN: 0-133847-01-2

5335 Let's Talk About Going to the Hospital
Rosen Publishing Group's PowerKids Press
29 E 21st Street
New York, NY 10010

212-777-3017
800-237-9932
Fax: 888-436-4643
e-mail: rosenpub@tribeca.ios.com
www.powerkidspress.com

If a child has to check into the hospital, chances are he or she is already upset about being ill. Knowing how a hospital functions and what the procedures are, such as when family members can visit, will help in what is already a stressful situation. Grades K-5.

24 pages
ISBN: 0-823950-36-0

5336 Living with Hearing Loss

Marcia B Dugan, author

Gallaudet University Press
800 Florida Avenue NE
Washington, DC 20002

202-651-5488
Fax: 202-651-5489
TTY: 888-630-9347
e-mail: gupress@gallaudet.edu
gupress.gallaudet.edu

192 pages
ISBN: 1-563681-34-0

5337 Screening for Hearing Loss and Other Otiti s Media

Jackson Roush PhD, author

AGB Association for the Deaf and Hard of Hearing
3417 Volta Place NW
Washington, DC 20007

202-337-5220
800-432-7543
Fax: 202-337-8314
TTY: 202-337-5221
e-mail: publications@agbell.org
www.agbell.org

2001 245 pages Softcover
ISBN: 0-769300-00-6

Pamphlets

5338 Otitis Media
Deafness Research Foundation
15 W 39th Street
New York, NY 10018

212-768-1181

Offers information on otitis media, prevention, causes, treatments and symptoms.

DESCRIPTION

5339 PASSIVE-AGGRESSIVE BEHAVIOR

Involves the following Biologic System(s):

Developmental/Behavioral/Psychiatric Disorders

Passive-aggressive behavior refers to a type of disruptive conduct that is apparent in approximately 20 percent of children and adolescents. Although seemingly compliant, affected individuals usually harbor negative, aggressive, or hostile feelings, but are unable to directly express them. These negative, hostile feelings are typically manifested indirectly and nonviolently through procrastination, forgetfulness, inefficiency, pouting or sullenness, stubbornness, obstructionism, and resistance to requests or demands. When infants and toddlers, passive-aggressive children and adolescents may have manifested their negativistic personalities through difficulties with feeding and toilet training.

Passive-aggressive individuals may be unaware that they are using their behavior to counteract or offset certain frustrations (e.g., feelings of inadequacy). They may persist in these behaviors in an attempt to regain control of a situation or to punish and retaliate. These stubbornly compliant behaviors are apparent in other situations that typically provoke direct displays of assertiveness, hostility, or other forms of aggression. Parents may be overly, but inconsistently, demanding and critical; conversely, affected individuals may, in some cases, be reared by parents or caregivers who are overly permissive and tolerant.

Treatment for passive-aggressive behavior includes the cooperation of parents or caregivers who are often in the best position to provide motivation for children to learn to appropriately express their assertiveness. Such motivation may be further supported by the establishment of firm rules and guidelines, the setting of realistic goals, and the prioritizing of responsibilities. Some parents or caregivers may benefit from direct management training that teaches the necessary skills to facilitate proper behavior and other social skills. Individual, group, and family psychotherapy may also be indicated. Other treatment is supportive.

See also **General Resources** on page 917

Government Agencies

5340 NIH/National Institute of Mental Health
6001 Executive Boulevard, Room 8184, MSC 9663
Bethesda, MD 20892

> 301-443-4513
> 866-615-6464
> Fax: 301-443-4279
> TTY: 301-443-8431
> e-mail: nimhinfo@nih.gov
> www.nimh.nih.gov

Conducts strategic planning for specific research areas as well as for the Institute as a whole.

Dr Thomas R Insel, Director

National Associations & Support Groups

5341 American Mental Health Foundation
1049 5th Avenue
New York, NY 10028
USA

> 212-639-1561
> Fax: 212-737-9027

Researches the theories and techniques of treatment of emotional illness and the implementation of reforms in the mental health system. Efforts have resulted in development of better and less expensive treatment methods. Findings are disseminated in English and other major languages.

Monroe W Spero, MD

5342 Christian Horizons
PO Box 3381
Grand Rapids, MI 49501

> 616-956-7063
> Fax: 616-956-7063
> e-mail: info@christianhorizonsinc.org
> www.christianhorizonsinc.org

Devoted to assisting individuals, with developmental disabilities, on a day-to-day basis.

5343 Federation of Families for Children's Mental Health
9605 Medical Center Drive, Suite 280
Rockville, MD 20850

> 240-403-1901
> Fax: 240-403-1909
> e-mail: ffcmh@ffcmh.org
> www.ffcmh.org

The National family run organization is dedicated exclusively to helping children with mental health needs and their families achieve a better quality of life.

Sandra Spencer, Executive Director

5344 NADD: National Association for the Dually Diagnosed
132 Fair Street
Kingston, NY 12401

> 845-331-4336
> 800-331-5362
> Fax: 845-331-4569
> e-mail: info@thenadd.org
> www.thenadd.org

Nonprofit organization designed to promote the interests of professional and parent development with resources for individuals who have the coexistence of mental illness and mental retardation. Provides conferences, educational services and training materials to professionals, parents, concerned citizens and service organizations.

Dr Robert Fletcher, CEO

5345 National Alliance for the Mentally Ill
2107 Wilson Blvd, Ste 300, Colonial Pplace Three
Arlington, VA 22201

703-524-7600
800-950-6264
Fax: 703-524-9094
TDD: 703-516-7227
e-mail: info@nami.org
www.nami.org

NAMI is a nonprofit, grassroots, self-help, support and advocacy organization of consumers, families and friends of people with severe mental illness, such as schizophrenia, bipolar disorder, major despressive disorder, obsessive compulsive disorder, anxiety disorders, autism and other severe and persistent mental illnesses that affect the brain.

Suzanne Vogel-Scibilia MD, President

5346 National Mental Health Association
2000 N Beauregard Street, 6th Floor
Alexandria, VA 22311

703-684-7722
800-969-6642
Fax: 703-684-5968
TTY: 800-433-5959
www.nmha.org

Addresses all aspects of mental health and mental illness. NMHA with over 340 affiliates works to improve the mental health of all Americans.

David L Shern PhD, President & CEO

5347 National Mental Health Consumers' Self-Help Clearinghouse
1211 Chestnut Street, Suite 1207
Philadelphia, PA 19107

215-751-1810
800-553-4539
Fax: 215-636-6312
e-mail: info@mhselfhelp.org
www.mhselfhelp.org

Offers information, support and appropriate referrals; and promotes public and professional education. Provides networking for those with special interests related to albinism. Promotes and supports research and funding that will improve diagnosis and management of albinism and hypopigmentation.

Joseph Rogers, Executive Director & Founder

State Agencies & Support Groups

5348 Center for Family Support
333 7th Avenue, 9th Floor
New York, NY 10001

212-629-7939
Fax: 212-239-2211
www.cfsny.org

The Center for Family (CFS) is a not-for-profit human service agency providing support and assistance to individuals with developmental disabilities and traumatic brain injuries throughout New York City, Long Island, the lower Hudson Valley region and New Jersey.

Steven Vernickofs, Executive Director

Web Sites

5349 Borderline Personality Disorder Sanctuary
www.mhsanctuary.com/borderline/

Offers a bookstore, resources, articles, hotlines and answers questions about mental health.

5350 CyberPsych
www.cyberpsych.org

CyberPsych presents information about psychoanalysis, psychotherapy, and special topics such as anxiety disorder, the problematic use of alcohol, homophobia, and the traumatic effects of racism. CyberPsych is a nonprofit network which offers free web hosting and technical support for internet communicatios, to nonprofit groups and individuals.

5351 Dual Diagnosis
www.toad.net/~arcturus/dd/papd.htm

Review of personality disorders including PAPD.

5352 El Rolphe Center
members.aol.com/elrolphe/PassiveAggressive.html

Description and overview of the Passive/Aggressive Personality by Dr Sidney Langston.

5353 I.D. Weeks Library
www.usd.edu/library/

5354 National Anxiety Foundation
www.lexington-on-line.com/naf.html

Offers information and help to persons with panic disorders, manic and depressive disorders and mental illness.

5355 New York Online Access to Health
www.noah-health.org

Provides access to high quality full-text consumer health information that is accurate, timely, relevant and unbiased.

5356 Planetpsych
www.planetpsych.com

Planetpsych is an online resource for mental health information.

5357 Psych Central
www.psychcentral.com

Offers free informational and educational articles and resources on psychology, support and mental health online.

Book Publishers

5358 Challenging Behaviour

Eric Emerson, author

Cambridge University Press
32 Avenue of the Americas
New York, NY 10013

212-924-3900
800-872-7423
Fax: 212-691-3239
e-mail: information@cup.org
www.cup.org

Analysis and intervention in people with severe intellectual disabilities

2nd Edition 232 pages Paperback
ISBN: 0-521794-44-7

5359 Clinical Assessment and Management of Severe Personality Disorders
American Psychiatric Press
1000 Wilson Boulevard, Suite 1825
Arlington, VA 22209

703-907-7322
800-368-5777
Fax: 703-907-1091
e-mail: appi@psych.org
www.appi.org

Focuses on issues relevant to the clinician in private practice, including the diagnosis of a wide range of personality disorders and alternative management approaches.

1996 250 pages Hardcover
ISBN: 0-880484-88-6

Paul S Links, Editor

5360 Personality and Psychopathology

American Psychiatric Press
1000 Wilson Boulevard, Suite 1825
Arlington, VA 22209

703-907-7322
800-368-5777
Fax: 703-907-1091
e-mail: appi@psych.org
www.appi.org

Compiles the most recent findings from more than 30 internationally recognized experts. Analyzes the association between personality and psychopathology from several interlocking perspectives: descriptive, developmental, etiological, and theraputic.

1999 544 pages Hardcover
ISBN: 0-880489-23-2

C Robert Cloninger MD, Editor

5361 Type A Behavior

Sage Publications
2455 Teller Road
Thousand Oaks, CA 91320

805-499-0721
Fax: 805-499-0871
e-mail: info@sagepub.com
www.sagepub.com

This important book brings together leading scholars to answer questions about enviromental and genetic factors roles in the development of Type A behavior, whether or not gender has an effect and if Type A parents raise Type A children. Presents current Type A research and discusses issues including theoretical advances, hostility, special populations, measurement and prediction refinements, work settings, medical and psychological refinements and extensions, and interventions.

1991 436 pages Hardcover

DESCRIPTION

5362 PATENT DUCTUS ARTERIOSUS

Synonym: PDA

Involves the following Biologic System(s):

Cardiovascular Disorders

Patent ductus arteriosus is characterized by the persistence of a fetal vessel that maintains a passageway between the major artery that carries oxygen-rich blood to the tissues of the body (descending aorta) and the artery that carries deoxygenated blood to the lungs (pulmonary artery). Before birth, fetal blood receives oxygen from the mother's blood rather than from its own lungs, making it unnecessary for fetal blood to pass from the right side of the heart to the lungs to be oxygenated. To accommodate this fetal blood flow, blood passes through an opening (foramen ovale) in the wall (septum) between the two upper chambers of the heart (atria). Fetal blood is diverted away from the lungs through a vessel known as the ductus arteriosus that connects the pulmonary artery and the aorta. Normally, both the foramen ovale and ductus arteriosus close soon after birth. The persistence of the opening (patency) of the ductus arteriosus causes some blood from the aorta to flow into the pulmonary artery to the lungs instead of moving away from the heart to nourish the tissues of the body.

Symptoms and physical findings associated with patent ductus arteriosus depend upon the size of the opening and the volume of the diverted blood. A small defect may result in no symptoms while a larger opening may result in difficulty in breathing (dyspnea), rapid heartbeat (tachycardia), failure to gain weight, inflammation of the lining of the heart (bacterial endocarditis), and inefficient pumping by the heart (heart failure). Physical findings may include enlargement of the heart (cardiomegaly); characteristic heart sounds; a machinery-like heart murmur; and, if left untreated, abnormally high pressure in the lung's circulatory system (pulmonary hypertension).

Premature infants may require early intervention through restriction of fluid intake, certain drug therapy, or surgery to prevent malfunctioning of the heart or lungs. However, if no immediate surgical or medicinal intervention is required or administered, this defect may spontaneously close in many premature newborns.

In full-term infants and children, a patent ductus arteriosus may require intervention (surgical or catheter closure). Such treatment may be helpful in preventing or alleviating associated complications. The exact cause of patent ductus arteriosus in the full-term infant is unknown. It is thought to result from different genetic and environmental factors (multifactorial). For example, this irregularity may be associated with maternal German measles (rubella) infection. In addition, patent ductus arteriosus is often accompanied by other congenital heart defects. This defect appears in approximately 60 of 100,000 births and is more prevalent in females than males by a ratio of about two to one. The patent ductus arteriosus is non routinely closed in a non-surgical, outpatient catheter procedure in otherwise healthy children.

See also **General Resources** on page 917

Government Agencies

5363 NIH/National Heart, Lung and Blood Institu te

National Institute of Health

31 Center Dr MSC 2486, Bldg 31, Room 5A48

Bethesda, MD 20892

301-592-8573

Fax: 240-629-3246

TTY: 240-629-3255

e-mail: NHLBIinfo@nhlbi.nih.gov

www.nhlbi.nih.gov

Primary responsibility of this organization is the scientific investigation of heart, blood vessel, lung and blood disorders. Oversees research, demonstration, prevention, education, control and training activities in these fields and emphasizes the prevention and control of heart diseases.

Elizabeth G Nabel, MD, Director

Susan Shurin, MD, Deputy Director

5364 NIH/National Institute of Child Health and Human Development

31 Center Drive, Building 31

Bethesda, MD 20892

301-496-5133

Fax: 301-496-1104

www.nichd.nih.gov

Established in 1962 by congress, today the institute conducts and supports research on topics related to the health of children, adults, families and populations. Some of these topics include: developmental disabilities, growth and development, infant death, reproductive health and birth defects.

Nancy D Wirth, Director

Lisa Kaeser, Program & Public Liaison

National Associations & Support Groups

5365 American Heart Association

7272 Greenville Avenue

Dallas, TX 75231

214-373-6300

800-242-8721

Fax: 214-706-1341

e-mail: inquire@amhrt.org

www.amhrt.org

Supports research, education and community service programs with the objective of reducing premature death and disability from cardiovascular diseases and stroke; coordinates the efforts of health professionals, and others engaged in the fight against heart and circulatory disease.

M Cass Wheeler, CEO

5366 Genetic Alliance
4301 Connecticut Avenue NW
Washington, DC 20008

202-966-5557
800-336-4363
Fax: 202-966-8553
e-mail: info@geneticalliance.org
www.geneticalliance.org

A coalition of voluntary genetic support groups, consumers and professionals addressing the needs of individuals and families affected by genetic disorders from a national perspective.

Sharon Terry, President/CEO

5367 March of Dimes Birth Defects Foundation
1275 Mamaroneck Avenue
White Plains, NY 10605

914-428-7100
888-663-4637
Fax: 914-428-8203
e-mail: resourcecenter@modimes.org
www.marchofdimes.com

Partnership of volunteers and professionals dedicates to improving the health of babies by preventing birth defects and infant mortality. Over 100 chapters are located across the country and can be located through the National Office.

Dr Jennifer Howse, President

Web Sites

5368 Congenital Heart Information Network
www.tchin.org

An international organization that provides reliable information, support services and resources to families of children with congenital heart defects and acquired heart disease, adults with congenital heart defects, and the professionals who work with them.

5369 Southern Illinois University School of Medicine
www.siumed.edu/peds/index.htm

Mission is to assist the people of central and southern Illinois in meeting their present and future health care needs through education, clinical service and research.

5370 Yale University School of Medicine
www.info.med.yale.edu/intmed/cardio/chd

A helpful site that explains the causes, symptoms and treatments for Patent Ductus Arteriosus.

Book Publishers

5371 Congenital Disorders Sourcebook
Omnigraphics
PO Box 625
Holmes, PA 19043

800-234-1340
Fax: 800-875-1340
e-mail: info@omnigraphics.com
www.omnigraphics.com

Basic consumer health information on disorders aquired during gestation, including spina bifida, hydrocephalus, cerebral palsy, heart defects, craniofacial abnormalities and fetal alcohol syndrome.

650 pages
ISBN: 0-780809-45-9

DESCRIPTION

5372 PEMPHIGUS

Involves the following Biologic System(s):

Dermatologic Disorders

Pemphigus refers to a group of chronic skin disorders that are characterized by the appearance of blisters on the skin and delicate mucous membranes that line the mouth, for example. Pemphigus most often occurs among the adult population, but may appear at any age. Associated findings include a phenomenon known as Nikolsky's sign, characterized by the tendency of the upper layer of the skin to separate or slough off from the lower layer upon rubbing or other minor trauma. Pemphigus is thought to result from an autoimmune reaction during which the body mistakenly attacks healthy cells. In this case, antibodies attack the cells that glue skin together, resulting in disruptions in contact between the cells.

Benign familial pemphigus is a relatively mild form of this disorder that is inherited as an autosomal dominant trait and is characterized by the persistent and recurrent formation of blisters mainly in the groin area, the armpit (axillary) region, the sides of the neck, and on the bending surfaces of the arms and legs. These localized or widespread lesions rupture, erode, and then crust over and heal. This form of pemphigus is also known as Hailey-Hailey disease.

Pemphigus foliaceus is a rare, usually mild form of the disorder that is characterized by small blisters that are usually localized and rupture easily, erode, and then heal by crusting over or scaling. These lesions most commonly appear on the scalp, neck, face, and trunk. The blisters may cause itching, pain, or burning in the affected areas. Affected individuals may also experience the sloughing off of the upper skin layer (Nikolsky's sign). Some affected individuals may develop a more generalized pattern of eruptions characterized by excessive shedding or peeling of the skin. Treatment for pemphigus foliaceus may include therapy with corticosteriod drugs. In some cases, topical application of corticosteroid ointments, salves, or creams proves beneficial.

Pemphigus vulgaris is a very severe form of disease that is manifested by eruptions of painful, ulcerative lesions in the delicate mucous membranes that line the mouth. Later findings include the appearance of large blisters on previously unaffected areas of the face, chest, abdomen, armpit region, groin area, and the various pressure points of the body. These lesions enlarge and rupture, leaving raw areas that may partially crust over, but have little or no tendency to heal. These raw or denuded areas sometimes give rise to wart-like granulations that emit a strong, offensive odor. This stage of pemphigus vulgaris is sometimes referred to as pemphigus vegetans. The folds of the skin are particularly susceptible to the development of these wart-like lesions. Individuals with pemphigus vulgaris also exhibit Nikolsky's sign. Life-threatening complications associated with pemphigus vulgaris may include secondary bacterial infections such as sepsis or debilitating conditions such as malnutrition and the loss of essential elements, known as electrolytes, in the fluid portion of the blood (e.g., sodium, potassium, and calcium). For this reason, early diagnosis and treatment of pemphigus vulgaris is essential to its successful management. Positive diagnosis may be determined through microscopic examination of a skin sample, obtained through biopsy, that indicates the presence of certain antibody deposits. Initial treatment may include high-dose corticosteroid therapy, followed by long-term administration of corticosteroid or other immunosuppressive drugs to control the disease. Antibiotic therapy may be indicated for treatment of skin or secondary bacterial infections.

Neonatal pemphigus vulgaris develops in the unborn fetus of an affected mother by transmission of the mother's antibodies through the placenta. In most cases, the severity of disease in the fetus is related to the severity of the mother's disease. If the mother is severely affected, the placental transmission of antibodies may potentially threaten the life of the unborn child.

See also **General Resources** on page 917

Government Agencies

5373 NIH/National Institute of Arthritis and Musculoskeletal and Skin Diseases
1 AMS Circle
Bethesda, MD 20892

301-402-4484
Fax: 301-718-6366
e-mail: ord@od.nih.gov
rarediseases.info.nih.gov

The mission of the National Institute of Arthritis and Musculoskeletal and Skin Diseases is to support research into the causes, treatment, and prevention of arthritis and musculoskeletal and skin diseases, the training of basic and clinical scientists to carry out this research, and the dissemination of information on research progress in these diseases.

Stephen I Katz MD PhD, Director

5374 NIH/National Institute of Child Health and Human Development
31 Center Drive, Building 31
Bethesda, MD 20892

301-496-5133
Fax: 301-496-1104
www.nichd.nih.gov

Established in 1962 by congress, today the institute conducts and supports research on topics related to the health of children, adults, families and populations. Some of these topics include: developmental disabilities, growth and development, infant death, reproductive health and birth defects.

Nancy D Wirth, Director
Lisa Kaeser, Program & Public Liaison

National Associations & Support Groups

5375 American Autoimmune Related Diseases Association
22100 Gratiot Avenue
E Detroit, MI 48021

586-776-3900
www.aarda.org

The American Autoimmune Related Diseases Association is dedicated to the eradication of autoimmune diseases and the alleviation of suffering and the socioeconomic impact of autoimmunity through fostering and facilitating collabration in the areas of education, public awareness, research,and patient in an effective, ethical and efficient manner.

Virginia Ladd, Director

5376 Genetic Alliance
4301 Connecticut Avenue NW
Washington, DC 20008

202-966-5557
800-336-4363
Fax: 202-966-8553
e-mail: info@geneticalliance.org
www.geneticalliance.org

A coalition of voluntary genetic support groups, consumers and professionals addressing the needs of individuals and families affected by genetic disorders from a national perspective.

Sharon Terry, President/CEO

5377 International Pemphigus Foundation
1540 River Park Drive, Suite 208
Sacramento, CA 95815

916-922-1298
Fax: 916-922-1458
e-mail: pemphigus@pemphigus.org
www.pemphigus.org

A nonprofit organization with these goals: to increase awareness of pemphigus and pemphigold among the public and the medical community; to provide information and emotional support to pemphigus and pemphigold patients and caregivers; to provide referrals to specialists and to support research into advanced treatments and a cure.

Janet Segall, Interim Executive Director
David A Sirois PhD, President

5378 March of Dimes Birth Defects Foundation
1275 Mamaroneck Avenue
White Plains, NY 10605

914-428-7100
888-663-4637
Fax: 914-428-8203
e-mail: resourcecenter@modimes.org
www.marchofdimes.com

Partnership of volunteers and professionals dedicates to improving the health of babies by preventing birth defects and infant mortality. Over 100 chapters are located across the country and can be located through the National Office.

Dr Jennifer Howse, President

5379 Society for Pediatric Dermatology
8365 Keystone Crossing, Suite 107
Indianapolis, IN 46240

317-202-0224
Fax: 317-205-9481
e-mail: spd@hp-assoc.com
www.pedsderm.net

Objective is to promote, develop and advance education, research and care of skin disease in all pediatric age groups.

Kent Lindeman, Executive Director

State Agencies & Support Groups

California

5380 International Pemphigus Foundation: Southe rn California Support Group

310-559-5462
e-mail: lynntg@prodigy.net

Lynn Glick

Maryland

5381 International Pemphigus Foundation: Baltim ore Support Group

410-750-1618
e-mail: byrnete@comcast.net

Erica Byrne

Massachusetts

5382 International Pemphigus Foundation: Massac husetts Support Group

978-463-0965
e-mail: alppy@comcast.net

Alan Papert

New York

5383 International Pemphigus Foundation: New Yo rk Support Group

Valley Stream, NY

516-825-4594
e-mail: mayykoe@aol.com

Matt Koenig

South Carolina

5384 International Pemphigus Foundation: South Carolina Support Group

Gray Court, SC

864-386-1620
e-mail: bubba2coggins@juno.com

Cheryl Jordan

Texas

5385 International Pemphigus Foundation
828 San Pablo Avenue
Albany, CA 94706

510-527-4970
Fax: 510-527-8497
e-mail: pemphigus@pemphigus.org
www.pemphigus.org

International Pemphigus Foundation is a 501(c)(3) nonprofit organization. Our goals are to increase awareness of pemphigus and pemphigoid among the public and the medical community; to provide information and emotional support to pemphigus and pemphigold patients and caregivers; to provide referrals to specialists and to support research into advanced treatments and a cure.

12 pages Newsletter/Qtr

Janet Segall, Executive Director

5386 International Pemphigus Foundation Dallas Support Group

817-557-9642
e-mail: angela.bob@netzero.net

Angela Vickers

5387 International Pemphigus Foundation: Housto n Support Group
5231 Kinglet Street
Houston, TX 77035

713-723-5647
Fax: 713-726-0286
e-mail: richardm@hal-pc.org

Richard M Schwartz

Audio Video

5388 International Pemphigus Foundation Promoti onal Video
International Pemphigus Foundation
1540 River Park Drive, Suite 208
Sacramento, CA 95815

916-922-1298
e-mail: pemphigus@pemphigus.org
www.pemphigus.org

Promotional video available ($5.00 S/H).

Free 15 Minutes

Web Sites

5389 Pemphigus FAQ
www.geocities.com/HotSprings/7445/

Offers information about pemphigus.

Newsletters

5390 IPF Quarterly
1540 River Park Drive, Suite 208
Sacramento, CA 95815

916-922-1298
e-mail: pemphigus@pemphigus.org
www.pemphigus.org

The International Pemphigus Foundation's newsletter. Dedicated exclusively to the subject of pemphigus and pemphigoid, providing the latest medical research news and reports on treatment, drugs and events.

12 pages Quarterly

5391 National Pemphigus Foundation Newsletter
1098 Euclid Avenue, PO Box 9606
Berkeley, CA 94709

510-527-4970
Fax: 510-527-8497
e-mail: PVnews@aol.com
www.pemphigus.org

Provides the latest medical research news and reports on treatment, drugs and events relating to pemphigus. Contains support group updates, as well as news on the Foundation's many activities.

Pamphlets

5392 An Introduction to Pemphigus
1540 River Park Drive, Suite 208
Sacramento, CA 95815

916-922-1298
Fax: 916-922-1458
e-mail: pemphigus@pemphigus.org
www.pemphigus.org/pubs.html

An overview of pemphigus

14 pages Handbook

5393 Pemphigus and Pemphigoid At a Glance
1540 River Park Drive, Suite 208
Sacramento, CA 95815

916-922-1298
Fax: 916-922-1458
e-mail: pemphigus@pemphigus.org
www.pemphigus.org/pubs.html

An introductory brochure designed for the doctors office. It provides a helpful overview of each disease.

2 pages Brochure

DESCRIPTION

5394 PHENYLKETONURIA (PKU)

Synonyms: Classic phenylketonuria, PKU

Involves the following Biologic System(s):

Genetic/Chromosomal/Syndrome/Metabolic Disorders

Phenylketonuria (PKU) is an inherited metabolic disorder characterized by the absence or deficiency of phenylalanine hydroxylase, an enzyme that assists in the metabolism of phenylalanine. This enzyme normally converts phenylalanine into tyrosine. The absence of phenylalanine hydroxylase results in the accumulation of excessive phenylalanine in the blood. This may lead to severe mental retardation that is frequently accompanied by seizures and other neurologic problems.

Initially, affected newborns usually have no symptoms; however, early symptoms may include severe vomiting and poor eating. Mental retardation develops slowly but progressively and may become apparent within the first few months of life. Untreated or undiagnosed children may develop neuromuscular irregularities such as involuntary, continuous, slow movements of the arms and legs (athetosis). Other findings may include seizures and hyperactivity, sometimes accompanied by rhythmic behaviors such as rocking. Affected infants usually have light-colored skin, blonde hair, and blue eyes. In addition, an eczema-type rash may develop that eventually disappears with age. Children with PKU often produce an unpleasant, musty odor that results from the presence of phenylacetic acid in the sweat and urine. Other findings in untreated children may include a small head (microcephaly), irregularities of the teeth and upper jaw (maxilla), and delayed growth.

Phenylketonuria is diagnosed by a blood test known as the Guthrie or PKU test. A small amount of blood is withdrawn from the newborn's heel. If blood levels of phenylalanine are elevated, further testing is done to confirm the presence of this disorder. Treatment for PKU is aimed toward reducing dietary intake of phenylalanine in order to prevent or lessen the effects of damage to the brain. This diet is administered and monitored under close supervision. Phenylalanine is not manufactured by the body and is obtained solely through diet. Certain levels of phenylalanine must be maintained to prevent life-threatening complications. Immediate dietary management is initiated upon diagnosis. It is recommended that pregnant women with PKU or affected women who are planning to become pregnant maintain a low phenylalanine diet to avoid the risk of miscarriage. In addition, infants born to women with PKU who are not on a special diet are at high risk of such irregularities as mental retardation, microcephaly, and congenital heart defects.

Phenylketonuria is transmitted as an autosomal recessive trait. In the United States, approximately one in 16,000 is affected by this disorder, however, routine blood screening performed shortly after birth should identify infants with this disorder.

See also **General Resources** on page 917

National Associations & Support Groups

5395 Association for Neuro-Metabolic Disorders
5223 Brookfield Lane
Sylvania, OH 43506

419-885-1497
e-mail: volk4olks@aol.com

Nonprofit organization that serves as an advocate organization for families of patients with the following neuro-metabolic disorders: phenylketonuria, maple syrup urine disease, galactosemia, and biotinidase deficiency. Provides educational information for parents and children; provides networking information on support groups for new parents; supports scientific research into the treatments of these four neuro-metabolic disorders.

Cheryl Volk, Contact Person

5396 Children's PKU Network
3790 Via De La Valle, Suite 120
Del Mar, CA 92014

858-509-0767
800-377-6677
Fax: 858-509-0768
e-mail: pkunetwork@aol.com
www.pkunetwork.org

Provides support services and treatment products to families affected by phenylketonuria (PKU). Services include referral, newborn express packages, digital scale sales and crises intervention aid.

Cindy Neptune, Executive Director

5397 March of Dimes Birth Defects Foundation
1275 Mamaroneck Avenue
White Plains, NY 10605

914-428-7100
888-663-4637
Fax: 914-428-8203
e-mail: resourcecenter@modimes.org
www.marchofdimes.com

Partnership of volunteers and professionals dedicates to improving the health of babies by preventing birth defects and infant mortality. Over 100 chapters are located across the country and can be located through the National Office.

Dr Jennifer Howse, President

State Agencies & Support Groups

Illinois

5398 PKU Organization of Illinois
PO Box 102
Palatine, IL 60078

630-415-2219
Fax: 208-978-8963
e-mail: info@pkuil.org
www.pkuil.org

Resource for families in Illinois and around the world dealing with phenylketonuria. Founded in 1969 for the benefit of patients and families.

Joseph Annunzio, President
Lisa Irgang, VP

Research Centers

5399 National Phenylketonuria (PKU) Foundation
6301 Tejas Drive
Pasadena, TX 77503

713-487-4802

Web Sites

5400 National Human Genome Research Institute
biotech.law.lsu.edu/research/fed/tfgt/appendix5.htm

Report on the history of phenylketonuria screening in newborns in the U.S.

5401 National Society for Phenylketonuria (UK)
www.nspku.org

Helps and supports people with PKU, their families and caregivers. The NSPKU actively promotes the care and treatment of PKU and works closely with medical professionals in the UK.

5402 Online Mendelian Inheritance in Man
www.ncbi.nlm.nih.gov

This database is a catalog of human genes and genetic disorders.

5403 PKU Kid Zone
www.pkuil.org/kidzone.htm

Provides activities for chidren to have fun online.

5404 PKU Mailing List
www.nspku.org/listserve

Worldwide mailing list making communication between families dealing with PKU easier.

5405 PKU Organization of Illinois
www.pkuil.org

Committed to the support of appropriate research initiatives to better understand PKU and eventually find a cure. Support services include: get togethers for kids and parents to express their concerns and share ways of coping with the disease, annual picnics throughout the state and family camp to get to know other PKU families, and activities on both state and national levels in protecting the interests of PKU families.

5406 Star-G: Screening, Technology and Research in Genetics
www.newbornscreening.info/pro/facts.html

General and newborn screening information for amino acid disorders including PKU.

Newsletters

5407 National PKU News
6869 Woodland Avenue NE, Suite 116
Seattle, WA 98115

206-525-8140
Fax: 206-525-5023
e-mail: schuett@pkunews.org
www.pkunews.org

Nonprofit organization dedicated to providing up-to-date, accurate news and information to families and professionals dealing with phenylketonuria through this newsletter.

2000+ 3 issues/year

Virginia Schuett, Director/Editor

5408 PKU Press
PKU Organization of Illinois
PO Box 102
Palatine, IL 60078

630-415-2219
Fax: 208-978-8963
e-mail: info@pkuil.org
www.pkuil.org

Provides information, support, and highlights achievements for the benefit of the PKU community.

20 pages 3x/year

Joseph Annunzio, President
Lisa Irgang, VP

Pamphlets

5409 PKU Information Sheet
March of Dimes
1275 Mamaroneck Avenue
White Plains, NY 10605

914-997-4488
www.marchofdimes.com/professionals/14332_1219.asp

DESCRIPTION

5410 PHOBIAS

Involves the following Biologic System(s):
Developmental/Behavioral/Psychiatric Disorders

A phobia is a persistent, exaggerated, unreasonable fear or dread of certain activities, situations, objects, or events. Exposure to the activity, situation, or object that arouses fear typically elicits signs of anxiety or panic reaction. Such symptoms may include nausea, abdominal pain, irregular pulsation or racing of the heart (palpitations), sweating, and dizziness. In contrast to adults, children, especially younger one, don't see their fear as excessive or unreasonable. Most children are fearful of particular things as they reach certain age plateaus. For example, young children are often afraid of monsters or of being alone in the dark. Older children may be fearful of death or other distressing situations. Children may become fearful of events or situations that they view on television. Others may have fear or dread related to conflicts in the home. These fears are not unusual and may often be alleviated by reassurances and comforting by parents and caregivers. However, a fear or phobia that interferes with normal, day-to-day functioning is considered pathologic.

Simple or specific phobias include fear of certain animals and insects or particular situations (e.g., fear of flying, etc.). Social phobias, often appearing in late childhood or adolescence, include fear and avoidance of certain social situations such as using public bathroom facilities or eating, speaking, performing, or writing in public. Researchers believe that some simple phobias may result from an associated, traumatic childhood experience or from the existence of a similar fear in a parent or caregiver. More complicated specific phobias (e.g., fear of attending school, etc.) may be associated with such conflicts as a hostile-dependent relationship between the parent or caregiver and the child.

Treatment for phobias is dependent upon the specific fear, the extent of the fear, and the effect of the phobias on day-to-day living. Parents or caregivers are counseled to remain calm and patient when confronted with a phobic episode. Behavioral therapy, including relaxation therapy for older children, may be indicated and may include the training of parents or caregivers in the use of supportive measures and techniques. Slow and orderly exposure to the activity, situation, or object of fear (desensitization) may help to alleviate the fear. Older children and adolescents with social phobias may learn to overcome their particular fear through social skills training. Other treatment is symptomatic and supportive.

See also **General Resources** on page 917

Government Agencies

5411 Center for Mental Health Services Knowledge Exchange Program
US Department of Health and Human Services
PO Box 42557
Washington, DC 20015

800-789-2647
Fax: 240-747-5470
TDD: 866-889-2647
http://mentalhealth.samhsa.gov

Supplies the public with expert responses to commonly asked questions about various mental health disorders, and directs the caller to appropriate resources.

5412 NIH/National Institute of Mental Health
6001 Executive Boulevard, Room 8184, MSC 9663
Bethesda, MD 20892

301-443-4513
866-615-6464
Fax: 301-443-4279
TTY: 301-443-8431
e-mail: nimhinfo@nih.gov
www.nimh.nih.gov

Conducts strategic planning for specific research areas as well as for the Institute as a whole.

Dr Thomas R Insel, Director

National Associations & Support Groups

5413 American Mental Health Foundation
1049 5th Avenue
New York, NY 10028

212-639-1561
Fax: 212-737-9027

Organization dealing with medical theory of emotional illness.

5414 Anxiety Disorders Association of America
8730 Georgia Avenue, Suite 600
Silver Spring, MD 20910

240-485-1001
Fax: 240-485-1035
e-mail: AnxDis@adaa.org
www.adaa.org

A national nonprofit organization dedicated exclusively to promoting the prevention, treatment, and cure of anxiety disorders and improving the lives of all people touched by these disorders. ADAA provides educational and advocacy services, supports research, self help, and access to care. ADAA serves consumers, health care professionals, researchers, educators and other interested individuals and organizations. The association publishes a bimonthly newsletter ands hosts an annual conference.

Francine Greenberg, Communications/PR Manager

5415 Anxiety Disorders Institute
1 Dunwoody Park Suite 112
Atlanta, GA 30338

770-395-6845

Provides support, training, and services for those suffering from anxiety disorders, and their families.

5416 Anxiety and Phobia Treatment Center
Whire Plains Hospital Center
Davis Avenue
White Plains, NY 10601

914-681-1038
Fax: 914-681-2284
e-mail: questions@phobia-anxiety.org
phobia-anxiety.com

Treatment groups for individuals suffering from phobias. Deals with fears through contextual therapy, a treatment and study of the phobia in the actual setting in which the phobic reactions occur. Conducts Intensive Courses, Phobia Self-Help Groups, 8-week Phobia Clinics and individual treatment. Publications: PM Newsletter, bimonthly. Articles and papers. Annual conference.

Fredrick J Neumen, MD, Director

5417 Federation of Families for Children's Mental Health
9605 Medical Center Drive, Suite 280
Rockville, MD 20850

240-403-1901
Fax: 240-403-1909
e-mail: ffcmh@ffcmh.org
www.ffcmh.org

The National family run organization is dedicated exclusively to helping children with mental health needs and their families achieve a better quality of life.

Sandra Spencer, Executive Director

5418 Freedom From Fear
308 Seaview Avenue
Staten Island, NY 10305

718-351-1717
Fax: 718-667-8893
freedomfromfear.com

The mission of Freedom From Fear is to aid and counsel individuals and their families who suffer from anxiety and depressive illness.

Mary Guardino, Founder

5419 National Alliance for the Mentally Ill
2107 Wilson Blvd, Ste 300, Colonial Place Three
Arlington, VA 22201

703-524-7600
800-950-6264
Fax: 703-524-9094
TDD: 703-516-7227
e-mail: info@nami.org
www.nami.org

NAMI is a nonprofit, grassroots, self-help, support and advocacy organization of consumers, families and friends of people with severe mental illness, such as schizophrenia, bipolar disorder, major despressive disorder, obsessive compulsive disorder, anxiety disorders, autism and other severe and persistent mental illnesses that affect the brain.

Suzanne Vogel-Scibilia MD, President

5420 National Anxiety Foundation
3135 Custer Drive
Lexington, KY 40517

859-272-7166
www.lexington-on-line.com/naf.html

Nonprofit organization that provides education to the public and professionals about anxiety through printed and electronic media.

Stephen Cox MD, President & Medical Director

5421 National Mental Health Association
2000 N Beauregard Street, 6th Floor
Alexandria, VA 22311

703-684-7722
800-969-6642
Fax: 703-684-5968
TTY: 800-433-5959
www.nmha.org

Addresses all aspects of mental health and mental illness. NMHA with over 340 affiliates works to improve the mental health of all Americans.

David L Shern PhD, President & CEO

5422 National Mental Health Consumers' Self-Help Clearinghouse
1211 Chestnut Street, Suite 1207
Philadelphia, PA 19107

215-751-1810
800-553-4539
Fax: 215-636-6312
e-mail: info@mhselfhelp.org
www.mhselfhelp.org

Offers information, support and appropriate referrals; and promotes public and professional education. Provides networking for those with special interests related to albinism. Promotes and supports research and funding that will improve diagnosis and management of albinism and hypopigmentation.

Joseph Rogers, Executive Director & Founder

5423 Phobia Society of America
133 Rollins Avenue, Suite 4B
Rockville, MD 20852

301-231-9350
Fax: 301-231-7392
www.adaa.org

Offers support for those suffering from phobia and panic attacks.

5424 Phobics Anonymous
PO Box 1180
Palm Springs, CA 92263

706-327-2148

Twelve-step program for panic disorders and anxiety. Publications available.

Marily Gellis PhD, Contact

5425 Selective Mutism Foundation
PO Box 450632
Sunrise, FL 33345

305-748-7714
Fax: 305-748-7714
personal.mia.bellsouth.net/mia/gla/garde

Promotes awareness and understanding for individuals and families affected by selective mutism, an inherited anxiety disorder in which children with normal or deficient language skills are unable to speak in school or social situations. SM is often mistaken for normal shyness and may go undetected for as long as two years. Encourages research and treatment. Maintains speakers' bureau. Publications: Let's Talk, annual newsletter. Selective Mutism, A Silent Cry for Help, brochure.

Sue Newman, Co-Founder & Director

5426 Special Interest Group on Phobias and Related Anxiety Disorders (SIGPRAD)
245 E 87th Street
New York, NY 10028

212-860-5560
Fax: 212-744-5751
e-mail: lindy@interport.net
www.cyberpsych.org

For psychologists, psychiatrists, social workers and other individuals interested in treatment of anxiety disorders. Objectives are to increase knowledge, facilitate communication, and support research and treatment of phobias and related anxiety disorders. Conducts programs at professional meetings. Affiliated with the Association for Advancement of Behavior Therapy. Periodic symposiums and workshops.

Carol Lindemann, PhD, CEO

5427 Territorial Apprehensiveness (TERRAP) Programs
932 Evelyn Street
Menlo Park, CA 94025

800-274-6242

To disseminate information concerning the recognition, causes, and treatment of anxieties, fears and phobias especially agoraphobia. Provides information and counseling for those with phobias. Sponsors service centers and training for psychotherapists and counselors. Publications: TERRAP Manual, audiotapes, booklets, monographs, and videos.

Crucita V Hardy, Director

State Agencies & Support Groups

5428 Center for Family Support
333 7th Avenue, 9th Floor
New York, NY 10001

212-629-7939
Fax: 212-239-2211
www.cfsny.org

The Center for Family (CFS) is a not-for-profit human service agency providing support and assistance to individuals with developmental disabilities and traumatic brain injuries throughout New York City, Long Island, the lower Hudson Valley region and New Jersey.

Steven Vernickofs, Executive Director

Research Centers

5429 UC Berkeley School of Social Welfare
Mental Health & Social Welfare Research Group
303 Haviland Hall
Berkeley, CA 94720

510-642-3949
e-mail: spsegal@berkeley.edu
socialwelfare.berkeley.edu/mhswrg/mhswrg.html

Steven P Segal, Director

Audio Video

5430 Acquiring Courage: Audio Cassette Program for the Rapid Treatment of Phobias
New Harbinger Publications
5674 Shattuck Avenue
Oakland, CA 94609

510-652-2002
800-748-6273
Fax: 510-652-5472
e-mail: customerservice@newharbinger.com
newharbinger.com

ISBN: 1-879237-03-2

5431 Anxiety Disorders
American Counseling Association
5999 Stevenson Avenue
Alexandria, VA 22304

703-823-9800
800-347-6647
Fax: 703-823-0252
e-mail: ryep@counseling.org
counseling.org

Increase your awareness of anxiety disorders, their symptoms, and effective treatments. Learn the effect these disorders can have on life and how treatment can change the quality of life for people presently suffering from these disorders. Includes 6 audiotapes and a study guide.

5432 Fear of Illness
New Harbinger Publications
5674 Shattuck Avenue
Oakland, CA 94609

510-652-2002
800-748-6273
Fax: 510-652-5472
e-mail: customerservice@newharbinger.com
harbinginger.com

120 minute videotape that reduces fears arising from unexplained pain or symptoms; learn to relax while you desensitize to strange body sensations.

ISBN: 1-572240-15-6

5433 Flying
New Harbinger Publications
5674 Shattuck Avenue
Oakland, CA 94609

510-652-2002
800-748-6273
Fax: 510-652-5472
e-mail: customerservice@newharbinger.com
newharbinger.com

120 minute videotape that reduces fear to the point where you can take longer and longer flights; desensitize to the sensations of flying.

ISBN: 1-879237-90-3

5434 Heights
New Harbinger Publications
5674 Shattuck Avenue
Oakland, CA 94609

510-652-2002
800-748-6273
Fax: 510-652-5472
e-mail: customerservice@newharbinger.com
newharbinger.com

120 minute videotape that makes you feel more comfortable in high - rise buildings, on bridges, and on mountain roads.

ISBN: 1-879237-91-1

Web Sites

5435 Answers to Your Questions about Panic Disorder
www.apa.org/pubinfo/panic.html

The objects of the APA shall be to advance psychology as a science and profession and as a means of promoting health, education, and human welfare by: encouragement of psychology in all its branches in the broadest and most liberal manner, the promotion of research in psychology and the improvement fo research methods and conditions, and the improvement of the qualifications and usefulness of psychologists through high standards of ethics, conduct, education, and achievement.

5436 Anxiety Panic Internet Resource
www.algy.com/anxiety/

It is the web's first and still best self-help resource for those with anxiety disorders, Panic attacks, phobias, extreme shyness, obsessive-compulsive behaviors, and generalized anxiety disrupt the lives of an estimated 15% of the population. It is a free grass-root website dedicated to providing information, relief, and support for those recovering from debilitating anxiety.

5437 Basic Guided Relaxation: Advanced Technique
www.dstress.com/guided.htm

A guide to relaxation.

5438 Causes of Anxiety and Panic Attacks
www.algy.com/anxiety/files/barlow.html

Provides information concerning phobias, what they are, the symptoms, and the effects of phobias.

5439 CyberPsych
www.cyberpsych.org

CyberPsych presents information about psychoanalysis, psychotherapy, and special topics such as anxiety disorder, the problematic use of alcohol, homophobia, and the traumatic effects of racism. CyberPsych is a nonprofit network which offers free web hosting and technical support for internet communication, to nonprofit groups and individuals.

5440 National Anxiety Foundation
www.lexington-on-line.com/naf.html

Endeavours to educate the public and professionals about anxiety through printed and electronic media. A volunteer, nonprofit entity.

5441 National Panic/Anxiety Disorder Newsletter
www.npadnews.com

We provide the most up to date material which is gathered from many resourced and contributors form all corners of the globe.

5442 Panic Disorder, Separation, Anxiety Disorder
www.klis.com/chandler/pamphlet/panic

Provides information about panic attacks and more, about what can be done and what medican treatments there are.

5443 Planetpsych
www.planetpsych.com

Planetpsych is an online resource for mental health information.

5444 Recovery Panic Anxiety
www.alt.recovery.panic.anxiety.self-help

An online support group t talk about anxiety recovery.

Book Publishers

5445 An End to Panic: Breakthrough Techniques for Overcoming Panic Disorder

Elke Zuercher-White, author

New Harbinger Publications
5674 Shattuck Avenue
Oakland, CA 94609

510-652-2002
800-748-6273
Fax: 510-652-5472
e-mail: customerservice@newharbinger.com
www.newharbinger.com

A state of the art treatment program covers breathing retraining, taking charge of fear-fueling thoughts, overcoming the fear of physical symptoms, coping with phobic situations, avoiding relapse, and living in the here and now.

232 pages Paperback
ISBN: 1-572241-13-6

5446 Anxiety & Phobia Workbook

Edmund J Bourne, author

New Harbinger Publications
5674 Shattuck Avenue
Oakland, CA 94609

510-652-2002
800-748-6273
Fax: 510-652-5472
e-mail: customerservice@newharbinger.com
www.newharbinger.com

This comprehensive guide is recommended to those struggling with anxiety disorders. Includes step-by-step instructions for the

crucial cognitive-behavioral techniques that have given real help to hundreds of thousands of readers struggling with anxiety disorders.

448 pages 4th Edition
ISBN: 1-572244-13-5

5447 Anxiety Cure: An Eight-Step Program for Ge tting Well
John Wiley & Sons
10475 Crosspoint Boulevard
Indianapolis, IN 46256

877-762-2974
Fax: 800-597-3299
www.wiley.com

A practical guide, written by a father and his two daughters, featuring a step-by-step program for curing the six main kinds of anxiety.

272 pages 2nd Edition
ISBN: 0-471464-87-2

5448 Anxiety Disorders
Cambridge University Press
40 W 20th Street
New York, NY 10011

212-924-3900
800-872-7423
Fax: 914-937-4712
e-mail: marketing@cup.org
cup.org

This comprehensive text covers all the anxiety disorders found in the latest DSM and ICD classifications. Provides detailed information about seven principal disorders, including anxiety in the medically ill. For each disorder, the book covers diagnosis criteria, epidemiology, etiology and pathogenesis, clinical features, natural history and different diagnoses. Describes treatment approaches, both psychological and pharmacological.

354 pages

5449 Anxiety Disorders: Practioner's Guide
John Wiley & Sons
605 3rd Avenue
New York, NY 10058

212-850-6000
Fax: 212-850-6008
e-mail: info@wiley.com
wiley.com

210 pages
ISBN: 0-471931-12-8

5450 Anxiety and Phobia Workbook
Anxiety Disorders Association of America
8730 Georgia Avenue
Silver Spring, MD 20910

301-231-9350
Fax: 301-231-7392
e-mail: AnxDis@adaa.org
adaa.org

Comprehensive guide offering help to anyone who is struggling with panic attacks, agoraphobia, social fears, generalized anxiety, obsessive-compulsive behavior or other anxiety disorders.

1995

Alies Muskin, COO
Michelle Alonso, Communications/Membership

5451 Encyclopedia of Phobias, Fears, and Anxieties
Facts on File
11 Penn Plaza, Room M274
New York, NY 10001

212-290-8090
800-322-8755

500 pages

5452 Helping Your Anxious Child
New Harbinger Publications
5674 Shattuck Avenue
Oakland, CA 94609

510-652-2002
800-748-6273
Fax: 510-652-5472
e-mail: customerservice@newharbinger.com
www.newharbinger.com

Step-by-step guide for parents of anxious children to help them overcome their fears and anxieties. Detailed strategies and techniques.

168 pages Paperback
ISBN: 1-572241-91-8

5453 It's Nobody's Fault: New Hope and Help for Difficult Children and Their Parents
ADD WareHouse
300 NW 70th Avenue
Plantation, FL 33317

954-792-8944
800-233-9273
Fax: 954-792-8545
addwarehouse.com

This book explains that neither the parents nor children are causes of mental disorders and related problems.

184 pages

5454 Perfectionism: What's Bad About Being Too Good
Free Spirit Pub

With help for superkids, workaholics, type A's. straight A's, procrastinators, overachievers, and caring adults, this book explains the differance between healthy ambition and unhealthy perfectionism and gives straight strategies for getting out of the perfectionist trap- from recognizing the symptoms to rewarding yourself for who you are, not what you do. It explains why some people become perfectionists, what it does to the body, and why girls are more prone to it, and more.

1999 144 pages

Miriam Adderholt, PhD, Author
Miriam Elliot, Author

5455 Psychological Trauma
American Psychiatric Press
1400 K Street, NW
Washington, DC 20005

202-682-6262
800-368-5777
Fax: 202-789-2648
e-mail: order@appi.org
www.appi.org

Epidemiology of trauma and post-tramatic stress disorder. Evaluation, neuroimaging, neuroendocrinology and pharmacology.

1998 206 pages

5456 Shy Children, Phobic Adults: Nature and Treatment of Social Phobia
American Psychological Press
1400 K Street, NW
Washington, DC 20005

202-682-6262
800-368-5777
Fax: 202-789-2648
e-mail: orders@appi.org
www.appi.org

Describes the simuliarities and differences in the syndrome across all ages. Draws from the clinical, social and developmental literatures, as well as from extensive clinical experience. Illustrates the impact of developmental stage on phenomenology, diagnosis and assessment and treatment of social phobia.

1998 321 pages

Pamphlets

5457 5 Smart Steps to Less Stress
ETR Associates
PO Box 1830
Santa Cruz, CA 95061

831-438-4060
800-321-4407
Fax: 800-435-8433

Steps to managing stress include: know what stresses you, manage your stress, take care of your body, take care of your feelings, ask for help.

5458 Anxiety Disorders
National Institute of Mental Health
6001 Executive Boulevard
Bethesda, MD 20892

301-443-4513
Fax: 301-443-4279
TTY: 301-443-8431
e-mail: nimhinfo@nih.gov
nih.gov/publicat

This brochure helps to identify the symptoms of anxiety disorders, explains the role of research in understanding the causes of these conditions, describes effective treatments, helps you learn how to obtain treatment and work with a doctor or therapist, and suggests ways to make treatment more effective.

5459 Anxiety Disorders Fact Sheet
Center for Mental Health Services
PO Box 42490
Washington, DC 20015

800-789-2647
Fax: 301-984-8796
e-mail: ken@mentalhealth.org
mentalhealth.org

This fact sheet presents basic information on the symptoms, formal diagnosis, and treatment for generalized anxiety disorder, panic disorders, phobias, and post traumatic stress disorder.

3 pages

5460 Anxiety Disorders in Children and Adolescents
Center for Mental Health Services
PO Box 42490
Washington, DC 20015

800-789-2647
Fax: 301-984-8796
e-mail: ken@mentalhealth.org
mentalhealth.org

This fact sheet defines anxiety disorders, identifies warning signs, discusses risk factors, describes types of help available, and suggests what parents or other caregivers can do.

3 pages

5461 Families Can Help Children Cope with Fear, Anxiety
Center for Mental Health Services
PO Box 42490
Washington, DC 20015

800-789-2647
Fax: 301-984-8796
e-mail: ken@mentalhealth.org
mentalhealth.org

This fact sheet defines conduct disorder, identifies risk factors, discusses types of help available, and suggests what parents or other caregivers responses should be to common signs of fear and anxiety.

5462 Panic Attacks
ETR Associates
PO Box 1830
Santa Cruz, CA 95061

831-438-4060
800-321-4407
Fax: 800-435-8433

Describes causes of panic attacks, including genetics, stress, and
drug use; prevention and treatment, and how to stop a panic attack
in its tracks.

DESCRIPTION

5463 PHOTOSENSITIVITY

Covers these related disorders: Photoallergic reaction, Phototoxic reaction

Involves the following Biologic System(s):

Dermatologic Disorders

Photosensitivity, sometimes referred to as sun allergy, is an abnormal reaction of the skin to sunlight or artificial light that is usually characterized by the rapid development of redness, swelling, tenderness, peeling, blistering, hives, or other skin irregularities. The skin reactions associated with photosensitivity are often induced by the interaction of light and certain substances known as photosensitizers that are ingested or applied directly to the skin. Such photosensitizers may include antibiotics, antifungal agents, and other drugs as well as some perfumes, soaps, dyes, and plants (e.g., buttercups, parsley, parsnips, mustard, etc.).

Particular wavelengths of light interact with photosensitizers to produce skin inflammations (dermatitis) that may be considered photoallergic or phototoxic. A photoallergic reaction is a delayed immune or allergic response of the skin that results from having been previously exposed to a photosensitizer and light. Such photosensitizers may include barbiturates, certain antibiotics such as tetracycline, and other medications as well as certain topical agents such as coal tar derivatives, perfume oils such as bergamot, etc. A phototoxic reaction is a nonimmune response to the accumulation of certain chemicals in the skin. This type of skin reaction may be similar in appearance to a severe sunburn; some individuals may develop hives or blisters. The initial inflammation is usually followed by abnormally increased skin pigmentation (hyperpigmentation). Phototoxic reactions result from high doses of certain photosensitizers that may cause photoallergic reactions in lower doses, as well as from additional chemical substances. Treatment includes the withdrawal of offending medications and other photosensitizers and sunlight avoidance. In addition, administration of antihistamines and topical corticosteroids may be effective in eliminating associated itching (pruritus).

Photosensitivity is also associated with certain disorders in children. Such disorders may include congenital erythropoietic porphyria (EPP), an autosomal recessive disorder that results from a deficiency of an enzyme. This particular enzyme is necessary for the synthesis of heme, which is the oxygen-carrying component of a certain protein (hemoprotein) found in the tissues of the body. Congenital erythropoietic porphyria develops within a few months of birth and is characterized by a severe sensitivity to light that may cause blistering eruptions on the skin, leading to severe scarring, abnormally increased skin pigmentation, and other skin irregularities. Children with this disorder may also have numerous other abnormalities. Erythropoietic protoporphyria is an autosomal dominant disorder that results from a deficiency of an enzyme that is also essential to the proper synthesis of heme. This disorder appears during early childhood and is characterized by pain, tingling, and a burning feeling upon exposure to sunlight. The skin may redden, swell, and form blisters or hives. In addition to having nail irregularities, children may develop fever and chills. Repeated exposure to sunlight may result in skin thickening and other chronic associated irregularities; however, some children experience improvement during their preadolescent years. Treatment for these types of disorders includes the avoidance of direct sunlight and the use of protective clothing and appropriate sunscreens. In addition, the administration of sufficient quantities of beta-carotene to cause a light yellowing of the skin may be effective in reducing sensitivity to sunlight. Photosensitivity is a feature of many other disorders that may include Cockayne syndrome, xeroderma pigmentosum, hydroa vacciniforme, Rothmund-Thomson syndrome, and other diseases.

Occasionally, some individuals experience an unusual photosensitive reaction to sunlight in the absence of any apparent photosensitizer or associated disease. This type of photosensitivity is called polymorphous light eruption and is one of the most common sun-related skin problems. It is characterized by the appearance of hives or other itchy, rash-type reactions on exposed areas. Polymorphous light eruption usually occurs after a prolonged initial sun exposure in the spring or summer. The eruption may occur within hours or days of the exposure and may remain for hours, days, or weeks. Treatment may include oral or topical corticosteroid therapy. In addition, susceptible people are counseled to avoid the sun, wear protective clothing, and use sunscreen.

Individuals with certain types of photosensitivity may benefit from the cautious administration of photosensitizing drugs that enhance pigmentation of the skin (psoralens). In addition, certain types of phototherapy may be effective. Other treatment is symptomatic and supportive.

See also **General Resources** on page 917

Government Agencies

5464 NIH/National Eye Institute
31 Center Drive MSC 2510
Bethesda, MD 20892

301-496-5248
e-mail: 2020@nei.nih.gov
www.nei.nih.gov

Conducts and supports research that helps prevent and treat eye diseases and other disorders of vision. This research leads to sight-saving treatments, reduces visual impairment and blindness, and improves the quality of life for people of all ages. NEI-supported research has advanced our knowledge of how the eye functions in health and disease.

Paul A Sieving M.D., Ph.D., Director

5465 NIH/National Institute of Arthritis and Mu sculoskeletal and Skin Diseases
1AMS Circle
Bethesda, MD 20892

301-402-4484
Fax: 301-718-6366
e-mail: ord@od.nih.gov
rarediseases.info.nih.gov

The mission of the National Institute of Arthritis and Musculoskeletal and Skin Diseases is to support research into the causes, treatment, and prevention of arthritis and musculoskeletal and skin diseases, the training of basic and clinical scientists to carry out this research, and the dissemination of information on research progress in these diseases.

Stephen l Katz MD PhD, Director

5466 NIH/National Institute of Child Health and Human Development
31 Center Drive, Building 31
Bethesda, MD 20892

301-496-5133
Fax: 301-496-1104
www.nichd.nih.gov

Established in 1962 by congress, today the institute conducts and supports research on topics related to the health of children, adults, families and populations. Some of these topics include: developmental disabilities, growth and development, infant death, reproductive health and birth defects.

Nancy D Wirth, Director
Lisa Kaeser, Program & Public Liaison

National Associations & Support Groups

5467 Genetic Alliance
4301 Connecticut Avenue NW
Washington, DC 20008

202-966-5557
800-336-4363
Fax: 202-966-8553
e-mail: info@geneticalliance.org
www.geneticalliance.org

A coalition of voluntary genetic support groups, consumers and professionals addressing the needs of individuals and families affected by genetic disorders from a national perspective.

Sharon Terry, President/CEO

5468 March of Dimes Birth Defects Foundation
1275 Mamaroneck Avenue
White Plains, NY 10605

914-428-7100
888-663-4637
Fax: 914-428-8203
e-mail: resourcecenter@modimes.org
www.marchofdimes.com

Partnership of volunteers and professionals dedicates to improving the health of babies by preventing birth defects and infant mortality. Over 100 chapters are located across the country and can be located through the National Office.

Dr Jennifer Howse, President

5469 Society for Pediatric Dermatology
8365 Keystone Crossing, Suite 107
Indianapolis, IN 46240

317-202-0224
Fax: 317-205-9481
e-mail: spd@hp-assoc.com
www.pedsderm.net

Objective is to promote, develop and advance education, research and care of skin disease in all pediatric age groups.

Kent Lindeman, Executive Director

Libraries & Resource Centers

California

5470 University of California, San Francisco Dermatology Drug Research
515 Spruce
San Francisco, CA 94143

415-476-2001
Fax: 415-476-6014
cc.ucsf.edu/people

Conducts clinical testing of new or existing pharmalogic agents used in the treatment of skin disorders.

John Koo, MD, Director

Delaware

5471 Delaware Division of Libraries for the Blind and Physically Handicapped
43 S Dupont Highway
Dover, DE 19901

302-736-4748
800-282-8676
Fax: 302-736-6787
TDD: 302-739-4748
e-mail: bedpg@lib.de.us

Braille readers receive service from Philadelphia and Pennsylvania, summer reading program, braille writer and cassettes.

Beth Landon, Librarian

Illinois

5472 Dermatology Information Network (DERMINFONET)
American Academy of Dermatology
PO Box 4014
Schaumburg, IL 60168

847-330-0230
Fax: 847-330-0050

Consists of a collection of dermatologic databases that are available to members on a subscription and/or purchase basis. These databases are designed to run on a wide variety of personal computers.

5473 National Library of Dermatologic Teaching Slides
American Academy of Dermatology
930 N Meacham Road
Shaumburg, IL 60173

847-330-0230
Fax: 847-330-0050
www.aad.org

A collection of dermatologic teaching slides offering the most comprehensive series ever assembled. Each set offers a realistic presentation of classic clinical skin conditions encountered by the dermatologist.

New York

5474 Laboratory of Dermatology Research
Memorial Sloan-Kettering Cancer Center
1275 York Avenue
New York, NY 10021

212-639-2000
Fax: 212-639-3576
www.mskcc.org

Specific studies on the identification of skin disorders and dermatology.

Biijan Safai, MD, Head

5475 Rockefeller University Laboratory for Investigative Dermatology
1230 York Avenue
New York, NY 10021

212-327-7458
Fax: 212-327-7459

Research into skin disorders and the whole specialty of dermatology in general.

D Martin Carter, MD, PhD, Head

Research Centers

5476 University of California, San Francisco Dermatology Drug Research
515 Spruce
San Francisco, CA 94143

415-476-2001
Fax: 415-221-4751

Conducts clinical testing of new or existing pharmacologic agents used in the treatment of skin disorders.

John Koo, MD, Director

Magazines

5477 International Journal of Dermatology
International Society of Dermatology
138 Palm Coast Parkway, NE No 333
Palm Coast, FL 32137

386-437-4405
Fax: 386-437-4427
e-mail: info@intsocdermatol.org
www.intsocderm.org

Focuses on information for dermatologists and the whole specialty of dermatology research and education.

10 times a year

5478 Journal of Dermatologic Surgery and Oncology
International Society for Dermatologic Surgery
930 N Meachan Road
Schaumburg, IL 60173

847-330-9830
Fax: 847-330-1135

Focuses on medical updates and information on dermatology.

Monthly

Newsletters

5479 Awareness
NAPVI
PO Box 317
Watertown, MA 02471

617-972-7441
800-562-6265
Fax: 617-972-7444
www.spedex.com/napvi

Newsletter offering regional news, sports and activities, conferences, camps, legislative updates, book reviews, audio reviews, professional question and answer column and more for the visually impaired and their families.

Quarterly

5480 DVH Quarterly
University of Arkansas at Little Rock
2801 S University Avenue
Little Rock, AR 72204

Fax: 501-663-3536

Offers information on upcoming events, conferences and workshops on and for visual disabilities. Book reviews, information on the newest resources and technology, educational programs, want ads and more.

Quarterly

Bob Brasher, Editor

5481 Dermatology Focus
Dermatology Foundation
1560 Sherman Avenue
Evanston, IL 60201

847-328-2256
Fax: 847-328-0509
dermatologyfoundation.org

Includes membership activities, research articles and lists recipients of foundation awards.

Quarterly

5482 Dermatology World
American Academy of Dermatology
PO Box 94020
Palatine, IL 60094

847-330-0230
Fax: 847-330-0050

Offers Academy members information outside the clinical realm. It carries news of government actions, reports of socioeconomic issues, societal trends and other events which impinge on the practice of dermatology.

Monthly

5483 Progress in Dermatology
Dermatology Foundation
1560 Sherman Avenue
Evanston, IL 60201

847-328-2256
Fax: 847-328-0509
dermatologyfoundation.org

Bulletin offering information on research reports and clinical trials.

Quarterly

DESCRIPTION

5484 PHYSICAL & SEXUAL ABUSE
Involves the following Biologic System(s):
Developmental/Behavioral/Psychiatric Disorders

Child abuse is a pervasive societal disease that has been gaining increasing recognition in the last 40 years. Maltreatment of children includes neglect, physical abuse and sexual abuse. In 1996, one million children were confirmed by protective US agencies as having been abused. Reporting figures since that time have been on the rise.

Neglect is the most common form of abuse, and covers a wide range of irresponsible behaviors that negatively impact the growth and well being of a child. Inadequate supervision may result in injury from falling, usage of a dangerous object such as a knife, scissors or other tools, or ingestion of toxic products and medications. Neglect may also include providing insufficient food, clothing and shelter for a child, which carries a high risk of malnutrition, illness, and poor emotional development. Parents or guardians who do not ensure proper medical care for their children are also negligent, particularly for children with chronic serious medical illnesses.

Physical abuse encompasses a wide range of symptoms but always involves purposeful injury inflicted on a child. Physical abuse can be difficult to identify, especially in toddlers, because children are prone to accidents and receive bruises and cuts as routine events. One key element in the diagnosis is ascertaining whether the injury could have happened the way it was reported. Another important clue is whether the child at a given developmental stage, could have performed the reported event. For example, a report of a six-month old who "fell" and broke his femur (thigh bone) should raise suspicion as a six-month old infant is too young to walk. Common abusive injuries include bruises from belts, hands or cords, burns from cigarettes or hot water immersion, fractures or brain injury from vigorous shaking and internal abdominal injuries from trauma to the back and abdomen. It is important for health care providers, or friends and family members, to record all injuries as a pattern may develop that will help diagnose the situation.

Sexual abuse occurs when a child is involved in sexual activities that he/she cannot fully comprehend, he/she cannot give consent to, or that violate societal norms. Common ages of abuse are between 9 and 12 years. Approximately 25 percent of women and 12 percent of men report histories of being sexually abused as children. Normal sexual play between children of similar age and developmental level can be distinguished from abuse by assessing disparity of age/development and the level of coercion involved. Abusive acts include fondling, intercourse, oral-genital and anal-genital contact, as well as voyeurism, exhibitionism and pornography. Perpetrators are more commonly male adults and adolescents, although women have been known to commit these crimes as well. This type of abuse is often very difficult to recognize because there are frequently no physical signs or symptoms and victims are reluctant and embarrassed to disclose the information. There is often a trusting and/or fearful relationship between the perpetrator and victim that binds the victim to secrecy. Certain telltale signs include inappropriate sexualized behaviors and language, and sexually transmitted diseases such as gonorrhea and chlamydia or symptoms such as discharge or bleeding. Physical evidence may include abrasions, hymenal tears, bruising, foul discharge or even pregnancy.

Professionals working with children, including teachers, social workers and health care providers are all mandated reporters, which means that if abuse is suspected they must report the family to the local protective service agency. It is critical to note that the burden of proof does not lie with the reporter, so even if there is a degree of uncertainty, one is required to act upon his or her concern.

See also **General Resources** on page 917

Government Agencies

5485 Administration for Children & Families-Chi ld Abuse and Neglect Prevention
Department of Health & Human Services
330 C Street SW, Room 2422
Washington, DC 20201

202-205-8618
Fax: 202-205-8221
www.acf.hhs.gov/programs/cb

Wade F Horn PhD, Assistant Secretary

National Associations & Support Groups

5486 AMT Children of Hope Foundation
c/o Nassau County Police Department
1490 Franklin Avenue
Mineola, NY 11501

516-781-3511
877-796-4673
Fax: 516-781-0691
www.amtchildrenofhope.com

Safe infant abandonment, nationwide, 24-hour crisis line. Confidential referrals to 'safe havens' and professional services.

Tinothy Jaccard, Founder & President

5487 American Professional Society on the Abuse of Children
PO Box 30669
Charleston, SC 29417

843-764-2905
877-402-7722
Fax: 803-753-9823
e-mail: apsac@comcast.net
www.apsac.org

Dedicated to providing professional education which promotes effective, culturally sensitive and interdisciplinary approaches to the identification, intervention, treatment and prevention of child abuse and neglect.

Daphne Wright, National Operations Manager

5488 Child Abuse Prevention Association
503 E 23rd Street
Independence, MO 64055

816-252-8388
Fax: 816-252-1337
e-mail: capa@childabuseprevention.org
www.childabuseprevention.org

Mission is to prevent and treat all forms of child abuse by creating changes in individuals, families and society which strengthen relationships and promote healing.

Jeanette Issa, CEO
Tamara Tucker, Program Director

5489 Child Welfare League of America
440 1st Street NW, 3rd Floor
Washington, DC 20001

202-638-2952
Fax: 202-638-4004
www.cwla.org

National nonprofit organization dedicated to developing and promoting policies and programs to protect America's children from harm and strengthen America's families.

Shay Bilchik, President/CEO
Joyce Johnson, Public Relations

5490 Childhelp
Childhelp National Headquarters
15757 N 78th Street
Scottsdale, AZ 85260

480-922-8212
Fax: 480-922-7061
TDD: 800-2AC-HILD
www.childhelp.org

Dedicated to meeting the physical, emotional and spiritual needs of abused and neglected children through focusing its efforts and resources upon treatment, prevention and research.

Sara O'Meara, Co-Founder/CEO
Yvonne Federson, Co-Founder/President

5491 Childhelp National Child Abuse Hotline
www.childhelp.org

800-4AC-HILD
TDD: 800-2AC-HILD
www.childhelp.org

Abuse crisis counseling and referral services available 24/7 with assistance in over 140 languages.

5492 Children's Defense Fund
25 E Street NW
Washington, DC 20001

202-628-8787
800-233-1200
e-mail: cdfinfo@childrensdefense.org
www.childrensdefense.org

Mission is to ensure every child a healthy start, a head start, a fair start, a safe start and a moral start in life.

William lynch, Jr., President
Carol Biondi, Child Advocate/Commissioner

5493 Heroes Great and Small
PO Box 705
Armuchee, GA 30105

706-235-4463
e-mail: heroesgreatandsmall@yahoo.com
www.heroesgreatandsmall.org

Free education and support groups for sexually-abused children, adolescents and non-offending family members. Referrals for areas with groups or assistance in starting local groups nationwide.

5494 IVAT: Institute on Violence, Abuse and Tra uma
6160 Cornerstone Court East
San Diego, CA 92121

858-623-2777
Fax: 858-646-0761
www.ivatcenters.org

Formerly the Family Violence & Sexual Assault Institute. Shares and disseminates vital information, improves networking among professionals, and assists with program evaluation, consultation and training that promotes violence-free living.

Robert Geffner PhD, President
Dawn Alley PhD, Community Relations & Outreach

5495 KidsPeace National Centers/Hospital
5300 KidsPeace Drive
Orefield, PA 18069

800-854-3123
e-mail: admissions@kidspeace.org
www.kidspeace.org

Counseling, info and referral services for children and youth in crisis.

C T O'Donnell, President & CEO

5496 KlaasKids Foundation for Children
PO Box 925
Sausalito, CA 94966

415-331-6867
Fax: 415-331-5633
e-mail: klaaskids@pacbell.net
www.klaaskids.org

Established in 1994 to give meaning to the death of twelve-year-old kidnap and murder victim Polly Hannah Klaas and to create a legacy in her name that would be protective of children for generations to come. The Foundation's mission is to stop crimes against children.

5497 National Center for Missing & Exploited Children
Charles B Wang International Children's Building
699 Prince Street
Alexandria, VA 22314

703-274-3900
800-843-5678
Fax: 703-274-2200
www.missingkids.com

Private, nonprofit organization, co-founded in 1984 by John Walsh, whose son Adam was abducted and murdered. NCMEC serves as a focal point in providing assistance to parents, children, law enforcement, schools and the community in recovering missing children and raising public awareness about ways to help prevent child abduction, molestation and sexual exploitation. NCMEC spends 94 cents of every dollar directly on programs and services.

John Walsh, Founder

5498 National Center for Missing and Exploited Children: 24-hour Hotline

800-843-5678
800-THE-LOST

The primary means by which NCMEC serves as an information clearinghouse and delivers technical assistance.

5499 National Child Pornography Tipline and Cyber Tipline
www.cybertipline.com

800-843-5678
www.cybertipline.com

The National Center for Missing and Exploited Children, in conjunction with the US Postal Inspection Service, US Customs Service and the Federal Bureau of Investigation, serves as the tipline, handling calls from individuals reporting the sexual exploitation of children through the production and distribution of pornography. For online reporting visit the website.

5500 National Children's Advocacy Center
210 Pratt Avenue
Huntsville, AL 35801

256-533-5437
Fax: 256-534-6883
www.nationalcac.org

A non profit organization that provides training, prevention, intervention and treatment services to fight child abuse and neglect.

Deborah Callins, Executive Director
JoAnn Jaco Plucker, Federal Programs Director

5501 National Children's Alliance
516 C Street NE
Washington, DC 20002

202-548-0090
800-239-9950
Fax: 202-548-0099
e-mail: info@nca-online.org
www.nca-online.org

Nationwide nonprofit membership organization which promotes and supports communities in providing a coordinated investigation and response to victims of severe child abuse.

Nancy Chandler, Executive Director
Julie Pape, Director Programs

5502 National Exchange Club Foundation
3050 Central Avenue
Toledo, OH 43606

419-535-3232
800-924-2643
Fax: 419-535-1989
www.preventchildabuse.com/cap.htm

Committed to making a difference in the lives of children, families and communities through its national project, the prevention of child abuse.

Charles Braddock, President

5503 Prevent Child Abuse America
500 N Michigan Avenue, Suite 200
Chicago, IL 60611

312-663-3520
Fax: 312-939-8962
e-mail: mailbox@preventchildabuse.org
www.preventchildabuse.org

Mission is to prevent the abuse and neglect of the nation's children. Supports education and research.

James M Hmurovich, Interim President/CEO

5504 Project Cuddle
2973 Harbor Boulevard, # 326
Costa Mesa, CA 92626

714-432-9681
888-628-3353
Fax: 714-433-6815
e-mail: info@projectcuddle.org
www.projectcuddle.org

Safe infant abandonment, nationwide, 24-hour crisis line. All calls are confidential. Help in finding a safe, legal alternative to abandonment.

Debbe Magnusen, Founder

5505 Rape, Abuse and Incest National Network (RAINN)
2000 L Street NW, Suite 406
Washington, DC 20036

202-544-1034
800-656-HOPE
Fax: 202-544-3556
e-mail: info@rainn.org
www.rainn.org

Operates a 24 hour national sexual assault hotline and carries out programs to prevent sexual assault, help victims and ensure that rapists are brought to justice.

Darcey West, Communications Manager
Chelsea Bowers, Membership Information

5506 Safe Place for Newborns
120 S 6th Street, Suite 1150
Minneapolis, MN 55402

612-317-2895
877-440-2229
Fax: 612-317-2899
e-mail: safeplace@safeplacefornewborns.com
www.safeplacefornewborns.com

Crisis line. Will provide a list of hospitals in Minnesota and Wisconsin which accept healthy babies up to three days old with no questions asked. Will provide information on other states with 'safe place' programs.

Laure Krupp, Executive Director

5507 Stop It Now!
351 Pleasant Street, Suite B-319
Northampton, MA 01060

413-587-3500
888-773-8368
Fax: 413-587-3505
e-mail: info@stopitnow.com
www.stopitnow.com

A nonprofit organization founded on the belief and experience that we as individuals and as a society can challenge the way we act. Mission is to call on all abusers and potential abusers to stop and seek help, to educate adults about the ways to stop sexual abuse, and to increase public awareness of the trauma of child sexual abuse.

Maxine J Stein, President/CEO

5508 The Kempe Center: For the Prevention & Treatment of Child Abuse and Neglect
1825 Marion Street
Denver, CO 80218

303-864-5300
e-mail: info@kempe.org
http://kempecenter.org

Provides education, clinical services and research on child abuse and neglect. Can provide referrals to local agencies.

Pat Loewi, President/CEO
Gene Liffick, Operations Director

5509 Youth Crisis Hotline
Youth Development International
PO Box 178408
San Diego, CA 92177

800-HIT-HOME
http://hometown.aol.com/garnierlaw/hithome.html

Services for runaway/homeless youth, referrals to resources for abuse and crisis counseling.

State Agencies & Support Groups

Alaska

5510 Rid Alaska of Child Abuse
PO Box 35595
Juneau, AK 99803

800-478-4444
e-mail: Help@RIDAlaskaOfChildAbuse
www.ridalaskaofchildabuse.org

Nonprofit organization dedicated to providing resources and information, raising public awareness of the occurrence of child abuse, lessening the stigma placed on child sexual abuse victims/survivors, promoting child safety and abuse prevention programs, researching and posting safety tips and maintaining a website.

Debra Gerrish, President/State Coordinator
Tia M Holley, VP

Arizona

5511 Crisis Nursery
2334 E Polk Street
Phoenix, AZ 85006

602-273-7363
Fax: 602-244-1316
e-mail: cninfo1@crisisnurseryphx.com
www.crisisnurseryphx.com

Offers hope and support, through prevention and protection, to children in our community threatened with abuse and neglect. Since 1977, over 13,000 children have found a safe refuge at Crisis Nursery. Its mission is to provide a last resort for parents and families who are simply overwhelmed, a safe and healthy place for children who can no longer remain with their families, a temporary home for children who haven't one to call their own and a transitional placement with follow up for services.

Marsha Porter, Executive Director

California

5512 Child Sexual Abuse Treatment Program (Giar retto)
EMQ Children & Family Services
232 E Gish Road
San Jose, CA 95112

408-453-7616
e-mail: csc@emq.org
www.emq.org

Sexual abuse treatment center

F Jerome Doyle, CEO
Kristine Austin, Director Public Relations

Georgia

5513 Prevent Child Abuse Georgia
1720 Peachtree Street NW, Suite 600
Atlanta, GA 30309

404-870-6543
800-244-5373
Fax: 404-870-6587
e-mail: dmiddleton@pcageorgia.org
www.preventchildabusega.org

Private, statewide, community-based nonprofit organization with the sole mission of preventing child abuse and neglect.

Doug Middleton, Executive Director

Illinois

5514 Prevent Child Abuse Illinois
528 S 5th Street, Suite 211
Springfield, IL 62701

217-522-1129
Fax: 217-522-0655
e-mail: rharley@preventchildabuseillinois.org
www.preventchildabuseillinois.org

Roy A Harley, Executive Director

Indiana

5515 Prevent Child Abuse Indiana
9130 E Otis Avenue
Indianapolis, IN 46216

317-542-7002
888-542-7064
Fax: 317-542-7003
e-mail: education@pcain.org
www.pcain.org

Sandra Runkle, Interim Executive Director

Iowa

5516 Prevent Child Abuse Iowa
505 11th Street, Suite 900
Des Moines, IA 50309

515-244-2200
Fax: 515-280-7835
e-mail: sscott@pcaiowa.org
www.pcaiowa.org

Steve Scott, Executive Director

New York

5517 Child Abuse Prevention Project: Be'ad HaYeled (For the Sake of the Child)
Board of Jewish Education of Greater New York
520 8th Avenue, 15th Floor
New York, NY 10018

646-472-5300
Fax: 646-472-5421
e-mail: info@bjeny.org
www.bjeny.org

Be'ad HaYeled was created in 1995 specifically for the Jewish community by the Board of Jewish Education of Greater New York and the Jewish Board of Family and Children's Services. Training workshops give educators, parents and communal workers the skills needed to recognize signs of abuse and to intervene in an effective and appropriate manner Halachically, clinically and legally. Additional programs deal with parenting methods, communication skills and other relevant family issues.

Phyllis Miller, Associate Special Education

5518 Prevent Child Abuse New York
134 S Swan Street
Albany, NY 12210

518-445-1273
Fax: 518-436-5889
e-mail: cdeyss@preventchildabuseny.org
www.preventchildabuseny.org

Not-for-profit agency whose singular mission is to prevent child abuse in all its forms. Prevent Child Abuse New York is a chartered state chapter of Prevent Child Abuse America.

Christine Deyss, Executive Director

North Carolina

5519 Prevent Child Abuse North Carolina
3725 National Drive, Suite 101
Raleigh, NC 27612

919-829-8009
Fax: 919-832-0308
e-mail: jtollewhiteside@preventchildabusenc.org
www.prventchildabusenc.org

Statewide not-for-profit organization with the mission of ending child abuse in the state of North Carolina.

Jennifer Tolle Whiteside, President/CEO

Virginia

5520 Childhelp Children's Center of Virginia
8415 Arlington Boulevard
Fairfax, VA 22031

703-208-1500
Fax: 703-208-1540
e-mail: mail@childhelpva.org
www.childhelpusa.org/regional/virginia2

Dedicated to meeting the physical, emotional and spiritual needs of abused and neglected children through focusing its efforts and resources upon treatment, prevention and research.

Libraries & Resource Centers

5521 Child Welfare Information Gateway
Children's Burea/ACYF
1250 Maryland Avenue SW, 8th Floor
Washington, DC 20024

703-385-7565
800-394-3366
Fax: 703-385-3206
e-mail: info@childwelfare.gov
www.childwelfare.gov

The National Clearinghouse on Child Abuse and Neglect Information and the National Adoption Information Clearinghouse have consolidated and expanded to create the Child Welfare Information Gateway. It is a service of the US DHHS and provides access to information and resources to help protect children and strengthen families.

Research Centers

5522 National Center on Child Abuse Prevention Research
500 N Michigan Avenue, Suite 200
Chicago, IL 60611

312-663-3520
Fax: 312-939-8962
www.preventchildabuse.org

Established with the support of the Skillman Foundation to increase understanding of the complex causes of child maltreatment, to evaluate the effectiveness of prevention programs, and to disseminate this information out into the field and public.

Conferences

5523 Annual New York State Child Abuse Prevention Conference
134 S Swan Street
Albany, NY 12210

518-445-1273
Fax: 518-436-5889
e-mail: rreyes@preventchildabuseny.org
www.preventchildabuseny.org/conf06/

Presented by Prevent Child Abuse New York, a not-for-profit agency whose singular mission is to prevent child abuse in all its forms. PCANY is a chartered state chapter of Prevent Child Abuse America. Conference attendees include those who work in home-based and center-based family support programs, child abuse prevention and child protective services, intervention and treatment, health care and mental health, schools, religious and civic organizations, and parents, themselves.

R Reyes, Contact

Audio Video

5524 Break the Silence: Kids Against Child Abuse
The Health Connection
55 W Oak Ridge Drive
Hagerstown, MD 21740

301-393-3270
800-548-8700
Fax: 888-294-8405
www.healthconnection.org

Jane Seymore explains physical abuse, sexual abuse and neglect. Animation illustrates each story. All the stories end happily, and the main point is that children should tell a trusted adult. 28 minutes. Grades 1-5.

1994

5525 I Am the Boss of My Body: Preventing Child Sexual Abuse
The Health Connection
55 W Oak Ridge Drive
Hagerstown, MD 21740

301-393-3270
800-548-8700
Fax: 888-294-8405
www.healthconnection.org

Children feel empowered when they see this video and learn that they have the authority and the right to say no to any touch that makes them feel strange. Grades 1-4.

1999 18 Minutes

Web Sites

5526 American Professional Society on the Abuse of Children
www.apsac.org

Dedicated to providing professional education which promotes effective, culturally sensitive and interdisciplinary approaches to the identification, intervention, treatment and prevention of child abuse and neglect.

5527 Bikers Against Child Abuse
www.bacausa.com

Has the intent to create a safer environment for abused children. An established, united body of bikers in a stand to empower children to not feel afraid of the world in which they live. They work in conjunction with local officials who are already in place to protect children.

5528 Child Abuse Legislation
www.childabuse.com/legislat.htm

Prevention through education and awareness.

5529 Child Abuse Prevention Network
child-abuse.com

For professionals in the field of child abuse and neglect. Child maltreatment, physical abuse, psychological maltreatment, neglect, sexual abuse and emotional abuse and neglect are the key areas of concern. Provides unique and powerful tools for all workers to support the identification, investigation, treatment, adjudication and prevention of child abuse and neglect.

5530 Child Abuse Quilts: Revealing and Healing the Pain of Child Abuse
mbgoodman.tripod.com/caq/caq1.html

Site shows 28 quilts made dealing with the subject of child abuse, child abuse prevention and violence against children. Some of the quiltmakers knew the pain of abuse first hand, others knew it through the eyes of others, often close family members. Quilts are displayed in the hope that each person who sees them will leave re-awakened to the tragedy of child abuse and resolved to prevent it.

5531 Child Abuse.com

www.childabuse.com

Comprehensive resource bringing awareness and education in preventing child abuse and related issues. The site was created to inform, support and encourage those dealing with any aspect of child abuse, in a positive non-threatening environment.

5532 Child Trauma Academy

www.childtraumaacademy.com

Provides information on free online courses that offer creative and practical approaches to understanding and working with maltreated children.

5533 Children's Bureau

www.acf.hhs.gov/programs/cb

Is responsible for programs that promote the economic and social well-being of families, chidren, individuals, and communities. Programs aim to achieve the following: families and individuals empowered to increase their own economic independence and productivity, and strong healthy, supportive commuties that have a positive impact on the quality of life and the development of children.

5534 Children's House

child-abuse.com/childhouse/

An interactive resource center and meeting place for the exchange of information that serves the well-being of children.

5535 Coalition for America's Children

www.usakids.org

The Coalition is an alliance of national, state and local nonprofit organizations working to call attention to the serious obstacles impeding children's well-being and to boost children's concerns to the top of the public policy agenda.

5536 Connect for Kids

Benton Foundation
www.connectforkids.org

Family-friendly politics and information on how to connect with hundreds of groups working on behalf of children.

5537 Intrafamilial (Incest) Abuse Resources

www.vachss.com/help_text/incest.html

Many resources on the subject of child abuse, both physical and sexual.

5538 KidsPeace

www.kidspeace.org

Counseling, info and referral services for children and youth in crisis.

5539 Making Daughters Safe Again

mdsasupport.homestead.com/index.html

Is the only organization in the world specializing in mother-daughter sexual abuse. We are also distinguished by the innovative online group experience we provide for survivors.

5540 National Council on Child Abuse & Family Violence

www.nccafv.org

Providing intergenerational violence prevention services since 1984.

5541 Pandora's Box

www.prevent-abuse-now.com

Offers more than 270 pages of resource information on child abuse prevention and child protection.

5542 Prevent Child Abuse America

www.preventchildabuse.org

Providing and inspiring hope to everyone involved in the effort to prevent the abuse and neglect of our nations children. Working with 40 statewide chapters to provide leadership in promoting and implementing prevention efforts at both the national and local levels.

5543 Prevent Child Abuse California

www.pca-ca.org

Mission is to prevent child abuse in all its forms by maximizing resources throughout the state of California.

5544 Rape, Abuse and Incest National Network (RAINN)

www.rainn.org

Operates a 24 hour national sexual assault hotline and carries out programs to prevent sexual assault, help victims and ensure that rapists are brought to justice.

5545 Sibling Abuse Survivors' Information & Advocacy Network

www.sasian.org

Provides information about problems associated with domestic sibling incest abuse.

5546 Stop Child Abuse Now

www.cfn.org/~scan/scan.html

Is a nonprofit organization dedicated to stopping child abuse of all forms, and improving the lives of survivors of all types of abuse and loss. By speaking out about abuse, we increase the public's awareness of the prevalence of abuse. Our goal is to join with other organizations and individuals who wish to ultimately put a stop to child abuse.

Book Publishers

5547 A Child Called It: One Child's Courage to Survive

Dave Pelzer, author

Health Communications, Inc (HCI)
3201 SW 15th Street
Deerfield Beach, FL 33442

954-360-0909
800-441-5569
Fax: 800-360-0034
www.hci-online.com

The author's true story of abuse he suffered as a child.

ISBN: 1-558743-66-9

5548 Body Language of the Abused Child

Jacqueline A Rankin, author

Rankin File/Signature Book Printing
8041 Cessna Avenue
Gaithersburg, MD 20879

301-258-8353
Fax: 301-670-4147
e-mail: book@sbpbooks.com
www.signaturebook.com/Books/rankin.htm

Uses body language to identify a suspected victim.

1999 271 pages Paperback
ISBN: 1-887711-06-6

5549 It's My Body

Lory Freeman, author

Parenting Press
PO Box 75267
Seattle, WA 98175

206-364-2900
800-992-6657
Fax: 206-364-0702
www.parentingpress.com

Helps adults and preschool children talk about sexual abuse together. Introduces touching codes children can use for their protection. Ages 3-8.

32 pages Paperback
ISBN: 1-403408-96-3

5550 My Body is Mine, My Feelings are Mine

Susan Hoke, author

YouthLight
714 Cove Trail, PO Box 115
Chapin, SC 29036

800-209-9774
Fax: 803-345-0888
e-mail: yl@sc.rr.com
www.youthlightbooks.com

For K-5th grade. First part to be read to children, the second part teaches adults how to educate children about body safety. Sexual victimization can be prevented through explanation of how to identify inappropriate touching and what to do about it.

77 pages Paperback

5551 Protect Your Child from Sexual Abuse: A Parent's Guide

Janie Hart-Rossi, author

Parenting Press
PO Box 75267
Seattle, WA 98175

206-364-2900
800-992-6657
Fax: 206-364-0702
www.parentingpress.com

Accompanies 'It's My Body.' Parents guide for information about sexual abuse and what to do to prevent it. Includes activities and games to use as teaching tools. 1-12 years.

64 pages Paperback
ISBN: 0-943990-06-8

5552 Something Happened and I'm Scared to Tell

Patricia Kehoe PhD, author

Parenting Press
PO Box 75267
Seattle, WA 98175

206-364-2900
800-992-6657
Fax: 206-364-0702
www.parentingpress.com

With the help of a friendly lion, a young sexual abuse victim is able to talk about sexual abuse and recover self-esteem. A gentle and positive approach to reassure children. Ages 3-7.

32 pages Paperback
ISBN: 0-943990-28-9

5553 Soul Murder Revisited

Leonard Shengold, author

Yale University Press
PO Box 209040
New Haven, CT 06520

203-432-0960
800-987-7323
Fax: 203-432-0948
yalepress.yale.edu/yupbooks

Further reflections on how abuse occurs and its consequences. Discusses the psychopathology of soul murder and appropriate therapy for victims.

2000 336 pages Paperback
ISBN: 0-300086-99-7

5554 Soul Murder: The Effects of Childhood Abuse and Deprivation

Yale University Press
PO Box 209040
New Haven, CT 06520

203-430-960
800-987-7323
www.yale.edu/yup

Discusses how abuse occurs and its consequences.

5555 Treating Abused Adolescents

Eliana Gil, author

Guilford Press
72 Spring Street
New York, NY 10012

800-365-7006
Fax: 212-966-6708
e-mail: info@guilford.com
www.guilford.com

Professional resource for clinicians treating abused adolescents. Explores the residual effects of earlier child abuse and current or cumulative abuse.

1996 228 pages Paperback
ISBN: 1-572301-15-5

5556 Trouble with Secrets

Karen Johnson, author

Parenting Press
PO Box 75267
Seattle, WA 98175

206-364-2900
800-992-6657
Fax: 206-364-0702
www.parentingpress.com

Helps children distinguish between secrets that should be kept and those that shouldn't.

32 pages Paperback
ISBN: 0-943990-22-X

Newsletters

5557 APSAC Advisor

American Profess. Society on the Abuse of Children
PO Box 30669
Charleston, SC 29417

843-764-2905
877-402-7722
Fax: 803-753-9823
e-mail: apsac@comcast.net
www.apsac.org

News journal for professionals in the field of child abuse and neglect. It provides succint, data-based articles that keep professionals informed of the latest developments in policy and practice in the field of child maltreatment.

Ronald C Hughes PhD, Editor-in-Chief

5558 Lookin' Up

Prevent Child Abuse America
500 N Michigan Avenue, Suite 200
Chicago, IL 60611

312-663-3520
Fax: 312-939-8962
www.preventchildabuse.org

Newsletter of Prevent Child Abuse America.

Quarterly

Pamphlets

5559 Understanding SBS/Shaken Impact Syndrome B rochure
National Center on Shaken Baby Syndrome
2955 Harrison Boulevard, #102
Ogden, UT 84403

801-627-3399
888-273-0071
Fax: 801-627-3321
e-mail: mail@dontshake.com
www.dontshake.com

Information brochure on shaken baby syndrome.

DESCRIPTION

5560 PICA

Involves the following Biologic System(s):
Developmental/Behavioral/Psychiatric Disorders

Pica is a type of eating disorder characterized by the recurrent or chronic ingestion of nonfood or nonnutritive substances such as dirt, flaking paint or plaster, clay, charcoal, ashes, wool, and other nonfoods. Although this psychological disorder usually commences during the first or second year of life, some children are affected during infancy. The pattern should last at least one month to fit the diagnosis of pica. Pica is often self-limiting with resolution occurring during the childhood years; however, sometimes it may persist into adolescence or adulthood. If the symptoms associated with pica occur initially in older children or adults (e.g., pregnant women), this is usually indicative of a nutritional deficiency, such as iron or zinc, rather than a psychological disorder.

Children who are mentally retarded are particularly susceptible to development of this unusual disorder. Other factors that may influence the evolution of pica include environmental influences such as family discord, lack of or ineffective nurturing, and nutritional and emotional neglect. In addition, pica is sometimes associated with certain psychiatric disorders.

Children who eat nonfood or nonnutritive substances may be at risk of developing certain types of parasitic infections. For example, the ingestion of dirt (geophagia) may result in toxocariasis, an infection resulting from the spread of the larvae of the common roundworm (Toxocara canis) throughout the body. Symptoms of toxocariasis are often mild and may include fever, weakness, and discomfort. Other children may develop a cough, wheezing, enlarged liver (hepatomegaly), and eye lesions. In addition, another parasitic infection known as toxoplasmosis may develop from dirt ingestion. This common parasitic infection is caused by Toxoplasma gondii and may produce no symptoms or may sometimes be characterized by rash, fever, and other mononucleosis-type symptoms. In individuals with compromised immune systems, toxoplasmosis may result in more serious, widespread disease. Children who eat paint, paint dust, or paint flakes are at risk of developing lead poisoning that may damage the central nervous system, red blood cells, and digestive system.

Any nutritional deficiencies and other medical problems, such as lead toxicity, should be addressed. Treatment emphasizes psychosocial, environmental, and family education approaches. Nutritional supplements may be considered.

See also **General Resources** on page 917

National Associations & Support Groups

5561 Eating Disorders and Family Crisis Center
3801 Connecticut Avenue NW
Washington, DC 20008

202-362-3009
Fax: 433-645-2420
e-mail: brockhansenlcsw@aol.com
shamebusters.com

5562 International Association of Eating Disorders Professionals Foundation
PO Box 1295
Pekin, IL 61555

309-346-3341
800-800-8126
Fax: 775-239-1597
e-mail: iaedpmembers@earthlink.net
www.iaedp.com

Well-known for providing first-quality education and high-level training standards to an international multidisciplinary group of healthcare treatment providers who treat the full spectrum of eating disorder problems.

Emmett R Bishop MD, President
Bonnie Harken, Managing Director

5563 NIH/National Institute of Mental Health Eating Disorders Program
Room 35231
Bethesda, MD 20892

301-496-1891
Fax: 301-402-1561

5564 National Alliance for the Mentally Ill
2107 Wilson Blvd, Ste 300, Colonial Place Three
Arlington, VA 22201

703-524-7600
800-950-6264
Fax: 703-524-9094
TDD: 703-516-7227
e-mail: info@nami.org
www.nami.org

NAMI is a nonprofit, grassroots, self-help, support and advocacy organization of consumers, families and friends of people with severe mental illness, such as schizophrenia, bipolar disorder, major despressive disorder, obsessive compulsive disorder, anxiety disorders, autism and other severe and persistent mental illnesses that affect the brain.

Suzanne Vogel-Scibilia MD, President

5565 National Eating Disorders Association (NED A)
603 Stewart Street, Suite 803
Seattle, WA 98101

206-382-3587
800-931-2237
Fax: 206-829-8501
e-mail: info@NationalEatingDisroders.org
www.NationalEatingDisorders.org

Dedicated to the elimination of eating disorders through prevention efforts, education, referral and support services, advocacy, training and research. Offers free information and referrals as well as educational curriculum and materials for sale. A toll free information & referral helpline is also available, linking more than 1,200 callers per month to vital information and life-saving treatment.

Kari M Augustyn, Director Programs
Lynn S Grefe, Chief Executive Officer

5566 National Mental Health Association
2000 N Beauregard Street, 6th Floor
Alexandria, VA 22311

703-684-7722
800-969-6642
Fax: 703-684-5968
TTY: 800-433-5959
www.nmha.org

Addresses all aspects of mental health and mental illness. NMHA
with over 340 affiliates works to improve the mental health of all
Americans.

David L Shern PhD, President & CEO

**5567 National Mental Health Consumers' Self-Help
Clearinghouse**
1211 Chestnut Street, Suite 1207
Philadelphia, PA 19107

215-751-1810
800-553-4539
Fax: 215-636-6312
e-mail: info@mhselfhelp.org
www.mhselfhelp.org

Offers information, support and appropriate referrals; and promotes
public and professional education. Provides networking for those
with special interests related to albinism. Promotes and supports research and funding that will improve diagnosis and management of
albinism and hypopigmentation.

Joseph Rogers, Executive Director & Founder

Web Sites

5568 Eating Disorder Referrals
www.eating-disorder-referral.com/pica.php

A free referral resource with listings across the nation. Can also access by phone, toll free at 866-323-5608

5569 KidsHealth for Parents
kidshealth.org/parent/emotions/behavior/pica.html

General overview of pica.

5570 Pica Information Page
www.tobacco.org/resources/health/pica.html

A small group of citizens that seeks to alert the public about a new
category of hazardous waste.

DESCRIPTION

5571 PINWORM (ENTEROBIUS VERMICULARIS)

Synonyms: Enterobiasis, Oxyuriasis, Threadworm

Involves the following Biologic System(s):

Infectious Disorders

Pinworm infection (enterobiasis) refers to a common condition in which small, white, parasitic worms (Enterobius vermicularis) infect the human intestinal tract. Such infection results from ingestion of parasitic eggs. The eggs hatch in the stomach, and the larvae then typically migrate to and grow within the upper part of the large intestine (cecum). On rare occasions, pinworms may migrate to the vagina of affected girls, potentially causing such symptoms as vaginal irritation or itching. Pinworms can also cause appendicitis, cystitis (infection of the urinary tract), and diverticulitis (inflammation from out-pouchings in the colon (large intestinal tract).

At night, pinworms migrate from the intestines to the anal region where they deposit their eggs, potentially causing itching (pruritus), irritation, and sleeplessness. Scratching often results in reinfestation from ingestion of eggs that become imbedded under the fingernails and are inadvertently deposited in the mouth. Parasitic eggs are also often deposited from the anal area onto clothing, bedding, furniture, or toys, where they may then be transferred from the fingers to the mouth, causing reinfection or infection of others. In addition, in some cases, eggs may be inhaled from the air and swallowed. Parasitic eggs may remain viable for up to three weeks at regular room temperature.

The diagnosis of enterobiasis is made by detecting parasitic eggs or pinworms. The eggs or worms may be obtained by pressing sticky tape against the perianal region of affected children during early morning hours before the children awaken. The tape is then examined under a microscope to verify the presence of pinworms or eggs. In addition, pinworms may sometimes be detected by the naked eye. Treatment may include the administration of drugs that destroy pinworms (anthelmintic drugs), such as pyrantel pamoate or mebendazole, and, in some patients, topical anti-itch ointments that help relieve itching and irritation. Anthelmintic medications should also be given to all other members of the household. Handwashing after going to the bathroom and before meals is critical. Linens should be washed thoroughly.

Enterobiasis is a very common infection that may occur in individuals of all ages. However, children between the ages of five to 14 years are most commonly affected.

See also **General Resources** on page 917

Government Agencies

5572 Centers for Disease Control
1600 Clifton Road
Atlanta, GA 30333

404-639-3311
www.cdc.gov

Mission is to promote health and quality of life by preventing and controlling disease, injury, and disability.

5573 NIH/National Institute of Allergy and Infectious Diseases
6610 Rockledge Drive, MSC 6612
Bethesda, MD 20892

301-496-5717
Fax: 301-402-3573
TDD: 800-877-8339
www.niaid.nih.gov

Conducts and supports basic and applied research to better understand, treat, and ultimately prevent infectious, immunologic, and allergic diseases.

Anthony S Fauci MD, Director

5574 NIH/National Institute of Child Health and Human Development
31 Center Drive, Building 31
Bethesda, MD 20892

301-496-5133
Fax: 301-496-1104
www.nichd.nih.gov

Established in 1962 by congress, today the institute conducts and supports research on topics related to the health of children, adults, families and populations. Some of these topics include: developmental disabilities, growth and development, infant death, reproductive health and birth defects.

Nancy D Wirth, Director
Lisa Kaeser, Program & Public Liaison

National Associations & Support Groups

5575 World Health Organization
Avenue Appia 20
CH-1211 Geneva 27,
Switzerland

www.who.int

WHO is the directing and coordinating authority for health within the United Nations system.

Dr Margaret Chan, Director General

Web Sites

5576 KidsHealth for Parents
www.kidshealth.org

Signs, symptoms, doagnosis, and treatment of pinworms.

5577 MayoClinic.com
www.mayoclinic.com/health/pinworm/DS00687

Introduction, risk factors, prevention and treatment of pinworms.

Pamphlets

5578 Pinworm Infection
CDC
1600 Clifton Road
Atlanta, GA 30333

800-311-3435
www.cdc.gov/ncidod/dpd/parasites/pinworm/

Pinworm infection factsheet provided by the CDC.

DESCRIPTION

5579 PITYRIASIS ROSEA

Involves the following Biologic System(s):
Dermatologic Disorders, Infectious Disorders

Pityriasis rosea is an inflammatory skin condition that may develop at any age but mostly commonly affects children and young adults. In some cases, the onset of the condition may be preceded by certain generalized symptoms, such as fever, inflammation of the throat (pharyngitis), and muscle and joint pain (myalgia and arthralgia). Pityriasis rosea typically begins with the development of a single oval or round patch known as a herald patch. This patch is usually red, pink, or light brown with a raised border and is covered with fine scales. A herald patch varies in diameter from one to 10 centimeters and may occur anywhere on the body. About five to 10 days after the appearance of the herald patch, there is a widespread eruption of similar, smaller patches (lesions), particularly on the torso and upper arms and thighs. These lesions, which are less than one centimeter in diameter, are usually slightly raised, oval or round, and red, pink, or light brown. In addition, they may be scaly and tend to peel. Lesions may continue to appear over several days and develop on other areas of the body, such as the forearms and calves, face, and scalp. The lesions are typically distributed along the subtle lines in the skin that indicate the direction of skin fibers (Langer's or cleavage lines). Some individuals with the condition may experience no associated symptoms (asymptomatic). Others may experience mild to severe itching (pruritus). Pityriasis rosea is a self-limited condition that has a duration of approximately two to 12 weeks, with an average of approximately four to five weeks. As skin lesions heal, affected areas may have abnormally increased or diminished pigmentation (postinflammatory hyperpigmentation or hypopigmentation) that gradually resolves after several weeks or months.

If individuals with pityriasis rosea experience no associated symptoms, treatment may not be necessary. Those with widespread lesions and scaling may benefit from using a cream that softens the skin (emollient). Associated itching may be relieved by lubricating lotions that contain the natural compounds camphor or menthol or medicated skin creams, such as a nonfluorinated topical corticosteroid. Certain medications taken by mouth such as oral antihistamines may help those who experience bothersome itching while attempting to sleep. Antihistamines, which are medications that often induce drowsiness, reduce the effects of histamine, a chemical that is released during allergic inflammatory reactions.

The cause of pityriasis rosea is unknown. However, many researchers speculate that the condition results from infection with a viral agent.

See also **General Resources** on page 917

Government Agencies

5580 NIH/National Institute of Arthritis and Mu sculoskeletal and Skin Diseases
1AMS Circle
Bethesda, MD 20892

301-402-4484
Fax: 301-718-6366
e-mail: ord@od.nih.gov
rarediseases.info.nih.gov

The mission of the National Institute of Arthritis and Musculoskeletal and Skin Diseases is to support research into the causes, treatment, and prevention of arthritis and musculoskeletal and skin diseases, the training of basic and clinical scientists to carry out this research, and the dissemination of information on research progress in these diseases.

Stephen I Katz MD PhD, Director

National Associations & Support Groups

5581 American Academy of Dermatology (AAD)
PO Box 4014
Schaumburg, IL 60168

847-240-1280
866-503-7546
Fax: 847-240-1859
e-mail: mrc@aad.org
www.aad.org

Dedicated to achieving high quality dermatologic care for everyone which encompasses: responsiveness, unification and representation of the specialty, and excellence in pateint care, education and research.

Stephen P Stone MD, President
William P Coleman III, MD, VP

5582 National Psoriasis Foundation
6600 SW 92nd Avenue, Suite 300
Portland, OR 97223

503-245-7404
800-723-9166
Fax: 503-245-0626
e-mail: getinfo@psoriasis.org
www.psoriasis.org

The NPF is committed through education and advocacy to improving the lives of people who have psoriasis and supporting research to cure the millions of people with the chronic skin disease. Provides free psoriasis, psoriatic arthritis and treatment information; assists with insurance/discrimination issues; sponsors community educational meetings; directs people to support groups and physicians; offers a pen-pal program; and provides credited phototherapy courses for medical professionals.

Kelly Coates, Patients Relations Manager

5583 Society for Pediatric Dermatology
8365 Keystone Crossing, Suite 107
Indianapolis, IN 46240

317-202-0224
Fax: 317-205-9481
e-mail: spd@hp-assoc.com
www.pedsderm.net

Objective is to promote, develop and advance education, research and care of skin disease in all pediatric age groups.

Kent Lindeman, Executive Director

Web Sites

5584 DermNet NZ: The Dermatology Resource
www.dermnetnz.org

Information about the skin from the New Zealand Dermatological Society.

Pamphlets

5585 Pityriasis Rosea
American Academy of Dermatology
PO Box 4014
Schaumburg, IL 60168

847-240-1280
866-503-7546
Fax: 847-240-1859
e-mail: mrc@aad.org
www.aad.org/public/publications

Discusses the appearance, symptoms, and causes of this common rash. Diagnosis and treatment are also explained.

Pkgs of 50

Stephen P Stone MD, President

DESCRIPTION

5586 PNEUMONIA

Involves the following Biologic System(s):

Infectious Disorders, Respiratory Disorders

Pneumonia refers to a group of disorders characterized by an acute inflammation of the lungs. The causes of pneumonia are many and may include infection by certain bacteria, viruses, bacteria-like organisms, fungi, yeasts, and protozoa. In addition, noninfectious causes include the inhalation (aspiration) of food or other substances into the airway and lungs, an abnormal response of the immune system to certain substances (hypersensitivity reaction), and an inflammatory response to radiation or certain drugs. Pneumonia may also result as a complication of surgery or injury, due to the impaired ability to cough, breathe deeply, or expel mucus.

Pneumonia in very young children is most commonly caused by certain respiratory viruses, such as RSV, or respiratory syncytial virus; influenza; parainfluenza (the virus that causes croup); and adenoviruses. Symptoms and findings associated with this type of pneumonia in infants and young children may include cough, nasal discharge, fever, rapid breathing (tachypnea), or a bluish color to the skin and mucous membranes (cyanosis). Antibiotics do not treat viral infections, though some viruses are susceptible to new antiviral therapies. Most infants and children recover from viral pneumonia with no complications. However, some may develop subsequent lung irregularities.

Although bacterial pneumonia is not common among children, certain conditions (e.g., viral respiratory illnesses, immune deficiency disorders, certain congenital defects, blood irregularities, etc.) may put them at increased risk for developing this type of pneumonia. The most common types of bacteria that cause pneumonia in children include Streptococcus pneumoniae (pneumococcus), Streptococcus pyogenes, Staphylococcus aureus, and Haemophilus influenzae type b. Symptoms associated with bacterial pneumonia vary according to age, type of bacteria involved, and other factors. Infants and young children may develop a stuffy nose and other signs of upper respiratory infection, loss of appetite, sudden onset of fever, restlessness, respiratory distress, and cyanosis. In addition, infants with Staphylococcus aureus infection, a more serious type of disease, may develop lethargy, increased irritability, difficulty breathing (dyspnea), vomiting, or diarrhea. Abscesses may form in the lungs and may lead to the development of air-containing cysts (pneumatoceles). Accumulation of pus,

or empyema, may occur in the space surrounding the lungs. Older children and adolescents with bacterial pneumonia may develop symptoms commonly associated with mild upper respiratory tract infection followed by chills, shaking, fever, drowsiness, rapid breathing, coughing, or chest pain. Treatment for bacterial pneumonia includes the use of appropriate antibiotics. In the case of Staphylococcus aureus infection, drainage of pus accumulations may be indicated. Other treatment is symptomatic and supportive. Vaccination is important for preventing pneumonia in children. Vaccinations against Haemophilus influenzae and Streptococcus pneumoniae in the first year of life have greatly reduced their role in pneumonia in children.

Atypical pneumonias include those resulting from infection by bacteria-like microorganisms such as Mycoplasma pneumoniae and Chlamydia pneumoniae. Symptoms associated with these types of infections include fatigue, sore throat, cough, joint pain, or rash. Treatment may include the use of certain antibiotics.

Children with compromised immune systems are at risk for developing certain types of pneumonia infections caused by fungi (e.g., histoplasmosis, coccidioidomycosis, cryptococcosis, etc.) and other common organisms such as Pneumocystis carinii. Pneumocystis pneumonia is particularly prevalent among individuals with AIDS. Choice of drug therapy relates to the appropriate identification of the causative organism. Other treatment is symptomatic and supportive.

See also **General Resources** on page 917

See also **General Resources** on page 917

Government Agencies

5587 NIH/National Institute of Allergy and Infectious Diseases
6610 Rockledge Drive, MSC 6612
Bethesda, MD 20892

301-496-5717
Fax: 301-402-3573
TDD: 800-877-8339
www.niaid.nih.gov

Conducts and supports basic and applied research to better understand, treat, and ultimately prevent infectious, immunologic, and allergic diseases.

Anthony S Fauci MD, Director

National Associations & Support Groups

5588 March of Dimes Birth Defects Foundation
1275 Mamaroneck Avenue
White Plains, NY 10605

914-428-7100
888-663-4637
Fax: 914-428-8203
e-mail: resourcecenter@modimes.org
www.marchofdimes.com

Partnership of volunteers and professionals dedicates to improving the health of babies by preventing birth defects and infant mortality. Over 100 chapters are located across the country and can be located through the National Office.

Dr Jennifer Howse, President

5589 World Health Organization
Avenue Appia 20
CH-1211 Geneva 27,
Switzerland

www.who.int

WHO is the directing and coordinating authority for health within the United Nations system.

Dr Margaret Chan, Director General

Research Centers

5590 National Jewish Medical & Research Center
1400 Jackson Street
Denver, CO 80206

303-388-4461
800-222-5864
www.njc.org

National Jewish is a nonsectarian, nonprofit independent clinical research, medical center that focuses on respiratory, immunologic, allergic, and infectious diseases.

Michael Salem MD, President/CEO
J Verne Singleton, COO

Web Sites

5591 American Lung Association
www.lungusa.org

Information regarding lung disease in all its forms, with special emphasis on asthma, tobacco control and environmental health. Includes information and a fact sheet on pneumonia.

5592 Department of Health and Human Services
www.ahcpr.gov/consumer/pneucons.htm

Pneumonia research findings for consumers.

5593 Kid's Health
kidshealth.org/parent/infections/

Kids health is the largest and most visited site on the web providing doctor-approved health information about children from before birth through adolescence. Kids health provides families with accurate, up to date and jargon free health information they can use.

5594 Mayo Clinic
www.mayoclinic.com/health/pneumonia/DS00135

5595 National Jewish Medical & Research Center
www.njc.org

National Jewish is a nonsectarian, nonprofit independent clinical research, medical center. Focusing on respiratory, immunologic, allergic, and infectious diseases. The Center's mission is to develop and provide innovative clinical programs for treating and rehabilitating patients of all ages and for preventing disease, discovering knowledge to enhance prevention, treatment and cures through an integrated program of basic and clinical research, and educating professionals and the public.

Book Publishers

5596 Let's Talk About Going to the Hospital
Rosen Publishing Group's PowerKids Press
29 E 21st Street
New York, NY 10010

212-777-3017
800-237-9932
Fax: 888-436-4643
e-mail: rosenpub@tribeca.ios.com
www.powerkidspress.com

If a child has to check into the hospital, chances are he or she is already upset about being ill. Knowing how a hospital functions and what the procedures are, such as when family members can visit, will help in what is already a stressful situation. Grades K-5.

24 pages
ISBN: 0-823950-36-0

DESCRIPTION

5597 POLYDACTYLY

Synonyms: Polydactylia, Polydactylism
Involves the following Biologic System(s):
Genetic/Chromosomal/Syndrome/Metabolic Disorders,
Orthopedic and Muscle Disorders

Poldactyly refers to an abnormality that is present at birth (congenital) in which an infant has more than the usual number of fingers or toes. Defects associated with this abnormality may range from simple skin tags or stumps of flesh to extra fingers or toes that are completely developed. In some families polydactyly is passed from generation to generation.

Polydactyly involving the toes occurs in approximately two out of every 1,000 births. Although the fifth toe is the digit most often duplicated, polydactyly sometimes affects the great or big toe. Careful evaluation is indicated so that treatment of possible associated abnormalities may be appropriately coordinated. However, if the extra digit is small or rudimentary, it may be tied off (ligated) at birth or soon thereafter. This method allows for the digit to spontaneously detach itself after a period of time. In those cases where the digit is jointed, treatment usually involves surgical amputation of the extra digit and repair of other associated structures and tissues. Surgical intervention of this type is usually performed at approximately one year of age.

Duplication of a finger usually appears near the small finger (pinky) or thumb. As in polydactyly of the toes, small, rudimentary digits may be tied off, while more complex deformities typically require surgical intervention at about one year of age.

Polydactyly may also occur in association with several genetic disorders. These disordersinclude acrocephalopolysyndactyly type II (Carpenter's syndrome), characterized by mental retardation and irregularities involving the head, hand, and genitalia; trisomy 13 syndrome (Patau's syndrome), characterized by cleft lip and palate, polydactyly, mental retardation, and irregularities of the central nervous system, heart, genitalia, and internal organs; chondroectodermal dysplasia (Ellis-van Creveld syndrome), a bone growth disorder characterized by short stature, cardiac defects, polydactyly, and developmental defects of the teeth, and nails (hypoplastic). The efficacy of treating polydactyly associated with these and other disorders depends upon the exact nature of the disorder in question.

See also **General Resources** on page 917

Government Agencies

5598 NIH/National Institute of Arthritis and Musculoskeletal and Skin Diseases
1AMS Circle
Bethesda, MD 20892

301-402-4484
Fax: 301-718-6366
e-mail: ord@od.nih.gov
rarediseases.info.nih.gov

The mission of the National Institute of Arthritis and Musculoskeletal and Skin Diseases is to support research into the causes, treatment, and prevention of arthritis and musculoskeletal and skin diseases, the training of basic and clinical scientists to carry out this research, and the dissemination of information on research progress in these diseases.

Stephen I Katz MD PhD, Director

5599 NIH/National Institute of Child Health and Human Development
31 Center Drive, Building 31
Bethesda, MD 20892

301-496-5133
Fax: 301-496-1104
www.nichd.nih.gov

Established in 1962 by congress, today the institute conducts and supports research on topics related to the health of children, adults, families and populations. Some of these topics include: developmental disabilities, growth and development, infant death, reproductive health and birth defects.

Nancy D Wirth, Director
Lisa Kaeser, Program & Public Liaison

National Associations & Support Groups

5600 CHERUB-Association of Families and Friends of Children with Limb Disorders
Children's Hospital of Buffalo
936 Delaware Avenue
Buffalo, NY 14209

716-762-9997
e-mail: pffdvsg@ohio.net
www.ohio.net

Offers support to families of juveniles diagnosed with a limb disorder.

Sandra Richenberg
Kathy Gura

5601 Genetic Alliance
4301 Connecticut Avenue NW
Washington, DC 20008

202-966-5557
800-336-4363
Fax: 202-966-8553
e-mail: info@geneticalliance.org
www.geneticalliance.org

A coalition of voluntary genetic support groups, consumers and professionals addressing the needs of individuals and families affected by genetic disorders from a national perspective.

Sharon Terry, President/CEO

5602 March of Dimes Birth Defects Foundation
1275 Mamaroneck Avenue
White Plains, NY 10605

914-428-7100
888-663-4637
Fax: 914-428-8203
e-mail: resourcecenter@modimes.org
www.marchofdimes.com

Partnership of volunteers and professionals dedicates to improving
the health of babies by preventing birth defects and infant mortality. Over 100 chapters are located across the country and can be located through the National Office.

Dr Jennifer Howse, President

5603 Shriners Hospitals for Children
Headquarters
2900 Rocky Point Drive
Tampa, FL 33607

813-281-0300
800-237-5055
Fax: 813-281-8496
www.shrinershq.org

Network of 22 hospitals that provide expert, no-cost orthopaedic
and burn care to children under 18.

Web Sites

5604 CliniWeb
www.ohsu.edu/cliniweb

Is one of the original catalogs of health and bimedical information
on the web.

5605 On The Other Hand
www.ontheotherhand.org

Provides information, support, and suggestions for parents, relatives. and friends of children with hand anomalies.

5606 Polydactyly
www.eatonhand.com/hw/hw024.htm

Explanation and general overview of the disorder.

DESCRIPTION

5607 PORPHYRIA

Synonyms: EPP, Erythrohepatic protoporphyria, Ferrochelatase deficiency, Protoporphyria

Involves the following Biologic System(s):
Hematologic and Oncologic Disorders

Porphyria is a rare group of hereditary metabolic disorders characterized by enzyme deficiencies that result in the abnormal accumulation of chemicals known as porphyrins in certain tissues of the body. Porphyrins are formed during the manufacture of heme, the pigmented, iron-containing component of hemoglobin, which is the oxygen-carrying protein in red blood cells. The porphyrias may be classified as erythropoietic or hepatic porphyrias. The erythropoietic porphyrias are characterized by overproduction of porphyrins in the blood-forming tissue of the bone marrow. In individuals with hepatic porphyrias, there is abnormally increased production of porphyrins in the liver. The range and severity of associated symptoms and the age at onset are variable and depend on the underlying enzyme deficiency and the form of porphyria present. Erythropoietic protoporphyria is the most common form of porphyria and is thought to affect approximately one in 5,000 to 10,000 individuals.

In patients with erythropoietic protoporphyria, also known as EPP, deficiency of the enzyme ferrochelatase results in excessive accumulation of protoporphyrin in red blood cells and the fluid portion of the blood (plasma). Excessive protoporphyrin is also concentrated in a liquid secreted by the liver (bile) and is eliminated in the feces. In some patients, abnormal accumulations of protoporphyrin also become deposited within the liver itself.

Symptoms associated with EPP usually begin in childhood before age 10. The most common symptom is an abnormal sensitivity of the skin to sunlight and certain forms of artificial light (photosensitivity). Affected children typically experience pain, burning, and itching of the skin within an hour of exposure to sunlight. Such symptoms are often followed hours later by redness and inflammation of the skin and abnormal accumulation of fluid (edema) beneath the skin in affected areas. However, abnormal burning sensations of the skin may occur in the absence of associated redness or fluid accumulation. Rarely, if sun exposure is prolonged, fluid-filled blisters (vesicles) may develop or there may be bleeding in the skin or mucous membranes, appearing as pinpoint purplish spots (petechiae) or small bluish-purple patches (purpura). Such blistering or bruising may persist for several days after exposure to the sun. In addition, prolonged, repeated sun exposure may cause mild scarring, abnormal thickening of the skin in certain areas, or an abnormality of the nails in which the nails become separated from the nail beds (onycholysis). Although symptoms associated with photosensitivity typically become apparent during infancy or early childhood, the condition sometimes does not occur until adolescence or adulthood.

Many patients with EPP may also develop lumps of solid matter in the gall bladder (gallstones or cholelithiasis) at an unusually early age. The gall bladder is a small, muscular sac under the liver that stores and concentrates bile from the liver. In addition, uncommonly, there may be mildly decreased levels of circulating red blood cells (anemia). Rarely, patients may develop progressive liver damage that may lead to liver failure.

EPP is caused by changes (mutations) in the gene that regulates the production of the enzyme ferrochelatase. This gene is located on the long arm of chromosome 18 (18q21.3). Several different mutations of the gene have been identified in individuals with the disorder. In most cases, EPP has autosomal dominant inheritance. However, there have been reports in which patients inherited two different mutations of the gene, one from each parent. In addition, some individuals who inherit one copy of the disease gene may have slightly elevated levels of protoporphyrin, yet do not experience symptoms associated with the disease.

Patients with EPP benefit from avoiding sunlight, using topical sunscreens, and wearing protective clothing, such as sunglasses, hats, long sleeves, and double layers. Administration of beta-carotene by mouth may help improve tolerance to sunlight. Therapy with cholestyramine, a medication that acts upon the liver's bile acids, may help to alleviate skin symptoms and liver disease. Additional treatment is symptomatic and supportive.

See also **General Resources** on page 917

Government Agencies

5608 NIH/National Institute of Child Health and Human Development
31 Center Drive, Building 31
Bethesda, MD 20892

301-496-5133
Fax: 301-496-1104
www.nichd.nih.gov

Established in 1962 by congress, today the institute conducts and supports research on topics related to the health of children, adults, families and populations. Some of these topics include: developmental disabilities, growth and development, infant death, reproductive health and birth defects.

Nancy D Wirth, Director
Lisa Kaeser, Program & Public Liaison

National Associations & Support Groups

5609 American Porphyria Foundation
4900 Woodway, Suite 780, PO Box 22712
Houston, TX 77227

713-266-9617
866-273-3635
Fax: 713-840-9552
e-mail: porphyrus@aol.com
www.porphyriafoundation.com

Dedicated to improving the health and wellness of individuals and families affected by porphyria through enhanced public awareness; support of research; and development of educational programs and educational material.

Karl E Anderson MD, Chairman

5610 Erythropoietic Protoporphyria Research & Education Fund
Brigham & Women's Hospital
Channing Laboratory, 181 Longwood Avenue
Boston, MA 02115

617-525-8249
Fax: 617-731-1541
e-mail: mmmathroth@rics.bwh.harvard.edu
www.brighamandwomens.org/eppref

A support group for patients with Erythropoietic Protoporphyria and their families and their physicians, providing information on this disease and publishing a bi-annual newsletter available online on the website.

Micheline Mathews Roth, MD, Medical Director

5611 Genetic Alliance
4301 Connecticut Avenue NW
Washington, DC 20008

202-966-5557
800-336-4363
Fax: 202-966-8553
e-mail: info@geneticalliance.org
www.geneticalliance.org

A coalition of voluntary genetic support groups, consumers and professionals addressing the needs of individuals and families affected by genetic disorders from a national perspective.

Sharon Terry, President/CEO

5612 March of Dimes Birth Defects Foundation
1275 Mamaroneck Avenue
White Plains, NY 10605

914-428-7100
888-663-4637
Fax: 914-428-8203
e-mail: resourcecenter@modimes.org
www.marchofdimes.com

Partnership of volunteers and professionals dedicates to improving the health of babies by preventing birth defects and infant mortality. Over 100 chapters are located across the country and can be located through the National Office.

Dr Jennifer Howse, President

Libraries & Resource Centers

5613 National Digestive Diseases Information Clearinghouse
2 Information Way
Bethesda, MD 20892

301-654-3810
800-891-5389
Fax: 703-738-4929
e-mail: nddic@info.niddk.nih.gov
www.digestive.niddk.nih.gov

The National Institute of Diabetes and Digestive and Kidney Diseases conducts and supports research on many of the most serious diseases affecting public health. The Institute supports much of the clinical research on the diseases of internal medicine and related subspecialty fields as well as many basic science disciplines.

Kathy Kranzfelder, Project Officer

Newsletters

5614 APF Newsletter
American Porphyria Foundation
PO Box 22712
Houston, TX 77227

713-266-9617
www.porphyriafoundation.com

The newsletter provides updates on treatment and reserach, as well as informative articles on patients and specialists who treat porphyria.

Quarterly

Pamphlets

5615 Porphyria Fact Sheet
Nat'l Digestive Diseases Information Clearinghouse
2 Information Way
Bethesda, MD 20892

800-891-5389
Fax: 703-738-4929
e-mail: nddic@info.niddk.nih.gov
www.niddk.nih.gov

DESCRIPTION

5616 POST-TRAUMATIC STRESS DISORDER

Synonym: PTSD

Involves the following Biologic System(s):

Developmental/Behavioral/Psychiatric Disorders

Traumatic events can stay with children for a long time. Such events can range from the rare and horrific, such as severe torture, to more common events such as an automobile accident or a violent crime. With immediate media coverage of violence in our world, children are often exposed to the violent acts of war and terror through the television. Moreover, children may be directly or indirectly affected by events of terror and violence that now pervade our society. Effects of some childhood experiences can last well into adulthood. When the after-effects of a traumatic event are so severe and so persistent that they impair normal childhood functioning, behavior or development, professional help should be considered.

Post-Traumatic Stress Disorder, or PTSD, is a diagnosis made to describe the psychological and physiological symptoms that arise from experiencing, witnessing or participating in a traumatic event. PTSD in a child may result from exposure to a traumatic event which the child experienced or witnessed. It may occur if the child was confronted by death or serious injury, or a threat to the physical integrity of self or others. Studies indicate that 15 to 43% of girls and 14 to 43% of boys have experienced at least one traumatic event in their lifetime. Of those children and adolescents who have experienced a trauma, 3 to 15% of girls and 1 to 6% of boys meet criteria for PTSD. Researchers and clinicians are beginning to recognize that PTSD may not present itself in children in the same way as it does in adults. The classical triad of symptoms includes re-experiencing, numbing of responsiveness, and hyperarousal. Other symptoms include regression, bedwetting, separation anxiety and new fears previously not expressed. Children are also more likely to exhibit their 're-experience' in play. Very young children may present with few PTSD symptoms. Instead, young children may report more generalized fears such as stranger or separation anxiety, avoidance of situations that may or may not be related to the trauma, sleep disturbances, and a preoccupation with words or symbols that may or may not be related to the trauma. Elementary school-aged children may be unable to recall the sequence of the events related to the trauma or believe that there were warning signs that predicted the trauma. PTSD in adolescents may begin to more closely resemble PTSD in adults. Adolescents are more likely to engage in traumatic reenactment in which they incorporate aspects of the trauma into their daily lives. In addition, adolescents are more likely than younger children or adults to exhibit impulsive and aggressive behaviors. Response to traumatic events can also vary from child to child. Some characteristics, however, are common among all children with PTSD. If a child has survived a life-threatening event, there may be a profound sense of guilt, particularly if others did not survive the event. These guilt feelings may be exacerbated if the child had to do extraordinary things to survive. In other cases, a child with PTSD may complain of physical symptoms that have no discernible anatomic or physiological explanation, but which are manifestations of psychic distress; these are known as somatic complaints. The child with PTSD is also liable to experience a range of feelings that make it difficult or impossible for him or her to carry on with life in a normal fashion. They may feel that the trauma they experienced damaged them permanently and irreparably. Children who suffer from PTSD may also experience depression, Obsessive-Compulsive Disorder, social phobia or in the adolescent population, substance abuse.

Therapies include medication and/or psychotherapy. Behavior therapy focuses on helping the child recognize the thought processes that result in traumatic stress reactions. Behavior therapy may involve exposing the patient in a safe and controlled environment to stimuli that prompt a stress reaction; through repeated exposures, the child slowly is desensitized and in time will be able to experience the stimuli without having a stress reaction. As with many psychiatric disorders, treatment often involves some combination of therapy and medication.

Early intervention with skilled providers is vital for successful treatment of children with PTSD.

See also **General Resources** on page 917

Government Agencies

5617 National Center for PTSD

www.ncptsd.va.gov/topics/children.html

A special center within the US Department of Veterans Affairs, which advances clinical care and social welfare through research, education, training and diagnosis.

National Associations & Support Groups

5618 Association of Traumatic Stress Specialist s
PO Box 246
Phillips, ME 04966

800-991-2877
Fax: 207-639-2434
e-mail: admin@atss.info
www.atss.info

An international membership organization which develops standards of service and education for qualified individuals who provide services, intervention and treatment in the field of traumatic stress.

Susy Sanders, President
Jo Halligan, Vice President

5619 International Critical Incident Stress Foundation
3290 Pine Orchard Lane, Suite 106
Ellicott City, MD 21042

410-750-9600
Fax: 410-750-9601
e-mail: info@icisf.org
www.icisf.org

Nonprofit, open membership foundation dedicated to the prevention and mitigation of disabling stress by education, training and support services for all emergency service professionals; Continuing education and training in emergency mental health services for psychologists, psychiatrists, social workers and licensed professional counselors.

Donald Howell, President & Executive Director
Stephanie Beam, General Information

5620 Traumatic Incident Reduction Association
5145 Pontiac Trail
Ann Arbor, MI 48105

734-761-6268
800-499-2751
Fax: 734-663-6861
e-mail: info@tir.org
www.tir.org

Devoted to reducing the affects of traumatic incidents and providing education on how to deal with traumatic events.

Marian Volkman, President
Ragnhild Malnati, VP

Research Centers

5621 International Society for Traumatic Stress Studies
60 Revere Drive, Suite 500
Northbrook, IL 60062

847-480-9028
Fax: 847-480-9282
e-mail: istss@istss.org
www.istss.org

Provides a forum for sharing research, clinical strategies, public policy concerns and theoretical formulation on trauma in the US and worldwide. Dedicated to discovery and dissemination of knowledge and to the stimulation of policy, program and service initiatives that seek to reduce traumatic stressors and their permanent and long-term consequences. Members include psychiatrists, psychologists, social workers, nurses, counselors, researchers, administrators, advocates, and others.

Rick Koepke, Executive Director
Nicki Patti, Education Manager

Audio Video

5622 Complex PTSD in Children
Sidran Institute
200 E Joppa Road, Suite 207
Towson, MD 21286

410-825-8888
888-825-8249
Fax: 410-337-0747
e-mail: sidran@sidran.org
www.sidran.org

Tape I: Etiology, Assessment, Advocacy; Tape II: Therapeutic Interventions

VHS 41 Minutes

5623 PTSD in Children: Move in the Rhythm of th e Child
Sidran Institute
200 E Joppa Road, Suite 207
Towson, MD 21286

410-825-8888
888-825-8249
Fax: 410-337-0747
e-mail: sidran@sidran.org
www.sidran.org

Trauma experts explain the circumstances, symptoms and therapy techniques for PTSD in children and the effect on our communities. Primarily for use by mental health professionals, it is an excellent resource for any who work with children.

VHS 58 Minutes

5624 Significant Event Childhood Trauma
Sidran Institute
200 E Joppa Road, Suite 207
Towson, MD 21286

410-825-8888
888-825-8249
Fax: 410-337-0747
e-mail: sidran@sidran.org
www.sidran.org

Topics discussed inlude: effects; targeting resources; in the classroom; single parents; divorce; violence; addiction; and intervention.

DVD

Web Sites

5625 Association of Traumatic Stress Specialist s
www.atss.info

An international membership organization which develops standards of service and education for qualified individuals who provide services, intervention and treatment in the field of traumatic stress.

5626 David Baldwin's Trauma Information Pages
www.trauma-pages.com

Brief summary of what is known about traumatic symptoms and responses including PTSD and coping strategies. Pages include additional links to more detailed references, online articles and web resources.

5627 Facts for Health: PTSD
ptsd.factsforhealth.org

5628 Helping Kids Cope With a New Threat
www.apa.org/monitor/apr02/helpingkids.html

An online article about the issues of traumatic stress in children in particular after the September 11 attacks.

5629 International Critical Incident Stress Foundation
www.icisf.org

Nonprofit, open membership foundation dedicated to the prevention and mitigation of disabling stress by education, training and support services for all emergency service professionals; Continuing education and training in emergency mental health services for psychologists, psychiatrists, social workers and licensed professional counselors.

5630 Madison Institute of Medicine
www.miminc.org

Disseminates innovative approaches to the education of professionals and the general public on many mental health topics such as PTSD, OCD, depression, SAD and others.

5631 PTSD Alliance
www.ptsdalliance.org

A group of professional and advocacy organizaions that have joined forces to provide educational resources to individuals diagnosed with PTSD and their loves ones; those at risk for developing PTSD; and medical, healthcare and other frontline professionals.

5632 Sidran Institute - Traumatic Stress Educat ion & Advocacy
www.sidran.org

Provides education, resources, information and advocacy, publications, training and consulting on traumatic stress.

Book Publishers

5633 Coping with Post-Traumatic Stress Disorder
Rosen Publishing Group
29 E 21st Street
New York, NY 10010

800-237-9932
Fax: 888-436-4643
www.rosenpublishing.com

Revised 2002 192 pages

5634 EMDR: Breakthrough Therapy for Overcoming Anxiety, Stress and Trauma
200 E Joppa Road
Baltimore, MD 21286

410-825-8888
888-825-8249
Fax: 410-337-0747
e-mail: sidran@sidran.org
sidran.org

EMDR-Eye Movement Desensitization and Reprocessing, has successfully relieved symptoms like depression, phobias and nightmares of PTSD survivors, with a rapidity that almost defies belief. In this book for general audiences, Shapiro, the originator of EMDR, explains how she created the groundbreaking therapy, how it works and how it can help people who feel stuck in negative reactions and behaviors. Included with the text are a variety of compelling case studies.

284 pages

5635 Effective Treatments for PTSD
Guilford Press
72 Spring Street
New York, NY 10012

800-365-7006
Fax: 212-966-6708
e-mail: info@guilford.com
www.guilford.com

Represents the collaborative work of experts across a range of theoretical orientations and professional backgrounds. Addresses general treatment considerations and methodological issues, reviews and evaluates literature on treatment approaches for children, adolescents and adults.

2004 388 pages Paperback
ISBN: 1-593850-14-0

5636 Helping Kids Heal - 75 Activities to Help Children Recover from Trauma & Loss
Rebecca Carman CSW, author

Sidran Institute
200 E Joppa Road, Suite 207
Towson, MD 21286

410-825-8888
888-825-8249
Fax: 410-337-0747
e-mail: sidran@sidran.org
www.sidran.org

75 activities to use with school-aged children after traumatic events. Broken down into 13 sections that follow the natural sequence of recovery.

117 pages Paperback

5637 PTSD Workbook
Courage to Change
PO Box 486
Wilkes-Barre, PA 18703

800-440-4003
Fax: 800-772-6499
www.couragetochange.com

Outlines simple and effective techniques employed by PTSD experts for trauma survivors in order to conquer their most distressing symptoms. Readers learn to evaluate their type of trauma and then learn the most effective strategies to overcome them.

5638 Post Traumatic Stress Disorder Sourcebook
Glenn R Schiraldi, author

McGraw Hill Publishers
books.mcgraw-hill.com

877-833-5524
books.mcgraw-hill.com

Offers help and hope for lasting recovery. A guide for sufferers and theor loved ones.

446 pages Paperback
ISBN: 0-737302-65-8

5639 Posttraumatic Stress Disorder in Children and Adolescents
Raul R Silva MD, author

Sidran Institute
200 E Joppa Road, Suite 207
Towson, MD 21286

410-825-8888
888-825-8249
Fax: 410-337-0747
e-mail: sidran@sidran.org
www.sidran.org

An expert guide to the most importatnt issues pertaining to PTSD, trauma, stress and concurrent conditions. Includes 15 chapters that address different aspects of childhood and adolescent trauma.

384 pages Paperback

5640 Saddest Time
Childs Work/Childs Play
135 Dupont Street
Plainville, NY 11803

800-962-1141
Fax: 800-262-1886
e-mail: info@Childswork.com
Childswork.com

Helps children ages 6 - 12 understand that death is sad and sometimes tragic, but it is also part of life.

5641 Traumatic Stress: The Effects of Overwhelm ing Experience on Mind, Body and Society
Guilford Press
72 Spring Street
New York, NY 10012

800-365-7006
Fax: 212-966-6708
e-mail: info@guilford.com
www.guilford.com

The current state of research and clinical knowledge on traumatic stress and its treatment. Contributions from leading authorities summarize emerging knowledge. Addresses the uncertainties and controversies that confront the field of traumatic stress, including the complexity of post-traumatic adaptations and the unproven effectiveness of some approaches to prevention and treatment.

596 pages Paperback
ISBN: 1-572304-57-0

5642 Treating Psychological Trauma and PTSD

John Wilson et al, author

Sidran Institute
200 E Joppa Road, Suite 207
Towson, MD 21286

410-825-8888
888-825-8249
Fax: 410-337-0747
e-mail: sidran@sidran.org
www.sidran.org

Identifies 65 PTSD symptoms contained within five symptom clusters, and then addresses 80 target objectives for treatment, which can be treated by 11 different psychotherapeutic approaches.

443 pages Paperback

Pamphlets

5643 Helping Children and Adolescents Cope with Violence and Disasters
National Institute of Mental Health
Public Info Branch, 6001 Executive Boulevard
Bethesda, MD 20892

301-443-4513
866-615-6464
Fax: 301-443-4279
TTY: 301-443-8431
e-mail: nimhinfo@nih.gov
www.nimh.nih.gov/publicat

Booklet that discusses children and adolescents' reactions to violence and disasters, emphasizing the wide range of responses and the role that parents, teachers and therapists can play in the healing process.

5644 Post Traumatic Stress Disorder: A Guide
Madison Institute of Medicine
www.miminc.org/shop/store/

Comprehensive overview, diagnosis and treatment of PTSD.

2000 69 pages

5645 Post-Traumatic Stress Disorder, A Real Ill ness
National Institute of Mental Health
Public Info Branch, 6001 Executive Boulevard
Bethesda, MD 20892

301-443-4513
866-615-6464
Fax: 301-443-4279
TTY: 301-443-8431
e-mail: nimhinfo@nih.gov
www.nimh.nih.gov/publicat

An easy-to-read pamphlet of simple information about what it is, when it starts, how long it lasts and how to get help.

9 pages

5646 What Is Post Traumatic Stress Disorder?
Sidran Institute
200 E Joppa Road, Suite 207
Towson, MD 21286

410-825-8888
888-825-8249
Fax: 410-337-0747
e-mail: sidran@sidran.org
www.sidran.org

Provides an introduction of PTSD as well as symptoms, possible treatment, and other helpful resources.

DESCRIPTION

5647 PRADER-WILLI SYNDROME

Synonym: PWS

Involves the following Biologic System(s):

Endocrinologic Disorders,
Genetic/Chromosomal/Syndrome/Metabolic Disorders

Prader-Willi syndrome is a genetic disorder characterized by severely diminished muscle tone (hypotonia) during early infancy, short stature, unusually small hands and feet, obesity, genital abnormalities, and mental retardation. The disorder is thought to affect approximately one in 15,000 individuals. In most cases of Prader-Willi syndrome, there is decreased fetal activity during the last months of pregnancy. After birth, most affected infants experience hypotonia, have feeding difficulties due to decreased swallowing and sucking reflexes, and fail to grow and gain weight at the expected rate (failure to thrive). Starting at approximately six months to six years of age, affected infants or children begin to have an excessive appetite (polyphagia), become obsessed with eating, or lack a sense of satisfaction after a meal and often engage in binge-type eating. As a result, patients develop an abnormally increased body weight (progressive obesity) due to an excessive accumulation of body fat, particularly over the thighs, buttocks, and lower abdomen.

Infants and children with Prader-Willi syndrome also may have characteristic abnormalities of the head and face (craniofacial area), such as almond-shaped eyes, upslanting eyelid folds (palpebral fissures), abnormal deviation of one eye in relation to the other (strabismus), a thin, tented upper lip, and full cheeks. In addition, affected males and females may have insufficient secretion of certain hormones that stimulate the gonads (hypogonadotropic hypogonadism). The gonads are the reproductive glands, such as the testes or ovaries, within which the reproductive cells (sperm or ova) are produced. Affected males typically have an abnormally small penis (micropenis) and undescended testes (cryptorchidism), potentially delayed or incomplete development of secondary sexual characteristics, insufficient production of the male sex hormone testosterone, decreased or absent sperm production, and infertility. Affected females often have abnormally small underdeveloped external genitalia (i.e., hypoplastic labia minor and clitoris), absence or abnormal cessation of menstrual cycles (primary or secondary amenorrhea), and infertility. Development of female secondary sexual characteristics may be normal or incomplete. Most children with Prader-Willi syndrome also have mild to moderate mental retardation; however, in some cases, severe mental retardation may be present. Many affected children experience difficulties with speech articulation and may have an abnormally high-pitched, nasal voice. Children with Prader-Willi syndrome may have behavioral problems that become apparent during later childhood, including outbursts of anger, rage-like episodes, and stubbornness.

Some individuals with Prader-Willi syndrome may develop diabetes mellitus during or soon after puberty. Diabetes mellitus is characterized by impaired fat, protein, and carbohydrate metabolism due to insufficient production of the hormone insulin or the body's inability to appropriately utilize insulin. Associated symptoms may include excessive thirst (polydipsia) and urination (polyuria). In addition, adolescents and young adults may be prone to experiencing cardiac insufficiency, potentially resulting in life-threatening complications during the second or third decade of life.

In children with Prader-Willi syndrome, treatment typically includes measures to help prevent progressive obesity or to ensure strict weight control, such as a low-calorie diet and a proper exercise program under a physician's direction. Nutritional behavioral modification methods may be implemented that require the cooperation and support of all family members, such as ensuring regular feeding habits (e.g., having meals at the same time and location on a daily basis) and the inaccessibility of food between meals. In young males with Prader-Willi syndrome, testosterone replacement therapy may result in enlargement of micropenis; in addition, testosterone therapy during adolescence or young adulthood may have beneficial effects on the development of secondary sexual characteristics. Treatment of children with Prader-Willi syndrome also may include special education and behavioral therapies to help manage behavioral problems.

Prader-Willi syndrome is caused by deletion or disruption of certain genes (contiguous gene syndrome) located on the long arm of chromosome 15 (15q11-13). Most affected individuals have missing genetic material or deletion of 15q11-13 that affects the chromosome received from the father (paternally derived chromosome).

See also **General Resources** on page 917

Government Agencies

5648 NIH/National Institute of Child Health and Human Development
National Institutes of Health
31 Center Drive
Bethesda, MD 20892

301-496-5133
www.nichd.nih.gov

Offers reprints, articles and various information on Prader-Willi Syndrome in children and adults.

Nancy D Wirth, Director
Lisa Kaeser, Program & Public Liaison

National Associations & Support Groups

5649 Foundation for Prader-Willi Research
6407 Bardstown Road, Suite 252
Louisville, KY 40291

502-384-8405
Fax: 502-749-9388
www.fpwr.org

Dedicated to the advancement of research on PWS. The Foundation chooses projects that are highly relevant for individuals with PWS and their familes and that are scientifically sound.

Rachel Tugon, Executive Director
Alice Viroslav, President

5650 Genetic Alliance
4301 Connecticut Avenue NW
Washington, DC 20008

202-966-5557
800-336-4363
Fax: 202-966-8553
e-mail: info@geneticalliance.org
www.geneticalliance.org

A coalition of voluntary genetic support groups, consumers and professionals addressing the needs of individuals and families affected by genetic disorders from a national perspective.

Sharon Terry, President/CEO

5651 March of Dimes Birth Defects Foundation
1275 Mamaroneck Avenue
White Plains, NY 10605

914-428-7100
888-663-4637
Fax: 914-428-8203
e-mail: resourcecenter@modimes.org
www.marchofdimes.com

Partnership of volunteers and professionals dedicates to improving the health of babies by preventing birth defects and infant mortality. Over 100 chapters are located across the country and can be located through the National Office.

Dr Jennifer Howse, President

5652 Prader-Willi Syndrome Association
5700 Midnight Pass Road, Suite 6
Sarasota, FL 34242

941-312-0400
800-926-4797
Fax: 941-312-0142
e-mail: national@pwsausa.org
www.pwsausa.org

Provides educational materials, support, and advocacy for parents, caregivers, medical professionals, educators and all others involved with persons in PWS community.

Janalee Heinemann, Executive Director
Diane Spencer, Support Coordinator

State Agencies & Support Groups

Alaska

5653 Prader-Willi Northwest Association
16208 SE 46th Place
Bellevue, WA 98006

424-641-9452
e-mail: jlunderwood@juno.com

Joane Underwood, Co-President

Arizona

5654 Prader-Willi Syndrome Arizona Association
13839 N Bentwater Drive
Tucson, AZ 85737

520-297-7025
e-mail: p.penta@comcast.net

Tammie Penta, President

Arkansas

5655 PWSA of Arkansas
Prader-Willi Syndrome Association
2504 S Drive
North Little Rock, AR 72118

501-753-8715

Jim Patton, President

California

5656 PWSA of California
Prader-Willi Syndrome Association
805 El Toro Drive
Bakersfield, CA 93304

805-831-7627

Wesley Crawford

5657 Prader-Willi California Foundation
3655 Torrance Boulevard, Suite 360
Torrance, CA 90503

310-316-3339
800-400-9994
Fax: 310-316-3730
e-mail: PWCF1@aol.com
www.pwcf.org

Lisa Graziano, Executive Director

Colorado

5658 Prader-Willi Colorado Association
PWSA
8290 South Yukon Way
Littleton, CO 80128

303-973-4780
e-mail: hosler@dynamicssolutions.com

Lynette Hosler, President

Connecticut

5659 PWSA of Connecticut (North Haven)
Prader-Willi Syndrome Association
35 Ansonia Drive
North Haven, CT 06473

203-744-4189
e-mail: bmaf@juno.com

Barb Farmer, President

5660 Prader-Willi Connecticut Association
PWSA
35 Ansonia Drive
North Haven, CT 06473

203-239-9902
e-mail: pwsactchapter@yahoo.com
www.angelfire.com/ct/pwsctchapter/

Eileen Fletcher
Vicki Knopf

Delaware

5661 Prader-Willi Delaware Association
PWSA
300 Bethel Circle Millwood
Middletown, DE 19709

302-378-7385
e-mail: swede455@aol.com

Karen Swanson, President

Florida

5662 PWSA Florida Chapter
PWSA
694 SE Ashley Oak Way
Stuart, FL 34997

772-287-2587
e-mail: pwfa2000@aol.com
http://members.aol.com/delchert/pwsa2.htm

Dan Krauer, President

5663 PWSA of Florida (Tampa)
Prader-Willi Syndrome Association
1914 W Carmen Street
Tampa, FL 33606

813-251-1259
e-mail: PWFA2000@aol.com

Debbie Peaton, President
Keith Peaton, President

Georgia

5664 PWSA Chapter - Atlanta
Prader-Willi Syndrome Association
3562 Hidden Acres Drive
Atlanta, GA 30340

404-892-8191

Greg Talley, President

5665 PWSA of Georgia
3577-A Chamblee Tucker, PMB 173
Atlanta, GA 30341

678-534-0724
877-534-0724
Fax: 678-534-0742
e-mail: pwsaga@earthlink.net
www.pwsaga.org

Debbie Lange, Executive Director

Hawaii

5666 Prader-Willi Northwest Association
269 Kaha Street
Kailua, HI 96734

808-263-8177
e-mail: Oncpa@pixi.com

Tami Ho, Contact Person

Idaho

5667 Prader-Willi Northwest Association-Idaho
550 Lodgepole Road
Athol, ID 83801

208-683-2993
e-mail: idaho4ts@aol.com

Gene Todhunter, Contact

Illinois

5668 PWSA of Illinois
PWSA
505 Drexel Avenue
Glencoe, IL 60022

847-242-9082
e-mail: illinois@pwsausa.org
www.pwsausa.org/IL/

Ron Bruns, President

Indiana

5669 PWSA of Indiana
Prader-Willi Syndrome Association
7458 Glendale Drive
Avon, IN 46123

317-823-5748
e-mail: pwsain@yahoo.com
www.pwsausa.org/IN/

Jaque McGuire

Iowa

5670 PWSA of Iowa
Prader-Willi Syndrome Association
15554 226th Street
Zwingle, IA 52079

319-686-4270
e-mail: Ktcaedav@netins.net

Tammy Davis, President

Kansas

5671 Prader-Willi Syndrome Advocates
14 NE Bayview Drive
Lees Summit, MO 64064

816-350-1375

Teri Douglas
Barry Douglas

Kentucky

5672 PWSA of Kentucky
Prader-Willi Syndrome Association
3207 Laurel Oak Court
Edgewood, KY 41017

859-331-5759
e-mail: frankandannette@fuse.net

Frank Beck, President

Louisiana

5673 PWSA Chapter - Louisiana
Prader-Willi Syndrome Association
742 Anicet Tauzin Road
Arnaudville, LA 70512

318-754-7263

Doris Richard, President

Maine

5674 Prader-Willi Association of New England (Maine, Mass, RI, NH, VT)
2 Ernest Street
Webster, MA 01570

508-943-1400
www.pwsane.org

Sherie Bombardier, Contact

Maryland

5675 PWSA of Maryland, Virginia & DC
Prader-Willi Syndrome Association
2601 Chriswell Place
Herndon, VA 20171

410-822-3752
e-mail: pwsamd@pwsausa.org
www.pwsausa.org/MD/

Linda Keder, President
Susaie Wood, Maryland Contact

Massachusetts

5676 Prader-Willi Association of New England (Maine, Mass, RI, NH, VT)
2 Ernest Street
Webster, MA 01570

508-943-1400
www.pwsane.org

Sherie Bombardier, Contact

Michigan

5677 PWSA of Michigan
Prader-Willi Syndrome Association
62 North Center Street
Saranac, MI 48881

616-642-0017
Fax: 941-313-0142
e-mail: mi@pwsausa.org
www.pwsausa.org/MI/

Jon Hendrick
Chris Hendrick

Minnesota

5678 PWSA Chapter - Minnesota
Prader-Willi Syndrome Association
7691 Iverson Avenue S
Cottage Grove, MN 55015

651-768-0045
e-mail: dwestenfield@datalink.com
www.pwsausa.org/MN/

Denise Westenfield, President
Kymm Salwasser, Treasurer

Missouri

5679 PWSA Missouri Chapter
Prader-Willi Syndrome Missouri Association
3233 Hedgetree Lane Street
St Louis, MO 63129

314-845-6910
Fax: 314-935-7461
e-mail: joleary@wustl.edu
www.pwsausa.org/MO/

Judy O'Leary, President

Montana

5680 Prader-Willi Northwest Association
3706 29th Street West
Seattle, WA 98199

206-285-7679
e-mail: susanlundh@yahoo.com

Nebraska

5681 PWSA of Nebraska
Prader-Willi Syndrome Association
302 S 49th Avenue
Omaha, NE 68132

402-551-9168
e-mail: jvarner@cox.net
www.pwsausa.org

Jennifer Varner, Contact

Nevada

5682 PWSA Las Vegas/Nevada Support Group
PWS NV S.H.A.R.E.
www.pwsnv.org

702-526-0630
e-mail: pwsnv.org@gmail.com
www.pwsnv.org

New Jersey

5683 PWSA - New Jersey Chapter
Prader-Willi Syndrome Association
514 Gatewood Road
Cherry Hill, NJ 08003

856-795-4229
e-mail: pwsa.nj@gmail.com
www.pwsausa.org/NJ/

Sybil Cohen, President

New Mexico

5684 PWS Project for New Mexico

505-332-6868
e-mail: claroque@arc-a.org

New York

5685 PWSA Chapter - Franklin Square
Prader-Willi Syndrome Association
175 Court House Road
Franklin Square, NY 11010

516-328-6982
800-442-1655
www.athenet.net/~pwsa-usa/WI/

Mary Cucciaia, President

5686 PWSA of New York
Prader-Willi Syndrome Association
190 Lincoln Place
Brooklyn, NY 11217

718-783-0181

Henry Singer, President

5687 Prader-Willi Alliance of New York
PWSA NY Chapter
PO Box 1114
Niagara Falls, NY 14304

585-442-1655
800-442-1655
e-mail: alliance@prader-willi.org
www.prader-willi.org

Hon. Daniel D Angiolillo, President

North Carolina

5688 PWSA of North Carolina
PWSA
4627 Mt Sinai Road
Durham, NC 27705

919-489-0390

Mary Jones Patterson

North Dakota

5689 PWSA Chapter - Bottineau
Prader-Willi Syndrome Association
818 7th Street E
Bottineau, ND 58318

701-228-5103

Barb Kruize, President

5690 PWSA Chapter - Fraser Ltd - Fargo
Prader-Willi Syndrome Association
2902 S University Drive
Fargo, ND 58103

701-232-3301
Fax: 701-237-5775
e-mail: fraser@fraserltd.org
www.fraserltd.org

Fraser provides services and supports to assist people to celebrate and live life as independently as possible. Residential homes are available with services that are individualized reflecting on the total person and centering around choice, empowerment, recreation and leisure activities at home and in the community. New to Fraser are Family Support Services, Representative Payee Services, and licensing for the Qualified Service Provider Programs.

Rikki Iverson, Residential Program Systems Coord

5691 PWSA of North Dakota
Prader-Willi Syndrome Association
8501 435th Avenue NE
Regan, ND 58477

701-286-6228
e-mail: shellysivak@yahoo.com

Michelle Sivak, President

Ohio

5692 PWSA of Ohio
State Office
1087 Dover Drive
Medina, OH 44256

330-723-0004
e-mail: pwsaohio@aol.com
www.pwsaohio.org

Steve Fetsko, President

5693 Prader-Willi Families of Ohio

330-896-0776
e-mail: pwfohio@aol.com

Johanna Costello, President

Oklahoma

5694 PWSA of Oklahoma
Prader-Willi Syndrome Association
3820 SE 89th Street
Oklahoma City, OK 73135

405-677-8089
Fax: 405-522-6256
e-mail: Rdmosley@swbell.net

Daphne Mosley, President
Curt Shacklett, Chairman

Oregon

5695 PWSA of Oregon
Prader-Willi Syndrome Association
456 Horn Lane
Eugene, OR 97404

541-688-2403
e-mail: wade175@juno.com
www.pwsausa.org

Lennae Elkington, President

Pennsylvania

5696 PWSA Chapter - Western Pennsylvania
Prader-Willi Syndrome Association
5890 Monogahela Avenue
Bethel Park, PA 15102

412-831-9291

Sandy Innekus, President

5697 PWSA of Pennsylvania
Prader-Willi Syndrome Association
104 Persimmon Place
Cranberry Township, PA 16066

724-779-4415
e-mail: debpwsapa@yahoo.com

Debbie Fabio, President

South Carolina

5698 PWSA - South Carolina
Prader-Willi Syndrome Association
912 Lake Spur Lane
Chapin, SC 29036

803-345-1379
e-mail: rleazer8@cs.com

Rhett Eleazer, Contact

Tennessee

5699 PWSA - Tennessee
Prader-Willi Syndrome Association
105 Foxwood Lane
Franklin, TN 37065

615-790-6659
e-mail: Tcbo333@aol.com

Terry Bolander

5700 PWSA Chapter - Nashville
Prader-Willi Syndrome Association
PO Box 40
Nashville, TN 37202

615-322-8086

Beth Joseph, President

5701 PWSA of Tennessee
Prader-Willi Syndrome Association
105 Foxwood Lane
Franklin, TN 37065

615-790-6659
e-mail: Tcbo333@aol.com

Terry Bolander, President

Texas

5702 PWSA Chapter - North Texas
Prader-Willi Syndrome Association
2302 Greenbriar Court
Grand Prairie, TX 75050

972-988-6928

Diane Smiley, President

5703 Texas Prader-Willi Syndrome Association
PO Box 578
Coppell, TX 75019

972-956-9957
e-mail: info@texaspwsa.com
www.pwsausa.org; www.texaspwsa.com

Derek Snitker

Utah

5704 PWSA Chapter - Orem
Prader-Willi Syndrome Association
235 S Palisades Drive
Orem, UT 84097

801-221-5964

Brent Tobler, President
Pamela Tobler

5705 PWSA Chapter - Pleasant Grove
Prader-Willi Syndrome Association
613 E 630 N
Pleasant Grove, UT 84062

801-785-3444

Dennis Smith, President
Glenda Smith

5706 Prader-Willi Utah Association
Prader-Willi Syndrome Association
722 East 300 North
Lehi, UT 84043

801-768-8851
Fax: 801-768-3924
e-mail: ccnms@networld.com
www.pwsausa.org/UT/

Michelle Holbrook, President

Virginia

5707 PWSA of Maryland, Virginia & DC
Prader-Willi Syndrome Association
2601 Chriswell Place
Herndon, VA 20171

703-716-4189
e-mail: pwsamd@pwsausa.org
www.pwsausa.org/MD/

Linda Keder, President
Sherri Planton, Virginia Contact

Washington

5708 PWSA Chapter - Northwest Washington
Prader-Willi Syndrome Association
22310 91st Avenue W
Edmonds, WA 98020

425-640-2473

Sean Doyle, President
Illona Doyle

5709 PWSA of Region Northwest
Prader-Willi Syndrome Association
3706 29th Avenue W
Seattle, WA 98199

206-285-2560
e-mail: slundh@ips.net

Serving patients and families with Prader-Willi syndrome in the Washington, Oregon, Idaho, Alaska, and Hawaii regions.

Billie McSwan, President

5710 PWSA of Washington
Prader-Willi Syndrome Association
5501 Birch Road
Pasco, WA 66301

509-547-4801

Janet Pearson, President

West Virginia

5711 PWSA of West Virginia
Prader-Willi Syndrome Association
717 Morgan Avenue
Morgantown, WV 26305

304-296-6412
e-mail: Lee@be.wvu.edu

Henry Lee, President
Lee President

Wisconsin

5712 PWSA of Wisconsin
Prader-Willi Syndrome Association
2701 N Alexander Street
Appleton, WI 54911

866-797-2947
e-mail: wisonsin@pwsausa.org
www.pwsausa.org/wi/

Mary Ann Larson, Program Director

5713 PWSA of Wisconsin - Madison
Prader-Willi Syndrome Association
115 Marinette Trail
Madison, WI 53593

608-238-6757

Pat LaBella, President

Research Centers

5714 Foundation for Prader-Willi Research
6407 Bardstown Road, Suite 252
Louisville, KY 40291

502-384-8405
Fax: 502-749-9388
www.fpwr.org

Dedicated to the advancement of research on PWS. The Foundation chooses projects that are highly relevant for individuals with PWS and their familes and that are scientifically sound.

Rachel Tugon, Executive Director
Alice Viroslav, President

Audio Video

5715 A Deadly Hunger
Prader-Willi Syndrome Association
5700 Midnight Pass Road, Suite 6
Sarasota, FL 34242

941-312-0400
800-926-4797
Fax: 941-312-0142
e-mail: national@pwsausa.org
www.pwsausa.org

A five part series of news segments that spotlight PWS.

2000 DVD

5716 A Tribute to PWS Children from Around the World
Prader-Willi Syndrome Association
5700 Midnight Pass Road, Suite 6
Sarasota, FL 34242

941-312-0400
800-926-4797
Fax: 941-312-0142
e-mail: national@pwsausa.org
www.pwsausa.org

A video of children with PWS of all ages. The presentation is set to music.

10 Minutes

Mark Ryan, Producer

5717 Food, Behavior and Beyond
Prader-Willi Syndrome Association
5700 Midnight Pass Road, Suite 6
Sarasota, FL 34242

941-312-0400
800-926-4797
Fax: 941-312-0142
e-mail: national@pwsausa.org
www.pwsausa.org

Comprehensive DVD as a joint project of PWSA and IPWSO. Can be used as a teaching tool for the staff of provider agencies and parents.

DVD

5718 Maribel

Prader-Willi Syndrome Association
5700 Midnight Pass Road, Suite 6
Sarasota, FL 34242

941-312-0400
800-926-4797
Fax: 941-312-0142
e-mail: national@pwsausa.org
www.pwsausa.org

Chronicles a family's struggle with their adult daughter with PWS.

2004 DVD/VHS

5719 PWS - The Early Years

Prader-Willi Syndrome Association
5700 Midnight Pass Road, Suite 6
Sarasota, FL 34242

941-312-0400
800-926-4797
Fax: 941-312-0142
e-mail: national@pwsausa.org
www.pwsausa.org

Practical suggestions for families with a young child newly diagnosed with PWS. Includes family interviews.

2002 Video 42 Mins

5720 Prader-Willi Syndrome - An Overview for He alth Professionals

Prader-Willi Syndrome Association
5700 Midnight Pass Road, Suite 6
Sarasota, FL 34242

941-312-0400
800-926-4797
Fax: 941-312-0142
e-mail: national@pwsausa.org
www.pwsausa.org

A medical overview of PWS for health care professionals. It handles all the major genetics and health care issues of the child with PWS.

2004 35 Minutes

Mark Ryan, Producer

Web Sites

5721 International Prader-Willi Syndrome Organi zation (IPWSO)
www.ipswo.org

5722 Online Mendelian Inheritance in Man
www.ncbi.nlm.nih.gov

This database is a catalog of human genes and genetic disorders.

5723 Prader-Willi Alliance of New York
www.prader-willi.org

A chapter of the PWSA, it represents the interests of individuals in New York State with Prader-Willi Syndrome, their families, and the professionals who provide services to the Prader-Willi population.

5724 Prader-Willi Syndrome Association
www.pwsausa.org

Dedicated to serving individuals affected by Prader-Willi Syndrome, their families, and interested professionals. To provide information, education, and support services to its members. PWSA offers a toll free telephone number for informationand referrals, a bimonthly newsletter, publications and audiovisual presentations about PWS, an annual national conference for families and professionals and a nationwide network of local chapters, parents, and professionals.

Book Publishers

5725 Cookbook for the PWS Diet

Donna Unterberger, author

Prader-Willi Syndrome Association
5700 Midnight Pass Road, Suite 6
Sarasota, FL 34242

941-312-0400
800-926-4797
Fax: 941-312-0142
e-mail: national@pwsausa.org
www.pwsausa.org

Low-fat, low-sugar recipes that are nutritious for the entire family. Includes a substitution list.

2003

Janalee Heinemann, Executive Director

5726 Growth Hormone and Prader-Willi Syndrome

Linda Keder, author

Prader-Willi Syndrome Association
5700 Midnight Pass Road, Suite 6
Sarasota, FL 34242

941-312-0400
800-926-4797
Fax: 941-312-0142
e-mail: national@pwsausa.org
www.pwsausa.org

Reference for families and care givers.

2001 52 pages Softcover

5727 Management of Prader-Willi Syndrome

Prader-Willi Syndrome Association
5700 Midnight Pass Road, Suite 6
Sarasota, FL 34242

941-312-0400
800-926-4797
Fax: 941-312-0142
e-mail: national@pwsausa.org
www.pwsausa.org

Comprehensive reference on the diagnosis and care of individuals with Prader-Willi Syndrome. Contributions by 32 experts in PWS.

550 pages 3rd Edition
ISBN: 0-387253-97-1

5728 Nutitional Care for Children with PWS, Inf ants and Toddlers

Prader-Willi Syndrome Association
5700 Midnight Pass Road, Suite 6
Sarasota, FL 34242

941-312-0400
800-926-4797
Fax: 941-312-0142
e-mail: national@pwsausa.org
www.pwsausa.org

Provides answers to frequently asked questions about nutrition and feeding of infants and toddlers with PWS.

Revised 2004 62 pages Softcover

5729 Overview of the Prader-Willi Syndrome

Lota Mitchell, MSW, author

Prader-Willi Syndrome Association
5700 Midnight Pass Road, Suite 6
Sarasota, FL 34242

941-312-0400
800-926-4797
Fax: 941-312-0142
e-mail: national@pwsausa.org
www.pwsausa.org

Offers a short introduction of the syndrome to parents and professionals.

1994 13 pages Softcover

5730 Prader-Willi Syndrome is What I Have Not W ho I Am!

Janalee Heinemnann, author

Prader-Willi Syndrome Association
5700 Midnight Pass Road, Suite 6
Sarasota, FL 34242

941-312-0400
800-926-4797
Fax: 941-312-0142
e-mail: national@pwsausa.org
www.pwsausa.org

A book of feelings written by children and young adults with PWS. A portion of the book discusses journal writing as an opportunity for readers to share their feelings.

2005

Janalee Heinemann, Executive Director

5731 Sometimes I'm Mad, Sometimes I'm Glad - A Sibling Booklet

Sarah Heinemann, author

Prader-Willi Syndrome Association
5700 Midnight Pass Road, Suite 6
Sarasota, FL 34242

941-312-0400
800-926-4797
Fax: 941-312-0142
e-mail: national@pwsausa.org
www.pwsausa.org

A voice of a sibling of someone with PWS, that displays the range of feelings that arise. Ages 5-13.

Revised 2005

5732 Supporting the Student/PWS for Teachers

Prader-Willi Syndrome Association
5700 Midnight Pass Road, Suite 6
Sarasota, FL 34242

941-312-0400
800-926-4797
Fax: 941-312-0142
e-mail: national@pwsausa.org
www.pwsausa.org

Offers educational information for the professional dealing with a child who has PWS. Contains a worksheet, brochure, and 27-minute audiotape.

5733 Teacher's Handbook for the Student with PW S (Educator's Resource)

Prader-Willi Syndrome Association
5700 Midnight Pass Road, Suite 6
Sarasota, FL 34242

941-312-0400
800-926-4797
Fax: 941-312-0142
e-mail: national@pwsausa.org
www.pwsausa.org

A resource manual that provides teachers with valuable information on working with students of all abilities.

2003

5734 Tool Box of Hope - For When Your Body Does n't Feel Good

Deva Joy Gouss, author

Prader-Willi Syndrome Association
5700 Midnight Pass Road, Suite 6
Sarasota, FL 34242

941-312-0400
800-926-4797
Fax: 941-312-0142
e-mail: national@pwsausa.org
www.pwsausa.org

An interactive workbook for parents and care givers to provide children with fun and practical ways to express their feelings, get along with others, take medicine and make friends.

2003 2003 pages Ages 3-adult

Newsletters

5735 Gathered View

Prader-Willi Syndrome Association
5700 Midnight Pass Road, Suite 6
Sarasota, FL 34242

941-312-0400
800-926-4797
Fax: 941-312-0142
e-mail: national@pwsausa.org
www.pwsausa.org

The official newsletter of PWSA USA. It offers current research findings, behavior and weight management techniques, educational news and more.

Bimonthly

Pamphlets

5736 An Early Prader-Willi Syndrome Diagnosis & How to Make it Easier on Parents

Prader-Willi Foundation
40 Holly Lane
Roslyn Hts, NY 11577

516-944-8136
Fax: 516-944-3173
e-mail: foundation@prader-willi.inter.net
www.prader-willi.org

A parent of a child with PWS and an advocate for others with the afflication speaks.

5737 Behavior Management - A Collection of Arti cles

Prader-Willi Syndrome Association
5700 Midnight Pass Road, Suite 6
Sarasota, FL 34242

941-312-0400
800-926-4797
Fax: 941-312-0142
e-mail: national@pwsausa.org
www.pwsausa.org

Booklet discusses behavior concerns, skin picking, social skills education and the use of psychotropic medications.

2000 49 pages

5738 Child With Prader-Willi Syndrome: Birth to Three

Prader-Willi Syndrome Association
5700 Midnight Pass Road, Suite 6
Sarasota, FL 34242

941-312-0400
800-926-4797
Fax: 941-312-0142
e-mail: national@pwsausa.org
www.pwsausa.org

A positive and helpful booklet for families, care providers, and physicians. It discusses the common concerns of the first three years and early intervention strategies.

Revised 2004 34 pages Softcover

5739 Growing Up with Prader-Willi Syndrome - Pe rsonal Reflections of a Mother

Janalee Heinemann, author

Prader-Willi Syndrome Association
5700 Midnight Pass Road, Suite 6
Sarasota, FL 34242

941-312-0400
800-926-4797
Fax: 941-312-0142
e-mail: national@pwsausa.org
www.pwsausa.org

A collection of seventeen articles including tips for managing family life.

Revised 2003 37 pages Booklet

5740 Ongoing Research on Family Functioning & Behavior Problems in Prader-Willi

Prader-Willi Foundation
40 Holly Lane
Roslyn Hts, NY 11577

516-944-8136
Fax: 516-944-3173
e-mail: foundation@prader-willi.inter.net
www.prader-willi.org

Discusses the results of a survey conducted by the authors among families of individuals with PWS.

5741 Physical Therapy Intervention for Individu als With Prader-Willi Syndrome

Prader-Willi Syndrome Association
5700 Midnight Pass Road, Suite 6
Sarasota, FL 34242

941-312-0400
800-926-4797
Fax: 941-312-0142
e-mail: national@pwsausa.org
www.pwsausa.org

5742 Prader-Willi Syndrome: A Guide for Familie s & Professionals

Moris Angulo, author

Prader-Willi Syndrome Association
5700 Midnight Pass Road, Suite 6
Sarasota, FL 34242

941-312-0400
800-926-4797
Fax: 941-312-0142
e-mail: national@pwsausa.org
www.pwsausa.org

A brief, nontechnical overview of PWS.

Revised 2005 12 pages

5743 Prader-Willi Syndrome: Medical Alerts

Prader-Willi Syndrome Association
5700 Midnight Pass Road, Suite 6
Sarasota, FL 34242

941-312-0400
800-926-4797
Fax: 941-312-0142
e-mail: national@pwsausa.org
www.pwsausa.org

Booklet that provides life saving documents for care providers, doctors, hospitals and parents.

2005

5744 Prader-Willi Syndrome: Some Reflections on Behavior

Prader-Willi Foundation
40 Holly Lane
Roslyn Heights, NY 11577

516-944-8136
Fax: 516-944-3173
e-mail: national@pwsausa.org
www.pwsausa.org

5745 Psychiatric Medicine & Prader-Willi Syndrome

Prader-Willi Foundation
40 Holly Lane
Roslyn Hts, NY 11577

516-944-8136
Fax: 516-944-3173
e-mail: foundation@prader-willi.inter.net
www.prader-willi.org

Child/adolescent psychiatrist and mother of a child with Prader-Willi syndrome speaks as an advocate of the use of psychiatric medicine in the treatment of certain aspects of PWS behaviors.

5746 Stuart H. Williams: Portrait of an Artist

Prader-Willi Foundation
40 Holly Lane
Roslyn Hts, NY 11577

516-944-8136
Fax: 516-944-3173
e-mail: foundation@prader-willi.inter.net
www.prader-willi.org

Features the life and work of an adult with Prader-Willi syndrome.

5747 Student with Prader-Willi Syndrome - Infor mation for Educators

Prader-Willi Syndrome Association
5700 Midnight Pass Road, Suite 6
Sarasota, FL 34242

941-312-0400
800-926-4797
Fax: 941-312-0142
e-mail: national@pwsausa.org
www.pwsausa.org

An information packet for educators of children with PWS. It includes a handbook, worksheets and brochures. Applicable for Pre-k through high school.

DESCRIPTION

5748 PRECOCIOUS PUBERTY

Synonym: Pubertas praecox

Covers these related disorders: Gonadotropin-dependent precocious puberty, Gonadotropin-independent precocious puberty

Involves the following Biologic System(s):

Endocrinologic Disorders

Precocious puberty refers to a condition in which the onset of sexual maturation occurs before the age of eight years in girls and nine years in boys. True precocious puberty refers to the premature sexual development of the sex glands (i.e., ovaries and testes) as well as the outward appearance of the child (secondary sexual characteristics). Precocious pseudopuberty refers to the early development of only the secondary sex characteristics with no involvement of the sex glands.

True precocious puberty results from the premature production and secretion by the pituitary gland of gonadotropin, a hormone that stimulates the ovaries and the testes. Because the release of hormones from the pituitary gland is controlled by another gland, the hypothalamus, functional abnormalities of or growth of a tumor in the pituitary or the hypothalamus may also result in premature sexual development. These abnormalities may include hormone-secreting tumors of the pituitary gland, brain lesions such as a hypothalamic hamartoma, and other lesions of the central nervous system that may activate the hypothalamus. True precocious puberty may also result from an underactive thyroid gland (hypothyroidism). However, for most children with precocious puberty, the exact cause is not known. More girls are affected by precocious puberty than boys. Although most cases appear sporadically, some patients have a family history of this condition. Sexual characteristics associated with true precocious puberty are always consistent with the sex of the affected child (isosexual characteristics). Such characteristics may include the early appearance of underarm and pubic hair, facial hair in boys, and breasts and menstrual cycles in girls. The penis, testes, and ovaries enlarge and acne may develop. Although height and weight may increase rapidly, advanced bone growth may result in premature closure of the growing ends of the bone (epiphyses) and, thus, slower linear growth leading to short stature.

Precocious pseudopuberty may be caused by a tumor of the ovary, testis, or adrenal gland. Such tumors may cause excessive production of sex hormones. This form of the disorder may also be inherited as an autosomal dominant trait. In addition, precocious pseudopuberty may be associated with other disorders such as McCune-Albright syndrome, which is a condition resulting from the overproduction of hormones of multiple glands. This syndrome is characterized by premature sexual development in girls, irregularities of skin color (pigmentation) and the skeletal system, and abnormalities of various glands. Physical characteristics associated with precocious pseudopuberty are similar to those of true precocious puberty, although the testes and ovaries are not usually involved. However, children affected with this form of the disorder may develop secondary sexual characteristics associated with those of the opposite sex (heterosexual characteristics). In addition, precocious pseudopuberty may prompt early maturation of the hormonal cycle that results in true precocious puberty.

Treatment for true precocious puberty may include the administration of gonadotropin-releasing hormones. These hormones work by diminishing the stimulatory response of the pituitary gland to the gonadotropin-releasing hormones produced naturally within the body until normal puberty begins. Treatment for precocious pseudopuberty may include the use of certain medications that reduce the levels of male and female sex hormones (i.e., testosterone and estrogen). In addition, surgery may be indicated in those patients who have precocious puberty as a result of certain types of tumors. Other treatment is symptomatic and supportive.

See also **General Resources** on page 917

Government Agencies

5749 NIH/National Institute of Child Health and Human Development

31 Center Drive, Building 31
Bethesda, MD 20892

301-496-5133
Fax: 301-496-1104
www.nichd.nih.gov

Established in 1962 by congress, today the institute conducts and supports research on topics related to the health of children, adults, families and populations. Some of these topics include: developmental disabilities, growth and development, infant death, reproductive health and birth defects.

Nancy D Wirth, Director
Lisa Kaeser, Program & Public Liaison

National Associations & Support Groups

5750 Genetic Alliance
4301 Connecticut Avenue NW
Washington, DC 20008

202-966-5557
800-336-4363
Fax: 202-966-8553
e-mail: info@geneticalliance.org
www.geneticalliance.org

A coalition of voluntary genetic support groups, consumers and professionals addressing the needs of individuals and families affected by genetic disorders from a national perspective.

Sharon Terry, President/CEO

5751 MAGIC Foundation: Major Aspects of Growth in Children
6645 W North Avenue
Oak Park, IL 60302

708-383-0808
800-362-4423
Fax: 708-383-0899
e-mail: mary@magicfoundation.org
www.magicfoundation.org

A national nonprofit organization providing support and education regarding growth disorders in children and related adult disorders. Provides educational information, networking, a national conference, a kids' program and an extensive medical library.

Mary Andrews, CEO
Dianne Tamburrino, Executive Director

5752 March of Dimes Birth Defects Foundation
1275 Mamaroneck Avenue
White Plains, NY 10605

914-428-7100
888-663-4637
Fax: 914-428-8203
e-mail: resourcecenter@modimes.org
www.marchofdimes.com

Partnership of volunteers and professionals dedicates to improving the health of babies by preventing birth defects and infant mortality. Over 100 chapters are located across the country and can be located through the National Office.

Dr Jennifer Howse, President

Web Sites

5753 KidsHealth: Precocious Puberty
www.kidshealth.org/parents/

General overview of precocious puberty including signs, causes, diagnosis and treatment.

5754 Online Mendelian Inheritance in Man
www.ncbi.nlm.nih.gov/entrez/dispomim.cgi?id=176400

This database contains textual information and references. It also contains copious links to MEDLINE and sequence records in the Entrez system, and links to additional related resources at NCBI and elsewhere.

5755 Society for Endocrinology
www.endocrinology.org

Aims to advance education and research in endocrinology for the benefit of the public. Lists resources such as journals, books, events, and training courses available.

5756 University of Michigan Health System
www.med.umich.edu/1libr/yourchild/puberty.htm

Information on early puberty or precocious puberty.

Pamphlets

5757 Precocious Puberty
Human Growth Foundation
997 Glen Cove Avenue, Suite 5
Glen Head, NY 11545

800-451-6434
Fax: 516-671-4055
e-mail: hgf1@hgfound.org
www.hgfound.org/publications_HGF.htm

Booklet

DESCRIPTION

5758 PREMATURITY

Involves the following Biologic System(s):

Neonatal and Infant Disorders

Premature birth (also known as preterm birth) refers to the birth of an infant before the 37-week gestational period. Most pregnancies last for 40 weeks. About 12 percent of babies in the United States — or 1 in 8 — are born prematurely each year. Although at least 40 percent of premature births occur for unknown reasons, prematurity may result from many different factors including a condition in which the mother develops high blood pressure, large quantities of protein in the urine, and an abnormal accumulation of fluid in the body (preeclampsia); maternal heart disease, kidney disease, or diabetes; acute infection; trauma; uterine irregularities (e.g., bicornate uterus); and placental abnormalities (e.g., placenta previa). Other contributing factors may include multiple pregnancy, maternal drug use, and fetal distress. Poor nutrition and lack of appropriate prenatal care may also put the unborn child at risk for premature birth.

Premature infants usually have a characteristic appearance in addition to their small size. For example, their heads often appear too large for their bodies and their skin may be very pink, smooth, translucent, and covered with downy hair (lanugo). They may have sparse hair and very little subcutaneous fat. In girls, the genitals may be incompletely developed such that the labia majora do not cover the labia minora. In affected boys, the testes may not fully descend into the scrotum. Other findings may include the absence of the creases on the palms and soles, incomplete development of the ear, and other irregularities. In addition, the survival or health of a premature infant may be compromised as a result of the incomplete development of certain body systems. The earlier the delivery, the more immature the organs. Common irregularities associated with prematurity include inadequate development of the lungs and subsequent deficiency in the production of a substance that allows the air sacs in the lungs to remain open (surfactant). This condition may lead to respiratory distress syndrome (also called hyaline membrane disease) and associated life-threatening oxygen deficiency in the blood. Immature organ development may affect the brain, resulting in deficiencies in spontaneous breathing, inadequate sucking, and difficulty in swallowing. There is also an increased risk of bleeding in the brain (intraventricular hemorrhage). Premature infants are also particularly susceptible to serious infection resulting from incomplete placental transfer of maternal antibodies. Immature liver function may result in

a temporary increase in blood levels of bilirubin causing yellowing of the eyes, skin, and mucous membranes (jaundice). Other complications of prematurity may include poor body temperature regulation, small stomach capacity, inadequacy of the intestinal tract that may result in injury or decreased blood flow to the intestines (necrotizing enterocolitis), immature kidney function, fluctuations in bloodsugar levels, reduced levels of calcium in the blood, and other irregularities related to underdevelopment of body systems. It has also been shown that premature babies are prone to developing depression as teenagers.

One of the most important steps to preventing prematurity is to receive prenatal care as early as possible in the pregnancy, and to continue such care until the baby is born. Statistics clearly show that early and good prenatal care reduces the chance of premature birth and related deaths. Two tactics are used to deal with a potential premature birth: delay the arrival of birth as much as possible, or prepare the premature fetus for arrival. Both of these tactics may be used simultaneously. Treatment for premature infants depends upon the maturity of the various organ systems at the time of birth. In many cases, these infants are cared for around the clock in a neonatal care unit where body temperature may be regulated in an incubator and respiration may be maintained through artificial ventilation, if necessary. Feeding may be accomplished through the use of intravenous feeding or through a feeding tube directly into the stomach. Nutritional supplementation may include the administration of iron and vitamins. In addition, liquids may be given to maintain fluid levels in the body. Antibiotics may be administered to help treat infection. Discharge from the hospital takes place once the infant has reached appropriate weight and certain functional criteria have been established. In addition, before discharge, parents or caregivers of these infants are given complete instructions in their proper care. Other treatment is symptomatic and supportive.

See also **General Resources** on page 917

Government Agencies

5759 NIH/National Institute of Child Health and Human Development

31 Center Drive, Building 31
Bethesda, MD 20892

301-496-5133
Fax: 301-496-1104
www.nichd.nih.gov

Established in 1962 by congress, today the institute conducts and supports research on topics related to the health of children, adults, families and populations. Some of these topics include: developmental disabilities, growth and development, infant death, reproductive health and birth defects.

Nancy D Wirth, Director
Lisa Kaeser, Program & Public Liaison

National Associations & Support Groups

5760 Alexis Foundation - Premature Infants and Children
PO Box 1126
Birmingham, MI 48012

248-543-4169
877-253-9470
e-mail: thealexisfoundation@prodigy.net
pages.prodigy.net/thealexisfoundation

Their mission is to raise public and political awareness of the problems facing prematurely-born infants; education on the problems faced and how they can be foreseen and handled; make essential premature accessories readily available; and promote strong communication between doctors, nurses, and parents.

Elaine Sayers, Founder

5761 March of Dimes Birth Defects Foundation
1275 Mamaroneck Avenue
White Plains, NY 10605

914-428-7100
888-663-4637
Fax: 914-428-8203
e-mail: resourcecenter@modimes.org
www.marchofdimes.com

Partnership of volunteers and professionals dedicates to improving the health of babies by preventing birth defects and infant mortality. Over 100 chapters are located across the country and can be located through the National Office.

Dr Jennifer Howse, President

5762 National Perinatal Association
2090 Linglestown Road, Suite 107
Harrisburg, PA 17110

888-971-3295
Fax: 717-920-1390
e-mail: npa@nationalperinatal.org
www.nationalperinatal.org

The National Perinatal Association promotes the health and well being of mothers and infants enriching families, communities and the world.

Sharon Chesna, President
Mary Jo Crosby, VP Development

5763 Ropard: Association for Retinopathy of Pre maturity & Related Diseases
PO Box 250425
Franklin, MI 48025

800-788-202
e-mail: ropard@yahoo.com
www.ropard.org

Funds clinically relevant basic science and clinical research to eliminate retinopathy of prematurity and associated retinal diseases; innovative work leading directly to the development of new low vision devices and teaching techniques and services for children who are visually impaired and their families.

5764 Sidelines-National High Risk Pregnancy Sup port Network
PO Box 1808
Laguna Beach, CA 92652

888-447-4754
Fax: 949-497-5598
e-mail: sidelines@sidelines.org
www.sidelines.org

Non profit organization that provides international support for women and their families experiencing premature births and complicated pregnancies.

Candace Hurley, Founder & Executive Director
Tracy Hoogenboom, Administrative Director

State Agencies & Support Groups

Georgia

5765 Georgia Perinatal Association
c/o Terri Negron
5607 Walden Farm Drive
Powder Springs, GA 30127

www.georgiaperinatal.org

Works to promote perinatal health through education, collaboration and influence of state public policy. It collaborates with others to improve pregnancy and infant outcomes.

Elizabeth Lambertz-Guima, President
Edward Clark

Texas

5766 Texas Perinatal Association
19 Cloister Parkway
Amarillo, TX 79121

e-mail: lisaplat@aol.com
www.txpa.org

Committed to achieving continuous improvement in the quality of health care to mothers and infants in the state of Texas.

Laura Street

Wisconsin

5767 Wisconsin Association for Perinatal Care
McConnell Hall
1010 Mound Street
Madison, WI 53715

608-267-6060
Fax: 608-267-6089
e-mail: wapc@perinatalweb.org
www.perinatalweb.org

Provides leadership and education for improved perinatal health outcomes of women, infants and their families through: increased public awareness; engaging the diverse community of perinatal health care advocates; and coordinating systems of perinatal care in Wisconsin.

Ann E Conway, Executive Director
Kristine E Casto, Learning Coordinator

Libraries & Resource Centers

5768 National Center for Education in Maternal and Child Health
Georgetown University
2115 Wisconsin Ave NW, Suite 601
Washington, DC 20007

202-784-9770
Fax: 202-784-9777
e-mail: mchlibrary@ncemch.org
www.ncemch.org

Information and advocacy resources for families and professionals. Includes listings of organizations providing general information and organizations focusing on more specific areas of concern to families and young adults who have disabilities.

Rochelle Mayer, Director

Research Centers

5769 NIH/National Institute of Child Health and Human Development
NICHD Clearinghouse
PO Box 3006
Rockville, MD 20847

800-370-2943
Fax: 301-984-1473
e-mail: NICHDclearinghouse@mail.nih.gov
www.nichd.nih.gov

The National Institute for Child Health and Human Development conducts and supports laboratory, clinical and epidemiological research on the reproductive, neurobiologic, developmental, and behavioral processes that determine and maintain the health of children, adults, families, and populations.

Web Sites

5770 Children's Medical Ventures
chmv.respironics.com

The company offers high quality products which meet the unique needs of these special babies, including appropriately sized items, safety equipment and specialty feeding and skin care products.

5771 March of Dimes - Prematurity
www.marchofdimes.com/prematurity/prematurity.asp

Information on prematurity provided by the March of Dimes.

5772 Newborns in Need
www.newbornsinneed.org

Charity organization for the care of sick and needy babies and their families.

5773 PREBIC-International Preterm Birth Collabo rative
www.prebic.org

Supports and enhances international networking among researchers in preterm birth.

5774 Preemie Ring
x.webring.com/hub?ring=preemie

A collection of home pages about premature infants and premature infant care, etc.

5775 Preemie Twins
www.preemietwins.com

Online resource for both parents of multiples and/or premature infants.

5776 Preemie World
www.preemie.info

A meeting place for family and friends of preemies.

5777 Premature Baby-Premature Child
www.prematurity.org

Preemie parent support for preemie special needs.

5778 Prematurely Yours
www.prematurelyyours.com

Special products for special babies.

Kim Bryant, RN, President
Becky Meloan, RN, VP

Book Publishers

5779 Prematurely Yours
6712 Townpoint Road
Suffolk, VA 23435

757-560-5574
Fax: 757-483-9557
e-mail: kbryant@prematurelyyours.com
www.prematurelyyours.com

Designed exclusively to record milestones for the premature infant, from birth to six years of age. Such milestones as maintaining their body temperature, nippling their feedings, and breathing without the aid of extra oxygen are, of course, taken for granted with a full term infant.

40 pages Hardcover

Kim Bryant, RN, President
Becky Meloan, RN, VP

Magazines

5780 Left Side Lines
Sidelines
PO Box 1808
Laguna Beach, CA 82652

888-447-4754
www.sidelines.org

Offers articles, insights and tips related to the challange of coping with a high-risk pregnancy. Specific information is provided on prematurity, NICU, multiples, and nutrition.

80 pages

5781 Preemie Magazine
6412 Brandon Avenue, Suite 274
Springfield, VA 22150

703-468-1005
www.preemiemagazine.com

Started by five preemie parents, it provides free information and an online community for preemie parents and professionals.

Deborah A Discenza, Founder & Publisher
Nicole Hutzul, Sales & Marketing

Pamphlets

5782 March of Dimes-Preterm Birth Fact Sheet
www.marchofdimes.com/prematurity/5196_5799.asp

Fact sheet discusses the possible causes of preterm birth, complications associated with, and current research.

DESCRIPTION

5783 PREVENTABLE CHILDHOOD INFECTIONS
Involves the following Biologic System(s):
Infectious Disorders

There are several infectious diseases that typically manifest in childhood, that are preventable with proper immunizations. This chapter will cover the following: Diphtheria; Tetanus; Pertussis; Rubella (German Measles); Measles; Mumps; Polio; Chickenpox.

Diphtheria is an acute, contagious disease characterized at its onset by sore throat and painful swallowing. One to 4 days after exposure, infected individuals may also develop a low-grade fever, headache, nausea and vomiting, chills, and a rapid heart rate. Other symptoms may include signs associated with upper respiratory tract infection. Within a few days, a grayish-brown pseudomembrane may form over the tonsils, voice box, trachea, and palate. The throat may swell causing difficulties with breathing, eating, and drinking. The lymph nodes in the neck may become swollen and enlarged. Occasionally, the bacterium may cause damage to the heart or central nervous system. Diphtheria vaccine is usually combined with those for whooping cough (pertussis) and tetanus. This DPT combination is routinely given in a series in the first few months of life. Booster doses are required. In most cases, diphtheria is transmitted through coughed or exhaled droplets. Treatment is with antibiotics and an antitoxin.

Pertussis (whooping cough) is a highly contagious infectious disease in which inflammation of the respiratory tract occurs as the result of a bacterial infection. Transmission of the disease usually occurs through inhalation of bacteria spread through coughing or sneezing. Pertussis usually affects infants and children, although the disease may occur at any age. Pertussis infection lasts about 6 weeks, occurring in 3 stages: moderate cold-like symptoms (catarrhal stage); severe coughing (paroxysmal stage); cessation of symptoms (convalescent stage). Treatment typically includes bed rest and measures to ensure proper nutition and fluid intake. Erythromycin or other antibiotics may be given.

Tetanus is an infectious disease of the central nervous system caused by a toxic bacteria. The toxin acts on nerves that control muscle activity, causing the symptoms associated with tetanus. The bacterium typically enters puncture wounds caused by dirty objects such as nails, splinters or glass fragments. It may also enter the body via drug injec-

tion, surgical wounds, burns, animal bites or the fetal umbilical cord stump after birth (neonatal tetanus). Symptoms usually appear from 2 to 14 days after infection, but sometimes take months to become apparent. Tetanus may be classified into general or localized. Initial symptoms of generalized tetanus often include: prolonged spasms of the muscles of the jaw (trismus or lockjaw); difficulties in opening the mouth, chewing and swallowing (dysphagia); irritability, headaches and restlessness. Patients may also experience prolonged spasms of facial muscles, profuse sweating, a mild fever, and a rapid pulse. Progressed disease includes severe muscle contractions. Treatment of tetanus includes the use of human antibodies against tetanus toxins (tetanus immune globulin) and antibiotic medications; surgical cleaning of the wound site; and the use of muscle relaxants. Children should receive the previously mentioned DPT vaccine and appropriate booster shots. Boosters should also be given to any patients with wounds who have an unknown or incomplete tetanus booster status.

German measles, or rubella, is a contagious viral disease characterized by swollen lymph nodes and a fine, reddish-pink rash that persists for 1 to 3 days. It is transmitted through inhalation of droplets coughed or exhaled into the air by infected individuals. Early symptoms may include swollen lymph nodes, especially in the neck and back of the head; joint pain (arthralgia); low-grade fever; cold symptoms; and redness and discomfort of the throat. Within 1 or 2 days, a mildly itchy rash appears on the face, spreading to the trunk, arms and legs. This is accompanied by a generalized spreading red flush. The rash usually subsides after 3 days. In some cases, enlargement of the spleen may occur. Measles symptoms range from slight to severe, the latter occuring primarily in older children and adults. In addition, pregnant women with German measles are at risk of transmitting the disease to the newborn (congentital rubella, see below). Protection against infection is provided through rubella immunization, usually in combination with measles and mumps vaccine.Immunization is generally recommended to women of child-bearing age who have not had German measles or have not been previously vaccinated. Treatment for rubella is symptomatic.

Measles is a highly contagious infection caused by the measles virus. Infection is characterized by a typical, spreading rash and other symptoms. Measles is typically a disease of the young, but may develop at any age. It is spread through airborne droplets from an infected individual. One measles infection usually imparts lifelong immunity. Early symptoms develop from 1 to 2 weeks after exposure and include low-grade fever; inflammation of the nasal mucous membranes; runny nose; hacking cough; conjunctivitis and increased sensitivity to light. These symptoms are followed 2 to 3 days later by the development of tiny, grayish-white specks, each surrounded by an irregular red ring (Koplik's spots), that appear on the inside of the cheeks, usually near the back teeth. A rash, accompanied by a high fever, may develop within 3 to 5 days after the onset of symptoms, characterized by faint, reddish flat spots that first appear behind the ears, at the hairline and on the neck, and then spread over the entire body. Certain lymph nodes and the spleen may become enlarged. Protection against measles is provided by immunization, usually in combination with mumps and rubella vaccines. A second immunization is usually given upon entering school. Treatment may include medication to reduce fever, antibiotics andincreased fluid intake. Bed rest in a warm, humidified room is also recommended. Other treatment is symptomatic and supportive.

Congenital rubella refers to a condition in which the virus that causes German measles is passed from an affected mother through the placenta to the fetus. Likelihood of transmission and the potential for miscarriage, stillbirth or severe developmental abnormalities is highest during the first 3 months of pregnancy. These abnormalities include growth retardation, heart defects, eye problems, an unusually small head (microcephaly), and purplish skin lesions. Many infants with congenital rubella have inner ear or auditory nerve defects that may result in hearing difficulties. Additional findings may include mental retardation and delays in motor development. There is also a risk of hepatitis, anemia, lowered levels of circulating blood platelets, pneumonia and bone irregularities. Prevention is directed toward immunization. Treatment is symptomatic and supportive.

Mumps is an acute, infectious viral disease caused by a paramyxovirus. It is characterized by enlargement of the salivary glands, particularly those that lie below and in front of the ears (parotid glands). Mumps usually affects children from 5 through 15 years. It is spread through airborne droplets or direct contact with saliva, or possibly, urine, from an infected individual. Outbreaks most often occur in late winter or early spring. Infection usually results in lifelong immunity. Symptoms of mumps may appear within 2 weeks to 24 days after exposure, and may include fever, neck pain, weakness, discomfort and headache. One or both parotid glands may become enlarged or tender to the touch. Chewing and swallowing may become increasingly painful. There may also be fever and swelling of other salivary glands and the throat. Swelling of the parotid glands usually resolves within 7 to 10 days. Possible complications include meningitis, as well as swelling of the joints, pancreas, heart muscle, kidneys and thyroid gland. Protection against mumps is typically administered in the previously mentioned combination vaccine from 12 to 15 months of age, and once again before entering school. Treatment is symptomatic and supportive.

Polio, or poliomyelitis, is an acute infectious disease caused by one of 3 polio viruses transmitted through fecal contamination or, occasionally, through the air. It may produce no symptoms, but will grant immunity to those infected. In most patients, especially young children, it is accompanied by only mild symptoms. These appear 3 to 5 days after infection, and may include fever, headache, sore throat, vomiting, weakness and abdominal discomfort. Recovery is often complete in 1 to 3 days. In some cases there is a brief recovery and symptoms reappear including brain and spinal cord involvement with neck and back stiffness and skin sensitivity. This reappearance constitutes major illness. Morecommon in older children and adults, the major illness may be paralytic or nonparalytic. Immunization to prevent polio is routinely administered. Treatment for the mild form includes bed rest and pain relievers. Paralysis usually requires physical therapy. Other treatment is symptomatic and supportive.

Chickenpox is a common, highly contagious viral disease caused by the varicella zoster virus. Most cases occur before the age of 10. Those who do not contract the virus during childhood remain susceptible during adulthood, when symptoms are typically more severe. Chickenpox is spread by inhalation of airborne droplets or direct contact with fluid from skin blisters. Older children particularly may experience generalized symptoms, including, fever, headache, mild abdominal pain, lack of appetite and malaise. A characteristic rash develops on the chest, abdomen, face or scalp, consisting of masses of small, red, extremely itchy spots that become fluid-filled blisters. As the first lesions dry, new crops form. Complications of chickenpox may include bacterial infection of the lesions, encephalitis and impaired control of voluntary movements. Newborns may also experience a particularly severe, progressive form of chickenpox (neonatal chickenpox). Treatment of children with mild cases of chickenpox is symptomatic and supportive. In more severe cases, the antiviral drug acyclovir may be administered. A vaccine is now available in the US to help prevent chickenpox.

See also **General Resources** on page 917

Government Agencies

5784 Centers for Disease Control
1600 Clifton Road
Atlanta, GA 30333

404-639-3311
www.cdc.gov

Mission is to promote health and quality of life by preventing and controlling disease, injury, and disability.

5785 NIH/National Institute of Allergy and Infectious Diseases
6610 Rockledge Drive, MSC 6612
Bethesda, MD 20892

301-496-5717
Fax: 301-402-3573
TDD: 800-877-8339
www.niaid.nih.gov

Conducts and supports basic and applied research to better understand, treat, and ultimately prevent infectious, immunologic, and allergic diseases.

Anthony S Fauci MD, Director

National Associations & Support Groups

5786 Polio Society
4200 Wisconsin Avenue NW, #106273
Washington, DC 20016

301-897-8180
Fax: 202-994-3153
e-mail: jsh1@mhg.edu

A chartered nonprofit organization primarily for polio survivors and family members. It provides educational resources and support group services.

5787 Polio Survivors Association
12720 La Reina Avenue
Downey, CA 90242

562-862-4508
Fax: 562-862-5018
e-mail: info@polioassociation.org
www.polioassociation.org

Nonprofit organization dedicated to education, advocacy, and support to promote the well being and improve the quality of life for severley disabled polio survivors.

Richard Dagget, President

5788 Post-Polio Health International
4207 Lindell Boulevard, Suite 110
Saint Louis, MO 63108

314-534-0475
Fax: 314-534-5070
e-mail: info@post-polio.org
www.post-polio.org

Provides information to Polio survivors, their families and the health care community and promotes networking among the post-polio community.

Joan L Headley, Executive Director

5789 World Health Organization
Avenue Appia 20
CH-1211 Geneva 27,
Switzerland

www.who.int

WHO is the directing and coordinating authority for health within the United Nations system.

Dr Margaret Chan, Director General

Web Sites

5790 Canadian Task Force on Preventive Health C are
www.ctfphc.org

This website is designed to serve as a practical guide to health care providers, planners and consumers for determining the inclusion or exclusion, content and frequency of a wide variety of preventive health interventions, using the evidence based recommendations of the Canadian Task Force on Preventice Health Care.

5791 Centers for Disease Control-Infection Cont rol
www.cdc.gov/ncidod/dhqp/index.html

Promotes health and quality of life by preventing and controlling disease, injury, and disability.

5792 Health Research Project (HaRP)
www.harpnet.org

A program by USAID, the project strives to improve the health status of infants, children, mothers and families through the development and research of new tools, technologies, policies and approaches.

5793 KidsHealth - Measles
kidshealth.org/parent/infections/lung/measles.html

KidsHealth provides doctor-approved health information about children from before birth through adolescence. KidsHealth provides families with accurate, up to date and jargon free health information they can use.

5794 KidsHealth - Rubella (German Measles)
kidshealth.org/parent/

KidsHealth provides doctor-approved health information about children from before birth through adolescence. KidsHealth provides families with accurate, up to date and jargon free health information they can use.

5795 KidsHealth - Tetanus
kidshealth.org/parent/

KidsHealth provides doctor-approved health information about children from before birth through adolescence. KidsHealth provides families with accurate, up to date and jargon free health information they can use.

5796 Pan American Health Organization (PAHO)
www.paho.org

The mission is to strengthen national and local health systems and improve the health of the peoples of the Americas, in collaboraton with Ministries of Health, other government and international agencies, nongovernmental organizations, universities, social security agencies, community groups, and many others. Health topics include measles, mumps, rubella and diptheria.

5797 Parent Zone
www.parentzonescotland.gov.uk

This site offers a broad range of information for parents, carers and others responsible for school age children. The website also provides a comprehensive list of links o useful organizations and recent publications.

5798 Polio Connection of America
www.geocities.com/w1066w/

For survivors of the Polio Survivors to chat and the site offers links to other polio sites.

5799 Polio Experience Network
www.polionet.org/

Offers information, inspiration, ideas and resources to help patients understand polio and post-poli syndrome, and to confidently manage life with it. Also helps loved ones cope with the effects of polio. Resources are also offered for students doing research on the disease as well as general resources available.

5800 Post Polio Awareness & Support Society of British Columbia
www.ppass.bc.ca

A non profit society formed as a network for polio survivors, those affected by polio, and any interested in polio.

5801 Slack Incorporated
www.slackinc.com

A leading provider of healthcare information, educational programs, and meeting and exhibit management services worldwide.

5802 Virtual Pediatric Hospital
www.virtualpediatrichospital.org

A digital library of pediatric information including resources for patients and health care professionals.

Book Publishers

5803 Everything You Need to Know About Measles and Rubella

Trisha Hawkins, author

Rosen Publishing/PowerKids Press
29 E 21st Street
New York, NY 10010
212-777-3017
800-237-9932
Fax: 888-436-4643
e-mail: rosenpub@tribeca.ios.com
www.powerkidspress.com

Examines the continuing threat of these highly infectious respiratory diseases. Grades 7-12.

2001 64 pages
ISBN: 0-823933-22-9

5804 IVUN Resource Directory
4207 Lindell Boulevard, Suite 110
Saint Louis, MO 63108
314-534-0475
Fax: 314-534-5070
e-mail: ventinfo@post-polio.org
www.post-polio.org/ivun

A networking tool for health professionals and both long-term and new ventilator users. Sections include health professionals, ventilator users, equipment and aids, manufacturers, service and repair, organizations, etc. Published annually in October.

34 pages Annually

Joan L Headley, Executive Director & Editor

5805 Let's Talk About Having Chicken Pox

Elizabeth Weitzman, author

Rosen Publishing/PowerKids Press
29 E 21st Street
New York, NY 10010
212-777-3017
800-237-9932
Fax: 888-436-4643
e-mail: rosenpub@tribeca.ios.com
www.powerkidspress.com

Highly contagious chicken pox is one of the childhood illnesses that few kids escape. This book tells kids how to handle the illness, where it comes from and how long it will take to recover. Grades K-5.

24 pages
ISBN: 0-823950-31-X

5806 Measles

Maxine Rosaler, author

Rosen Publishing/PowerKids Press
29 E 21st Street
New York, NY 10010
212-777-3017
800-237-9932
Fax: 888-436-4643
e-mail: rosenpub@tribeca.ios.com
www.powerkidspress.com

An examination of the history of this once thought to be harmless disease, from its ancient origins to near eradication.

2005 64 pages
ISBN: 1-404202-56-0

5807 Post-Polio Directory
4207 Lindell Boulevard, Suite 110
Saint Louis, MO 63108
314-534-0475
Fax: 314-534-5070
e-mail: info@post-polio.org
www.post-polio.org

Over 32 pages of post polio clinics, health professionals, support groups, and other useful contacts. The directory includes international listings. Published annually in March.

Joan L Headley, Executive Director & Editor

Newsletters

5808 Infectious Diseases in Children
Slack Incorporated
6900 Grove Road
Thorofare, NJ 08086
800-257-8290
e-mail: customerservice@slackinc.com
idinchildren.com

Pediatric news source.

Monthly

Philip A Brunell MD, Chief Medical Editor

5809 Post-Polio Health
4207 Lindell Boulevard, Suite 110
Saint Louis, MO 63108
314-534-0475
Fax: 314-534-5070
e-mail: editor@post-polio.org

Provides information to polio survivors, their families, and the health care community and promotes networking among the post-polio community.

12 pages Quarterly
ISSN: 1066-5331

Joan L Headley, Editor & Executive Director

Pamphlets

5810 Tetanus and Diptheria Vaccine
Centers for Disease Control & Prevention
1600 Clifton Road
Atlanta, GA 30333
404-639-3311
800-311-3435
www.cdc.gov/Nip/publications/VIS/vis-td.pdf

Factsheet about the diseases and the vaccines.

DESCRIPTION

5811 PROTEIN C DEFICIENCY

Synonyms: PC deficiency, PROC deficiency

Covers these related disorders: Protein C deficiency Type I, Protein C deficiency Type II

Involves the following Biologic System(s):
Hematologic and Oncologic Disorders

Protein C deficiency is a blood clotting (thrombotic) disorder characterized by the recurrent formation of blood clots within the veins of the body (venous thrombosis). Protein C, which is formed in the liver, is a specialized protein that helps to prevent the formation of blood clots. When activated, protein C helps to dissolve fibrin, the semisolid portion of blood clots, thus inhibiting the formation of a clot. A deficiency of this protein, therefore, results in abnormal clot formation. Some signs of this disorder may become apparent during adolescence. Associated symptoms depend upon the organ or tissue affected by clot formation that leads to reduced or absent blood flow. Affected individuals may develop blood clots and inflammation in the veins of the legs (thrombophlebitis). This can occur when the blood moves slowly in the veins, such as from prolonged bed rest during an illness, surgery, or hospital stay. In some patients, these clots may dislodge from the vein and travel through the blood stream (embolus) to different parts of the body including the heart, lungs, or brain, potentially leading to life-threatening complications. However, not all patients with protein C deficiency experience all the signs associated with this disorder.

In the event of a blood clotting episode, the antithrombin factor heparin may be administered through injection into a vein (intravenous) or under the skin (subcutaneous). Other treatment may include continuing oral administration of the anti-coagulant drug warfarin to prevent a recurrence of thrombotic activity

Two types of protein C deficiency have been described in the general population. The more common form is Type I in which both protein C levels and activity are deficient. In the less common Type II, the amount of protein is normal but its activity or performance is impaired. The inherited form of protein C deficiency may be transmitted as an autosomal dominant trait. The gene for this disorder is located on the long arm of chromosome 2 (2q13-14). Protein C deficiency may also be acquired in connection with infection.

See also **General Resources** on page 917

Government Agencies

5812 NIH/National Heart, Lung and Blood Institu te
National Institute of Health
31 Center Dr MSC 2486, Bldg 31, Room 5A48
Bethesda, MD 20892

301-592-8573
Fax: 240-629-3246
TTY: 240-629-3255
e-mail: NHLBInfo@nhlbi.nih.gov
www.nhlbi.nih.gov

Primary responsibility of this organization is the scientific investigation of heart, blood vessel, lung and blood disorders. Oversees research, demonstration, prevention, education, control and training activities in these fields and emphasizes the prevention and control of heart diseases.

Elizabeth G Nabel, MD, Director
Susan Shurin, MD, Deputy Director

National Associations & Support Groups

5813 Genetic Alliance
4301 Connecticut Avenue NW
Washington, DC 20008

202-966-5557
800-336-4363
Fax: 202-966-8553
e-mail: info@geneticalliance.org
www.geneticalliance.org

A coalition of voluntary genetic support groups, consumers and professionals addressing the needs of individuals and families affected by genetic disorders from a national perspective.

Sharon Terry, President/CEO

5814 March of Dimes Birth Defects Foundation
1275 Mamaroneck Avenue
White Plains, NY 10605

914-428-7100
888-663-4637
Fax: 914-428-8203
e-mail: resourcecenter@modimes.org
www.marchofdimes.com

Partnership of volunteers and professionals dedicates to improving the health of babies by preventing birth defects and infant mortality. Over 100 chapters are located across the country and can be located through the National Office.

Dr Jennifer Howse, President

5815 Med Help International
6300 North Wickham Road, Suite 130
Melbourne, FL 32940

321-259-7505
Fax: 321-751-0858
e-mail: office@medhelp.org
www.medhelp.org

A not-for-profit organization dedicated to helping patients find the highest quality medical information in the world today. Patients are offered the tools necessary to make informed treatment decisions within the short time lines dictated by their illness or disease.

Cynthia ThompsonD, President & Co-Founder
Philip A Garfinkel, VP & Co-Founder

State Agencies & Support Groups

Texas

5816 Vitamin C Foundation
PO Box 73172
Houston, TX 77273

281-443-3634
888-443-3634
Fax: 630-416-1309
e-mail: ascorbade@aol.com
www.vitamincfoundation.org

A Texas nonprofit organization devoted to preserving and distributing knowledge about ascorbic acid and its vital role in the life process.

Owen R Fonorow, Co-Founder
M S Till Sr, Co-Founder

Web Sites

5817 AllRer Health
www.health.allrer.com

A medical and health information resource containing outstanding database of health articles and reference materials.

5818 Factor V Leiden: Thrombophilia Support Pag e
www.fvleiden.org

Factor V Leiden is the most common hereditary blood coagulation disorder in the US. It is present in 3-7% of the population in Europe and America. It is associated with Venous thrombosis, DVT, unexplained miscarriage, blood clots in the lungs, gall bladder dysfunction, preeclampsia and/or eclapsia, stroke and/or heart attack.

5819 HealthCentral.com
www.healthcentral.com

Offering information on health issues for children, women, men and seniors. Information on Protein C Deficiency includes a description, causes, symptoms, diagnosis, treatment and questions that can be asked of the doctor.

5820 MedicineNet
www.medicinenet.com

An online, healthcare media publishing company. It provides easy to read, in-depth, authoritative medical information for consumers via an interactive web site.

5821 Merck
www.merck.com

A site that offers research driven pharmaceutical products and services to improve human and animal health, directly and through its joint ventures.

5822 Online Mendelian Inheritance in Man
www.ncbi.nlm.nih.gov

This database is a catalog of human genes and genetic disorders.

Book Publishers

5823 Merck Manual of Diagnosis and Therapy
Merck Publishing Group
PO Box 2000 RY84-15
Rahway, NJ 07065

732-594-4600
Fax: 732-388-3610
www.merckbooks.com

Since it was first published in 1899, The Merck Manual has set the standard for excellence in the medical community for current, complete, and comprehensive information for all healthcare professionals. Written by more than 300 medical experts in all fields of medicine from around the world.

2006 18th Ed 2832 pages Hardcover
ISBN: 0-911910-18-2

Mark H Beers MD, Editor-in-Chief
Robert S Porter MD, Editor

5824 Protein Deficiency and Pesticide Toxicity

Eldon M Boyd, author

Charles C Thomas
2600 South First Street
Springfield, IL 62704

800-258-8980
Fax: 217-789-9130
e-mail: books@ccthomas.com
www.ccthomas.com

Discusses the approaches for analyzing Protein Deficiency and Pesticide Toxicity.

468 pages Hardcover
ISBN: 0-398024-76-6

DESCRIPTION

5825 PSORIASIS

Involves the following Biologic System(s):

Dermatologic Disorders

Psoriasis is a common, chronic skin disease characterized by red patches of skin that are covered by dry, thick, silvery scales. This disorder may occur at any age, but most commonly appears from the ages of 10 to 40 years. Although males and females are affected equally, females are more prone to development of this disorder when it appears during childhood. In addition, approximately half of those individuals who develop psoriasis in childhood have a family history of the disorder, but the pattern of transmission has not been determined. Individuals with psoriasis appear to produce new skin cells at a greatly accelerated rate while shedding their old cells at a normal rate. The subsequent buildup of new cells produces thickened areas of new skin that are covered by old skin, thus forming the characteristic dry, thickened, silvery patches associated with psoriasis.

Psoriatic lesions may appear anywhere on the body, but most commonly form on the scalp, elbows, knees, back, buttocks, navel area, and genitalia. In addition, relatively smaller lesions may appear on the face and pitting may develop on the nails. Peeling away a scale produces specks of bleeding from the capillaries (Auspitz's sign). Itching of the skin (pruritus) is common and scratching leads to more lesions (Koebner's phenomenon). On rare occasions, severe psoriasis may develop in newborns, accompanied by lesion formation in the diaper area.

There are different types of psoriasis. The most common form is called discoid psoriasis and is characterized by patches that form mainly on the elbows, knees, scalp, and other areas of the arms, legs, and trunk. Other findings may include nail irregul|arities such as pitting, thickening, and separation from the nail beds. In addition, psorasis is sometimes accompanied by painful swelling of the joints (arthritis). Guttate psoriasis occurs primarily in children and young adults and is characterized by the sudden appearance of small, oval, drop-like lesions on the trunk and upper portions of the arms and legs. Guttate psoriasis often develops following a streptococcal infection, viral infection, or sunburn. In addition, this form of the disorder sometimes follows the conclusion or withdrawal of corticosteroid treatment. Pustular psoriasis may be localized or generalized. In its localized form, eruptions of pustules develop over individual reddish patches that are present, usually, on the palms of the hands and the soles of the feet. Psoriasis is usually apparent on other parts of the body. Affected individuals may also experience localized discomfort. Generalized pustular psoriasis is an acute, severe, sometimes life-threatening form of the disorder that is characterized by the widespread eruption of small pustules in individuals with mild, moderate, or other types of psoriasis. Generalized pustular psoriasis is sometimes accompanied by high fever, pain in the joints, elevated levels of white blood cells (leukocytosis), low levels of blood calcium (hypocalcemia), and other irregularties.

Treatment of psoriasis is dependent upon age, area of involvement, and the type and severity of the disease. Many treatment protocols that are effective for adults may be too toxic for children; therefore, most treatment for children with psoriasis is conservative and mainly directed toward comfort and alleviation of pain. Such treatment may include the use of tar preparations in the form of gels, ointments, or bath emulsions. Additional topical treatments may include the cautious use of corticosteroid preparations, vitamin D analogs, and other ointments. Treatment for scalp lesions may include the use of a phenol and saline solution followed by tar shampoo and, when lesions are reduced, the application of a corticosteroid preparation. Severe psoriasis in children may indicate the use of various drugs such as methotrexate and certain oral retinoids; however, this therapy may be accompanied by severe side effects. Other treatment is symptomatic and supportive.

See also **General Resources** on page 917

National Associations & Support Groups

5826 National Psoriasis Foundation
6600 SW 92nd Avenue, Suite 300
Portland, OR 97223

503-244-7404
800-723-9166
Fax: 503-245-0626
e-mail: getinfo@psoriasis.org
www.psoriasis.org

Promotes awareness and understanding of psoriasis and psoriatic arthritis through education and advocacy. The foundation also ensures access to treatment and supports research that leads to effective management of the condition.

Gail M Zimmerman, President/CEO
Pam Field, VP Operations

Research Centers

5827 Psoriasis Research Association
107 Vista del Grande
San Carlos, CA 94070

415-593-1392

5828 University of California, San Francisco Dermatology Drug Research
515 Spruce
San Francisco, CA 94143

415-476-2001
Fax: 415-221-4751

Conducts clinical testing of new or existing pharmacologic agents used in the treatment of skin disorders.

John Koo, MD, Director

Audio Video

5829 National Library of Dermatologic Teaching Slides
American Academy Of Dermatology
PO Box 94020
Palatine, IL 60094

847-330-0230
Fax: 847-330-0050

A collection of dermatologic teaching slides offering the most comprehensive series ever assembled. Each set offers a realistic presentation of classic clinical skin conditions encountered by the dermatologist.

Web Sites

5830 American Academy of Dermatology (AAD)
www.aad.org/aadpamphrework/Psoriasis.html

The American Academy of Dermatoloy is dedicated to achieving the highest quality of dermatologic care for everyone. Acheivement of this vision requires a dynamic organization whose mission embodies: Excellence in patient care, education and research, adherence to eithical conduct, respinsiveness to its members and to the public unification and representation of the specialty.

5831 National Psoriasis Foundation
www.psoriasis.org

Promotes awareness and understanding of psoriasis and psoriatic arthritis through education and advocacy. The foundation also ensures access to treatment and supports research that leads to effective management of the condition.

5832 Psoriasis Association
www.psoriasis-association.org.uk

Formed with these aims in view: to raise awareness of psoriasis; support those who have psoriasis; and fund research into the causes of and treatments for psoriasis.

4000 members

5833 Psoriasis Connections
www.psoriasisconnect.com

Connects people with medical experts on psoriasis, those affected by the condition, family and friends, and other relevant resources.

5834 Psoriasis Help Group
tatoonic.fortunecity.com/mothership/498/

Offers a forum, chat room, and information about the disease.

5835 Skin Page
pinch.com/skin/

Noncommercial site that provides shortcuts to search past messages in the skin diseases newsgroups and other databases. Includes a psoriasis information page and other resources.

5836 UnderstandingPsoriasis.org by Healthology
www.understandingpsoriasis.org

Current information on psoriasis gathered and presented by leaders in the field of dermatology.

Book Publishers

5837 Handbook of Psoriasis

Charles Camisa, author

Blackwell Publishing
Commerce Place, 350 Main Street
Malden, MA 02148

781-388-8200
800-216-2522
Fax: 781-388-8210
www.blackwellpublishing.com

Reference for health care professionals, easy to read, yet detailed information.
2005 2nd Ed Paperback
ISBN: 1-405109-27-7

5838 Managing Your Psoriasis
MasterMedia
16 E 72nd Street
New York, NY 10021

212-260-5600

1993 Softcover
ISBN: 0-942361-83-0

5839 Psychological Approaches to Dermatology

Linda Papadopoulos, author

Blackwell Publishing
Commerce Place, 350 Main Street
Malden, MA 02148

781-388-8200
800-216-2522
Fax: 781-388-8210
www.blackwellpublishing.com

References all the main skin conditions - psoriasis, eczema, vitiligo, dermatitis, alopecia, and others. The book blends theory and practical experience, making it a highly recommended read.
1999 176 pages Paperback
ISBN: 1-854332-92-9

5840 Textbook of Psoriasis

Peter Van de Kerkhof, author

Blackwell Publishing
Commerce Place, 350 Main Street
Malden, MA 02148

781-388-8200
800-216-2522
Fax: 781-388-8210
www.blackwellpublishing.com

Written for dermatologists, it is a concise and clinical account of psoriasis, divided into three sections: morphology of the skin, etiology and pathogenesis, and current treatments.
2003 2nd Ed Hardback
ISBN: 1-405107-17-4

Magazines

5841 International Journal of Dermatology
International Society of Dermatology
138 Palm Coast Parkway, NE No 333
Palm Coast, FL 32137

386-437-4405
Fax: 386-437-4427
e-mail: info@intsocdermatol.org
www.intsocderm.org

Focuses on information for dermatologists and the whole specialty of dermatology research and education.

10 times a year

5842 Journal of Dermatologic Surgery and Oncology
International Society for Dermatologic Surgery
930 N Meachan Road
Schaumburg, IL 60173
847-330-9830
Fax: 847-330-1135

Focuses on medical updates and information on dermatology.

Monthly

5843 Psoriasis Advance
National Psoriasis Foundation
6600 SW 92nd Avenue, Suite 300
Portland, OR 97223
503-244-7404
800-723-9166
Fax: 503-245-0626
e-mail: getinfo@psoriasis.org
www.psoriasis.org

Member magazine that evolved from two formerly published newsletters (Bulletin & Psoriasis Resource) connecting the psoriasis community.

36 pages Bi-monthly

Gail M Zimmerman, President/CEO
Sharon DeBusk, Editor/Writer

Journals

5844 Psoriasis Forum
National Psoriasis Foundation
6600 SW 92nd Avenue, Suite 300
Portland, OR 97223
503-244-7404
800-723-9166
Fax: 503-245-0626
e-mail: getinfo@psoriasis.org
www.psoriasis.org

Journal for professional members of the foundation. It is dedicated to providing up-to-date, practical information to health care providers on the front line of psoriasis treatment.

Gail M Zimmerman, President/CEO
Paula Fasano, Director Marketing/Communications

Newsletters

5845 Awareness
NAPVI
PO Box 317
Watertown, MA 02471
617-972-7441
800-562-6265
Fax: 617-972-7444
www.spedex.com/napvi

Newsletter offering regional news, sports and activities, conferences, camps, legislative updates, book reviews, audio reviews, professional question and answer column and more for the visually impaired and their families.

Quarterly

5846 Bulletin
National Psoriasis Foundation
6600 SW 92nd Avenue, Suite 300
Portland, OR 97223
503-244-7404
800-723-9166
Fax: 503-245-0626
e-mail: getinfo@psoriasis.org
www.psoriasis.org

Published for 35 years by the National Psoriasis Foundation, past issues are available online in pdf form. It covered both traditional and alternative treatments, self-help techniques, research and a wide variety of human-interest topics. Please refer to the foundation's magazine Psoriasis Advance for updated information and resources.

5847 DVH Quarterly
University of Arkansas at Little Rock
2801 S University Avenue
Little Rock, AR 72204
Fax: 501-663-3536

Offers information on upcoming events, conferences and workshops on and for visual disabilities. Book reviews, information on the newest resources and technology, educational programs, want ads and more.

Quarterly

Bob Brasher, Editor

5848 Dermatology Focus
Dermatology Foundation
1560 Sherman Avenue
Evanston, IL 60201
847-328-2256
Fax: 847-328-0509
dermatologyfoundation.org

Includes membership activities, research articles and lists recipients of foundation awards.

Quarterly

5849 Dermatology World
American Academy of Dermatology
PO Box 94020
Palatine, IL 60094
847-330-0230
Fax: 847-330-0050

Offers Academy members information outside the clinical realm. It carries news of government actions, reports of socioeconomic issues, societal trends and other events which impinge on the practice of dermatology.

Monthly

5850 Progress in Dermatology
Dermatology Foundation
1560 Sherman Avenue
Evanston, IL 60201
847-328-2256
Fax: 847-328-0509
dermatologyfoundation.org

Bulletin offering information on research reports and clinical trials.

Quarterly

5851 Psoriasis Resource
National Psoriasis Foundation
6600 SW 92nd Avenue, Suite 300
Portland, OR 97223
503-244-7404
800-723-9166
Fax: 503-245-0626
e-mail: getinfo@psoriasis.org
www.psoriasis.org

Published from 1999 to 2002, three times a year, by the National Psoriasis Foundation, past issues are available online in pdf form. It helped people make educated decisions about medication, therapy and product choices available for skin and joints. Please refer to the foundation's magazine Psoriasis Advance for updated information and resources.

Pamphlets

5852 Alternative Approaches
National Psoriasis Foundation
6600 SW 92nd Avenue, Suite 300
Portland, OR 97223

503-244-7404
800-723-9166
Fax: 503-245-0626
e-mail: getinfo@psoriasis.org
www.psoriasis.org

Non-traditional therapies and treatments for both psoriasis and psoriatic arthritis including stress management, topical preparations and Chinese medicine.

2005 13 pages

Gail M Zimmerman, President/CEO

5853 Conception, Pregnancy and Psoriasis
National Psoriasis Foundation
6600 SW 92nd Avenue, Suite 300
Portland, OR 97223

503-244-7404
800-723-9166
Fax: 503-245-0626
e-mail: getinfo@psoriasis.org
www.psoriasis.org

Overview of the effect of pregnancy on psoriasis and treatment, risks and other considerations during conception.

2006 9 pages

Gail M Zimmerman, President/CEO
Paula Fasano, Director Marketing/Communications

5854 Phototherapy: Light Treatment for Psoriasi s
National Psoriasis Foundation
6600 SW 92nd Avenue, Suite 300
Portland, OR 97223

503-244-7404
800-723-9166
Fax: 503-245-0626
e-mail: getinfo@psoriasis.org
www.psoriasis.org

Light treatment options: PUVA, lasers, broad-band UVB, and narrow-band UVB.

2006 13 pages

Gail M Zimmerman, President/CEO

5855 Psoriasis 101: Learning to Live in the Ski n You're In
National Psoriasis Foundation
6600 SW 92nd Avenue, Suite 300
Portland, OR 97223

503-244-7404
800-723-9166
Fax: 503-245-0626
e-mail: getinfo@psoriasis.org
www.psoriasis.org

Designed to educate young people, teens and college-age young adults about psoriasis. It is written from a young person's standpoint with bytes of information.

2006 12 pages

Gail M Zimmerman, President/CEO
Paula Fasano, Director Marketing/Communications

5856 Psoriasis Research: Progress & Promise
National Psoriasis Foundation
6600 SW 92nd Avenue, Suite 300
Portland, OR 97223

503-244-7404
800-723-9166
Fax: 503-245-0626
e-mail: getinfo@psoriasis.org
www.psoriasis.org

Overview of present research and the foundation's role in supporting it. Includes new treatments and progress being made in genetics.

2004 11 pages

Gail M Zimmerman, President/CEO

5857 Psoriasis on Specific Skin Sites
National Psoriasis Foundation
6600 SW 92nd Avenue, Suite 300
Portland, OR 97223

503-244-7404
800-723-9166
Fax: 503-245-0626
e-mail: getinfo@psoriasis.org
www.psoriasis.org

Information on the disease affecting nails, ears, eyelids, face, mouth and lips, hands, feet and skin folds.

2005 9 pages

Gail M Zimmerman, President/CEO
Paula Fasano, Director Marketing/Communications

5858 Psoriasis: Common Questions & Their Answers
National Psoriasis Foundation
6600 SW 92nd Avenue, Suite 300
Portland, OR 97223

503-244-7404
800-723-9166
Fax: 503-245-0626
e-mail: getinfo@psoriasis.org
www.psoriasis.org

Gail M Zimmerman, President/CEO
Paula Fasano, Director Marketing/Communications

5859 Psoriasis: How it Makes You Feel
National Psoriasis Foundation
6600 SW 92nd Avenue, Suite 300
Portland, OR 97223

503-244-7404
800-723-9166
Fax: 503-245-0626
e-mail: getinfo@psoriasis.org
www.psoriasis.org

Living with psoriasis and the emotional impact.

Gail M Zimmerman, President/CEO
Paula Fasano, Director Marketing/Communications

5860 Psoriatic Arthritis
National Psoriasis Foundation
6600 SW 92nd Avenue, Suite 300
Portland, OR 97223

503-244-7404
800-723-9166
Fax: 503-245-0626
e-mail: getinfo@psoriasis.org
www.psoriasis.org

Overview of the joint disease that affects about 10-30% of psoriasis sufferers. Includes diagnosis and treatment details.

2005 11 pages

Gail M Zimmerman, President/CEO
Paula Fasano, Director Marketing/Communications

5861 Questions and Answers About Psoriasis
NAMSIC, National Institutes of Health
1 AMS Circle
Bethesda, MD 20892

301-495-4484
Fax: 301-587-4352
TTY: 301-565-2966
www.niams.nih.gov

Offers various information for the psoriasis patient and their family regarding treatments, risks, nutrition and more.

2003 22 pages

5862 Scalp Psoriasis
National Psoriasis Foundation
6600 SW 92nd Avenue, Suite 300
Portland, OR 97223

503-244-7404
800-723-9166
Fax: 503-245-0626
e-mail: getinfo@psoriasis.org
www.psoriasis.org

Possible treatment, tips and regimens for psoriasis of the scalp.

2005 9 pages

Gail M Zimmerman, President/CEO
Paula Fasano, Director Marketing/Communications

5863 Skin Cancer Risks from Psoriasis Treatments
National Psoriasis Foundation
6600 SW 92nd Avenue, Suite 300
Portland, OR 97223

503-244-7404
800-723-9166
Fax: 503-245-0626
e-mail: getinfo@psoriasis.org
www.psoriasis.org

Gail M Zimmerman, President/CEO
Paula Fasano, Director Marketing/Communications

5864 Specific Forms of Psoriasis
National Psoriasis Foundation
6600 SW 92nd Avenue, Suite 300
Portland, OR 97223

503-244-7404
800-723-9166
Fax: 503-245-0626
e-mail: getinfo@psoriasis.org
www.psoriasis.org

Plaque, Pustular, guttate, inverse, and erythrodermic: overview and treatment considerations for each type of the disease.

2006 7 pages

Gail M Zimmerman, President/CEO
Paula Fasano, Director Marketing/Communications

5865 Sun and Water Therapy
National Psoriasis Foundation
6600 SW 92nd Avenue, Suite 300
Portland, OR 97223

503-244-7404
800-723-9166
Fax: 503-245-0626
e-mail: getinfo@psoriasis.org
www.psoriasis.org

Provides information on climatotherapy sites as well as an overview of natural sunlight and water treatment options.

2005 11 pages

Gail M Zimmerman, President/CEO
Paula Fasano, Director Marketing/Communications

5866 Things to Consider
National Psoriasis Foundation
6600 SW 92nd Avenue, Suite 300
Portland, OR 97223

503-244-7404
800-723-9166
Fax: 503-245-0626
e-mail: getinfo@psoriasis.org
www.psoriasis.org

Discusses making treatment decisions, talking with your physician and knowing your rights.

5867 Your Diet & Psoriasis
National Psoriasis Foundation
6600 SW 92nd Avenue, Suite 300
Portland, OR 97223

503-244-7404
800-723-9166
Fax: 503-245-0626
e-mail: getinfo@psoriasis.org
www.psoriasis.org

An overview of diet-related research and therapies.

2005 9 pages

Gail M Zimmerman, President/CEO
Paula Fasano, Director Marketing/Communications

Camps

5868 Camp Discovery
American Academy of Dermatology
930 E Woodfield Road
Schaumburg, IL 60173

847-240-1737
866-503-7546
Fax: 847-330-8907
e-mail: jmueller@aad.org
www.campdiscovery.org

A camp for young people with serious skin conditions. There is no fee and transportation is provided. Two locations: Camp Horizon in Millville, PA and Camp Knutson in Crosslake, MN.

Stephen P Stone MD, President
Julie Mueller, Camp Information

DESCRIPTION

5869 PTOSIS

Synonym: Blepharoptosis

Covers these related disorders: Acquired ptosis, Congenital ptosis

Involves the following Biologic System(s):

Neurologic Disorders, Ophthalmologic Disorders

Ptosis, or blepharoptosis, refers to a condition in which one or both of the upper eyelids droop or sag as a result of an irregularity that is present at birth or an acquired weakness in the muscles of the upper eyelid that are responsible for movement. This condition may also be the result of irregularities of the nerve response for regulating muscle movements of the upper eyelids (third cranial nerve or oculomotor nerve). Congenital ptosis varies in severity; therefore, treatment depends upon the extent of the defect. If the eyelid droop is sufficient to cover the pupil, the ability to see is impaired. In some infants and children, the development of the affected eye may be slowed, resulting in reduced or lost vision (amblyopia) in that eye. In such cases, early intervention through surgery may aid in preventing the development of impaired vision. However, surgery to correct ptosis strictly for cosmetic reasons is often postponed until the affected child reaches the age of three or four years.

In some cases, ptosis is accompanied by an abnormality of certain eye muscles, resulting in irregular movements of the eyes. Other ocular irregularities often associated with congenital ptosis include misalignment of the eyes in relation to each other (strabismus) or an imbalance in the way each eye deflects light (anisometropia). Medical specialists recommended early treatment of any accompanying abnormalities to avert complications. Ptosis may also occur as a characteristic feature of several syndromes including congenital fibrosis syndrome, Horner syndrome, or Sturge-Weber syndrome. Congenital ptosis is transmitted as an autosomal dominant trait.

Acquired ptosis may develop secondary to several disorders or conditions including myasthenia gravis, a muscular disorder; botulism, a severe type of food poisoning; progressive lesions within the skull that impact on the third cranial nerve; inflammation or growths that impact the eye orbit or lid. Treatment for acquired ptosis depends upon and may be directed toward the underlying cause.

See also **General Resources** on page 917

Government Agencies

5870 NIH/National Eye Institute
31 Center Drive MSC 2510
Bethesda, MD 20892

301-496-5248
e-mail: 2020@nei.nih.gov
www.nei.nih.gov

Conducts and supports research that helps prevent and treat eye diseases and other disorders of vision. This research leads to sight-saving treatments, reduces visual impairment and blindness, and improves the quality of life for people of all ages. NEI-supported research has advanced our knowledge of how the eye functions in health and disease.

Paul A Sieving M.D., Ph.D., Director

National Associations & Support Groups

5871 Genetic Alliance
4301 Connecticut Avenue NW
Washington, DC 20008

202-966-5557
800-336-4363
Fax: 202-966-8553
e-mail: info@geneticalliance.org
www.geneticalliance.org

A coalition of voluntary genetic support groups, consumers and professionals addressing the needs of individuals and families affected by genetic disorders from a national perspective.

Sharon Terry, President/CEO

5872 March of Dimes Birth Defects Foundation
1275 Mamaroneck Avenue
White Plains, NY 10605

914-428-7100
888-663-4637
Fax: 914-428-8203
e-mail: resourcecenter@modimes.org
www.marchofdimes.com

Partnership of volunteers and professionals dedicates to improving the health of babies by preventing birth defects and infant mortality. Over 100 chapters are located across the country and can be located through the National Office.

Dr Jennifer Howse, President

5873 National Association for Visually Handicapped
22 W 21st Street, 6th Floor
New York, NY 10010

212-889-3141
Fax: 212-727-2931
e-mail: navh@navh.org
www.navh.org

Serves as a clearinghouse for information about all services available to the partially-sighted from public and private sources. Conducts self-help groups. Provides information on large print books, textbooks and educational tools.

Dr Lorraine Marchi, Founder & CEO

5874 National Eye Research Foundation
910 Skokie Boulevard, Suite 207A
Northbrook, IL 60062

847-564-4652
800-621-2258
Fax: 847-564-0807
e-mail: info@nerf.org
www.nerf.org

Devoted to the enhancement of care and study of eye related diseases.

Web Sites

5875 National Association for Visually Handicapped
www.navh.org

Helps to cope with the difficulties of vision impairment.

5876 Online Mendelian Inheritance in Man
www.ncbi.nlm.nih.gov

This database is a catalog of human genes and genetic disorders.

5877 Royal National Institute of the Blind
www.rnib.org.uk

A leading UK charity offering information, support and advice to over two million people with sight problems.

DESCRIPTION

5878 PULMONARY HYPERTENSION

Covers these related disorders: Persistent fetal circulation (PFC)

Involves the following Biologic System(s):
Cardiovascular Disorders, Respiratory Disorders

Primary pulmonary hypertension is a condition in which the blood pressure within the pulmonary artery is abnormally high (hypertension). The pulmonary artery arises from the base of the lower right chamber of the heart (ventricle) and carries oxygen-poor blood to the lungs, where the exchange of oxygen and carbon dioxide occurs. When this occurs in newborn infants, it is known as persistent fetal circulation or more appropriately, persistent pulmonary hypertension in the newborn (PPHN).

PPHN is a condition in newborns in which blood continues to circulate through certain fetal openings or channels which usually close shortly after birth. These include the fetal opening between the left and right upper chambers of the heart (foramen ovale) and the fetal channel that joins the major artery of the body (aorta) and the pulmonary artery (ductus arteriosus). PPHN may occur in newborns for unknown reasons (idiopathic) or may result from a lack of oxygen during the birth process (birth asphyxia); certain abnormalities during pregnancy (e.g., amniotic fluid leak); certain birth defects (e.g., underdevelopment of the lungs seen in a diaphragmatic hernia); or other conditions, such as meconium aspiration, polycythemia (excess number of red blood cells, etc. PPHN affects approximately one in 500 t0 700 newborns.

Newborns with PPHN often experience symptoms immediately after birth or within the first 12 hours of life. Some may have bluish discoloration of the skin and mucous membranes (cyanosis) and increasing difficulties breathing (respiratory distress). Symptoms associated with respiratory distress may include rapid breathing (tachypnea), grunting upon exhalation, drawing in of the chest wall during inhalation, and a rapid heart rate (tachycardia).

In newborns with PPHN, immediate measures may be necessary to prevent or treat potentially life-threatening complications. Additional therapy is directed toward treating the underlying cause of the condition and providing ongoing supportive measures to increase the supply of oxygen to bodily tissues. Oxygen therapies may include the use of measures to mechanically assist breathing (mechanical ventilation), administration of certain medications (e.g.,

surfactant therapy; inhalation of nitric oxide to help widen pulmonary blood vessels), or use of a device known as an extracorporeal membrane oxygenator (ECMO). This device delivers oxygen to an infant's blood as it is circulated outside of the body and then returns the oxygenated blood to the body.

In contrast to PPHN, primary pulmonary hypertension is a progressive condition that often becomes apparent between the ages of 10 to 20 years. Females appear to be slightly more affected than males. Researchers suspect that th|e condition may be the result of the interactions of different genes, possibly in association with the involvement of certain environmental factors (multifactorial inheritance).

In patients with primary pulmonary hypertension, abnormal thickening and loss of elasticity of pulmonary arterial walls may cause abnormal obstruction and increased resistance of the blood flow from the right ventricle to the lungs. Consequently, the heart muscle must pump harder and at a higher pressure to adequately propel blood through the pulmonary artery, leading to enlargement of the right ventricle. Affected individuals may experience exercise intolerance (inability to do physical exercise at the level that would be expected of someone in his or her general physical condition), easy fatigability, and, in some cases, dizziness, fainting episodes (syncope), headaches, and chest pain. In addition, as the right ventricle begins to weaken in its ability to pump blood efficiently (right ventricular failure), patients may experience cyanosis, coldness of the affected limbs, enlargement of the liver (hepatomegaly), and an abnormal accumulation of fluid in body tissues (edema). Patients with severe pulmonary hypertension may experience sudden abnormalities in the rhythm or rate of the heartbeat (arrhythmias), resulting in life-threatening complications. Supportive therapies for the treatment of primary pulmonary hypertension may include intravenous administration of the medication prostacyclin to help widen pulmonary arteries (vasodilation) and increase blood flow. In addition, in some patients, the administration of calcium channel blocking agents by mouth may be beneficial. In many patients with severe primary pulmonary hypertension, heart-lung or lung transplantation may be required.

See also **General Resources** on page 917

Government Agencies

5879 NIH/National Heart, Lung and Blood Institu te
National Institute of Health
31 Center Dr MSC 2486, Bldg 31, Room 5A48
Bethesda, MD 20892

301-592-8573
Fax: 240-629-3246
TTY: 240-629-3255
e-mail: NHLBIinfo@nhlbi.nih.gov
www.nhlbi.nih.gov

Primary responsibility of this organization is the scientific investigation of heart, blood vessel, lung and blood disorders. Oversees research, demonstration, prevention, education, control and training activities in these fields and emphasizes the prevention and control of heart diseases.

Elizabeth G Nabel, MD, Director
Susan Shurin, MD, Deputy Director

5880 NIH/National Institute of Child Health and Human Development
31 Center Drive, Building 31
Bethesda, MD 20892

301-496-5133
Fax: 301-496-1104
www.nichd.nih.gov

Established in 1962 by congress, today the institute conducts and supports research on topics related to the health of children, adults, families and populations. Some of these topics include: developmental disabilities, growth and development, infant death, reproductive health and birth defects.

Nancy D Wirth, Director
Lisa Kaeser, Program & Public Liaison

National Associations & Support Groups

5881 American Heart Association
7272 Greenville Avenue
Dallas, TX 75231

214-373-6300
800-242-8721
Fax: 214-706-1341
e-mail: inquire@amhrt.org
www.amhrt.org

Supports research, education and community service programs with the objective of reducing premature death and disability from cardiovascular diseases and stroke; coordinates the efforts of health professionals, and others engaged in the fight against heart and circulatory disease.

M Cass Wheeler, CEO

5882 American Lung Association
61 Broadway, 6th Floor
New York, NY 10006

212-315-8700
800-586-4872
www.lungusa.org

The American Lung Association fights lung disease in all its forms, with special emphasis on asthma, tobacco control and environmental health. The American Lung Association is funded with contributions from the public, along with gifts and grants from corporations, foundations and government agencies. The association achieves its many successes through the work of thousands of committed volunteers and staff.

Terri E Weaver, PhD RN CS FAAN, Chairman

5883 Foundation for Pulmonary Hypertension
PO Box 61540
New Orleans, LA 70161

504-533-5888
Fax: 504-533-2447

5884 Genetic Alliance
4301 Connecticut Avenue NW
Washington, DC 20008

202-966-5557
800-336-4363
Fax: 202-966-8553
e-mail: info@geneticalliance.org
www.geneticalliance.org

A coalition of voluntary genetic support groups, consumers and professionals addressing the needs of individuals and families affected by genetic disorders from a national perspective.

Sharon Terry, President/CEO

5885 March of Dimes Birth Defects Foundation
1275 Mamaroneck Avenue
White Plains, NY 10605

914-428-7100
888-663-4637
Fax: 914-428-8203
e-mail: resourcecenter@modimes.org
www.marchofdimes.com

Partnership of volunteers and professionals dedicates to improving the health of babies by preventing birth defects and infant mortality. Over 100 chapters are located across the country and can be located through the National Office.

Dr Jennifer Howse, President

5886 Pulmonary Hypertension Association
801 Roeder Road, Suite 400
Silver Spring, MD 20910

301-565-3004
800-748-7274
Fax: 301-565-3994
e-mail: pha@phassociation.org
www.phassociation.org

PHA's mission is to seek a cure; provide hope, support and education; promote awareness, and advocate for the pulmonary hypertension community.

Rino Aldrighetti, President
Adrienne Dern, VP

Web Sites

5887 MayoClinic.com - Pulmonary Hypertension
mayoclinic.com/health/pulmonary-hypertension/DS00430

Introduction to the disorder, signs, symptoms, treatment, etc.

DESCRIPTION

5888 PULMONARY VALVE STENOSIS

Covers these related disorders: Critical pulmonic stenosis
Involves the following Biologic System(s):
Cardiovascular Disorders

Pulmonary valve stenosis is a congenital heart defect characterized by abnormal narrowing (stenosis) of the valve between the lower right-sided, pumping chamber of the heart (right ventricle) and the pulmonary artery. Situated where the pulmonary artery arises from the base of the right ventricle, the pulmonary valve enables blood to flow from the right ventricle to the lungs while preventing the backward flow of blood. The pulmonary artery carries oxygen-depleted (deoxygenated) blood to the lungs, where the exchange of oxygen and carbon dioxide occurs. In infants and children with pulmonary valve stenosis, narrowing of the pulmonary valve opening increases resistance of the blood flow from the right ventricle to the pulmonary artery. As a result, the heart muscle must pump harder and at a higher pressure to propel blood to the pulmonary artery, potentially leading to thickening of the heart muscle (hypertrophy) of the right ventricle. Pulmonary valve stenosis affects approximately one in 1,250 individuals in the general population, comprising approximately 10 percent of all heart defects that are present at birth (congenital heart defects). Less commonly, pulmonary stenosis may be due to structural abnormalities other than a restricted valvular opening, such as narrowing within the upper region of the right ventricle or a portion of the pulmonary artery (e.g., isolated infundibular stenosis, branch pulmonary artery stenosis).

In infants and children with pulmonary valve stenosis, the severity of associated symptoms may vary, depending on the size of the restricted valvular opening and, in some patients, the presence of additional heart defects. For example, some affected children may also have relatively small septal defects, such as an abnormal opening in the fibrous partition (septum) that divides the ventricles or the two upper chambers (atria) of the heart (ventricular or atrial septal defects). Infants and children with mild pulmonary valve stenosis usually have no associated symptoms (asymptomatic), do not experience hypertrophy of heart muscle, and have normal growth and development. In such patients, the condition is usually initially suspected due to detection of characteristic, abnormal heart sounds (heart murmurs) during a physician's examination with a stethoscope. In patients with moderate pulmonary valve stenosis, the right ventricle may be of normal size or mildly thickened. Although such patients are usually asymptomatic, others may experience some symptoms, such as easy fatigability and exercise intolerance.

In newborns or young infants with severe pulmonary valve stenosis, the right ventricle may be unable to pump blood adequately (right ventricular failure) and become moderately or severely enlarged. Findings associated with right ventricular failure may include poor feeding, enlargement of the liver (hepatomegaly), an abnormal accumulation of fluid in body tissues (edema) or other abnormalities. In addition, blood may begin to circulate through a previously closed fetal opening in the heart (foramen ovale) between the left and right atria that closes shortly after birth. Abnormal opening of the foramen ovale in those with pulmonary valve stenosis may cause oxygen-depleted blood to pass from the right to the left side of the atria (right-to-left shunting), into the left ventricle and into the aorta for transport to the body's tissues. Because this oxygen-depleted blood bypasses the lungs and instead recirculates throughout the body, bodily tissues receive less oxygenated blood (hypoxia). In such cases, affected newborns or infants are said to have critical pulmonic stenosis. In addition, in some infants, certain associated heart (cardiac) defects, such as atrial or ventricular septal defects, may also allow some mixing of oxygen-poor and oxygen-rich blood. Due to recirculation of oxygen-poor blood to the body's tissues, affected newborns or infants may experience mild to moderate bluish discoloration of the skin and mucous membranes (cyanosis), shortness of breath (dyspnea), and other serious symptoms and findings.

In these newborns or infants, emergency procedures are performed to widen the restricted valvular opening. Such procedures may include inflation of a balloon-tipped cathet|er (valvuloplasty) or surgical correction or resection of the valve (valvotomy). Although corrective measures may not be required in those with mild stenosis, such patients should receive regular follow-up evaluations. Such monitoring is necessary to ensure appropriate intervention for patients who may potentially experience increasing obstruction across the pulmonary valve or increasing hypertrophy of the right ventricle requiring surgical intervention. Other treatment is symptomatic and supportive.

Pulmonary valve stenosis may occur as a spontaneous, isolated finding; with other congenital heart defects; or in association with certain underlying disorders (e.g., Noonan syndrome). In some patients, the condition is thought to be determined by the interactions of several different genes, possibly in association with the involvement of certain environmental factors (multifactorial inheritance).

See also **General Resources** on page 917

Government Agencies

5889 NIH/National Heart, Lung and Blood Institu te
National Institute of Health
31 Center Dr MSC 2486, Bldg 31, Room 5A48
Bethesda, MD 20892

301-592-8573
Fax: 240-629-3246
TTY: 240-629-3255
e-mail: NHLBIinfo@nhlbi.nih.gov
www.nhlbi.nih.gov

Primary responsibility of this organization is the scientific investigation of heart, blood vessel, lung and blood disorders. Oversees research, demonstration, prevention, education, control and training activities in these fields and emphasizes the prevention and control of heart diseases.

Elizabeth G Nabel, MD, Director
Susan Shurin, MD, Deputy Director

5890 NIH/National Institute of Child Health and Human Development
31 Center Drive, Building 31
Bethesda, MD 20892

301-496-5133
Fax: 301-496-1104
www.nichd.nih.gov

Established in 1962 by congress, today the institute conducts and supports research on topics related to the health of children, adults, families and populations. Some of these topics include: developmental disabilities, growth and development, infant death, reproductive health and birth defects.

Nancy D Wirth, Director
Lisa Kaeser, Program & Public Liaison

National Associations & Support Groups

5891 American Heart Association
7272 Greenville Avenue
Dallas, TX 75231

214-373-6300
800-242-8721
Fax: 214-706-1341
e-mail: inquire@amhrt.org
www.amhrt.org

Supports research, education and community service programs with the objective of reducing premature death and disability from cardiovascular diseases and stroke; coordinates the efforts of health professionals, and others engaged in the fight against heart and circulatory disease.

M Cass Wheeler, CEO

5892 Division of Pediatric Pulmonology
New York Medical College
Pediatric Specialty Ctr, 19 Bradhurst Avenue
Hawthorne, NY 10532

914-493-7585
Fax: 914-594-4336
e-mail: pedpulm@nymc.edu
www.nymc.edu

The division is dedicated to teaching and patient care.

5893 Genetic Alliance
4301 Connecticut Avenue NW
Washington, DC 20008

202-966-5557
800-336-4363
Fax: 202-966-8553
e-mail: info@geneticalliance.org
www.geneticalliance.org

A coalition of voluntary genetic support groups, consumers and professionals addressing the needs of individuals and families affected by genetic disorders from a national perspective.

Sharon Terry, President/CEO

5894 March of Dimes Birth Defects Foundation
1275 Mamaroneck Avenue
White Plains, NY 10605

914-428-7100
888-663-4637
Fax: 914-428-8203
e-mail: resourcecenter@modimes.org
www.marchofdimes.com

Partnership of volunteers and professionals dedicates to improving the health of babies by preventing birth defects and infant mortality. Over 100 chapters are located across the country and can be located through the National Office.

Dr Jennifer Howse, President

Web Sites

5895 Congenital Heart Information Network
www.tchin.org

An international organization that provides reliable information, support services and resources to families of children with congenital heart defects and acquired heart disease, adults with congenital heart defects, and the professionals who work with them.

5896 Southern Illinois University School of Medicine
www.siumed.edu/peds/index.htm

The mission of SUI School of Medicine is to assist the people of central and southern Illinois in meeting their present and future health care needs through education, clinical service and research.

Book Publishers

5897 Congenital Disorders Sourcebook
Omnigraphics
PO Box 625
Holmes, PA 19043

800-234-1340
Fax: 800-875-1340
e-mail: info@omnigraphics.com
www.omnigraphics.com

Basic consumer health information on disorders aquired during gestation, including spina bifida, hydrocephalus, cerebral palsy, heart defects, craniofacial abnormalities and fetal alcohol syndrome.

650 pages
ISBN: 0-780809-45-9

DESCRIPTION

5898 PYLORIC STENOSIS

Synonym: Infantile pyloric stenosis

Involves the following Biologic System(s):

Gastrointestinal Disorders

Pyloric stenosis refers to a condition in which the passageway (pyloric canal) that leads from the stomach to the first part of the small intestine known as the duodenum is narrowed or obstructed due to the thickening of the muscle that surrounds this opening (pyloric sphincter). Although the specific cause for this thickening is not known, many factors may be responsible, including breast-feeding, irregularities in nerve distribution to the muscle, and certain disorders such as Turner syndrome, Cornelia de Lange syndrome, trisomy 18 syndrome, and eosinophilic gastroenteritis. Pyloric stenosis is also commonly associated with certain birth defects of the gastrointestinal tract such as tracheoesophageal fistula.

Symptoms and findings associated with this disorder may develop as early as the first week of life; however, in some infants, this abnormality does not cause noticeable symptoms until the fourth or fifth month. At about the third week of life, episodes of forceful and explosive vomiting (projectile vomiting) may occur. After eating, rhythmic, wave-like movements (peristalsis) may be visible in the infant's abdominal area. Prolonged vomiting may result in excessive fluid loss (dehydration) and loss of essential elements known as electrolytes in the fluid portion of the blood (e.g., sodium, potassium, and calcium).

Treatment for infantile pyloric stenosis includes the administration of fluids to counteract the effects of dehydration. Once body fluids andelectrolytes stabilize, a surgical procedure known as a pyloromyotomy may be performed. During this procedure, a lengthwise incision is made along the thickened pyloric muscle to correct the defect.

Pyloric stenosis affects approximately three in every 1,000 infants in the United States. Boys are more often affected than girls by a ratio of four to one. Children of parents who had pyloric stenosis are approximately 10 to 20 percent more likely to be affected. Infants with types B or O blood develop this defect more often than those with other blood types.

See also **General Resources** on page 917

National Associations & Support Groups

5899 American College of Gastroenterology
PO Box 342260
Bethesda, MD 20827

301-263-9000
www.acg.gi.org

Founded to advance the scientific study and medical practice of diseases of the gastrointestinal (GI) tract.

Jack A DiPalma, President
Amy E Foxx-Orenstein, VP

5900 Cyclic Vomiting Syndrome Association
3585 Cedar Hill Road NW
Canal Winchester, OH 43110

614-837-2586
Fax: 614-837-2586
e-mail: waitesd@cvsaonline.org
www.cvsaonline.org

A volunteer organization serving the needs of CVS patients, their families around the world and the growing medical community studying CVS. The network has grown to over 37 medical advisors and over 90 volunteers in over 32 countries.

$75/year

Kathleen Adams, President/Research Liaison

5901 Digestive Disease National Coalition
507 Capitol Court NE, Suite 200
Washington, DC 20002

202-544-7497
Fax: 202-546-7105
www.ddnc.org

Advocacy organization comprised of 22 voluntary and professional societies concerned with the many diseases of the digestive tract and liver.

Nancy Norton, Chairperson
Dr. Maurice Cerulli, President

5902 International Foundation for Functional Gastrointestinal Disorders
PO Box 170864
Milwaukee, WI 53217

414-964-1799
888-964-2001
Fax: 414-964-7176
e-mail: iffgd@iffgd.org
www.iffgd.org

Nonprofit education and research organization founded in 1991. IFFGD addresses the issues surrounding life with gastrointestinal (GI) functional and mobility disorders and increases the awareness about these disorders among the general public, researchers and the clinical care community.

Nancy J Norton, Founder
William Norton, VP

5903 Intestinal Disease Foundation
100 W Station Square Drive
Pittsburgh, PA 15219

412-261-5888
877-587-9606
Fax: 412-471-2722
e-mail: info@intestinalfoundation.org
www.intestinalfoundation.org

Nonprofit organization whose mission is to improve the quality of life of adults and children affected by chronic digestive illness through information, guidance and support. IDF offers a quarterly newsletter, Intestinal Fortitude, educational seminars, volunteer phone network, and Pittsburgh area support groups.

5904 March of Dimes Birth Defects Foundation
1275 Mamaroneck Avenue
White Plains, NY 10605

914-428-7100
888-663-4637
Fax: 914-428-8203
e-mail: resourcecenter@modimes.org
www.marchofdimes.com

Partnership of volunteers and professionals dedicates to improving the health of babies by preventing birth defects and infant mortality. Over 100 chapters are located across the country and can be located through the National Office.

Dr Jennifer Howse, President

5905 North American Society for Pediatric Gastroenterology/Hepatology/Nutrition
PO Box 6
Flourtown, PA 19031

215-233-0808
Fax: 215-233-3918
e-mail: naspghan@naspghan.org
www.naspghan.org

Strives to improve the care of infants, children and adolescents with digestive disorders by promoting advances in clinical care of children with chronic abdominal pain, diarrhea, constipation, vomiting, bleeding from the GI tract, inflammatory bowel disease, liver diseases, diseases of the pancreas, poor weight gain and nutritional problems.

Philip Sherman, President
Margaret K Stallings, Executive Director

5906 Pediatric/Adolescent Gastroesophageal Reflux Association (PAGER)
PO Box 486
Buckeystown, MD 21717

301-601-9541
e-mail: GERGROUP@aol.com
www.reflux.org

Non profit organization providing information and support to parents and children dealing with gastroesophageal reflux.

Beth Anderson, Director
Jan Gambino-Burns, Associate Director

Libraries & Resource Centers

5907 National Digestive Diseases Information Clearinghouse
2 Information Way
Bethesda, MD 20892

301-654-3810
800-891-3810
Fax: 703-738-4929
e-mail: nddic@info.niddk.nih.gov
www.digestive.niddk.nih.gov

The National Institute of Diabetes and Digestive and Kidney Diseases conducts and supports research on many of the most serious diseases affecting public health. The Institute supports much of the clinical research on the diseases of internal medicine and related subspecialty fields as well as many basic science disciplines.

Kathy Kranzfelder, Project Officer

Web Sites

5908 American Pediatric Surgical Association
www.eapsa.org/parents/pyloric.htm

For parents: an overview of Pyloric Stenosis including symptoms, treatment and complications.

5909 Common Pediatric Conditions- Pyloric Stenosis
www.surgery.vcu.edu/content/pylostenosis.htm

Information on causes and surgery from Virginia Commonwealth University Department of Surgery.

5910 Dr. Koop
www.drkoop.com/ency/93/000970.html

Information on the condition, causes, symptoms, tests and treatment.

5911 KidsHealth-Pyloric Stenosis
www.kidshealth.org/parent/

Definition, causes, symptoms, treatment and complications.

5912 MEDLINEplus Medical Encyclopedia: Pyloric Stenosis
www.nlm.nih.gov/medlineplus/ency/article/000970.htm

Definitions, causes, symptoms, treatment, prognosis and complications.

5913 National Digestive Diseases Information Clearinghouse
www.digestive.niddk.nih.gov

The National Institute of Diabetes and Digestive and Kidney Diseases conducts and supports research on many of the most serious diseases affecting public health. The Institute supports much of the clinical research on the diseases of internal medicine and related subspecialty fields as well as many basic science disciplines.

5914 Online Mendelian Inheritance in Man
www.ncbi.nlm.nih.gov

This database is a catalog of human genes and genetic disorders.

5915 Southern Illinois University School of Medicine
www.siumed.edu/peds/index.htm

The mission of SUI School of Medicine is to assist the people of central and southern Illinois in meeting their present and future health care needs through education, clinical service and research.

Journals

5916 Journal of Pediatric Gastroenterology and Nutrition

NASPGHAN, author

Lippincott Williams & Wilkins
530 Walnut Street
Philadelphia, PA 19106

215-521-8300
Fax: 215-521-8902
www.lww.com

Publication of the North American Society for Pediatric Gastroenterolgy, Hepatology and Nutrition, which strives to improve the care of infants, children and adolescents with digestive disorders by promoting advances in clinical care of children with chronic abdominal pain, diarrhea, constipation, vomiting, bleeding from the GI tract, inflammatory bowel disease, liver diseases, diseases of the pancreas, poor weight gain and nutritional problems.

Newsletters

5917 NASPGHAN News
PO Box 6
Flourtown, PA 19031

215-233-0808
Fax: 215-233-3939
e-mail: naspghan@naspghan.org
www.naspgn.org

Publication of the North American Society for Pediatric Gastroenterolgy and Nutrition, which strives to improve the care of infants, children and adolescents with digestive disorders by promoting advances in clinical care of children with chronic abdominal pain, diarrhea, constipation, vomiting, bleeding from the GI tract, inflammatory bowel disease, liver diseases, diseases of the pancreas, poor weight gain and nutritional problems.

DESCRIPTION

5918 REFRACTION DISTURBANCES

Synonym: Ametropia

Disorder Type: Vision

Covers these related disorders: Anisometropia, Astigmatism, Hyperopia (Farsightedness), Myopia (Nearsightedness)

Involves the following Biologic System(s):
Ophthalmologic Disorders

Refraction abnormalities are defects in the cornea and the lens of the eye to focus visual images appropriately on the nerve-rich membrane at the back of the eye (retina). The cornea is the convex, transparent area in front of the eye. The lens, which is located behind the pupil, is held in place by a circular muscle that changes the shape of the lens to make appropriate adjustments in focus (ciliary muscle). As light passes through the cornea and the lens, it is bent (refracted) so that it is properly focused on the retina, which contains millions of tiny nerve cells that respond to light (photoreceptors). However, in individuals with refraction defects, light rays are not properly focused on the retina (ametropia) due to abnormalities of the cornea, the lens, or the size of the eye. These refraction defects lead to visual abnormalities.

There are three primary types of refraction abnormalities: namely, farsightedness (hyperopia), nearsightedness (myopia), and astigmatism. In farsightedness, parallel light rays come to focus behind rather that on the retina. This may be due to shortness of the eyeball from front to back, abnormally reduced refractive power of the cornea or lens, or backward displacement of the lens. If farsightedness is mild or moderate, affected children may be able to clearly visualize near and far objects due to accommodation, a process by which the shape of the lens changes and brings the area of focus forward. The range and extent of accommodation is highest durign childhood and gradually decreases with age. With greater degrees of farsightedness, affected children may experience blurring of vision, eyestrain, fatigue, and recurrent headaches. They may also engage in repeated eye rubbing and squinting and appear uninterested in reading or schoolwork. Children with farsightedness may achieve clear vision with glasses or contact lenses with convex lenses.

In children with nearsightedness (myopia), parallel light rays come to focus in front of the retina due to increased length of the eyeball from front to back, abnormally increased refractive power of the cornea or lens, or forward displacement of the lens. Affected children experience blurring of vision when focusing on distant objects, tend to hold reading material and other objects close to their face, and often squint in an effort to improve clearness and clarity of vision. Nearsightedness usually becomes apparent during school age, particularly in the years prior to and up to adolescence. The degree of nearsightedness typically becomes more severe until early adulthood, when it tends to stabilize. Many affected children have a hereditary predisposition for nearsightedness; in addition, the condition may occur in association with the other eye abnormalities (e.g., glaucoma, keratoconus) or other underlying disorders. Clear vision may be attained with glasses or contact lenses with concave lenses. Until the degree of nearsightedness stabilizes, prescriptions may need to be periodically increased in strength (e.g., varying from every few months to once every one or two years).

In children with astigmatism, parallel light rays are not clearly focused in a point on the retina due to unequal curvature of refractive surfaces of the eye. Astigmatism may result from irregularities in curvature of the cornea or, in some cases, abnormalities of the lens. Many individuals have minor degrees of astigmatism and have no associated symptoms. With more severe degrees of astigmatism, affected children may experience blurring and distortion of vision, fatigue, eyestrain, and recurrent headaches. In many cases, they may also engage in frequent eye rubbing, squint in an attempt to improve clearness and clarity of vision, hold reading materials and other objects close, and appear uninterested in schoolwork. In children with astigmatism, visual correction may be achieved with the part-time or ongoing use of glasses with cylindric or spherocylindric lenses. In some cases, contact lenses may be used to help correct vision.

Some children may also have a visual condition known as anisometropia in which the refractive or focusing ability of one eye significantly differs from the other. For example, one eye may have normal focusing ability, whereas the other may be affected by nearsightedness, farsightedness, and astigmatism. For proper vision to develop during infancy and early childhood, corresponding visual images mustform on both retinas to ensure the transmission of compatible nerve impulses (via the optic nerves) to the brain. If the images from one eye differ dramatically from the other, one may be suppressed, causing impaired visual development in one eye (amblyopia). Therefore, in infants and children with anisometropia, prompt detection and appropriate visual correction is essential to ensure proper visual development in both eyes.

See also **General Resources** on page 917

Government Agencies

5919 NIH/National Eye Institute
31 Center Drive MSC 2510
Bethesda, MD 20892

301-496-5248
e-mail: 2020@nei.nih.gov
www.nei.nih.gov

Conducts and supports research that helps prevent and treat eye diseases and other disorders of vision. This research leads to sight-saving treatments, reduces visual impairment and blindness, and improves the quality of life for people of all ages. NEI-supported research has advanced our knowledge of how the eye functions in health and disease.

Paul A Sieving MD, PhD, Director

National Associations & Support Groups

5920 Division on Visual Impairments
Council for Exceptional Children
1110 North Glebe Road, Suite 300
Arlington, VA 22201

800-224-6830
Fax: 703-264-9494
TTY: 866-915-5000
www.ed.arizona.edu/dvi/welcome.htm; www.cec.sped.org

A division within the CEC, it handles concerns for Federal, state and local issues and policies related to education of youths, children and infants with visual impairments.

Ellyn Ross, President
Shirley J Wilson, Secretary

5921 Lighthouse International
111 E 59th Street
New York, NY 10022

212-821-9200
800-829-0500
Fax: 212-821-9707
TTY: 212-821-9713
e-mail: info@lighthouse.org
www.lighthouse.org

Provides services, information, resource contacts, education and research related to the needs of children who are visually impaired and their families.

Tara A Cortes RN, PhD, President/CEO
Cynthia Stuen, Senior VP Services/Education

5922 National Alliance of Blind Students
c/o Terry Pacheco
1155 15th Street NW, Suite 1004
Washington, DC 20005

202-467-5081
800-424-8666
Fax: 202-467-5085
e-mail: rj.hodson@verizon.net
www.blindstudents.org

An advocacy and consumer organization for high school and college students who are blind or visually impaired. It works to facilitate progress toward full accessibility of college programs and facilities, provides opportunities for discussion of issues important to students and assists with National Student Seminars.

Rebecca Hodson, President

5923 National Association for Parents of Childr en with Visual Impairments
PO Box 317
Watertown, MA 02471

617-972-7441
800-562-6265
Fax: 617-972-7444
e-mail: napvi@perkins.org
www.spedex.com/napvi/

Offers emotional support for parents of blind or visually impaired children. Provides information, training and assistance, and help in understanding and using available resources.

5924 National Association for Visually Handicapped
22 W 21st Street, 6th Floor
New York, NY 10010

212-889-3141
Fax: 212-727-2931
e-mail: navh@navh.org
www.navh.org

Serves as a clearinghouse for information about all services available to the partially-sighted from public and private sources. Conducts self-help groups. Provides information on large print books, textbooks and educational tools.

Dr Lorraine Marchi, Founder & CEO

State Agencies & Support Groups

Alabama

5925 Alabama Institute for the Deaf & Blind
PO Box 698
Talladega, AL 35160

256-761-3200
Fax: 256-761-3344
www.nectas.unc.edu

Services include central directory, representatives of agencies, service providers, families, and coordinators of infant, toddler, and preschool special education programs.

Joseph Busta, Interagency Coordinating Council

Arizona

5926 National Association for Parents of the Visually Impaired
Po Box 317
Watertown, MA 02471

617-972-7441
800-562-6265
Fax: 617-972-7444
www.spedex.com/napvi

Mary Ellen Simmons

California

5927 Blind Childrens Center
4120 Marathon Street
Los Angeles, CA 90029

323-664-2153
Fax: 323-665-3828
www.blindchildrenscenter.org

Family-centered agency that serves children with visual impairments from birth to school age. The center-based programs and services help the children acquire skills and build their independence.

5928 Helen Keller National Center SW Region
6160 Cornerstone Court E
San Diego, CA 92121

858-623-2777
Fax: 858-642-0266
TTY: 858-646-0784
e-mail: ckirscher@cspp.edu
www.helenkeller.org

Cathy Kircher, SW Regional Representative

Connecticut

5929 Region 1 of the National Association for Parents of the Visually Impaired
252 Rye Street
Broad Brook, CT 06016

860-623-4129

Susan Ellsworth

Georgia

5930 Southeastern Region-Helen Keller National Center
1003 Virginia Avenue, Suite 104
Atlanta, GA 30354

404-766-9625
Fax: 404-766-3447
TTY: 404-766-2820

Susan Lascek, Supervisor Of Reg Representatives

Illinois

5931 Helen Keller National Center - North Central Region
485 42nd Avenue, Suite 5
East Moline, IL 61244

309-755-0024
Fax: 309-755-0025
TTY: 309-755-0021
e-mail: hknc5ljt@aol.com
www.helenkeller.org

Information and referral services for people who have a vision and a hearing loss combination, contact our regional office. We serve Illinois, Indiana, Ohio, Minnesota, Wisconsin and Michigan.

Laura Thomas, Regional Representative
Tara Upton, Administrative Assistant

5932 National Association for Parents of the Visually Impaired
16 Thornfield Lane
Hawthorn Woods, IL 60047

847-438-0705

Kevin O'Connor

5933 Region 3 of the National Association for Parents of the Visually Impaired
16 Thornfield Lane
Hawthorn Woods, IL 60047

847-438-0705

Kevin O'Connor

Kansas

5934 Great Plains Region-Helen Keller National Center
4330 Shawnee Mission Parkway
Mission, KS 66205

913-677-4562
Fax: 913-677-1544
e-mail: hknc7bj@aol.com
www.helenkeller.org

Services are free and offer client advocacy, consultation and technical assistance to schools and agencies; assistance in developing local services information and referral; public education and awareness; maintenance of the National Registry.

Beth Jordan, Regional Representative

Maryland

5935 National Organization of Parents of Blind Children
1800 Johnson Street
Baltimore, MD 21230

410-659-9314
Fax: 410-685-5653
e-mail: nfb@iamdiyrx.net
www.nfh.org

Informational and emotional support to parents who have a child, adolescent, or adult family member with blindness or visual impairment.

Massachusetts

5936 New England Region-Helen Keller National Center
313 Washington Street
Newton, MA 02158

617-630-1580
Fax: 617-630-1579
e-mail: hkncmeb@aol.com

New Mexico

5937 Region 5 of the National Association for Parents of the Visually Impaired
PO Box 1337
Alamogordo, NM 88311

505-682-2693

Ohio

5938 Region 2 of the National Association for Parents of the Visually Impaired
3910 Pocahontas Avenue
Cincinnati, OH 45227

513-561-8542

Victoria Gorman Miller

Pennsylvania

5939 East Central Region-Helen Keller National Center
4351 Garden City Drive
New Carrollton, MD 20785

301-459-5474
Fax: 301-459-5070
e-mail: hkncreg3cl@aol.com
www.helenkeller.org

South Carolina

5940 Region 4 of the National Association for Parents of the Visually Impaired
1032 Trail Road
Belton, SC 29627

864-338-9593

Washington

5941 Northwestern Region-Helen Keller National Center
2366 Eastlake Avenue E
Seattle, WA 98102

206-324-9120
e-mail: nwhknc@juno.com

Libraries & Resource Centers

Alabama

5942 Mobile Association for the Blind
2440 Gordon Smith Drive
Mobile, AL 36617

334-473-3585

Offers work adjustment training, activities of daily living, mobility, communication skills and sheltered employment for adults and children who are visually impaired.

Mahlon McCracken, Executive Director

Arizona

5943 Educational Services for the Visually Impaired
PO Box 668
Little Rock, AR 72203

501-371-5710

Offers textbooks, braille books and more to the visually impaired grades K-12 in the Arkansas area.

David Beavers, Director

Arkansas

5944 Arkansas Regional Library for the Blind and Physically Handicapped
1 Capitol Mall
Little Rock, AR 72201

501-682-1155
Fax: 501-682-1529
TDD: 501-682-1002
e-mail: nlsbooks@asl.lib.ar.us
www.asl.lib.ar.us/ASL_LBPH.htm

Public library books in recorded or braille format. Popular fiction and nonfiction books for all ages, books and players are on free loan, sent to patrons by mail and may be returned postage free. Anyone who cannot see well enough to read regular print with glasses on or who has a disability that makes it difficult to hold a book or turn the pages is eligible.

John D Hall, Director

California

5945 American Action Fund for Blind Children and Adults
18440 Oxnard Street
Tarzana, CA 91356

818-343-2022
www.actinfund.org

Offers a charitable and educational fund, braille assistive devices and a lending library for the visually impaired.

5946 Blind Children's Center
4120 Marathon Street
Los Angeles, CA 90029

323-664-2153
Fax: 323-665-3828
www.blindcntr.org

Offers support and informational groups.

5947 Braille Institute Desert Center
70-251 Ramon Road
Rancho Mirage, CA 92270

760-321-2555

Dedicated to providing blind and visually impaired men, women and children with the training, programs and services they need to enjoy productive lives. Services offered include child development, youth programs, library services and adult education.

5948 Braille Institute Sight Center
741 N Vermont Avenue
Los Angeles, CA 90029

213-663-1111
e-mail: bils@brailib.org

Offers help, programs, services and information to the blind and visually impaired children and adults.

Dr. Henry Chang, Librarian

5949 Braille Institute Youth Center
3450 Cahuenga Boulevard W
Los Angeles, CA 90068

213-851-5695

Offers various youth programs and services for the blind and visually impaired youngster.

5950 New Beginnings - Blind Children's Center
4120 Marathon, Street
Los Angeles, CA 90029

323-664-2153
800-222-3566
Fax: 323-665-3828

Helps children and their families become independent by creating a climate of safety and trust. Services include an infant stimulation program, educational preschool, interdisciplinary assessment services, family services, correspondence program, toll-free national hotline and a publication and research service.

5951 San Francisco Public Library for the Blind and Print Disabled
100 Larkin Street
San Francisco, CA 94102

415-557-4293
Fax: 415-557-4375
e-mail: lbphmgr@sfpl.lib.ca.us
www.library.ca.us

Foreign-language books on cassette, children's books on cassettes and more.

Martin Maqid, Librarian

5952 Variety Audio
PO Box 5731
San Jose, CA 95150

408-277-4839

Summer reading programs, braille writer, magnifiers, closed-circuit TV, large-print photocopier, cassette books and magazines, children's books on cassette, home visits and other reference materials on blindness and other handicaps.

Louisa Griehshammer

District of Columbia

5953 Council of Families with Visual Impairment
1155 15th Street NW
Washington, DC 20005

202-467-5081

Members are sighted parents of blind or visually impaired children. Offers a forum for support and outreach, sharing of experiences in parent-child relationships, and educational and cultural information about child development. Monitors developments in technical and legislative arenas.

Nola Webb, President

Florida

5954 Florida Bureau of Braille and Talking Book Library Services
420 Platt Street
Daytona Beach, FL 32114

386-239-6000
Fax: 386-239-6069
TDD: 800-226-6079
e-mail: mike_gunde@dbs.doe.state.fl.us
www.state.fl.us/dbs/lswel.html

Discs, cassettes, closed-circuit TV, large-print photocopier, films, children's books on cassettes and more.

Michael Gunde, Librarian

5955 Talking Book Library, Jacksonville Public Library
1755 Edgewood Avenue W, Suite 1
Jacksonville, FL 32208

904-765-5588
Fax: 904-768-7404
TDD: 904-768-7822
e-mail: jerryr@coj.net
neflin.org/neflin/members/jackspub.html

Discs, cassettes and reference materials on blindness and other disabilities.

Jerry Reynolds, Librarian Senior

5956 Talking Book Service - Manatee County Central Library
6081 26th Street W
Bradenton, FL 34207

941-742-5914
Fax: 941-751-7089
TDD: 941-742-5951
e-mail: patricia.schubert@co.manatee.fl.us
www.co.manatee.fl.us

Offers children's books on disc and cassette and more reference materials for the blind and physically handicapped.

Patricia Schubert, Librarian

Georgia

5957 Albany Library for the Blind and Physical Handicapped
300 Pine Avenue
Albany, GA 31701

229-420-3220
Fax: 229-420-3240
e-mail: sinquefk@mail.dougherty.public.lib.ga.us
www.docolib.org/LBPH/index.html

Offers discs, cassettes, reference materials on blindness and other handicaps, large-print photocopiers, summer reading programs, cassette books and more.

Kathryn Sinquefield, Librarian

5958 Bainbridge Subregional Library for the Blind and Physically Handicapped
301 S Monroe Street
Bainbridge, GA 31717

912-248-2680
800-795-2680
Fax: 912-248-2670
TDD: 912-248-2665
e-mail: lbph@mail.deccatur.public.lib.ga.us
www.deccatur.public.lib.ga.us/local/lbph/lbph1.htm

Discs, cassettes, summer reading programs, closed-circuit TV, magnifiers and more.

Kathy Hutchins, Librarian

5959 CEL Subregional Library for the Blind and Physically Handicapped
2708 Mechanics
Savannah, GA 31401

912-354-5864
Fax: 912-354-5534
TDD: 912-652-3635
e-mail: stokesl@cel.co.chatman.ga.us

Summer reading programs, braille writer, magnifiers, closed-circuit TV, large-print photocopier, cassette books and magazines, children's books on cassette, home visits and other reference materials on blindness and other handicaps.

Linda Stokes, Librarian

Idaho

5960 Idaho State Talking Book Library
325 W State Street
Boise, ID 83702

208-334-2117
Fax: 208-334-4016
TDD: 800-377-1363
e-mail: tblbooks@isl.state.id.us
www.lili.org/isl/tblinfo.htm

Summer reading programs, braille writer, magnifiers, closed-circuit TV, large-print photocopier, cassette books and magazines, children's books on cassette, home visits and other reference materials on blindness and other handicaps.

Sue Walker, Librarian

Illinois

5961 Chicago Library Service for the Blind
1055 W Roosevelt Road
Chicago, IL 60608

312-746-9210

Summer reading programs, braille writer, magnifiers, closed-circuit TV, large-print photocopier, cassette books and magazines, children's books on cassette, home visits and other reference materials on blindness and other handicaps.

Carol Pellish, Librarian

5962 Illinois State Library, Talkng Book and Braille Service
300 S 2nd Street
Springfield, IL 62701

217-782-9435
Fax: 217-782-8261
TDD: 800-665-5576
e-mail: sruda@ilsos.net
www.cyberdriveillinois.com/library/isl/bph/bph.html

Summer reading programs, braille writer, magnifiers, closed-circuit TV, large-print photocopier, cassette books and magazines, descriptive videos, children's books on cassette, home visits and other reference materials on blindness and other handicaps.

Sharon Ruda, Librarian

5963 Mid Illinois Talking Book System
515 York Street
Quincy, IL 62301

217-224-6619
Fax: 217-224-9818

Summer reading programs, braille writer, magnifiers, closed-circuit TV, large-print photocopier, cassette books and magazines, children's books on cassette, home visits and other reference materials on blindness and other handicaps.

5964 Mid-Illinois Talking Book Center
845 Brenkman Drive
Pekin, IL 61554

309-353-4110
Fax: 309-353-8281
e-mail: hitbc@darkstar.rsa.lib.il.us
www.mitbc.org

Summer reading programs, braille writer, magnifiers, closed-circuit TV, large-print photocopier, cassette books and magazines, children's books on cassette, home visits and other reference materials on blindness and other handicaps.

Eileen Sheppard, Librarian

5965 Talking Book Center of Northwest Illinois
PO Box 125
Coal Valley, IL 61240

309-799-3137
Fax: 309-799-7916
e-mail: kodean@libby.rbls.lib.il.us
www.rbls.lib.il.us

Subregional library provides Talking Book and Braille Book programs to eligible persons unable to use standard print materials due to visual or physical disabilities. Includes cassette books and magazines; summer reading program.

Indiana

5966 Northwest Indiana Subregional Library for Blind and Physically Handicapped
1919 W Lincoln Highway
Merrillville, IN 46410

219-769-3541
Fax: 219-769-0690

Summer reading programs, braille writer, magnifiers, closed-circuit TV, large-print photocopier, cassette books and magazines, children's books on cassette, home visits and other reference materials on blindness and other handicaps.

Renee Lewis

Iowa

5967 Iowa Library for the Blind and Physically Handicapped
Iowa Department for the Blind
524 4th Street
Des Moines, IA 50309

515-281-1333
Fax: 515-281-1378
TDD: 515-281-1355
e-mail: keninger.karen@blind.state.ia.us
www.blind.state.ia.us

Summer reading programs, magnifiers, closed-circuit TV, large-print photocopier, children's books on cassette, children's books in Braille and Print Braille, cassette magazines, home visits and reference materials on blindness and other handicaps.

Karen Keninger, Program Manager/Librarian

Kansas

5968 CKLS Headquarters
1409 Williams Street
Great Bend, KS 67530

316-792-2393
800-362-2642
Fax: 316-792-5495
e-mail: cenks@ink.org
www.macular.org

Summer reading programs, braille writer, magnifiers, closed-circuit TV, large-print photocopier, cassette books and magazines, children's books on cassette, home visits and other reference materials on blindness and other handicaps.

Jerri Robinson, Librarian

5969 Services for the Visually Disabled
629 Poyntz Avenue
Manhattan, KS 66502

785-776-4741
Fax: 785-776-1545
e-mail: marionr@manhattan.lib.ks.us

Summer reading programs, braille writer, magnifiers, closed-circuit TV, large-print photocopier, cassette books and magazines, children's books on cassette, home visits and other reference materials on blindness and other handicaps.

Marion Rice, Librarian

Kentucky

5970 Kentucky Library for the Blind and Physically Handicapped
PO Box 818
Frankfort, KY 40602

502-564-8300
800-372-2968
Fax: 502-564-5773
e-mail: richard.feindel@kdla.net
www.kdla.net/libserv/ktbl.htm

Large-print photocopier, cassette books and magazines, children's books on cassette, and other reference materials on blindness and other handicaps.

5,200 members

Richard Feindel, Librarian

Maryland

5971 Maryland State Library for the Blind and Physically Handicapped
415 Park Avenue
Baltimore, MD 21201

410-230-2424
Fax: 410-333-2095
TTY: 800-934-2541
TDD: 410-333-8679
e-mail: recept@lbta.lib.md.us
www.lbph.lib.md.us

Summer reading programs, braille writer, magnifiers, large-print photocopier, cassette books and magazines, children's books on cassette, and other reference materials on blindness and other handicaps.

5972 Prince George's County Memorial Library Talking Book Center
6530 Adelphi Road
Hyattsville, MD 20782

301-779-9330

Summer reading programs, braille writer, magnifiers, closed-circuit TV, large-print photocopier, cassette books and magazines, children's books on cassette, home visits and other reference materials on blindness and other handicaps.

Shirley Tuthill, Librarian

Massachusetts

5973 Braille and Talking Book Library Perkins School for the Blind
175 N Beacon Street
Watertown, MA 02472

617-924-3434
Fax: 617-926-2027
e-mail: perkins@bpl.org
www.perkins.org

Patricia Kirk

5974 Carroll Center for the Blind
770 Centre Street
Newton, MA 02158

617-969-6200
800-852-3131
Fax: 617-969-6204
www.carroll.org

Assists blind and visually impaired adults and adolescents to adjust to loss of vision. The goal of this dynamic program is to help the person become more independent, to restore self-confidence, prepare for employment and improve the quality of life. Programs of individual counseling are offered as part of the program.

Rachel Rosenbaum, President

Michigan

5975 Downtown Detroit Subregional Library for the Blind and Handicapped
121 Gratiot Avenue
Detroit, MI 48226

313-224-0580
Fax: 313-965-1977
TDD: 313-224-0584
e-mail: deveans@cms.xx.wayne.edu
www.detroit.lib.mi.us

Summer reading programs, braille writer, magnifiers, closed-circuit TV, large-print photocopier, cassette books and magazines, children's books on cassette, home visits and other reference materials on blindness and other handicaps.

Deborah Evans, Librarian

5976 Kent County Library for the Blind
775 Ball Avenue NE
Grand Rapids, MI 49503

616-336-3250
Fax: 616-336-3201
e-mail: kdlem@lakeland.lib.mi.us

Summer reading programs, braille writer, magnifiers, closed-circuit TV, large-print photocopier, cassette books and magazines, children's books on cassette, home visits and other reference materials on blindness and other handicaps.

Claudya Muller, Librarian

5977 Library of Michigan Service for the Blind
PO Box 30007
Lansing, MI 48909

517-373-5614
Fax: 517-373-5865
e-mail: info@sbph.libomich.lib.mi.us

Summer reading programs, braille writer, magnifiers, closed-circuit TV, large-print photocopier, cassette books and magazines, children's books on cassette, home visits and other reference materials on blindness and other handicaps.

5978 Macomb Library for the Blind and Physically Handicapped
16480 Hall Road
Clinton Township, MI 48038

586-286-1580
Fax: 586-286-0634
TDD: 810-869-40
e-mail: macbld@libcoop.net
www.macomb.lib.mi.us/macspe/

Summer reading programs, braille writer, closed-circuit TV, cassette books and magazines, children's books on cassette, reference materials on blindness and other handicaps.

Beverlee Babcock, Librarian

5979 Mideastern Michigan Library Co-op
G-4195 W Pasadena Avenue
Flint, MI 48504

810-732-1120
Fax: 810-732-1715
e-mail: cnash@genesse.freeret.org
www.fakon.edu/gdl/talking.htm

Summer reading programs, braille writer, magnifiers, closed-circuit TV, large-print photocopier, cassette books and magazines, children's books on cassette, home visits and other reference materials on blindness and other handicaps.

Carolyn Nash, Librarian

5980 Muskegon County Library for the Blind
635 Ottawa Street
Muskegon, MI 49442

231-724-6248
Fax: 231-724-6675
TDD: 231-722-4103
www.muskcolib.org

Summer reading programs, braille typewriter, magnifiers, closed-circuit TV, large-print photocopier, cassette books and magazines, children's books on cassette, home visits and other reference materials on blindness and other handicaps, The Reading Edge, Perkins Brailler and large print books.

Linda Clapp, Librarian

5981 Upper Peninsula Library for the Blind Physically Handicapped
1615 Presque Isle Avenue
Marquette, MI 49855

906-228-7697
Fax: 906-228-5627
e-mail: uproc.lib.mi.us
www.upesc.lib.mi.us/uplbph

Summer reading programs, braille writer, magnifiers, closed-circuit TV, large-print photocopier, cassette books and magazines, children's books on cassette, home visits and other reference materials on blindness and other handicaps.

Suzanne Dees, Librarian

5982 Washtenaw County Library
PO Box 8645
Ann Arbor, MI 48107

734-222-4357
Fax: 734-222-6715
e-mail: contact us@ewashtenaw.org
www.ewashtenaw.org

Summer reading programs, braille writer, magnifiers, closed-circuit TV, large-print photocopier, cassette books and magazines, children's books on cassette, home visits and other reference materials on blindness and other handicaps.

Margeret Wolfe, Librarian

5983 Washtenaw County Library for the Blind and Physically Disabled
PO Box 8645
Ann Arbor, MI 48107

734-971-6059
Fax: 734-971-3892
e-mail: lbpd@co.washtennaw.mi.us
www.co.washten.ml.us/depts/lib/liblbpd.h

Book lovers club.adaptive technology,cassette equipment, cassette books and magazines, described videos, low vision aids reference and referral services.

Margaret Wolfe, Coordinator

5984 Wayne County Regional Library for the Blind
30555 Michigan Avenue
Westland, MI 48186

734-727-7300
Fax: 734-727-7333
TTY: 734-727-7330
e-mail: werlbph@tln.lib.mi.us
www.wayneregional.lib.mi.us

Summer reading programs, braille writer, magnifiers, closed-circuit TV, large-print photocopier, cassette books and magazines, children's books on cassette, home visits and other reference materials on blindness and other handicaps.

Reginald Williams, Wayne County Librarian

Minnesota

5985 Minnesota Library for the Blind & Physically Handicapped
Highway 298, PO Box 68
Fairbault, MN 55021

507-333-4828
800-722-0550
Fax: 507-333-4832
e-mail: libblnd@state.mn.us

Summer reading programs, braille writer, magnifiers, closed-circuit TV, large-print photocopier, cassette, large print, braille books and magazines, children's books on cassette, and other reference materials on blindness and other handicaps.

Catherine A Durivage, Program Director

Missouri

5986 Adriene Resource Center for Blind Children
1445 Boonville Avenue
Springfield, MO 65802

417-862-2781
Fax: 417-862-7566
e-mail: blind@ag.org
www.gospelpublishing.com

Offers braille and cassette lending library, braille and cassette Sunday school materials for all ages, braille and cassette periodicals and resource assistance, and resources for blind children and children of blind parents.

Paul Weingariner, Director

5987 Assemblies of God National Center for the Blind
1445 Boonville Avenue
Springfield, MO 65802

417-862-2781
Fax: 417-862-7566
e-mail: blind@ag.org
www.gospelpublishing.com

Offers braille and cassette lending library, braille and cassette Sunday school materials for all ages, braille and cassette periodicals and resource assistance, and resources for blind children and children of blind parents.

Paul Weingariner, Director

5988 Wolfner Memorial Library for the Blind
PO Box 387
Jefferson City, MO 65102

573-751-8720
Fax: 573-526-2985
TDD: 800-347-1379
e-mail: beckles@mail.sos.state.mo.us

Summer reading programs, braille writer, magnifiers, closed-circuit TV, large-print photocopier, cassette books and magazines, children's books on cassette, home visits and other reference materials on blindness and other handicaps.

Elizabeth Eckles, Librarian

Nebraska

5989 Nebraska Library Commission Talking Book & Braille Services
1200 N Street
Lincoln, NE 68508

402-471-4038
800-742-7691
Fax: 402-471-6244
TDD: 402-471-4038
e-mail: doertli@nlc.state.ne.us
www.ncl.state.ne.us/tbbs/tbbsl/html

Free loan of books and magazines on cassette and in Braille, including children's materials, along with specially designed playback equipment. Summer reading program for children, Braille embossing, closed circuit TV, large-print copier. Reference materials on blindness and other disabilities.

David Oerti, Librarian

New Jersey

5990 New Jersey Library for the Blind and Handicapped
2300 Stuyvesant Avenue
Trenton, NJ 08618

609-292-6450
800-792-8322
Fax: 609-530-6384
TDD: 877-882-5593
e-mail: nglbh@njstatelib.org
www.mjstatelib.org

Summer reading programs, braille writer, magnifiers, closed-circuit TV, large-print, cassette braille books and magazines, children's books on cassettes in braille and other reference materials on blindness and other handicaps.

Deborah Rutledeger, Director

New Mexico

5991 New Mexico State Library for the Blind and Physically Handicapped
1209 Camino Carlos Ray
Santa Fe, NM

505-476-9700
Fax: 505-476-9701
e-mail: jbrewstr@stlib.state.nm.us
www.stlib.state.nm.us

Summer reading programs, braille writer, magnifiers, closed-circuit TV, large-print photocopier, cassette books and magazines, children's books on cassette, home visits and other reference materials on blindness and other handicaps.

Glee Wenzel, Librarian

New York

5992 Helen Keller National Center
111 Middle Neck Road
Sands Point, NY 11050

516-944-8900
Fax: 516-944-7302

Provides diagnostic, evaluation, short term comprehensive rehabilitation and personal adjustment training. A technical assistance center is offered providing assistance to public and private agencies and to parent groups who work towards community integration and the enhancement of the quality of life. A national parent network is also provided that develops and shares information about advocacy, legislation, new services and achievements.

5993 New York State Talking Book & Braille Library
Empire State Plaza, CEC
Albany, NY 12230

518-474-5801
Fax: 518-474-5786
TDD: 518-474-7121
e-mail: jane@unix2.nysed.gov
www.suffolk.lib.ny.us

Books on audio cassette, cassette players, braille books, summer reading programs, braille writer, magnifiers, closed-circuit TV, large-print photocopier, cassette books and magazines, children's books on cassette, reference materials on blindness and other handicaps.

Jane Somers, Director

North Carolina

5994 North Carolina Library for the Blind
1811 Capital Boulevard
Raleigh, NC 27635

919-733-4376
Fax: 919-733-6910
TDD: 919-733-1462
e-mail: nclbph@ncsl.der.state.nc

Summer reading programs, braille writer, magnifiers, closed-circuit TV, large-print photocopier, cassette books and magazines, children's books on cassette, home visits and other reference materials on blindness and other handicaps.

Francine Martin, Librarian

Ohio

5995 American Council of Blind Parents
34400 Cedar Road, Apartment 108
University Heights, OH 44121

800-424-8666

Members are sighted parents of blind or visually impaired children. Offers a forum for support and outreach, sharing of experiences in parent-child relationships, and educational and cultural information about child development. Monitors developments in technical and legislative arenas.

Nola Webb, President

Oregon

5996 Oregon State Library, Talking Book and Braille Services
250 Winter Street NW
Salem, OR 97310

503-378-4243
Fax: 503-588-7119
TDD: 503-378-4276
e-mail: tbabs@sparkie.osl.state.or.us

Cassette books and magazines, children's books on cassette, home visits and other reference materials on blindness and other handicaps.

Donna Bensen, Regional Librarian

Virginia

5997 Alexandria Library Talking Book Service
5005 Duke Street
Alexandria, VA 22304

703-519-5900
Fax: 703-519-5915
TDD: 703-838-4568
e-mail: emccaffr@lea.eda
www.www.alexandria.lib.va.us

Summer reading programs, braille writer, magnifiers, closed-circuit TV, large-print photocopier, cassette books and magazines, children's books on cassette, home visits and other reference materials on blindness and other handicaps.

Patricia Bates, Librarian

5998 Division for the Visually Handicapped
1920 Association Drive
Reston, VA 20191

703-620-3660

Members are teachers, college faculty members, administrators, supervisors and others concerned with the education and welfare of visually handicapped and blind children and youth. This is a division of the Council For Exceptional Children.

Dr. Kay Ferrell, President

5999 Division on Visual Impairments
Council for Exceptional Children
1110 North Glebe Road, Suite 300
Arlington, VA 22201

800-224-6830
Fax: 703-264-9494
TTY: 866-915-5000
www.ed.arizona.edu/dvi/welcome.htm; www.cec.sped.org

A division within the CEC, it handles concerns for Federal, state and local issues and policies related to education of youths, children and infants with visual impairments.

Ellyn Ross, President
Shirley J Wilson, Secretary

6000 Virginia State Library for the Visually and Physically Handicapped
1901 Roane Street
Richmond, VA 23222

804-367-0014

Summer reading programs, braille writer, magnifiers, closed-circuit TV, large-print photocopier, cassette books and magazines, children's books on cassette, home visits and other reference materials on blindness and other handicaps.

Mary Ruth Halapatz, Librarian

Washington

6001 Washington Library for the Blind and Physically Handicapped
821 Lenora Street
Seattle, WA 98129

206-386-4636
Fax: 206-386-4685
e-mail: wtbbl@spl.lib.wa.us
www.spl.lib.wa.us

Summer reading programs, braille writer, magnifiers, closed-circuit TV, large-print photocopier, cassette books and magazines, children's books on cassette, home visits and other reference materials on blindness and other handicaps.

Jan Ames, Librarian

West Virginia

6002 West Virginia School for the Blind
301 E Main Street
Romney, WV 26757

304-822-3521
Fax: 304-822-4896
e-mail: cjohn@access.mountain.net

Summer reading programs, braille writer, magnifiers, closed-circuit TV, large-print photocopier, cassette books and magazines, children's books on cassette, home visits and other reference materials on blindness and other handicaps.

Cynthia Johnson, Librarian

Research Centers

6003 Arlene R Gordon Research Institute
Lighthouse International
111 E 59th Street
New York, NY 10022

212-821-9525
800-829-0500
Fax: 212-821-9707
TTY: 212-821-9713
e-mail: research@lighthouse.org
www.lighthouse.org

The institute is the only research institute within a vision rehabilitation agency. Trainees can come and acquire research skills in both laboratory and field settings. It is comprised on these major divisions: Evaluation research; Vision research; and Psychosocial research.

Amy Horowitz, Director
Joann P Reinhardt PhD, Director Psychosocial Research

6004 Center for the Partially Sighted
12301 Wilshire Boulevard, Suite 600
Los Angeles, CA 90025

310-458-3501
Fax: 310-458-8179
e-mail: info@low-vision.org
www.low-vision.org

Provides professional, comprehensive vision rehabilitation services to visually impaired people of all ages. For those whose sight is severely limited due to macular degeneration, diabetic retinopathy, glaucoma, retinal detachment, stroke or other conditions not correctable medically or surgically.

6005 Helen Keller National Center
111 Middle Neck Road
Sands Point, NY 11050

516-944-8900
Fax: 516-944-7302

Provides diagnostic evaluation, short term comprehensive rehabilitation and personal adjustment training. A technical assistance center is offered providing assistance to public and private agencies and to parent groups who work towards community integration and the enhancement of the quality of life. A national parent network is also provided that develops and shares information about advocacy, legislation, new services and achievements.

6006 Mobile Association for the Blind
2440 Gordon Smith Drive
Mobile, AL 36617

251-473-3585
877-292-5463
Fax: 251-470-8622
e-mail: sales@mobile.blind.com
www.mobileblind.com

Offers work adjustment training, activities of daily living, mobility, communication skills and sheltered employment for adults and children who are visually impaired.

Mahlon McCracken, Executive Director

6007 National Eye Research Foundation
910 Skokie Boulevard, Suite 207A
Northbrook, IL 60062

847-564-4652
800-621-2258
Fax: 847-564-0807
e-mail: info@nerf.org
www.nerf.org

Devoted to the enhancement of care and study of eye related diseases.

6008 New Beginnings - The Blind Children's Center
4120 Marathon Street
Los Angeles, CA 90029

213-664-2153

The purpose of the Center is to turn initial fears into hope. Helps children and their families become independent by creating a climate of safety and trust. Children learn to develop self confidence and to master a wide range of skills. Services include an infant stimulation program, educational preschool, interdisciplinary assessment services, family services, correspondence program, toll free national hotline and a publication and research service.

6009 Research to Prevent Blindness
645 Madison Avenue
New York, NY 10022

212-752-4333
800-621-0026
www.rpbusa.org

Provides research grants to scientists interested in eye disease and vision disorders.

Audio Video

6010 Heart to Heart
Blind Children's Center
4120 Marathon Street
Los Angeles, CA 90029

323-644-2153
Fax: 323-665-3828
www.blindcntr.org

Parents of blind and partially sighted children talk about their feelings.

Videotape

6011 Let's Eat
Blind Children's Center
4120 Marathon Street
Los Angeles, CA 90029

213-664-2153
Fax: 213-665-3828

Teaches competent feeding skills to children with visual impairments.

Videotape

6012 See What I Feel
Britannica Film Co.
345 4th Street
San Francisco, CA 94107

415-597-5555

A blind child tells her friends about her trip to the zoo. Each experience was explained as a blind child would experience it. A teacher's guide comes with this video.

Films

Web Sites

6013 Lighthouse International
www.lighthouse.org

The mission is to overcome vision impairment for people of all ages through worldwide leadership in rehabilitation services, education, research, prevention and advocacy.

6014 National Alliance of Blind Students
www.blindstudents.org

The leading national advocacy and consumer organization for students in high school or college who are blind or visually impaired.

6015 National Association for Visually Handicapped
www.navh.org

Helps to cope with the difficulties of vision impairment.

Book Publishers

6016 Children with Visual Impairments: A Parents' Guide
Peytral Publications
PO Box 1162
Minnetonka, MN 55345

952-949-8707
877-739-8725
Fax: 952-906-9777
www.peytral.com

Covers visual impairments ranging from low vision to total blindness. Offers authoritative information and empathy, parental insight on diagnosis and treatment, orientation and mobility, literacy, legal issues and more. Valuable to parents, educators and support staff.

395 pages

M Cay Holbrook PhD, Editor

6017 Mainstreaming the Visually Impaired Child: Blind & Partially Sighted Students

Michael D Oralnsky PhD, author

Nat'l Assn for Parents of Children with Visual
PO Box 317
Watertown, MA 02471

617-972-7441
800-562-6265
Fax: 617-972-7444
www.spedex.com/napvi

121 pages

6018 Ophthalmic Disorders Sourcebook
Omnigraphics
615 Griswold
Detroit, MI 48226

313-961-1340
800-234-1340
Fax: 800-875-1340
e-mail: info@omnigraphics.com
www.omnigraphics.com

Basic consumer information about glaucoma, cataracts, macular degeneration, strabismus, refractive disorders and more.

1996 631 pages
ISBN: 0-780800-81-8

Magazines

6019 Journal of Visual Impairment and Blindness
American Foundation for the Blind
11 Penn Plaza, Suite 300
New York, NY 10001

212-502-7600
Fax: 212-502-7777
e-mail: afbinfo@afb.net
www.afb.org

Published in braille, regular print and on cassette this journal contains a wide variety of subjects including rehabilitation, psychology, education, legislation, medicine, technology, employment, sensory aids and childhood development as they relate to visual impairments.

10x Year

6020 Reaching, Crawling, Walking - Let's Get Moving

Blind Children's Center
4120 Marathon Street
Los Angeles, CA 90029

323-664-2153
Fax: 323-665-3828
e-mail: info@blindchildrenscenter.org
www.blindchildrenscenter.org

Orientation and mobility for visually impaired preschool children.

24 pages

6021 Seeing Candy

National Association for Visually Handicapped
22 W 21st Street, 6th Floor
New York, NY 10010

212-889-3141
Fax: 212-727-2931
e-mail: staff@navh.org
www.navh.org

This newsletter offers short stories, news, medical updates, assistive device information, poems, resources, crossword puzzles and more for the visually impaired.

Biannually

6022 Tactic

Clovernook Home and School for the Blind
7000 Hamilton Avenue
Cincinnati, OH 45231

513-522-3860
Fax: 513-728-3950
e-mail: clovernook@aol.com

Quarterly

Newsletters

6023 Awareness

Nat'l Assn for Parents of Children with Visual
PO Box 317
Watertown, MA 02471

617-972-7441
800-562-6265
Fax: 617-972-7444
www.spedex.com/napvi/awareness.html

Contains NAPVI regional news, commentary, letters to the editor, legislative updates, and information on conferences and events.

32 pages Quarterly

6024 National Library Service for the Blind & Physically Handicapped

Library of Congress Reference Section
1291 Taylor Street NW
Washington, DC 20542

202-707-5100
800-424-8567
Fax: 202-707-0712
TTY: 202-707-0744
TDD: 202-707-0744
e-mail: nis@loc.gov
www.loc.gov/nls

Provides information and advocacy resources for families and professionals, including listings of organizations focusing on more specific areas of concern to families and young adults who have disabilities. Administers a natural library service that provides recorded and braille reading materials to eligible children and adults who cannot read standard print.

12 pages Quarterly
ISSN: 1046-1663

Vicki Fitzpatrick, Editor

6025 Talking Book Topics

National Library Services for the Blind
1291 Taylor Street NW
Washington, DC 20542

202-707-5100
Fax: 202-707-0712
www.loc.gov/nls

Offers hundreds of listings of books, fiction and nonfiction, for adults and children on cassette. Also offers listings on foreign language books on cassette, talking magazines and reviews.

Bimonthly

Pamphlets

6026 Dancing Cheek to Cheek

Blind Children's Center
4120 Marathon Street
Los Angeles, CA 90029

213-664-2153
Fax: 213-665-3828
www.blindchildrenscenter.org

Discusses beginning social, play and language interactions.

33 pages

6027 Family Guide - Growth and Development of the Partially Seeing Child

National Association for Visually Handicapped
22 W 21st Street, 6th Floor
New York, NY 10010

212-889-3141
Fax: 212-727-2931
e-mail: staff@navh.org
www.navh.org

Offers information for parents and guidelines in raising a partially seeing child.

6028 Family Guide to Vision Care

American Optometric Association
243 N Lindbergh Boulevard
Saint Louis, MO 63141

314-991-4100
Fax: 314-991-4101
www.aoanet.org

Offers information on the early developmental years of your vision, finding a family optometrist and how to take care of your eyesight through the learning years, the working years and the mature years.

6029 Heart to Heart

Blind Children's Center
4120 Marathon Street
Los Angeles, CA 90029

213-664-2153
Fax: 213-665-3828
www.blindchildrenscenter.org

Parents of blind and partially sighted children talk about their feelings.

12 pages

6030 Learning to Play

Blind Children's Center
4120 Marathon Street
Los Angeles, CA 90029

213-664-2153
Fax: 213-665-3828
www.blindchildrenscenter.org

Discusses how to present play activities to the visually impaired preschool child.

12 pages

6031 Let's Eat

Blind Children's Center
4120 Marathon Street
Los Angeles, CA 90029

213-664-2153
Fax: 213-665-3828
www.blindchildrenscenter.org

Teaches competent feeding skills to children with visual impairments.

28 pages

6032 Move with Me

Blind Children's Center
4120 Marathon Street
Los Angeles, CA 90029

213-664-2153
Fax: 213-665-3828
www.blindchildrenscenter.org

A parent's guide to movement development for visually impaired babies.

12 pages

6033 Selecting a Program

Blind Children's Center
4120 Marathon Street
Los Angeles, CA 90029

213-664-2153
Fax: 213-665-3828
www.blindchildrenscenter.org

A guide for parents of infants and preschoolers with visual impairments.

28 pages

6034 Standing on My Own Two Feet

Blind Children's Center
4120 Marathon Street
Los Angeles, CA 90029

323-664-2153
Fax: 323-665-3828
e-mail: info@blindchildrenscenter.org
www.blindchildrenscenter.org

A step-by-step guide to designing and constructing simple, individually tailored adaptive mobility devices for preschool-age children who are visually impaired.

36 pages

6035 Talk to Me

Blind Children's Center
4120 Marathon Street
Los Angeles, CA 90029

213-664-2153
Fax: 213-665-3828
www.blindchildrenscenter.org

A language guide for parents of deaf children.

11 pages

6036 Talk to Me II

Blind Children's Center
4120 Marathon Street
Los Angeles, CA 90029

213-664-2153
Fax: 213-665-3828
www.blindchildrenscenter.org

A sequel to Talk To Me, available in English and Spanish.

15 pages

Camps

6037 Bloomfield

5300 Angeles Vista Boulevard
Los Angeles, CA 90043

323-295-4555
800-352-2290
Fax: 323-296-0424
e-mail: info@juniorblind.org
www.junoirblind.org

This camp is dedicated to serving blind and developmentally disabled children and adults.

6038 Florida School-Deaf and Blind

207 San Marco Avenue
Saint Augustine, FL 32084

800-800-344
www2.kidscamps.com

6039 National Camps for Blind Children

Christian Record
4444 S 52nd Street
Lincoln, NE 68516

402-488-0981
Fax: 402-488-7582
e-mail: info@christianrecord.org
www.christianrecord.org

Camps throughout the US and Canada are offered at no cost to the legally blind, ages 9-65. Activities include archery, beeper basketball, water sports, hiking and rock climbing and horseback riding. $35 registration fee.

Keith Elliott, Director

6040 VISIONS/Vacation Camp for the Blind

500 Greenwich Street, 3rd Floor
New York, NY 10013

212-625-1616
888-245-8333
Fax: 212-219-4078
e-mail: tmdecker@visionvcb.org
www.visionvcb.org

Family programs at Vacation Camp for the Blind in Rockland County, NY for children who are blind, severely visually impaired or multi-handicapped. Parent or guardian must attend winter weekends and summer session.

Thomas M Decker, Camp Director
Nancy D Miller, Executive Director

DESCRIPTION

6041 RESPIRATORY DISTRESS SYNDROME OF THE NEWBORN

Synonyms: Hyaline membrane disese (HMD), RDS

Covers these related disorders: Meconium aspiration syndrome

Involves the following Biologic System(s):

Neonatal and Infant Disorders, Respiratory Disorders

Respiratory distress syndrome of the newborn (RDS) is a breathing disorder characterized by insufficient production of surfactant, which consists of substances produced by certain cells in the lungs. Surfactant contributes to the elasticity of lung (pulmonary) tissue and enables the air sacs (alveoli) of the lungs to remain open between breaths. The exchange of oxygen and carbon dioxide takes place across the thin walls of the air sacs. Due to insufficient surfactant in newborns with RDS, greater pressure is required to expand the lungs' airways and air sacs. As a result, the air sacs may collapse and the lungs may become unable to properly provide oxygenated blood to the body.

Surfactant is produced as the lungs mature during fetal development. Sufficient levels of surfactant are often present after approximately 35 weeks of pregnancy (gestation). RDS primarily occurs in newborns who are born prior to 37 weeks of gestation (premature newborns), affecting up to 80 percent of those who are born before 28 weeks' gestation and up to 30 percent of infants born between 32 and 36 weeks' gestation. The condition also occurs with increased frequency in infants who are born to mothers with diabetes or those who are delivered by Cesarean section. In other newborns, RDS may occur in the absence of known predisposing factors or may be due to certain birth defects or other conditions, such as meconium aspiration syndrome.rome, or persistent fetal circulation. Respiratory distress syndrome of the newborn is sometimes referred to as hyaline membrane disease, because insufficient surfactant production may cause the formation of a fibrous membrane known as hyaline membrane lining the lungs' small airways (bronchioles), ducts (alveolar ducts), and air sacs (alveoli).

Symptoms associated with RDS usually occur within minutes of birth, although they may not be recognized for several hours. These symptoms may vary in severity, depending upon the degree of prematurity or other underlying causes responsible for the condition. Newborns may experience increasing difficulty breathing (dyspnea), characterized by rapid, labored, shallow breaths (tachypnea); grunting upon exhalation; drawing in of the chest wall during inhalation; and bluish discoloration of the skin and mucous membranes (cyanosis) due to lack of sufficient oxygen supply to bodily tissues (hypoxia). Air may leak into the chest cavity surrounding the lungs (pneumothorax), causing collapse of the lungs and further breathing difficulties. Without appropriate treatment, cyanosis and breathing difficulties may progressively worsen and body temperature and blood pressure may fall. As infants with severe RDS tire, grunting upon exhalation may subside, breathing becomes irregular, and life-threatening complications may result. Depending upon the severity of the condition, infants with RDS may begin to gradually improve in about three days or may experience life-threatening symptoms within approximately two to seven days after birth.

Meconium aspiration syndrome is characterized by blockage and irritation of the airways of the lungs due to passage of meconium before birth and inhalation of meconium before or during delivery. Meconium is the thick, sticky material that forms a newborn's first stools, and is typically passed during the first 24 to 48 hours after birth. In some cases, a fetus may pass meconium into the amniotic fluid before birth and then inhale this into the lungs before or right after birth. The skin of newborns with meconium aspiration is usually stained with meconium. In severe cases, symptoms include diminished muscle tone, an abnormally slow heartbeat, or absence of spontaneous respiration at birth.

In newborns with meconium aspiration syndrome, treatment may include immediate suctioning of an affected infant's mouth, throuat, and nose and placement of a tube into the windpipe to remove meconium from the airways. In most affected newborns, imporvement usually occurs in approximately three days.

If physicians suspect that a newborn may be born prematurely, steps may be taken to delay delivery in order to help decrease the risk of RDS. If delivery cannot be delayed, some women may be given certain corticosteroid medications (e.g., dexamethasone or betamethasone) approximately 48 to 72 hours before the delivery of premature newborns to help stimulate the production of surfactant before birth. In addition, an artificial surfactant may be administered into the windpipe of affected newborns immediately after birth or within 24 hours, to help reduce the severity of RDS and associated symptoms or complications. Additional treatment may include symptomatic and supportive measures, such as use of an oxygen hood or support with a ventilator.

See also **General Resources** on page 917

Government Agencies

6042 NIH/National Heart, Lung and Blood Institu te
National Institute of Health
31 Center Dr, Bldg 31 Rm 5A48
Bethesda, MD 20892

301-592-8573
Fax: 301-629-3246
TTY: 240-629-3255
e-mail: NHLBIinfo@nhlbi.nih.gov
www.nhlbi.nih.gov

Primary responsibility of this organization is the scientific investigation of heart, blood vessel, lung and blood disorders. Oversees research, demonstration, prevention, education, control and training activities in these fields and emphasizes the prevention and control of heart diseases.

Elizabeth G Nabel, MD, Director
Susan Shurin, MD, Deputy Director

6043 NIH/National Institute of Child Health and Human Development
31 Center Drive, Building 31
Bethesda, MD 20892

301-496-5133
Fax: 301-496-1104
www.nichd.nih.gov

Established in 1962 by congress, today the institute conducts and supports research on topics related to the health of children, adults, families and populations. Some of these topics include: developmental disabilities, growth and development, infant death, reproductive health and birth defects.

Nancy D Wirth, Director
Lisa Kaeser, Program & Public Liaison

National Associations & Support Groups

6044 American Lung Association
61 Broadway, 6th Floor
New York, NY 10006

212-315-8700
800-586-4872
www.lungusa.org

The American Lung Association fights lung disease in all its forms, with special emphasis on asthma, tobacco control and environmental health. The American Lung Association is funded with contributions from the public, along with gifts and grants from corporations, foundations and government agencies. The association achieves its many successes through the work of thousands of committed volunteers and staff.

Hallema Sharif Clyburn, Director Media Relations

6045 Genetic Alliance
4301 Connecticut Avenue NW
Washington, DC 20008

202-966-5557
800-336-4363
Fax: 202-966-8553
e-mail: info@geneticalliance.org
www.geneticalliance.org

A nonprofit tax exempt organization founded in 1986 as a national coalition of consumers, professionals and genetic support groups to voice the common concerns of children and adults and families living with, and at risk of, genetic conditions. The Alliance builds partnerships among consumers and professionals and the private and public sectors to promote optimum healthcare and enhanced quality of life for individuals identified with genetic conditions.

Sharon Terry, President/CEO

6046 March of Dimes Birth Defects Foundation
1275 Mamaroneck Avenue
White Plains, NY 10605

914-428-7100
888-663-4637
Fax: 914-428-8203
e-mail: resourcecenter@modimes.org
www.marchofdimes.com

Partnership of volunteers and professionals dedicated to improving the health of babies by preventing birth defects and infant mortality. Over 100 chapters are located across the country and can be located through the National Office.

Dr Jennifer Howse, President

Web Sites

6047 American Lung Association
www.lungusa.org

The American Lung Association fights lung disease in all its forms, with special emphasis on asthma, tobacco control and environmental health.

6048 KidsHealth
www.kidshealth.org

KidsHealth provides doctor-approved health information about children from before birth through adolescence.

6049 RSV Info Center
www.rsvinfo.com

A comprehensive overview about the most common cause of lower respiratory tract infections in children.

DESCRIPTION

6050 RESPIRATORY SYNCYTIAL VIRUS INFECTION

Synonym: RSV infection

Involves the following Biologic System(s):

Infectious Disorders, Respiratory Disorders

The respiratory syncytial virus (RSV) is the most common cause of lower respiratory tract infections in infants and young children. RSV is primarily spread by the inhalation of virus-containing airborne droplets. The virus is present worldwide and causes annual epidemics of RSV infection in late autumn, winter, or as late as May or June. Such outbreaks typically peak from January through March. Nearly every child is affected by RSV infection by age two, and many experience recurrent reinfection throughout childhood.

In older children and adults, RSV infection may cause no apparent symptoms (asymptomatic) or may result in mild to moderate lung infection and associated cold-like symptoms. However, RSV infection may be severe in others, particularly infants, young children, children with heart or lung disease, or individuals with compromised immune systems. In such patients, RSV infection may lead to inflammation of the lungs' small airways (bronchiolitis), inflammation of the airways and lung tissue (bronchopneumonia), or, in extremely severe cases, potentially life-threatening complications. RSV infection is known to be the leading cause of bronchiolitis or bronchopneumonia in children younger than one year of age.

In infants and young children with RSV infection, symptoms typically begin approximately four days after infection. Initial symptoms include a runny nose (rhinorrhea) and sore throat (pharyngitis). Patients may then develop a low fever, begin to cough and sneeze, and soon experience wheezing, which is the production of a whistling sound during breathing due to inflammation and associated narrowing of the airways. If RSV infection progresses, patients may develop additional symptoms, including increasing wheezing and coughing, an abnormally rapid rate of breathing (tachypnea), drawing in of the chest wall during inhalation, and bluish discoloration of the skin and mucous membranes (cyanosis). Patients with extremely severe disease progression may develop increasingly rapid breathing, temporary cessation of breathing (apnea), listlessness, and potentially life-threatening complications. In other infants or young children with RSV infection, initial running of the nose and coughing may be followed by poor feeding, listlessness, and difficulties breathing (dyspnea) with little or no wheezing.

As mentioned above, many children experience reinfection with RSV. Reinfection usually causes less severe symptoms than those associated with initial disease. However, depending upon the age of patients and other factors, secondary infections may also sometimes be associated with severe lower respiratory tract infections. Older children who experience reinfection with RSV generally have more mild symptoms.

In children with mild or moderate RSV infection without associated bronchiolitis or bronchopneumonia, treatment typically includes symptomatic and supportive measures. Affected infants, young children, children with heart or lung disease, or those with compromised immune systems may require hospitalization. Treatment may include providing respiratory therapy with humidified air to help supply adequate oxygen to bodily tissues; ensuring an adequate intake of fluids; or administering certain medications to relax the smooth muscles of the small airways (bronchodilators). Certain infants and children are at high risk for severe RSV disease, such as those with lung disease, congenital heart disease, or immunodeficiency. In these children, certain preventive or prophylactic therapies such as RSV-specific antibodies may be recommended to help reduce (or even prevent) the severity of RSV infection in these at-risk infants and young children.

See also **General Resources** on page 917

Government Agencies

6051 Centers for Disease Control
1600 Clifton Road
Atlanta, GA 30333

404-639-3311
www.cdc.gov

Mission is to promote health and quality of life by preventing and controlling disease, injury, and disability.

6052 NIH/National Institute of Allergy and Infectious Diseases
6610 Rockledge Drive, MSC 6612
Bethesda, MD 20892

301-496-5717
Fax: 301-402-3573
TDD: 800-877-8339
www.niaid.nih.gov

Conducts and supports basic and applied research to better understand, treat, and ultimately prevent infectious, immunologic, and allergic diseases.

Anthony S Fauci MD, Director

6053 NIH/National Institute of Child Health and Human Development
31 Center Drive, Building 31
Bethesda, MD 20892

301-496-5133
Fax: 301-496-1104
www.nichd.nih.gov

Established in 1962 by congress, today the institute conducts and supports research on topics related to the health of children, adults, families and populations. Some of these topics include: developmental disabilities, growth and development, infant death, reproductive health and birth defects.

Nancy D Wirth, Director
Lisa Kaeser, Program & Public Liaison

National Associations & Support Groups

6054 American Lung Association
61 Broadway, 6th Floor
New York, NY 10006

212-315-8700
www.lungusa.org

Founded in 1904 to fight tuberculosis, the American Lung Association today fights lung disease in all its forms, with special emphasis on asthma, tobacco control and environmental health.

Hallema Sharif Clyburn, Director Media Relations

6055 World Health Organization
Avenue Appia 20
CH-1211 Geneva 27,
Switzerland

www.who.int

WHO is the directing and coordinating authority for health within the United Nations system.

Dr Margaret Chan, Director General

Web Sites

6056 American Lung Association
www.lungusa.org

Information regarding lung disease in all its forms, with special emphasis on asthma, tobacco control and environmental health.

6057 KidsHealth
www.kidshealth.org/parent/infections/lung/rsv.html

Provides an explanation of the disorder as well as treatment and prevention.

6058 MediConsult
www.mediconsult.com/kids/shareware/rsv/

Is an independent firm of experienced consultants. Provides excellent consulting services and have successfully worked with private and public stakeholders in the healthcare system both locally and internationally. Our focus is to provide expertise and counsel and we encourage formation of teams with partners, clients and their staff, to jointly take a project from inception to implementation. Through this philosophy we have been able to achieve identifiable client benefits.

6059 RSV Info Center
www.rsvinfo.com

An information center where anyone can find a comprehensive overview about the most common cause of lower respiratory tract infections in children.

DESCRIPTION

6060 RETINITIS PIGMENTOSA

Synonym: RP

Involves the following Biologic System(s):

Ophthalmologic Disorders

Retinitis pigmentosa (RP) refers to a group of inherited disorders in which changes occur in the light-sensitive, nerve-rich tissue membrane (retina) at the rear of the eye. This process is a slow, progressive degeneration leading to blindness. Changes in the retina include clumping (aggregation) or scattering (dispersion) of the retinal pigment, thinning or weakening of the vessels that supply the retina with oxygen-rich blood, and shrinking of the retina and the area where the optic nerve enters the retina (optic disk). Characteristic findings and symptoms of RP include difficulty in seeing at night or in dim light (night blindness; nyctalopia), a progressive reduction in the visual field with gradual loss of central vision, tunnel vision associated with loss of the peripheral visual field, and accompanying reduction of retinal function. Retinitis pigmentosa usually becomes apparent in childhood, progressing to blindness during middle age. However, the onset, severity, and rate of this progressive degeneration are widely variable.

Leber congenital retinal amaurosis (amaurosis congenita; congenital amaurosis) is a form of retinitis pigmentosa that occurs at birth or shortly thereafter and is characterized by shrinking of the optic disk (optic atrophy), thinning or weakening of the blood vessels of the retina, and widespread irregularities of retinal pigmentation. Leber congenital retinal amaurosis is transmitted as an autosomal recessive trait. In addition, retinitis pigmentosa-like degenerative changes may be associated with several metabolic, neurodegenerative, and multifold disorders.

Treatment for retinitis pigmentosa is supportive and may include the use of visual devices to enhance remaining vision. This disorder may appear as a sporadic occurrence or may be inherited, usually as an autosomal dominant disorder. There is also evidence of autosomal recessive and X-linked genetic transmission.

See also **General Resources** on page 917

Government Agencies

6061 NIH/National Eye Institute
31 Center Drive MSC 2510
Bethesda, MD 20892

301-496-5248
e-mail: 2020@nei.nih.gov
www.nei.nih.gov

Conducts and supports research that helps prevent and treat eye diseases and other disorders of vision. This research leads to sight-saving treatments, reduces visual impairment and blindness, and improves the quality of life for people of all ages. NEI-supported research has advanced our knowledge of how the eye functions in health and disease.

Paul A Sieving M.D., Ph.D., Director

National Associations & Support Groups

6062 National Association for Visually Handicapped
22 W 21st Street, 6th Floor
New York, NY 10010

212-889-3141
Fax: 212-727-2931
e-mail: navh@navh.org
www.navh.org

Serves as a clearinghouse for information about all services available to the partially-sighted from public and private sources. Conducts self-help groups. Provides information on large print books, textbooks and educational tools.

Dr Lorraine Marchi, Founder & CEO

6063 National Eye Health Education Program
National Eye Institute
31 Center Drive, MSC 2510
Bethesda, MD 20892

301-496-5248
Fax: 301-496-1065
www.nei.nih.gov/nehep

A program conducted by the National Eye Institute for large-scale professional and public education programs in partnership with national organizations.

Rosemary Janiszewski, Director
Karen Silver, Health Education Coordinator

6064 National Eye Research Foundation
910 Skokie Boulevard, Suite 207A
Northbrook, IL 60062

847-564-4652
800-621-2258
Fax: 847-564-0807
e-mail: info@nerf.org
www.nerf.org

Devoted to the enhancement of care and study of eye related diseases.

6065 National Retinitis Pigmentosa Foundation Helpline
11350 McCormick Road, #800
Hunt Valley, MD 21031

800-638-2300

Provides information and referral services to persons suffering from retinitis pigmentosa.

6066 RP International
PO Box 900
Woodland Hills, CA 91365

818-992-0500
800-344-4877
Fax: 818-992-3265
e-mail: info@rpinternational.org
www.rpinternational.org

Dedicated to promoting and supporting research to find effective treatments and cures for retinitis pigmentosa, macular degeneration, and other degenerative diseases. Provides referrals to genetic counselors and support groups and offers a variety of educational materials including a regular newsletter and brochures.

Helen Harris, President/Founder

Research Centers

6067 UIC Eye Center
Department of Ophthalmology & Visual Sciences
1855 W Taylor Street
Chicago, IL 60612

312-996-6590
Fax: 312-996-7770
e-mail: eyeweb@uic.edu
www.uic.edu/com/eye/department

Offers help, support, information and research for persons with vision problems, including retinitis pigmentosa.

Web Sites

6068 British Retinitis Pigmentosa Society
www.brps.org.uk/

Website aims to provide a better understanding of the inherited retinal disorders. The content of this website has been written by people who have many years experience of living with RP and by very knowledgeable professionals in the field of opththalmology.

6069 Foundation Fighting Blindness
www.blindness.org/retinitis-pigmentosa.asp

Searches for treatments and cures for macular degeneration, retinitis pigmentosa (RP), usher syndrome and the entire spectrum of retinal degenerative diseases.

6070 National Association for Visually Handicapped
www.navh.org

Helps to cope with the difficulties of vision impairment.

6071 Retina South Africa - Fighting Blindness
www.rpsa.org.za/retinitis.htm

Represents retinitis pigmentosa, macular degeneration, usher syndrome and over 200 other rare conditions. Offers supports, education and counseling to affected people and their families. Self employment skills are also provided by unemployed sufferers to encourage financial independence and self esteem.

6072 Royal National Institute of the Blind
www.rnib.org.uk

A leading UK charity offering information, support and advice to over two million people with sight problems.

6073 Texas Association of Retinitis Pigmentosa
www.geocities.com/HotSprings/7815/front.htm

Nonprofit organization based in Texas serving as a national information-sharing center to provide human services to persons with progressive vision loss from retinitis pigmentosa and other retinal degenerative disorders.

Book Publishers

6074 Children with Visual Impairments: A Parents' Guide
Peytral Publications
PO Box 1162
Minnetonka, MN 55345

952-949-8707
877-739-8725
Fax: 952-906-9777
www.peytral.com

Covers visual impairments ranging from low vision to total blindness. Offers authoritative information and empathy, parental in-sight on diagnosis and treatment, orientation and mobility, literacy, legal issues and more. Valuable to parents, educators and support staff.

395 pages

M Cay Holbrook PhD, Editor

Newsletters

6075 RP Messenger
Texas Association of Retinitis Pigmentosa
PO Box 8388
Corpus Christi, TX 78468

512-852-8515
Fax: 361-852-8515
www.jwen.com/rp

A biannual newsletter offering information on retinitis pigmentosa.

Biannual

DESCRIPTION

6076 RETINOBLASTOMA

Involves the following Biologic System(s):

Hematologic and Oncologic Disorders, Ophthalmologic Disorders

Retinoblastoma is a malignant tumor of the nerve-rich membrane at the back of the eye known as the retina. This membrane converts light waves into nerve impulses and transmits them to the brain via the optic nerve (the second cranial nerve), resulting in vision. Retinoblastoma occurs in approximately one in 18,000 live births. In most cases, one eye is affected (unilateral). However, both eyes may be involved (bilateral) in about 30 percent of affected children. In some severe cases, the tumor may spread to other parts of the body (metastasize), particularly when there is tumor invasion of the middle layer of the eye (choroid) or the optic nerve. If tumor growth occurs along the optic nerve, the brain may be affected. However, in most children with retinoblastoma, metastasis rarely occurs before the tumor is detected.

Unilateral retinoblastoma is usually detected at approximately 21 months to two years of age, whereas bilateral retinoblastoma is typically diagnosed at about 11 to 12 months. Rarely, the tumor may be detected at birth, during later childhood or adolescence, or adulthood. In most cases, the first sign associated with retinoblastoma is the appearance of a yellowish-white mass in the pupil area (leukokoria) due to the presence of the tumor behind the lens of the eye and reflection of light off the tumor. Additional symptoms and findings often include abnormal deviation of the affected eye in relation to the other (strabismus) and impaired or absent vision. In some cases, affected children experience secondary complications, such as detachment of the retina or abnormally increased pressure of the fluid of the eye (glaucoma). Children who have more advanced retinoblastoma may also experience bleeding (hemorrhaging) within the chamber of the eye in front of the iris (hyphema), irregularities of the pupil, pain, or other symptoms. In cases of severely advanced disease or metastasis, associated findings may include protusion of the eye ball (proptosis) and abnormally increased pressure within the skull (intracranial pressure).

A gene responsible for retinoblastoma (RB gene) has been located on the long arm chromosome 13 (13q14). Many cases of unilateral retinoblastoma are thought to be due to deletions or abnormal changes (mutations) of the gene that occur randomly, for unknown reasons (sporadic). In familial cases, the exact mechanisms of inheritance are not understood. However, bilateral retinoblastoma and some cases of unilateral disease are thought to result from deletion of the gene from one chromosome and inheritance of one mutated disease gene (hemizygous state) or inheritance of two mutated RB genes (homozygous state of RB gene). Individuals with familial retinoblastoma may also have an increased risk for other malignancies. About one percent of children treated for familial retinoblastoma eventually develop a malignant bone tumor (osteosarcoma) by 10 years of age. In addition, estimates in medical literature indicate that about 30 percent of those with familial retinoblastoma are affected by a second malignancy within 30 years after their initial diagnosis.

In some rare cases, affected children may have retinoblastoma in association with an underlying chromosomal deletion syndrome (chromosome 13, monosomy 13q syndrome) that is characterized by deletion (monosomy) of a portion of chromosome 13q including the RB gene at band 13q14. Although associated symptoms and findings may vary, affected children may have characteristic abnormalities of the head and facial (craniofacial) area including a high forehead, prominent eyebrows, a rounded (bulbous) tip of the nose and broad nasal bridge, prominent earlobes, a large mouth, and a thin upper lip.

The treatment of children with retinoblastoma is directed toward preserving vision. In children with unilateral retinoblastoma, treatment typically includes surgical removal of the affected eye and a portion of the optic nerve. However, if the tumor is very small, other measures may be indicated, such as the use of radiation or extremely cold temperatures (cryotherapy) to destroy the tumor. In children with bilateral retinoblastoma, treatment is directed toward preserving useful vision in at least one eye. Therefore, initial therapy may include cryotherapy or radiotherapy of one or both eyes. Bilateral therapy may be recommended since there have been cases in which the more severely affected eye has responded more dramatically to such measures. When one eye has no remaining vision or is affected by painful complications, removal of the eye may be advised. If tumor growth has begun to extend beyond the eye, radiation therapy may also be conducted. Therapy with anticancer drugs, such as cyclophosphamide and doxorubicin, may be considered with radiation therapy. Children and adults who have been affected by familial retinoblastoma should be carefully monitored for secondary malignancies. In addition, family members of affected children should be examined by an eye specialist to detect or help rule out the presence of retinoblastoma.

See also **General Resources** on page 917

Government Agencies

6077 NIH/National Cancer Institute
6116 Executive Boulevard, Room 3036A
Bethesda, MD 20892

800-422-6237
www.cancer.gov

The National Cancer Institute coordinates the National Cancer Program, which conducts and supports research, training, health information dissemination, and other programs with respect to the cause, diagnosis, prevention, and treatment of cancer, rehabilitation from cancer, and the continuing care of cancer patients and the families of cancer patients.

John E Niederhuber MD, Director

National Associations & Support Groups

6078 Candlelighters Childhood Cancer Foundation
PO Box 498
Kensington, MD 20895

301-962-3520
800-366-2223
Fax: 310-962-3521
e-mail: staff@candlelighters.org
www.candlelighters.org

The Candlelighters Childhood Cancer Foundation National Office was founded in 1970 by concerned parents of children with cancer. Today our membership of over 50,000 members of the national office and more than 100,000 members across the across the country, including Candlelighters affiliate groups, includes, parents of children who are being treated or have been treated for cancer.

Ruth Hoffman, Executive Director

6079 Division on Visual Impairments
Council for Exceptional Children
1110 N Glebe Road, Suite 300
Arlington, VA 22201

800-224-6830
Fax: 703-264-9494
TTY: 866-915-5000
www.ed.arizona.edu/dvi/welcome.htm; www.cec.sped.org

A division within the CEC, it handles concerns for Federal, state and local issues and policies related to education of youths, children and infants with visual impairments.

Ellyn Ross, President
Shirley J Wilson, Secretary

6080 Genetic Alliance
4301 Connecticut Avenue NW
Washington, DC 20008

202-966-5557
800-336-4363
Fax: 202-966-8553
e-mail: info@geneticalliance.org
www.geneticalliance.org

A coalition of voluntary genetic support groups, consumers and professionals addressing the needs of individuals and families affected by genetic disorders from a national perspective.

Sharon Terry, President/CEO

6081 Institute for Families
4650 Sunset Blvd, MS#111
Los Angeles, CA 90027

323-669-4649
Fax: 323-665-7869
e-mail: info@instituteforfamilies.org
www.instituteforfamilies.org

A non-profit organization providing free of charge support and services to professionals and families of visually impaired children.

6082 Lighthouse International
111 E 59th Street
New York, NY 10022

212-821-9200
800-829-0500
Fax: 212-821-9707
TTY: 212-821-9713
e-mail: info@lighthouse.org
www.lighthouse.org

Provides services, information, education, resource contacts and research related to the needs of children who are visually impaired and their families.

Tara A Cortes RN, PhD, President/CEO
Cynthia Stuen, Senior VP Services/Education

6083 National Alliance of Blind Students
c/o Terry Pacheco
1155 15th Street NW, Suite 1004
Washington, DC 20005

202-467-5081
800-424-8666
Fax: 202-467-5085
e-mail: rj.hodson@verizon.net
www.blindstudents.org

An advocacy and consumer organization for high school and college students who are blind or visually impaired. It works to facilitate progress toward full accessibility of college programs and facilities, provides opportunities for discussion of issues important to students and assists with National Student Seminars.

Rebecca Hodson, President

6084 National Association for Parents of Childr en with Visual Impairments
PO Box 317
Watertown, MA 02471

617-972-7441
800-562-6265
Fax: 617-972-7444
e-mail: napvi@perkins.org
www.spedex.com/napvi/

Offers emotional support for parents of blind or visually impaired children. Provides information, training and assistance, and help in understanding and using available resources.

6085 National Childhood Cancer Foundation
4600 East West Highway, Suite 600
Bethesda, MD 20814

800-458-6223
e-mail: info@curesearch.org
www.curesearch.org

CureSearch unites the world's largest childhood cancer research organization, the Children's Oncology Group, and the National Childhood Cancer Foundation through our mission to cure childhood cancer. Research is the key to the cure.

6086 National Support & Information Network
NAPVI
PO Box 317
Watertown, MA 02272

617-972-7441
800-562-6265
www.spedex.com/napvi/network.html

Nationwide support group that provides direct support, information and referral services for parents of children with vision impairments and or multiple related disabilities.

6087 Retinoblastoma International
4650 Sunset Blvd, MS#88
Los Angeles, CA 90027

323-669-2299
Fax: 323-660-8541
e-mail: info@retinoblastoma.net
www.retinoblastoma.net

Retinoblastoma information for parents, family and friends of retinoblastoma patients, as well as online medical education and training for health care professionals.

Christina S Ashford, President
Robin Einstein, Treasurer

State Agencies & Support Groups

Connecticut

6088 Parents Association of Connecticut Childre n with Visual Impairments (PACVI)
PO Box 455
Newtown, CT 06470

203-364-1450
www.spedex.com/napvi/chapters.html

Sabeena Ali, Co-President

Florida

6089 Florida Families of Children with Visual I mpairments

Ormond Beach, FL 32174

386-677-7760
e-mail: ffcvi@yahoo.com

Sue Townsend, President

Massachusetts

6090 Massachusetts Association for Parents of t he Visually Impaired (MAPVI)

Maynard, MA 01754

978-897-3005
e-mail: mapvi-info@viguide.com

Judy Westgate, President

New Hampshire

6091 New England Retinoblastoma Support Group (NERSG)

Salem, NH 03079

603-893-3908

Tom Gelinas, Treasurer

Web Sites

6092 A Parent's Guide to Understanding Retinobl astoma
www.retinoblastoma.com/frameset1.htm

Dr David H Abramson

6093 Children's Cancer Web
www.cancerindex.org/ccw

An independent nonprofit site, established to provide a directory of childhood cancer resources.

6094 Life With Retinoblastoma
www.mrmegabyte.net/rb/retino.html

A support site written by the parent of a child with retinoblastoma.

6095 Online Mendelian Inheritance in Man
www.ncbi.nlm.nih.gov

This database is a catalog of human genes and genetic disorders.

6096 Retinoblastoma Solutions
www.retinoblastomasolutions.org

Dedicated to advancing retinoblastoma research and making available molecular diagnostic tests to families that cannot afford it.

Book Publishers

6097 Children with Visual Impairments: A Parents' Guide
Peytral Publications
PO Box 1162
Minnetonka, MN 55345

952-949-8707
877-739-8725
Fax: 952-906-9777
www.peytral.com

Covers visual impairments ranging from low vision to total blindness. Offers authoritative information and empathy, parental insight on diagnosis and treatment, orientation and mobility, literacy, legal issues and more. Valuable to parents, educators and support staff.

395 pages

M Cay Holbrook PhD, Editor

6098 Let's Talk About Going to the Hospital
Rosen Publishing Group's PowerKids Press
29 E 21st Street
New York, NY 10010

212-777-3017
800-237-9932
Fax: 888-436-4643
e-mail: rosenpub@tribeca.ios.com
www.powerkidspress.com

If a child has to check into the hospital, chances are he or she is already upset about being ill. Knowing how a hospital functions and what the procedures are, such as when family members can visit, will help in what is already a stressful situation. Grades K-5.

24 pages
ISBN: 0-823950-36-0

6099 Let's Talk About When Kids Have Cancer

Melanie Apel Gordon, author

Rosen Publishing Group's PowerKids Press
29 E 21st Street
New York, NY 10010

212-777-3017
800-237-9932
Fax: 888-436-4643
e-mail: customerservice@rosenpub.com
www.powerkidspress.com

In a straightforward yet comforting way, this book explains what cancer is, what kinds of treatments surround the disease and how to cope if a child or the friend of a child has cancer.

24 pages Paperback
ISBN: 0-823951-95-2

6100 My Fake Eye, The Story of My Prosthesis
Institute for Families
4650 Sunset Blvd, MS#111
Los Angeles, CA 90027

323-669-4649
Fax: 323-665-7869
e-mail: info@instituteforfamilies.org
www.instituteforfamilies.org

A full color book and comforting tool for children, siblings and parents dealing with eye enucleation. Available in Spanish.

6101 My New Eye Patch
Institute for Families
4650 Sunset Blvd, MS#111
Los Angeles, CA 90027

323-669-4649
Fax: 323-665-7869
e-mail: info@instituteforfamilies.org
www.instituteforfamilies.org

A book for describing the feelings and experiences surrounding wearing an eye patch, for children and parents. Available in Spanish.

6102 Surviving Childhood Cancer: A Guide for Families
New Harbinger Publications
5674 Shattuck Avenue
Oakland, CA 94609

510-652-0215
800-748-6273
Fax: 510-652-5472
e-mail: customerservice@newharbinger.com
www.newharbinger.com

Cancer in a child is an overwhelming experience for a family. This book explains common medical procedures and offers readers practical advice about how to cope with emotions and stress during this time.

232 pages Paperback
ISBN: 1-572241-02-0

Newsletters

6103 Awareness
NAPVI
PO Box 317
Watertown, MA 02272

617-972-7441
800-562-6265
www.spedex.com/napvi/awareness.html

Contains regional NAPVI news and announcements, legislative updates, upcoming events and conferences and articles and letters to the editor.

32 pages Quarterly

6104 DVI Quarterly
Division on Visual Impairments (CEC)
1110 N Glebe Rd, Suite 300
Arlington, VA 22201

561-541-2296
www.cec.sped.org/mb/

News on the Division of Visual Impairments, articles and announcements having to do with the education of students with visual impairmnets.

1000+ Quarterly

Sheila Amato, Editor

6105 Retinoblastoma Support News
Institute for Families
4650 Sunset Blvd, MS#111
Los Angeles, CA 90027

323-669-4649
Fax: 323-665-7869
e-mail: info@instituteforfamilies.org
www.instituteforfamilies.org

Newsletter for educational professionals and the families of children with retinoblastoma.

Quarterly

Pamphlets

6106 A Parent's Guide to Understanding Retinobl astoma
IRIS Medical Instruments/IRIDEX Corp
1212 Terra Bella Ave
Mountain View, CA 94043

650-962-8100
800-388-4747
Fax: 650-962-0486
www.retinoblastoma.com/frameset1.htm

Dr David H Abramson

6107 Early Detection
Retinoblastoma International
4650 Sunset Blvd, MS#88
Los Angeles, CA 90027

323-669-2299
Fax: 323-660-8541
e-mail: info@retinoblastoma.net
www.retinoblastoma.net

A brochure promoting the early detection and treatment of retinoblastoma.

2 pages

DESCRIPTION

6108 RETINOPATHY OF PREMATURITY

Synonym: ROP

Involves the following Biologic System(s):

Neonatal and Infant Disorders, Ophthalmologic Disorders

Retinopathy of prematurity (ROP) is a condition characterized by improper development of blood vessels within the retinas of both eyes. The retinas are the nerve-rich membranes at the back of the eyes that contain specialized, light-sensitive nerve cells (rods and cones). The rods and cones convert visual images into nerve impulses that are transmitted to the brain via the optic nerve (second cranial nerve). ROP primarily occurs in newborns of low birth weight who are born at less than 37 weeks after conception (premature newborns). Premature infants who weigh less than approximately three pounds, are delivered before 33 weeks of pregnancy, and develop abnormally high levels of oxygen in the blood (hyperoxia) as a result of oxygen therapy for breathing difficulties are considered to be particularly at risk for retinopathy of prematurity. Less commonly, other factors may play some role in contributing to the condition, such as heart disease, infection, abnormally low levels of circulating red blood cells (anemia), or other conditions. Generally, the lower an infant's birthweight and the greater the degree of prematurity, the higher the risk for the development of ROP.

During fetal development, the blood vessels that will supply the retinas grow from the center of the retinas, gradually extending to their outer edges shortly after birth. However, in premature newborns, the retinal blood vessels are incompletely developed, potentially causing abnormalities in subsequent retinal growth and function. In infants with ROP, associated findings may range from mild or temporary changes of the outer edges of the retina to severe abnormalities affecting the entire retina. During the active or acute stage of ROP, which typically occurs within the first month or so of life, associated findings may include abnormal narrowing of certain retinal blood vessels and subsequent widening or abnormal twisting of other retinal vessels. In addition, there is an apparent lack of blood vessel growth in certain areas of the retina, particularly of the outer rim. There may also be a gradual development of new blood vessels outside the normal area of retinal blood vessel growth, such as over the surface of the retina or into the jelly-like fluid behind the lens of the eye (vitreous humor). These vessels may tend to bleed (hemorrhage) into the retina, and some patients may develop retinal scarring as well as the formation of retinal folds or breaks or detachment of the outer portion of the retina. In severe cases, patients may undergo chronic disease progression, leading to complete retinal detachment and progressive retinal degeneration. The retina may eventually appear as an abnormal whitish membrane behind the lens of the eye (leukokoria). As the condition continues to progress, infants may develop increased fluid pressure within the eye (glaucoma), gradual degeneration and shrinkage of the eye (phthisis bulbi), and associated visual impairment leading to blindness.

In many infants with ROP, the condition spontaneously subsides and regresses. Such children may have an increased risk of progressive nearsightedness (myopia) or other eye abnormalities. However, in fewer than 10 percent, there may be ongoing disease progression, potentially causing total retinal detachment and severe visual impairment or blindness. In fact, it is retinal detachment that is the main cause of visual impairment and blindness in ROP.

The prevention of ROP depends upon proper prenatal care and other measures to help prevent premature births. In addition, infants who are born prematurely are monitored closely to ensure prompt detection of ROP and appropriate treatment as required. In severe cases of ROP, a technique that freezes affected areas of the retina (cryotherapy) may help to reduce potentially severe complications. Laser therapy can "burn away" the periphery of the retina, which has no normal blood vessels. Both laser treatment and cryotherapy, only used in infants with advanced ROP, destroy the peripheral areas of the retina, slowing or reversing the abnormal growth of blood vessels. Unfortunately, the treatments also destroy some side vision but saves central vision.In some patients with total retinal detachment, surgical techniques may be used to help reattach the retina.

See also **General Resources** on page 917

Government Agencies

6109 NIH/National Eye Institute

31 Center Drive MSC 2510
Bethesda, MD 20892

301-496-5248
e-mail: 2020@nei.nih.gov
www.nei.nih.gov

Conducts and supports research that helps prevent and treat eye diseases and other disorders of vision. This research leads to sight-saving treatments, reduces visual impairment and blindness, and improves the quality of life for people of all ages. NEI-supported research has advanced our knowledge of how the eye functions in health and disease.

Paul A Sieving M.D., Ph.D., Director

6110 NIH/National Institute of Child Health and Human Development
31 Center Drive, Building 31
Bethesda, MD 20892

301-496-5133
Fax: 301-496-1104
www.nichd.nih.gov

Established in 1962 by congress, today the institute conducts and supports research on topics related to the health of children, adults, families and populations. Some of these topics include: developmental disabilities, growth and development, infant death, reproductive health and birth defects.

Nancy D Wirth, Director
Lisa Kaeser, Program & Public Liaison

National Associations & Support Groups

6111 Association for Retinopathy of Prematurity and Related Diseases
PO Box 250425
Franklin, MI 48025

800-788-2020
e-mail: ropard@yahoo.com
www.ropard.org

Funds clinically relevant basic science and clinical research to eliminate retinopathy of prematurity and associated retinal diseases.

Susan Campbell, Administrative Director
Paula Korelitz, Outreach Director

6112 Division on Visual Impairments
Council for Exceptional Children
1110 North Glebe Road, Suite 300
Arlington, VA 22201

800-224-6830
Fax: 703-264-9494
TTY: 866-915-5000
www.ed.arizona.edu/dvi/welcome.htm; www.cec.sped.org

A division within the CEC, it handles concerns for Federal, state and local issues and policies related to education of youths, children and infants with visual impairments.

Ellyn Ross, President
Shirley J Wilson, Secretary

6113 Lighthouse International
111 E 59th Street
New York, NY 10022

212-821-9200
800-829-0500
Fax: 212-821-9707
TTY: 212-821-9713
e-mail: info@lighthouse.org
www.lighthouse.org

Provides information, services, education, resource contacts and research related to the needs of children who are visually impaired and their families.

Tara A Cortes RN, PhD, President/CEO
Cynthia Stuen, Senior VP Services/Education

6114 National Alliance of Blind Students
c/o Terry Pacheco
1155 15th Street NW, Suite 1004
Washington, DC 20005

202-467-5081
800-424-8666
Fax: 202-467-5085
e-mail: rj.hodson@verizon.net
www.blindstudents.org

An advocacy and consumer organization for high school and college students who are blind or visually impaired. It works to facilitate progress toward full accessibility of college programs and facilities, provides opportunities for discussion of issues important to students and assists with National Student Seminars.

Rebecca Hodson, President

6115 National Association for Parents of Childr en with Visual Impairments
PO Box 317
Watertown, MA 02471

617-972-7441
800-562-6265
Fax: 617-972-7444
e-mail: napvi@perkins.org
www.spedex.com/napvi/

Offers emotional support for parents of blind or visually impaired children. Provides information, training and assistance, and help in understanding and using available resources.

6116 National Association for Visually Handicapped
22 W 21st Street, 6th Floor
New York, NY 10010

212-889-3141
Fax: 212-727-2931
e-mail: navh@navh.org
www.navh.org

Serves as a clearinghouse for information about all services available to the partially-sighted from public and private sources. Conducts self-help groups. Provides information on large print books, textbooks and educational tools.

Dr Lorraine Marchi, Founder & CEO

6117 National Eye Research Foundation
910 Skokie Boulevard, Suite 207A
Northbrook, IL 60062

847-564-4652
800-621-2258
Fax: 847-564-0807
e-mail: info@nerf.org
www.nerf.org

Devoted to the enhancement of care and study of eye related diseases.

Audio Video

6118 Management of Retinopathy of Prematurity V ideo
ROPARD
PO Box 250425
Franklin, MI 48025

800-788-2020
e-mail: ropard@yahoo.com
www.ropard.org

Information on ROP related diseases including long term treatment considerations.

Web Sites

6119 National Association for Visually Handicapped
www.navh.org
Helps to cope with the difficulties of vision impairment.

Book Publishers

6120 Children with Visual Impairments: A Parents' Guide
Peytral Publications
PO Box 1162
Minnetonka, MN 55345

952-949-8707
877-739-8725
Fax: 952-906-9777
www.peytral.com

Covers visual impairments ranging from low vision to total blindness. Offers authoritative information and empathy, parental insight on diagnosis and treatment, orientation and mobility, literacy, legal issues and more. Valuable to parents, educators and support staff.

395 pages

M Cay Holbrook PhD, Editor

Newsletters

6121 Sight Lines
ROPARD
PO Box 250425
Franklin, MI 48025

800-788-2020
e-mail: ropard@yahoo.com
www.ropard.org

Susan Campbell, Editor

Pamphlets

6122 Looking Ahead:A Parents Guide to the Devel opment Child w/ Retinopathy Prematurity
ROPARD
PO Box 250425
Franklin, MI 48025

800-788-2020
e-mail: ropard@yahoo.com
www.ropard.org

Visual stimulation activity suggestions for the development of children up to five years of age with retinopathy of prematurity.

DESCRIPTION

6123 SARCOIDOSIS

Synonyms: Sarcoid of Boeck, Schaumann's disease
Involves the following Biologic System(s):
Connective Tissue Disorders

Sarcoidosis is a multisystem disorder that is characterized by the abnormal development of inflammatory growths or nodules (i.e., epithelioid granulomas) in various organs in the body. The cause of this inflammatory disorder is unknown; however, it is believed that granuloma formation associated with sarcoidosis may result from infection or an exaggerated immune response to specific agents (antigens). In addition, researchers believe that some people may be genetically predisposed to sarcoidosis and develop the disease only if triggered by environmental or other factors. Although this disorder most commonly occurs during young adulthood, it may occur in children and in the elderly. Symptoms and physical findings associated with sarcoidosis are dependent upon the organ(s) involved and, in children, the age of onset. Most affected children, however, share the common symptoms of fatigue, weight loss, cough, pain in the bones and joints, and abnormally low levels of circulating red blood cells (anemia).

The nodules or granulomas associated with sarcoidosis may develop in almost any organ of the body, but most commonly affect the lungs, upper respiratory tract, lymph nodes, skin, eyes, liver, bones, joints, bone marrow, skeletal muscles, heart, liver, spleen, or the central and peripheral nervous systems. In older children and adults, the lungs are most often affected (90 percent of patients), while younger children experience less lung involvement. Characteristic findings in older children may include swelling of the lymph nodes near the blood vessels that enter and exit the lungs (hilar lymphadenopathy) as well as the lymph nodes near the windpipe (paratracheal lymphadenopathy) and those under the skin (peripheral lymphadenopathy). In addition, nodule formation may cause inflammations in the eye (e.g., uveitis and iritis) and other eye lesions, skin lesions, and liver changes. Younger children may develop a reddish, combination-type rash consisting of waxy pimples and flat, discolored lesions (maculopapular erythematous rash) as well as inflammation of the joints (arthritis).

Diagnosis of sarcoidosis is usually a challenge as it is often difficult to distinguish from other disorders with similar symptoms and findings. Therefore, differential diagnosis often involves a physical examination, medical and environmental history, and the comprehensive evaluation of laboratory tests and chest x-rays, biopsy of tissue samples, and specialized testing. Laboratory findings may show excessive levels of calcium in the blood (hypercalcemia) and in the urine (hypercalciuria), abnormally high levels of protein in the blood (hyperproteinemia), excessive levels of certain granular white cells in the blood (eosinophilia), and other blood irregularities. For example, the cells of the nodules secrete a substance called angiotensin-converting enzyme, which, in some patients, is elevated to detectable levels in the blood. Testing for this enzyme may also be employed to measure disease activity. In addition, pulmonary function tests may be used to measure progress of the disease in those children with lung involvement, and repeat chest x-rays may also be indicated to monitor progress.

In some children, sarcoidosis may resolve spontaneously within a period of months or years; however, some children may have a more chronic form of the disease that may result in progressive lung involvement, eye disease that may cause blindness, and other prolonged symptoms and findings. Treatment for sarcoidosis may include the use of corticosteroid drops or ointments to alleviate eye inflammations and oral corticosteroids to alleviate acute symptoms such as resistant inflammatory lesions of the eyes, joint pain, fever, shortness of breath, and other symptoms. Approximately 90 percent of cases are responsive to corticosteroids and can be controlled with modest maintenance doses. If no symptoms are present, corticosteroid treatment is usually not advised. Other treatment is symptomatic and supportive.

See also **General Resources** on page 917

National Associations & Support Groups

6124 American Autoimmune Related Diseases Association
22100 Gratiot Avenue
E Detroit, MI 48021

586-776-3900
www.aarda.org

The American Autoimmune Related Diseases Association is dedicated to the eradication of autoimmune diseases and the alleviation of suffering and the socioeconomic impact of autoimmunity through fostering and facilitating collabration in the areas of education, public awareness, research,and patient in an effective, ethical and efficient manner.

Virginia Ladd, Director

6125 National Sarcoidosis Resource Center and Networking Program
PO Box 1593
Piscataway, NJ 08854

732-699-0733
Fax: 732-699-0882
www.nsrc-global.net

Formed to heighten public awareness and to educate people about this often chronic and disabling disease; offers information and support. The center serves the United States, Canada, Europe.

Sandra Conroy, President

6126 Sarcoid Networking Association
6424 151st Ave E
Sumner, WA 98390

253-891-6886
e-mail: sarcoidosis_network@prodigy.net
www.sarcoidosisnetwork.org

A nonprofit organization dedicated to improving the lives of those affected by sarcoidosis through providing support, eduation and other resources.

Dolores O'Leary, Executive Director

6127 Sarcoid Registry
5239 SW Lance St
Roseburg, OR 97470

541-905-2092
e-mail: admin@snaregistry.org
www.snaregistry.org

Operates under the laedership of SNA-Sarcoid Networking Association to bring the Sarcoidosis community together.

Kristi Anderson, Director

6128 Sarcoidosis Network Foundation
11428 E Artesia Blvd, Suite 10
Artesia, CA 90701

562-809-8500
Fax: 562-809-8182
www.sarcoid-network.org

A nonprofit organization that promotes awareness and education; supports research to find a cure; and supports those affected by sarcoidosis and their families.

Ruth Jacobs, President
Charles Walker, VP

6129 Sarcoidosis Research Institute
3475 Central Avenue
Memphis, TN 38111

901-766-6951
Fax: 901-774-7294
e-mail: sarcoidosis@bellsouth.net
www.sarcoidosisresearch.org

Provides patient and professional education that will result in enhanced methods of diagnosis and treatment of the disease; information that will assist patients and their support network in the management of the disease; and engages in research initiatives that will result in a cure for the debilitating disease.

State Agencies & Support Groups

California

6130 REACH - Sarcoidosis Support
10843 Kenney St
Norwalk, CA 90650

714-739-4023

Ruth Jacobs

Colorado

6131 Denver Sarcoidosis Awareness Support Group
4351 Ireland St
Denver, CO 80249

303-375-9376
e-mail: contacts@denversarcoidosisawareness.org
www.denversarcoidosisawareness.org

Provides support through sharing of experiences, discussing feeling and emotions, and sharing coping strategies.

Shirley R Holley, Founder

Georgia

6132 Sarcoidosis Support Group
St Joseph's/Chandler Health System
5353 Reynolds St
Savannah, GA 31405

912-819-8032
e-mail: balkstra@sjchs.org

Cindy Balkstra RN

Indiana

6133 Central Indiana Sarcoidosis Support Group
Kindred Hospital
1700 W 10th St
Indianapolis, IN 46202

317-335-2981
e-mail: indysarcoid@aol.com

Robbie Darden

Maryland

6134 Sarcoidosis Awareness Network
1031 Farrar Ave
Cheltenham, MD 20623

301-372-2885
e-mail: tsan4w@aol.com

Linda Lanier, President

Michigan

6135 Sarcoidosis Awareness Foundation
14540 Whitcomb St
Detroit, MI 48227

e-mail: SarcoidAwareness@aol.com

Janie L Chuney

6136 Sarcoidosis Resource Support Group
PO Box 3231
Highland Park, MI 48203

315-575-4852
e-mail: pmullins@detroitsworkplace.org

Pam Mullins
Dot Lawrence

6137 Sarcoidosis Support - Beaumont
William Beaumont Hospital
300 W 13 Mile Rd
Royal Oak, MI 48073

248-545-0320
e-mail: jaynie04@aol.com

Victoria Rice

New Jersey

6138 Sarcoidosis Support Resource Central New Jersey
National Sarcoidosis Resource Center
PO Box 1593
Piscataway, NJ 08855

732-699-0733
Fax: 732-699-0882

Sandra Conroy

New York

6139 Long Island Sarcoidosis Support
1989 N Jerusalem Rd
E Meadow, NY 11554

516-483-2666

Robert Schoenfeld, Facilitator

North Carolina

6140 Sarcoidosis Support Group
1021 Fitzgerald Dr
Wilmington, NC 28405

910-395-0154

Uldridge Galloway

6141 University of North Carolina Sarcoidosis Support Group
Div. of Pulmonary Medicine
130 Mason Farm Rd, CB# 7020
Chapel Hill, NC 27599

919-966-4675
e-mail: juliem@med.unc.edu

Julie Montenegro RN

Pennsylvania

6142 Sarcoidosis Self-Help
2112 Highland Avenue
New Castle, PA 16105

412-652-6089

Della Emmanuel

South Carolina

6143 Sarcoidosis Support
MUSC Medical Center
171 Ashley Ave
Charleston, SC 29425

803-792-0280

Kathy Lanza

Tennessee

6144 Middle Tennessee Sarcoidosis Support Group
PO Box 1342
Cookesville, TN 38503

931-528-7826

Becky Robertson

6145 Sarcoidosis Patient Forum
Sarcoidosis Research Institute-SRI
3475 Central Avenue
Memphis, TN 38111

901-774-5511

Paula Polite, President

Virginia

6146 Sarcoidosis Support Group
704 Woodnote Land
Newport News, VA 23608

804-988-3065

Beverly Moses

Libraries & Resource Centers

6147 National Sarcoidosis Resource Center
PO Box 1593
Piscataway, NJ 08854

908-699-0733
Fax: 908-699-0882
www.nscr-global.net

Provides general information about special services for sarcoidosis patients; strives to increase public awareness about this unknown disease, and to generate interest in sarcordosis and support research, leading to easy diagnosis, better treatments and, ultimately, a cure.

Sandra Conroy

6148 Sarcoidosis Center
Baptist Hospital East
6005 Park Avenue, Suite 501
Memphis, TN 38119

901-761-5877
Fax: 901-761-2280
e-mail: sarcoid@sarcoidcenter.com
www.sarcoidcenter.com

A nonprofit organization providing an exchange of information regarding sarcoidosis for patients and professionals.

Norman T Soskel MD

Research Centers

6149 National Jewish Medical & Research Center
1400 Jackson St
Denver, CO 80206

303-388-4461
800-222-5864
www.nationaljewish.org/disease-info

Information on ongoing sarcoidosis research and available treatment programs at the center.

Dr Kevin Brown, Vice Chair/Associate Professor

6150 Sarcoidosis Research Institute
3475 Central Avenue
Memphis, TN 38111

901-766-6951
Fax: 901-774-7294
e-mail: sarcoidosis@bellsouth.net
www.sarcoidosisresearch.org

Provides patient and professional education that will result in enhanced methods of diagnosis and treatment of the disease; information that will assist patients and their support network in the management of the disease; and engages in research initiatives that will result in a cure for the debilitating disease.

Audio Video

6151 Dialogue with Doris
PC Publications
PO Box 1593
Piscataway, NJ 08855

732-699-0733
Fax: 732-699-0882

6152 Help with a Hidden Disease Update
PC Publications
PO Box 1593
Piscataway, NJ 08855

732-699-0733
800-223-6429
Fax: 732-699-0882

6153 International World Conference on Sarcoidosis-Patient Symposium
PC Publications
PO Box 1593
Piscataway, NJ 08855

732-699-0733
Fax: 732-699-0882

Cassette.

6154 Of Their Own-Person To Person Show
PC Publications
PO Box 1593
Piscataway, NJ 08855

732-699-0733
Fax: 732-699-0882

6155 Sarcoidosis Conference 2
PC Publications
PO Box 1593
Piscataway, NJ 08855

732-699-0733
Fax: 732-699-0882

6156 Sarcoidosis Conference 3
PC Publications
PO Box 1593
Piscataway, NJ 08855

732-699-0733
Fax: 732-699-0882

6157 Sarcoidosis and Lyme Disease
PC Publications
PO Box 1593
Piscataway, NJ 08855

732-699-0733
Fax: 732-699-0882

6158 Sarcoidosis-What's That?
PC Publications
PO Box 1593
Piscataway, NJ 08855

732-699-0733
Fax: 732-699-0882

Web Sites

6159 Foundation for Sarcoidosis Research
www.stopsarcoidosis.org

Takes the lead as a nonprofit organization in funding research in finding a cure for sarcoidosis and improving patient care.

6160 Health Answers
www.healthanswers.com

HealthAnswers offers a breadth of services in medical education, sales force training, patient support solutions, professional promotion and consumer solutions.

6161 NIH/National Heart, Lung and Blood Institu te
www.nhlbi.nih.gov/health/dci/Index/s.html

A part of the National Institutes of Health, this NHLBI site offers general information and answers to questions about Sarcoidosis.

6162 National Sarcoidosis Resource Center
www.nsrc-global.net

The center provides information to people throughout the U.S., Canada, and Europe. They have an ongoing research study of the symptoms and demographics of Sarcoidosis patients.

6163 Online Mendelian Inheritance in Man
www.ncbi.nlm.nih.gov

This database is a catalog of human genes and genetic disorders.

6164 Sarcoid Life
www.sarcoidlife.org

6165 Sarcoidosis
www.epler.com/wsarc.html

General information and answers to questions about Sarcoidosis.

6166 Sarcoidosis Center
www.sarcoidcenter.com

A nonprofit corporation designed to provide information for patients and physicians regarding sarcoidosis. The site includes a list of sarcoidosis experts by country.

6167 Sarcoidosis Research Institute
www.sarcoidosisresearch.org

Provides patient and professional education that will result in enhanced methods of diagnosis and treatment of the disease.

Book Publishers

6168 Sarcoidosis Resource Guide and Directory
PC Publications
PO Box 1593
Piscataway, NJ 08855

732-699-0733
Fax: 732-699-0882

1993 304 pages Paperback
ISBN: 0-963122-25-8

Newsletters

6169 Online Sarcoidosis Newsletter
National Sarcoidosis Resource Center
PO Box 1593
Piscataway, NJ 08855

732-699-0733
Fax: 732-699-0882

Offers information on the center's activities and events, medical and legislative updates for the patients and their families.

Quarterly

6170 Sarcoidosis Networking
Sarcoid Networking Association
6424 151st Avenue E
Sumner, WA 98390

253-891-6886
e-mail: sarcoidosis_network@prodigy.net
www.sarcoidnetwork.org

Helps those affected by sarcoidosis network with one another and the medical community.

Quarterly

Dolores O'Leary, Executive Director

Pamphlets

6171 A Sarcoidosis Questionnaire: Demographics and Symptomatology-Patients Respond
PC Publications
PO Box 1593
Piscataway, NJ 08855

732-699-0733
800-223-6429
Fax: 732-699-0882

6172 Anemia of Sarcoidosis
PC Publications
PO Box 1593
Piscataway, NJ 08855

732-699-0733
Fax: 732-699-0882

6173 Bronchoalveolar Lymphocytes in Sarcoidosis
PC Publications
PO Box 1593
Piscataway, NJ 08855

732-699-0733
Fax: 732-699-0882

6174 Case Report-MR Imaging of Myocardial Sarcoidosis
PC Publications
PO Box 1593
Piscataway, NJ 08855

732-699-0733
Fax: 732-699-0882

6175 Case Report-Osseous Sarcoidosis and Chronic Polyarthritis
PC Publications
PO Box 1593
Piscataway, NJ 08855
732-699-0733
Fax: 732-699-0882

6176 Coping with Sarcoidosis
National Sarcoidosis Resource Center
PO Box 1593
Piscataway, NJ 08855
732-699-0733
Fax: 732-699-0882

A pamphlet offering information on how to manage and live with sarcoidosis.

6177 Drugs That Have Been Used for the Treatment of Sarcoidosis
PC Publications
PO Box 1593
Piscataway, NJ 08855
732-699-0733
Fax: 732-699-0882

6178 Effects of Sarcoid and Steroids on Angiotensin-Converting Enzyme
PC Publications
PO Box 1593
Piscataway, NJ 08855
732-699-0733
Fax: 732-699-0882

6179 Masqueraders of Sarcoidosis
PC Publications
PO Box 1593
Piscataway, NJ 08855
732-699-0733
Fax: 732-699-0882

6180 Multidisciplinary Clinico-Pathologic Conference
PC Publications
PO Box 1593
Piscataway, NJ 08855
732-699-0733
Fax: 732-699-0882

6181 National Sarcoidosis Resource Center
PC Publications
PO Box 1593
Piscataway, NJ 08855
732-699-0733
Fax: 732-699-0882
www.nsrc-global.net

A booklet offering a brief introduction to the illness and information on the role of the Center in finding a cure and educating the public on Sarcoidosis.

6182 Neurosarcoidosis
PC Publications
PO Box 1593
Piscataway, NJ 08855
732-699-0733
Fax: 732-699-0882

6183 Neurosarcoidosis or Multiple Sclerosis?
National Sarcoidosis Resource Center
PO Box 1593
Piscataway, NJ 08855
732-699-0733
Fax: 732-699-0882

6184 Paranoid Psychosis Due to Neurosarcoidosis
PC Publications
PO Box 1593
Piscataway, NJ 08855
732-699-0733
800-223-6429
Fax: 732-699-0882

6185 Patient Information Package
National Sarcoidosis Resource Center
PO Box 1593
Piscataway, NJ 08855
732-699-0733
Fax: 732-699-0882

Contains various brochures and pamphlets offering information about sarcoidosis.

6186 Presidential Proclamation-National Sarcoidosis Awareness Day
PC Publications
PO Box 1593
Piscataway, NJ 08855
732-699-0733
Fax: 732-699-0882

6187 Psychological Factors in Sarcoidosis
PC Publications
PO Box 1593
Piscataway, NJ 08855
732-699-0733
Fax: 732-699-0882

6188 Pulmonary Sarcoidosis: Evaluation with High Resolution
PC Publications
PO Box 1593
Piscataway, NJ 08855
732-699-0733
Fax: 732-699-0882

6189 Pulmonary Sarcoidosis: What We Are Learning
PC Publications
PO Box 1593
Piscataway, NJ 08855
732-699-0733
Fax: 732-699-0882

6190 Right & Left Ventricular Function At Rest In Patients with Sarcoidosis
PC Publications
PO Box 1593
Piscataway, NJ 08855
732-699-0733
Fax: 732-699-0882

6191 Sarcoidosis
PC Publications
PO Box 1593
Piscataway, NJ 08855
732-699-0733
Fax: 732-699-0882

Offers information on the illness, causes, symptoms and treatments.

6192 Sarcoidosis Questionnaire: Demographics and Symptomatology-The Patients Respond
PC Publications
PO Box 1593
Piscataway, NJ 08855
732-699-0733
Fax: 732-699-0882

6193 Sarcoidosis and Other Granulatomous
PC Publications
PO Box 1593
Piscataway, NJ 08855

732-699-0733
800-223-6429
Fax: 732-699-0882

6194 Sarcoidosis and You-A Listing of Possible Symptoms
PC Publications
PO Box 1593
Piscataway, NJ 08855

732-699-0733
Fax: 732-699-0882

6195 Sarcoidosis-International Review
PC Publications
PO Box 1593
Piscataway, NJ 08855

732-699-0733
Fax: 732-699-0882

6196 Sarcoidosis-Pleural Involvement Mimicking a Coin Lesson
PC Publications
PO Box 1593
Piscataway, NJ 08855

732-699-0733
Fax: 732-699-0882

6197 Sarcoidosis: A Multisystem Disease
PC Publications
PO Box 1593
Piscataway, NJ 08855

732-699-0733
Fax: 732-699-0882

Explains the effects of the illness on the lungs and joints.

6198 Sarcoidosis: Usual and Unusual Manifestations
PC Publications
PO Box 1593
Piscataway, NJ 08855

732-699-0733
Fax: 732-699-0882

6199 Seasonal Clustering of Sarcoidosis
National Sarcoidosis Resource Center
PO Box 1593
Piscataway, NJ 08855

732-699-0733
Fax: 732-699-0882

6200 Successful Treatment of Myocardial Sarcoidosis with Steriods
PC Publications
PO Box 1593
Piscataway, NJ 08855

732-699-0733
Fax: 732-699-0882

6201 Support Group Listing
PC Publications
PO Box 1593
Piscataway, NJ 08855

732-699-0733
Fax: 732-699-0882

6202 World Association Sarcoidosis Other Granulatomous
PC Publications
PO Box 1593
Piscataway, NJ 08855

732-699-0733
Fax: 732-699-0882

DESCRIPTION

6203 SCLERODERMA

Covers these related disorders: Linear scleroderma, Morphea, Systemic sclerosis

Involves the following Biologic System(s):
Connective Tissue Disorders

Scleroderma is a connective tissue disease characterized by the build up of collagen (connective tissue) resulting in thickening and hardening of the skin and underlying tissues or, in some forms of scleroderma, other organs of the body. In patients with morphea, a form of the disease that primarily affects the skin and its underlying (subcutaneous) tissues, lesions appear as limited or localized patches. In linear scleroderma, lesions appear in a band-like pattern. In other patients, particularly in adults, scleroderma may occur as a generalized, systemic disease affecting the skin and subcutaneous tissues, blood vessels, and internal organs, such as the heart, lungs, kidneys, and certain parts of the digestive tract. Although the underlying cause of scleroderma is not known, some researchers speculate that it may be an autoimmune disease in which there is an abnormal immune response against the body's own tissues. During childhood, scleroderma is more common in girls than boys.

Children with scleroderma are primarily affected by morphea or linear scleroderma. Associated symptoms and findings usually become apparent at age two or older. Patients initially develop patchy skin lesions that are dry, red or violet, and shiny in appearance. These lesions may cause associated pain or unusual sensations, such as prickling feelings in affected areas. In some children, the lesions may have a linear distribution and develop primarily on one side of the body. The lesions gradually become hard (indurated) and develop waxy, pale centers and elevated borders. As the disease continues to progress, the lesions become larger and merge, potentially involving a large area, such as an entire arm or leg. Affected areas may eventually develop deep scar tissue and firmly bind to underlying tissues, potentially resulting in pain and permanent bending of affected joints in fixed postures (joint contractures). In children with morphea or linear scleroderma, active disease may spontaneously subside over months or years or may slowly progress over many years.

Rarely, children may develop generalized, systemic scleroderma (systemic sclerosis). In such cases, associated symptoms and findings usually become apparent at age four or older. Children with systemic sclerosis often initially experience Raynaud's phenomenon, a condition characterized by sudden contraction of blood vessels supplying the fingers or toes, causing an interruption of blood flow and a subsequent excess of blood in affected areas following the restoration of blood flow (reactive hyperemia). Such episodes are usually triggered by exposure to cold temperatures and are characterized by numbness, tingling, and bluish or whitish discoloration of the fingers or toes (cyanosis) due to lack of blood flow and subsequent reddening and pain.

Children with systemic sclerosis also often develop skin lesions on the hands and feet and, in some cases, the torso and facial area. These lesions may include groups of permanently widened (dilated) blood vessels (telangiectasias). As the disease progresses, skin lesions typically become hard, develop unusually light or dark pigmentation, and gradually bind to underlying tissues and structures. Children may also experience joint swelling, discomfort, and inflammation (arthritis) as well as degenerative changes of various organs, including those of the digestive tract, particularly the esophagus; the heart; the lungs and the kidneys. Associated symptoms may be extremely variable, depending upon the rate of disease progression and the specific bodily tissues and organs affected. In some patients, such abnormalities may include difficulty swallowing (dysphagia); chronic inflammation of the lungs due to unintended inhalation of foreign matter into the airways (aspiration pneumonia); high blood pressure (hypertension); or respiratory, heart, or kidney failure. Active disease may be gradually progressive or include periods during which symptoms temporarily subside (remit).

The treatment of children with scleroderma is symptomatic and supportive. Such measures may include the use of steroids, such as cortisone or prednisone, to decrease inflammation in muscles, joints or rarely in the skin itself. Non-steroidal anti-inflammatory drugs (NSAIDs) such as ibuprofen and naproxen are sometimes used for children who have arthritis to decrease joint inflammation early physical therapy to help prevent or minimize the development of joint contractures; systemic therapy with methotrexate or other medications (e.g., cytotoxic drugs), if appropriate; careful control of high blood pressure in those with systemic disease; and other measures as required. In addition, patients with Raynaud's phenomenon| should avoid cold temperatures whenever possible and dress warmly before such exposure. Scleroderma is a chronic and slowly progressive disease, lasting for months or years. The outlook depends on the type of scleroderma, where and how much skin is involved and whether or not internal organs are affected.

See also **General Resources** on page 917

Government Agencies

6204 NIH/National Institute of Arthritis and Musculoskeletal and Skin Diseases
1AMS Circle
Bethesda, MD 20892

301-402-4484
Fax: 301-718-6366
e-mail: ord@od.nih.gov
rarediseases.info.nih.gov

The mission of the National Institute of Arthritis and Musculoskeletal and Skin Diseases is to support research into the causes, treatment, and prevention of arthritis and musculoskeletal and skin diseases, the training of basic and clinical scientists to carry out this research, and the dissemination of information on research progress in these diseases.

Stephen I Katz MD PhD, Director

National Associations & Support Groups

6205 American Autoimmune Related Diseases Association
22100 Gratiot Avenue
E Detroit, MI 48021

586-776-3900
www.aarda.org

The American Autoimmune Related Diseases Association is dedicated to the eradication of autoimmune diseases and the alleviation of suffering and the socioeconomic impact of autoimmunity through fostering and facilitating collabration in the areas of education, public awareness, research,and patient in an effective, ethical and efficient manner.

Virginia Ladd, Director

6206 International Scleroderma Network
7455 France Ave S, #266
Edina, MN 55435

952-831-3091
800-564-7099
e-mail: isn@sclero.org
www.scerlo.org

Nonprofit organization for the research, education, support, and awareness for scleroderma and related illnesses. Website available in 20 languages.

Shelley Ensz, Founder/President

6207 Juvenile Scleroderma Network
1204 W 13th Street
San Pedro, CA 90731

310-519-9511
866-338-5892
Fax: 800-369-8309
e-mail: outreachJSDN@aol.com
www.jsdn.org

A nonprofit organization that provides support and friendship to children who have Juvenile Scleroderma.

6208 Scleroderma Foundation
300 Rosewood Dr, Suite 105
Danvers, MA 01923

978-463-5843
800-722-4673
Fax: 978-463-5809
e-mail: sfinfo@scleroderma.org
www.scleroderma.org

Nonprofit national organization for people with scleroderma and their family and friends. Provides support and promotes education and research.

Joseph Camerino PhD, Chair
David Parker, Secretary

6209 Scleroderma Society
1725 York Avenue, Suite 29-F
New York, NY 10128

212-427-7040

Mark Flagan, PhD, President

6210 United Scleroderma Foundation
PO Box 399
Watsonville, CA 95077

978-463-5843
800-722-4673
Fax: 978-463-5809
e-mail: outreach@scleroderma.com
www.unitedsclerodermafoundation

Nonprofit organization.

State Agencies & Support Groups

Florida

6211 Scleroderma Foundation Southeast Florida Chapter
5506 NW 61st Ave
Coral Springs, FL 33067

954-255-8335
e-mail: sclerodermasofl@bellsouth.net
Jodi Danois, Executive Director

Illinois

6212 Scleroderma Foundation Chicago Chapter
203 N Wabash St, #2219
Chicago, IL 60601

312-660-1131
Fax: 312-660-1133
e-mail: montana9932@msn.com

Ann Peterson, Executive Director

Nevada

6213 Scleroderma Foundation Nevada Chapter
5720 S Arville St, Suite 102
Las Vegas, NV 89118

702-368-1572
Fax: 702-368-1582
e-mail: sfnvchapter@gmail.com
www.scleroderma.org/chapter/nevada

Sheila Gray, President

New Jersey

6214 Scleroderma Foundation New Jersey Chapter
PO Box 285
Haddon Heights, NJ 08035

856-547-5010
866-675-5545
Fax: 856-547-5010
e-mail: sfdv1@verizon.net

Liz Van Dzura, Executive Director

New York

6215 Scleroderma Foundation Tri-State, Inc (NY, NJ, CT)
59 Front St
Binghamton, NY 13905

607-723-2239
800-867-0885
Fax: 607-723-2039
e-mail: sdtristate@aol.com
www.scleroderma.org/chapter/tristate/

Rosemary Markoff, Executive Director
Tom Knapp, Assistant

Rhode Island

6216 Rhode Island Scleroderma Support Group
Roger Williams Medical Ctr
825 Chalkstone Ave
Providence, RI 02908

401-781-5013
e-mail: scleroderma@hotmail.com

Carole Cowell, Contact

Texas

6217 Scleroderma Foundation Texas Bluebonnet Ch apter
PO Box 84344
Pearland, TX 77584

713-436-1640
866-532-7673
Fax: 713-436-1668
e-mail: ritakirkup@sbcglobal.net

Rita Kirkup, Executive Director

Virginia

6218 Scleroderma Foundation Greater Washington DC Chapter
2010 Corporate Ridge, 7th Fl, PMB 126
McLean, VA 22102

888-233-4779
e-mail: csod@t-grp.com

Carol Sodetz, Contact

Washington

6219 Scleroderma Foundation Evergreen Chapter
PO Box 84506
Seattle, WA 98116

206-285-9822
e-mail: bunny@garthefamily.comm

Bunny Garthe, President

Research Centers

6220 National Registry for Childhood Onset Scle roderma (NRCOS)
University of Pittsburgh School of Medicine
www.sctc-online.org/studies/nrcos.htm

412-383-8674
800-603-8960
e-mail: jablonj@msx.dept-med.pitt.edu
www.sctc-online.org/studies/nrcos.htm

An opportunity to study various aspects of scleroderma and coordinate a multi-center effort to accumulate information, thus launching new research investigations. Sponsored by the Scleroderma Foundation.

Jennifer Jablon, Research Coordinator
Thomas A Medsger Jr, MD, Principal Investigator

6221 Scleroderma Research Foundation
220 Montgomery St, Suite 1411
San Francisco, CA 94104

415-834-9444
800-441-2873
Fax: 415-834-9177
e-mail: info@sclerodermaresearch.org
www.srfcure.org

Since being founded in 1987 by the late Sharon Monsky, the Scleroderma Research Foundation's mission has been to find a cure for scleroderma, a life-threatening and degenerative illness, by funding and facilitating the most promising, highest quality re-

search and placing the disease and its need for a cure in the public eye.

Stephanie K Marrus, President
Charles Spaulding, Vice President, Communications

Alabama

6222 University of Alabama - Birmingham Arthrit is Clinical Intervention Program
1717 6th Ave S
Birmingham, AL 35249

205-937-7754
866-876-2247

Sheree Carter

Arizona

6223 Mayo Clinic Scleroderma Service
13400 E Shea Blvd
Scottsdale, AZ 85259

480-301-4342
www.mayoclinic.org/rheumatology-sct/

Heidi Garcia, Research Info

District of Columbia

6224 Georgetown University
Dept of Rheumatology
PHC Bldg, 3800 Reservoir Rd, 6th Fl
Washington, DC 20007

202-687-6317
e-mail: sy86@georgetown.edu

For adult and pediatric patients with localized and systemic scleroderma.

Suria Yesmin, Research Contact

Web Sites

6225 Health Answers
www.healthanswers.com

HealthAnswers offers a breadth of services in medical education, sales force training, patient support solutions, professional promotion and consumer solutions.

6226 Online Mendelian Inheritance in Man
www.ncbi.nlm.nih.gov

This database is a catalog of human genes and genetic disorders.

6227 Scleroderma A to Z
www.scerlo.org/a-to-z.html

Presented by the International Scleroderma Network, it has over 1000 pages of scleroderma and scleroderma related information, resources, and links in over 20 languages.

6228 Scleroderma Foundation
www.scleroderma.org

The national organziation for people with scleroderma and their families and friends.

6229 Scleroderma Message Board
disc.server.com/Indices/7571.html

An online message board about scleroderma and related conditions.

6230 Scleroderma Support
health.groups.yahoo.com/group/sclerodermasupport2/

A place where people who live with scleroderma can talk online.

Book Publishers

6231 Cooking Up A Storm for Scleroderma: Recipe s from the Scleroderma Foundation

Scleroderma Foundation
300 Rosewood Dr, Suite 105
Danvers, MA 01923

978-463-5843
800-722-4673
Fax: 978-463-5809
e-mail: sfinfo@scleroderma.org
www.scleroderma.org

Over 480 recipes contributed by the foundations members, including patients, friends and family.

6232 It's Not Just Growing Pains

Thomas J.A. Lehman, PhD, author

Oxford University Press
198 Madison Ave
New York, NY 10016

212-726-6000
800-445-9714
Fax: 919-677-1303
e-mail: custserv.us@oup.com
www.oup.com/usa

2004 Hardback
ISBN: 0-195157-28-1

6233 Let's Talk About Going to the Hospital

Rosen Publishing Group's PowerKids Press
29 E 21st Street
New York, NY 10010

212-777-3017
800-237-9932
Fax: 888-436-4643
e-mail: rosenpub@tribeca.ios.com
www.powerkidspress.com

If a child has to check into the hospital, chances are he or she is already upset about being ill. Knowing how a hospital functions and what the procedures are, such as when family members can visit, will help in what is already a stressful situation. Grades K-5.

24 pages
ISBN: 0-823950-36-0

6234 Medifocus Guidebook on Scleroderma

Medifocus.com, Inc
11529 Daffodil Lane, Suite 200
Silver Spring, MD 20902

301-649-9300
800-965-3002
Fax: 301-649-7809
e-mail: info@medifocus.com
www.medifocus.com

This guidebook has four sections: an overview for patients; a guide to medical literature; research centers; and a resource and organization guide. Updates are available online for a year with purchase of the book. Also available in electronic format.

105 pages

6235 Scleroderma

NAMSIC, National Institutes of Health
1 AMS Circle
Bethesda, MD 20892

301-495-4484
Fax: 301-587-4352
TTY: 301-565-2966
www.nih.gov/niams/

143 pages

6236 Scleroderma Book (The)

Maureen Mayes, MD, author

Oxford University Press
198 Madison Ave
New York, NY 10016

212-726-6000
800-445-9714
Fax: 919-677-1303
e-mail: custserv.us@oup.com
www.oup.com/usa

2005 Hardback
ISBN: 0-195169-40-9

Magazines

6237 Scleroderma Voice

Scleroderma Foundation
300 Rosewood Dr, Suite 105
Danvers, MA 01923

978-463-5843
800-722-4673
Fax: 978-463-5809
e-mail: sfinfo@scleroderma.org
www.scleroderma.org

Includes articles and stories, answers to medical questions, updates on research and treatments, and advice on dealing with scleroderma.

Quarterly

Journals

6238 Scleroderma Care and Research

Scleroderma Clinical Trials Consortium
715 Albany St, E-5
Boston, MA 02118

617-638-4486
e-mail: trials@blackmule.com
www.sclero.org/medical/journals/scar/a-to-z.html

Published by a group of international scleroderma researchers, it covers topics of interest to rheumatologists and others involved in scleroderma care, worldwide.

Pamphlets

6239 Handout on Health: Scleroderma

NIAMS, National Institutes of Health
31 Center Dr, Bldg 31, Rm 4C02
Bethesda, MD 20892

301-496-8190
Fax: 301-480-2814
www.niams.nih.gov/hi

Information including current research efforts for scleroderma.

Revised 7/2006

Camps

6240 Camp Discovery

American Academy of Dermatology
930 E Woodfield Road
Schaumburg, IL 60173

847-240-1737
866-503-7546
Fax: 847-330-8907
e-mail: jmueller@aad.org
www.campdiscovery.org

A camp for young people with serious skin conditions. There is no fee and transportation is provided. Two locations: Camp Horizon in Millville, PA and Camp Knutson in Crosslake, MN.

Stephen P Stone MD, President
Julie Mueller, Camp Information

6241 Camp Wonder
Children's Skin Disease Foundation
712 Bancroft Rd, #511
Walnut Creek, CA 94598

925-947-3825
Fax: 925-947-0677
www.csdf.org/camp/

Established by the CSDF for young people who suffer from skin diseases. Medically staffed camps are free to children, ages 7-17 with skin diseases that are serious or life threatening.

DESCRIPTION

6242 SCOLIOSIS

Synonym: Rachioscoliosis

Covers these related disorders: Compensatory scoliosis, Congenital scoliosis, Idiopathic kyphosis (Scheuermann's disease), Idiopathic scoliosis, Kyphosis, Neuromuscular scoliosis, Syndrome-associated scoliosis

Involves the following Biologic System(s):
Orthopedic and Muscle Disorders

The term scoliosis refers to a condition characterized by a sideward (lateral) curvature of the spine. Idiopathic scoliosis is the most common form of this disorder and occurs for no known reason in otherwise healthy individuals who range in age from infancy to adolescence. Adolescent scoliosis is the most common form and accounts for 80 percent of idiopathic scoliosis. Approximately 20 percent of people with scoliosis report at least one other affected family member. Therefore, in these cases, scoliosis is thought to have a genetic component. Idiopathic scoliosis that develops during infancy often corrects itself, but it may become progressive in older children. Treatment is dependent upon age and the degree of curvature progression. Mild curvatures may require little or no treatment, while more severe involvement may require surgery or the use of braces, etc. (orthotics). Although men and women are affected in about equal numbers, women are more at risk for more significant curvature progression. Girls between onset of puberty growth spurt and cessation of spinal growth are at the greatest risk for idiopathic scoliosis. Physical examination reveals asymmetry in the height of the shoulder and hip, with forward bending.

Congenital scoliosis, apparent at birth or soon thereafter, results from the improper or incomplete development of the vertebrae during the first trimester of pregnancy. This condition may appear singularly or in association with abnormalities of other systems of the body including the heart (i.e., congenital heart disease) and genitourinary tract (e.g., absence of one kidney, duplication of the tubes that carry urine, horseshoe kidney, and other malformations). Congenital scoliosis is often accompanied by other spinal cord defects (spinal dysraphism) that may range from mild to severe. In addition, children born with certain genetic disorders such as Klippel-Feil syndrome may experience associated scoliosis. The progression of the curvature is dependent upon the specific underlying vertebral malformation, its particular growth potential, and its location. About one quarter of affected children experience no progression of the curvature and, therefore, require no treatment. Ap-

proximately half of those remaining may require early treatment, such as spinal fusion of the affected area, to stop progression of the curvature.

Neuromuscular scoliosis is associated with certain childhood diseases (e.g., cerebral palsy, Duchenne muscular dystrophy, polio, and other disorders). This type of scoliosis tends to be progressive, with the degree of deformity dependent upon many factors. Those affected children who are unable to walk (nonambulatory) often develop additional skeletal irregularities involving the pelvis and spine. In severe cases, respiratory difficulties may develop. Early evaluation and intervention through surgery and other means help to alter the progression of the spinal deformity and its associated complications.

Kyphosis is characterized by an exaggerated backward curvature of the spine. Children with poor posture resulting in mild kyphosis who have no associated spinal irregularities may be treated by maintaining good posture. Congenital kyophosis, however, results from various malformations in the spinal column and may range from mild to severe deformity. Scoliosis also is present in one-third of patients with kyphosis. When several vertebrae are involved, there is a round back appearance; when only one vertebra is involved, there is an angular curve. As affected children grow, progression of the spinal abnormality may continue until growth is complete, possibly resulting in partial paralysis. Idiopathic kyphosis or Scheuermann's disease is common to both adolescent boys and girls; cause remains unknown. Examination and x-ray screening may determine whether kyphosis is postural or a result of a spinal malformation. Symptoms of Scheuermann's disease may include mild but chronic back pain and a round-shouldered appearance.

Children with mild kyphosis may be advised to refrain from strenuous activities, while those with more severe symptoms may benefit from sleeping on a very firm mattress, or using a brace or cast. Surgery is rarely indicated.

Certain syndromes (e.g., Marfan syndrome, neurofibromatosis) place affected children at risk for spinal irregularities such as scoliosis and kyphosis. Treatment for these children includes regular orthopedic examination and intervention to prevent progression of the irregularity.

Scoliosis sometimes results from unequal leg length resulting from an irregular tilt (obliquity) of the pelvis. Treatment for this compensatory scoliosis may include the use of special orthopedic shoes.

See also **General Resources** on page 917

Government Agencies

6243 NIH/National Institute of Arthritis and Mu sculoskeletal and Skin Diseases
1AMS Circle
Bethesda, MD 20892

301-402-4484
Fax: 301-718-6366
e-mail: ord@od.nih.gov
rarediseases.info.nih.gov

The mission of the National Institute of Arthritis and Musculoskeletal and Skin Diseases is to support research into the causes, treatment, and prevention of arthritis and musculoskeletal and skin diseases, the training of basic and clinical scientists to carry out this research, and the dissemination of information on research progress in these diseases.

Stephen I Katz MD PhD, Director

National Associations & Support Groups

6244 International Federation of Spine Associations
Howard M Shulman
9908 Cape Scott Court
Raleigh, NC 27614

919-846-2204
e-mail: ifousa@aol.com
www.ifosa.org

IFOSA is a federation of various national Spine Associations from countries in North America, Europe and Australia. These organizations principally represent the spine patients and their families. At the annual meetings of IFOSA, representatives from each of these member organizations are invited to attend and discuss the emotional and social problems which face the spine patient and his or her family.

6245 National Dissemination Center for Children with Disabilities
PO Box 1492
Washington, DC 20013

202-884-8200
800-695-0285
Fax: 202-884-8441
e-mail: nichcy@aed.org
www.nichcy.org

A national information and referral center for families, educators and other professionals on: disabilities in children and youth; programs and services; IDEA, the nation's special education law; and research-based information on effective practices.

Suzanne Ripley, Executive Director

6246 National Scoliosis Foundation
5 Cabot Place
Stoughton, MA 02072

781-341-6333
800-673-6922
Fax: 781-341-8333
e-mail: nsf@scoliosis.org
www.scoliosis.org

Promotes school screening, offers public awareness materials to promote public education, maintains a resource center for professional information, conducts scoliosis conferences, and offers support groups to people affected by the disease.

Joseph O'Brien, President/CEO

6247 Scoliosis Association
PO Box 811705
Boca Raton, FL 33481

561-994-4435
800-800-0669
Fax: 561-994-2455
e-mail: normlipin@aol.com
www.scoliosis-assoc.org

Sponsors and encourages spinal screening programs. Disseminates information throughout the country, and raises funds for scoliosis research. Membership fee of $20.00 includes subscription to newsletter. Videos and printed information available.

Norm Lipin

Libraries & Resource Centers

6248 Johns Hopkins Department of Orthopaedics Surgery
601 N Caroline Street
Baltimore, MD 21287

410-955-1830
Fax: 410-955-1719
www.hopkinsmedicine.org/orthopedicsurgery/

Scoliosis is a three-dimensional curvature of the spine, best appreciated on an anteroposterior radiograph and physical examination. Many different causes have been identified. The most common type is idiopathic scoliosis.

Research Centers

6249 Scoliosis Research Society
555 E Wells Street, Suite 1100
Milwaukee, WI 53202

414-289-9107
Fax: 414-276-3349
e-mail: info@srs.org
www.srs.org

An international society that is committed to research and education for health care professionals in the field of spinal deformities. It is recognized as one of the world's premier spine societies. Current membership includes over 800 of the world's leading spine surgeons as well as researchers, physician assistants and orthotists.

George H Thompson MD, President
Tressa Goulding, Executive Director

6250 Shriners Hospital for Children
Headquarters
2900 Rocky Point Drive
Tampa, FL 33607

813-281-0300
800-237-5055
Fax: 813-281-8496
www.shrinershq.org

Shrine's official philanthropy is Shriners Hospital for Children, a network of 22 hospitals that provide expert, no-cost orthopaedic and burn care to children under 18.

Audio Video

6251 Cutting Edge Medical Report
National Scoliosis Foundation
5 Cabot Place
Stoughton, MA 02072

781-341-6333
800-673-6922
Fax: 781-341-8333
e-mail: nsf@scoliosis.org
www.scoliosis.org

As seen on the Discovery Channel, this video is an in-depth examination of the latest developments in the diagnosis and treatment of scoliosis.

18 Minutes

6252 Dealing with Scoliosis: A Patient Guide to Diagnosis and Treatment

National Scoliosis Foundation
5 Cabot Place
Stoughton, MA 02072

781-341-6333
800-673-6922
Fax: 781-341-8333
e-mail: nsf@scoliosis.org
www.scoliosis.org

An upbeat video featuring Miss North Carolina Michelle Mauney and that explains diagnosis and treatment of scoliosis through the experience of several teenagers and young adults.

20 Minutes

6253 Ellie's Back

National Scoliosis Foundation
5 Cabot Place
Stoughton, MA 02072

781-341-6333
800-673-6922
Fax: 781-341-8333
e-mail: nsf@scoliosis.org
www.scoliosis.org

An eight-year-old, and her mother team up together to produce a film that portrays life with scoliosis through the eyes of a young child.

15 Minutes

6254 Growing Straighter and Stronger

National Scoliosis Foundation
5 Cabot Place
Stoughton, MA 02072

781-341-6333
800-673-6922
Fax: 781-341-8333
e-mail: nsf@scoliosis.org
www.scoliosis.org

Produced for the pre-screening education of students in grades 5-9. It emphasizes the importance of follow-up screening, encourages peer support and prescribed follow-up treatment. Video is also available on loan for a refundable deposit plus shipping and handling.

15 Minutes

6255 Preparing Yourself for Spinal Surgery (For Teenagers with Severe Scoliosis)

National Scoliosis Foundation
5 Cabot Place
Stoughton, MA 02072

781-341-6333
800-673-6922
Fax: 781-341-8333
e-mail: nsf@scoliosis.org
www.scoliosis.org

Patient educational video helping to reduce the anxiety for teenagers facing surgery by giving a sense of what to expect before, during, and after surgery.

18 Minutes

6256 School Screening with Dr. Robert Keller

National Scoliosis Foundation
5 Cabot Place
Stoughton, MA 02072

781-341-6333
800-673-6922
Fax: 781-341-8333
e-mail: nsf@scoliosis.org
www.scoliosis.org

A training video that teaches the proper technique for doing spinal screening. Defines scoliosis and kyphosis. Four teenagers, three with curves and one without, are examined and the findings explained.

60 Minutes

6257 Sharing Scoliosis: You're Not Alone

National Scoliosis Foundation
5 Cabot Place
Stoughton, MA 02072

781-341-6333
800-673-6922
Fax: 781-341-8333
e-mail: nsf@scoliosis.org
www.scoliosis.org

The Missouri chapter of the NSF, shares their experience with scoliosis including diagnosis, wearing a brace, surgery, and recovery. It is a good source of support for patients of all ages and their families.

26 Minutes

6258 Taking the Mystery Out of Spinal Deformities

Children's Hospital of LA, Div. of Orthopaedics
4650 Sunset Boulevard
Los Angeles, CA 90027

323-660-2450
www.childrenshospitalla.org

Answers questions most often asked by screeners, patients and parents.

Videotape

6259 Understanding Scoliosis

National Scoliosis Foundation
5 Cabot Place
Stoughton, MA 02072

781-341-6333
800-673-6922
Fax: 781-341-8333
e-mail: nsf@scoliosis.org
www.scoliosis.org

A Kaiser Permanente educational video that clearly and positively addresses the patient community. In this video four teenagers at various stages of treatment talk about their life with scoliosis.

8 Minutes

6260 What's This Thing Called Scoliosis

Dr Charles Ray, author

National Scoliosis Foundation
5 Cabot Place
Stoughton, MA 02072

781-341-6333
800-673-6922
Fax: 781-341-8333
e-mail: nsf@scoliosis.org
www.scoliosis.org

A comprehensive overview of scoliosis using the latest computer technology. The anatomical spine and animated model work together to truly show the 3D aspects of scoliosis and the corresponding impact on the patient.

17 Minutes

6261 You Are Not Alone
Minnesota Spine Center
606 24th Avenue S
Minneapolis, MN 55454

612-332-3843

A video presenting two women's experiences with surgery. Personal life, concerns, hospital experience, recovery and improved lifestyle are openly discussed.

Videotape

Web Sites

6262 American Academy of Orthopaedic Surgeons
www.aaos.org

Provides an informational fact sheet on scoliosis in children and adolescents.

6263 Health Answers
www.healthanswers.com

HealthAnswers offers a breadth of services in medical education, sales force training, patient support solutions, professional promotion and consumer solutions.

6264 John Hopkins Department of Orthopaedics Surgery
www.hopkinsmedicine.org/orthopedicsurgery/

The orthopaedics faculty works together as a team to provide optimum patient care, seeking out a role in patient care as both educators and treating physicians working together with you and your community health care providers to offer you the best possible medical and surgical care available.

6265 Natalie's Brace
www.nataliesbrace.com/scoliosis/

Personal website offering personal details and photos on scoliosis braces, general information and support.

6266 North Ameerican Spine Society
www.spine.org/fsp/prob_action-injury-scoliosis.cfm

Provides information on adolescent idiopathic scoliosis, including a description of, common problems associated with the curvature, and possible treatments.

6267 Online Mendelian Inheritance in Man
www.ncbi.nlm.nih.gov

This database is a catalog of human genes and genetic disorders.

6268 Scoliosis Help
www.scoliosishelp.org

6269 Scoliosis Message Forum
www.scoliosis.org/forum/index.php

An independent list maintained by people who have scoliosis. You can find people with whom you can share your experiences and ask questions.

6270 Scoliosis Research Society
www.srs.org

An international society that is committed to research and education for health care professionals in the field of spinal deformities. It is recognized as one of the world's premier spine societies. Current membership includes over 800 of the world's leading spine surgeons as well as researchers, physician assistants and orthotists.

6271 Wheeless' Textbook of Orthopaedics
www.wheelessonline.com

Derives from a variety of sources, including journals, articles, national meetings lectures and other textbooks.

Book Publishers

6272 Adult Scoliosis Surgery...It Can Be Done
Saint Luke's Spine Center
11311 Shaker Boulevard
Cleveland, OH 44104

216-368-7000

Describes various types of surgery and procedures used in adult scoliosis patients.

21 pages

6273 Coalition Index
American School Health Association
PO Box 708
Kent, OH 44240

330-678-1601
Fax: 330-678-4526
e-mail: asha@asahweb.org
www.ashaweb.org

Helps plan health education curriculums with information on materials obtained from nearly 20 national health-related organizations.

6274 Deenie
Simon & Schuster/Atheneum Books
866 3rd Avenue
New York, NY 10022

212-698-2808
877-989-0009
Fax: 212-698-4350
www.simonsays.com

Deenie, a beautiful thirteen-year-old girl, had a mother who was pushing her to become a model. The agency representatives told Deenie she had the looks but walked differently. Deenie's main wish was to become a cheerleader. Her close friend, Janet, made the cheerleading squad but Deenie didn't make the finalist list. After this her gym teacher noticed her posture and called her family. After seeing therapists, the diagnosis of adolescent idiopathic scoliosis was made.

159 pages Hardcover
ISBN: 0-689866-10-0

6275 Getting Ready, Getting Well
Mary Knapp, author

National Scoliosis Foundation
5 Cabot Place
Stoughton, MA 02072

781-341-6333
Fax: 781-341-8333
e-mail: scoliosis@aol.com

A guide for those anticipating surgery; divided into three sections: Making Up Your Mind, Taking Charge, and Home Again.

73 pages

6276 Growing Up with Scoliosis: A Young Girl's Story
Michelle Spray, author

National Scoliosis Foundation
5 Cabot Place
Stoughton, MA 02072

781-341-6333
800-673-6922
Fax: 781-341-8333
e-mail: nsf@scoliosis.org
www.scoliosis.org

A personal account of growing up with scoliosis and the different stages of treatment, progression and surgery.

6277 Handbook of Scoliosis

Scoliosis Research Society
555 East Wells Street, Suite 1100
Milwaukee, WI 53202

414-289-9107
Fax: 414-276-3349
www.srs.org

6278 Nothing Hurts But My Heart

Linda Barr, author

National Scoliosis Foundation
5 Cabot Place
Stoughton, MA 02072

781-341-6333
800-673-6922
Fax: 781-341-8333
e-mail: nsf@scoliosis.org
www.scoliosis.org

For every boy, girl, and their parents who learn that bracing may be needed to treat their scoliosis. The story is of a young gymnast dealing with the issues of wearing a brace.

6279 Scoliosis Surgery, The Definitive Patient's Reference: Second Edition

Dave Wolpert, author

National Scoliosis Foundation
5 Cabot Place
Stoughton, MA 02072

781-341-6333
800-673-6922
Fax: 781-341-8333
e-mail: nsf@scoliosis.org
www.scoliosis.org

For all those contemplating surgery or that know someone who is; it explains in detail everything you need to know, written in layman's terms by someone who has gone through it.

6280 Scoliosis: What Young People and Parents Need to Know

American Physical Therapy Association
1111 N Fairfax Street
Alexandria, VA 22314

703-684-2782
800-999-2782
Fax: 703-684-7343
www.apta.org

A physical therapist's perspective about what scoliosis is and what parents and young people should look for to detect scoliosis. Also available in Spanish.

12 pages Packet of 25

6281 Stopping Scoliosis

Nancy Schommer, author

National Scoliosis Foundation
5 Cabot Place
Stoughton, MA 02072

781-341-6333
800-673-6922
Fax: 781-341-8333
e-mail: nsf@scoliosis.org
www.scoliosis.org

Filled with accurate, currently researched information for adults concerned with their condition or that of a young person.

6282 Textbook of Scoliosis & Other Spinal Deformities

WB Saunders Company
Independence Square W
Philadelphia, PA 19104

215-238-7800

1994
ISBN: 0-721655-33-5

6283 There's an S on My Back: S is for Scoliosis

Mary Mahony, author

National Scoliosis Foundation
5 Cabot Place
Stoughton, MA 02072

781-341-6333
800-673-6922
Fax: 781-341-8333
e-mail: nsf@scoliosis.org
www.scoliosis.org

The medical journey of a fifth grader diagnosed with idiopathic scoliosis at a school screening. A realistic fiction, the story gives us a day-by-day account of what a preadolescent experiences.

6284 Tina's Story...Scoliosis and Me

Alfred I DuPont Institute
PO Box 269
Wilmington, DE 19899

302-651-4000

Suggested for parents of children anticipating surgery. This outstanding book, written as an eighth grade project by a thirteen-year-old scoliosis patient, relates her experiences and emotions while wearing a brace for three years prior to surgery.

6285 Twenty Years At Hull House

Jane Addams, author

New American Library/Penguin Group
375 Hudson Street
New York, NY 10014

212-366-2000
800-631-8571
us.penguingroup.com

336 pages
ISBN: 0-451527-39-4

6286 What Can I Give You?

Mary Mahony, author

National Scoliosis Foundation
5 Cabot Place
Stoughton, MA 02072

781-341-6333
800-673-6922
Fax: 781-341-8333
e-mail: nsf@scoliosis.org
www.scoliosis.org

A wounderful story of a loving mother's care for her daughter. The medical saga of Erin and Mary offers insight and inspiration to families living with congenital scoliosis and valuable guidance to the physicians who treat them.

Newsletters

6287 Backtalk

Scoliosis Association
PO Box 811705
Boca Raton, FL 33481

561-994-4435
Fax: 561-994-2455
e-mail: normlipin@aol.com
www.scoliosis-assoc.org

Information for families, patients and health care professionals. Includes a section for pen pals, an Ask the Doctor column, and a highlighted personal story.

3-4/yr

6288 Spinal Connection
National Scoliosis Foundation
5 Cabot Place
Stoughton, MA 02072

781-341-6333
800-673-6922
Fax: 781-341-8333
e-mail: nsf@scoliosis.org
www.scoliosis.org

Offers updated information, the latest medical advances, and new research studies in the area of abnormal spinal curvatures.

8 pages Bi-annual

Pamphlets

6289 1 in Every 10 Persons Has Scoliosis
National Scoliosis Foundation
5 Cabot Place
Stoughton, MA 02072

781-341-6333
800-673-6922
Fax: 781-341-8333
e-mail: nsf@scoliosis.org
www.scoliosis.org

Explains what scoliosis is and illustrates how to screen for it. It also contains facts about the Foundation.

6290 Adolescent Idiopathic Scoliosis-Prevalence ,Natural History, Treatments
National Scoliosis Foundation
5 Cabot Place
Stoughton, MA 02072

781-341-6333
800-673-6922
Fax: 781-341-8333
e-mail: nsf@scoliosis.org
www.scoliosis.org

6291 Boston Bracing System for Idiopathic Scoli osis
National Scoliosis Foundation
5 Cabot Place
Stoughton, MA 02072

781-341-6333
800-673-6922
Fax: 781-341-8333
e-mail: nsf@scoliosis.org
www.scoliosis.org

6292 Brace & Her Brace is No Handicap
National Scoliosis Foundation
5 Cabot Place
Stoughton, MA 02072

781-341-6333
800-673-6922
Fax: 781-341-8333
e-mail: nsf@scoliosis.org
www.scoliosis.org

Contains two illustrated short stories, each about a teenage girl coping successfully with scoliosis.

6293 Getting a Second Opinion
National Scoliosis Foundation
5 Cabot Place
Stoughton, MA 02072

781-341-6333
800-673-6922
Fax: 781-341-8333
e-mail: nsf@scoliosis.org
www.scoliosis.org

Reprinted from Health Tips.

6294 Medical Update Column
National Scoliosis Foundation
5 Cabot Place
Stoughton, MA 02072

781-341-6333
800-673-6922
Fax: 781-341-8333
e-mail: nsf@scoliosis.org
www.scoliosis.org

Reprints from past issues of the Spinal Connections Medical Update Column available on various topics.

6295 NSF Packets
National Scoliosis Foundation
5 Cabot Place
Stoughton, MA 02072

781-341-6333
800-673-6922
Fax: 781-341-8333
e-mail: nsf@scoliosis.org
www.scoliosis.org

Packet contains information for parents and young people, adults, and health care professionals.

6296 Postural Screening Program
National Scoliosis Foundation
5 Cabot Place
Stoughton, MA 02072

781-341-6333
800-673-6922
Fax: 781-341-8333
e-mail: nsf@scoliosis.org
www.scoliosis.org

Guidelines for physicians and school nurses.

6297 Questions Most Often Asked the NSF
National Scoliosis Foundation
5 Cabot Place
Stoughton, MA 02072

781-341-6333
800-673-6922
Fax: 781-341-8333
e-mail: nsf@scoliosis.org
www.scoliosis.org

Answers the most frequently asked questions about scoliosis and the foundation in general.

6298 Questions and Answers About Scoliosis
Federal Citizen Information Center

Pueblo, CO 81009

888-878-3256
www.pueblo.gsa.gov

6299 Scoliosis Research Society
555 East Wells Street, Suite 1100
Milwaukee, WI 53202

414-289-9107
Fax: 414-276-3349
e-mail: tjackson@execinc.com
www.srs.org/

The Scoliosis Research Society is a professional organization, made up of physicians and allied health personnel. The primary focus is on providing continuing medical education for health care professionals and on funding/supporting research in spinal deformities. Founded in 1966, the SRS has gained recognition as one of the world's leading spine societies. Current membership includes over 800 of the world's leading spine surgeons as well as some researchers, physician assistants and orthotists.

Tressa Goulding, Executive Director
Tiffany Ann Jackson, Membership Manager

6300 Scoliosis and Kyphosis
Scoliosis Research Society
611 East Wells Street, Suite 1100
Milwaukee, WI 53202

414-289-9107
Fax: 414-276-3349
www.srs.org

Information and advice from parents.

6301 Scoliosis: A Handbook for Patients
National Scoliosis Foundation
5 Cabot Place
Stoughton, MA 02072

781-341-6333
800-673-6922
Fax: 781-341-8333
e-mail: nsf@scoliosis.org
www.scoliosis.org

Information on detection and treatment of adolescent scoliosis, kyphosis and lordosis and adult scoliosis.

6302 When the Spine Curves
National Scoliosis Foundation
5 Cabot Place
Stoughton, MA 02072

781-341-6333
800-673-6922
Fax: 781-341-8333
e-mail: nsf@scoliosis.org
www.scoliosis.org

Camps

6303 Hemlocks Easter Seals Recreation
85 Jones Street
Hebron, CT 06248

860-228-9496
800-832-4409
Fax: 860-228-2091
e-mail: info@eastersealscamphemlocks.org
www.eastersealscamphemlocks.org

Accepts campers, ages 6 and under, whose major disability is orthopedic. First preference is given to Connecticut residents. A computer camp is also available.

Carl Larson

DESCRIPTION

6304 SEIZURES

Synonyms: Convulsions, Epilepsy

Covers these related disorders: Absence (petit mal) seizures, Complex partial seizures, Generalized (grand mal) tonic-clonic seizures, Simple partial seizures, Epilepsy

Involves the following Biologic System(s):

Neurologic Disorders

Seizures are a neurologic condition characterized by sudden episodes of uncontrolled electrical activity in the brain. These electrical disturbances may cause abnormal motor activities, lost or impaired consciousness, impaired control of certain involuntary functions (autonomic dysfunction), or sensory or behavioral abnormalities. Seizures are a common neurologic condition of childhood, affecting approximately six in 1,000 children. Approximately 70 percent of children who experience one seizure never experience another, whereas about 30 percent develop recurring seizures, which is referred to as epilepsy. Seizures may result from many different causes, including fever, head injury, infection or inflammation of the brain, insufficient oxygen supply to the brain, or certain metabolic imbalances. Seizures may also be caused by brain tumors, particular degenerative metabolic or neurological diseases, abnormal reactions to certain medications, or drug intoxication. There are also a number of syndromes and genetic disorders in which seizures are a primary feature. In many children, the exact underlying cause of recurrent seizures cannot be determined and the disorder is termed idiopathic epilepsy.

The specific form that a seizure takes and its associated symptoms may depend upon a number of factors, including the region of the brain in which the electrical disturbance arises and how widely it spreads from its point of origin. Epileptic seizures may be broadly classified into two groups: partial and generalized seizures. Partial seizures often result due to damage or impairment of a limited area of the brain, whereas generalized seizures may affect a wide area of the brain. In addition, some partial seizures may begin in a particular brain region but spread to affect most of the brain, ultimately becoming a generalized seizure. Because different seizure types may cause similar symptoms, specialized techniques that record brain wave activity (electroencephalography or EEG) and other neurologic imaging tests (such as MRI or CT scans) may play an important role in classifying certain seizure disorders.

Partial seizures, which may account for up to 40 percent of childhood seizures, may be subdivided into simple partial seizures, during which consciousness is retained, and complex partial seizures, during which consciousness is impaired. Simple partial seizures are characterized by abnormal, rhythmic muscle contractions and relaxations (clonic activity) and increased muscle tone and rigidity (tonic activity), particularly affecting muscles of the neck, face, arms, and legs. Simple partial seizures, which usually last about 10 to 20 seconds, are frequently associated with abnormal eye movements and head turning. In many child|ren, simple partial seizures may be preceded by an aura consisting of headache, chest discomfort, and a feeling of anxiety, fear, or dread.

Complex partial seizures are characterized by a sudden pause in activity and a blank stare and may be preceded by an aura that consists of a vague feeling of fear or unpleasantness, headache, and chest discomfort. Most patients also perform certain involuntary actions following loss of consciousness. In infants, such actions may include lip smacking, swallowing, or chewing, whereas older children may conduct incoordinated, semipurposeful actions, such as rubbing objects or pulling at clothing. Such seizures may last approximately one to two minutes.

Generalized seizures may be subdivided into nonconvulsive (petit mal, absence) seizures and convulsive (grand mal or tonic-clonic) seizures. Absence seizures, which rarely occur before the age of five, usually last from a few seconds up to half a minute. During an episode, children experience a momentary loss of consciousness during which they cease speaking or performing other motor activities. They typically have a blank facial expression, their eyelids may flicker, and the head may fall forward. Patients typically have no awareness of the episode and resume the activity they were performing before the seizure.

Generalized tonic-clonic seizures may be preceded by an aura and occasionally begin with a shrill cry as patients lose consciousness. During an episode, the eyes roll back, muscles of the entire body stiffen, and all muscle groups begin to rhythmically contract and relax. If temporary cessation of breathing (apnea) occurs, patients may quickly develop an abnormal, bluish discoloration of the skin and mucous membranes (cyanosis). Bladder and bowel control may be temporarily lost. After an episode, patients are typically semiconscious and disoriented and may remain in a deep sleep for up to two hours (postictal state). During such a seizure episode, patients should be placed on one side, tight clothing around the neck should be loosened, and the jaw should be gently extended to enhance breathing. However, the mouth should not be forcibly opened nor should an object be placed between the teeth.

Generalized seizures also include a form of epilepsy known as infantile spasms, which typically begin between the ages of four and eight months and continue to approximately 18 months. Infantile spasms are characterized by sudden, brief, symmetric contractions of the arms and legs, neck, and torso. Spasms may occur for several minutes with brief intervals between each spasm. Episodes tend to occur when children are drowsy or immediately upon awakening. Depending upon the underlying cause, the condition may evolve into different forms of epilepsy later in life and may be associated with an increased risk of mental retardation.

Seizures that occur in association with a rapidly rising fever, known as febrile seizures, are the most common seizure disorder of childhood. Febrile seizures most commonly occur between nine months to five years of age and may affect up to four percent of all children. This type of seizure rarely develops into epilepsy. In many cases, there is a history of such seizures among siblings and parents, indicating that genetic factors may play some causative role. Febrile seizures often occur in association with certain upper respiratory infections and acute inflammation of the middle ear (otitis media). However, because convulsions may result from serious infections of the brain (e.g., meningitis), a thorough medical evaluation must be conducted to determine the cause of the fever. Febrile seizures are typically characterized by muscle rigidity followed by abnormal, rhythmic contractions and relaxations of muscle groups (generalized tonic-clonic seizures). The seizure may last from seconds up to about 10 minutes and is often followed by a brief period of drowsiness.

Generalized or partial seizures that continue for more than 30 minutes without a return to consciousness are known as status epilepticus. Such seizures may occur due to underlying metabolic abnormalities, neurologic disorders, congenital brain malformations, or inflammation of the brain. They may also represent prolonged febrile seizures, develop due to sudden withdrawal of antiseizure (anticonvulsant) medication, or result from unknown causes. Status epilepticus may result in life-threatening complications and is considered a medical emergency, requiring hospitalization. Treatment may include supplemental oxygen, intravenous fluids, physical and neurologic evaluations, intravenous medications including appropriate antiseizure drugs, and other measures as required. Children affected by the condition before one year of age are more likely to have mental retar-

dation and other long-term effects, secondary to an underlying CNS disorder.

The treatment of seizures depends on the underlying cause, the type of seizure present, and other factors. If a treatable condition or disorder is identified, such as a fever, abnormal blood sugar levels, or certain tumors, measures are taken as required to treat the underlying cause. For example, in the case of febrile seizures, thorough evaluations are conducted to determine the fever's cause and measures are then taken as necessary to control the fever. If an underlying cause cannot be identified or adequately treated or controlled, treatment typically includes the administration of antiseizure (anticonvulsant) medications to help prevent, reduce, or control seizures. The specific anticonvulsant medication prescribed may depend on several factors, including the classification of the seizure, patient history, and possible side effects. Anticonvulsant drugs used to treat certain types of seizures may include carbamazepine, phenobarbital, primidone, phenytoin, gabapentin, or valproate. In addition, adrenocorticotropic hormone (ACTH) is often used to treat children with infantile spasms. If seizure control is not obtained with a particular medication, other anticonvulsants may be substituted. In some patients, combination drug therapy may be necessary to adequately control seizures. If seizure control is not obtained with anticonvulsant medications, surgery may be considered. Additional treatment is symptomatic and supportive.

See also **General Resources** on page 917

National Associations & Support Groups

6305 American Epilepsy Society
342 N Main Street
W Hartford, CT 06117

860-586-7505
Fax: 860-568-7550
www.aesnet.org

A society of clinicians, researchers, and health care professionals which promotes education and research of epilepsy.

Suzanne C Berry, Executive Director
Martin Rotblatt, Associate Director

6306 C.A.N.D.L.E.
4414 McCampbell Drive
Montgomery, AL 36106

334-271-3947
Fax: 334-271-3947

Networking, referrals to local resources, and local chapters.

6307 Cleveland Clinic Children's Hospital & Epilepsy Center
9500 Euclid Avenue
Cleveland, OH 44195

216-444-2200
800-223-2273
Fax: 216-445-7792
TTY: 216-444-0261
cms.clevelandclinic.org/childrenshospital/

Provides innovative care for infants, children, and adolescents with complex medical problems. Includes medical, surgical, rehabilitation, psychiatric and intensive care, latest technology, including a computerized epilepsy monitoring unit, a consolidated pediatric intensive care unit and operating suites. Physicians are known for their expertise in treating major medical problems, such as cardiovascular disease, cancer, digestive disorders, musculoskeletal problems and neurosensory disorders.

Imad Najm MD, Director
Prakash Kotagal MD, Pediatric Epilepsy Head

6308 Epilepsy Concern International Service Group
1282 Wynnewood Drive
West Palm Beach, FL 33417

407-683-0044

Epilepsy Concern, founded in 1978, strives to start and maintain small self-help groups of caring people who are seeking help in dealing with epilepsy. The organization is comprised of self-supporting units called area councils that represent geographic areas. Members of the groups are mostly people with epilepsy and their families.

6309 Epilepsy Foundation
8301 Professional Place
Landover, MD 20785

301-459-3700
800-332-1000
Fax: 301-577-2684
e-mail: postmaster@efa.org
www.epilepsyfoundation.org

A national, charitable, nonprofit, volunteer agency dedicated to the welfare of people with epilepsy and their families. Its goals are the prevention and cure of seizure disorders, the alleviation of their effects, and the promotion of independence and optimal quality of life for people who have these disorders. The organization offers education, advocacy, service and research support groups, and has a network of local affiliates serving nearly 100 communities.

Tony Coelho, Chair
Eric R Hargis, President/CEO

6310 Epilepsy Foundation of America Helpline
Epilepsy Foundation
8301 Professional Place
Landover, MD 20785

301-459-3700
800-332-1000
Fax: 301-577-2684
e-mail: postmaster@efa.org
www.epilepsyfoundation.org

A toll free information and referral service staffed by specially trained people who will answer questions and discuss concerns about seizure disorders and their treatment. Staff will direct callers to local affiliates of the EFA and tell about a broad range of medical services that respond to the needs of people with seizure disorders.

Eric Hargis, CEO

6311 Epilepsy Institute
257 Park Avenue S, Suite 302
New York, NY 10010

212-677-8550
Fax: 212-677-5825
e-mail: website@epilepsyinstitute.org
www.epilepsyinstitute.org

Program services are available to residents of NYC and Westchester County. The institute is a nonprofit social service organization with information available in Spanish, French, Chinese and Russian.

6312 FACES: Finding a Cure for Epilepsy & Seizures
724 Second Ave, LL
New York, NY 10016

212-871-0245
Fax: 212-871-1823
e-mail: nyufaces@yahoo.com
www.nyufaces.org

Nonprofit organization affiliated with NYU Medical Center and its Comprehensive Epilepsy Center. It strives to accomplish its mission through research, clinical programs, awareness, and community education and events.

Valerie Luscuzek, Executive Director
Althea Morris, Education Coordinator

6313 Genetic Alliance
4301 Connecticut Avenue NW
Washington, DC 20008

202-966-5557
800-336-4363
Fax: 202-966-8553
e-mail: info@geneticalliance.org
www.geneticalliance.org

A coalition of voluntary genetic support groups, consumers and professionals addressing the needs of individuals and families affected by genetic disorders from a national perspective.

Sharon Terry, President/CEO

6314 National Association of Epilepsy Centers
5775 Wayzata Blvd, Suite 200
Minneapolis, MN 55416

952-525-4526
888-525-6232
Fax: 952-525-1560
e-mail: info@naec-epilepsy.org
www.naecepilepsy.org

A nonprofit organization that encourages and supports professional and technical education in the treatment of epilepsy. Over 60 centers nationwide are members of the trade association, which will make referrals to its member centers.

Robert J Gumnit, MD, President
Gregory L Barkley MD, VP

6315 Parents Against Childhood Epilepsy (PACE)
7 E 85th St, Suite A3
New York, NY 10028

212-665-7223
Fax: 212-327-3075
e-mail: pacenyemail@aol.com
www.paceusa.org

Research and education fund for severe seizure disorders and epilepsy.

Susan Fahey, Chair
Lauren Beck, President

State Agencies & Support Groups

Arkansas

6316 Epilepsy Education Association of Arkansas
2902 E Kiehl, Suite 1B
Sherwood, AR 72120

501-833-8680
e-mail: sharon@epilepsyarkansas.com
www.epilepsyarkansas.com

A resource and provider of support and education in Arkansas for those with epilepsy.

Sharon Wingo McGinn, Director
Judy Hess RN, Co-Director

California

6317 Epilepsy Foundation of Northern California
5700 Stoneridge Mall Rd. Suite 295
Pleasanton, CA 94588

925-224-7760
800-632-3532
Fax: 925-224-7770
e-mail: efnca@epilepsynorcal.org
www.epilepsynorcal.org

Nonprofit center serving families affected by epilepsy since 1953.

William J Marks Jr, MD, President
Neva Hirschkorn, Executive Director

Florida

6318 Epilepsy Association of Big Bend
1215 Lee Ave, Suite M-4
Tallahassee, FL 32303

850-222-1777
Fax: 850-222-7440
e-mail: epilepsyassoc@earthlink.net

Services include: case management, prevention education, counseling and advocacy, information and referral.

6319 Epilepsy Foundation of Florida
7300 N Kendall Drive, Suite 700
Miami, FL 33156

305-670-4949
Fax: 305-670-0904
e-mail: information@epilepsysofla.org
www.epilepsysofla.org

The Epilepsy Foundation of Southern Florida and of Northeast Florida merged to formed one organization.

Patricia Dean, President
A.G. Newmyer III, VP

6320 Epilepsy Services of Northeast Florida
6028 Chester Avenue
Jacksonville, FL 32217

904-731-3751
e-mail: efnefjohn@aol.com

Services include : program case management, program prevention and education, employment services, children's summer camp, counseling and advocacy, and information and referrals.

6321 Florida Epilepsy Services Providers Association
11200 NW 8th Avenue
Gainesville, FL 32601

352-392-6449
800-330-9746
Fax: 352-392-5792
e-mail: fespa@floridaepilepsy.org
www.floridaepilepsy.org

A nonprofit membership organization of epilepsy services providers in the state of Florida, that serve the needs of those with epilepsy and their families. Local offices for services can be found for different regions and counties of Florida.

Jim Lyons, Program Director

New Jersey

6322 Epilepsy Foundation New Jersey
429 River View Plaza
Trenton, NJ 08611

609-392-4900
Fax: 609-392-5621
TDD: 800-852-7899
e-mail: efnj@efnj.com
www.efnj.com

A nonprofit organization providing support services for those with seizure disorders and their families.

Eric M Joice, Executive Director
Liza Grundell, Deputy Director

New York

6323 Chrissy & Friends
930 Willowbrook Rd
Staten Island, NY 10314

718-698-1800
e-mail: info@chrissyandfriends.org
www.chrissyandfriends.org

Offers children with epilepsy an opportunity to develop friendships through a variety of activities and tutoring programs.

RoseAnne DeRenzo, President
RoseAnne Zielechowski, VP

6324 Epilepsy Foundation of Long Island
506 Stewart Avenue
Garden City, NY 11530

516-739-7733
888-672-7154
Fax: 516-739-1861
e-mail: info@efli.org
www.epilepsyfoundation.org/longisland/

Richard E Daly, Executive Director
Paul Giotis, Program Operations

Pennsylvania

6325 Epilepsy Foundation Eastern Pennsylvania
919 Walnut Street, Suite 700
Philadelphia, PA 19107

215-629-5003
800-887-7165
Fax: 215-629-4997
e-mail: epilepsy@efsepa.org
www.efsepa.org

Caren B Anders, Board President
Jeanette K Chelius, Executive Director

6326 Epilepsy Foundation of Western/Central Pennsylvania
1323 Forbes Avenue, Suite 102
Pittsburgh, PA 15219

412-261-5880
800-316-5585
Fax: 412-261-5361
e-mail: staff@efwp.org
www.efwp.org

Judith K Painter, Executive Director
Peggy Beem, Associate Director

Washington

6327 Epilepsy Foundation Northwest
3800 Aurora Avenue N, Suite 370
Seattle, WA 98103

206-547-4551
800-752-3509
e-mail: msterling@epilepsynw.org
www.epilepsynw.org

Serves all of Oregon & Washington.

Krista C Sandberg, Executive Director
Altae Hancock, Associate Director/Manager

Research Centers

California

6328 EpiCenter
University of California, Irvine

Irvine, CA 92697

949-824-5011
www.ucihs.uci.edu/epilepsyresearch/index.htm

Researchers, scientists and physicians studying the mechanisms and consequences of epilepsies through a variety of scientific approaches and research.

Tallie Z Baram, Chair

Illinois

6329 Citizens United for Research in Epilepsy (CURE)
730 N Franklin Street, Suite 404
Chicago, IL 60610

312-255-1801
800-765-7118
Fax: 312-255-1809
e-mail: info@CUREepilepsy.org
www.cureepilepsy.org

Susan Axelrod, President/Founder
Susan Green, Executive Director

Maryland

6330 Epilepsy Research Laboratory, Department of Neurology
Johns Hopkins University
Meyer 2-147, 600 N Wolfe St
Baltimore, MD 21287

e-mail: pfranasz@jhimi.edu
www.hopkinsneuro.org/epilepsy/

The Epilepsy Center evaluates and cares for seizure disorder patients from pediatric through adult.

Gregory K Bergey MD, Director

Missouri

6331 Pediatric Epilepsy Center
St Louis Children's Hospital
One Children's Place, Suite 12E47
St Louis, MO 63110

314-454-4089
Fax: 314-454-4225
www.neuro.wustl.edu/epilepsy/pediatric/

A comprehensive and one of the largest centers for epilespy and seizure disorder care and research in the nation. It includes dedicated staff and an inpatient Epilepsy Monitoring Unit.

Edwin Trevathan MD, Director Pediatric Division

New York

6332 Center for Neural Recovery & Rehabilitation Research
Helen Hayes Hospital
Route 9W
West Haverstraw, NY 10993

845-786-4225
888-707-3422
Fax: 845-947-3097
www.helenhayeshospital.org/research/

Helen E Scharfman PhD, Director

North Carolina

6333 Duke University Comprehensive Epilepsy Center
Box 3807
Durham, NC 27710

919-684-6936
Fax: 919-681-6566
e-mail: haglu001@mc.duke.edu
neuro.surgery.duke.edu

Evaluation of potential surgical candidates by epilepsy specialists.

Dr Michael Haglund, Director

Tennessee

6334 Neuroscience Institute, University of Tenn essee Health Science Center
855 Monroe Ave, Suite 515
Memphis, TN 38163

901-448-5957
Fax: 901-448-7193
www.utmem.edu/neuroscience/

Epilepsy research and studies.

Brenda Smith, Contact

Texas

6335 Baylor Comprehensive Epilepsy Center
Baylor College of Medicine
One Baylor Plaza
Houston, TX 77030

713-798-8259
Fax: 713-798-7533
www.bcm.edu/neurol/research/epilep/epilep8.html

Individualized care for those with seizure disorders.

Eli M Mizrahi MD, Director

Wisconsin

6336 Regional Epilepsy Center
Aurora St. Luke's Medical Center
2801 W Kinnickic River Pkwy, Ste 570
Milwaukee, WI 53215

414-385-8780
www.aurorahealthcare.org/services/epilepsy/

Dr George Morris, Director

Audio Video

6337 Because You Are My Friend
Epilepsy Foundation
8301 Professional Place
Landover, MD 20785

301-459-3700
800-332-1000
Fax: 301-577-2684
e-mail: postmaster@efa.org
www.epilepsyfoundation.org

Video tape for children that provides a clear explanation of epilepsy, first aid and the importance of friendship. Cartoon slide presentation with child narration.

6338 Comprehensive Clinical Management of the Epilepsies
Epilepsy Foundation
8301 Professional Place
Landover, MD 20785

301-459-3700
800-332-1000
Fax: 301-577-2684
e-mail: postmaster@efa.org
www.epilepsyfoundation.org

Excellent reference on the treatment of epilepsy.

17 minutes

6339 Epilepsy: The Untold Story
Fanflight Productions
4196 Washington Street
Boston, MA 02131

617-469-4999
800-937-4113
Fax: 617-469-3379
e-mail: info@fanlight.com
www.fanlight.com

This video tells the story of six people with Temporal Lobe Epilepsy.

1993 Video - 27 mins
ISBN: 1-572951-37-0

Nicole Johnson, Publicity Coordinator

6340 How to Recognize and Classify Seizures
Epilepsy Foundation
8301 Professional Place
Landover, MD 20785

301-459-3700
800-332-1000
Fax: 301-577-2684
www.epilepsyfoundation.org

Discusses the classification of seizures and epileptic syndromes.

25 minutes

6341 Just Like You and Me
WellMe/State of the Art
2201 Wisconsin Ave NW, Ste 350
Washington, DC 20008

202-537-0818
Fax: 202-537-0828
e-mail: contact@wellme.com
wellme.stateart.com/productions/health/epilepsy/

A video/patient info guide package on successfully living with epilepsy.

6342 Rest of the Family
Epilepsy Foundation
8301 Professional Place
Landover, MD 20785

301-459-3700
800-332-1000
Fax: 301-577-2684
www.epilepsyfoundation.org

Presents the feelings and concerns of other family members, including siblings, of children with epilepsy.

Videocassette

6343 Seizure First Aid
Epilepsy Foundation
8301 Professional Place
Landover, MD 20785

301-459-3700
800-332-1000
Fax: 301-577-2684
www.epilepsyfoundation.org

This video combines footage of real seizures with reenactments to demonstrate proper first aid procedures. In addition, people with epilepsy talk about how they feel when they have a seizure, and discuss how they would like friends, family and the general public to react when a seizure occurs. 10 minutes.

Video & DVD

6344 Understanding Seizures & Epilepsy
Epilepsy Foundation
8301 Professional Place
Landover, MD 20785

301-459-3700
800-332-1000
Fax: 301-577-2684
www.epilepsyfoundation.org

Provides an explanation of seizure disorders in everyday language and dispels many misconceptions about epilepsy with medically accurate information.

Videocassette

Web Sites

6345 American Epilepsy Society
www.aesnet.org

The society promotes research and education of professionals in the field of epilepsy and related disorders. The site includes a comprehensive listing of postgraduate training opportunities in the fields related to epilepsy.

6346 Curing Epilepsy: Focus on the Future/Bench marks for Epilepsy Research
www.ninds.nih.gov/funding/research/epilepsyweb/

Summary of March 2000, White House-initiated conference.

6347 Epilepsy Foundation of America
www.epilepsyfoundation.org

Through its efforts the organization ensures that people with seizures are able to participate in all life experiences. Its goals are to eventually prevent, control and cure epilepsy through research, education, advocacy, and services.

6348 Epilepsy.com
www.epilepsy.com

Epilepsy resources made available through an initiative by the Epilepsy Therapy Development Project.

6349 HealingWell.com
www.healingwell.com/epilepsy/

Offers information and resources including books, newsletters, and videos on a variety of diseases and chronic illnesses including epilepsy.

6350 NIH/National Institute of Neurological Dis orders and Stroke (NINDS)
www.ninds.nih.gov

The mission of NINDS is to reduce the burden of neurological disease - a burden borne by every age group, by every segment of society, by people all over the world.

6351 North Pacific Epilepsy Research
www.seizures.net/

Provides information to the public and health care professionals.

Book Publishers

6352 A Bomb in the Brain: A Heroic Tale of Science, Surgery and Survival
MacMillan Publishing Company
866 3rd Avenue
New York, NY 10022

212-702-2000

The autobiographical account of this author's struggle with epilepsy and the debilitating effects it has on health, emotions, and mental stability.

Grades 10-12

6353 A Season of Secrets
Little, Brown & Company
34 Beacon Street
Boston, MA 02108

617-227-0730

Grades 4-6

6354 Brainstorms Companion: Epilepsy in Our Vie w

Steven C Schachter MD, author

Epilepsy Foundation
8301 Professional Place
Landover, MD 20785

301-459-3700
800-332-1000
Fax: 301-577-2684
www.epilepsyfoundation.org

Family members, friends and coworkers of those with seizure disorders describe their feelings and observations.

1994 160 pages Paperback
ISBN: 0-781702-30-5

6355 Brainstorms: Epilepsy in Our Words

Steven C Schachter MD, author

Epilepsy Foundation
8301 Professional Place
Landover, MD 20785

301-459-3700
800-662-6922
Fax: 301-577-2684
www.epilepsyfoundation.org

Patients describe their experiences with seizures. Sixty-eight in-depth personal accounts of actual seizures are followed by a short section on how epilepsy affects the lives of the patients.

1993 197 pages Paperback
ISBN: 0-802774-65-2

6356 Children with Seizures: A Guide For Parent s, Teachers and Other Professionals

Epilepsy Foundation
8301 Professional Place
Landover, MD 20785

301-459-3700
800-332-1000
Fax: 301-577-2684
www.epilepsyfoundation.org

6357 Dotty the Dalmatian Has Epilepsy

Tim Peters & Company, Inc
87 Main St, PO Box 370
Peapack, NJ 07977

908-234-2050
800-543-2230
Fax: 908-234-1961
e-mail: info@timpetersandcompany.com
www.timpetersandcompany.com

Part of the Dr. Wellbook® series, this is the story of Dotty the Dalmatian who discovers she has epilepsy.

16 pages Softcover
ISBN: 1-879874-35-0

6358 Embrace the Dawn

Andrea Davidson, author

Epilepsy Foundation
8301 Professional Place
Landover, MD 20785

301-459-3700
800-332-1000
Fax: 301-577-2684
www.epilepsyfoundation.org

A moving biographical account of one person's lifelong experience with epilepsy.

127 pages Softcover

6359 Epilepsy

Franklin Watts c/o Grolier
90 Old Sherman Turnpike
Danbury, CT 06816

203-797-3500
Fax: 203-797-3197
www.grolier.com

This book explains what epilepsy is, causes of epileptic seizures, diagnosis and treatments.

96 pages Grades 7-12
ISBN: 0-531108-07-4

6360 Epilepsy A to Z

Demos Medical Publishing
386 Park Avenue South, Suite 301
New York, NY 10016

212-683-0072
800-532-8663
Fax: 212-683-0118
e-mail: orderdept@demosmedpub.com
www.demosmedpub.com

Easy reference in finding brief answers to questions regarding epilepsy terminology.

1995 322 pages Softcover
ISBN: 0-939957-75-0

6361 Epilepsy, A Guide to Balancing Your Life

Ilo E Leppik MD, author

Demos Medical Publishing
386 Park Avenue South, Suite 301
New York, NY 10016

212-683-0072
800-532-8663
Fax: 212-683-0118
e-mail: orderdept@demosmedpub.com
www.demosmedpub.com

Part of the Quality of Life Guide Series from the American Academy of Neurology Press. Provides reliable and practical information for those diagnosed with epilepsy and seizure disorders.

2006 192 pages Softcover
ISBN: 1-932603-20-0

6362 Epilepsy: 199 Answers

Andrew N Wilner MD, author

Demos Medical Publishing
386 Park Avenue South, Suite 301
New York, NY 10016

212-683-0072
800-532-8663
Fax: 212-683-0118
e-mail: orderdept@demosmedpub.com
www.demosmedpub.com

Helps to better understand conversations with the doctor and empowers the patient/caregiver to ask the right questions, resulting in optimal care.

2003 180 pages Softcover
ISBN: 1-888799-70-5

6363 Epilepsy: Frequency, Causes and Consequenc es

Epilepsy Foundation
8301 Professional Place
Landover, MD 20785

301-459-3700
800-332-1000
Fax: 301-577-2684
www.epilepsyfoundation.org

Statistical study that addresses the causes, natural history, prevalence and risk factors of epilepsy in certain populations and the impact on the community.

1990

6364 Epilepsy: I Can Live with That

Sue Goss, author

Epilepsy Foundation
8301 Professional Place
Landover, MD 20785

301-459-3700
800-332-1000
Fax: 301-577-2684
www.epilepsyfoundation.org

The experience of epilepsy as recorded by a group of ordinary men and women living in Australia. Each story focuses on personal growth, triumph over disability and emphasizes individual courage and hope.

1995 Softcover

6365 Growing Up With Epilepsy

Lynn Bennett Blackburn MD, author

Demos Medical Publishing
386 Park Avenue South, Suite 301
New York, NY 10016

212-683-0072
800-532-8663
Fax: 212-683-0118
e-mail: orderdept@demosmedpub.com
www.demosmedpub.com

Guidance in raising a child with epilepsy, including navigating the educational system, discipline, and social development.

2003 168 pages Softcover
ISBN: 1-888799-74-3

6366 Keto Kid, Helping Your Child to Succeed on the Ketogenic Diet

Deborah Ann Snyder DO, author

Demos Medical Publishing
386 Park Avenue South, Suite 301
New York, NY 10016

212-683-0072
800-532-8663
Fax: 212-683-0118
e-mail: orderdept@demosmedpub.com
www.demosmedpub.com

2006 176 pages Softcover
ISBN: 1-932603-29-3

6367 Lee the Rabbit with Epilepsy

Deborah M. Moss, author

Epilepsy Foundation
8301 Professional Place
Landover, MD 20785

301-459-3700
800-332-1000
Fax: 301-577-2684
www.epilepsyfoundation.org

Written for children ages three to six, this illustrated picture book follows the adventures of a small rabbit who has seizures. It follows her journey from the first seizure, the initial doctors visit through to treatment.

1989 21 pages Hardcover

6368 Living Well with Epilepsy

Robert Gumnit MD, author

Demos Medical Publishing
386 Park Avenue South, Suite 301
New York, NY 10016

212-683-0072
800-532-8663
Fax: 212-683-0118
e-mail: orederdept@demosmedpub.com
www.demosmedpub.com

Designed to help both health-care professionals and patients to understand all aspects of diagnosis and management; to enable patients to participate more knowledgeably in interactions with their health care team and to help steer them toward a more normal, fulfilling life.

1997 249 pages Soft / 2nd Ed
ISBN: 1-888799-11-0

6369 Missing Michael - A Mother's Story of Love

Epilepsy Foundation
8301 Professional Place
Landover, MD 20785

301-459-3700
800-332-1000
Fax: 301-577-2684
www.epilepsyfoundation.org

A mother's story of her struggle with raising her son with epilepsy. Deatils in dealing with the health care system, the school system, and the complications of medication.

Paperback

6370 Mom I Have a Staring Problem

Epilepsy Foundation
8301 Professional Place
Landover, MD 20785

301-459-3700
800-332-1000
Fax: 301-577-2684
www.epilepsyfoundation.org

Tiffany, a seven-year old, describes her experiences with petit mal seizures; her feelings, wishes and fears. Written to help adults recognize a hidden problem that could be occuring with a child who has learning problems.

1994 24 pages Softcover
ISBN: 0-802774-65-2

6371 My Friend Matty: A Story About Living with Epilepsy

Epilepsy Foundation
8301 Professional Place
Landover, MD 20785

301-459-3700
800-332-1000
Fax: 301-577-2684
www.epilepsyfoundation.org

A comic-book style publication for educating children written by parents whose 5-year old boy passed away.

Paperback

6372 Pediatric Epilepsy

Demos Medical Publishing
386 Park Avenue South, Suite 301
New York, NY 10016

212-683-0072
800-532-8663
Fax: 212-683-0118
e-mail: orderdept@demosmedpub.com
www.demosmedpub.com

Covers the diagnosis, treatment, classification and management of childhood epilepsies.

2001 666 pages Hardcover
ISBN: 1-888799-30-9

6373 Pediatric Epilepsy Resource Handbook
FACES/NYU Medical Center
724 Second Ave, LL
New York, NY 10016

212-871-0245
Fax: 212-871-1823
e-mail: nyufaces@yahoo.com
www.nyufaces.org

3rd Edition

6374 School Planning
Epilepsy Foundation
8301 Professional Place
Landover, MD 20785

301-459-3700
800-332-1000
Fax: 301-577-2684
TDD: 800-332-2070
www.epilepsyfoundation.org

This guide describes some epilepsy-related problems that children and youth may face in the areas of academics, school achievement and social development. Suggests ways parents can take a proactive approach to ensure appropriate testing, placement and achievement of educational goals for their children.

125 pages Hardcover
ISBN: 0-802774-65-2

6375 Seizures and Epilepsy In Childhood: A Guid e
Johns Hopkins University Press
2715 N Charles Street
Baltimore, MD 21218

410-516-6900
800-537-5487
Fax: 410-516-6968
www.press.jhu.edu

A standard resource for parents in need of comprehensive medical information about their child with epilepsy.

2002 432 pages 3rd Ed / Hard
ISBN: 0-801870-50-x

6376 Your Child and Epilepsy
Roger J Gumnit MD, author

Demos Medical Publishing
386 Park Avenue South, Suite 301
New York, NY 10016

212-683-0072
800-532-8663
Fax: 212-683-0118
e-mail: orderdept@demospub.com
www.demosmedpub.com

Provides information to help parents understand their child's epilepsy, suggestions on how to evaluate health care, to find better care if necessary and advice on how to help children with epilepsy to develop self-confidence and self-motivation.

1995 256 pages Softcover
ISBN: 0-939957-76-0

Kathy Gonzalez, Order Dept/Fulfillment Coordinator

Magazines

6377 Epilepsy Foundation
Epilepsy Foundation
8301 Professional Place
Landover, MD 20785

301-459-3700
800-332-1000
Fax: 301-577-2684
www.epilepsyfoundation.org

Catalog of epilepsy information materials, including pamphlets, books, manuals, videotapes and other items is available upon request.

6378 EpilepsyUSA
Epilepsy Foundation
8301 Professional Place
Landover, MD 20785

301-459-3700
800-332-1000
Fax: 301-577-2684
TDD: 800-332-2070
e-mail: postmaster@efa.org
www.epilepsyfoundation.org

Information on concerns about seizure disorders and epilepsy and new developments in treatment.

24 pages 6 issues/yr

Journals

6379 Epilepsy & Behavior
Elsevier
6277 Sea Harbor Drive
Orlando, FL 32887

407-345-4020
877-839-7126
Fax: 407-363-1354
e-mail: usjcs@elsevier.com
www.elsevier.com

An international journal that offers current information on the behavioral aspects of seizures and epilepsy.

Bi-monthly
ISSN: 1525-5050

Newsletters

6380 AES News
American Epilepsy Society
342 N Main Street
W Hartford, CT 06117

860-586-7505
Fax: 860-568-7550
www.aesnet.org

16 pages 3x/year

Deepak K Lachhwani, Editor
Suzanne C Berry, Executive Director

6381 Epilepsia: Journal of the International League Against Epilepsy
Blackwell Publishing
350 Main Street
Malden, MA 02148

781-388-8200
888-661-5800
Fax: 781-388-8210
www.blackwellpublishing.com

A leading international journal on the epilepsies for more than 30 years, Epilepsia provides comprehensive coverage of current clinical and research results.

12 per year
ISSN: 0013-9580

Philip A Schwartzkroin, Co-Editor
Simon Shorvon, Co-Editor

6382 Epilepsy Services of West Central Florida Newsletter
4023 N Armenia Avenue
Tampa, FL 33607

813-870-3414
Fax: 813-870-1321
e-mail: eswcf@gte.net
www.epilepsyservices.com

Information on medical, case management, employment services for persons with a seizure disorder, education and prevention programs for professional and community groups.

4 pages 3 times a year

Thomas Orth, Executive Director
Barbara Bowman

6383 FACES: Finding a Cure for Epilepsy & Seizu res
724 Second Ave, LL
New York, NY 10016

212-871-0245
Fax: 212-871-1823
e-mail: nyufaces@yahoo.com
www.nyufaces.org

Covers new studies, research, events and special interest stories.

Quarterly

Melissa Murphy, Research Coordinator
Mark Farley, Education Coordinator

6384 THRESHOLD
2150 Highway 35 N, Suite 207C
Sea Grit, NJ 08750

732-974-1144
800-336-5843
TTY: 800-852-7889
e-mail: fscnj@aol.com
www.cfnj.com

Provides information and support to parents of children with uncontrolled seizure disorders. Also provides parent-to-parent support information.

Pamphlets

6385 Child with Epilepsy at Camp
Epilepsy Foundation
8301 Professional Place
Landover, MD 20785

301-459-3700
800-332-1000
Fax: 301-577-2684
www.epilepsyfoundation.org

Written for camp counselors, it helps parents explain to them the specific needs of children with epilepsy at camp to ensure a safe camping experience.

14 pages Pamphlet

6386 Child's Guide To Seizure Disorders
Epilepsy Foundation
8301 Professional Place
Landover, MD 20785

301-459-3700
800-332-1000
Fax: 301-577-2684
www.epilepsyfoundation.org

A pamphlet for children, brightly-colored and explains seizures, why medication should be taken, etc.

6387 Epilepsy in Children: The Teacher's Role
Epilepsy Foundation
8301 Professional Place
Landover, MD 20785

301-459-3700
800-332-1000
Fax: 301-577-2684
www.epilepsyfoundation.org

Provides an explanation for teachers on handling seizures in the classroom, the need for good communication between students and first aid procedures.

6388 Epilepsy: You and Your Child
Epilepsy Foundation
8301 Professional Place
Landover, MD 20785

301-459-3700
800-332-1000
Fax: 301-577-2684
www.epilepsyfoundation.org

This instructional booklet offers information on emotional aspects of epilepsy, how to handle seizures, medication, diet and nutrition, and offers referral organizations for parents.

6389 Febrile Seizures Fact Sheet
NINDS/NIH Neurological Institute
PO Box 5801
Bethesda, MD 20824

301-496-5751
800-352-9424
TTY: 301-468-5981
www.ninds.nih.gov/disorders/febrile_seizures/

Also available in Spanish.

6390 Finding Out About Seizures: A Guide to Medical Tests
Epilepsy Foundation
8301 Professional Place
Landover, MD 20785

301-459-3700
800-332-1000
Fax: 301-577-2684
www.epilepsyfoundation.org

Introduces adults and children with epilepsy to the types of tests they may have to undergo.

6391 H.O.P.E. Series: Seizures in Childhood
Epilepsy Foundation
8301 Professional Place
Landover, MD 20785

301-459-3700
800-332-1000
Fax: 301-577-2684
www.epilepsyfoundation.org

Provides an overview of the challenges associated with living with epilepsy and other seizure disorders, including potential hazards, first aid procedures, and overall help in daily living.

6392 H.O.P.E. Series: Seizures in the Teen Year s
Epilepsy Foundation
8301 Professional Place
Landover, MD 20785

301-459-3700
800-332-1000
Fax: 301-577-2684
www.epilepsyfoundation.org

Provides general information specifically for teens with epilepsy and seizure disorders.

6393 Infantile Spasms
NINDS/NIH Neurological Institute
PO Box 5801
Bethesda, MD 20824

301-496-5751
800-352-9424
TTY: 301-468-5981
www.ninds.nih.gov/disorders/infantilespasms/

Information sheet on infantile spasms (West Syndrome).

6394 Kids and Seizures: Know the Hidden Signs
Epilepsy Foundation
8301 Professional Place
Landover, MD 20785

301-459-3700
800-332-1000
Fax: 301-577-2684
www.epilepsyfoundation.org

Written for camp counselors, it helps parents explain to them the specific needs of children with epilepsy at camp to ensure a safe camping experience.

6395 Managing Seizures, Information for Caregivers

Epilepsy Foundation
8301 Professional Place
Landover, MD 20785

301-459-3700
800-332-1000
Fax: 301-577-2684
www.epilepsyfoundation.org

Explains seizures, routine and special care, emergency aid and first aid for caregivers. Includes a poster size chart for medicines and general guidance in handling a seizure.

6396 Me and My World Storybook

Epilepsy Foundation
8301 Professional Place
Landover, MD 20785

301-459-3700
800-332-1000
Fax: 301-577-2684
TDD: 800-332-2070
www.epilepsyfoundation.org

An excellent pamphlet for explaining epilepsy to children and their friends. It also discusses various types of epilepsy and its effects on family members. Ages 4-8.

6397 Medicines for Epilepsy

Epilepsy Foundation
8301 Professional Place
Landover, MD 20785

301-459-3700
800-332-1000
Fax: 301-577-2684
www.epilepsyfoundation.org

Offers information on medication and treatments, generic drugs, side effects, drug abuse and more. Contains a color chart with pictures of the most common medications for epilepsy.

6398 Safety and Seizures

Epilepsy Foundation
8301 Professional Place
Landover, MD 20785

301-459-3700
800-332-1000
Fax: 301-577-2684
www.epilepsyfoundation.org

6399 Seizures and Epilepsy: Hope Through Research

NINDS/NIH Neurological Institute
PO Box 5801
Bethesda, MD 20824

301-496-5751
800-352-9424
TTY: 301-468-5981
www.ninds.nih.gov/disorders/epilepsy/

Also available in Spanish.

6400 Seizures, Epilepsy and Your Child

Epilepsy Foundation
8301 Professional Place
Landover, MD 20785

301-459-3700
800-332-1000
Fax: 301-577-2684
www.epilepsyfoundation.org

A pamphlet for parents, providing guidance on daily life, first aid and treatment for children with epilepsy.

6401 Surgery for Epilepsy

Epilepsy Foundation
8301 Professional Place
Landover, MD 20785

301-459-3700
800-332-1000
Fax: 301-577-2684
www.epilepsyfoundation.org

Describes current surgical treatment and the testing that precedes it.

12 pages

6402 Talking to Your Doctor About Seizure Disorders

Epilepsy Foundation
8301 Professional Place
Landover, MD 20785

301-459-3700
800-332-1000
Fax: 301-577-2684
www.epilepsyfoundation.org

Designed to help the patient talk with medical personnel about treatment of epilepsy.

6403 The ADA: Questions and Answers

Epilepsy Foundation
8301 Professional Place
Landover, MD 20785

301-459-3700
800-332-1000
Fax: 301-577-2684
www.epilepsyfoundation.org

Offers a brief overview of the Americans with Disabilities Act and how it covers those with epilepsy.

6404 What Everyone Should Know About Epilepsy

Epilepsy Foundation
8301 Professional Place
Landover, MD 20785

301-459-3700
800-332-1000
Fax: 301-577-2684
www.epilepsyfoundation.org

6405 When Seizures Don't Look Like Seizures

Epilepsy Foundation
8301 Professional Place
Landover, MD 20785

301-459-3700
800-332-1000
Fax: 301-577-2684
www.epilepsyfoundation.org

Describes and helps with the subtle signs of a seizure for parents, child care providers and school personnel.

ISBN: 0-802774-65-2

Camps

6406 Camp Frog

1323 Forbes Avenue, Suite 102
Pitsburgh, PA 15219

412-261-5880
800-316-5585
Fax: 412-261-3561
e-mail: staff@cfwp.org
www.cfwp.org

Summer camp for children and teens with epilepsy/seizure disorders. It is a nationally recognized program with around the clock medical supervision during the week long program.

Kate Wilsom, Coordinator

DESCRIPTION

6407 SICKLE CELL DISEASE

Synonyms: Homozygous Hb S, Sickle cell anemia
Involves the following Biologic System(s):
Hematologic and Oncologic Disorders

Sickle cell disease is an inherited blood disorder that primarily affects African Americans and is characterized by the presence of crescent or sickle-shaped red cells in the blood and the chronic premature destruction of red blood cells (hemolytic anemia). In this disorder, the red blood cells contain an abnormal form of the oxygen-carrying protein (hemoglobin) called hemoglobin S (Hgb S). This abnormality reduces the level of available oxygen (ischemia) in the blood cells and results in their characteristic sickle shape. These irregular cells tend to block the tiny blood vessels of various tissues and organs; they may cause restricted or obstructed blood flow resulting in tissue or organ damage (infarction). In addition, their unusual shape renders them fragile, leading to their premature destruction and thus anemia.

The symptoms of sickle cell disease tend to appear at or around six months of age and may include headaches; shortness of breath (dyspnea); paleness; fatigue; and a yellowish hue of the eyes, skin, and mucous membranes (jaundice). Any activity that would normally reduce the blood oxygen levels (e.g., exercise, exertion, illness, or high-altitude flying) may induce a sickle cell crisis or sudden worsening of the anemic condition accompanied by abdominal and bone pain, dyspnea, and vomiting. Infarction or a blocked blood vessel (vaso-occlusion) may also result in sickle cell crisis with the affected child experiencing chest pain and increased dyspnea. By adolescence most of those affected develop an enlarged spleen (splenomegaly) that is no longer capable of assisting in fighting certain infections, leaving the body more vulnerable to certain types of infections (encapsulated organisms, notably pneumococcal pneumonia). Other symptoms may include skin changes resulting from poor circulation, stroke resulting from insufficient oxygen reaching the brain, or blood in the urine (hematuria) resulting from kidney damage. As the affected child grows to adulthood, the liver and heart may enlarge (hepatosplenomegaly) and a heart murmur may develop. The lungs, intestines, and gall bladder may also be affected. In addition, affected children may develop such distinct characteristics as a short torso with long extremities, fingers, and toes.

Because there is no known cure for sickle cell disease, treatment is geared toward prevention, control, and pain management. Such treatment may include the avoidance of activities that reduce blood oxygen levels, a full immunization regimen, and prompt medical intervention for any illness or viral infection. Other treatment may include folic acid supplementation, antibiotic medication for treatment and prevention of infection, oxygen therapy to improve the level of oxygen in the blood, and acetaminophen or other medication to relieve pain. To manage a sickle cell crisis, as well as the pain associated with it, affected children may be given intravenous fluids, pain-relieving drugs, and possibly blood transfusions. Other treatments being studied include certain drugs, gene therapy, and bone marrow transplantation.

Sickle cell disease is inherited as an autosomal recessive trait. In this case, the defective gene for hemoglobin S is transmitted by both parents. If a child inherits this gene from only one parent (and one normal gene from the other parent, that child will usually be symptom-free, but will be a carrier of the sickle cell trait. The incidence of this disorder in the United States is approximately 150 African American children in 100,000; however, approximately one in 12 black children carries the sickle cell trait.

See also **General Resources** on page 917

Government Agencies

6408 NIH/National Heart, Lung and Blood Institu te
National Institute of Health
31 Center Dr MSC 2486, Bldg 31, Room 5A48
Bethesda, MD 20892

301-592-8573
Fax: 240-629-3246
TTY: 240-629-3255
e-mail: NHLBIinfo@nhlbi.nih.gov
www.nhlbi.nih.gov

Primary responsibility of this organization is the scientific investigation of heart, blood vessel, lung and blood disorders. Oversees research, demonstration, prevention, education, control and training activities in these fields and emphasizes the prevention and control of heart diseases.

Elizabeth G Nabel, MD, Director
Susan Shurin, MD, Deputy Director

6409 NIH/National Institute of Child Health and Human Development
31 Center Drive, Building 31
Bethesda, MD 20892

301-496-5133
Fax: 301-496-1104
www.nichd.nih.gov

Established in 1962 by congress, today the institute conducts and supports research on topics related to the health of children, adults, families and populations. Some of these topics include: developmental disabilities, growth and development, infant death, reproductive health and birth defects.

Nancy D Wirth, Director
Lisa Kaeser, Program & Public Liaison

National Associations & Support Groups

6410 American Sickle Cell Anemia Association
10300 Carnegie Avenue
Cleveland, OH 44106

216-229-8600
Fax: 216-229-4500
e-mail: irabragg@ascaa.org
www.ascaa.org

Provides education, testing, counseling, supportive services to the population at risk for sickle cell anemia and its hemoglobin variants. Bilingual educator on staff, educational materials and distribution of literature is provided by ASCAA. Referrals for children and families with special needs.

Ira Bragg-Grant, Executive Director

6411 Genetic Alliance
4301 Connecticut Avenue NW
Washington, DC 20008

202-966-5557
800-336-4363
Fax: 202-966-8553
e-mail: info@geneticalliance.org
www.geneticalliance.org

A coalition of voluntary genetic support groups, consumers and professionals addressing the needs of individuals and families affected by genetic disorders from a national perspective.

Sharon Terry, President/CEO

6412 Keon Paschal Perry Sickle Cell Anemia Disease Awareness
7510 Granby Street, Perry Building
Norfolk, VA 23505

888-406-5111
e-mail: keon4u@aol.com
www.keon.qpg.com

International Sickle Cell Anemia Disease Awareness Campaign.

Roy L Perry-Bey, CEO/Executive Direct

6413 Sickle Cell Disease Association of America
231 E Baltimore St, Suite 800
Baltimore, MD 21202

410-528-1555
800-421-8453
Fax: 410-528-1495
e-mail: scdaa@sicklecelldisease.org
www.sicklecelldisease.org

Promotes the finding of a universal cure for sickle cell disease while improving the quality of life for individuals and families where sickle cell related conditions exists. It also assists in the organization and development of local chapters.

Willarda V Edwards MD, President/COO
Sonya I Ross, VP Programs/Services

6414 Sickle Cell Information Center
Grady Memorial Hospital
80 Jesse Hill Jr Drive, PO Box 109
Atlanta, GA 30303

404-616-3572
Fax: 404-616-5998
e-mail: aplatt@emory.edu
www.scinfo.org

Sickle cell resources, education, news and research updates for caregivers, patients and professionals.

6415 Sickle Cell Parent and Family Network
PO Box 19854
Cincinnati, OH 45219

513-641-5683
Fax: 513-398-9620
e-mail: muhjahmarshall@sprintmail.com
www.cintishares.com/sicklecellparent.htm

Support and education for families affected by sickle cell disease, and interested professionals.

State Agencies & Support Groups

Alabama

6416 Sickle Cell Foundation of Greater Montgomery
3180 US Highway 80 W
Montgomery, AL 36108

334-286-9122
800-742-5534
Fax: 334-286-4804
e-mail: sickle2@aol.com
www.scfgm.org

Willie Owens, Executive Director

California

6417 Sickle Cell Disease Foundation of California
6133 Bristol Parkway, Suite 240
Culver City, CA 90230

310-693-0247
877-288-2873
Fax: 310-693-0266
e-mail: info@scdfc.org
www.scdfc.org

Educates, screens and offers counsel to those at risk for having children with sickle cell disease and other hemoglobin disorders.

Mary E Brown, President/CEO
Roger Brown, Director Development/Public Affairs

Connecticut

6418 Sickle Cell Disease Association of America - Connecticut Chapter
Hartford Regional Office
Gengras Amb Ctr, 114 Woodland St, Suite 2101
Hartford, CT 06105

860-527-0119
800-379-0119
Fax: 860-714-8007
www.sicklecellct.org

Regional office loactions in Hartford, New Haven and New London.

Georgia

6419 Sickle Cell Foundation of Georgia
2391 Benjamin E Mays Drive
Atlanta, GA 30311

404-755-1641
800-326-5287
Fax: 404-755-7955
e-mail: n_nichols@sicklecellatlaga.org
www.sicklecellatlaga.org

Provides education, screening, and counseling programs for sickle cell and other abnormal hemoglobins. The Foundation has a deep-rooted commitment to making strides in monitoring the occurrence of sickle cell, improving the quality of life for those with the disease and cooperating with individuals conducting research.

D Jean Brannan, President/CEO
Harold Dobbs, Outreach Coordinator

Louisiana

6420 NE Louisiana Sickle Cell Anemia Foundation
1604 Winnsboro Road
Monroe, LA 71202

318-322-0896
Fax: 318-387-4740
e-mail: sickle@bayou.com

The Northeast Louisiana Sickle Cell Anemia Foundation is a community based tax exempt organization that assists victims with the inherited blood disease sickle cell anemia.

LeSandre R Starks, Executive Director

Massachusetts

6421 Community Sickle Cell Support Group
1542 Tremont St
Roxbury, MA 02120

617-427-4100
e-mail: cscsginc@aol.com
www.cscsginc.org

Jackie Rodriguez, Executive Director

New Mexico

6422 Sickle Cell Council of New Mexico
7800 Marble NE
Albuquerque, NM 87110

505-254-9550
e-mail: victoria@sicklecellnm.org
www.sicklecellnm.org

Blood screening, education, and genetic counseling.

Victoria Jones, Executive Director

New York

6423 Sickle Cell Disease Foundation of Greater New York
127 W 127th Street
New York, NY 10027

212-865-1500

A voluntary health organization formed to support and conduct research and educational programs aimed at the control of sickle cell anemia.

Dick Campbell, Executive Director

North Carolina

6424 Eastern North Carolina Chapter (SCDAA)
344 Center Street
Jacksonville, NC 28546

910-346-2510
800-826-1314
Fax: 910-346-2614
e-mail: sickle@bizec.rr.com

Marcia M Wright, Executive Director

6425 Sickle Cell Disease Association of the Piedmont
1102 E Market Street
Greensboro, NC 27401

336-274-1507
800-733-8297
Fax: 336-275-7984
e-mail: grobinson@scdap.org
www.scdap.org

Dedicated to educating the public and providing support to people affected by sickle cell disease. Serving the following counties: Alamance, Forsyth, Caswell, Guilford, Randolph, and Rockingham.

Gladys A Robinson, Executive Director

6426 Sickle Cell Regional Network
821 Baxter St, Suite 312
Charlotte, NC 28202

704-332-4184
800-435-6004
Fax: 704-332-2246
e-mail: plambright@sc-cnc.org

Patricia Lambright, Executive Director

Pennsylvania

6427 Lehigh Valley Sickle Cell Support Group
PO Box 1711
Allentown, PA 18105

610-706-0636
e-mail: SororW@aol.com
www.members.aol.com/SororW/index.html

For anyone affected/effected by Sickle Cell and all interested persons. Learn more about sickle cell disease and how you can help.

6428 Sickle Cell Disease Association of America , Philadelphia/Delaware Valley Chapter
4601 Market Street
Philadelphia, PA 19139

215-471-8686
Fax: 215-471-7441
e-mail: scdaa.pdvc@verizon.net
www.sicklecelldisorder.com

A support group for parents of a child or children with sickle cell disease.

Stanley A Simpkins, Executive Director

South Carolina

6429 James R Clark Memorial Sickle Cell Foundation
1420 Gregg Street
Columbia, SC 29201

803-765-9916
800-506-1273
Fax: 803-799-6471
e-mail: jrcsc@bellsouth.net
www.midnet.sc.edu/jrcsc/

The mission of the foundation is to optimize the social and psychological well being of residents with sickle cell disease within the fifteen county area of South Carolina. This mission is accomplished through the provision of comprehensive services to individuals, families, and communities and is further enhanced by collaboration with appropriate federal, state, and local resources and through the involvement of volunteers and contributors.

Lena Stevenson, Executive Director

Texas

6430 Sickle Cell Association of Austin - Marc Thomas Chapter
1 Highland Ctr, 314 E Highland Mall Blvd, Ste 108
Austin, TX 78752

512-458-9767
Fax: 512-458-9714
e-mail: info@marcthomas.org
www.marcthomas.org

To raise awareness, resources and support for clients with sickle cell disease.

Linda Thomas, Executive Director
Nora Bouie-Burleson, Office Manager

6431 Sickle Cell Association of the Texas Gulf Coast
6300 West Loop S, Suite 340
Bellaire, TX 77401

713-400-2355
888-908-2355
Fax: 713-400-2360
e-mail: nbrowning@sicklecell-texas.org
www.sicklecell-texas.org

Nicole Browning, Executive Director
Tosca Davis, Community Relations Manager

Libraries & Resource Centers

South Carolina

6432 Children's Center for Cancer and Blood Disorders
University of South Carolina School of Medicine
5 Richland Memorial Park
Columbia, SC 29203

803-777-7000

Joint clinical and basic research of juvenile cancer and blood disorders.

Dr. Robert S Ettinger, Director

Research Centers

California

6433 Northern California Comprehensive Sickle C ell Center
Children's Hospital at Oakland
747 52nd St
Oakland, CA 94609

510-450-5647
e-mail: evichinsky@mail.cho.org

Sickle cell disease research.

Elliott Vichinsky MD, Director

6434 University of Southern California Comprehensive Sickle Cell Center
2025 Zonal Avenue, Room 304
Los Angeles, CA 90033

323-442-1259
Fax: 323-442-1255
e-mail: cagejohn@hsc.usc.edu

Cage S Johnson MD, Director

District of Columbia

6435 Howard University Center for Sickle Cell Disease
2121 Georgia Avenue NW
Washington, DC 20059

202-865-8292
Fax: 202-806-4517
www.huhosp.org/sicklecell/default.htm

Dr. Oswaldo Castro, Director

Georgia

6436 Comprehensive Sickle Cell Center
Medical College of Georgia
1521 Pope Ave
Augusta, GA 30912

706-721-0174
Fax: 706-721-2643
www.mcg.edu/center/sicklecell/

New York

6437 Bronx Comprehensive Sickle Cell Center
Albert Einstein College of Medicine
Ullman Bldg, 1300 Morris Park Ave
Bronx, NY 10461

718-430-2088
Fax: 718-824-3153
e-mail: nagel@aecom.yu.edu

Ronald L Nagel MD, Director

North Carolina

6438 Duke University Comprehensive Sickle Cell Center
Medical Center
Box 2615
Durham, NC 27710

919-684-5378
Fax: 919-681-7688
e-mail: telen002@mc.duke.edu

Research into sickle cell disease including molecular and organ studies.

Marilyn Telen MD, Director

Ohio

6439 Comprehensive Sickle Cell Center
Cincinnati Children's Hospital Medical Ctr
3333 Burnet Avenue
Cincinnati, OH 45229

513-636-4541
800-344-2462
Fax: 513-636-5562
e-mail: blood@cchmc.org
www.cincinnatichildrens.org

Offers research and statistical information in the area of sickle cell disease.

Clinton Joiner MD, Pediatric Director

Texas

6440 Center for Cancer and Blood Disorders
Children Medical Center Dallas
1935 Motor Street
Dallas, TX 75235

214-456-2382
Fax: 214-456-6133
e-mail: ccbdinfo@childrens.com
www.childrens.com/ccbd/

A comprehensive program for diagnosis, patient/family education and management of sickle cell diseases in childhood and adolesance. Offers access to state-of-the art research projects and clinical management.

George R Buchanan, Medical Director
Zora R Rogers, MD, Associate Medical Director

6441 Southwestern Comprehensive Sickle Cell Cen ter
UT Southwestern Medical Ctr/Pediatrics Dept
5323 Harry Hines Blvd
Dallas, TX 75390

214-648-8594
Fax: 214-648-3122
e-mail: George.Buchanan@UTsouthwestern.edu

State-of-the-art patient care, clinical and basic lab research, education and advocacy programs.

Dr George Buchanan, Director

Web Sites

6442 American Sickle Cell Anemia Association
www.ascaa.org

The mission of the American Sickle Cell Anemia Association is to ensure the availability and accessibility of quality, comprehensive sickle cell services, and promote the public professional awareness about sickle cell anemis an it's hemoglobin diseases ad trait variants.

6443 Information Center for Sickle Cell and Tha lassemic Disorders
sickle.bwh.harvard.edu

Free online information to the biomedical community, health care personnel and patients. The information can be of particular help to patients in enabling them to have a fuller and more knowledgeable role in their care.

6444 International Association of Sickle Cell Nurses and Physician Assistants
www.iascnapa.org

The association is made up of over 300 sickle cell nurses and physician assistants worldwide. It recognizes its responsibility to maintain high standards in the provision of quality and accessible health care services for individuals with sickle cell disease.

6445 Online Mendelian Inheritance in Man
www.ncbi.nlm.nih.gov

This database is a catalog of human genes and genetic disorders.

6446 Sickle Cell Disease Association of America
www.sicklecelldisease.org

Promotes the finding of a universal cure for sickle cell disease while improving the quality of life for individuals and families where sickle cell related conditions exists.

6447 Sickle Cell Disease Forum
www.sicklecelldisease.org/forum/

Online forum for sickle cell disease discussion/chat sponsored by the Sickle Cell Disease Association of America.

6448 Sickle Cell Kids
www.sicklecellkids.org

Teaches children how to stay healthy and answers questions about sickle cell disease. A joint venture of the Georgia Comprehensive Sickle Cell Center at Grady Health System and Cynthia Gentry, artist.

Book Publishers

6449 Blood & Circulatory Disorders Sourcebook
Omnigraphics
615 Griswold
Detroit, MI 48226

610-461-3548
800-234-1340
Fax: 800-875-1340
e-mail: info@omnigraphics.com
www.omnigraphics.com

Basic consumer health information on blood and its components, anemias, leukemias, bleeding disorders, and circulatory disorders, including sickle cell disease, aplastic anemia, thalassemia, and hemophilia.

2005 659 pages 2nd Edition
ISBN: 0-780807-46-4

6450 Let's Talk About Going to the Hospital
Rosen Publishing Group's PowerKids Press
29 E 21st Street
New York, NY 10010

212-777-3017
800-237-9932
Fax: 888-436-4643
e-mail: rosenpub@tribeca.ios.com
www.powerkidspress.com

If a child has to check into the hospital, chances are he or she is already upset about being ill. Knowing how a hospital functions and what the procedures are, such as when family members can visit, will help in what is already a stressful situation. Grades K-5.

24 pages
ISBN: 0-823950-36-0

6451 Let's Talk About Sickle Cell Anemia
Melanie Apel Gordon, author

Rosen Publishing Group's PowerKids Press
29 E 21st Street
New York, NY 10010

212-777-3017
800-237-9932
Fax: 888-436-4643
e-mail: rosenpub@tribeca.ios.com
www.powerkidspress.com

Explains why sickle cell anemia is a disease that strikes more African Americans than any other people in the country. Describes symptoms and explains how a kid can help take care of himself during a pain crisis. Grades K-5.

24 pages
ISBN: 0-823954-17-X

6452 Sickle Cell Anemia
Franklin Watts c/o Grolier
90 Old Sherman Turnpike
Danbury, CT 06816

203-797-3500
Fax: 203-797-3197
www.grolier.com

1994 76 pages
ISBN: 0-531125-10-6

6453 Sickle Cell Disease: Basic Principles & Clinical Practice
Raven Press
1185 Avenue of the Americas
New York, NY 10036

212-930-9500

1994 928 pages
ISBN: 0-781701-42-2

6454 Understanding Sickle Cell Disease
Miriam Bloom PhD, author

University Press of Mississippi
3825 Ridgewood Road
Jackson, MS 39211

601-432-6205
800-737-7788
Fax: 601-432-6217
e-mail: press@ihl.state.ms.us
www.upress.state.ms.us

Part of the Understanding Health and Sickness Series. For general readers, a guide to understanding a debilitating genetic disease that affects tens of thousands who are of African heritage.

128 pages Paperback
ISBN: 0-878057-45-5

Pamphlets

6455 Sickle Cell Disease
March of Dimes Resource Center
1275 Mamaroneck Avenue
White Plains, NY 10605

888-663-4637
914-997-4488
Fax: 914-997-4763
TTY: 914-977-4764
e-mail: resourcecenter@modimes.org
www.marchofdimes.org/professionals/681_1221.asp

Fact Sheets: one to two page review written for the general public. Also available electronically from website www.modimes.org. Brochures: 3 panel color brochures written for the general public.

Camps

6456 Camp Crescent Moon
Sickle Cell Disease Foundation of California
6133 Bristol Parkway, Suite 240
Culver City, CA 90230

310-693-0247
877-288-2873
Fax: 310-693-0266
e-mail: info@scdfc.org
www.scdfc.org/program_services/

A specialized camp for children with sickle cell disease between the ages of 8 and 14 in southern & central California.

Mary E Brown, Camp Director
Deborah Green, Assistant Camp Director

DESCRIPTION

6457 SLEEP APNEA

Involves the following Biologic System(s):

Respiratory Disorders

Obstructive sleep apnea (OSA) is a breathing disorder that is commonly seen in the pediatric population. Specifically, it is when normal ventilation during sleep is disrupted because of upper airway obstruction. This process occurs intermittently throughout sleep and causes significant disruptions in normal sleep patterns. Although in adults this can result in excessive daytime sleepiness, children typically manifest changes in behavior or deficits in attention, thus affecting school performance.

Studies indicate that roughly 2% of children between the ages of 2-18 years are affected by this disorder. Girls and boys are equally likely to have OSA and African American children are more commonly affected than children of other ethnicities. OSA is also more common in children with obesity, craniofacial abnormalities and/or neurologic disorders. Children with Down syndrome are at especially increased risk.

The cause of obstructive sleep apnea is not well understood. Adenotonsillar (adenoids and tonsils) hypertrophy (increase in size) seems to be part of the process but even after tonsillectomy and adenoidectomy (removal of these tissues) many patients relapse, implying other processes involved.

The clinical features commonly seem with OSA include noisy breathing during sleep, prominent snoring often in a crescendo pattern that ends with a pause in respirations for performance, nocturnal enuresis (bed wetting) and frequent daytime napping. Complications of OSA can be failure to thrive or gain weight appropriately, pulmonary hypertension which cause stress on the right side of the heart and neurological sequelae.

Diagnosis should not be based solely on a history of snoring. Many children snore who do not suffer from OSA, however, a careful history focusing on some of the clinical features mentioned above should raise the suspicion of OSA and further evaluation can be considered. The physical exam of tonsillar hypertrophy may help support the diagnosis but often a polysomnography test, commonly called sleep study, is the most accurate way to diagnose OSA. The sleep study is a comprehensive diagnostic tool involving monitoring a patient during sleep using multiple parameters including the visual surveillance, monitoring of the heart rate and rhythm, monitoring of the respiratory rate, measurement of expired lung gases, oxygen saturation in the blood, chest wall rise with breathing and others. While the necessity of this study in children may be debated, it is considered a definitive way to establishthe diagnosis of OSA.

In general, nonsurgical therapy is very limited for the typical patient with OSA. Treatment of childhood OSA is primarily surgical. Removal of the tonsils and adenoids are often the first line of treatment as well as targeting weight reduction when relevant. Most children respond well to tonsillectomy and adenoidectomy, but for those who do not improve, nasal continued positive airway pressure (NCPAP) is another effective option which enhances the infant's respiratory function.

OSA is an important cause of health, emotional and behavioral problems in school aged children and effective and timely treatment can significantly improve school performance, and productivity and well-being of these children.

See also **General Resources** on page 917

National Associations & Support Groups

6458 American Academy of Sleep Medicine
1 Westbrook Corporate Center, Suite 920
Westchester, IL 60154

708-492-0930
Fax: 708-492-0943
www.aasmnet.org

National not-for-profit professional membership organization dedicated to the advancement of sleep medicine. The Academy's mission is to assure quality care for patients with sleep disorders, promote the advancement of sleep research and provide public and professional education. The AASM delivers programs, information and services to and through its members and advocates sleep medicine supportive policies in the medical community and the public sector.

Jerome Barrett, Executive Director
Jennifer Markkanen, Assistant Executive Director

6459 American Narcolepsy Association
PO Box 26230
San Francisco, CA 94126

800-222-6085
Fax: 415-788-4795

Provides information and referrals to people with sleep disorders.

Michelle Auerbach, Contact

6460 American Sleep Apnea Association
1424 K Street NW, Suite 302
Washington, DC 20005

202-293-3650
Fax: 202-293-3656
e-mail: asaa@sleepapnea.org
www.sleepapnea.org

Offers help and information to persons with sleep apnea and their families.

Rochelle Goldberg, MD, President & CMO
Dave Hargett, Chair

6461 National Sleep Foundation
1522 K Street NW, Suite 500
Washington, DC 20005

202-347-3471
Fax: 202-347-3472
e-mail: nsf@sleepfoundation.org
www.sleepfoundation.org

An independent, nonprofit organization dedicated to improving public health and safety by achieving public understanding of sleep and sleep disorders, and by supporting public education, sleep-related research, and advocacy. Actively collaborates with sleep centers and support groups for patients with sleep disorders and safety organizations.

Richard Gelula, CEO

State Agencies & Support Groups

6462 Center for Disabilities and Development
University of Iowa Hospitals and Clinics
100 Hawkins Drive
Iowa City, IA 52242

319-353-6900
877-686-0031
e-mail: cdd-webmaster@uiowa.edu
www.healthcare.uiowa.edu/cdd

A trusted resource for healthcare, training, research and information for people with disabilities that include: behavior disorders, brain injury, cerebral palsy, diabetes, down syndrome, learning disabilities, mental retardation, sleep disorders and spina bifida.

Elayne Sexsmith, Administrator
Amy Mikelson, Supervisor Info Resource Service

Libraries & Resource Centers

6463 American Academy of Somnology
PO Box 27077
Las Vegas, NV 89126

702-371-0947
e-mail: somnology@aol.com
www.hopperinstitute.com/aas_intro.html

Covers about 75 physicians, dentists, nurses, psychologists, technicians, and students and sponsoring organizations, including associations, institutions, and corporations, with a special interest in sleep. Newsletter, published yearly.

Research Centers

6464 Sleep Disorders Center
Beth Israel Deaconess Medical Ctr
330 Brookline Avenue
Boston, MA 02215

617-667-3237
Fax: 617-975-5506
www.bidmc.harvard.edu

Provides testing and treatment for those with sleep disorders and offers educational workshops, plus support for their families.

Jean K Matheson, MD, Division Chief

Web Sites

6465 About.com on Sleep Disorders
www.sleepdisorders.about.com

Well-organized information including new developments and a chat room.

6466 American Academy of Sleep Medicine
www.aasmnet.org

The mission is to assure quality care for patients with sleep disorders, promote the advancement of sleep research and provide public and professional education.

6467 American Sleep Apnea Association
www.sleepapnea.org

Is dedicated to reducing injury, disbility, and death from sleep apnea and to enhancing the well being of those affected by this common disorder. The ASAA promotes education and awareness, the ASAA A.W.A.K.E. Network of voluntary mutual suport groups, research, and continuous improvement of care.

6468 MEDLINEplus on Sleep Apnea
www.nlm.nih.gov/medlineplus/sleepapnea.html

Offers information about Sleep Apnea.

6469 NIH/National Center on Sleep Disorders Research
www.nhlbi.nih.gov/about/ncsdr/index.htm

Coordinates sleep research, training and education supported by the government.

6470 National Sleep Foundation
www.sleepfoundation.org

Is an independent nonprofit organization dedicated to improving public health and safety by achieving understanding of sleep and slepp disorders, and by supporting education, sleep-related research, and advocacy.

6471 Sleepdisorders.com
www.sleepdisorders.com

Provides a full range of internet communications and technology solutions from strategic consulting to concept design, content development, software engineering, and ongoing enhancements and maintenance. Our projects have encompassed direct-to-consumer marketing, direct-to-patient education, healthcare professional training, corporate intranets and database management systems, dynamic database-driven websites and hospital training.

6472 Sleepnet.com
www.sleepnet.com/sleepapnea2000.html

Categorizes sleep disorders for research, forums are up-dated frequently and posts are thoughtful and insightful.

Book Publishers

6473 Concise Guide to Evaluation and Management of Sleep Disorders
American Psychiatric Publishing
1000 Wilson Boulevard, Suite 1825
Arlington, VA 22209

703-907-7322
800-368-5777
Fax: 703-907-1091
e-mail: appi@psych.org
www.appi.org

Overview of sleep disorders medicine, sleep physiology and pathology, insomnia complaints, excessive sleepiness disorders, parasomnias, medical and psychiatric disorders and sleep, medications with sedative - hypnotic properties, special problems and populations.

2002 296 pages Paper 3rd Ed
ISBN: 1-585620-45-6

6474 Consumer's Guide to Psychiatric Drugs
New Harbinger Publications
5674 Shattuck Avenue
Oakland, CA 94609

510-652-2002
800-748-6273
Fax: 510-652-5472
e-mail: customerservice@newharbinger.com
newharbinger.com

Helps consumers understand what treatment options are available and what side effects to expect. Covers possible interactions with other drugs, medical conditions and other concerns. Explains how each drug works, and offers detailed information about treatments for depression, bipolar disorder, anxiety and sleep disorders, as well as other conditions.

340 pages
ISBN: 1-572241-11-X

6475 Let's Talk About Going to the Hospital
Rosen Publishing Group's PowerKids Press
29 E 21st Street
New York, NY 10010

212-777-3017
800-237-9932
Fax: 888-436-4643
e-mail: rosenpub@tribeca.ios.com
www.powerkidspress.com

If a child has to check into the hospital, chances are he or she is already upset about being ill. Knowing how a hospital functions and what the procedures are, such as when family members can visit, will help in what is already a stressful situation. Grades K-5.

24 pages
ISBN: 0-823950-36-0

6476 Principles and Practice of Sleep Medicine
Elsevier Health Sciences Division
1600 John F Kennedy Blvd, Suite 1800
Philadelphia, PA 19103

215-239-3900
800-545-2522
Fax: 215-239-3990
www.us.elsevierhealth.com

Covers the recent advances in basic sciences as well as sleep pathology in adults. Encompasses developments in this rapidly advancing field and also includes topics related to psychiatry, circadian rhythms, cardiovascualr diseases and sleep apnea diagnosis and treatment. Hardcover.

2005 1552 pages 4th Edition
ISBN: 0-721607-97-7

6477 Restless Nights
Yale University Press
PO Box 209040
New Haven, CT 06520

203-432-0960
800-987-7323
Fax: 203-432-0948
yalepress.yale.edu/yupbooks

This book provides an explanation of sleep apnea symptoms, risk-factors, advice on diagnosis and consultation, and current available treatments.

2003 288 pages
ISBN: 0-300085-44-0

6478 Sleep Disorders Diagnosis and Treatment: Current Clinical Practice Series
American Psychiatric Publishing
1400 K Street NW
Washington, DC 20005

202-682-6262
800-368-5777
Fax: 202-789-2648
e-mail: appi@psych.org
appi.org

250 pages
ISBN: 0-896035-27-1

Katie Duffy, Marketing Assistant

6479 Sleep Disorders Sourcebook
Omnigraphics
PO Box 625
Holmes, PA 19043

800-234-1340
Fax: 800-875-1340
e-mail: info@omnigraphics.com
omnigraphics.com

Basic consumer health information about sleep and its disorders, including sleep apnea, insomnia, sleepwalking, restless leg syndrome and narcolepsy.

567 pages 2nd Edition
ISBN: 0-780807-43-0

6480 Sleeping Like a Baby

Avi Sadeh, author

Yale University Press
PO Box 209040
New Haven, CT 06520

203-432-0960
800-987-7323
Fax: 203-432-0948
yalepress.yale.edu/yupbooks

A practical and sensitive guide to solving your child's sleep problems.

2001 224 pages
ISBN: 0-300088-24-3

6481 Snoring From A to Zzzz
Spencer Press
2525 NW Lovejoy Street, Suite 402
Portland, OR 97210

503-223-4959
Fax: 503-223-1608
e-mail: dereklipman@aol.com

Covers organizations, associations, support groups, and manufactorers of sleep-related medical products relevant to sleep disorders. Discussess every aspect of snoring and sleep apnea from causes to cures.

256 pages Paperback
ISBN: 0-965070-81-6

Derek S Lipman, MD, Author/Editor

6482 Snoring and Sleep Apnea
Demos Medical Publishing
386 Park Avenue S
New York, NY 10016

212-683-0072
800-532-8663
Fax: 212-683-0118
e-mail: orderdept@demosmedpub.com
www.demosmedpub.com

A straightforward, jargon-free approach to dealing with snoring and sleep problems.

286 pages 3rd Ed/Soft
ISBN: 1-888799-29-3

Pamphlets

6483 Get the Facts About Sleep Apnea

American Sleep Apnea Association
1424 K Street NW, Suite 302
Washington, DC 20005

202-293-3650
Fax: 202-293-3656
e-mail: asaa@sleepapnea.org
www.sleepapnea.org

Brochures are also available in bulk.

6484 Sleep Apnea

National Sleep Foundation
1522 K Street NW, Suite 500
Washington, DC 20005

202-347-3471
Fax: 202-347-3472
e-mail: nsf@sleepfoundation.org
www.sleepfoundation.org

A brochure about sleep apnea, a breathing disorder characterized
by brief interruptions of breathing during sleep. Brochure explains
what it is, who gets it, and how it is diagnosed and treated.

DESCRIPTION

6485 SLEEPWALKING

Synonym: Somnambulism

Involves the following Biologic System(s):

Developmental/Behavioral/Psychiatric Disorders

Sleepwalking, also known as somnambulism, is a condition where the child engages in activities that are normally associated with wakefulness while asleep or in a sleeplike state. It occurs most commonly in children, particularly those from approximately four to six years of age. About 10 to 15 percent of children experience at least one episode of sleepwalking during childhood. In addition, approximately one in five children who sleepwalk has a family history of the condition. In many patients, sleepwalking occurs in association with bed-wetting (nocturnal enuresis) or night terrors (sleep disturbances that typically occur shortly after the onset of sleep). In some cases, a stressful event may lead to an episode of sleepwalking.

In children, sleepwalking occurs during stage four of NREM (nonrapid eye movement) sleep. NREM sleep consists of four progressively deeper stages of sleep that are typically characterized by slow, deep brain waves, muscle relaxation and slowed breathing rate, slowed heart rate, and lowered blood pressure. In contrast, REM (rapid eye movement) sleep, which is associated with dreaming, is characterized by increased levels of brain activity, rapid eye movements, and involuntary muscle jerks.

During an episode of sleepwalking, affected children may simply sit up in bed or move to the edge of the bed, without engaging in actual sleepwalking. In other cases, however, children may get out of bed and walk through their home. They may also perform certain routine acts, such as turning on a hallway light. Unless children are simultaneously experiencing night terrors, they usually do not have associated anxiety. During an episode, most children have their eyes open and are guided by their vision. Therefore, they typically move around familiar obstacles; however, some children may make no effort to avoid certain objects in their path, potentially resulting in injury. In addition, some children may mumble simple words or phrases or repeatedly perform certain acts, such as turning a doorknob back and forth. If children are urged to return to bed during such an episode, they may sometimes follow such instruction; however, they usually must be gently steered back to their beds. Sleepwalking episodes typically last only a few minutes, and children usually have little or no memory of the experience. In children, sleepwalking is rarely associated with

psychologic abnormalities, and the number of episodes usually decreases by early adolescence. However, the persistence of sleepwalking episodes into adulthood is thought to be associated with a significant risk of psychiatric disease. Parents or caregivers of children who sleepwalk should take precautions to help protect them against injury. Possible obstacles or breakable objects should be removed from their paths. It may be advisable to block staircases and to have children sleep on the ground floor of the house, if possible.

See also **General Resources** on page 917

Government Agencies

6486 NIH/National Institute of Mental Health
6001 Executive Boulevard, Room 8184, MSC 9663
Bethesda, MD 20892

301-443-4513
866-615-6464
Fax: 301-443-4279
TTY: 301-443-8431
e-mail: nimhinfo@nih.gov
www.nimh.nih.gov

Conducts strategic planning for specific research areas as well as for the Institute as a whole.

Dr Thomas R Insel, Director

National Associations & Support Groups

6487 American Academy of Sleep Medicine
1 Westbrook Corporate Center, Suite 920
Westchester, IL 60154

708-492-0930
Fax: 708-492-0943
www.aasmnet.org

National not-for-profit professional membership organization dedicated to the advancement of sleep medicine. The Academy's mission is to assure quality care for patients with sleep disorders, promote the advancement of sleep research and provide public and professional education. The AASM delivers programs, information and services to and through its members and advocates sleep medicine supportive policies in the medical community and the public sector.

Jerome Barrett, Executive Director
Jennifer Markkanen, Assistant Executive Director

6488 Center for Disabilities and Development
University of Iowa Hospitals and Clinics
100 Hawkins Drive
Iowa City, IA 52242

319-353-6900
877-686-0031
e-mail: cdd-webmaster@uiowa.edu
www.healthcare.uiowa.edu/cdd

A trusted resource for healthcare, training, research and information for people with disabilities that include: behavior disorders, brain injury, cerebral palsy, diabetes, down syndrome, learning disabilities, mental retardation, sleep disorders and spina bifida.

Elayne Sexsmith, Administrator
Amy Mikelson, Supervisor Info Resource Service

6489 Federation of Families for Children's Mental Health
9605 Medical Center Drive, Suite 280
Rockville, MD 20850

240-403-1901
Fax: 240-403-1909
e-mail: ffcmh@ffcmh.org
www.ffcmh.org

The National family run organization is dedicated exclusively to helping children with mental health needs and their families achieve a better quality of life.

Sandra Spencer, Executive Director

6490 National Mental Health Consumers' Self-Help Clearinghouse
1211 Chestnut Street, Suite 1207
Philadelphia, PA 19107

215-751-1810
800-553-4539
Fax: 215-636-6312
e-mail: info@mhselfhelp.org
www.mhselfhelp.org

Offers information, support and appropriate referrals; and promotes public and professional education. Provides networking for those with special interests related to albinism. Promotes and supports research and funding that will improve diagnosis and management of albinism and hypopigmentation.

Joseph Rogers, Executive Director & Founder

6491 National Sleep Foundation
1522 K Street NW, Suite 500
Washington, DC 20005

202-347-3471
Fax: 202-347-3472
e-mail: nsf@sleepfoundation.org
www.sleepfoundation.org

An independent, nonprofit organization dedicated to improving public health and safety by achieving public understanding of sleep and sleep disorders, and by supporting public education, sleep-related research, and advocacy. Actively collaborates with sleep centers, support groups for patients with sleep disorders and safety organizations.

Richard Gelula, CEO

Libraries & Resource Centers

6492 American Academy of Somnology
PO Box 27077
Las Vegas, NV 89126

702-371-0947
e-mail: somnology@aol.com
www.hopperinstitute.com/aas_intro.html

Covers about 75 physicians, dentists, nurses, psychologists, technicians, and students and sponsoring organizations, including associations, institutions, and corporations, with a special interest in sleep.

Web Sites

6493 About.com on Sleep Disorders
www.sleepdisorders.about.com

Well-organized information including new developments and a chat room.

6494 National Sleep Foundation
www.sleepfoundation.org

Is an independent nonprofit organization dedicated to improving public health and safety by achieving understnading of sleep and sleep disorders, and by supporting education, sleep-related research, and advocacy.

6495 Online Mendelian Inheritance in Man
www.ncbi.nlm.nih.gov

This database is a catalog of human genes and genetic disorders.

6496 Sleep Walking in Children
familydoctor.org/160.xml

Brief overview of possible parental concerns of sleep walking in children.

6497 SleepEducation.com
www.sleepeducation.com

Online resources on sleep related topics and sleep disorders including sleepwalking.

6498 Sleepdisorders.com
www.sleepdisorders.com

Provides a full range of internet communications and technology solutions from strategic consulting to concept design, content development, software engineering, and ongoing enhancements and maintenance. Our projects have encompassed direct-to-customer marketing, direct-to-patient education, healthcare professional training, corporate intranets and database management systems, dynamic database-driven web sites and hospital training.

Book Publishers

6499 Concise Guide to Evaluation and Management of Sleep Disorders
American Psychiatric Publishing
1000 Wilson Boulevard, Suite 1825
Arlington, VA 22209

703-907-7322
800-368-5777
Fax: 703-907-1091
e-mail: appi@psych.org
www.appi.org

Over view of sleep disorders medicine, sleep physiology and pathology, insomnia complaints, excessive sleepiness disorders, parasomnias, medical and psychiatric disorders and sleep, medications with sedative-hypnotic properties, special problems and populations.

2002 296 pages Paper 3rd Ed
ISBN: 1-585620-45-6

6500 Depression and Sleep
American Psychiatric Press
1400 K Street NW
Washington, DC 20005

202-682-6262
800-368-5777
Fax: 202-789-2648
e-mail: order@appi.com
www.appi.com

Contents include normal sleep, neurochemistry of sleep, sleep in depression, neurochemistry of depression, antidepressent drugs and sleep, and clinical management of sleep disorders in depression.

1996 64 pages

6501 Sleep Disorders Diagnosis and Treatment: Current Clinical Practice Series
American Psyciatric Publishing Group
1400 K Street NW
Washington, DC 20005

202-682-6262
800-368-5777
Fax: 202-789-2648
e-mail: order@appi.com
www.appi.com

1998 250 pages

6502 Sleep Disorders Sourcebook

Omnigraphics
PO Box 625
Holmes, PA 19043

800-234-1340
Fax: 800-875-1340
e-mail: info@omnigraphics.com
omnigraphics.com

Basic consumer health information about sleep and its disorders, including insomnia, sleepwalking, sleep apnea, restless leg syndrome and narcolepsy.

567 pages 2nd Edition
ISBN: 0-780807-43-0

6503 Sleep: The Brazelton Way

T Berry Brazelton; Joshua D Sparrow, author

Perseus Books Group-Da Capo Press
11 Cambridge Center
Cambridge, MA 02142

617-252-5200
www.perseusbooksgroup.com

Pediatrician provide highly effective and affordable guides to lead parents through struggles of getting babies and toddlers to sleep.

2003 Paperback
ISBN: 0-738207-82-9

6504 Snoring From A to Zzzz

Spencer Press
2525 NW Lovejoy Street, Suite 402
Portland, OR 97210

503-223-4959
Fax: 503-223-1608
e-mail: dereklipman@aol.com

Covers organizations, associations, support groups, and manufactorers of sleep-related medical products relevant to sleep disorders. Discussess every aspect of snoring and sleep apnea from causes to cures.

256 pages Paperback
ISBN: 0-965070-81-6

Derek S Lipman, MD, Author/Editor

DESCRIPTION

6505 SPEECH IMPAIRMENT

Synonym: Speech dysfunction

Involves the following Biologic System(s):

Neurologic Disorders

Speech impairment refers to the decreased ability or inability to effectively communicate through vocalizations or uttered sounds. Difficulty speaking or more profound dysfunctions of speech may result from many different factors that include neurologic influences; muscular defects, injuries, or paralysis; structural irregularities of the vocal cords; psychologic influences; mental retardation; and other factors.

In some children, speech impairment may be classified as a dysfunction of articulation characterized by the inability to articulate or produce words properly (dysarthria) as a result of damage to the part of the brain responsible for regulation of the muscles that control the speech apparatus (e.g., mouth, lips, and voice box or larynx). Such damage may result from head or brain injuries, tumors, strokes, and certain diseases. Characteristic speech patterns of children with dysarthria are varied and may be described as unintelligible, slow, slurred, halting, tremulous, hoarse, or possessing a nasal quality. Additional causes of articulation dysfunction or delay include structural defects such as cleft lip or palate, hearing impairment or deafness, and other nervous system irregularities. In addition, speech impairment may result from irregularities directly related to the vocal cords that may affect the quality of the voice.

Impaired ability to communicate (aphasia or dysphasia) may also result from injury to the part of the brain responsible for language comprehension, resulting in the reduced ability or inability to express, write, or understand language. Such injury may be caused by head trauma, brain lesions, infection, or other factors. This type of impairment may be present in many different variations such as garbled sentences, extremely slow and difficult speech, absence of speech (mutism), and other irregularities. In addition, children with behavioral, emotional, or psychologic irregularities as well as those with hearing impairment may also experience delays in language comprehension and development.

It is important to identify the underlying cause of any dysfunction of speech or delay in speech development in order to allow for the most favorable educational and social outcome. Specialists in the diagnosis and treatment of these types of disorders (e.g., otolaryngologists and speech therapists) may base their treatment plans on the evaluation of family and medical histories, physical examination of essential speech structures, and specialized testing that may include speech, language, and hearing assessments. Treatment is directed toward the specific cause of impairment and may include exercises tailored to the specific patient's needs, as well as the cooperation of parents or caregivers, pediatricians, educators, and others to provide a supportive environment.

See also **General Resources** on page 917

Government Agencies

6506 NIH/National Institute on Deafness and Oth er Communication Disorders (NIDCD)
31 Center Drive, MSC 2320
Bethesda, MD 20892

e-mail: nidcdinfo@nidcd.nih.gov
www.nidcd.nih.gov

A National Institute of Health, the NIDCD supports research and provides education and information on these following health topics: voice, speech, language, hearing, ear infections, deafness, balance, smell and taste.

Dr James F Battey JrD, Director
Judith A Cooper PhD, Deputy Director

National Associations & Support Groups

6507 American Speech Language Hearing Associati on (ASHA)
10801 Rockville Pike
Rockville, MD 20852

301-897-5700
800-638-8255
Fax: 301-571-0457
e-mail: pr@asha.org
www.asha.org

A professional and credentialing association made up of more than 123,000 international pathologists, audiologists and scientists. The association promotes the interests of and provides services for those in the hearing, speech, and language field, and advocates for people with communication disorders.

Arlene A Pietranton, Executive Director
Maureen E Thompson, Director Governance Operations

6508 Auditory-Verbal Learning Institute
7205 North Habana Ave
Tampa, FL 33614

813-227-8766
Fax: 813-932-9583
e-mail: info@avli.org
www.avli.org

Promotes and teaches Auditory-Verbal Therapy.

Pamela Sullins, Director/CEO
Alisa Jenkins, Marketing/Product Consultant

State Agencies & Support Groups

New York

6509 Brooklyn College Speech and Hearing Center
2900 Bedford Ave, 4400 Boylan Hall
Brooklyn, NY 11210

718-951-5186
Fax: 718-951-4363
e-mail: mbergen@brooklyn.cuny.edu
depthome.brooklyn.cuny.edu/speech/center/

Provides diagnostic and rehabilitative services to children and
adults with speech, language, hearing and voice impairments.

Dr Michael Bergen, Director
Susan Bohne, Assistant Director

North Carolina

**6510 North Carolina Speech, Hearing and Languag e
Association**
PO Box 28359
Raleigh, NC 27611

919-833-3984
Fax: 919-832-0445
www.ncshla.org

Promotes the professional practice of speech, language and hearing
sciences and works to enhance the lives of those who are communicatively impaired, through a variety of programs and opportunities.

G Peyton Maynard, Executive VP
AJ Jacques, Executive Secretary

Ohio

6511 Cleveland Hearing and Speech Center
11206 Euclid Avenue
Cleveland, OH 44106

216-231-8787
Fax: 216-231-7141
www.chsc.org

A nonprofit organization in Northeast Ohio dedicated to serving
the needs of those with special communication needs.

Bernard P Henri, Executive Director
Michael Lerner, Marketing/Communications Manager

6512 Speech and Hearing Clinic
Kent State University
A104 Music & Speech Bldg, PO Box 5190
Kent, OH 44242

330-672-2672
Fax: 330-672-2643
www.chhs.kent.edu/spa/speech.htm

Services provided include: full-service clinic diagnoses, therapy,
treatment and hearing aid repair.

Carol Sommer, Director

Oklahoma

6513 Oklahoma Speech Language Hearing Associati on
PO Box 53217, State Capitol Station
Oklahoma City, OK 73152

405-271-4214
Fax: 405-271-3360
e-mail: oslha@hotmail.org
www.oslha.org

Suzanne Stanton, President
Linda Doss, Membership Contact

Oregon

6514 Reading and Speech Clinic
243 SW Scalehouse Loop, Suite 2B
Bend, OR 97702

541-389-3302
800-283-0818
e-mail: ellen@readingandspeechclinic.com
www.readingandspeechclinic.com

Provides alternate therapies for improving speech, language, spelling and reading difficulties.

Ellen Jacobs PhD, Director

Tennessee

**6515 Memphis State University, Center for the
Communicatively Impaired**
807 Jefferson Avenue
Memphis, TN 38105

901-678-2009
Fax: 901-525-1282
www.ausp.memphis.edu

Offers research into hearing loss, deafness, and speech impairments.

Maurice I Mendel, Director

Texas

6516 Callier Center for Communication Disorders
University of Texas at Dallas
1966 Inwood Road
Dallas, TX 75235

214-905-3000
Fax: 214-905-3022
TDD: 214-905-3012
e-mail: barbara.cmber@utdallas.edu
www.callier.utdallas.edu

Multidisciplinary center serving infants through adults with all
types of communcation disorders: diagnostic and treatment; hearing aid services; cochlear implant evalution and follow-up; N
Texas Cochlear Implant Summer Listening Camp; aural rehabilitation services; assistive listening device program; tinnitus and hyperacusis clinic; speech-language pathology and psychological
diagnostic and therapy services; research.

Dr Thomas Campbell, Director
Christine A Dollaghan, Child Language Development

**6517 Texas Tech University Speech-Language -Hearing
Clinic**
Lubbock, TX 79409

806-742-3907

Sherry Sancribian, Director

Virginia

6518 Speech Simulation Research Foundation
Cedar Hall, Box 824
Nassawadox, VA 23413

757-442-2755

Focuses on hearing and speech disorders.

Monte Penney, Director

Washington

**6519 Scottish Rite Centers for Childhood Langua ge
Disorders**
1155 Broadway E
Seattle, WA 98102

206-324-6293
www.srccld.org

Association offering speech-language evaluations and treatment,
hearing screening and consultation and referrals to children ages
birth to 18 years with hearing or speech disorders. Seven loca-
tions/clinincs are offered throughout the state of Washington.

Martin Fischer

6520 University of Washington Department of Spe ech & Hearing Sciences
1417 NE 42nd Street
Seattle, WA 98105

206-685-7400
Fax: 206-543-1093
e-mail: sphscadv@u.washington.edu
www.depts.washington.edu/sphsc/

Committed to understanding the basic processes and mechanisms involved in human speech, hearing, language, their disorders and to improving the quality of life for individuals affected by communication disorders across the life span.

Stacy Betz, Child Language Disorders

Research Centers

6521 Boys Town National Research Hospital
555 N 30th Street
Omaha, NE 68131

402-498-6511
Fax: 402-498-6638
TTY: 402-498-6543
www.boystownhospital.org

An internationally recognized center for state-of-the-art research, diagnosis, treatment of patients with ear diseases, hearing and balance disorders, cleft lip and palate, and speech/language problems.

6522 Gallaudet University, Cued Speech Team
800 Florida Avenue NE
Washington, DC 20002

202-651-5000

Transmission of spoken languages are researched.

Elizabeth L Kiplia, Coordinator

Arizona

6523 National Center for Neurogenic Communicati on Disorders
University of Arizona
Speech & Hearing Sciences Bldg, Rm 500
Tucson, AZ 85721

520-621-1472
cnet.shs.arizona.edu

The center is supported by a grant from the NIDCD, a National Institute of Health, and is staffed by scientists, educators and students who are concerned with speech and language disorders caused by diseases of the nervous system.

Thomas J Hixon PhD, Director
Kathryn A Bayles PhD, Associate Director

Colorado

6524 Speech, Language, and Hearing Center
University of Colorado, Boulder
2501 Kittregde Loop Rd
Boulder, CO 80309

303-492-5375
www.colorado.edu/CDSS/slhs/slhcenter.html

Focuses on communication disorders including speech and hearing impairments.

Susan M Moore, Director

Michigan

6525 University Center for the Development of L anguage & Literacy
University of Michigan
1111 E Catherine Street
Ann Arbor, MI 48109

734-764-8440
Fax: 734-647-2489
www.languageexperts.org/research/

Focuses on communicative disorders including hearing impairments and speech disorders. Provides intensive language intervention for adults with aphasia as well as children with language disorders. Clinic offers residential program for adults and school liasion for children.

Holly Craig PhD, Director
Joanne Marttila Pierson PhD, Associate Director

Nevada

6526 University of Nevada - Department of Speec h-Language Pathology
School of Medicine
Redfield Bldg, MS 152
Reno, NV 89557

775-784-4887
Fax: 775-784-4095
e-mail: lgoldberg@medicine.nevada.edu
www.unr.edu/spa/

The department includes an active clinic and nine faculty for research in language, speech and hearing.

Thomas Watterson, Chair
Leslie Goldberg, Clinical Director

New York

6527 Henry Youngerman Center for Communication Disorders
SUNY Fredonia/Dept Speech Pathology & Audiology
Thompson Hall W121
Fredonia, NY 14063

716-673-3202
Fax: 716-673-3235
e-mail: SpeechPathology.Audiology@fredonia.edu
www.fredonia.edu/department/SpeechPathology/

Studies communications disorders including hearing and speech. It features a newly constructed research lab.

Dr Michelle Nottella, Director

North Carolina

6528 Communications Disorders Clinic
Reich College of Education
730 Rivers St, PO Box 32041
Boone, NC 28608

828-262-2185
Fax: 828-262-6766
www.cdclinic.appstate.edu

The clinic provides prevention, assessment, and treatment of speech, language and hearing disorders for all ages. It also provides several outreach programs.

Mary Ruth Sizer, Director

Washington

6529 University of Washington Speech and Hearin g Clinic
4131 15th Avenue NE
Seattle, WA 98105

206-543-5440
Fax: 206-616-1185
e-mail: shclinic@u.washington.edu
depts.washington.edu/sphsc/

A center for education and research serving speech, language, and hearing needs within the university and the community. Serves as a teaching facility in the fields of speech-language pathology and audiology, with state of the art technology, innovative diagnostic and treament methods, and internationally and nationally recognized areas of research.

Nancy Alarcon MS, CCC-SLP, Director
Joan Hanson, Manager

Wisconsin

6530 Waisman Center - Auditory Physiology Resea rch Laboratory

University of Wisconsin, Madison
1500 Highland Ave
Madison, WI 53705

608-262-0818
www.physiology.wisc.edu/BruggeLab.html

The research laboratory is part of the Waisman Center which is dedicated to advancing the knowledge about human development, developmental disabilities, and neurodegenerative disorders.

Dr John Brugge, Director

Web Sites

6531 Auditory-Verbal International

The goal is for children who are deaf or hard of hearing to grow up in typical learning and living environments and to become independent, participating citizens in mainstream society. The philosophy supports the option for children with all degrees of hearing impairment to develop the ability to listen and to use verbal communication within their own family and community constellations.

6532 Parent Pals

parentpals.com/gossamer/pages/Speech_and_Language

Their goal is to provide special education and gifted information, continuing education, support, weekly tips, games, book resources, and news and views for parents and professionals.

Book Publishers

6533 Assisting Survivors of Traumatic Brain Inj ury

Karen Hux, author

Pro-Ed
8700 Shoal Creek Boulevard
Austin, TX 78757

512-451-3246
800-897-3202
Fax: 512-451-8542
e-mail: info@proedinc.com
www.proedinc.com

For speech-language pathologists, it is divided into three sections: understanding TBI, understanding the role of speech-language pathologists, and understanding reintegration.

2003 359 pages Softcover
ISBN: 0-890798-95-8

6534 Listen Little Star

Auditory-Verbal Learning Institute
7205 North Habana Ave
Tampa, FL 33614

813-227-8766
Fax: 813-932-9583
e-mail: info@avli.org
www.avli.org

A family activity kit for parents designed to help their babies develop listening and speaking skills. It includes 12 activities, a workbook, checklist, plush toy, and note-taking section.

6535 Management of Motor Speech Disorders in Children and Adults

Pro-Ed
8700 Shoal Creek Boulevard
Austin, TX 78757

512-451-3246
800-897-3202
Fax: 800-397-7633
e-mail: info@proedinc.com
www.proedinc.com

Second edition of this popular text incorporates information about both dysarthria and apraxia of speech in children and adults and reviews techniques for physical and motor speech examination and treatment techniques.

618 pages Hardcover
ISBN: 0-890797-84-6

6536 Preschool Motor Speech Evaluation & Interv ention

Pro-Ed
8700 Shoal Creek Boulevard
Austin, TX 78757

512-451-3246
800-897-3202
Fax: 800-397-7633
e-mail: info@proedinc.com
www.proedinc.com

Comprehensive resource manual for evaluating and treating oral motor and motor speech disorders in children 18 months to six years of age.

6537 Visible Speech

SRC Software Research Corp.
Box 4277, Station A
Victoria, BC, V8X 3X8, IT

250-727-3744

Computerized speech culture, analysis and computer-based speech training.

6 pages

AE Wright, Publisher

Journals

6538 American Journal of Speech-Language Pathol ogy

American Speech Language Hearing Association
10801 Rockville Pike
Rockville, MD 20852

301-897-5700
888-498-6699
e-mail: subscriptions@asha.org
www.asha.org

For speech-language pathologists and researchers.

Quarterly

Jeannette D Hoit, Editor

6539 Communication Disorders Quarterly

Pro-Ed
8700 Shoal Creek Boulevard
Austin, TX 78757

512-451-3246
800-897-3202
Fax: 800-397-7633
e-mail: info@proedinc.com
www.proedinc.com

It is the official journal of the Division for Communicative Disabilities and Deafness of the CEC. It provides research, intervention, and practice in speech, language and hearing.

Quarterly
ISSN: 1528-7401

Kathy Coufal PhD, Editor

6540 Journal of Speech, Language, and Hearing R esearch

American Speech Language Hearing Association
10801 Rockville Pike
Rockville, MD 20852

301-897-5700
888-498-6699
e-mail: subscriptions@asha.org
www.asha.org

Basic and applied research in communication processes, both normal and disordered.

Bi-monthly

Katherine Verdolini, Editor, Speech
Alan G Kamhi, Editor, Language

6541 Language, Speech, and Hearing in Schools
American Speech Language Hearing Association
10801 Rockville Pike
Rockville, MD 20852

301-897-5700
888-498-6699
e-mail: subscriptions@asha.org
www.asha.org

Focuses on research for speech-language pathologists and audiologists in the school setting.

Quarterly

Brian Goldstein, Editor

Newsletters

6542 Callier Communications
Callier Center - University of Texas at Dallas
1966 Inwood Road
Dallas, TX 75235

214-905-3000
Fax: 214-905-3022
TDD: 214-905-3012
www.callier.utdallas.edu

Eloyce Newman, Public Information Officer

6543 Communique
NCSHLA Publications
PO Box 28359
Raleigh, NC 27611

919-833-3984
Fax: 919-832-0445
e-mail: ncshla@bellsouth.net
www.ncshla.org

The official newsletter of NCSHLA.

Quarterly

G Peyton Maynard, Executive VP
AJ Jacques, Executive Secretary

Pamphlets

6544 Speech and Voice Impairment
United Parkinson Foundation
833 W Washington Boulevard
Chicago, IL 60607

312-733-1893

1983

Camps

6545 Boys Town National Research Hospital
555 N 30th Street
Omaha, NE 68131

402-498-6511
Fax: 402-498-6638
TTY: 402-498-6543

An internationally recognized center for state-of-the-art research, diagnosis, treatment of patients with ear diseases, hearing and balance disorders, cleft lip and palate, and speech/language problems. Also includes programs such as Parent/Child Workshops, Center for Childhood Deafness, Register for Heredity Hearing Loss, Center for Hearing Research, Center for Abused Handicapped, and summer programs for gifted deaf teens and college students.

Patrick E Brookhouser, MD, Director

6546 Central Michigan University Summer Clinics
444 Moore
Mount Pleasant, MI

517-774-3803

Designed for children, ages 6 and up, with speech, language and hearing disorders who can benefit from intensive clinical work. A wide range of recreational and social activities form part of the clinical program and promote the social use of skills learned in class.

6547 Meadowood Springs Speech and Hearing Camp
PO Box 1025
Pendleton, OR

541-276-2752
Fax: 541-276-7227
e-mail: meadowoodcamp@uci.ne
www.meadowoodsprings.org

On 143 acres in the Blue Mountains of Eastern Oregon, this camp is designed to help young people who have diagnosed clinical disorders of speech, hearing or language. A full range of activities in recreational and clinical areas is available. For cabin reservations 541-566-2191.

Rosemarie Atfield, Executive Director
Marie Story, Camp Manager

6548 University of Iowa - Wendell Johnson Speech and Hearing Clinic
Wendell Johnson Speech And Hearing Center
Iowa City, IA 52242

319-335-1845
Fax: 319-335-8851

The clinic offers assessment and remediation for disordered communication in adults and children. The clinic also offers an Intensive Summer Residential Clinic for school age children needing intervention services because of speech, language, hearing and/or reading problems.

Richard Hurtig, Professor/Chair
Ann L Michael, Clinic Director

6549 University of Texas at Dallas, Callier Center for Communication Disorders
1966 Inwood Road
Dallas, TX 75235

214-905-3000
Fax: 214-905-3022
TDD: 214-905-3012
e-mail: eloyce@utdallas.edu
www.callier.utdallas.edu

Multidisciplinary center serving infants through adults with all types of communcation disorders: diagnostic and treatment; hearing aid services; cochlear implant evalution and follow-up; North Texas Cochlear Implant Summer Listening Camp; aural rehabilitation services; assistive listening device program; tinnitus and hyperacusis clinic; speech-language pathology and psychological diagnostic and therapy services; research.

Eloyce Newman, Public Information

DESCRIPTION

6550 SPINA BIFIDA

Covers these related disorders: Encephalocele, Meningocele, Myelocele (Myelomeningocele, Meningomyelocele), Spina bifida occulta

Involves the following Biologic System(s): Neurologic Disorders, Orthopedic and Muscle Disorders

Spina bifida, literally meaning "cleft spine," is a congenital abnormality, known as a neural tube defect, which is characterized by the failure during embryonic development of one or more of the developing vertebrae to develop completely or fuse. This frequently results in the exposure of part of the spinal cord. It is the most common neural tube defect in the United States—affecting 1,500 to 2,000 of the more than 4 million babies born in the country each year. Spina bifida occulta, the most common and least severe form of this defect, is characterized by a dimpling, dark tufts of hair, spider-like fine lines (telangiectasia), or a benign fatty tumor (lipoma) on the lower back or lumbosacral area. There is no protrusion or exposure of the spinal cord and it rarely involves problems with the nervous system. Some affected children, however, may experience weakness in the legs and feet and difficulty in bladder and bowel control resulting from an adhesion of the spinal cord to the area of the abnormality.

Meningocele occurs when the three membranes surrounding the spinal cord (meninges) protrude through the vertebral defect. Most meningoceles are covered by skin and contain cerebrospinal fluid. Although most affected children have no apparent neurologic involvement, some children may experience nerve dysfunction and associated irregularities (e.g., tethered spinal cord, diastematomyelia, and syringomyelia). If cerebrospinal fluid is leaking from the meningocele, immediate surgery is usually required to avoid infection or inflammation of the meninges (meningitis). Surgery to correct the meningocele may be performed at a later date in those children who are not at risk for such infection.

Myelocele is a severe form of spina bifida that affects one in 1,000 newborns. This form of the disorder is characterized by a protrusion of the spinal cord and meninges through the vertebral canal, covered by a raw swelling. Most myeloceles are located in the lumbosacral region. This abnormality may result in impaired function of the skeletal system, the skin, the genitourinary tract, and the peripheral and central nervous systems. Physical findings associated with myelocele are widely variable and depend upon the portion of the spinal cord affected and may include the inability to control the bladder and bowel functions, lack of muscle tone in the legs, and other irregularities of the lower extremities. Some children with myelocele develop an unusual accumulation of cerebrospinal fluid in the skull, resulting in enlargement of the head (hydrocephalus) and associated symptoms that may include choking and difficulty in feeding and breathing. The insertion of a tube or shunt is often indicated to relieve fluid buildup. Treatment of myelocele often involves a team of medical specialists working closely to manage care for the affected child. This care usually involves surgery to repair the myelocele. Other approaches to treatment are geared toward correction, alleviation, or management of symptoms. For example, training children or their parents how to empty the bladder through catheterization may help to avoid ur|inary tract infections and kidney disease. Also, laxatives or enemas may be used to relieve the constipation often associated with this abnormality. Other treatment may include the use of braces and canes or crutches and physical therapy to maintain joint mobility and to strengthen muscular function. Further treatment is supportive. The exact cause of myelocele is unknown; however, it is thought that environmental and nutritional influences may be contributing factors.

Encephalocele, a very severe and rare type of spina bifida, is characterized by the protrusion of the brain through a defect in the cranium. Affected children often experience visual difficulties, mental retardation, and seizures.

A common screening method used to look for spina bifida during pregnancy is a second trimester maternal serum alpha fetoprotein (MSAFP) screening. The MSAFP screen measures the level of a protein called alpha-fetoprotein (AFP), which is made naturally by the fetus and placenta. During pregnancy, a small amount of AFP normally crosses the placenta and enters the mother's bloodstream. But if abnormally high levels of this protein appear in the mother's bloodstream it may indicate that the fetus has a neural tube defect. Amniocentesis, an exam in which a sample of fluid is obtained from the amniotic sac that surrounds the fetus, may also be used to diagnose spina bifida. Research has shown that supplementation with folic acid, starting before pregnancy, reduces the risk of neural tube defects. It is recommended that all women of childbearing age consume 400 micrograms of folic acid daily.

See also **General Resources** on page 917

Government Agencies

6551 NIH/National Institute of Arthritis and Mu sculoskeletal and Skin Diseases
1AMS Circle
Bethesda, MD 20892

301-402-4484
Fax: 301-718-6366
e-mail: ord@od.nih.gov
rarediseases.info.nih.gov

The mission of the National Institute of Arthritis and Musculoskeletal and Skin Diseases is to support research into the causes, treatment, and prevention of arthritis and musculoskeletal and skin diseases, the training of basic and clinical scientists to carry out this research, and the dissemination of information on research progress in these diseases.

Stephen I Katz MD PhD, Director

National Associations & Support Groups

6552 Easter Seals Disability Services
230 West Monroe Street, Suite 1800
Chicago, IL 60606

312-726-6200
800-221-6827
Fax: 312-726-1494
TDD: 312-726-4258
e-mail: info@easterseals.com
www.easterseals.com

Helps individuals with special needs and disabilities and their families to lead better lives through a variety of services including job training, development centers, rehabilitation, and education.

Lou Lowenkron, Chairman
James E Williams Jr, President/CEO

6553 Genetic Alliance
4301 Connecticut Avenue NW
Washington, DC 20008

202-966-5557
800-336-4363
Fax: 202-966-8553
e-mail: info@geneticalliance.org
www.geneticalliance.org

A coalition of voluntary genetic support groups, consumers and professionals addressing the needs of individuals and families affected by genetic disorders from a national perspective.

Sharon Terry, President/CEO

6554 March of Dimes Birth Defects Foundation
1275 Mamaroneck Avenue
White Plains, NY 10605

914-428-7100
888-663-4637
Fax: 914-428-8203
e-mail: resourcecenter@modimes.org
www.marchofdimes.com

Partnership of volunteers and professionals dedicated to improving the health of babies by preventing birth defects and infant mortality. Over 100 chapters are located across the country and can be located through the national office.

Dr Jennifer Howse, President

6555 National Center for Education in Maternal and Child Health
Georgetown University
2115 Wisconsin Ave NW, Suite 601
Washington, DC 20007

202-784-9770
Fax: 202-784-9777
e-mail: mchlibrary@ncemch.org
www.ncemch.org

Provides leadership in disseminating information, program development, and education to individuals with an interest in maternal and child health (MCH), public health policy, and systems of care.

Rochelle Mayer, Director
Olivia Pickett, Director Library Services

6556 National Dissemination Center for Children with Disabilities
PO Box 1492
Washington, DC 20013

202-884-8200
800-695-0285
Fax: 202-884-8441
e-mail: nichcy@aed.org
www.nichcy.org

A national information and referral center for families, educators and other professionals on: disabilities in children and youth; programs and services; IDEA, the nation's special education law; and research-based information on effective practices.

Suzanne Ripley, Executive Director

6557 National Rehabilitation Information Center
4200 Forbes Blvd, Suite 202
Lanham, MD 20706

301-459-5900
800-346-2742
Fax: 301-459-4263
TTY: 301-459-5984
e-mail: naricinfo@heitechservices.com
www.naric.com

An online gateway to over 70,000 disability and rehabilitation related documents and journal articles, and other resources.

Mark Odum, Director

6558 Spina Bifida Association of America
4590 MacArthur Boulevard NW, Suite 250
Washington, DC 20007

202-944-3285
800-621-3141
Fax: 202-944-3295
e-mail: sbaa@sbaa.org
www.sbaa.org

Serves as the national office representing approximately 60 chapters of parents and other members of families having children born with spina bifida, individuals with spina bifida, and health professionals who work with them. Operates a national information and referral service, periodic public awareness campaigns, scholarships and an annual meeting.

Cindy Brownstein, CEO
Caroline Alston, Director, Programs/Field Initiative

State Agencies & Support Groups

Alabama

6559 Spina Bifida Association of Alabama
PO Box 661424
Birmingham, AL 35266

256-325-8600
e-mail: Al_spina_bifida_support@hotmail.com
www.sbaa.org

Providing medical, social, and financial support to those afflicted with spina bifida.

Patricia Switzer, President

Arizona

6560 Arizona Spina Bifida Association
1001 E Fairmount Avenue
Phoenix, AZ 85014

602-274-3323
Fax: 602-274-7632
e-mail: office@azspinabifida.org
www.azspinabifida.org

Arkansas

6561 Spina Bifida Association of Arkansas
PO Box 24663
Little Rock, AR 72221

501-978-7222
Fax: 501-296-1787
e-mail: sigmondr@attwb.net
www.sbaar.typepad.com

Providing medical, social, and financial support to those afflicted with spina bifida.

Vicki Rucker, Executive Director

California

6562 Spina Bifida Association of Greater Bay Ar ea
100 West South Street
Tracy, CA 95376

925-215-1503
Fax: 209-830-1903
e-mail: spinabifidasupport@comcast.net
www.sbaa.org

Providing medical, social, and financial support to those afflicted with spina bifida.

Traci Whittemore, President

6563 Spina Bifida Association of Greater San Di ego
PO Box 232272
San Diego, CA 92193

619-491-9018
Fax: 619-275-3361
e-mail: sbaofgsd@hotmail.com
www.sbaa.org

Providing medical, social, and financial support to those afflicted with spina bifida.

Mary Robbins Wade, President

Colorado

6564 Spina Bifida Association of Colorado
PO Box 22994
Denver, CO 80222

303-797-7870
e-mail: mhys1@juno.com
www.coloradospinabifida.org

Providing medical, social, and financial support to those afflicted with spina bifida.

Margaret Hays, President

Connecticut

6565 Spina Bifida Association of Connecticut
PO Box 2545
Hartford, CT 06146

800-574-6274
e-mail: sbac@sbac.org
www.sbac.org

Providing medical, social, and financial support to those afflicted with spina bifida.

Fred Liguori, President

Florida

6566 Spina Bifida Association of Central Florid a
7643 Persian Drive
Orlando, FL 32819

407-248-9210
Fax: 407-248-9227
e-mail: info@sbacfl.org
www.sbacfl.org

Providing medical, social, and financial support to those afflicted with spina bifida.

Beccy Hosoda, President

6567 Spina Bifida Association of Florida Space Coast
3744 Grand Meadows Blvd
Melbourne, FL 32934

321-757-6977
Fax: 321-454-9737
e-mail: mlk1984@earthlink.net
www.sbafsc.org

Providing medical, social, and financial support to those afflicted with spina bifida.

Leslie Krysinel, President

6568 Spina Bifida Association of Jacksonville N emours Childrens Clinic
807 Children's Way
Jacksonville, FL 32207

904-390-3686
800-722-6355
Fax: 904-390-3466
e-mail: Sbaj@sbaj.org
www.sbaj.org

Providing medical, social, and financial support to those afflicted with spina bifida.

Stephanie King, Executive Director
Margaret Quintana, Treasurer

6569 Spina Bifida Association of Southeast Florida
PO Box 559046
Miami, FL 33255

305-220-2559
e-mail: SBAofSEFL@bellsouth.net
www.sbaa.org

Providing medical, social, and financial support to those afflicted with spina bifida.

Irene Ballart, President

6570 Spina Bifida Association of Tampa Bay
PO Box 290527
Tampa, FL 33687

813-933-4827
e-mail: sbatampabay@aol.com

Providing medical, social, and financial support to those afflicted with spina bifida.

Dianne Gore, President

Georgia

6571 Spina Bifida Association of Georgia
1448 McLendon Dr, Suite B
Decatur, GA 30033

770-939-1044
Fax: 770-939-1049
e-mail: Jokula@spinabifida.org
www.spinabifidaga.org

Jim Okula, Executive Director

Illinois

6572 Spina Bifida Association of Illinois
8765 W Higgins Rd, Suite 403
Chicago, IL 60631

800-969-4722
Fax: 773-444-0327
e-mail: sbail@sbail.org
www.sbail.org

The Illinois Spina Bifida Association is dedicated to improving the quality of life of people with spina bifida through direct services, information and referral and public awareness. Direct services include family outreach, education advocacy and more.

Adam Rappaport, Executive Director
Rebecca May, Program Director

Indiana

6573 Spina Bifida Association of Central Indian a
PO Box 19814
Indianapolis, IN 46219

317-592-1630
e-mail: membership@sbaci.org
www.sbaci.org

Providing medical, social, and financial support to those afflicted with spina bifida.

Lisa Jones, President

6574 Spina Bifida Association of Northern Indiana
PO Box 2437
Elkhart, IN 46515

574-293-4976
e-mail: katieandjacobsmom@yahoo.com
www.sbaa.org

Providing medical, social, and financial support to those afflicted with spina bifida.

Tim Yoder, President

Iowa

6575 Center for Disabilities and Development
University of Iowa Hospitals and Clinics
100 Hawkins Drive
Iowa City, IA 52242

319-353-6900
877-686-0031
e-mail: cdd-webmaster@uiowa.edu
www.healthcare.uiowa.edu/cdd

A trusted resource for healthcare, training, research and information for people with disabilities that include: behavior disorders, brain injury, cerebral palsy, diabetes, down syndrome, learning disabilities, mental retardation, sleep disorders and spina bifida.

Elayne Sexsmith, Administrator
Amy Mikelson, Supervisor Info Resource Service

6576 Spina Bifida Association of Iowa
PO Box 1456
Des Moines, IA 50305

515-986-9088
e-mail: SpinaBifidaIowa@yahoo.com
www.SpinaBifidaIA.com

Providing support, a reimbursement program, quarterly newsletter and public awareness campaigns.

Rod Tressel, President

Kansas

6577 Spina Bifida Association of Kansas
1605 N Robin Circle
Wichita, KS 67212

316-516-7225
e-mail: mlubbers@kscable.com
www.sbaa.org

Providing medical, social, and financial support to those afflicted with spina bifida.

Tim Wolke, President

Kentucky

6578 Spina Bifida Association of Kentucky
Kosair Charities Centre
982 Eastern Parkway, Box 18
Louisville, KY 40217

866-340-7225
Fax: 502-637-1010
e-mail: sbak@sbak.org
www.sbak.org

Providing support to those afflicted with spina bifida.

Patty Dissell, Executive Director

Louisiana

6579 Spina Bifida Association of Greater New Orleans
PO Box 1346
Kenner, LA 70063

504-737-5181
e-mail: sbagno@sbagno.org
www.sbagno.org

Providing support to those afflicted with spina bifida.

Julie Johnston, Coordinator

Maryland

6580 Spina Bifida Association of Chesapeake-Pot omac
PO Box 1750
Annapolis, MD 21404

888-733-0988
Fax: 410-295-9744
e-mail: Shumate@kennedykrieger.org
www.chesapeakespinabifida.org

Providing support to those afflicted with spina bifida.

Toni Shumate, Executive Director

Massachusetts

6581 Spina Bifida Association of Massachusetts
733 Turnpike St, #282
N Andover, MA 01845

888-479-1900
Fax: 978-649-8725
e-mail: packard44@comcast.net
www.msbaweb.org

Ellen Dugan, Operations

Michigan

6582 Grand Rapids Spina Bifida & Hydrocephalus Association
1204 E 8th Street
Holland, MI 49423

616-392-1358
Fax: 616-394-1166
www.sbaa.com

Providing medical, social, and financial support to those afflicted with spina bifida and hydrocephalus.

6583 SW Michigan SB & Hydrocephalus Association
PO Box 212
Mattawan, MI 49071

269-385-3959
Fax: 269-342-9765
www.sbaa.org

Dedicated to improving the quality of life of individuals with spina bifida and/or hydrocephalus and their families through awareness, education, and research. Offers a variety of educational guides and materials for schools, professionals, parents, and the general public.

6584 Spina Bifida Association of Upper Peninsula Michigan
1220 N 3rd Street
Ishpeming, MI 49849

906-485-5127
e-mail: cbengson@chartermi.net
www.sbauppermichigan.org

Providing support to those affected by spina bifida.

Lois Bengson, President

6585 Spina Bifida Association of West Michigan
681 Spaulding Ave SE
Ada, MI 49301

616-949-3428
e-mail: thelees3@yahoo.com

Providing support to those afflicted with spina bifida.

Carol Carpenter, Interim President

Minnesota

6586 Spina Bifida Association of Minnesota
PO Box 29323
Brooklyn Center, MN 55429

651-222-6395
Fax: 651-228-0914
e-mail: sbamn@hotmail.com
www.sbamn.org

Providing support to those afflicted with spina bifida.

James Thayer, Executive Director

Mississippi

6587 Spina Bifida Association of Mississippi
PO Box 180594
Richland, MS 39218

601-420-0030
Fax: 601-420-0300
e-mail: sbafms@yahoo.com
www.spinabifidams.com

Providing support to those afflicted with spina bifida.

Amy Wilkinson, Executive Director

Missouri

6588 Spina Bifida Association of Greater Saint Louis
8050 Watson Road, Suite 115
St. Louis, MO 63119

314-843-2244
800-784-0983
Fax: 314-765-6246
e-mail: sbastl@charter.net
www.sbastl.com

Providing support to those afflicted with spina bifida.

Mark Abbott, Chairman

Nebraska

6589 Spina Bifida Association of Nebraska
7101 Newport Avenue, Suite 206
Omaha, NE 68152

402-572-3570
Fax: 402-572-3002
e-mail: sbamom@cox.net
www.spinabifidanebraska.org

Providing support to those afflicted with spina bifida.

Megan Sorensen, President

New Jersey

6590 Spina Bifida Association of Bergen and Passaic Counties
181 Glen Avenue
Midland Park, NJ 07432

201-670-0590
Fax: 201-670-6381
e-mail: TJA84@aol.com
www.sbaa.org

Providing medical, social, and financial support to those afflicted with spina bifida.

Shirl Cichewicz, President

6591 Spina Bifida Association of the Tri-State Region
84 Park Avenue
Flemington, NJ 08822

908-782-7475
Fax: 908-782-6102
e-mail: info@sbatsr.org
www.sbatsr.org

Serves New Jersey, New York metro area and Southern Connecticut. Providing medical, social, and financial support to those afflicted with spina bifida.

Jane Horowitz, Executive Director
Haley Hopper, Director Development

New Mexico

6592 Spina Bifida Association of New Mexico
1127 University Boulevard NE
Albuquerque, NM 87102

505-242-1184
e-mail: SBANM@aol.com
www.sbaa.org

Providing medical, social, financial support to those afflicted with spina bifida.

Rey Garduno, President
Gordon Hendrickson, Executive Director

New York

6593 Spina Bifida Association of Albany/Capital District
109 Spring Road
Scotia, NY 12302

518-399-9151
e-mail: Sbaalbany102@aol.com
www.sbaalbany.org

Providing support to those afflicted with spina bifida.

Karen Wentworth, Director

6594 Spina Bifida Association of Greater Roches ter
PO Box 3
Fairport, NY 14450

585-388-7450
e-mail: pritch50@yahoo.com

Providing support to those afflicted with spina bifida.

Mary Pritchard, Chair

6595 Spina Bifida Association of Nassau County
12 Hampton Rd
South Beach, NY 11789

631-821-9028
e-mail: kid3418@optonline.net
www.sbancny.org

Providing support to those afflicted with spina bifida.

Leslieann Sussman, President

6596 Spina Bifida Association of Western New York
137 Warner Ave
N Tonawanda, NY 14120

716-446-5595
Fax: 716-735-7561
e-mail: pmorris@sbawny.org
www.sbawny.org

Providing support to those living with spina bifida.

Cynthia Carlson, President

North Carolina

6597 Spina Bifida Association of North Carolina
3915 Grace Court
Indian Trail, NC 28079

800-847-2262
Fax: 800-847-2262
e-mail: sbanc@mindspring.com
sbanc.home.mindspring.com

Providing support to those afflicted with spina bifida. There are five regional support groups in the state.

Kim Gates, Charlotte/Piedmont Contact
Jolyne Wagner, Raleigh Area Contact

Ohio

6598 Spina Bifida Association of Canton
PO Box 9024
Canton, OH 44711

330-863-2531
e-mail: cmgriffin@neo.rr.com
www.sbacanton.org

Providing support to those afflicted with spina bifida.

Connie Griffin, President

6599 Spina Bifida Association of Central Ohio
7574 Danbridge Way
Westerville, OH 43082

614-818-3840
e-mail: lauriedvm@sbcglobal.net
www.sbaco.blogspot.com

Providing support to those afflicted with spina bifida.

Laurie Schulze, President

6600 Spina Bifida Association of Cincinnati
3245 Deborah Lane
Cincinnati, OH 45239

513-923-1378
e-mail: sbacincy@excel.com
www.sbacincy.org

Providing support to those afflicted with spina bifida.

Diane Burns, President

6601 Spina Bifida Association of Greater Dayton
4801 Springfield St
Dayton, OH 45431

937-236-1122
Fax: 937-434-4899
e-mail: sbadayton@yahoo.com
www.sbadayton.org

Providing support to those afflicted with spina bifida.

David Skinner, President

6602 Spina Bifida Association of North West Ohio
15518 County Rd F
Holgate, OH 43527

419-264-1131
e-mail: clark_ginnette@yahoo.com
www.sbaa.org

Providing support to those afflicted with spina bifida.

Ginnette Clark, President

6603 Spina Bifida Association of Tri-County Ohio
PO Box 8701
Warren, OH 44484

330-793-8544
e-mail: jchappel@sbcglobal.net
www.spaa.org

Providing support to those living with spina bifida, from youth into adulthood. Also places an emphasis on parent support groups.

Julie Solomon, President

Pennsylvania

6604 Spina Bifida Association Pittsburgh
361 Princeton Drive
Pittsburgh, PA 15235

412-829-4719
e-mail: davenshan1@juno.com
www.sbaa.org

Providing medical, social, and financial support to those afflicted with spina bifida.

Shannon Williams, President

6605 Spina Bifida Association of Delaware Valley
PO Box 72109
Thorndale, PA 19372

215-412-9396
800-223-0222
e-mail: President@sbadv.org
www.sbadv.org

Providing medical, social, and financial support to those living with spina bifida.

Keri Mascaro, President

6606 Spina Bifida Association of Greater Pennsylvania
215 E State St, Suite D
Quarryville, PA 17566

717-786-9280
Fax: 717-786-8821
e-mail: SBAofPA@aol.com
www.geocities.com/sbaofpa/

Providing medical, social, and financial support to those afflicted with spina bifida.

Pat Fulvio, Executive Director

Rhode Island

6607 Spina Bifida Association of Rhode Island
PO Box 6948
Warwick, RI 02887

401-732-7862
Fax: 401-732-7862
e-mail: rid24703@ride.ri.net
www.sbaa.org

Providing medical, social, and financial support to those afflicted with spina bifida.

Cindy Ponte, Presdient

Tennessee

6608 Spina Bifida Association of Tennessee
PO Box 23056
Nashville, TN 37202

615-791-8117
e-mail: lynnhess56@comcast.net
www.sbaa.org

Providing medical, social, and financial support to those living with spina bifida.

Lynn Hess, President

Texas

6609 Spina Bifida Association of Austin
8710 Tallwood Drive
Austin, TX 78759

512-794-8156

Providing medical, social, and financial support to those afflicted with spina bifida.

Carol Bowen, President

6610 Spina Bifida Association of Houston-Gulf Coast
624 Pasadena Blvd, Suite 305
Pasadena, TX 77506

713-473-8035
Fax: 281-997-2378
e-mail: president@sbahgc.org
www.sbahgc.org

Providing medical, social, and financial support to those afflicted with spina bifida.

David Enderli, President

6611 Spina Bifida Association of North Texas
705 Ave B, Suite 409
Garland, TX 75040

972-238-8755
Fax: 972-414-3772
e-mail: sbnorthtexas@aol.com

Providing medical, social, and financial support to those living with spina bifida.

Carol Barrett, Contact

6612 Spina Bifida Association of Texas
10615 Perrin Beitel Rd, Suite 701
San Antonio, TX 78217

866-597-2289
e-mail: sbinfo@sbatx.org
www.sbatx.org

Providing medical, social, and financial support to those afflicted with spina bifida.

Nora Oyler, Executive Director

Utah

6613 Spina Bifida Association of Utah
900 S 1500 East, Apt C124
Clearfield, UT 84015

801-663-3120
e-mail: irhall@csolutions.net
www.sbautah.org

Providing medical, social, and financial support to those living with spina bifida.

Ilene Hall, President

Virginia

6614 Spina Bifida Association of the Roanoke Valley
PO Box 7652
Roanoke, VA 24019

540-342-1231
Fax: 540-890-1244
e-mail: sbaroanokevalley@yahoo.com
www.sbarv.org

Providing medical, social, and financial support to those living with spina bifida.

Millie Wilson, President

Washington

6615 Evergreen Spina Bifida Association
PO Box 642
Sumner, WA 98390

253-589-3700
e-mail: evergreensba@yahoo.com
www.evergreenspinabifida.org

Providing medical, social, and financial support to those afflicted with spina bifida.

Ed Kennedy, President

Wisconsin

6616 Spina Bifida Association of Greater Fox Valley
325 N John Street
Kimberly, WI 54136

920-687-0801
Fax: 920-982-3783
e-mail: fus1234@athenet.net
www.sbaa.org

Providing support to those living with spina bifida.

Kelly Richard

6617 Spina Bifida Association of Northern Wisconsin
PO Box 421
Schofield, WI 54476

715-359-9674
e-mail: dtackley@cheqnet.net

Providing medical, social, and financial support to those afflicted with spina bifida.

David Bouchard, President

6618 Spina Bifida Association of Wisconsin
830 N 109th Street, Suite 6
Wauwatosa, WI 53226

414-607-9061
Fax: 414-607-9602
e-mail: sbawi@sbawi.org
www.sbawi.org

SBAWI is made up of those with spina bifida, as well as family, friends and health care providers. The association is dedicated to helping its membership emotionally, educationally, and financially.

Rita Flores, Executive Director

Audio Video

6619 Challenge (The)
Spina Bifida Association of America
4590 MacArthur Boulevard NW, Suite 250
Washington, DC 20007

202-944-3285
800-621-3141
Fax: 202-944-3295
e-mail: sbaa@sbaa.org
www.sbaa.org

A human look of how people come to grips with and overcome the challenges related to living with Spina Bifida.

1992 14 minutes

6620 How to Guide Your Child Through Special Education
Spina Bifida Association of America
4590 MacArthur Boulevard NW
Washington, DC 20007

202-944-3285
800-621-3141
Fax: 202-944-3295
e-mail: spinabifida@aol.com
www.infohiway.com/spinabifida

Enlightens and encourages viewers, and informs parents on special education, planning for the future, and laws designed to protect children with disabilities.

6621 Teaching the Student with Spina Bifida Video
Paul H Brookes Publishing Company
PO Box 10624
Baltimore, MD 21285

410-337-8539

A compelling companion to the book by the same name, this heartening videotape draws viewers into the inclusive classroom for a first-hand look.

Web Sites

6622 Association for Spina Bifida and Hydroceph alus
www.asbah.org

A UK charity that provides information and advice to those with spina bifida and their families.

6623 Children with Spina Bifida: A Resource Page for Parents
www.waisman.wisc.edu/~rowley/sb-kids/

A resource page for parents with children with Spina Bifida.

6624 Harvard Web Forum for Spina Bifida
neuro-www.mgh.harvard.edu/forum/spinabifidamenue

A web forum to discuss and comment on Spina Bifida.

6625 International Federation for Spina Bifida and Hydrocephalus
www.ifglobal.org

The world-wide umbrella organization for spina bifida and hydracephalus organizations. It's primary goal is prevention through the dissemination of information and education.

6626 LFSN: Lipomyelomeningecele Family Support Network
www.lfsn.org

A network of families providing support and information sharing to those affected by Occult Spinal Dysraphisms.

6627 March of Dimes Birth Defects Foundation
www.marchofdimes.com

March of Dimes researchers, columnteers, educators, outreach workers and advocates work together to give all babies a fighting chance against the threats to their health: prematurity, birth defects, low birthweight.

6628 Online Mendelian Inheritance in Man
www.ncbi.nlm.nih.gov

This database is a catalog of human genes and genetic disorders.

6629 Spina Bifida Association of America
www.sbaa.org

The mission is to promote the prevention os spina bifida and to enhance the lives of all affected. The association was founded to address the specific needs of the spina bifida community and serves as the national representative of almost 60 chapters. SBAA's efforts benefit thousands of infants, children, adults, parents and professionals each year.

6630 Wheeless' Textbook of Orthopaedics
www.wheelessonline.com

Derives from a variety of sources, imcluding journals, articles, national meetings lectures and other textbooks.

Book Publishers

6631 All Kinds of Friends, Even Green!

Ellen B Sensi, author

Spina Bifida Association of America
4590 MacArthur Boulevard NW, Suite 250
Washington, DC 20007

202-944-3285
800-621-3141
Fax: 202-944-3295
e-mail: sbaa@sbaa.org
www.sbaa.org

Moses has spina bifida and a lot of friends. Which one will he choose to write about for his school project?

6632 Answering Your Questions About Spina Bifida
Spina Bifida Association of America
4590 MacArthur Boulevard NW, Suite 250
Washington, DC 20007

202-944-3285
800-621-3141
Fax: 202-944-3295
e-mail: sbaa@sbaa.org
www.sbaa.org

Provides information to help people understand the basic medical, educational and social issues which commonly affect people with Spina Bifida.

6633 Bowel Continence and Spina Bifida
Spina Bifida Association of America
4590 MacArthur Boulevard NW, Suite 250
Washington, DC 20007

202-944-3285
800-621-3141
Fax: 202-944-3295
e-mail: sbaa@sbaa.org
www.sbaa.org

An excellent book aimed at anyone (infant or adult) trying to attain bowel continence. Focuses on continence programs, bowel management development and includes a chart and glossary of terms.

6634 COLT
Association for the Care of Children's Health
19 Mantua Road
Mountain Royal, NJ 08061

609-224-1742
Fax: 609-423-3420
e-mail: amkent@tmg.smathub.com
www.acch.org

An adolescent boy with spina bifida becomes involved in a therapeutic riding program and uses skills learned there to cope with the challenges of everyday life.

Hardcover

6635 Children with Spina Bifida: A Parent's Gui de
Spina Bifida Association of America
4590 MacArthur Boulevard NW, Suite 250
Washington, DC 20007

202-944-3285
800-621-3141
Fax: 202-944-3295
e-mail: sbaa@sbaa.org
www.sbaa.org

Comprehensive publication provides easy-to-understand coverage of neurosurgery, physical therapy, emotional health, education, urological concerns, orthopedic concerns, childhood development and more. Valuable for parents, educators and libraries.

6636 Complete IEP Guide: How to Advocate for Your Special Ed Child
Spina Bifida Association of America
4590 MacArthur Boulevard NW, Suite 250
Washington, DC 20007

202-944-3285
800-621-3141
Fax: 202-944-3295
e-mail: sbaa@sbaa.org
www.sbaa.org

This all-in-one guide will help you understand special education law, identify your child's needs, prepare for meetings, develop the IEP and resolve disputes.

6637 Confronting the Challenges of Spina Bifida
Spina Bifida Association of America
4590 MacArthur Boulevard NW, Suite 250
Washington, DC 20007

202-944-3285
800-621-3141
Fax: 202-944-3295
e-mail: sbaa@sbaa.org
www.sbaa.org

A group curriculum addressing self-care, self-esteem, and social skills in eight to 13 year olds.

6638 Congenital Disorders Sourcebook
Omnigraphics
PO Box 625
Holmes, PA 19043

800-234-1340
Fax: 800-875-1340
e-mail: info@omnigraphics.com
www.omnigraphics.com

Basic consumer health information on disorders aquired during gestation, including spina bifida, hydrocephalus, cerebral palsy, heart defects, craniofacial abnormalities and fetal alcohol syndrome.

650 pages
ISBN: 0-780809-45-9

6639 Featherless/Desplumado
Juan Felipe Herrera, author

Spina Bifida Association of America
4590 MacArthur Boulevard NW, Suite 250
Washington, DC 20007

202-944-3285
800-621-3141
Fax: 202-944-3295
e-mail: sbaa@sbaa.org
www.sbaa.org

Tomasito, although confined to a wheelchair, feels free when on the soccer field.

6640 Friends No Matter What
Rose Blivins, author

Spina Bifida Association of America
4590 MacArthur Boulevard NW, Suite 250
Washington, DC 20007

202-944-3285
800-621-3141
Fax: 202-944-3295
e-mail: sbaa@sbaa.org
www.sbaa.org

The story of two boys, one in a wheelchair and one who loves to play basketball. How will it work out?

6641 Guidelines for Spina Bifida and Health Car e Services Throughout Life
Spina Bifida Association of America
4590 MacArthur Boulevard NW, Suite 250
Washington, DC 20007

202-944-3285
800-621-3141
Fax: 202-944-3295
e-mail: sbaa@sbaa.org
www.sbaa.org

Guidelines designed to help spina bifida sufferers throughout their entire lives.

6642 Introduction to Spina Bifida
Spina Bifida Association of America
4590 MacArthur Boulevard NW, Suite 250
Washington, DC 20007

202-944-3285
800-621-3141
Fax: 202-944-3295
e-mail: sbaa@sbaa.org
www.sbaa.org

An aid and guide for those who care for someone with spina bifida, written in non-medical terms and language.

6643 Looking for Goodwill
Patt & Scott Price, author

Spina Bifida Association of America
4590 MacArthur Boulevard NW, Suite 250
Washington, DC 20007

202-944-3285
800-621-3141
Fax: 202-944-3295
e-mail: sbaa@sbaa.org
www.sbaa.org

An inspirational read, the result of a trek across the US and random interviews showing the heart and attitude of America.

6644 Margaret's Moves
Dutton Children's Books
375 Hudson Street
New York, NY 10014

212-366-2000

This story deals with all the nuances and impairments that children afflicted with spina bifida must encounter and succeed in overcoming.

Grades 4-6

6645 Negotiating the Special Education Maze: A Guide for Parents and Teachers
Spina Bifida Association of America
4590 MacArthur Boulevard NW, Suite 250
Washington, DC 20007

202-944-3285
800-621-3141
Fax: 202-944-3295
e-mail: sbaa@sbaa.org
www.sbaa.org

An excellent aid for the development of an effective special education program.

6646 New Language of Toys: Teaching Communicati on Skills to Children with Special Needs
Spina Bifida Association of America
4590 MacArthur Boulevard NW, Suite 250
Washington, DC 20007

202-944-3285
800-621-3141
Fax: 202-944-3295
e-mail: sbaa@sbaa.org
www.sbaa.org

A guide for parents and teachers, this reader-friendly resource guide provides a wealth of information on how play activities affect a child's language development (with a focus on special needs) and where to get the toys and materials to use in these activities.

6647 Nick Joins In

Joe Lasker, author

Spina Bifida Association of America
4590 MacArthur Boulevard NW, Suite 250
Washington, DC 20007

202-944-3285
800-621-3141
Fax: 202-944-3295
e-mail: sbaa@sbaa.org
www.sbaa.org

When Nick, who is in a wheelchair, enters a regular classroom, for the first time he realizes that he has much to contribute.

6648 Princess Pooh

Spina Bifida Association
4590 Macarthur Boulevard NW
Washington, DC 20007

202-944-3285
e-mail: sbaa@sbaa.org
www.sbaa.org

Jealous of her disabled sister's royal treatment as she sits on her 'throne with wheels,' Patty Jean borrows it and discovers that life in a wheelchair isn't so easy.

6649 Rolling Along with Goldilocks and the Three Bears

Cindy Meyers, author

Spina Bifida Association of America
4590 MacArthur Boulevard NW, Suite 250
Washington, DC 20007

202-944-3285
800-621-3141
Fax: 202-944-3295
e-mail: sbaa@sbaa.org
www.sbaa.org

The familiar folktale with a special-needs twist.

6650 SPINAbilities: A Young Person's Guide to Spina Bifida

Spina Bifida Association of America
4590 MacArthur Boulevard NW, Suite 250
Washington, DC 20007

202-944-3285
800-621-3141
Fax: 202-944-3295
e-mail: sbaa@sbaa.org
www.sbaa.org

Practical suggestions and tips for young people on becoming independent and managing their healthcare.

6651 Sexuality and the Person with Spina Bifida

Stephen Sloan PhD, author

Spina Bifida Association of America
4590 MacArthur Boulevard NW, Suite 250
Washington, DC 20007

202-944-3285
800-621-3141
Fax: 202-944-3295
e-mail: sbaa@sbaa.org
www.sbaa.org

Focuses on sexuality, sexual development, sexual activity, and other important issues.

6652 Steps to Independence: Teaching Everyday Skills to Children with Special Needs

Spina Bifida Association of America
4590 MacArthur Boulevard NW, Suite 250
Washington, DC 20007

202-944-3285
800-621-3141
Fax: 202-944-3295
e-mail: sbaa@sbaa.org
www.sbaa.org

A guide to help parents teach life skills to their disabled child.

6653 Taking Charge

Spina Bifida Association of America
4590 Macarthur Boulevard NW
Washington, DC 20007

202-944-3285
Fax: 202-944-3295
e-mail: sbaa@sbaa.org
www.sbaa.org

Teenagers talk about life and physical disabilities.

6654 Teaching Students with Spina Bifida

BOSC Books-Books on Special Children
PO Box 3378
Amherst, MA 01004

413-256-8164
Fax: 413-256-8896
www.boscbooks.com

Explores the vital issues of concern to students with spina bifida including aspects of their social, personal and cognitive development. The book is sensitively written and abounds with useful tips covering such things as crutch storage, work space organization, etc.

460 pages Softcover

6655 Unlocking Potential: College and Other Choices for People with LD and AD/HD

Spina Bifida Association of America
4590 MacArthur Boulevard NW, Suite 250
Washington, DC 20007

202-944-3285
800-621-3141
Fax: 202-944-3295
e-mail: sbaa@sbaa.org
www.sbaa.org

An indispensible tool for high school students with learning disabilities and AD/HD. Includes a comprehensive listing of resources.

6656 Views from Our Shoes: Growing Up with a Brother or Sister with Special Needs

Spina Bifida Association of America
4590 MacArthur Boulevard NW, Suite 250
Washington, DC 20007

202-944-3285
800-621-3141
Fax: 202-944-3295
e-mail: sbaa@sbaa.org
www.sbaa.org

A balanced view of the positives and negatives of living with a disabled sibling. Written for siblings ages nine and up.

6657 You Are Special - You Are the One

Spina Bifida Association of America
4590 Macarthur Boulevard NW
Washington, DC 20007

202-944-3285
800-621-3141
Fax: 202-944-3295
e-mail: spinabifida@aol.com
www.infohiway.com/spinabifida

A coloring storybook about Holly, a little girl with Spina Bifida.

Newsletters

6658 Insights into Spina Bifida
Spina Bifida Association of America
4590 MacArthur Boulevard NW, Suite 250
Washington, DC 20007

202-944-3285
800-621-3141
Fax: 202-944-3295
e-mail: sbaa@sbaa.org
www.sbaa.org

Includes articles on the latest research, legislation, features, emotional aspects, educational information, and information on the Association's national conference.

Bimonthly

6659 NASS News
222 S Prospect Avenue
Park Ridge, IL 60068

847-698-1628

Association activities newsletter.

Pamphlets

6660 Educational Issues Among Children With Spina Bifida
Spina Bifida Association of America
4590 MacArthur Boulevard NW, Suite 250
Washington, DC 20007

202-944-3285
800-621-3141
Fax: 202-944-3295
e-mail: sbaa@sbaa.org
www.sbaa.org

6661 Learning Among Children with Spina Bifida
Spina Bifida Association of America
4590 MacArthur Boulevard NW, Suite 250
Washington, DC 20007

202-944-3285
800-621-3141
Fax: 202-944-3295
e-mail: sbaa@sbaa.org
www.sbaa.org

6662 Monetary Allowance, Health Care and Vocational Training & Rehabilitation
National Veterans Services Fund
PO Box 2465
Darien, CT 06820

203-656-0003
800-521-0198
Fax: 203-656-1957
e-mail: NatVetSvc@optonline.net
www.nvsf.org

Monetary allowance, health care, vocational training and rehabilitation for Vietnam Veterans' children with spine bifida.

Pamphlet

6663 SBAA General Information Brochure
Spina Bifida Association of America
4590 Macarthur Boulevard NW
Washington, DC 20007

202-944-3285
800-621-3141
Fax: 202-944-3295
e-mail: spinabifida@aol.com
www.infohiway.com/spinabifida

6664 SBAA General Information Packet
Spina Bifida Association of America
4590 MacArthur Boulevard NW, Suite 250
Washington, DC 20007

202-944-3285
800-621-3141
Fax: 202-944-3295
e-mail: sbaa@sbaa.org
www.sbaa.org

6665 Social Development and the Person With Spina Bifida
Spina Bifida Association of America
4590 MacArthur Boulevard NW, Suite 250
Washington, DC 20007

202-944-3285
800-621-3141
Fax: 202-944-3295
e-mail: sbaa@sbaa.org
www.sbaa.org

20 pages

6666 Urologic Care of the Child with Spina Bifida
David Joseph MD, author

Spina Bifida Association of America
4590 MacArthur Boulevard NW, Suite 250
Washington, DC 20007

202-944-3285
800-621-3141
Fax: 202-944-3295
e-mail: sbaa@sbaa.org
www.sbaa.org

2001

Camps

6667 Mountaineer Spina Bifida Camp
350 Capital Street
Charleston, WV 800-6

304-558-7098
800-800-642
Fax: 304-558-2866
www2.kidscamps.com

DESCRIPTION

6668 SPINAL MUSCULAR ATROPHIES

Synonym: SMA

Covers these related disorders: Fazio-Londe disease (Progressive bulbar palsy of childhood), SMA type I (Werdnig-Hoffmann disease; Acute SMA), SMA type II (Intermediate SMA), SMA type III (Kugelberg-Welander disease)

Involves the following Biologic System(s):
Neurologic Disorders, Orthopedic and Muscle Disorders

The spinal muscular atrophies (SMAs) refer to a group of progressive, inherited neuromuscular disorders characterized by the progressive degeneration of motor neurons. Motor neurons are nerves that originate in the spinal cord and stimulate and control muscle movement (motor neurons). Spinal muscular atrophy type I, also called Werdnig-Hoffmann disease, usually becomes apparent between the second and fourth month of life; however, some infants may have symptoms at birth, including difficult breathing and the inability to feed. Other characteristic symptoms and findings include lack of muscle tone (hypotonia), muscle weakness, the inability to control head movements, absence of tendon stretch reflexes, and uncontrollable twitching or small movements (fasciculations) of the tongue and possibly other muscles. Within two to three years of age, continued breathing and feeding difficulties, along with other progressive problems, may lead to life-threatening complications. Treatment is symptomatic and supportive.

Children with SMA type II usually show signs of progressive muscle weakness of the legs and, to a lesser degree, the arms during the first or second year of life. As the disease progresses, many affected children develop side-to-side curvature of the spine (scoliosis), difficulty swallowing, and a nasal quality to their speech. Children with SMA type II may be severely physically handicapped and are usually of average or above average intelligence. Affected chidren are prone to repeated respiratory infections and breathing difficulties. Life-threatening complications may occur during adolescence or early adulthood.

SMA type III or chronic spinal muscular atrophy may become apparent between the ages of two to 17 years. This is the mildest form of SMA. Progressive weakness associated with chronic SMA is most apparent in the trunk area of the body, especially in the muscles of the shoulder girdle area. There is muscle weakness and loss of muscle mass (atrophy). In addition, deep tendon reflexes may be decreased or absent and muscle twitching (fasciculations) may be present. Some affected children may also have a tremor when the hands are outstretched. Repeated respiratory infections are common.

Fazio-Londe disease, also called progressive bulbar palsy of childhood, is a rare type of spinal muscular atrophy that results from degeneration of motor neurons located, for the most part, in the brain stem. This rare disorder is characterized by progressive palsy or paralysis of the nerves that emerge from the skull (cranial nerves). Symptoms and physical findings associated with Fazio-Londe disease include progressive loss of muscle mass (atrophy) and paralysis of the muscles of the tongue, mouth, lips, throat (pharynx), and voice box (larynx).

A team approach involving specialists such as neurologists, orthopedists, and physical therapists, in cooperation with parents or caregivers, may be helpful in providing care for children with spinal muscular atrophies. Other treatment is symptomatic and supportive.

SMA is usually inherited as an autosomal recessive trait, although some cases of autosomal dominant transmission have been reported. This disorder occurs in approximately one out of every 25,000 births. The genes for SMA types I, II, and III seem to be related and are located on the long arm of chromosome 5 (5q11-13).

See also **General Resources** on page 917

National Associations & Support Groups

6669 Association for Neuro-Metabolic Disorders
5223 Brookfield Lane
Sylvania, OH 43506

419-885-1497
e-mail: volk4olks@aol.com

A nonprofit organization that serves as an advocate organization for families of patients with the following neuro-metabolic disorders: phenylketonuria, maple syrup urine disease, galactosemia, and biotinidase deficiency. Provides educational information for parents and children; provides networking information on support groups for new parents; supports scientific research into the treatments of these four neuro-metabolic disorders.

Cheryl Volks, Contact Person

6670 Families of Spinal Muscular Atrophy
PO Box 196
Libertyville, IL 60048

847-367-7620
800-886-1762
Fax: 847-357-7623
e-mail: info@fsma.org
www.curesma.org

Families of SMA was founded for the purpose of encouraging support and raising funds to promote research into the causes and cure of spinal muscular atrophy. Funds are specifically directed to scientific, educational, or literary purposes in keeping with a charitable organization. It has more than 24 chapters worldwide and over 5000 member families.

Kenneth Hobby, Executive Director
Lenna Silberman Scott, Media Relations/PR

6671 Fight SMA / Andrew's Buddies
1807 Libbie Ave, Suite 104
Richmond, VA 23226

804-515-0080
Fax: 804-515-0081
e-mail: heatherlennon@fightsma.com
www.andrewsbuddies.org

Corporation with 15 US chapters that works to raise awareness of SMA and accelerate treatment and a cure.

Martha Slay, President
Sarah Williams, Treasurer

6672 Genetic Alliance
4301 Connecticut Avenue NW
Washington, DC 20008

202-966-5557
800-336-4363
Fax: 202-966-8553
e-mail: info@geneticalliance.org
www.geneticalliance.org

A coalition of voluntary genetic support groups, consumers and professionals addressing the needs of individuals and families affected by genetic disorders from a national perspective.

Sharon Terry, President/CEO

6673 March of Dimes Birth Defects Foundation
1275 Mamaroneck Avenue
White Plains, NY 10605

914-428-7100
888-663-4637
Fax: 914-428-8203
e-mail: resourcecenter@modimes.org
www.marchofdimes.com

Partnership of volunteers and professionals dedicated to improving the health of babies by preventing birth defects and infant mortality. Over 100 chapters are located across the country and can be located through the national office.

Dr Jennifer Howse, President

6674 Muscular Dystrophy Association
3300 E Sunrise Drive
Tucson, AZ 85718

520-529-2000
800-572-1717
Fax: 520-529-5300
e-mail: mda@mdausa.org
www.mdausa.org

Bob Mackle, Director Public Information

6675 Spinal Muscular Atrophy Coalition (SMA Coa lition)
119 W 72nd Street, PO Box 187
New York, NY 10023

212-589-0800
Fax: 212-247-3079
e-mail: smacoalition@wswdc.org
www.smacoalition.org

A group of nonprofit organizations that stand together to raise awareness and advocate for progress towards the treatment and cure of SMA.

6676 Spinal Muscular Atrophy Foundation
119 W 72nd St, #187
New York, NY 10023

646-253-7100
Fax: 212-247-3079
e-mail: info@smafoundation.org
www.smafoundation.org

Loren Eng, President
Cynthia Joyce, Executive Director

State Agencies & Support Groups

Arizona

6677 Families of SMA - Arizona Chapter
PO Box 641
Queen Creek, AZ 85242

480-752-8093
e-mail: arizona@fsma.org

Karey Kaler, President

California

6678 Families of SMA - Northern California Chap ter
PO Box 9014
Santa Rosa, CA 95405

707-571-8990
e-mail: ncalif@fsma.org

David Sereni, President

Connecticut

6679 Families of SMA - Connecticut Chapter
PO Box 185744
Hamden, CT 06518

203-288-1488
e-mail: conn@fsma.org

Jonathan Goldsberry, President

Indiana

6680 SMA Support Inc
PO Box 6301
Kokomo, IN 46904

317-536-6063
Fax: 801-460-2813
www.smasupport.com

Laura Stants, Contact

New York

6681 Families of SMA - Long Island NY Chapter
PO Box 322
Rockville Center, NY 11571

516-214-0348
e-mail: longisland@fsma.org

Debbie Cuevas, President

Tennessee

6682 Families of SMA - Tennessee Chapter
PO Box 7025
Knoxville, TN 37921

865-945-7636
e-mail: tennessee@fsma.org

Lise Murphy, President

Research Centers

6683 SMA Research Group
Stanford University School of Medicine
300 Pasteur Dr, Rm A343
Stanford, CA 94305

650-498-7658
Fax: 650-725-7459
e-mail: sma@stanfordmed.org
sma.stanford.edu

SMA clinical trials.

Ching Wang MD, PhD, Director
Tony Trela, Division Coordinator

6684 Spinal Muscular Atrophy Clinic
Columbia Pediatric Neuromuscular Disease Ctr
180 Ft Washington Ave, Harkness Pavilion, Ste 525
New York, NY 10032

212-342-0263
Fax: 212-342-2893
e-mail: kidsmda@columbia.edu
www.columbiasma.org

Dr Darryl De Vivo, Director
Dr Petra Kaufmann, Associate Director

6685 Spinal Muscular Atrophy Project
NINDS
PO Box 5801
Bethesda, MD 20824

301-496-5751
800-352-9424
e-mail: smaproject-fd@saic.com
www.smaproject.org

Research program established by NINDS (National Institute of
Neurological Disorders and Stroke) as a model of developing a
safe and effective treatment for SMA. The program adopts the
methods used by the pharmaceutical industry to carry out drug discovery according to accepted standards.

Audio Video

6686 Living with SMA
Families of SMA
PO Box 196
Libertyville, IL 60048

847-367-7620
800-886-1762
Fax: 847-357-7623
e-mail: info@fsma.org
www.curesma.org

Tapes 3 and 4 are available and are part of the Living with SMA
video series. Overview of Type II and Type III/Kennedy's.

18 pages

Web Sites

6687 Families of Spinal Muscular Atrophy
www.curesma.org

Families of SMA was founded for the purpose of encouraging support and raising funds to promote research into the causes and cure
of spinal muscular atrophy.

6688 Online Mendelian Inheritance in Man
www.ncbi.nlm.nih.gov

This database is a catalog of human genes and genetic disorders.

6689 SMA Net
www.affari.com/smanet

Is to provide a source of information for research, prevention and
treatment of spinal muscular atrophy.

6690 Spinal Muscular Atrophy Information Page
www.ninds.nih.gov/disorders/sma/

6691 Spinal Muscular Atrophy Project
www.smaproject.org

Research program established by NINDS (National Institute of
Neurological Disorders and Stroke) as a model of developing a
safe and effective treatment for SMA. The program adopts the
methods used by the pharmaceutical industry to carry out drug discovery according to accepted standards.

Newsletters

6692 Compass
Families of SMA
PO Box 196
Libertyville, IL 60048

847-367-7620
800-886-1762
Fax: 847-357-7623
e-mail: info@fsma.org
www.curesma.org

Newsletter dedicated solely to SMA research updates and information.

42 pages Quarterly

Jill Jarecki PhD, Research Director

6693 Directions
Families of SMA
PO Box 196
Libertyville, IL 60048

847-367-7620
800-886-1762
Fax: 847-357-7623
e-mail: info@fsma.org
www.curesma.org

32 pages Quarterly

6694 SMA Newsletter
Columbia Pediatric Neuromuscular Disease Ctr
180 Ft Washington Ave, Harkness Pavilion, Ste 525
New York, NY 10032

212-342-0263
Fax: 212-342-2893
e-mail: kidsmda@columbia.edu
www.columbiasma.org

Research updates, upcoming events and conferences, news, and a
kids page.

Jessica Rascoll DPT, Newsletter Contact

Pamphlets

6695 Facts About Spinal Muscular Atrophy
Muscular Dystrophy Association
3300 E Sunrise Drive
Tucson, AZ 85718

520-529-2000
800-572-1717
Fax: 520-529-5300
www.mda.org/publications/fa-sma-qa.html

Covers the four forms of the disease and outlines the characteristics and genetic patterns of the SMAs. Research efforts aimed at
finding the causes, treatments, and cures are also described.

6696 Understanding SMA
Families of SMA
PO Box 196
Libertyville, IL 60048

847-367-7620
800-886-1762
Fax: 847-357-7623
e-mail: info@fsma.org
www.curesma.org

This booklet is for the educaton and support of those with SMA.

18 pages

DESCRIPTION

6697 STRABISMUS

Synonyms: Heterotropia, Manifest deviation, Squint
Covers these related disorders: Accommodation strabismus, Nonparalytic strabismus, Paralytic strabismus
Involves the following Biologic System(s):
Neurologic Disorders, Ophthalmologic Disorders, Orthopedic and Muscle Disorders

Strabismus refers to a condition in which the eyes are not aligned properly in relation to each other and are focused on different objects simultaneously. Approximately four percent of all children under six years of age are affected by some form of strabismus. The eye deviations associated with this condition are classified according to the direction of the deviation. An eye that is turned inward is considered esotropic or convergent; an eye turned outward is exotropic or divergent; an eye turned upward is hypertropic; and an eye turned downward is hypotropic. In normal vision, both eyes focus as a unit to produce a single, three-dimensional image. In children with strabismus, the divergent images sent to the brain from the eyes may produce double vision (diplopia). In many cases, the brain will compensate for this error by blocking the image from the deviated eye, often resulting in poor vision or loss of vision in that eye (suppression amblyopia).

The most common type of strabismus is nonparalytic, in which this often-inherited ocular deviation is constant and results from a defect in the actual positioning of the eyes. Approximately 50 percent of individuals with nonparalytic strabismus have one eye turned inward. These inward-turned or esotropic deviations that appear before six months of age are classified as congenital or infantile esotropia. Outward-turned or exotropic deviations, the second most common type of strabismus, usually occur in children between six months and four years of age. Some outward deviations may result from neurologic disorders and craniofacial abnormalities.

Paralytic strabismus results from dysfunction of an eye muscle as the result of ocular muscle paralysis or a deficit of the nerves that supply the muscles. This resultant muscular imbalance causes the degree of deviation in the affected eye to vary as the eyes move.

Farsighted children are at particular risk for developing accommodative strabismus (accommodative esotropia), in which the lens of the eye tries to compensate for blurred images received by the brain by focusing the eyes inward (converging). If the compensation or accommodation demands are too great, some children may develop this additional eye abnormality.

Strabismus may result from many different factors; therefore, medical specialists make every effort to determine and treat the underlying cause as soon as possible after diagnosis. Such factors may include hereditary influences; trauma; neurologic abnormalities resulting from intracranial tumors or weaknesses in the walls of blood vessels in the brain (aneurysms); infection; systemic disorders; blood vessel malformations; structural abnormalities; and association with certain syndromes such as Duane syndrome.

Permanent loss of vision can occur if strabismus and its attendant amblyopia are not treated before age 4 to 6 years. Interventions may include wearing a patch over the normal eye in order to compel the brain to receive images from the affected eye. Patching often improves the vision in the deviating eye. Upon improvement, surgery may be performed to equalize the pull of the eye muscles. Children affected with paralytic strabismus may also benefit from wearing glasses with special lenses (prisms) that deflect light, thus altering positioning of objects seen through the lenses. In addition, children with paralytic strabismus with significant ocular deviation may benefit from eye muscle surgery to improve alignment. Farsighted children with accommodative strabismus may be treated with prescription glasses that lessen the need for ocular accommodation when focusing on objects that are far away. Certain medications in the form of eye drops may also aid in focusing on objects that are nearby. Other treatment is aimed toward the underlying cause of the ocular deviation.

See also **General Resources** on page 917

Government Agencies

6698 NIH/National Eye Institute
31 Center Drive MSC 2510
Bethesda, MD 20892

301-496-5248
e-mail: 2020@nei.nih.gov
www.nei.nih.gov

Conducts and supports research that helps prevent and treat eye diseases and other disorders of vision. This research leads to sight-saving treatments, reduces visual impairment and blindness, and improves the quality of life for people of all ages. NEI-supported research has advanced our knowledge of how the eye functions in health and disease.

Paul A Sieving M.D., Ph.D, Director

National Associations & Support Groups

6699 American Association for Pediatric Ophthalmology and Strabismus
PO Box 193832
San Francisco, CA 94119

415-561-8505
Fax: 415-561-8531
e-mail: aapos@aao.org
www.aapos.org

A membership organization of pediatric opthalmologists providing leadership for comprehensive medical and surgical eye care of children and adults with stabismus.

Christie L Morse, President

6700 Genetic Alliance
4301 Connecticut Avenue NW
Washington, DC 20008

202-966-5557
800-336-4363
Fax: 202-966-8553
e-mail: info@geneticalliance.org
www.geneticalliance.org

A coalition of voluntary genetic support groups, consumers and professionals addressing the needs of individuals and families affected by genetic disorders from a national perspective.

Sharon Terry, President/CEO

6701 National Association for Visually Handicapped
22 W 21st Street, 6th Floor
New York, NY 10010

212-889-3141
Fax: 212-727-2931
e-mail: navh@navh.org
www.navh.org

Serves as a clearinghouse for information about all services available to the partially-sighted from public and private sources. Conducts self-help groups. Provides information on large print books, textbooks and educational tools.

Dr Lorraine Marchi, Founder & CEO

Research Centers

6702 Emory Eye Center - Strabismus Research
1365B Clinton Rd NE
Atlanta, GA 30322

404-778-3431
www.eyecenter.emory.edu/strabismus_research.htm

Clinical strabismus research.

Scott R Lambert MD
Amy K Hutchinson MD

6703 National Eye Research Foundation
910 Skokie Boulevard, Suite 207A
Northbrook, IL 60062

847-564-4652
800-621-2258
Fax: 847-564-0807
e-mail: info@nerf.org
www.nerf.org

Devoted to the enhancement of care and study of eye related diseases.

Web Sites

6704 National Association for Visually Handicapped
www.navh.org

Helps to cope with the difficulties of vision impairment.

6705 Online Mendelian Inheritance in Man
www.ncbi.nlm.nih.gov

This database is a catalog of human genes and genetic disorders.

6706 Royal National Institute of the Blind
www.rnib.org.uk

A leading UK charity offering information, support and advice to over two million people with sight problems.

6707 Strabismus Web Book
www.smbs.buffalo.edu/oph/ped/webbook.htm

Is an online book about Strabismus.

Book Publishers

6708 Ophthalmic Disorders Sourcebook
Omnigraphics
615 Griswold
Detroit, MI 48226

313-961-1340
800-234-1340
Fax: 313-961-1383
e-mail: info@omnigraphics.com
www.omnigraphics.com

Basic consumer information about glaucoma, cataracts, macular degeneration, strabismus, refractive disorders and more.

1996 631 pages
ISBN: 0-780800-81-8

Journals

6709 Journal of AAPOS
Elsevier
360 Park Ave South
New York, NY 10010

212-633-3719
800-654-2452
Fax: 212-633-3820
e-mail: usjcs@elsevier.com
journals.elsevierhealth.com/periodicals/ympa

The official publication of the American Association for Pediatric Ophthalmology and Strabismus. Includes article by ledaing experts in their fields, new diagnostic techniques, and general expert information for all ages.

6 issues/yr
ISSN: 1091-8531

David G Hunter MD, PhD, Editor-in-Chief
T D Kozachek PhD, Managing Editor

DESCRIPTION

6710 STUTTERING

Involves the following Biologic System(s):

Developmental/Behavioral/Psychiatric Disorders, Neurologic Disorders

Stuttering refers to a type of speech dysfunction that interferes with the normal flow of speech (dysfluency). This dysfunction is characterized by difficulty in uttering certain sounds, letters, syllables, words, or phrases and is usually manifested by frequent hesitations, stumbling, or delay in enunciation, as well as prolongation of certain sounds. As young children develop language skills, they typically experience hesitations in speech as a result of still-developing muscle coordination and limited vocabulary. If excessive attention is given to these temporary speech deficiencies, some children may become self-conscious, anxious, and fearful of speaking. These types of emotional reactions may be manifested as persistent and compulsive movements of certain muscle groups that interfere with the normal flow of speech. Children who stutter may have difficulty with only particular letters, sounds, or words. In addition, the severity of the stutter is often related to the amount of stress evoked by the particular situation. Some affected children and adults may have associated tremors or tics. It is estimated that over three million Americans stutter. Stuttering affects individuals of all ages but occurs most frequently in young children between the ages of 2 and 6 who are developing language. Boys are three times more likely to stutter than girls.R

Although most stuttering results from psychological causes, this speech dysfunction may sometimes occur as a result of certain disorders of the central nervous system, neuromuscular abnormalities, or injury to organs related to speech. Stuttering that results from behavioral influences is often self-limited and, in 80 percent of those affected, resolves during childhood.

There are a variety of treatments available for stuttering. Any of the methods may improve stuttering to some degree, but there is at present no cure for stuttering. Stuttering therapy, however, may help prevent developmental stuttering from becoming a life-long problem. In young children, treatment for stuttering is mainly supportive. Parents or caregivers are often counseled not to place undue emphasis on speech irregularities. Additional supportive care may include recognition of accomplishments and other gestures that will contribute to the development of self-worth. If stuttering persists beyond early childhood or into adulthood, speech therapy is usually indicated.

See also **General Resources** on page 917

Government Agencies

6711 NIH/National Institute on Deafness and Oth er Communication Disorders (NIDCD)
31 Center Drive, MSC 2320
Bethesda, MD 20892

800-241-1044
TTY: 800-241-1055
e-mail: nidcdinfo@nidcd.nih.gov
www.nidcd.nih.gov

Conducts and supports biomedical research and research training on normal mechanisms, as well as diseases and disorders of hearing, balance, smell, taste, voice, speech and language.

Dr James F Battey Jr, Director
Judith A Cooper PhD, Deputy Director

National Associations & Support Groups

6712 American Speech Language Hearing Associati on (ASHA)
10801 Rockville Pike
Rockville, MD 20852

301-897-5700
800-638-8255
Fax: 301-571-0457
e-mail: pr@asha.org
www.asha.org

A professional and credentialing association made up of more than 123,000 international pathologists, audiologists and scientists. The association promotes the interests of and provides services for those in the hearing, speech, and language field, and advocates for people with communication disorders.

Arlene A Pietranton, Executive Director
Maureen E Thompson, Director Governance Operations

6713 Genetic Alliance
4301 Connecticut Avenue NW
Washington, DC 20008

202-966-5557
800-336-4363
Fax: 202-966-8553
e-mail: info@geneticalliance.org
www.geneticalliance.org

A coalition of voluntary genetic support groups, consumers and professionals addressing the needs of individuals and families affected by genetic disorders from a national perspective.

Sharon Terry, President/CEO

6714 National Center for Stuttering
388 2nd Ave, Suite 136
New York, NY 10010

800-221-2483
Fax: 212-683-1372
e-mail: executivedirector@stuttering.com
www.stuttering.com

Distributes information for parents of young children showing early signs of stuttering. For older children and adults, free information is available on treatment programs nationwide.

Martin F Schwartz, Executive Director

6715 National Stuttering Association
119 W 40th Street, 14th Fl
New York, NY 10018

212-944-4050
800-937-8888
Fax: 212-944-8244
e-mail: info@westutter.org
www.westutter.org

A self-help support organization for people who stutter. It maintains a toll-free hotline on stuttering and a nationwide resource list for individuals seeking a speech-language pathologist who specializes in stuttering. Several publications are also directed toward medical professionals who serve the stuttering community.

Elaine Saitta, Executive Director
Katia Skowronska, Assistant Director

6716 Speak Easy International Foundation
233 Concord Drive
Paramus, NJ 07562

201-262-0895
Fax: 201-262-0895

A self-help support group for stutters.

Bob Gathman, Founder/President

6717 Stuttering Foundation of America
3100 Walnut Grove Road, Suite 603, PO Box 11749
Memphis, TN 38111

901-452-7343
800-992-9392
Fax: 901-452-3931
e-mail: info@stutteringhelp.org
www.stutteringhelp.org

Provides free online resources, services and support to those who stutter and their families, as well as support for research into the causes of stuttering. Extensive educational programs on stuttering for professionals are also offered.

Jane H Fraser, President

6718 Stuttering Resource Foundation
123 Oxford
New Rochelle, NY 10804

800-232-4773

State Agencies & Support Groups

Colorado

6719 Speech, Language, & Hearing Center University of Colorado
2501 Kittredge Loop Rd., Campus Box 409
Boulder, CO 80309

303-492-5375
Fax: 303-492-3274
e-mail: susan.moore@colorado.edu
www.colorado.edu/slhs

Informational and emotional support to parents who have a child, adolescent, or adult family member with special needs.

Web Sites

6720 NIH/National Institute on Deafness and Oth er Communication Disorders (NIDCD)
www.nidcd.nih.gov/health/voice/stutter.asp

Fact sheet and information page on stuttering and other resources.

6721 Online Mendelian Inheritance in Man
www.ncbi.nlm.nih.gov

This database is a catalog of human genes and genetic disorders.

6722 Parent Pals
parentpals.com/gossamer/pages/Speech_and_Language

Their goal is to provide special education and gifted information, continuing education, support, weekly tips, games, book resources, and news and views for parents and professionals.

Book Publishers

6723 Child Psychotherapy Treatment Planner
Courage to Change
PO Box 1268
Newburgh, NY 12551

800-440-4003
Fax: 800-772-6499

Provides treatment planning guidelines and pre-written treatment plan components for 30 child behavioral and psychological problems, including blended family problems, divorce, communication disorder, attachment disorder, academic problems, stuttering, underachievement and more.

288 pages Softcover

6724 Early Childhood Stuttering
Pro-Ed
8700 Shoal Creek Boulevard
Austin, TX 78757

512-451-3246
800-897-3202
Fax: 512-451-8542
e-mail: info@proedinc.com
www.proedinc.com

Written for clinicians, students and other speech-language professionals. It discusses the history of stuttering, the different classifications and highlights the prevalence of the disorder in very young children.

6725 Programmed Therapy for Stuttering in Child ren and Adults
Charles C Thomas Publisher
2600 S 1st Street
Springfield, IL 62704

217-789-8980
800-258-8980
Fax: 217-789-9130
e-mail: books@ccthomas.com
www.ccthomas.com

This book highlights the systematic scientific approach to studying and treating stuttering by way of learning theory, single-subject research design and operant conditioning.

2001 360 pages 2nd Edition
ISBN: 0-398071-07-3

6726 Straight Talk on Stuttering: Information, Encouragement, and Counsel

Lloyd M Hulit, author

Charles C Thomas Publisher
2600 S 1st Street
Springfield, IL 62704

217-789-8980
800-258-8980
Fax: 217-789-9130
e-mail: books@ccthomas.com
www.ccthomas.com

Written for stutterers and those who interact with stutterers, including parents, caregivers, teachers, and speech-language pathologists. The author dispels myths, corrects the misperceptions and creates a message of hope for all people who have this fascinating communication disorder.

338 pages 2nd Ed/ Hard
ISBN: 0-398075-19-4

6727 Stutter No More

Dr Martin F Schwartz, author

National Center for Stuttering
388 2nd Ave, Suite 136
New York, NY 10010

800-221-2483
Fax: 212-683-1372
e-mail: executivedirector@stuttering.com
www.stuttering.com

The book covers a simple learning technique to stop stuttering in 9-12 months.

6728 Stuttering

Pro-Ed
8700 Shoal Creek Boulevard
Austin, TX 78757

512-451-3246
800-897-3202
Fax: 512-451-8542
e-mail: info@proedinc.com
www.proedinc.com

Written by a practicing clinician and a recovering stutterer, this text supplies a detailed description of the development of the disorder in school-age children and a description of the demands and capacities model that has proven so useful in planning therapy for pre-school children.

233 pages
ISBN: 0-890796-99-8

6729 Stuttering Intervention: A Collaborative Journey to Fluency Freedom

David A Shapiro, author

Pro-Ed
8700 Shoal Creek Boulevard
Austin, TX 78757

512-451-3246
800-897-3202
Fax: 512-451-8542
e-mail: info@proedinc.com
www.proedinc.com

An individualized, collaborative approach to the assessment and treatment of those who stutter and their families, written for speech-language professionals.

6730 Stuttering Prediction Instrument for Young Children

Pro-Ed
8700 Shoal Creek Boulevard
Austin, TX 78757

512-451-3246
800-897-3202
Fax: 512-451-8542
e-mail: info@proedinc.com
www.proedinc.com

The SPI is designed for children ages three to eight years and assesses a child's history, reactions, part-word repetitions, prolongations, and frequency of stuttered words to assist in measuring severity and predicting chronicity.

3-8 pages

6731 Stuttering Severity Instrument for Children and Adults, Third Edition

Pro-Ed
8700 Shoal Creek Boulevard
Austin, TX 78757

512-451-3246
800-897-3202
Fax: 512-451-8542
e-mail: info@proedinc.com
www.proedinc.com

Measures the stuttering severity of both children and adults for clinical and research use. Complete SSI-3 kit includes examiner's manual and picture plates and 50 test record and frequency computation forms all in a sturdy storage box.

Newsletters

6732 Stuttering Foundation of America

Stuttering Foundation of America
3100 Walnut Grove Road, Suite 603, PO Box 11749
Memphis, TN 38111

901-452-7343
800-992-9392
Fax: 901-452-3931
e-mail: info@stutteringhelp.org
www.stutteringhelp.org

Quarterly newsletter.

Jane H Fraser, President

Camps

6733 Meadowood Springs Speech and Hearing Camp

PO Box 1025
Pendleton, OR

541-276-2752
Fax: 541-276-7227
e-mail: meadowoodcamp@uci.ne
www.meadowoodsprings.org

On 143 acres in the Blue Mountains of Eastern Oregon, this camp is designed to help young people who have diagnosed clinical disorders of speech, hearing or language. A full range of activities in recreational and clinical areas is available. For cabin reservations 541-566-2191.

Rosemarie Atfield, Executive Director
Marie Story, Camp Manager

6734 University of Iowa - Wendell Johnson Speech and Hearing Clinic

Wendell Johnson Speech And Hearing Center
Iowa City, IA 52242

319-335-1845
Fax: 319-335-8851

The clinic offers assessment and remediation for disordered communication in adults and children. The clinic also offers an Intensive Summer Residential Clinic for school age children needing intervention services because of speech, language, hearing and/or reading problems.

Richard Hurtig, Professor/Chair
Ann L Michael, Clinic Director

DESCRIPTION

6735 SUBACUTE SCLEROSING PANENCEPHALITIS (SSPE)

Synonyms: Dawson's encephalitis, Van Bogaert's encophalitis

Involves the following Biologic System(s):

Immunologic and Rheumatologic Disorders, Neurologic Disorders

Subacute sclerosing panencephalitis (SSPE) is a rare, life-threatening, slow viral infection of the brain caused by a measles-like virus. SSPE appears months or years after a typical mild or severe measles infection and occurs most frequently in children and adolescents between the ages of five and 15 years. This disease occurs more often in children who develop measles before 18 months of age and is twice as prevalent in boys as it is in girls. Symptoms develop gradually and may commence with subtle behavorial changes such as forgetfulness or outbursts of temper, deterioration in school performance, sleeplessness, and hallucinations. These symptoms are often followed by more bizarre behavior, seizures, repetitive muscular jerks (myoclonic jerks) and other abnormal movements, eye irregularities, and mental deterioration (dementia). Late findings may include muscular rigidity or, in some patients, weak muscles, difficulty swallowing, blindness, or coma. In addition, due to generalized weakness and impaired muscle control associated with SSPE, life-threatening complications such as pneumonia may occur. Subacute sclerosing panencephalitis is incompatible with life; its usual duration is from one to three years.

The diagnosis of SSPE may be confirmed through laboratory tests that detect the presence of antibodies to the measles virus in the cerebrospinal fluid and the presence of large numbers of measles antibodies in the serum. In most cases, subacute sclerosing pnencephalitis may be prevented by immunization with attenuated measles virus vaccine.

Treatment of SSPE is geared toward chronic care. Over the last decade, however, stabilization of disease and in clinical progression has been observed with medications that alter the body's immune system response to this virus (immunomodulators), such as interferon and certain antiviral drugs including ribavirin and isoprinosine. Studies of other therapeutic programs are ongoing. Other treatment is symptomatic and supportive.

See also **General Resources** on page 917

Government Agencies

6736 Centers for Disease Control
1600 Clifton Road
Atlanta, GA 30333

404-639-3311
www.cdc.gov

Mission is to promote health and quality of life by preventing and controlling disease, injury, and disability.

6737 NIH/National Institute of Allergy and Infectious Diseases
6610 Rockledge Drive, MSC 6612
Bethesda, MD 20892

301-496-5717
Fax: 301-402-3573
TDD: 800-877-8339
www.niaid.nih.gov

Conducts and supports basic and applied research to better understand, treat, and ultimately prevent infectious, immunologic, and allergic diseases.

Anthony S Fauci MD, Director

6738 NIH/National Institute of Neurological Dis orders and Stroke (NINDS)
PO Box 5801
Bethesda, MD 20824

301-496-5751
800-352-9424
www.ninds.nih.gov/disorders/subacute_panencephalitis

National Associations & Support Groups

6739 Genetic Alliance
4301 Connecticut Avenue NW
Washington, DC 20008

202-966-5557
800-336-4363
Fax: 202-966-8553
e-mail: info@geneticalliance.org
www.geneticalliance.org

A coalition of voluntary genetic support groups, consumers and professionals addressing the needs of individuals and families affected by genetic disorders from a national perspective.

Sharon Terry, President/CEO

6740 World Health Organization
Avenue Appia 20
CH-1211 Geneva 27,
Switzerland

www.who.int

WHO is the directing and coordinating authority for health within the United Nations system.

Dr Margaret Chan, Director General

Web Sites

6741 Centers for Disease Control
www.cdc.gov/epo/mmwr/preview/mmwrhtml/00001185.htm
Mission is to promote health and quality of life by preventing and controlling disease, injury, and disability.

6742 Encephalitis Information Resource

www.encepahlitis.info

Site is provided by the Encephalitis Society

6743 MedlinePlus

www.nlm.nih.gov/Medlineplus/ency/article/001419.htm

Information on the condition, causes, symptoms, tests, and treatment.

6744 NIH/National Institute of Neurological Dis orders and Stroke (NINDS)

www.ninds.nih.gov/disorders/subacute_panencephalitis

Information fact sheet on the disorder.

Book Publishers

6745 Let's Talk About Going to the Hospital

Rosen Publishing Group's PowerKids Press
29 E 21st Street
New York, NY 10010

212-777-3017
800-237-9932
Fax: 888-436-4643
e-mail: rosenpub@tribeca.ios.com
www.powerkidspress.com

If a child has to check into the hospital, chances are he or she is already upset about being ill. Knowing how a hospital functions and what the procedures are, such as when family members can visit, will help in what is already a stressful situation. Grades K-5.

24 pages
ISBN: 0-823950-36-0

DESCRIPTION

6746 SUDDEN INFANT DEATH SYNDROME

Synonyms: Cot death, Crib death, SIDS

Involves the following Biologic System(s):

Neonatal and Infant Disorders

Sudden infant death syndrome (SIDS) refers to the sudden, unexpected, and unexplained death of an apparently healthy infant. This syndrome may occur from the ages of two weeks to one year, but most commonly occurs between the ages of two to four months. Approximately 75 to 95 percent of all deaths related to SIDS occur by the age of six months. Sudden infant death syndrome is responsible for approximately half of all infant deaths that occur between the ages of 1 month and one year and, in the United States, affects approximately 1.3 of every 1,000 infants in that age group. SIDS is somewhat more common in boys and in infants born to individuals of African-American or Native American descent. In addition, sudden infant death syndrome occurs more often during the winter months.

Very little is sure about the exact cause of SIDS, but researchers believe that certain brain stem abnormalities may be a contributing factor to its occurrence. Such irregularities may affect the regulation of body temperature, cardiorespiratory function, and associated sleep and arousal mechanisms. Although the relationship is not fully understood, brain stem abnormalities, especially sleep and arousal deficit, may interact with certain other influencing factors (epidemiologic risk factors) to put infants at risk for SIDS. Such epidemiologic risk factors may include prematurity, low birth weight, bottle feeding, exposure to smoking, recent illness with fever and previous near death episodes requiring resuscitation. Also, mothers with abnormally low levels of circulating red blood cells (anemia) or those who smoke or use drugs during pregnancy may be at increased risk for having an infant with SIDS. Other factors may include insufficient prenatal care and low socioeconomic status. In addition, recent studies have shown that putting infants to sleep on their stomachs is a significant risk factor, as is the use of soft bedding or extra linens and toys (e.g., comforters, quilts, stuffed animals, etc.) in the crib.

To alleviate certain risk factors, appropriate prenatal care is essential in the possible prevention of SIDS. Also, after birth, parents are counseled to be alert to any respiratory changes or distress and to closely observe infants during and after any illness. In addition, new guidelines recommend that infants be placed in the crib on their backs, as statistics have shown declines in SIDS rates among those who have complied with this recommendation. Sleeping on the back has been recommended for some time to avoid SIDS, with the catchphrase "Back To Bed" and "Back to Sleep." Other guidelines include the advice that crib mattresses should be firm and should fit tightly within the crib frame; that comforters, quilts, pillows, toys, etc. should be removed from the crib; that, if possible, sleeper-type pajamas be used instead of blankets; that if a blanket must be used, it should be thin, should reach no further than the infant's chest, and shou ld be tucked around the infant's chest and mattress; and that the baby's head should be uncovered at all times during sleep. Infants who die from SIDS tend to have higher concentrations of nicotine and cotinine (a biological marker for secondhand smoke exposure) in their lungs than those who die from other causes. Parents who smoke can significantly reduce their children's risk of SIDS by either quitting or smoking only outside and leaving their house completely smoke-free. In the event of the death of an infant from SIDS, counseling by trained specialists is strongly advised for parents and remaining siblings. In addition, support groups composed of families who have been affected by SIDS may be comforting and helpful.

See also **General Resources** on page 917

Government Agencies

6747 National Center for Health Statistics
1600 Clifton Road
Atlanta, GA 30333

404-639-3534
800-311-3435
www.cdc.gov

National Associations & Support Groups

6748 American SIDS Institute
509 Augusta Drive
Marietta, GA 30067

770-426-8746
800-232-7437
Fax: 770-426-1369
e-mail: prevent@sids.org
www.sids.org

A national nonprofit organization dedicated to the prevention of sudden infant death syndrome and the promotion of infant health.

Marc Peterzell, Chairman
Betty McEntire PhD, Executive Director

6749 Compassionate Friends
PO Box 3696
Oak Brook, IL 60522

630-990-0010
877-969-0010
Fax: 630-990-0246
e-mail: nationaloffice@compassionatefriends.org
www.compassionatefriends.org

Compassionate Friends assists families toward the positive resolution of grief following the death of a child of any age and provides information to help others be supportive. A national nonprofit, self-help support organization that offers friendship, understanding, and hope to bereaved parents, grandparents and siblings.

Rick Yotti, President
Ronald Haynes, VP

6750 Council of Guilds for Infant Survival
PO Box 3586
Davenport, IA 52808

319-322-4870

Conducts research and provides information on SIDS.

Chris Elliott

6751 First Candle/SIDS Alliance
1314 Bedford Avenue, Suite 210
Baltimore, MD 21208

410-653-8226
800-221-7437
Fax: 410-653-8709
e-mail: info@firstcandle.org
www.sidsalliance.org; www.firstcandle.org

First Candle started as the National SIDS Foundation focusing on supporting families that experienced SIDS. In 2002, it broadened its scope to include other areas of infant death, committing its resources in hopes of having an impact on all these areas. It's mission is to help babies survive and thrive.

Marian Sokol, President
Deborah M Boyd, Executive Director

6752 National Center for Education in Maternal and Child Health
Georgetown University
2115 Wisconsin Ave NW, Suite 601
Washington, DC 20007

202-784-9770
Fax: 202-784-9777
e-mail: mchlibrary@ncemch.org
www.ncemch.org

6753 National Center for the Prevention of SIDS
1314 Bedford Avenue Suite 210
Baltimore, MD 21208

800-221-7437
Fax: 410-653-8709

Offers medical updates and information on prevention of SIDS and other disorders to parents and professionals.

6754 National SIDS/Infant Death Resource Center
8280 Greensboro Drive, Suite 300
McLean, VA 22102

703-821-8955
866-866-7437
Fax: 703-821-2098
e-mail: sids@circlesolutions.com
www.sidscenter.org

NSIDRC provides resources, referrals, and technical assistance to SIDS families, public health and other professionals, and the general public. Produces both consumer and professional educational materials on SIDS/Infant Death and related issues such as risk reduction and grief and bereavement for distribution to its requestors.

Olivia Cowdrill, Project Coordinator
Laura Randall, Information Specialist

6755 National Sudden Infant Death Syndrome Foundation
31 Center Drive, Room 2A32
Bethesda, MD 20892

301-496-5133
Fax: 301-496-7101

6756 Parents Helping Parents - A Family Resource Center
3041 Olcott Street
Santa Clara, CA 95054

408-727-5775
Fax: 408-727-0182
e-mail: general@php.com
www.php.com

A group of parents and professionals committed to alleviating some of the problems, hardships and concerns of families with children having special needs.

Candy Smith, Director

6757 Pregnancy and Infant Loss Center
163 Freelon Street
San Francisco, CA 94107

612-473-9372
866-710-2229
www.babycenter.com

Offers support, resources, and education on miscarriage, stillbirth and newborn death. Nonprofit organization, membership and quarterly newsletter $20 per year.

6758 SHARE National Headquarters
Saint Elizabeth's Hospital
211 S 3rd Streete
Belleville, IL 62222

618-234-2120

6759 SIDS Educational Services
PO Box 2426
Hyattsville, MD 20784

301-322-2620
Fax: 301-322-9822
e-mail: SIDSES@aol.com
www.sidssurvivalguide.org

Suports families gieving the loss of children to Sudden Infant Death Syndrome and other infant death causes. Information and support services are also provided to children grieving any type of death.

6760 SIDS Information and Referral Hotline
SIDS Alliance
1314 Bedord Avenue
Baltimore, MD 21208

410-653-8226
800-221-7437
Fax: 410-653-8709

24 hour information and referral line for parents who wish to discuss their concerns with a SIDS counselor, request additional information about SIDS and to receive referrals to the local SIDS affiliate in their area.

State Agencies & Support Groups

Alabama

6761 Bureau of Family Health Services-Alabama C hild Death Review
Alabama Department of Public Health
201 Monroe Street, Suite 1354
Montgomery, AL 36104

334-206-2953
Fax: 334-206-2972
www.adph.org/cdr/

Bob Hinds, Director

Alaska

6762 SIDS Information & Counseling Program Alaska Department of Health
1231 Gambell Street, Suite 302
Anchorage, AK 99501

907-272-1534
Fax: 907-274-1384
sid-network.org/map

Linda D Vlastuin, RN, MPH, Program Consultant

Arizona

6763 Office of Women's & Children's Health
Arizona Department of Health Services
150 N 18th Ave, Suite 320
Phoenix, AZ 85007

602-542-1875
Fax: 602-542-1843
e-mail: newbers@azdhs.gov
www.hs.state.az.us

The Unexplained Infant Death Council comes under the OWCH and assists the department to develop unexplained infant death training and educational programs.

Susan Newberry, Manager

Arkansas

6764 Arkansas Department of Health - SIDS Information & Counseling Program
4815 W Markham Street
Little Rock, AR 72205

501-661-2321

Deborah Frazier, RN, Project Coordinator

California

6765 Bereavement Group for Children
The Center for Attitudinal Healing
33 Buchanan Drive
Sausalito, CA 94965

415-331-6161
Fax: 415-331-4545

For children who have suffered the loss of a close loved one. Parent group meets separately at the same time.

Jimmy Pete

6766 California SIDS Program
PO Box 11447
Berkeley, CA 94712

510-849-4111
800-369-7437

Sally Jacober, MSW, MPH, Program Director

6767 Region IX Office Program Consultants for Maternal and Child Health
50 United Nations Plaza
San Francisco, CA 94102

415-437-8101
Fax: 415-437-8105
nrc.uchsc.edu

Lyn Headley, MD

Colorado

6768 Colorado SIDS Program
425 S Cherry Street, Suite 890
Denver, CO 80246

303-320-7771
888-285-7437
Fax: 303-320-7827
e-mail: shelia@coloradosids.org
www.coloradosids.org

Sheila Marquez, RN, Executive Director

6769 Region VIII Office Program Consultants for Maternal and Child Health
1961 Stout Street
Denver, CO 80294

303-844-7854
Fax: 303-844-2019
e-mail: laurie.konsella@hhs.gov

Laurie Konsella, M.P.A

Connecticut

6770 SIDS Program-Connecticut Department of Health
410 Capitol Avenue, MS 11 MAT
Hartford, CT 06134

860-509-8074
Fax: 860-509-7720
www.sidscenter.org

Jann Dalton, MSW

Delaware

6771 SIDS Information & Counseling - Division of Public Health
501 Ogletown Road
Newark, DE 19711

302-368-6840

Elaine Markell, LCSW, BCD, Program Coordinator

District of Columbia

6772 Division of Community Health Nursing
825 N Capitol Street, NE
Washington, DC 20002

202-698-0705
Fax: 202-645-7030

Mary Breach, RN, MSN, Nursing Coordinator

Florida

6773 Children's Medical Services Program Florida SIDS Program
Bin A-13 4025 Bald Cypress Way
Tallahassee, FL 32399

850-245-4444
Fax: 850-245-4047
e-mail: susann-arbor@doh.state.fl.us
www.doh.state.fl.us

Georgia

6774 Georgia Department of Human Resources Children's Health Services
2 Peach Tree Street NW
Atlanta, GA 30303

404-656-6750
www.legis.state.ga.us

Linette Jackson Hunt, MD, MPH, Chief

6775 Georgia Department of Human Resources - Center for Family Resource Planning
2 Peach Tree Street NW
Atlanta, GA 30319

404-656-7660
www.legis.states.ga.us

Provides grief support for parents.

Lee Hackel

6776 Region IV Office Program Consultants For Maternal and Child Health
Atlanta Federal Center
61 Forsyth Street, SW, Suite 3M60
Atlanta, GA 30303

404-562-7980
Fax: 404-562-7974
e-mail: kgonzalez@hrsa.gov
nrc.uchsc.edu

Dorothy Redfern, RN, MSPH

Hawaii

6777 Hawaii SIDS Information & Counseling Project
Kapiolani Children's Medical Center
1319 Punahou Street #1100
Honolulu, HI 96826

808-983-8368

Sharon Morton, RN, Nurse Consultant

Idaho

6778 Child Health Improvement Program Idaho Department of Health
450 W State Street 6th Floor
Boise, ID 83720

208-334-5957

Simonne deGlee, MS, PNP, SIDS Coordinator

Illinois

6779 Region V Office Program Consultants for Maternal and Child Health
233 N Michigan Avenue
Chicago, IL 60603

312-353-4042
Fax: 312-886-3770
e-mail: dparker@hrsa.gov

Kathryn Vedder, MD, MPH

6780 Statewide SIDS Program - Illinois Department of Public Health
535 W Jefferson Street
Springfield, IL 62761

217-785-4528
www.illinois.gov

Lori Bennett, Coordinator

Indiana

6781 Indiana State Board of Health - SIDS Project
2 N Meridian Street
Indianapolis, IN 46204

317-233-1325
e-mail: opac@isdh.state.in.us
www.in.gov/isdh/

Larry Humbert, Project Director

Iowa

6782 Iowa SIDS Program
Iowa Department of Public Health
321 E 12th Street
Des Moines, IA 50319

515-281-7689
www.idph.state.ia.us

Beverly Richardson, MA, MCH Consultant

Kansas

6783 Kansas Department of Health & Environment Bureau of Family Health
1000 SW Jackson Street, Suite 220
Topeka, KS 66612

785-291-3368
800-332-6262
Fax: 785-296-6553
www.kdheks.gov

Azzie N Young, PhD, Director

Kentucky

6784 Kentucky Department of Human Resources Bureau of Health Services
275 E Main Street
Frankfort, KY 40621

502-564-7042
governor.ky.gov

Ida Lyons, RN, SIDS Coordinator

Louisiana

6785 Public Health Services of Louisiana
628 N 4th Street
Baton Rouge, LA 70802

225-342-9500
Fax: 225-342-5568
e-mail: webadmin@dhh.state.la.us
www.dhh.state.la.us/

Jamie Roques, RNC, SIDS Coordinator

Maine

6786 Department of Human Services
221 State Street
Augusta, ME 04333

207-287-3707
Fax: 207-287-3005
TTY: 800-606-0215
www.maine.gov/dhhs

Kathleen Jewett, Program Coordinator

Maryland

6787 Center for Infant & Child Loss
630 W Fayette Street, Room 5-684
Baltimore, MD 21201

410-706-5062
800-808-7437
Fax: 410-706-0146
e-mail: caring@infantandchildloss.org
www.infantandchildloss.org

Donna C Becker, RN, MSN, Director

6788 Maryland SIDS Information & Counseling Program
2905 64th Avenue
Cheverly, MD 20785

301-773-9671
sids-network.org

Daniel Timmel, MSW, Project Director

Massachusetts

6789 Massachusetts Chapter of SIDS Alliance
Boston Medical Center
1 Boston Medical Place
Boston, MA 02118

617-414-SIDS
800-641-7437
www.bmc.org

State chapter offering educational resources and information on SIDS, parent groups, support networks, monthly meetings and workshops to the community.

Penny Begley, Chapter President
Mary McClain, RN, MS

6790 Region I Office Program Consultants For Maternal and Child Health
John F Kennedy Building
Room 1826
Boston, MA 02203

617-565-1433
Fax: 617-565-3044
e-mail: btausey@hrsa.gov
www.mchb.hrsa.gob

Shirley A Smith, RN, MS

Michigan

6791 Apnea Identification Program
Children's Hospital of Michigan
3901 Beaubien Street
Detroit, MI 48201

313-745-5437
888-DMC-2500
www.chmkids.org

Karen Braniff, RN, MSW, Nurse Specialist

6792 Genesee County Health Department
630 S Saginaw Street
Flint, MI 48502

810-257-3612
Fax: 810-257-3147
www.gchd.us

Bonnie Haun, RN, MS

6793 Kent County Health Department
700 Fuller Avenue NE
Grand Rapids, MI 49503

616-632-7100
Fax: 616-632-7083
www.accesskent.com

Colleen Jillson, RN, SIDS Coordinator

6794 Oakland County Health Division - SIDS Project
1200 N Telegraph Road
Pontiac, MI 48341

248-858-1280
Fax: 248-858-0178
www.oakgov.com/health

Peggy Conrad, PHN, SIDS Coordinator

6795 SIDS LEAD - Children's Special Health Care Services
Michigan Department of Public Health
3423 N Martin Luther King Jr Boulevard
Lansing, MI 48906

517-373-3500
e-mail: arias@state.mi.us
www.mdmh.state.mi.us/

Cheryl Lauber, MSN

6796 SIDS Nursing Intervention Program
43525 Elizabeth Road
Mount Clemens, MI 48053

810-469-5520

Loretta Lindsay, RN, Coordinator

Minnesota

6797 Minnesota Sudden Infant Death Center
Minneapolis Children's Medical Center
2525 Chicago Avenue
Minneapolis, MN 55404

612-863-6107

Kathleen Farnbach, PHN, Project Coordinator

Mississippi

6798 Mississippi State Department of Health and Child Health Services
570 East Woodrow Wilson Drive
Jackson, MS 39216

601-576-7400
www.msdh.state.ms.us

Geneva Cannon, Nurse Consultant

Missouri

6799 Region VII Office Program Consultants for Maternal and Child Health
Federal Building
601 E 12th Street
Kansas City, MO 64106

816-426-5291
Fax: 816-426-3633
e-mail: bappelbaum@hrsa.gov

Bradley Appelbaum, MD, MPH

6800 SIDS Resources
929 De Mun Avenue
Saint Louis, MO 63105

314-862-3033
800-421-3511
www.sidsresources.org

Helen Fuller, MSW, Executive Director

Montana

6801 Montana Department of Health & Environmental Sciences
Family & Maternal & Child Health Bureau
Cogswell Building
Helena, MT 59620

406-444-4740

Maxine Ferguson, RN, MN, Bureau Chief

Nebraska

6802 Nebraska SIDS Foundation
University of Nebraska Medical Center
600 S 42nd Street
Omaha, NE 68198

402-559-4212

Valerie Ciciulla, Coordinator

Nevada

6803 Nevada State Division of Health, Maternal & Child Health
505 E King Street, Room 205
Carson City, NV 89710

702-687-4885

Luana Ritch, Health Educator

New Hampshire

6804 New Hampshire SIDS Program
New Hampshire Division of Public Health Services
6 Hazen Drive
Concord, NH 03301

603-271-4533
800-852-3345
Fax: 603-271-3745

Audrey Knight, MSN, CPNP, SIDS Coordinator

New Jersey

6805 New Jersey Department of Health - Child Health Program
CN 364, 363 W State Street
Trenton, NJ 08625

609-292-5616

Judith Hall, BSN, RNC, Evaluator

6806 New Jersey SIDS Resource Center
254 Easton Avenue
New Brunswick, NJ 08901

732-249-2160

New York

6807 New York City Information & Counseling Program for SIDS
520 1st Avenue, Room 506
New York, NY 10016

212-757-1051
800-522-5006

Judith Gaines, CSW, PhD, SIDS Program Director

6808 Region II Office Program Consultants for Maternal and Child Health
26 Federal Plaza
New York, NY 10278

212-264-2571
Fax: 212-264-2673
e-mail: ssmith@hrsa.gov

Margaret Lee, MD

6809 SIDS Regional Center for Eastern New York State
State University of New York at Stony Brook
Health Sciences Center, Level 2
Stony Brook, NY 11794

516-444-8365
www.sidscenter.org

Marie Chandick, CSW, Director

6810 Western New York SIDS Center
200 Fairport Village Lane
Fairport, NY 14450

716-223-5110

Gabrielle Weiss, BPS, Director

North Carolina

6811 North Carolina SIDS Information and Counseling Program
North Carolina Department Of Environmental Health
900 Boxter Street
Charlotte, NC 28204

704-334-7242
800-868-8777
Fax: 704-334-7854
www.safetync.org

Dianne Tyson, BSW, Administrative Assistant

North Dakota

6812 North Dakota SIDS Management Program
600 E Boulevard Avenue
Bismarck, ND 58505

701-328-4464
Fax: 701-328-1412

Bertie Hagberg, RN, Coordinator

Ohio

6813 Perinatal and Infant Health Unit - SIDS Information and Counseling Program
Ohio Department Of Health
246 N High Street
Columbus, OH 43266

614-466-4716
e-mail: webmaster@ghodh.state.oh.us
www.adh.state.oh.us/

Ben Chukwumah, MD, MPH, Project Director

Oklahoma

6814 Oklahoma State Department of Health - Maternal and Child Health Services
1000 NE 10th Street
Oklahoma City, OK 73117

405-271-4480
e-mail: cddr@health.state.ok.us
www.health.state.ok.us/program/mchs/

Edd D Rhoades, MD, MPH, Director

Oregon

6815 Oregon State Health Division - SIDS Information and Counseling Program
1400 SW 5th Avenue
Portland, OR 97201

503-229-6617

Sue Omel, RN, MPH, Child Coordinator

6816 SIDS Resource of Oregon
4035 NE Sandy Boulevard, Suite 209
Portland, OR 97212

503-287-8265
800-221-7437
Fax: 503-287-8693
e-mail: sidsor@teleport.com
www.teleport.com/~sidsor

Todd Llinchliffer

Pennsylvania

6817 Pennsylvania SIDS Center
834 Chesnut Street Suite 200
Philadelphia, PA 19107

215-955-1400
800-258-7437
Fax: 215-923-2989

Rosanne English, RN, Executive Director

6818 Region III Office Program Consultants for Maternal and Child Health
Public Ledger Building
150 S Independence Mall West, Suite 1172
Philadelphia, PA 19106

215-861-4379
Fax: 215-861-4338
e-mail: valos@hrsa.gov

Jane Coury, MSN, RN

Rhode Island

6819 Rhode Island Department of Health National SIDS Foundation
377 Spring Green Road
Warwick, RI 02888

401-453-1646
Fax: 401-444-3422

Anne M Roach, RN, SIDS Coordinator

South Carolina

6820 South Carolina Department of Health & Environmental Control - SIDS Information
2600 Bull Street
Columbia, SC 29201

803-252-9250

Brenda Creswell, ACSW, LMSW, SIDS Coordinator

South Dakota

6821 South Dakota Department of Health
Health Building
600 E Capitol
Pierre, SD 57501

605-773-3737
800-738-2301
Fax: 605-773-5683
e-mail: dolt.info@state.sd.us
www.state.sd.us

Nancy Hoyme, SIDs Coordinator

Tennessee

6822 Tennessee SIDS Program
Tennessee Department Of Health
425 5th Ave, N Cordell Hull Bldg, 3rd Fl
Nashville, TN 37243

615-741-7335
Fax: 615-741-1063
e-mail: tn.health@state.tn.us
www2.state.tn.us

Judith Womack, RN, Director Child Health

Texas

6823 Harris County Health Department
PO Box 25249
Houston, TX 77265

713-620-6895
e-mail: publicinfo@hd.co.harris.tx.us
www.hd.co.harris.tx.us/phs/

Kathleen Ingrando, RN, BSN, Program Coordinator

6824 North Texas SIDS Information And Counseling Program
5000 Harry Hines
Dallas, TX 75235

214-590-0135
Fax: 214-590-0173

Leslie U Malone, SIDS Coordinator

6825 Region VI Office Program Consultants For Maternal and Child Health
1301 Young Street 10th Floor
Dallas, TX 75202

214-767-3003
Fax: 214-767-3038
e-mail: twells@hrsa.gov

Marianne Davenport, CPNP, MPH

6826 Texas Department of Health - SIDS Information and Counseling Program
1100 W 49th Street
Austin, TX 78756

512-458-7111
888-963-7111
Fax: 512-458-7238
e-mail: kathy.clement@tdh.state.tx.us
www.dshs.state.tx.us

Linda G Prentice, MD, Program Coordinator

Utah

6827 Utah Department of Health
Child Health Bureau
PO Box 1016
Salt Lake City, UT 84116

801-538-6140
hlunix.hl.state.ut.us

Karen Nash, RN, MS, PNP, SIDS Director

Vermont

6828 Vermont Department of Health - SIDS Information and Counseling Program
108 Cherry Street
Burlington, VT 05401

802-652-4174
Fax: 802-656-8170
e-mail: sshepar@udh.state.ut.us

Cindy Indham, RN, BSN, Director

Virginia

6829 Virginia SIDS Program - Virginia Department of Health
Virginia Department of Health
P.O. Box 2448
Richmond, VA 23218

804-864-7001
Fax: 804-864-7001
e-mail: schuettd@aol.com
www.vdh.state.va.us

Arlethia V Rogers, RN, Nurse Consultant

Washington

6830 Region X Office Program Consultants for Maternal and Child Health
2201 6th Avenue
Seattle, WA 98121

206-553-0215

Kay Girl, RNC, MN, Acting

6831 SIDS Northwest Regional Center
Washington Department of Health
4800 Sand Point Way NE
Olympia, WA 98504

360-236-3560
800-441-4392
www.doh.wa.gov

Lauren Valk Lawson, MN, Program Director

West Virginia

6832 West Virginia Department of Health and Human Services
WV Department Of Health & Human Resources
State Capitol Complex, Bldg 3 Rm 206
Charleston, WV 25305

304-558-0684
Fax: 304-558-1130
www.wvdhhr.org

Joan R Kenny, RN, SIDS Director

Wisconsin

6833 Counseling and Research Center for SIDS
PO Box 1997
Milwaukee, WI 53201

218-739-5252
www.chw.org

Kathy Geracie, BSW, Program Coordinator

Wyoming

6834 Wyoming Department of Health
Division of Health and Medical Services
401 Hathaway Building
Cheyenne, WY 82002

307-777-7656
Fax: 307-777-7439
e-mail: wdh@state.wy.us
www.wdh.state.wy.us

J Richard Hillman, MD, PhD, Administrator

Libraries & Resource Centers

6835 National Sudden Infant Death Syndrome Resource Center

Circle Solutions, Inc
8280 Greensboro Drive, Suite 300
McLean, VA 22102

703-821-8955
Fax: 703-821-2098
e-mail: info@circlesolutions.com
www.circlesolutions.com

6836 Sudden Infant Death Syndrome (SIDS) Network

6 Gonch Farm Road
Ledyard, CT 06339

Fax: 860-887-7309
sids-network.org/

Research Centers

6837 American SIDS Institute

509 Augusta Drive
Marietta, GA 30067

770-426-8746
800-232-7437
Fax: 770-426-1369
e-mail: prevent@sids.org
www.sids.org

A national nonprofit organization dedicated to the promotion of infant health and the prevention of sudden infant death syndrome.

Marc Peterzell, Chairman
Betty McEntire PhD, Executive Director

6838 CJ Foundation for SIDS

Don Imus WFAN Pediatric Center
30 Prospect Ave
Hackensack, NJ 07601

973-783-2592
800-620-7832
Fax: 201-996-5326
e-mail: info@sudc.org
www.sudc.org/page.asp

6839 Center for Research for Mothers & Children

National Institute of Child Health & Development
Building 31, Center Drive
Bethesda, MD 20892

301-496-5575
e-mail: NICHDClearinghouse@mail.nih.gov
www.nichd.nih.gov

This institute conducts and supports research on all stages of human development, from the preconception to adulthood, to better understand the health of children, adults, families, and communities.

6840 Massachusetts Sudden Infant Death Syndrome

Boston City Hospital
818 Harrison Avenue
Boston, MA 02118

617-638-8131

A joint program of Boston City Hospital and Children's Hospital. Services provided include around-the-clock availability for consultation to health professionals and families, counseling of families, parent group meetings and supportive home visits.

6841 National Sudden Infant Death Syndrome Research Center

Circle Solutions, Inc
8280 Greensboro Drive, Suite 300
McLean, VA 22102

703-821-8955
Fax: 703-821-2098
e-mail: info@circlesolutions.com
www.circlesolutions.com

Provides information services and technical assistance concerning SIDS and related topics in order to promote understanding of SIDS and to comfort those affected by a SIDS loss. Offers its services to parents, family members, caregivers, counselors, medical and legal professionals, and the general public.

6842 Pathology Department SIDS/SUDC Research Project

Children's Hospital San Diego
3020 Children's Way, MC5007
San Diego, CA 92123

858-966-5944

Dr Henry Krous, Director
Amy Chadwick, Project Manager

6843 Pediatric Pulmonary Unit

Massachusetts General Hospital
55 Fruit Street
Boston, MA 02114

617-726-2000
www.massgeneral.org

Sudden infant death syndrome and childhood disorders research.

Dorothy Kelly, MD, Associate Director

6844 Southwest SIDS Research Institute

Brazosport Memorial Hospital
100 Medical Drive
Lake Jackson, TX 77566

409-297-4411
e-mail: admin@brazosportmemorial.com
www.brazosportmemorial.com

6845 Sudden Infant Death Syndrome Institute of The University of Maryland

1314 Bedford Ave, Suite 210
Baltimore, MD 21208

410-653-8226
Fax: 410-653-8709

Dr. M John O'Brien, MB, Director

6846 USC - Neonatology Research Units

1240 Mission Road
Los Angeles, CA 90033

323-266-3813
Fax: 323-266-5049
www.usc.edu

Focuses on clinical problems of the newborn and premature infant.

Paul YK Wu, MD, Director

Conferences

6847 National Sudden Infant Death Syndrome Alliance Conference

www.healthyplace.com

800-221-7437
www.healthyplace.com

Unites parents, caregivers, and researchers with government, business, and community service groups in a nationwide movement to advance the support of SIDS families and hasten the elimination of SIDS through medical research. Funds medical research and offers emotional support nationally and locally.

Audio Video

6848 A Cradle Song: The Families of SIDS

Fanlight Productions
47 Halifax Street
Boston, MA 02131

617-469-4999
Fax: 617-469-3379
e-mail: fanlight@tiac.net
www.fanlight.com

SIDS parents share the pain and anger which have dominated their lives, but they also offer hope to others coping with grief. Provides much-needed information about this mysterious illness.

29 minutes
ISBN: 1-572950-63-3

6849 SIDS: Reducing the Risk

InJoy Productions, Inc
7107 La Vista Place
Longmont, CO 80503

303-447-2082
800-326-2082
Fax: 303-449-8788
e-mail: custserv@injoyvideos.com
www.injoyvideos.com

An informative video in which leading medical experts explain practical measures parents can take to reduce the risk of Sudden Infant Death Syndrome.

27 minutes

Web Sites

6850 American SIDS Institute

www.sids.org

A national nonprofit health care organization that is dedicated to the prevention of sudden infant death and the promotion of infant health through an aggresive, comprehensive nationwide program of: Research, Clinical Services, Education and Family Support.

6851 Center for Research for Mothers & Children

www.nichd.nih.gov

Composed of several branches the principle NIH source of support for research and research training in maternal and child health, through grants, contracts, and cooperative agreements. Through this research, CRMC-supported scientists are advancing fundamental and clinical knowledge concerning maternal health and child development problems such as low birth wieght, mental retardation and developmental disabilities, specific learning disabilities, congenital and genetic defects and others.

6852 Compassionate Friends

www.compassionatefriends.org

Assists families toward the positive resolution of grief following the death of a child of any age and provides information to help others be supportive.

6853 Health Answers

www.healthanswers.com

HealthAnswers offers a breadth of services in medical education, sales force training, patient support solutions, professional promotion and consumer solutions.

6854 National Center for Education in Maternal and Child Health

www.ncemch.org

The National Center for Education in Maternal and Child Health provides national leadership to the maternal and child health community in three key areas - program development, policy analysis and education, and knowledge to improve the health and well-being of the nation's children and families.

6855 Online Mendelian Inheritance in Man

www.ncbi.nlm.nih.gov

This database is a catalog of human genes and genetic disorders.

6856 SID Network

sids-network.org/net.htm

Nonprofit voluntary agency that is dedicated to eliminate sudden infant death syndrome through the support of SIDS research projects, provide support for those who have been touched by the tragedy of sudden Infant Death Syndrome and to raise public awareness of sudden infant death syndrome through education.

Book Publishers

6857 Apparent Life - Threatening Event and Sudden Infant Death Syndrome

Circle Solutions, Inc
8280 Greensboro Drive, Suite 300
McLean, VA 22102

703-821-8955
866-866-7437
Fax: 703-821-2098
e-mail: info@circlesolutions.com
www.circlesolution.com

Provides information about ALTE and its relationship to SIDS.

1992 29 pages

Olivia Cowdrill, Project Coordinator
Kelly Kenneally, Information Specialist

6858 Crib Death: The Sudden Infant Death Syndrome

Futura Publishing Company
135 Bedford Road
Armonk, NY 10504

914-273-1014
Fax: 914-273-1015
www.growinghealthcare.com

A thorough book, that discusses the theories of SIDS and their implications. Athough it is aimed at the medical professional, lay people will also gain a clearer understanding of SIDS.

1995 456 pages Hardcover

6859 Death Investigations and Sudden Infant Death Syndrome

Circle Solutions, Inc
8280 Greensboro Drive, Suite 300
McLean, VA 22102

703-821-8955
Fax: 703-821-2098
e-mail: info@circlesolutions.com
www.circlesolutions.com

Contains abstracts of articles on autopsies, death certification, and infant death scene investigation and SIDS.

1991 104 pages

6860 Death of a Child, the Grief of the Parents A Lifetime Journey

Circle Solutions, Inc
8280 Greensboro Drive, Suite 300
McLean, VA 22102

703-821-8955
Fax: 703-821-2098
e-mail: info@circlesolutions.com
www.circlesolutions.com

1997 38 pages

6861 Grief, Bereavement and Sudden Infant Death Syndrome
Circle Solutions, Inc
8280 Greensboro Drive, Suite 300
McLean, VA 22102

703-821-8955
Fax: 703-821-2098
e-mail: info@circlesolutions.com
www.circlesolutions.com

Contains abstracts of selected materials on the grief and bereavement process specific to the loss of a child to SIDS.

1991 28 pages

6862 SIDS Research
Circle Solutions, Inc
8280 Greensboro Drive, Suite 300
McLean, VA 22102

703-821-8955
Fax: 703-821-2098
e-mail: info@circlesolutions.com
www.circlesolutions.com

Contains abstracts of relevant articles published during 1993.

1995 146 pages

6863 SIDS Survival Guide
Independent Publishers Group
814 N Franklin Street
Chicago, IL 60610

312-337-0747
800-888-4741
Fax: 312-337-5985
e-mail: frontdesk@ipgbook.com
www.ipgbook.com

Offers information and comfort for grieving family, friends and professionals who seek to help them.

1994 290 pages Paperback
ISBN: 0-964121-87-5

6864 SIDS: A Parents Guide to Understanding & Preventing SIDS
Hachette Book Group USA
322 South Enterprise Blvd
Lebanon, IN 46052

800-759-0190
Fax: 800-286-9471
e-mail: customer.service@hbgusa.com
www.hbgusa.com

1995
ISBN: 0-316779-12-1

6865 Smoking and Sudden Infant Death Syndrome
Circle Solutions, Inc
8280 Breensboro Drive, Suite 300
McLean, VA 22102

703-821-8955
Fax: 703-821-2098
e-mail: info@circlesolutions.com
www.circlesolutions.com

Contains abstracts of materials about tobacco use, its relationship to SIDS, and the dangers to the unborn and the newly born from passive and secondary smoking.

1992 34 pages

6866 Sudden Death in Infancy, Childhood & Adolescence
Cambridge University Press
32 Avenue Of The Americas
New York, NY 10013

212-924-3900
Fax: 212-691-3239
e-mail: newyork@cambridge.org
www.cambridge.org/us

1994 400 pages
ISBN: 0-521420-31-8

6867 Sudden Infant Death Syndrome Risk Factors
Circle Solutions, Inc
8280 Greensboro Drive, Suite 300
McLean, VA 22102

703-821-8955
Fax: 703-821-2098
e-mail: info@circlesolutions.com
www.circlesolutions.com

Contains selected articles published between 1989 and 1993 on the risk factors for SIDS.

1994 131 pages

Newsletters

6868 Illuminations
First Candle/SIDS Alliance
1314 Bedford Avenue, Suite 210
Baltimore, MD 21208

410-653-8226
800-221-7437
Fax: 410-653-8709
e-mail: info@firstcandle.org
www.sidsalliance.org; www.firstcandle.org

Quarterly

6869 Network
Parent Care
9041 Colgate Street
Indianapolis, IN 46268

317-872-9913
Fax: 317-872-0795

Offers information on support groups, meetings, organizations and resources for parents and professionals dealing with the chronically ill child.

6870 Newsletter: SIDS
Massachusetts Center For SIDS
1 Boston Medical Center Place
Boston, MA 02118

617-638-8000
www.bmc.org/program/sids/

Offers information on SIDS, articles pertaining to the latest information available on the mystery condition, latest research and fund-raising news and professional resources available.

Monthly

Pamphlets

6871 After Sudden Infant Death Syndrome
Circle Solution, Inc
8280 Greensboro Drive, Suite 300
McLean, VA 22102

703-821-8955
Fax: 703-821-2098
e-mail: info@circlesolutions.com
www.circlesolutions.com

1993 16 pages

6872 Bilingual Risk Reduction Brochure
First Candle/SIDS Alliance
1314 Bedford Avenue, Suite 210
Baltimore, MD 21208

410-653-8226
800-221-7437
Fax: 410-653-8709
e-mail: info@firstcandle.org
www.sidsalliance.org; www.firstcandle.org

Provides an understanding of the risk of SIDS and the steps that can be taken to help the baby survive and thrive.

2 pages

6873 Facts About Apnea and Other Apparent Life-Threatening Events
Circle Solution, Inc
8280 Greensboro Drive, Suite 300
Vienna, VA 22102

703-821-8955
Fax: 703-821-2098
e-mail: info@circlesolutions.com
www.circlesolutions.com

Explains apparent life-threatening events in infants, their relationship to SIDS and current views on home monitoring.

1987 2 pages

6874 Facts About SIDS
Sudden Infant Death Syndrome Alliance
1314 Bedford Avenue
Baltimore, MD 21208

410-653-8226
Fax: 410-653-8709

Offers information on basic facts, answers to the most frequently asked questions about SIDS and information on numbers to call and referral centers for more help.

6875 Infant Positioning and Sudden Infant Death Syndrome
Circle Solutions, Inc
8280 Greensboro Drive, Suite 300
McLean, VA 22102

703-821-8955
Fax: 703-821-2098
e-mail: info@circlesolutions.com
www.circlesolutions.com

Contains abstracts of selected articles on the topic of sleep position and SIDS.

1994

6876 National SIDS Resource Center Brochure
Circle Solutions, Inc
8280 Greensboro Drive, Suite 300
McLean, VA 22102

703-821-8955
Fax: 703-821-2098
e-mail: info@circlesolutions.com
www.circlesolutions.com

1994

6877 Nationwide Survey of Sudden Infant Death Syndrome (SIDS) Service
Circle Solutions, Inc
8280 Greensboro Drive, Suite 300
McLean, VA 22102

703-821-8955
Fax: 703-821-2098
e-mail: info@circlesolutions.com
www.circlesolutions.com

Analysis of availability of SIDS services.

1994

6878 Pacifiers and SIDS: Reducing the Risk
First Candle/SIDS Alliance
1314 Bedford Avenue, Suite 210
Baltimore, MD 21208

410-653-8226
800-221-7437
Fax: 410-653-8709
e-mail: info@firstcandle.org
www.sidsalliance.org; www.firstcandle.org

A brochure for parents and caregivers.

6879 SIDS Prevention
Corporate Office
4 Carbonero Way
Scotts Valley, CA 95099

831-438-4060
800-321-4407
Fax: 800-435-8433
www.ctr.org

Gives overview, risk factors, prevention of Sudden Infant Death Syndrome.

50 pamphlets

6880 SIDS: Toward Prevention and Improved Infant Health
American SIDS Institute
509 Augusta Drive
Marietta, GA 30067

770-426-8746
800-232-sids
Fax: 770-426-1369
e-mail: prevent@sids.org
www.sids.org

Practical guide for those planning a pregnancy, for parents-to-be and for new parents.

6881 Surviving the Death of a Baby
First Candle/SIDS Alliance
1314 Bedford Avenue, Suite 210
Baltimore, MD 21208

410-653-8226
800-221-7437
Fax: 410-653-8709
e-mail: info@firstcandle.org
www.sidsalliance.org; www.firstcandle.org

13 pages

DESCRIPTION

6882 SYNCOPE

Involves the following Biologic System(s):

Cardiovascular Disorders

Syncope is a medical term describing a phenomenon more commonly known as fainting. Specifically, syncope is a brief loss of consciousness that resolves without intervention. In the pediatric population most episodes of syncope are uncomplicated without neurologic or cardiac aftereffects (sequelae).

The true incidence of syncope is difficult to ascertain since many episodes are not reported to a medical provider. Roughly 15-25% of all children experience at least one episode of syncope or near-syncope, although adolescents are are the most common segment of the pediatric population to experience syncope and the most likely to have recurrent episodes.

The most common cause of fainting in pediatrics is neurocardiogenic (related to a problem of the nervous system and the heart) syncope, also known as vasovagal or vasodepressor syncope. The other cases of syncope can be divided into neurologic, cardiac, metabolic, toxin (drug abuse), and psychogenic. While greater than 95% of syncopal episodes have a benign etiology (cause), such as the simple vasovagal syncope, there are several rare causes that are fatal, accounting for 4-5 deaths per 100,000 pediatric patients. The possibility of a fatal etiology necessitates the need for a thorough investigation into any syncopal episode.

An appropriate evaluation begins with a thorough history and physical exam. The history should focus on details around the event, change in position (from sitting to standing, for instance), exercise, trauma, and past history of similar events. Family history is critical when evaluating unexplained sudden deaths, hearing loss, cardiac disease, recurrent fainting, seizure disorders or arrhythmias. The physical exam should include a careful neurologic exam as well as a thorough cardiac exam looking for murmurs, clicks or gallops (unusual heart sounds) and careful blood pressure measurements including orthostatic measurements (when the patient is sitting and then stands up. In individuals who have fainted, the blood pressure can drop significantly upon standing, indicating at least one possible cause of the syncopal episode.

The diagnostic evaluation continues with an electrocardio-

gram looking at abnormal rhythms as well as signs of cardiomyopathy (heart disease). If the physical examination and ECG are normal and the history is consistent with a simple 'faint', no further workup may be necessary. If the history is inconsistent with vasovagal syncope or if there are any abnormalities on the physical or ECG, referral to a specialist, usually a pediatric cardiologist or adult cardiologist, is appropriate. Further testing may include a tilt table test, 24-hour holter monitor, echocardiography, exercise stress testing or electrophysiology testing.

Treatment for syncope varies depending on the etiology. For simple vasodepressor syncope, management is often focused on increasing fluid and salt intake in an effort to improve blood volume and pressure. Often discovering the triggers for these patients enables them to avoid them or anticipate their response more effectively (i.e. lying on the ground with feet up before syncope occurs). Medication is an option if the syncopal episodes are frequent and impacton the patient's lifestyle. The most widely used and successfully used medication class has been beta-blockers. More serious cardiac causes of syncope may need to be treated with antiarrhythmics, pacemakers or defibrillators. These interventions can be life-saving and allow patients to lead full productive lives.

See also **General Resources** on page 917

National Associations & Support Groups

6883 NIH/National Heart, Lung and Blood Institu te

National Institute of Health
31 Center Dr MSC 2486, Bldg 31, Rm5A48
Bethesda, MD 20892

301-592-8573
Fax: 301-629-3246
TTY: 240-629-3255
e-mail: NHLBIinfo@nhlbi.nih.gov
www.nhlbi.nih.gov

Primary responsibility of this organization is the scientific investigation of heart, blood vessel, lung and blood disorders. Oversees research, demonstration, prevention, education, control and training activities in these fields and emphasizes the prevention and control of heart diseases.

Elizabeth G Nabel, MD, Director
Susan Shurin, MD, Deputy Director

6884 NIH/National Institute of Neurological Dis orders and Stroke (NINDS)

PO Box 5801
Bethesda, MD 20824

301-496-5751
800-352-9424
Fax: 301-496-0296
TTY: 301-468-5981
www.ninds.nih.gov

Information and advocacy resources for families and professionals. Includes listings of organizations providing general information and organizations focusing on more specific areas of concern to families and young adults who have disabilities.

Story C Landis PhD, Director
Audrey C Penn MD, Deputy Director

Research Centers

6885 Syncope Center at Columbia Presbyterian Medical Center
Harkness Pavilion, Room 342, 180 Ft Washington Ave
New York, NY 10032

212-305-8053
Fax: 212-305-3137

Web Sites

6886 EMedicine Journal: Syncope
www.emedicine.com/med/topic3385.htm

Syncope information covering background, pathophysiology, frequency, mortality/morbidity, causes, lab studies and tests, diet, activity, drugs used in treatment, complications and patient education. Authored by Dr Jatin Dave and co-authored by Dr John Michael Gaziano.

6887 Exercise-Related Syncope in the Young Athlete
www.findarticles.com

Article from American Family Physician about young athletes and syncope.

6888 NINDS Syncope Information Page
www.ninds.nih.gov/disorders/syncope/

6889 Syncope Information Page
americanheart.org/presenter.jhtml?identifier=4749

American Heart Association information page about Syncope such as what it is and what causes it.

DESCRIPTION

6890 SYNDACTYLY

Synonyms: Syndactylia, Syndactylism
Involves the following Biologic System(s):
Orthopedic and Muscle Disorders

Syndactyly refers to an abnormality that is present at birth (congenital) and characterized by the joining together (fusing) of two or more fingers or toes. This relatively common abnormality seems to occur more frequently in boys than in girls. It is often inherited as an autosomal dominant trait. Syndactyly often results from incomplete or abnormal embryonic development of the fingers or toes. In some infants, it occurs spontaneously as the hands or feet of the developing fetus may be unnaturally constricted within the uterus. Classification of syndactyly is based on the severity of the clinical presentation. Defects associated with syndactyly may range from a simple or incomplete joining or webbing of the skin between two digits to fusion from the base to the tip of the digits, complete with fusion of the bones and nails.

Syndactyly of the foot may involve complete or incomplete webbing that usually affects the second and third toes. This simple condition is referred to as zygosyndactyly and often requires no treatment. Syndactyly may also involve webbing and bone fusion (synostosis) of the fourth and fifth toes with duplication of the fifth toe in a condition called syndactyly/polysyndactyly.

As in the foot, syndactyly of the hand may involve a simple webbing. However, in some cases, the fusion of certain fingers may be more complex and involve shared nerves and blood supply. Syndactyly of the fingers should be carefully evaluated to determine the best method of treatment, allowing for growth and dexterity of the fingers.

Syndactyly may also occur in association with several genetic disorders. Such disorders include acrocephalopolysyndactyly type II (Carpenter's syndrome), characterized by mental retardation and irregularities involving the head, hand, and genitalia; acrocephalosyndactyly type I (Apert's syndrome), characterized by craniofacial irregularities and syndactyly of the hands and feet; trisomy 18 syndrome, a chromosomal abnormality characterized by multiple craniofacial abnormalities, irregularities of the hands and feet, and severe mental retardation; and other inherited diseases. Treatment of syndactyly associated with these and other inherited disorders depends upon the nature of the underlying disorder. In itself, a minor incomplete syndactyly is not an indication for surgery if the only issue is its appearance. However, a syndactyly that prevents full range of motion in the involved fingers warrants surgical release to increase the fingers' ability to function. The timing of surgery is variable. However, as more fingers are involved and as the syndactyly becomes more complex, release should be performed earlier.

See also **General Resources** on page 917

Government Agencies

6891 NIH/National Institute of Arthritis and Musculoskeletal and Skin Diseases
1 AMS Circle
Bethesda, MD 20892

301-402-4484
Fax: 301-718-6366
e-mail: ord@od.nih.gov
rarediseases.info.nih.gov

The mission of the National Institute of Arthritis and Musculoskeletal and Skin Diseases is to support research into the causes, treatment, and prevention of arthritis and musculoskeletal and skin diseases, the training of basic and clinical scientists to carry out this research, and the dissemination of information on research progress in these diseases.

Stephen I Katz MD PhD, Director

National Associations & Support Groups

6892 CHERUB-Association of Families and Friends of Children with Limb Disorders
Children's Hospital of Buffalo
936 Delaware Avenue
Buffalo, NY 14209

716-762-9997

Answers the questions and problems that families of juveniles diagnosed with a disorder may be experiencing.

Sandra Richenberg
Kathy Gura

6893 Genetic Alliance
4301 Connecticut Avenue NW
Washington, DC 20008

202-966-5557
800-336-4363
Fax: 202-966-8553
e-mail: info@geneticalliance.org
www.geneticalliance.org

A coalition of voluntary genetic support groups, consumers and professionals addressing the needs of individuals and families affected by genetic disorders from a national perspective.

Sharon Terry, President/CEO

6894 March of Dimes Birth Defects Foundation
1275 Mamaroneck Avenue
White Plains, NY 10605

914-428-7100
888-663-4637
Fax: 914-428-8203
e-mail: resourcecenter@modimes.org
www.marchofdimes.com

Partnership of volunteers and professionals dedicated to improving the health of babies by preventing birth defects and infant mortality. Over 100 chapters are located across the country.

Dr Jennifer Howse, President

6895 Shriners Hospitals for Children

Headquarters
2900 Rocky Point Drive
Tampa, FL 33607

813-281-0300
800-237-5055
Fax: 813-281-8496
www.shrinershq.org

Network of 22 hospitals that provide expert, no-cost orthopaedic and burn care to children under 18.

Web Sites

6896 A-to-Z Health & Disease Information
www.hmc.psu.edu/healthinfo/pq/poly.htm

Information page on polydactyly and syndactyly provided by Penn State Medical Center. Information includes a listing of physicians who treat the disorder, causes, symptoms, a general overview, diagnosis and treatment.

6897 CliniWeb
www.ohsu.edu/cliniwebC5/C5.660.585.html

Is one of the original catalogs of health and bimedical information on the web.

6898 Online Mendelian Inheritance in Man
www.ncbi.nlm.nih.gov

This database is a catalog of human genes and genetic disorders.

6899 Pediatric Plastic Surgery
surgery.missouri.edu/peds/conditions/syndactyly.php

Answers to questions about syndactyly and surgery provided by the University of Missouri Children's Hospital.

6900 Syndactyly
www.pncl.co.uk/~belcher/information/Syndactyly.pdf

Information sheet on syndactyly.

DESCRIPTION

6901 SYSTEMIC LUPUS ERYTHEMATOSUS

Synonyms: Lupus, SLE

Involves the following Biologic System(s):

Immunologic and Rheumatologic Disorders

Systemic lupus erythematosus (SLE) is a chronic, inflammatory, multisystem disorder of connective tissue that may affect many organ systems in the body including the skin, joints, membranes that line the walls of certain bodily cavities (serosal membranes), or kidneys. In children with the disorder, associated symptoms are often progressive and, without appropriate treatment, may result in life-threatening complications. However, in some patients, symptoms may spontaneously subside and periodically recur with varying levels of severity (relapsing-remitting). SLE usually becomes apparent during late adolescence or a patient's 20s or 30s. However, in up to 20 percent of patients, symptoms may begin during childhood, usually after the age of eight. Females are more commonly affected than males in all age groups.

The specific underlying cause of SLE is unknown. However, the disorder is thought to result from abnormalities in the regulating mechanisms of the immune system that normally prevent it from attacking the body's own cells and tissues. In addition, researchers speculate that certain microorganisms or other environmental factors may play some role in causing SLE. Familial cases have also been reported, suggesting potential genetic mechanisms. In some individuals, SLE-like symptoms may also occur after exposure to certain medications, such as particular antiseizure drugs or certain antibiotics known as sulfonamides. Drug-induced symptoms are usually relatively mild and subside when the responsible medication is removed.

The range and severity of associated symptoms and findings may vary. Although associated symptoms may begin suddenly or gradually, most children with SLE tend to have more acute, severe symptoms than adults. In some children, symptoms may tend to recur or worsen in association with certain infections. In addition, exposure to sunlight may worsen associated skin or other symptoms. Many children with SLE initially experience generalized symptoms, such as a fever, a general feeling of ill health (malaise), joint swelling and inflammation (arthritis) or pain (arthralgia), loss of appetite (anorexia), and weight loss. Most children also have associated skin abnormalities, including a scaly, reddish or bluish rash that is in a distinctive butterfly distribution across the cheeks and the bridge of the nose (butter-fly rash). The affected area may be abnormally sensitive to sunlight (photosensitive), and the rash may gradually spread to other facial areas, the neck, scalp, chest, and arms. Additional skin symptoms may include flat, reddish, dot-like spots (punctate lesions) on the fingertips, palms, soles, arms, legs, and torso; abnormal changes of the tissues beneath the fingernails and toenails (nail beds); tender, reddish-purple swellings or nodules on the legs (erythema nodosum); and itchy, reddish, flat or raised lesions of the skin and mucous membranes (erythema multiforme). Patients may also develop painless sores of the mucous membranes of the mouth and nose. The hair may be abnormally coarse and dry, and some children may have patchy areas of baldness on the scalp (alopecia).

Many children with SLE may also experience joint stiffness; inflammation of muscles (myositis), causing muscle pain and weakness; abnormal changes and localized loss of bone in certain areas (aseptic necrosis), particularly the head of the thigh bone (femur); and Raynaud's phenomenon. This condition is characterized by sudden contraction of the relatively small blood vessels supplying the fingers and toes (digits), causing an interruption of blood flow to the digits and a subsequent excess of blood in affected areas following restoration of blood flow (reactive hyperemia). Such episodes are usually triggered by exposure to cold temperatures and are characterized by numbing, tingling, and bluish or whitish discoloration of the digits due to lack of blood flow and subsequent reddening and pain as blood flow is reestablished. Many children with SLE may also develop inflammation of the membranes that line the lungs and chest cavity (pleurisy), surround the heart (pericarditis), and line the wall of the abdomen and cover the abdominal organs (peritonitis). Additional heart abnormalities may also be present, such as abnormal heart murmurs, inflammation of heart muscle (myocarditis), enlargement of the heart (cardiomegaly), a decreased ability of the heart to pump blood effectively to the lungs and the rest of the body (heart failure), and, in some severe cases, heart attacks (myocardial infarctions), potentially causing life-threatening complications.

Kidney involvement is common among children with SLE and may be the only disease manifestation. Associated inflammation of the filtering units of the kidneys (glomerulonephritis) may be mild, moderate, or severe. Symptoms and findings may range from small amounts of blood in the urine (hematuria) of mildly increased levels of protein in the urine (proteinuria) to kidney failure that causes potentially life-threatening complications. Some children with SLE may also experience symptoms due to involvement of the brain and spinal cord (central nervous system). Associated neurologic abnormalities may include personality changes, episodes of abnormally increased electrical activity in the brain (seizures), or other findings. In addition, in some children, disease progression may also affect other tissues and organs, causing additional symptoms and findings.

The treatment of SLE is individualized and based upon the severity of the disease and the specific organ systems affected. Episodes of active disease should be considered emergencies that require immediate evaluation and aggressive treatment to help prevent damage to affected tissues and organs. In addition, careful follow-up and ongoing monitoring is required to detect worsening disease and to ensure prompt, appropriate treatment as required. Therapy may include the use of nonsteroidal antiinflammatory drugs (NSAIDs)s or salicylates (aspirin) to help alleviate joint pain and antimalarial agents or topical corticosteroid creams to treat skin symptoms. In severe cases, immunosuppressive drugs may also be administered; however, such agents must be used with great caution in children. Treatment of kidney inflammation may also include the use of certain corticosteroids, such as prednisone, and in some patients, the addition of immunosuppressive agents, such as azathioprine. Children with severe kidney disease may require regular dialysis or kidney transplantation. Dialysis is a medical procedure that removes excess fluid from the body and waste products from the blood. Additional treatment is symptomatic and supportive.

See also **General Resources** on page 917

National Associations & Support Groups

6902 American Autoimmune Related Diseases Association
22100 Gratiot Avenue
E Detroit, MI 48021

586-776-3900
www.aarda.org

The American Autoimmune Related Diseases Association is dedicated to the eradication of autoimmune diseases and the alleviation of suffering and the socioeconomic impact of autoimmunity through fostering and facilitating collabration in the areas of education, public awareness, research,and patient in an effective, ethical and efficient manner.

Virginia Ladd, Director

6903 American Juvenile Arthritis Organization
2970 Peachtree Road NW, Suite 200
Atlanta, GA 30305

404-237-8771
800-933-7023
Fax: 404-237-8153
e-mail: info.ga@arthritis.org
www.arthritis.org

Devoted to serving the special needs of children, teens, and young adults with childhood rheumatic diseases and their families. Offers both support and information through national and local programs that serve the needs of families, friends and health professionals. Serves as a clearinghouse of information, sponsors an annual national conference, monitors and promotes legislation, sponsors research, and offers training to both parents and health professionals.

Sage Rhodes, President

6904 American Lupus Society
260 Ample Street, Suite 123
Ventura, CA 93003

805-339-0443
800-331-1802
Fax: 805-339-0467

Devoted to meeting the needs of people touched by lupus through education, support, and research.

6905 Children's Hospital Boston
300 Longwood Avenue
Boston, MA 02115

617-355-6000
TTY: 617-355-0443
www.childrenshospital.org

Mission is to provide the highest quality care; be the leading source of reseach and discovery; educate the next generation of leaders in child health and enhance the health and well-being of the children and families in our local community.

James Mandell, MD, President & CEO
Sandra Fenwick, Chief Operating Officer

6906 Genetic Alliance
4301 Connecticut Avenue NW
Washington, DC 20008

202-966-5557
800-336-4363
Fax: 202-966-8553
e-mail: info@geneticalliance.org
www.geneticalliance.org

A coalition of voluntary genetic support groups, consumers and professionals addressing the needs of individuals and families affected by genetic disorders from a national perspective.

Sharon Terry, President/CEO

6907 Lupus Foundation of America
2000 L Street NW, Suite 710
Washington, DC 20036

202-349-1155
800-558-0121
Fax: 202-349-1156
e-mail: LupusInfo@aol.com
www.lupus.org/newsite/

The LFA mission is to educate and support those affected by lupus. It supports research into the cause and cure of lupus. Information resources are available on request, including free pamphlets, brochures (English/Spanish), and articles for people seeking an understanding of lupus. Books and materials on lupus are also available through the LFA. There are nearly 300 chapters, branches, and support groups in 32 states throughout the US.

Sandra C Raymond, President/CEO
Cindy Coney, Board Secretary

6908 Lupus Information Network
230 Ranch Drive
Bridgeport, CT 06606

203-372-5795

Seeks to foster better understanding of the disease among patients and the general public, educators and professionals through the distribution of educational materials.

Linda Rosinsky, President

Research Centers

6909 Hahnemann University Lupus Study Center
221 N Broad Street
Philadelphia, PA 19107

215-854-8100

Raphael J DeHoratius, Director

6910 Lupus Research Institute
330 Seventh Ave, Suite 1701
New York, NY 10001

212-812-9881
Fax: 212-545-1843
e-mail: lupus@LupusNY.org
www.lupusresearchinstitute.org

Established exclusively for lupus research. It has invested almost $20 million in new research and has funded 73 studies in 22 states.

Robert J Ravitz, Co-Chair
John A Luke, Treasurer

6911 SLE Lupus Foundation
330 Seventh Ave, Suite 1701
New York, NY 10001

212-685-4118
800-745-8787
Fax: 212-545-1843
e-mail: lupus@LupusNY.org
www.lupusny.org

Purpose is to raise funds for research grants, provide information and services to lupus patients, and educate the public about lupus. Patient services include self-help groups, orientation meetings, referrals, publications, and counseling on personal and financial problems related to the disease.

Richard K DeScherer, President
Margaret G Dowd, Executive Director

Web Sites

6912 Children's Hospital Boston
www.childrenshospital.org

Mission is to provide the highest quality care; be the leading source of reseach and discovery; educate the next generation of leaders in child health and enhance the health and well-being of the children and families in our local community.

Book Publishers

6913 Are You Tired Again...I Understand

Marilyn Deutsch PhD, author

Lupus Foundation of America
PO Box 932615
Atlanta, GA 31193

866-484-3532
Fax: 770-442-9742
e-mail: orders@lupus.org
www.lupus.org

An activity workbook for children to help them understand and what to expect when living with someone with lupus.

1996 42 pages Paperback

6914 Coping with Lupus

Robert Phillips PhD, author

Lupus Foundation of America
PO Box 932615
Atlanta, GA 31193

866-484-3532
Fax: 770-442-9742
e-mail: LupusInfo@aol.com
www.lupus.org

A practicing psychologist offers sound, meaningful and compassionate advice to individuals who must live with lupus.

2001 373 pages Softcover

6915 Disability Handbook for Social Security Applicants

Douglas Smith, author

Lupus Foundation of America
PO Box 932615
Atlanta, GA 31193

866-484-3532
e-mail: LupusInfo@aol.com
www.lupus.org

The handbook also includes the Disability Evaluation Guide for People with Systemic Lupus Erythematosus: Writing Medical Reports to the Social Security Administration. It helps people get their disability benefits promptly, without unnecessary appeals. Tells what you have to prove and how to prove it.

1995 137 pages Softcover

6916 Embracing the Wolf: A Lupus Victim and Her Family Learn to Live
Cherokee Publishing Company
PO Box 1730
Marietta, GA 30061

770-438-7366
800-653-3952

This book gives a very detailed accout of the effects of the disease that include emotions and moods for the victim and the way in which these attributes affect loved ones.

192 pages
ISBN: 0-877971-66-8

Kenneth W Boyd, Publisher

6917 Get to Sleep! How To Sleep Well...Despite Lupus

Robert Phillips PhD, author

Lupus Foundation of America
PO Box 932615
Atlanta, GA 31193

770-280-4177
866-484-3532
Fax: 770-442-9742
e-mail: orders@lupus.org
www.lupus.org

Written in a simple, straightforward style, this easy to follow action guide teaches you the most effective strategies for enabling you to get the sleep you want and need.

1995 14 pages
ISBN: 0-895294-75-3

6918 Immune System Disorders Sourcebook
Omnigraphics
PO Box 625
Holmes, PA 19043

800-234-1340
Fax: 800-875-1340
e-mail: info@omnigraphics.com
www.omnigraphics.com

Basic information about lupus, multiple sclerosis, guillain-barre syndrome and other disorders of the immune system.

671 pages 2nd Edition
ISBN: 0-780807-48-0

6919 In Search of the Sun: A Woman's Courageous Victory Over Lupus

Scribner
866 3rd Avenue
New York, NY 10022

212-702-2000
800-257-5755

This book is a revision of Henrietta Aladjem's book, The Sun Is My Enemy. In this book, with Peter Schur, she discusses her fight with this deadly and widespread disease.

6920 Let's Talk About Going to the Hospital

Rosen Publishing Group's PowerKids Press
29 E 21st Street
New York, NY 10010

212-777-3017
800-237-9932
Fax: 888-436-4643
e-mail: rosenpub@tribeca.ios.com
www.powerkidspress.com

If a child has to check into the hospital, chances are he or she is already upset about being ill. Knowing how a hospital functions and what the procedures are, such as when family members can visit, will help in what is already a stressful situation. Grades K-5.

24 pages
ISBN: 0-823950-36-0

6921 Loopy Lupus Helps Tell Scott's Story

Lupus Foundation of America
PO Box 932615
Atlanta, GA 31193

770-280-4177
866-484-3532
Fax: 770-442-9742
e-mail: orders@lupus.org
www.lupus.org

Written by a boy named Scott and his 3rd grade class explaining what it is like to live with lupus.

2002 34 pages Paperback

6922 Lupus Book

Daniel J Wallace MD, author

Lupus Foundation of America
PO Box 932615
Atlanta, GA 31193

770-280-4177
866-484-3532
Fax: 770-442-9742
e-mail: orders@lupus.org
www.lupus.org

Packed with useful, easy to understand information and practical guidance for people with lupus, their family members, friends and physicians. This hardcover book explains virtually every aspect of the disease and will help people better manage their day to day fight with lupus.

2005 271 pages 3rd Edition
ISBN: 0-195181-81-4

6923 Lupus Erythematosus: A Patient's Guide

Lupus Foundation of America
PO Box 932615
Atlanta, GA 31193

770-280-4177
866-484-3532
Fax: 770-442-9742
e-mail: orders@lupus.org
www.lupus.org

A popular LFA publication, the handbook provides a brief but detailed overview of the disease and guide for living well with lupus.

2000 27 pages

6924 Lupus Q&A: Everything You Need To Know

Lupus Foundation of America
PO Box 932615
Atlanta, GA 31193

770-280-4177
866-484-3532
Fax: 770-442-9742
e-mail: orders@lupus.org
www.lupus.org

Resource written for patients that want to learn more about lupus than what their doctors may or may not tell them.

2004 240 pages Paperback

6925 Sick and Tired of Feeling Sick and Tired

Lupus Foundation of America
PO Box 932615
Atlanta, GA 31193

770-280-4177
866-484-3532
Fax: 770-442-9742
e-mail: orders@lupus.org
www.lupus.org

Written in simple terms, the author offers understanding and practical guidance to people who live with ICI's and those who care for and about them.

2000 304 pages New Ed/ Paper
ISBN: 0-393320-65-0

6926 When Mom Gets Sick

Rebecca Samuels, author

Lupus Foundation of America
PO Box 932615
Atlanta, GA 31193

770-280-4177
866-484-3532
Fax: 770-442-9742
e-mail: orders@lupus.org
www.lupus.org

Written and illustrated by a nine-year-old, this is a compelling story based on the experiences of a sensitive and insightful young girl who makes the best from what could be a devastating situation.

27 pages

Magazines

6927 Lupus Now®

Lupus Foundation of America
2000 L Street NW, Suite 710
Washington, DC 20036

202-349-1155
888-385-8787
Fax: 202-349-1156
e-mail: info@lupus.org
www.lupus.org/newsite/

National and official magazine of the LFA. It includes lifestyle and wellness features and articles, research news, upcoming events, and other timely information for people with lupus, their families and health professionals.

48 pages 3x/year

DESCRIPTION

6928 TAY-SACHS DISEASE

Synonyms: GM2 gangliosidosis, type I, Hexa deficiency, Hexosaminidase A deficiency, Tay-Sachs disease, infantile type, TSD

Covers these related disorders: Tay-Sachs disease, juvenile type (GM2 gangliosidosis, type III)

Involves the following Biologic System(s):
Genetic/Chromosomal/Syndrome/Metabolic Disorders

Tay-Sachs disease, also known as GM2 gangliosidosis type I or infantile type, is a progressive degenerative metabolic disorder that occurs when two copies of the disease gene are inherited from the parents (autosomal recessive trait). The disorder, which belongs to a group of diseases known as lysosomal storage disorders, results from insufficient activity of the enzyme beta-hexosaminidase A. Enzymes within lysosomes, which are the major digestive units of cells, break down particles of nutrients such as certain fats and carbohydrates. In individuals with Tay-Sachs disease, insufficient activity of the enzyme hbeta-exosaminidase A causes an abnormal accumulation of particular fats (i.e., gangliosides) in certain tissues of the body, particularly nerve cells of the brain. Tay-Sachs disease affects approximately one in 3,500 to 4,000 newborns. The disease occurs predominantly in people of Ashkenazi Jewish (i.e., northeastern European Jewish) descent. About one in 30 individuals of Ashkenazi Jewish ancestry carries a single copy of the disease gene (heterozygous carrier).

Infants with Tay-Sachs disease appear to develop as expected until approximately four to six months of age, except for a marked startle reaction to sudden noises (hyperacusis) that may be apparent soon after birth. From four to six months of age, affected infants may begin to have decreased focusing and eye contact and appear listless and irritable. As the disease progresses, infants have delays in the acquisition of skills requiring the coordination of mental and physical activities (psychomotor delays) and lose previously acquired skills. By about one year of age, most affected children lose the ability to roll over, sit, stand, or vocalize sounds. In addition, muscle tone is severely diminished (hypotonia). With continuing disease progression, children experience increasing muscle rigidity and associated restrictions of movement (spasticity); uncontrolled electrical disturbances in the brain (seizures) that may be accompanied by prolonged contractions and relaxations of certain muscles (tonic-clonic convulsions); development of abnormal red circular areas of the middle layer of the eyes (cherry-red spots or Tay's sign); blindness; deafness; and loss of cognitive abilities (dementia). In many affected children, there is also enlargement of the brain (metabolic megalencephaly) due to abnormal accumulation of gangliosides in brain cells. Life-threatening complications often develop by approximately two to four years of age.

There are also variants of Tay-Sachs disease in which the onset of symptoms occurs later in life. For example, in children with the variant known as Tay-Sachs disease, juvenile type (GM2 gangliosidosis, type III), symptoms typically become apparent during mid-childhood although they may sometimes develop as early as the second year of life. This disease variant, which is characterized by varying levels of hexosaminidase deficiency, is also inherited as an autosomal recessive trait. Associated symptoms may include progressive impairment of voluntary movements (ataxia); involuntary movements characterized by rapid, jerking or slow, repetitive, writhing movements (choreoathetosis); loss of speech; seizures; and visual loss. Patients may experience life-threatening complications by approximately 15 years of age.

The disease gene responsible for Tay-Sachs disease is located on the long arm of chromosome 15 (15q23-24). Several distinct changes (mutations) in this disease gene have been identified in individuals with Tay-Sachs disease. In addition, different mutations are responsible for the infantile and juvenile forms of the disorder. Tests have been developed to help confirm carrier status in individuals who may carry a single copy of the disease gene (e.g., serum or leukocyte hexosaminidase A testing). It is recommended that individuals of Askenazi Jewish descent obtain testing prior to starting a family. In addition, genetic counseling is provided for those individuals who are heterozygous carriers and desire to start a family or have additional children. Specialized testing is also available that may confirm a diagnosis of Tay-Sachs disease before birth (e.g., chorionic villus sampling). The treatment of infants and children with Tay-Sachs disease includes symptomatic and supportive measures. Even with the best of care, children with Tay-Sachs disease usually die by age 4, from recurring infection.

See also **General Resources** on page 917

Government Agencies

6929 NIH/National Institute of Child Health and Human Development
31 Center Drive, Building 31
Bethesda, MD 20892

301-496-5133
Fax: 301-496-1104
www.nichd.nih.gov

Established in 1962 by congress, today the institute conducts and supports research on topics related to the health of children, adults, families and populations. Some of these topics include: developmental disabilities, growth and development, infant death, reproductive health and birth defects.

Nancy D Wirth, Director
Lisa Kaeser, Program & Public Liaison

6930 NIH/National Institute of Neurological Dis orders and Stroke (NINDS)
PO Box 5801
Bethesda, MD 20824

301-496-5751
800-352-9424
Fax: 301-496-0296
TTY: 301-468-5981
www.ninds.nih.gov

Works to reduce the burden of neurological disease by conducting, fostering, coordinating and guiding research on the causes, prevention, diagnosis and treatment of neurological disorders and stroke, while supporting basic research in related scientific areas.

Story C Landis Ph.D., Director
Audrey S Penn M.D., Deputy Director

National Associations & Support Groups

6931 Association for Neuro-Metabolic Disorders
5223 Brookfield Lane
Sylvania, OH 43506

419-885-1497
e-mail: volk4olks@aol.com

A nonprofit organization that serves as an advocate organization for families of patients with the following neuro-metabolic disorders: phenylketonuria, maple syrup urine disease, galactosemia, and biotinidase deficiency. Provides educational information for parents and children; provides networking information on support groups for new parents; supports scientific research into the treatments of these four neuro-metabolic disorders.

Cheryl Volk, Contact Person

6932 Canadian Society for Mucopolysaccharid e & Related Diseases Inc
PO Box 30034, RPO Parkgate, North Vancouver
Britich Columbia,
Canada

604-924-5130
800-667-1846
Fax: 604-924-5131
www.mpssociety.ca

Committed to supporting families affected with MPS and related diseases, educating medical professionals and the general public about MPS and related diseases, and raising funds for research.

Kirsten Harkins, Executive Director

6933 Chicago Center for Jewish Genetic Disorder
Ben Gurion Way, 30 South Wells Street
Chicago, IL 60606

312-357-4718
e-mail: jewishgeneticsctr@juf.org
www.jewishgeneticscenter.org

Provides public and professional education and to empower community members to seek out information and prevention strate-

gies.Represents the blending of science with religious, cultural and historical sensitivity and awareness.

Karen Litwack, Director
Rachel Sacks, Community Outreach Coordinator

6934 Conner's Way Foundation for Tay-Sachs Dise ase
7746 Rockburn Drive
Ellicott City, MD 21043

410-379-0568
www.connersway.com

Provides support for parents and families with Tay-Sachs disease. Also, provides fundraising events.

Desiree Hopf, Co-Chair
Carl Hopf, Co-Chair

6935 Genetic Alliance
4301 Connecticut Avenue NW
Washington, DC 20008

202-966-5557
800-336-4363
Fax: 202-966-8553
e-mail: info@geneticalliance.org
www.geneticalliance.org

A coalition of voluntary genetic support groups, consumers and professionals addressing the needs of individuals and families affected by genetic disorders from a national perspective.

Sharon Terry, President/CEO

6936 Genetic Alliance, Inc
4301 Connecticut Avenue NW, Suite 404
Washington, DC 20008

202-966-5557
Fax: 202-966-8553
e-mail: info@geneticalliance.org
www.geneticalliance.org

Dedicated to improving the quality of life for everyone living with genetic conditions. Provide accuracy organizations results in measurable growth: increased funding for research, access to services, and support for emerging technologies.

Sharon Terry, President/CEO
James O'Leary, Program Manager

6937 Jewish Genetic Disease Consortium
315 West 39th Street, Suite 701
New York, NY 10018

866-370-4363
e-mail: info@jewishgeneticdiseases.org
www.jewishgeneticdiseases.org

Created as a means by which a number of smaller, individual organizations could join together to heighten awareness of Jewish genetic diseases with a strong and unified voice.

Lois Neufeld, Co-Chair
Stan Michelman, Co-Chair

6938 March of Dimes Birth Defects Foundation
1275 Mamaroneck Avenue
White Plains, NY 10605

914-997-4488
www.marchofdimes.com

Mission is to improve the health of babies by preventing birth defects, premature birth, and infant mortality. Provide research, community services, education and advocacy to save babies' lives, to give all babies a fighting chance against the threats to their health: prematurity, birth defects, low birthweight.

6939 NIH/National Institute of Neurological Dis orders and Stroke (NINDS)
PO Box 5801
Bethesda, MD 20824

301-496-5751
800-352-9424
Fax: 301-496-0296
TTY: 301-468-5981
www.ninds.nih.gov

Mission is to reduce the burden of neuroligical disease - a burden borne by every age group, by every segment of society, by people all over the world.

Story C. Landis Ph.D., Director
Walter J. Koroshetz M.D., Deputy Director

6940 National Foundation for Jewish Genetic Diseases
250 Park Avenue, Suite 1000
New York, NY 10017

212-371-1030

Provides the information regarding this and related disorders for the people suffering from them.

6941 National Tay-Sachs and Allied Diseases Association
2001 Beacon Street, Suite 204
Boston, MA 02135

617-277-4463
800-906-8723
Fax: 617-277-0134
e-mail: info@ntsad.org
www.ntsad.org

Dedicated to the treatment and prevention of Tay-Sachs and related diseases, and to provide information and support services to individuals and families affected by these diseases through education, research, genetic screening, family services and advocacy.

Diana Pangonis, Interim Executive Director

Web Sites

6942 Chicago Center for Jewish Genetic Disorder
www.jewishgeneticscenter.org

e-mail: jewishgeneticsctr@juf.org
www.jewishgeneticscenter.org

Provides public and professional education and to empower community members to seek out information and prevention strategies.Represents the blending of science with religious, cultural and historical sensitivity and awareness.

6943 Genetic Alliance, Inc
www.geneticalliance.org

Dedicated to improving the quality of life for everyone living with genetic conditions. Provide accuracy organizations results in measurable growth: increased funding for research, access to services, and support for emerging technologies.

6944 Health Answers
www.healthanswers.com

HealthAnswers offers a breadth of services in medical education, sales force training, patient support solutions, professional promotion and consumer solutions.

6945 Healthfinder
www.healthfinder.gov

A key resource for finding the best government and nonprofit health and human services information on the internet. Links to carefully selected information and web sites from over 1,500 health-related organizations.

6946 Jewish Genetic Disease Consortium
www.jewishgeneticdiseases.org

Created as a means by which a number of smaller, individual organizations could join together to heighten awareness of Jewish genetic diseases with a strong and unified voice.

6947 Kansas University Medical Center
www.kumc.edu

Is a nationally recognized biomedical research center, offers education programs through its Schools of Allied Health, Medicine, Nursing, Pharmacy and Graduate Studies.

6948 March of Dimes Birth Defects Foundation
www.marchofdimes.com

Mission is to improve the health of babies by preventing birth defects, premature birth, and infant mortality. Provide research, community services, education and advocacy to save babies' lives, to give all babies a fighting chance against the threats to their health: prematurity, birth defects, low birthweight.

6949 NIH/National Institute of Neurological Dis orders and Stroke (NINDS)
www.ninds.nih.gov

Mission is to reduce the burden of neuroligical disease - a burden borne by every age group, by every segment of society, by people all over the world.

6950 National Tay-Sachs and Allied Disease Foundation
www.ntsad.org

Dedicated to the treatment and prevention of Tay-Sachs and related diseases, and to provide information and support services to individuals and families affected by these diseases through education, research, genetic screening, family services and advocacy.

6951 Online Mendelian Inheritance in Man
www.ncbi.nlm.nih.gov

This database is a catalog of human genes and genetic disorders.

6952 The Canadian Society for Mucopolysaccharid e & Related Diseases Inc
www.mpssociety.ca

Committed to supporting families affected with MPS and related diseases, educating medical professionals and the general public about MPS and related diseases, and raising funds for research.

Book Publishers

6953 Home Care Book
National Tay-Sachs and Allied Diseases Association
2001 Beacon Street, Suite 204
Boston, MA 02135

617-277-4463
800-906-8723
Fax: 617-277-0134
e-mail: info@ntsad.org
www.ntsad.org

written by parents for parents and professionals, the Home Care Book is a guide to caring for children with progressive neurological disorders at home.

Diana Pangonis, Contact

6954 Home-Care Book
National Tay-Sachs and Allied Diseases Association
2001 Beacon Street, Room 204
Brookline, MA 02146

617-277-4463

A guide for caring for children with progressive neurological diseases.

6955 International Quality for Adult Tay-Sachs Carrier Testing
National Tay-Sachs and Allied Diseases Association
2001 Beacon Street, Room 204
Boston, MA 02135

617-277-4463
800-906-8723
Fax: 617-277-0134
e-mail: info@ntsad.org
www.ntsad.org

6956 Let's Talk About Going to the Hospital
Rosen Publishing Group's PowerKids Press
29 E 21st Street
New York, NY 10010

212-777-3017
800-237-9932
Fax: 888-436-4643
e-mail: rosenpub@tribeca.ios.com
www.powerkidspress.com

If a child has to check into the hospital, chances are he or she is already upset about being ill. Knowing how a hospital functions and what the procedures are, such as when family members can visit, will help in what is already a stressful situation. Grades K-5.

24 pages
ISBN: 0-823950-36-0

6957 Lifting of Canavan's Carrier Testing Facilities
National Tay-Sachs and Allied Diseases Association
2001 Beacon Street, Room 204
Boston, MA 02135

617-277-4463
800-906-8723
Fax: 617-277-0134
e-mail: info@ntsad.org
www.ntsad.org

6958 Monograph on Canavan's Disease
National Tay-Sachs and Allied Diseases Association
2001 Beacon Street, Room 204
Boston, MA 02135

617-277-4463
800-906-8723
Fax: 617-277-0134
e-mail: info@ntsad.org
www.ntsad.org

6959 Tay-Sachs Carrier Testing Directory
National Tay-Sachs and Allied Diseases Association
2001 Beacon Street, Room 204
Brookline, MA 02146

617-277-4463

6960 Tay-Sachs Disease
Rosen Publishing
29 East 21st Street
New York, NY 10010

212-777-3017
800-237-9932
Fax: 888-436-4643
e-mail: rosenpub@tribeca.ios.com
www.powerkidspress.com

With colorful graphics and photographs, and a clear presentation of a tragic genetic disease, this title looks at gentic inheritance, dominant and recessive genes, and the carrier screening programs working to prevent Tay-Sachs.

6-12 64 pages 2007
ISBN: 1-404206-97-3

6961 Tay-Sachs Disease-A Bibliography, Medical Dictionary, & Annotated Research Guide
ICON Health Publications/ICON Group International
7404 Trade Street
San Diego, CA 92121

Fax: 858-635-9414
e-mail: orders@icongroupbooks.com
www.icongrouponline.com

A 3-in-1 reference book that provides a complete medical dictionary covering hundreds of terms and expressions relationg to Tay-Sachs disease. Also gives extensive lists of bibliographic citations. Provides information to users on how to update their knowledge using various internet resources.

132 pages

6962 The Official Parent's Sourcebook on Tay-Sachs Disease
ICON Health Publications/ICON Group International
7404 Trade Street
San Diego, CA 92121

Fax: 858-635-9414
e-mail: orders@icongroupbooks.com
www.icongrouponline.com

A comprehensive manual for anyone interested in self-directed research on tay-Sachs. Fully referenced with ample Internet listings and glossary.

128 pages

6963 There is Only One Child
National Tay-Sachs and Allied Diseases Association
2001 Beacon Street, Room 204
Brookline, MA 02146

617-277-4463

Newsletters

6964 Breakthrough
National Tay-Sachs and Allied Diseases Association
2001 Beacon Street, Room 204
Boston, MA 02135

617-277-4463
800-906-8723
Fax: 617-277-0134
e-mail: info@ntsad.org
www.ntsad.org

Annual newsletter for friends and supporters that focuses on the latest advances in research, profiles of families and individuals helped by NTSAD and disease profiles.

6965 The Connection
The Canadian MPS Society
PO Box 30034, RPO Parkgate, North Vancouver
British Columbia,
Canada

604-924-5130
800-667-1846
Fax: 604-924-5131
www.mpssociety.ca

Members only quarterly newsletter, a valuable resource filled with information on MPS-related news, including updates on new treatments and care options, current research and clinical trials, MPS-related events, and family news.

Pamphlets

6966 Late Onset Tay-Sachs Fact Sheet
National Tay-Sachs and Allied Diseases Association
2001 Beacon Street, Room 204
Boston, MA 02135

617-277-4463
800-906-8723
Fax: 617-277-0134
e-mail: info@ntsad.org
www.ntsad.org

Quick reference information sheet on the chronic or late onset of Tay-Sachs is available for no charge.

6967 Services to Families
National Tay-Sachs And Allied Diseases Association
2001 Beacon Street, Room 204
Boston, MA 02135

617-277-4463
800-906-8723
Fax: 617-277-0134
e-mail: info@ntsad.org
www.ntsad.org

Offers information on the Association parent peer groups, referrals and advocacy services to families and patients.

6968 Tay-Sachs & Sandhoff Disease

The Canadian MPS Society
PO Box 30034, RPO Parkgate, North Vancouver
British Columbia,
Canada

604-924-5130
800-667-1846
Fax: 604-924-5131
www.mpssociety.ca

6969 Tay-Sachs Information Sheet

March of Dimes Public Health Education Materials
1275 Mamaroneck Avenue
White Plains, NY 10605

914-428-7100
888-663-4637
Fax: 914-428-8203
e-mail: resourcecenter@modimes.org
www.modimes.org

Offers a brief overview of the illness, causes, symptoms and treatments.

6970 Tay-Sachs Is

National Tay-Sachs and Allied Diseases Association
2001 Beacon Street, Room 204
Brookline, MA 02146

617-277-4463

Information on the history of the disease, what a victim of the disease should know and what they can do as far as resources and referrals.

6971 What Every Family Should Know

National Tay-Sachs & Allied Diseases Association
2001 Beacon Street, Room 204
Boston, MA 02135

617-277-4463
800-906-8723
Fax: 617-277-0134
e-mail: info@ntsad.org
www.ntsad.org

50 page booklet detailing lysosomal storage and leukodystrophy disorders, with sections on Tay-Sachs, Sandhoff, Niemann-Pick, Gaucher, Canavan, Fabry, Pompe, therapeutic approaches and unique disease table.

6972 What is Tay-Sachs?

National Tay-Sachs and Allied Diseases Association
2001 Beacon Street, Room 204
Boston, MA 02135

617-277-4463
800-906-8723
Fax: 617-277-0134
e-mail: info@ntsad.org
www.ntsad.org

Informative educational pamphlet describing Infantile tay-Sachs, its inheritance and prevention is available for no charge.

DESCRIPTION

6973 TELANGIECTASIA

Synonym: Telangiectasis

Covers these related disorders: Ataxia-telangiectasia (AT), Phlebectasia, Cutis marmorata, Hereditary hemorrhagic telangiectasia, Rendu-Osler-Weber disease, Spider Angioma

Involves the following Biologic System(s): Dermatologic Disorders

Telangiectasia refers to the permanent widening or dilation of small blood vessels near the surface of the skin (superficial capillaries, arterioles, and venules). This results in the appearance of relatively small, red, well-defined skin lesions that have fine or coarse red lines or a spider-like network of red lesions that radiate from a central point (spider telangiectasia). Telangiectasias may develop as the result of an underlying disorder such as lupus erythematosus, dermatomyositis, rosacea, or psoriasis. These skin lesions may also result from exposure to sunlight, x-rays, or other forms of radiation.

Ataxia-telangiectasia (AT) is a rare, inherited, progressive disorder of the nervous system involving degenerative changes in the central nervous system along with defects in the immune system. AT is transmitted as an autosomal recessive trait and is characterized by the appearance during early childhood of telangiectasias involving the ears, face, the membranes that line the white outer coat of the eyes (bulbar conjunctiva), or other areas. Affected children are at risk for recurrent respiratory infections. Degeneration of the cerebellum, which is the part of the brain responsible for the regulation and coordination of voluntary movement and other vital functions, also occurs in children with AT.

Congenital generalized phlebectasia, sometimes called cutis marmorata telangiectatica congenita, is a benign telangiectasia that is apparent at birth and is characterized by red or purple-hued net-like lesions that may have a somewhat marbled appearance. These telangiectasias may be localized to an arm or leg or the trunk of the body; however, sometimes these skin lesions are more widely spread. In addition, the lesions may become more prominent with changes in outside temperature, crying, or exertion. This condition often resolves spontaneously by adolescence. Treatment is supportive.

Generalized essential telangiectasia is a rare condition that may affect children or adults and is characterized by the appearance of solitary or convergent patches of network-like telangiectasias. These lesions may appear on large but localized areas of the body such as the arms or legs or may sometimes involve or progress to the entire body. This disorder is limited to the skin with no health-associated irregularities. Treatment is supportive.

Hereditary benign telangiectasia is a rare, genetic disorder that is inherited as an autosomal dominant trait and is characterized by the appearance of telangiectasias on the skin of the face, arms, and upper portion of the trunk. This progressive disorder is limited to the skin.

Hereditary hemorrhagic telangiectasia, also called Rendu-Osler-Weber disease, is an inherited disorder that is transmitted as an autosomal dominant trait and is characterized by recurrent nosebleeds and the development of small telangiectasias of the skin and mucous membranes. These lesions range in color from red to purple and most often appear on the face, lips, and the membranes of the nose and mouth. In addition, the gastrointestinal tract, genitourinary tract, liver, brain, lungs, throat, voice box (larynx), and the membrane that lines the eyelids and whites of the eyes (conjunctiva) may be involved. Because the affected blood vessels may be fragile, they often break resulting in bleeding or hemorrhage from the gastrointestinal and genitourinary tracts, lungs, mouth, and nose.

Spider angioma, sometimes called spider nevus, is a telangiectasia characterized by the central, elevated, red lesion that is surrounded by a radiating, spider-like network of small blood vessels. Although these types of telangiectasias are often associated with conditions in which levels of circulating estrogen are elevated (e.g., pregnancy and liver disease), spider angiomas may also occur in preschool and school-age children. These lesions usually appear on the face, ears, forearms, and hands and often resolve on their own. Treatment is directed toward the removal of persistent angiomas and may include various methods such as freezing with liquid nitrogen (cryotherapy), the use of electric current to promote coagulation (electrocoagulation), or certain laser techniques such as intensed pulse light using a specially constructed flash lamp and focusing optics.

Telangiectasias can result in naevus flammeus (port-wine stain), which is a flat birthmark on the head or neck that spontaneously regresses. A port-wine stain, if present, will grow proportionally with the child. There is a high association with Sturge-Weber syndrome, a nevus formation in the skin and is associated with glaucoma, meningeal angiomas, and mental retardation. Unilateral nevoid telangiectasia refers to the appearance of telangiectasias on one side of the body in conjunction with an increase in the levels of circulating estrogen. These lesions sometimes develop in adolescent girls when they begin menstruation. Pregnancy may also prompt their development. When apparent in men, telangiectasias are the result of circulating estrogen secondary to liver disease. If this condition results from pregnancy, the lesions often fade or resolve during the postpartum period. Chronic treatment with corticosteroids may also lead to telangiectasias.

See also **General Resources** on page 917

Government Agencies

6974 NIH/National Institute of Arthritis and Mu sculoskeletal and Skin Diseases
1AMS Circle
Bethesda, MD 20892

301-402-4484
Fax: 301-718-6366
e-mail: ord@od.nih.gov
rarediseases.info.nih.gov

The mission of the National Institute of Arthritis and Musculoskeletal and Skin Diseases is to support research into the causes, treatment, and prevention of arthritis and musculoskeletal and skin diseases, the training of basic and clinical scientists to carry out this research, and the dissemination of information on research progress in these diseases.

Stephen I Katz MD PhD, Director

National Associations & Support Groups

6975 A-T Project: Cancer Research for Children with A-T
3002 Enfield Road
Austin, TX 78703

512-472-4892
Fax: 512-472-4892
e-mail: A-TProject@austin.rr.com
www.atproject.org

A nonprofit foundation organized to support biomedical research for the disease of ataxia-telangiectasia.

Robert Howard, President

6976 American Academy of Dermatology (AAD)
PO Box 4014
Schaumburg, IL 60168

847-240-1280
866-503-7546
Fax: 847-240-1859
e-mail: mrc@aad.org
www.aad.org

Dedicated to achieving high quality dermatologic care for everyone which encompasses: responsiveness, unification and representation of the specialty, and excellence in pateint care, education and research.

Stephen P Stone MD, President
William P Coleman III, MD, VP

6977 American Skin Association
346 Park Avenue South, 4th Floor
New York, NY 10010

212-889-4858
800-499-7546
Fax: 212-889-4959
e-mail: AmericanSkin@compuserve.com
www.americanskin.org

The American Skin Association is the only volunteer led health organization dedicated through research, education and advocacy to saving lives and alleviating human suffering caused by the full spectrum of skin disorders.

Howard P Milstein, Chairman
George W Hambrick, Jr, President/Founder

6978 Ataxia-Telangiectasia Children's Project
668 S Military Trail
Deerfield Beach, FL 33442

954-481-6611
800-543-5728
Fax: 954-725-1153
e-mail: info@atcp.org
www.atcp.org

A non-profit organization that raises funds to support and coordinate biomedical research projects, scientific conferences and a clinical center aimed at finding a cure for ataxia-telagiectasia, a lethal genetic disease that attacks childre, causing progressive loss of muscle control, cancer and immune system problems.

Brad Margus, Founder
Vicki Margus, Founder

6979 Children's Hospital Boston
300 Longwood Avenue
Boston, MA 02115

617-355-6000
TTY: 617-355-0443
www.childrenshospital.org

Mission is to provide the highest quality care; be the leading source of reseach and discovery; educate the next generation of leaders in child health and enhance the health and well-being of the children and families in our local community.

James Mandell, MD, President & CEO
Sandra Fenwick, Chief Operating Officer

6980 Hereditary Hemorrhagic Telangiectasia (HHT) Foundation International
PO Box 329
Monkton, MD 21111

410-357-9932
800-448-6389
Fax: 410-357-9931
e-mail: hhtinfo@hht.org
www.hht.org

Dedicated to increasing public and professional awareness and understanding of hereditary hemorrhagic telangiectasia (HHT). Supports ongoing medical research into the cause, prevention, and treatment of HHT; and offers a variety of materials including informational brochures and a quarterly newsletter.

Marianne Clancy, Executive Director

6981 NIH/National Institute of Neurological Dis orders and Stroke (NINDS)
PO Box 5801
Bethesda, MD 20824

301-496-5751
800-352-9424
Fax: 301-496-0296
TTY: 301-468-5981
www.ninds.nih.gov

Mission is to reduce the burden of neuroligical disease - a burden borne by every age group, by every segment of society, by people all over the world.

Story C. Landis Ph.D., Director
Walter J. Koroshetz M.D., Deputy Director

6982 National Ataxia Foundation
2600 Fernbrook Lane N
Minneapolis, MN 55447

763-553-0020
Fax: 763-553-0167
e-mail: naf@ataxia.org
www.ataxia.org

Objectives of this organization are to make an early diagnosis of ataxia by locating all potential victims and encouraging them to have an examination, public information and professional education materials and basic research on the disease.

6983 Society for Pediatric Dermatology
8365 Keystone Crossing, Suite 107
Indianapolis, IN 46240

317-202-0224
Fax: 317-205-9481
e-mail: spd@hp-assoc.com
www.pedsderm.net

Objective is to promote, develop and advance education, research and care of skin disease in all pediatric age groups.

Kent Lindeman, Executive Director

Web Sites

6984 American Academy of Dermatology (AAD)
www.aad.org

Dedicated to achieving high quality dermatologic care for everyone which encompasses: responsiveness, unification and representation of the specialty, and excellence in pateint care, education and research.

6985 American Skin Association
www.americanskin.org

The American Skin Association is the only volunteer led health organization dedicated through research, education and advocacy to saving lives and alleviating human suffering caused by the full spectrum of skin disorders.

6986 Ataxia-Telangiectasia Children's Project
www.atcp.org

A non-profit organization that raises funds to support and coordinate biomedical research projects, scientific conferences and a clinical center aimed at finding a cure for ataxia-telagiectasia, a lethal genetic disease that attacks childre, causing progressive loss of muscle control, cancer and immune system problems.

6987 Children's Hospital Boston
www.childrenshospital.org

Mission is to provide the highest quality care; be the leading source of reseach and discovery; educate the next generation of leaders in child health and enhance the health and well-being of the children and families in our local community.

6988 Hereditary Hemorrhagic Telangiectasia (HHT) Foundation International
www.hht.org

Dedicated to increasing public and professional awareness and understanding of hereditary hemorrhagic telangiectasia (HHT). Supports ongoing medical research into the cause, prevention, and treatment of HHT; and offers a variety of materials including informational brochures and a quarterly newsletter.

6989 NIH/National Institute of Neurological Dis orders and Stroke (NINDS)
www.ninds.nih.gov

Mission is to reduce the burden of neuroligical disease - a burden borne by every age group, by every segment of society, by people all over the world.

6990 National Ataxia Foundation
www.ataxia.org

Objectives of this organization are to make an early diagnosis of ataxia by locating all potential victims and encouraging them to have an examination, public information and professional education materials and basic research on the disease.

6991 Online Mendelian Inheritance in Man
www.ncbi.nlm.nih.gov

This database is a catalog of human genes and genetic disorders.

6992 Society for Pediatric Dermatology
www.pedsderm.net

Objective is to promote, develop and advance education, research and care of skin disease in all pediatric age groups.

Newsletters

6993 A-T Project: Cancer Research for Children with A-T Newsletter
3002 Enfield Road
Austin, TX 78703

512-472-4892
Fax: 512-472-4892
e-mail: A-TProject@austin.rr.com
www.atproject.org

A newsletter of the nonprofit foundation organized to support biomedical research for the diseases of ataxia-telangiectasia.

Robert Howard, President

6994 Hereditary Hemorrhagic Telangiectasia Foundation International Newsletter
PO Box 329
Monkton, MD 21111

410-357-9932
800-448-6389
Fax: 410-357-9931
e-mail: hhtinfo@hht.org
www.hht.org

The Foundation is dedicated to increasing public and professional awareness and understanding of hereditary hemorrhagic telangiectasia (HHT). Supports ongoing medical research into the cause, prevention, and treatment of HHT.

Quarterly

Pamphlets

6995 Ataxia-Telangiectasia and Cancer Risk
668 S Military Trail
Deerfield Beach, FL 33442

954-481-6611
800-543-5728
Fax: 954-725-1153
e-mail: info@atcp.org
www.atcp.org

6996 Ataxia-Telangiectasia and Estrogen Replace ment in Females
668 S Military Trail
Deerfield Beach, FL 33442

954-481-6611
800-543-5728
Fax: 954-725-1153
e-mail: info@atcp.org
www.atcp.org

6997 Ataxia-Telangiectasia and Immune Function
668 S Military Trail
Deerfield Beach, FL 33442

954-481-6611
800-543-5728
Fax: 954-725-1153
e-mail: info@atcp.org
www.atcp.org

6998 Ataxia-Telangiectasia and Swallowing Probl ems
668 S Military Trail
Deerfield Beach, FL 33442

954-481-6611
800-543-5728
Fax: 954-725-1153
e-mail: info@atcp.org
www.atcp.org

6999 Ataxia-Telangiectasia and X-Rays
668 S Military Trail
Deerfield Beach, FL 33442

954-481-6611
800-543-5728
Fax: 954-725-1153
e-mail: info@atcp.org
www.atcp.org

DESCRIPTION

7000 TETRALOGY OF FALLOT

Synonym: Fallot's syndrome

Involves the following Biologic System(s):

Cardiovascular Disorders

Tetralogy of Fallot is a combination of four specific heart malformations that are present at birth (congenital heart defects). Normally, oxygen-poor blood that returns from the body to the heart into the right upper chamber of the heart (right atrium), is pumped into the right lower chamber (right ventricle), and is then pumped into the pulmonary artery and on to the lungs, where the exchange of oxygen and carbon dioxide occurs. Oxygen-rich blood returns from the lungs to the heart via the left atrium, is pumped into the left ventricle, and is subsequently pumped into the major artery of the body (aorta) for circulation to the body's tissues. However, newborns with tetralogy of Fallot typically have four coexisting cardiac defects: i.e., (1) obstruction of the normal outflow of blood from the right ventricle due to abnormal narrowing (stenosis) of the opening between the right ventricle and the pulmonary artery (pulmonary stenosis); (2) an abnormal opening in the partition (septum) that separates the ventricles of the heart (ventricular septal defect or VSD); (3) displacement or override of the aorta, allowing oxygen-poor blood to flow directly from the right ventricle into the aorta; and (4) abnormal thickness of the right ventricle (right ventricular hypertrophy). Tetralogy of Fallot is thought to affect approximately one in 1,000 infants and children.

In patients with tetralogy of Fallot, the onset and severity of associated symptoms depend, in part, upon the degree of right ventricular outflow obstruction. Primary symptoms and findings in mild cases may be only a an unusual heart sound (murmur) heard through the stethoscope. In other cases, there may be a bluish discoloration of the skin and mucous membranes (cyanosis) due to decreased levels of oxygen in the blood; an insufficient supply of oxygen to bodily cells (hypoxia); and difficulties feeding. In infants with tetralogy of Fallot, cyanosis is typically most apparent in the nail beds of the fingers and toes and in the mucous membranes of the mouth and lips. In severe cases, cyanosis may be apparent soon after birth. In such newborns, pulmonary blood flow may primarily depend upon the fetal vascular channel that joins the pulmonary artery and the aorta (ductus arteriosus). Because this fetal vascular channel closes shortly after birth, severe cyanosis may develop within the first hours or days after birth. In other patients, cyanosis may not become apparent until later during the first year of life.

Some affected infants experience periodic attacks or spells during which cyanosis worsens (hypoxic or blue spells). During such hypoxic spells, patients may become restless and cyanotic; develop extreme shortness of breath;|and potentially lose consciousness (syncope). Although the onset of these attacks is unpredictable, they may tend to occur after severe crying episodes or upon awakening (Tet spells). The duration of the spells may range from a few minutes to a few hours, and they should be considered life-threatening and an indication for surgical repair.

Tetralogy of Fallot may be diagnosed based upon a complete clinical examination and patient history, detection of distinctive heart murmurs, and various specialized tests (e.g., x-ray studies, echocardiogram, electrocardiogram, cardiac catheterization). Surgery is performed in the first year of life, and often in the first six months of life, depending upon the severity of right ventricular outflow obstruction. Corrective open-heart surgery patches the ventricular septal defect, and enlarges the opening between the pulmonary artery and right ventricle. In many cases, corrective open-heart surgery may be recommended during the neonatal or infant period to avoid the risk of cyanotic spells later in infancy. Before and after corrective open-heart surgery, patients may be susceptible to bacterial infection of certain areas of the heart (e.g., bacterial endocarditis). Therefore, patients should be provided with antibiotic medication (antibiotic prophylaxis) with dental visits and certain surgical procedures. Additional treatment is symptomatic and supportive.

Tetralogy of Fallot may occur as an isolated condition, with other congenital heart defects, or in some cases, in association with certain chromosomal abnormalities (e.g., DiGeorge syndrome — a partial gene deletion that results in heart defects, low calcium levels, and immune deficiency — and Down syndrome.) Prenatal factors associated with higher than normal risk for this condition include maternal rubella (German measles) or other viral illnesses during pregnancy, poor prenatal nutrition, maternal alcoholism, mother over 40 years old, and diabetes. Researchers indicate that, in some patients, tetralogy of Fallot may be due to the interaction of one or more genes v(22q11). As with patients that have undergone any heart surgery, antibiotic prophylaxis (prevention) is indicated during dental treatment in order to prevent infective endocarditis, inflammation of the heart's inner lining or the heart valves.

See also **General Resources** on page 917

Government Agencies

7001 NIH/National Heart, Lung and Blood Institu te
National Institute of Health
31 Center Dr MSC 2486, Bldg 31, Room 5A48
Bethesda, MD 20892

301-592-8573
Fax: 240-629-3246
TTY: 240-629-3255
e-mail: NHLBIinfo@nhlbi.nih.gov
www.nhlbi.nih.gov

Primary responsibility of this organization is the scientific investigation of heart, blood vessel, lung and blood disorders. Oversees research, demonstration, prevention, education, control and training activities in these fields and emphasizes the prevention and control of heart diseases.

Elizabeth G Nabel, MD, Director
Susan Shurin, MD, Deputy Director

7002 NIH/National Institute of Child Health and Human Development
31 Center Drive, Building 31
Bethesda, MD 20892

301-496-5133
Fax: 301-496-1104
www.nichd.nih.gov

Established in 1962 by congress, today the institute conducts and supports research on topics related to the health of children, adults, families and populations. Some of these topics include: developmental disabilities, growth and development, infant death, reproductive health and birth defects.

Nancy D Wirth, Director
Lisa Kaeser, Program & Public Liaison

National Associations & Support Groups

7003 American Heart Association
7272 Greenville Avenue
Dallas, TX 75231

214-373-6300
800-242-8721
Fax: 214-706-1341
e-mail: inquire@amhrt.org
www.amhrt.org

Supports research, education and community service programs with the objective of reducing premature death and disability from cardiovascular diseases and stroke; coordinates the efforts of health professionals, and others engaged in the fight against heart and circulatory disease.

M Cass Wheeler, CEO

7004 Children's Hospital Boston
300 Longwood Avenue
Boston, MA 02115

617-355-6000
TTY: 617-355-0443
www.childrenshospital.org

Mission is to provide the highest quality care; be the leading source of reseach and discovery; educate the next generation of leaders in child health and enhance the health and well-being of the children and families in our local community.

James Mandell, MD, President & CEO
Sandra Fenwick, Chief Operating Officer

7005 Congenital Heart Anomalies, Support, Education & Resources (CHASER)
2112 N Wilkins Road
Swanton, OH 43558

419-825-5575
Fax: 419-825-2880
e-mail: chaser@compuserve.com
www.csun.edu/~hcmth011/chaser/

National organization for support, education and resources for families and patients who deal with children born with congenital heart malformations.

Anita Myers, Executive Director

7006 Genetic Alliance
4301 Connecticut Avenue NW
Washington, DC 20008

202-966-5557
800-336-4363
Fax: 202-966-8553
e-mail: info@geneticalliance.org
www.geneticalliance.org

A coalition of voluntary genetic support groups, consumers and professionals addressing the needs of individuals and families affected by genetic disorders from a national perspective.

Sharon Terry, President/CEO

7007 Little Hearts
110 Court Street, Suite 3A, PO Box 171
Cromwell, CT 06416

860-635-0006
866-435-4673
e-mail: info@littlehearts.org
www.littlehearts.org

Provides support, resources, networking, and hope to families affected by congenital heart defects. Membership consists of families nationwide who have or are expecting a child with a congenital heart defect.

Lenore Cameron, Director

Web Sites

7008 American Heart Association
www.amhrt.org

Supports research, education and community service programs with the objective of reducing premature death and disability from cardiovascular diseases and stroke; coordinates the efforts of health professionals, and others engaged in the fight against heart and circulatory disease.

7009 Children's Hospital Boston
www.childrenshospital.org

Mission is to provide the highest quality care; be the leading source of reseach and discovery; educate the next generation of leaders in child health and enhance the health and well-being of the children and families in our local community.

7010 Congenital Heart Anomalies, Support, Education & Resources (CHASER)
www.csun.edu/~hcmth011/chaser/

National organization for support, education and resources for families and patients who deal with children born with congenital heart malformations.

7011 Congenital Heart Information Network
www.tchin.org

An international organization that provides reliable information, support services and resources to families of children with congenital heart defects and acquired heart disease, adults with congenital heart defects, and the professionals who work with them.

7012 Little Hearts
www.littlehearts.net

Provides support, resources, networking, and hope to families affected by congenital heart defects. Membership consists of families nationwide who have or are expecting a child with a congenital heart defect.

7013 Southern Illinois University School of Medicine
www.siumed.edu/peds/index.htm

The mission of SUI School of Medicine is to assist the people of central and southern Illinois in meeting their present and future health care needs through education, clinical service and research.

Book Publishers

7014 Congenital Disorders Sourcebook
Omnigraphics
PO Box 625
Holmes, PA 19043

800-234-1340
Fax: 800-875-1340
e-mail: info@omnigraphics.com
www.omnigraphics.com

Basic consumer health information on disorders aquired during gestation, including spina bifida, hydrocephalus, cerebral palsy, heart defects, craniofacial abnormalities and fetal alcohol syndrome.

650 pages
ISBN: 0-780809-45-9

DESCRIPTION

7015 THALASSEMIAS

Covers these related disorders: Alpha-thalassemia, Beta-thalassemia, Beta-thalassemia minor, Beta-thalassemia major

Involves the following Biologic System(s):
Genetic/Chromosomal/Syndrome/Metabolic Disorders, Hematologic and Oncologic Disorders

The term thalassemia refers to a group of inherited blood disorders that includes the alpha-thalassemias and the more common beta-thalassemias. The thalassemias are characterized by the faulty production of hemoglobin, the protein that carries oxygen within the red blood cells. Hemoglobin is composed of two pairs of amino acid chains (globins), the alpha chains and the beta chains. The improper synthesis of hemoglobin is caused by a defect within the globin genes and results in abnormal, fragile red blood cells. Beta-thalassemia minor, a less severe form of the disease, is inherited when the defective gene is transmitted by one parent, while beta-thalassemia major is inherited through the defective genes of both parents.

A mild anemia is usually present in individuals with beta-thalassemia minor; however, it is not unusual for affected individuals to be symptom-free. Symptoms of beta-thalassemia major include fatigue; shortness of breath (dyspnea); and yellowing of the skin, eyes, and mucous membranes (jaundice). Other symptoms, usually associated with the premature destruction of red blood cells (hemolytic anemia) and subsequent release of iron, may include bronzed or freckled skin and enlargement of the spleen (splenomegaly). In severe cases, iron that gets deposited in the heart, liver, and pancreas may eventually lead to impaired function. In addition, extreme activity of the bone marrow may result in thickened and enlarged bones in the skull and face, while normal growth may be retarded.

Alpha-thalassemia, far less common than beta-thalassemia, ranges in severity from a carrier state with no symptoms to the most severe form that is incompatible with life. The severity of symptoms is dependent upon the level of alpha-chain involvement. The most severe form of alpha-thalassemia involves the complete absence of alpha-chain production.

Thalassemia patients vary a lot in their treatment needs depending on the severity of their anemia. Treatment for symptomatic thalassemias includes blood transfusion therapy to ensure normal growth. However, repeated blood transfusions may exacerbate iron deposition into the internal organs (hemosiderosis), necessitating treatment with iron-chelating drugs that increase iron excretion. Other treatment may include bone marrow transplantation.

Thalassemia is inherited as an autosomal recessive trait and is most prevalent among people living in or originating from the Mediterranean, the Middle East, and Southeast Asia. As with other genetically acquired disorders, aggressive birth screening and genetic counseling is recommended.

See also **General Resources** on page 917

Government Agencies

7016 NIH/National Heart, Lung and Blood Institu te
National Institute of Health
31 Center Dr MSC 2486, Bldg 31, Rm5A48
Bethesda, MD 20892

301-592-8573
Fax: 301-629-3246
TTY: 240-629-3255
e-mail: NHLBIinfo@nhlbi.nih.gov
www.nhlbi.nih.gov

Primary responsibility of this organization is the scientific investigation of heart, blood vessel, lung and blood disorders. Oversees research, demonstration, prevention, education, control and training activities in these fields and emphasizes the prevention and control of heart diseases.

Elizabeth G Nabel, MD, Director
Charles Peterson, MD, MBA, Director, Blood Diseases/Resources

---

National Associations & Support Groups

7017 AHEPA Cooley's Anemia Foundation
1909 Q Street NW, Suite 500
Washington, DC 20009

202-232-6300
Fax: 202-232-2140
e-mail: ahepa@ahepa.org

Dedicated to advancing the treatment and cure of cooley's anemia, an inherited blood disorder. Provides information, referrals to local medical sources, medical supplies to people in need, and listings of informational materials available from the Foundation.

7018 Children's Blood Foundation
333 East 38th Street, Suite 380
New York, NY 10016

212-297-4336
Fax: 212-297-4340
e-mail: info@childrensbloodfoundation.org
www.childrensbloodfoundation.org

Mission is to support the comprehenisve clinical care of children living with blood disorders; to foster research to help understand the causes of childhood blood disorders; and to sponsor the fellowship training of pediatricians of the subspecialty of pediatric hematology and oncology.

1952

John Calicchio, Chairman

7019 Children's Hospital Boston
300 Longwood Avenue
Boston, MA 02115

617-355-6000
TTY: 617-355-0443
www.childrenshospital.org

Mission is to provide the highest quality care; be the leading source of reseach and discovery; educate the next generation of leaders in child health and enhance the health and well-being of the children and families in our local community.

James Mandell, MD, President & CEO
Sandra Fenwick, Chief Operating Officer

7020 Cooley's Anemia Foundation
330 Seventh Avenue, #900
New York, NY 10001

800-522-7222
Fax: 212-279-5999
e-mail: info@cooleysanemia.org
www.cooleysanemia.org

The only US-based voluntary health organization that aids in patient services, medical research, education and public information to fight thalassemia, a blood disease also known as Cooley's anemia. Members of CAF work alongside the Thalassemia Action Group (TAG) to provide national support, encouragement and friendship to other patients and families.

1954

Frank Somma, National President
Gina Cioffi, Esq., National Executive Director

7021 Genetic Alliance
4301 Connecticut Avenue NW
Washington, DC 20008

202-966-5557
800-336-4363
Fax: 202-966-8553
e-mail: info@geneticalliance.org
www.geneticalliance.org

A coalition of voluntary genetic support groups, consumers and professionals addressing the needs of individuals and families affected by genetic disorders from a national perspective.

Sharon Terry, President/CEO

7022 March of Dimes Birth Defects Foundation
1275 Mamaroneck Avenue
White Plains, NY 10605

914-997-4488
www.marchofdimes.com

Mission is to improve the health of babies by preventing birth defects, premature birth, and infant mortality. Provide research, community services, education and advocacy to save babies' lives, to give all babies a fighting chance against the threats to their health: prematurity, birth defects, low birthweight.

7023 Thalassemias Action Group (TAG)
330 Seventh Avenue, #900
New York, NY 10001

800-522-7222
Fax: 212-279-5999
e-mail: tag@cooleysanmeia.org
www.cooeysanemia.org

Promotes positive attidtude toward life; stresses the importance of compliance and chelation therapy; and provides patients with a channel of communication and information.

1985

Jesal Kapasi, President
Kathy Hatzinas, First Vice President

7024 X-Linked Alpha Thalassemia Family Support Network
1437 Cool Springs Drive
Mesquite, TX 75181

972-222-0050
e-mail: nordtx@earthlink.net

State Agencies & Support Groups

California

7025 Cooley's Anemia Foundation-California
2629 Foothill Boulevard, #319
La Crescenta, CA 91214

800-601-2821
e-mail: ca_chapter@hotmail.com

Robert Yamashita, President
Christine Giannamore, Coordinator

Georgia

7026 Cooley's Anemia Foundation-Buffalo Chapter
781 Eagle Crossing Drive
Lawrenceville, GA 30044

678-357-4021
Fax: 678-969-0367
e-mail: supermom2kids@earthlink.net

Tahseen Mahmood, President

Illinois

7027 Cooley's Anemia Foundation-Illinois
Oakbrook Towers
40 N Tower Road #2A
Oakbrook, IL 60521

630-268-8775

Pat Matarrese, President

Maryland

7028 Cooley's Anemia Foundation-Capital Area (DC, VA, MD)
15321 Peach Orchard Road
Silver Spring, MD 20905

301-989-8947
e-mail: cvitaliti@aol.com

Carl C Vitaliti, President

Massachusetts

7029 Cooley's Anemia Foundation-Massachusetts Chapter
44 Joseph Road
Newton, MA 02160

617-332-5952
e-mail: rvscomi@comcast.net

Rudi Viscomi, President

New Jersey

7030 Cooley's Anemia Foundation - New Jersey Chapter
1 Engle Street
Englewood, NJ 07631

201-569-2193
Fax: 201-569-2613

Vincent D'Elia Esq

New York

7031 Cooley's Anemia Foundation - Rochester
19 Devenwood Lane
Pittsford, NY 14534

716-248-3385

Peter Paradiso, President

7032 Cooley's Anemia Foundation - Staten Island
2136 E 4th Street
Brooklyn, NY 11223
718-627-7469

Terri DiFilippo, President

7033 Cooley's Anemia Foundation-Buffalo
135 Wellington Road
Buffalo, NY 14216
716-832-3055

Dennis Locurto, President

7034 Cooley's Anemia Foundation-Long Island/Bro oklyn Chapter
PO Box 190
Franklin Square, NY 11010
516-358-9100
Fax: 516-358-9101
e-mail: trotolo@optonline.net

Thomas Rotolo, President

7035 Cooley's Anemia Foundation-Queens
157-26 9th Avenue
Beachurst, NY 11357
718-746-7677
Fax: 718-746-7678
e-mail: cafqueens@verizon.net

Paul Tucci-President, tuccman63@yahoo.com
Abbey Chakalis-Events Manager, abbeycaf@verizon.net

7036 Cooley's Anemia Foundation-Suffolk Chapter
740 Smithtown Bypass #201
Smithtown, NY 11787
631-863-0532
Fax: 631-863-0535
e-mail: ruthscaf@optonline.net

Kevin O'Hare, President

7037 Cooley's Anemia Foundation-Westchester/Roc kland Chapter
3 Sammuel Purdy Lane
Katonah, NY 10536
914-232-1808
e-mail: anemia@optonline.net

Peter Chicco, President
Janet Manning, Executive Director

Texas

7038 Cooley's Anemia Foundation - Texas
1004 Field Trail
Mesquite, TX 75150
214-324-6147
Fax: 214-324-0612

Mateen Shah, President

Conferences

7039 TAG Conference
Thalassemia Action Group
330 Seventh Avenue, #900
New York, NY 10001
800-522-7222
Fax: 212-279-5999
e-mail: info@cooleysanemia.org
www.cooleysanemia.org

Held annually around March-April, look at website for more information.

Audio Video

7040 Tag Surfing
Cooley's Anemia Foundation
330 Seventh Avenue, #900
New York, NY 10001
800-522-7222
Fax: 212-279-5999
e-mail: info@cooleysanemia.org
www.cooleysanemia.org

Video

7041 To Live
Cooley's Anemia Foundation
330 Seventh Avenue, #900
New York, NY 10001
800-522-7222
Fax: 212-279-5999
e-mail: info@cooleysanemia.org
www.cooleysanemia.org

16 minute version.
Video

7042 You're Not Alone
Cooley's Anemia Foundation
330 Seventh Avenue, #900
New York, NY 10001
800-522-7222
Fax: 212-279-5999
e-mail: info@cooleysanemia.org
www.cooleysanemia.org

Video

Web Sites

7043 Children's Blood Foundation
www.childrensbloodfoundation.org

Mission is to support the comprehenisve clinical care of children living with blood disorders; to foster research to help understand the causes of childhood blood disorders; and to sponsor the fellowship training of pediatricians of the subspecialty of pediatric hematology and oncology.

7044 Children's Hospital Boston
www.childrenshospital.org

Mission is to provide the highest quality care; be the leading source of reseach and discovery; educate the next generation of leaders in child health and enhance the health and well-being of the children and families in our local community.

7045 Cooley's Anemia Foundation
www.cooleysanemia.org

The only US-based voluntary health organization that aids in patient services, medical research, education and public information to fight thalassemia, a blood disease also known as Cooley's anemia. Members of CAF work alongside the Thalassemia Action Group (TAG) to provide national support, encouragement and friendship to other patients and families.

7046 March of Dimes Birth Defects Foundation
www.marchofdimes.com

Mission is to improve the health of babies by preventing birth defects, premature birth, and infant mortality. Provide research, community services, education and advocacy to save babies' lives, to give all babies a fighting chance against the threats to their health: prematurity, birth defects, low birthweight.

7047 NIH/National Heart, Lung and Blood Institu te
www.nhlbi.nih.gov

Primary responsibility of this organization is the scientific investigation of heart, blood vessel, lung and blood disorders. Oversees research, demonstration, prevention, education, control and training activities in these fields and emphasizes the prevention and control of heart diseases.

7048 Online Mendelian Inheritance in Man
www.ncbi.nlm.nih.gov

This database is a catalog of human genes and genetic disorders.

7049 Thalassemias Action Group (TAG)
www.cooeysanemia.org

Promotes positive attitdude toward life; stresses the importance of compliance and chelation therapy; and provides patients with a channel of communication and information.

Book Publishers

7050 Blood & Circulatory Disorders Sourcebook
Omnigraphics
PO Box 625
Holmes, PA 19043

800-234-1340
Fax: 800-875-1340
e-mail: info@omnigraphics.com
www.omnigraphics.com

Basic consumer health information on blood and its components, anemias, leukemias, bleeding disorders, and circulatory disorders, including aplastic anemia, thalassemia, sickle-cell disease and hemophilia.

2005 659 pages
ISBN: 0-780807-46-4

7051 Coloring Book on Thalassemia
Cooley's Anemia Foundation
330 Seventh Avenue, #900
New York, NY 10001

800-522-7222
Fax: 212-279-5999
e-mail: info@cooleysanemia.org
www.cooleysanemia.org

Available in English, Italian, Greek and Chinese.

7052 Cooley's Anemia 7th Annual Symposium
Cooley's Anemia Foundation
330 Seventh Avenue, #900
New York, NY 10001

800-522-7222
Fax: 212-279-5999
e-mail: info@cooleysanemia.org
www.cooleysanemia.org

Published by the New York Academy of Sources.
1997

7053 Genes, Blood & Courage
Cooley's Anemia Foundation
330 Seventh Avenue, #900
New York, NY 10001

800-522-7222
Fax: 212-279-5999
e-mail: info@cooleysanemia.org
www.cooleysanemia.org

7054 Let's Talk About Going to the Hospital
Rosen Publishing Group's PowerKids Press
29 E 21st Street
New York, NY 10010

212-777-3017
800-237-9932
Fax: 888-436-4643
e-mail: rosenpub@tribeca.ios.com
www.powerkidspress.com

If a child has to check into the hospital, chances are he or she is already upset about being ill. Knowing how a hospital functions and what the procedures are, such as when family members can visit, will help in what is already a stressful situation. Grades K-5.

24 pages
ISBN: 0-823950-36-0

7055 Mom, I'll Stop Crying, If You Stop Crying
Cooley's Anemia Foundation
129-09 26th Avenue
Flushing, NY 11354

718-321-2873
800-522-7222
Fax: 718-321-3340
e-mail: ncaf@aol.com
www.thalassemia.org

A courageous battle against a deadly disease.

7056 What is Cooley's Anemia
Cooley's Anemia Foundation
129-09 26th Avenue
Flushing, NY 11354

718-321-2873
800-522-7222
Fax: 718-321-3340
e-mail: ncaf@aol.com
www.thalassemia.org

Patient and family handbook.

Gina Cioffi, National Executive Director

7057 What is Thalassemia?
Cooley's Anemia Foundation
129-09 26th Avenue
Flushing, NY 11354

718-321-2873
800-522-7222
Fax: 718-321-3340
e-mail: ncaf@aol.com
www.thalassemia.org

A guide to help thalassemics and their parents understand thalassemia, the reasons for treatment and hope for the future.
Rino Vullo

Newsletters

7058 CAF Medical Update
Cooley's Anemia Foundation
330 Seventh Avenue, #900
New York, NY 10001

800-522-7222
Fax: 212-279-5999
e-mail: info@cooleysanemia.org
www.cooleysanemia.org

Medical information.
Biannual

7059 Lifeline
Cooley's Anemia Foundation
330 Seventh Avenue, #900
New York, NY 10001

800-522-7222
Fax: 212-279-5999
e-mail: info@cooleysanemia.org
www.cooleysanemia.org

Cooley's Anemia Foundation

Biannual

7060 TAG Newsletter
Thalassemia Action Group
330 Seventh Avenue, #900
New York, NY 10001

800-522-7222
Fax: 212-279-5999
e-mail: tag@cooleysanemia.org
www.cooleysanemia.org

Pamphlets

7061 Cooley's Anemia Fact Cards
Cooley's Anemia Foundation
330 Seventh Avenue, #900
New York, NY 10001

800-522-7222
Fax: 212-279-5999
e-mail: info@cooleysanemia.org
www.cooleysanemia.org

7062 Cooley's Anemia Foundation (CAF) Pamphlet
Cooley's Anemia Foundation
330 Seventh Avenue, #900
New York, NY 10001

800-522-7222
Fax: 212-279-5999
e-mail: info@cooleysanemia.org
www.cooleysanemia.org

7063 Desferal Q & A
Cooley's Anemia Foundation
330 Seventh Avenue, #900
New York, NY 10001

800-522-7222
Fax: 212-279-5999
e-mail: info@cooleysanemia.org
www.cooleysanemia.org

Guidelines for home infusion.

7064 Sibling Donor Cord Blood Program Pamphlet
Cooley's Anemia Foundation
330 Seventh Avenue, #900
New York, NY 10001

800-522-7222
Fax: 212-279-5999
e-mail: info@cooleysanemia.org
www.cooleysanemia.org

7065 Thalassemia Action Group (TAG) Patient Support Group Brochure
Cooley's Anemia Foundation
330 Seventh Avenue, #900
New York, NY 10001

800-522-7222
Fax: 212-279-5999
e-mail: info@cooleysanemia.org
www.cooleysanemia.org

7066 What is Thalassemia Trait?
Cooley's Anemia Foundation
330 Seventh Avenue, #900
New York, NY 10001

800-522-7222
Fax: 212-279-5999
e-mail: info@cooleysanemia.org
www.cooleysanemia.org

This booklet offers information on the thalassemia trait.

DESCRIPTION

7067 THROMBOCYTOPENIAS

Covers these related disorders: Idiopathic thrombocytopenia purpura (ITP)

Involves the following Biologic System(s):
Hematologic and Oncologic Disorders

Thrombocytopenia is a term that describes a condition in which the level of circulating platelets in the blood is reduced, resulting in a tendency to bleed. By changing shape and adhering to each other and the walls of broken blood vessels, platelets, also known as thrombocytes, play an essential role in the clotting process. Normal blood levels usually demonstrate 150,000 to 350,000 platelets per microliter. When the platelet count is reduced to 30,000 per microliter or lower, abnormal bleeding under the skin may occur and result in purple bruising or spots (purpura). Nosebleeds (epistaxis), bleeding of the gums , and blood in the urine (hematuria) are also common. Often, low platelet levels do not lead to clinical problems; rather, they are picked up on a routine full blood count.

Thrombocytopenia may result from a slowdown in platelet production or the rapid destruction of these cells. Certain diseases such as anemia, leukemia, lymphoma, bone marrow disorders, or autoimmune diseases may cause thrombocytopenia. Other causes include enlargement of the spleen (splenomegaly), cirrhosis, certain drugs, viral infection, and x-ray or radiation exposure.

The treatment of thrombocytopenia is based upon its underlying cause. For example, if the low platelet count is caused by a specific underlying disease, treatment is geared toward that disease. Low platelet counts caused by a specific drug necessitate the withdrawal of that drug. If bleeding is severe, platelet transfusions may be administered.

Idiopathic thrombocytopenia purpura (ITP) is a term used to describe thrombocytopenia of unknown origin. This condition often follows a viral infection and, in children, usually disappears within a month or so with no treatment. The duration of ITP in adolescents and adults is often more prolonged, and close medical follow up and avoidance of contact sports and activities is essential.

See also **General Resources** on page 917

Government Agencies

7068 NIH/National Heart, Lung and Blood Institu te
National Institute of Health
31 Center Dr MSC 2486, Bldg 31, Room 5A48
Bethesda, MD 20892

301-592-8573
Fax: 240-629-3246
TTY: 240-629-3255
e-mail: NHLBIinfo@nhlbi.nih.gov
www.nhlbi.nih.gov

Primary responsibility of this organization is the scientific investigation of heart, blood vessel, lung and blood disorders. Oversees research, demonstration, prevention, education, control and training activities in these fields and emphasizes the prevention and control of heart diseases.

Elizabeth G Nabel, MD, Director
Susan Shurin, MD, Deputy Director

National Associations & Support Groups

7069 American Heart Association
7272 Greenville Avenue
Dallas, TX 75231

214-373-6300
800-242-8721
Fax: 214-706-1341
e-mail: inquire@amhrt.org
www.amhrt.org

Our mission is to reduce disability and death from cardiovascular diseases and stroke. Parents will find education and support to you better care for a child with arrhythmias.

M Cass Wheeler, CEO

7070 Children's Blood Foundation
333 East 38th Street, Suite 380
New York, NY 10016

212-297-4336
Fax: 212-297-4340
e-mail: info@childrensbloodfoundation.org
www.childrensbloodfoundation.org

Promotes the welfare of and addresses the issues that affect people with immune or idiopathic thrombocytopenic purpura. Goals are to provide patient support, ongoing medical research to advance the knowledge and treatment and educate the public and medical communities about the disorder. Provides educational and support materials including fact sheets, brochures, and a booklet entitled 'What's It Called Again?'

John Calicchio, Chairman

7071 Children's Hospital Boston
300 Longwood Avenue
Boston, MA 02115

617-355-6000
TTY: 617-355-0443
www.childrenshospital.org

Mission is to provide the highest quality care; be the leading source of research and discovery; educate the next generation of leaders in child health and enhance the health and well-being of the children and families in our local community.

James Mandell, MD, President & CEO
Sandra Fenwick, Chief Operating Officer

7072 Genetic Alliance
4301 Connecticut Avenue NW
Washington, DC 20008

202-966-5557
800-336-4363
Fax: 202-966-8553
e-mail: info@geneticalliance.org
www.geneticalliance.org

A coalition of voluntary genetic support groups, consumers and professionals addressing the needs of individuals and families affected by genetic disorders from a national perspective.

Sharon Terry, President/CEO

7073 Platelet Disorder Support Association
PO Box 61533
Potomac, MD 20859

301-770-6636
877-528-3538
Fax: 301-770-6638
e-mail: pdsa@pdsa.org
www.itppeople.com

Our organization is devoted to bringing you the most timely, accurate and comprehensive information about ITP and assisting you in meeting others who share your interests.

Joan Young, President

Web Sites

7074 American Heart Association
www.amhrt.org

Our mission is to reduce disability and death from cardiovascular diseases and stroke. Parents will find education and support to you better care for a child with arrhythmias.

7075 Children's Blood Foundation
www.childrensbloodfoundation.org

Promotes the welfare of and addresses the issues that affect people with immune or idiopathic thrombocytopenic purpura. Goals are to provide patient support, ongoing medical research to advance the knowledge and treatment and educate the public and medical communities about the disorder. Provides educational and support materials including fact sheets, brochures, and a booklet entitled 'What's It Called Again?'

7076 Children's Hospital Boston
www.childrenshospital.org

Mission is to provide the highest quality care; be the leading source of reseach and discovery; educate the next generation of leaders in child health and enhance the health and well-being of the children and families in our local community.

7077 Online Mendelian Inheritance in Man
www.ncbi.nlm.nih.gov

This database is a catalog of human genes and genetic disorders.

7078 Platelet Disorder Support Association
www.itppeople.com

Our organization is devoted to bringing you the most timely, accurate and comprehensive information about ITP and assisting you in meeting others who share your interests.

Book Publishers

7079 Harrison's Principles of Inernal Medicine 15th Edition
McGraw-Hill
PO Box 182604
Columbus, OH 43272

877-833-5524
Fax: 614-759-3749
www.mcgraw-hill.com

Raises the bar for internal medicine references. Features over 90 new chapters, Harrison's continues to provide authoritative record of internal medicine as practiced by the leading experts in the field.

7080 Let's Talk About Going to the Hospital
Rosen Publishing Group's PowerKids Press
29 E 21st Street
New York, NY 10010

212-777-3017
800-237-9932
Fax: 888-436-4643
e-mail: rosenpub@tribeca.ios.com
www.powerkidspress.com

If a child has to check into the hospital, chances are he or she is already upset about being ill. Knowing how a hospital functions and what the procedures are, such as when family members can visit, will help in what is already a stressful situation. Grades K-5.

24 pages
ISBN: 0-823950-36-0

DESCRIPTION

7081 THUMBSUCKING

Involves the following Biologic System(s):

Developmental/Behavioral/Psychiatric Disorders

Thumbsucking is a common habit that is prevalent among infants and young children. This behavior is usually used as a device for providing pleasure, amusement, comfort, oral gratification, and release of stress or tension. Sometimes a security object, such as a blanket, may become part of the thumbsucking habit. In most children, thumbsucking reaches a plateau between the ages of 18 months to two years and then slowly but steadily decreases until it disappears at about five to six years of age. One reason to encourage children to give up the habit before they enter school is to prevent the teasing they would otherwise receive. By adolescence, most normal children abandon thumbsucking because of peer pressure.

Although it is generally thought that thumbsucking does not cause any long-term developmental irregularities, thumbsucking that continues beyond age six may lead to acquired problems with the bones and tissues of the thumb and an abnormal bite or contact pattern between upper and lower teeth (malocclusion). The longer the habit persists, the more likely affected children are to develop these types of problems. Conversely, the earlier this habit comes to an end, the more likely that irregular positioning of the teeth will improve without intervention.

Many physicians agree that, as a general rule, the best treatment for thumbsucking is to ignore the behavior and wait patiently for the children to outgrow the habit or to discontinue the behavior on their own. Treatment is generally supportive as punishing or reprimanding often adds to stress levels, becomes a power struggle with the parent, and may actually worsen the problem. Other treatment may include the use of certain appliances that are fitted with small projections that alert children to their behavior when they attempt to suck their thumbs. Older children may require the use of orthodontic appliances to correct irregularities associated with malocclusion.

See also **General Resources** on page 917

Government Agencies

7082 NIH/National Institute of Dental and Crani ofacial Research (NIHDCR)

National Institutes of Health
31 Center Drive, MSC 2290, Building 31
Bethesda, MD 20892

301-496-4261
Fax: 301-402-2185
e-mail: nidcrinfo@mail.nih.gov
www.nidcr.nih.gov

The mission is to promote the general health of American people by improving their oral, dental and craniofacial health. Through the conduct and support of research and training of researchers, the NIDCR aims to promote health, prevent diseases and conditions, and develop new diagnostic and therapeutics.

Dr Lawrence A Tabak, Director
Thomas G Murphy, Acting Executive Director

7083 National Oral Health Information Clearinghouse

1 NOHIC Way
Bethesda, MD 20892

301-402-7364
Fax: 301-480-4098
TDD: 301-656-7581
e-mail: nidcrinfo@mail.nih.gov
www.nidcr.nih.gov

Produces and distributes patient and professional education materials including fact sheets, brochures, information packets and provides referrals to other organizations dealing with special care in oral health. Special care is an approach to oral health management that is tailored to the specific needs of persons with a variety of medical, disabling or mental conditions.

National Associations & Support Groups

7084 American Dental Association

211 East Chicago Avenue
Chiacgo, IL 60611

312-440-2500
www.ada.org

Committed to the public's oral health, ethics, science and professional advancement; leading a unified profession through initiatives in advocacy, education, research and the development of standards.

7085 C.S. Mott Children's Hospital

1500 East Medical Center Drive
Ann Arbor, MI 48109

734-936-4000
www.med.umich.edu/mott

Provides information on how to handle a child's thumbsucking. Why they do it; how long it will last; how to help overcome the issue?

7086 Children's Hospital Boston

300 Longwood Avenue
Boston, MA 02115

617-355-6000
TTY: 617-355-0443
www.childrenshospital.org

Mission is to provide the highest quality care; be the leading source of reseach and discovery; educate the next generation of leaders in child health and enhance the health and well-being of the children and families in our local community.

James Mandell, MD, President & CEO
Sandra Fenwick, Chief Operating Officer

Web Sites

7087 American Dental Association
www.ada.org

Committed to the public's oral health, ethics, science and professional advancement; leading a unified profession through initiatives in advocacy, education, research and the development of standards.

7088 C.S. Mott Children's Hospital
www.med.umich.edu/mott

Provides information on how to handle a child's thumbsucking. Why they do it; how long it will last; how to help overcome the issue?

7089 Children's Hospital Boston
www.childrenshospital.org

Mission is to provide the highest quality care; be the leading source of reseach and discovery; educate the next generation of leaders in child health and enhance the health and well-being of the children and families in our local community.

7090 NIH/National Institute of Dental and Crani ofacial Research (NIHDCR)
www.nidcr.nih.gov

The mission is to promote the general health of American people by improving their oral, dental and craniofacial health. Through the conduct and support of research and training of researchers, the NIDCR aims to promote health, prevent diseases and conditions, and develop new diagnostic and therapeutics.

7091 National Oral Health Information Clearinghouse
www.nidcr.nih.gov

Produces and distributes patient and professional education materials including fact sheets, brochures, information packets and provides referrals to other organizations dealing with special care in oral health. Special care is an approach to oral health management that is tailored to the specific needs of persons with a variety of medical, disabling or mental conditions.

Pamphlets

7092 A Healthy Mouth for Your Baby
National Oral Health Information Clearinghouse
1 NOHIC Way
Bethesda, MD 20892

301-402-7364
Fax: 301-480-4098
TDD: 301-656-7581
e-mail: nidcrinfo@mail.nih.gov
www.nidcr.nih.gov

7093 Seal Out Tooth Decay
National Oral Health Information Clearinghouse
1 NOHIC Way
Bethesda, MD 20892

301-402-7364
Fax: 301-480-4098
TDD: 301-656-7581
e-mail: nidcrinfo@mail.nih.gov
www.nidcr.nih.gov

7094 Thumbsucking
Nat'l Institute of Dental & Craniofacial Research
31 Center Drive, MSC 2290
Bethesda, MD 20892

301-496-4261
Fax: 301-496-9988
www.nidr.nih.gov/

DESCRIPTION

7095 TICS

Covers these related disorders: Chronic motor tic disorder, Tourette syndrome, Transient tics of childhood
Involves the following Biologic System(s):
Neurologic Disorders

Tics are repetitive or stereotypical, compulsive, abrupt (spasmodic) movements of a muscle or muscle groups. Although any muscle may be affected, tics most commonly involve muscles of the eyes, face, neck, or shoulders. Movements may include blinking, sniffing, facial grimacing, lip smacking, tongue thrusting, or shoulder shrugging. Tics may begin as intentional movements to relieve perceived tension. However, they may rapidly become unintentional or involuntary in nature. Although tics are extremely difficult to suppress, most patients are able to do so for short periods. Tics are often worsened by stress or any perceived attention to the condition; in contrast, they typically disappear during sleep.

In most patients, tics become apparent between approximately five to 10 years of age. According to some estimates, as many as 25 percent of children may be affected. Most children may experience a spontaneous disappearance of tics within a few weeks or less than one year after onset. In such patients, the condition is referred to as transient tics of childhood. Supportive measures that may be helpful in alleviating transient tics include providing children with a tranquil environment as well as additional rest.

Some children may experience chronic motor tics that persist throughout adult life. In such patients, the condition is known as chronic motor tic disorder. Chronic motor tics may simultaneously affect muscles in up to three different muscle groups.

In contrast to transient tics of childhood and chronic motor tics, which are considered relatively benign, restricted tic disorders, a genetic, neurologic disorder known as Tourette syndrome is characterized by multiple, chronic, complex tics. Tourette syndrome usually becomes apparent in children between the ages of two to 14 years. Initial symptoms typically include motor tics of the face, eyelids, shoulders, and neck. Movements may include grimacing, excessive eye blinking, or stretching of the neck. Vocal (phonic) tics, such as involuntary coughing, grunting, barking, or throat clearing, are also common. Additional symptoms may include involuntary repetition of obscene words (coprolalia) or words spoken by other individuals (echolalia); aggressive behaviors; the performance of repetitive actions or impulses in response to recurrent, persistent thoughts (obsessive-compulsive behaviors); and secondary learning, emotional, or social difficulties. Researchers suggest that variable expression of the disease gene responsible for Tourette syndrome may cause transient tics of childhood or chronic motor tics in other individuals, indicating possible overlap between the conditions. Several studies have demonstrated that immediate (first-degree) relatives of patients with Tourette syndrome have an increased frequency of such tic conditions.

In some patients with severe chronic motor tic disorder, treatment may include therapy with certain medications (e.g., certain benzodiazepines or haloperidol). The treatment of Tourette syndrome is symptomatic and supportive and may include therapy with certain medications, such as haloperidol, pimozide, clonidine, clonazepam, or carbamazepine. In addition, for those with learning, behavioral, and social difficulties, multidisciplinary management and the provision of special social, academic, and vocational services may be important in helping patients achieve their potential. (Please refer to the section entitled Tourette Syndrome for further information on this disorder.)

See also **General Resources** on page 917

Government Agencies

7096 NIH/National Institute of Neurological Dis orders and Stroke (NINDS)
PO Box 5801
Bethesda, MD 20824

301-496-5751
800-352-9424
Fax: 301-496-0296
TTY: 301-468-5981
www.ninds.nih.gov

Works to reduce the burden of neurological disease by conducting, fostering, coordinating and guiding research on the causes, prevention, diagnosis and treatment of neurological disorders and stroke, while supporting basic research in related scientific areas.

Story C Landis Ph.D., Director
Audrey S Penn M.D., Deputy Director

National Associations & Support Groups

7097 American Academy of Child & Adolescent Psy chiatry
3615 Wisconsin Avenue NW
Washington, DC 20016

202-966-7300
Fax: 202-966-2891
www.aacap.org

Mission is to promote mentally healthy children, adolescents and families through research, training, advocacy, prevention, comprehensive diagnosis and treatment, peer support and collaboration.

Thomas F Anders M.D., President

7098 Genetic Alliance
4301 Connecticut Avenue NW
Washington, DC 20008

202-966-5557
800-336-4363
Fax: 202-966-8553
e-mail: info@geneticalliance.org
www.geneticalliance.org

A coalition of voluntary genetic support groups, consumers and professionals addressing the needs of individuals and families affected by genetic disorders from a national perspective.

Sharon Terry, President/CEO

7099 NADD: National Association for the Dually Diagnosed
132 Fair Street
Kingston, NY 12401

845-331-4336
800-331-5362
Fax: 845-331-4569
e-mail: info@thenadd.org
www.thenadd.org

Nonprofit organization designed to promote the interests of professional and parent development with resources for individuals who have the coexistence of mental illness and mental retardation. Provides conferences, educational services and training materials to professionals, parents, concerned citizens and service organizations.

Dr Robert Fletcher, CEO

7100 Tourette Syndrome Association
42-40 Bell Boulevard, Suite 205
Bayside, NY 11361

718-224-2999
888-486-8738
Fax: 718-279-9596
e-mail: ts@tsa-usa.org
www.tsa-usa.org

Dedicated to identifying the cause, finding the cure and controlling the effects of TS. Strives to improve the quality of life for all people with Tourette syndrome.

7101 WE MOVE (Worldwide Education and Advocacy for Movement Disorders)
204 W 84th Street
New York, NY 10024

212-241-8567
800-437-6682
Fax: 212-987-7363
e-mail: wemove@wemove.org
www.wemove.org

Provides movement disorder information and education materials to physicians, patients, the media and the public via its comprehensive web sites, training courses, and more. It's goal is to make early diagnosis, up-to-date treatment and patient support a reality for all people living with movement disorders.

Susan Bressman, President

Audio Video

7102 Dakota
Tourette Syndrome Association
42-40 Bell Boulevard
Bayside, NY 11361

718-224-2999
888-486-8738
Fax: 718-279-9596
e-mail: ts@tsa-usa.org
tsa-usa.org

A happy eleven year old baseball playing, video game whiz, Dakota is diagnosed with Tourette's Syndrome and ADHD.

7 minutes

7103 Family Life with Tourette Syndrome... Personal Stories
Tourette Syndrome Association
42-40 Bell Boulevard
Bayside, NY 11361

718-224-2999
888-486-8738
Fax: 718-279-9596
e-mail: ts@tsa-usa.org
tsa-usa.org

In extended, in-depth interviews, all the people engagingly profiled in After the Diagnosis...The Next Steps, reveal the individual ways they developed to deal with TS. Each shows us that the key to leading a successful life in spite of having TS, is having a loving, supportive network of family and friends. Available in its entirety or as separate vignettes.

58 minutes

7104 Ryan
Tourette Syndrome Association
42-40 Bell Boulevard
Bayside, NY 11361

718-224-2999
888-486-8738
Fax: 718-279-9596
e-mail: ts@tsa-usa.org
tsa-usa.org

Ryan's family first thought his behavior was a deliberate way to get attention, later educate themselves and others about Ryan's Tourette's Syndrome.

11 minutes

7105 The Turners
Tourette Syndrome Association
42-40 Bell Boulevard
Bayside, NY 11361

718-224-2999
888-486-8738
Fax: 718-279-9596
e-mail: ts@tsa-usa.org
tsa-usa.org

Three of the four Turner daughters have Tourette's Syndrome in varying degress.

12 minutes

Web Sites

7106 American Academy of Child & Adolescent Psychiatry
www.aacap.org

Mission is to promote mentally healthy children, adolescents and families through research, training, advocacy, prevention, comprehensive diagnosis and treatment, peer support and collaboration.

7107 MHG Neurology Web Forums
www.mgh.harvard.edu/forum

7108 NADD: National Association for the Dually Diagnosed
www.thenadd.org

Nonprofit organization designed to promote the interests of professional and parent development with resources for individuals who have the coexistence of mental illness and mental retardation. Provides conferences, educational services and training materials to professionals, parents, concerned citizens and service organizations.

7109 NIH/National Institute of Neurological Disorders and Stroke (NINDS)
www.ninds.nih.gov

Works to reduce the burden of neurological disease by conducting, fostering, coordinating and guiding research on the causes, prevention, diagnosis and treatment of neurological disorders and stroke, while supporting basic research in related scientific areas.

7110 Online Mendelian Inheritance in Man
www.ncbi.nlm.nih.gov

This database is a catalog of human genes and genetic disorders.

7111 Parents Helping Parents
php.com

Mission is to help children with special needs revive the resources, love, hope, respect, health care, education, and other services they need to reach their full potential by providing them with strong families, dedicated professionals and responsive systems to serve them.

7112 Tourette Spectrum Disorder Association
www,tourettesyndrome.org

The Tourette Spectrum Disorder Association (TSDA) mission is to promote awareness, greater understanding and to increase education about TS and it's spectrum of manifestations among professionals, the general public, and individuals with TS in order to facilitate the early accurate diagnosis of TS and its associated disorders and to promote sympathetic, appropriate treatment for those with this disorder.

7113 Tourette Syndrome Association
www.tsa-usa.org

Dedicated to identifying the cause, finding the cure and controlling the effects of TS. Strives to improve the quality of life for all people with Tourette syndrome.

7114 Tourette Syndrome Online
www.tourette-syndrome.com

Devoted to children and adults with Tourette syndrome disorder and their families, friends, teachers and medical professionals.

7115 WE MOVE (Worldwide Education and Advocacy for Movement Disorders)
www.wemove.org

Provides movement disorder information and education materials to physicians, patients, the media and the public via its comprehensive web sites, training courses, and more. It's goal is to make early diagnosis, up-to-date treatment and patient support a reality for all people living with movement disorders.

Book Publishers

7116 A Mind of its Own, Tourette's Syndrome: A Story and a Guide
Oxford University Press
198 Madison Avenue
New York, NY 10016

212-726-6000
800-451-7556
Fax: 919-677-1303
oup-usa.org/orbs/

Composed of two parts which interrelate with each other. One part is an on-going story about Michael, a boy with TS, and his family and friends. Michael is a fictional composite character drawn from experience with many patients. Portrays a relatively mild case because the majority of the cases are mild. The second part consists of factual information which we have tried to present in a clear and readable manner. Includes illustration, some tables and other materials that may be of interest.

174 pages
ISBN: 0-195065-87-5

7117 Cognitive-Behavioral Management of Tic Disorders
John Wiley & Sons
111 River Street
Hoboken, NJ 07030

201-748-6000
Fax: 201-748-6088
e-mail: info@wiley.com
www.wiley.com

Provides a comprehensive review of what is known about the occurance and diagnosis of Tics.

2005 Paperback
ISBN: 0-470093-80-1

7118 Hi, I'm Adam
Hope Press
PO Box 188
Duarte, CA 91009

800-321-4039
Fax: 626-358-3520
www.hopepress.com

Adam Buehrens is ten years old and has Tourette syndrome. Adam wrote and illustrated this book because he wants everyone to know he and other children with Tourette syndrome are not crazy. They just hava a common neurological disorder. If you know a child that has tics, temper tantrums, unreasonable fears, or problems dealing with school, you will find this a reassuring story.

7119 Teaching the Tiger
Hope Press
PO Box 188
Duarte, CA 91009

800-321-4039
Fax: 626-358-3520
www.hopepress.com

A handbook for innovative methods of teaching children with ADD, Tourette Syndrome, and Obsessive-Compulsive Disorders.

ISBN: 1-878267-34-5

7120 Tourette Syndrome
Dilligaf Publishing for Awareness Project
64 Court Street
Ellsworth, ME 04605

207-667-5031

Includes an overview on the syndrome and tips of how to recognize traditional tics in the classroom; evaluation and referral are the basic components of this easy-to-read, basic book for the classroom teacher.

20 pages

7121 Tourette's Syndrome - Tics, Obsession, Com pulsions: Developmental Psychopathology
John Wiley & Sons
111 River Street
Hoboken, NJ 07030

201-748-6000
Fax: 201-748-6088
e-mail: info@wiley.com
www.wiley.com

Once thought to be rare, Tourette's Syndrome is now seen as a relatively common childhood disorder either in its complete or partial incarnations. Drawing on the work of contributors hailing from the prestigeous Yale University Child Psychiatry Department, this edited volume explores the disorder from many perspectives, mapping out the diagnosis, genetics, phenomenology, natural history, and treatment of Tourette's syndrome.

1998 600 pages Hardcover
ISBN: 0-471160-37-7

7122 What Makes Ryan Tic?
Hope Press
PO Box 188
Duarte, CA 91009

800-321-4039
Fax: 626-358-3520
www.hopepress.com

A moving and informative story of how a mother struggled with the many behavioral problems presented by her son with Tourette syndrome, ADHD and oppostional defiant disorder.

Journals

7123 Movement Disorders
John Wiley & Sons
111 River Street
Hoboken, NJ 07030

201-748-6000
Fax: 201-748-6088
e-mail: info@wiley.com
www.wiley.com

Publishes reviews, viewpoints, full length articles, historical reports, brief reports, clinical/scientific notes, videotape briefs, patient/imaging briefs, and letters. ISSN: 0885-3185

Vol 22 13 Issues

Pamphlets

7124 Matthew and Tics
Tourette Syndrome Association
42-40 Bell Boulevard
Bayside, NY 11361

718-224-2999
888-486-8738
Fax: 718-279-9596
e-mail: ts@tsa-usa.org
tsa-usa.org

A story for young children with Tourette's Syndrome and their peers; promotes acceptance and understanding.

7125 Tics and Tourette's Syndrome Fact Sheet
Movement Disorder Resource Center - WE MOVE
204 E 84th Street
New York, NY 10024

212-241-8567
800-437-6682
Fax: 212-987-7363
www.life-in-motion.org

Provides overviews of both diseases.

DESCRIPTION

7126 TOURETTE SYNDROME

Synonyms: Gilles de la Tourette syndrome, GTS
Involves the following Biologic System(s):
Neurologic Disorders

Tourette syndrome is a neurologic disorder that typically becomes apparent in children between the ages of two to 14 years, with approximately 50 percent of cases occurring before seven years of age. The disorder, which is thought to affect about one in 2,000 individuals, is approximately three times more prevalent in males than females and is more common among Caucasians than other populations. In children with Tourette syndrome, associated symptoms and findings vary greatly in range and severity. Initial symptoms may include involuntary, repetitive (stereotypical) muscle movements (motor tics) of the face, eyelids, shoulders, and neck, such as grimacing, abrupt head turning, excessive eye blinking, or stretching of the neck. In some patients with severe symptoms, motor tics may evolve to include self-mutilating behaviors, such as nail biting, lip biting, or facial punching. Children with Tourette syndrome may also develop vocal tics, such as involuntary coughing, grunting, barking, sniffling, or throat clearing. As the disease progresses, additional symptoms may develop including involuntary repetition of obscene words (coprolalia), words spoken by other individuals (echolalia), or one's own words (palilalia) or imitation of other individuals' behaviors (echokinesis or echopraxia). The symptoms associated with Tourette syndrome may periodically decrease or increase in intensity; may subside during high levels of concentration, such as when reading or studying; and may worsen with stress. Tourette syndrome is considered a life-long disorder; however, in approximately 50 to 66 percent of patients, symptoms significantly decrease about 10 to 15 years after initial diagnosis and treatment.

Children with Tourette syndrome may also experience associated behavioral abnormalities, such as aggressive behavior or the performance of repetitive actions or impulses in response to recurrent, persistent thoughts (obsessive-compulsive behaviors). Obsessive-compulsive behaviors are typically performed to help neutralize obsessive thoughts and relieve anxieties. Many affected children may also develop learning, emotional, or social difficulties. The treatment of Tourette syndrome is symptomatic and supportive and may include therapy with certain medications, such as haloperidol, pimozide, clonidine, clonazepam, or carbamazepine. In addition, for those with learning, behavioral, and social difficulties, multidisciplinary management and the provision of special social, academic, and vocational services may be important in helping patients achieve their potential.

Although the exact cause of Tourette syndrome is unknown, studies suggest that the disorder may result due to abnormalities of neurotransmitter (dopamine) activity within a certain area of the brain (basal ganglia). In most cases, Tourette syndrome is thought to be inherited as an autosomal dominant trait that occurs as the result of changes (mutations) in a gene located on the long arm (q) of chromosome 18 (18q22.1). Some children with mutations of this disease gene may not have symptoms associated with the disorder (incomplete penetrance). In addition, in those children with the defective gene who do have symptoms associated with Tourette syndrome, such symptoms may vary in range and severity from case to case (variable expressivity). Such variability of gene expression and penetrance may be suggested by the fact that immediate (first-degree) relatives of patients have an increased frequency of Tourette syndrome, tic conditions, and obsessive-compulsive disorder. In addition, some researchers suspect that Tourette syndrome may result from inheritance of a disease gene in combination with certain environmental factors that may trigger the gene's expression (multifactorial inheritance). Research suggests that individuals who have two copies of a disease gene for Tourette syndrome (homozygotes) typically express the disorder, whereas some who inherit one disease gene (heterozygotes) may not develop the disorder unless particular environmental factors (e.g., infection, such as due to exposure to Group A beta-hemolytic streptococcus) trigger its expression. Tourette syndrome is associated with a vary of misconceptions, for instance, that people with Tourette syndrome are mentally disturbed and that they always exhibit coprolalia. Tourette's is a neurological condition that (according to the most recent research) is primarily genetic in nature. Although there may be learning disabilities associated with Tourette's, the brain is wholly undamaged in respect to intellectual functioning. Statistically, coprolalia is present in less than 5% of TS patients.

See also **General Resources** on page 917

National Associations & Support Groups

7127 American Academy of Child & Adolescent Psy chiatry
3615 Wisconsin Avenue NW
Washington, DC 20016

202-966-7300
Fax: 202-966-2891
www.aacap.org

Mission is to promote mentally healthy children, adolescents and families through research, training, advocacy, prevention, comprehensive diagnosis and treatment, peer support and collaboration.

Thomas F Anders M.D., President

7128 Children's Hospital Boston
300 Longwood Avenue
Boston, MA 02115

617-355-6000
TTY: 617-355-0443
www.childrenshospital.org

Mission is to provide the highest quality care; be the leading source of reseach and discovery; educate the next generation of leaders in child health and enhance the health and well-being of the children and families in our local community.

James Mandell, MD, President & CEO
Sandra Fenwick, Chief Operating Officer

7129 Genetic Alliance
4301 Connecticut Avenue NW
Washington, DC 20008

202-966-5557
800-336-4363
Fax: 202-966-8553
e-mail: info@geneticalliance.org
www.geneticalliance.org

A coalition of voluntary genetic support groups, consumers and professionals addressing the needs of individuals and families affected by genetic disorders from a national perspective.

Sharon Terry, President/CEO

7130 Tourette Syndrome Association
42-40 Bell Boulevard, Suite 205
Bayside, NY 11361

718-224-2999
888-486-8738
Fax: 718-279-9596
e-mail: ts@tsa-usa.org
http://tsa-usa.org

Dedicated to identifying the cause, finding the cure and controlling the effects of TS. Strives to improve the quality of life for all people with Tourette syndrome.

7131 Tourette Syndrome Association - Massachusetts Chapter
PO Box 653
Marston's Mills, MA 02648

617-277-7589

Offers a newsletter and an educator's conference.

7132 Tourette Syndrome Association of New Jersey
26 W High Street
Somerville, NJ 08876

732-972-4459
e-mail: NJTSA@AOL.COM
www.tsanj.org

7133 WE MOVE (Worldwide Education and Advocacy for Movement Disorders)
204 W 84th Street
New York, NY 10024

212-241-8567
800-437-6682
Fax: 212-987-7363
e-mail: wemove@wemove.org
www.wemove.org

A nonprofit organization dedicated to educating and informing patients, professionals and the public about the latest clinical advances, managment and treatment options for neurologic movement disorders.

Susan Bressman, President

State Agencies & Support Groups

Arizona

7134 Tourette Syndrome Association-Arizona Chap ter
PO Box 41406
Tucson, AZ 85717

520-620-2288
www.tsaarizona.org

Bill Peterson, President

Connecticut

7135 Tourette Syndrome Association-Connecticut Chapter
915 Brickyard Road
Woodstock, CT 06281

203-912-7310
e-mail: ts@tsact.org
www.tsact.org

Donna Blain, Director

Florida

7136 Tourette Syndrome Association-Florida Chap ter
PO Box 7123
St. Petersburg, FL 33734

727-418-0249
e-mail: tsafleducation@yahoo.com
www.tsa-fl.org

Donna Sakuta, Executive Director

Georgia

7137 Tourette Syndrome Association-Georgia and South Carolina Chapter
PO Box 568112
Atlanta, GA 31156

770-901-9998
888-799-2101
e-mail: tsageorgia@bellsouth.net
www.tsaofga-sc.org

Illinois

7138 Tourette Syndrome Association-Illinois Cha pter
800 Roosevelt Road, Building A, Suite 10
Glen Ellyn, IL 60137

630-790-8083
877-TSA-IL55
www.tsa-illinois.org

Sande S Shamash, Executive Director

Indiana

7139 Tourette Syndrome Association-Indiana Chap ter
PO Box 49
Clear Creek, IN 47426

812-333-7076
e-mail: admin@tsaindiana.org
www.tsaindiana.org

Maryland

7140 Tourette Syndrome Association-Greater Wash ington
33 University Boulevard East
Silver Spring, MD 20901

301-681-4133
877-295-2148
Fax: 301-576-4527
e-mail: tsagw@aol.com
www.tsagw.org

Serving Washington, D.C., Maryland, Virginia, and West Virginia

Sue Jacob, Executive Director

Minnesota

7141 Tourette Syndrome Association-Minnesota Ch apter
2233 University Avenue, Suite 338
St. Paul, MN 55114

651-646-0099
e-mail: director@tsa-mn.org
www.tsa-mn.org

Maureen Kenney, Executive Director

New Jersey

7142 Tourette Syndrome Association-New Jersey C hapter
50 Division Street, Suite 205
Somerville, NJ 08876

908-575-7350
Fax: 908-575-8699
www.tsanj.org

Tim Omaggio, President

New York

7143 Tourette Syndrome Association-Greater New York State Chapter
20 Thomas Jefferson Lane
Synder, NY 14226

716-839-4430
Fax: 716-839-1956
e-mail: conners@adelphia.net
www.tsa-gnys.org

Susan Conners, President

7144 Tourette Syndrome Association-Long Island Chapter
PO Box 615
Jericho, NY 11753

516-876-6947
www.li-tsa.org

Lisa Filippi, Chair

7145 Tourette Syndrome Association-New York Cit y Chapter
www.tsa-nyc.org

646-202-9683
www.tsa-nyc.org

7146 Tourette Syndrome Association-New York Hud son Valley Chapter
PO Box 517
Ardsley, NY 10502

914-378-5025
e-mail: info@tsa-nyhv.org
www.tsa-nyhv.org

Serves Westchester, Rockland, Orange, Putnam, Dutchess and Ulster Counties in New York.

7147 Tourette Syndrome Association-Rochester Ch apter
PO Box 129
Penfield, NY 14526

585-987-5196
e-mail: tsa@touretterochester.org
www.touretterochester.org

Ohio

7148 Tourette Syndrome Association-Ohio Chapter
PO Box 28345
Columbus, OH 43228

614-539-1795
800-543-2675
e-mail: admin@tsaohio.org
www.tsaohio.org

Pennsylvania

7149 Tourette Syndrome Association-Pennsylvania Chapter
132 W Middle Street
Gettysburg, PA 17325

717-337-1134
800-990-3300
Fax: 717-337-1960
e-mail: info@patsainc.org
www.patsainc.org

Laura Umbrell, Administrator

Utah

7150 Tourette Syndrome Association-Utah Chapter
PO Box 701312
West Valley City, UT 84170

801-967-2125
866-274-0700
e-mail: maren@tsa-utah.org
www.tsa-utah.org

Maren Farmer, Chairman

Washington

7151 Tourette Syndrome Association-Washington State Chapter
318 West Galer Street
Seattle, WA 98119

206-621-2108
e-mail: tsawashingtonchapter@yahoo.com
www.tourette.net/wa

Includes Oregon

Research Centers

7152 Tourette Syndrome Clini
Yale Child Study Center
230 S Frontage Road
New Haven, CT 06510

203-785-2513
info.med.yale.edu

Clinical care center offering research solely into the causes, symptoms and treatments for persons with Tourette syndrome.

James F Leckman, MD

7153 Tourette Syndrome Clinic
Cincinnati Children's Hospital Medical Center
333 Burnet Avenue
Cincinnati, OH 45229

513-636-4200
800-344-2462
TTY: 513-636-4900
e-mail: tics@cchmc.org
www.cincinnatichildrens.org

Clinic that specializes in evaluating, diagnosing and treating kids, adolescents and adults with Tourette's Syndrome symptoms, including tics, hyperactivity, attention deficits, obsessive compulsive behaviors and other symptoms of Tourette Syndrome.

Donald L Gilbert, MD, MS, Director

Audio Video

7154 After the Diagnosis...The Next Steps
Tourette Syndrome Association
42-40 Bell Boulevard, Suite 205
Bayside, NY 11361

718-224-2999
888-486-8738
Fax: 718-279-9596
e-mail: ts@tsa-usa.org
www.tsa-usa.org

When the diagnosis is Tourette syndrome, what do you do first? How do you sort out the complexities of the disorder? Whose advice do you follow? What steps do you take to lead a normal life? Six people with TS—as different as any six people can be—relate the sometimes difficult, but finally triumphant path each took to lead the rich, fulfilling life they now enjoy. Narrated by Academy Award-winning actor, Richard Dreyfuss, the stories are refreshing blends of poignancy, fact and inspiration.

35 Minutes

7155 Clinical Counseling: Toward a Better Understanding of TS

Tourette Syndrome Association
42-40 Bell Boulevard, Suite 205
Bayside, NY 11361

718-224-2999
888-486-8738
Fax: 718-279-9596
e-mail: ts@tsa-usa.org
www.tsa-usa.org

Certain key issues often surface during the counseling sessions of people with TS and their families. These important areas of concern are explored for counselors, social workers, educators, psychologists and other allied professionals. Expert clinical practitioners offer invaluable insights for those working with people affected by Tourette syndrome.

14 Minutes

7156 Complexities of TS Treatment: A Physician's Roundtable

Tourette Syndrome Association
42-40 Bell Boulevard, Suite 205
Bayside, NY 11361

718-224-2999
888-486-8738
Fax: 718-279-9596
e-mail: ts@tsa-usa.org
www.tsa-usa.org

Three of the most highly regarded experts in the diagnosis and treatment of Tourette syndrome offer insight, advice and treatment strategies to fellow physicians and other healthcare professionals.

15 Minutes

7157 Dakota

Tourette Syndrome Association
42-40 Bell Boulevard
Bayside, NY 11361

718-224-2999
888-486-8738
Fax: 718-279-9596
e-mail: ts@tsa-usa.org
www.tsa-usa.org

A happy eleven year old baseball playing, video game whiz, Dakota is diagnosed with Tourette's Syndrome and ADHD.

7 minutes

7158 Echolalia

Hope Press
PO Box 188
Duarte, CA 91009

800-321-4039
Fax: 626-358-3520
www.hopepress.com

A story about a best selling writer who is diagnosed at age 35 with having Tourette syndrome.

David E Comings, MD, Presenter

7159 Family Life with Tourette Syndrome

Tourette Syndrome Association
42-40 Bell Boulevard, Suite 205
Bayside, NY 11361

718-224-2999
888-486-8738
Fax: 718-279-9596
e-mail: ts@tsa-usa.org
www.tsa-usa.org

In extended, in-depth interviews, all the people engagingly profiled in After the Diagnosis...The Next Steps, reveal the individual ways they developed to deal with TS. Each show us that the key to leading a successful life in spite of having TS, is having a loving, supportive network of family and friends.

7160 Family Life with Tourette Syndrome... Personal Stories

Tourette Syndrome Association
42-40 Bell Boulevard
Bayside, NY 11361

718-224-2999
888-486-8738
Fax: 718-279-9596
e-mail: ts@tsa-usa.org
tsa-usa.org

In extended, in-depth interviews, all the people engagingly profiled in After the Diagnosis...The Next Steps, reveal the individual ways they developed to deal with TS. Each shows us that the key to leading a successful life in spite of having TS, is having a loving, supportive network of family and friends. Available in its entirety or as separate vignettes.

58 minutes

7161 Gift of Hope

Tourette Syndrome Association
42-40 Bell Boulevard, Suite 205
Bayside, NY 11361

718-224-2999
Fax: 718-279-9596
www.tsa-usa.org

The cause of Tourette syndrome lies in the brain. This video offers five people who have TS explaining their reasons for agreeing to register with TSA's Brain Bank Program.

14 minutes

7162 Kevin and Me

Hope Press
PO Box 188
Duarte, CA 91009

800-321-4039
Fax: 626-358-3520
www.hopepress.com

A memoir of a single moter who struggled with her son's Tourette syndrome and discovered music therapy as a magincal influence on him and their relationship.

David E Comings, MD, Presenter

7163 Ryan

Tourette Syndrome Association
42-40 Bell Boulevard
Bayside, NY 11361

718-224-2999
888-486-8738
Fax: 718-279-9596
e-mail: ts@tsa-usa.org
tsa-usa.org

Ryan's family first thought his behavior was a deliberate way to get attention, lateer educate themselves and others about Ryan's Tourette's Syndrome.

11 minutes

7164 The Turners
Tourette Syndrome Association
42-40 Bell Boulevard
Bayside, NY 11361

718-224-2999
888-486-8738
Fax: 718-279-9596
e-mail: ts@tsa-usa.org
tsa-usa.org

Three of the four Turner daughters have Tourette's Syndrome in varying degress.

12 minutes

7165 Understanding and Treating the Hereditary Psychiatric Spectrum Disorders
Hope Press
PO Box 188
Duarte, CA 91009

800-321-4039
Fax: 626-358-3520
www.hopepress.com

Learn with ten hours of audio tapes from a two day seminar given in May 1997 by David E Comings, MD. Tapes cover: ADHD, Tourette syndrome, obsessive-compulsive disorder, conduct disorder, oppositional defiant disorder, autism and other hereditary psychiatric spectrum disorders. Eight Audio tapes.

David E Comings, MD, Presenter

Web Sites

7166 American Academy of Child & Adolescent Psy chiatry
www.aacap.org

Mission is to promote mentally healthy children, adolescents and families through research, training, advocacy, prevention, comprehensive diagnosis and treatment, peer support and collaboration.

7167 American Academy of Neurology: Tourette Syndrome
www.aan.com/public/tour.html

A specialty medical society established to advance the art and science of neurology and therby promote the best possible care for patients with neurological disorders by: ensuring appropriate access to neurological care, supporting and advocating for an environment which ensures ethical, high quality neurological care, and providing excellence in professional education by offering a variety of programs in the clinical aspects of neurology and the basic neuroscience to healh professionals.

7168 Children's Hospital Boston
www.childrenshospital.org

Mission is to provide the highest quality care; be the leading source of reseach and discovery; educate the next generation of leaders in child health and enhance the health and well-being of the children and families in our local community.

7169 Health Answers
www.healthanswers.com

HealthAnswers offers a breadth of services in medical education, sales force training, patient support solutions, professional promotion and consumer solutions.

7170 MHG Neurology Web Forums
www.mgh.harvard.edu/forum

7171 NIH/National Institute of Neurological Dis orders and Stroke (NINDS)
www.ninds.nih.gov

The mission of NINDS is to reduce the burden of neurological disease - a burden borne by every age group, by every segment of society, by people all over the world.

7172 Online Mendelian Inheritance in Man
www.ncbi.nlm.nih.gov

This database is a catalog of human genes and genetic disorders.

7173 Parents Helping Parents
www.php.com

Mission is to help children with special needs revive the resources, love, hope, respect, health care, education, and other services they need to reach their full potential by providing them with strong families, dedicated professionals, and responsive systems to serve them.

7174 Tourette Spectrum Disorder Association
www.tourettesyndrome.org

Mission is to promote awareness, greater understanding and to increase education about TS and its spectrum of manifestations among professionals, the general public and individuals with TS in order to facilitate the early accurate disgnosis of TS and its associated disorders to promote sympathetic. appropriate treatment for those with this disorder.

7175 Tourette Syndrome Association
www.tsa-usa.org

Is the only voluntary nonprofit membership organization in this field. Its mission is to identify the cause of, find the cure for and control the effects of this disorder.

7176 Tourette Syndrome Global Awareness Program
home.c2i.net/tourette

We work for an exchange of information between people in all countries - in order to make a bond between people working for TS in all parts of the world.

7177 Tourettes Syndrome Online
www.tourettes-syndrome.com

Devoted to children and adults with Tourette Syndrome disorder and their families, friends, teachers and medical professionals.

Book Publishers

7178 Adam and the Magic Marble
Hope Press
PO Box 188
Duarte, CA 91009

800-321-4039
Fax: 626-358-3520
www.hopepress.com

7179 Children With Tourette Syndrome: A Parents Guide
Peytral Publications
P.O. Box 1162
Minnetonka, MN 55345

952-949-8707
877-739-8725
Fax: 952-906-9777
www.peytral.com

Informative handbook for parents of children and teens; covers medical, educational, legal, family life, daily care, emotional issues and more.

352 pages

7180 Children with Tourette Syndrome: A Parent's Guide-2nd Edition
ADD WareHouse
300 NW 70th Avenue, Suite 102
Plantation, FL 33317

954-792-8100
800-233-9273
Fax: 954-792-8545
www.addwarehouse.com

The first guide written specifically for parents and other family members is a collaboration by a team of medical specialists, therapists, people with TS, and parents. It provides a complete introduction to TS and how it's diagnosed and treated. Also, chapters on family life, emotions, education and legal rights

2007 361 pages

7181 Don't Think About Monkeys: Extraordinary Stories Written by People with Tourette
Hope Press
PO Box 188
Duarte, CA 91009

800-321-4039
Fax: 626-358-3520
www.hopepress.com

Collection of fourteen stories written by teenager and adults with Tourette syndrome, describing how they have managed to cope and live with disorder. Especially inspiring to others with this and similar disorders.

200 pages
ISBN: 1-878267-33-7

7182 Hi! I'm Adam!
Hope Press
PO Box 188
Duarte, CA 91009

800-321-4039
Fax: 626-358-3520
www.hopepress.com

7183 Living with Tourette Syndrome
Simon & Schuster
611 W Bay Street
Tampa, FL 33606

888-793-9972

Provides valuable advice for children and adults with TS, their families, co-workers, teachers and friends. Describes the symptoms and related disorders, exposes many myths surrounding the disease, and advises adults on business and personal relationships.

256 pages
ISBN: 0-684811-60-0

7184 Matthew and the Tics
Tourette Syndrome Association
42-40 Bell Boulevard, Suite 205
Bayside, NY 11361

718-224-2999
Fax: 718-279-9596
e-mail: ts@tsa-usa.org
www.tsa-usa.org

A story for young children with TS and their peers.

2 pages

7185 Mind of It's Own: Tourette Syndrome
Oxford University Press
2001 Evans Road
Cary, NC 27513

212-726-6000
Fax: 919-677-1303
www.oup-usa.org

1994 192 pages
ISBN: 0-195065-87-5

7186 RYAN: A Mother's Story of Her Hyperactive/ Tourette Syndrome Child
Hope Press
PO Box 188
Duarte, CA 91009

800-321-4039
Fax: 626-358-3520
www.hopepress.com

A moving and informative story of how a mother struggled with the many behavioral problems presented by her son with Tourette syndrome, ADHD and oppositional defiant disorder.

7187 Raising Joshua
Hope Press
PO Box 188
Duarte, CA 91009

800-321-4039
Fax: 626-358-3520
www.hopepress.com

A mothers story of Josh, a boy with Tourette syndrome and attention deficit hyperactivity disorder.

7188 Teaching the Tiger
Hope Press
PO Box 188
Duarte, CA 91009

800-321-4039
Fax: 626-358-3520
www.hopepress.com

A handbook for individuals involved with the education of children with Tourette Syndrome, ADD, and OCD.

Handbook
ISBN: 1-878267-34-5

7189 Tourette Syndrome and Human Behavior
Hope Press
PO Box 188
Duarte, CA 91009

800-321-4039
Fax: 626-358-3520
www.hopepress.com

Available in hardcover.

7190 Tourette Syndrome: Advances in Neurology, Volume 58
Tourette Syndrome Association
42-40 Bell Boulevard, Suite 205
Bayside, NY 11361

718-224-2999
888-4TO-URET
Fax: 718-279-9596

In this single-volume reference, more than 90 of the foremost research and clinical leaders in the field review the current state of knowledge about this disorder.

400 pages

Thomas N Chase, MD, Editor
Arnold J Friedhoff, MD

7191 Tourette Syndrome: The Facts
Oxford University Press
2001 Evans Road
Cary, NC 27513

212-726-6000
Fax: 919-677-1303
www.oup-usa.org

A guide for clinicians, general practitioners, school teachers, and anyone seeking an accsible introduction the disorder.

1998 122 pages
ISBN: 0-198523-98-X

7192 Tourette's Syndrome
ADD WareHouse
300 NW 70th Avenue, Suite 102
Plantation, FL 33317

954-792-8100
800-233-9273
Fax: 954-792-8545
www.addwarehouse.com

Provides any information needed on Torette's Syndrome.

2001 400 pages
ISBN: 0-596500-07-6

7193 Unwelcome Companion: An Insider's View of Tourette Syndrome
Silver Run Publications
124 Partridge Lane
Athens, GA 30606

706-549-7463

This book is full of medical information about the causes and treatments of TS, making it a valuable resource for patients, families and doctors.

1995 135 pages
ISBN: 0-964637-61-8

7194 What Makes Ryan Tic?
Hope Press
PO Box 188
Duarte, CA 91009

800-321-4039
Fax: 626-358-3520
www.hopepress.com

Newsletters

7195 Tourette Syndrome Association Newsletter
42-40 Bell Boulevard, Suite 205
Bayside, NY 11361

718-224-2999
Fax: 718-279-9596
e-mail: ts@tsa-usa.org
tsa-usa.org

Offers information, articles and news on the latest technology and advancements for persons with Tourette syndrome.

Quarterly

Pamphlets

7196 Commentary on Alternative Therapies for Tourette Syndrome
Tourette Syndrome Association
42-40 Bell Boulevard, Suite 205
Bayside, NY 11361

718-224-2999
Fax: 718-279-9596

Summarizes physician/patient reports of symptom management through nonpharmacological interventions.

2 pages

7197 Consumer's Guide to Tourette Syndrome Medications
Tourette Syndrome Association
42-40 Bell Boulevard, Suite 205
Bayside, NY 11361

718-224-2999
Fax: 718-279-9596

Covers common medications used for the control of TS motor and vocal tics as well as those traditionally prescribed for associated behaviors.

1992 12 pages

7198 Coping with Tourette Syndrome in the Classroom
Tourette Syndrome Association
42-40 Bell Boulevard, Suite 205
Bayside, NY 11361

718-224-2999
Fax: 718-279-9596

Includes practical guidelines for education developed from a study about cognitive effects on learning.

7199 Coping with Tourette Syndrome, A Parent's Viewpoint
Tourette Syndrome Association
42-40 Bell Boulevard, Suite 205
Bayside, NY 11361

718-224-2999
Fax: 718-279-9596

An acclaimed medical writer and mother of three children with TS, the author sensitively addresses common concerns and feelings of parents.

7200 Current Pharmacology of Tourette Syndrome
Tourette Syndrome Association
42-40 Bell Boulevard, Suite 205
Bayside, NY 11361

718-224-2999
Fax: 718-279-9596

Covers all current medications used to treat TS with specific information about clinical evaluations and diagnosis.

12 pages

7201 Dental Treatment of Patients with Gilles de la Tourette Syndrome
Tourette Syndrome Association
42-40 Bell Boulevard, Suite 205
Bayside, NY 11361

718-224-2999
Fax: 718-279-9596

Discusses TS movements and possible adverse interactions of dentistry and TS medications.

5 pages

7202 Development of Behavioral and Emotional Problems in Tourette Syndrome
Tourette Syndrome Association
42-40 Bell Boulevard, Suite 205
Bayside, NY 11361

718-224-2999
Fax: 718-279-9596

Using the Child Behavior Checklist, 78 male children were assessed for a variety of behavioral problems. Relation to tic severity covered.

7203 Discipline and the Child with Tourette Syndrome
Tourette Syndrome Association
42-40 Bell Boulevard, Suite 205
Bayside, NY 11361

718-224-2999
Fax: 718-279-9596

Helps children redirect impulses and compulsions through teaching cause and effect relationships.

7204 Educator's Guide to Tourette Syndrome
Tourette Syndrome Association
42-40 Bell Boulevard, Suite 205
Bayside, NY 11361

718-224-2999
Fax: 718-279-9596

Covers symptoms, treatments and techniques for classroom management, attentional, writing and language problems.

16 pages

7205 Genetics of Tourette's Syndrome: Who it Affects and How it Occurs in Families
Tourette Syndrome Association
42-40 Bell Boulevard, Suite 205
Bayside, NY 11361

718-224-2999
Fax: 718-279-9596

10 pages

7206 Georges Gilles de la Tourette-The Man and His Times
Tourette Syndrome Association
42-40 Bell Boulevard, Suite 205
Bayside, NY 11361

718-224-2999
Fax: 718-279-9596

Rare historical biography of the famous French neurologist G. Gilles De La Tourette.

7207 Getting Into College: Strategies for the Student with Tourette Syndrome
Tourette Syndrome Association
42-40 Bell Boulevard, Suite 205
Bayside, NY 11361

718-224-2999
Fax: 718-279-9596

7208 Gift of Hope
Tourette Syndrome Association
42-40 Bell Boulevard, Suite 205
Bayside, NY 11361

718-224-2999
Fax: 718-279-9596

TSA Brain Bank Program registration information. Includes donor cards.

7209 Grandparents Club
Tourette Syndrome Association
42-40 Bell Boulevard, Suite 205
Bayside, NY 11361

718-224-2999
Fax: 718-279-9596

A flyer describing how to join with other grandparents to support TS research to benefit future generations.

7210 Guide to Diagnosis & Treatment
Tourette Syndrome Association
42-40 Bell Boulevard, Suite 205
Bayside, NY 11361

718-224-2999
Fax: 718-279-9596

Covers symptoms, pharmacology and clinical assessments.

7211 Health Insurance Issues and Solutions for People with Torette Syndrome
Tourette Syndrome Association
42-40 Bell Boulevard, Suite 205
Bayside, NY 11361

718-224-2999
Fax: 718-279-9596

Detailed, up-to-date packet of medical information for obtaining health insurance as well as information for submission to insurance carriers.

7212 Helpful Techniques to Aid the Student with Tourette Syndrome
Tourette Syndrome Association
42-40 Bell Boulevard, Suite 205
Bayside, NY 11361

718-224-2999
Fax: 718-279-9596

Helpful hints for teacher with specific suggestions for test taking, math computation, and note taking.

1 pages

7213 Just Right
Tourette Syndrome Association
42-40 Bell Boulevard, Suite 205
Bayside, NY 11361

718-224-2999
Fax: 718-279-9596

Details data gathered about the awareness and perceptions their subjects had immediately prior to the onset of tic and obses-sive-compulsive symptoms, which are important to the implication of certain brain regions that may be involved in processing sensorimotor information in tic disorder pathology.

1997 6 pages

7214 Learning Problems & the Student with Tourette Syndrome
Tourette Syndrome Association
42-40 Bell Boulevard, Suite 205
Bayside, NY 11361

718-224-2999
Fax: 718-279-9596

Report on learning problems identified through a study of 200 children with TS.

7215 NINDS Seeks Patients with Tourette Syndrome
National Inst. of Neurological Disorders/Stroke
PO Box 5801
Bethesda, MD 20824

301-496-5751
800-352-9424

New program announcements and requests for applications.

7216 Need to Know
Tourette Syndrome Association
42-40 Bell Boulevard, Suite 205
Bayside, NY 11361

718-224-2999
Fax: 718-279-9596

Recollections of a young woman who was diagnosed with TS in her 20s.

7217 Peer Problems in Tourette's Disorder
Tourette Syndrome Association
42-40 Bell Boulevard, Suite 205
Bayside, NY 11361

718-224-2999
Fax: 718-279-9596

Detailed research findings of peer problems in children with TS. Includes statistical results obtained from these studies.

7218 Pharmacotherapy of Tourette Syndrome and Associated Disorders
Tourette Syndrome Association
42-40 Bell Boulevard, Suite 205
Bayside, NY 11361

718-224-2999
Fax: 718-279-9596

Overview with emphasis on the complexities of prescribing TS medications.

19 pages

7219 Problem Behaviors & Tourette Syndrome
Tourette Syndrome Association
42-40 Bell Boulevard, Suite 205
Bayside, NY 11361

718-224-2999
Fax: 718-279-9596

Describes recent research and what is now known about the relationship of a variety of behaviors and TS.

7220 Recognizing Tourette Syndrome in the Classroom
Tourette Syndrome Association
42-40 Bell Boulevard, Suite 205
Bayside, NY 11361

718-224-2999
Fax: 718-279-9596

Provides an overview offering detailed symptoms checklist, post-diagnosis advice and covers special education needs.

4 pages

7221 Risperidone as a Treatment for Tourette Syndrome
Tourette Syndrome Association
42-40 Bell Boulevard, Suite 205
Bayside, NY 11361

718-224-2999
Fax: 718-279-9596

6 pages

7222 Specific Classroom Strategies and Techniqu es for Students with TS-2nd Edition
Tourette Syndrome Association
42-40 Bell Boulevard, Suite 205
Bayside, NY 11361

718-224-2999
Fax: 718-279-9596

An educator with TS spells out concrete methods for managing students with TS. She outlines many valuable classroom interventions to help youngsters deal with tic symptons, ADHD, visual motor and fine motor integration, and behavioral difficulties.

7223 TS: A Look at the Interface Between Tourette Syndrome and the Law
Tourette Syndrome Association
42-40 Bell Boulevard, Suite 205
Bayside, NY 11361

718-224-2999
Fax: 718-279-9596

Summarizes important legislation protecting the rights of students with TS. Also covers resources and hints about how to prepare for dealing successfully with educators and school systems.

7224 TSA Medical Letters
Tourette Syndrome Association
42-40 Bell Boulevard, Suite 205
Bayside, NY 11361

718-224-2999
Fax: 718-279-9596

Annual publication of TSA's Medical Committe covering recent, significant findings from scientific articles.

16 pages

7225 Teens and Tourette Syndrome
Tourette Syndrome Association
42-40 Bell Boulevard, Suite 205
Bayside, NY 11361

718-224-2999
Fax: 718-279-9596
e-mail: ts@tsa-usa.org
tsa-usa.org

Covers self esteem, friends, dating, drugs and alcohol, stress, depression, academic and vocational planning, sibling relationships and medication.

7226 Tourette Syndrome Fact Sheet
National Inst. of Neurological Disorders/Stroke
31 Center Drive, MSC 2540, Building 31, Room 8A06
Bethesda, MD 20892

301-496-5751
800-352-9424

Also available in Spanish.

7227 Tourette Syndrome and Other Tic Disorders
Tourette Syndrome Association
42-40 Bell Boulevard, Suite 205
Bayside, NY 11361

718-224-2999
Fax: 718-279-9596

Comprehensive overview of the complexities of TS. Includes tic syndrome classifications, epidemiology, genetics, behavioral aspects, and summary.

17 pages

7228 Tourette Syndrome and the School Psychologist
Tourette Syndrome Association
42-40 Bell Boulevard, Suite 205
Bayside, NY 11361

718-224-2999
Fax: 718-279-9596

The role of the school psychologist is covered including testing procedures, counseling strategies and social implications.

7229 Tourette Syndrome and the School Nurse
Tourette Syndrome Association
42-40 Bell Boulevard, Suite 205
Bayside, NY 11361

718-224-2999
Fax: 718-279-9596

Comprehensive professional guide to educational, social and medical implications.

7230 What School Bus Drivers Need to Know About Students with Tourette Syndrome
Tourette Syndrome Association
42-40 Bell Boulevard, Suite 205
Bayside, NY 11361

718-224-2999
Fax: 718-279-9596
e-mail: ts@tsa-usa.org
tsa-usa.org

Includes a description of the disorder, as well as related disorders and suggestions as to what school bus drivers can do for students with TS.

Camps

7231 Tourette Syndrome Camp Organization
6933 N Kedzie, #816
Chicago, IL 60645

773-465-7536
www.tourettecamp.com

Dedicated to promoting camping opportunities for children with Tourette Syndrome and its assocaited disorders, Obsessive Compulsive Disorder (OCD) and Attention Deficit/Hyperactivity Disorder (ADD/ADHD).

DESCRIPTION

7232 TOXOPLASMOSIS

Covers these related disorders: Congenital toxoplasmosis
Involves the following Biologic System(s):
Infectious Disorders

Toxoplasmosis is a common infection caused by the single-celled parasite Toxoplasma gondii. This parasite multiplies in the intestines of cats, and its eggs (oocysts) are shed in cat feces. Humans may acquire toxoplasmosis due to contact with cat feces (e.g., in litter boxes), from exposure to contaminated soil, or by eating undercooked or raw meat (lamb, pork, and beef) that contains a form of the parasite (tissue cysts). In addition, if a woman acquires toxoplasmosis during pregnancy, the developing fetus may be affected (congenital toxoplasmosis) due to transmission via the placenta.

Most children who acquire toxoplasmosis after birth and have normally functioning immune systems do not have any apparent symptoms (asymptomatic). However, some children may experience enlargement of one or more lymph nodes (lymphadenopathy). More rarely, such patients may also have other, variable symptoms and findings, such as fever; joint or muscle pain; enlargement of the liver (hepatomegaly); or inflammation of the lungs (pneumonia), the liver (hepatitis), or the middle layer of and the nerve-rich membrane at the back of the eyes (chorioretinitis). Most children with normal immune systems who acquire toxoplasmosis after birth recover spontaneously. However, others may require treatment with certain medications.

Toxoplasmosis is typically more severe in children who acquire the disease during fetal development or who have compromised immune systems. When the infection is transmitted via the placenta during pregnancy (or, in some cases, during vaginal delivery), patients are said to have congenital toxoplasmosis. The disease is typically more severe if the infection is acquired during early pregnancy (first trimester), but the risk of disease transmission is greatest during later pregnancy (third trimester). Approximately 50 percent of women who acquire toxoplasmosis during pregnancy and do not receive treatment transmit the infection to the developing fetus. In the United States, congenital toxoplasmosis affects approximately one in 1,000 newborns.

Without treatment, almost all patients demonstrate certain findings associated with toxoplasmosis by adolescence,

particularly chorioretinitis. Chorioretinitis may cause blurred vision, abnormal sensitivity to light (photophobia), and possible visual impairment. In some affected infants, findings may include short height and low weight at birth (intrauterine growth retardation); persistent yellowish discoloration of the skin, whites of the eyes, and mucous membranes (jaundice); retinal scarring; skin rash; lymphadenopathy; decreased levels of circulating blood platelets (thrombocytopenia); hepatitis; hearing loss; or other findings. Severely affected infants may have an abnormally small head (microcephaly), an abnormal accumulation of cerebrospinal fluid around the brain (hydrocephalus), chorioretinitis, episodes of abnormally increased electrical activity in the brain (seizures), delays in the acquisition of skills requiring the coordination of physical and mental activities (psychomotor retardation), and calcium deposits in the brain. Life-threatening complications may occur shortly after birth.

In children who have compromised immune systems, such as those with acquired immunodeficiency syndrome (AIDS), toxoplasmosis often occurs suddenly and is extremely severe (fulminant). In such patients, infection may rapidly affect the lungs, heart, and brain. In fulminant toxoplasmosis, the most common symptoms are often neurological and may include headache, impaired cognition (thinking), seizures, and impaired control of voluntary movement (ataxia). Without treatment, life-threatening complications result.

The treatment of newborns with congenital toxoplasmosis, affected children with compromised immune systems, and other patients with acquired toxoplasmosis may include the use of combination drug therapies with such medications as pyrimethamine, folinic acid, sulfadiazine or triple sulfonamides, leukovorin, or spiramycin. Additional treatment is symptomatic and supportive. It is important to note that all newborns with congenital toxoplasmosis should receive appropriate drug therapy, regardless of whether they have severe, mild, or no associated symptoms. Appropriate drug therapy for women who contract toxoplasmosis any time during pregnancy may reduce the risk of congenital toxoplasmosis by approximately 60 percent. Such therapy may includeclindamycin and pyrimethamine combined trimethoprim-sulfamethoxasole or sulfadiazine. Pyrimethamine is not given during early pregnancy since it may increase the risk of birth defects during early fetal development. Treatment in AIDS patients is continued as long as the immune system is weak, to prevent reactivation of the disease.In addition, certain measures may be helpful in preventing toxoplasmosis, such as thoroughly cooking all meat, washing hands after handling raw meat, and avoiding direct contact with cat feces.

See also **General Resources** on page 917

See also **General Resources** on page 917

Government Agencies

7233 Centers for Disease Control
1600 Clifton Road
Atlanta, GA 30333

404-639-3311
www.cdc.gov

Mission is to promote health and quality of life by preventing and controlling disease, injury, and disability.

7234 Centers for Disease Control and Prevention
1600 Clifton Road NE
Atlanta, GA 30333

404-639-3534
www.cdc.gov

Mission is to promote health and quality of life by preventing and controlling disease, njury, and disability.

Julie Louise Gerberding, M.D., M.P.H., Director

7235 NIH/National Institute of Allergy and Infectious Diseases
6610 Rockledge Drive, MSC 6612
Bethesda, MD 20892

301-496-5717
Fax: 301-402-3573
TDD: 800-877-8339
www.niaid.nih.gov

Conducts and supports basic and applied research to better understand, treat, and ultimately prevent infectious, immunologic, and allergic diseases.

Anthony S Fauci MD, Director

7236 NIH/National Institute of Allergy and Infe ctious Diseases
6610 Rockledge Drive, MSC 6612
Bethesda, MD 20892

301-496-5717
Fax: 301-402-3573
TDD: 800-877-8339
www.niaid.nih.gov

Conducts and supports basic and applied research to better understand, treat, and ultimately prevent infectious, immunologic, and allergic diseases.

Anthony Fauci MD, Director

National Associations & Support Groups

7237 Arc of the United States
National Organization Mental Retardation
1010 Wayne Avenue, Suite 650
Silver Spring, MD 20910

301-565-3842
800-433-5255
Fax: 301-565-5342
e-mail: info@thearc.org
www.thearc.org

The Arc of the United States works to include all children and adults with congnitive, intellectual, developmental disabilities in every community. We are a national organization of and for the people with mental retardation and related developmental disabilities and their families. It is devoted to promoting and improving

supports and services for people with mental retardation and their families. The ARC was founded by a small group of parents and other concerned individuals.

Adam Aaronson, Public Inquiries Director
Suzette Crim, Operations Director

7238 Children's Hospital Boston
300 Longwood Avenue
Boston, MA 02115

617-355-6000
TTY: 617-355-0443
www.childrenshospital.org

Mission is to provide the highest quality care; be the leading source of reseach and discovery; educate the next generation of leaders in child health and enhance the health and well-being of the children and families in our local community.

James Mandell, MD, President & CEO
Sandra Fenwick, Chief Operating Officer

7239 World Health Organization
Avenue Appia 20
CH-1211 Geneva 27,
Switzerland

www.who.int

WHO is the directing and coordinating authority for health within the United Nations system.

Dr Margaret Chan, Director General

Web Sites

7240 Children's Hospital Boston
www.childrenshospital.org

Mission is to provide the highest quality care; be the leading source of reseach and discovery; educate the next generation of leaders in child health and enhance the health and well-being of the children and families in our local community.

7241 Toxoplasmosis Fact Sheet
www.thebody.com/treat/toxo.html

Offers information about what the disease is, how to treat it, what treatments to use, and if it can be prevented.

Pamphlets

7242 Toxoplasmosis
March of Dimes Resource Center
1275 Mamaroneck Avenue
White Plains, NY 10605

888-663-4637
Fax: 914-997-4763

7243 Toxoplasmosis Fact Sheet
Division of Parasitic Diseases
1600 Clifton Road NE
Atlanta, GA 30333

404-639-3534
www.cdc.gov

DESCRIPTION

7244 TRANSPOSITION OF THE GREAT ARTERIES

Synonym: Transposition of the great vessels

Involves the following Biologic System(s):

Cardiovascular Disorders

Transposition of the great arteries is a heart defect that is present at birth (congenital) in which the major blood vessels that transport blood away from the heart (aorta and pulmonary artery) are switched (transposed) from their normal position. The pulmonary artery normally arises from the base of the lower right-sided pumping chamber (right ventricle) of the heart and carries oxygen-poor blood to the lungs, where the exchange of oxygen and carbon dioxide occurs. The aorta, the main artery of the body, normally arises from the base of the left ventricle and carries oxygen-rich (oxygenated) blood to the body's tissues. However, in infants with transposition of the great arteries, the aorta arises from the right ventricle and the pulmonary artery arises from the left ventricle. As a result, oxygenated blood recirculates to the lungs, while the oxygen-poor blood recirculates throughout the body, and bodily tissues receive insufficient levels of oxygenated blood (hypoxia).

Transpositon of the great arteries is not compatible with life unless there is some communication between the pulmonary and systemic circulation, thus allowing for some mixing of deoxygenated and oxygenated blood. Certain fetal shunts may provide such mixing. These include persistence of the fetal channel that joins the pulmonary artery and the aorta (ductus arteriosus), an opening in the fibrous partition (septum) between the upper chambers (atria) of the heart (patent foramen ovale). Some patients with transposition have mixing of blood through openings in the septum between the ventricles (ventricular septal defect, VSD) or atria (atrial septal defects, ASD)

In newborns with transposition of the great arteries, symptoms are primarily cyanosis (bluish discoloration of fingers and toes and mucous membranes). Shortly after birth, affected infants may experience abnormally rapid and deep breathing (tachypnea, hyperpnea) and cyanosis. Without treatment, life-threatening complications will result. Medical treatment includes a medication called prostaglandin E to open the ductus arteriosus and allow mixing. A cardiac catheterization to place a balloon catheter across the atrial septum (balloon septostomy) may be necessary to allow for mixing of blood. Permanent treatment of infants with transposition of the great arteries includes surgery to switch the aorta and coronary arteries and pulmonary artery back to their normal positions (arterial switch operation). This operation is done in the first weeks of life.

Transposition of the great arteries is more common in males than females and affects approximately one in 2,000 newborns. Infants are most often normal sized, full term, and otherwise healthy. The condition is thought to result from the interactions of several different genes, possibly in association with the involvement of environmental factors (multifactorial inheritance). Although the exact underlying cause of this heart defect is unknown, rese archers suggest that it may result from an error during the development of an embryonic structure that later divides the aorta and pulmonary artery.

See also **General Resources** on page 917

Government Agencies

7245 NIH/National Heart, Lung and Blood Institu te

National Institute of Health
31 Center Dr MSC 2486, Bldg 31, Room 5A48
Bethesda, MD 20892

301-592-8573
Fax: 240-629-3246
TTY: 240-629-3255
e-mail: NHLBIinfo@nhlbi.nih.gov
www.nhlbi.nih.gov

Primary responsibility of this organization is the scientific investigation of heart, blood vessel, lung and blood disorders. Oversees research, demonstration, prevention, education, control and training activities in these fields and emphasizes the prevention and control of heart diseases.

Elizabeth G Nabel, MD, Director
Susan Shurin, MD, Deputy Director

7246 NIH/National Heart, Lung, and Blood Instit te

PO Box 30105
Bethesda, MD 20824

301-592-8573
Fax: 301-629-3246
TTY: 240-629-3255
e-mail: nhlbinfo@nhlbi.nih.gov
www.nhlbi.nih.gov

Provides leadership for a national program in diseases of the heart, blood vessels, lungs, and blood; blood resources; and sleep disorders.

Elizabeth G Nabel MD, Director

7247 NIH/National Institute of Child Health and Human Development

31 Center Drive, Building 31
Bethesda, MD 20892

301-496-5133
Fax: 301-496-1104
www.nichd.nih.gov

Established in 1962 by congress, today the institute conducts and supports research on topics related to the health of children, adults, families and populations. Some of these topics include: developmental disabilities, growth and development, infant death, reproductive health and birth defects.

Nancy D Wirth, Director
Lisa Kaeser, Program & Public Liaison

National Associations & Support Groups

7248 American Academy of Pediatrics
141 NW Point Boulevard
Elk Grove Village, IL 60007

847-434-4000
Fax: 847-434-8000
e-mail: kidsdocs@aap.org
www.aap.org

The American Academy of Pediatrics and its member pediatricians dedicate their efforts and resources to the health, safety and well-being of infants, children, adolescents and young adults.

Jay E Berkelhamer MD, FAAP, President

7249 American Heart Association
7272 Greenville Avenue
Dallas, TX 75231

214-373-6300
800-242-8721
Fax: 214-706-1341
e-mail: inquire@amhrt.org
www.amhrt.org

Supports research, education and community service programs with the objective of reducing premature death and disability from cardiovascular diseases and stroke; coordinates the efforts of health professionals, and others engaged in the fight against heart and circulatory disease.

M Cass Wheeler, CEO

7250 Congenital Heart Information Network
600 North 3rd Street, First Floor
Philadelphia, PA 19123

215-627-4034
Fax: 215-627-4036
e-mail: mb@tchin.org
www.tchin.org

CHIN is an international organization that provides reliable information, support services and resources to families of children with congenital heart defects and acquired heart disease.

Mona Barmash, President

7251 Genetic Alliance
4301 Connecticut Avenue NW
Washington, DC 20008

202-966-5557
800-336-4363
Fax: 202-966-8553
e-mail: info@geneticalliance.org
www.geneticalliance.org

A coalition of voluntary genetic support groups, consumers and professionals addressing the needs of individuals and families affected by genetic disorders from a national perspective.

Sharon Terry, President/CEO

7252 United Network for Organ Sharing
700 N 4th Street
Richmond, VA 23219

804-782-4800
Fax: 804-782-4817
www.unos.org

Our mission is to advance organ availability and transplantation by uniting and supporting our communities for the benefit of patients through education, technology and policy development.

Walter K Graham, Executive Director/President/CEO
Vicki F Sauer, Executive VP/COO

Web Sites

7253 American Academy of Pediatrics
www.aap.org

The American Academy of Pediatrics and its member pediatricians dedicate their efforts and resources to the health, safety and well-being of infants, children, adolescents and young adults.

7254 American Heart Association
www.amhrt.org

Supports research, education and community service programs with the objective of reducing premature death and disability from cardiovascular diseases and stroke; coordinates the efforts of health professionals, and others engaged in the fight against heart and circulatory disease.

7255 Congenital Heart Information Network
www.tchin.org

An international organization that provides reliable information, support services and resources to families of children with congenital heart defects and acquired heart disease and adults with congenital heart defects, and the professionals who work with them.

7256 NIH/National Heart, Lung and Blood Institu te
www.nhlbi.nih.gov

Provides leadership for a national program in diseases of the heart, blood vessels, lungs, and blood; blood resources; and sleep disorders.

7257 Southern Illinois University School of Medicine
www.siumed.edu/peds/index.htm

The mission of SUI School of Medicine is to assist the people if Central and Southern Illinois in meeting thier present and future health care needs through education, clinical service and research.

7258 United Network for Organ Sharing
www.unos.org

Our mission is to advance organ availability and transplantation by uniting and supporting our communities for the benefit of patients through education, technology and policy development.

7259 Yale University School of Medicine
www.info.med.yale.edu/intmed/cardio/chd

A site that offers information on Transposition of the Great Arteries and other congenital heart conditions.

DESCRIPTION

7260 TRISOMY 18 SYNDROME

Synonyms: Chromosome 18, trisomy 18, Edwards syndrome

Covers these related disorders: Trisomy 18 mosaicism

Involves the following Biologic System(s):
Genetic/Chromosomal/Syndrome/Metabolic Disorders

Trisomy 18 syndrome is a chromosomal disorder that affects about one in 300 newborns. With the exception of reproductive cells, cells of the body normally have 23 pairs of chromosomes that are numbered from 1 to 22 (with a 23rd pair consisting of one X chromosome from the mother and an X or a Y chromosome from the father). However, in infants with trisomy 18 syndrome, all or a portion of chromosome 18 is present three times (trisomy) rather than twice in cells of the body. In some affected infants, only a percentage of cells may contain the trisomy 18 chromosomal abnormality (mosaicism).

The symptoms and physical findings associated with trisomy 18 syndrome are variable and depend upon the exact location, and percentage, of body cells containing the additional chromosomal material from chromosome 18. However, infants with trisomy 18 syndrome experience development delays, usually severe mental retardation, low birth weight, difficulties feeding and breathing, and a failure to gain weight and grow at the expected rate (failure to thrive). In addition, almost all infants with trisomy 18 have complex structural heart defects, failure of one or both testes to descend into the scrotum (cryptorchidism) in affected males, malformations of the hands and feet, additional skeletal abnormalities, and characteristic malformations of the head and facial (craniofacial) area.

In infants with trisomy 18 syndrome, defects of the hands and feet of ten include closed fists with overlapping, abnormally bent fingers; underdeveloped or absent thumbs; and webbing between certain fingers or toes (syndactyly). Affected infants also often have additional skeletal abnormalities, such as a small pelvis, narrow hips with limited movements, fusion of certain bones of the spinal column (vertebrae), or sideways curvature of the spine (scoliosis). Characteristic craniofacial abnormalities associated with trisomy 18 syndrome typically include an abnormally small head (microcephaly); a prominent back portion of the head (occiput); a small mouth (microstomia) and a small jaw (micrognathia); malformed, low-set ears; and short, narrow eyelid folds (palpebral fissures). Additional craniofacial malformations may be present, such as incomplete closure of the roof of the mouth (cleft palate), an abnormal groove in the upper lip (cleft lip), and drooping of the upper eyelids (ptosis). Some infants may have kidney defects . The abnormalities of trisomy 18 are generally not compatible with more than a few months of life. Fifty percent of the affected infants do not survive beyond the first week of life. Although the exact cause of trisomy 18 syndrome is unknown, it is thought to result from errors during division of a parent's reproductive cells (meiosis) and, in some cases of mosaicism, errors during cellular division after fertilization (e.g., postzygotic nondisjunction). Parents who have a child with translocational trisomy 18 and want additional children should have chromosome studies, because they are at increased risk to have another child with trisomy 18.

See also **General Resources** on page 917

See also **General Resources** on page 917

Government Agencies

7261 NIH/National Institute of Child Health and Human Development
31 Center Drive, Building 31
Bethesda, MD 20892

301-496-5133
Fax: 301-496-1104
www.nichd.nih.gov

Established in 1962 by congress, today the institute conducts and supports research on topics related to the health of children, adults, families and populations. Some of these topics include: developmental disabilities, growth and development, infant death, reproductive health and birth defects.

Nancy D Wirth, Director
Lisa Kaeser, Program & Public Liaison

National Associations & Support Groups

7262 Chromosome 18 Registry & Research Society
7155 Oakridge Drive
San Antonio, TX 78229

210-657-4968
Fax: 210-657-4968
e-mail: office@chromosome18.org
www.chromosome18.org

The purpose of the Chromosome 18 Registry & Research Society is to offer support to patients and families, to educate the public about different available treatments and to connect families and doctors to the research community.

500 Members

Claudia Traa, Executive Director
Ben Flowe Jr, VP Public Relations

7263 Congenital Heart Anomalies, Support, Education & Resources (CHASER)
2112 N Wilkins Road
Swanton, OH 43558

419-825-5575
Fax: 419-825-2880
e-mail: chaser@compuserve.com
www.csun.edu/~hcmth011/chaser/

National organization for support, education and resources for families and patients who deal with children born with congenital heart malformations.

Anita Myers, Executive Director

7264 Genetic Alliance
4301 Connecticut Avenue NW, Suite 404
Washington, DC 20008

202-966-5557
Fax: 202-966-8553
e-mail: info@geneticalliance.org
www.geneticalliance.org

The Genetic Alliance promotes healthy living by working to speed the translation of genetic advances into quality and affordable healthcare, public awareness and consumer-centered public policies.

Sharon Terry, President/CEO

7265 MUMS: National Parent to Parent Network
150 Custer Street
Green Bay, WI 54301

920-336-5333
877-336-5333
Fax: 920-339-0995
e-mail: mums@netnet.net
www.netnet.net/mums

A national parent-to-parent organization for parents or care providers of a child with any disability, rare or not so rare disorder, chromosomal abnormality or health condition.

Julie J Gordon, Director

7266 Support Organization for Trisomy 18, 13, and Related Disorders (SOFT)
2982 S Union Street
Rochester, NY 14624

585-594-4621
800-716-7638
e-mail: barbsoft@rochester.rr.com
www.trisomy.org

SOFT is a network of families and professional dedication to provide support and understanding to families involved in the issue and decision surrounding the diagnosis and care related to chromosome disorders. Support is provided throughout prenatal diagnosis, the child's life and after their passing. It is committed to the support of families and personal decisions in alliance with a parent-professional partnership. Includes listings of local chapters in 25 states.

Barb Vanherreweghe, Contact

7267 Trisomy 18 Foundation
4491 Cheshire Station Plaza, Suite 157
Dale City, VA 22193

e-mail: t18info@trisomy18.org
www.trisomy18.org

The foundation's mission is to search for a cure and treatments; to educate and support medical professionals; and to create a worldwide caring community for those affected.

Victoria Miller, Executive Director
Mindy Wilsford, Operations Director

Research Centers

7268 Trisomy 18 Foundation
4491 Cheshire Station Plaza, Suite 157
Dale City, VA 22193

e-mail: t18info@trisomy18.org
www.trisomy18.org

The foundation's mission is to search for a cure and treatments; to educate and support medical professionals; and to create a worldwide caring community for those affected.

Victoria Miller, Executive Director
Mindy Wilsford, Operations Director

Book Publishers

7269 Introduction to Trisomy 18
SOFT
2982 S Union Street
Rochester, NY 14624

585-594-4621
800-716-7638
e-mail: barbsoft@rochester.rr.com
www.trisomy.org

Addresses parent question regarding the disorder as well as explains the chromosomes, diagnosis and characteristics.

Revised 1998

Barb Vanherreweghe, Contact

DESCRIPTION

7270 TRISOMY 13 SYNDROME

Synonyms: Chromosome 13, trisomy 13, D1 trisomy syndrome, Patau syndrome

Covers these related disorders: Trisomy 13 mosaicism

Involves the following Biologic System(s):

Genetic/Chromosomal/Syndrome/Metabolic Disorders

Trisomy 13 syndrome is a chromosomal disorder that is thought to affect approximately one in 5,000 newborns. With the exception of reproductive cells, cells of the body normally have 23 pairs of chromosomes that are numbered from 1 to 22. The 23rd pair includes one X chromosome from the mother and an X or a Y chromosome from the father. In infants with trisomy 13 syndrome, all or a portion of chromosome 13 is present three times (trisomy) rather than twice. In some affected infants, a certain percentage of cells contain the extra chromosome 13, whereas other cells have the normal two. This finding is known as chromosomal mosaicism.

In infants with trisomy 13 syndrome, associated symptoms and physical findings are pronounced and depend upon the specific length and location of the duplicated portion of chromosome 13 as well as the percentage of the body cells containing the defect.

Abnormalities associated with trisomy 13 syndrome include severe developmental delays, profound mental retardation, incomplete closure of the roof of the mouth (cleft palate), an abnormal groove in the upper lip (cleft lip), and unusually small eyes (microphthalmia). Additional characteristic symptoms and findings include abnormal bending of the fingers, the presence of extra fingers and toes (polydactyly), failure of the testes to descend into the scrotum (cryptorchidis in affected males, and malformation of the uterus in affected females, i.e., bicornuate uterus). Many infants have severe feeding difficulties, abnormally diminished muscle tone (hypotonia), and episodes of temporary cessation of breathing (apnea).

Defects in the brain can result in seizure activity and deafness. Most infants with trisomy 13 syndrome also have additional physical malformations, including an abnormally small head (microcephaly) with a sloping forehead; widely set eyes (ocular hypertelorism); a broad, flat nose; low-set, malformed ears; and a small jaw (micrognthia). Reddish, purplish benign growths (hemangiomas) may be present on the forehead or other areas due to an abnormal distribution of minute blood vessels (capillaries). Many affected infants may also have additional skeletal abnormalities, heart defects, and brain malformations. More than 80% of children with trisomy 13 die in the first month.. Because of the severity of congenital defects, life-sustaining procedures are generally not attempted. Parents of infants with trisomy 13 caused by a translocation should have genetic testing and counseling, which may help them prevent recurrence. The exact cause of trisomy 13 syndrome is unknown.

See also **General Resources** on page 917

Government Agencies

7271 NIH/National Institute of Child Health and Human Development

31 Center Drive, Building 31
Bethesda, MD 20892

301-496-5133
Fax: 301-496-1104
www.nichd.nih.gov

Established in 1962 by congress, today the institute conducts and supports research on topics related to the health of children, adults, families and populations. Some of these topics include: developmental disabilities, growth and development, infant death, reproductive health and birth defects.

Nancy D Wirth, Director
Lisa Kaeser, Program & Public Liaison

National Associations & Support Groups

7272 Congenital Heart Anomalies, Support, Education & Resources (CHASER)

2112 N Wilkins Road
Swanton, OH 43558

419-825-5575
Fax: 419-825-2880
e-mail: chaser@compuserve.com
www.csun.edu/~hcmth011/chaser/

National organization for support, education and resources for families, patients and professionals who deal with children born with congenital heart malformations. Information on hospitals, medical assistance, and schooling. Offers Chaser News, an international newsletter and Chaser's Pediatric Heart Surgeons Facility Directory.

Anita Myers, Executive Director

7273 Genetic Alliance

4301 Connecticut Avenue NW
Washington, DC 20008

202-966-5557
800-336-4363
Fax: 202-966-8553
e-mail: info@geneticalliance.org
www.geneticalliance.org

A coalition of voluntary genetic support groups, consumers and professionals addressing the needs of individuals and families affected by genetic disorders from a national perspective.

Sharon Terry, President/CEO

7274 National Dissemination Center for Children with Disabilities
PO Box 1492
Washington, DC 20013

> 202-884-8200
> 800-695-0285
> Fax: 202-884-8441
> e-mail: nichcy@aed.org
> www.nichcy.org

A national information and referral center for families, educators and other professionals on: disabilities in children and youth; programs and services; IDEA, the nation's special education law; and research-based information on effective practices.

Suzanne Ripley, Executive Director

7275 Support Organization for Trisomy 18, 13, and Related Disorders (SOFT)
2982 S Union Street
Rochester, NY 14624

> 585-594-4621
> 800-716-7638
> e-mail: barbsoft@rochester.rr.com
> www.trisomy.org

SOFT is a network of families and professional dedication to providing support and understanding to families involved in the issue and decision surrounding the diagnosis and care in related chromosome disorders. Support is provided throughout pre-natal diagnosis, the child's life and after their passing. It is committed to the support of families personal decision in alliance with a parent-professional partnership. Site includes a listing of local chapters in 25 states.

Barb Vanherreweghe, Contact

Web Sites

7276 Living with Trisomy 13
www.livingwithtrisomy13.org

Brings together families of children diagnosed with Trisomy 13 Syndrome through the use of photos and videos.

Book Publishers

7277 Introduction to Trisomy 13
SOFT
2982 S Union Street
Rochester, NY 14624

> 585-594-4621
> 800-716-7638
> e-mail: barbsoft@rochester.rr.com
> www.trisomy.org

Addresses parent question regarding the disorder as well as explains the chromosomes, diagnosis and characteristics.

Revised 1998

Barb Vanherreweghe, Contact

DESCRIPTION

7278 TUBERCULOSIS

Synonym: TB

Involves the following Biologic System(s):

Infectious Disorders, Respiratory Disorders

Tuberculosis (TB) is an infectious disease that is most often caused by the bacterium Mycobacterium tuberculosis, but may sometimes result from infection with Mycobacterium bovis or Mycobacterium africanum. As a result of improvements in living conditions, the number of people in the United States infected with this disease declined dramatically throughout most of the twentieth century. However, tuberculosis rates once again began to rise in the mid-1980s in association with such factors as immigration of individuals from countries that had high incidence rates of TB, poverty, poor access to health care among groups at high risk, the increase in AIDS infections, overcrowded and sometimes unsanitary conditions in certain institutional settings, and the development of antibiotic-resistant strains of tuberculosis bacteria. The neglect of TB control programs has also contributed to the resurgence of TB. This disease is most prevalent among the elderly, people with compromised immune systems, and those of low socioeconomic status.

Tuberculosis is usually transmitted through airborne droplets coughed or sneezed into the air by an infected person. The droplets are inhaled into the lungs where the bacteria multiply and travel to the lymph nodes that are responsible for draining the lungs; however, in the vast majority of cases, the immune system either destroys or seals off the bacteria. If this primary pulmonary tuberculosis infection is not completely resolved, the bacteria may become dormant within certain white blood cells called macrophages and be later reactivated. This reemergence of symptoms at a later date may be due to influences such as an impaired immune system, corticosteroid drug usage, or advancing age. In addition to the lungs, the tuberculosis bacteria may sometimes spread throughout the body via the bloodstream and affect other parts of the body (extrapulmonary tuberculosis). This type of disseminated disease may infect the lymph nodes, upper respiratory tract, skin, liver, spleen, kidneys, gastrointestinal tract, bones, joints, brain, spine, the sac surrounding the heart (pericardium), and other organs.

Symptoms and physical findings associated with primary pulmonary tuberculosis in children may include enlargement of the lymph nodes and the subsequent compression and obstruction of the large air passages of the lungs (bronchial tubes). This obstruction may result in lung collapse, cough, and less commonly wheezing, rapid breathing (tachypnea), and respiratory distress. Other symptoms may be absent or mild, but more pronounced in infants, and may include moderate difficulty in breathing (dyspnea), a nonproductive cough, and occasionally fever, loss of appetite (anorexia), and night sweats. In addition, some infants may have failure to thrive, a condition in which the current weight or rate of weight gain is significantly below that of other children of similar age and sex. Pneumonia may develop and, in rare instances, blister-type lesions may develop in the lungs that sometimes rupture, resulting in the presence of air between the lungs and the chest wall (pneumothorax) and possible associated lung collapse.

On rare occasions, tuberculosis may be transmitted from mother to fetus through a placental lesion or by the inhalation or swallowing of infected amniotic fluid by the baby before or during birth. Congenital tuberculosis is rare and more commonly occurs soon after birth, usually through inhalation of airborne droplets from an infected person. Symptoms and findings associated with congenital tuberculosis may not develop for two or three weeks and may include drowsiness, fever, difficulty in breathing, poor feeding, drainage from the ears, enlarged lymph glands, enlarged liver and spleen (hepatosplenomegaly), abdominal swelling, skin lesions, and failure to thrive.

Diagnosis of tuberculosis may be established through evaluation of family and medical history, physical examination, skin and sputum testing, chest x-ray, and sometimes testing of cerebrospinal and other fluids as well as microscopic examination of tissue samples (biopsy).

Treatment for tuberculosis includes the prolonged administration of at least two different types of antibiotics to assure that all bacteria are destroyed. The antibiotics most often used for children with this disease include combinations of isoniazid, rifampin, pyrazinamide as well as streptomycin, and ethionamide that are especially effective for drug-resistant disease. The primary difference between treatment of TB in adults and children is ethambutol since one of the side effects is impaired vision. Because this effect is difficult to monitor in young children, ethambutol is not routinely recommended for children less then five years old. Corticosteroids may also be administered, especially in children with associated inflammatory irregularities that adversely affect organ function. In addition, the medication isoniazid may sometimes be preventively administered to those at high risk of tuberculosis infection, such as other members of the household, or to those with positive skin test results but no symptomatic or x-ray evidence of disease. The best method to prevent cases of pediatric tuberculosis is to find, diagnose, and treat cases of active tuberculosis among adults. Routine testing for TB with a tuberculin skin test is now only recommended in children who are at high risk for having the illness.

See also **General Resources** on page 917

Government Agencies

7279 Centers for Disease Control and Prevention Division: Tuberculosis Elimination
National Center For Prevention Services
1600 Clifton Road NE, MS E-10
Atlanta, GA 30333

404-639-8135
e-mail: cdcinfo@cdc.gov
www.cdc.gov/nchstp/tb/contact.html

Kenneth G. Castro, MD, Director
Phillip Talboy, Deputy Director

7280 NIH/National Institute of Allergy and Infectious Diseases
6610 Rockledge Drive, MSC 6612
Bethesda, MD 20892

301-496-5717
Fax: 301-402-3573
TDD: 800-877-8339
www.niaid.nih.gov

Conducts and supports basic and applied research to better understand, treat, and ultimately prevent infectious, immunologic, and allergic diseases.

Anthony S Fauci MD, Director

7281 New York City Department of Health Bureau of Tuberculosis Control
125 Worth Street
New York, NY 10012

212-788-4204
www.nyc.gov/html

Michael R Bloomberg, Mayor
Desiree Kim, Executive Director

National Associations & Support Groups

7282 American Lung Association
61 Broadway, 6th Floor
New York, NY 10006

212-315-8700
800-586-4872
www.lungusa.org

The American Lung Association fights lung disease in all its forms, with special emphasis on asthma, tobacco control and environmental health. The American Lung Association is funded by contributions from the public, along with gifts and grants from corporations, foundations and government agencies. The association achieves its many successes through the work of thousands of committed volunteers and staff.

Hallema Sharif Clyburn, Director Media Relations
Bruce A Herring, Board Chair Elect

7283 National Tuberculosis Center at New Jersey Medical School
University of Medicine and Dentistry of New Jersey
185 South Orange Avenue
Newark, NJ 07103

973-972-4631
Fax: 973-972-3268
e-mail: njmsadmiss@umdnj.edu
www.umdnj.edu

The National Tuberculosis Center was established in 1993 in response to the resurgence of tuberculosis in the United States. The center operates under the direction of Lee B. Reichman, MD, MPH. The center operates a toll-free information line to provide state-of-the-art information to health care professionals and the public. Senior medical staff and nurses are available to respond to calls Monday-Friday from 9am-5pm.

Lee B Reichman MD, Executive Director
Reynard J McDonald MD, Medical Director

7284 World Health Organization
Avenue Appia 20
CH-1211 Geneva 27,
Switzerland

www.who.int

WHO is the directing and coordinating authority for health within the United Nations system.

Dr Margaret Chan, Director General

Research Centers

7285 Francis J. Curry National Tuberculosis Center
3180 Eighteenth Street, Suite 102
San Francisco, CA 94110

415-502-4600
Fax: 415-502-4620
e-mail: tbcenter@nationaltbcenter.edu
www.nationaltbcenter.edu

7286 University of Illinois at Chicago Institute for Tuberculosis Research
904 W Adams Street
Chicago, IL 60607

202-318-2476

Michael J Groves, PhD, Director

Web Sites

7287 American Lung Association
www.lungusa.org

Information regarding lung disease in all its forms, with special emphasis on asthma, tobacco control and environmental health.

7288 Centers for Disease Control
www.cdc.gov

Mission is to promote health and the quality of life by preventing and controlling disease, injury, and disability.

7289 Columbia University
www.cpmc.columbia.edu

Provides what you need to know about tuberculosis, and what kind of treatment to prevent tuberculosis.

7290 Health Answers
www.healthanswers.com

HealthAnswers offers a breadth of services in medical education, sales force training, patient support solutions, professional promotion and consumer solutions.

7291 NOAH

www.noah.cuny.edu/tb/nycdoh/nycdohtb1.html

Provides access to high quality full-text consumer health information in English and Spanish that is accurate, timely, relevant and unbaised.

7292 National Tuberculosis Center

www.nationaltbcenter.edu/

Creates, enhances and disseminates state of the art resources and models of excellence to control and eliminate tuberculosis nationally and internationally. We are committed to the belief that everyone deserves the highest quality of care in a manner consistent with his or her culture, values and language. We develop and deliver highly versatile, culturally appropriate trainings and educational products, provide technical assistance and facilitate regional, state and national initiatives.

Book Publishers

7293 Forgotten Plague: How the Battle Against Tuberculosis Was Won & Lost

Hachette Book Group USA
1271 Avenue Of The Americas
New York, NY 10020

617-227-0730
Fax: 617-227-4633
www.hachettebookgroupusa.com

1994 Paperback
ISBN: 0-316763-81-0

Alison Lindsay, Director Of Marketing

7294 Know About Tuberculosis

Walker & Company
104 5th Avenue
New York, NY 10011

212-727-8300
Fax: 212-727-0984
e-mail: orders@walkerbooks.com
www.walkerbooks.com

1994 hardcover
ISBN: 0-802783-38-4

7295 Lung Disorders Sourcebook

Omnigraphics
615 Griswold
Detroit, MI 48226

800-234-1340
Fax: 800-875-1340
e-mail: info@omnigraphics.com
omnigraphics.com

Basic consumer health information on lung disorders including tuberculosis, asthma and cystic fibrosis.

678 pages
ISBN: 0-780803-39-6

Pamphlets

7296 Classification of Tuberculosis and Other Mycrobacterial Diseases

American Lung Association
1740 Broadway
New York, NY 10019

212-315-8700

Chart listing different classes of tuberculosis and other mycrobacterial diseases.

7297 Facts About Tuberculosis

American Lung Association
1740 Broadway
New York, NY 10019

212-315-8700

Primary public information leaflet on TB as well as on its impact and treatment.

8 pages

7298 Global Epidemic Multi-Drug Resistant Tuberculosis

American Lung Association
61 Broadway, 6th Floor
New York, NY 10006

212-315-8700
www.lungusa.org

Bruce A Herring, Board Chair Elect
Harold Wimmer, CLAS President

7299 TB Skin Test

American Lung Association
1740 Broadway
New York, NY 10019

212-315-8700

Primary public information leaflet on the TB skin test.

8 pages

7300 TB: What You Should Know

American Lung Association
45 Ash Street
East Hartford, CT 06108

860-289-5401
www.lungusa.org

Offers a brief overview of tuberculosis, how transmission is possible, and TB skin testing.

7301 This Is Mr. TB Germ

American Lung Association
1740 Broadway
New York, NY 10019

212-315-8700

Lively booklet of drawings and very brief text giving a basic description of TB and its treatments.

20 pages

DESCRIPTION

7302 TUBEROUS SCLEROSIS

Synonyms: Epiloia, TS
Involves the following Biologic System(s):
Dermatologic Disorders, Neurologic Disorders

Tuberous sclerosis (TS) is a hereditary multisystem disorder that is one of a group of diseases described as neuro-cutaneous syndromes, because of large involvement of both the skin and the central nervous system (brain and/or spinal cord). It is characterized by multiple, wart-like, raised areas (papules) on the skin of the face (adenoma sebaceum); benign, tumor-like nodules (hamartomas) of the brain, the heart, the kidneys, the nerve-rich membrane at the back of the eyes (retinas), or other organs; episodes of abnormally increased, uncontrolled electrical activity in the brain (seizures); and mental retardation. Associated symptoms and findings may vary greatly from patient to patient, including among members of the same family. TS is caused by abnormal changes (mutations) in a gene or genes. These mutations may occur randomly for unknown reasons (sporadically) or may be inherited as an autosomal dominant trait. At least two genes have been identified that may cause TS. One disease gene, known as TSC1 gene, is located on the long arm (q) of chromosome 9 (9q34). A second gene, called the TSC2 gene, is on the short arm (p) of chromosome 16 (16p13.3). Tuberous sclerosis affects approximately one in 30,000 individuals.

TS is often apparent shortly after birth and presents as distinctive skin abnormalities and the development of either infantile spasms (hypsarrhythmia) or partial seizures characterized by sudden, repeated flexion or extension of the muscles of the neck, torso, arms, and legs. Seizures may later take the form of myoclonic epilepsy, in which there are sudden, shock-like contractions of a muscle or muscle groups. As many as 90 percent of infants with TS also have sharply defined areas of abnormally diminished skin coloration (hypopigmentation) on the torso, face, arms, or legs. These areas typically have an ashleaf-like appearance.

Seizures that begin during later childhood are often characterized by prolonged muscle contractions and alternating relaxation and contraction of muscles (generalized tonic-clonic seizures). Seizures tend to become progressively more severe and are often difficult to treat. In addition, approximately 60 to 70 percent of children with TS experience mental retardation, almost all of whom also have seizure disorders. However, seizures also occur in most of those without mental retardation. Generally, the younger a patient experiences symptoms associated with TS, the greater the risk for mental retardation.

Beginning at about age two to six, about 80 percent of children with TS also develop red, shiny nodules (lesions) over the cheeks and nose. These nodules gradually become larger and assume a wart-like, fleshy appearance (adenoma sebaceum). Similar nodules may also develop on the forehead. Many children have additional, distinctive skin lesions. These may include raised, knobby, skin-colored lesions with an orange-peel consistency (shagreen patches) primarily located onthe lower back; firm, skin-colored nodules that develop around the nails of the fingers and toes during puberty, and rarely, coffee-colored discolorations of the skin (cafe-au-lait spots).

In patients with TS, the characteristic tumor-like nodules that develop in the brain are known as tubers. These growths often become hardened due to an abnormal accumulation of calcium salts (calcification). In addition, depending upon their size and location, tubers may block the normal flow of cerebrospinal fluid (CSF), causing an abnormal accumulation of CSF in the brain (hydrocephalus). The severity of neurologic impairment typically increases with the number of tubers within the brain. Rarely, a tuber may differentiate into a malignant brain tumor (astrocytoma).

Approximately 50 percent of affected children also have benign tumors of the heart muscle (rhabdomyoma). Although rhabdomyomas may disrupt the normal rhythm or rate of the heartbeat (arrythmias), these tumors tend to gradually resolve on their own. Benign, tumor-like nodules or multiple cysts may also develop in the kidneys, causing blood in the urine (hematuria), pain, or, in severe cases, kidney failure. Hamartomas may also develop in other tissues and organs of the body, such as the retinas and the lungs. In patients with severe TS, life-threatening complications may occur by adulthood.

The management of patients with TS is symptomatic and supportive, including therapy with anticonvulsant medications to help control seizures. In addition, physicians may regularly monitor patients to detect certain serious conditions potentially associated with TS, such as abnormal accumulations of cerebrospinal fluid or malignant transformation of hamartomas in the brain. If such conditions are confirmed, immediate surgical intervention or other measures are performed as required. Medications are required for controlling seizures, which is often difficult.

The need for special schooling or care is determined by the severity of mental retardation.

See also **General Resources** on page 917

National Associations & Support Groups

7303 Epilepsy Foundation
8301 Professional Place
Landover, MD 20785

> 301-459-3700
> 800-332-1000
> Fax: 301-577-2684
> e-mail: postmaster@efa.org
> www.epilepsyfoundation.org

An organization works to ensure that people with seizures are able to participate in all life experiences; and to prevent, control and cure epilepsy through research, education, advocacy and services.

7304 Family Support Network
Tuberous Sclerosis Alliance
801 Roeder Road Suite 750
Silver Spring, MD 20910

> 800-255-6872
> Fax: 301-562-9870
> e-mail: info@tsalliance.org
> www.tsalliance.org

The Support Network is an organized partnership of individuals whose lives have been affected by Tuberous Sclerosis. Across the nation, the Support Network is providing the latest medical information, education and support to those individuals who are seeking understanding about the genetic disease and offering them words of encouragement and empowerment.

Nancy L Taylor, Chief Executive Officer
Kari L Carlson, Executive Vice President

7305 Genetic Alliance
4301 Connecticut Avenue NW
Washington, DC 20008

> 202-966-5557
> 800-336-4363
> Fax: 202-966-8553
> e-mail: info@geneticalliance.org
> www.geneticalliance.org

A coalition of voluntary genetic support groups, consumers and professionals addressing the needs of individuals and families affected by genetic disorders from a national perspective.

Sharon Terry, President/CEO

7306 National Tuberous Sclerosis Association
8181 Professional Place, Suite 110
Landover, MD 20785

> 301-459-9888
> 800-225-6872
> Fax: 301-459-0394
> e-mail: ntsa@ntsa.org
> www.ntsa

Nonprofit organization.

Carolyn Wilson, Contact

7307 Tuberous Sclerosis Alliance
801 Roeder Road, Suite 750
Silver Spring, MD 20910

> 301-562-9890
> 800-225-6872
> Fax: 301-562-9870
> e-mail: info@tsalliance.org
> www.tsalliance.org

National voluntary organization dedicated to finding a cure for the many aspects of tuberous sclerosis complex.

Web Sites

7308 AGSA Newsletter
www.dirsca.org.au/pub/docs/facttube.txt

7309 Health Answers
www.healthanswers.com

HealthAnswers offers a breadth of services in medical education, sales force training, patient support solutions, professional promotion and ocnsumer solutions.

7310 Online Mendelian Inheritance in Man
www.ncbi.nlm.nih.gov

This database is a catalog of human genes and genetic disorders.

7311 TS International
www.stsn.nl/tsi/tsi.htm

Goals and objectives are to increase the knowledge of TS throughout the world, to stimulate, co-ordinate and originate research on TS, to interest statutory international organizations in the welfare of TS sufferers, to support national TS associations in the work, to initiate the realistation of new TS associatons, to exchange information of mutual interest between TS associations.

Book Publishers

7312 Early Years Guide of the Life Stage Program
Tuberous Sclerosis Alliance
801 Roeder Road, Suite 750
Silver Spring, MD 20910

> 301-562-9890
> 800-225-6872
> Fax: 301-562-9870
> e-mail: info@tsalliance.org
> www.tsalliance.org

A resource guide for families of infants and young children with tuberous sclerosis.

7313 School-Aged Guide of the Life Stages Program
Tuberous Sclerosis Alliance
801 Roeder Road, Suite 750
Silver Spring, MD 20910

> 301-562-9890
> 800-225-6872
> Fax: 301-562-9870
> e-mail: info@tsalliance.org
> www.tsalliance.org

A resource guide for parents of school-aged children with Tuberous Sclerosis.

Michael Coburn, President/CEO
Becky Bull, VP Development/Communications

7314 Tuberous Sclerosis: 3rd Edition
Oxford University Press
2001 Evans Road
Cary, NC 27513

> Fax: 919-677-1303
> www.oup-usa.org

A revision offering up-to-date medical information to families, researchers, and professionals on TS.

ISBN: 0-195122-10-0

Newsletters

7315 Perspective

National Tuberous Sclerosis Association
8181 Professional Place, Suite 110
Landover, MD 22265

301-459-9888
800-225-6872
Fax: 301-459-0394
e-mail: ntsa@ntsa.org
www.ntsa.org

Offers the latest research and medical information on tuberous sclerosis to physicians and health care professionals.

Bimonthly

Holly Knorr, Managing Editor

Pamphlets

7316 Living with Tuberous Sclerosis

National Tuberous Sclerosis Association
8181 Professional Place, Suite 110
Landover, MD 20785

301-459-9888
800-225-6872
Fax: 301-459-0394
e-mail: ntsa@ntsa.org
www.ntsa.org

True stories of people living with Tuberous Sclerosis.

Softcover

7317 Tuberous Sclerosis: Fact Sheet

National Inst. of Neurological Disorders/Stroke
31 Center Drive, MSC 2540, Building 31, Room 8A06
Bethesda, MD 20892

301-496-5751
800-352-9424

Story C Landis, Director
Walter J Koroshetz, Deputy Director

DESCRIPTION

7318 TURNER SYNDROME

Synonyms: Chromosome 45,X syndrome, XO syndrome
Involves the following Biologic System(s):
Genetic/Chromosomal/Syndrome/Metabolic Disorders

Turner syndrome is a chromosomal disorder that affects only females. In most cases, females have two X chromosomes and males have one X and one Y chromosome in cells of the body. However, in females with Turner syndrome, one of the X chromosomes is deleted (missing) from cells or is functionally defective; some cells have the normal pair of X chromosomes whereas others do not (mosaicism). Although associated symptoms and findings may be variable, the most consistent abnormalities associated with the disorder include short stature and defective development of the ovaries (gonadal dysgenesis).

Many newborns with Turner syndrome have an abnormal accumulation of fluid in and associated swelling of the backs of the hands and the tops of the feet (peripheral lymphedema). Additional features that may be apparent at birth include an abnormally short, webbed neck (pterygium colli) with a low hairline; a narrow roof of the mouth (palate) or a small jaw (micrognathia); abnormal outward deviation of the elbows upon extension (cubitus valgus); a broad chest with widely spaced, underdeveloped, and/or inverted nipples; or deeply set, narrow, and/or outwardly curved (convex) nails. In most cases, females with Turner syndrome also have kidney (renal) malformations (e.g., horseshoe kidney and/or cleft or double renal pelvis). In addition, in some cases, heart (cardiac) defects may be present, such as abnormalities affecting the major artery (aorta) that arises from the lower left chamber (ventricle) of the heart (e.g., bicuspid aortic valve, coarctation of the aorta). In almost all affected females, there is also defective development of the ovaries (ovarian dysgenesis), i.e., the paired glands within which the female reproductive cells are produced (ova or eggs) and from which certain female hormones are secreted. Consequently, in most cases, female secondary sexual characteristics fail to develop (e.g., breast development, appearance of hair in the pubic area and under the arms, menstruation) and most affected females are infertile. In addition, although intelligence is typically normal, some females with Turner syndrome may experience learning disabilities (e.g., difficulty with visual-spatial relationships) and may have poor coordination. The treatment of children with Turner syndrome may include hormone replacement therapy (e.g., estrogen therapy, human growth hormone therapy); surgical intervention for congenital heart defects, renal malformations, webbing of the neck, or other abnormalities; special education for those with learning disabilities; and other treatment measures as required. Turner syndrome is thought to result from errors during the division of a parent's reproductive cells (meiosis). According to estimates in the medical literature, the disorder may affect from approximately one in 2,000 to one in 4,000 female newborns.

See also **General Resources** on page 917

Government Agencies

7319 NIH/National Institute of Child Health and Human Development
31 Center Drive, Building 31
Bethesda, MD 20892

301-496-5133
Fax: 301-496-1104
www.nichd.nih.gov

Established in 1962 by congress, today the institute conducts and supports research on topics related to the health of children, adults, families and populations. Some of these topics include: developmental disabilities, growth and development, infant death, reproductive health and birth defects.

Nancy D Wirth, Director
Lisa Kaeser, Program & Public Liaison

National Associations & Support Groups

7320 American Society for Reproductive Medicine
1209 Montgomery Highway
Birmingham, AL 35216

205-987-5000
Fax: 205-978-5005
e-mail: asrm@asrm.org
www.asrm.org

The American Society for Reproductive Medicine is an organization devoted to advancing knowledge and expertise in infertility, reproductive medicine and biology. The ASRM is a voluntary non-profit organization.

Robert W Rebar, MD, Executive Director
Sue Prescott, General Services Director

7321 Genetic Alliance
4301 Connecticut Avenue NW
Washington, DC 20008

202-966-5557
800-336-4363
Fax: 202-966-8553
e-mail: info@geneticalliance.org
www.geneticalliance.org

A coalition of voluntary genetic support groups, consumers and professionals addressing the needs of individuals and families affected by genetic disorders from a national perspective.

Sharon Terry, President/CEO

7322 Human Growth Foundation
997 Glen Cove Avenue, Suite 5
Glen Head, NY 11545

516-671-4041
800-451-6434
Fax: 516-671-4055
e-mail: hgf1@hgfound.org
www.hgfound.org

A voluntary, nonprofit organization whose mission is to help children and adults with disorders of growth and growth hormones through research, education, support and advocacy. The foundation is dedicated to helping medical science to better understand the process of growth. It is composed of concerned parents and friends of children and adults with growth problems and interested health professionals.

Patricia D Costa, Executive Director

7323 MAGIC Foundation: Major Aspects of Growth in Children: Turner's Syndrome Division
6645 W North Avenue
Oak Park, IL 60302

708-383-0808
Fax: 708-383-0899
www.magicfoundation.org

A national nonprofit organization providing support and education regarding growth disorders in children and related adult disorders. Provides educational information, networking, a national conference, a kids' program and an extensive medical library.

Dianne Tamburrino, Executive Director
Susan Smith, Director Medical Education

7324 Turner's Syndrome Society of the US
14450 TC Jester, Suite 260
Houston, TX 77014

823-249-9988
800-365-9944
Fax: 832-249-9987
e-mail: tssus@turner-syndrome-us.org
www.turner-syndrome-us.org

More than 38 chapters across the country. Goals are to promote public awareness of the disease, support those affected by the condition and aid in continuing research. Membership dues for a single person are $40, a family, $60, and for professionals, $60.

2,500 members

Frances A McAnear, Program Coordinator
Merriott J Terry, Executive Director, Chomosome Dis.

State Agencies & Support Groups

Alaska

7325 Turner's Syndrome Society of Alaska
1334 N Street
Anchorage, AK 99501

907-279-3202
e-mail: marytullius@hotmail.com
www.turner-syndrome-us.org

Mary Tullius

Arizona

7326 Turner's Syndrome Society of Arizona
2215 Wickenburg Road
Ponopah, AZ 85354

602-443-3805
www.turner-syndrome-us.org

Tracie Holley

California

7327 Turner's Syndrome Society Central And Northern

Bay Point, CA 94565

925-299-7729
e-mail: rosie1038@attbi.com
www.turner-syndrome-us.org

Rosemary Morris

7328 Turner's Syndrome Society of Southern California
8902 Heil Avenue #24
Westminster, CA 92683

714-847-1102
e-mail: ccurby@meritlending.com
www.turner-syndrome-us.org

Colleen Curby, President

Colorado

7329 Turner's Syndrome Society of Rocky Mountain
4972 S Garland
Littleton, CO 80123

720-981-2632
www.turner-syndrome-us.org

Donna Landrum

Connecticut

7330 Turner's Syndrome Society of Connecticut
57 Cianci Drive
Southington, CT 06489

860-628-8729
e-mail: barry1157@aol.com
www.turner-syndrome-us.org

Sandra Gittleman

Florida

7331 Turner's Syndrome Society - Tampa Support Group
3202 W Fair Oaks Avenue
Tampa, FL 33611

813-837-0582
e-mail: heddyb@gateway.net
www.turner-syndrome-us.org

Heddy Brown

7332 Turner's Syndrome Society of Northern Florida
6447 Cooper Lane
Jacksonville, FL 32210

904-786-1420
e-mail: sebri448@cs.com
www.turner-syndrome-us.org

Kim Brown

7333 Turner's Syndrome Society of South Florida
235 NE 23rd Street #204
Ft. Lauderdale, FL 33305

954-567-2380
e-mail: tigger3927@aol.com
www.turner-syndrome-us.org

Rachel Nowak

Iowa

7334 Turner's Syndrome Society of Iowa/New Found Friends
2615 Meadow Glen Road
Ames, IA 50014

515-292-2757
e-mail: epolashek@aol.com
www.turner-syndrome-us.org

Cathie Berglund

Kentucky

7335 Turner's Syndrome Society of Kentucky
380 Bob-O-Link Drive
Lexington, KY 40503

606-278-5935
www.turner-syndrome-us.org

Elizabeth Howard

Louisiana

7336 Turner's Syndrome Society of Gulf Coast
7731 Butterfield Road
New Orleans, LA 70126

334-476-7940
www.turner-syndrome-us.org

Donna Baudier

Maryland

7337 Turner's Syndrome Society of Maryland
2206 229th Street
Pasadena, MD 21122

410-360-5571
e-mail: jmatts@erols.com
users.erols.com/jmatts/

Kathy Mattson

Massachusetts

7338 Turner's Syndrome Society of New England
60 Joy Street, Apartment 303
Boston, MA 02114

617-557-4837
Fax: 617-636-6131
www.turner-syndrome-us.org

Geralyn Dwyer

Michigan

7339 Turner's Syndrome Society of Southeastern Michigan
7490 Drew Circle, Apartment 8
Westland, MI 48185

734-421-1192
e-mail: ksemrau@aol.com
www.turner-syndrome-us.org

Kim Semrau

7340 Turner's Syndrome Society of West Michigan
1569 Sibley Street NW
Grand Rapids, MI 49504

616-735-3931
www.turner-syndrome-us.org

Mary Dawson

Minnesota

7341 Turner's Syndrome Society of Minnesota
7109 Autumn Terrace
Eden Prairie, MN 55346

612-937-9725
www.turner-syndrome-us.org

Becky Mobarry

Missouri

7342 Turner's Syndrome Society of St. Louis/ West Illinois
1514 Azalia Drive
Saint Louis, MO 63119

314-892-2635
www.turner-syndrome-us.org

Cheryl Jost

Nevada

7343 Turner's Syndrome Society of Nevada
PO Box 94002
Las Vegas, NV 89193

702-731-3452
www.turner-syndrome-us.org

Joelle Barnes

New Hampshire

7344 Turner's Syndrome Society of Northern New England
1261 Old North Main Street
Laconia, NH 03246

603-528-3510
www.turner-syndrome-us.org

Lori Ann Pawlowski
Dawn And Matt Dragon

New Jersey

7345 Turner's Syndrome Society of New Jersey
238 Hempstead Drive
Somerset, NJ 08873

732-249-3727
www.turner-syndrome-us.org

Linda Kalb

New York

7346 Turner's Syndrome Society of Central New York
476 Ford Hill Road
Berkshire, NY 13736

607-657-8425
e-mail: tlkwwjd@aol.com
www.turner-syndrome-us.org

Tammy Kozak

7347 Turner's Syndrome Society of Rochester
88 Moreland Road
Rochester, NY 14612

716-473-7181
www.turner-syndrome-us.org

Susan Sponseller

7348 Turner's Syndrome Society of Upstate New York
115 Union Avenue #205
Saratoga Springs, NY 12866

518-209-1793
e-mail: saratogatif@aol.com
www.turner-syndrome-us.org

Tiffany Festo

North Carolina

7349 Turner's Syndrome Society of North Carolina
1223 Pine Springs Drive
Hendersonville, NC 28739

828-692-4975
e-mail: rich02@msn.com
www.turner-syndrome-us.org

Cheryl Tuttle

Ohio

7350 Turner's Syndrome Society of Southwestern Ohio
8530 Gateview Court
Dayton, OH 45424

937-667-5276
e-mail: schwando@email.msn
www.turner-syndrome-us.org

Barb Schwandner

Oklahoma

7351 Turner's Syndrome Society of Oklahoma
5904 East Lattimer
Tulsa, OK 74115

918-838-7355
www.turner-syndrome-us.org

Jean Radtke

Pennsylvania

7352 Turner's Syndrome Society of Philadelphia
2322 Taggart Court
Wilmington, DE 19810

302-475-5780
e-mail: jmkurze@aol.com
www.turner-syndrome-us.org

Joann Kurzeknabe

Rhode Island

7353 Turner's Syndrome Society of Rhode Island
24 Turner Street, Unit 3
Warwick, RI 02886

401-732-2136
e-mail: deb pomerantz@hotmail.com
www.turner-syndrome-us.org

South Carolina

7354 Turner's Syndrome Society of South Carolina
153 Gannet Point Road
Beaufort, SC 29902

843-522-8508
www.turner-syndrome-us.org

Robin Butler

Tennessee

7355 Turner's Syndrome Society of Mid-South
2541 Clydes Place Cove
Memphis, TN 38133

901-385-1720
e-mail: hmschlmom3@yahoo.com
www.turner-syndrome-us.org

Penny Williams

7356 Turner's Syndrome Society of Tennessee
9202 Shady Bend Lane
Knoxville, TN 37922

423-539-2210
www.turner-syndrome-us.org

Kathy Blackbourne

Texas

7357 Turner's Syndrome Society of Houston
11602 Bexhil
Houston, TX 77065

281-469-3810
e-mail: hou-tss@swbell.net
www.turner-syndrome-us.org

Cindy Dunnam

7358 Turner's Syndrome Society of North Texas
3211 W Division #28
Arlington, TX 76012

817-460-2443
e-mail: smithar1@earthlink.org
www.turner-syndrome-us.org

Patricia Burton

7359 Turner's Syndrome Society of San Antonio
923 Escalon Avenue
San Antonio, TX 78221

210-621-0073
www.turner-syndrome-us.org

Carolyn Braden

Utah

7360 Turner's Syndrome Society of Salt Lake City
2337 Chateau Drive
Roy, UT 84067

801-825-4118
e-mail: kristyne70@hotmail.com
www.turner-syndrome-us.org

Kristyne Rudolph

Virginia

7361 Turner's Syndrome Society of National Capitol Area
6200 Westchester Park Drive #406
College Park, MD 20740

301-345-3136
www.turner-syndrome-us.org

Deb Shoup

Washington

7362 Turner's Syndrome Society of Inland Northwest
5317 N Washington Street
Spokane, WA 99205

509-326-3703
www.turner-syndrome-us.org

Nancy Owen

Wisconsin

7363 Turner's Syndrome Society of Southeastern Wisconsin
10122 63rd Street
Kenosha, WI 53142

262-857-9528
e-mail: thejohnsonact@earthlink.net
www.turner-syndrome-us.org

Amy Johnson

Libraries & Resource Centers

7364 Turner's Syndrome Society Resource Center
Turner Syndrome Society of the United States
14450 TC Jester, Suite 260
Houston, TX 77014

832-249-9988
800-365-9944
Fax: 832-249-9987
www.turner-syndrome-us.org

Allows members to have access to the most recent articles being published in the area of Turner Syndrome, a listing of local chapters, physician referrals and booklets and videos offering guidance to families and physicians.

Frances A McAnear, Program Coordinator

Web Sites

7365 Endocrine Society
www.endo-society.org

Is the worlds largest and most active professional organization of endocrinologists in the world. The society is internationally known as the leading source of state of the art research and clinical advancements in endocrinology and metabolism. The society is dedicated to promoting excellence in research, education and clinical practice in the field of endocriniology.

7366 Health Answers
www.healthanswers.com

HealthAnswers offers a breadth of services in medical education, sales force training, patient support solutions, professional promotion and consumer solutions.

7367 Human Growth Foundation
www.hgfound.org

A voluntary nonprofit organization whose mission is to help chidren, and adults with disorders of growth and growth hormones through research, education, support and advocacy.

7368 MAGIC Foundation: Major Aspects of Growth in Children: Turner's Syndrome Division
www.magicfoundation.org

Is a national nonprofit organization created to provide support services for the families of children afflicted with a wide variety of chronic and or critical disorders, syndromes and diseases that affected a child's growth.

7369 Online Mendelian Inheritance in Man
www.ncbi.nlm.nih.gov

This database is a catalog of human genes and genetic disorders.

7370 Turner's Syndrome Society of the United States
www.turner-syndrome.us.org

A nonprofit organization that provides assistance, support, and education to girls and women with turner syndrome, their families, physicians, and the interested public.

Newsletters

7371 Turner's Syndrome News
Turner's Syndrome Society of the United States
14450 TC Jester, Suite 260
Houston, TX 77014

800-365-9944
Fax: 832-249-9987
www.turner-syndrome-us.org

Includes articles addressing current issues in turner syndrome, updates on national and local activities and letters from girls and women with Turner's syndrome and their families.

Quarterly

Frances A McAnear, Program Coordinator

Pamphlets

7372 Answers to Some Commonly Asked Questions
Turner Syndrome Society of the United States
14450 TC Jester, Suite 260
Houston, TX 77014

800-365-9944
Fax: 832-249-9987
www.turner-syndrome-us.org

Offers information on the Society's activities and the role they play in supporting people with Turner Syndrome.

Frances A McAnear, Program Coordinator

7373 Facing the Challenges of Turner Syndrome Together
Turner Syndrome Society of the United States
14450 TC Jester, Suite 260
Houston, TX 77014

800-365-9944
Fax: 832-249-9987
www.turner-syndrome-us.org

Brochure offering information on Turner's syndrome, statistics on how widespread the disease is and the Society's role in conquering this disease and supporting its members.

Frances A McAnear, Program Coordinator

7374 Facts About Turner Syndrome
Turner Syndrome Society of the United States
14450 TC Jester, Suite 260
Houston, TX 77014

800-365-9944
Fax: 832-249-9987
www.turner-syndrome-us.org

Offers statistical and factual information on the disease of Turner Syndrome, causes, symptoms, prevention and treatment.

Frances A McAnear, Program Coordinator

7375 How to Start a Turner Syndrome Support Group
Turner Syndrome Society of the United States
14450 TC Jester, Suite 260
Houston, TX 77014

800-365-9944
Fax: 832-249-9987
www.turner-syndrome-us.org

Offers information to the lay person on how to obtain material from medical professionals, and publicity aspects and funding aspects in pertaining to starting a support group.

Frances A McAnear, Program Coordinator

7376 Turner's Syndrome
Human Growth Foundation
7777 Leesburg Pike, Suite 202S
Falls Church, VA 22043

703-883-1773
800-451-6434
www.turner-syndrome-us.org

Background of a tremendous need for further information about Turner's Syndrome.

7377 Turner's Syndrome Society Resource Bibliographies
Turner's Syndrome Society of the United States
14450 TC Jester, Suite 260
Houston, TX 77014

800-365-9944
Fax: 832-249-9987
www.turner-syndrome-us.org

These fact sheets offer information on books, videos and other resources available on Turner Syndrome.

Frances A McAnear, Program Coordinator

7378 Turner's Syndrome: A Personal Perspective
Turner's Syndrome Society of the United States
14450 TC Jester, Suite 260
Houston, TX 77014

800-365-9944
Fax: 832-249-9987
www.turner-syndrome-us.org

A reprint from the Adolescent and Pediatric Gynecology Journal offering a personal account of a woman with Turner Syndrome and her experiences.

Frances A McAnear, Program Coordinator

7379 Turner's Syndrome: Guide for Families
Turner's Syndrome Society of the United States
14450 TC Jester, Suite 260
Houston, TX 77014

800-365-9944
Fax: 832-249-9987
www.turner-syndrome-us.org

Offers information to parents on the causes, symptoms, diagnosis and prognosis of Turner's syndrome, includes resources of where to go for help and support.

Frances A McAnear, Program Coordinator

7380 Turner's Syndrome: The Hows and Whys of the Missing X Chromosome
Human Growth Foundation
7777 Leesburg Pike, Suite 2020S
Falls Church, VA 22043

703-883-1773
800-451-6434
www.turner-syndrome-us.org

Women with Turner's Syndrome lack one of the X chromosomes. This carries genes for conditions relating to the development of ovaries, sex hormone production, and physical development in general.

DESCRIPTION

7381 ULCERATIVE COLITIS
Involves the following Biologic System(s):
Gastrointestinal Disorders

Ulcerative colitis is an inflammatory bowel disease (IBD) characterized by chronic inflammation and ulceration of the lining of the colon, the major part of the large intestine. The disease initially affects the lowest region of the large intestine (rectum) and gradually progresses to involve varying lengths or all of the colon. The range and severity of associated symptoms is extremely variable and may depend in part on the amount of the colon that is affected. Ulcerative colitis usually becomes apparent during adolescence or young adulthood. However, in some patients, associated symptoms may occur as early as the first year of life. The frequency of the disorder varies greatly in different countries and is thought to be higher in urban areas. In the United States and northern Europe, ulcerative colitis affects approximately 100 to 200 per 100,000 individuals in the general population. In developed countries, inflammatory bowel disease, including ulcerative colitis, is the most common cause of chronic intestinal inflammation during mid-childhood. The exact cause of ulcerative colitis is unknown. However genetic, immune, and environmental factors are thought to be contributing factors.

In patients with ulcerative colitis, the onset of symptoms may be gradual (insidious) or sudden, rapid, and severe (fulminant). Most patients experience episodes of watery diarrhea with varying amounts of blood, mucus, or pus. Associated findings may include abdominal cramping and pain; persistant, inability or difficulty emptying the bowel at defecation (tenesmus); and an urgent, compelling urge to defecate. Fulminant colitis is characterized by over six daily bowel movements, a high fever, chills, abnormally low levels of iron or the protein albumin in the blood, an increase in certain circulating white blood cells (leukocytosis), and other findings. In some children, additional findings include failure to grow and gain weight at the expected rate and lack of appetite (anorexia). The frequency of episodes may vary greatly. Most patients experience periods of remission during which symptoms subside and eventual, periodic recurrences (exacerbations). However, some patients may have infrequent episodes and others may experience severe, ongoing symptoms.

Certain complications may occur in association with ulcerative colitis. For example, because of blood loss during episodes, there may be inadequate levels of iron and ab-

normally reduced levels of the oxygen-carrying protein of the blood (iron-deficiency anemia). Some individuals with ulcerative colitis may develop sudden massive enlargement of the colon (toxic megacolon). Without prompt, appropriate treatment, toxic megacolon may result in tearing or perforation of the colon, potentially causing life-threatening complications. In addition, patients who have ulcerative colitis for more than 10 years have an increased risk of colon cancer. Regular examination of the colon (colonoscopies) and biopsies are recommended beginning at eight to 10 years after disease onset to help ensure prompt detection and treatment. During a colonoscopy, tissue inside the colon is examined using a flexible viewing instrument. To obtain a biopsy, small samples of tissue are removed from the colon for examination under a microscope.

Many patients with ulcerative colitis may also eventually experience more generalized, systemic symptoms. By the third decade of life, some patients may develop ankylosing spondylitis (AS), a chronic, progressive, inflammatory disease that affects joints of the spine and results in pain, stiffness, and possible loss of spinal mobility. In patients with ulcerative colitis, AS most commonly affects joints of the back and the hips and may cause lower back pain and stiffness, particularly in the morning. Some patients with ulcerative colitis may also develop a chronic skin condition characterized by irregular, bluish-red skin sores (pyoderma gangrenosum); chronic inflammation of the liver (chronic active hepatitis); and inflammation of the bile ducts (primary sclerosing cholangitis).

Since ulcerative colitis cannot be cured, the goals of treatment with medication are to induce remissions, maintain remissions, minimize side effects of treatment, and improve the quality of life. In patients with mild colitis, treatment often includes administration of anti-inflammatory drugs, such sulfasalazine, which may alleviate symptoms and potentially prevent recurrences. Patients with moderate to severe colitis who do not respond to such treatment may receive corticosteroid therapy, such as with the drug prednisone or immunomodulators that suppress the body's immune system, thus reducing inflammation. If affected individuals have fulminant colitis or colitis that is unresponsive to drug therapy, treatment may include surgical removal of the colon (colectomy). Additional treatment is symptomatic and supportive. An interesting new treatment uses nicotine. It has long been observed that the risk of ulcerative colitis appears to be higher in nonsmokers and in ex-smokers. In certain circumstances, patients improve when treated with nicotine where other medications have not been effective.

See also General Resources on page 917

Government Agencies

7382 NIH/National Institute of Diabetes and Dig estive and Kidney Disease
9000 Rockville Pike
Building 31, Room 904A
Bethesda, MD 20892

301-496-4000
TTY: 301-402-9612
e-mail: NIHinfo@od.nih.gov
www.nih.gov

Offers information and referrals to persons afflicted with ulcerative colitis.

National Associations & Support Groups

7383 Crohn's & Colitis Foundation of America
386 Park Avenue South
New York, NY 10016

212-685-3440
800-932-2423
Fax: 212-779-4098
e-mail: info@ccfa.org
www.ccfa.org

Supports basic and clinical research into a cure and prevention for Crohn's disease and ulcerative colitis; conducts professional and patient education activities; produces public service programs and a wide variety of literature about inflammatory bowel disease for patients and their families, professionals and the public; and sponsors chapters nationwide.

James V Romano, PhD, President/CEO

7384 Digestive Disease National Coalition
507 Capitol Court NE, Suite 200
Washington, DC 20002

202-544-7497
Fax: 202-546-7105
www.ddnc.org

Advocacy organization comprised of 22 voluntary and professional societies concerned with the many diseases of the digestive tract and liver.

Nancy Norton, Chairperson
Dr. Maurice Cerulli, President

7385 Genetic Alliance
4301 Connecticut Avenue NW
Washington, DC 20008

202-966-5557
800-336-4363
Fax: 202-966-8553
e-mail: info@geneticalliance.org
www.geneticalliance.org

A coalition of voluntary genetic support groups, consumers and professionals addressing the needs of individuals and families affected by genetic disorders from a national perspective.

Sharon Terry, President/CEO

7386 International Foundation for Functional Gastrointestinal Disorders
PO Box 170864
Milwaukee, WI 53217

414-964-1799
888-964-2001
Fax: 414-964-7176
e-mail: iffgd@iffgd.org
www.iffgd.org

Nonprofit education and research organization founded in 1991. IFFGD addresses the issues surrounding life with gastrointestinal (GI) functional and mobility disorders and increases the awareness about these disorders among the general public, researchers and the clinical care community.

Nancy J Norton, Founder
William Norton, VP

7387 Intestinal Disease Foundation
1323 Forbes avenue Suite 200
Pittsburgh, PA 15219

416-261-5888
877-587-9606
Fax: 412-471-2722
e-mail: info@intestinalfoundation.org
www.intestinalfoundation.org

Nonprofit organization whose mission is to improve the quality of life of adults and children affected by chonic digestive illness through information, guidance and support. IDF offers a quarterly newsletter, Intestinal Fortitude, educational seminars, volunteer phone network, and Pittsburgh area support groups.

Linda Schurr, Executive Director

7388 Pediatric Crohn's & Colitis Association
PO Box 188
Newton, MA 02468

617-489-5854
e-mail: questions@pcca.hypermart.net
pcca.hypermart.net

Focuses on all aspects of pediatric and adolescent Crohn's disease and ulcerative colitis, including medical, nutritional, psychological and social factors. Activities include information sharing, educational forums, newsletters and hospital outreach programs, as well as support of research.

7389 United Ostomy Association Hotline
P.O. Box 66
Fairview, TN 37062

949-660-8624
800-826-0826
Fax: 949-660-9262
e-mail: info@uoa.org
www.uoa.org

An advocate for ostomy and alternative procedure patients answering questions from employment issues to insurability practices. Also publishes magazines, patient care guides, conducts conferences and youth rally summer camps. We sponsor networks and resources for children, teens young adults, and parents.

Nancy Italia, Executive Director
Ken Aukett, President Of Mgmt Board Of Director

Libraries & Resource Centers

7390 National Digestive Diseases Information Clearinghouse
2 Information Way
Bethesda, MD 20892

301-654-3810
800-891-5389
Fax: 703-738-4929
e-mail: nddic@info.niddk.nih.gov
www.digestive.niddk.nih.gov

The National Institute of Diabetes and Digestive and Kidney Diseases conducts and supports research on many of the most serious diseases affecting public health. The Institute supports much of the clinical research on the diseases of internal medicine and related subspecialty fields as well as many basic science disciplines.

Kathy Kranzfelder, Project Officer

Research Centers

7391 Center for Digestive Disorders
Central Dupage Hospital
25 N Winfield Road
Winfield, IL 60190

630-933-1600
www.cdh.org

Web Sites

7392 Ask NOAH About: Stomach and Intestinal (Gastrointestinal) Disorders
noah-health.org/english/illness/gastro/gastro.html

Provides access to high quality full-text consumer health information in English and Spanish that is accurate, timely, relevant and unbiased.

7393 Colitis Cookbook
www.colitiscookbook.com/

A cookbook for people with colitis and other diseases.

7394 Crohn's & Colitis Foundation of America
www.ccfa.org

Our mission is to prevent Crohn's disease and ulcerative colitis through research, and to improve the quality of life of children and adults affected by these digestive diseases through eduation and support.

7395 Health Answers
www.healthanswers.com

HealthAnswers offers a breadth of services in medical education, sales force training, patient support solutions, professional promotion and consumer solutions.

7396 IBS Self-help group
www.ibsgroup.org/

Works to educate those who are living with IBS and to increase awareness about his and other functional gastrointesinal disorders. The group was founded in support for those who suffer from IBS, those who are looking for support for someone who has IBS, and medical professionals who want to learn more about IBS.

7397 National Digestive Diseases Information Clearinghouse
www.digestive.niddk.nih.gov

The National Institute of Diabetes and Digestive and Kidney Diseases conducts and supports research on many of the most serious diseases affecting public health. The Institute supports much of the clinical research on the diseases of internal medicine and related subspecialty fields as well as many basic science disciplines.

7398 Online Mendelian Inheritance in Man
www.ncbi.nlm.nih.gov

This database is a catalog of human genes and genetic disorders.

7399 Pediatric Crohn's & Colitis Association
pcca.hypermart.net

We are committed to helping children with IBD and their families better understand the Crohn's disease and ulcerative colitis.

Book Publishers

7400 Angry Gut, The: Coping with Colitis and Crohn's Disease
Plenum Publishing Corporation
10 E 53 Street
New York, NY 10022

212-207-7600
Fax: 212-463-0742
e-mail: info@plenum.com
www.springerlink.com

Overview of the symptoms, diagnosis, complications, and treatment of IBD.

1993 364 pages
ISBN: 0-306444-70-4

7401 Ask Audrey
7466 Pebble Lane
West Bloomfield, MI 48322

248-626-6960

A compilation of material and the personal story of a medical psychotherapist who has inflammatory bowel disease. Includes practical tips on issues such as handling diarrhea, sexuality, relationships, traveling, coping with hospital stays, ostomies, and TPN.

7402 Digestive Diseases & Disorders Sourcebook
Omnigraphics
PO Box 625
Holmes, PA 19043

800-234-1340
Fax: 800-875-1340
e-mail: info@omnigraphics.com
omnigraphics.com

Basic consumer health information including celiac disease, crohn's disease, diarrhea, hernias, irritable bowel syndrome and ulcers.

335 pages
ISBN: 0-780803-27-2

7403 IBD Nutrition Book
John Wiley & Sons
432 Elizabeth Avenue
Somerset, NJ 08875

800-225-5945
Fax: 732-302-2300
e-mail: custserv@wiley.com
www.wiley.com

Clinical dietitian/nutritionist's overview of the role of diet in IBD, including recipes and meal plans.

7404 Inflammatory Bowel Disease
Lippincott Williams & Wilkins
351 W Camden Street
Baltimore, MD 21201

410-528-4000
800-638-3030
www.lww.com

Detailed information on every aspect of IBD. Topics include medical and surgical management, epidemiology, fertility and pregnancy, psychosocial factors, and diagnostic techniques. Written for medical professionals and laypersons who are comfortable with medical terminology.

7405 Inflammatory Bowel Disease - From Bench to Bedside
Williams & Wilkins
351 W Camden Street
Baltimore, MD 21201

301-528-4000
www.lww.com

Offers in-depth information on the impact of basic research developments on the management of Crohn's disease and ulcerative colities. Written for medical professionals and laypersons who are comfortable with medical terminology.

7406 New People Not Patients: A Source Book for Living with IBD

Crohn's and Colitis Foundation of America
386 Park Avenue S
New York, NY 10016

212-685-3440
www.gastro.org/public/ibd.html

7407 Ostomy Book: Living Comfortably with Colostomies, Ileostomies and Urostomies

United Ostomy Association
19772 Macarthur Boulevard
Irvine, CA 92612

949-660-8624
Fax: 949-660-9262
www.uoa.org

An in-depth resource on how to adapt to an ostomy.

7408 Treating IBD: A Patient's Guide to the Medical and Surgical Management

Crohn's and Colities Foundation of America
386 Park Avenue S
New York, NY 10016

212-685-3440
www.gastro.org/public/ibd.html

7409 You're Bigger than It

Hotel Dieu Hospital
Ontario, Canada,

613-544-3310

This cartoon book offers a lively, brief introduction to the basics of living with IBD. Contact can be reached at extension 2400.

Newsletters

7410 Inner Circle

Reach Out for Youth with Ileitis and Colitis
15 Chemung Place
Jericho, NY 11753

516-822-8010
e-mail: reachoutforyouth@reachoutforyouth.org
www.reachoutforyouth.org

Newsletter for youth with ileitis and colitis.

Pamphlets

7411 Bleeding in the Digestive Tract

Nat'l Digestive Diseases Information Clearinghouse
9000 Rockville Pike
Bethesda, MD 20892

301-496-3583
www.niddik.nih.gov

Informational fact sheet.

7412 Crohn's Disease, Ulcerative Colitis, and Your Child

Crohn's and Colitis Foundation of America
386 Park Avenue S
New York, NY 10016

212-685-3440
www.ccfa.org

7413 Guide for Children & Teenagers

Crohn's and Colitis Foundation of America
386 Park Avenue S
New York, NY 10016

212-685-3440
www.ccfa.org

7414 Inside Story

Reach Out for Youth with Illeitis and Colitis
15 Chemung Place
Jericho, NY 11753

516-822-8010

Educational brochure for youth with illeitis and colitis.

7415 Living with IBD: A Guide for Teenagers

Crohn's and Colitis Foundation of America
386 Park Avenue S
New York, NY 10016

212-685-3440
www.ccfa.org

7416 Questions and Answers About Ulcerative Colitis

Crohn's and Colitis Foundation of America
386 Park Avenue S
New York, NY 10016

212-685-3440
www.ccfa.org

7417 Teacher's Guide to Crohn's Disease & Ulcerative Colitis

Crohn's & Colitis Foundation of America
386 Park Avenue S, 17th Floor
New York, NY 10016

212-665-3440
800-932-2423
Fax: 212-779-4098
e-mail: info@ccfa.org
www.ccfa.org

7418 Ulcerative Colitis

National Organization for Rare Disorders
PO Box 8923
New Fairfield, CT 06812

203-746-6518
800-999-6673
e-mail: orphan@rarediseases.org
www.rarediseases.org

Informational fact sheet.

DESCRIPTION

7419 URTICARIA

Synonym: Hives

Involves the following Biologic System(s):

Dermatologic Disorders

Urticaria, more commonly known as hives, is a skin condition characterized by the development of raised, usually itchy (pruritic), white or reddish lesions (wheals). The wheals associated with urticaria vary in size and may sometimes blend together to form large, patchy skin lesions. Although individual lesions may disappear within minutes, hours, or days, new eruptions may continue to appear for weeks. Urticaria is considered to be a chronic skin disorder if wheals continue to appear for six weeks or longer.

Although the cause of urticaria is sometimes unknown, it often results as an immune or allergic response during which histamine or other substances are released causing small blood vessels in the upper skin layer to widen and release fluid, thus producing the characteristic wheals associated with hives. These allergic reactions may be caused by ingestion of certain foods such as shellfish, strawberries, nuts, eggs; drugs such as aspirin, penicillin, or codeine; and food dyes or other additives. In addition, allergic responses may be triggered by contact with certain plant substances, insects, animals or animal saliva, or topical skin preparations. Other causative agents may include injection of certain drugs, blood transfusions, insect bites or stings, and inhalation of pollen and other allergens. The rash derived from poison-ivy is commonly mistaken for urticaria. Poison-ivy is caused by urushiol toxin. This resin can be spread by contact, but it is easily washed off.

Urticaria may also develop in association with certain viral infections such as infectious mononucleosis or hepatitis, certain bacterial or parasitic infections, or in response to the cold, the sun, or exercise. Hives are also associated with many other disorders. For example, hives may develop in conjunction with swelling of certain areas of soft tissue (angioedema or angioneurotic edema). Angioedema involves deeper layers of the skin as well as the upper respiratory tract, the gastrointestinal tract, the face and neck, the hands and feet, and genitalia. A distinct disorder known as urticaria pigmentosa may develop during early childhood and is characterized by reddish-brown skin lesions that are spread over the body and change into hive-like lesions when stroked, rubbed, or scratched. Hives may be associated with other systemic disorders and with certain inherited disorders such as amyloidosis, familial cold urticaria, and hereditary angioedema, which is a severe and potentially life-threatening form of angioedema.

Hives often disappear quickly with no intervention; however, the application of calamine lotion or the administration of antihistamines may be helpful in relieving associated itching and swelling. Children with acute, severe urticaria or those who experience difficulty in breathing or swallowing require immediate medical attention. Other treatment for urticaria is often dependent upon the underlying cause. If one's triggers can be id entified, however, then outbreaks can often be managed by limiting one's exposure to these situations. For example, the administration of two specific types of antihistamines is often indicated for the control of chronic urticaria, while sunscreen protection is the treatment of choice for those individuals with urticaria resulting from sun exposure (solar urticaria). Stress reduction is often effective in reducing symptoms associated with hives. Other treatment is symptomatic and supportive.

See also **General Resources** on page 917

Government Agencies

7420 NIH/National Institute of Allergy and Infectious Diseases
6610 Rockledge Drive, MSC 6612
Bethesda, MD 20892

301-496-5717
Fax: 301-402-3573
TDD: 800-877-8339
www.niaid.nih.gov

Conducts and supports basic and applied research to better understand, treat, and ultimately prevent infectious, immunologic, and allergic diseases.

Anthony S Fauci MD, Director

7421 NIH/National Institute of Arthritis and Mu sculoskeletal and Skin Diseases
1AMS Circle
Bethesda, MD 20892

301-402-4484
Fax: 301-718-6366
e-mail: ord@od.nih.gov
rarediseases.info.nih.gov

The mission of the National Institute of Arthritis and Musculoskeletal and Skin Diseases is to support research into the causes, treatment, and prevention of arthritis and musculoskeletal and skin diseases, the training of basic and clinical scientists to carry out this research, and the dissemination of information on research progress in these diseases.

Stephen I Katz MD PhD, Director

7422 NIH/National Institute of Child Health and Human Development
31 Center Drive, Building 31
Bethesda, MD 20892

301-496-5133
Fax: 301-496-1104
www.nichd.nih.gov

Established in 1962 by congress, today the institute conducts and supports research on topics related to the health of children, adults, families and populations. Some of these topics include: developmental disabilities, growth and development, infant death, reproductive health and birth defects.

Nancy D Wirth, Director
Lisa Kaeser, Program & Public Liaison

National Associations & Support Groups

7423 Genetic Alliance
4301 Connecticut Avenue NW
Washington, DC 20008

202-966-5557
800-336-4363
Fax: 202-966-8553
e-mail: info@geneticalliance.org
www.geneticalliance.org

A coalition of voluntary genetic support groups, consumers and professionals addressing the needs of individuals and families affected by genetic disorders from a national perspective.

Sharon Terry, President/CEO

7424 Society for Pediatric Dermatology
8365 Keystone Crossing, Suite 107
Indianapolis, IN 46240

317-202-0224
Fax: 317-205-9481
e-mail: spd@hp-assoc.com
www.pedsderm.net

Objective is to promote, develop and advance education, research and care of all skin disease in all pediatric age groups.

Kent Lindeman, Executive Director

Web Sites

7425 Allergy Web
www.allergyweb.com

Provides information that may help you learn more about allergies and asthma.

7426 InteliHealth
www.intelihealth.com

Our mission is to empower people with trusted solutions for healthier lives. We accomplish this by providing credible information for the most trusted sources, and have become one of the leading on-line health information companies in the world.

DESCRIPTION

7427 VENTRICULAR SEPTAL DEFECTS

Synonym: VSDs

Involves the following Biologic System(s):

Cardiovascular Disorders

Ventricular septal defects (VSDs) are considered the most common structural heart malformations, comprising up to 20 percent of all heart defects that are present at birth (congenital). VSDs are characterized by the presence of an abnormal opening in the fibrous muscular partition (septum) that separates the two lower pumping chambers (ventricles) of the heart. The ventricles are the chambers that pump blood out of the heart via large blood vessels (arteries). The pulmonary artery arises from the base of the right ventricle and carries oxygen-poor (deoxygenated) blood to the lungs, where the exchange of oxygen and carbon dioxide occurs. The aorta, the main artery of the body, arises from the base of the left ventricle and carries oxygen-rich (oxygenated) blood to the body's tissues.

In infants with ventricular septal defects, the abnormal opening in the septum between the two ventricles allows oxygenated blood in the left ventricle to flow into the right ventricle and recirculate to the lungs rather than to the rest of the body's tissues. Symptoms and findings may vary, depending upon the size and location of the ventricular septal defect and the associated effects on pulmonary blood pressure and flow. If the VSD is large, it may result in significantly increased blood flow through the lungs' blood vessels.

Small VSDs usually cause no associated symptoms and, in up to 50 percent of patients, may close spontaneously before school age. Small ventricular septal defects may be detected during a routine physical examination based upon a characteristic heart sound (heart murmur) heard with a stethoscope. In infants with larger VSDs, too much blood is pumped to the lungs. This may result in persistent elevation of blood pressure in the pulmonary circulation (pulmonary hypertension), enlargement of the heart (cardiomegaly), and abnormally rapid breathing (tachypnea). Additional symptoms and findings may include difficulty with lower respiratory tract infections, increased sweating, difficulties feeding, and failure to grow and gain weight at the expected rate (failure to thrive). When these symptoms and findings occur, the infant is said to have congestive heart failure (CHF). Large VSDs may be diagnosed upon a complete clinical examinationand various specialized tests, such as x-ray studies, echocardiogram (ultrasound of the heart),

electrocardiogram, or cardiac catheterization.

Children and adolescents with unclosed VSDs may be at an increased risk of bacterial infection of the lining of the heart (endocarditis). Such infection is rare before the age of two years. Due to the increased risk of bacterial endocarditis, affected individuals are cautioned to take antibiotic medication before dental visits and surgical procedures. After the VSD is successfully closed, preventive treatment is needed only during a six-month healing period. Closing small ventricular septal defects may not be needed. They often close on their own in childhood or adolescence. But if the opening is large, even in patients with few symptoms, closing the hole in the first two years of life is recommended to prevent serious problems later.

In some patients, VSDs may occur in association with certain underlying genetic syndromes, chromosomal abnormalities, or malformation syndromes that are caused by exposure to certain infectious agents, medications, or other environmental factors (teratogenic syndromes).

See also **General Resources** on page 917

National Associations & Support Groups

7428 American Heart Association
7272 Greenville Avenue
Dallas, TX 75231

> 214-373-6300
> 800-242-8721
> Fax: 214-706-1341
> e-mail: inquire@amhrt.org
> www.amhrt.org

Supports research, education and community service programs with the objective of reducing premature death and disability from cardiovascular diseases and stroke; coordinates the efforts of health professionals, and others engaged in the fight against heart and circulatory disease.

M Cass Wheeler, CEO

Web Sites

7429 Congenital Heart Information Network
www.ohsu.edu

An international organization that provides reliable information, support services and resources to families of children with congenital heart defects and acquired heart disease and adults with congenital heart defects, and the professionals who work with them.

7430 Southern Illinois University School of Medicine
www.siumed.edu

The mission of SUI School of Medicine is to assist the people of central and southern Illinois in meeting their present and future needs through education, clinical service and research.

7431 Yale University School of Medicine
www.info.med.yale.edu

A site that offers information on Ventricular Septal Defects and other congenital heart conditions.

DESCRIPTION

7432 WILLIAMS SYNDROME

Synonyms: WBS, Williams-Beuren syndrome, WMS, WS

Involves the following Biologic System(s):

Cardiovascular Disorders,

Genetic/Chromosomal/Syndrome/Metabolic Disorders

Williams syndrome is a genetic disorder characterized by mild growth delays before birth (prenatal growth retardation); growth delays after birth (postnatal growth retardation); mild short stature; characteristic abnormalities of the head and face (craniofacial area); and variable levels of mental deficiency. Unusual features of the head and face may result in a distinctive appearance that becomes more pronounced with advancing age. Characteristic features include a rounded face with full cheeks; full, thick lips and a large mouth that is typically in an open position, prominent ears; flared eyebrows; short eyelid folds (palpebral fissures); and a broad nasal bridge with a wide tip and nostrils that flare forward (anteverted). Dental abnormalities are often present, such as small teeth (hypodontia) with underdeveloped (hypoplastic) tooth enamel. Distinctive abnormalities of the eyes may also occur, including divergence of one eye in relation to the other (strabismus) and an unusual star-like (stellate) pattern in the colored portions of the eyes (irides).

Most children and adults with Williams syndrome also have mild to moderate mental retardation. Affected individuals may have an intelligence quotient (I.Q.) ranging from 80, which is considered the low end of average, to 40, which is considered moderate mental retardation. The average I.Q. is approximately 56, which is considered at the lower end of the range for mild mental retardation. Other findings associated with Williams syndrome may include a short attention span, easy distractibility, a poor relationship between visual stimuli and resultant movements (motor-visual integration skills), and strong general language skills as opposed to general cognitive abilities. Most affected children and adults have a friendly personality and a talkative, outgoing manner of speech.

Some infants and children with Williams syndrome may also have additional physical abnormalities, such as heart defects, musculoskeletal abnormalities, or unusually increased blood calcium levels during infancy (transient infantile hypercalcemia). For example, affected infants may develop narrowing (stenosis) in the area above the valve leading from the lower left-sided pumping chamber (ventricle) of the heart to the main artery (aorta) of the body (supravalvular aortic stenosis); obstruction of normal blood flow from the right ventricle of the heart to the lungs (branch pulmonary stenosis); high blood pressure (hypertension); or other cardiovascular abnormalities including narrowing of the blood vessels to the head and abdominal organs. Musculoskeletal defects may include limited movements of certain joints; abnormal curvature of the spine (e.g., scoliosis, kyphosis, lordosis); and an awkward gait. Some individuals with Williams syndrome also have abnormalities affecting the urinary tract, such as the return flow of urine from the urinary bladder back into a ureter (vesicoureteral reflux), recurrent urinary tract infections, and other findings (e.g., nephrocalcinosis, bladder diverticula). Digestive problems may also occur, including chronic constipation. Depending upon the specific abnormalities present, treatment may include limitation of calcium in and elimination of vitamin D from the diet in those with high levels of calcium in the blood; heart surgery for those with certain structural cardiac defects; and special educational and supportive services, such as physical therapy, individualized educational programs, speech therapy, and occupational therapy. Other treatment is symptomatic and supportive.

Most cases of Williams syndrome appear to occur randomly (sporadically) for unknown reasons; however, some familial cases have been reported. Sporadic and inherited cases of the disorder appear to occur due to missing genetic material (deletion) from genes located next to one another (contiguous genes) on the long arm (q) of chromosome 7 (7q11.23). The syndrome is thought to affect approximately one in 10,000 newborns.

See also **General Resources** on page 917

Government Agencies

7433 NIH/National Institute of Child Health and Human Development

31 Center Drive, Building 31
Bethesda, MD 20892

301-496-5133
Fax: 301-496-1104
www.nichd.nih.gov

Established in 1962 by congress, today the institute conducts and supports research on topics related to the health of children, adults, families and populations. Some of these topics include: developmental disabilities, growth and development, infant death, reproductive health and birth defects.

Nancy D Wirth, Director
Lisa Kaeser, Program & Public Liaison

National Associations & Support Groups

7434 Cincinnati Center for Developmental Disorders
Cincinnati Children's Hospital Medical Center
3333 Burnet Avenue, Pavilion Building
Cincinnati, OH 45229

513-636-4200
800-344-2462
Fax: 513-636-7361
TTY: 513-636-4900
www.chmcc.org

Cincinnati Center for Developmental Disorders provides diagnosis, evaluation, treatment, training and education for infants, children and adolescents with a variety of developmental disorders.

Sonya G Oppenheimer, MD, Director
Melinda Chalfonte-Evans, PhD, Treatment Director

7435 Genetic Alliance
4301 Connecticut Avenue NW
Washington, DC 20008

202-966-5557
800-336-4363
Fax: 202-966-8553
e-mail: info@geneticalliance.org
www.geneticalliance.org

A coalition of voluntary genetic support groups, consumers and professionals addressing the needs of individuals and families affected by genetic disorders from a national perspective.

Sharon Terry, President/CEO

7436 Williams Syndrome Association
PO Box 297
Clawson, MI 48017

284-244-2229
800-806-1871
Fax: 248-244-2230
e-mail: info@williams-syndrome.org
www.williams-syndrome.org

Devoted to improving the lives of individuals with Williams Syndrome and their families. The WSA supports research into all facets of the syndrome, and the development of the most up to date educational materials regarding Williams Syndrome.

Terry Monkaba, Executive Director
Erin Cunningham, Assistant Director

7437 Williams Syndrome Foundation
University of California

Irvine, CA 92697

949-824-7259
e-mail: hlenhoff@uci.edu
www.wsf.org

The WSF offers support for those affected with the condition through opportunities in education, housing, employment and recreation.

Gordon Biescar, Treasurer/President
Patrick S Smith, Secretary

Research Centers

7438 Patient Recruitment & Public Liaison Office Clinical Center
10 Cloister Court, Building 61
Bethesda, MD 20892

800-411-1222
Fax: 301-480-9793
e-mail: prpl@cc.nih.gov
www.cc.nih.gov

The NIH Clinical Center is a federally funded biomedical research facility that supports clinical investigations conducted by the institutes of the National Institute of Health.

Web Sites

7439 Healthfinder
www.healthfinder.gov

A guide for health information.

7440 Kansas University Medical Center
www.kumc.edu

A nationally recognized biomedical research center, offers educational programs through its Schools of Allied Health, Medicine, Nursing, Pharmacy and Graduate Studies.

7441 Lili Claire Foundation
www.liliclairefoundation.org/

Helps to ease the challenges families face by providing a unique and comprehensive blend of programs and support services.

7442 Online Mendelian Inheritance in Man
www.ncbi.nlm.nih.gov

This database is a catalog of human genes and genetic disorders.

7443 Rare Genetic Diseases in Children (NYU)
www.med.nyu.edu/rgdc/homenow.htm

We target issues arising from rare genetic diseases affecting children, and to assist in the endeavor to bring knowledge and hope to those for whom there is, at present, so little.

7444 Williams Syndrome Foundation Home Page
www.williamssyndrome.org/

Seeks to create or enhance opportunities in education, housing, employment and recreation for people who have Willimas Syndrome and other related or similar conditions. The WSF identifies, initiates, funds and provides strategic guidance for major, long range development projects, either by itself, or by cooperating with other organizations.

7445 Williams Syndrome Monthly Medline Alert
www.geocities.com/HotSprings/8172/

DESCRIPTION

7446 WILMS TUMOR

Synonyms: Nephroblastoma, Renal Tumor, Kidney Tumor
Involves the following Biologic System(s):
Hematologic and Oncologic Disorders

Wilms tumor (also known as nephroblastoma) is a rare malignant tumor of the kidney that accounts for about eight percent of childhood cancers. It occurs with equal frequency among males and females. Wilms tumor may develop in any region of either kidney. In most cases, tumor development occurs in one kidney (unilateral). However, both kidneys may be involved (bilateral) in about five to 10 percent of affected children. In some severe cases, the tumor may spread to other parts of the body (metastasize), particularly the lungs.

Wilms tumor typically becomes apparent by approximately three to five years of age. The most common sign is the presence of a smooth, firm mass in the abdominal area. Approximately 50 percent of affected children experience associated abdominal pain or vomiting (emesis) and about 10 to 25 percent have blood in their urine (microscopic or gross hematuria). In addition, up to 60 percent of children with Wilms tumor have high blood pressure (hypertension) due to the tumor's pressure on an artery near the kidney (renal artery). In severe cases, long-term hypertension may result in the inability of the heart to pump blood effectively throughout the body (cardiac failure).

Selection of treatment is based on the stage of the cancer and whether the histology (appearance of the Wilms tumor under the microscope) is favorable or unfavorable. In children with Wilms tumor in one kidney, treatment typically includes immediate surgical removal of the affected kidney (nephrectomy). During surgery, the remaining kidney is examined to exclude tumor development. After surgery, therapy may include the use of certain anticancer drugs (chemotherapy). According to the National Wilms Tumor Study Group, the preferred chemotherapy regimen consists of therapy with dactinomycin and vincristine that may be combined with doxorubicin. Those with advanced disease may also receive radiation therapy through the use of x-rays or other sources of radioactivity. In children with Wilms tumor in both kidneys, chemotherapy and radiation therapy may be considered before surgery.

The exact cause of Wilms tumor is not understood. However, missing genetic material (deletion) from one of at least three different chromosomal locations has been noted in affected individuals. Such deletions have been located on the short arm of chromosome 11 (at 11p13 or 11p15.5) and on the long arm of chromosome 16 (16q). These genetic changes may appear to occur randomly for unknown reasons (sporadic) or may be inherited as an autosomal dominant trait. In rare cases, deletions at one of these locations (i.e., 11p13) may be associated with two rare disorders that are characterized by Wilms tumor. These include Denys-Drash syndrome and WAGR syndrome. Denys-Drash syndrome is characterized by Wilms tumor, abnormal kidney function (nephropathy leading to renal failure), and severe malformations of the reproductive and urinary tracts (e.g., pseudohermaphroditism). WAGR syndrome is characterized by Wilms tumor, absence of all or a portion of the pigmented area (iris) of the eyes at birth (aniridia), genitourinary malformations, and mental retardation.

See also **General Resources** on page 917

Government Agencies

7447 Cancer Information Service
National Cancer Institute
6116 Executive Boulevard, Suite 3036A
Bethesda, MD 20892

800-422-6237
Fax: 301-330-7968
TTY: 800-332-8615
http://cis.nci.nih.gov

The Cancer Information Service provides the latest and most accurate cancer information to patients, their families, the public, and health professionals. Through its network of regional offices, the CIS serves the United States, Puerto Rico, the U.S. Virgin Islands, and the Pacific Islands.

Andrew C Von Eschenback, Director

7448 National Cancer Institute
6116 Executive Boulevard, Room 3036A
Bethesda, MD 20892

800-422-6237
www.cancer.gov

The National Cancer Institute coordinates the National Cancer Program, which conducts and supports research, training, health information dissemination, and other programs with respect to the cause, diagnosis, prevention, and treatment of cancer, rehabilitation from cancer, and the continuing care of cancer patients and the families of cancer patients.

John E Niederhuber MD, Director

National Associations & Support Groups

7449 American Cancer Society
2970 Clairmont Road
Atlanta, GA 840

404-315-1123
800-282-4914
Fax: 404-315-9348
e-mail: angelina.veal@cancer.org
www.cancer.org

The American Cancer Society is a nationwide, community-based voluntary health organization. Headquartered in Atlanta, Georgia, the ACS has state divisions and more than 3,400 local offices. For more than 80 years, ACS has led the way in cancer research. The goal is to prevent cancer, save lives, and diminish suffering from cancer.

Shannon Mejri, Program Assistant
Virginia Krawiec, Program Director

7450 Candlelighters Childhood Cancer Foundation
PO Box 498
Kensington, MD 20895

301-962-3520
800-366-2223
Fax: 310-962-3521
e-mail: staff@candlelighters.org
www.candlelighters.org

The Candlelighters Childhood Cancer Foundation National Office was founded in 1970 by concerned parents of children with cancer. Today our membership of over 50,000 members of the national office and more than 100,000 members across the across the country, including Candlelighters affiliate groups, includes, parents of children who are being treated or have been treated for cancer.

Ruth Hoffman, Executive Director

7451 Children's Cancer Research Institute
University of Texas Health Science Ctr
8403 Floyd Curl Drive
San Antonio, TX 78229

210-562-9000
Fax: 210-562-9014
e-mail: chessher@uthscsa.edu
ccri.uthscsa.edu

The Children's Cancer Research Institute was created by the State of Texas with $200 million from the State's tobacco settlement. Fulfilling its legislative mandate, it is CCRI's mission to advance scientific knowledge relevant to childhood cancer, to accelerate the translation of knowledge into novel therapies, and to eliminate cancer at all ages through discovery, development, and dissemination of scientific knowledge relevant to childhood cancer.

Sharon Murphy MD, Director
Bill Chessher, Administrator

7452 Children's Hopes and Dreams
Wish Fulfillment Foundation
280 Route 46
Dover, NJ 07801

706-482-2248
Fax: 706-482-2289
e-mail: chdfdover@juno.com
www.childrenswishes.org

Children's Hopes & Dreams has been serving children with serious childhood illnesses since 1983. We are one of the oldest wish fulfillment organizations in the world.

10,000 Members

Mariann Oswald, Program Director

7453 Children's Wish Foundation International
8615 Roswell Road
Atlanta, GA 30350

770-393-9474
800-323-9474
Fax: 770-393-0683
e-mail: wish@childrenswish.org
www.childrenswish.org

A nonprofit organization that fulfills wishes for children with life threatening illnesses. The criteria for wish fulfillment are: the child must be under the age of eighteen, and have been diagnosed with a life threatening illness.

Arthur Stein, President
Linda Dozoretz, Founder/Executive Director

7454 National Childhood Cancer Foundation
4600 East West Highway, Suite 600
Bethesda, MD 20814

800-458-6223
e-mail: info@curesearch.org
www.curesearch.org

CureSearch unites the world's largest childhood cancer research organization, the Children's Oncology Group, and the National Childhood Cancer Foundation through our mission to cure childhood cancer. Research is the key to the cure.

Research Centers

7455 National Wilms Tumor Study
Fred Hutchinson Cancer Research Center
1100 Fairview Avenue N, PO Box 19024
Seattle, WA 98109

206-667-4842
Fax: 206-667-6623
e-mail: nwtsg@fhcrc.org
www.nwtsg.org

To improve the survival of children with Wilms tumor and other renal tumors, to study the long-term outcome of children with successfully treated by identifying adverse effects of treatment, to study the epidemiology and biology of Wilms tumor and to make information regarding successful treatment strategies for Wilms tumor available to physicians around the world.

Web Sites

7456 CancerCare
www.cancercare.org

A national nonprofit organization dedicated to providing free, professional support services to those affected by cancer.

7457 Children's Cancer Web
www.cancerindex.org/ccw

An independent nonprofit site, established to provide a directory of childhood cancer resources.

7458 OncoLink: The University of Pennslyvania Cancer Center Resource
www.oncolink.upenn.edu/about/index

Mission to help cancer patients, families, health care professionals, and the general public get accurate cencer-related information at no charge.

7459 Online Mendelian Inheritance in Man
www.ncbi.nlm.nih.gov

This database is a catalog of human genes and genetic disorders.

Book Publishers

7460 Let's Talk About Going to the Hospital
Rosen Publishing Group's PowerKids Press
29 E 21st Street
New York, NY 10010

212-777-3017
800-237-9932
Fax: 888-436-4643
e-mail: senpub@tribeca.ios.com
www.powerkidspress.com

If a child has to check into the hospital, chances are he or she is already upset about being ill. Knowing how a hospital functions and what the procedures are, such as when family members can visit, will help in what is already a stressful situation. Grades K-5.

24 pages
ISBN: 0-823950-36-0

7461 Let's Talk About When Kids Have Cancer

Melanie Apel Gordon, author

Rosen Publishing Group's PowerKids Press
29 E 21st Street
New York, NY 10010

212-777-3017
800-237-9932
Fax: 888-436-4643
e-mail: customerservice@rosenpub.com
www.powerkidspress.com

In a straightforward yet comforting way, this book explains what
cancer is, what kinds of treatments surround the disease and how to
cope if a child or the friend of a child has cancer.

24 pages Paperback
ISBN: 0-823951-95-2

7462 Surviving Childhood Cancer: A Guide for Families

New Harbinger Publications
5674 Shattuck Avenue
Oakland, CA 94609

510-652-0215
800-748-6273
Fax: 510-652-5472
e-mail: customerservice@newharbinger.com
www.newharbinger.com

Cancer in a child is an overwhelming experience for a family. This
book explains common medical procedures and offers readers
practical advice about how to cope with emotions and stress during
this time.

232 pages Paperback
ISBN: 1-572241-02-0

DESCRIPTION

7463 WILSON DISEASE

Synonyms: Hepatolenticular degeneration, WD, WND
Involves the following Biologic System(s):
Gastrointestinal Disorders

Wilson disease is a genetic disorder in which a defect in copper metabolism causes an abnormal accumulation of copper in the liver, brain, kidneys, corneas, and other tissues of the body. The disorder is often characterized by progressive liver disease, degenerative changes of the brain, kidney failure, and the presence of characteristic grayish-green or reddish-gold rings at the outer margins of the corneas (Kayser-Fleischer rings). If untreated, Wilson disease can cause severe brain damage, liver failure, and death. Wilson disease is a progressive disorder in which the age at onset may vary from patient to patient. Symptoms and findings may not become apparent until five or six years of age and most commonly begin during mid-adolescence. However, in some patients, the disease may not become apparent until adulthood. Wilson disease is thought to have a prevalence of approximately one in 30,000 individuals worldwide.

In individuals with Wilson disease, copper progressively accumulates in the liver and is released into other organs and tissues of the body, particularly the brain, corneas, and kidneys. Associated symptoms and findings may be variable; however, individuals within certain multigenerational families typically have similar clinical presentations. Affected children under 10 years of age tend to have associated liver abnormalities. Neurologic symptoms rarely affect those under 10 years of age; however, young adults tend to have neurologic involvement. Individuals with Wilson disease, liver disease is characterized by enlargement of the liver (hepatomegaly) with or without enlargement of the spleen (splenomegaly); acute or chronic inflammation of the liver (hepatitis); and internal scarring (fibrosis) and impaired functioning of the liver (cirrhosis). Those with cirrhosis may have yellowish discoloration of the skin, mucous membranes, and whites of the eyes (jaundice); unusually high blood pressure (hypertension) in certain veins near the liver (portal hypertension); an abnormal accumulation of fluid in certain body tissues (edema) and the abdominal cavity (ascites); and enlargement of blood vessels in the wall of the esophagus (esophageal varices), potentially causing them to rupture and bleed. In severe cases, affected individuals may develop fulminant hepatitis, a severe form of liver disease characterized by localized loss of liver tissue (necrosis), defects of blood clotting (coagulation), coma

(hepatic encephalopathy), and potentially life-threatening complications.

Neurologic symptoms associated with Wilson disease may appear to develop suddenly or may occur gradually. Many such symptoms are thought to result from progressive involvement of a region of the brain that assists in regulating muscular movements (basal ganglia). Neurologic symptoms often initially include abnormalities of muscle tone (progressive dystonia), muscle stiffness and rigidity. In addition, patients may experience involuntary, rhythmic, quivering movements of the extremities on one side of the body (unilateral) that may eventually become generalized. Additional neurologic symptoms include difficulties speaking (dysphonia), drooling, a fixed smile due to drawing back of the upper lip, and involuntary, rapid, jerky movements in association with slow, writhing movements (choreoathetosis). Wilson disease may also result in the premature breakdown of red blood cells (hemolysis). This condition may progress to a chronic condition known as hemolytic anemia. In this form of anemia, premature destruction of red blood cells causes reduced levels of the protein that enables red blood cells to transport oxygen to cells (hemoglobin). In addition, the kidneys may become unable to regulate the appropriate balance between water and salt content, filter waste products from the blood and excrete them in urine, and perform other vital functions (progressive renal failure).

Wilson disease is an autosomal recessive disorder that results from changes (mutations) of a gene on the long arm of chromosome 13 (13q14.3-q21.1).

The goal in treating Wilson disease is twofold: to remove excess copper and to prevent the mineral from building up again. It often consists of the administration of penicillamine, a medication that binds with copper (chelation) and enables it to be excreted from the body. This treatment is accompanied by supplementation of vitamine B6. If affected individuals are unable to tolerate penicillamine, the medications trientine and zinc acetate may be appropriate substitutes. Physicians and other health care professionals may also recommend a diet that is low in copper intake (less than one mg/day), suggesting avoidance of such foods as chocolate, liver, shellfish, and nuts. Liver transplantation may be considered in those with fulminant hepatitis. Other treatment for individuals with Wilson disease is symptomatic and supportive.

See also **General Resources** on page 917

National Associations & Support Groups

7464 American Liver Foundation
75 Maiden Lane, Suite 603
New York, NY 10038

212-668-1000
800-465-4837
Fax: 212-483-8179
e-mail: info@liverfoundation.org
www.liverfoundation.org

Nonprofit, national voluntary health organization dedicated to the prevention, treatment and cure of hepatitis and other liver diseases through research, education, and advocacy on behalf of those affected by or at risk of liver disease.

Frederick G Thompson, President/CEO
Marie P Bresnahan, VP Programs

7465 Children's Liver Alliance
3835 Richmond Avenue, Suite 190
Staten Island, NY 10312

718-987-6200
Fax: 718-987-6200
e-mail: organtrans@msn.com
www.transweb.org

Aids in easing the physical and emotional strains that the child is experiencing, so they can better deal with the disorder through different media resources that are also available to family and friends.

Kathie DeLuca, Office Manager

7466 Children's Liver Association for Support Services
27023 McBean Parkway, #126
Valencia, CA 91355

661-263-9099
877-679-8256
Fax: 661-263-9099
e-mail: supportsru@aol.com
www.classkids.org

CLASS is an all volunteer, nonprofit organization dedicated to serving the emotional, educational and financial needs of families coping with childhood liver disease and transplantation. Our goal is to be both a service to families and a valuable resource for the medical community.

Diane Sumner, President
Ann Whitehead, VP

7467 Genetic Alliance
4301 Connecticut Avenue NW
Washington, DC 20008

202-966-5557
800-336-4363
Fax: 202-966-8553
e-mail: info@geneticalliance.org
www.geneticalliance.org

A coalition of voluntary genetic support groups, consumers and professionals addressing the needs of individuals and families affected by genetic disorders from a national perspective.

Sharon Terry, President/CEO

7468 United Liver Foundation
5777 W Century Boulevard
Los Angeles, CA 90045

310-670-4624
Fax: 310-670-4672
e-mail: pbrady@liver411.com
www.liver411.com

A national organization that promotes research and cures for hepatitis and other liver diseases.

Pam Brady, Contact Person
Donna Gracon, Chapter Director

7469 Wilson's Disease Association
1802 Brookside Drive
Wooster, OH 44691

330-264-1450
888-264-1450
Fax: 330-264-0974
e-mail: info@wilsondisease.org
www.wilsonsdisease.org

Provides patients and their families with a membership list, e-mail correspondence, meetings for support and education, and a newsletter. Supports patients with financial assistance for medication and travel, and develops centers of excellence.

800 Members

Libraries & Resource Centers

7470 National Digestive Diseases Information Clearinghouse
2 Information Way
Bethesda, MD 20892

301-654-3810
800-891-5389
Fax: 703-738-4929
e-mail: nddic@info.niddk.nih.gov
www.digestive.niddk.nih.gov

The National Institute of Diabetes and Digestive and Kidney Diseases conducts and supports research on many of the most serious diseases affecting public health. The Institute supports much of the clinical research on the diseases of internal medicine and related subspecialty fields as well as many basic science disciplines.

Kathy Kranzfelder, Project Officer

Research Centers

7471 National Center for the Study of Wilson's Disease
432 W 58th Street, Suite 614
New York, NY 10019

212-523-8717
Fax: 212-523-8708
www.wilsonsdisease.org

Web Sites

7472 Children's Liver Alliance
www.livertx.org

Offers a fact sheet on liver conditions.

7473 Children's Liver Association for Support Services
www.classkids.org

CLASS is an all volunteer, nonprofit organization dedicated to serving the emotional, educational and financial needs of families coping with childhood liver disease and transplantation. Our goal is to be both a service to families and a valuable resource for the medical community.

7474 Wilson's Disease Association International
www.wilsondisease.org/

Funds research and facilitates and promotes the identification, education, treatment, and support of patients and other individuals affected by Wilson's Disease.

7475 Wilson's Disease Patient Information Exchange
www.gourmandizer.com/wilsons/indexx.html

Pages provide Wilson's Disease patients and their families a forum to share and compare their symptoms, treatments and to tell how the disease has affected thier lives.

Newsletters

7476 Children's Liver Alliance Newsletter
3835 Richmond Avenue, Suite 190
Staten Island, NY 10312

718-987-6200
Fax: 718-987-6200
www.transweb.org

Aids in easing the physical and emotional strains that the child is experiencing, so they can better deal with the disorder through different media resources that are also available to both friends and family.

4-12 pages

Kathie DeLuca, Office Manager

Pamphlets

7477 Wilson's Disease
Nat'l Digestive Diseases Information Clearinghouse
2 Information Way
Bethesda, MD 20892

301-654-3810
Fax: 301-907-8906
e-mail: nddic@info.niddk.nih.gov
www.niddk.nih.gov

Government Agencies

7478 Administration on Developmental Disabilities
Department of Health and Human Services
150 S. Independence
W. Philadelphia, PA 19106

215-861-4000
Fax: 215-861-4070
TTY: 202-690-6415
www.acf.hhs.gov

Information and advocacy resources for families and professionals. Includes listings of organizations providing general information and organizations focusing on more specific areas of concern to families and young adults who have disabilities.

7479 Agency for Health Care Research
Department of Health and Human Services
540 Gaither Road
Rockville, MD 20850

301-427-1364
Fax: 301-427-1364
www.ahrq.gov

Healthcare information and advocacy resources for families and professionals.

7480 Centers for Disease Control
Department of Health and Human Services
1600 Clifton Road
Atlanta, GA 30333

404-639-3311
www.cdc.gov

Federal agency that protects America's health and safety, provides information to guide health decisions, and builds strong partnerships to promote health.

7481 Educational Help for the Handicapped
Nat'l Info Center for Children and Youth
PO Box 1492
Washington, DC 20013

800-999-5599

Offers Federal assistance at many levels to enable children, youth and adults to receive education and training. Under the provisions of the Education for All Handicapped Children Act (EHA) of 1975, state and local school districts must provide an appropriate elementary and secondary education for disabled children from age 6 through 21. Presently, some states provide educational and related services for preschool age children.

7482 NIH/National Cancer Institute
Department of Health and Human Services
9000 Rockville Pike, Building 31, Room 10A16
Bethesda, MD 20892

301-496-5583
800-422-6237
www.nci.nih.gov/

Leads a national effort to reduce the burden of cancer morbidity and mortality and ultimately to prevent the disease. Through basic and clinical biomedical research and training, NCI conducts and supports programs to understand the causes of cancer; prevent, detect, diagnose, treat, and control cancer; and disseminate information to the practitioner, patient, and public.

7483 NIH/National Eye Institute
31 Center Drive MSC 2510
Bethesda, MD 20892

301-496-5248
e-mail: 2020@nei.nih.gov
www.nei.nih.gov

Conducts and supports research that helps prevent and treat eye diseases and other disorders of vision. This research leads to sight-saving treatments, reduces visual impairment and blindness, and improves the quality of life for people of all ages. NEI-supported research has advanced our knowledge of how the eye functions in health and disease.

Paul A Sieving M.D., Ph.D, Director

7484 NIH/National Genome Research Institute (NH GRI)
31 Center Drive, Building 31, Room 4B09
Bethesda, MD 20892

301-402-0911
Fax: 301-402-2218
www.genome.gov

Supports the NIH component of the Human Genome Project, a worldwie research effort designed to analyze the structure of human DNA and determine the location of the estimated 30,000 to 40,000 human genes. The NHGRI Intramural Research Program develops and implements understanding, diagnosing, and treating of genetic diseases.

7485 NIH/National Heart, Lung and Blood Institu te
Department of Health and Human Services
31 Center Drive, MSC 2480, Building 31, Room 5A52
Bethesda, MD 20892

301-594-1348
301-480-4907
TTY: 123-019-9912
e-mail: nihinfo@od.nih.gov
www.nhbli.nih.gov/nhlbi/nhlbi.htm

Provides leadership for a national research program in diseases of the heart, blood vessels, lungs, and blood and in transfusion medicine through support of innovative basic, clinical, population-based and health education research. NHLBI also maintains an information clearinghouse.

Elizabeth Nabel MD, Director

7486 NIH/National Insitute of Allergy and Infectious Diseases
Department of Health and Human Services
31 Center Drive, MSC 2480, Building 31, Room 5A52
Bethesda, MD 20892

301-496-4634
e-mail: nihinfo@od.nih.gov
www.niaid.nih.gov

NIAID's research strives to understatnd, treat and ultimately prevent the many infectious, immunologic and allergic diseases that threaten millions of American lives.

7487 NIH/National Institute of Arthritis and Mu suloskelatal and Skin Diseases
Department of Health and Human Services
1 AMS Circle
Bethesda, MD 20892

301-495-4484
877-226-4267
Fax: 301-718-6366
TDD: 301-565-2966
e-mail: niamsinfo@mail.nih.gov
www.nih.gov/niams

The mission of the NIAMS, a part of the NIH, is to support research into the causes, treatment, and prevention of arthritis and musculoskeletal and skin diseases, the training of basic and clinical scientists to carry out this research, and the dissemination of information on research progress in these diseases. The Institute also maintains an information clearinghouse.

Lillian Hatch, Librarian

7488 NIH/National Institute of Child Health and Human Development
Department of Health and Human Services
PO Box 3006
Rockville, MD 20847

800-370-2943
Fax: 301-496-7101
e-mail: nihinfo@od.nih.gov
www.nih.gov/nichd

The National Institute for Child Health and Human Development conducts and supports laboratory, clinical and epidemiological research on the reproductive, neurobiologic, developmental, and behavioral processes that determine and maintain the health of children, adults, families, and populations.

7489 NIH/National Institute of Dental and Crani ial Research (NIHDCR)

National Institutes of Health
31 Center Drive, MSC 2290, Building 31
Bethesda, MD 20892

301-496-4261
Fax: 301-402-2185
e-mail: nidcrinfo@mail.nih.gov
www.nidcr.nih.gov

The National Institute of Dental and Craniofacial Research promotes the general health of the American people by improving their oral, dental and craniofacial health. The NIDCR aims to promote health, to prevent diseases and conditions, and to develop new diagnostics and therapeutics.

Dr Lawrence A Tabak, Director
Thomas G Murphy, Acting Executive Director

7490 NIH/National Institute of Diabetes and Dig estive and Kidney Diseases

Department of Health and Human Services
2 Information Way
Bethesda, MD 20892

301-654-3810
Fax: 301-907-8906
e-mail: nddic@info.niddk.nih.gov
www.niddk.nih.gov

Conducts and supports basic and applied research and provides leadership for a national program in diabetes, endrocrinology, and metabolic diseases; digestive diseases and nutrition and kidney, urologic and hemotologic diseases. Several of these diseases are among the leading causes of disability and death; all seriously affect the quality of life of those who have them. NIDDK also maintains an information clearinghouse.

7491 NIH/National Institute of Mental Health

Department of Health and Human Services
5600 Fishers Lane
Rockville, MD 20857

301-443-4513
e-mail: nihinfo@odnih.gov
www.nimh.nih.gov

NIMH provides national leadership dedicated to understanding, treating, and preventing mental illnesses through basic research on the brain and through clinical, epidemiological, and services research.

7492 NIH/National Institute of Neurological Dis rs and Stroke (NINDS)

PO Box 5801
Bethesda, MD 20824

301-496-5751
800-352-9424
Fax: 301-496-0296
TTY: 301-468-5981
www.ninds.nih.gov

Information and advocacy resources for families and professionals. Includes listings of organizations providing general information and organizations focusing on more specific areas of concern to families and young adults who have disabilities.

7493 NIH/National Institute on Alcohol Abuse an d Alcoholism (NIAAA)

5635 Fishers Land
Bethesda, MD 20892

www.niaaa.nih.gov

NIAAA conducts research focused on improving the treatment and prevention of alcoholism and alcohol-related problems to reduce the enormous social and economic consequences of this disease.

7494 NIH/National Institute on Deafness and Oth er Communication Disorders (NIDCD)

31 Center Drive, MSC 2320
Bethesda, MD 20892

301-496-7243
800-241-1044
Fax: 301-402-0018
TTY: 800-241-1055
e-mail: nidcdinfo@nidcd.nih.gov
www.nidcd.nih.gov

The National Institute on Deafness and Other Communication Disorders (NIDCD) is a national resource center for health information about hearing, balance, smell, taste, voice, speech, and language for health professionals, patients, industry, and the public.

Dr James F Battey Jr, Director
Judith A Cooper PhD, Deputy Director

7495 NIH/Office of Rare Diseases (ORD)

Department of Health and Human Services
31 Center Drive, Room 1B03
Bethesda, MD 20892

301-402-4336
e-mail: sg18b@nih.gov
rarediseases.info.nih.gov/org

Information and advocacy resources for families and professionals. Includes listings of organizations providing general information and organizations focusing on more specific areas of concern to families and young adults who have disabilities.

7496 National Center for Education in Maternal and Child Health

Georgetown University
2115 Wisconsin Ave NW, Suite 601
Washington, DC 20007

202-784-9770
Fax: 202-784-9777
e-mail: mchlibrary@ncemch.org
www.ncemch.org

Information and advocacy resources for families and professionals. Includes listings of organizations providing general information and organizations focusing on more specific areas of concern to families and young adults who have disabilities.

7497 National Center for Health Statistics

Department of Health and Human Services
6525 Belcrest Road
Hyattsville, MD 20782

301-458-4636
e-mail: nchsquery@cdc.gov
www.cdc.gov/nchswww

Information and advocacy resources for families and professionals. Includes listings of organizations providing general information and organizations focusing on more specific areas of concern to families and young adults who have disabilities.

7498 National Clearinghouse on Postsecondary Education: HEATH Resource Center

Department of Health and Human Services
1 Dupont Circle NW, Suite 800
Washington, DC 20036

Fax: 202-401-2608
TTY: 202-205-8241
www.ed.gov/offices/osers

Provides information for individuals with disabilities and resources for families and professionals. Includes listings of organizations providing general information and organizations focusing on more specific areas of concern to families and young adults who have disabilities.

7499 National Coalition of Title 1 Chapter 1 Parents
3609 Georgia Avenue
Washington, DC 20010

202-291-8100
Fax: 202-291-8200

Information and advocacy resources for parents and professionals. Includes listings of organizations providing general information and organizations focusing on more specific areas of concern to families and young adults who have disabilities.

7500 National Council on Disability
Department of Health and Human Services
1331 F Street NW, Suite 1050
Washington, DC 20004

202-272-2004
Fax: 202-272-2022
TTY: 202-272-2074
www.ncd.gov

Information and advocacy resources for families and professionals. Includes listings of organizations providing general information and organizations focusing on more specific areas of concern to families and young adults who have disabilities.

7501 National Council on Patient Information and Education
4915 Saint Elmo Avenue, Suite 505
Bethesda, MD 20814

301-656-8565
Fax: 301-656-4464
e-mail: ncpie@erols.com
www.talkaboutrx.org

7502 National Health Council
1730 M Street NW, Suite 500
Washington, DC 20036

202-785-3910
Fax: 202-785-5923
e-mail: info@nhcouncil.org
www.healthanswers.com

Information and advocacy resources for families and professionals. Includes listings of organizations providing general information and organizations focusing on more specific areas of concern to families and young adults who have disabilities.

7503 National Health Information Center
PO Box 1133
Washington, DC 20013

301-565-4137
800-336-4797
Fax: 301-984-4256
e-mail: info@nhif.org
www.nhic.org

The National Health Information Center can put you in touch with organizations that can answer your health-related questions. The National Health Information Center can provide you with names and addresses of appropriate organizations.

7504 National Library Service for the Blind and Physically Handicapped
Library of Congress Reference Section
1291 Taylor Street NW
Washington, DC 20542

202-707-5100
800-424-8567
Fax: 202-707-0712
TTY: 202-707-0744
TDD: 202-707-0744
e-mail: nis@loc.gov
www.loc.gov/nls

Administers a national library service that provides recorded and braille reading materials to eligible children and adults who cannot read standard print.

Frank Kurt Cylke, Director

7505 National Maternal & Child Health Clearinghouse
2070 Chain Bridge Road, Suite 450
Vienna, VA 22182

703-821-8955
Fax: 703-821-2098
e-mail: nmchc@circsol.com
www.circsol.com

Information and advocacy resources for families and professionals. Includes listings of organizations providing general information and organizations focusing on more specific areas of concern to families and young adults who have disabilities.

7506 National Mental Health: Knowledge Exchange Network
Department of Health and Human Services
11426-28 Rockville Pike, Suite 405
Rockville, MD 20852

800-789-2647
Fax: 301-984-8796
e-mail: ken@mentalhealth.com
www.mentalhealth.org

Information and advocacy resources for families and professionals. Includes listings of organizations providing general information and organizations focusing on more specific areas of concern to families and young adults who have disabilities.

7507 National Oral Health Information Clearinghouse
Institute of Dental and Craniofacial Research
1 NOHIC Way
Bethesda, MD 20892

301-402-7364
Fax: 301-480-4098
TTY: 301-656-7581
e-mail: nidcrinfo@mail.nih.gov
www.nidcr.nih.gov

Produces and distributes patient and professional education materials including fact sheets, brochures, information packets and provides referrals to other organizations dealing with special care in oral health. Special Care is an approach to oral health management that is tailored to the specific needs of persons with a variety of medical, disabling, or mental conditions. Database includes bibliographic citations, abstracts, and availability information for a variety of printed materials.

7508 National Prevention Information Network
Center for Disease Control
PO Box 6003
Rockville, MD 20849

301-562-1098
800-458-5231
Fax: 888-282-7681
TTY: 800-243-7012
e-mail: info@cdcnac.org
www.cdcnpin.org

Information and advocacy resources for families and professionals. Includes listings of organizations providing general information and organizations focusing on more specific areas of concern to families and young adults who have disabilities.

7509 National Recreation and Park Association
22377 Belmont Ridge Road
Ashburn, VA 20148

703-858-0784
e-mail: info@nrpa.org

Information on adaptive sports and recreation activities for people of many abilities. Includes local chapters, referrals, fun and social interaction and support groups.

7510 National Rehabilitation Information Center
4200 Forbes Blvd, Suite 202
Lanham, MD 20706

301-459-5900
800-346-2742
Fax: 301-459-4263
TTY: 301-459-5984
e-mail: naricinfo@heitechservices.com
www.naric.com

Resources for families and professionals dealing with the rehabilitation of people with disabilities.

Mark Odum, Director

7511 Office for Fair Housing & Equal Opportunity
Department of Housing & Urban Development
451 7th Street SW
Washington, DC 20002

202-708-1112
TTY: 202-708-1455
e-mail: nis@loc.gov
www.loc.gov/nls

Information and advocacy resources for families and professionals. Includes listings of organizations providing general information and organizations focusing on more specific areas of concern to families and young adults who have disabilities.

7512 Office of Special Education and Rehabilitation Services
330 C Street SW, Switzer Building, Room 3132
Washington, DC 20202

202-205-8723
Fax: 202-401-2608
TTY: 202-205-8241
www.ed.gov/offices/osers

Information and advocacy resources for families and professionals. Includes listings of organizations providing general information and organizations focusing on more specific areas of concern to families and young adults who have disabilities.

7513 President's Committee on Employment of People with Disabilities
1331 F Street NW, 3rd Floor
Washington, DC 20004

202-376-6200
Fax: 202-376-6868
www.pcepd.gov

Information and advocacy resources for families and professionals. Includes listings of organizations providing general information and organizations focusing on more specific areas of concern to families and young adults who have disabilities.

7514 President's Committee on Mental Retardation
370 L'Enfant Promenade SW, Suite 701
Washington, DC 20447

202-619-0634
Fax: 202-205-9519
e-mail: prma@acp.dhhs.govprograms/pcmr
www.acf.dhhs.gov/

Information and advocacy resources for families and professionals. Includes listings of organizations providing general information and organizations focusing on more specific areas of concern to families and young adults who have disabilities. Serves in an advisory capacity to the President of the U.S. and the Secretary of the Dept. of Health and Human Services.

National Associations & Support Groups

7515 AASK: Adopt A Special Kid
8201 Edgewater Drive, Suite 103
Oakland, CA 94621

510-553-1748
888-680-7349
Fax: 510-553-1747
e-mail: info@aask.org
www.adoptaspecialkid.org

AASK provides complete, no-fee foster and adoption services to families interested in parenting children in the California foster care system. AASK also offers fee _ for -service home studies and other services for families wishing to adopt children from outside of the system.

Vali Ebert, Executive Director
Andrea Schneider, Family Coordinator

7516 ABLEDATA
8630 Fenton Street, Suite 930
Silver Spring, MD 20910

301-608-8998
800-227-0216
Fax: 301-608-8958
TTY: 301-608-8912
e-mail: abledata@orcmacro.com
www.abledata.com

ABLEDATA provides objective information on assistive technology and rehabilitation equipment available from domestic and international source to consumers, organizations, professionals,and caregivers within the United States. We serve the nation's disability, and senior communities.

David Johnson, Publications Director
Katherine Belknap, Project Director

7517 ACRMD:Lifespire
350 5th Avenue, Suite 301
New York, NY 10118

212-741-0100
Fax: 212-242-0696
e-mail: info@lifespire.org
www.acrmd.com

Life is committes to the principle that all individuals with a development disability are able to become contributing members of their family and community. It is Lifespire's aim to provide these indiviuals with the assistance and support necessary so that they can attain the skills necessary to maintain themselves in their community in the most integrated and independent manner possible.

Mark Van Voorst, CEO/President

7518 ADARA
PO Box 480
Myersville, MD 21773

501-224-6678
Fax: 501-868-8812
TTY: 501-868-8850
e-mail: ADARAorgn@aol.com
www.adara.org

Our mission is to facilitat excellence in human service delivery with individuals who are Deaf or Hard of Hearing. This mission is accomplished by enhancing the professional competencies of the membership, expanding opportunities for networking among ADARA colleagues and supporting positive public policies for individuals who are Deaf or Hard of Hearing.

Steve Hamerdinger, President

7519 AIM for the Handicapped Adventures in Movement
945 Danbury Road
Dayton, OH 45420

937-294-4611
800-332-8210
Fax: 937-294-3783
e-mail: aimforthehandicapped@aim

To help individuals achieve their highest potentential through the AIM Method of Specialized Movement Education.

Jean Collett, President
Emilie Hounshell, Secretary

7520 ARC of the United States
1010 Wayne Avenue, Suite 650
Silver Spring, MD 20910

301-565-3842
Fax: 301-565-5342
e-mail: info@thearc.org
www.thearc.org

The ARC is the national organization of and for people with mental retardation and related developmental disabilities and their families. Devoted to promoting and improving supports and services for people with mental retardation and their families. The association also fosters research and education regarding the prevention of mental retardation in infants and young children. The ARC was founded in 1950 by a small group of parents and other concerned individuals.

Sue Swenson, Executive Director
Adam Aaronson, Public Inquiries Director

7521 Academy for Guided Imagery
30765 Pacific Coast Highway, Suite 369
Malibu, CA 90265

800-726-2070
Fax: 800-727-2070
www.academygorguidedimagery.com

The Academy for Guided Imagery is dedicated to educating and supporting practicing clinicians in their uses of imagery and imagery related approaches to therapy and healing. The Academy is an accredited Post-graduate training provider for health professionals, and a source of self-care products an programsfor those struggling with a chronic, difficult, or painful illness.

David E. Bresler PhD,LAc, President

7522 Academy of Rehabilitative Audiology
PO Box 952
DeSoto, TX 75123

952-920-0484
Fax: 952-920-6098
e-mail: ara@incnet.com
www.audrehab.org

The primary purpose of ARA is to promote excellence in hearing care through the provision of comprehensive rehabilitative and habilitative services.

350 Members

Sheila R Pratt, President
John A Nelson, Secretary

7523 Access Board
1331 F Street NW, Suite 1000
Washington, DC 20004

202-272-0080
Fax: 800-872-2253
TTY: 800-993-2822
e-mail: info@access-board.gov
www.access-board.gov

The Access Board is an independent Federal agency devoted to accessibility for people with disabilities.Created in 1973 to ensure access to federally funded facilities,the Board is now a leading source of information on accessible design. The Board develops and maintains design criteria for the built environment,transit vehicles, telecommunications equipment, and for electronic and information technology.

David L. Bidd, Chairman
Douglas Anderson, Vice Chairman

7524 Adoptive Families of America
42 W 38th Street, Suite 901
New York, NY 10018

646-366-0830
Fax: 646-366-0842
e-mail: letters@adoptivefamilies.com
www.adoptivefamilies.com

Information and advocacy resources for families and professionals interested in adoption.

7525 Advocates Across America
PO Box 754
Chandler, AZ 85244

602-750-0004
Fax: 480-814-9404
e-mail: twk@axa.org
www.axa.org

Dedicated to teaching parents and other interested people how to effectively advocate for the educational rights of children with special needs. Special needs includes: ADD/ADHD, learning disabilities, severe health conditions or any other physical, mental or emotional disability.

7526 Advocates for Deaf & Hard of Hearing Youth
PO Box 75949
Washington, DC 20013

301-589-8444
Fax: 301-589-8444
e-mail: sponlts@juno.com

Information on deafness, hearing impairments, child welfare and advocacy.

Catherine Moses, President

7527 Alexander Graham Bell Association for the Deaf and Hard of Hearing
3417 Volta Place NW
Washington, DC 20007

202-337-5220
800-432-7543
Fax: 202-337-8314
TTY: 202-337-5221
e-mail: agbell2@aol.com
www.agbell.org

Gathers and disseminates information on pediatric hearing loss, and educational issues for hearing impaired children, promotes better public understanding of hearing loss in children and adults, provides scholarships and financial aid to families of children with hearing loss, and promotes early detection of hearing loss in infants. Publishes magazine for parents and professionals who work with children.

Donna Sorkin, Executive Director

7528 Alliance for Technology Access (ATA)
1304 Southpoint Boulevard, Suite 240
Petaluma, CA 94954

707-778-3011
800-914-3017
Fax: 707-765-2080
TTY: 707-778-3015
TDD: 707-778-3015
e-mail: ATAinfo@ATAcess.org
www.ataccess.org

The mission of the Alliance for Technology Access (ATA) is to increase the use of technology be children and adults with disabilities and functional limitations.

Mary Lester, Executive Director
Todd Plummer, Executive Director

7529 Ambulatory Pediatric Association
6728 Old McLean Village Drive
McLean, VA 22101

703-556-9222
Fax: 703-556-8729
e-mail: info@ambpeds.org
info@ambped.org

The Ambulstory Pediatric Association fosters the health of children, adolescents,and families by promoting generalism in academic pediatrics and acacademics in general pediatrics.

Robert Needlman, MD, Director, Continuity Care
Alice A. Kuo MD, Program Director

7530 American Academy of Audiology
11730 Plaza America Drive, Suite 300
Reston, VA 20190

703-790-8466
800-222-2336
Fax: 703-790-8631
e-mail: info@audiology.org
www.audiology.org

A professional organization dedicated to providing high quality and balanced hearing care to the public. Provides professional development, education and research and provides increased public awareness of hearing disorders and audiologic services.

Laura Fleming Doyle, CAE, Executive Director
Sydney Hawthorne Davis, Director Communications

7531 American Academy of Child and Adolescent Psychiatry
3615 Wisconsin Avenue NW
Washington, DC 20016

202-966-7300
Fax: 202-966-2891
aacap.org

The AACAP (American Academy of Child and Adolescent Psychiatry) is the leading national professional medical association dedicated to treating and improving the quality of life for children, adolescents, and families affected by these disorders. The AACAP is a 501 (c)(3) nonprofit organization established in 1953.

Richard Sarles, MD, President
Sandy Marts, Administrator

7532 American Academy of Dermatology (AAD)
PO Box 4014
Schaumburg, IL 60168

847-240-1280
866-503-7546
Fax: 847-240-1859
e-mail: MRC@aad.org
www.aad.org

Largest, most influential and most representative of all dermatologic associations. Committed to the highest quality standards in continuing medical education. Developed a platform to promote and advance the science and art of medicine and surgery related to the skin; promotes the highest possible standards in clinical practice, education and research in dermatology and related disciplines; and supports and enhances patient care and promotes the public interest relating to dermatology.

Stephen P Stone MD, President
William P Coleman III, MD, VP

7533 American Academy of Pediatrics
141 NW Point Boulevard
Elk Grove Village, IL 60007

847-434-4000
Fax: 847-434-8000
e-mail: kidsdocs@aap.org
www.aap.org

The American Academy of Pediatrics and its member pediatricians dedicate their efforts and resources to the health, safety and well-being of infants, children, adolescents and young adults.

Jay E Berkelhamer MD, FAAP, President

7534 American Amputee Foundation
PO Box 250218
Little Rock, AR 72225

501-666-2523
Fax: 501-666-8367
e-mail: american_amputee_foundation@hotmail.com
www.americanamputee.org

AAF empowers amutees, their families, and care providers to make informed decisions be providing them information, referral, peer counseling, literature, and education.

Catherine J. Walden, Executive Director
Shelly Soderlund, Executive Assistant

7535 American Association for Leisure and Recreation
1900 Association Drive
Reston, VA 20191

703-476-3400
800-213-7193
Fax: 703-476-9527
e-mail: aair@aahperd.org
www.aahperd.org/aair

American Association for Leisure and Recreation serves recreation professionals practitioners, educators, and students who advance the profession and enhance the quality of life of all Americans

through creative and meaningful leisure and recreation experiences.

Christine Tipps, President
Judy Brookhiser, District Representative

7536 American Association of Children's Residential Centers (AACRC)
11700 W. Lake Park Drive
Milwaukee, WI 53224

877-33A-ACRC
877-332-2272
Fax: 877-332-2272
e-mail: mskarich@alliance1.org
www.aacrc-dc.org

The American Association of Children's Residential Centers brings professionals together to advance the frontiers of knowledge pertaining to the spectrum of therapeutic living environments for children and adolescents with behavioral health disorders.

Brian Carroll, President
William Powers, Secretary

7537 American Association of the Deaf-Blind
814 Thayer Avenue, Suite 302
Silver Spring, MD 20910

301-495-4403
Fax: 301-495-4404
TTY: 301-495-4402
e-mail: info@aadb.org
www.aadb.org

The American Association of the Deaf-Blind is a national consumer organization of, by, and for deaf-blind Americans. Deaf-blind does not necessarily mean totally deaf and totally blind. It is a broad term that describes people who have varying degrees and types of both vision and hearing loss together. Our mission is to endeavor to enable deaf-blind persons to achieve their maximum potential through increased independence, productivity and integration into the community.

600 Members

Harry Anderson, President
Arthur Roehrig, VP

7538 American Association on Intellectual and Developmental Disabilities
444 North Capitol Street NW, Suite 846
Washington, DC 20001

202-387-1968
800-424-3688
Fax: 202-387-2193
e-mail: aamr@access.digex.net
www.aamr.org

American Association on Intellectual and Developmental Disabilitiess' mission is to promote progressive policies, sound research, effective practices, and universal human rights for people with intellectual disabilities.

Hank Bersani Jr, President
Doreen Croser, Executive Director

7539 American Auditory Society
352 Sundial Ridge Circle
Dammeron Valley, UT 84783

435-574-0062
Fax: 435-574-0063
e-mail: amaudsoc@aol.com
www.amauditorysoc.org

The primary aims of the Society are to increase knowledge and understanding of the ear, hearing and balance; disorders of the ear, hearing and balance, and preventions of these disorders; and habilitation and rehabilitation of individuals with hearing and balance dysfunction.

Thomas Powers, PhD, President
Wayne J Staab, PhD, Executive Director

7540 American Autoimmune Related Diseases Association
22100 Gratiot Avenue
E Detroit, MI 48021

586-776-3900
www.aarda.org

Dedicated to the eradiction of autoimmune diseases and the alleviation of suffering and the socio-economic impact of autoimmunity through fostering and facilitating collaboration in the areas of education, public awareness, research and patient services in an effective, ethical and efficient manner.

Virginia Ladd, Director

7541 American Blind Bowling Association
315 N Main Street
Houston, PA 15342

724-745-5986
www.acb.org

Information on adaptive bowling activities for people who are blind.

Judy Refosco, Contact Person

7542 American Blind Skiing Foundation
2228 Grand Trail
Aurora,, IL 60504

847-255-1739
e-mail: ABSF@absf.org
www.absf.org

ABSF is committed to serving visually impaired children & adults,giving them the opportunities and experiences that build confidence & independencethat can last a lifetime.....

7543 American Board of Dermatology
Henry Ford Health System
1 Ford Place
Detroit, MI 48202

313-874-1088
Fax: 313-872-3221
e-mail: abderm@hfhs.org
www.abderm.org

Sole mission is to ensure competence for patients with cutaneous diseases through board representation.

Stephen B Webster, MD, Association Executive Director
Antoinette F Hood, MD, Executive Director

7544 American Board of Pediatrics
111 Silver Cedar Court
Chapel Hill, NC 27514

919-929-0461
Fax: 919-929-9255
e-mail: abpeds@abpeds.org
abp.org

The American Board os Pediatrics cerifies general pediaiatricians and pediatric subspecialists based on standards of exellence that lead to high quality health care for infants, children and adolescents.

7545 American Camping Association
5000 State Road, 67 N
Martinsville, IN 46151

765-342-8456
800-428-2267
Fax: 765-342-2065
e-mail: bookstore@acacamps.org
www.acacamps.org

The American Camping Association is a community of camp professionals who, for nearly 100 years, have joined together to share our knowladge and expxerience and to ensure the quality of camp program.

Melary Irvin, Customer Service Specialist

7546 American Cancer Society
2200 Century Parkway, Suite 950
Atlanta, GA 30345

800-282-4914
Fax: 404-315-9348
e-mail: angelina.veal@cancer.org
www.cancer.org

The American Cancer Society is a nationwide, community-based voluntary health organization. Headquartered in Atlanta, Georgia, the ACS has state divisions and more than 3,400 local offices. For more than 80 years, ACS has led the way in cancer research. The goal is to prevent cancer, save lives, and diminish suffering from cancer.

Virginia Krawiec, Program Director
Shannon Mejri, Program Assistant

7547 American Canoe Association
7432 Alban Station Boulevard, Suite B-232
Springfield, VA 22150

703-451-0141
Fax: 703-451-2245
e-mail: aca@acanet.org
www.acanet.org

The mission of the American Canoe Association is to promote the health, social and personal benefits of canoeing, kayaking and rafting and to servethe needs off all paddlers for safe, enjoyable and quality paddling opportunities.

Pamela Dillon, Executive Director
Rochelle Luckey, Insurance Coordinator

7548 American Dermatological Association
PO Box 554
Millwood, NY 10546

847-330-9830
Fax: 847-330-1135
e-mail: info@amer-derm-assn.org
www.amer-derm-assn.org

Professional society of physicians specializing in dermatology. Promotes teaching, practice, public education and research into dermatology.

Dr. Darrell S Riegel, President

7549 American Epilepsy Society
342 N Main Street
W Hartford, CT 06117

860-586-7505
Fax: 860-586-7550
e-mail: info@aesnet.org
www.aesnet.org

The purpose of the American Epilepsy Society is to encourage education and research for the prevention, treatment and cure of epilepsy.

Suzanne C Berry, Executive Director
Martin Rotblatt, Associate Director

7550 American Hearing Research Foundation
8 S Michigan Avenue, Suite 814
Chicago, IL 60603

312-726-9670
Fax: 312-726-9695
e-mail: ahrf@american-hearing.org
www.american-hearing.org

A nonprofit foundation serving two vital roles — funding significant research in hearing and balance disorders and helping educate the public.

William L Lederer, Executive Director
Lorraine L Koch, Assistant Director

7551 American Heart Association
7272 Greenville Avenue
Dallas, TX 75231

214-373-6300
800-242-8721
Fax: 214-706-1341
e-mail: inquire@amhrt.org
www.amhrt.org

Supports research, education and community service programs
with the objective of reducing premature death and disability from
cardiovascular diseases and stroke; coordinates the efforts of health
professionals, and others engaged in the fight against heart and circulatory disease.

M Cass Wheeler, CEO

7552 American Juvenile Arthritis Organization
2970 Peachtree Road NW, Suite 200
Atlanta, GA 30305

404-237-8771
800-933-7023
Fax: 404-237-8153
e-mail: info.ga@arthritis.org
www.arthritis.org

Devoted to serving the special needs of children, teens, and young
adults with childhood rheumatic diseases and their families. Offers
both support and information through national and local programs
that serve the needs of families, friends and health professionals.
Serves as a clearinghouse of information, sponsors an annual national conference, monitors and promotes legislation, sponsors research, and offers training to both parents and health professionals.

Sage Rhodes, President

7553 American Liver Foundation
75 Maiden Lane, Suite 603
New York, NY 10038

212-668-1000
800-465-4837
Fax: 212-483-8179
e-mail: info@liverfoundation.org
www.liverfoundation.org

National, voluntary, nonprofit organization dedicated to the prevention, treatment and cure of liver diseases. The foundation offers
support groups, advocacy, medical research support and education.

Frederick G Thompson, President/CEO
Marie P Bresnahan, VP Programs

7554 American Lung Association
61 Broadway, 6th Floor
New York, NY 10006

212-315-8700
800-586-4872
www.lungusa.org

The American Lung Association fights lung disease in all its forms,
with special emphasis on asthma, tobacco control and environmental health. The American Lung Association is funded with contributions from the public, along with gifts and grants from
corporations, foundations and government agencies. The association achieves its many successes through the work of thousands of
committed volunteers and staff.

Hallema Sharif Clyburn, Director Media Relations

7555 American Pediatrics Society
3400 Research Forest Drive, Suite B-7
The Woodlands, TX 77381

281-419-0052
Fax: 281-419-0082
e-mail: info@aps-spr.org
aps-spr.org

The objects of the Society shall be to bring together men and
womenfor the advancement of the study of children and their diseases, for the prevention of illness and the promotion of health in
childhood, for the promotion of pediatric education and research,
and to honor those who, by their contributions to pediatrics, have
aided in its advancement.

Debbie Anagnostelis, Executive Director
Kathy Cannon, Associate Executive Director

7556 American Red Cross
2025 E Street NW
Washington, DC 20006

202-303-4498
800-797-8022
Fax: 202-303-0044
e-mail: info@usa.redcross.org
www.redcross.org

The American Red Cross has been the nation's premier emergency
response organization. As part of a worldwide movement that offers neutral humanitarian care to the victims of war, the American
Red Cross distinguished itself by also aiding victims of devastating
natural disasters.

7557 American Skin Association
346 Park Avenue South, 4th Floor
New York, NY 10010

212-889-4858
800-499-7546
Fax: 212-889-4959
e-mail: AmericanSkin@compuserve.com
www.americanskin.org

The American Skin Association is the only volunteer led health organization dedicated through research, education and advocacy to
saving lives and alleviating human suffering caused by the full
spectrum of skin disorders.

Howard P Milstein, Chairman
George W Hambrick, Jr, President/Founder

7558 American Society for Deaf Children
3820 Hartzdale Drive
Camp Hill, PA 17011

717-703-0073
800-942-2732
Fax: 717-909-5599
e-mail: asdc@deafchildren.org
www.deafchildren.org

A nonprofit, parent-helping-parent organization promoting a positive attitude toward signing and deaf culture. Also provides support, encouragement, and current information about deafness to
families with deaf and hard of hearing children.

Sandy Harvey, Executive Director

7559 American Speech Language Hearing Associati on (ASHA)
10801 Rockville Pike
Rockville, MD 20852

301-897-5700
800-638-8255
Fax: 301-571-0457
TTY: 301-897-0157
e-mail: pr@asha.org
www.asha.org

A professional organization made up of over 123,000 hearing,
speech and language professionals. It is a credentialing organization as well promotes the interests of provides services and information for those with communication disorders.

Arlene A Pietranton, Executive Director

7560 American Wheelchair Table Tennis Association
P.O. Box 5266
Kendall Park, NJ 08824

914-937-3932
Fax: 732-422-4546
e-mail: johnsonjennifer@yahoo.com
www.wsusa.org/wsusa/directories

AWTTA is the National Governing Body of Wheelchair Sports,
U.S.A., for table tennis. Information on adaptive table tennis activities for people of many abilities. Includes local chapters, referrals,
fun and social interaction and support groups.

Jennifer Johnson, Contact Person

7561 Association for Children's Mental Health
100 W. Washtenaw St. Suite 4
Lansing, MI 48933

517-372-4016
Fax: 517-372-4032
www.acmh-mi.org

ACMH is a family organization with statewide staff and membership who support activities to enhance the system or services which address the needs of children with serious emotional disorders and their families. ACMH is a statewide chapter of the national Federation of families for Children's Mental Health and our membership of over 1200 individuals is comprised of family members, professionals and concerned.

Amy Winans, Executive Director
Mary Porter, Business Manager

7562 Association for Education & Rehabilitation of the Blind & Visually Impaired
1703 N Beauregard Street, Suite 440
Alexandria, VA 22311

703-671-4500
877-492-2708
Fax: 703-671-6391
e-mail: markr@aerbvi.org
www.aerbvi.org

This association is the only international membership organization dedicated to rendering all possible support and assistance to the professionals who work in all phases of education and rehabilitation of blind and visually impaired children and adults.

Mark Richert, Executive Director
Barbara Sherr, Executive Assistant

7563 Association for Persons with Severe Handicaps (TASH)
1025 Vermont Avenue, Floor 7
Washington, DC 20005

202-263-5600
Fax: 202-637-0138
e-mail: nweiss@tash.org
www.tash.org

An international association of people with disabilities, their family members, other advocates, and professionals fighting for a society in which inclusion of all people in all aspects of society is the norm.

Barbara Trader, Executive Director
Rose Holsey, Director Of Operation

7564 Association for the Gifted Child
Council for Exceptional Children
1110 N Glebe Road, Suite 300
Arlington, VA 22201

703-620-3660
888-232-7733
Fax: 703-264-9494
TTY: 703-264-9446
e-mail: service@cec.sped.org
www.cec.sped.org

Focuses on the delivery of information to both professionals and parents about gifted and talented children and their needs.

Dr Drew Allbritten, Executive Director

7565 Association for the Handicapped
350 5th Avenue, Suite 3304
New York, NY 10118

212-868-1217
Fax: 212-868-1219

Information on adaptive sports and recreation activities for people of many abilities. Includes local chapters, referrals, fun and social interaction and support groups.

7566 Association for the Help of Retarded Children
83 Maiden Lane
New York, NY 10038

212-780-2690
Fax: 212-777-5893
e-mail: ahrcnyc@dti.net
www.ahrcnyc.org

Developmentally disabled children and adults, their families, and interested individuals. Provides support services, training programs, clinics, schools and residential facilities to the developmentally disabled. Publications: The Chronicle, quarterly newsletter.

Shirley Berenstein, Editor

7567 Association of Blind Athletes
33 N Institute Street
Colorado Springs, CO 80903

719-630-0422
Fax: 719-630-0616
e-mail: usaba@usa.net
www.usaba.org

The mission of the United States Association of Blind Athletes is to increase the number and quality of grassroots through competitive, world-class athletic opportunities for Americans who are blind or visually impaired. We value the life enhancing aspects of sports and the opportunity to demonstrate the abilities of people who are blind and visually impaired.

Mark Lucas, Executive Director
Nicole Jomantas, Communications Director

7568 Association of Children's Prosthetic/ Orthotic Clinics
6300 N River Road, Suite 727
Rosemont, IL 60018

847-698-1637
Fax: 847-823-0536
e-mail: king@aaos.org
www.acpoc.org

An association of professionals who are involved in clinics which provide prosthetic-orthotic care for children with limb loss or orthopaedic disabilities.

7569 Association of University Centers on Disabilities
1010 Wayne Avenue, Suite 920
Silver Spring, MD 20910

301-588-8252
800-424-3410
Fax: 301-588-2842
TTY: 301-588-3319
e-mail: gjesien@aucd.org
www.aucd.org

The Association of University Centers on Disabilities (formerly the American Association of University Affiliated Programs) is a nonprofit organization that promotes and supports the national network of university centers on disabilities, which includes University Centers for Excellence in Developmental Disabilities Education, Research, and Service Leadership Education in Neurodevelopmental and Related Disabilities Programs and Developmental Disabilities Research Centers.

David R. Johnson Ph.D, Pesident
Jan Nisbet Ph.D, Secretary

7570 Barbara DeBoer Foundation
2069 S Busse Road
Mount Prospect, IL 60056

800-895-8478
foundationcenter.org

Offers a variety of programs that include advocacy services, donor awareness, referral information, medication and medical center information.

7571 Beneficial Designs
2240 Meridian Boulevard, Suite C
Minden, NV 89423

776-783-8822
Fax: 775-783-8823
e-mail: mail@beneficialdesigns.com
www.beneficialdesign.com

Beneficial Designs works towards universal access through research, design, and education. We believe all individuals should have access to the physical, intellectual, and spiritual aspects of life. We seek to enhance the quality of life for people of all abilities, and work to achieve this aim by developing and marketing technology for daily living, vocational, and leisure activities.

Peter Axelson, Founder/Research Director
Denise Yamada Axelson, Research Coordinator

7572 Benetech
480 S California Avenue, Suite 201
Palo Alto, CA 94306

650-644-3400
Fax: 650-475-1066
e-mail: info@benetech.org
www.benetech.org

Benetech (formerly Arkenstone) is a nonprofit venture that combines the impact of technological solutions with the social entrepreneurship business model to help disadvantaged communities in our society and across the world.

Jim Fruchterman, President/CEO
Marc Levine, Senior Project Manager

7573 Birth Defect Research for Children
930 Woodcock Road, Suite 225
Orlando, FL 32803

407-895-0802
Fax: 407-895-0824
e-mail: staff@birthdefects.org
www.birthdefects.org

A nonprofit organization that provides information about birth defects of all kinds to parents and professionals. Offers a library of medical books and files of information on less common categories of birth defects and is involved in research to discover possible links between environmental exposures and birth defects.

Betty Mekdeci, Executive Director

7574 Boundless Playgrounds
45 Wintonbury Avenue
Bloomfield, CT 06002

860-243-8315
877-268-6353
Fax: 860-243-5854
e-mail: info@boundlessplaygrounds.org
www.boundlessplaygrounds.org

Boundless Playgrounds helps communities create extraordinary playgrounds where all children,with and without disabilities,can develop essential skills for life as they learn together together through play.

Amy Jaffe Barzach, Co-Founder/Executive Director
Jean Schappet, Co-Founder/Creative Director

7575 Boy Scouts of America National Council
PO Box 152079
Irving, TX 75015

972-580-2000
Fax: 972-580-2502
www.scouting.org

The mission of the Boy Scouts of America is to prepare young peopleto make ethical and moral choices over their lifetimes by instilling in them the values of the values of the Scouts Oath and Law.

7576 Braille Revival League
American Council of the Blind
1155 15th Street NW, Suite 1004
Washington, DC 20005

202-467-5081
800-424-8666
Fax: 202-467-5085
e-mail: info@acb.org
www.acb.org

Encourages blind people to read and write in braille, advocates for mandatary braille instruction in educational facilities for the blind, strives to make available a supply of braille materials from libraries and printing houses and more.

7577 Brass Ring Society
500 Macaw Lane, #5
Fern Park, FL 32730

407-339-6188
800-666-9474
Fax: 407-339-6369
www.brassring.org

Society that seeks to fulfill the dreams of children with life-threatening illnesses.

Ray Esposito, Director

7578 Breckenridge Outdoor Education Center
PO Box 697
Breckenridge, CO 80424

970-453-6422
800-383-2632
Fax: 970-453-4676
e-mail: boec@boec.org
www.boec.org

The Breckenridge outdoor Education Center is a non-profit organization whose mission is to expand the potential of people with disabilities and special needs through meaningful,educational,and inspiring outdoor experiences.

Bruce Fitch, Executive Director
Carol Padlick, Finance Director

7579 CANDU Parent Group
Riverwalk Community Center
1403 North Main Street, Suite 301
Wheaton, IL 60187

630-752-0066
Fax: 630-752-1064
e-mail: il@namidupage.org
www.namidupage.org

Support and advocacy group for parents of children with serious emotional disturbance, behavioral disorders, or mental illness.

7580 CHERUB-Association of Families and Friends of Children with Limb Disorders
Children's Hospital of Buffalo
936 Delaware Avenue
Buffalo, NY 14209

716-762-9997

Answers the questions and problems that families of juveniles diagnosed with a disorder may be experiencing.

Sandra Richenberg
Kathy Gura

7581 Cancer Information Service
National Cancer Institute
6116 Executive Boulevard, Suite 3036A
Bethesda, MD 20892

800-422-6237
Fax: 301-330-7968
TTY: 800-332-8615
www.cis.nic.nih.gov

The Cancer Information Service provides the latest and most accurate cancer information to patients, their families, the public, and health professionals. Through its network of regional offices, the

CIS serves the United States, Puerto Rico, the U.S. Virgin Islands, and the Pacific Islands.

Andrew C Von Eschenback, Director

7582 Candlelighters Childhood Cancer Foundation
PO Box 498
Kensington, MD 20895

301-962-3520
800-366-2223
Fax: 301-962-3521
e-mail: staff@candlelighters.org
www.candlelighters.org

The Candlelighters Childhood Cancer Foundation was founded by concerned parents of children with cancer. The foundation is a national nonprofit membership organization whose mission is to educate, support, serve, and advocate for families of children with cancer, survivors of childhood cancer, and the professionals who care for them.

Ruth Hoffman, Executive Director

7583 Center for Best Practices in Early Childhood
College of Education and Human Services
1 University Circle
Macomb, IL 61455

309-298-1390
Fax: 309-298-1414
e-mail: robinson1@wiu.edu
www.wiu.edu/thecenter

Operates the following: Early Childhood Interactive Technology Literacy Curriculum Project; Disseminating and Replicating an Effective Early Childhood Comprehensive Technology System; Expressive Arts Outreach; ECCSPLOR-IT; LiTECH Interactive Outreach; STARNET Regions I and III; and Provider Connections.

Joyce Johanson, Associate Director
Linda Robinson, Assistant Director

7584 Center for Literacy and Disability Studies
301A South Columbia Street, Suite 1100
Chaple Hill, NC 27599

919-966-8566
Fax: 919-843-3250
e-mail: literacy@acpub.duke.edu
www.med.unc.edu/ahs/clds

The Center for Literacy and Disability Studies is a unit within the Department of Allies Health Sciences,school of Medicine, at the University of North Carolina at Chapel Hill.

7585 Center for Mental Health Services Knowledge Exchange Network
US Department of Health and Human Services
PO Box 42557
Washington, DC 20015

800-789-2647
Fax: 240-747-5470
TDD: 866-889-2647
http://mentalhealth.samhsa.gov

Supplies the public with responses to their commonly asked questions about mental health issues and services.

7586 Chai Lifeline/Camp Simcha National Office
151 W 30th Street
New York, NY 10001

212-465-1300
800-242-4543
Fax: 212-465-0949
e-mail: eschwartz@childlifeline.org
www.chailifeline.org

Chai Life is a not for profit organization dedicated to helping children suffering from serous illness as well as their family members. We ofeer a comprehensive range os services to addess the multiple needs of patients,parents,and siblings.

Esther Schwartz, Director of Hospital Services

7587 Child Care Plus+
Univ. of Montana Rural Institute on Disabilities
634 Eddy Avenue
Missoula, MT 59812

406-243-6355
800-235-4122
Fax: 406-243-4730
TDD: 406-243-5467
e-mail: ccplus@selway.umt.edu
www.ccplus.org

Provides inclusion information and resources for child care providers and other professionals: written materials (newsletter, curriculum, articles), training, workshops, technical assistance and various other resources.

Sandra L. Morris, Center Co-Director
Sara McCorkle, Center Coordinator

7588 Children's Defense Fund
25 E Street NW
Washington, DC 20001

202-628-8787
800-233-1200
Fax: 202-662-3510
e-mail: cdfinfo@childrensdefense.org
www.childrensdefense.org

Information and advocacy resources for families and professionals. Includes listings of organizations providing general information and organizations focusing on more specific areas of concern to families and young adults who have disabilities.

David W Hornbeck, President/CEO
Marian Wright Edelman, Founder/President

7589 Children's Hopes and Dreams
Wish Fulfillment Foundation
280 Route 46
Dover, NJ 07801

973-361-7366
Fax: 973-361-6627
e-mail: chdfdover@juno.com
www.childrenswishes.org

Three programs: Dream fulfillment program is for children age four through seventeen with life threatening illness who have not received a dream before; Pen Pal Program matches children five through seventeen with chronic or life threatening illnesses, conditions, disabilities or major trauma to other ill children by their age, sex and illness category; Kid's Kare Package program supplies new donated items to children through Pen Pal Program and/or health care professionals.

10,000 Members

Mariann Oswald, Program Director

7590 Children's Hospice International
901 North Pitt Street, Suite 230
Alexandria, VA 22314

800-242-4453
Fax: 703-684-0330
e-mail: info@chionline.org
www.chionline.org

This nonprofit organization works to improve hospice care for children. Free services include information and referral service for child care, counseling, support groups, pain management, professional education, and research. This is a membership group, with a membership fee for other services.

Ann Armstrong-Dailey, Founding Director/CEO
Martin Doblmeier, Director

7591 Children's Hospital Boston
300 Longwood Avenue
Boston, MA 02115

617-355-6000
Fax: 617-277-4832
TTY: 617-355-0443
e-mail: webteam@tch.harvard.edu
www.childrenshospital.org

Children's Hospital Boston is a 325 bed comprehensive center for pediatric health care. As the largest pediatric medical center in the United States, Children's offers a complete range of health care services for children from 15 weeks gestation through 21 years of age (and older in some cases).

Michelle Davis, Public Affairs VP
Susan Craig, Media Relations Manager

7592 Children's Organ Transplant Association
2501 Cota Drive
Bloomington, IN 47403

800-366-2682
e-mail: cota@cota.org
www.cota.org

The association provides fundraising assistance for children needing life-saving transplants and promotes organ, marrow and tissue donation.

Rick Lofgren, President/CEO

7593 Children's Wish Foundation International
8615 Roswell Road
Atlanta, GA 30350

770-393-9474
800-323-9474
Fax: 770-393-0683
e-mail: wish@childrenswish.org
www.childrenswish.org

A nonprofit organization that fulfills wishes for children with life threatening illnesses. The criteria for wish fulfillment are: The child must be under the age of eighteen, and have been diagnosed with a life threatening illness.

Arthur Stein, President
Linda Dozoretz, Founder/Executive Director

7594 Chill: Straight Talk About Stress
Childs Work/Childs Play
135 Dupont Street, PO Box 760
Plainview, NY 11803

516-349-5520
800-962-1141
Fax: 800-262-1886
e-mail: info@Childswork.com
www.Childswork.com

Childswork/Childsplay uses a prevention and intervention model when creating its high-quality products. These programs focus on the behavioral,social,and emotional issues children deal with at home and at school. Through the use of games, print materials and visual media,counselors and educators have a superior array of counseling tools at their disposal.

7595 Christian Horizons
PO Box 3381
Grand Rapids, MI 49501

616-956-7063
Fax: 616-956-7063
e-mail: info@christianhorizonsinc.org
www.christianhorizonsinc.org

Devoted to assisting individuals, with developmental disabilities, on a day-to-day basis.

7596 Compassionate Friends
PO Box 3696
Oak Brook, IL 60522

630-990-0010
877-969-0010
Fax: 630-990-0246
e-mail: nationaloffice@compassionatefriends.org
www.compassionatefriends.org

Compassionate Friends assists families toward the positive resolution of grief following the death of a child of any age and provides information to help others be supportive. A national nonprofit, self-help support organization that offers friendship, understanding, and hope to bereaved parents, grandparents and siblings.

Rick Yotti, President
Ronald Haynes, VP

7597 Cooperative Wilderness Handicapped Outdoor Group
Idaho State University
921 South 8th Avenue
Pocatello, ID 83209

208-282-3912
Fax: 208-282-2127
e-mail: krindavi@isu.edu
www.isu.edu/cwhog

A regional self-help group to provide recreational opportunities for people of all disabilities. The program is part of the Idaho State University.

Dr. Michael McCurry, Professor Of Geosciences
Dr. Leslie Devaud, Associate Professor Of Ph Sciences

7598 Council for Educational Diagnostic Services (CEDS)
Council for Exceptional Children
1110 N Glebe Road, Suite 300
Arlington, VA 22201

703-620-3660
888-232-7733
Fax: 703-264-9494
TTY: 703-264-9446
www.unr.edu

Promotes the highest quality of diagnostic and prescriptive procedures involoved in the education of individuals with disabilities and/or who are gifted. Members include educational diagnosticians, psychologists, social workers, speech and language specialists, physcians, and other professionals and related service professionals.

Nancy Halmhuber, President
Jennifer Goldblatt, VP

7599 Council for Exceptional Children
1920 Association Drive
Reston, VA 22091

703-620-3660
888-232-7733
Fax: 703-264-9494
TTY: 866-915-5000
www.cec.sped.org

Advocates appropriate policies, standards and development for students with special needs.

Lynda Van Kuren, Contact

7600 Council of Administrators of Special Education
Council for Exceptional Children
1110 N Glebe Road, Suite 300
Arlington, VA 22201

703-620-3660
888-232-7733
Fax: 703-264-9494
TTY: 703-264-9446
www.casecec.org

A international professional educational organization which is affiliated with the Council for Exceptional Children (CEC) whose members are dedicated to the enhancement of the worth, dignity, potential, and uniqueness of each individual in society. The mission is to provide leadership and support to members by shaping policies and practices which impact the quality of education.

7601 Council of Families with Visual Impairments
American Council of the Blind
1155 15th Street NW, Suite 1004
Washington, DC 20005

202-467-5081
800-424-8666
Fax: 202-467-5085
e-mail: info@acb.org
www.acb.org

A network of parents with blind or visually impaired children that offers support and outreach, shares experiences in parent/child relationships, exchanges educational, cultural and medical information about child development and more.

7602 Courage Center
3915 Golden Valley Road
Golden Valley, MN 55422

763-520-0312
888-846-8253
Fax: 612-520-0577
TTY: 763-520-0245
e-mail: courageinfo@courage.org
www.courage.org

The mission of Courage Center is to empower people with physical disabilities to reach for their full potential in every aspect of life. We are guided by the vision that one day, all people will live, work, learn and play in a community based on abilities, not disabiliries.

Paula Hart, VP/COO
Eric Stevens, CEO

7603 CureSearch: The National Childhood Cancer Foundation
440 E Huntington Drive, PO Box 60012
Arcadia, CA 91066

800-458-6223
Fax: 301-718-0047
e-mail: info@curesearch.org
www.curesearch.org

Cure Search unites the Children's Oncology Group (COG) and the National Childhood Center Foundation (NCCF) through a shared mission to cure and prevent childhood and adolescent cancer through scientific discovery and compassionate care.

Sally Charney, Public Education Director

7604 Deafness Research Foundation
641 Lexington Avenue Floor 15
New Yorkon, NY 10022

212-328-9480
800-535-3323
e-mail: susan@drf.org
www.drf.org

The nation's largest voluntary health organization entirely committed to public awareness and support for basic and clinical research into deafness and hearing disabilities. Sponsors a broad program of innovative research and education into the causes, treatments and prevention of nerve deafness, increases the number of young scientists entering and engaged in otologic studies, increases the nation's awareness and creates an understanding of serious hearing dysfunctions.

Susan Greco, Executive Director

7605 Developmental Delay Resources
5801 Beacon St.
Pittsburgh, PA 15217

800-497-0944
Fax: 412-422-1374
www.devdelay.org

A nonprofit organization dedicated to meeting the needs of those working with children who have developmental delays in sensory motor, language, social, and emotional areas. DDR provides a net-

work for parents and professionals and current information after the diagnosis to support children with special needs.

7606 Developmental Disabilities Nurses Association
Po Box 536489
Orlando, FL 32853

407-835-0642
800-888-6733
Fax: 407-426-7440
e-mail: ddnahq@aol.com
www.ddna.org

A nonprofit professional nursing organization founded to meet the professional needs of nurses serving individuals with developmental disabilities.

Mary Kay Moore, President
Norma Lester, Secretary

7607 Disability Rights Education & Defense Fund
2212 6th Street
Berkeley, CA 94710

510-644-2555
Fax: 510-841-8645
e-mail: info@dredf.org
www.dredf.org

Nonprofit law and public policy center that specializes in laws affecting more than 45 million Americans with disabilities. DREDF was founded 16 years ago to challenge the barriers that exclude people with disabilities from participating in all aspects of society.

Mary Lou Breslin, Co-Founder

7608 Disabled Shooting Services
National Rifle Association of America
11250 Waples Mill Road
Fairfax, VA 22030

703-267-1495
e-mail: info@nrpa.org
www.nrahq.org/compete/disabled.asp

Information on adaptive shooting activities for people of many abilities. Includes local chapters, referrals, fun and social interaction and support groups.

Dave Baskin, Department Head

7609 Disabled Sports USA
451 Hungerford Drive, Suite 100
Rockville, MD 20850

301-217-0960
Fax: 301-217-0968
e-mail: information@dsusa.org
www.dsusa.org

A national nonprofit, organization established in 1967 by disabled Vietnam veterans to serve the war injured. DS/USA now offers nationwide sports rehabilitation programs to anyone with a permanent disability.

7610 Division for Early Childhood
27 Fort Missoula Road, Suite 2
Missoula, MT 59804

406-543-0872
Fax: 406-543-0887
TTY: 703-264-9446
e-mail: dec@dec-sped.org
www.dec-sped.org

This division is one of seventeen divisions of the Council for Exceptional Children, the largest international professional organization dedicated to improving educational outcomes for individuals with exceptionalities, students with disabilities, and/or the gifted.

7611 Division for Physical and Health Disablities

Council for Exceptional Children
1110 N Glebe Road, Suite 300
Arlington, VA 22201

703-620-3660
888-232-7733
Fax: 703-264-9474
TTY: 703-264-9446
www.cec.spec.org

Advocates for quality education for individuals with physical disabilities and special health care needs in schools, hospitals, or home settings.

Elisabeth Cohen, President
Alison Stafford, Vice President

7612 Division of Birth Defects & Developmental Disabilities

National Center for Environmental Health
4770 Buford Highway NE
Atlanta, GA 30341

770-488-7150
888-232-6789
Fax: 770-488-7156
www.cdc.gov

Information and advocacy resources for families and professionals dealing with children with birth defects and developmental disabilities.

7613 Division on Career Development and Transition

Council for Exceptional Children
1110 N Glebe Road, Suite 300
Arlington, VA 22201

703-620-3660
888-232-7733
Fax: 703-264-9474
TTY: 866-915-5000
www.cec.spec.org

Focuses on the career development of individuals with disablilities and their transition from school to adult life.

7614 ERIC Clearinghouse on Disabilities & Gifted Children

Council for Exceptional Children
1110 N Glebe Road Suite 300
Arlington, VA 22201

703-620-3660
888-232-7733
Fax: 703-264-9494
TTY: 866-915-5000
e-mail: ericec@cec.sped.org
www.cec.sped.org/ericec.htm

Information and advocacy resources for families and professionals. Includes listings of organizations providing general information and organizations focusing on more specific areas of concern to families and young adults who have disabilities.

7615 Easter Seals Disability Services

230 West Monroe Street, Suite 1800
Chicago, IL 60606

312-726-6200
800-221-6827
Fax: 312-726-1494
TDD: 312-726-4258
e-mail: info@easterseals.com
www.easterseals.com

Easter Seals mission is to create solutions that change lives for children and adults with disabilities and to provide appropriate developmental and rehabilitation services. Services provided include early intervention, after-school programs, preschool, tutoring, medical rehabilitation, vocational services, adult and senior day services, respite and in home care, camping and recreation, residential housing, support services, support groups, transportation and referrals.

Loe Lowenkron, Chairman
James E Williams Jr, President/CEO

7616 Endocrine Society

8401 Connecticut Avenue, Suite 900
Chevy Chase, MD 20815

301-941-0200
Fax: 301-941-0259
e-mail: endostaff@endo-society.org
www.endo-society.org/

To advance exellence in endocrinology and promote its essentail role as an integrative force in scientifc research and medical practice.

7617 Family Caregiver Alliance

690 Market Street, Suite 102
San Francisco, CA 94104

415-434-3388
Fax: 415-434-3508

Good information with resources and hotline numbers.

7618 Family Voices

2340 Alamo SE, Suite 102
Albuquerque, NM 87106

505-872-4774
Fax: 505-872-4780
e-mail: kidshealth@familyvoices.org
www.familyvoices.org

Family Voices,a national grassroots network of families and friends, advocates for health care services that are famliy-centered,community-based, comprehensive. coordinated and culturally competent for all children and youth with special health care needs; promotes the inclusion of all families as decision makers at all levels of health care; and supports essential partnerships between families and professionals.

7619 Federation for Children with Special Needs Center

1135 Tremont Street, Suite 420
Boston, MA 02120

617-236-7210
800-331-0688
Fax: 617-572-2094
e-mail: fcsninfo@fcsn.org
www.fcsn.org

The Federation is a center for parents and parent organizations to work together on behalf of children (up to age 22) with special needs and their families. The Federation operates a Parent Center in Massachusetts that offers a variety of services to parents, parent groups and others who are concerned with children with special needs.

Pat Blake, Associate Executive Director
Sara Miranda, Associate Executive Director

7620 Federation of Families for Children's Mental Health

9605 Medical Center Drive, Suite 280
Rockville, MD 20850

240-403-1901
Fax: 240-403-1909
e-mail: ffcmh@ffmh.org
www.ffcmh.org

The National family run organization is dedicated exclusively to helping children with mental health needs and their families achieve a better quality of life.

Sandra Spencer, Executive Director

7621 Foundation for Exceptional Children

16 Lake Shore Road
Grosse Poimte Farm, MI 48236

313-885-8660

To improve the well-being of children and families by providing theapeutic,social and educational services.

7622 Friends' Health Connection
PO Box 114
New Brunswick, NJ 08903

732-418-1811
800-483-7436
Fax: 732-249-9897
e-mail: info@friendshealthconnection.org
www.friendshealthconnection.org

Organization Mission Friends' Health Connection is a nonprofit organization that connects people who are currently experiencing or who have overcome the same disease,illness, handicap or injury in oder to communicate for mutualsupport.

1989

7623 Genetic Alliance
4301 Connecticut Avenue NW, Suite 404
Washington, DC 20008

202-966-5557
800-336-4363
Fax: 202-966-8553
e-mail: info@geneticalliance.org
www.geneticalliance.org

A nonprofit tax exempt organization founded in 1986 as a national coalition of consumers, professionals and genetic support groups to voice the common concerns of children and adults and families living with, and at risk of, genetic conditions. The Alliance builds partnerships among consumers and professionals and the private and public sectors to promote optimum healthcare and enhanced quality of life for individuals identified with genetic conditions.

Sharon Terry, President/CEO

7624 Girl Scouts of the USA
Membership and Program Group
420 5th Avenue
New York, NY 10018

212-852-8000
800-223-0624
Fax: 212-852-6515
www.girlscouts.org

Girl Scout of the USA is the world's preeminent organization dedicated solely to girls-all girls-where, in an accepting and nurturing envirment, girls build character and skills for success in the real world.

7625 Handicapped Scuba Association
1104 El Prado
San Clemente, CA 92672

949-498-4540
800-673-5084
Fax: 949-498-6128
e-mail: hsahdq@compuserve.com
www.hsascuba.com

Information on adaptive scuba diving activities for people of many abilities. Includes local chapters, referrals, fun and social interaction and support groups.

7626 Handle with Care
PO Box 1569
Wimberly, TX 78676

512-842-5049
888-590-5049
Fax: 512-847-6257

Information and advocacy resources for families and professionals. Includes listings of organizations providing general information and organizations focusing on more specific areas of concern to families and young adults who have disabilities.

7627 Helen Keller Center's National Parent Network
141 Middle Neck Road
Sands Point, NY 11050

516-944-8900
800-255-0411
Fax: 516-944-7302

Establishes a coalition of state parent organizations to promote the exchange of information among parents of deaf-blind youth. Provides training to parents to develop their legislative advocacy skills, empowers parents and their families to obtain services and ensures parents a meaningful life for their sons and daughters.

7628 Helen Keller International
352 Park Avenue S, 12th Floor
New York, NY 10010

212-532-0544
877-535-5374
Fax: 212-532-6014

Nonprofit organization that directly addresses the causes of preventable blindness. Also provides rehabilitation services to blind people, and we help reduce the micronutrient malnutrition which can cause blindness and death in children.

Kathy Spahn, President
Shawn K. Baker, Vice President

7629 Heriditary Disease Foundation
3960 Broadway, 6th Floor
New York, NY 10032

212-928-2121
Fax: 212-928-2172
e-mail: cures@hdfoundation.org
www.hdfoundation.org

Conducts interdisciplinary workshop program that recruits scientists to develop and apply new technologies, supports basic research on genetic illness through grant and postdoctural fellowship programs at major universities, and provides research tissue to medical investigators.

Nancy Wexler, President

7630 Houston Challengers TIRR Sports
1475 W Gray
Houston, TX 77019

713-521-3737

Information on adaptive sports and recreation activities for people of many abilities. Includes local chapters, referrals, fun and social interaction and support groups.

7631 Human Growth Foundation
997 Glen Cove Avenue, Suite 5
Glen Head, NY 11545

516-671-4041
800-451-6434
Fax: 516-671-4055
e-mail: hgfl@hgfound.org
www.hgfound.org

Provides referrals to support groups, services, and genetic counseling on its toll-free telephone line. Encourages communication among support groups and continuing education.

Patricia D Costa, Executive Director

7632 Independent Living Research Utilization Program
2323 S Shepard, Suite 1000
Houston, TX 77019

713-520-0232
Fax: 713-520-5785
TTY: 713-520-5136

Information and advocacy resources for families and professionals on independent living for people with disabilities.

7633 Indian Health Service
Mental Health/Social Service Programs Branch
801 Thompson Avenue, Suite 400
Rockville, MD 20852

301-443-1083

Includes listings of organizations providing general information and organizations focusing on more specific areas of concern to Native American families and young adults who have disabilities.

7634 Institute for Families of Blind Children
PO Box 54700, Mail Stop 111
Los Angeles, CA 90054

213-669-4649
800-669-4549
e-mail: info@instituteforfamilies.org
www.instituteforfamilies.org

Offers support and information to families of blind children. Provides direct counseling and nation-wide telephone counseling.

7635 International Braille and Technology Center for the Blind
National Federation of the Blind
1800 Johnson Street
Baltimore, MD 21230

410-659-9314
Fax: 410-685-5653
e-mail: nfb@nfb.org
www.nfb.org

World's largest and most complete evaluation and demonstration center of all assistive technology used by the blind from around the world. Includes all Braille, synthetic speech, print-to-speech scanning, internet and portable devices and programs. Available for tours by appointment to blind persons, employers, technology manufacturers, teachers, parents and those working in the assistive technology field.

Cartis Chong, Director Technology

7636 International Society of Dermatology
138 Palm Coast Parkway NE, No.333
Palm Coast, FL 32137

386-437-4405
Fax: 386-437-4427
e-mail: info@IntSocDermatol.org
www.intsocderm.org

Promotes interest, education and research in dermatology.

Coleman Jacobson MD, President

7637 International Wheelchair Aviators
1117 Rising Hill Way
Escondido, CA 92029

619-746-5018

Provides information for pilots or future pilots who have a disability.

7638 Iron Overload Diseases Assocation
433 Westwind Drive
North Palm Beach, FL 33408

561-840-8412
Fax: 561-842-9881
e-mail: iod@ironoverload.org
www.ironoverload.org

Committed to providing information and support to affected individuals and their families, educating the general public, promoting and supporting research, and pressing for earlier diagnosis and more effective treatment. Acts as a clearinghouse for affected individuals and family members, provides telephone consultations, offers referrals to genetic counseling and support groups. Provides a variety of educational and support materials including books, newsletters, pamphlets, and fact sheets.

7639 Jewish Children's Adoption Network
PO Box 147016
Denver, CO 80214

303-573-8113
Fax: 303-893-1447
e-mail: jcan@qwest.net
www.users.qwest.net/~jcan

Information and advocacy resources for families and professionals. Includes listings of organizations providing general information.

Stephen Krausz, PhD, President

7640 Job Opportunities for the Blind
1800 Johnson Street
Baltimore, MD 21230

410-659-9314
Fax: 410-685-5653
e-mail: nfb@iamdigex.net.net
www.nfb.org

Information and resources for those with visual impairments.

7641 Just One Break
570 Seventh Avenue, 6th Floor
New York, NY 10018

212-785-7300
Fax: 212-785-4513
TTY: 212-785-4515
e-mail: justonebreak@interactive.net
www.justonebreak.com

Information and advocacy resources for families and professionals dealing with families and young adults who have disabilities.

7642 Learning Disabilities Association of Ameri ca
4156 Library Road
Pittsburgh, PA 15234

412-341-1515
888-300-6710
Fax: 412-344-0224
e-mail: info@LDAAmerica.org
www.LDAAmerica.org

Helps families of the affected individual through information and referral to professionals in their area. A membership organization with affiliates in 43 states.

Sheila Buckley, Executive Director

7643 MUMS: National Parent to Parent Network
150 Custer Street
Green Bay, WI 54301

920-336-5333
877-336-5333
Fax: 920-339-0995
e-mail: mums@netnet.net
www.netnet.net/mums/

Matches parents of children with rare disorders. Provides information and advocacy resources for families and professionals. Includes listings of organizations providing general information and organizations focusing on more specific areas of concern to families and young adults who have disabilities.

Julie Gordon, Director

7644 Make Today Count
101 1/2 S Union Street
Alexandria, VA 22314

703-548-9674

An organization that helps patients and their families cope with cancer and other serious diseases and improve their quality of life.

7645 March of Dimes Birth Defects Foundation
1275 Mamaroneck Avenue
White Plains, NY 10605

914-428-7100
888-663-4637
Fax: 914-428-8203
e-mail: resourcecenter@modimes.org
www.marchofdimes.com

Partnership of volunteers and professionals dedicated to the misson of the March of Dimes to improve the health of babies by preventing birth defects and infant mortality. Chapters are situated across the country and can be located through the web site, National Office, or telephone book. The Resource Center answers questions relating to preconception health, pregnancy, childbirth and birth defects.

Dr Jennifer Howse, President

7646 March of Dimes Nursing Modules
1275 Mamaroneck Avenue
White Plains, NY 10605

914-428-7100
888-663-4637
Fax: 914-428-8203
e-mail: resourcecenter@modimes.org
www.marchofdimes.com

Nursing modules are self-directed learning monographs designed for registered nurses and nurse-midwives. Created to help nurses meet the challenges posed by a rapidly changing world of technological advances, evolving demographics and greater cultural diversity, they focus on effective care delivery during the pre-conceptional, prenatal, intrapartum, postpartum and inter-conceptional periods.

7647 NADD: National Association for the Dually Diagnosed
132 Fair Street
Kingston, NY 12401

845-331-4336
800-331-5362
Fax: 845-331-4569
e-mail: info@thenadd.org
www.thenadd.org

Nonprofit organization designed to promote the interests of professional and parent development with resources for individuals who have the coexistence of mental illness and mental retardation. Provides conferences, educational services and training materials to professionals, parents, concerned citizens, and service organizations.

Dr Robert Fletcher, CEO

7648 NAEYC: National Association for the Education of Young Children
1313 L Street, NW, Suite 500
Washington, DC 20005

202-232-8777
800-424-2460
Fax: 202-328-1846
e-mail: pubaff@aeyc.org
www.naeyc.org

Information and advocacy resources for families and professionals. Includes listings of organizations providing general information and organizations focusing on more specific areas of concern to families and young adults who have disabilities.

7649 National Ability Center
PO Box 682799
Park City, UT 84068

435-649-3991
Fax: 435-658-3992
TDD: 435-649-3991
e-mail: info@nac1985.org
www.nac1985.org

Information on adaptive sports and recreation activities for people of many abilities. Includes local chapters, referrals, fun and social interaction and support groups.

Michele Depalma, Program Administrator
Brooke Hafets, Outreach Manager

7650 National Academy for Child Development (NACD)
549 25th Street
Ogden, UT 84401

801-621-8606
Fax: 801-621-8389
e-mail: info@nacd.org
www.nacd.org

International organization of parents and professionals dedicated to helping children and adults reach their full potential.

7651 National Adoption Center
1500 Walnut Street, Suite 701
Philadelphia, PA 19102

215-735-9988
800-862-3678
Fax: 215-735-9410
e-mail: nac@nationaladoptioncenter.org
www.adopt.org/adopt

Information and advocacy resources for families and professionals interested in or dealing with adoption. Includes listings of organizations providing general information and organizations focusing on specific areas of concern.

7652 National Alliance for the Mentally Ill
2107 Wilson Blvd, Ste 300, Colonial Place Three
Arlington, VA 22201

703-524-7600
800-950-6264
Fax: 703-524-9094
TDD: 703-516-7227
e-mail: info@nami.org
www.nami.org

NAMI is a nonprofit, grassroots, self-help, support and advocacy organization of consumers, families and friends of people with severe mental illness, such as schizophrenia, bipolar disorder, major despressive disorder, obsessive compulsive disorder, anxiety disorders, autism and other severe and persistent mental illnesses that affect the brain.

Suzanne Vogel-Scibilia MD, President

7653 National Amputee Golf Association
PO Box 23285
Milwaukee, WI 53223

414-376-1268
800-633-6242
Fax: 414-376-1268
e-mail: naga@execpc.com
www.amputee-golf.org

Information on adaptive golf activities for people of many abilities. Includes local chapters, referrals, fun and social interaction and support groups.

7654 National Archery Association
One Olympic Plaza
Colorado Springs, CO 80909

719-578-4576
Fax: 719-632-4733
e-mail: naa-ofc@ix.netcom.com
www.usarchery.org

Information on adaptive archery activities for people of many abilities. Includes local chapters, referrals, fun and social interaction and support groups.

7655 National Arts and Disability Center
300 UCLA Medical Plaza, Suite 3330
Los Angeles, CA 90095

310-794-1141
Fax: 310-794-1143
TTY: 310-267-2356
e-mail: oraynor@mednet.ucla.edu
www.dcp.ucla.edu/nadc/

Information and advocacy resources for families and professionals. Includes listings of organizations providing general information on art and disabilities.

7656 National Association for Parents of Childr en with Visual Impairments
PO Box 317
Watertown, MA 02471

617-972-7441
800-562-6265
Fax: 617-972-7444
e-mail: napvi@perkins.org
www.spedex.com/napvi/

7657 National Association of Blind Students
National Federation of the Blind
1800 Johnson Street
Baltimore, MD 21230

410-659-9314
Fax: 410-685-5653

Provides support, information and encouragement to blind college and university students. Leads the way in offering resources for national testing, accessible textbooks and materials, overcoming negative attitudes about blindness from school personnel, developing new techniques of accomplishing laboratory or field assignments and many other college experiences. Offers strong advocacy and motivational support.

7658 National Association of Protection and Advocacy Systems
900 2nd Street NE, Suite 211
Washington, DC 20002

202-408-9514
Fax: 202-408-9520
TTY: 202-408-9521
e-mail: NAPAS@earthlink.net
www.napas.org

Information and advocacy resources for families and professionals. Includes listings of organizations providing general information and organizations focusing on more specific areas of concern to families and young adults who have disabilities.

Curtis L Decker, Executive Director

7659 National Association of the Dually Diagnosed
132 Fair Street
Kingston, NY 12401

845-331-4336
800-331-5362
Fax: 845-331-4569
e-mail: nadd@ulster.net
www.thenadd.org

Seeks to stimulate the public and professional awareness regarding the dually diagnosed population, and to encourage the exchange of pertinent information, promoting educational and training programs, advocating for appropriate governmental policies, supporting research focusing on indentification, diagnosis, and treatment.

7660 National Center for Learning Disabilities
381 Park Avenue S, Suite 1401
New York, NY 10016

212-545-7510
888-575-7373
Fax: 212-545-9665
www.ncld.org

Works to ensure that the ntaion's 15 million children, adolescents and adults with learning disabilites have every opportunity to succeed in school, work and life. NCLD provides essential information to parents, professionals and individuals with learning disabilities, promotes research and programs to foster effective learning and advocates for policies to protect and strengthen educational rights and opportunities.

Sheldon Horowitz MD, Director, Professional Services
James H Wendorf, Executive Director

7661 National Center for Sight
National Society To Prevent Blindness
500 Remington Road
Schaumburg, IL 60173

847-843-2020
Fax: 847-843-8458

A toll-free line offering information on a broad range of vision, eye health and safety topics including sports eye safety, lazy eye, diabetic retinopathy, glaucoma, cataracts, children's eye disorders, and more.

7662 National Center for Vision and Child Development
Lighthouse
111 E 59th Street
New York, NY 10022

212-821-9200
800-829-0500
Fax: 212-821-9707
TTY: 212-821-9713
www.lighthouse.org

The mission is to overcome vision impairment for people of all ages through worldwide leadership in rehabilitation services, education, research, prevention and advocacy.

7663 National Center on Accessbility
University of Indiana
2805 E 10th Street, Suite 190
Bloomington, IN 47408

812-856-4422
800-424-1877
Fax: 812-856-4480
e-mail: nca@indiana.cdu
www.indiana.edu

Information on adaptive activities for people of many abilities. Includes local chapters, referrals, fun and social interaction and support groups.

7664 National Children's Cancer Society
1015 Locust Street, Suite 600
Saint Louis, MO 63101

314-241-1600
800-532-6459
Fax: 314-241-6949
e-mail: nccs@children-cancer.com
www.children-cancer.com

NCCS offers a multifaceted outreach program, which includes financial assistance, education, information, and emotional support. They provide financial assistance for bone marrow transplantation, donor harvest, donor search, donor recruitment, and family emergency expenses (such as travel, hotel, food). They also have an active advocacy program to help families with insurance companies and hospitals.

Mark Stolze, President
Julie Komanetsky, Director Patient/Family Services

7665 National Christian Resource Center
Bethesda Lutheran Homes
600 Hoffman Drive
Watertown, WI 53094

920-261-3050
800-369-4636
Fax: 920-261-8441
www.blhs.org

Information and advocacy resources for families and professionals. Includes listings of organizations providing general information and organizations focusing on more specific areas of concern to families and young adults who have disabilities.

7666 National Disability Sports Alliance
25 W Independence Way
Kingston, RI 02882

401-792-7130
Fax: 401-792-7132
e-mail: info@ndsaonline.org
www.ndsaonline.org

Nonprofit organization. Coordinates sports, recreation and fitness activities for individuals with physical disabilities. Main focus is on cerebral palsy, traumatic brain injury and stroke.

Jerry McCole, Executive Director

7667 National Dissemination Center for Children with Disabilities
PO Box 1492
Washington, DC 20013

202-884-8200
800-695-0285
Fax: 202-884-8441
e-mail: nichcy@acd.org
www.nichcy.org

A national information and referral center that provides information on disabilities and disability-related issues for families, educators and other professionals.

Suzanne Ripley, Executive Director

7668 National Early Childhood Technical Assistance System
Campus Box 8040 UNC-CH
Chapel Hill, NC 27599

919-962-2001
Fax: 919-966-7463
e-mail: nectas@unc.edu
www.nectas.unc.edu

Assists states and other designated governing jurisdictions as they develop multidisciplinary, coordinated and comprehensive services for children with special needs.

7669 National Family Caregivers Association
10400 Connecticut Avenue, Suite 500
Kensington, MD 20895

301-942-6430
800-896-3650
Fax: 301-942-2302
e-mail: info@nfcacares.org
www.nfcacares.org

The only not-for-profit organization dedicated to making life better for all of America's family caregivers. Services include information support and validation, public awareness and advocacy; NFCA strives to minimize the disparity between a caregivers quality of life and that of mainstream Americans.

7670 National Father's Network
Kindering Center
16120 NE 8th Street
Bellevue, WA 98008

425-747-4004
800-224-6827
Fax: 425-284-9664
e-mail: jmay@fathersnetwork.org
fathersnetwork.org

Information and advocacy resources for fathers. Includes listings of organizations providing general information and organizations focusing on more specific areas of concern to fathers and young adults who have disabilities.

7671 National Foundation for Facial Reconstruction
317 E 34th Street, Room 901
New York, NY 10016

212-263-6656
Fax: 212-263-7534
e-mail: info@nffr.org
www.nffr.org

The National Foundation for Facial Reconstruction, founded in 1951 by the late Dr. John Marquis Converse, to enable patients with facial disformities to lead productive fulfilling lives. NFFR lends its support to the mulidisciplinary craniofacial team at the Institute of Reconstructive Plastic Surgery at NYU Medical Center. An assembly of world-reowned surgeons, mental health professionals, research specialists and staff, give their time and expertise, using the latest reconstructive techniques.

Whitney Burnett, Executive Director

7672 National Foundation for Transplants
5350 Poplar Avenue, Suite 430
Memphis, TN 38119

901-684-1697
800-489-3863
Fax: 901-684-1128
e-mail: jhill@transplants.org
www.transplants.org

Nonprofit organization that assists transplant canidates and recipients nationwide when public or private insurance does not cover all their transplant-related costs. Offers a fund raising program for patients who need to raise $10,000 or more, and grant program that helps patients with smaller, one-time needs.

Donna Noelker, Director of Patient Services

7673 National Foundation of Wheelchair Tennis
940 Calle Amanecer, Suite B
San Clemente, CA 92673

714-361-3663
Fax: 714-361-6603
e-mail: nfwt@aol.com
www.nfwt.org

Information on adaptive tennis for people of many abilities. Includes local chapters, referrals, fun and social interaction and support groups.

7674 National Handicapped Sports
451 Hungerford Drive, Suite 100
Rockville, MD 20850

301-217-0960
Fax: 301-217-0968
e-mail: dsusa@dsusa.org
www.dsusa.org

Information on adaptive sports and recreation activities for people of many abilities, including local chapters, referrals, fun and social interaction and support groups.

7675 National Hospice Organization
1901 N Moore Street, Suite 901
Arlington, VA 22209

703-243-5900
800-338-8898

The nation's only advocate for terminally ill children, patients and their families. Provides member programs, represents hospice care interests in Congress, regulatory agencies and the public.

7676 National Industries for the Blind
1901 N Beauregard Street, Suite 200
Alexandria, VA 22311

703-998-0770
Fax: 703-998-8268

A nonprofit organization that represents over 100 associated industries serving people who are blind in thirty-six states. These agencies serve people who are blind or visually impaired and help them to reach their full potential. Services include job and family counseling, job skills training, instruction in Braille and other communication skills, children's programs and more.

7677 National Industries for the Severely Handicapped
2235 Cedar Lane
Vienna, VA 22182

703-560-6800
Fax: 703-849-8916
e-mail: info@nish.org
www.nish.org

Information and advocacy resources for families and professionals. Includes listings of organizations providing general information and organizations focusing on more specific areas of concern to families and young adults who have disabilities.

7678 National Mental Health Consumers' Self-Help Clearinghouse
1211 Chestnut Street, Suite 1207
Philadelphia, PA 19107

215-751-1810
800-553-4539
Fax: 215-636-6312
e-mail: info@mhselfhelp.org
www.mhselfhelp.org

Offers information, support, and appropriate referrals and promotes public and professional education. Provides networking for those with special interest related to albinism and management of albinism and hypopigmentation.

Joseph Rogers, Executive Director

7679 National Organization on Disability
910 16th Street NW, Suite 600
Washington, DC 20006

202-293-5960
Fax: 202-293-7999
TDD: 202-293-5968
e-mail: ability@nod.org
www.nod.org

The mission of the National Organization on Disability (N.O.D.) is to expand the participation and contribution of America's 54 million men, women and children with disabilities in all aspects of life, by raising awareness through programs and information.

Tom Ridge, Chairman
Michael R Deland, President

7680 National Parent Network on Disabilities
1130 17th Street NW, Suite 400
Washington, DC 20036

202-463-2299
Fax: 202-463-9403

Information and advocacy resources for families and professionals. Includes listings of organizations providing general information and organizations focusing on more specific areas of concern to families and young adults who have disabilities.

7681 National Parent Resource Center
Federation for Children with Special Needs
95 Berkeley Street, Suite 104
Boston, MA 02116

617-482-2915
800-695-2939
Fax: 617-572-2094
e-mail: fcsninfo@fcsn.org
www.fcsn.org

A parent-run resource system designed to further the needs and goals of family-centered, community-based coordinated care for children with special health needs and their families. Offers written materials, training packages, workshops and presentations for parents and professionals on special education, health care financing and other topics.

7682 National Parent to Parent Support and Information System
PO Box 907
Blue Ridge, GA 30513

706-632-8822
800-651-1151
Fax: 706-632-8830
e-mail: judd103w@wonder.em.cdc.gov
www..nppsis.org

NPPSIS is a nonprofit organization established to support, strengthen, and empower families through one-on-one parent contacts. Links families nationally whose children have special health care needs and rare disorders, and provides parents with heath care information, resources and referrals to allow them to identify appropriate services.

7683 National Perinatal Association (NPA)
3500 E Fletcher Avenue, Suite 205
Tampa, FL 33613

813-971-1008
800-971-1008
Fax: 813-971-9306
e-mail: npaonline@aol.com
www.nationalperinatal.org

Information and advocacy resources for families and professionals. Includes listings of organizations providing general information and organizations focusing on more specific areas of concern to families and young adults who have disabilities.

7684 National Rehabilitation Information Center
8201 Corporate Drive, Suite 600
Landover, MD 20785

301-459-5900
800-346-2742
Fax: 301-459-4263
TTY: 301-459-5984
e-mail: naricinfo@heitechservices.com
www.naric.com

NARIC is a library and information center focusing in disability and rehabilitation research. Information specialists provide quick information and referrals free of charge. Other services include customized searches of REHABDATA, the premier database of disability and rehabilitation literature, and documents from NARIC's collection of more than 70,000 documents are available for nominal fee.

Mark Odum, Director

7685 National Respite Locator Service
800 Eastowne Drive, Suite 105
Chapel Hill, NC 27514

800-773-5433
Fax: 919-490-4905
www.respitelocator.org

Information for families and professionals interested in repite care. Includes listings of organizations that provide respite services to families.

7686 National Self-Help Clearinghouse
365 5th Avenue, Suite 3300
New York, NY 10016

212-817-1822
e-mail: info@selfhelpweb.org
www.selfhelpweb.org

Information and advocacy resources for families and professionals. Includes listings of organizations providing general information and organizations focusing on more specific areas of concern to families and young adults who have disabilities.

Frank Riessman, Executive Director

7687 National Skeet & Sporting Clay Headquarters
5931 Roft Road
San Antonio, TX 78253

210-688-3371
800-877-5338
Fax: 210-688-3014

Information on adaptive skeet and sporting clay activities for people of many abilities.

7688 National Sleep Foundation
1522 K Street NW, Suite 500
Washington, DC 20005

202-347-3471
Fax: 202-347-3472
e-mail: nsf@sleepfoundation.org
www.sleepfoundation.org

Works to improve the quality of life for millions of Americans who suffer from sleep disorders, and to prevent the catastrophic accidents that are related to poor or disordered sleep through research, education and the dissemination of information towards the cause of Narcolepsy Project. Seeks patients to aid new research project targeting the cause of the disorder.

Richard Gelula, CEO

7689 National Technical Assistance Center for Children's Mental Health
Georgetown University Child Development Center
3307 M Street NW
Washington, DC 20007

202-687-5000
Fax: 202-687-8899
e-mail: gucdc@georgetown.edu
dml.georgetown.edu/depts/pediatrics/gucdc

Provides services to children experiencing emotional and mental problems.

7690 National Vaccines Information Center
204 Mill Street, Suite B1
Vienna, VA 22180

703-938-DPT3
Fax: 703-938-5768
www.909shot.com

Information and advocacy resources for families and professionals. Includes listings of organizations providing general information and organizations focusing on more specific areas of concern to families and young adults who have disabilities.

Kathi Williams, VP

7691 National Wheelchair Racquetball Association
2380 McGinley Road
Monroeville, PA 15146

412-856-2400
Fax: 412-856-2437

Information on adaptive racquetball activities for people of many abilities.

7692 National Wheelchair Shooting Federation
102 Park Avenue
Rockledge, PA 19111

215-379-2359
Fax: 215-663-9662

Information on adaptive shooting activities for people of many abilities.

7693 National Wheelchair Softball Association
1616 Todd Court
Stamford, CT 55033

651-437-1792
Fax: 612-437-3889

Information on adaptive softball activities for people of many abilities.

7694 National Youth Crisis Hotline
5331 Mount Alifan Drive
San Diego, CA 92111

800-448-4663

Information and referral for runaways; also youth and parents with problems.

7695 NineLine
460 W 41st Street
New York, NY 10036

800-999-9999
www.nineline.org

Nationwide crisis/suicide hotline.

7696 North American Riding for the Handicapped
7475 Dakin Street, Suite 600
Denver, CO 80223

303-452-1212
800-369-7433
Fax: 303-252-4610
e-mail: narha.org
www.narha.org

Information on adaptive riding activities for people of many abilities. Includes local chapters, referrals, fun and social interaction and support groups. NARHA is a membership organization that promotes and supports equine activities for the disabled. Membership dues are $50 - $150.

7697 Pan American Health Organization (PAHO)
525 23rd Street NW
Washington, DC 20037

202-974-3000
Fax: 202-974-3663
e-mail: postmaster@paho.org
www.paho.org

Acts as the directing and co-ordinating authority on international health work; aids in the prevention and control of epidemic, endemic and other diseases; promotes the improvement of nutrition, housing, sanitation, recreation, economic or working conditions; promotes improved standards of teaching and training in the health, medical and related professions; and fosters activities in the field of mental health.

7698 Parents Information Network FFCMH
1926 1700th Avenue
Lincoln, IL 62656

217-735-1662
ffcmh.org/local.htm

Bridget Schneider

7699 Pathways Awareness Foundation
150 N Michigan Avenue, Suite 2100
Chicago, IL 60601

800-955-2445
Fax: 888-795-8154
TTY: 800-326-8154
e-mail: friends@pathwaysawareness.org
www.pathwaysawareness.org

Established in 1988, Pathways Awareness Foundation is a national, nonprofit organization dedicated to raising awareness about the gift of early detection and early therapy for infants and children with physical movement differences. PAF provides informational materials to raise awareness of subtle indicators of physical development problems in infants and young children. We also have a parent answered toll-free phone. Our activities are based upon the expertise of our Medical Round Table.

Kathy O'Brien, Resource Director
Jan Stevens, Outreach Coordinator

7700 Pharmaceutical Manufacturers Association
1100 15th Street NW
Washington, DC 20005

800-762-4636
www.oncolink.com/specialty/chemo/indigen

Many drug companies have programs to provide free medicines (including chemotherapy) to needy patients. Eligibility requirements vary, but most are available to those not covered by private or public insurance programs. Ask your physician to request, on letterhead, a free copy of the Directory of Pharmaceutical Indigent Programs.

7701 Pike Institute on Law and Disability
Boston University School of Law
765 Commonwealth Avenue
Boston, MA 02115

Fax: 617-353-2906
TTY: 617-353-2904
e-mail: pikeinst@bu.edu
www.bu.edu/law/pike

Information and advocacy resources for families and professionals.
Includes listings of organizations providing general information
and organizations focusing on more specific areas of concern to
families and young adults who have disabilities.

7702 Pilot Parents (PP)
1941 S 42nd Street, Suite 122
Omaha, NE 68105

402-346-5220
Fax: 402-346-5253
e-mail: aadamson@olliewebb.org
www.olliewebb.org

Parents, professionals and others concerned with providing emotional and peer support to new parents of children with special
needs. Sponsors a parent-matching program which allows parents
who have had sufficient experience and training in the care of their
own children to share their knowledge and expertise with parents
of children recently diagnosed as disabled. Publications: The Ga-
zette, newsletter, published 6 times a year.

Laurie Ackermann, Executive Director
Jennifer Varner, Coordinator

7703 Pioneers Division of CEC
Council for Exceptional Children
1920 Association Drive
Reston, VA 20191

703-620-3660
800-873-8255
Fax: 703-264-9474
TTY: 703-264-9446
www.cec.spec.org

Promotes activities and programs to increase awareness of the educational needs of children with disablties and/or who are gifted,
and the services that are available to them.

7704 Planetree Health Information Service
2040 Webster Street
San Francisco, CA 94115

415-923-3680

A nonprofit consumer-oriented resource for health information, including relaxation and visualization techniques. Write or call for a
catalog and price list.

7705 Prevent Blindness America
500 E Remington Road
Schaumburg, IL 60173

847-843-2020
800-331-2020
www.preventblindness.org

Produces educational materials, offers guidance regarding current
available teatments, eye care facilities and programs, and current
eye research findings through the National Center for Sight. Administers a research program.

7706 Rainbows
1111 Tower Road
Schaumburg, IL 60173

708-310-1880

Peer support groups for adults and children who are grieving.

7707 Resources for Children with Special Needs
116 E 16th Street, 5th Floor
New York, NY 10003

212-677-4650
Fax: 212-254-4070
e-mail: info@resourcesnyc.org
www.resourcesnyc.org

A not for profit agency providing information, referrals, advocacy,
training and support for New York City parents of children with
learning, developmental, emotional and physical disabilities and
special needs and the professionals who serve them. Publishers of
The Comprehensive Directory: Programs and Services for
Children and Youth with Disabilities and their Families in the
Metro New York Area, Camps 2004, Schools and services for
Children with Autism Spectrum Disorders.

Karen Schlesinger, Executive Director
Helena Craner, Associate Director

7708 Roeher Institute
York University
Kinsmen Building, 4700 Keele Street
North York, ON, M3J
Canada

416-661-9611
Fax: 416-661-5701
TDD: 416-661-2023
e-mail: info@roeher.ca
www.indie.ca/roeher

Conducts research for various pediatric disabilities.

7709 Ronald McDonald Houses
One Kroc Drive
Oak Brook, IL 60523

603-623-7048
Fax: 630-623-7488
www.rmhc.org

Provides national programs, funding and other support to network
of 150 local Ronald McDonald Houses, homes-away-from-homes
for families of seriously ill children

7710 Rural Institute on Disabilities
University of Montana
52 Corbin Hall
Missoula, MT 59812

406-243-5467
800-732-0323
Fax: 406-243-4730
TTY: 403-243-5467
e-mail: rural@ruralinstitute.umt.edu
www.ruralinstitute.umt.edu

Information and advocacy resources for families and professionals.
Includes listings of organizations providing general information
and organizations focusing on more specific areas of concern to
families and young adults who have disabilities.

**7711 Sexuality Information and Education Council of the US
(SIECUS)**
130 W 42nd Street, Suite 350
New York, NY 10036

212-819-9770
Fax: 212-819-9776
e-mail: siecus@siecus.org
www.siecus.org/

Information and advocacy resources for families and professionals.
Includes listings of organizations providing general information
and organizations focusing on more specific areas of concern to
families and young adults who have disabilities.

7712 Sibling Support Project
Children's Hospital and Regional Medical Center
PO Box 5371 CL-09
Seattle, WA 98105

206-987-2000
Fax: 206-527-5705
e-mail: dmeyer@chmc.org
www.seattlechildren.org

Information and advocacy resources for families and professionals. Includes listings of organizations providing general information and organizations focusing on more specific areas of concern to families and young adults who have disabilities.

7713 Ski for Light
1455 W Lake Street
Minneapolis, MN 55408

612-827-3232

Nonprofit organization founded in 1975 to promote the physical fitness of visually and movility impaired adults.

7714 Society for Pediatric Dermatology
8365 Keystone Crossing, Suite 107
Indianapolis, IN 46240

317-202-0224
Fax: 317-205-9481
e-mail: spd@hp-assoc.com
www.pedsderm.net

Objective is to promote, develop and advance education, research and care of skin disease in all pediatric age groups.

Kent Lindeman, Executive Director

7715 Sparrow Foundation
1155 N 130th, Suite 310
Seattle, WA 98104

206-745-5403
www.sparrow-fdn.org

This nonprofit charitable and educational organization was started by the family of a child who needed a bone marrow transplant, for which their insurance carrier refused to pay. The foundation provides seed money to schools, youth organizations, service clubs, and churches which help persons with medical needs.

7716 Spaulding for Children
16250 Northland Drive, Suite 100
Southfield, MI 48075

248-443-7080
Fax: 248-443-7099
www.spaulding.org

Information and advocacy resources for families and professionals. Includes listings of organizations providing general information and organizations focusing on more specific areas of concern to families and young adults who have disabilities.

7717 Special Needs Advocate for Parents (SNAP)
3029 Wilshire Blvd. Suite 200
Santa Monica, CA 90403

310-452-3759
888-310-9889
Fax: 310-450-5769
e-mail: info@spapinfo.org
www.snapinfo.org

Nonprofit organization with advisors nationwide and information and advocacy resources for families and professionals. Includes listings of organizations providing general information and organizations focusing on more specific areas of concern to families and young adults who have disabilities, support groups, educational advocates and medical insurance problem solving. Quarterly newsletter with articles of interest.

Marla Kraus, Executive Director

7718 Special Olympics
1133 19th Street, NW
Washington, DC 20036

202-628-3630
Fax: 202-824-0200
e-mail: info@specialolympics.org
www.specialolympics.org

Information on adaptive sports and recreation activities and related health issues for people of many abilities. Including local chapters, referrals, fun and social interaction and support groups.

7719 Specialized Training of Military Parents (STOMP)
Washington PAVE
6316 S 12th Street
Tacoma, WA 98465

253-565-2266
800-572-7368
Fax: 253-566-8052
TTY: 253-565-2266
e-mail: stomp@washingtonpave.com
www.stompproject.org

Information and advocacy resources for military families who have children with special education or health needs. Includes listings of organizations providing general information and organizations focusing on more specific areas of concern and family to family connections.

Heather Hedbon, Founder & Director
Luz Adriana Martinez, Parent Education Coordinator

7720 Starbright
5757 Wilshire Boulevard, Suite M100
Los Angeles, CA 90036

310-479-1212
800-315-2580
Fax: 310-479-1235

The Foundation is dedicated to the development of projects that empower seriously ill children to combat the medical and emotional challenges they face on a daily basis. STARBRIGHT projects do more then educate and entertain, address the core issues that accompany illness, the pain, fear and lonliness and depression that can be as damaging as the sickness itself.

7721 Tech Connection
Family Resource Associates
35 Haddon Avenue
Shrewsbury, NJ 07702

732-747-5310
Fax: 732-747-1896
e-mail: techhorin@aol.com
www.techconnection.org

Tech Connection is a resource center to help children and adults who have disabilities gain access to the benefits of technology. Includes nationwide network of community-based assistive technology, resource centers, hands on consultants and product demonstrations and evaluations.

7722 Technology Assistance for Special Consumers
PO Box 443
Huntsville, AL 35804

256-532-5996
Fax: 256-532-2355
TDD: 256-532-5996
e-mail: tasc@travellers.com

Technology group of parents, consumers and professionals; provides resources to help children and adults who have disabilities gain access to the benefits of technology. Includes nationwide network of community-based assistive technology, resource centers, hands on consultants and product demonstrations.

7723 US Paralympics
U.S. Olympic Committee
1 Olympic Plaza
Colorado Springs, CO 80909

719-866-2030
Fax: 719-866-2029
e-mail: alison.nicholas@usoc.org
www.usparalympics.com

A division of the United States Olympic Committee, we focus our efforts on enhancing programs, funding and opportunities for persons with physical disabilities to participate in Paralympic sport. The Paralympic Games are the second largest sporting event in the world, conceding top honors only to the Olympics. The multi-sport competition showcases the talents and abilities of the world's most elite athletes with physical disabilities.

Alison Nicholas, Program Coordinator
Beth Bason, Communications Coordinator

7724 Vision of Children Foundation
12730 High Bluff Drive, Suite 250
San Diego, CA 92130

858-799-0810
Fax: 858-794-2348
e-mail: darlalopez@aol.com
www.visionofchildren.org

Provides information, promotes research and assists the families of blind and visually impaired children in locating organizations and service providers who can give support.

Samuel A Hardage, Chairman
Andrea Carter, Executive Director

7725 WE MOVE (Worldwide Education and Advocacy for Movement Disorders)
Mt. Siani Medical Center
204 W 84th Street
New York, NY 10024

212-241-8567
800-437-6682
Fax: 212-875-8389
e-mail: wemove@wemove.org
www.wemove.org

WE MOVE provides movement disorder information and educational materials to physicians, patients, the media, and the public via its comprehensive web site, training courses, patient support group and more. Its goal is to make early diagnosis, up-to-date treatment and patient support a reality for all people living with movement disorders.

Susan Bressman, President

7726 World Institute on Disability
510 16th Street, Suite 100
Oakland, CA 94612

510-763-4100
Fax: 510-763-4109
TTY: 510-208-9493
e-mail: wid@wid.org
www.wid.org

Information and advocacy resources for families and professionals. Includes listings of organizations providing general information and organizations focusing on more specific areas of concern to families and young adults who have disabilities.

Stanley K Yarnell MD, Chairman
Martin B Schulter, Vice Chair

7727 World Research Foundation
41 Bell Rock Plaza
Sedona, AZ 86351

928-284-3300
Fax: 928-248-3530
e-mail: info@wrf.org
www.wrf.org

Nonprofit organization. Your global source of information on illnesses and therapies used around the world.

LaVerne Ross, Co-Founder
Steven Ross

7728 Young Adult Institute
61 W 23rd Street
New York, NY 10010

212-924-0511

A nonprofit professional organizations serving developmentally disabled children and adults in many programs throughout the New York metropolitan area. Provides over 50 program sites for thousands of participants.

Joel Levy, Executive Director

7729 Zero to Three
2000 M Street NW, Suite 200
Washington, DC 20036

202-638-1144
800-899-4301
Fax: 202-638-0851
zerotothree.org

The mission is to promote the healthy development of our nation's infants and toddlers by supporting and strengthening families, communities and those who work on their behalf. We are dedicated to advancing current knowledge , promoting beneficial policies and practices and providing training, technical assistance, and leadership development. A nonprofit organization.

Matthew E Melmed, Executive Director

State Agencies & Support Groups

Alabama

7730 ARC of Morgan County
401 14th Street, Suite 4-E
Decatur, AL 35601

205-355-6192
Fax: 256-350-4502
e-mail: arc@hiwaay.net

Informational and emotional support to parents who have a child, adolescent, or adult family member with special needs.

7731 Early Intervention Program
2129 East South Blvd
Montgomery, AL 36111

334-281-8780
Fax: 334-281-1973
e-mail: oholder@rehab.state.al.us
www.nectas.unc.edu

Services include central directory, representatives of agencies, service providers, families, and coordinators of infant, toddler, and preschool special education programs.

Ouidah Holder, Infant/Toodler Program Coordinator

7732 Friends for Life Auburn United Methodist Church
137 S Gay Street
Auburn, AL 36830

334-826-8800

Informational and emotional support to parents who have a child, adolescent, or adult family member with special needs.

7733 Special Education Action Committee Huntsville Outreach Office
3322 S Memorial Parkway, Suite 25
Huntsville, AL 35801

256-882-3911
Fax: 256-882-3974
e-mail: seach@traveler.com
www.hsv.tis.net/~seachsv

Informational and emotional support to parents who have a child, adolescent, or adult family member with special needs.

7734 Special Education Services
Department of Education
PO Box 302101
Montgomery, AL 36104

334-242-8114
Fax: 334-242-9192
e-mail: jwaid@sdenet.alsde.edu
www.nectas.unc.edu

Services include central directory, representatives of agencies, service providers, families, and coordinators of infant, toddler, and preschool special education programs.

Phyllis Mayfield, Preschool Specialist

7735 Statewide Technology Access & Response System for Alabamians with Disabilities
2125 E South Boulevard, PO Box 20752
Montgomery, AL 36120

334-613-3480
800-782-7656
Fax: 334-613-3485
TDD: 334-613-3519
e-mail: tgannaway@rehab.state.al.us
www.mindspring.com/alstar/

State assisted programs and support group information for people of many abilities. Includes local chapters, referrals, fun and social interaction and support groups.

Alaska

7736 Alaska Department of Education
801 W 10th Street, Suite 200
Juneau, AK 99801

907-465-2831
Fax: 907-465-2441
e-mail: dbrown@educ.state.ak.us
www.nectas.unc.edu

Individuals with Disabilities Education Act requires early intervention and preschool special education for children with disabilities and special health care needs. Services include central directory, representatives of agencies, service providers, families, and coordinators of infant, toddler, and preschool special education programs.

Diann Brown, Preschool Special Ed. Coordinator

7737 Assistive Technologies of Alaska
1016 W 6th Street, Suite 205
Anchorage, AK 99501

907-563-0138
Fax: 907-269-3632
TDD: 907-269-3569
e-mail: atadvr@corecom.net
www.labor.state.ak.us

State assisted programs and support group information for people of many abilities. Includes local chapters, referrals, fun and social interaction and support groups.

7738 Maternal, Child & Family Health, Early Intervention/Infant Learning Program
State of Alaska Department of Health
1231 Gambell Street
Anchorage, AK 99501

907-269-3419
Fax: 907-269-3465
e-mail: jbatuk@health.state.ak.us

Early intervention and preschool special education for children with disabilities and special health care needs. Services include administration of statewide early intervention programs for infants and toddlers with developmental delays or disabilities and their families.

Jane Atuk, Part C Coordinator
Karen Martinek, Special Needs Services Unit

7739 PARENTS
4743 E Northern Lights Boulevard
Anchorage, AK 99508

907-337-7678
800-478-7678
Fax: 907-337-7671
TDD: 907-337-7678
e-mail: parentsss@alaska.com
www.parentsinc.org

Parent Training and Information (PTI) programs help parents to understand their children's specific needs, communicate more effectively with professionals, participate in the educational planning process, and obtain information about relevant programs, services and resources.

Arizona

7740 Arizona Early Intervention Program Department of Economic Security
3839 N. 3rd St, Suite 304 Site Code No. 801 A-6
Phoenix, AZ 85012

602-532-9960
Fax: 602-200-9820
e-mail: azeip@aztec.asu.edu
www.de.state.az.us

Early intervention and preschool special education for children with disabilities and special health care needs. Services include central directory, representatives of agencies, service providers, families, and coordinators of infant, toddler, and preschool special education programs.

Diane Renne, Infant/Toodler Program Coordinator

7741 Arizona Technology Access Program Institute for Human Development
2400 N. Central Avenue, Suite 300
Pheonix, AZ 85004

602-728-9534
800-477-9921
Fax: 602-728-9353
TTY: 602-728-9536
e-mail: Daniel.Davidson@nau.edu
www.nau.edu/ihd/aztap

State assisted programs and support group information for people of many abilities. Includes local chapters, referrals, fun and social interaction and support groups.

7742 Blake Foundation Children's Achievement Center
3825 E 2nd Street
Tucson, AZ 85716

520-325-0611
Fax: 520-327-5414
www.nectas.unc.edu

Services include central directory, representatives of agencies, service providers, families, and coordinators of infant, toddler, and preschool special education programs.

Annabell Rose, Interagency Coordinating Council

7743 Division of Special Education State Department of Education
1535 W Jefferson
Phoenix, AZ 85007

602-542-3852
Fax: 602-542-5404
e-mail: lbusenb@mail1.ade.state.az.us
www.nectas.unc.edu

Individuals with Disabilities Education Act requires all states and territories to provide early intervention and preschool special education for children with disabilities and special health care needs. Services include central directory, representatives of agencies, service providers, families, and coordinators of infant, toddler, and preschool special education programs.

Lynn Busenbark, Preschool Special Ed. Coordinator

7744 Pilot Parents of Southern Arizona
2600 N Wyatt Drive
Tucson, AZ 85712

520-324-3150
Fax: 520-324-3154
e-mail: ppsa@pilotparents.org
www.pilotparents.org

Parent Training and Information (PTI) programs help parents to understand their children's specific needs, communicate more effectively with professionals, participate in the educational planning process, and obtain information about relevant programs, services and resources.

7745 Raising Special Kids
2400 N. Central Ave., Suite 200
Phoenix, AZ 85004

602-242-4366
800-237-3007
Fax: 602-242-4306
e-mail: info@raisingspecialkids.org
www.raisingspecialkids.org

Provides support and training to families of children who have disabilities and special health needs, helps parents communicate more effectively with professionals, participate in the educational planning process and obtain information about programs and resources available to them. Offers training to professionals in health, education and social services.

Joyce Millard-Hoie, Executive Director
Marla Urbina, Director Family Support

7746 Southwest Human Development
2850 North 24th Street
Phoenix, AZ 85008

602-266-5976
Fax: 602-274-8952
e-mail: gward@swhd.org
www.swhd.org

Services include central directory, representatives of agencies, service providers, families, and coordinators of infant, toddler, and preschool special education programs.

Ginger Mach-Ward, Interagency Coordinating Council

Arkansas

7747 Arkansas Disability Coalition
1123 S University, Suite 225
Little Rock, AR 72204

501-614-7020
800-223-1330
Fax: 501-614-9082
TDD: 501-614-7020
e-mail: adc@alltel.net
www.adcpti.org

Parent Training and Information (PTI) programs help parents to understand their children's specific needs, communicate more effectively with professionals, participate in the educational planning process, and obtain information about relevant programs, services and resources.

Wanda Stovall, Director
Christy Bell, Parent Trainer

7748 DD Services, Department of Human Services
PO Box 1437, Slot 2520
Little Rock, AR 72203

501-682-8699
Fax: 501-682-8890
e-mail: dds1@aristotle.net
www.nectas.unc.edu

Individuals with Disabilities Education Act requires all states and territories to provide early intervention and preschool special education for children with disabilities and special health care needs. Services include central directory, representatives of agencies, service providers, families, and coordinators of infant, toddler, and preschool special education programs.

Sherry Cobb, Infant/Toddler Program Coordinator

7749 FOCUS
305 W Jefferson Avenue
Jonesboro, AR 72401

870-935-2750
Fax: 870-931-3755
e-mail: focusinc@ipa.net
www.taalliance.org

Parent Training and Information (PTI) programs help parents to understand their children's specific needs, communicate more effectively with professionals, participate in the educational planning process, and obtain information about relevant programs, services and resources.

7750 Increasing Capabilities Access Network
Dept of Education/Arkansas Rehabilitation Services
26 Corporate Hill Drive
Little Rock, AR 72205

Fax: 501-666-5319
TTY: 501-666-8868
TDD: 800-828-2799
e-mail: 102503.3602@compuserve.com
www.arkansas-ican.org

State assisted programs and support group information for people of many abilities. Includes local chapters, referrals, fun and social interaction and support groups.

Barry Vuletich, Program Administrator

7751 Parent to Parent Arc of Arkansas
2004 Main Street
Little Rock, AR 72206

501-375-7770
Fax: 501-372-4621

Informational and emotional support to parents who have a child, adolescent, or adult family member with special needs.

7752 Special Education Section State Department of Education
4 Capitol Mall, Room 105-C
Little Rock, AR 72201

501-682-4225
Fax: 501-682-4313
e-mail: sreifeiss@arkedu.k12.ar.us
www.nectas.unc.edu

Individuals with Disabilities Education Act requires all states and territories to provide early intervention and preschool special education for children with disabilities and special health care needs. Services include central directory, representatives of agencies, service providers, families, and coordinators of infant, toddler, and preschool special education programs.

Sandra Reifeissk, Preschool Special Ed. Coordinator

California

7753 ARC Family Resource Project
2421 Lomitas Avenue, PO Box 219
Santa Rosa, CA 95402

877-694-4335
Fax: 707-578-8601
e-mail: arcsoco@sonic.net

Parent Training and Information (PTI) programs help parents to understand their children's specific needs, communicate more effectively with professionals, participate in the educational planning process, and obtain information about relevant programs, services and resources.

Traci N Turner, Program Coordinator
Elvis Bozarth, President

7754 CARE Family Resource Center
1350 Arnold Drive, Suite 203
Martinez, CA 94553

925-313-0999
Fax: 925-370-8651

Informational and emotional support to parents who have a child, adolescent, or adult family member with special needs.

7755 Carolyn Kordich Family Resource Center
1135 W. 257th Street
Harbor City, CA 90710

310-325-7288
Fax: 310-325-7288
e-mail: ckfrc@worldnet.att.net

Informational and emotional support to parents who have a child, adolescent, or adult family member with special needs.

7756 Challenged Family Resource Center
827 West 20th Street
Merced, CA 95340

209-385-5314
Fax: 209-385-5317
e-mail: dkuneck@aol.com
www.challengedfrc.com

Informational and emotional support to parents who have a child, adolescent, or adult family member with special needs.

7757 Children Living with Illness
The Center for Attitudinal Healing
33 Buchanan Drive
Sausalito, CA 94965

415-331-6161
Fax: 415-331-4545

For children who are ill, have an ill sibling, or an ill parent. Parent group meets separately at the same time.

Jimmy Pete

7758 Comfort Connection Family Resource Center
12361 Lewis Street, Suite 101
Garden Grove, CA 92840

714-748-7491
Fax: 714-748-8149

Informational and emotional support to parents who have a child, adolescent, or adult family member with special needs.

7759 Department of Developmental Services of Early Start Program
1600 Ninth Street
Sacramento, CA 94244

916-654-1690
800-515-2229
Fax: 916-654-2054
TDD: 916-654-2054
e-mail: earlystart@dds.ca.gov
www.dds.ca.gov

Individuals with Disabilities Education Act requires all states and territories to provide early intervention and preschool special education for children with disabilities and special health care needs. Services include central directory, representatives of agencies, service providers, families, and coordinators of infant, toddler, and preschool special education programs.

Rick Ingraham, Manager

7760 Early Start Family Resource Network
1855 Business Center Drive
San Bernadino, CA 92412

909-890-4791
800-974-5553
Fax: 909-890-4709
www.irclibrary.com/csfrn/

Informational and emotional support to parents who have a child, adolescent, or adult family member with special needs.

7761 Exceptional Family Resource Center
9245 Sky Park Court, Suite 130
San Diego, CA 92123

619-594-7416
800-281-8252
Fax: 858-268-4275
e-mail: efro@cybergate.com
www.efrconline.org

Informational and emotional support to parents who have a child, adolescent, or adult family member with special needs.

7762 Exceptional Family Support, Education and Advocacy Center
6402 Skyway
Paradise, CA 95969

530-876-8321
Fax: 530-876-0346
e-mail: sea@sunset.net
www.taalliance.org

Parent Training and Information (PTI) programs help parents to understand their children's specific needs, communicate more effectively with professionals, participate in the educational planning process, and obtain information about relevant programs, services and resources.

7763 Exceptional Parents
Family Resource Center
4440 N 1st Street
Fresno, CA 93726

559-229-2000
Fax: 559-229-2956
TTY: 559-225-6059
e-mail: epu1@cybergate.com
www.exceptionalparents.org

Informational and emotional support to parents who have a child, adolescent, or adult family member with special needs.

7764 Families Caring for Families
Family Resource Center
113 W Pillsbury Street, Suite A1
Lancaster, CA 93534

661-949-1746
Fax: 661-948-7266

Informational and emotional support to parents who have a child, adolescent, or adult family member with special needs.

7765 Family First Program Alpha Resource Center
4501 Cathedral Oaks Road, Suite A1
Santa Barbara, CA 93110

805-683-2145
Fax: 805-967-3647
e-mail: arcofsb@slcom.com

Informational and emotional support to parents who have a child, adolescent, or adult family member with special needs.

7766 Family Focus Resource Center
18111 Nordhoff Street
Northridge, CA 91330

818-677-5675
Fax: 818-677-5574
e-mail: family.focus@csun.edu
www.csun.edu/~ffrc/family-html.html

Informational and emotional support to parents who have a child, adolescent, or adult family member with special needs.

Ann R Bisno, PhD, Project Director
Judith F Sultan, Coordinator

7767 Family Resource Center
5250 Claremont Avenue
Stockton, CA 95207

209-472-3674
Fax: 209-472-3673

Informational and emotional support to parents who have a child, adolescent, or adult family member with special needs.

7768 H.E.A.R.T.S. Connection Family Resource Center
3101 N Sillect Avenue, Suite 115
Bakersfield, CA 93308

661-328-9055
Fax: 661-328-9940

Informational and emotional support to parents who have a child, adolescent, or adult family member with special needs.

7769 Harbor Regional Center Family and Professional Resource Center
21231 Hawthorne Boulevard
Torrance, CA 90503

310-543-0691
Fax: 310-316-8843
e-mail: familyresourcecntr@hddf.com
www.hddf.com

Informational and emotional support to parents who have a child, adolescent, or adult family member with special needs.

7770 MATRIX: Parent Network and Family Resource Center
94 Galli Drive, Suite C
Novato, CA 94949

415-884-3535
800-578-2592
Fax: 415-884-3555
e-mail: info@matrixparents.orgrg
www.matrixparents.org

Informational and emotional support to parents who have a child, adolescent, or adult family member with special needs.

Noris Thompson, Executive Director

7771 Matrix Parents Network and Resource Center
5350 Commerce Boulevard, Suite J
Rohnert Park, CA 94928

707-586-3314
Fax: 707-586-3145
e-mail: SonomaCo@matrixparents.org
www.matrixparents.org

Matrix is a nonprofit agency that serves families of children with special needs and disabilities. Provides information and referral, individual support, technical assistance, support groups, training about special education and services, and direction to appropriate early start services.

7772 Parents Helping Parents of San Francisco
594 Monterey Boulevard
San Francisco, CA 94127

415-841-8820
Fax: 415-841-8824
www.taalliance.org

Parent Training and Information (PTI) programs help parents to understand their children's specific needs, communicate more effectively with professionals, participate in the educational planning process, and obtain information about relevant programs, services and resources.

7773 Parents Helping Parents of Santa Clara
3041 Olcott Street
Santa Clara, CA 95054

408-727-5775
Fax: 408-727-0182
e-mail: info@php.com
www.php.com

Informational and emotional support to parents who have a child, adolescent, or adult family member with special needs.

Helena Cohen, Program Coordinator
Kathy Weitsman, Parent Liaison

7774 Peaks and Valleys Family Resource Center
20 Sherwood Place No. 4
Salinas, CA 93906

831-755-1450
800-400-2937
Fax: 831-755-1470
e-mail: peaks@montereyk12.ca.us

Informational and emotional support to parents who have a child, adolescent, or adult family member with special needs.

7775 San Gabriel/Pomona Parents' Place
1500 W Covina Parkway, Suite 207
West Covina, CA 91790

626-856-8861
800-422-2022
Fax: 626-337-2736
e-mail: empower@gte.net
www.parentsplacefrc.com

Family Resource Center committed to supporting, promoting and enhancing family focused services in a parent driven atmosphere for families who have children with special needs. Family Resource Centers are part of the California Early Start Program which addresses the unique and individual needs of families raising a child with a disability. The Parent's Place is dedicated to empowering families through information/education, referrals and parent to parent support.

Sona Baghdassarian, Director
Judy Kyne, Administrative Secretary

7776 South Central Los Angeles Regional Center for Devlopmentally Disabled Persons
6500 W Adams Boulevard
Los Angeles, CA 90007

213-744-7000
Fax: 213-744-8494
TTY: 213-763-5634

Informational and emotional support to parents who have a child, adolescent, or adult family member with special needs.

7777 Special Connections Family Resource Center
809-H Bay Avenue
Capitola, CA 95010

831-464-0669
Fax: 831-465-9177

Informational and emotional support to parents who have a child, adolescent, or adult family member with special needs.

7778 Special Education Division State Department of Education
PO Box 944272
Sacramento, CA 94244

916-327-3696
Fax: 916-327-8878
e-mail: cbourne@mail515a.cde.ca.gov
www.nectas.unc.edu

Individuals with Disabilities Education Act requires all states and territories to provide early intervention and preschool special education for children with disabilities and special health care needs. Services include central directory, representatives of agencies, service providers, families, and coordinators of infant, toddler, and preschool special education programs.

Constance J Bourne, Preschool Special Ed. Coordinator

7779 Starlight Children's Foundation
5757 Wilshire Boulevard, Suite M-100
Los Angeles, CA 90036

310-479-1212
800-274-7827
Fax: 323-634-0090
e-mail: Jenny@starlight.org
www.starlight.org

International nonprofit organization dedicated to improving the quality of life for seriously ill children and their families. Working with more than 850 hospitals worldwide, the Foundation provides an impressive menu of both in-hospital and outpatient programs and services. A leader in delivering distractive entertainment therapies, over 85,000 children benefit from Starlight's programs each month.

Jenny Issacson, Communications Director
Jasmine Moir, Communications Manager

7780 Support for Families of Children with Disabilities
2601 Mission, Suite 710
San Francisco, CA 94110

415-282-7494
Fax: 415-282-1226
e-mail: sfcdmiss@aol.com
www.taalliance.org

Parent Training and Information (PTI) programs help parents to understand their children's specific needs, communicate more effectively with professionals, participate in the educational planning process, and obtain information about relevant programs, services and resources.

7781 Team Advocates for Special Kids, Anaheim
100 W Cerritos Avenue
Anaheim, CA 92805

714-533-8275
Fax: 714-533-2533
e-mail: taskca@aol.com
www.taalliance.org

Programs help parents to understand their children's specific needs, communicate more effectively with professionals, participate in the educational planning process, and obtain information about relevant programs, services and resources.

7782 Team Advocates for Special Kids, San Diego
4550 Kearney Villa Road, #102
San Diego, CA 92123

858-874-2386
Fax: 858-874-2375

Programs help parents to understand their children's specific needs, communicate more effectively with professionals, participate in the educational planning process, and obtain information about relevant programs, services and resources.

7783 Warmline Family Resource Center
2035 Hurley Way Suite 290
Sacramento, CA 95825

916-922-9276
800-660-7995
Fax: 916-922-9341
e-mail: warmlinefrc@warmlinefrc.com
www.warmlinefrc.org

Informational and emotional support to parents who have a child, adolescent, or adult family member with special needs.

Colorado

7784 Assistive Technology Partners
601 E 18th Avenue, Suite 130
Denver, CO 80203

303-315-1280
800-255-3477
Fax: 303-837-1208
TTY: 303-864-5110
e-mail: cathy.bodine@uCHSC.edu
www.uchsc.edu/catp

State assisted programs and support group information for people of many abilities. Focuses on assitive technology devices and services for persons with disabilities, training and technical assistance available.

7785 Colorado Consortium of Intensive Care Nurseries United Parents (UP)
1056 E 19th Avenue, B535
Denver, CO 80218

303-861-6557
Fax: 303-764-8092
e-mail: McGinley.Pandora@ex.tchden.org

Informational and emotional support to parents who have a child, adolescent, or adult family member with special needs.

7786 Delta/Montrose Parent to Parent
2091 E Locust Road
Montrose, CO 81401

970-249-2878
Fax: 970-252-0544
e-mail: children@gj.net

Informational and emotional support to parents who have a child, adolescent, or adult family member with special needs.

7787 Denver Early Childhood Connections
2727 W 92nd Avenue
Denver, CO 80204

303-458-0852
Fax: 303-744-9502

Provides resource coordination for children eligible for Part C services and referrals to other agencies for children with needs outside of the Part C realm. Parent to parent support, parent education and community playgroups are some of the services that are conducted. Forums are hosted on varied topics relevant to parents of young children as well as inservice and pre-service workshops on child development. IFSP development, parent's rights under IDEA, and other resource packets are available.

Newsletter

Judith Persoff, Executive Director

7788 Disability Connection and RAFT, Larimer County's Early Childhood Connection
PO Box 270714
Fort Collins, CO 80527

970-229-0224
Fax: 970-229-0242
e-mail: bstuts@fornet.org

Informational and emotional support to parents who have a child, adolescent, or adult family member with special needs.

7789 Effective Parent Project
255 Main Street
Grand Junction, CO 81501

970-241-4068
Fax: 970-241-3725

Informational and emotional support to parents who have a child, adolescent, or adult family member with special needs.

7790 El Groupo Vida
777 Bannock, Mail Code 1701
Denver, CO 80204

303-295-0628
Fax: 303-295-7850

Informational and emotional support to parents who have a child, adolescent, or adult family member with special needs.

7791 Helen Keller National Center - Rocky Mount ain Center
1880 S Pierce Street, #5
Lakewood, CO 80329

303-934-9037
Fax: 303-934-2939
www.hknc.org

7792 Help Parent Support Group Hope & Education for Loving Parents
378 S Falcon
Pueblo West, CO 81007

719-545-2282
Fax: 719-547-1282
e-mail: fastgram@aol.com

Informational and emotional support to parents who have a child, adolescent, or adult family member with special needs.

7793 Oasis
1120 N Circle Drive, Suite 19
Colorado Springs, CO 80909

719-635-8722
Fax: 719-577-9482
e-mail: oasis@juno.com

Informational and emotional support to parents who have a child, adolescent, or adult family member with special needs.

7794 PEAK Parent Center
611 N Weber, Suite 200
Colorado Springs, CO 80903

719-531-9400
800-284-0251
Fax: 719-531-9452
TDD: 719-531-9403
e-mail: info@peakparent.org
www.peakparent.org

Parent Training and Information (PTI) programs help parents to understand their children's specific needs, communicate more effectively with professionals, participate in the educational planning process, and obtain information about relevant programs, services and resources.

7795 Parent Support Group of Littleton & Auora
7600 E Arapahoe, Suite 219
Englewood, CO 80112

303-773-0044
Fax: 303-773-8780

Informational and emotional support to parents who have a child, adolescent, or adult family member with special needs.

7796 Parents Supporting Parents of Eagle County
PO Box 2656
Vail, CO 81658

970-926-6015
Fax: 970-926-6015

Informational and emotional support to parents who have a child, adolescent, or adult family member with special needs.

7797 Parents Supporting Parents of Garfield and Pitkin County
PO Box 784
Silt, CO 81652

970-876-5768
Fax: 970-876-5204

Informational and emotional support to parents who have a child, adolescent, or adult family member with special needs.

7798 Prevention Initiatives State Department of Education
210 E Colfax, Room 301
Denver, CO 80203

303-866-6709
Fax: 303-866-6662
e-mail: smith_s@cde.state.co.us
www.nectas.unc.edu

Provides early intervention and preschool special education for children with disabilities and special health care needs. Services include central directory, representatives of agencies, service providers, families, and coordinators of infant, toddler, and preschool special education programs.

Susan Smith, Infant/Toddler Program Coordinator

7799 Resources for Young Children and Families
1120 N Circle Drive, Suite 19
Colorado Springs, CO 80909

719-577-9190
Fax: 719-577-9482
e-mail: partc@rycf.org

Informational and emotional support to parents who have a child, adolescent, or adult family member with special needs.

7800 Wilderness on Wheels Foundation
3131 S Vaughn Way, Suite 305
Aurora, CO 80014

303-751-3959

State assisted programs and support group information for people of many abilities. Includes local chapters, referrals, fun and social interaction and support groups.

Connecticut

7801 Assistive Technology Project
Department of Social Services, BRS
25 Sigourney Street, 11th Floor
Hartford, CT 06106

860-424-4881
800-537-2549
Fax: 860-424-4850
TDD: 860-424-4850
e-mail: cttap@aol./com
www.tachact.uconn.edu

State assisted programs and support group information for people of many abilities. Includes local chapters, referrals, fun and social interaction and support groups.

7802 CPAC
338 Main Street
Niantic, CT 06357

860-739-3089
Fax: 860-739-7460
e-mail: cpacino@aol.com
www.cpacinc.org

Programs help parents to understand their children's specific needs, communicate more effectively with professionals, participate in the educational planning process, and obtain information about relevant programs, services and resources.

7803 Department of Mental Retardation
460 Capital Avenue
Hartford, CT 06106

860-418-6134
Fax: 860-418-6003
e-mail: lbgood993@aol.com
www.birth23.org

Individuals with Disabilities Education Act requires all states and territories to provide early intervention and preschool special education for children with disabilities and special health care needs. Services include central directory, representatives of agencies, service providers, families, and coordinators of infant, toddler, and preschool special education programs.

Linda Goodman, Infant/Toddler Program Coordinator

7804 Division of Child & Family Studies
National Early Childhood Technical Assistance Ctr
263 Farmington Avenue
Farmington, CT 06030

860-679-1500
Fax: 860-679-1571
e-mail: bruder@nso1.uchc.edu
www.nectas.unc.edu

Individuals with Disabilities Education Act requires all states and territories to provide early intervention and preschool special education for children with disabilities and special health care needs. Services include central directory, representatives of agencies, service providers, families, and coordinators of infant, toddler, and preschool special education programs.

Mary Beth Bruder, Interagency Coordinator

7805 Parent to Parent Network of Connecticut the Family Center
Dept. of Connecticut Children's Medical Center
282 Washington
Hartford, CT 06106

860-545-9021
Fax: 860-545-9201
TTY: 860-545-9002
e-mail: mcole@ccmckids.org
www.ccmkids.org

Informational and emotional support to parents who have a child, adolescent, or adult family member with special needs.

7806 State Department of Education
25 Industrial Park Road
Middletown, CT 06457

860-807-2054
Fax: 860-807-2062
www.nectas.unc.edu

Individuals with Disabilities Education Act requires all states and territories to provide early intervention and preschool special education for children with disabilities and special health care needs. Services include central directory, representatives of agencies, service providers, families, and coordinators of infant, toddler, and preschool special education programs.

Maria Synodi, Preschool Special Ed. Coordinator

Delaware

7807 Delaware Assisstive Technology Initiative (DATI)
University of Delaware
PO Box 269
Wilmington, DE 19899

302-651-6790
800-870-3284
Fax: 302-651-6793
TDD: 302-651-6794
e-mail: dati@asel.udel.edu
www.dati.org

The Delaware Assistive Technology Initiative (DATI) connects Delawareans who have disabilities with the tools they need in order to learn, work, play and participate in community life safely and independently. DATI services include: Equipment demonstration center in each county; no-cost, short-term equipment loans that let you try before you buy; Equipment Exchange Program; AT workshops and other training sessions; advocacy for improved AT access policies and funding and several more.

7808 Department of Public Instruction
PO Box 1402
Dover, DE 19703

302-739-4667
Fax: 302-739-2388
e-mail: mtoomey@state.de.us
www.nectas.unc.edu

Individuals with Disabilities Education Act requires all states and territories to provide early intervention and preschool special education for children with disabilities and special health care needs. Services include central directory, representatives of agencies, service providers, families, and coordinators of infant, toddler, and preschool special education programs.

Martha Toomey, Preschool Special Ed. Coordinator

7809 Parent Information Center of Delaware
700 Barksdale Road, Suite 3
Newark, DE 19711

302-366-0152
Fax: 302-366-0276
e-mail: PEP700@aol.com
www.taalliance.org

Programs help parents to understand their children's specific needs, communicate more effectively with professionals, participate in the educational planning process, and obtain information about relevant programs, services and resources.

District of Columbia

7810 Advocates for Justice and Education
2041 Martin Luther King Jr Avenue
Washington, DC 20020

202-678-8060
888-327-8060
Fax: 202-678-8062
e-mail: aje.qpg.com
www.taalliance.org

Programs help parents to understand their children's specific needs, communicate more effectively with professionals, participate in the educational planning process, and obtain information about relevant programs, services and resources.

7811 DC Arc
900 Vamum Street, NE
Washington, DC 20017

202-636-2950
Fax: 202-636-2996
www.taalliance.org

Programs help parents to understand their children's specific needs, communicate more effectively with professionals, participate in the educational planning process, and obtain information about relevant programs, services and resources.

7812 DC-EIP Services
609 H Street NW, 5th Floor
Washington, DC 20002

202-727-5930
Fax: 202-737-0725
TDD: 202-727-2114
www.nectas.unc.edu

Provides early intervention and preschool special education for children with disabilities and special health care needs. Services include central directory, representatives of agencies, service providers, families, and coordinators of infant, toddler, and preschool special education programs.

Joan Christopher, Infant/Toddler Program Coordinator

7813 Georgetown University Child Development Center
National Early Childhood Technical Assistance Ctr
3307 M Street NW
Washington, DC 20007

202-687-8635
Fax: 202-687-8899
www.nectas.unc.edu

Individuals with Disabilities Education Act requires all states and territories to provide early intervention and preschool special education for children with disabilities and special health care needs. Services include central directory, representatives of agencies, service providers, families, and coordinators of infant, toddler, and preschool special education programs.

Tawara Taylor, Interagency Coordinating Council

7815 Partnership for Assistive Technology
220 I Street NE, Suite 202
Washington, DC 20002

202-547-0198
Fax: 202-547-2662
TDD: 202-547-2657

State assisted programs and support group information for people of many abilities. Includes local chapters, referrals, fun and social interaction and support groups.

Florida

7816 Alliance for Assistive Service and Technology (FAAST)
325 John Knox Road, Building 400, Suite 402
Tallahassee, FL 32301

850-487-3278
888-788-9216
Fax: 850-487-2805
TDD: 850-922-5951
e-mail: faast@faast.org
www.faast.org

State assisted programs and support group information for people of many abilities. Includes local chapters, referrals, fun and social interaction and support groups.

2-8 pages Newsletter

7817 Early Intervention Unit, Division of Children's Medical Services
1309 Winewood Boulevard
Tallahassee, FL 32399

850-488-6005
Fax: 850-921-5241
e-mail: Fran_L_Wilber@dcf.state.fl.us
www.nectas.unc.edu

Individuals with Disabilities Education Act requires all states and territories to provide early intervention and preschool special education for children with disabilities and special health care needs. Services include central directory, representatives of agencies, service providers, families, and coordinators of infant, toddler, and preschool special education programs.

Fran Wilber, Infant/Toddler Program Coordinator

7818 Family Network on Disabilities
2735 Whitney Road
Clearwater, FL 33760

727-523-1130
800-825-5736
Fax: 727-523-8687
TDD: 727-523-1130
e-mail: fnd@gate.net
www.fndfl.org

Parent Training and Information (PTI) programs help parents to understand their children's specific needs, communicate more effectively with professionals, participate in the educational planning process, and obtain information about relevant programs, services and resources.

7819 Florida Department of Education
325 W Gaines Street
Tallahassee, FL 32399

850-245-0505
Fax: 850-245-9667
e-mail: westc@mail.doe.state.fl.us
www.fldoe.org

Individuals with Disabilities Education Act requires all states and territories to provide early intervention and preschool special education for children with disabilities and special health care needs. Services include central directory, representatives of agencies, service providers, families, and coordinators of infant, toddler, and preschool special education programs.

Carale West, Preschool Special Ed. Coordinator

7820 Florida's Collaboration for Young Children and their Families Head State
1310 Cross Creek Circle, Suite A
Tallahassee, FL 32301

850-487-8871
Fax: 850-487-0045
e-mail: kkamiya@com1.med.usf.edu
www.nectas.unc.edu

Provides early intervention and preschool special education for children with disabilities and special health care needs. Services include central directory, representatives of agencies, service providers, families, and coordinators of infant, toddler, and preschool special education programs.

Katherine Kamiya, Interagency Coordinator

7821 US Blind Golfers Association
3093 Shamrock Street N
Tallahassee, FL 32308

904-893-4511
Fax: 904-893-4511
e-mail: nightgolf@concentric.net

State assisted programs and support group information for people of many abilities. Includes local chapters, referrals, fun and social interaction and support groups.

Georgia

7822 DHR/Division of Public Health - Babies Can 't Wait Program
2 Peachtree Street NE, Room 7-315
Atlanta, GA 30303

404-657-2726
888-651-8224
Fax: 404-657-2763
e-mail: skmoss@dhr.state.ga.us
www.health.state.ga.us/programs/bcw

Babies Can't Wait (BCW) Program is Georgia's Part C Early Intervention Program under Part C of the federal Individuals with Disabilities Education Improvement Act (IDEA). Services include a comprehensive, coordinated, multidisciplinary, interagency system of early intervention supports for infants and toddlers with disabilities from birth to age 3 and their families.

Stephanie Moss, BCW Infant Toddler Program Manager

7823 Department for Exceptional Students Georgia Department of Education
205 Jessie Hill Jr. Drive, SE, Suite 1870
Atlanta, GA 30334

404-657-9965
Fax: 404-651-6457
e-mail: tbowen@doe.k12.ga.us
www.nectas.unc.edu

Provides early intervention and preschool special education for children with disabilities and special health care needs. Services include central directory, representatives of agencies, service providers, families, and coordinators of infant, toddler, and preschool special education programs.

Toni Waylor Bowen, Preschool Special Ed. Coordinator

7824 Department of Counseling and Educational Leadership-Columbus State University
4225 University Avenue, Suite 754
Columbus, GA 31907

706-568-2222
Fax: 706-569-3134
www.nectas.unc.edu

Individuals with Disabilities Education Act requires all states and territories to provide early intervention and preschool special education for children with disabilities and special health care needs. Services include central directory, representatives of agencies, service providers, families, and coordinators of infant, toddler, and preschool special education programs.

Katherine McCormick, Interagency Coordinating Council

7825 Parent to Parent of Georgia
3805 Presidential Parkway, Suite 207
Atlanta, GA 30340

770-451-5484
800-229-2038
Fax: 770-458-4091
e-mail: parenttoparent@fga.org
www.parenttoparentofga.org

Statewide informational and emotional support to families and individuals affected by disability.

7826 Parents Educating Parents and Professional for All Children (PEPPAC)
8318 Durelee Lane, Suite 101
Douglasville, GA 30134

770-577-7771
Fax: 770-577-7774
e-mail: peppac@bellsouth.net
www.taalliance.org

Parent Training and Information (PTI) programs help parents to understand their children's specific needs, communicate more effectively with professionals, participate in the educational planning process, and obtain information about relevant programs, services and resources.

7827 Tools for Life Division of Rehabilitation Services
1700 Century Circle B-4
Atlanta, GA 30345

404-894-4960
800-578-8665
Fax: 404-894-9320
TDD: 404-657-3085
e-mail: 102476.1737@compuserve.com
www.gatfl.org

State assisted programs and support group information for people of many abilities. Includes local chapters, referrals, fun and social interaction and support groups.

Hawaii

7828 AWARE
200 N Vineyard Boulevard, Suite 310
Honolulu, HI 96817

808-536-9684
Fax: 808-537-6780
e-mail: LDAH@gte.net
www.taalliance.org

Parent Training and Information (PTI) programs help parents to understand their children's specific needs, communicate more effectively with professionals, participate in the educational planning process, and obtain information about relevant programs services, and resources.

7829 Assistive Technology Resource Centers of H awaii (ATRC)
414 Kuiwii Street, Suite 104
Honolulu, HI 96817

808-532-7110
800-645-3007
Fax: 808-532-7120
e-mail: atrc-info@atrc.org
www.atrc.org

State assisted programs and support group information for people of many abilities. Includes local chapters, referrals, fun and social interaction and support groups.

7830 Parents and Children Together (PACT)
1475 Linapuni #117A
Honolulu, HI 96819

808-847-3285
Fax: 808-841-1485
www.nectas.unc.edu

Individuals with Disabilities Education Act requires all states and territories to provide early intervention and preschool special education for children with disabilities and special health care needs. Services include central directory, representatives of agencies, service providers, families, and coordinators of infant, toddler, and preschool special education programs.

Ha'Aheo Mansfield, Interagency Coordinating Council

7831 Special Needs Branch Department of Education
637 18th Avenue, Building C, Room 102
Honolulu, HI 96816

808-733-4840
Fax: 808-733-4404
e-mail: michael_fahley@notes.k12.hi.us
www.nectas.unc.edu

Individuals with Disabilities Education Act requires all states and territories to provide early intervention and preschool special education for children with disabilities and special health care needs. Services include central directory, representatives of agencies, service providers, families, and coordinators of infant, toddler, and preschool special education programs.

Michael Fahey, Preschool Special Ed. Coordinator

7832 Zero-To-3 Hawaii Project
1600 Kapiolani Boulevard, Suite 1401
Honolulu, HI 96814

808-942-8223
Fax: 808-946-5222
e-mail: jeanj@hawaii.edu
www.nectas.unc.edu

Services include central directory, representatives of agencies, service providers, families, and coordinators of infant, toddler, and preschool special education programs.

Jean Johnson, Infant/Toddler Program Coordinator

Idaho

7833 Assistive Technology Project
129 W 3rd Street
Moscow, ID 83843

208-885-3573
Fax: 208-885-3628
TDD: 208-855-3559
e-mail: seile861@uidaho.edu
www.educ.uidaho.edu/idatech

State assisted programs and support group information for people of many abilities. Includes local chapters, referrals, fun and social interaction and support groups.

7834 Department of Education
PO Box 83720
Boise, ID 83720

208-332-6915
Fax: 208-334-4664
e-mail: jkbrenn@sde.state.id.us
www.nectas.unc.edu

Individuals with Disabilities Education Act requires all states and territories to provide early intervention and preschool special education for children with disabilities and special health care needs. Services include central directory, representatives of agencies, service providers, families, and coordinators of infant, toddler, and preschool special education programs.

Jane Brennan, Preschool Special Ed. Coordinator

7835 Idaho Parents Unlimited
600 N Curtis Road, Suite 100
Boise, ID 83706

208-342-5884
800-242-4785
Fax: 208-342-1408
TDD: 208-342-5884
e-mail: pul@rmci.net
www.ipulidaho.org

Parent Training and Information (PTI) programs help parents to understand their children's specific needs, communicate more effectively with professionals, participate in the educational planning process, and obtain information about relevant programs services, and resources.

7836 Infant/Toddler Program
PO Box 83720
Boise, ID 83720

208-334-5523
Fax: 208-334-6664
e-mail: jonesm@dhw.state.id.us
www.idahochild.org

Services include central directory, representatives of agencies, service providers, families, and coordinators of infant, toddler, and preschool special education programs.

Mary Jones, Infant/Toddler Program Coordinator

7837 Palouse Area Parent To Parent
317 17th Avenue
Lewiston, ID 83501

208-746-8599
TTY: 208-746-8599
e-mail: irel102w@wonder.em.cdc.gov

Informational and emotional support to parents who have a child, adolescent, or adult family member with special needs.

7838 Parent Reaching Out to Parents
2195 Ironwood Court
Coeur d'Alene, ID 83814

208-769-1409
Fax: 208-769-1430
parentsreachingout.com

Informational and emotional support to parents who have a child, adolescent, or adult family member with special needs.

Lorena Freund, Coordinator
Kathy Dalberg, Secretary/Treasurer

Illinois

7839 Archway
PO Box 1180, 2751 W Main
Carbondale, IL 62903

618-549-4442
Fax: 618-549-0231

Informational and emotional support to parents who have a child, adolescent, or adult family member with special needs.

7840 Assistive Technology Project
1 W Old State Capitol Plaza, Suite 100
Springfield, IL 62701

217-522-7985
Fax: 217-522-8067
TDD: 217-522-9966
e-mail: iatp@fgi.net
www.ittech.org

State assisted programs and support group information for people of many abilities. Includes local chapters, referrals, fun and social interaction and support groups.

7841 Child and Family Connections
9455 S Hoyne Street
Chicago, IL 60620

773-233-1799
Fax: 773-233-2011

Informational and emotional support to parents who have a child, adolescent, or adult family member with special needs.

7842 Developmental Services Center
1304 W Bradley
Champaign, IL 61821

217-359-0287
Fax: 217-356-9851
www.dsc-illinois.org

Informational and emotional support to parents who have a child, adolescent, or adult family member with special needs.

7843 Family Resource Center on Disabilities
20 E Jackson Boulevard, Room 900
Chicago, IL 60604

312-939-3513
Fax: 312-939-7297
TTY: 312-939-3519
TDD: 312-939-3519
www.frcd.com

Parent Training and Information (PTI) programs help parents to understand their children's specific needs, communicate more effectively with professionals, participate in the educational planning process, and obtain information about relevant programs, services and resources.

7844 Family T.I.E.S. Network
830 S Spring Street
Springfield, IL 62704

217-544-5809
800-865-7842
Fax: 217-544-6018
e-mail: FTIESN@aol.com
www.taalliance.org

Parent Training and Information (PTI) programs help parents to understand their children's specific needs, communicate more effectively with professionals, participate in the educational planning process, and obtain information about relevant programs, services and resources.

7845 Greater Interagency Council Parent to Parent Support Network
925 W 175th Street
Homewood, IL 60430

708-799-2718
Fax: 708-799-7974

Informational and emotional support to parents who have a child, adolescent, or adult family member with special needs.

7846 Leukemia Research Foundation
2700 Patriot Boulevard, Suite 100
Glenview, IL 60026

847-424-0600
Fax: 847-424-0606
e-mail: info@lrfmail.org
www.leukemia-research.org

Founded to conquer leukemia by funding research into the causes and cures of the disease and to enrich the quality of life by those touched by leukemia.

Janie Weisenberg, Executive Director

7847 National Center for Latinos with Disabilities
1921 S Blue Island Avenue
Chicago, IL 60608

312-666-3393
800-532-3393
Fax: 312-666-1787
TTY: 312-666-1788
e-mail: ncld@ncld.com
homepage.interaccess.com/~ncld/

Parent Training and Information (PTI) programs help parents to understand their children's specific needs, communicate more effectively with professionals, participate in the educational planning process, and obtain information about relevant programs, services and resources.

Everardo Franco, Executive Director
Nancy Perez, Coordinator Info and Referral

7848 Next Steps - Parents Reaching Parents
100 W Randolph, Suite 8-100
Chicago, IL 60601

312-814-4042
Fax: 312-814-5849
TTY: 312-814-4042
e-mail: caroldors@aol.com

Informational and emotional support to parents who have a child, adolescent, or adult family member with special needs.

7849 Office of Community Health and Prevention Bureau of Early Intervention, DHR
222 South College, 2nd Floor
Springfield, IL 62704

217-782-1981
Fax: 217-782-7849
www.dhs.state.il.us/ei

Provides early intervention and preschool special education for children with disabilities and special health care needs. Services include central directory, representatives of agencies, service providers, families, and coordinators of infant, toddler, and preschool special education programs.

Mary Miller, Infant/Toddler Program Coordinator

7850 Parent to Parent Network
1530 Lincoln Avenue
Charleston, IL 61920

217-348-0127
Fax: 217-348-0740

Informational and emotional support to parents who have a child, adolescent, or adult family member with special needs.

7851 Southern IL Child and Family Connections
2751 W Main Street
Carbondale, IL 62903

888-340-6702
Fax: 618-549-8137

Informational and emotional support to parents who have a child, adolescent, or adult family member with special needs.

7852 State Board of Education Department of Special Education
National Early Childhood Technical Assistance Ctr
100 N 1st Street, Suite 233
Springfield, IL 62777

217-782-4835
Fax: 217-782-7849
e-mail: preising@smtp.isbe.state.il.us
www.nectas.unc.edu

Individuals with Disabilities Education Act requires all states and territories to provide early intervention and preschool special education for children with disabilities and special health care needs. Services include central directory, representatives of agencies, service providers, families, and coordinators of infant, toddler, and preschool special education programs.

Pam Reising-Rechner, Preschool Special Ed. Coordinator

Indiana

7853 ATTAIN: Assistive Technology Through Action in Indiana
32 E Washington Street, Suite 1400
Indianapolis, IN 46204

317-486-8808
800-527-8246
Fax: 317-486-8809
TDD: 800-743-3333
e-mail: attaininfo@attaininc.org
www.attanic.org

State assisted programs and support group information for people of many abilities. Includes local chapters, referrals, fun and social interaction and support groups.

7854 Assistive Technology Training and Information Center
3354 Pine Hill Drive, PO Box 2441
Vincennes, IN 47591

812-886-0575
800-962-8842
Fax: 812-886-1128
e-mail: inattic1@aol.com
www.theattic.org

Technology group of parents, consumers and professionals that provides resources to help children and adults who have disabilities gain access to the benefits of technology. Includes nationwide network of community-based assistive technology, resource centers, hands on consultants and product demonstrations.

7855 Division of Exceptional Learners Indiana Department of Education
State House, Room 229
Indianapolis, IN 46204

317-232-0570
Fax: 317-232-0589
e-mail: scochran@doe.state.in.us
www.doe.state.in.us/exceptional

Individuals with Disabilities Education Act requires all states and territories to provide preschool special education for children with disabilities. Special Education and related services are provided through the public schools.

Sheron Cochran, Preschool Special Ed Coordinator

7856 Down Syndrome Association of Central Indiana
10792 Downing Street
Carmel, IN 46033

317-574-9757
Fax: 317-574-9757

Provides informational and emotional support to parents who have a child, adolescent, or adult family member with special needs. Program offers an important connection for a parent who is seeking support for a special disability issue, by matching him or her with a trained veteran parent.

7857 Family Resource Center of Southeast Indiana
4101 Timberview Road
West Harrison, IN 47060

812-637-1445

Informational and emotional support to parents who have a child, adolescent, or adult family member with special needs.

7858 First Direction
PO Box 4234
Lafayette, IN 47903

765-423-1460

Informational and emotional support to parents who have a child, adolescent, or adult family member with special needs.

7859 First Steps
402 W Washington Street, Suite W-386
Indianapolis, IN 46204

317-232-2429
Fax: 317-232-7948
e-mail: mgreer@fssa.state.in.us
www.nectas.unc.edu

Individuals with Disabilities Education Act requires all states and territories to provide early intervention and preschool special education for children with disabilities and special health care needs. Services include central directory, representatives of agencies, service providers, families, and coordinators of infant, toddler, and preschool special education programs.

Maureen Greer, Infant/Toddler Program Coordiantor

7860 First Steps for Families
500 8th Avenue
Terre Haute, IN 47804

812-231-8419
Fax: 812-231-8208
e-mail: famnetwork@aol.com

Informational and emotional support to parents who have a child, adolescent, or adult family member with special needs.

7861 First Steps, Early Interventions, New Horizons Rehabilitation
PO Box 98
Batesville, IN 47006

812-934-4528
Fax: 812-934-2522
TTY: 812-934-4528

Informational and emotional support to parents who have a child, adolescent, or adult family member with special needs.

7862 Future Choices
309 N High Street
Muncie, IN 47305

765-741-3494
Fax: 765-741-8333
e-mail: futurechoicesinc@aol.com

Informational and emotional support to parents who have a child, adolescent, or adult family member with special needs.

7863 Indiana Parent Information Network (IPIN)
4755 Kingsway Drive, Suite 105
Indianapolis, IN 46205

317-257-8683
Fax: 317-251-7488
e-mail: familynetw@aol.com
www.ai.org/ipin

Informational and emotional support to parents who have a child, adolescent, or adult family member with special needs.

7864 Knox County Advocates
1806 Indiana Avenue
Vincennes, IN 47591

812-882-0375
Fax: 812-886-1128
e-mail: INATTIC1@aol.com

Informational and emotional support to parents who have a child, adolescent, or adult family member with special needs.

7865 NEO Fight
4363 Idlewild Lane
Carmel, IN 46033

317-255-5242
www.member.tripod.com/-neofight

Informational and emotional support to parents who have a child, adolescent, or adult family member with special needs.

7866 Project Special Care
4755 Kinsway Drive, Suite 105
Indianapolis, IN 46205

317-257-8683
Fax: 317-251-7488
www.ipin.org

Informational and emotional support to parents who have a child, adolescent, or adult family member with special needs.

7867 US Rowing Assocation
201 S Capitol Avenue, Suite 400
Indianapolis, IN 46225

317-237-5656
Fax: 317-237-5646
e-mail: members@usrowing.org
www.usrowing.org

State assisted programs and support group information for people of many abilities. Includes local chapters, referrals, fun and social interaction and support groups.

Iowa

7868 ARC of East Central Iowa Pilot Parents
680 2nd Street SE, Suite 200
Cedar Rapids, IA 52404

319-365-0487
800-843-0272
Fax: 319-365-9938

Informational and emotional support to parents who have a child, adolescent, or adult family member with special needs.

7869 Bureau of Children, Family, and Community Services
Grimes State Office Building, 3rd Floor
Des Moines, IA 50319

515-281-5502
Fax: 515-242-6019
e-mail: dee.gethman@ed.state.ia.us
www.nectas.unc.edu

Individuals with Disabilities Education Act requires all states and territories to provide early intervention and preschool special education for children with disabilities and special health care needs. Services include central directory, representatives of agencies, service providers, families, and coordinators of infant, toddler, and preschool special education programs.

Dee Gethmann, Preschool Special Ed. Coordinator

7870 Family Educator Connection Program
3706 Cedar Heights Drive
Cedar Falls, IA 50613

319-273-8265
Fax: 319-273-8275
TTY: 319-273-8291
e-mail: dhansen@aea7.k12.ia.us
www.aea7.k12.ia.us

Informational and emotional support to parents who have a child, adolescent, or adult family member with special needs.

7871 Iowa Program for Assistive Technology
University Hospital School
100 Hawkins Drive
Iowa City, IA 52242

800-331-3027
Fax: 319-356-8284
TDD: 800-331-3027
e-mail: jane_gay@uiowa.edu
www.uiowa.edu/infotech

State assisted programs and support group information for people of many abilities. Includeslocal chapters, referrals, fun and social interaction and support groups.

7872 Iowa's System of EI Services
Grimes State Office Building, 3rd Floor
Des Moines, IA 50319

515-281-7145
Fax: 515-242-6019
e-mail: lynda.pletcher@ed.state.ia.us
www.nectas.unc.edu

Individuals with Disabilities Education Act requires all states and territories to provide early intervention and preschool special education for children with disabilities and special health care needs. Services include central directory, representatives of agencies, service providers, families, and coordinators of infant, toddler, and preschool special education programs.

Lynda Pletcher, Infant/Toddler Program Coordinator

7873 Parent Educator Connection
Grimews State Office Bldg
Des Moines, IA 50318

515-242-5295
800-572-5073
Fax: 712-722-1643
e-mail: bjones@aea5.k12.ia.uss

Informational and emotional support to parents who have a child, adolescent, or adult family member with special needs.

7874 Parent Educator Connection Program
Heartland AEA 11, 6500 Corporate Drive
Johnston, IA 50131

515-270-9030
800-362-2720
Fax: 515-270-5383
www.aea11.k12.ia.us/pareduc/

Provides informational and emotional support to parents who have a child, adolescent, or adult family member with special needs. Program offers an important connection for a parent who is seeking support for special disability issue, by matching him or her with a trained veteran parent.

Terry Mendell, Lead Coordinator

Kansas

7875 Assistive Technology for Kansas Project
2601 Gabriel, PO Box 738
Parsons, KS 67357

316-421-8367
Fax: 620-421-8367
TDD: 316-421-0954
e-mail: ssack@parsons.lsi.ukans.edu
www.atk.lsi.ukans.edu

State assisted programs and support group information for people of many abilities. Includes local chapters, referrals, fun and social interaction and support groups.

7876 Department of Health & Environment
1000 Sw Jackson
Topeka, KS 66612

785-296-1500
Fax: 785-368-6368
e-mail: info@kdhe.state.ks.us
www.kdhe.state.ks.us

Individuals with Disabilities Education Act requires all states and territories to provide early intervention and preschool special education for children with disabilities and special health care needs. Services include central directory, representatives of agencies, service providers, families, and coordinators of infant, toddler, and preschool special education programs.

Jayne Garcia, Infant/Toddler Program Coordinator

7877 Families Together
3033 West 2nd, Suite 106
Witchita, KS 67203

316-945-7747
888-815-6364
Fax: 316-945-7795
e-mail: witchita@familiestogetherinc.org
www.familiestogetherinc.org

Parent Training and Information (PTI) programs help parents to understand their children's specific needs, communicate more effectively with professionals, participate in the educational planning process, and obtain information about relevant programs, services and resources.

Connie Zienkewicz, Director
Marita McDaniel, Executive Assistant

7878 Families Together/Parent to Parent of KS
501 Jackson, Suite 400
Topeka, KS 66603

785-233-4777
800-264-6343
Fax: 756-233-4787
TTY: 785-233-4777
e-mail: family@inlandnet.net

Informational and emotional support to parents who have a child, adolescent, or adult family member with special needs.

7879 Special Education Administration State Department of Education
120 E 10th Avenue
Topeka, KS 66612

785-296-1944
Fax: 785-296-6715
e-mail: cdermyer@ksbe.state.ks.us
www.kansped.org

Individuals with Disabilities Education Act requires all states and territories to provide early intervention and preschool special education for children with disabilities and special health care needs. Services include central directory, representatives of agencies, service providers, families, and coordinators of infant, toddler, and preschool special education programs.

Carol Dermyer, Preschool Special Ed. Coordinator

Kentucky

7880 Assistive Technology Services Network
8412 Westport Road
Louisville, KY 40242

502-327-0022
800-346-2115
Fax: 502-327-9974
TDD: 502-327-9855
www.katsnet.org

State assisted programs and support group information for people of many abilities. Includes local chapters, referrals, fun and social interaction and support groups.

7881 College of Education - Western Kentucky University
Interdisciplinary Early Childhood Education
#1 Big Red Way, Western Kentucky University
Bowling Green, KY 42101

270-745-5414
Fax: 270-745-6474
e-mail: vicki.stayton@wku.edu
www.nectas.unc.edu

Individuals with Disabilities Education Act requires all states and territories to provide early intervention and preschool special edu-

cation for children with disabilities and special health care needs. Services include central directory, representatives of agencies, service providers, families, and coordinators of infant, toddler, and preschool special education programs.

Vicki Stayton, Interagency Coordinating Council

7882 Division of Preschool Services
1711 Capotol Plaza Tower
Frankfort, KY 40601

502-564-7056
Fax: 502-564-6771
e-mail: bsinglet@kde.state.ky.us
www.nectas.unc.edu

Provides early intervention and preschool special education for children with disabilities and special health care needs. Services include central directory, representatives of agencies, service providers, families, and coordinators of infant, toddler, and preschool special education programs.

Barbara Singleton, Preschool Special Ed. Coordinator

7883 Infant-Toddler Program, Division of Mental Retardation
275 E Main Street
Frankfort, KY 40621

502-564-7722
Fax: 502-564-0438
e-mail: jhenson@mail.state.ky.us
www.nectas.unc.edu

Individuals with Disabilities Education Act requires all states and territories to provide early intervention and preschool special education for children with disabilities and special health care needs. Services include central directory, representatives of agencies, service providers, families, and coordinators of infant, toddler, and preschool special education programs.

Jim Henson, Infant/Toddler Program Coordinator

7884 Special Parent Involvement Network
10301-B Deering Road
Louisville, KY 40272

502-937-6894
Fax: 502-937-6464
e-mail: FamilyTmg@aol.com
www.kyspin.com

Parent Training and Information (PTI) programs help parents to understand their children's specific needs, communicate more effectively with professionals, participate in the educational planning process, and obtain information about relevant programs, services and resources.

Louisiana

7885 Division of Special Populations
PO Box 94064
Baton Rouge, LA 70804

225-342-3631
Fax: 225-342-5880
e-mail: edjohnson@mail.doe.state.la.us
www.nectas.unc.edu

Individuals with Disabilities Education Act requires all states and territories to provide early intervention and preschool special education for children with disabilities and special health care needs. Services include central directory, representatives of agencies, service providers, families, and coordinators of infant, toddler, and preschool special education programs.

Evelyn Johnson, Infant/Toddler Program Coordinator

7886 Families Helping Families of Greater New Orleans
1323 Division Street, Suite 110
Metairie, LA 70002

504-888-9111
800-766-7736
Fax: 504-888-0246
e-mail: fhfgno@ix.netcom.com
www.fhfgno.org

Informational and emotional support to parents who have a child, adolescent, or adult family member with special needs.

7887 Louisiana Assistive Technology Access Network
3042 Old Forge Drive, Suite D
Baton Rouge, LA 70898

225-925-9500
800-270-6185
Fax: 225-925-9560
TDD: 225-925-9500
e-mail: latanstate@aol.com
www.latan.org

State assisted programs and support group information for people of many abilities. Includes local chapters, referrals, fun and social interaction and support groups.

7888 Preschool Programs - Division of Special Populations
PO Box 94064
Baton Rouge, LA 70804

225-342-1190
Fax: 225-342-5880
e-mail: jzube@mail.doe.state.la.us
www.nectas.unc.edu

Individuals with Disabilities Education Act requires all states and territories to provide early intervention and preschool special education for children with disabilities and special health care needs. Services include central directory, representatives of agencies, service providers, families, and coordinators of infant, toddler, and preschool special education programs.

Janice Zube, Preschool Special Ed. Coordinator

7889 Project PROMPT
4323 Division Street, Suite 110
Metairie, LA 70002

504-888-9111
800-766-7736
Fax: 504-888-0246
e-mail: thsgno@ix.netcom.com
www.taalliance.org

Parent Training and Information (PTI) programs help parents to understand their children's specific needs, communicate more effectively with professionals, participate in the educational planning process, and obtain information about relevant programs, services and resources.

Maine

7890 CDC Lincoln County
PO Box 1114
Damariscotta, ME 04543

207-563-1411
Fax: 207-563-6312
www.nectas.unc.edu

Individuals with Disabilities Education Act requires all states and territories to provide early intervention and preschool special education for children with disabilities and special health care needs. Services include central directory, representatives of agencies, service providers, families, and coordinators of infant, toddler, and preschool special education programs.

Jean Eaton, Interagency Coordinating Council

7891 Child Department Services
146 State House Station
Augusta, ME 04333

207-287-3272
Fax: 207-287-5900
e-mail: jaci.holmes@state.me.us

Provides early intervention and preschool special education for children with disabilities and special health care needs. Services include central directory, representatives of agencies, service providers, families, and coordinators of infant, toddler, and preschool special education programs.

Joanne C Holmes, Infant/Toddler Program Coordinator

7892 Child Department Services, Department of Education
146 State House Station
Augusta, ME 04333

207-287-3272
Fax: 207-287-5900
e-mail: jaci.holmes@state.me.us
www.nectas.unc.edu

Provides early intervention and preschool special education for children with disabilities and special health care needs. Services include central directory, representatives of agencies, service providers, families, and coordinators of infant, toddler, and preschool special education programs.

Joanne C Holmes, Preschool Special Ed. Coordiantor

7893 Consumer Information and Technology Training Exchange (Maine CITE)
46 University Drive
Augusta, ME 04330

207-621-3195
Fax: 207-621-3193
TDD: 207-621-3195
e-mail: powers@maine.maine.edu
www.mainecite.org

State assisted programs and support group information for people of many abilities. Includes local chapters, referrals, fun and social interaction and support groups.

7894 Special Needs Parent Info Network
12 Shuman Ave., Suite 7
Augusta, ME 04330

207-623-2144
800-870-7746
Fax: 207-623-2148
e-mail: jlachnace@mpg.org
www.mpf.org

Parent Training and Information (PTI) programs help parents to understand their children's specific needs, communicate more effectively with professionals, participate in the educational planning process, and obtain information about relevant programs, services and resources.

7895 York County Parent Awareness
150 Main Street, Midtown Mall
Sanford, ME 04027

207-324-2337
Fax: 207-324-5621
e-mail: ycpa@mmp.org

Informational and emotional support to parents who have a child, adolescent, or adult family member with special needs.

Maryland

7896 ARC Family Connection Parent to Parent Program
11600 Nebel Street
Rockville, MD 20852

301-984-5777
Fax: 301-816-2429

Informational and emotional support to parents who have a child, adolescent, or adult family member with special needs.

7897 Developmental Pediatrics School of Medicine, University of Maryland
630 W Fayette Street, Room 5686
Baltimore, MD 21201

410-706-3542
Fax: 410-706-0835
www.nectas.unc.edu

Individuals with Disabilities Education Act requires all states and territories to provide early intervention and preschool special education for children with disabilities and special health care needs. Services include central directory, representatives of agencies, service providers, families, and coordinators of infant, toddler, and preschool special education programs.

Renee Wachtel, Interagency Coordinating Council

7898 MD Infant/Toddler/Preschool Services Division
200 W Baltimore Street
Baltimore, MD 21201

410-767-0261
800-535-0182
Fax: 410-333-2661
TDD: 410-333-0781
e-mail: dmetzger@msde.state.md.us
www.nectas.unc.edu

Individuals with Disabilities Education Act requires all states and territories to provide early intervention and preschool special education for children with disabilities and special health care needs. Services include central directory, representatives of agencies, service providers, families, and coordinators of infant, toddler, and preschool special education programs.

Deborah Metzger, Infant/Toddler Program Coordinator

7899 Maryland Infant and Toddlers Program Family Support Network
200 W Baltimore, 4th Floor
Baltimore, MD 21201

410-767-0652
Fax: 410-333-8165

Informational and emotional support to parents who have a child, adolescent, or adult family member with special needs.

7900 Parents Place of Maryland
7484 Candlewood Road, Suite S
Hanover, MD 21076

410-859-5300
Fax: 410-859-5301
e-mail: parplace@aol.com
www.somerset.net/ParentsPlace

Parent Training and Information (PTI) programs help parents to understand their children's specific needs, communicate more effectively with professionals, participate in the educational planning process, and obtain information about relevant programs, services and resources.

7901 Partners in Intensive Care
PO Box 41043
Bethesda, MD 20824

301-681-2708
Fax: 301-681-2707

Informational and emotional support to parents who have a child, adolescent, or adult family member with special needs.

7902 Technology Assistance Program Maryland Rehabilitation Center
2301 Argonne Drive, Room T-17
Baltimore, MD 21218

410-554-9230
800-832-4827
Fax: 410-554-9237
e-mail: mdtap.org
www.mdtap.org

State assisted programs and support group information for people of many abilities. Includes local chapters, referrals, fun and social interaction and support groups.

Massachusetts

7903 Bureau of Early Childhood Programs
350 Main Street
Malden, MA 02148

781-388-3300
Fax: 781-388-3394
e-mail: eschaefer@doe.mass.edu
www.nectas.unc.edu

Individuals with Disabilities Education Act requires all states and territories to provide early intervention and preschool special education for children with disabilities and special health care needs. Services include central directory, representatives of agencies, service providers, families, and coordinators of infant, toddler, and preschool special education programs.

Elisabeth Schaefer, Preschool Special Ed. Coordinator

7904 Children's Happiness Foundation
858 Plain Street
Marshfield, MA 02050

781-837-9609
Fax: 781-837-5229
e-mail: rsvpmktg@aol.com

Serves New England children ages three to eighteen with life-threatening or chronic degenerative diseases.

7905 Early Intervention Services
250 Washington Street
Boston, MA 02108

617-624-5969
Fax: 617-624-5990
e-mail: Ron.Benham@state.ma.us

Individuals with Disabilities Education Act requires all states and territories to provide early intervention and preschool special education for children with disabilities and special health care needs. Services include central directory, representatives of agencies, service providers, families, and coordinators of infant, toddler, and preschool special education programs.

Ron Benham, Infant/Toddler Program Coordinator

7906 Education Development Center - EDC
55 Chapel Street
Newton, MA 02458

617-969-7100
800-225-4276
Fax: 617-969-3440
e-mail: pprintz@edc.org
www.edc.org

One of the largest nonprofit education and health organizations. With programs for children and families combining research and practice, promoting professional development and systematic change, forging community links, and influencing the policies and legislation that affect the lives of children. The New England RAP incorporates proven strategies to enhance the efforts of organizations servicing children with disabilities and their families.

Philip Printz, Project Director

7907 Family Ties at Massachusetts Department of Public Health
109 Rhode Island Rd.
Lakeville, MA 02347

508-947-1231
Fax: 617-727-9296
TDD: 508-947-0977
e-mail: division.CSHCN@state.ma.us
www.massfamilyties.org

Informational and emotional support to parents who have a child, adolescent, or adult family member with special needs.

7908 Federation for Children with Special Needs
1135 Tremont Street Suite 420
Boston, MA 02120

617-236-7210
800-331-0688
Fax: 617-572-2094
TDD: 617-482-2915
e-mail: fcsninfo@fcsn.org
www.fcsn.org/

Parent Training and Information (PTI) programs help parents to understand their children's specific needs, communicate more effectively with professionals, participate in the educational planning process, and obtain information about relevant programs, services and resources.

Richard J Robinson, Executive Director

7909 Greater Boston Arc Parent Support
1505 Commonwealth Avenue
Boston, MA 02135

617-783-3900
Fax: 617-783-9190
e-mail: bostonarc@aol.com
gbarc.org

Informational and emotional support to parents who have a child, adolescent, or adult family member with special needs.

7910 Massachusetts Assistive Technology Partnership
1295 Boylston Street, Suite 310
Boston, MA 02215

617-355-7153
Fax: 617-355-6345
TDD: 617-355-7301
e-mail: matp@matp.net
www.matp.org

State assisted programs and support group information for people of many abilities. Includes local chapters, referrals, fun and social interaction and support groups.

7911 National Birth Defects Center
40 2nd Avenue, Suite 520
Waltham, MA 02451

781-466-9555
Fax: 781-487-2361

Treats patients with birth defects, mental retardation and genetic diseases.

Michigan

7912 CAUSE
2365 Woodlake Frive, Suite 100
Okemos, MI 48864

517-347-2283
800-221-9105
Fax: 517-886-9366
TTY: 517-347-2283
TDD: 517-886-9167
www.causeonline.org

Parent Training and Information (PTI) programs help parents to understand their children's specific needs, communicate more effectively with professionals, participate in the educational planning process, and obtain information about relevant programs, services and resources.

7913 Early on Michigan
PO Box 30008
Lansing, MI 48909

517-335-4865
Fax: 517-373-7504
e-mail: banfieldj@state.mi.us
www.1800earlyon.org

Provides early intervention and preschool special education for children with disabilities and special health care needs. Services include central directory, representatives of agencies, service providers, families, and coordinators of infant, toddler, and preschool special education programs.

Julie Banfield, Infant/Toddler Program Coordinator

7914 Family Support Network of Michigan Parent Participation Program-MDCH
200 6th Street, 3rd Fl., S Tower, Suite 315
Detroit, MI 48226

517-373-3740
Fax: 313-256-2605
TDD: 517-373-3573

Informational and emotional support to parents who have a child, adolescent, or adult family member with special needs.

7915 Livingston County CMH Services
2280 East Grand River
Howell, MI 48843

517-546-4126
Fax: 517-546-1300
www.nectas.unc.edu

Provides early intervention and preschool special education for children with disabilities and special health care needs. Services include central directory, representatives of agencies, service providers, families, and coordinators of infant, toddler, and preschool special education programs.

Mac Miller, Interagency Coordinating Council

7916 Office of Special Education
PO Box 30008
Lansing, MI 48909

517-241-6354
Fax: 517-373-7504
e-mail: banfieldj@state.mi.us
www.nectas.unc.edu

Individuals with Disabilities Education Act requires all states and territories to provide early intervention and preschool special education for children with disabilities and special health care needs. Services include central directory, representatives of agencies, service providers, families, and coordinators of infant, toddler, and preschool special education programs.

Julie Banfield, Preschool Special Ed. Coordinator

7917 Parents are Experts
23077 Greenfield Road, Suite 205
Southfield, MI 48075

248-557-5070
800-827-4843
Fax: 248-557-4456
TDD: 248-557-5070
e-mail: ucp@ameritech.net
www.taalliance.org

Parent Training and Information (PTI) programs help parents to understand their children's specific needs, communicate more effectively with professionals, participate in the educational planning process, and obtain information about relevant programs, services and resources.

7918 TECH 2000 Project-Michigan Disability Rights Coalition
740 W Lake Lansing Road, Suite 400
East Lansing, MI 48823

517-333-2477
800-760-4600
Fax: 517-333-2677
TDD: 517-333-2477
e-mail: roanne@match.org
www.discoalition.org

State assisted programs and support group information for people of many abilities. Includes local chapters, referrals, fun and social interaction and support groups.

Minnesota

7919 ARC Suburban
1526 E 122nd Street
Burnsville, MN 56337

612-890-3057
Fax: 612-890-3527

Informational and emotional support to parents who have a child, adolescent, or adult family member with special needs.

7920 Department of Children, Family, & Learning
1500 Highway 36 W
Roseville, MN 55113

651-582-8200
Fax: 651-582-8872
e-mail: michael.eastman@state.mn.us

Individuals with Disabilities Education Act requires all states and territories to provide early intervention and preschool special education for children with disabilities and special health care needs. Services include central directory, representatives of agencies, service providers, families, and coordinators of infant, toddler, and preschool special education programs.

Michael Eastman, Preschool Special Ed. Coordinator

7921 Family to Family Network ARC of Hennepin County
4301 Highway 7, Suite 104
Minneapolis, MN 55416

612-920-0855
Fax: 612-920-1480

Informational and emotional support to parents who have a child, adolescent, or adult family member with special needs.

7922 Interagency Early Intervention Project
550 Cedar Street
Saint Paul, MN 55101

612-296-7032
Fax: 612-296-5076
e-mail: jan.rubenstein@state.mn.us
www.pediatricservices.com

Individuals with Disabilities Education Act requires all states and territories to provide early intervention and preschool special education for children with disabilities and special health care needs. Services include central directory, representatives of agencies, service providers, families, and coordinators of infant, toddler, and preschool special education programs.

Jan Rubenstein, Infant/Toddler Program Coordinator

7923 Parents for Parents
345 N Smith Avenue, MS 70-403
Saint Paul, MN 55102

651-220-6731
Fax: 651-220-6125
e-mail: pat.schaffner@childrenshc.org

Informational and emotional one-to-one support to parents who have a child or adolescent with special needs.

Pat Schaffner, Parent to Parent Specialist

7924 Pilot Parents in Anoka and Ramsey Counties
1201 89th Avenue NE, Suite 305
Blaine, MN 55434

612-783-4958
Fax: 612-783-4900

Informational and emotional support to parents who have a child, adolescent, or adult family member with special needs.

7925 Pilot Parents of Northeast Minnesota
201 Ordean Building
Duluth, MN 55802

218-726-4725
Fax: 218-726-4722

Informational and emotional support to parents who have a child, adolescent, or adult family member with special needs.

7926 Vinland Center
PO Box 308
Loretto, MN 55357

763-479-3555
Fax: 763-479-2605
e-mail: vinland@vinldancenter.org
www.vinlandcenter.org

State assisted programs and support group information for people of many abilities. Includes local chapters, referrals, fun and social interaction and support groups.

7927 Voyageur Outward Bound School
101 E Chapman, Suite 120
St. Ely, MN 55731

218-365-7790
800-321-4453
Fax: 218-365-7079
www.vobs.com

State assisted programs and support group information for people of many abilities. Includes local chapters, referrals, fun and social interaction and support groups.

7928 Wilderness Inquiry
808 14th Avenue SE
Minneapolis, MN 55414

612-676-9400
800-728-0719
Fax: 612-676-9475
TTY: 800-728-0719
e-mail: winquiry@aol.com
www.wildernessinquiry.org

State assisted programs and support group information for people of many abilities. Includes local chapters, referrals, fun and social interaction and support groups.

Mississippi

7929 First Steps Program
570 East Woodrow Wilson
Jackson, MS 39215

601-576-7816
Fax: 601-576-7540
www.nectas.unc.edu

Individuals with Disabilities Education Act requires all states and territories to provide early intervention and preschool special education for children with disabilities and special health care needs. Services include central directory, representatives of agencies, service providers, families, and coordinators of infant, toddler, and preschool special education programs.

Roy Hart, Infant/Toddler Program Coordinator

7930 Office of Special Education
359 NW Street, Suite 337, PO Box 771
Jackson, MS 39205

601-359-3498
Fax: 601-359-2078
e-mail: dbowman@mdek12.state.ms.us
www.nectas.unc.edu

Individuals with Disabilities Education Act requires all states and territories to provide early intervention and preschool special education for children with disabilities and special health care needs. Services include central directory, representatives of agencies, service providers, families, and coordinators of infant, toddler, and preschool special education programs.

Dot Bowman, Preschool Special Ed. Coordinator

7931 Parent Partners
5 Old River Place, Suite 101
Jackson, MS 39202

601-354-3302
800-366-5707
Fax: 601-354-2426
e-mail: ptiofms@misnet.com
www.parentpartners.org

Parent Training and Information (PTI) programs help parents to understand their children's specific needs, communicate more effectively with professionals, participate in the educational planning process, and obtain information about relevant programs, services and resources.

7932 Project Start
PO Box 1698
Jackson, MS 39215

601-987-4872
800-852-8328
Fax: 601-364-2349
e-mail: spower@netdoor.com
www.msprojectstart.org

State assisted programs and support group information for people of many abilities. Includes local chapters, referrals, fun and social interaction and support groups.

Missouri

7933 Assistance Technology Project
4731 S Cochise, Suite 114
Independence, MO 64055

816-373-5193
Fax: 816-373-9314
TTY: 816-373-9315
e-mail: matpmo@gni.com
www.doir.state.mo.us/matp/

State assisted programs and support group information for people of many abilities. Includes local chapters, referrals, fun and social interaction and support groups.

7934 Children's Therapy Center
600 E 14th Street
Sedalia, MO 65301

660-826-4400
Fax: 660-826-4420
www.nectas.unc.edu

Services include central directory, representatives of agencies, service providers, families, and coordinators of infant, toddler, and preschool special education programs.

Roger Garlich, Interagency Coordinating Council

7935 Department of Elementary and Secondary Education
PO Box 480
Jefferson City, MO 65102

573-751-2965
Fax: 573-526-4404
e-mail: pgoff@mail.dese.state.mo.us
www.nectas.unc.edu

Individuals with Disabilities Education Act requires all states and territories to provide early intervention and preschool special education for children with disabilities and special health care needs. Services include central directory, representatives of agencies, service providers, families, and coordinators of infant, toddler, and preschool special education programs.

Paula Goff, Preschool Special Ed. Coordinator

7936 Disabilities Advocacy & Support Network
The Network 1515 E Pythian , PO Box 5030
Springfield, MO 65801

417-895-7464
Fax: 417-895-7412
TTY: 417-895-7430
e-mail: sdasn@aol.com
www.disabilitiesnetwork.org

Informational and emotional support to parents who have a child, adolescent, or adult family member with special needs.

7937 Family Resource Network
Park A Plaza
601 Business Loop 70 W, Suite 2161
Columbia, MO 65203

573-449-8663
e-mail: betty@ccc.missouri.edu

Informational and emotional support to parents who have a child, adolescent, or adult family member with special needs.

7938 Missouri Parents Act
8301 State Line Road, Suite 204
Kansas City, MO 64114

816-531-7070
800-743-7634
Fax: 816-531-4777
www.ptimpact.com

Parent Training and Information (PTI) programs help parents to understand their children's specific needs, communicate more effectively with professionals, participate in the educational planning process, and obtain information about relevant programs, services and resources.

7939 Parent Act
1 W Armour Boulevard, Suite 301
Kansas City, MO 64111

816-531-7070
Fax: 816-531-4777
e-mail: impactes@coop.cm.org
www.taalliance.org

Parent Training and Information (PTI) programs help parents to understand their children's specific needs, communicate more effectively with professionals, participate in the educational planning process, and obtain information about relevant programs, services and resources.

7940 Positive Solutions for Life Challenges
Route 3, Box 441
Warswaw, MO 65355

660-438-6990

Informational and emotional support to parents who have a child, adolescent, or adult family member with special needs.

7941 United Services
4140 Old Mill Parkway
Saint Peters, MO 63376

636-926-2700
Fax: 636-447-4919
e-mail: ssalmo@unitedsrvcs.org
www.unitedsrvcs.org

Provides services to children ages infant to five-years-old with special needs. Preschool and daycare onsite. We also offer support groups for siblings and family members, parent library available.

Suzanne Salmo, Social Worker

Montana

7942 CO-TEACH/Division of Educational Research and Service
School of Education
University of Montana
Missoula, MT 59812

406-243-5344
Fax: 406-243-2797
e-mail: coteach@selway.umt.edu

Informational and emotional support to parents who have a child, adolescent, or adult family member with special needs.

7943 Developmental Disabilities Program
PO Box 4210
Helena, MT 59604

406-444-5647
Fax: 406-444-0230
e-mail: jspiegle@mt.gov
www.nectas.unc.edu

Individuals with Disabilities Education Act requires all states and territories to provide early intervention and preschool special education for children with disabilities and special health care needs. Services include central directory, representatives of agencies, service providers, families, and coordinators of infant, toddler, and preschool special education programs.

Jan Spiegle, Infant/Toddler Program Coordinator

7944 Division of Special Education
PO Box 202501
Helena, MT 59620

406-444-4425
Fax: 406-444-3924
e-mail: dmccarthy@opi.mt.gov
www.nectas.unc.edu

Individuals with Disabilities Education Act requires all states and territories to provide early intervention and preschool special education for children with disabilities and special health care needs. Services include central directory, representatives of agencies, service providers, families, and coordinators of infant, toddler, and preschool special education programs.

Daniel McCarthy, Preschool Special Ed. Coordinator

7945 MonTECH
634 Eddy Avenue, Rural Inst on Disab
Missoula, MT 59812

406-243-5676
800-732-0323
Fax: 406-243-4730
TDD: 800-732-0323
e-mail: montech@selway.umt.edu
www.rudi.montech.umt.edu/

State assisted programs and support group information for people of many abilities. Includes local chapters, referrals, fun and social interaction and support groups.

7946 Parents Let's Unite for Kids
516 N 32nd Street
Billings, MT 59101

406-255-0540
e-mail: plukmt@aol.com
www.taalliance.org

Parent Training and Information (PTI) programs help parents to understand their children's specific needs, communicate more effectively with professionals, participate in the educational planning process, and obtain information about relevant programs, services and resources.

7947 Quality Life Concepts
PO Box 2506
Great Falls, MT 59403

406-452-9531
Fax: 406-453-5930

Informational and emotional support to parents who have a child, adolescent, or adult family member with special needs.

Nebraska

7948 Assistive Technology Partnership
301 Centennial Mall South, Po Box 94987
Lincoln, NE 68516

402-471-0734
Fax: 402-471-6052
TDD: 402-471-0734
e-mail: atp@nde4.rde.state.ne.us
www.nde.state.ne.us/atp/ATPECHome.html

State assisted programs and support group information for people of many abilities. Includes local chapters, referrals, fun and social interaction and support groups.

7949 Individual and Family Support Arc of Lincoln & Lancaster County
645 M Street, Suite 19
Lincoln, NE 68508

402-477-6925
Fax: 402-477-6927

Informational and emotional support to parents who have a child, adolescent, or adult family member with special needs.

7950 Nebraska Parents Center
1941 S 42nd Street, Suite 122
Omaha, NE 68105

402-346-0525
800-284-8520
Fax: 402-346-5253
TDD: 402-346-0525
e-mail: npc@uswest.ne.net
www.neparentcenter.org

Parent Training and Information (PTI) programs help parents to understand their children's specific needs, communicate more effectively with professionals, participate in the educational planning process, and obtain information about relevant programs, services and resources. The Nebrask Parent Center services families statewide. There is no fee for services. Call for additional information.

Glenda Davis, Project Director

7951 Parent Assistance Network
310 W 24th
Kearney, NE 68847

308-237-6025
Fax: 308-237-6014

Informational and emotional support to parents who have a child, adolescent, or adult family member with special needs.

7952 Parent Support Group
123 S Webb Road
Grand Island, NE 68802

308-385-5925
Fax: 308-385-5797
e-mail: msheen@genie.esu10.k12.ne.us

Informational and emotional support to parents who have a child, adolescent, or adult family member with special needs.

7953 Parents Encouraging Parents
NE Department of Education
301 Centennial Mall Street, PO Box 94987
Lincoln, NE 68509

Fax: 402-471-0117
TTY: 402-471-2471
e-mail: ginny_w@nde4.nde.state.ne.us

Informational and emotional support to parents who have a child, adolescent, or adult family member with special needs.

7954 Special Education Office State Department of Education
301 Centennial Mall South
Lincoln, NE 68509

402-471-4319
Fax: 402-471-0117
e-mail: jan_t@nde4.nde.state.ne.us
www.nectas.unc.edu

Individuals with Disabilities Education Act requires all states and territories to provide early intervention and preschool special education for children with disabilities and special health care needs. Services include central directory, representatives of agencies, service providers, families, and coordinators of infant, toddler, and preschool special education programs.

Jan Thelen, Preschool Special Ed. Coordinator

Nevada

7955 Assistive Technology Collaborative
711 S Stewart Street, Rehab Division
Carson City, NV 89701

775-687-4452
Fax: 775-687-3292
TTY: 702-687-3388
e-mail: pgowins@govmail.state.nv.us
www.state.nv.us.80

State assisted programs and support group information for people of many abilities. Includes local chapters, referrals, fun and social interaction and support groups.

7956 Early Intervention Services Division of Child & Family Services
3987 S McCarren Boulevard
Reno, NV 89502

775-688-2284
Fax: 775-688-2558
e-mail: mkwalter@govmail.state.nv.us
www.nectas.unc.edu

Provides early intervention and preschool special education for children with disabilities and special health care needs. Services include central directory, representatives of agencies, service providers, families, and coordinators of infant, toddler, and preschool special education programs.

Marilyn K Walter, Infant/Toddler Program Coordinator

7957 Educational Equity, Special Education Branch
700 E 5th Street, Suite 113
Carson City, NV 89701

775-687-9171
Fax: 775-687-9123
e-mail: gdopf@nsn.scs.unr.edu
www.nectas.unc.edu

Individuals with Disabilities Education Act requires all states and
territories to provide early intervention and preschool special education for children with disabilities and special health care needs.
Services include central directory, representatives of agencies, service providers, families, and coordinators of infant, toddler, and
preschool special education programs.

Gloria Dopf, Preschool Special Ed. Coordinator

7958 Nevada Parent Network
University of Nevada-Reno
COE, REPC/285
Reno, NV 89557

702-784-4921
800-216-7988
Fax: 702-702-4997
e-mail: cdinnell@scs.unr.edu
www.iser.com/npn-NV.html

Informational and emotional support to parents who have a child,
adolescent, or adult family member with special needs.

7959 Nevada Parents Encouraging Parents (PEP)
2355 Red Rock Street, Suite 106
Las Vegas, NV 89146

702-388-8899
800-216-5188
Fax: 702-388-2966
e-mail: pepinfo@nvpep.org
www.nvpep.org

Parent Training and Information (PTI) programs help parents to
understand their children's specific needs, communicate more effectively with professionals, participate in the educational planning
process, and obtain information about relevant programs, services
and resources.

Karen Taycher, Executive Director

7960 Parents Encouraging Parents
2355 Red Roack Street Suite 106
Las Vegas, NV 89146

702-388-8899
Fax: 702-388-2966
www.nvpep.org

Informational and emotional support to parents who have a child,
adolescent, or adult family member with special needs.

New Hampshire

7961 Bureau of Early Learning
101 Pleasant Street
Concord, NH 03301

603-271-2178
Fax: 603-271-1953
e-mail: rlittlefield@ed.state.nh.us
www.nectas.unc.edu

Individuals with Disabilities Education Act requires all states and
territories to provide early intervention and preschool special education for children with disabilities and special health care needs.
Services include central directory, representatives of agencies, service providers, families, and coordinators of infant, toddler, and
preschool special education programs.

Ruth Littlefield, Preschool Special Ed. Coordinator

7962 Division of Special Education
101 Pleasant Street
Concord, NH 03301

603-271-3776
Fax: 603-271-1099
www.nectas.unc.edu

Individuals with Disabilities Education Act requires all states and
territories to provide early intervention and preschool special education for children with disabilities and special health care needs.
Services include central directory, representatives of agencies, service providers, families, and coordinators of infant, toddler, and
preschool special education programs.

Jane Weisman, Interagency Coordinating Council

7963 Family Center Early Supports & Services
105 Pleasant Street
Concord, NH 03301

603-271-5122
Fax: 603-271-5166
e-mail: cohara@dhhs.state.nh.us
www.familyvoices.org

Services include central directory, representatives of agencies, service providers, families, and coordinators of infant, toddler, and
preschool special education programs.

Carolyn O'Hara, Infant/Toddler Program Coordiantor

7964 High Hopes Foundation of New Hampshire
416k Daniel Webster Highway
Merrimacl, NH 03054

603-529-1010
800-639-6804
Fax: 603-529-0037
e-mail: HighHopeNH@aol.com
www.highhopesnh.org

Volunteer organization dedicated to granting wishes of seriously ill
New Hampshire children from three through 18 years old.

60+ members

Linda Bennett, President
Patricia Bouley, Director Marketing

7965 Parent Information Center
PO Box 2405
Concord, NH 03302

603-224-7005
Fax: 603-224-4365
TDD: 603-224-7005
e-mail: picnh@aol.com
www.taalliance.org/ptis/nhpic

Parent Training and Information (PTI) programs help parents to
understand their children's specific needs, communicate more effectively with professionals, participate in the educational planning
process, and obtain information about relevant programs, services
and resources.

7966 Parent to Parent of New Hampshire
12 Flynn Street
Lebanon, NH 03766

603-448-6393
800-698-5465
Fax: 603-448-6311
www.p2pnh.org

Informational and emotional support to parents who have a child,
adolescent, or adult family member with special needs.

**7967 Technology Partnership Project Institute on
Disability/UAP**
The Concord Center
10 Ferry Street Suite 317
Concord, NH 03301

603-224-0630
Fax: 603-228-3470
TDD: 603-224-0630
e-mail: institute.disability@unh.edu
iod.unh.edu

State assistive programs funded by the National Institute on Disability and Rehabilitation Research. Includes directories, support
group information, training and project information.

New Jersey

7968 Division of Student Services
Riverview Executive Plaza, Building 100
Trenton, NJ 08625

609-984-4950
Fax: 609-292-5558
e-mail: btkach@doh.state.nj.us
www.nectas.unc.edu

Individuals with Disabilities Education Act requires all states and territories to provide early intervention and preschool special education for children with disabilities and special health care needs. Services include central directory, representatives of agencies, service providers, families, and coordinators of infant, toddler, and preschool special education programs.

Barbara Tkach, Preschool Special Ed. Coordinator

7969 Early Intervention System
PO Box 364
Trenton, NJ 08625

609-777-7734
Fax: 609-292-3580
e-mail: Terry.Harrison@dob.state.nj.us
www.state.nj-us/health/8hs/eiphome.htm

Individuals with Disabilities Education Act requires all states and territories to provide early intervention and preschool special education for children with disabilities and special health care needs. Services include central directory, representatives of agencies, service providers, families, and coordinators of infant, toddler, and preschool special education programs.

Terry Harrison, Infant/Toddler Program Coordinator

7970 Family Support Center of New Jersey
Lion's Head Office Park
35 Beaverson Boulevard, Suite 8 A
Brick, NJ 08723

732-262-8020
800-372-6510
Fax: 732-262-4373
e-mail: FSCNJ@aol.com
www.efnj.com

Informational and emotional support to parents who have a child, adolescent, or adult family member with special needs.

7971 New Jersey Self-Help Clearinghouse
100 E Hanover Avenue, Suite 202
Cedar Knolls, NJ 07297

973-326-6789
800-367-6274
Fax: 973-326-9467
TTY: 973-625-9053
e-mail: info@selfhelpgroups.org
www.njgroups.org

The NJ Self-Help Group Clearinghouse provides contacts for over 4,500 New Jersey support groups and over 1,100 national support networks for most illnesses, addictions, disabilities, bereavement, parenting and other stressful life situations. The organization also helps individuals wanting to start a group.

7972 New Jersey Statewide Parent to Parent
2150 Highway 35, Suite 207C
Sea Girt, NJ 08750

800-372-6510
Fax: 973-642-8080

Informational and emotional support to parents who have a child, adolescent, or adult family member with special needs.

7973 Statewide Parent Advocacy Network
35 Halsey Street, 4th Floor
Newark, NJ 07102

973-642-8100
Fax: 973-642-8080
e-mail: span@bellatlantic.net
www.taalliance.org/ptis/nj

Parent Training and Information (PTI) programs help parents to understand their children's specific needs, communicate more ef-

fectively with professionals, participate in the educational planning process, and obtain information about relevant programs, services and resources.

New Mexico

7974 EPICS Project-SW Communication Resources
PO Box 788
Bernalilo, NM 87004

505-867-3396
800-765-7320
Fax: 505-867-3398
TDD: 505-867-3396
www.disabilityrights.org

Parent Training and Information (PTI) programs help parents to understand their children's specific needs, communicate more effectively with professionals, participate in the educational planning process, and obtain information about relevant programs, services and resources.

7975 Long Term Services Division
PO Box 26110
Santa Fe, NM 87502

505-827-0103
Fax: 505-827-2455
www.nectas.unc.edu

Individuals with Disabilities Education Act requires all states and territories to provide early intervention and preschool special education for children with disabilities and special health care needs. Services include central directory, representatives of agencies, service providers, families, and coordinators of infant, toddler, and preschool special education programs.

Cathy Stevenson, Infant/Toddler Program Coordiantor

7976 Parents Reaching Out
1920 B Columbia Drive SE
Albuquerque, NM 87106

505-247-0192
800-524-5176
Fax: 505-247-1345
TDD: 505-865-3700
e-mail: nmproth@aol.com
www.parentsreachingout.org

Provides peer support, technical assistance and information statewide to families in New Mexico who have family member with unique or special needs and professionals who care for them.

7977 Special Education Unit
300 Don Gaspar Avenue
Santa Fe, NM 87501

505-827-6788
Fax: 505-827-6791
e-mail: mlandazuri@sde.state.nm.us
www.nectas.unc.edu

Individuals with Disabilities Education Act requires all states and territories to provide early intervention and preschool special education for children with disabilities and special health care needs. Services include central directory, representatives of agencies, service providers, families, and coordinators of infant, toddler, and preschool special education programs.

Maria Landazuri, Preschool Special Ed. Coordinator

7978 Technology Assistance Program
435 St Michael's Drive, Building D
Santa Fe, NM 87505

505-954-8539
800-866-2253
Fax: 505-954-8562
TDD: 800-866-2253
e-mail: nmdvrtap@aol.com

State assisted programs for people of many abilities. Includes local chapters, referrals, fun and social interaction and support groups.

New York

7979 Advocacy Center
277 Alexander Street, Suite 500
Rochester, NY 14607

716-546-1700
800-650-4967
Fax: 716-546-7069
e-mail: advocacy@frontiernet.net
www.advocacycenter.com

Parent Training and Information (PTI) programs help parents to understand their children's specific needs, communicate more effectively with professionals, participate in the educational planning process, and obtain information about relevant programs, services and resources.

7980 Advocates for Children of New York
151 W 30th Street, 5th Floor
New York, NY 10001

212-947-9779
Fax: 212-947-9790
e-mail: info@advocatesforchildren.org
www.advocatesforchildren.org

Parent Training and Information (PTI) programs help parents to understand their children's specific needs, communicate more effectively with professionals, participate in the educational planning process, and obtain information about relevant programs, services and resources.

Elisa Hyman, Executive Director

7981 Aurora of Central New York
518 James Street, Suite 100
Syracuse, NY 13203

315-422-7263
Fax: 315-422-4792
TDD: 315-422-4792
e-mail: auroracny@auroraofcny.org
www.auroraofcny.org

Professional counseling services to assist individuals and their families deal with the trauma of hearing or vision loss.

7982 Early Intervention Program
Corning Tower Room 208, Empire Street Plaza
Albany, NY 12237

518-473-7016
Fax: 518-473-8673
e-mail: dmn02@health.state.ny.us
www.nectas.unc.edu

Individuals with Disabilities Education Act requires all states and territories to provide early intervention and preschool special education for children with disabilities and special health care needs. Services include a central directory, representatives of agencies, service providers, families, and coordinators of infant, toddler, and preschool special education programs.

Donna Noyes, Infant/Toddler Program Coordinator

7983 Friends of Karen
118 Titicus Road, PO Box 190
Purdys, NY 10578

845-277-4547
800-637-2774
www.friendsofkaren.org

Dedicated to helping terminally and catastrophically ill children and their families in the New York metropolitan area only. They provide assistance with payments for physicians, hospitals and medications, help with extra expenses beyond medical bills, provide home nursing services and equipment, supplies for loans, and offers emotional support.

7984 Marty Lyons Foundation
326 W 48th Street
New York, NY 10036

212-977-9474
877-560-9474
Fax: 212-977-1752
e-mail: mlf_hq@martylyonsfoundation.org
martylyonsfoundation.org

Chapters in New Jersey, New York, Massachussets, Connecticut, Maryland, North Carolina, South Carolina, Georgia, Texas, Pennsylvania and Florida provide a special wish to children ages three to seventeen who are terminally ill or have a life-threatening disease.

300 volunteers

Pamela Pfarr, Manager, Program Services

7985 New York Department of Education
1 Commerce Plaza
Albany, NY 12234

518-473-4823
Fax: 518-486-4154
e-mail: mplotzke@mail.nysed.gov

Individuals with Disabilities Education Act requires all states and territories to provide early intervention and preschool special education for children with disabilities and special health care needs. Services include central directory, representatives of agencies, service providers, families, and coordinators of infant, toddler, and preschool special education programs.

Michael Plotzker Vesid, Preschool Special Ed. Coordinator

7986 Parent Network Center
250 Delaware Avenue, Suite 3
Buffalo, NY 14202

716-853-1570
800-724-7408
Fax: 716-853-1574
TDD: 716-853-1573
www.taalliance.org

Parent Training and Information (PTI) programs help parents to understand their children's specific needs, communicate more effectively with professionals, participate in the educational planning process, and obtain information about relevant programs, services and resources.

7987 Parent to Parent of New York State
500 Balltown Road
Schenectady, NY 12304

518-381-4350
800-305-8817
Fax: 518-382-1959
e-mail: parent2par@aol.com
www.parenttoparentnys.org

Informational and emotional support to parents who have a child, adolescent, or adult family member with special needs.

1500 Members

Carolyn Schimanski, Executive Director

7988 Resources for Children with Special Needs
200 Park Avenue S, Suite 816
New York City, NY 10003

212-667-4650
Fax: 212-254-4070
e-mail: resourcenyc@prodigy.net
www.epsty.com/resourcenyc

Parent Training and Information (PTI) programs help parents to understand their children's specific needs, communicate more effectively with professionals, participate in the educational planning process, and obtain information about relevant programs, services and resources.

7989 Saint Mary's Healthcare System for Children
One Penn Plaze Suite 2420
New York, NY 10119

212-586-8723
Fax: 212-586-5170
www.nycharities.org

Information and advocacy resources for families and professionals. Includes listings of organizations providing general information and organizations focusing on more specific areas of concern to families and young adults who have disabilities.

7990 Sinergia/Metropolitan Parent Center
15 W 65th Street, 6th Floor
New York, NY 10023

212-496-1300
Fax: 212-496-5608
e-mail: Sinergia@panix.com
www.panic.com/~sinergia

Parent Training and Information (PTI) programs help parents to understand their children's specific needs, communicate more effectively with professionals, participate in the educational planning process, and obtain information about relevant programs, services and resources.

7991 TRIAD Project-Advocates for Persons with Disabilities
One Empire State Plaza, Suite 1001
Albany, NY 12223

518-474-2825
800-522-4369
Fax: 518-473-6005
TTY: 518-473-4231
e-mail: leffingw@emi.com

State assisted programs and support group information for people of many abilities. Includes local chapters, referrals, fun and social interaction and support groups.

7992 Ulster County Social Services
7 Cicero Avenue
New Paltz, NY 12561

845-255-1713
Fax: 845-255-3202
www.nectas.unc.edu

Individuals with Disabilities Education Act requires all states and territories to provide early intervention and preschool special education for children with disabilities and special health care needs. Services include central directory, representatives of agencies, service providers, families, and coordinators of infant, toddler, and preschool special education programs.

Thomas Roach, Interagency Coordinating Council

North Carolina

7993 Assistive Technology Project, Human Resources, Voc. and Rehab. Services
1110 Navaho Drive, Suite 101
Raleigh, NC 27609

919-850-2787
800-852-0042
Fax: 919-850-2792
TTY: 919-850-2787
e-mail: rickic@mindspring.com
www.ncatp.org

State assisted programs and support group information for people of many abilities. Includes local chapters, referrals, fun and social interaction and support groups.

7994 ECAC
907 Barra Row, Suites 102/103
Davidson, NC 28036

704-892-1321
Fax: 704-892-5028
TDD: 704-892-1321
e-mail: ecac@ecac.org
www.ecac-parentcenter.org

Parent Training and Information (PTI) programs help parents to understand their children's specific needs, communicate more effectively with professionals, participate in the educational planning process, and obtain information about relevant programs, services and resources.

7995 Exceptional Children Division
301 N Wilmington Street
Raleigh, NC 27601

919-807-3300
Fax: 919-807-3482
e-mail: kbaars@state.nc.us
www.ncpublicschools.org

Individuals with Disabilities Education Act requires all states and territories to provide early intervention and preschool special education for children with disabilities and special health care needs. Services include central directory, representatives of agencies, service providers, families, and coordinators of infant, toddler, and preschool special education programs.

Kathy Baars, Preschool Special Ed. Coordinator

7996 Family Support Network of North Carolina
University of North carolina
200 N Greensboro St, Carr Mill Mall, 2nd Fl Ste D9
Carrboro, NC 27510

919-966-2841
800-852-0042
Fax: 919-966-2916
e-mail: cdr@med.unc.edu
www.fsnnc.org

Family Support Network of North Carolina promotes and provides support for families with children who have special needs. Families are in a unique position to offer information and support to other families. An experienced family member can share the most practical advice and help a parent navigate the complex service systems. Having support can make it easier for families to experience the joy and satisfaction that can come from parenting a child with special needs.

Laura Curtis, Education & Outreach Coordinator
Irene Nathan Zipper, Director

7997 Partnerships for Inclusion
2415 W Vernon Avenue
Kingston, NC 28501

919-559-5156
e-mail: msteele@greenvillenc.com
www.nectas.unc.edu

Individuals with Disabilities Education Act requires all states and territories to provide early intervention and preschool special education for children with disabilities and special health care needs. Services include central directory, representatives of agencies, service providers, families, and coordinators of infant, toddler, and preschool special education programs.

Sandy Steele, Interagency Coordinating Council

7998 Rockingham County Schools
511 Harrington Highway
Eden, NC 27288

336-627-2615
Fax: 336-627-2660
e-mail: speele@greenvillenc.com
www.ncpublicschools.org/success/regionalcontacts

Individuals with Disabilities Education Act requires all states and territories to provide early intervention and preschool special education for children with disabilities and special health care needs. Services include central directory, representatives of agencies, service providers, families, and coordinators of infant, toddler, and preschool special education programs.

Susan Peele, Interagency Coordinating Council

North Dakota

7999 Developmental Disabilities Unit
1237 W Divide Avenue, Suite 1A
Bismarck, ND 58501

701-328-8936
800-755-8529
Fax: 701-328-8969
e-mail: sobald@nd.gov
www.nectas.unc.edu

Individuals with Disabilities Education Act requires all states and territories to provide early intervention and preschool special education for children with disabilities and special health care needs. Services include central directory, representatives of agencies, service providers, families, and coordinators of infant, toddler, and preschool special education programs.

Debra Balsdon, Infant/Toddler Program Coordinator

8000 Interagency Program Assistive Technology
PO Box 743
Cavalier, ND 58220

701-265-4807
Fax: 701-265-3150
TDD: 701-265-4807
e-mail: lee@pioneer.state.nd.us
www.ndipat.org

State assisted programs and support group information for people of many abilities. Includes local chapters, referrals, fun and social interaction and support groups.

8001 Special Education Division
600 E Boulevard
Bismarck, ND 58505

701-328-2271
Fax: 701-328-4149
www.nectas.unc.edu

Individuals with Disabilities Education Act requires all states and territories to provide early intervention and preschool special education for children with disabilities and special health care needs. Services include central directory, representatives of agencies, service providers, families, and coordinators of infant, toddler, and preschool special education programs.

Brenda Oas, Preschool Special Ed. Coordinator
Jeanette Kolberg, Preschool Special Ed. Coordinator

Ohio

8002 Bureau of EI Services
246 N High Strees, PO Box 118
Columbus, OH 43266

614-644-9164
Fax: 614-728-9163
e-mail: coser@gw.odh.state.oh.us
www.ohiohelpmegrow.org

Individuals with Disabilities Education Act requires all states and territories to provide early intervention and preschool special education for children with disabilities and special health care needs. Services include central directory, representatives of agencies, service providers, families, and coordinators of infant, toddler, and preschool special education programs.

Cindy Oser, Infant/Toddler Program Coordinator

8003 Celebrating Families of Children & Adults with Special Needs
16 Vassar Drive
Dayton, OH 45406

937-275-0990
800-432-2199
Fax: 937-275-0277
e-mail: families@erinet.com
www.eparent.com

Informational and emotional support to parents who have a child, adolescent, or adult family member with special needs.

8004 Division of Early Childhood Education
65 S Front Street, Room 309
Columbus, OH 43215

614-466-0224
Fax: 614-728-2338
www.nectas.unc.edu

Individuals with Disabilities Education Act requires all states and territories to provide early intervention and preschool special education for children with disabilities and special health care needs. Services include central directory, representatives of agencies, ser-

vice providers, families, and coordinators of infant, toddler, and preschool special education programs.

Jane Wiechel, Preschool Special Ed. Coordinator

8005 East Central Regional Office
170 W High Avenue
New Philadelphia, OH 44663

330-364-5567
Fax: 330-343-3038
e-mail: ECE_Greer@ode.ohio.gov@inet
www.nectas.unc.edu

Individuals with Disabilities Education Act requires all states and territories to provide early intervention and preschool special education for children with disabilities and special health care needs. Services include central directory, representatives of agencies, service providers, families, and coordinators of infant, toddler, and preschool special education programs.

Edith Greer, Preschool Special Ed. Coordinator

8006 Family Information Network
143 NW Avenue, Building A
Tallmadge, OH 44278

330-633-2055
Fax: 330-633-2658

Informational and emotional support to parents who have a child, adolescent, or adult family member with special needs.

8008 OCECD
165 W Center Street, Suite 302
Marion, OH 43302

614-382-5452
800-374-2806
Fax: 614-383-6421
e-mail: ocecd@edu.gte.net
www.ocecd.org

Parent Training and Information (PTI) programs help parents to understand their children's specific needs, communicate more effectively with professionals, participate in the educational planning process, and obtain information about relevant programs, services and resources.

8009 Ohio Protection and Advocacy Organization
5350 Brookpark Avenue
Cleveland, OH 44134

216-398-5501
800-672-1220
Fax: 216-398-5505

Informational and emotional support to parents who have a child, adolescent, or adult family member with special needs.

8010 Operation Liftoff of Ohio
PO Box 1094
Gallipolis, OH 45631

Fulfills a dream for children in Ohio and surrounding states who have a life-threatening illness.

8011 Society for Rehabilitation
9521 Lake Shore Boulevard
Mentor, OH 44060

440-352-8993
Fax: 440-352-6632
e-mail: info@societyhelps.org
www.societyhelps.org

Individuals with Disabilities Education Act requires all states and territories to provide early intervention and preschool special education for children with disabilities and special health care needs. Disability therapy is provided for children and adults.

Richard J Kessler, Executive Director

8012 Train-Ohio Super Computer Center
1224 Kinnear Road
Columbus, OH 43212

614-292-9248
Fax: 614-292-7168
TDD: 614-292-2426
www.osc.edu

State assisted programs and support group information for people of many abilities. Includes local chapters, referrals, fun and social interaction and support groups.

Oklahoma

8013 Oklahoma ABLE Tech-Wellness Center
1514 W Hall of Fame
Stillwater, OK 74078

405-744-9748
800-257-1705
Fax: 405-744-7670
TTY: 800-257-1705
e-mail: mljwell@okway.okstate.edu
www.okstate.edu/wellness/athome.htm

State assisted programs and support group information for people of many abilities. Includes local chapters, referrals, fun and social interaction and support groups.

8014 Parents Reaching Out in Oklahoma
1917 S Harvard Avenue
Oklahoma City, OK 73128

405-681-9710
Fax: 405-685-4006
TDD: 405-681-9710
e-mail: prook@aol.com
www.ucp.org/probase.htm

Parent Training and Information (PTI) programs help parents to understand their children's specific needs, communicate more effectively with professionals, participate in the educational planning process, and obtain information about relevant programs, services and resources.

8015 Special Education Office
2500 N Lincoln Boulevard
Oklahoma City, OK 73105

405-522-4513
Fax: 405-522-3503
e-mail: mark_sharp@mail.sde.state.ok.us
www.nectas.unc.edu

Individuals with Disabilities Education Act requires all states and territories to provide early intervention and preschool special education for children with disabilities and special health care needs. Services include central directory, representatives of agencies, service providers, families, and coordinators of infant, toddler, and preschool special education programs.

Mark Sharp, Infant/Toddler Program Coordinator

Oregon

8016 Early Childhood CARES Program
1895 E 15th Avenue
Eugene, OR 97403

541-346-2639
Fax: 541-343-5650
e-mail: Judy_Newman@ccmail.uoregon.edu

Individuals with Disabilities Education Act requires all states and territories to provide early intervention and preschool special education for children with disabilities and special health care needs. Services include central directory, representatives of agencies, service providers, families, and coordinators of infant, toddler, and preschool special education programs.

Judy Newman, Interagency Coordinating Council

8017 Early Intervention Programs
255 Capitol Street NE
Salem, OR 97301

503-378-3598
Fax: 503-373-7968
e-mail: jane.mulholland@odeexl.ode.state.or.us
www.nectas.unc.edu

Individuals with Disabilities Education Act requires all states and territories to provide early intervention and preschool special education for children with disabilities and special health care needs. Services include central directory, representatives of agencies, service providers, families, and coordinators of infant, toddler, and preschool special education programs.

Jane Mulholland, Infant/Toddler Program Coordinator

8018 Oregon Parent Training and Information Center
2295 Liberty Street NE
Salem, OR 97303

503-581-8156
888-505-2673
Fax: 503-391-0429
e-mail: orpti@orpti.org
www.orpti.org

Informational and emotional support to parents who have a child, adolescent, or adult family member with special needs.

8019 Special Education Programs
255 Capitol Street NE
Salem, OR 97301

503-378-3598
Fax: 503-373-7968
e-mail: nancy.johnson-dorn@state.or.us
www.nectas.unc.edu

Provides early intervention and preschool special education for children with disabilities and special health care needs. Services include central directory, representatives of agencies, service providers, families, and coordinators of infant, toddler, and preschool special education programs.

Nancy Johnson-Dorn, Preschool Special Ed. Coordinator

8020 Technology Access for Life Needs Project
1257 Ferry Street, Se
Salem, OR 97310

503-361-1201
Fax: 503-370-4530
TDD: 503-361-1201
e-mail: ati@orednet.org

State assisted programs and support group information for people of many abilities. Includes local chapters, referrals, fun and social interaction and support groups.

Pennsylvania

8021 Bureau of Special Education
333 Market Street, 7th Floor
Harrisburg, PA 17126

717-783-6882
800-874-2301
Fax: 717-783-6139
TDD: 717-787-7367
e-mail: ebeck@state.pa.us
rprice@state.pa.us

Services include central directory, representatives of agencies, service providers, families, and coordinators of infant, toddler, and preschool special education programs.

Esther Beck, Educational Supervisor
Rick Price, Division Chief

8022 Division of Early Intervention Services
PO Box 2675
Harrisburg, PA 17105

717-783-8302
Fax: 717-772-0012
e-mail: jackiee@dpw.state.pa.us
www.nectas.unc.edu

Individuals with Disabilities Education Act requires all states and territories to provide early intervention and preschool special education for children with disabilities and special health care needs. Services include central directory, representatives of agencies, service providers, families, and coordinators of infant, toddler, and preschool special education programs.

Jacqueline Epstein, Infant/Toddler Program Coordinator

8023 Montgomery County Intermediate Unit #23
1605 B W Main Street
Norristown, PA 19403

610-539-8550
Fax: 610-539-5973
www.nectas.unc.edu

Services include a central directory, representatives of agencies, service providers, families, and coordinators of infant, toddler, and preschool special education programs.

Dennis Harkin, Interagency Coordinating Council

8024 Parent Education Network
2107 Industrial Highway
York, PA 17402

717-600-0100
800-522-5827
Fax: 717-600-8101
TDD: 717-600-0100
e-mail: pen@parentednet.org
www.parentednet.org

Parent Training and Information (PTI) programs help parents to understand their children's specific needs, communicate more effectively with professionals, participate in the educational planning process, and obtain information about relevant programs, services and resources.

8025 Parent to Parent ARC Allegheny
711 Bingham Street
Pittsburgh, PA 15203

412-995-5001
e-mail: ptparc@arcallegheny.org
www.arcallegheny.org

Informational and emotional support to parents who have a child, adolescent, or adult family member with special needs.

8026 Parent to Parent of Pennsylvania
150 S Progress Avenue
Harrisburg, PA 17109

717-540-4722
Fax: 717-540-7603
e-mail: bril1134@cdc.gov
www.nauticom.net/www/eita

Informational and emotional support to parents who have a child, adolescent, or adult family member with special needs.

8027 Parents Union for Public Schools
1315 Walnut Street, Suite 1124
Philadelphia, PA 19107

215-546-1166
Fax: 215-731-1688
e-mail: Parents@aol.com
www.nyfac.org

Parent Training and Information (PTI) programs help parents to understand their children's specific needs, communicate more effectively with professionals, participate in the educational planning process, and obtain information about relevant programs, services and resources.

8028 Pennsylvania's Initiative on Assistive Technology, Institute on Disabilities
University Affliated Program
423 Ritter Annex, Temple University
Philadelphia, PA 19122

215-204-5966
800-204-7428
Fax: 215-204-9371
TTY: 800-750-7428
e-mail: piat@astro.temple.edu
www.temple.edu/inst_disabilities

Most of PAIT's activities are free to Pennsylvania residents, and are focused on the provision of public awareness of the benefit and scope of assistive technology (AT), information and referral, advocacy and funding, and training. PAIT is the state's contractor for the implementation of Pennsylvania's Assistive Technology Lending library.

8029 US Wheelchair Weightlifting Association
39 Michael Place
Levittown, PA 19057

215-945-1964

State assisted programs and support group information for people of many abilities. Includes local chapters, referrals, fun and social interaction and support groups.

Rhode Island

8030 Assistive Technology Access Partnership
40 Fountain Street
Providence, RI 02903

401-421-7005
Fax: 401-222-3574
TTY: 401-421-7016
e-mail: reginac@ors.state.ri.us
www.atap.state.ri.us

State assisted programs and support group information for people of many abilities. Includes local chapters, referrals, fun and social interaction and support groups.

8031 Central Region Early Intervention Program
J Arthur Trudeau Memorial Center
250 Commonwealth Avenue
Warwick, RI 02886

401-823-1731
Fax: 401-823-1849

Informational and emotional support to parents who have a child, adolescent, or adult family member with special needs.

8032 Office Integrated Social Services
255 Westminister Road
Providence, RI 02903

401-222-4600
Fax: 401-222-4979
e-mail: abcohen@ride.ri.net
www.nectas.unc.edu

Individuals with Disabilities Education Act requires all states and territories to provide early intervention and preschool special education for children with disabilities and special health care needs. Services include central directory, representatives of agencies, service providers, families, and coordinators of infant, toddler, and preschool special education programs.

Amy Cohen, Preschool Special Ed. Coordinator

8033 Rhode Island Arc
99 Bald Hill Road
Cranston, RI 02920

401-463-9191
Fax: 401-463-9244
www.nectas.unc.edu

Individuals with Disabilities Education Act requires all states and territories to provide early intervention and preschool special education for children with disabilities and special health care needs. Services include central directory, representatives of agencies, service providers, families, and coordinators of infant, toddler, and preschool special education programs.

James Healey, Interagency Coordinating Council

8034 Rhode Island Department of Health
600 New London Avenue
Cranston, RI 02920

401-462-0318
Fax: 401-462-6253
www.nectas.unc.edu

Individuals with Disabilities Education Act requires all states and territories to provide early intervention and preschool special education for children with disabilities and special health care needs. Services include central directory, representatives of agencies, service providers, families, and coordinators of infant, toddler, and preschool special education programs.

Ron Caldarone, Infant/Toddler Program Coordinator

8035 Rhode Island Parent Information Network
175 Main Street
Pawtucket, RI 02860

401-727-4144
800-464-3399
Fax: 401-727-4040
www.ripin.org

Nonprofit organization providing information, training, support and advocacy to parents.

South Carolina

8036 Assistive Technology Project
Center for Developmental Disabilities
USC School of Medicine
Columbia, SC 29208

Fax: 803-935-5342
TDD: 803-935-5263
e-mail: scatp@scsn.net
www.scsn.net/users/scatp

State assisted programs and support group information for people of many abilities. Includes local chapters, referrals, fun and social interaction and support groups.

8037 BabyNet
1751 Calhoun Street
Columbia, SC 29201

803-898-0784
Fax: 803-898-0613
e-mail: strickll@dhec.sc.gov
www.scdhec.net/babynet

Individuals with Disabilities Education Act requires all states and territories to provide early intervention and preschool special education for children with disabilities and special health care needs. Services include central directory, representatives of agencies, service providers, families, and coordinators of infant, toddler, and preschool special education programs.

Kathy Hart, Infant/Toddler Program Coordinator

8038 Office of Exceptional Children South Carolina Department of Education
1429 Senate Street, Room 808
Columbia, SC 29201

803-734-8811
Fax: 803-734-4824
e-mail: njenkins@sde.state.sc.us
www.myschools.com/offices/ec

Individuals with Disabilities Education Act requires all states and territories to provide early intervention and preschool special education for children with disabilities and special health care needs. Services include central directory, representatives of agencies, service providers, families, and coordinators of infant, toddler, and preschool special education programs.

Norma Donaldson-Jenkins, Preschool Special Ed. Coordinator
Susan Duranti, Director

8039 PRO-Parents
652 Bush River Road
Columbia, SC 29210

803-772-5688
800-759-4776
Fax: 803-772-5341
e-mail: proparents@proparents.org
www.proparents.org

Parent Training and Information (PTI) programs help parents to understand their children's specific needs, communicate more effectively with professionals, participate in the educational planning process, and obtain information about relevant programs, services and resources.

3500 Members

South Dakota

8040 DakotaLink
1925 Plaza Boulevard
Rapid City, SD 57702

605-394-1876
Fax: 605-394-5315
TTY: 800-645-0673
e-mail: rreed@sdtie.sdserv.org
www.tie.net/dakotalink

State assisted programs and support group information for people of many abilities. Includes local chapters, referrals, fun and social interaction and support groups.

8041 Office of Special Education
700 Governors Drive
Pierre, SD 57501

605-773-4478
Fax: 605-773-6846
e-mail: barbh@deca.state.sd.us
www.nectas.unc.edu

Individuals with Disabilities Education Act requires all states and territories to provide early intervention and preschool special education for children with disabilities and special health care needs. Services include central directory, representatives of agencies, service providers, families, and coordinators of infant, toddler, and preschool special education programs.

Barb Hemmelman, Infant/Toddler Program Coordinator

8042 South Dakota Parent Connection
3701 W 49th, Suite 2008
Souix Falls, SD 57106

605-361-3171
Fax: 605-361-2928
e-mail: bschreck@dakota.net
www.taalliance.org

Parent Training and Information (PTI) programs help parents to understand their children's specific needs, communicate more effectively with professionals, participate in the educational planning process, and obtain information about relevant programs, services and resources.

8043 University Affiliated Program, School of Medicine
414 E Clark Street
Vermillion, SD 57069

605-677-5311
Fax: 605-677-6274
e-mail: jwounded@used.edu
www.nectas.unc.edu

Individuals with Disabilities Education Act requires all states and territories to provide early intervention and preschool special education for children with disabilities and special health care needs. Services include central directory, representatives of agencies, service providers, families, and coordinators of infant, toddler, and preschool special education programs.

Joanne Wounded Head, Interagency Coordinating Council

Tennessee

8044 Center for Early Childhood
E Tennessee State University, Box 70434
Johnson City, TN 37614

423-439-7555
Fax: 423-439-7561
child.etsu.edu

Individuals with Disabilities Education Act requires all states and territories to provide early intervention and preschool special education for children with disabilities and special health care needs. Services include central directory, representatives of agencies, service providers, families, and coordinators of infant, toddler, and preschool special education programs.

Wesley Brown, Interagency Coordinating Council

8045 Office of Special Education, State Department of Education
710 James Robertson Parkway
Nashville, TN 37243

615-532-6319
Fax: 615-532-9412
e-mail: dmattraw@mail.state.tn.us
www.nectas.unc.edu

Individuals with Disabilities Education Act requires all states and territories to provide early intervention and preschool special education for children with disabilities and special health care needs. Services include central directory, representatives of agencies, service providers, families, and coordinators of infant, toddler, and preschool special education programs.

Doris Mattraw, Preschool Special Ed. Coordinator

8046 STEP
424 E Bernard Avenue, Suite 3
Greenvilles, TN 37745

423-639-0125
Fax: 423-636-8217
TDD: 423-636-8217
e-mail: tnstep@aol.com
www.taalliance.org

Parent Training and Information (PTI) programs help parents to understand their children's specific needs, communicate more effectively with professionals, participate in the educational planning process, and obtain information about relevant programs, services and resources.

8047 Technology Access Center of Middle Tennessee
2222 Metrocenter Boulevard, Suite 126
Nashville, TN 37228

615-248-6733
800-368-4651
Fax: 615-259-2536
e-mail: tactn@nashville.com
tac.ataccess.org

Technology group of parents, consumers and professionals; provides resources to help children and adults who have disabilities gain access to the benefits of technology. Includes nationwide network of community-based assistive technology, resource centers, hands on consultants and product demonstrations.

Texas

8048 Department of Assistive and Rehabilitation Services
4900 N Lamar Boulevard
Austin, TX 78751

512-424-6754
800-250-2246
Fax: 512-424-6749
e-mail: marytbetho'hanlon@dars.state.tx.us
www.eci.state.tx.us

Individuals with Disabilities Education Act part C requires all states and territories to provide early intervention to infants and toddlers with disabilities. Services include a full array of infant intervention fields and disciplines.

MaryBeth O'Hanlon, Assistant Commissioner

8049 Office of the Dean, University of Texas at Austin
College of Education, EBB 210
Austin, TX 78712

512-471-7255
Fax: 512-471-0846
www.nectas.unc.edu

Individuals with Disabilities Education Act requires all states and territories to provide early intervention and preschool special education for children with disabilities and special health care needs. Services include central directory, representatives of agencies, service providers, families, and coordinators of infant, toddler, and preschool special education programs.

Alba Ortiz, Interagency Coordinating Council

8050 Parent Case Management
4601 Hartford
Abilene, TX 79605

915-793-3500
Fax: 915-793-3549

Support network for parents of children with disabilities and/or chronic illness. Veteran parents offer support to parents who are just learning of their child's diagnosis. Offers support and insight into parenting a child with special needs, as well as referrals to trained veteran parents.

8051 Partners Resource Network
1090 Longfellow Drive, Suite B
Beaumont, TX 77706

409-898-4684
800-866-4726
Fax: 409-898-4869
TTY: 409-898-4816
e-mail: partnersresource@shegioml.net
www.partnerstx.org

Support network for parents of children with disabilities and/or chronic illness. Veteran parents offer support to parents who are just learning of their child's diagnosis. Offers support and insight into parenting a child with special needs, as well as referrals to trained veteran parents.

8052 Project PODER
1017 N Main Avenue, Suite 207
San Antonio, TX 78212

210-222-2637
Fax: 210-475-9283
TDD: 800-682-9747
e-mail: poder@world-net.com
www.tfepoder.org/poder

Parent Training and Information (PTI) programs help parents to understand their children's specific needs, communicate more effectively with professionals, participate in the educational planning process, and obtain information about relevant programs, services and resources.

8053 South Central Region-Helen Keller National Center
4230 Lyndon B Johnson
Dallas, TX 75244

972-490-9677
Fax: 972-490-6042
e-mail: ccfutbol@aol.com

8055 Texas Assistive Technology Partnership
Texas University Affiliated Program
4030-2 W Baker Lane Building 2, Suite 220
Austin, TX 78759

512-232-0740
800-828-7839
Fax: 512-232-0761
TTY: 512-232-0762
tcds.edb.utexas.edu

State assisted programs and support group information for people of many abilities. Includes local chapters, referrals, fun and social interaction and support groups.

Utah

8056 Baby Watch Early Intervention Program
44 N Medical Drive, PO Box 144720
Salt Lake City, UT 84114

801-584-8226
Fax: 801-584-8496
e-mail: sord@doh.state.ut.us
www.utahbabywatch.org

Individuals with Disabilities Education Act requires all states and territories to provide early intervention and preschool special education for children with disabilities and special health care needs. Services include central directory, representatives of agencies, service providers, families, and coordinators of infant, toddler, and preschool special education programs.

Susan Ord, Infant/Toddler Program Coordinator

8057 Computer Center for Citizens with Disabilities
UT Center for Assistive Technology
1595 W 500 Street
Salt Lake City, UT 84104

801-887-9533
888-866-5550
Fax: 801-887-9382
e-mail: cboogaar@usoe.k12.ut.us
www.usor.utah.gov/ucat/computers

Technology group of parents, consumers and professionals; provides resources to help children and adults who have disabilities gain access to the benefits of technology. Includes nationwide network of community-based assistive technology, resource centers, hands on consultants and product demonstrations.

8058 Special Education Services Unit
250 E 500 S
Salt Lake City, UT 84111

801-538-7708
Fax: 801-538-7991
e-mail: Brenda.Broadbent@usoe.k12.ut.us
www.nectas.unc.edu

Individuals with Disabilities Education Act requires all states and territories to provide early intervention and preschool special education for children with disabilities and special health care needs. Services include central directory, representatives of agencies, service providers, families, and coordinators of infant, toddler, and preschool special education programs.

Brenda Broadbent, Preschool Special Ed. Coordiantor

8059 US Disabled Ski Team
Box 100
Park City, UT 84060

435-649-9090
Fax: 435-649-3613
e-mail: info@usaa.org

State assisted programs and support group information for people of many abilities. Includes local chapters, referrals, fun and social interaction and support groups.

8060 Utah Center for Assistive Technology
Center for Persons with Disabilities
UMC 6855
Logan, UT 84322

801-797-1982
Fax: 801-797-2355
TDD: 801-797-2096
e-mail: sharon@cpo2.usu.edu

State assisted programs and support group information for people of many abilities. Includes local chapters, referrals, fun and social interaction and support groups.

8061 Utah Parent Center
2290 E 4500 S, Suite 110
Salt Lake City, UT 84117

801-272-1051
800-468-1160
Fax: 801-272-8907
e-mail: upc@inconnect.com
www.parentcenter.org

Parent Training and Information (PTI) programs help parents to understand their children's specific needs, communicate more effectively with professionals, participate in the educational planning process, and obtain information about relevant programs, services and resources. Offers free written materials, workshops, individual consultations, newsletter, statewide volunteer network, parent to parent support.

Helen Post, Director

Vermont

8062 Assistive Technology Project
103 S Main Street, Weeks Building, 1st Floor
Waterbury, VT 05671

Fax: 802-241-2174
TTY: 802-241-2620
TDD: 801-797-2096
e-mail: lynnec@dad.state.vt.us
www.uvm.edu/uapvt/cats.html

State assisted programs and support group information for people of many abilities. Includes local chapters, referrals, fun and social interaction and support groups.

8063 Center on Disabilities and Community Inclusion
101 Cherry Street, Suite 450
Burlington, VT 05401

802-656-4031
Fax: 802-656-1357
TDD: 802-656-4031
e-mail: ccloning@zoo.uvm.edu
www.uvm.edu/~cdci

In collaboration with individuals with disabilities, their families and communities, will promote the independence, inclusion, participation and personal choice of individuals with disabilities of all ages in all environments through the development and enhancement of culturally sensitive, responsive services and supports, interdisciplinary training, technical assistance, exemplary service models, research, dissemination of information and advocacy for the legal and civil rights of the disabled.

Chigee Cloninger, Executive Director

8064 Family, Infant, and Toddler Project
208 Colchester Avenue
Burlington, VT 05405

802-656-8112
Fax: 802-656-1357
e-mail: bmccar@vdh.state.vt.us
www.nectas.unc.edu

Individuals with Disabilities Education Act requires all states and territories to provide early intervention and preschool special education for children with disabilities and special health care needs. Services include central directory, representatives of agencies, service providers, families, and coordinators of infant, toddler, and preschool special education programs.

Beverly MacCarty, Infant/Toddler Program Coordinator

8065 Special Education Unit
120 State Street
Montpelier, VT 05620

802-828-5115
Fax: 802-828-3140
e-mail: kandrews@doe.state.vt.us
www.nectas.unc.edu

Individuals with Disabilities Education Act requires all states and territories to provide early intervention and preschool special education for children with disabilities and special health care needs. Services include central directory, representatives of agencies, service providers, families, and coordinators of infant, toddler, and preschool special education programs.

Kathy Andrews, Preschool Special Ed. Coordinator

8066 Vermont Parent Information Center
600 Blair Park Road, Suite 301
Williston, VT 05495

802-658-5315
800-639-7170
Fax: 802-658-5395
TDD: 802-658-5315
e-mail: vpic@vtpic.com
www.vtpic.com

Dedicated to increasing and expanding educational and developmental opportunities that improve the quality of life for children with special needs and their families. We believe that we can achieve this goal only when we provide families with the chance to build on their own strengths, and to feel respected for their values and beliefs.

Connie Curtain, Executive Director

Virginia

8067 Infant & Toddler Program
PO Box 1797
Richmond, VA 23218

804-371-6592
Fax: 804-371-7959
e-mail: alucas@dmhmrsas.state.va.us
www.nectas.unc.edu

Provides early intervention and preschool special education for children with disabilities and special health care needs. Services include central directory, representatives of agencies, service providers, families, and coordinators of infant, toddler, and preschool special education programs.

Anne Lucas, Infant/Toddler Program Coordinator

8068 Office of Special Education, Virginia
101 N 14th Street
Richmond, VA 23219

804-225-2675
Fax: 804-371-8796
e-mail: prnondak@mail.vak12ed.edu
www.pen.k12.va.us

Individuals with Disabilities Education Act requires all states and territories to provide early intervention and preschool special education for children with disabilities and special health care needs. Services include central directory, representatives of agencies and coordinators preschool special education programs.

Phyllis Mondak, Preschool Special Ed. Coordinator

8069 Parent Educational Advocacy Training Cente r
2922 West Marshall Street
Richmond, VA 23230

703-923-0010
800-869-6782
Fax: 800-693-3514
TDD: 703-923-0010
e-mail: partners@peatc.org
www.peatc.org

Parent Training and Information (PTI) programs help parents to understand their children's specific needs, communicate more effectively with professionals, participate in the educational planning process, and obtain information about relevant programs, services and resources.

Cheryl Takemoto, Executive Director
Suzanne Wolfe, Director Programs & Operations

8070 Tidewater Center for Technology Access
1413 Laskin Road
Virginia Beach, VA 23451

757-437-6524
Fax: 757-474-6540
e-mail: tcta@aol.com.vi
www.tcta.ataccess.org

Technology group of parents, consumers and professionals; provides resources to help children and adults who have disabilities gain access to the benefits of technology. Includes nationwide net-

work of community-based assistive technology, resource centers, hands on consultants and product demonstrations.

8071 Virginia Assistive Technology System
8004 Franklin Farms Drive
PO Box K300
Richmond, VA 23288

804-662-9990
800-552-5019
Fax: 804-662-9478
TTY: 757-662-9990
e-mail: vatskhk@aol.com
www.vats.org

State assisted programs and support group information for people of many abilities. Includes local chapters, referrals, fun and social interaction and support groups.

Washington

8072 Infant Toddler Early Intervention Program
640 Woodland Square Loop, SE
Olympia, WA 98504

360-725-3516
Fax: 360-725-3523
e-mail: LoereSK@dshs.wa.govt
www.nectas.unc.edu

Early intervention and preschool special education for children with disabilities and special health care needs. Services include central directory, representatives of agencies, service providers, families, and coordinators of infant, toddler, and preschool special education programs.

Sandy Loerch, Infant/Toddler Program Coordinator

8073 Office of the Superintendent of Public Instruction
PO Box 47200
Olympia, WA 98504

360-753-0317
Fax: 360-586-0247
e-mail: ashureen@inspire.ospi.wednet.edu
www.nectas.unc.edu

Services include central directory, representatives of agencies, service providers, families, and coordinators of infant, toddler, and preschool special education programs.

Anne Shureen, Preschool Special Ed. Coordinator

8074 Washington Leukemia and Lymphoma Society Alaska Chapter
Leukemia Society of America
530 Dexter Avenue North, Suite 300
Seattle, WA 98109

206-628-0777
888-345-4572
Fax: 206-292-9791
www.leukemia-lymphoma.org

Dedicated to finding cures for leukemia and related cancers and to improving the quality of life for patients and their families.

Kathryn Bennett, Executive Director

8075 Washington PAVE
6316 S 12th Street
Tacoma, WA 98465

253-565-2266
800-572-7368
Fax: 253-566-8052
TTY: 800-572-7368
e-mail: wapave9@washingtonpave.org
www.washingtonpave.org

Parent Training and Information (PTI) programs help parents to understand their children's specific needs, communicate more effectively with professionals, participate in the educational planning process, and obtain information about relevant programs, services and resources.

Joanna S Butts, Executive Director

West Virginia

8076 Early Intervention Program
350 Capitol Street, Room 427
Charleston, WV 25301

304-558-1069
Fax: 304-558-2866
www.nectas.unc.edu

Individuals with Disabilities Education Act requires all states and territories to provide early intervention and preschool special education for children with disabilities and special health care needs. Services include central directory, representatives of agencies, service providers, families, and coordinators of infant, toddler, and preschool special education programs.

Pam Roush, Infant/Toddler Program Coordinator

8077 Office of Special Education Administration
1900 Kawanha Boulevard E
Charleston, WV 25305

304-558-2696
Fax: 304-558-3741
e-mail: pcarte@access.k12.wv.us
www.nectas.unc.edu

Individuals with Disabilities Education Act requires all states and territories to provide early intervention and preschool special education for children with disabilities and special health care needs. Services include central directory, representatives of agencies, service providers, families, and coordinators of infant, toddler, and preschool special education programs.

Ginger Huffman, Preschool Special Ed. Coordinator

8078 West Virginia Assistive Technology System
Airport Research and Office Park
955 Hartman Run Road
Morgantown, WV 26505

800-841-8436
Fax: 304-293-7294
TDD: 304-293-4692
e-mail: stewiat@wvnvm.wvnet.edu

State assisted programs and support group information for people of many abilities. Includes local chapters, referrals, fun and social interaction and support groups.

8079 West Virginia Parent Training and Information
371 Broaddus Avenue
Clarksburg, WV 26301

304-624-1436
Fax: 304-624-1438
e-mail: WVPTI@aol.com
www.taalliance.org/ptis/wv/index.htm

Parent Training and Information (PTI) programs help parents to understand their children's specific needs, communicate more effectively with professionals, participate in the educational planning process, and obtain information about relevant programs, services and resources.

Wisconsin

8080 Birth to 3 Program
1 West Wilson St, Room 418, PO Box 7851
Madisonton, WI 53370

608-266-7469
Fax: 608-261-6752
e-mail: kremema@dhfs.state.wi.us
www.nectas.unc.edu

Early intervention and preschool special education for children with disabilities and special health care needs. Services include central directory, representatives of agencies, service providers, families, and coordinators of infant, toddler, and preschool special education programs.

Mitchell Kremer, Infant/Toddler Program Coordinator

8081 Development and Training Center
2125 3rd Street
Eau Circle, WI 54703

715-833-7755
Fax: 715-833-7757
www.nectas.unc.edu

Individuals with Disabilities Education Act requires all states and territories to provide early intervention and preschool special education for children with disabilities and special health care needs. Services include central directory, representatives of agencies, service providers, families, and coordinators of infant, toddler, and preschool special education programs.

Stacy H Wigfield, Interagency Coordinating Council

8082 Division of Community Services
1 Wilson Street, Room 418, PO Box 7851
Madison, WI 53707

608-267-3270
Fax: 608-267-6752
dhfs.wisconsin.gov/bdds/birthto3

Individuals with Disabilities Education Act requires all states and territories to provide early intervention and preschool special education for children with disabilities and special health care needs. Services include central directory, representatives of agencies, service providers, families, and coordinators of infant, toddler, and preschool special education programs.

Beth Wroblewski, Preschool Special Ed. Coordinator

8083 Early Childhood Handicapped Prgrams
PO Box 7841
Madison, WI 53707

608-267-9172
Fax: 608-267-3746
e-mail: langejr@mail.state.wi.us
www.nectas.unc.edu

Services include central directory, representatives of agencies, service providers, families, and coordinators of infant, toddler, and preschool special education programs.

Jenny Lange, Preschool Special Ed. Coordinator

8084 Parent Education Project of Wisconsin
2192 S 60th Street
West Allis, WI 53219

414-328-5520
Fax: 414-328-5530
TDD: 414-328-5520
e-mail: pmcolletti@aol.com
www.members.aol.com/pepofwi

Parent Training and Information (PTI) programs help parents to understand their children's specific needs, communicate more effectively with professionals, participate in the educational planning process, and obtain information about relevant programs, services and resources.

8085 WisTech
1 West Wilson Street, Room 951, PO Box 7851
Madison, WI 53707

608-266-8905
Fax: 608-267-3203
TTY: 608-267-9880
dhfs.wisconsin.gov/disablilities

State assisted programs and support group information for people of many abilities. Includes local chapters, referrals, fun and social interaction and support groups.

Wyoming

8086 Division of Developmental Disabilities
6101 Yellowstone Road
Cheyenne, WY 82002

307-777-7115
Fax: 307-777-3337
www.nectas.unc.edu

Provides early intervention and preschool special education for children with disabilities and special health care needs. Services include central directory, representatives of agencies, service providers, families, and coordinators of infant, toddler, and preschool special education programs.

Mitch Brauchie, Interagency Coordinating Council

8087 Parent Information Center
5 N Lobban
Buffalo, WY 82834

307-684-2277
Fax: 307-684-5314
TDD: 307-684-2277
e-mail: tdawsonpic@vci.com
www.taalliance.org

Parent Training and Information (PTI) programs help parents to understand their children's specific needs, communicate more effectively with professionals, participate in the educational planning process, and obtain information about relevant programs, services and resources.

8088 Special Education Unit
2300 Cheyenne Avenue, 2nd Floor
Cheyenne, WY 82002

307-777-6236
Fax: 307-777-6234
e-mail: smofie@educ.state.wy.uss
www.nectas.unc.edu

Individuals with Disabilities Education Act requires all states and territories to provide early intervention and preschool special education for children with disabilities and special health care needs. Services include central directory, representatives of agencies, service providers, families, and coordinators of infant, toddler, and preschool special education programs.

Sara Mofield, Preschool Special Ed. Coordinator

8089 Wyoming's New Options in Technology (WYNOT)
University of Wyoming
1000 East University Avenue
Laramie, WY 82072

307-766-2084
Fax: 307-721-2084
TTY: 800-861-4312
e-mail: wynot.uw@uwyo.edu
www.uwyo.edu/wynot

State assisted programs and support group information for people of many abilities. Includes local chapters, referrals, fun and social interaction and support groups.

Libraries & Resource Centers

Arizona

8090 Special Needs Center/Phoenix Public Library
12 E McDowell Road
Phoenix, AZ 85004

602-261-8690
e-mail: choh@lib.ci.phoenix.az.us
www.ci.phonix.az.us

Offers talking books and records, braille books and magazines, large print books, video print enlarger, video magnifier and VersaBraille software with synthetic speech for the blind, visually handicapped, physically/mentally handicapped and speech and hearing impaired children and adults.

Mary Roatch, Supervisor

8091 Technology Access Center of Tucson
PO Box 13178
Tucson, AZ 85732

520-745-5588
Fax: 520-790-7637
e-mail: tactaz@aol.com

Technology group of parents, consumers and professionals; provides resources to help children and adults who have disabilities gain access to the benefits of technology. Includes nationwide net-

work of community-based assistive technology, resource centers, hands on consultants and product demonstrations.

Arkansas

8092 Arkansas Easter Seals Technology Resource Center
3920 Woodland Heights Road
Little Rock, AR 72212

501-227-3602
Fax: 501-227-3601
e-mail: atrce@aol.com
www.arkeasterseals.org

Technology group of parents, consumers and professionals; provides resources to help children and adults who have disabilities gain access to the benefits of technology. Includes nationwide network of community-based assistive technology, resource centers, hands on consultants and product demonstrations.

8093 Crowley Ridge Regional Library
315 W Oak
Jonesboro, AR 72401

870-935-5133

Offers a children's summer reading program, large print and books on cassette.

Ruth Ball

8094 Educational Services for the Visually Impaired
PO Box 668
Little Rock, AR 72203

501-371-5710

Offers textbooks, braille books and more to the visually impaired grades K-12 in the Arizona area.

David Beavers, Director

8095 Library for the Blind and Handicapped, Southwest
PO Box 668
Magnolia, AR 71754

870-234-0399
Fax: 870-234-5077
e-mail: lbph@hotmail.com

Offers a children's summer reading program and a book collection featuring discs and casettes.

Susan Walker, Librarian

California

8096 Alliance for Technology Access (ATA)
1304 Southpoint Boulevard, Suite 240
Petaluma, CA 94954

707-778-3011
Fax: 707-765-2080
TDD: 707-778-3015
e-mail: atainfo@ataccess.org
www.ataccess.org

Technology group of parents, consumers and professionals; provides resources to help children and adults who have disabilities gain access to the benefits of technology. Includes nationwide network of community-based assistive technology, resource centers, hands on consultants and product demonstrations.

Mary Lester, Executive Director

8097 Assistive Technology Center Simi Valley Hospital
Rehabilatation Unit North
PO Box 1325
Simi Valley, CA 93062

805-582-1881
Fax: 805-582-2855
e-mail: dssacca@aol.com

Technology group of parents, consumers and professionals; provides resources to help children and adults who have disabilities gain access to the benefits of technology. Includes nationwide network of community-based assistive technology, resource centers, hands on consultants and product demonstrations.

8098 Center for Accessible Technology
2547 8th Street, 112-A
Berkeley, CA 94710

510-841-3224
Fax: 510-841-7956
TDD: 510-841-5621
e-mail: info@cforat.org
www.cforat.org

Provides resources to help children and adults who have disabilities gain access to the benefits of technology.

8099 Clearinghouse for Specialized Media and Technology (CSMT)
California Department of Education
1430 N Street, Suite 3207
Sacramento, CA 95814

916-445-5103
Fax: 916-323-9732
e-mail: rbrawley@cde.ca.gov
http://csmt.cde.ca.gov

Assists California schools and students in the identification and acquisition of textbooks, reference books and study materials in aural media, braille, large print and electronic media access technology.

Rod Brawley, Manager

8100 Sacramento Center for Assistive Technology
701 Howe Avenue, Suite E-5
Sacramento, CA 95825

916-927-7228
e-mail: scatca@quicknet.com
www.quicknet.com/~scat

Technology group of parents, consumers and professionals; provides resources to help children and adults who have disabilities gain access to the benefits of technology. Includes nationwide network of community-based assistive technology, resource centers, hands on consultants and product demonstrations.

District of Columbia

8101 Georgetown University Child Development Center
3307 M Street NW
Washington, DC 20007

202-687-8635
Fax: 202-687-8899

8102 HEATH Resource Center
1 DuPont Circle, Suite 800
Washington, DC 20036

920-939-9320
800-544-3284
Fax: 202-833-5696
TTY: 202-939-9320
e-mail: heath@ace.nche.edu
www.HEATH-Resource-Center.org

Dan Gardner, Information Specialist

Florida

8103 Center for Independence Technology and Education, (CITE)
215 E New Hampshire Street
Orlando, FL 32804

407-898-2483
Fax: 407-895-5255
e-mail: comcite@aol.com

Technology group of parents, consumers and professionals; provides resources to help children and adults who have disabilities gain access to the benefits of technology. Includes nationwide network of community-based assistive technology, resource centers, hands on consultants and product demonstrations.

8104 University of Miami, Mailman Center for Child Development
1601 NW 12th Avenue
Miami, FL 33136

305-243-6631
Fax: 305-284-4911
pediatrics.med.miami.edu/mccd1

Focuses on birth defects and children's illnesses.

Dr. Robert Stempfel, Jr, Director

8105 West Florida Regional Library
200 W Gregory Street
Pensacola, FL 32501

850-436-5065
Fax: 850-436-5039
TDD: 850-435-1763
e-mail: tlambert@ci.pensacola.fl.us
www.ocls.lib.fl.us/Site/TalkingBooks.html

Offers children's print/braille books.

Tamatha Lambert, Librarian

Georgia

8106 Augusta-Richmond County Public Library
425 9th Street
Augusta, GA 30901

706-821-2625
Fax: 706-724-5403
e-mail: talkbook@mail.richmond.public.lib.ga.us
www.scescape.net/~ecgrl/lbph.htm

Discs, cassettes, braille writer, films, large print books, summer reading program, magnifiers and reference materials on blindness and other handicaps.

Gary Swint, Librarian

8107 Gainesville Subregional LBPH Hall County Public Library
2434 Old Cornelia Highway
Gainesville, GA 30507

770-531-2500
Fax: 770-531-2502
TDD: 770-531-2530
e-mail: kevans@mail.hall.public.lib.ga.us
www.hall.public.lib.ga.us/ehmap.htm#program

Summer reading programs, braille writer, magnifiers, closed-circuit TV, large-print photocopier, cassette books and magazines, children's books on cassette, home visits and other reference materials on blindness and other handicaps.

Kathy Evans, Librarian

8108 La Fayette Subregional Library for the Blind and Physically Disabled
305 S Duke Street
La Fayette, GA 30728

706-638-2992
Fax: 706-638-4028
e-mail: stubblec@mail.walker.public.lib.ga.us
www.walker.public.lib.ga.us

Summer reading programs, braille writer, magnifiers, closed-circuit TV, large-print photocopier, cassette books and magazines, children's books on cassette, home visits and other reference materials on blindness and other handicaps.

Charles Stubblefield, Librarian

8109 Macon Subregional Library for the Blind and Handicapped, Washington Memorial
1180 Washington Avenue
Macon, GA 31201

912-744-0877
800-805-7613
Fax: 912-742-3161
TDD: 912-744-0877
e-mail: shherrilr@mail.bbib.public.lib.ga.us

Summer reading programs, braille writer, magnifiers, closed-circuit TV, large-print photocopier, cassette books and magazines, children's books on cassette, home visits and other reference materials on blindness and other handicaps.

Rebecca Sherrill, Librarian

8110 Oconee Regional Library, Library for the Blind and Physically Handicapped
801 Bellevue Avenue, PO Box 100
Dublin, GA 31040

478-275-5382
Fax: 478-272-0524
TDD: 478-275-3821
www.laurens.public.lib.ga.us/lbph.htm

Summer reading programs, braille writer, magnifiers, closed-circuit TV, large-print photocopier, cassette books and magazines, children's books on cassette, home visits and other reference materials on blindness and other handicaps.

Betty Schlid, Librarian

8111 Rome Subregional Library for the Blind and Physically Handicapped
205 Riverside Parkway NE
Rome, GA 30161

706-236-4618
Fax: 706-236-4631
TDD: 706-236-4618
e-mail: dianam@mail.floyd.public.lib.ga.us
www.floyd.public.lib.ga.us/tbc.htm

Summer reading programs, braille writer, magnifiers, closed-circuit TV, large-print photocopier, cassette books and magazines, children's books on cassette, home visits and other reference materials on blindness and other handicaps.

Diana Mills, Librarian

8112 Special Needs Library of NE Georgia Athens-Clarke County Regional Library
2025 Baxter Street
Athens, GA 30606

706-613-3655
Fax: 706-613-3660
TDD: 706-613-3655
e-mail: burnsp@mail.clarke.public.lib.ga.us
www.clarke.public.lib.ga.us/tbc.htm

Discs, cassettes, large print books, reference materials on blindness, films, closed-circuit TV, magnifiers, braille writer, summer reading programs, cassette books and magazines and more.

Paige Burns, Librarian

8113 Subregional Library for the Blind and Physically Handicapped
1120 Bradley Drive
Columbus, GA 31906

706-649-0780
Fax: 706-649-1914
TDD: 706-649-0974
e-mail: barness@mail.muscogee.public.lib.ga.us

Braille writer, magnifiers, closed-circuit TV, large-print photocopier, cassette books and magazines, children's books on cassette, home visits and other reference materials on blindness and other handicaps.

Suzanne Barnes, Librarian

8114 Tech-Able
1112A Brett Drive
Conyers, GA 30094

770-922-6768
Fax: 770-922-6769
e-mail: techable@america.net
www.gatfl.org

Technology group of parents, consumers and professionals; provides resources to help children and adults who have disabilities gain access to the benefits of technology. Includes nationwide network of community-based assistive technology, resource centers, hands on consultants and product demonstrations.

Hawaii

8115 Aloha Special Technology Access Center
710 Green Street
Honolulu, HI 96813

808-523-5547
Fax: 808-536-3765
e-mail: gstachi@yahoo.com
www.geocities.com/astachi/index.html

Technology group of parents, consumers and professionals; provides resources to help children and adults who have disabilities gain access to the benefits of technology. Member of nationwide network of community-based assistive technology, resource centers, hands on consultants and product demonstrations.

8116 Library for the Blind and Physically Handicapped, Hawaii State Library
402 Kapahulu Avenue
Honolulu, HI 96815

808-733-8444
Fax: 808-733-8449
TDD: 808-733-8444
e-mail: olbcirc@state.lib.hi.us
www.hcc.hawaii.edu/hspls/oahu/lbph.html

Summer reading programs, braille writer, magnifiers, closed-circuit TV, large-print photocopier, cassette books and magazines, children's books on cassette, home visits and other reference materials on blindness and other handicaps.

Fusako Miyashiro, Librarian

Illinois

8117 Northern Illinois Center for Adaptive Technology
3615 Louisiana Road
Rockford, IL 61108

815-229-2163
Fax: 815-229-2135
e-mail: davegrass@earthlink.net
www.nicat.ataccess.org

Technology group of parents, consumers and professionals; provides resources to help children and adults who have disabilities gain access to the benefits of technology. Includes nationwide network of community based assistive technology, resource centers, hands on consultants and product demonstrations.

Dave Grass, Director

8118 Parents Alliance Employment Project
Illinois Employment and Training Center
837 S Westmore Drive
Lombard, IL 60148

630-495-4345
Fax: 630-495-0387
TDD: 630-495-6055

Information and advocacy resources for families and professionals. Includes listings of organizations providing general information and organizations focusing on more specific areas of concern to families and young adults who have disabilities.

8119 Professional Assistance Center for Education (PACE)
National-Louis University
2840 Sheridan Road
Evanston, IL 60201

847-475-1100
Fax: 847-256-5190
e-mail: cbur@evan1.nl.edu

A two-year, noncredit certification program servicing students with learning disabilities. The program provides a rare opportunity for students from all parts of the country to continue their education in an age appropriate environment. Committed to an instructional approach that integrates both group and individual teaching for career preparation, academics, life skills, and socialization. Transitional program offered to qualified graduates.

Carol Burns, Director

8120 Shawnee Library System
607 S Greenbriar Road
Carterville, IL 62918

618-985-3711
800-445-2665
Fax: 618-985-4211
e-mail: dbrawley@shawls.lib.il.us
www.shawls.lib.il.us

Lends recorded books and magazines, descriptive videos, and braille to adults and children unable to read standard print due to blindness, visual impairment, physical disablity and reading disability. Information on blindness and disabilities. Public presentations.

Diana Brawley Sussman, Director

8121 Suburban Audio Visual Service
920 Barnsdale Road
La Grange Park, IL 60526

630-352-7671

Summer reading programs, braille writer, magnifiers, closed-circuit TV, large-print photocopier, cassette books and magazines, children's books on cassette, home visits and other reference materials on blindness and other handicaps.

Leon Drolet, Jr, Librarian

Indiana

8122 Allen County Public Library
PO Box 2270
Fort Wayne, IN 46802

260-421-1200
Fax: 260-421-1386
e-mail: webmaster@acpl.lib.in.us
www.acpl.lib.in.us

Summer reading programs, braille writer, magnifiers, closed-circuit TV, large-print photocopier, cassette books and magazines, children's books on cassette, home visits and other reference materials on blindness and other handicaps.

Joyce Misner, Librarian

8123 Assistive Technology Training and Information Center
3354 Pine Hill Drive
Vincennes, IN 47591

812-886-0575
800-962-8842
Fax: 812-886-1128
TTY: 800-962-8842
e-mail: inattic2@aol.com

Informational and emotional support to parents who have a child, adolescent, or adult family member with special needs.

8124 Bartholomew County Public Library
5th at Lafayette
Columbus, IN 47201

812-379-1277
Fax: 812-379-1275

Summer reading programs, braille writer, magnifiers, closed-circuit TV, large-print photocopier, cassette books and magazines, children's books on cassette, home visits and other reference materials on blindness and other handicaps.

Wilma Perry, Librarian

8125 Elkhart Public Library
300 S 2nd Street
Elkhart, IN 46516

219-522-2665
www.elkhardt.lib.in.us

Summer reading programs, braille writer, magnifiers, closed-circuit TV, large-print photocopier, cassette books and magazines, children's books on cassette, home visits and other reference materials on blindness and other handicaps.

Pat Ciancio, Librarian

8126 Special Services Division - Indiana State Library
140 N Senate Avenue
Indianapolis, IN 46204

317-232-3684
800-622-4970
Fax: 317-232-3728
e-mail: bph@statelib.lib.in.us

Summer reading programs, braille writer, magnifiers, closed-circuit TV, braille and large print books and magazines, children's books on cassette and in braiile, and other reference materials on blindness and other handicaps.

Lissa Shanahan, Librarian
Carole Rose, Childrens/Braille Services

Kansas

8127 Kansas State Library
State Capitol Building
Topeka, KS 66612

785-296-3296
800-432-3919
Fax: 785-296-6650
e-mail: ksst16lb@ink.org
skywyas.lib.ks.us/KSL/

Summer reading programs, braille writer, magnifiers, closed-circuit TV, large-print photocopier, cassette books and magazines, children's books on cassette, home visits and other reference materials on blindness and other handicaps.

Caroline Lang, Librarian

8128 Manhattan Public Library
629 Poyntz Avenue
Manhattan, KS 66502

785-776-4741
Fax: 785-776-1545
e-mail: marionr@manhaHan.lib.ks.us

Summer reading programs, braille writer, magnifiers, closed-circuit TV, large-print photocopier, cassette books and magazines, children's books on cassette, home visits and other reference materials on blindness and other handicaps.

Lois Hartley, Librarian

8129 Prenatal Diagnostic and Genetic Center
HCA Wesley Medical Center
550 N Hillside
Wichita, KS 67214

316-688-2362

Sechin Cho, MD

8130 South Central Kansas Library System
901 N Main Street
Hutchinson, KS 67501

620-336-5441
800-234-0529
Fax: 620-663-1215
e-mail: nwks11b@ink.org
skyways.lib.ks.us/sckls/

Summer reading programs, braille writer, magnifiers, closed-circuit TV, large-print photocopier, cassette books and magazines, children's books on cassette, home visits and other reference materials on blindness and other handicaps.

Karen Socha, Librarian

8131 Technology Resource Solutions for People
1710 W Schilling Road
Salina, KS 67401

785-827-9383
800-526-9731
Fax: 785-823-2015
TDD: 785-827-9383
e-mail: trspks@midusa.net
www.occk.com/generalinfor

Technology group of parents, consumers and professionals; provides resources to help children and adults who have disabilities gain access to the benefits of technology. Includes nationwide network of community-based assistive technology, resource centers, hands on consultants and product demonstrations.

8132 Wesley Medical Research Institutes
3306 E Central
Wichita, KS 67208

316-686-7172

Respiratory and birth defects disorders research.

Dr. Sechin Cho, MD, Director

8133 Wichita Public Library
223 S Main Street
Wichita, KS 67202

316-262-0611
Fax: 316-262-4540

Summer reading programs, braille writer, magnifiers, closed-circuit TV, large-print photocopier, cassette books and magazines, children's books on cassette, home visits and other reference materials on blindness and other handicaps.

Brad Reha, Librarian

Kentucky

8134 Bluegrass Technology Center
196 Beasley Street, Suite 103A
Lexington, KY 40505

859-294-4343
800-209-7767
Fax: 859-294-0704
e-mail: office@bluegrass.org
www.bluegrass-tech.org

Technology group of parents, consumers and professionals; provides resources to help children and adults who have disabilities gain access to the benefits of technology. Includes nationwide network of community-based assistive technology, resource centers, hands on consultants and product demonstrations.

8135 EnTech: Enabling Technologies of Kentuckiana
301 York Street
Louisville, KY 40203

502-574-1637
e-mail: entech@iglou.org

Technology group of parents, consumers and professionals; provides resources to help children and adults who have disabilities gain access to the benefits of technology. Includes nationwide network of community-based assistive technology, resource centers, hands on consultants and product demonstrations.

8136 Louisville Talking Book Library
301 York Street
Louisville, KY 40203

502-574-1625
Fax: 502-574-1657
e-mail: denning@lfpl.org
lfpl.org

Summer reading programs, braille writer, magnifiers, closed-circuit TV, large-print photocopier, cassette books and magazines, children's books on cassette, home visits and other reference materials on blindness and other handicaps.

Tom Denning, Coordinator

8137 Northern Kentucky Talking Book Library
502 Scott Boulevard
Covington, KY 41011

859-962-4095
Fax: 859-962-4096
www.kenton.lib.ky.us/information/talking

Summer reading programs, braille writer, magnifiers, closed-circuit TV, large-print photocopier, cassette books and magazines, children's books on cassette, home visits and other reference materials on blindness and other handicaps.

Jama Rooney, Librarian

8138 Western Kentucky Assistive Technology Consortium
607 Poplar Street, Suite 211, PO Box 266
Murray, KY 42071

270-759-4233
Fax: 270-759-4208
e-mail: wkatc@cablecomm-ky.net

Technology group of parents, consumers and professionals; provides resources to help children and adults who have disabilities gain access to the benefits of technology. Includes nationwide network of community-based assistive technology, resource centers, hands on consultants and product demonstrations.

Louisiana

8139 Louisiana State Library
701 N 4th Street
Baton Rouge, LA 70802

225-342-4923
Fax: 225-219-8404
e-mail: sbph@pelican. state.lib.la.us
www.state.lib.la.us/thelibrary/index.htm

Summer reading programs, braille writer, magnifiers, closed-circuit TV, large-print photocopier, cassette books and magazines, children's books on cassette, home visits and other reference materials on blindness and other handicaps.

Jennifer Anjier, Librarian

8140 Louisiana State University Genetics Section of Pediatrics
1501 Kings Highway
Shreveport, LA 71130

318-675-5681

TF Thurman, MD, Director

Maine

8141 Bangor Public Library
145 Harlow Street
Bangor, ME 04401

207-947-8336
Fax: 207-945-6694
e-mail: bplill@bpl.lib.me.us
www.bpl-lib.me.us

Summer reading programs, braille writer, magnifiers, closed-circuit TV, large-print photocopier, cassette books and magazines, children's books on cassette, home visits and other reference materials on blindness and other handicaps.

Judith Leighton, Librarian

8142 Cary Library
107 Main Street
Houlton, ME 04730

207-532-1302
Fax: 207-532-4350
www.cary.lib.me.us

Summer reading programs, braille writer, magnifiers, closed-circuit TV, large-print photocopier, cassette books and magazines, children's books on cassette, home visits and other reference materials on blindness and other handicaps.

Norma Watson, Librarian

8143 Lewiston Public Library
200 Lisbon Street
Lewiston, ME 04240

207-784-0135
Fax: 207-784-3011
e-mail: webmaster@lpl.avenet.org
www.avenet.org

Summer reading programs, braille writer, magnifiers, closed-circuit TV, large-print photocopier, cassette books and magazines, children's books on cassette, home visits and other reference materials on blindness and other handicaps.

Muriel Landry, Librarian

8144 Maine State Library
64 State House Station
Augusta, ME 74333

207-287-5650
Fax: 207-287-5624
e-mail: benitad@ursus3.ursus.maine.edu

Summer reading programs, braille writer, magnifiers, closed-circuit TV, large-print photocopier, cassette books and magazines, children's books on cassette, home visits and other reference materials on blindness and other handicaps.

Benita Davis, Librarian

8146 Portland Public Library
5 Monument Square
Portland, ME 04101

207-871-1700
Fax: 207-871-1703
www.portlandlibrary.org

Summer reading programs, braille writer, magnifiers, closed-circuit TV, large-print photocopier, cassette books and magazines, children's books on cassette, home visits and other reference materials on blindness and other handicaps.

Janice Littlefield, Librarian

8147 Waterville Public Library
73 Elm Street
Waterville, ME 04901

207-872-5433
e-mail: wpl@borg.com
www.borg.com

Summer reading programs, braille writer, magnifiers, closed-circuit TV, large-print photocopier, cassette books and magazines, children's books on cassette, home visits and other reference materials on blindness and other handicaps.

Meta Vigue, Librarian

Maryland

8148 Learning Independence Through Computers
1001 Eastern Avenue, 3rd Floor
Baltimore, MD 21202

410-659-5462
Fax: 410-659-5472
e-mail: lincmd@aol.com

Technology group of parents, consumers and professionals; provides resources to help children and adults who have disabilities gain access to the benefits of technology. Includes nationwide network of community-based assistive technology, resource centers, hands on consultants and product demonstrations.

Massachusetts

8149 Resources for Rehabilitation
33 Bedford Street, Suite 19A
Lexington, MA 02420

781-862-6455
800-621-0026

Provides training and information to professionals who serve individuals with vision loss and other disabilities. Publishes a variety of resource guides on coping with visual impairment.

8150 Talking Book Library at Worcester Public Library
3 Salem Square
Worcester, MA 01608

508-799-1730
800-762-0085
Fax: 508-799-1656
TDD: 508-799-1731
e-mail: talkbook@cwmars.org
www.worcpublib.org/talkingbook

Massachusetts subregional library within the Library of Congress National Library Service for the Blind and Physically Handicapped network. Provides audiocassette books, large print books, described videos and print/braille books to registered partons. Has

adapted computers and other assistive technology for on-site use. Offers reference and referral service.

James L Izatt, Librarian

8151 Worcester Public Library
3 Salem Square
Worcester, MA 01608

508-799-1655
Fax: 508-799-1652
e-mail: jizatt@site.cwmars.org

Summer reading programs, braille writer, magnifiers, closed-circuit TV, large-print photocopier, cassette books and magazines, children's books on cassette, home visits and other reference materials on blindness and other handicaps.

James L Izatt, Librarian

Michigan

8152 Frederick Douglas Branch for Specialized Services and Physically Handicapped
3666 Grand River/Trumbull
Detroit, MI 48226

313-883-9414
Fax: 313-833-9717
TDD: 313-833-5492
www.detroit.lib.mi.us

Summer reading programs, braille writer, magnifiers, closed-circuit TV, large-print photocopier, cassette books and magazines, children's books on cassette, home visits and other reference materials on blindness and other handicaps.

Deborah Evans, Librarian

Minnesota

8153 PACER Center
8167 Normandale Boulevard
Minneapolis, MN 55437

952-838-9000
Fax: 952-838-0199
TTY: 952-838-0190
e-mail: pacer@pacer.org
www.pacer.org

Parent Training and Information (PTI) programs help parents to understand their children's specific needs, communicate more effectively with professionals, participate in the educational planning process, and obtain information about relevant programs, services and resources.

8154 Star Center for Family Health
University of Minnesota Gateway
200 Oak Street SE, Suite 160
Minneapolis, MN 55455

612-626-4260
Fax: 612-626-2134
www.peds.umn.edu/peds-adol/

Helps children, youth, and families develop new and enhanced ways of coping with stress, learn strategies for adjusting to living with a chronic illness, and discover new ways of finding health, balance and well-being.

Elizabeth Latts, MSW, Resource Coordinator

Missouri

8155 Technology Access Center
12110 Clayton Road
Saint Louis, MO 63130

314-569-8404
Fax: 314-569-8449
TTY: 314-569-8446
e-mail: mostltac@aol.com

Technology group of parents, consumers and professionals; provides resources to help children and adults who have disabilities gain access to the benefits of technology. Includes nationwide network of community-based assistive technology, resource centers, hands on consultants and product demonstrations.

8156 Whitney Library for the Blind
1445 Boonville Avenue
Springfield, MO 65802

417-862-2781
Fax: 417-862-7566
e-mail: blind@ag.org
www.gospelpublishing.com

Offers braille and cassette lending library, braille and cassette Sunday school materials for all ages, braille and cassette periodicals and resource assistance, and resources for blind children and children of blind parents.

Paul Weingariner, Director

Montana

8157 Montana State Library
1515 E 6th Avenue
Helena, MT 59601

406-444-3009
Fax: 406-444-5612
TDD: 406-444-5431

Summer reading programs, braille writer, magnifiers, closed-circuit TV, large-print photocopier, cassette books and magazines, children's books on cassette, home visits and other reference materials on blindness and other handicaps.

Sandra Jarvie, Librarian

Nebraska

8158 North Platte Public Library
120 W 4th Street
North Platte, NE 69101

308-535-8036
www.northplattechamber.com

Summer reading programs, braille writer, magnifiers, closed-circuit TV, large-print photocopier, cassette books and magazines, children's books on cassette, home visits and other reference materials on blindness and other handicaps.

Brenda Behsman, Librarian

Nevada

8159 Las Vegas-Clark County Library District
1401 E Flamingo Road
Las Vegas, NV 89119

702-507-3400
Fax: 702-507-3482
www.lvccd.org

Summer reading programs, braille writer, magnifiers, closed-circuit TV, large-print photocopier, cassette books and magazines, children's books on cassette, home visits and other reference materials on blindness and other handicaps.

Mary Anne Morton, Librarian

8160 Nevada State Library and Archives
100 N Stewart Street
Carson City, NV 89701

775-684-3360
800-922-2880
Fax: 775-684-3330
TDD: 775-687-8338
dmla.clan.lib.nv.us

Summer reading programs, braille writer, magnifiers, closed-circuit TV, large-print photocopier, cassette books and magazines, children's books on cassette, home visits and other reference materials on blindness and other handicaps.

Kevin E Putnam, Librarian

New Hampshire

8161 New Hampshire State Library
117 Pleasant Street
Concord, NH 03301

603-271-3429
e-mail: talking@lilac.nhsh.lib.nh.us
www.state.nh.us

Summer reading programs, braille writer, magnifiers, closed-circuit TV, large-print photocopier, cassette books and magazines, children's books on cassette, home visits and other reference materials on blindness and other handicaps.

Eileen Keim, Librarian

New Jersey

8162 Center for Enabling Technology
622 Route 10 W, Suite 22B
Whippany, NJ 07981

973-428-1455
Fax: 973-560-9751
TTY: 973-428-1450
e-mail: cetnj@aol.com

Technology group of parents, consumers and professionals; provides resources to help children and adults who have disabilities gain access to the benefits of technology. Includes nationwide network of community-based assistive technology, resource centers, hands on consultants and product demonstrations.

New York

8163 Institute for Basic Research in Developmental Disabilities
1050 Forest Hill Road
Staten Island, NY 10314

718-494-0600
Fax: 718-494-0837

Conducts research into neurodegenerative diseases, Alzheimer's disease, developmental disabilities, fragile X syndrome, Down syndrome, autism, epilepsy and basic science issues underlying all developmental disabilities.

Dr. Krystyna Wisniewski

8164 JGB Cassette Library International
Jewish Guild for the Blind
15 W 65th Street
New York, NY 10023

212-769-6331

Summer reading programs, braille writer, magnifiers, closed-circuit TV, large-print photocopier, cassette books and magazines, children's books on cassette, home visits and other reference materials on blindness and other handicaps.

Bruce Massis

8165 Keren-Or Jerusalem Center for Multi- Handicapped Blind Children
350 7th Avenue, Suite 200
New York, NY 10010

212-279-4070
Fax: 212-279-4043
e-mail: info@keren-or.org
www.keren-or.org

Center houses and cares for over 85 resident and day students who in addition to blindness or very low vision suffer from other severe physical and or mental disabilities. Provides training in daily living skills, as well as therapy, rehabilitation and education. Funds aquired through government stipends, contributions, bequests and legacies. Keren-OR is an IRS 501(C)(3) tax exempt organization.

Dr. Edward L Steinburg, Chairman
Dr. Albert Hornblass, President

8166 Nassau Library System
900 Jerusalem Avenue
Uniondale, NY 11553

516-292-8920
Fax: 516-481-4777
e-mail: nls@lilrc.org

Summer reading programs, braille writer, magnifiers, closed-circuit TV, large-print photocopier, cassette books and magazines, children's books on cassette, home visits and other reference materials on blindness and other handicaps.

Dorothy Pruyear, Librarian

8167 Techspress Resource Center for Independent Living
401-409 Columbia Street, PO Box 210
Utica, NY 13503

315-797-4642
Fax: 315-797-4747
e-mail: lana.gossin@rcil.com

Technology group of parents, consumers and professionals; provides resources to help children and adults who have disabilities gain access to the benefits of technology. Includes nationwide network of community-based assistive technology, resource centers, hands on consultants and product demonstrations.

North Carolina

8168 Carolina Computer Access Center
401 E 9th Street
Charlotte, NC 28202

704-342-3004
Fax: 704-342-1513
e-mail: ccacnc@aol.com
ccac.ataccess.org

Enabling individuals with disabilities to control and direct their own lives by providing information about demonstrations of, and access to assistive technology tools.

Linda Schilling, Executive Director

Ohio

8169 Blick Clinic for Developmental Disabilities
640 W Market Street
Akron, OH 44303

330-762-5425
Fax: 330-762-4019
e-mail: blickclinic@blickclinic.com
www.blickclinic.com

Dr. Jane Holan

8170 Cleveland Public Library
325 Superior Avenue N.E.
Cleveland, OH 44114

216-623-2800
Fax: 216-623-7015
e-mail: lbphmgr1@library.cpl.org
www.cpl.org

Summer reading programs, braille writer, magnifiers, closed-circuit TV, large-print photocopier, cassette books and magazines, children's books on cassette, home visits and other reference materials on blindness and other handicaps.

Barbara Mates, Librarian

8171 Ohio Regional Library for the Blind and Physically Handicapped
800 Vine Street, Library Square
Cincinnati, OH 45202

513-369-6999
Fax: 513-369-3111
TDD: 513-369-6072

Summer reading programs, braille writer, magnifiers, closed-circuit TV, large-print photocopier, cassette books and magazines, children's books on cassette, home visits and other reference materials on blindness and other handicaps.

Donna Foust, Librarian

8172 Technology Resource Center
1133 Edwin C. Moses Boulevard, #370
Dayton, OH 45408

937-461-3305
Fax: 937-461-6304
TDD: 937-236-6110
e-mail: trcdoh@aol.com
www.trcd.org

Technology group of parents, consumers and professionals; provides resources to help children and adults who have disabilities gain access to the benefits of technology. Includes nationwide network of community-based assistive technology, resource centers, hands on consultants and product demonstrations.

Kevin Leonard, Coordinator
Judy Havens, Community Based Rehab Technologist

Oklahoma

8173 Oklahoma Library for the Blind & Physically Handicapped
300 NE 18th Street
Oklahoma City, OK 73105

405-521-3514
Fax: 405-521-4582
e-mail: olbph@oltn.odl.state.ok.us
www.state.ok.us/library

Summer reading programs, braille writer, magnifiers, closed-circuit TV, large-print photocopier, cassette books and magazines, children's books on cassette, home visits and other reference materials on blindness and other handicaps.

Geraldine Adams, Director

8174 Tulsa City-County Library System
400 Civic Center
Tulsa, OK 74103

918-596-7977
www.tulsalibrary.org

Summer reading programs, braille writer, magnifiers, closed-circuit TV, large-print photocopier, cassette books and magazines, children's books on cassette, home visits and other reference materials on blindness and other handicaps.

Ellen Ontko, Librarian

Oregon

8175 Oregon State Library
250 Winter Street NW
Salem, OR 97310

503-378-4243
Fax: 503-588-7119
TDD: 503-378-4276
e-mail: mary.c.mohr@state.or.us

Summer reading programs, braille writer, magnifiers, closed-circuit TV, large-print photocopier, cassette books and magazines, children's books on cassette, home visits and other reference materials on blindness and other handicaps.

Mary Mohr, Librarian

Pennsylvania

8176 Free Library of Philadelphia
1901 Vine Street
Philadelphia, PA

215-686-5322
e-mail: flpblind@library.phila.gov
www.library.phila.gov

Summer reading programs, braille writer, magnifiers, closed-circuit TV, large-print photocopier, cassette books and magazines, children's books on cassette, home visits and other reference materials on blindness and other handicaps.

Vickie Lange Collins, Librarian

8177 Library for the Blind & Physically Handicapped, Leonard C. Staisey Building
Carnegie Library of Pittsburgh
4724 Baum Boulevard
Pittsburgh, PA 15213

412-687-2440
800-242-0586
Fax: 412-687-2442
e-mail: clbph@clpgh.org
www.clpgh.org/clp/lbph

Provides on loan recorded books and magazines, large print books, and described videos to Western Pennsylvania residents unable to use standard printed materials due to visual, physically-based reading disabilities. Also loans special cassette and disc machines; does not loan equipment to play described videos. Information about disabilities and related agencies is also available.

Sue Murdock, Agency Head
Kathleen Kappel, Assistant Agency Head

Rhode Island

8178 TechACCESS of Rhode Island
100 Jefferson Boulevard
Warwick, RI 02888

401-463-0202
800-916-8324
Fax: 401-463-3433
TTY: 401-273-0202
e-mail: techaccess@techaccess-ri.org
www.trcd.org

Technology group of parents, consumers and professionals; provides resources to help children and adults who have disabilities gain access to the benefits of technology. Includes nationwide network of community-based assistive technology, resource centers, hands on consultants and product demonstrations.

South Carolina

8179 Family Connection of South Carolina
2712 Middleburg Drive, Suite 103-B
Columbia, SC 29204

803-252-0914
800-578-8750
Fax: 803-799-8017
e-mail: famconn@mindspring.org

Support network for parents of children with disabilities and/or chronic illness. Veteran parents offer support to parents who are just learning of their child's diagnosis. Offers support and insight into parenting a child with special needs, as well as referrals to trained veteran parents.

8180 South Carolina State Library
P.O. Box 11469
Columbia, SC 29211

803-734-8666
Fax: 803-734-8676
TDD: 803-734-7298
e-mail: guynell@leo.scsl.state.sc.us
www.state.sc.us.

Summer reading programs, braille writer, magnifiers, closed-circuit TV, large-print photocopier, cassette books and magazines, children's books on cassette, home visits and other reference materials on blindness and other handicaps.

Guynell Williams, Librarian

South Dakota

8181 South Dakota State Library
800 Governors Drive
Pierre, SD 57501

605-773-3131
Fax: 605-773-4950
TDD: 605-773-4950
e-mail: darn@stlib.state.sd.us

Summer reading programs, braille writer, magnifiers, closed-circuit TV, large-print photocopier, cassette books and magazines, children's books on cassette, home visits and other reference materials on blindness and other handicaps.

Daniel Boyd, Librarian

Tennessee

8182 East Tennessee Technology Access Center
4918 N Broadway
Knoxville, TN 37918

865-219-0130
Fax: 865-219-0137
e-mail: etstactn@aol.com
www.discoveret.org/ettac

Assistive technology group of parents, consumers and professionals; provides resources to help children and adults who have disabilities gain access to the benefits of technology. Includes nationwide network of community-based assistive technology, resource centers, hands on consultants and product demonstrations.

Dr Lois Symington, Executive Director
Alice Wershing, Educational Technology Coordinator

8183 Saint Jude Children's Research Hospital
332 N Lauderdale Street
Memphis, TN 38101

901-495-3300

Texas

8184 Baylor College of Medicine Birth Defects Center
One Baylor Plaza
Houston, TX 77030

713-798-4951
www.bcm.tmc.edu

Frank Greenberg, MD, Director

8185 Texas State Library
PO Box 12927
Austin, TX 78711

512-463-5460
Fax: 512-463-5436
TDD: 512-463-5449
e-mail: dale.propp@tsl.state.tx.us

Summer reading programs, braille writer, magnifiers, closed-circuit TV, large-print photocopier, cassette books and magazines, children's books on cassette, home visits and other reference materials on blindness and other handicaps.

Dale Propp, Librarian

Utah

8186 Utah State Library Commission
2150 S 300 W
Salt Lake City, UT 84115

801-468-6789

Summer reading programs, braille writer, magnifiers, closed-circuit TV, large-print photocopier, cassette books and magazines, children's books on cassette, home visits and other reference materials on blindness and other handicaps.

Gerald Buttars, Librarian

Vermont

8187 Vermont Department of Libraries
Box 1870, RD #4
Montpelier, VT 05602

802-828-3273
Fax: 802-828-2199
e-mail: ssu@dol.state.vt.us

Summer reading programs, braille writer, magnifiers, closed-circuit TV, large-print photocopier, cassette books and magazines, children's books on cassette, home visits and other reference materials on blindness and other handicaps.

S Francis Woods, Librarian

Virginia

8188 Arlington County Department of Libraries
1015 N Quincy Street
Arlington, VA 22201

703-228-5990
Fax: 703-228-5962
TDD: 703-358-6320
www.co.arlington.va.us/lib/

Summer reading programs, braille writer, magnifiers, closed-circuit TV, large-print photocopier, cassette books and magazines, children's books on cassette, home visits and other reference materials on blindness and other handicaps.

Roxanne Barnes, Librarian

8189 ERIC Clearinghouse on Disabilities and Gifted Education
1110 N Glebe Road
Arlington, VA 22201

703-264-9474
800-328-0272
Fax: 703-620-2521
TTY: 703-264-9449
e-mail: ericec@cec.speed.org
ericec.org

Offers educational materials and bibliographic information on topics such as ADD, gifted, behavior disorders, early childhood, inclusion and learning.

Susan Elting

8190 Fairfax County Public Library
12000 Government Center Parkway
Fairfax, VA 22035

703-324-3100
Fax: 703-222-5921
TDD: 703-660-8524
e-mail: sjapikse@leo.vsla.edu
www.co.fairfax.va.us/library/defaylt

Summer reading programs, braille writer, magnifiers, closed-circuit TV, large-print photocopier, cassette books and magazines, children's books on cassette, home visits and other reference materials on blindness and other handicaps.

Jeanette Studley, Librarian

8191 Newport News Public Library System
112 Main Street
Newport News, VA 23601

757-591-4821
Fax: 757-591-7425
e-mail: shalswin@leo.vsla.edu

Summer reading programs, braille writer, magnifiers, closed-circuit TV, large-print photocopier, cassette books and magazines, children's books on cassette, home visits and other reference materials on blindness and other handicaps.

Sue Balswin, Librarian

8192 Roanoke City Public Library System
2607 Salem Turnpike NW
Roanoke, VA 24017

540-853-2648
Fax: 540-853-1030

Summer reading programs, braille writer, magnifiers, closed-circuit TV, large-print photocopier, cassette books and magazines, children's books on cassette, home visits and other reference materials on blindness and other handicaps.

Rebecca Cooper, Librarian

8193 Virginia Beach Public Library
930 Independence Boulevard
Virginia Beach, VA 23455

757-523-9452
Fax: 757-523-9452

Summer reading programs, braille writer, magnifiers, closed-circuit TV, large-print photocopier, cassette books and magazines, children's books on cassette, home visits and other reference materials on blindness and other handicaps.

Susan Head, Librarian

West Virginia

8194 Cabell County Public Library
455 9th Street
Huntington, WV 25701

304-528-5700
Fax: 304-528-5701
e-mail: tbooks@cabell.libwv.us

Summer reading programs, braille writer, magnifiers, Arkenstone reader/scanner, cassette books and magazines, children's books on cassette, home visits and other reference materials on blindness and other handicaps.

Donna Cushman, Talking Books Coordinator

8195 Kanawha County Public Library
123 Capitol Street
Charleston, WV 25301

304-558-2323
Fax: 304-348-6530

Summer reading programs, braille writer, magnifiers, closed-circuit TV, large-print photocopier, cassette books and magazines, children's books on cassette, home visits and other reference materials on blindness and other handicaps.

Dixie Smith, Librarian

8196 West Virginia Library Commission
1900 Kanawha Boulevard E
Charleston, WV 25305

304-340-2041
800-642-9021
Fax: 304-558-2044
e-mail: fesenmf@mars.wrlc.wvnet.edu
librarycommission.lib.wv.us

Summer reading programs, braille writer, magnifiers, closed-circuit TV, large-print photocopier, cassette books and magazines, children's books on cassette, home visits and other reference materials on blindness and other handicaps.

Francis Fesenmainer, Librarian

Wisconsin

8197 Brown County Library
515 Pine Street
Green Bay, WI 54301

920-448-4400
www.co.brown.wi.us

Summer reading programs, braille writer, magnifiers, closed-circuit TV, large-print photocopier, cassette books and magazines, children's books on cassette, home visits and other reference materials on blindness and other handicaps.

Angela Basten, Librarian

Research Centers

8198 Association for Research of Childhood Cancer
PO Box 251
Buffalo, NY 14225

716-681-4433

A nonprofit organization staffed by volunteers and formed in 1971 by parents who had lost children to pediatric cancer. Chapter members raise funds by various projects in order to provide seed money to various pediatric research centers in order to find a cure and, ultimately, prevent the types of cancers that attack children.

8199 Baylor College of Medicine Birth Defects Center
6621 Fannin Street
Houston, TX 77030

713-770-3013
Fax: 713-770-4294

Frank Greenberg, MD, Director

8200 Children's Cancer Research Institute
University of Texas Health Science Ctr
8403 Floyd Curl Drive
San Antonio, TX 78229

210-562-9000
Fax: 210-562-9014
e-mail: chessher@uthscsa.edu
ccri.uthscsa.edu

A specialized cancer research center established by the largest single oncology endowment of $200 million from Texas' tobacco settlement. Through discovery, development and dissemination of scientific knowledge relevant to childhood cancer, the overall aim of the CCRI is to impact cancer at all ages.

Sharon Murphy MD, Director
Bill Chessher, Administrator

8201 Computer Access Center
5901 Green Valley Circle, Suite 320
Culver City, CA 90230

310-338-1597
Fax: 310-338-9318
e-mail: cac@cac.org
www.cac.org

Includes nationwide network of community-based assistive technology, resource centers, hands on consultants and product demonstrations.

8202 Division for Research (CEC-DR)
Council for Exceptional Children
1920 Association Drive
Reston, VA 20191

703-620-3660
Fax: 703-264-9474
TTY: 703-264-9446
www.cec.spec.org

Devoted to the advancement of research related to the education of individuals with disabilities and/or who are gifted. Members include university, public, and private school teachers, researchers, administrators, psychologists, speech/language clinicians, parents of children with special learning needs.

8203 Division of Birth Defects and Genetic Diseases
4770 Buford Highway
Chamblee, GA 30341

770-488-7150
Fax: 770-488-7156

Muin J Khoury, MD

8204 Early Intervention Research Institute, Developmental Center
Utah State University
9510 Old Main Hill
Logan, UT 84322

435-750-1172

8205 Georgetown University Child Development Center
3307 Main Street, NW
Washington, DC 20007

202-687-8899
Fax: 202-687-5000
e-mail: gucdc@georgetown.edu
gucdc.georgetown.edu

8206 Institute for Basic Research in Developmental Disabilities
1050 Forest Hill Road
Staten Island, NY 10314

718-494-0600
Fax: 718-494-0837

Conducts research into neurodegenerative diseases, Alzheimer's disease, developmental disabilities, fragile X syndrome, Down's syndrome, autism, epilepsy and basic science issues underlying all developmental disabilities.

8207 Keren-Or Jerusalem Center for Multi- Handicapped Blind Children
350 7th Avenue, Suite 200
New York, NY 10001

212-279-4070
Fax: 212-279-4043
e-mail: info@keren-or.org
www.karen-or.org

Center houses and cares for over 85 resident and day students who in addition to blindness or very low vision, suffer from other severe physical and or mental disabilities. Provides training in daily living skills, as well as therapy, rehabilitation and education. Funds aquired through government stipends, government contributions, grants, bequests and legacies. Keren-Or is an IRS 501 (C)(3) tax exempt organization.

Dr. Edward L Steinburg, Chairman
Dr. Albert Hornblass, President

8208 Louisiana State University Genetics Section of Pediatrics
1501 Kings Highway
Shreveport, LA 71103

318-675-5681

TF Thurman, MD, Director

8209 New England Regional Genetics Group
PO Box 920288
Needham, MA 02492

781-444-0126
Fax: 781-444-0127
e-mail: mfgnergg@verizon.net
www.nergg.org

Human genetic services and educational planning pertaining to birth defects.

Mary-Frances Garber, Coordinator

8210 Parent and Information Center
5 N Lobban
Buffalo, WY 82834

307-684-2277
800-660-9742
Fax: 307-684-5314
e-mail: tdawsonpic@vcn.com

Support network for parents of children with disabilities and/or chronic illness. Veteran parents offer support to parents who are just learning of their child's diagnosis. Offers support and insight into parenting a child with special needs, as well as referrals to trained veteran parents.

8211 Prenatal Diagnostic and Genetic Center
HCA Wesley Medical Center
550 N Hillside Street
Wichita, KS 67214

316-962-2000
Fax: 316-962-7076
www.wesleymc.com

Sechin Cho, MD

8212 Primary Children's Medical Center
Graduate Parents
100 N Medical Drive
Salt Lake City, UT 84113

801-588-3899
Fax: 801-588-3869
e-mail: PCSWAR2@jhc.com

8213 Research and Training Center for Children' Mental Health
Univerity of South Florida
13303 Bruce B Downs Boulevard
Tampa, FL 33612

813-974-4661
Fax: 813-974-6257
rtckids.usf.edu

Dedicated to promoting effective community based culturally competent family centered services for familes and thier children who are affeed by mental, emotional or behavioral disorders.

Bob Frieman, PhD, Department Chairman

8214 Research and Training Center on Family Support and Children's Mental Health
Portland State University/Regional Research Instit
PO Box 751
Portland, OR 97207

503-725-4040
Fax: 503-725-4180
e-mail: rtcinfo@rri.pdx.edu
rtc.pdx.edu

Dedicated to promoting effective community based, culturally competent, family centered services for families and their children who are or may be affected by mental, emotional or behavioral disorders. This goal is accomplished through collaborative research partnerships with family members, service providers, policy makers, and other concerned persons. Major efforts in dissemination and training include an annual conference and comprehensive web site.

Rachel Elizabeth, Public Information/Outreach

8215 TIES, The Children's Hospital
1056 E 19th Avenue
Denver, CO 80218

303-861-6395
800-332-2082
Fax: 303-861-3992

Karen Prescott, MS

8216 Team of Advocates for Special Kids
100 W Cerritos Avenue
Anaheim, CA 92805

714-533-8275
Fax: 714-533-2533
e-mail: taskca@aol.com

Technology group of parents, consumers and professionals; provides resources to help children and adults who have disabilities gain access to the benefits of technology. Includes nationwide network of community-based assistive technology, resource centers, hands on consultants and product demonstrations.

8217 Teratogen and Birth Defects Information Project
University of South Dakota
414 E Clark Street
Vermillion, SD 57069

605-677-5011
www.usd.edu

8218 UC Berkeley School of Social Welfare
Mental Health & Social Welfare Research Group
303 Haviland Hall
Berkeley, CA 94720

510-642-3949
e-mail: spsegal@berkeley.edu
socialwelfare.berkeley.edu/mhswrg/mhswrg.html

Steven P Segal, Director

8219 University of Alaska, Fairbanks
College of Rural Alaska
PO Box 7565000
Fairbanks, AK

907-474-7143
www.uaf.edu/rural/

8220 University of Iowa Birth Defects and Genetic Disorders Unit
2614 JCP
Iowa City, IA 52242

319-335-9901
e-mail: val-sheffield@uiowa.edu
www.uiowa.edu

James M Smith, Director

8221 University of Miami, Mailman Center for Child Development
PO Box 16820
Miami, FL 33101

305-585-2703
Fax: 305-547-6309

Focuses on birth defects and children's illnesses.

Dr. Robert Stempfel Jr, Director

8222 Wesley Medical Research Institutes
3306 E Central Avenue
Wichita, KS 67208

316-686-7172
www.wesleyme.com

Respiratory and birth defects disorders research.

Dr. Sechin Cho, MD, Director

Audio Video

8223 A Mind of Your Own
Fanlight Productions
4196 Washington Street, Suite 2
Boston, MA 02131

617-469-4999
Fax: 617-469-3379
e-mail: fanlight@fanlight.com
www.fanlight.com

Learning disabilities can make children feel lonely, confused, hopeless and worthless, even if they know they are smart, but it doesn't have to feel that way. Meet Henry, Matthew, Max and Stephanie, four incredible kids who don't let learning differences hold them back or get them down.

38 Minutes

Nicole Johnson, Publicity Coordinator

8224 Assisting Parents Through the Mourning Process
Hope
55 E 100 N
Logan, UT 84321

435-752-9533
Fax: 435-752-9533

Describes the mourning process experienced by some parents of children with disabilities and ways in which the professional can help them through the process.

20 minutes

8225 CANCER
Rosen Publishing Group
29 E 21st Street
New York, NY 10010

800-237-9932
Fax: 888-436-4643
e-mail: rosenpub@tribeca.ios.com
www.rosenpublishing.com

Interviews with experts and cancer patients reveal the many types, causes, and treatments for cancer. Recommended for grades seven-twelve.

30 Minutes
ISBN: 0-823921-76-0

8226 Disability Awareness
Active Parenting Publishers
810 Franklin Court, Suite B
Marietta, GA 30067

800-825-0060
Fax: 770-429-0334
www.activeparenting.com

Helps viewers think about how they feel when confronted by people with disabilities. Close-captioned with study guide.

19 minutes

8227 It's Just Part of My Life
National Kidney Foundation
30 E 33rd Street
New York, NY 10016

212-889-2210
800-622-9010
Fax: 212-689-9261
www.kidney.org

A 15-minute program for adolescent dialysis patients and their families.

8228 Kid's Health: TV Late Breaking News Video About Broken Bones and Cast Care
Aquarius Health Care Videos
5 Powderhouse Lane, PO Box 1159
Sherborn, MA 01770

508-651-2963
888-440-2963
Fax: 508-650-4216
e-mail: info@aquariusproductions.com
www.aquariusproductions.com

You probably have lots of questions. How do doctors know if a bone is really broken? What are casts and what do they do? What are some ways to take good care of your cast so you won't need a new one? The Kids Health TV News Tem answer these questions and more in an entertaining format.

Donna Kaufman

8229 Laughter Therapy
PO Box 827
Monterey, CA 93942

408-625-3788

These people can supply tapes of old Candid Camera movies to patients. Maintains a library of 50 topics.

8230 Meeting the Challenge: Parenting Children with Disabilities
Active Parenting Publishers
810 Franklin Court, Suite B
Marietta, GA 30067

800-825-0060
Fax: 770-429-0334
www.activeparenting.com

Award-winning video for parents of special-needs children. Other parents share their stories.

94 minutes

8231 My Body Is Not Who I Am
Aquarius Health Care Videos
5 Powderhouse Lane, PO Box 1159
Sherborn, MA 01770

508-651-2963
888-440-2963
Fax: 508-650-4216
e-mail: info@aquariusproductions.com
www.aquariusproductions.com

Children host this video and educate themselves and the viewer about disabilities. While profiling adults and children who talk candidly about their disabilites, they learn that people are more alike than different. This video is crafted to foster senitivity toward others and acceptance of people with disabilities. It provides general disability etiquette guidelines that both children and adults can benefit from. The video is fast paced and designed to keep children's attention. Closed caption.

K - 12 25 Minutes

Donna Kaufman

8232 No Fears, No Tears
Fanlight Productions
4196 Washington Street, Suite 2
Boston, MA 02131

617-469-4999
800-937-4113
Fax: 617-469-3379
e-mail: fanlight@fanlight.com
www.fanlight.com

Dr. Leora Kuttner explores the pioneer pain management project for children with cancer. The film proves the strenth of the human spirit and mind's ability to ease away excrutiating pain. See No Fears, No Tears - 13 Years Later.

1985 28 Minutes VHS

Nicole Johnson, Publicity Coordinator

8233 No Fears, No Tears - 13 Years Later
Fanlight Productions
4196 Washington Street, Suite 2
Boston, MA 02131

617-469-4999
800-937-4113
Fax: 617-469-3379
e-mail: fanlight@fanlight.com
www.fanlight.com

Dr. Leora Kuttner explore the effects of children's pain management therapies 13 years after use. See original No Fears, No Tears.

1998 47 Minutes VHS
ISBN: 1-572952-77-6

Nicole Johnson, Publicity Coordinator

8234 Not Just a Cancer Patient
Fanlight Productions
4196 Washington Street, Suite 2
Boston, MA 02131

617-469-4999
800-937-4113
Fax: 617-469-3379
e-mail: info@fanlight.com
www.fanlight.com

Focuses on several articulate teenagers who are undergoing cancer treatment to help caregivers understand the needs and feelings of this very special population.

1991 23 Minutes VHS
ISBN: 1-572950-86-2

Nicole Johnson, Publicity Coordinator

8235 Operation Sneek-a-Peek
Aquarius Health Care Videos
5 Powderhouse Lane, PO Box 1159
Sherborn, MA 01770

508-651-2963
888-440-2963
Fax: 508-650-4216
e-mail: info@aquariusproductions.com
www.aquariusproductions.com

Helps children feel more comfortable and safe in a hospital environment. The puppets in the video take the children on an educational, comforting and at times, humorous tour of the hospital operating and recovery rooms. This video eases children's concerns and fears with factual information and truthful demonstrations. Closed captioned.

20 Minutes

Donna Kaufman

8236 Recognizing Children with Special Needs
Aquarius Health Care Videos
5 Powderhouse Lane, PO Box 1159
Sherborn, MA 01770

508-651-2963
888-440-2963
Fax: 508-650-4216
e-mail: info@aquariusproductions.com
www.aquariusproductions.com

A great overview for caregivers of children on how to recognize special needs. Often times it is the little things children do every-day to compensate for, or express, a disability that can be observed by their caregiver. All types of disabilities are addressed, emotional, physical, psychological, and chonic illness. A wonderful tool for teachers, childcare staff, and students who play a vital role in our children's development. Closed captioned.

18 Minutes

Donna Kaufman

8237 Stress Reduction Tapes, Stress Reduction Clinic
University Massachusetts Medical
PO Box 547
Lexington, MA 02173

508-856-2656
www.mindfulnesstapes.com

There are two tapes sold separately that are appropriate for pre-teens or adolescents. Tapes may be ordered from the website.

8238 They're Just Kids
Aquarius Health Care Videos
5 Powderhouse Lane, PO Box 1159
Sherborn, MA 01770

508-651-2963
888-440-2963
Fax: 508-650-4216
e-mail: info@aquariusproductions.com
www.aquariusproductions.com

This documentary explores the advantages of the inclusion of disabled children in the classroom, Cub Scouts and other extracurricular activities. Unfortunately, there is a great deal of fear, apprehension and concern regarding mainstreaming. This film is an excellent tool to expedite and ease that integration of children and adults into the community as well as into recreational, social and educational programs. Closed captioned, for schools, parents and those working with disabled children.

27 Minutes

Donna Kaufman

8239 When Parents Can't Fix It
Fanlight Productions
4196 Washington Street, Suite 2
Boston, MA 02131

617-469-4999
Fax: 617-469-3379
e-mail: fanlight@fanlight.com
www.fanlight.com

Looks at the stresses and rewards in the lives of five families who are raising children with diabilities. Offers a realistic look and different family strengths and coping styles.

1997 58 minutes VHS
ISBN: 1-572952-55-5

Nicole Johnson, Publicity Coordinator

Web Sites

8240 Adolescent Health On-Line
www.ama-assn.org

Includes state-to-state guide to poison control centers, database of pediatrician and hospitals, basic home care instructions and immunizations.

8241 American Academy of Pediatrics
www.aap.org

Committed to the attainment of optimal physical, mental, and social health and well-being for all infants, children, adolescents, and young adults.

8242 American Board of Pediatrics
www.abp.org

Is an independent, nonprofit organization whose certificate is recognized throughout the world signifying a high level of physician competence. It consists of distinguished pediatricians in education, research, and clinical practice, as well as one or more nonphysicians who have a professional interest in the health and welfare of children and adolescents.

8243 American College of Medical Genetics
www.acmg.net

Provides education, resources and a voice for the medical genetics profession. To make genetic services available to and improve the health of the public, the ACMG promoted the development and implementation of methods to diagnose, treat and prevent genetic disease.

8244 American Society of Pediatric Neurosurgeons
www.aspn.org

The society is dedicated to the advancement of the subspecialty of Pediatric Neurosugery and to assure superlative care for children with neurosurgical disorders. It holds an annual meeting where recent advances in clinical and basic research into pediatric neurosurgical disorders are presented and discussed, and sponsors a journal, Pediatric Neurosurgery.

8245 Archives of Pediatric and Adolescent Medicine
www.ovid.com/site/cataloge/journal

It provides a forum for dialogue on a range of scientific, clinical, and humanistic issues relevant to the care of pediatric patients, from infancy to young adulthood. The journal's core articles are original clinical studies and reviews by experts.

8246 Association for Children with Hand or Arm Deficiency (REACH)
www.reach.org.uk/

Provides the means by which parents and professionals share experiences, information, and support.

8247 Birth Defect Research for Children
www.birthdefects.org

Nonprofit organization that provides parents and expectant parents with information about birth defects and support services for their children, including the National Birth Defect Registry.

8248 Cedars-Sinai Medical Center
www.cedars-siniai.edu

Focused on providing the finest healthcare available, resulting in advances in all areas of healthcare for both children and adult disorders.

8249 CenterWatch Clinical Trials Listings
www.centerwatch.com

CenterWatch is a Boston-based publishing and information services company. We provide information services used by patients, pharmaceutical, biotechnology and medical device companies, CRO's and research centers involved in clinical research around the world.

8250 Council for Exceptional Children
www.cec.sped.org

The worldwide mission of The Council for Exceptional Children is to improve education outcomes for individuals with exceptionalities. CEC, a nonprofit association, accomplishes its mission in support of special education professionals and others working on behalf of individuals with exceptionalities, by advocating for appropriate governmental policies, by setting professional standards, and by providing continuing professional development.

8251 CyberPsych
www.cyberpsych.org

CyberPsych presents information about psychoanalysis, psychotherapy, and special topics such as anxiety disorder, the problematic use of alcohol, homophobia, and the traumatic effects of racism. CyberPsych is a nonprofit network which offers free web hosting and technical support for internet communication, to nonprofit groups and individuals.

8252 Dermatology Foundation
www.dermfind.org

Committed to advancing dermatologic through research and education. The foundation is a charitable organization that has the primary service to fund research in skin cancer and other diseases of the skin, hair, and nails.

8253 Easter Seals Disability Services
www.easterseals.com

For more than 80 years, Easter Seals has helped people with disabilities in communities nationwide, from creating the first national voluntary act for children with disabilities in the 1920's to leading the creation and implementation of the Americans with Disabilities Act in the 1990's. Easter Seals child development services build strong foundations for children of all abilities.

8254 European Society for Pediatric Urology
www.espu.org/

Is a nonprofit society whose main purpose is to promote pediatric urology, appropriate practice, education as well as exchanges between practitioners involved in the treatment of genitourinary disorders in children.

8255 Federation for Children with Special Needs
www.fscn.org

Mission is to provide information, support, and assistance to parents of children with disabilites, their professional partners, and their communities. We are committed to listening to and learning from families and encouraging full participation in community life by all people, especially those with disabilities.

8256 GeneTest
www.geneclinics.org

By providing current, authoritative information on genetic testing and its use in diagnosis, management, and genetic couseling, GeneTests promots the appropriate use of genetic services in patient care and personal decision making.

8257 ICAN (International Child Amputee Network)
www.amp-info.net/childamp.htm

Is an internet mailing list to provide information and support contacts to children with absent or underdeveloped limbs and their parents.

8258 International Foundation for Functional Gastrointestinal Disorders
www.iffgd.org

Is a nonprofit education and research organization whoes mission is to inform, assist and support people affected by gastrointestinal disorders.

8259 KidsHealth at the AMA
www.ama-assn.org

Includes state-to-state guide to poison control centers, database of pediatricians and hospitals, basic home-care instructions and immunizations.

8260 LSUMC Family Medicine Patient Education
lib-sh.lsumc.edu

Offers databases, E-journals, E-books, and a library catalog.

8261 Low Vision Gateway
www.lowvision.org

Devoted to issues of vision loss, low vision aids, vision rehabilitation and the role of the doctor.

8262 MUMS: National Parent to Parent Network
www.netnet.net/mums

A national parent-to-parent organization for parents or care providers of a child with any disability, rare or not so rare disorder, chromosomal abnormality or health condition. MUM's main purpose is to provide support to parents in the form of a networking system that matches them with other parents whose children have the same or similar condition.

8263 March of Dimes Birth Defects Foundation
www.marchofdimes.com

March of Dimes researchers, volunteers, educators, outreach workers and advocated work together to give all babies a fighting chance against the threats to their health: prematurity, birth defects, low birthweight.

8264 Medical Economics Company
www.medec.com

Full text for non-prescription drugs and the PDR Guide to Drug Interactions.

8265 Medical Matrix: Pediatrics
www.medmatrix.org/SPages/Pediatric.asp

8266 Mental Help Net
mentalhelp.net

Seeks to advance the state of online mental health communications. We wish to provide the following: to discuss, develop and debate in an open forum the future of the mental health field in America and throughout the world, to help coordinate various componenets of the mental health field.

8267 NIH/National Institute on Disability and Rehabilitative Research (NIDRR)
www.ed.gov/offices/list/osers/nidrr/index.html

Is committed to improving results and outcomes for people with dsiabilities of all ages. It supports programs that serve millions of children, youth and adults with disablities.

8268 National Arthritis and Musculoskeletal & Skin Disease Info. Clearinghouse
www.nih.gov/niams

Supports and provides clinical and public information and research to increase understanding of the many skin diseases and related disorders. Also provides lists and order forms for their resources and materials.

8269 National Association for Visually Handicapped
www.navh.org

Helps to cope with the difficulties of vision impairment.

8270 National Dissemination Center for Children with Disabilities
www.nichcy.org

Provides information to the nation on: disabilities in children and youth; programs and services for infants, children, and youth with disabilities; IDEA, the nation's special education law; No Child Left Behind, the nation's general education law; and research-based information on effective practices for children with disabilities.

8271 National Library Service for the Blind and Physically Handicapped
www.loc.gov/nls

A free library program of braille and audio materials circulated to eligible borrowers in the United States by postage-free mail.

8272 National Newborn Screening and Genetic Resources Center
genes-r-us.uthscsa.edu

The mission is to provide a forum for interaction between consumers, health care professionals, researchers, organizations, and policy-makers in-refining and developing public health, newborn screening and geneting programs, and to serve as a national resource center for information and education in the areas of new-born screening and genetics.

8273 National Organization of Parents of Blind Children
www.nfb.org

Is a national membership organization of parents and friends of blind chilren reaching out to each other to give support, encouragement and information. We believe the real problem of blindness is not the loss of eyesight, but the misunderstanding and lack of information which exists. With proper training opportunity, blindness can be reduced to a physical nuisance.

8274 National Resource Library on Youth With Disabilities
www.cyfc.umn.edu/NRL/

Brings together comprehensive sources of information related to youth with chrionic or disabling conditions and their families. Topics include psychosocial issues, disability awareness, developmental processes, family, sexuality, education, employment, independent living, cultural issues, gender issues, service delivery, professional issues, advocacy and legal issues, and health issues.

8275 Nuclear Medicine at Children's Hospital, Boston
www.jpnm.org/contentch.html

8276 Office of Special Education and Rehabilitative Services
www.ed.gov/offices/list/osers/index

Mission is to strengthen the federal commitment to assuring access to equal opportunity for every individual; to supplement and complement the efforts of states, the local school systems and other instrumentalities of the states, the private nonprofit educational research institutions, community-based organizations, parents, and students to improve the quality of education; and to encourage the increased involvement of the public, parents, and students in federal education programs.

8277 Online Mendelian Inheritance in Man
www.ncbi.nlm.nih.gov

Conducts research on fundamental biomedical problems at the molecular level using mathematical and computational methods, maintains collaborations with several NIH institutes, academia, industry, and other governmental agencies, fosters scientific communication by sponsoring meetings, workshops, and lecture series, and supports training on basic and applied research in computational biology for postdoctoral fellows through the NIH Intramural Research Program.

8278 PDR - Physicians' Desk Reference
www.pdr.net

8279 PEDINFO: An index of the Pediatric Internet
www.pedinfo.org

Collection of links to pediatric information.

8280 Pediatric Behavior and Development
www.dbpeds.org

Is an independent web site created to promote better care and outcomes for children and families affected by developmental, learning, and behavioral problems by providing access to clinically relevant information and educational materials for physicians, fellows, resident physicians, and students. The site may also be of interest to psychologists, nurses, nurse practitioners, social workers, therapists, educators, and parents.

8281 Pediatric Points of Interest
www.pslgroup.com/dg/20112

Are a collection of updated links for pediatricians, parents and children to medical sources on the internet.

8282 Planetpsych
www.planetpsych.com

Planetpsych is an online resource for mental health information.

8283 Pregnancy and Child Health Resource Center from Mayo Health Oasis
www.mayohealth.org

Our mission is to empower people to manage their health. We accomplish this by providing useful and up-to-date information and

tools that reflect the expertise and standard of excellence of Mayo Clinic.

8284 Psych Central
www.psychcentral.com

Offers free informational and educational articles and resources on psychological support and mental health online.

8285 PubMed
www.ncbi.nlm.nih.gov/

Creates public databases, conducts research in computational biology, develops software tools for analyzing genome data, and disseminates biomedical information - all for better understanding molecular processes affecting human health and disease.

8286 Rare Genetic Diseases in Children (NYU)
www.med.nyu.edu/rgdc/homenow.htm

We target issues arising from rare genetic diseases affecting children, and to assist in the endeavor to bring knowledge and hope to those for whom there is, at present, so little.

8287 Save Babies Through Screening Foundation
www.savebabies.org

Is a national nonprofit public charity run by volunteers. Its mission is to improve the lives of babies by working to prevent disabilities and early death resulting from disorders detectable through newborn screening.

8288 Society for Adolescent Medicine
www.adolescenthealth.org

A multidisciplinary organization of professionals committed to improving the physical and psychosocial health and well-being of all adolescents.

8289 Southern Illinois University School of Medicine
www.siumed.edu/peds/index.htm

The mission of SUI School of Medicine is to assist the people of central and southern Illinois in meeting their present and future health care needs through education, clinical service and research.

8290 TRIP Database
www.tripdatabase.com

The TRIP Database allows users to rapidly and easily identify high quality medical literature from a wide range of sources.

8291 TransWeb
www.transweb.org

Mission is to provide information about donation and transplantation to the general public in order to improve organ and tissue procurement efforts worldwide, to provide transplant patients and families world wide with information specifically dealing with transplant-related issues and concerns and to provide and index sources for transplant-related information available through the internet and otherwise.

8292 Virtual Childrens Hosptial
www.vh.org

Is dedicated to helping patients find the highest quality medical information in the world today. We offer patients the tools necessary to make informed treatment decisions within the short timlines dictated by their illness or disease.

8293 WebMD Community Services
my.webmd.com

Provides valuable health information, tools for managing youth health, and support to those who seek information.

Magazines

8294 Childswork Childsplay
135 Dupont Street, PO Box 760
Plainview, NY 11803

800-431-1934
Fax: 888-803-3908
www.childswork.com

Full of training tools for children of all ages.

63 pages

8295 Exceptional Parent
209 Harvard Street, Suite 303
Brookline, MA 02146

617-730-5800
Fax: 617-730-8742
www.eparent.com

Provides information and support for families, parents, physicians and professionals in the special needs community. Published 11 times monthly plus a special January issue.

Monthly
ISSN: 0046-9157

Rick Rader MD, Editor-in-Chief

8296 Future Reflections
National Federation of the Blind
1800 Johnson Street
Baltimore, MD 21230

410-659-9314
Fax: 410-685-5653
e-mail: nfb@nfb.org
www.nfb.org

National magazine written specifically for parents and educators of blind children. Each issue addresses various topics important to blind children, their families and to school personnel.

Quarterly

Barbara Cheadle, Editor

8297 Journal of the Academy of Dermatology
American Academy of Dermatology
PO Box 94020
Palatine, IL 60094

847-330-0230
Fax: 847-330-0050

A scientific publication serving the clinical needs of the specialty and providing a wide selection of articles on various topics important to continuing medical education of Academy members and the international dermatologic community.

Monthly

Journals

8298 International Journal of Nursing in Intellectual & Developmental Disabilities
Developmental Disabilities Nurses Association
1685 H Street, PMB 1214
Blaine, WA 98230

800-888-6733
Fax: 360-332-2280
e-mail: ddnahq@aol.com
www.ddna.org

Electronic journal for nurses, individuals, families and others interested in promoting health and nursing supports for individuals with intellectual and developmental disabilities. Provides information and resources, educational strategies and policy development on a variety of clinical topics.

Ann Smith MSN, RN, CDDN, Editor

Newsletters

8299 ABDC Newsletter
Association of Birth Defect Children
800 Celebration Avenue, Suite 225
Celebration, FL 34747

407-566-8304
Fax: 407-566-8341
www.birthdefects.org

Offers updated information on the association activities, events and medical updates. Back issues available.

8 pages Quarterly

8300 BDRC Newsletter
Association of Birth Defect Children
800 Celebration Avenue, Suite 225
Celebration, FL 34747

407-566-8304
Fax: 407-566-8341
e-mail: info@birthdefects.org
www.birthdefects.org

Offers updated information on the association activities, events and medical updates.

8 pages Quarterly

8301 Child Life Council Newsletter
Child Life Council
11820 Parklawn Drive, Suite 202
Rockville, MD 20852

301-881-7090
800-252-4515
Fax: 301-881-7092
e-mail: clcstaff@childlife.org
www.childlife.org

The Child Life Council newsletter provides information to promote the well-being of children and families in health care settings. Newsletter is provided to members only.

12 pages Quarterly

Elizabeth Wanjau, Program Assistant

8302 Children's Hopes and Dreams
Wish Fulfillment Foundation
280 Route 46
Dover, NJ 07801

973-361-7366
Fax: 973-361-6627
e-mail: chdfdover@juno.com
childrenscharities.org/childrens_wisheso

Dream Newsletter (describes dreams recently fulfilled, events, request and info about programs) available upon request; at no cost. 4 times per year.

10,000 Members

8303 Connecting
2400 N. Central Avenue, Suite 200
Phoenix, AZ 85004

602-242-4366
800-237-3007
Fax: 602-242-4306
TDD: 602-242-4366
e-mail: info@specialkids.org
www.raisingspecialkids.org

Presenting informational and personal articles, calendar of events and news relevant to Arizona families of children with special needs. Subscription is free to families.

Bimonthly

Patricia Savieo, Editor/Communications Coordinator

8304 For Siblings Only

Family Resource Associates
35 Haddon Avenue
Shrewsbury, NJ 07702

732-747-5310
Fax: 732-747-1896

Quarterly newsletter for siblings of children with disabilities, aged four through 10.

S Levine, Editor

8305 Matchmaker

MUMS: National Parent to Parent Network
150 Custer Street
Green Bay, WI 54301

920-336-5333
877-336-5333
Fax: 920-339-0995
e-mail: mums@netnet.net
www.netnet.net/mums/

Matches parents of children with rare disorders. Provides information and advocacy resources for families and professionals. Includes listings of organizations providing general information and organizations focusing on more specific areas of concern to families and young adults who have disabilities.

Quarterly

Julie Gordon, Director

8306 Newsline

Federation for Children with Special Needs
1135 Tremonts Street, Suite 420
Boston, MA 02120

617-236-7210
800-331-0688
TDD: 800-331-0688
e-mail: kidinfo@fcsn.org
www.fcsn.org

Carolyn Romano, Editor
Janet Vohs, Editor

8307 PAL News

Parent Professional Advocacy League
95 Berkeley Street
Boston, MA 02116

617-482-2915
www.fcsn.org

Offers information on medical and technological updates in the area of research on birth defects, support groups and family resources for persons with disabled children.

Quarterly

8308 Sibling Forum

Family Resource Associates
35 Haddon Avenue
Shrewsbury, NJ 07702

732-747-5310
Fax: 732-747-1896
www.frainc.org

Quarterly newsletter for siblings of children with disabilities, aged 10 and up.

S Levine, Editor

Pamphlets

8309 AAP Education Resource Guide

American Academy of Pediatrics
141 NW Point Boulevard
Elk Grove Village, IL 60007

847-434-4000
800-433-9016
Fax: 847-434-8000
e-mail: cme@aap.org
www.aap.org

8310 About Children's Eyes

National Association for Visually Handicapped
22 W 21st Street, 6th Floor
New York, NY 10010

212-889-3141
Fax: 212-727-2931
e-mail: staff@navh.org
www.navh.org

How to identify the child with a visual problem.

8311 About Children's Vision: A Guide for Parents

National Association for Visually Handicapped
22 W 21st Street
New York, NY 10010

212-889-3141
Fax: 212-727-2931
e-mail: staff@navh.org
www.navh.org

Offers a better understanding of the normal and possible abnormal development of a child's eyesight.

Eva Cohen, Assistant to the Director

8312 Advanced Cancer: Coping with Advanced Canc er

National Cancer Institute
6116 Executive Blvd, Room 3036A
Bethesda, MD 20892

800-422-6237
800-422-6237
TTY: 800-332-8615

Booklet delving into all aspects of everyday living with cancer. Offers information on coping, how children react, facing the unknown, living wills, additional resources and making treatment decisions.

30 pages

8313 Amyloidosis and Kidney Disease

Information Clearinghouse
2 Information Way
Bethesda, MD 20892

301-654-3810
Fax: 301-907-8906
e-mail: nddic@info.niddk.nih.gov
www.niddk.nih.gov

8314 BDRC Newsletter Volume Reprints

Association of Birth Defect Children
930 Woodcock Road, Suite 225
Orlando, FL 32803

407-895-0802
Fax: 407-895-0824
e-mail: info@birthdefects.org
www.birthdefects.org

Offers a variety of reprints from the ABCD newsletter on birth defects.

8315 Basic Family Library

Candlelighters' Childhood Cancer Foundation
7910 Woodmont Avenue, Suite 460
Bethesda, MD 20814

301-657-8401
800-366-2223

A bibliography of materials on childhood cancers, medical support, death and bereavement and materials for children.

8316 Birth Defects: A Brighter Future

March of Dimes Resource Center
1275 Mamaroneck Avenue
White Plains, NY 10605

888-663-4637
Fax: 914-997-4763
www.marchofdimes.org

8317 Camps for Children with Cancer and Their Siblings

Candlelighters' Childhood Cancer Foundation
7910 Woodmont Avenue, Suite 460
Bethesda, MD 20814

301-657-8401
800-366-2223

A listing by state of day and overnight camp programs, children served and programs.

8318 Candlelighters Guide to Bone Marrow Transplants in Children

Candlelighters Childhood Cancer Foundation
PO Box 498
Kensington, MD 20895

301-962-3520
800-366-2223

For parents who are contemplating a BMT or harvest for their child or whose child is undergoing the procedure.

8319 Heart Disease, High Blood Pressure, Stroke and Diabetes

Information Clearinghouse
2 Information Way
Bethesda, MD 20892

301-654-3810
Fax: 301-907-8906
e-mail: nddic@info.niddk.nih.gov
www.niddk.nih.gov

8320 Helping Children Cope While a Sibling Undergoes Bone Marrow Transplant

Bone Marrow Foundation
981 1st Avenue, Suite 129
New York, NY 10022

212-838-3029
e-mail: thebmf@aol.com
www.bonemarrow.org

Discusses the wide array of emotions felt by the entire family as a child receives a bone marrow transplant.

8321 How to Find Out More About Your Child's Bi rth Defect or Disability

Association of Birth Defect Children
930 Woodcock Road, Suite 225
Orlando, FL 32803

407-895-0802
Fax: 407-895-0824
e-mail: info@birthdefects.org
www.birthdefects.org

An informational fact sheet that encourages parents who have a child with a birth defect or disability to become the expert on the child's disability with some suggestions on how to educate themselves.

8322 Hypoglycemia

Information Clearinghouse
2 Information Way
Bethesda, MD 20892

301-654-3810
Fax: 301-907-8906
e-mail: nddic@info.niddk.nih.gov
www.niddk.nih.gov

8323 Interstitial Cyctitis

Information Clearinghouse
1 Information Way
Bethesda, MD 20892

301-654-3820
Fax: 301-907-8906
e-mail: ndoc@info.niddk.nih.gov
www.niddk.nih.gov

8324 Liver Transplant Fund

American Liver Foundation
1425 Pompton Avenue
Cedar Grove, NJ 07009

973-857-2550
800-223-0179

8325 Liver Transplantation

American Liver Foundation
1425 Pompton Avenue
Cedar Grove, NJ 07009

973-857-2626
800-223-0179

8326 Managing Your Child's Eating Problems During Cancer Treatment

National Cancer Institute
Building 31, Room 10A24
Bethesda, MD 20892

800-422-6237

Contains information about the importance of nutrition, side-effects of cancer and its treatment.

32 pages

8327 Medullary Sponge Kidney

2 Information Way
Bethesda, MD 20892

301-654-3810
Fax: 301-907-8906
e-mail: nddic@info.niddk.nih.gov
www.niddk.nih.gov

8328 NPF Benefits of Membership Pamphlets

National Psoriasis Foundation
6600 SW 92nd Avenue
Portland, OR 97223

503-244-7404
Fax: 503-245-0626
e-mail: getinfo@npfusa.org
www.psoriasis.org

Offers all the pamphlets that are published through the foundation for members. Includes NPF 800 number and reply tear-off card.

8329 New Challenge: Responding to Families

Federation for Children with Special Needs
95 Berkeley Street
Boston, MA 02116

617-482-2915
www.fcsn.org

Addresses the needs of children with emotional, behavioral and mental disorders and their families.

8330 Nutrition for Early Chronic Kidney Disease

Information Clearing House
2 Information Way
Bethesda, MD 20892

301-654-3810
Fax: 301-907-8906
e-mail: nddic@info.niddk.nih.gov
www.niddk.nih.gov

8331 Nutrition for Later Chronic Disease
Information Clearinghouse
2 Information Way
Bethesda, MD 20892

301-654-3810
Fax: 301-907-8906
e-mail: nddic@info.niddk.nih.gov
www.niddk.nih.gov

8332 Pain, Pain Go Away: Helping Children with Pain
Association for the Care of Children's Health
7910 Woodmont Avenue, Suite 300
Bethesda, MD 20814

301-654-6549
800-808-2224
Fax: 301-986-4553

This booklet teaches parents about pain in children.

1993

8333 Preparing Your Child for a Bone Marrow Transplant
Bone Marrow Foundation
981 1st Avenue, Suite 129
New York, NY 10022

212-838-3029
e-mail: thebmf@aol.com
www.bonemarrow.org

Discusses the wide array of emotions felt by the entire family as a child receives a bone marrow transplant.

8334 Proteinuria
Information Clearinghouse
2 Information Way
Bethesda, MD 20892

301-654-3810
Fax: 301-907-8906
e-mail: nddic@info.niddk.nih.gov
www.niddk.nih.gov

8335 Renal Tubular Acidosis
Information Clearinghouse
2 Information Way
Bethesda, MD 20892

301-654-3810
Fax: 301-907-8906
e-mail: nddic@info.niddk.nih.gov
www.niddk.nih.gov

8336 Students with Cancer: A Resource for the Educator
National Cancer Institute
Building 31, Room 10A24
Bethesda, MD 20892

800-422-6237

Designed for teachers who have students with cancer in their classrooms or schools.

22 pages

8337 Talking with Your Child About Cancer
National Cancer Institute
Building 31, Room 10A24
Bethesda, MD 20892

800-422-6237

Designed for the parent whose child has been diagnosed with cancer.

16 pages

8338 Urethritis
2 Information Way
Bethesda, MD 20892

301-654-3810
Fax: 301-907-8906
e-mail: nddic@info.niddk.nih.gov
www.niddk.nih.gov

8339 When Someone In Your Family Has Cancer
National Cancer Institute
Building 31, Room 10A24
Bethesda, MD 20892

800-422-6237

Written for young people whose parent or sibling has cancer.

28 pages

8340 When Your Child Has a Life-Threatening Illness
Association for the Care of Children's Health
7910 Woodmont Avenue
Bethesda, MD 20814

301-654-6549
Fax: 301-986-4553

A concise, supportive booklet for parents. Sections include initial reactions, hope, communication, other children, impact on marriage, and single parent families.

1983

8341 Wish Fulfillment Organizations
Candlelighters' Childhood Cancer Foundation
7910 Woodmont Avenue, Suite 460
Bethesda, MD 20814

301-657-8401
800-366-2223

A list of groups granting wishes of children with life-threatening, chronic or terminal illnesses, with criteria and contacts.

8342 Young People with Cancer: A Handbook for Parents
National Cancer Institute
6116 Executive Blvd, R3036A
Bethesda, MD 20892

800-422-6237
TTY: 800-332-8615

Discusses the most common types of childhood cancer, treatments, and side effects and issues that may arise when a child is diagnosed with cancer.

86 pages

8343 Your Kidneys and How They Work
Information Clearinghouse
1 Information Way
Bethesda, MD 20892

301-654-3820
Fax: 301-907-8906
e-mail: ndoc@info.niddk.nih.gov
www.niddk.nih.gov

Camps

Alabama

8344 Camp ASCCA/Easter Seals
PO Box 21
Jackson's Gap, AL 800-T

256-825-9226
800-800-THE
Fax: 256-825-8332
e-mail: ascca@webshoppe.net
www.campascca.org

Camp for children and adults with disabilities, ages 6+.

Tom Collier, Camp Director

Arkansas

8345 Camp Aldersgate
Med Camps Coordinator
2000 Aldersgate Road
Little Rock, AR

501-225-1444
Fax: 501-225-2019
e-mail: info@campaldersgate.net
www.campaldersgate.net

A private nonprofit social service agency allied with the United Methodist Church which co-sponsors a series of summer medical camps with Med Camps of Arkansas, Inc., and thirteen various health agencies. The camps allow children and youth, ages 6-16, who have various medical conditions and physical disabilities to enjoy traditional camping experiences adapted to their abilities. The Camp also offers respite care, senior citizens programs, west side clinic and the children's center.

Ruth M Eyres, Coordinator

California

8346 Ability First
1300 E Green Street
Pasadena, CA 91106

626-396-1010
877-768-4600
Fax: 626-396-1021
e-mail: bstarkins@abilityfirst.org
www.abilityfirst.org

Services include residential camping programs, aquatics, lifespan programs and housing.

Brenda Starkins, Social Service Coordinator

8347 Ability First, Camp Paivika
600 Playground Drive
Cedarpines Park, CA 92332

909-338-1102
Fax: 909-338-2502
e-mail: kkunsek@abilityfirst.org
www.abilityfirst.com

Nonprofit camp owned and operated by Ability First to provide outdoor, recreational camping services for children and adults with physical and/or developmental disabilities. Located in the San Bernadino mountains, the camp has a dining lodge and rec room, four cabins, infirmary, program building and pool that are all fully accessible. Camp is available to rent during winter/spring for up to 80 people.

Brenda Starkins, Social Service Coordinator

8348 All Nations Camp
PO Box 2828
Wrightwood, CA

760-249-3822
Fax: 760-249-4492
www.gbod.org

Camp for children with disabilities, ages 8 to 18.

Ismael Nieto

8349 Camp Alex A. Krem
Camping Unlimited
PO Box 20774
El Sobrante, CA 94820

510-222-6662
Fax: 510-223-3046
e-mail: campkrem@campingunlimited.com
www.campingunlimited.com

Camp serves people of all ages and all handicaps. Summer Program: five two-week sessions of residential or travel camp. Year-round: weekend outings throughout the year. Vendorized by the California Regional Centers; camperships are available. Member of the American Camping Association.

Gary Breland, Executive Director
Leon Wong, Program Director

8350 Camp Joan Mier
Ability First
11677 E Pacific Coast Highway
Malibu, CA

310-457-9863
Fax: 310-457-6374
www2.kidscamps.com

8351 Camp Ronald McDonald at Eagle Lake
PO Box 172
Susanville, CA

530-825-3158
Fax: 530-825-3158
www.campronald.org

8352 Camp-A-Lot
5384 Linda Vista Road
San Diego, CA 800-7

800-800-748
Fax: 619-574-0317

Residential camping program for children and adults, ages 7 and up. San Diego locals offered transportation.

Jaculin Taylor

8353 Easter Seal Summer Camp Programs
2645 Pleasant Hill Road
Pleasant Hill, CA

925-689-1777

Offers education, adventure and the experience and enjoyment of living-out-of-doors in a striking and challenging wilderness environment. Serves ages 6 to 60, male and female.

Beverly Mayhall

8354 Enchanted Hills Camp
Lighthouse
214 Van Ness Avenue
San Francisco, CA 94102

415-431-1481
Fax: 415-863-7568
TTY: 415-431-4572

For blind, deaf/blind children and adults, ages 5 and up. This program offers a basic camping experience. Activities include music, art, dance, hiking and riding. Camperships are available to California residents.

Paul Reid

8355 Gloriana Opera Company
721 N Franklin Street, PO Box 273
Fort Bragg, CA 95437

707-964-7469
Fax: 707-965-9653
e-mail: info@gloriana.org
www.gloriana.org

Since 1977 superlative music theater productions all year long, plus concerts, childrens workshops and classes.

Diane Larson, President
Ana Lucas, Artistic Director

8356 Junior Wheelchair Sports Camp
Santa Barbara Parks and Recreation Department
PO Box 1990
Santa Barbara, CA

805-564-5318
Fax: 805-564-5475
www.ci.omaha.ne.us/parks

This five-day camp is for children 5-19 years old that are physically disabled. Sports instruction in aquatics, tennis, track and field, basketball, archery and new sports activities introduced each year. The camp counselors and instructors are also physically disabled to provide the children with a role model. Fee based on fundraising efforts.

8357 Okizu Foundation Camps
16 Digital Drive
Novato, CA 94948

415-382-8384
www.okizu.org

This foundation runs family camp programs for children who have cancer and their families, and for children who have or had a parent with cancer.

Colorado

8358 Magic of Music and Dance
PO Box M
Aspen, CO 800-5

970-923-0578
Fax: 970-923-7338
www2.kidscamps.com

8359 Rocky Mountain Village
Easter Seals Colorado
PO Box 115
Empire, CO

313-569-2333
Fax: 303-569-3857
e-mail: campinfo@cess.org
www.eastersealsco.org

Sessions are conducted for both developmentally and physically disabled children and adults. Activities include swimming, horseback riding, outdoor education, zigline challenge course elements.

Roman Kratczyk, Director

Connecticut

8360 Mansfield's Holiday Hill
41 Chaffeeville Road
Mansfield Center, CT

860-423-1375
Fax: 860-456-2444

A home not far from home where beautiful fields, forests, facilities and a caring staff support the activities and relationships of our camp families. The camp offers many programs such as: Outdoor Adventure; Tumbling; Dance; Adventure Ropes Course; Swimming; Arts & Crafts; Archery; Tennis and more to thirty boys and girls.

Dudley Hamlin

Florida

8361 Camp Thunderbird
909 E Welch Road
Apopka, FL

407-889-8088
Fax: 407-889-8072
e-mail: campthun@aol.com
www.questinc.com

Residential summer camping program for children and adults with a developmental disability. Campers enjoy swimming, sports, nature hikes, canoeing, etc.

Dr. Shirley O'Brien, Camp Director

8362 Easter Seals Camp Challenge
31600 Camp Challenge Road
Sorrento, FL

352-383-4711
Fax: 352-383-0744
e-mail: camp@fl.easter-seals.org
www2.kidscamps.com

Micheal Currence, Director Camping/Recreation
Melissa Guinta, Summer Camp Director

8363 VACC Camp
Miami Children's Hospital
3200 SW 60th Center
Miami, FL

305-662-8222
Fax: 305-663-8417
www.vacccamp.com

Georgia

8364 Squirrel Hollow
5665 Milam Road
Fairburn, GA 30213

770-774-8001
Fax: 770-774-8005
e-mail: bbox@thebedfordschool.org
www.thebedfordschool.org

A remedial summer program of The Bedford School; serves children with academic needs due to learning difficulties. For students ages 6-16 and held on the campus of The Bedford School in Fairburn, GA. Campers participate in an individualized academic program as well as recreational activities. Students receive the proper academic remediation as well as specific remedial help with physical skills, peer interaction and self-esteem.

Betsy E Box, Director
Jeff James, Assistant Director

Hawaii

8365 Camp Erdman YMCA
69-385 Farrington Highway
Waialua, HI

808-637-4615
Fax: 808-637-8874
www.camperdman.net

A specialized youth camp serving the needs of the disabled.

Josh Hermowitz, Executive Director

Illinois

8366 Camp Discovery
American Academy of Dermatology
930 E Woodfield Road
Schaumburg, IL 60173

847-240-1737
866-503-7546
Fax: 847-330-8907
e-mail: jmueller@aad.org
www.campdiscovery.org

A camp for young people with serious skin conditions. There is no fee and transportation is provided. Two locations: Camp Horizon in Millville, PA and Camp Knutson in Crosslake, MN.

Stephen P Stone MD, President
Julie Mueller, Camp Information

8367 Easter Seals - Timber Pointe Outdoor Center
20 Timber Pointe Lane
Hudson, IL 61748

309-365-8021
Fax: 309-365-8934
www.easterseals-acp.org

Handicapable camping for kids.

Kurt Fodeszwa, Director Camping

8368 Jewish Council for Youth Services
JCYS Camp Red Leaf
26710 West Nippersink Road
Ingleside, IL 60041

847-740-5010
Fax: 847-740-5014
e-mail: cmiller@jcys.org
www.campredleaf.bunkl.com

Overnight summer camp for youth and adults with developmental disabilites. Family Camps, respite weekends, trips, and other special events are offered throughout the year.

Carissa Miller, CTRS, Director
Diane Gould, LCSW, Director Special Services

8369 Olympia

Southern Illinois University
Mail Code 6519
Carbondale, IL

618-453-1423
Fax: 618-453-1445

Located on 6,500 acres of forests and meadows on the shores of Little Grassy Lake, Olympia Camp is for mentally and physically handicapped children and adults. Among the activities offered are arts and crafts, hay wagon rides, canoeing and swimming.

Craig Dittmar

8370 Peacock Camp

38685 N Deep Lake Road
Lake Villa, IL

847-356-3931

A residential summer camp for individuals ages 7-17 with a physical disability. Activities include swimming, arts and crafts, recreational game, nature activities and large group activities (such as campfires, carnivals, talent shows, etc.). There are four 12-day sessions per summer.

David Bogenschutz, Camp Director

8371 Summer Wheelchair Sports Camp

University of Illinois
1207 S Oak Street, Division of Rehab Education
Champaign, IL

217-333-4606
Fax: 217-333-0248
TTY: 217-333-1970
www2.kidscamps.com

8372 Touch of Nature Environmental Center

Southern Illinois University
Carbondale, IL

618-453-1121
Fax: 618-453-1188
www.pso.siu.edu

Providing a traditional camping experience for non-traditional campers, including recreational and outdoor programs for adults and children with various developmental, mental and physical disabilities as well as learning and behavioral disorders.

Randy Osborn, Camp Director
Chilang Lawless, Camp Registrant

Indiana

8373 Camp Isanogel

7601 W Isanogel Road
Muncie, IN

765-288-1073
Fax: 765-288-3103
e-mail: isanogel@iquest.net
www.isanogelcenter.og

Thirty-two years of programs for special needs of children through adults.

Karen Kovaen, Executive Director
Monica Sauter, Recreation Director

8374 Camp Millhouse

25600 Kelly Road
South Bend, IN

219-287-9833
Fax: 812-358-4381
www2.kidscamps.com

8375 Easter Seal Society

4251 S 600 E
Columbus, IN

812-342-0134
www2.kidscamps.com

8376 Happiness Bag Incorporated

3833 Union Road
Terre Haute, IN 47802

812-234-8867
www.happinessbag.org

Serves developmentally disabled age 5-adult; day and residential camp program; after school program; scouting; Special Olympic anticipation (basketball, athletics, bowling, softball and aquatics); and a bowling league.

Jodi Moan, Program Director
Patricia Porter, Executive Director

8377 Happy Hollow Children's Camp

3049 Happy Hollow Road
Nashville, IN

812-988-4900
Fax: 812-988-7505
e-mail: hhcdir@aol.com
www.happyhollowcamp.net

Accepts disabled campers.

Bernard Schrader

8378 Kiwanis Twin Lakes Camp

15543 12th Road
Plymouth, IN

219-941-2750

Serving the orthopedically handicapped children and young adults.

8379 Worthmore Academy

5220 E Fall Creek Parkway N Drive
Indianapolis, IN

317-253-5367

A center for learning disabilities providing educational assessments, alternative educational programs, academic guidance and public awareness services available as follows: full-time day school, K-8th, 1 to 1 teacher student ratio; six week summer school, K-12th, 1 to 1 teacher student ratio; after school tutoring; adult tutoring, educational assessments, counseling and educational seminars.

Brenda J Jackson, Director
Diana Buser, Assistant

Iowa

8380 Camp Courageous

PO Box 418
Monticello, IA 52310

319-465-5916
www.campcourageous.org

Over 3,500 disabled campers have attended this recreational and respite care facility. The camp is open 24 hours a day, 365 days a year and operates entirely on donations.

8381 Camp Courageous of Iowa

12007 190th Street
Monticello, IA

319-465-5916
Fax: 319-465-5919
e-mail: camp@campcourageous.org
www.campcourageous.com

A year round residential and respite care facility for individuals with special needs. Campers range in age from 3-80 years old. Activities include traditional activities like canoeing, hiking, swimming, nature and crafts plus adventure activities like caving, rock climbing, etc. Campers with disabilities have opportunities to succeed at challenging activities. This feeling of self-worth can transfer to home, work or school environments.

Jeanne Muellerleile, Camp Director

8382 Camp Tanager
1614 W Mount Vernon Road
Mount Vernon, IA

319-363-0681
Fax: 319-365-6411

Nonprofit camp for children with disabilities.

Robin Butler

8383 Des Moines YMCA Camp
1192 166th Drive
Boone, IA

515-432-7558
Fax: 515-432-5414
e-mail: ycamp@dmymca.org
www.y-camp.org

For boys and girls with cancer, diabetes, asthma, cystic fibrosis, hearing impaired and other disabilities.

Dan Breitbach, Executive Director

8384 Easter Seals Camp Sunnyside
Easter Seals Iowa
PO Box 4002
Des Moines, IA

515-289-1933
Fax: 515-289-1281
e-mail: essia@netins.net
www.easterseals.com

Each summer from June through August, campers with disabilities ages five and up, take part in one week camping sessions, gaining skills and independence by participating in activities like swimming, horseback riding, canoeing, fishing, camping and more. Financial assistance available.

Martha Wittkowski, President/CEO
Paul Thorne, Director Camping/Recreation

Kentucky

8385 Bethel Mennonite Camp
2773 Bethel Church Road
Clayhole, KY 41317

606-666-4911
Fax: 606-666-4911
e-mail: grow@bethelcamp.org
www.bethelcamp.org

8386 Easter Seal Kysoc
1902 Easterday Road
Carrollton, KY 800-8

502-732-5333
800-800-888
Fax: 502-732-0783
e-mail: ek1@cardinalhill.org
www.cardinalhill.org

Designed for the fullest camping experience for children or adults with physical disabilities, blind, deaf, behavior disorders, mental retardation, diabetes and multiple handicaps, ages 7 and up.

Heide Miller, CCD, CTRS, Director

Louisiana

8387 Camp Bon Coeur
PO Box 53765
Lafeyette, LA

337-233-8437
Fax: 337-233-4160
www.heartcamp.com

8388 Louisiana Lions Camp for Crippled Children
PO Box 171
Leesville, LA

337-239-0782
Fax: 318-239-9975
e-mail: lalions@lionscamp.org
www.lionscamp.org

Camp for disabled children.

Raymond Cecil III

8389 Med-Camps of Louisiana
102 Thomas Road Suite 615
West Monroe, LA 71291

318-329-8405
Fax: 318-329-8407
www.medcamps.com

Maine

8390 Camp Waban
5 Dunaway Drive
Sanford, ME

207-324-7955
Fax: 207-324-6050
www2.kidscamps.com

8391 Pine Tree Camp Children - Adults
149 Front Street
Bath, ME 04530

207-397-2141
Fax: 207-397-5324
e-mail: ptcamp@pinetreesociety.org
www.pinetreesociety.org

Peter D Phair, Director Services
Harvey Chesley, Director Operations

Maryland

8392 Easter Seals Camp Fairlee Manor
22242 Bay Shore Road
Chestertown, MD

410-778-0566
Fax: 410-778-0567
www2.kidscamps.com

8393 Kamp-A-Kom-Plish
9035 Ironsides Road
Nanjemoy, MD 20662

301-870-3226
Fax: 301-870-2620
www.kampakomplish.org

8394 The League at Camp Greentop and The Therapeutic Recreation
League: Serving People with Disabilities
1111 E Cold Spring Lane
Baltimore, MD 21239

410-323-0500
Fax: 410-323-3298
TTY: 410-435-4298
e-mail: jrondeau@leagueforpeople.org
www.campgreentop.org

Summer residential camp located in the Catoctin Mountain National Park. Since 1937, Greentop has been serving children and adults with physical, cognitive, emotional and multiple disabilities in a completely accessible camp setting. Campers enjoy a traditional camping program. Medical facilities, staffed with registered nurses 24 hours a day. ACA/MD Youth Camp. Year round travel programs also offered.

Jonathon Rondeau, Director
Katrina Johnson, Executive Director

Massachusetts

8395 Camp Paul for Exceptional Children
PO Box 53
Chelmsford, MA

Speech and occupational therapy.

Stephen Gannon

8396 Camp Ramah in New England (Summer)
39 Bennett Street
Palmer, MA 01069

413-283-9771
Fax: 413-283-6661
www.campramahane.org

8 week sleep-away camp for Jewish adolescents with developmental disabilities. Full camping program includes swimming, Hebrew singing and dancing, sports, arts and crafts, daily services, Kosher food, and Jewish studies classes.

Howard Blas, Director

8397 Camp Ramah in New England (Winter)
35 Highland Circle
Needham Heights, MA

701-449-7090
Fax: 413-283-6661
www.campramahane.org

8 week sleep-away camp for Jewish adolescents with developmental disabilities. Full camping program includes swimming, Hebrew singing and dancing, sports, arts and crafts, daily services, Kosher food, and Jewish studies classes.

Howard Blas, Director

8398 Carroll School Summer Programs
25 Baker Bridge Road
Lincoln, MA

781-259-8342
Fax: 781-259-8852
www.carrollschool.org

Academic and recreational programs designed to improve learning skills and build self-confidence. The school is a tutorial program for students not achieving their potential due to poor skills in reading, writing and math. The summer camp complements the summer school offering outdoor activities in a supportive, non-competitive environment.

8399 Handi-Kids/King Solomon Foundation
470 Pine Street
Bridgewater, MA

508-697-7557
Fax: 508-697-1529
e-mail: handi7557@aol.com
www.handikids.com

A therapeutic recreational facility in Bridgewater, Massachusetts offering after-school programs, special events, school vacation full-week and summer day camp programs. Every individual is welcome regardless of the severity of a child's disability.

Mary L Gallant, Program Director

8400 Massachusetts Easter Seals Camping Program
484 Main Street
Worcester, MA 01608

800-922-8290
Fax: 508-831-9768
TTY: 800-564-9700
www2.kidscamps.com

8401 New England Experience
22 Addington Road
Brookline, MA

617-244-1200

Held at Avon Old Farms School, campers may attend for 2, 4, 6 or 8 weeks. Highlights are circus training, computers, electronic music, sports and courses in creative writing and desktop publishing. Tutoring and SAT preparation are available.

Clark Adams

Michigan

8402 Camp Barakel
PO Box 159
Fairview, MI 48621

989-848-2279
Fax: 979-848-2280
www.campbarakel.org

Five-day Christian camp experience in mid-August for campers ages 13-55 who are physically disabled, visually impaired, upper trainable mentally impaired or educable mentally impaired, bus transportation provided from locations in Lansing, Flint, Bay City, and Marshall, Michigan.

Lee Brown, Program Director

8403 Camp Catch-A-Rainbow
American Cancer Society
1205 E Saginaw Street
Lansing, MI 800-A

517-371-2920

Open to any child who has, or has had, cancer.

8404 Camp Fish Tales
2177 Erickson Road
Pinconning, MI

517-879-5199
www.campfishtales.org

8405 Camp O' Fair Winds
2300 Austins Parkway
Flint, MI 48507

810-230-0244
800-482-6734
Fax: 810-230-0955
e-mail: tplotz@gsfwc.org
www.gsfwc.org/camps.htm

Outdoor program for all girls, ages 7-11. Our goal is to build confidence by giving girls a chance to voice their opinions and make their own decisions. We are able to accommodate girls with diabetes, ADHD, and learning disabilities. We are willing to make special accommodations - including hiring individual assistants for girls with hearing impairments and physical disabilities.

Therese Plotz, Camp Director
Olga Recio, Camp Secretary

8406 Discovery Center of Michigan
1450 E Brown Road
Mayville, MI

Accepts learning disabled campers ages 8-18.

Alan Zsolzai, Executive Director

8407 Indian Trails Camp
0-1859 Lake Michigan Drive NW
Grand Rapids, MI

616-677-5251
Fax: 616-677-2955
www.indiantrails-camp.org

Year round residential camping program for children and adults with physical disabilities.

Lynn Gust, Executive Director

Minnesota

8408 Camp Eden Wood
Friendship Ventures
10509 108th Street NW
Annandale, MN 55302

952-852-0101
800-450-8376
Fax: 952-852-0123
e-mail: fv@friendshipventures.org
www.friendshipventures.org

Camp Eden Wood offers resident camp programs for children, teenagers, and adults with developmental, physical or multiple disabilities, special medical conditions, Down syndrome, Williams syndrome, autism or other conditions. Summer camp offers archery, sailing, horseback riding, biking, fishing, creative arts, adventure challenge programs and other activities. Weekend camps and longer available. Other services available throughout the year.

Georgann Rumsey, President/CEO
Laurie Tschetter, Program Director

8409 Camp Friendship
Friendship Ventures
10509 108th Street NW
Annandale, MN 55302

952-852-0101
800-450-8376
Fax: 952-852-0123
e-mail: fv@friendshipventures.org
www.friendshipventures.org

Camp Friendship offers resident camp programs for children, teenagers, and adults with developmental, physical or multiple disabilities, special medical conditions, Down syndrome, Williams syndrome, autism or other conditions. Summer camp offers archery, sailing, horseback riding, biking, fishing, creative arts, adventure challenge programs and other activities. Weekend camps and longer available. Other services available throughout the year.

Georgann Rumsey, President/CEO
Laurie Tschetter, Program Director

8410 Camp Winnebago
19708 Camp Winnebago Road
Caledonia, MN

507-724-2351
Fax: 507-724-3786
e-mail: campwinn@means.net
www.campwinnebago.org

We offer one week summer sessions for children and adults with developmental disabilities. We also do integrated youth sessions to allow friends and siblings to attend with our traditional campers. Respite week-ends are offered monthly throughout the year. Travel vacations are also offered as an option. We also publish a newsletter and have a video available.

8-12 pages

Cathy Greeley, Executive Director
Marsha Dowe, Program Director

8411 Courage Camps
Courage Center
3915 Golden Valley Road
Golden Valley, MN 55422

612-588-0811
888-888-846
Fax: 612-520-0577
e-mail: camping@mtn.org
www.couragecamps.org

Summer resident camp serving children and adults who have physical or sensory disabilities. Also for children who need the help of a speech clinician. Special sessions include those for children who have been burned, children who have cancer and their siblings, and children who have hemophilia or sickle cell anemia. Offers special outdoor education or leadership sessions for deaf, or physically disabled teens and a sports camp for physically disabled and blind teens.

Eric Stevens, Executive Director

8412 Courage North
PO Box 1626
Lake George, MN 56458

218-266-3658
Fax: 218-266-3458
www.couragecamps.org

8413 Eden Wood Center
Friendship Ventures
6350 Indian Chief Road
Eden Prairie, MN

952-852-0101
Fax: 952-852-0123
e-mail: fv@friendshipventures.org
www.friendshipventures.org

Offers resident camp programs for children, teenagers and adults with developmental, physical or multiple disabilities, Down Syndrome, special medical conditions, Williams Syndrome, autism and/or other conditions. Fishing, creative arts, golf, sports and other activities are available. Creative Options Respite Care offers weekend camps year round for children, teenagers and adults. Ventures Travel offers guided vacations for teens and adults with developmental disabilities or other unique needs.

Georgann Rumsey, President/CEO
Laurie Tschetter, Program Director

8414 Knutson
523 N 3rd Street
Brainerd, MN

218-828-7610

Provides a camping program for mentally and physically disabled and emotionally disturbed children and adults. Campers must come with an established group that brings its own counselors. Swimming, sailing, archery, nature study and hiking are among the non-competitive activities.

Robert Larson

8415 Search Beyond Adventures
400 S Cedar Lake Road
Minneapolis, MN 800-8

612-374-4845
800-800-800
www2.kidscamps.com

Mississippi

8416 Tik-A-Witha
PO Box 126
Van Vleet, MS

662-844-7577
Fax: 662-680-3164
www2.kidscamps.com

Missouri

8417 Camp Wee-Y
Rural Route 2
Potosi, MO 800-3

573-438-2724
800-800-323

The YMCA day camp for children ages 6-8. Children are under the direction and supervision of their counselors and engage in small group and camp-wide activities and work on developing their skills and self-confidence.

Jean Jencks

8418 Sidney R. Baer Day Camp
2 Millstone Drive
Saint Louis, MO

Co-ed day camp serving campers ages 5-12 years old.

Astrid Balzer, Special Needs
Andy Brown, Camp Director

Nebraska

8419 Camp Easter Seals
609 N 60th Road
Nebraska City, NE 800-6

402-578-3992
800-800-650
www2.kidscamps.com

New Hampshire

8420 Camp Allen
56 Camp Allen Road
Bedford, NH 03110

603-622-8471
www.campallennh.org

A summer camp for individuals with disabilities.

8421 Camp Dartmouth-Hitchcock
Dartmouth-Hitchcock Medical Center Pediatrics
1 Medical Center Drive
Lebanon, NH

603-650-5597
Fax: 603-650-8980
www2.kidscamps.com

8422 Crotched Mountain School & Rehabilitation Center
1 Verney Drive
Greenfield, NH 800-9

603-547-3311
800-800-966
Fax: 603-547-3232
e-mail: info@cmf.org
www.cmf.org

Currently serves children ages 6-22 with multiple-handicaps including: Cerebral Palsy, Spina Bifida, visual and hearing impairments and neurological disabilities, developmental disorders, mental retardation, autism, behavioral and emotional disorders, seizure disorders, spinal cord and head injuries. Member of the National Association of Independent Schools and accredited with the NE Association of Schools and Colleges, Independent Schools of Northern NE.

Rita Phinney, Director Admissions
John Young, Registrar

New Jersey

8423 Bancroft Camp
425 Kings Highway East
Haddonfield, NJ 08033

856-429-0010
Fax: 207-729-1603
www.bancroft.org

Has served as a summer camp for children and adults enrolled in Bancroft programs. The camp recognizes the need for individuals with developmental disabilities to vacation with their families. The camp offers a resort program for people wishing to explore the fascinating coast of Maine or to relax in the clean New England air. Accommodations include accessible rustic cabins and bayfront cottages.

Joseph Kuhn, Director

8424 Camp Chatterbox
150 New Providence Road
Mountainside, NJ 07092

908-301-5451
www.campchatterbox.org

8425 Camp Merry Heart/Easter Seals Easter Seal Society
RD 21 O'Brian Road
Hackettstown, NJ

908-852-3896
Fax: 908-852-9263

An organized program of swimming, arts and crafts, boating, nature study and travel offered to the physically disabled, developmentally disabled, cerebral palsied, brain damaged and head injured children, ages 5-18, adults 19-75+. Fall and spring travel programs for adults.

Mary Ellen Ross, Camping Director

8426 Camp Oakhurst
111 Monmouth Road
Oakhurst, NJ

908-531-0215
www2.kidscamps.com

8427 Camp Vacamas
256 Macopin Road
West Milford, NJ

973-838-1394
Fax: 973-838-7534
e-mail: info@vacamas.org
www.vacamas.org

Disadvantaged children with asthma or sickle cell anemia, ages 8-16, are offered special programs in canoeing, backpacking, camping, music and leadership training. Sliding scale tuition. Year round programs for groups.

Michael Friedman, Executive Director
Philip Smith, Camp Director

8428 Cross Roads Outdoor Ministries
29 Pleasant Grove Road
Port Murray, NJ 07865

908-832-7264
Fax: 908-832-6593
e-mail: crossroadsom@yahoo.com
www.crossroadsretreat.com

Program for ages 6-15 offers Bible study, worship, swimming, crafts, hiking, canoeing and campfires. Special education program for those with developmental disabilities.

Jonathan Winters, Retreat Coordinator

8429 Easter Seals Camp Merry Heart
21 O'Brian Road
Hackettstown, NJ

908-852-3896
Fax: 908-852-9263

An organized program of swimming, arts and crafts, boating, nature study and travel offered to the physically disabled, developmentally disabled, cerebral palsied, brain damaged and head injured children, ages 5-18, adults 19-75+. Fall and spring travel programs for adults plus respite weekends.

Mary Ellen Ross, Director Camping

New Mexico

8430 Santa Fe Mountain Center
PO Box 449
Tesuque, NM

505-983-6158
Fax: 505-983-0460
www.sf-mc.com

Camp sessions offered to disabled campers from the ages of 1-20.

Skye Gray, Director

New York

8431 Advocates for Children of New York
151 W 30th Street, 5th Floor
New York, NY 10001

212-947-9779
Fax: 212-947-9790
e-mail: info@advocatesforchildren.org
www.advocatesforchildren.org

Camp fair.

Elisa Hyman, Executive Director

8433 Camp Huntington
56 Bruceville Road
High Falls, NY 12440

845-687-7840
Fax: 845-687-7211
e-mail: camohtgtn@aol.com
www.camphuntington.com

Summer activities include recreational, academic and vocational programs for the learning disabled, neurologically impaired and mildly ADA to mild/moderately retarded. An Olympic pool, horse riding and a special work training program are featured. Programs are tailored to meet individual needs, ages 6-21, and campers may enroll for 4 to 8 weeks.

Dr. Bruria Falik, Director

8435 Freedom Camp
Carr Bldg, 188 Genesee St, Suite 109
Auburn, NY 13021

315-253-5465

A summer day camp for youths with disabilities sponsored by Freedom Recreational Services. Freedom Camp is offered in two-week sessions at Casey Park in Auburn, New York.

Mary Ellen Perry, Executive Director

8436 Gow School Summer Programs
2491 Emery Road
South Wales, NY 14139

716-652-3450
Fax: 716-652-3457
e-mail: summer@gow.org
www.gow.org

Co-ed summer programs for ages 8-16, offer a balanced blend of morning academics, afternoon/evening traditional camp activities and weekend overnight trips (teen-tours). The primary purpose of these programs is to provide a positive experience while balancing these three elements. Committed to the creation of a positive and enjoyable experience for each participant, by defining and merging the goals of the camp and the school, with those of camper students, their families and educators.

Bekah D Atkinson, Admissions Director

8437 Marist Brothers Mid-Hudson Valley Camp
1455 Broadway
Esopus, NY 12429

845-384-6620
Fax: 845-384-6479

Serves special people: deaf, retarded and children with cancer; HIV positive children.

Brother Don Nugent, Administrator

8438 Oakhurst
853 Broadway
New York, NY

212-253-8680

Accepts children and young adults who are physically handicapped, ages 8-18. The program includes physical therapy, recreational activities and a work program for teenagers.

Marvin Raps

8439 Programs for Children with Disabilities: Ages 3 through 5
1 Commerce Plaza
Albany, NY

518-473-6108
e-mail: mpltzke@mail.nysed.gov

Michael C Noyes, PhD, Director

8440 Programs for Children with Special Health Care Needs
Tower Building
Albany, NY

518-474-2084
e-mail: cx104@health.state.ny.us

Claudia Lee, Acting Director

8441 Programs for Infants and Toddlers with Disabilities: Ages Birth Through 2
Empire State Plaza
Albany, NY

518-473-7016
e-mail: dmn02@health.state.ny.us

Donna M Noyes, PhD, Director

8442 Ramapo Anchorage Camp
PO Box 266
Rhinebeck, NY

845-876-8403
Fax: 845-876-8414

Residential program which serves children, ages 4-16, with a wide range of emotional, behavoral, and learning problems. A one-to-one ratio of counselors-to-campers enables children to build healthy relationships, increase self-esteem and improve learning skills. Character values such as honesty, concern for others, responsibility, and the courage to do one's best are encouraged. Campers demonstrate significant gains in their ability to maintain relationships, control impulses and adjust.

Bernie Kosberg, Executive Director
Michael Kunin, Associate Director

8443 Triangle
9 Camp Road
Rexford, NY

For learning disabled children, ages 7-18, with the emphasis on recreation and socialization skills. Vocational training, academics and speech therapy are available.

Shirley Schofield

8444 Wagon Road
Children's Aid Society
431 Quaker Road
Chappaqua, NY

914-238-4761
Fax: 914-238-0714
www.childrensaidsociety.org

Provides residential respite services to developmentally disabled children ages 7-18. At its 50 acre campus which is entirely wheelchair accessible, 24 hour RN and MD services are provided.

North Carolina

8445 Camp Winding Gap
Rural Route 1, Box 56
Lake Toxaway, NC

828-966-4520
Fax: 828-883-8720
www.campwindinggap.com

For boys and girls ages 8-16, with facilities for up to 75 campers. A high staff-camper ratio (less than 1 to 3) of carefully selected counselors provides a nurturing family atmosphere. A few children with disabilities are mainstreamed each session. Must be able to handle horseback riding and rugged terrain, this is a ranch type camp in a farm setting with many animals. Program includes regular camp activities.

Ann Hertzberg, Director

8446 Talisman Programs
64 Gap Creek Road
Zirconia, NC 28790

828-669-8639
888-458-8226
Fax: 828-669-2521
e-mail: summer@stonemountainschool.com
www.talismansummercamp.com

Talisman Programs offers summer programs for kids ages 8-17 with ADHD, learning disabilities, high functioning autism, or Aspergers Syndrome. Our high-adventure programs include paddling, hiking, rock climbing, an Alpine Tower, swimming, arts and crafts, and many other activities designed to promote communication and cooperation skills. We focus on building social skills and self esteem in 2 and 3 week programs. One session of academics.

Linda Tatsapaugh, Director

Ohio

8447 Camp Allyn
1414 Lake Allyn Road
Batavia, OH

513-732-0240
Fax: 513-735-1461
e-mail: ssc@one.net
www.steppingstonecenter.org

A camp for children and adults with disabilities.

Dennis Carter, Associated Director

8448 Highbrook Lodge Camp
12944 Aquilla Road
Chardon, OH

216-791-8118
Fax: 216-791-1101
e-mail: mmullin@clevelandsightcenter.org
www.clevelandsightcenter.org

A summer residential camp for blind and disabled children, adults and families.

Mike Mullin, Director

Oregon

8449 Easter Seals Oregon Camping Program
5757 SW Macadam Avenue
Portland, OR 800-5

503-228-5108
Fax: 503-228-1352
e-mail: camp@oregonseals.org
www2.kidscamps.com

8450 Mt Hood Kiwanis Camp
9320 SW Barbur Blvd, Suite 165
Portland, OR 97219

503-272-3288
Fax: 503-452-0062
www2.kidscamps.com

Pennsylvania

8451 Briarwood Day Camp
1380 Creek Road
Furlong, PA 18925

215-598-7143
Fax: 215-497-0587
www.briarwood-camp.com

A comprehensive day camp providing lunch and transportation for children with disabilities.

Ted Levin

8452 Camp Lee Mar
450 Route 590
Lackawaxen, PA

215-658-1788
Fax: 215-658-1710
e-mail: gtour400@aol.com
www.leemar.com

A camp for children with developmental challenges, ages 5-21. Offers a program of academics, speech therapy, vocational training and recreation. The academic program is designed to help each child develop skills in the areas of communication, reading and math. Activities include swimming, boating, team sports, tennis and perceptual motor training.

Lee Morrone, Director
Ariel J Segal, Assistant Director

8453 Keystone Community Resources
406 N Washington Avenue
Scranton, PA

570-346-7561
Fax: 570-342-3461
e-mail: LCunningham@keycommres.com
www.keycommres.com

Keystone serves both children and adults with developmental disabilities in a variety of residential settings. Support services include 24 hour supervision, on site nursing services, special and therapeutic recreation programs and psychological and psychiatric services.

Robert Fleese, President
Lisa Cunningham, Director Admissions

8454 Summer Experience
Vanguard School
PO Box 730
Paoli, PA

610-296-6700

For students who are experiencing learning difficulties due to neurological impairment, social/emotional disturbance and/or autism/pervasive developmental disorder.

Susan Snyder, Admissions Director
John D Wilson, Education Director

8455 Variety Club Camp & Development Center
Variety Club
PO Box 609
Worcester, PA

610-584-4366
Fax: 610-584-5586
e-mail: djfindley@msn.com
www.varietyphila.org

Year-round camping and recreation facility for children with special needs and their families. Includes summer camping, aquatics, weekend retreats and other specialty programs.

Daniel Findley, Executive Director

8456 Wesley Woods
1 Fiddlegreen Road
Grand Valley, PA

814-430-7802
Fax: 814-436-7669
www.wesleywoods.com

Exceptional children's camp for children with emotional and intellectual handicaps.

Herb West

8457 Yomeca
75 Hill School Road
Douglassville, PA

The YMCA day camp for children ages 9-13. Small group and camp-wide activities are offered. Streams, woods and trails to explore. Children ages 10-12 also have several overnights offered to them during the summer. Children continue to build upon established skills from earlier years, take on more leadership, challenge and responsibility and strengthen past friendships.

South Carolina

8458 Burnt Gin Camp
SC Department of Health and Environmental Control
Box 101106
Columbia, SC

803-898-0455
Fax: 803-898-0613
e-mail: aimonemi@columb60.dhec.state.sc.us
www.scdhec.net/hs/mch/burntgin/hsbgin5.htm

A residental camp for children who have physical disabilities and/or chronic illnesses. Camper/staff ratio is 2:1. Four seven-day sessions for 7-15 year olds and two six-day sesssions for 16-19 year olds. Limited to residents of South Carolina.

Marie I Aimone, Camp Director

Tennessee

8459 Camp Easter Seal
6300 Benders Ferry Road
Mount Juliet, TN 37122

615-444-2829
Fax: 615-444-8576
www.tn.easter-seals.org

Texas

8460 Children's Association for Maxiumum Potential CAMP
PO Box 27086
San Antonio, TX 78227

210-671-2598
www.campcamp.org

Overnight camping, day-care, respite and rehabilitation to children with severe medical, physical or mental disabilities. Large medical staff enables nationwide acceptance of children with severe problems.

8461 Hughen Center
2849 9th Avenue
Port Arthur, TX

409-983-6659
Fax: 409-983-6408

The Center provides a therapeutic, educational, and recreational program for children with physical disabilities. Physical and occupational therapy are featured. Day and residential.

Jeff Kuchar, Executive Director

8462 Texas Lions Camp
Lions Clubs of Texas
PO Box 290247
Kerrville, TX

830-896-8500
Fax: 830-896-3666
e-mail: tlc@ktc.com
www.lionscamp.com

The primary purpose of the League shall be to provide, without charge, a camp for physically disabled, hearing/vision impaired and diabetic children from the State of Texas, regardless of race, religion, or national origin. Our goal is to create an atmosphere wherein campers will learn the can do philosophy and be allowed to achieve maximum personal growth and self esteem. The camp welcomes boys and girls ages 7-16.

Stephen Mabry, Executive Director
Amber Schrank, Program Director

Utah

8463 Camp Kostopulos
2500 Emigration Canyon
Salt Lake City, UT

801-582-0700
Fax: 801-583-5176
www.campk.org

One of only a few camps in the Intermountain region that provides recreational opportunities for individuals of all ages with mental or physical disabilities. Activities include fifteen days of swimming, fishing, fieldtrips, nature study, arts and crafts and traditional outdoor adventure games. Five year-round programs offered.

Gary Ethington, Director

Vermont

8464 Farm and Wilderness Camps
HCR 70, Box 27
Plymouth, VT

802-422-3761
802-422-3761
Fax: 802-422-8660
www2.kidscamps.com

8465 Thorpe Camp
680 Capen Hill Road
Goshen, VT 05733

802-247-6611
www2.kidscamps.com

Virginia

8466 Camp Baker Services
7600 Beach Road
Chesterfield, VA

804-748-4789
Fax: 804-796-6880

Year round support services for children and adults with disabilities. Operated by the Richmond Area ARC, programs include: an 8-week summer camp program; weekend congregate respite services; summer day camp (8 wks); spring fling (spring break).

Melissa Wahers, Director
Jolene Loving, Assistant Director

8467 Camp Easter Seal East, Camp Easter Seal We st
201 E Main Street
Salem, VA 800-3

540-362-1656
Fax: 540-563-8928
www.campeasterseal-va.org

Six and 12 day summer camp sessions for children and adults ages 5 and older with physical disabilities, cognitive disabilities, sensory impairments. Therapeutic recreation activities including swimming, fishing, sports, horseback riding, rock climbing, and more. 26 speech therapy camp children with disabilities ages 8-16. 12 day Spina Bifida Self Help Skills Camp.

Deborah Duerk, Director
Devin Brown, Director

8468 Camp Fantastic
Special Love
117 Youth Development Court
Winchester, VA 22602

703-667-3774

Nonprofit organization that provides enriching programs for children with cancer, including Camp Fantastic.

8469 Camp Holiday Trails
400 Holiday Trails Lane
Charlottesville, VA 22903

434-977-3781
Fax: 434-977-8814
e-mail: Cht@firstva.com
www.summer-camps.virginia.cc

Private, nonprofit camp for children with special health needs, various chronic illnesses. Residential, 2 week sessions are open July 1 - August 10, $500 per 2 weeks; camperships are available. Coed 7-17, nationwide and international. Canoeing, swimming, horseback riding, arts and crafts, drama, ropes course, etc. 24-hr. medical supervision by doctor and nursing staff. Air conditioned cabins.

Mark D Andersen, Executive Director

8470 Makemie Woods Camp Conference Center
PO Box 39
Barhamsville, VA 23089

757-566-1496
800-566-1496
Fax: 757-566-8003
www.makemiewoods.org

Counselors serve as teachers, friends and activity leaders. The individual is important within the small group. No camper is lost in the crowd, but is an integral partner in the group process. Residential Christian Camp and conference center. Summer camp for children 8-18 special camp for children with diabetes.

Michelle Burcher, Director

8471 Overlook
RR 1, Box 203
Keezletown, VA

540-269-2267

A Christian life experience for youth and children, located at the base of the scenic Massanutten Mountains.

Ronald Robey

8472 Triangle D Camp for Children
1701 North Beauregard Street
Alexandria, VA 22311

414-248-1330
800-342-2383

Disabled campers.

Marilyn Caras

West Virginia

8473 Mountain Milestones Stepping Stones
15 Cottage Street
Morgantown, WV 800-9

304-296-0150
800-800-982
Fax: 304-296-0194
e-mail: stepping@westco.net
www2.kidscamps.com

A nonprofit organization.

Missy Weimex, Recreation Coordinator

Wisconsin

8474 Camp Joy
W7725 Kettle Moraine Drive
Whitewater, WI 53190

262-473-3132
Fax: 262-473-0941
www.campjoy.org

A year round residential camping program for children and adults with mental retardation and physical disabilities. Brochure, video, and application available upon request.

Shannon Durante, Camp Director

8475 Timbertop Nature Adventure Camp
1000 Division Street
Stevens Point, WI 54481

715-342-2980
Fax: 715-342-2987

For children who can benefit from an individualized program of learning in a non-competitive outdoor setting under the skilled leadership of people who understand the environment and the unique potential of these children.

8476 Wisconsin Lions Camp
3834 County Road A
Rosholt, WI

715-677-4761
Fax: 715-677-3297
TTY: 715-677-6999
e-mail: lioncamp@wi-net.com
www.wisconsinlionscamp.com

Serves children who have either a visual, hearing or mild cognitive disability. Many of the children also have multiple disabilities or medical conditions. Program activities include sailing, ropes course, bike and canoe trips, environmental education, swimming, camping, canoeing, outdoor living skills and handicrafts. ACA accredited, located in central Wisconsin, near Stevens Point.

Russell Link, Camp Director

Wish Foundations

8477 Children's Dream Factory of Maine
400 US Route 1, ATTN: Doris Simard
Falmouth, ME 04105

207-781-3406
800-639-1492
www.cureourchildren.org

Grants wishes for chronically or seriously ill children from Maine.

8478 Children's Wish Foundation
100 E Sybelia, Suite 300
Maitland, FL 32751

407-629-8920
Fax: 407-629-7206
www.childrenswish.org

Orlando-based organization that grants wishes for children with life-threatening illnesses who have not yet reached their 18th birthday. Focuses primarily on children who reside in Florida, but has also granted wishes to children from other parts of the US, Canada, England, and Russia.

8479 Dream Factory
200 W Broadway, Suite 504
Louisville, KY 40202

502-561-3001
800-456-7556
Fax: 502-561-3004
e-mail: DFHQTRS@aol.com
www.dreamfactoryinc.com

The Dream Factory grants dreams to children disagnosed with critical or chronic illnesses who are 3 through 18 years of age.

Stan Adler, Director Of Operations
Jennifer Habig, Directir Of Development

8480 Famous Fone Friends
9101 Sawyer Street
Los Angeles, CA 90035

310-204-5683
e-mail: fonefriends@aol.com

Offers the ability for a sick child's doctor or nurse to arrange for a well-known actor, athlete or other celebrity to call the child.

8481 Freedom's Wings International
PO Box 7076
East Brunswick, NJ 08816

732-432-8342
800-382-1197
www.freedomswings.org

Freedom's Wings International (FWI) is a non-profit organization run by and for people with physical disabilities. We provide the opportunity for those who are physically challenged to fly in specially adapted sailplanes, either as a passenger or as a member of the flight training program.

8482 Give Kids the World
210 S Bass Road
Kissimmee, FL 34746

407-396-1114
800-995-5437
Fax: 407-396-1207
e-mail: dream@gktw.org
www.gktw.org

Makes dreams come true for terminally ill children and their families with a six-day, cost-free visit to Walt Disney World area.

8483 Grant A Wish Foundation
6601 Frederick Road
Baltimore, MD 21228

410-242-1549
800-933-5470
Fax: 410-744-1984
www.grant-a-wish.org

We grant the wishes of children with life-threatening medical conditions to enrich the human experience with hope, strength and joy.

8484 Kids
9300-D Old Keene Mill Road
Burke, VA 22015

703-455-KIDS

Grants unfulfilled wishes to gravely ill children 16 and younger anywhere in the U.S.

8485 Magic Moments- Children's Hospital of Alabama
1600 7th Avenue S
Birmingham, AL 35233

205-939-9372
Fax: 205-939-6717
e-mail: info@magicmoments.org
www.magicmoments.org

Grants wishes to children four to nineteen living or being treated in Alabama, who have chronic, life-threatening diseases, or who have severe trauma (burns, spinal cord, head trauma).

8486 Make A Wish Foundation of America
4041 N Central Avenue, Suite 555
Pheonix, AZ 85012

602-230-9900
800-722-9474
Fax: 602-230-9627
www.wish.org

Information and advocacy resources for families and professionals. Includes listings of organizations providing general information and organizations focusing on more specific areas of concern to families and young adults who have disabilities.

8487 Sunshine Foundation
1041 Mill Creek Drive
Feasterville, PA 19053

215-396-4770
800-767-1976
Fax: 215-396-4774
e-mail: philly@sunshinefoundation.org
www.sunshinefoundation.org

Grants dreams and wishes of terminally and chronically ill children whose parents are under financial strain due to the child's illness. Original wish granting organization.

Patricia C Radecke, Executive Assistant

8488 Teddi Project
Camp Good Days and Special Times
356 North Midler Avenue
Syracuse, NY 13206

315-434-9477
Fax: 315-595-6153
www.campgooddays.org

Priority given to children from Central Florida and the upstate New York area, especially Buffalo, Rochester, Syracuse, Albany, and Binghamton. Services chronically or terminally ill children ages seven to seventeen.

8489 Thursday's Child
PO Box 259279
Madison, WI 53725

608-988-4234
e-mail: dorothyf@pciinet

Grants wishes to seriously ill children who live in or are being treated in southwest and south central Wisconsin.

8490 Wish Upon a Star
California Law Enforcement
PO Box 4000
Visalia, CA 93278

209-733-7753

Serves children in the state of California. Nonprofit, law enforcement effort designed to grant wishes of children afflicted with high-risk and terminal illnesses.

8491 Wish with Wings
917 W Sanford Street
Arlington, TX 76012

817-469-9474
Fax: 817-275-6005
e-mail: wish@awishwithwings.org
www.awishwithwings.org

Founded in 1982, grants wishes for children ages three-eighteen years of age who have life threatening diseases. The organization serves children who reside in or are receiving treatment in the state of Texas.

Kim Christian, Executive Director

8492 Wishing Star Foundation
915 W 2nd Avenue
Spokane, WA 99201

509-744-3411
Fax: 509-744-3414
e-mail: info@wishingstar.org
www.wishingstar.org

Serves Idaho, eastern Washington, and some areas of Oregon and Nevada. Grants wishes to children three to nineteen with life-threatening diseases.

Holly Stetson, Executive Director

8493 Wishing Well Foundation
PO Box 717, Jim Reid
Saint Louis, MO 63188

314-272-6190
www.wishingwellusa.org

Grants wishes to children in the St. Louis area only who are chronically or terminally ill.

DESCRIPTION

Cardiovascular

The cardiovascular system, also known as the circulatory system, consists of the heart and the blood vessels. The functions of the cardiovascular system include the following:

- To maintain the continual flow of blood throughout the body to provide cells with oxygen and vital nutrients

- To assist in the removal of carbon dioxide and other waste products from cells

The Heart

Anatomy

The heart, a hollow, muscular organ the approximate size and shape of a clenched fist, is an efficient pump that maintains the continuous flow of blood through the vessels to all areas of the body. It is located between the lungs in approximately the center of the chest, with its right margin located under the right side of the breastbone (sternum) and the remaining areas pointing toward the left. The "tip" or the lowest point of the heart, known as the apex, rests on the diaphragm and is situated beneath the left nipple.

The heart consists of four chambers and is divided into left and right sides by a thick, fibrous, central partition known as the septum. The upper chambers of the heart are known as atria, and the lower chambers are called ventricles. Each chamber is referred to by its location: i.e., the left and right atria and the left and right ventricles. The atria are smaller and have thinner walls than the ventricles. The walls of the chambers of the heart are composed of specialized cardiac muscle known as the myocardium, and their internal surfaces are lined with a thin layer of smooth membrane tissue called the endocardium.

The heart and the roots of its major blood vessels are surrounded by a membrane (pericardium) that consists of two fibrous layers. The pericardium has a tough outer layer (fibrous pericardium) that surrounds the heart like a loose-fitting bag, providing space for the heart to beat. The inner layer (serous pericardium) consists of an innermost "sheet" (visceral layer) that is attached to the heart and an outermost layer (parietal layer) that lines the inside of the fibrous pericardium. A space between the inner layers contains a thin film of fluid that lubricates the opposing surfaces of the inner membranes, enabling the heart to beat without friction.

Cardiac Function

Contraction of the heart muscle is termed systole, whereas relaxation is known as diastole. The atria and ventricles beat in a precise rhythmic pattern. One cycle of this pattern is known as a heartbeat. As the atria contract, they force blood into the ventricles. Once the ventricles fill with blood, they contract, pumping blood either to the lungs or out to the rest of the body.

The pumping action of the heart also involves the heart valves at the entrance to and exit from the ventricles. These valves control and direct the flow of blood through the heart. Two heart valves separate the atria from the ventricles (atrioventricular valves), preventing the backward flow of blood into the atria during ventricular contraction. The valves include the mitral or bicuspid valve, situated between the left atrium and left ventricle, and the tricuspid valve, located between the right atrium and right ventricle. In addition, two heart valves (semilunar valves) are situated between the two ventricles and the large blood vessels that transport blood away from the heart during ventricular contractions. The aortic semilunar valve, located where the major artery of the body (aorta) arises from the base of the left ventricle, enables blood to flow from the left ventricle into the aorta while preventing the backward flow of blood into the ventricle. The pulmonary semilunar valve, situated where the pulmonary artery arises from the base of the right ventricle, enables blood to flow from the right ventricle to the lungs while preventing the backward flow of blood.

"Oxygen-poor" or deoxygenated blood that has circulated through the body enters the right side of the heart into the right atrium through two large veins (the superior and inferior vena cava). The blood is then pumped through the tricuspid valve into the right ventricle. When the ventricle contracts, blood is pumped through the pulmonary semilunar valve into the pulmonary artery and on to the lungs, where the exchange of oxygen and carbon dioxide occurs. Oxygen-rich blood is returned to the left atrium by way of four pulmonary veins and is pumped through the bicuspid valve into the left ventricle. When the ventricle contracts, blood is pumped through the aortic semilunar valve into the aorta for circulation to the body's tissues.

The heart muscle or myocardium requires an ongoing supply of oxygen and other nutrients to function efficiently; thus, the coronary circulation transports vital oxygen-rich (oxygenated) and nutrient-rich arterial blood to the heart muscle and returns deoxygenated, nutrient-poor blood back to the venous system. Blood is transported to the myocardium by way of the left and right coronary arteries, which are the first branches of the aorta. Once blood is circulated to the myocardium, supplying the heart with oxygen and other nutrients, it passes into the cardiac veins, which then empty into the coronary sinus and into the right atrium.

Each heartbeat, also known as a cardiac cycle, consists of the contraction (systole) and relaxation (diastole) of the atria and ventricles. In order for the heart to pump efficiently, the different areas of the heart and the cardiac muscle fibers must work together in an exact sequence. Precise coordination is achieved through the transmission of electrical impulses originating from the heart's "pacemaker" (the sinoatrial node at the apex of the right atrium). These signals are then relayed to the various areas of the heart via a complex system of fibers (atrioventricular node, bundle of His, and Purkinje fibers). The electrical transmissions are delivered with precision timing to various areas of the heart, resulting in a rhythmic beat.

The Blood Vessels

Blood vessels are like a system of complex tubing of different sizes through which blood flows to various parts of the body. Different types of blood vessels have different purposes. For example:

- Some vessels ensure the movement of blood from one part of the body to another.

- Other much smaller vessels (i.e., the capillaries) facilitate the exchange of certain nutrients and waste products between the blood and the fluid surrounding cells within bodily tissues.

Function

There are several types of blood vessels including arteries, arterioles, capillaries, venules, and veins. The arteries, which carry blood away from the heart, progressively subdivide into smaller and smaller vessels known as arterioles, which control blood flow into the minute vessels known as capillaries. The arterioles help to regulate proper arterial blood distribution and pressure by constricting or expanding as necessary. The thin walls of microscopic capillaries facilitate the exchange of nutrients and waste products between the blood and tissue fluid surrounding the cells. For example, oxygen and glucose move from the blood in the capillaries to the fluid surrounding cells and then into the cells themselves; in contrast, carbon dioxide and other waste products move from the cells into the blood within the capillaries. The oxygen-poor blood then flows from the capillaries into the small blood vessels known as venules. The venules join with other venules and progressively increase in size, becoming larger veins that transport the blood toward the heart.

The systemic circulation also includes a specialized group of vessels known as the hepatic portal circulation, within which blood flow follows a somewhat different route. Veins from certain organs, such as the stomach, intestines, spleen, pancreas, and gallbladder, do not transport blood directly into the inferior vena cava but, rather, into the hepatic portal vein, which carries blood to veins, venules, and capillaries within the liver. Nutrients pass from the blood in the capillaries into liver cells where various toxic substances are filtered from the blood. Hepatic veins carry blood from the liver and rejoin the systemic circulation via the inferior vena cava.

Structure

Arteries and veins consist of three layers including an outermost layer (tunica adventitia), a middle layer of smooth muscle (involuntary muscle) tissue (tunica media), and an inner lining (tunica intima or endothelium). The middle layer of arteries is thicker than that of veins, enabling the arteries to withstand the pressure of ventricular contractions. In contrast, blood returning to the heart via the veins remains at a relatively low pressure. The passage of blood through the veins is assisted by involuntary muscle that compresses the walls of the veins; in addition, veins have one-way valves that prevent the backward flow of blood.

Capillaries have extremely thin walls and cannot be seen by the naked eye. They consist of only one layer (tunica intima), enabling oxygen and certain wastes to easily pass through them.

Fetal Blood Circulation

Because the developing fetus must obtain nutrients and oxygen from the mother's blood, the fetal circulation differs somewhat from the circulation after birth. During pregnancy, blood vessels carry fetal blood to the placenta, where oxygen and nutrients are exchanged between the fetal and maternal blood supply, and then return blood to the fetus. Two relatively small umbilical arteries carry deoxygenated blood, whereas a larger umbilical vein carries oxygen-rich blood. The fetal circulation also includes vascular channels or openings (e.g., ductus venosus, ductus arteriosus, foramen ovale), enabling most blood to bypass the developing liver and lungs. In most cases, once an infant is born and the pulmonary circulation is established, such vascular channels close and the umbilical blood vessels collapse soon after birth.

DESCRIPTION

Cells

The human body consists of literally trillions of atoms, molecules, and cells that are organized in several "structural levels."

Atoms and molecules. Atoms of oxygen, sodium, nitrogen, and carbon, for example, are the infinitesimal components of the most basic level of living matter of the body. Atoms link to one another to form molecules.

Cells. These are the smallest structural units that are able to live independently. The human body has billions of cells that are functionally integrated to perform the complex, vital tasks necessary for sustaining life. Cells are organized in the following ways:

- Tissues. Bodily tissues are organizations of structurally similar, specialized cells that carry out a common function.

- Organs. The organs of the body are groupings of two or more different types of tissues incorporated into a functional, structural unit to perform certain, specialized functions.

- Bodily systems. These comprise the final level of structural organization within the body. Bodily systems consist of several, interdependent organs that work together to perform integrated functions.

Certain mechanisms enable cells of the body to conduct activities that are vital for ongoing growth and survival. These include the processes of metabolism and homeostasis.

Metabolism
Metabolism refers to all the physical and chemical processes occurring within the body's tissues and includes catabolism and anabolism. Catabolism refers to the breakdown of large, complex substances into simpler, smaller substances, usually resulting in the release of energy. During anabolism, complex substances are built up from simpler substances, usually resulting in consumption of energy. The processes of respiration, circulation, digestion, and excretion, for example, collectively enable the body to provide those substances required for metabolism and remove the byproducts or waste products of metabolism. Abnormal changes in genetic material (mutations) or inherited defective genes may cause inborn errors of metabolism, affecting the body's ability to function properly.

Homeostasis
Homeostasis refers to the processes by which the body maintains a balanced internal environment (equilibrium). In order to maintain homeostasis, the body requires oxygen, water, other nutrients, and regulated atmospheric pressure and body temperature, for example. Because disturbances from the external environment as well as cellular activity continually challenge internal equilibrium, the body has on-going self-regulating systems (feedback systems) that induce the responses necessary to maintain or restore homeostasis. For example, abnormally decreased levels of oxygen in the blood are counteracted by increased breathing rates that restore normal blood oxygen levels.

Cells
Cells are extremely complex, containing several subcellular structures vital to life. Human cells vary greatly in size and shape and are adapted for their specific functions. However, most cells are similar in structure. They contain fluid material known as cytoplasm surrounded by a thin, outer membrane (plasma membrane). The plasma membrane separates the fluid and specialized structures (organelles) within each cell from the fluid that surrounds and bathes the cells of the body. The cytoplasm of most human cells contains a circular, membrane-bound structure known as the nucleus.

Plasma Membrane
The plasma membrane serves to keep cells intact. In addition, it regulates the entry of oxygen and certain vital nutrients into cells and enables the passage of carbon dioxide and other waste materials out of cells. Certain protein molecules on the surface of the plasma membrane also bind with other protein molecules, activating particular cellular functions.

Cytoplasm
The cytoplasm is essentially the "living matter" of the cell, containing the fluid that comprises the cell's inner environment and the specialized parts known as organelles. The organelles include the following:

- Ribosomes are relatively tiny particles that function as "protein factories." They produce proteins, which are large molecules consisting of combinations of certain chemical "building blocks" (amino acids). Proteins play an essential role in the body. Particular proteins serve as the source of "building materials" for certain tissues and organs of the body (e.g., muscle, skin, blood, etc.). Other protein compounds known as enzymes accelerate the rate of chemical reactions in the body. Proteins also play an essential role in the elimination of waste materials and have many other functions.

- Endoplasmic reticulum (ER) is a complex network of small tubular membranes arranged in complex folds. This network winds throughout the cytoplasm of a cell. Passageways within the endoplasmic reticulum transport proteins and other substances to different areas within a cell. Rough ER has a rough texture due to the presence of ribosomes attached to its outer surface. Carbohydrates, fats, and certain types of proteins are manufactured within smooth ER.

- The Golgi apparatus, which is located near the nucleus, is a system of microscopic, stacked membranous sacs and spaces. Small "bubbles" or sacs (vesicles) from the smooth ER transport newly produced proteins to the Golgi apparatus, where they fuse with the Golgi sacs. The Golgi apparatus then processes and modifies the proteins and packages them into small vesicles. These vesicles break away and eventually fuse with the plasma membrane, at which point they break open and release their contents outside of the cell for transport to other cells.

- Centrioles are typically paired rod-like structures that participate in cell division.

- Mitochondria are tiny organelles that have double membranes and sacs with inner, folded partitions. Known as the "power plants" of the cells, the mitochondria serve as the major source of cellular energy production due to their complex, ongoing chemical reactions.

- Lysosomes are the major digestive units of cells. Enzymes within lysosomes break down (digest) particles of nutrients as well as certain invading particles such as bacteria.

- Cilia are hair-like projections on the surfaces of certain cells that move together in a wave-like manner. For example, cilia within the mucous membranes of the respiratory tract (respiratory mucosa) propel mucus upward and out of the tract.

Nucleus

The nucleus regulates cellular activities by controlling the functions of the organelles and cell reproduction. It is surrounded by a nuclear envelope that encloses a cellular material within the nucleus known as nucleoplasm. Pores within the nuclear envelope's membranes enable the interior of the nucleus to "communicate" with the cell's cytoplasm. The nucleoplasm of the nucleus contains several structures including the nucleolus and chromatin.

The nucleolus regulates the formation of ribosomes within the nucleus. Ribosomes then move through the nuclear envelope to the cell's cytoplasm where they engage in protein production.

Chromatin, the material within the nucleus from which chromosomes are created, consists of thread-like structures comprised of protein and deoxyribonucleic acid (DNA). DNA is the carrier of the genetic code and is described as a "double helix" because of its relatively long, spiraling, ladder-like structure. It consists of strands of certain chemical groups that are linked by pairs of substances known as

"bases." There are four types of bases including adenine, which always pairs with thymine, and the base cytosine, which always pairs with guanine. Therefore, the sequence of bases on one strand of the helix coincides with the sequence on the other strand, enabling DNA molecules to duplicate before cell division.

Chromosomes

During the division and reproduction of cells, DNA condenses and gradually forms into the rod-like structures known as chromosomes. The DNA of the chromosomes carries the genetic information that controls the ultimate growth, development, and functioning of the body and determines the expression of certain inherited traits, such as blood groups, various physical characteristics (e.g., hair color, eye color, height), etc.

The cell that is produced when an egg (ovum) is fertilized by a sperm is known as a zygote. With the first and each subsequent division of the zygote, chromosomes within the zygote's nucleus are duplicated. Therefore, in most cases, all cells in the human body contain the same chromosomal material. In rare cases, some individuals may have some cells that contain differences in certain genetic material (mosaicism) due to an error in cellular division.

The nuclei of cells (except for ova and sperm) normally contain 46 individual chromosomes, one of each pair from the mother and the other from the father. Chromosome pairs are numbered from 1 to 22 with a 23rd pair consisting of one X chromosome from the mother and an X or a Y chromosome from the father. Males have an X and a Y chromosome and females have two X chromosomes within the 23rd pair. Each chromosome has a long arm designated "q" and a short arm designated "p." Both arms are further divided into numbered bands. Every individual chromosome contains thousands of genes, which are the hereditary units that contain segments of DNA. Genes function within cells by regulating the production of proteins. The 46 human chromosomes collectively contain approximately 100,000 genes that, together, are referred to as the "human genome."

Chromosomal Disorders

In some cases, due to certain abnormalities during cellular division (meiosis or mitosis), individuals may have abnormalities in the structure or number of chromosomes in the nuclei of cells of the body. There may be extra or missing whole chromosomes or chromosomal material within all or some of the body's cells. Because chromosomes contain many genes, the range and severity of associated symptoms and physical findings may vary greatly, depending upon the exact nature and location of the chromosomal abnormality.

RNA

Genes, which are sections of DNA, regulate the production of certain proteins. Ribonucleic acid or RNA is essential in "decoding" the inherited instructions within genes. RNA is similar in structure to one strand of DNA, with some differences-e.g., replacement of the base thymine with uracil. During the formation of RNA, a strand of DNA "unwinds" and a duplicate copy of a gene sequence is created. This copy is known as messenger RNA or mRNA. The mRNA migrates from the nucleus to the cytoplasm, promoting protein production in the ribosomes and endoplasmic reticulum. The ribosomes use information within the mRNA molecule to translate chemical "building blocks" known as amino acids into a properly sequenced protein strand.

Cellular Reproduction: Mitosis
Most cells of the body are replicated or reproduced during a complex process known as mitosis. During mitosis, a single cell divides in order to form two "daughter cells" with chromosomes identical to those within the original cell. The process of mitosis enables the body to produce new cells, to replace cells that have been damaged or lost due to injury or disease, and to replace cells that have aged and no longer function efficiently.

Sometimes mitosis may become uncontrolled, resulting in the development of an abnormal mass of replicating cells known as a neoplasm. Such growths may be noncancerous (benign tumors) or cancerous (malignant).

Cellular Reproduction: Meiosis
Reproductive cells in the male and female sex glands (gonads, including the testes and ovaries) carry out a different form of cell division known as meiosis. During mitosis, one cell division occurs, creating two daughter cells-each of which contains 46 chromosomes. Unlike mitosis, two cellular divisions occur during meiosis, resulting in four daughter cells-each of which contains half of the chromosomes (i.e., 23 chromosomes).

Genetic Mutations
During the processes of mitosis and meiosis, the chromosomes within an original cell and thus its genetic material (DNA) are replicated and passed along to its daughter cells. Sometimes, errors may occur during this replication process, resulting in small changes or mutations in genetic composition. Such genetic mutations are passed along with every subsequent division of the daughter cell. For example, a genetic mutation may occur during the production of a reproductive cell (ovum or sperm). If that cell is eventually involved in fertilization, the resultant zygote and all of its reproduced cells will contain the same genetic error. Thus, every cell of the developing embryo and fetus will contain the identical mutant gene.

Genes function within cells by directing the manufacture of a particular protein. Therefore, mutations of a particular gene may impair the appropriate production of its protein. The effects of a particular gene mutation depend upon the function of its protein within the body. Disorders that result due to such mutations are termed genetic disorders.

Genetic Disorders
Human traits are the result of the interaction of two genes, one received from the mother and one received from the father. There are typically two genes engaged in the regulation of a particular protein. If one such gene changes or mutates and "overrides" the instructions of the normal gene on the other chromosome, the abnormal gene is said to be dominant. If the mutated gene is not expressed and is "masked" by the normal gene on the other chromosome, the mutated gene is termed recessive. In such cases, two copies of the mutated gene are required for possible expression of the disease trait.

Genetic disorders may be classified into unifactorial and multifactorial defects. Unifactorial genetic disorders result due to abnormalities of a single gene or gene pair. Such disorders may be autosomal or X-linked.

In autosomal dominant disorders, the presence of a single copy of the disease gene results in the disorder. The mutated gene "overrides" or dominates the other normal gene. An affected individual may have inherited the disease gene from one of his or her parents, or the disease may arise as a result of an abnormal change (mutation) that occurred randomly, for unknown reasons (sporadically). If an individual with an autosomal dominant disorder has children, all offspring have a 50 percent risk of inheriting the defective gene.

In autosomal recessive disorders, two copies of the same disease gene are necessary for an individual to potentially develop the disorder. If both parents carry a single copy of the disease gene, all offspring have a 25 percent risk of inheriting both disease genes and expressing the disorder. Fifty percent of their children risk being carriers, and 25 percent may receive both normal genes for that trait.

In X-linked disorders, the disease gene is located on the X chromosome. As discussed earlier, females have two X chromosomes, whereas males have one X chromosome from the mother and one Y chromosome from the father. In females, certain disease traits on the X chromosome may be "masked" by the presence of a normal gene on the other X chromosome. In other cases, certain disease traits may not be fully masked by the normal gene; as a result, some females who carry a single copy of such a disease gene (heterozygous carriers) may express some of the symptoms associated with the disorder. In such cases, heterozygous females often have more variable, less severe symptoms than affected males. Because males have only one X chromosome, if they inherit such a disease gene, they generally express the physical characteristics or other findings associated with the disease and are typically more severely affected than females. Males with X-linked disorders transmit the disease gene to their daughters but not to their sons. Females with one copy of such a disease gene have a 50 percent risk of transmitting the gene to their daughters and their sons.

In multifactorial disorders, susceptibility to a disorder is determined by the interaction of several different genes, possibly in association with the involvement of certain environmental factors.

Tissues

As mentioned above, tissues are groups of structurally similar cells that perform a common function. Different tissues within the human body may vary greatly in terms of the size, shape, and specific functioning of their cells.

There are four main types of tissue in the human body including epithelial tissue, connective tissue, muscle tissue, and nervous tissue.

Epithelial tissue or epithelium covers the surfaces of the body, lines most of its hollow structures or cavities, and serves to provide protection and support. In addition, some epithelial tissues permit the absorption of certain nutrients (e.g., oxygen into the blood); help to protect the body against invading microorganisms; or produce and release certain secretions. The cells within epithelial tissue are tightly packed together and contain no blood vessels; however, blood vessels within underlying connective tissue provide epithelial cells with nutrients. Different types of epithelial tissue are categorized based upon cellular shape and thickness.

Connective Tissue

Connective Tissue

The purpose of connective tissue, the most widely distributed tissue of the body, is to bind together and, along with the skeleton, provide a supporting framework to bodily tissues and organs. The shape and arrangement of connective tissue cells and the intercellular substance between such cells differ depending upon the type of connective tissue. There are several major forms of connective tissue in the body including the following:

- Areolar tissue, which consists of cells embedded in webs of loosely arranged fibers, supports and provides form to most internal organs of the body.

- Adipose tissue, which consists of fat cells within a mesh of areolar tissue, serves to insulate the body against heat loss, protect and cushion certain areas of the body, and store fat as a future energy source.

- Fibrous connective tissue, which consists primarily of parallel rows of white collagen fibers, are the cords of strong, dense, flexible tissue that connect muscle to

bone (tendons). Collagen is the major structural protein of the body.

- Bone, the hardest connective tissue of the body, provides a supportive framework, assists in movement, and houses bone marrow.

- Cartilage, which has the consistency of firm or gel-like plastic, helps to absorb shock and provides flexibility.

- Blood, interestingly, is considered to be a type of connective tissue. Even though it has a different function in comparison to other connective tissues, it does have an extracellular liquid matrix (plasma). Plasma has several functions including providing a defense against invading microorganisms, repairing damage to blood vessels and tissues through blood clotting, and transporting oxygen, vital nutrients, and waste products.

The purpose of the body's muscle tissue is to enable movement through muscle contraction and relaxation. The nervous tissue of the body includes specialized cells that ensure ongoing, rapid communication between structures of the body and the control of bodily functions necessary to maintain life.

DESCRIPTION

Dermatologic

The dermatologic system includes the skin, the largest organ of the body, and its derivatives, such as the skin glands, the hair, and the nails. The skin, the sheet-like, outermost covering of body tissue, has several vital functions:

- To serve as a sensory organ. The skin's millions of sensory nerve endings (receptors) serve as somatic sense organs, enabling the body to respond to pain, variations in temperature, pressure or touch sensations, and other important changes in the surrounding environment.

- To help protect the human body from the harmful effects of the sun, chemicals, invading microorganisms, injuries, fluid loss, and other hazards.

- To assist in normalizing the body's temperature through the regulation of blood flow close to the body's surface and sweat secretion. For example, when the body is too cold, blood vessels within the skin constrict to help conserve body heat. When the body is too hot, blood vessels within the inner layer of the skin (dermis) widen (dilate) and the sweat glands secrete perspiration to cool the body.

The skin comprises several tissue layers including a thin, outermost layer (epidermis); a thicker, inner layer (dermis); and a thick underlying layer of subcutaneous tissue, which is a loose layer of connective tissue and fat. The subcutaneous tissue helps to insulate the body from extremes in temperature, protects underlying tissues from injury, and serves as a stored energy source.

Epidermis

The epidermis, which serves as the protective outer layer of skin, is made up of tightly packed cells (epithelial cells) that are arranged in layers. The thickness of the epidermis is variable, depending on its function; for example, it is relatively thick on the palms of the hands, yet comparatively thin on the eyelids.

The outermost layer of the epidermis (stratum corneum epidermidis) consists of dead cells that create a tough, protective covering. As the dead cells are sloughed off, they are replaced by new cells that are produced by rapidly dividing cells within the innermost layer of the epidermis (stratum germinativum). As new cells rise upward though cellular layers (strata) and approach the surface, their cytoplasm-i.e., the inner substance of cells other than the nucleus-is replaced by the tough protein keratin. In addition, specialized cells (melanocytes) within the deepest layer of the epidermis produce melanin, a pigment that gives coloration to the skin.

Dermis

The dermis, the innermost layer of skin, consists of connective tissue; lymph vessels, blood vessels, sensory nerve endings (skin receptors), and muscle fibers; as well as other specialized structures, including sweat glands, sebaceous glands, and hair follicles.

The uppermost portion of the dermis contains rows of peg-like projections (dermal papillae) that help bind together the dermal and epidermal layers (dermal-epidermal junction) and form the characteristic grooves and ridges (dermatoglyphic patterns) on the skin of the palms and tips of the fingers. Such ridges, which are unique to each individual, develop before birth.

The deeper portion of the dermis contains a network of fibers including those that provide the skin with the necessary toughness (collagen fibers) as well as elasticity and the ability to stretch (elastic fibers). The number of elastic fibers decreases with advancing age and the level of fat stored within the subcutaneous tissue is also reduced. Consequently, the skin loses its elasticity.

Skin Glands

The sweat glands within the dermis are classified according to their location and type of secretion. These glands include the eccrine and apocrine glands.

The eccrine glands are the most widespread sweat glands in the body. Their function is to produce sweat or perspiration, which helps to eliminate certain waste products (e.g., uric acid, etc.) and to maintain a constant body temperature.

The apocrine glands, larger glands that produce a thicker secretion than that of the eccrine glands, are primarily located under the arms (axilla) and around the genitals. Such glands begin to function during puberty.

The dermis also contains sebaceous glands, tiny glands that open into hair follicles. They produce an oily secretion known as sebum that helps to lubricate the hair and skin and protect the skin from drying. Sebum secretion increases during adolescence (due to increased levels of certain sex hormones); however, it decreases during later adulthood, contributing to skin wrinkling and cracking.

Hair

When epidermal cells grow into the dermis, a small tube called a hair follicle may be formed. The growth of a hair begins from a tiny cluster of cells (hair papilla) at the base of the follicle. New hair replaces any that has been cut or plucked, for example, as long as the hair papilla is alive. The hair itself is a threadlike structure consisting of dead cells filled with keratin. The root is that portion of the hair that remains hidden within the follicle, whereas the shaft is the visible portion of the hair. A particular hair color results from the amount and specific form of the pigment melanin that has been produced by melanocytes at the base of the hair follicle. The straightness or curliness of the hair depends upon the shape of the hair follicle.

A few areas of the body are hairless, including the palms of the hands, the soles of the feet, and the lips. Most hair on the body is fine and barely visible, with the most visible hair typically including that on the scalp, the eyebrows, and the eyelashes. Coarse hair also typically develops under the arms and in the pubic area during puberty (i.e., in response to the secretion of certain hormones). In addition, most males also develop coarser hair in the facial area, on the trunk, and on the arms and legs.

Skin Receptors

The dermis also has sensory nerve endings (skin receptors) that function as sense organs (i.e., somatic sense organs), transmitting messages to the brain concerning temperature, touch, pressure, and pain. For example, Pacini's corpuscle receptors, which are located deep within the dermis, detect pressure on the surface of the skin. Meissner's corpuscle receptors, which are usually close to the skin's surface, detect light touch sensations. Other skin receptors include those that detect other touch sensations, cold, heat, vibration, or pain.

Nails

The nails are produced when epidermal cells on the ends of the fingers and toes fill with the tough protein keratin. The nail body is the visible portion of the nail, whereas the remainder of the nail, known as the nail root, is hidden by a fold of skin (cuticle). A portion of the nail body that is closest to the root has a white, crescent-shaped area called the lunula. Tissue underneath the nail, known as the nail bed, contains many blood vessels, causing it to appear pinkish in color.

DESCRIPTION

Digestive

The digestive system consists of organs that break down food into small chemical components that ultimately may be used by cells of the body for energy (metabolism), growth, and repair. It includes the alimentary canal or gastrointestinal (GI) tract, which is the long, hollow passageway through which food passes, as well as associated organs, such as glands whose secreted juices help to break down (digest) food. Organs that comprise the GI tract include the mouth, pharynx, esophagus, stomach, small intestine, large intestine, and anus. Associated organs include the tongue, teeth, gallbladder, and digestive glands, such as the salivary glands, pancreas, and liver.

Nutrients

The foods of an individual's diet primarily include water as well as other nutrients necessary for growth and development. These include proteins, which play an essential role in cell repair and replacement; vitamins; carbohydrates, which serve as the primary energy source and assist in the breakdown and metabolism of other nutrients; fats; and minerals. Most minerals and vitamins may be absorbed into the blood circulation from the digestive system with no change in structure. However, other nutrients must be broken down into smaller, simpler (less complex) food molecules. Food is broken down (digested) through physical and chemical processes. Physical breakdown of food materials is performed by the chewing and grinding actions of the teeth, for example. The actions of certain digestive enzymes (i.e., substances that act as catalysts in the breakdown of proteins and other nutrients) as well as other substances (e.g., acids) chemically break down food as it travels through the GI tract. Thus, the nutrients are reduced into smaller molecules that may be absorbed through the lining of the intestinal wall for distribution to body cells.

Layers of the GI Tract

The hollow internal space within the alimentary canal or GI tract is known as the lumen. The walls of the GI tract consist of four layers of tissue, including an outermost covering (serosa); the mucous membrane (mucosa), which produces the mucus that lines the canal; the submucosa, a layer of connective tissue beneath the mucosa; and underlying layers of muscle tissue (muscularis). Regular, rhythmic contractions of involuntary (smooth) muscle within these layers of underlying muscle tissue propel food through the GI tract in a process known as peristalsis.

Mouth

Digestion begins in the mouth. The roof of the mouth, known as the palate, has a hard, bony, front portion (hard palate) and a soft, fleshy area (soft palate) that consists primarily of muscle. The tongue, which forms most of the floor of the mouth, is a flexible, muscular organ that helps manipulate food during chewing. It also contains the microscopic chemical receptors (taste receptors) that produce the nerve impulses necessary for taste (taste buds).

The teeth, which assist in the chewing and grinding of food, are firmly attached to the upper and lower jaws. The gums (gingiva), which consist of a mucous membrane and supporting fibrous tissues, surround the teeth, serving as "shock absorbers" and keeping the teeth tightly set into the jaws. Enclosing the oral cavity are the cheeks and the upper and lower lip. In addition, as with all of the GI tract, the mouth is lined by a mucous membrane. Saliva, a thin, watery fluid that is secreted by the salivary glands and the mucosa of the mouth, assists in the process of swallowing by moistening the oral mucosa; lubricating food; initiating the breakdown of certain food products through its digestive enzymes; and promoting the sense of taste.

Teeth

The teeth are essential for the chewing, tearing, and grinding of food (mastication) as it mixes with saliva. Humans typically have two sets of teeth including the primary (deciduous) teeth and the permanent (secondary) teeth. There are usually 20 primary teeth that erupt between the ages of six months and two to three years. The primary teeth are gradually replaced by the permanent teeth beginning at about six years of age. Adults typically have 32 permanent teeth.

There are four major types of teeth that are classified based upon their shape and location:

- Incisors are chisel shaped and have sharp edges for cutting during mastication. The incisors are the eight front teeth (i.e., four in the upper jaw and four in the lower jaw).

- Canines or cuspids are sharp, pointed teeth that tear or pierce food. The four canines (i.e., two in the upper jaw and two in the lower jaw) are situated next to the incisors.

- Premolars or bicuspids have large, flat surfaces with two grinding "cusps" to assist in the breakdown of food during mastication. The eight premolars are situated next to and in back of the canines. The primary teeth include no premolars.

- Molars or tricuspids also have large, flat surfaces, yet have three grinding "cusps." The 12 molars are located in back of the premolars. The primary teeth typically include only four molars in the upper jaw and four in the lower jaw. Wisdom teeth are typically known as third molars. They usually erupt in the late teens and early twenties.

The interior of each tooth contains living pulp, which includes connective tissue, sensory nerves, and blood and lymphatic vessels. The pulp is surrounded by the dental tissue known as dentin. In addition, each tooth is divided into a crown, neck, and root. The crown, the exposed portion of a tooth, is covered by enamel, the hardest tissue in the human body. The neck, which is the narrow portion of the tooth surrounded by the gums, and the root, which fits into the bony socket of the lower or upper jaw, are covered by the sensitive dental tissue cementum. A fibrous membrane (periodontal membrane) connects the cementum to the jaw and gums.

Salivary Glands

The salivary glands are the three pairs of glands that secrete saliva. Their secretions are released into ducts that empty into the mouth. Because the salivary glands release their secretions into ducts, they are exocrine glands. The salivary glands include the parotid, submandibular, and sublinqual. The parotid glands, the largest of the salivary glands, are located below and in front of the ears at the angle of the jaws. Their ducts open inside the cheeks. The submandibular glands are located toward the back of the mouth, and their ducts open under the tongue. The ducts of the sublingual glands secrete saliva onto the floor of the mouth. Saliva contains digestive enzymes (salivary amylase) that initiate the chemical digestion of certain foods (e.g. carbohydrates).

Pharynx

The pharynx, also known as the throat, is a muscular tube lined with mucous membranes and is part of the digestive and respiratory systems. Food and fluids enter the throat from the mouth and exit via the esophagus. However, air normally enters the pharynx from the nasal cavities and exits via the larynx. (For more information, please see the section entitled The Respiratory System.)

Esophagus

The esophagus is a muscular tube that transports food from the pharynx to the stomach. It is also lined with mucous membrane. The upper portion of the esophagus is encircled by a ring-shaped muscle (sphincter) that opens to allow the passage of food products. A similar muscle (cardiac sphincter) is located where the esophagus joins the stomach. The walls of the esophagus contain strong smooth muscles fibers, and rhythmic wavelike contractions of these involuntary muscles (peristalsis) propel food toward the stomach.

Stomach

The stomach is a hollow, pouch-like organ located in the upper portion of the abdominal cavity. It continues the breakdown of food that began in the mouth. Once food passes through the cardiac sphincter from the esophagus, it is contained in the stomach by contraction of the ring-shaped muscle at the end of the stomach (pyloric sphincter).

The walls of the stomach consist of three layers of smooth muscle and are lined with mucous membrane containing specialized cells that secrete gastric juices. These juices contain hydrochloric acid and digestive enzymes (e.g., rennin, pepsin) that are necessary for the breakdown of proteins. Rhythmic contractions of the stomach's smooth muscle layers mix digesting food with gastric juices, forming a semiliquid mixture known as chyme. Once partially digested food has been mixed into the chyme, relaxation of the pyloric sphincter and contractions of the stomach propel the chyme into the duodenum of the small intestine.

Small Intestine

The small intestine has three sections: the duodenum, jejunum, and the ileum. The function of the small intestine is to continue the breakdown of food products as they travel through the GI tract and to promote the absorption of nutrients into the bloodstream.

As rhythmic contractions of smooth muscles (peristalsis) propel food through the small intestine, digestive juices from the pancreas and bile from the liver are added to partially digested food within the duodenum. In addition, the mucus lining of the small intestine contains tiny glands that secrete intestinal digestive juice. Mucus, the enzymes within the intestinal digestive juice (e.g., maltase, sucrase, lactase, peptidase), and the secretions from the pancreas and liver serve to further break down food into smaller food molecules that may be more easily absorbed.

The mucosa of the small intestine is organized into several circular folds (plicae) covered with minute projections known as villi. Each villus contains finger-like lymphatic vessels (lacteals that absorb fat soluble nutrients (lipids) from the small intestine for transport to the blood circulation. Such fats are absorbed in the form of chyle, a cloudy milky substance containing products of digestion. The villi also contain blood capillaries that absorb certain products of digestion (e.g., amino acids, sugars).

Pancreas

The pancreas, an elongated gland located across the back of the abdomen, functions as both an exocrine and endocrine gland. It primarily consists of exocrine tissues that secrete pancreatic juice into ducts entering the duodenum. Pancreatic juice is an essential digestive juice that contains enzymes (e.g., trypsin, lipase, amylase) necessary for the breakdown of proteins, fats, carbohydrates, and certain acids. The pancreas also contains tiny clumps of endocrine cells (pancreatic islets) that secrete certain hormones, directly into the bloodstream.

The exocrine cells of the pancreas secrete their enzymes into several ducts that combine to form the main pancreatic duct. This duct joins with the common bile duct, which conveys bile from the gallbladder, and then opens into the duodenum. Most of the digestive enzymes secreted by the exocrine cells are activated by enzymes within the duodenum. In addition, exocrine cells of the pancreas secrete sodium bicarbonate, a substance that neutralizes the hydrochloric acid within the stomach's gastric juice as it enters the duodenum.

Liver, Bile Ducts, and Gallbladder

The liver, one of the largest organs of the body, is located within the upper right abdominal cavity. As part of the digestive system, the liver functions as an exocrine gland whose cells secrete the substance known as bile into a network of ducts (bile ducts). Bile, a liquid that consists of waste products, cholesterol, and bile salts, carries waste products from the liver and assists in the digestion and absorption of fats within the small intestine. The bile ducts transport bile from the liver to the gallbladder and on to the uppermost region of the small intestine (duodenum). The gallbladder, a small, muscular sac located under the liver, stores and concentrates bile from the liver. When chyme that contains fats (lipids) enters the duodenum from the stomach, the fats stimulate the secretion of a hormone (cholecystokinin) from the mucous membrane of the duodenum; in turn, the hormone stimulates contraction of the gallbladder, forcing bile into the small intestine.

The liver also has several additional essential functions in the body. These include regulating the blood levels of amino acids, the building blocks of proteins; helping to filter toxic substances from the blood; and producing certain proteins within the fluid portion of the blood (plasma). Such proteins include certain components that play a role in blood clotting (coagulation factors); particular blood proteins (complement system) that, when activated, destroy invading microorganisms; and the protein albumin, which helps to regulate the exchange of water between the bloodstream and bodily tissues. In addition, the liver produces cholesterol and certain proteins that transport fats in the bloodstream to cells throughout the body and processes hemoglobin for use of its iron content. Hemoglobin is the protein that enables red blood cells to transport large amounts of oxygen to cells.

Large Intestine

The large intestine is the organ that forms the lower portion of the GI tract. This organ, which has a larger diameter than the small intestine, consists of several areas. These include a pouch-like area (cecum); the ascending, transverse, descending, and sigmoid colons, the latter of which descends into the pelvic area and terminates in the rectum; and the end of the rectum known as the anal canal, which terminates at the external opening known as the anus. In addition, the appendix, a small, tubular structure, hangs from the cecum. Because the appendix contains lymphatic tissue, it may play a small role in helping to protect the body against infection; however, it has no known role in the body's digestive system.

As food matter that has not been broken down or absorbed moves through the lower region of the small intestine (ileum), it passes into the large intestine through the ileocecal valve. Bacteria within the large intestine act upon the undigested material, potentially resulting in the release and absorption of additional nutrients. Water, vitamins, fats and minerals are absorbed into the bloodstream through the lining of the large intestine. Remaining undigested material is expelled through the rectum, anal canal, and anus as feces. Swelling (distension) of the rectum typically stimulates the desire to defecate, i.e., empty feces from the rectum. Two ring-shaped muscles (sphincters) usually remain contracted to keep the anus closed except during the process of defecation. The inner anal sphincter consists of involuntary (smooth) muscle, where the outer anal sphincter is composed of voluntary muscle.

DESCRIPTION

Endocrine

The term "endocrine system" is used to describe a group of specialized tissues, glands, and other structures that have the ability to produce and secrete certain complex chemical substances (hormones) into the bloodstream or lymphatic circulation for transport to particular tissues or ogans. These hormones have specific effects on certain bodily functions. Hormones assist in regulating the body's growth; controlling the rate of chemical processes in the body (metabolism); promoting the maturation and function of reproductive organs and the development of secondary sexual characteristics (puberty); and regulating many other bodily activities. Each hormone molecule may eventually combine with (or bind to) a specific area (receptor) on the surface of a cell within its "target organ," triggering the appropriate response. In contrast, exocrine glands are "outwardly secreting glands"-i.e., they secrete certain substances into ducts for emptying into a particular cavity or onto a bodily surface. (For example, the salivary glands of the digestive system secrete saliva via ducts that empty into the mouth.)

The endocrine glands include the pituitary gland, gonads (ovaries and testes), thyroid gland, parathyroid glands, adrenal glands, pancreatic islets, thymus, pineal gland, and placenta.

Pituitary Gland

The pituitary gland, also known as the "master gland," is a relatively small structure located deep in a saddle-shaped cavity in the skull (sella turcica). The gland is connected to a region of the brain known as the hypothalamus by a stalk of nerve fibers (pituitary stalk). The hypothalamus controls the functioning of the pituitary gland through direct nerve stimulation as well as through the actions of certain nerve cells that secrete hormones (hormone-releasing and hormone-inhibiting factors) into the bloodstream for transport directly to the pituitary. Hormone-releasing factors cause the secretion of certain hormones by the pituitary gland, whereas hormone-inhibiting factors inhibit the production and release of such hormones.

The pituitary gland is divided into two main regions: i.e., the anterior pituitary gland (adenohypophysis) and the posterior pituitary gland (neurohypophysis). Each region is responsible for producing different hormones. The anterior lobe of the pituitary gland produces the following hormones, most of which are considered tropic hormones, i.e., hormones that stimulate the growth of another endocrine gland and the secretion of its hormones.

- Prolactin stimulates the growth of the female breasts (mammary glands) during pregnancy and the secretion of milk by the mammary glands after birth.

- Growth hormone serves to stimulate body development.

- Melanocyte-stimulating hormone (MSH) controls the amount of dark brown or black pigment (melanin) produced by certain specialized skin cells (melanocytes).

- Thyroid-stimulating hormone (TSH) stimulates the production of thyroid hormones.

- Adrenocorticotropic hormone (ACTH) stimulates the growth of the outer regions of the adrenal glands (adrenal cortex) and their production of hormones.

- Follicle-stimulating hormone (FSH) and luteinizing hormone (LH), which are known as gonadotropins, stimulate the gonads, i.e., the sex glands (ovaries and testes) within which the reproductive cells (ova and sperm) are produced.

In addition, the posterior region of the pituitary gland releases two hormones:

- Antidiuretic hormone (ADH) decreases urine production by increasing the reabsorption of water from urine into the blood.

- Oxytocin stimulates powerful contractions of involuntary (smooth) muscle within the uterus during labor. This hormone also stimulates the secretion of milk (lactation) by the female mammary glands during breast-feeding.

Gonads

In females, the paired glands, known as the ovaries, produce the female sex cells (ova or eggs), and, in males, the paired structures, called the testes, produce the male sex cells (spermatozoa or sperm). Follicle-stimulating hormone produced by the pituitary gland promotes the growth and maturation of the cavities in the ovaries (follicles) within which the ova develop and mature; in addition, it stimulates the ovarian follicles' production of the female hormone estrogen. In males, FSH promotes the growth and maturation of and production of sperm by the long, coiled tubules (seminiferous tubules) that form the bulk of the testes. In addition, in females, luteinizing hormone produced by the pituitary gland stimulates the maturation of ovarian follicles and their eggs, the follicles' secretion of estrogen, and the monthly release of ova from the follicles (ovulation). LH stimulates the formation of glandular structures (corpus luteum) within the ruptured follicles that secrete the female hormones progesterone and estrogen. In males, LH stimulates the cells located between the seminiferous tubules in the testes to produce and secrete the male sex hormone testosterone.

Thyroid Gland

The horseshoe-shaped thyroid gland consists of two lobes on either side of the windpipe (trachea) that are joined by a narrow region of tissue (isthmus). Tissue within the thyroid gland consists of follicular cells and parafollicular cells. The follicular cells, which comprise most of the thyroid gland, secrete the thyroid hormones thyroxine (T4) and triiodothyronine (T3). Certain amounts of the thyroid hormones are stored as a semifluid material within the follicular cells, from which they are released into the bloodstream as required. The parafollicular cells secrete the hormone calcitonin.

Secretion of the thyroid hormones T4 and T3 is controlled by the pituitary gland. These hormones assist in regulation of the metabolic rate, i.e., chemical activities within cells that release energy from nutrients or consume energy to create certain substances. The thyroid hormones also play a vital role in the normal mental and physical development and growth of infants and children.

Release of the hormone calcitonin occurs independently of the pituitary gland and hypothalamus. This hormone-in coordination with parathyroid hormone released by the parathyroid glands-helps to regulate the concentrations of calcium in the body. Calcium is a mineral that is important for proper functioning of the cells, blood clotting, muscle contraction, nerve impulse transmission, and other vital functions. Most calcium in the body is stored in bones of the skeleton. Calcitonin has the ability to decrease blood levels of calcium. It suppresses resorption of bone by inhibiting the activity of cells that "digests" bone matrix (osteoclasts), releasing calcium and phosphorus into blood.

Parathyroid Glands

The parathyroid glands are the two pairs of small, oval glands on the back of both lobes of the thyroid gland. These glands produce parathyroid hormone, which serves to increase levels of calcium in the blood by stimulating osteoclasts to reabsorb bone mineral, thus liberating calcium into blood.

Adrenal Glands

The adrenal glands are small, triangular organs that curve over the top of each kidney. The outer region (adrenal cortex) and inner region (adrenal medulla) of the glands have different functions.

The secretion of hormones by the adrenal cortex is regulated by hormones produced by the pituitary gland (e.g., adrenocorticotropic hormone [ACTH]). The adrenal cortex consists of three distinct zones of cells. The outer zone secretes hormones known as mineralocorticoids that help to regulate the levels of certain mineral salts (e.g., sodium) in the blood. The main mineralocorticoid, known as aldosterone, assists in maintaining the delicate balance between sodium and potassium-ultimately helping to regulate blood pressure and blood volume.

The middle and inner zones of the adrenal cortex together secrete hormones known as glucocorticoids, such as hydrocortisone. Glucocorticoids help to regulate the body's use of carbohydrates, fats, and proteins; maintain normal blood pressure; produce certain anti-inflammatory effects; and decrease the production of certain white blood cells that produce antibodies (anti-allergic effect). The middle and inner zones of the adrenal cortex also secrete small amounts of sex hormones (androgens) that stimulate the development of male secondary sexual characteristics and the female sexual drive.

The adrenal medulla or inner region of the adrenal glands releases the hormones epinephrine and norepinephrine in response to nerve impulses from sympathetic nerve fibers. The release of such hormones into the bloodstream serves to increase the heart rate, widen the air passages of the lungs, and dilate blood vessels that supply the skeletal muscles of the body.

Pancreatic Islets

The pancreas, an elongated gland that is located across the back of the abdomen, is divided into a head, body, and tail. It primarily consists of exocrine tissue that secretes digestive enzymes necessary for the breakdown of proteins, fats, carbohydrates, and certain acids.

The endocrine tissue of the pancreas, known as pancreatic islets or islets of Langerhans, consists of tiny clumps of cells among the exocrine cells. The alpha cells of the pancreatic islets secrete glucagon, whereas the beta cells secrete insulin. Glucagon promotes a chemical process (glycogenolysis) during which glycogen, a carbohydrate that is stored in the liver, is broken down into glucose and released into the bloodstream. Insulin serves to regulate and stabilize blood glucose levels by promoting the movement of energy-rich glucose into the cells of the body. The secretion of glucagon increases blood glucose levels. In contrast, secretion of insulin decreases levels of glucose in the blood.

Thymus

The thymus, a small lymphoid organ located behind the breastbone (sternum) in the upper portion of the chest, consists of two lobes that join in front of the windpipe (trachea). This organ functions as an essential part of the immune system, beginning its functions at approximately the twelfth week of fetal development until puberty. The thymus serves as a source of certain white blood cells (lymphocytes) before birth. In addition, the organ secretes hormones (e.g., thymosin) that promote the development of specialized lymphocytes, known as T lymphocytes, which defend the body against certain microorganisms (i.e., during cell-mediated immunity.)

Pineal Gland

The pineal gland is a small, cone-shaped gland that is located deep in the brain. It secretes the hormone melatonin, which is thought to play a role in regulating puberty, ovarian cycles, mood, sleep, and the body's "internal clock" (e.g., 24-hour circadian cycle).

Placenta

The placenta, the organ that develops in the uterus during pregnancy, serves to connect the blood supplies of the mother and the developing fetus. It develops from the chorion, i.e., the outermost layer of cells from the fertilized egg (zygote). The placenta produces chorionic gonadotropin hormone, which stimulates the ovaries to produce the female sex hormones estrogen and progesterone. Both of these hormones are necessary for the functioning of the placenta during pregnancy.

DESCRIPTION

Growth and Development

Human growth and development may be encompassed in two broad categories: namely, prenatal growth and postnatal growth.

Prenatal Growth

The prenatal period, which means the "period before birth," begins when the male reproductive cell (sperm) fertilizes the female reproductive cell (egg or ovum). The fertilized egg (zygote) is a single cell containing all the genetic information (DNA) necessary for the growth and development of a human being. Half of the genetic information (in the form of 23 chromosomes) comes from the egg and half is from the sperm (for a total of 46 chromosomes).

As the zygote begins to travel down the mother's fallopian tube, its single cell immediately begins to divide (in the process called mitosis). (Please see the section entitled Cells for more information.) In approximately three days, the zygote has become a solid mass of cells known as a morula. About a week to 10 days after fertilization, what has become a hollow cellular "ball" (blastocyst) becomes implanted in the lining of the mother's uterus. During the zygote's journey to the uterus for implantation, the ovum supplies nutrients necessary for development of the embryo. The "embryonic phase" of development extends from fertilization until the end of the eighth week of pregnancy (gestation).

As the blastocyst continues to develop, its walls form an outer layer of membranes (chorion) that surround and protect the embryo. In addition, an inner layer of membranes (amnion) forms the amniotic sac, the fluid-filled sac within which the embryo grows and develops, protecting it from injury.

The chorion develops into the placenta, the organ attached to the lining of the uterus that serves to connect the blood supplies of the mother and the developing embryo, enabling the exchange of vital nutrients (including oxygen) and waste products. Blood from the embryo flows through a cord-like structure (umbilical cord) to the placenta and passes into tiny, finger-like blood vessels (chorionic villi) surrounded by maternal blood. The umbilical cord contains three blood vessels: two umbilical arteries that carry oxygen-poor (deoxygenated) blood and a larger umbilical vein that carries oxygen-rich (oxygenated) blood.

Teratogens and Birth Defects

A thin layer of tissue separates the developing embryo's blood and the mother's blood, thus providing protection from certain harmful substances that may circulate in the mother's bloodstream. However, in some cases, particular substances, such as certain infectious agents or drugs (teratogens), may cross this barrier, potentially interfering with prenatal growth and causing developmental abnormalities. The specific abnormalities that may result depend upon a number of factors, including the stage of development during which such exposure occurred, certain genetic influences, the specific teratogen in question, and other environmental factors. Birth defects are abnormalities that are apparent at birth (congenital) or early infancy. Such malformations may occur due to prenatal exposure to teratogens, genetic factors, or a combination of both (multifactorial).

As mentioned above, the embryonic stage of development takes place from fertilization until the end of the eighth week of gestation. The fetal stage of development extends from the ninth week of gestation until birth. Pregnancy is usually approximately 39 weeks in duration and is divided into three phases known as trimesters, each of which is about three months in length.

By approximately the third week of gestation, the head of the developing embryo begins to form and the region that will later become the brain and spinal cord (neural crest) starts to develop. At about four weeks, "buds" of tissue have begun to form that will later develop into certain organs (e.g., liver, lungs, pancreas, etc.) and into the arms, hands, legs, and feet (limb buds); the neural tube continues to develop; and rudimentary eyes form. By approximately five weeks, all internal organs have begun to develop, the jaws form, and the limb buds continue to grow. And by six weeks, the nose, mouth, and ears are beginning to develop and fingers and toes are becoming apparent.

Early during the first trimester, the growing embryo develops three layers of cells known as primary germ layers: an inner layer (endoderm), a middle layer (mesoderm), and an outer layer (ectoderm). Specific tissues and organs develop from each of these layers. For example, the lining of the lungs, gastrointestinal tract, and thyroid arise from the endoderm; the dermis of the skin, the muscles, most bones, the kidneys, and the circulatory system arise from the mesoderm; and the facial bones, the brain and spinal cord, the sensory organs such as the eyes and ears, and the epidermis of the skin arise from the ectoderm. By approximately the fourth month of gestation, the internal organs and organ systems are formed and almost mature. Growth and development continues until approximately nine months' gestation, when birth typically occurs.

Labor and Birth

Birth is the process during which the fetus moves from the uterus down through the cervix and passes out through the vagina. During the end of pregnancy, the uterus begins to contract in preparation for birth. The process known as labor begins when contractions become regular and occur at progressively shorter intervals. In addition, strong uterine muscular contractions cause the cervix to open and widen (dilate), and the membranes surrounding the amniotic fluid rupture, resulting in the release of the amniotic fluid through the vagina ("breaking of the waters"). The process of labor includes the following stages:

- First stage, which begins with the onset of contractions and ends with full dilation of the cervix

- Second stage, during which the baby exits through the vagina

- Third stage, during which the placenta is expelled through the vagina

Postnatal Growth and Development

The postnatal period, which means "the period after birth," begins at birth and extends until death. The most rapid rate of growth during one's development occurs prenatally-during embryonic and fetal development. Although the rate of growth decreases after birth, it remains high during childhood, particularly during the first year of life. Individuals also experience a "growth spurt" at the onset of puberty that progresses until their adult height is obtained.

During the first five months of life, infants grow approximately 30 percent in height and their weight usually doubles. By the age of one year, their height has increased by about 50 percent from birth and their weight has typically tripled. Height and weight are carefully measured and recorded during regular visits to pediatricians to ensure that growth is progressing at a predictable, steady rate. Physicians use measurements known as percentiles to compare the height and weight of infants who are of the same age. If an infant is said to be at the "fiftieth percentile" for weight, 50% of infants weigh more and 50% weigh less. If an infant is at the "tenth percentile" for height, 90% of infants have a higher height and 10% have a lower height. When assessing growth and development, physicians consider the actual percentile as well as changes in percentiles between visits.

Between birth and adolescence, the relative proportions of the head, limbs, and trunk change dramatically. For example, an infant's head tends to be about one quarter of the height of the body; however, an adult's head is approximately one eighth that of the height of the body. In addition, from childhood to adulthood, the trunk tends to become proportionally shorter and the legs proportionally longer.

Different organs have varying rates of growth. For example, the human brain is about one quarter of its adult size at birth. The brain grows primarily during the first year of life and is typically three quarters of its adult size by the age of one year. In contrast, the small lymphoid organ known as the thymus gradually enlarges until puberty, at which time it begins to decrease in size (involution).

Developmental Milestones

Infants and children develop mental, physical, and behavioral skills in certain stages known as developmental milestones. Although the particular rate of development may vary from child to child, most children typically acquire such skills at certain ages. The development of these skills depends upon a number of factors including the following:

Genetic factors-e.g., certain developmental patterns, such as developing the ability to speak earlier than otherwise expected, may be present in particular families.

Physical factors-e.g., visual or hearing impairment may interfere with the ability to learn certain skills, potentially necessitating the use of special supportive techniques or services to ensure that children have the best chance to reach their developmental potential.

Environmental factors-e.g., appropriate levels of stimulation are important in helping children to develop certain skills, such as receiving regular verbal stimulation to promote language development.

When infants are born, they primarily communicate any needs (e.g., hunger, thirst, etc.) by crying. In addition, certain essential reflex reactions are typically present at birth. For example, when any objects touch newborns' lips, they usually respond by sucking (sucking reflex). When a side of the mouth is touched, newborns typically move their head toward that side, enabling them to locate the mother's nipple for breast-feeding (rooting reflex). And when newborns are startled, they stretch their arms and legs forward and out and extend their fingers (startle or Moro's reflex). These reflex reactions gradually fade as infants develop muscle strength and the ability to conduct and coordinate certain voluntary movements. For example, hand-eye coordination skills include watching objects, developing the ability to focus, tracking moving objects, and forming an association between seeing and performing certain actions by focusing on hand movements.

Development is typically assessed by evaluating the acquisition of skills in the areas of vision and fine movement, hearing and speech, locomotion, and social behavior. The following is a description of developmental milestones that are generally acquired during the first year of life:

By approximately one month of age, infants are usually able to:

- Focus on faces

- Bring their hands toward the face (e.g., mouth, eyes)

- Look at objects directly in front of them

- Turn toward familiar voices and respond to other sounds

- Move their head from side to side while lying on their stomach

At about three months, infants are usually able to:

- Track objects that move approximately 180 degrees

- Grasp objects placed in their hands

- Smile at familiar voices (e.g., mother's or father's)

- Make sounds that begin to resemble speech

- Raise their head 45 degrees when lying on their stomach

At approximately five months, infants are usually able to:

- Reach for objects

- Listen carefully to certain voices

- Hold their head steady while upright

- Roll from the stomach to the back

- Spontaneously smile

At about six months, infants are usually able to:

- Reach out for and move objects from one hand to another

- Turn their head to locate sounds

- Laugh, make certain vowel sounds, and babble to toys

- Roll from back to front and vice versa

- Sit with support

- Bear weight on their legs with support

At the age of nine months, infants are usually able to:

- Look for toys that have been hidden

- Grasp for toys that are out of reach

- Manipulate objects with both hands

- Listen to and comprehend certain sounds

- Occasionally utter strings of syllables (e.g., "mama" or "dada")

- Attempt to crawl, sit without support, and pull themselves to a sitting or standing position

- Step on alternative feet with support

By 12 months of age, infants are usually able to:

- Grasp and release objects

- Say several words

- Respond when they hear their names

- Wave good-bye

- Move from their stomach to a sitting position

- Crawl on their hands and knees

- Walk by holding furniture

- Walk without support for a few steps or with one hand held

DESCRIPTION

Hematologic

The blood is a circulating tissue composed of fluid and other formed elements such as red blood cells, white cells, and platelets. The study of the blood, its components, and blood-forming tissues is known as hematology. Blood is pumped by the heart through the body's arteries, veins, and capillaries. The noncellular, fluid portion of the blood is a pale, yellowish liquid known as plasma. The blood has several functions including:

- To serve as a transport system, carrying oxygen and other vital nutrients to body tissues and promoting the exchange and removal of carbon dioxide and other waste products from cells

- To help provide a defense against invading microorganisms, foreign tissue cells, and certain abnormal cells

- To help repair damage to blood vessels and tissues through the process of blood clotting

Blood Plasma
Approximately half of the blood's volume consists of plasma. This liquid, noncellular portion of the blood is approximately 95 percent water. In addition, the blood plasma also contains dissolved sugars (e.g., glucose, etc.), fats, salts, vitamins and minerals, amino acids necessary for the production of cellular proteins, and chemical messengers (such as hormones) that regulate specific cellular activities. Plasma also contains certain plasma proteins including globulins (e.g., antibodies, which are produced in response to a particular foreign protein [antigen]); albumin, which plays an important role in maintaining the balance of pressure from inside and outside the cell, ; and fibrinogen, a protein that is essential for blood clotting. In addition, certain waste products are dissolved in plasma and transported to the kidneys for excretion.

Formed Elements
The formed elements of the blood include red blood cells (erythrocytes), white blood cells (leukocytes), and platelets (thrombocytes). Red blood cells, platelets, and some white blood cells are produced in the bone marrow. However, most white blood cells are produced by lymphatic tissue (e.g., lymph nodes, spleen, thymus).

Red Blood Cells
The red blood cells (RBCs) are mostly rounded, double concave cells with thin centers and thicker edges. A cubic millimeter of blood contains approximately five million red blood cells. The relatively large surface area of the red blood cells because they are concave allows them to absorb and release oxygen molecules, and their shape facilitates their movement through narrow blood vessels. As mentioned above, red blood cells are produced in the bone marrow, where the rate of their formation is regulated by erythropoietin, a hormone produced by the kidneys. They typically circulate in the blood for approximately four months, at which time they break apart and are removed from the blood by the liver.

The red blood cells perform several essential functions. For example, RBCs transport carbon dioxide from the body's cells to the lungs for release into the environment. Carbon dioxide is a harmful waste product that is generated by normal cellular activities. The red blood cells also carry hemoglobin, an essential protein that contains iron. This red pigmented protein chemically combines (binds) with oxygen, producing oxyhemoglobin, which enables the red blood cells to transport oxygen to cells.

The various blood groups, such as blood types A, B, AB, and O, are classified based upon the presence or absence of certain antigens (or "marker proteins"). Antigens are proteins that stimulate the body to produce antibodies. The red blood cells may have two types of antigens: namely, A and/or B. The different A or B blood types are classified according to whether the red blood cells have both, one or the other, or neither antigen. In individuals with type B blood, for example, the body does not produce antibodies to inactivate or destroy the type B antigen; however, the blood plasma contains anti-A antibodies. In individuals with type A blood, the red blood cells contain type A antigen and the blood plasma has anti-B antibodies. In type O blood, the red blood cells contain neither type A nor type B antigens, whereas the blood plasma has both anti-A and anti-B antibodies. In contrast, in individuals with type AB blood, the red blood cells have both type A and type B antigens, and the blood plasma contains neither anti-A nor anti-B antibodies.

In approximately 85 percent of individuals, red blood cells also contain an antigen called Rh factor. Those with this antigen are said to have Rh-positive blood, whereas those without the antigen have Rh-negative blood.

White Blood Cells
White blood cells (WBCs) are larger than red blood cells; however, they are present in the blood in lower quantities. A cubic millimeter of blood contains approximately 7,500 white blood cells.

The white blood cells include two major categories: granular leukocytes, which have granules in the substance of the cell outside the nucleus (cytoplasm), and nongranular leukocytes. Granular leukocytes include neutrophils, eosinophils, and basophils, and nongranular leukocytes include lymphocytes and monocytes.

Neutrophils and monocytes, which are also known as phagocytes, are responsible for isolating, engulfing, and destroying microorganisms that have invaded the bloodstream. These cells engulf the microorganisms and digest them in a process known as phagocytosis.

Lymphocytes originate in the bone marrow and mature in lymphatic tissue. They become active immune cells in response to the presence of invading microorganisms. Lymphocytes known as B lymphocytes produce specific antibodies to inhibit certain microorganisms, whereas those known as T lymphocytes may actively destroy microorganisms or assist in the functions of the B lymphocytes.

Eosinophils help protect the body from various irritants that may cause allergies and are able to participate in phagocytosis. In addition, white blood cells known as basophils also play a role in allergic reactions and secrete certain chemicals such as heparin, which assists in the prevention of clotting as the blood circulates through the blood vessels (intravascular clotting).

Although granular leukocytes may have a lifespan of only a few days, nongranular leukocytes may survive for over six months. In fact, in some cases, certain individual lymphocytes may remain in the bloodstream for years.

Platelets

Platelets, which are the smallest blood cells, are produced in the bone marrow by specialized cells known as megakaryocytes and typically survive for approximately nine days. A cubic millimeter of blood contains approximately 250,000 platelets.

Platelets usually circulate in the bloodstream in an inactive state. However, when a blood vessel wall is injured, platelets respond through a complex process by clumping at the injury site and sticking to one another. The platelets and damaged tissue cells also release certain chemicals that stimulate blood clotting (coagulation) factors in the blood plasma. Due to a series of complex reactions, known as a cascade, long filaments of fibrin, a fibrous gel, are produced that capture circulating platelets, red blood cells, and white blood cells. Once the damaged blood vessel is "plugged," the filaments contract, forming a solid blood clot.

In some cases, blood clots may form in undamaged blood vessels, potentially blocking vital blood supply to certain tissues and organs. A stationary blood clot is called a thrombus. If a portion of such a clot dislodges and circulates in the bloodstream, it is known as an embolus. Healthy blood vessel walls secrete the chemical prostacyclin, which helps to prevent the unnecessary activation of platelets and clot formation. However, under certain circumstances, emboli travel from their origin to other parts of the body, notably the lungs, heart, and brain.

Measurement of Blood Components

The complete blood count (CBC) is a calculation of the cellular (formed elements) of blood. These calculations are generally determined by specially designed machines that analyze the different components of blood in less than a minute. A major portion of the complete blood count is the measure of the concentration of white blood cells, red blood cells, and platelets in the blood. The complete blood count (also called CBC) is generated by testing a simple blood sample.

White Blood Count (WBC), also called leukocyte count. Normal range varies slightly between laboratories but is generally between 4,300 and 10,800 cells per cubic millimeter (cmm).

Automated white cell differential. A machine generated percentage of the different types of white blood cells, usually split into granulocytes, lymphocytes, monocytes, eosinophils, and basophils.

Red cell count (RBC), also called erythrocyte count. Normal range varies slightly between laboratories but is generally between 4.2 - 5.9 million cells/cmm.

Hemoglobin (Hb). Hemoglobin is the protein molecule within red blood cells that carries oxygen and gives blood its red color. Normal range for hemoglobin is different between the sexes and is approximately 13 - 18 grams per deciliter (g/dl) for men and 12 - 16 g/dl for women.

Platelet count, also called thrombocyte count. Normal range varies slightly between laboratories but is in the range of 150,000 - 400,000 per cubic millimeter.

DESCRIPTION

Immune System

The body's immune system consists of specialized proteins, cells, and tissues that function to protect the body against...

- Invading microorganisms (e.g., bacteria, viruses, etc.) that may cause disease

- Foreign tissue cells (such as those that may have been transplanted from a donor)

- Toxins (such as harmful chemicals)

- Cells that have become cancerous

Nonspecific Immunity
Certain mechanisms provide the body with general protection from invading cells and toxins, maintaining "nonspecific immunity." For example, nonspecific immunity is provided by the presence of certain physical barriers that may prevent the entry of invading cells or toxins or expel them-as well as chemical barriers that may destroy invading cells or toxins. Such barriers include certain enzymes within the saliva of the mouth, tears, and sweat; the protective barrier of the skin; the cough reflex; hairs within the nose and the sneeze reflex; the presence of harmless bacteria within the intestines that help to control harmful microorganisms; and secretion of mucus by cells lining certain organs of the respiratory tract.

In addition, tissue injury results in an inflammatory response, which consists of a series of nonspecific immune reactions. During an inflammatory response-which produces characteristic swelling, discomfort, and redness-the blood vessels widen (dilate), increasing the blood supply and enabling certain white blood cells to move from the vessels to the site of injury. For example, invading microorganisms typically encounter white blood cells known as phagocytes, which contain the infection by engulfing and destroying the microbes (phagocytosis). Invading microorganisms may also encounter certain naturally produced substances, such as a group of blood proteins (complement system) that, when activated, serve to destroy such microbes, or interferon, proteins that are produced in response to viral infection.

Specific Immunity
Specific immunity consists of particular defenses against certain invading microorganisms or toxins and includes inborn and acquired immunity. From birth, individuals are immune to certain diseases that affect other animals (inborn immunity). Acquired immunity is obtained when certain protective proteins known as antibodies are passed to a developing fetus via the mother's placenta or to an infant via the mother's breast milk. Acquired immunity also results from casual exposure to certain disease-causing agents and immunization (stimulation of the immune system to provide protection against a particular disease, such as through vaccination).

Humoral or Cellular Immune Responses
Specific immunity, which relies on the actions of the white blood cells known as lymphocytes, includes the humoral- and cell-mediated immune responses.

Humoral Response
A humoral-mediated immune response, also known as an antibody-mediated response, primarily consists of the production of antibodies by cells called B lymphocytes or B cells. B lymphocytes initially arise from primitive cells in the bone marrow known as stem cells. Shortly before and after birth, certain stem cells develop into immature B cells.

When immature B cells recognize a disease-causing agent as foreign (antigen), they develop into activated B cells. Activated B cells rapidly divide into two lines of cells (clones): plasma cells, which secrete large amounts of antibodies into the blood, and memory cells, which are stored within the lymph nodes until they are stimulated by the same antigen that prompted their formation. They then also develop into plasma cells, secreting antibodies into the blood in response to the recognized antigen.

When antibodies are secreted into the blood, they bind to their specific antigens (antibody-antigen complex), making the antigens or the cells on which they are located harmless. Phagocytes then engulf and destroy large numbers of such antibody-antigen complexes. The binding of antibodies and antigens may stimulate the complement system, thereby improving the efficiency of phagocytosis.

Cellular Response
Cell-mediated immunity defends the body against certain microorganisms and possibly cancerous cells through the actions of particular white blood cells known as T lymphocytes or T cells. These cells initially develop within the thymus before birth. They arise from stem cells that migrate from the bone marrow to the thymus, where their development is facilitated by certain hormones. Newly formed T cells then migrate from the thymus to other lymphatic tissues, primarily the lymph nodes.

There are two main types of T lymphocytes involved in cell-mediated immunity including the helper cells and killer cells. Helper cells assist in the recognition of certain antigens and help to activate killer cells. The killer cells bind to cells invaded by viruses or other microbes and destroy them. It is thought that killer cells may function similarly against cancerous cells or foreign tissue cells.

Allergies and Autoimmune Disease
In some cases, humoral- or cell-mediated immune responses may inappropriately occur against the body's own

tissues. Such "autoimmunity" may result in hypersensitivity or autoimmune diseases. A hypersensitivity reaction is characterized by an excessive immune response to a substance that the body perceives as foreign (sensitizing antigen). For example, an allergic reaction is a hypersensitive response that occurs upon exposure to previously encountered, usually environmental substances (allergens), such as pollen, dust, or certain foods. Autoimmune diseases may be caused by the production of antibodies against the body's own cells (autoantibodies) and inappropriate cell-mediated immune responses against self antigens (autoantigens). One proposed theory suggests that certain viruses or bacteria may play some role in provoking an abnormal autoimmune reaction. For example, when a foreign protein from an invading bacterium or virus is very similar to one of the body's proteins, the immune system may be unable to distinguish between the invading and the "self" protein, potentially triggering an autoimmune response. It is not known what role genetic, hormonal, or other environmental factors may play in contributing to such a response. Autoimmune diseases may be localized, affecting a particular tissue, or may involve many tissues and organs of the body (systemic).

Infectious Diseases and Vaccination

The purpose of immunization is to induce immunity to provide protection against a certain disease. In response to a vaccine, the body's immune system produces certain immune defenses, such as antibodies or particular white blood cells that should protect against infection upon exposure to the disease-causing organism.

There are two major types of vaccination. In passive vaccination, antibodies obtained from a donor who was previously exposed to the microorganism are introduced into the body, thereby providing short-term protection against the disease-causing organism. In active vaccination, noninfectious portions of bacteria or viruses are introduced into the body, stimulating the production of antibodies against the foreign protein, resulting in longer-term immunity.

Some vaccines are intended for the general population, particularly infants and young children, such as immunization against the infectious diseases diphtheria, pertussis (whooping cough), and tetanus (DPT); measles, mumps, and rubella (German measles); hepatitis B; and polio. The recommended ages for immunization may vary from case to case. A child's pediatrician can recommend an appropriate immunization schedule.

Other vaccines are available for individuals who are at risk for certain infectious diseases due to their work situations (e.g., health care workers); their living situations or age groups (e.g., students living in dormitories, elderly individuals in nursing homes); local outbreaks of dangerous infectious diseases; or travel in certain countries.

Some individuals should not receive certain vaccinations, such as people with deficient immune systems. In individuals who have a fever or a preexisting infection, immunizations should be delayed. In addition, particular vaccines should not be given to young children or pregnant women.

DESCRIPTION

Musculoskeletal

Neuromuscular Activities

The muscles of the body, collectively referred to as the muscular system, consist of bundles of specialized cells that, unlike other cells, have the ability to contract and relax, resulting in movement of body parts and organs. There are two main types of muscles: namely, skeletal muscle and smooth muscle. In addition, the cardiac muscle is a highly specialized muscle that is sometimes referred to as a third muscle type.

Skeletal Muscle

The skeletal muscles, so named because they attach to bones of the skeleton, are the most prominent muscles in the body and typically contribute to approximately 40 to 45 percent of an individual's body weight. These muscles may also be referred to as striated ("cross striped") muscles or called voluntary muscles because their movements are under voluntary control.

Each skeletal muscle consists of groups of threadlike muscle cells, known as muscle fibers, in a highly organized arrangement. Each muscle fiber is made up of slender, striated strands called myofibrils that, in turn, are composed of bunches of microscopic, threadlike structures known as myofilaments. The myofilaments contain minute fibers or threads of proteins known as myosin and actin. The interactions of these proteins are essential for muscle contraction. During voluntary movement, skeletal muscle contracts and the bone to which it is attached (via tendons) moves in response to the contraction.

Neuromuscular Activities and Voluntary Movement:

The brain regulates voluntary movements of skeletal muscles by sending impulses to the nerve fibers that supply the muscle fibers (motor neurons). The area where nerve endings and muscle fibers join is known as the neuromuscular junction. When the brain sends such impulses, nerve endings release a specialized chemical (the neurotransmitter acetylcholine) that serves to stimulate the muscle fibers. A complex series of electrical and chemical processes is initiated resulting in muscle contraction.

When voluntary movements occur, there are coordinated contractions and simultaneous relaxations of several muscles. In other words, as several muscles contract, one muscle is primarily responsible for producing the particular movement (prime mover or agonist) and the others (synergists) contract in order to assist the prime mover in making the movement in question. While such muscles contract, other muscles known as antagonists simultaneously relax, producing movements that oppose those of the prime mover

and synergists. Such coordination of skeletal muscle movements helps to ensure smooth rather than jerky motions.

In addition to producing movement, the skeletal muscles also function to maintain posture and to produce body heat. For example, skeletal muscles are typically maintained at a level of slight, continuous contraction (muscle tone). Such muscle tone helps the body to maintain proper posture-i.e., the specific positioning of body parts to support their optimum function, place the least strain on different areas of the body, and maintain proper weight distribution. In addition, muscle fiber contraction creates most of the heat that the body needs to maintain its proper temperature.

Smooth Muscle

Smooth muscle cells have a smooth appearance when viewed under a microscope, lacking the striations of skeletal muscle cells. Rather, they consist of elongated, "spindle-shaped" cells that are typically organized parallel to one another. Also known as involuntary muscles since their movements are not under voluntary control, the smooth muscles help to regulate certain functional movements of internal organs. For example, in the process known as peristalsis, the rhythmic contractions of smooth muscle propel food forward through the digestive tract. Smooth muscle is also located within the blood vessel walls and several other areas of the body.

The actions of the smooth muscles are regulated by the autonomic nervous system, the portion of the nervous system that controls involuntary activities of blood vessels, organs, and other tissues and organ systems. Neurotransmitters released at nerve endings contribute to the series of events that lead to contraction of smooth muscles. As with the skeletal muscles, smooth muscle contractions rely upon the interactions between the myosin and actin filaments. In addition, smooth muscle cell activities may be affected by changes in the chemical composition of the fluid surrounding the cells as well as the release of certain hormones.

Cardiac Muscle

Cardiac muscle, also known as the myocardium, is a special type of striated muscle that is located only in the heart. Like the cells within the skeletal muscles, cardiac muscle cells also have cross striations. In addition, there are dark bands or disks (intercalated disks) at the junctures of adjacent cardiac fibers. These disks enable the fibers to contract as a unit, thereby ensuring the heart's efficiency in pumping blood throughout the circulatory system.

As with the smooth muscles, contraction of cardiac muscle is regulated by the autonomic nervous system. Cardiac muscle activities may also be affected by the release of specific hormones. Electrical impulses that stimulate a regulated, coordinated sequence of contractions originate from the heart's "pacemaker" (sinoatrial node), an area within the upper right chamber of the heart (right atrium).

DESCRIPTION

Nervous System

The nervous system is a complex network of structures that function to...

- obtain information about the body's internal environment and the external environment

- relay and analyze such "data"

- initiate, integrate, and control appropriate responses to this information

The nervous system includes the brain and spinal cord, known as the central nervous system; nerves that extend from the brain and spinal cord to all areas of the body, referred to as the peripheral nervous system; somatic sense organs, which are distributed in almost every area of the body but concentrated primarily in the skin; and special sensory organs, such as the eyes. In addition, the peripheral nervous system is further subdivided into the autonomic nervous system, which includes structures that regulate involuntary functions of the body.

Nervous System Cells

Cells of the nervous system ensure ongoing, rapid communications between different structures of the body and the control of bodily functions necessary to maintain life. There are two main types of cells within the nervous system:

- Nerve cells, also known as neurons, which conduct (transmit) impulses

- Glia, which are the connective tissue cells of the nervous system

Neurons contain a cell body, one or more slender, branching projections (dendrites) that transmit impulses toward the cell body, and a slender extension (axon or nerve fiber) that carries nerve impulses away from the cell body. A whitish, fatty substance known as myelin forms a protective "wrapping" or insulating sheath around certain axons, serving as an electrical insulator and ensuring the efficient conduction of nerve impulses.

There are three types of neurons:

- Sensory neurons (afferent ["toward"] neurons) carry impulses to the brain and spinal cord from all areas of the body.

- Motor neurons (efferent ["away from"] neurons) transmit impulses away from the brain and spinal cord to certain tissues (e.g., muscle or glandular tissues).

- Interneurons (connecting or central neurons) carry impulses from sensory neurons to motor neurons.

Glia hold together and protect neurons. The different types of glia include the following:

- Astrocytes are relatively large cells with thread-like projections. These "branches" connect with blood capillaries and neurons, holding them in proximity to one another. The walls of the capillaries and the projections of the astrocytes are said to form the "blood-brain barrier," which functions to separate systemic blood circulation from the central nervous system. This barrier prevents or slows the passage of certain toxic substances or infectious agents from the blood to the central nervous system.

- Oligodendroglia produce myelin and hold together nerve fibers.

- Microglia are relatively small cells with slender projections. When brain tissue becomes inflamed, these cells migrate toward the affected tissue, surround invading microorganisms or waste products, and digest them (phagocytosis).

Nerves and Nerve Impulses

Nerves consist of one or more bundles of impulse-carrying fibers known as axons that extend from the brain and spinal cord to all areas of the body. Certain nerves transmit impulses from particular receptor organs to the brain and spinal cord (afferent impulses) or from the CNS to certain specialized tissues (efferent impulses). White matter within the central nervous system and peripheral nervous system consists of bundles of axons that are myelinated; in contrast, gray matter of the nervous system primarily includes neuron cell bodies, dendrites, and unmyelinated axons.

The pathways by which nerve impulses are transmitted by neurons are known as neuron pathways. Nerve signals are electrical impulses or waves of electrical disturbances that result due to complex electrochemical changes in a neuron's environment. Such nerve impulses travel from the axon of one neuron (presynaptic neuron) to the dendrite of another neuron (postsynaptic neuron). The junction between two neurons is known as a synapse. As an electrical impulse reaches a synapse, the presynaptic neuron's axon releases small amounts of chemical substances known as neurotransmitters, which bind to certain areas (receptors) of the postsynaptic neuron. Consequently, the electrical impulse is conducted across the synapse to the postsynaptic neuron's dendrite. Thus, neurotransmitters are the chemical substances that enable neurons to communicate with one another.

Central Nervous System

The central nervous system includes the brain and the spinal cord. Bones of the skull enclose the brain, and bones of the spinal column (vertebrae) surround the spinal cord. In addition, a three-layered membrane (meninges) provides additional protection for the brain and spinal cord. The tough, fibrous outermost layer is known as the dura mater. The delicate middle layer, called the arachnoid mater, is separated from the elastic innermost layer (pia mater) by a space (subarachnoid space) that contains cerebrospinal fluid (CSF). This fluid, which acts as a protective "shock absorber," flows through the cavity within the vertebrae containing the spinal cord (spinal canal), the four cavities of the brain (ventricles), and the subarachnoid space.

Brain

The brain controls and regulates the many functions of the central nervous system including muscle control and coordination, sensory reception and response, and speech production as well as elaboration of thought and emotions. It consists of several major regions including the brain stem, diencephalon, cerebellum, and cerebrum.

Brain Stem

The brain stem consists of three structures: the medulla oblongata, pons, and midbrain. All regions of the brain stem serve as "two-lane" conduction "highways," with motor fibers relaying impulses from the brain to the spinal cord, and sensory fibers conducting messages from the spinal cord to other areas of the brain.

The medulla oblongata, a thick extension of the spinal cord, is located above the large opening (foramen magnum) in the bone that forms the back of the skull (occipital bone). It primarily consists of white matter mixed with bits of gray matter (reticular formation). The medulla contains groups of nerve cells (nuclei) of the ninth, eleventh, and twelfth cranial nerves (see below), thereby receiving and sending impulses involved in the sensation of taste and sending messages to muscles involved in swallowing, speech, and movements of the neck, shoulders, and tongue, for example. This region of the brain stem also contains nuclei of the tenth cranial nerve (vagus nerve) and thus receives and relays information concerning the regulation of blood vessel diameter (thus affecting blood pressure), beating of the heart, breathing, and digestion.

The pons and the midbrain both also contain white matter mixed with bits of gray matter. The pons has bundles of nerve fibers that connect with the region of the brain known as the cerebellum. In addition, it contains nuclei of the fifth, sixth, seventh, and eighth cranial nerves, thus relaying messages involved in movement of the eyes, jaws, and muscles of facial expression as well as receiving and transmitting sensory impulses from the face and ears. The midbrain contains nuclei of the third and fourth cranial nerves and therefore relays messages to muscles involved in controlling the reactions of the pupils of the eyes as well as five of the six muscles that move the eyes.

Diencephalon

The diencephalon is the region of the brain located between the midbrain and the cerebrum. It includes the hypothalamus and the thalamus.

The hypothalamus, a relatively small area of the brain, is situated under the thalamus and above the pituitary gland. One of its functions is to regulate the sympathetic nervous system, a division of the autonomic nervous system. The sympathetic nervous system controls certain involuntary activities during times of stress, such as raising blood pressure, increasing the heart rate and the breathing rate, and widening (dilating) the pupils. The hypothalamus is also involved in regulating body temperature, appetite, moods and emotions (such as anger, fear, etc.), and the sleep cycle.

Sleep and the Brain

Sleep is a natural state characterized by reduced consciousness and metabolic activity. During sleep, the brain typically engages in two main cycles, known as REM (rapid eye movement) and NREM (nonrapid eye movement) sleep. NREM sleep, which makes up approximately 80 percent of sleep in adults (and about 50 percent of sleep in infants), consists of four progressively deeper stages of sleep characterized by slow, deep brain waves; muscle relaxation; and regular, reduced autonomic activities (e.g., slowed breathing and heart rate; lowered blood pressure; etc.). Episodes of REM sleep periodically alternate with NREM sleep. REM sleep, which is associated with dreaming, includes increased levels of brain activity, irregular autonomic activities, rapid eye movements, and involuntary muscle jerks. A complete sleep cycle is usually approximately 90 minutes. Most individuals experience approximately four or five sleep cycles each night. It is not completely understood why sleep is a necessity, although most scientists agree that the brain requires regular rest to ensure optimum functioning-and that dreaming may help the brain to sort, manipulate, and store information obtained during waking activities. Many different areas of the brain, including the hypothalamus, are thought to play a role in regulating sleep.

The hypothalamus also controls the functions of the pituitary gland, an endocrine gland also known as the "master gland." The hypothalamus is attached to the pituitary gland by a stalk of nerve fibers known as the pituitary stalk. It regulates the gland's activities through direct nerve stimulation as well as through the actions of certain nerve cells whose axons secrete chemicals (hormone-releasing and hormone-inhibiting factors) into the bloodstream for transport directly to the pituitary. Hormone-releasing factors cause the secretion of certain hormones by the pituitary gland, whereas hormone-inhibiting factors halt the production and release of such hormones. The balance of these factors, via a feedback mechanism, is crucial in maintaining effective function of many of the body's activities.

The thalamus consists of two masses of gray matter located above the hypothalamus. The neurons within the thalamus relay impulses from sense organs of the body to the outer region of the cerebrum (cerebral cortex); transmit motor impulses from the cerebral cortex toward the spinal cord; associate certain sensations with emotions (e.g., unpleasant or pleasant feelings); and play a role in the body's state of responsiveness to sensory stimulation (arousal or alerting mechanisms).

Cerebellum

The cerebellum, a two-lobed, rounded region of the brain, has a "wrinkled" surface and is located under the back portion of the cerebrum and behind the brain stem. The surface (cortex) of the cerebellum contains parallel ridges that are separated by deep fissures. Three stalks of nerve fibers (peduncles) that arise from the inner side of each cerebellar hemisphere link to different areas of the brain stem. Messages between the cerebellum and other regions of the brain travel along these nerve stalks. Through messages transmitted via the brain stem, the cerebellum receives information concerning muscle contraction and relaxation and posture. The cerebellum works in conjunction with the basal ganglia and the thalamus, adjusting messages relayed to muscle groups from a certain area of the cerebrum (motor cortex) in order to maintain normal postures, sustain balance, and produce smooth and coordinated movements.

Cerebrum

The cerebrum is the largest area of the brain and is responsible for voluntary movements, sensory perception, emotions, memory, and comprehensive thought. The cerebrum contains several ridges (gyri) and grooves (sulci or fissures) and one deep groove known as the longitudinal fissure that divides the cerebrum into two halves (cerebral hemispheres). The left cerebral hemisphere controls the right side of the body, whereas the right hemisphere controls the left side of the body due to crossing of nerve fibers in the medulla of the brain stem. A thick band of myelinated nerve fibers known as the corpus callosum joins the lower midportions of and carries messages between the cerebral hemispheres. In addition, each hemisphere contains a fluid-filled cavity known as a ventricle (first and second or lateral ventricles). These ventricles communicate with a third ventricle in the center of the brain, and a fourth ventricle is located between the brain stem and the cerebellum.

Two sulci divide each hemisphere into four lobes that are designated by the bones over them: i.e., frontal, temporal, parietal, and occipital lobes. The surface of the cerebrum, called the cerebral cortex, consists of a thin layer of gray matter, whereas most of the interior of the cerebrum contains bundles of myelinated nerve fibers (white matter) known as tracts. In addition, deep within the white matter of the cerebrum are paired nerve cell clusters of gray matter known as the basal ganglia. Their function includes assist-

ing in the regulation of muscular actions as well as initiating and ceasing movements.

The cerebrum has various areas that are responsible for particular complex functions. These areas include the following:

- Sensory areas, which receive sensory information from somatic sense organs (e.g., in the skin, muscles, internal organs) and special sense organs (e.g., ears, eyes, etc.) and analyze and sort such information

- Motor areas, which transmit messages that control muscles, resulting in movement

- Association areas, which link sensory and motor areas, integrate information received from the various sense organs, and engage in memory storage, recall, recognition, decision making, judgment, comprehensive thought, and the experience of emotions.

Spinal Cord

The spinal cord is housed inside a central canal within the spinal column and extends from the foramen magnum at the base of the skull to the bottom of the first vertebra of the lower back. It is a long, cylindrical structure of nerve tissue and is an extension of the medulla oblongata of the brain stem. As mentioned above, the spinal cord is enclosed and protected by a three-layered membrane (meninges) and is bathed by cerebrospinal fluid.

The inner core of the spinal cord consists of gray matter (i.e., primarily containing nerve cell bodies and dendrites). Its outer portion is composed of columns of white matter that contain bundles of myelinated nerve fibers (spinal tracts). These pathways transmit sensory impulses from the spinal cord to the brain (ascending tracts) and motor impulses from the brain to the spinal cord (descending tracts). Certain ascending tracts transmit impulses that produce sensations of temperature and pain, and certain descending tracts convey impulses that control specific voluntary movements.

Peripheral Nervous System

The peripheral nervous system refers to those nerves outside the central nervous system. This part of the nervous system establishes communications between the brain and spinal cord and outlying (peripheral) parts of the body, such as muscles, glands, and internal organs. Nerves of the peripheral nervous system include the cranial nerves and the spinal nerves.

The cranial nerves are the 12 nerve pairs that arise directly from the brain and emerge through various openings in the skull (foramen). The cranial nerve pairs...

- Carry sensory impulses to the brain that are analyzed, sorted, and integrated, resulting in vision, smell, taste, hearing, and/or balance.

- Transmit motor and/or sensory information to particular areas of the head and neck.

- Convey impulses to glands and organs, resulting in certain involuntary (autonomic) activities.

The cranial nerve pairs include the...
- First cranial nerves or olfactory nerves
- Second cranial nerves or optic nerves
- Third cranial nerves or oculomotor nerves
- Fourth cranial nerves or trochlear nerves
- Fifth cranial nerves or trigeminal nerves
- Sixth cranial nerve or abducens nerves
- Seventh cranial nerves or facial nerves
- Eighth cranial nerves or vestibulocochlear nerves
- Ninth cranial nerves or glossopharyngeal nerves
- Tenth cranial nerves or vagus nerves
- Eleventh cranial nerves or accessory nerves
- Twelfth cranial nerves or hypoglossal nerves

The spinal nerves are the 31 pairs of nerves that emerge from either side of the spinal cord through gaps between adjacent bones (vertebrae) in the spinal column. The nerves are assigned a specific letter and number based upon the level of the spinal column from which they emerge. Eight pairs of spinal nerves are attached to the cervical segments; 12 pairs to the thoracic segments; five pairs to the lumber segments; five pairs to the sacrospinal segments; and one pair to the coccygeal segment. The designation "C2," for example, refers to the pair of spinal nerves attached to the second segment of the cervical region of the spinal cord. The spinal nerves that emerge from the spinal cord branch to form many of the nerves supplying the trunk and limbs. The function of the spinal nerves is to transmit sensory and motor impulses between the spinal cord to those areas of the body that are not supplied (innervated) by the cranial nerve pairs. More specifically, the sensory nerve fibers of the spinal nerves transmit impulses from sensory receptors in muscles, internal organs, and the skin to the spinal cord, whereas the motor nerve fibers convey motor impulses from the spinal cord to glands and muscles.

Autonomic Nervous System

The autonomic nervous system (ANS) is that portion of the peripheral nervous system responsible for regulation of the involuntary functioning of certain tissues and organs. The ANS includes specialized motor neurons that transmit impulses from the brain stem or the spinal cord to involuntary muscle tissue, cardiac muscle tissue, and specialized glandular cells that produce and secrete certain chemical substances (e.g., hormones, enzymes).

The autonomic nervous system includes two groups of motor neurons (preganglionic and postganglionic neurons) and a group of nerve cell bodies (ganglia) located between them. The cell bodies and dendrites of preganglionic neurons are located in gray matter of the brain stem or spinal cord, and their axons extend to a set of ganglia in the peripheral nervous system. Within the ganglia, the endings of preganglionic neuron axons join with cell bodies or dendrites of postganglionic neurons, which, in turn, convey nerve impulses from ganglia to smooth muscle, cardiac muscle, or glandular tissue. The tissues to which postganglionic neurons transmit impulses are known as visceral effectors.

Autonomic Nervous System Neurotransmitters
There are four distinct types of nerve fibers (axons) in the autonomic nervous system that release certain neurotransmitters (i.e., acetylcholine or norepinephrine). The sympathetic and parasympathetic nervous systems work somewhat, although not completely, in opposition to each other (antagonistic), since each division may inhibit certain visceral effectors and activate others.

The autonomic nervous system is further subdivided into the sympathetic and the parasympathetic nervous systems.

Sympathetic Nervous System

The sympathetic nervous system functions to prepare the body for an emergency. When the body is affected by stress, such as occurs during strong emotions (fear, anger) or exercise, sympathetic nerve impulses increase to many of the body's visceral effectors, resulting in what is sometimes called the "fright-or-flight response." During this response, the heart and breathing rates increase; the pupils of the eyes widen (dilate); and secretions of certain glands increase, while those of other glands decrease. In addition, most blood vessels constrict, resulting in raised blood pressure; blood vessels that supply skeletal muscle widen, supplying additional blood; and the digestive process slows due to a reduction in the rate of the wave-like contractions of smooth muscle within the GI tract.

Parasympathetic Nervous System

The parasympathetic nervous system controls most visceral nerve transmission under normal circumstances, thus slowing and steadying certain bodily activities. For example, impulses conducted by parasympathetic neurons tend to increase peristalsis, speeding the digestive process; slow the heart and breathing rates; contract the pupils; and stimulate the salivary glands.

1029

DESCRIPTION

Reproductive

The female reproductive system includes those organs that enable females to produce the specialized reproductive or sex cells (gametes) known as eggs (ova); engage in reproductive activity; provide nourishment to a fertilized ovum (zygote) during embryonic and fetal development; and give birth. The male reproductive system consists of those organs that enable males to produce and store the reproductive cells (gametes) known as sperm, engage in reproductive activity, and fertilize ova with sperm. The production and secretion of certain chemical substances (hormones) by glands of the endocrine system promote the maturation and normal functioning of reproductive organs and the development of secondary sexual characteristics (puberty) in males and females.

Female Reproductive System

The female reproductive system includes several organs, including the ovaries, fallopian tubes, uterus, vagina, and vulva. With the exception of the vulva (external genitalia), the female reproductive organs are located within the pelvic cavity. In addition, the female breasts (mammary glands) are supportive glands of the female reproductive system.

Ovaries

The female reproductive cells are produced in the paired structures known as the ovaries. These small, egg-shaped glands contain cavities known as follicles in which the female sex cells develop and mature (oogenesis). As females reach puberty (i.e., which typically has an onset between approximately nine to 13 years of age), the follicles begin to release eggs (ovulation) on a regular monthly cycle. This cycle is regulated by female sex hormones (estrogen and progesterone) that are also secreted by the ovaries.

The hormone estrogen promotes the development of female secondary sexual characteristics and normal functioning of reproductive organs (i.e., puberty). It promotes the development and maturation of female reproductive organs; development of the breasts; development of female body contours caused by fat deposition in the breasts and hip area, for example; and initiation (menarche) and regulation of the menstrual cycle. The menstrual cycle is the recurring monthly cycle during which the mucous membrane lining of the uterus (endometrium) is shed; begins to regrow, becoming thick and supplied with blood; is maintained in the uterus, and is again shed. The thickening of the endometrium is stimulated by the hormone progesterone in preparation for implantation of a fertilized egg (zygote). If such fertilization does not occur, progesterone and estrogen production decrease, causing the uterine lining and the unfertilized egg to be shed (menstruation). Progesterone also plays an essential role in the normal functioning of the placenta, the organ that nourishes the developing embryo and fetus during pregnancy.

Fallopian Tubes

A funnel-shaped duct, known as a fallopian tube, uterine tube, or oviduct, extends from each ovary to the uterus. Each tube ends in a structure shaped like a funnel whose edge has finger-like projections. When an egg is released from an ovary, it enters the fallopian tube with the assistance of the beating motions of these projections and microscopic hairs (cilia) on their surfaces. These motions help to propel the egg toward the uterus. In addition, the fallopian tubes serve as the passageways within which the male sex cells (sperm) move toward the ovaries.

Uterus

The uterus, a hollow, pear-shaped organ composed almost entirely of muscle (myometrium), is the organ within which a fertilized egg (zygote) becomes implanted and the developing embryo and fetus is nourished and grows during pregnancy. The organ consists of a lower narrow section known as the cervix and an upper portion called the body. The uterus usually lies in the pelvic cavity behind the bladder. However, during pregnancy, the uterus expands in size as the developing fetus grows and may eventually extend to the top of the abdominal cavity. During the end of pregnancy, strong uterine muscular contractions cause the cervix to open and widen (dilate) and expel the fetus through the vagina.

Other Components of the Female Reproductive System

The vagina is the muscular passage that connects the cervix and the external genitalia and is the portion of the female reproductive tract that opens to the exterior of the body. The vulva is the external, visible portion of the external genitalia.

Breasts

The female breasts, which are supportive glands of the female reproductive system, produce milk to nourish infants after birth (lactation). The female breast consists of approximately 15 to 20 divisions or lobes embedded within fatty tissue. Each lobe is comprised of smaller lobules of milk-secreting glandular cells that are organized in grape-like clusters (alveoli). The small ducts that drain the alveoli have their outlet within the nipple. The circular, colored (pigmented) area of skin surrounding the nipple is known as the areola. Due to secretion of the hormones progesterone and estrogen by the placenta and the ovaries during pregnancy, the milk-secreting glandular cells become active, causing the nipple to become enlarged. Before and after birth, the glands initially produce a thin, watery fluid (colostrum) containing antibodies and proteins that help to protect the newborn from certain infections. Another hormone known as prolactin is responsible for the secretion of milk.

Male Reproductive System

The male reproductive system also includes several organs, including the testes, reproductive ducts, seminal vesicles, bulbourethral glands, prostate gland, and penis.

Testes

In males, the gonads, i.e., the sex glands within which the reproductive cells are produced, are the paired oval-shaped structures known as the testes. The male sex cells produced by the testes, known as spermatozoa or sperm, are responsible for fertilizing the female ova. The testes are located in pouch-like structures called the scrotum.

Each testis is surrounded by a tough, fibrous membrane (tunica albuginea) and contains a long, narrow, coiled structure known as a seminiferous tubule. Sperm develop within the walls of the tubules in a process known as spermatogenesis. In addition, cells located between the tubules produce the male sex hormone testosterone. This male hormone and certain hormones produced in the pituitary gland (gonadotropin hormones) are responsible for the development and production of sperm.

As males reach puberty (i.e., which typically has an onset between approximately 12 to 14 years of age), increased secretion of testosterone promotes muscle and bone growth, stimulates the development of male secondary sexual characteristics, and promotes the normal functioning of the reproductive organs. More specifically, it stimulates sperm production; the development and maturation of male reproductive organs (e.g., seminal vesicles, prostate gland); and the development of male characteristics (e.g. deepening of the voice due to enlargement of the larynx and the vocal cords, growth of facial and body hair, etc.).

Reproductive Ducts

Sperm develop within the walls of the seminiferous tubules of the testes and pass through several reproductive ducts: i.e., the epididymis, ductus (vas) deferens, ejaculatory duct, and urethra. The first of these is the epididymis, a tightly coiled tube that runs along the top and behind the testes. The ductus or vas deferens is the muscular, movable tube that enables sperm to pass from the testes and the epididymis. The ductus deferens joins the duct from the seminal vesicles to form the ejaculatory duct. This duct enables sperm to empty into the urethra, the tube that passes along the length of the penis and carries sperm to the exterior of the body. In males, the urethra also serves as the passageway through which urine is excreted from the body.

Other Components of the Male Reproductive System

Semen (seminal fluid) is a fluid consisting of sperm as well as the secretions of certain supportive sex glands of the male reproductive tract. Such glands include the seminal vesicles, the prostate gland, and the bulbourethral glands.

Semen serves to protect sperm from the acidic environment within the female reproductive tract.

The seminal vesicles, a pair of pouch-like glands, produce the largest portion of the semen's volume. The secretions of the seminal vesicles contain the sugar fructose, which provides a source of energy promoting the mobility of the sperm. The prostate gland, the chestnut-shaped organ under the bladder and in front of the rectum, secretes a thin fluid that forms a portion of the semen's volume and helps sperm to maintain their mobility. The bulbourethral glands, also known as Cowper's glands, are two relatively small, pea-shaped organs located below the prostate gland. The glands produce mucus-like fluids that form a small portion of the semen's volume. In addition, such secretions help to lubricate the end of the urethra. The penis is the portion of the male genitalia through which semen and urine pass.

DESCRIPTION

Respiratory

The respiratory system, comprising the air passages from the nose, throat, bronchial tubes, and lungs, is responsible for filtering the air that enters the body, supplying oxygen to the body, and removing carbon dioxide from the blood. This process is known as respiration. Certain organs of the respiratory (pulmonary) system also influence speech and help to produce the sense of smell (olfaction).

The organs of the respiratory system are often classified into the upper and lower respiratory tract. The upper respiratory tract, which consists of organs that are located outside the actual chest cavity (thorax), includes the nose, pharynx, and larynx. The organs within the lower respiratory tract are located primarily within the thorax and include the trachea, the bronchial tree, and the lungs.

Nose
The nose functions as the uppermost portion of the respiratory tract. This hollow passage, which connects the naval cavities and the upper portion of the throat (nasopharynx), serves to filter, warm, and moisten the air entering the respiratory tract. Mucous membranes (respiratory mucosa) covered by microscopic hairs (cilia) line the entire nasal passage-as well as most passageways of the respiratory tract. Located within the nasal mucosa are specialized nerve receptors necessary for the sense of smell.

During inspiration, air enters the respiratory tract through the nostrils (external nares). Small hairs within the nostrils trap foreign particles, such as dust, pollen, or microorganisms, thus protecting against infection and allergic responses. Filtered air passes into the nasal cavities, which have moist surfaces due to mucus production. The nasal cavities are divided by a structure made of cartilage (nasal septum). Bones surrounding the nose contain hollow, air-filled cavities (paranasal sinuses) that affect the resonance of sound (e.g., during speech). In addition, these mucous-membrane lined cavities, which drain into the nasal cavities, assist in producing mucus for the respiratory tract.

As air passes through the nasal cavities, it is warmed, humidified, and filtered by three thin, mucosa-covered structures (conchae). Mucus on the surface of the conchae and other organs of the respiratory tract flows toward the nasopharynx due to the beating action of the cilia, thereby helping to move trapped foreign particles out of the respiratory tract.

Pharynx
The pharyx, also known as the throat, is a muscular tube lined with mucous membranes. The throat is part of both the respiratory and digestive systems and is divided into three regions: an uppermost portion (nasopharynx) that serves as an air passage; an area of the throat behind the mouth (oropharynx) that is a passage for food and air; and a lower segment (laryngopharynx) that functions as a passage for food only. Air normally enters the pharynx from the nasal cavities (although it may sometimes enter through the mouth) and exits via the larynx. However, food enters the pharynx from the mouth and continues through the digestive system via the esophagus.

The eustachian or auditory tubes also open into the nasopharynx, connecting the middle ears and the throat. In addition, the masses of lymphoid tissue that serve as the "front line" against invading microorganisms (tonsils) are located under the mucous membranes at the back of the pharynx.

Larynx
The larynx, also known as the voice box, connects the pharynx with the trachea. It consists of several areas of fibrous, flexible connective tissue (cartilage) and is also lined with mucous membranes. The larynx is responsible for producing the voice and preventing food from entering the airway during swallowing.

The opening of the larynx is partially covered by a "lid-like" flap of cartilage known as the epiglottis. This structure normally remains open, maintaining the larynx as part of the airway. However, when swallowing occurs, the epiglottis closes, sealing off the opening of the larynx and preventing food from passing into the larynx and the trachea. In addition, two strong, fibrous sheets of tissue known as the vocal cords stretch across the interior of the larynx. Passage of air over the vocal cords results in vibrations that help to create speech.

Trachea
The trachea, also known as the windpipe, extends from the larynx to an area behind the upper breastbone (sternum), where it then divides to form the two bronchi. The windpipe is a tube-like structure composed of elastic and fibrous tissues, smooth (involuntary) muscle, and rings of cartilage that help to keep the trachea open (patent). As with other organs of the respiratory tract, the trachea is also lined with mucous membranes (respiratory mucosa) covered by cilia. The secreted mucus helps to trap tiny foreign particles remaining in the inhaled air of the trachea, and the beating action of the cilia propels the mucus upward toward the pharynx and out of the respiratory tract.

Bronchial Tree
Because the numerous air passages of the lungs resemble an upside-down, tree-like structure, the bronchi and their branching airways are known as the bronchial tree. The trachea branches to form the main bronchi (primary bronchi) of the left and right lungs. Both of the primary bronchi then branch into smaller bronchi (secondary bronchi). The bron-

chi walls consist of three layers including an outer layer of fibrous, dense tissue; a middle layer of smooth muscle; and an inner layer of mucous membranes. In addition, the walls of the primary and secondary bronchi, like the trachea, are kept open by rings of cartilage, allowing the passage of air.

The bronchi divide into progressively smaller airways that eventually branch into tiny passages known as bronchioles. The walls of the bronchioles include only smooth muscle. The bronchioles then branch into microscopic tubes known as alveolar ducts that lead to the alveolar sacs. The walls of the alveolar sacs consist of many microscopic, grape-like structures called alveoli. The alveoli lie in contact with microscopic blood vessels (capillaries). The exchange of oxygen and carbon dioxide takes place across the thin walls of the alveoli, i.e., oxygen moves from the alveoli to the blood while carbon dioxide moves from the blood to the alveoli.

Lungs

The lungs, which are spongy, elastic organs located in the chest cavity, are divided into lobes: the left lung has two lobes, whereas the right lung has three. The narrow, rounded, upper area of each lung is known as the apex, and the broad, concave, lower portion of each lung that rests on the diaphragm is referred to as the base. In addition, a thin, moist, two-layered membrane known as the pleura lines the outside of the lungs and the inside of the chest cavity. A small amount of fluid separates the two layers of the pleura, serving as a lubricant as the lungs contract and expand during respiration.

The act of breathing (pulmonary ventilation) consists of two phases: inspiration and expiration. During inspiration, the chest and lungs expand, and air is drawn into the lungs. During expiration, the chest and lungs contract and air is forced out of the lungs.

Pulmonary Circulation

Pulmonary circulation refers to the movement of blood through vessels between the heart and the lungs for the removal of carbon dioxide and the addition of oxygen (oxygenation) to the blood. When the right lower chamber of the heart (ventricle) contracts, "oxygen-poor" (deoxygenated) blood is pumped to the lungs via the pulmonary artery. From there, the blood flows through the capillaries that lie in contact with the air-filled alveoli. Oxygen moves across the thin walls of the alveoli into the blood, whereas carbon dioxide is transported by the blood to the alveoli. Carbon dioxide exits the lungs during expiration. Oxygenated blood is returned to the left upper chamber of the heart (atrium) via four pulmonary veins and is propelled into the left ventricle. When the left ventricle contracts, the blood is pumped into the major artery of the body (aorta) for circulation to the body's tissues. In addition, the blood that nourishes the lungs themselves is supplied by the bronchial arteries.

DESCRIPTION

Sensory Organs

Certain specialized components of the nervous system, known as sense organs, are able to recognize specific stimuli in the external environment that affect the body, such as light, sound, temperature, or pressure. When the specialized microscopic structures that comprise the sensory organs (sensory receptors) recognize certain stimuli, they produce nervous impulses that are sent to the brain, the spinal cord, or both. The sense organs may be classified into two general categories: the somatic sense organs and the special sense organs.

Special Sense Organs

Sensory receptors for the special senses of hearing, vision, smell, and taste, are collected in the special sense organs, including the eyes (i.e., in the retinas), the ears (within the hearing apparatus), the nose (smell receptors), and the tongue (taste receptors). Sensory information received by these special sense organs travels to the brain via the cranial nerves, the 12 nerve pairs that arise from the brain and emerge through various openings in the skull. Most sensory information is transmitted to the sensory cortex of the brain.

Ears, Hearing, and Balance

The ear is the special sensory organ involved in hearing and balance. It consists of three major parts including
- external ear
- middle ear
- inner ear

The External Ear

The external ear includes the visible portion of the ear (pinna or auricle) and the external auditory canal. The pinna consists of folds of cartilage and skin surrounding the opening of the auditory canal, which is the tube that extends into the lower cranium bone (temporal bone) and ends at the partition between the external and middle ear (eardrum or tympanic membrane). The skin of the auditory canal contains specialized glands (ceruminous glands) that produce cerumen, a waxy substance that traps dust and other foreign bodies. Sound waves pass through the auditory canal and strike the eardrum, causing it to vibrate.

The Middle Ear

The middle ear, a tiny cavity between the eardrum and the inner ear, contains three minute, movable bones (ossicles) that conduct sound to the inner ear. The names of the bones essentially describe their shapes: i.e., the malleus (hammer), incus (anvil), and stapes (stirrup). When the eardrum vibrates in response to sound waves, the vibrations are transmitted and amplified by the three ear bones. The stapes' movement against a membrane-covered opening to the inner ear results in movement of the fluid within the inner ear.

The eustachian or auditory tube connects the middle ear to the uppermost region of the throat (nasopharynx). Although the eustachian tube is usually closed at rest, it opens due to muscle contractions associated with swallowing or yawning. The eustachian tube is shorter in infants and young children than in older children and adults. As a result, when an upper respiratory tract infection occurs, infants and young children have an increased likelihood of experiencing the backward flow of secretions from the nasopharynx into the middle ear space and associated infection of the middle ear (otitis media).

The Inner Ear

The inner ear contains a maze of complex, winding passages (known as the labyrinth) deep within the temporal bone. The major parts of the inner ear include the organ of hearing, known as the cochlea, and the organ of balance, the semicircular canals.

The cochlea, a hollow, coiled passage that resembles a snail's shell, contains the organ of Corti and thick fluid. The organ of Corti has tiny cells with hair-like extensions projecting into the fluid. Vibrations transmitted to the inner ear cause the fluid and the hair-like extensions to vibrate. As a result, the hair cells are stimulated to generate nerve impulses that are transmitted by the vestibulocochlear nerve (acoustic nerve or eighth cranial nerve) to the brain.

The three semicircular canals are fluid-filled tubes containing specialized hair cells that respond to movement of the fluid. When movements of the head cause fluid movement within a canal, the cells initiate nerve impulses to the brain via the vestibulocochlear nerve, resulting in necessary adjustments to maintain balance.

The Eyes and Vision

The eye is a specialized sensory organ that is actually part of the central nervous system. It focuses light waves to create an image on the nerve-rich membrane at the back of the eye (retina). The retina, in turn, converts the image into nerve impulses that are transmitted to the brain via the optic nerve (second cranial nerve).

Anatomy and Function of the Eye

The eye is embedded in pads of fat within the bony socket in the skull. Movements of the eye are regulated by a network of six muscles, each of which moves the eye in a particular direction or directions.

The outermost layer of the eye, known as the sclera, is a tough, fibrous tissue that includes the "white" of the eye and the cornea, which is the front, circular, transparent area that serves as the eye's primary lens. A flexible mucous membrane, the conjunctiva, covers the sclera and lines the eyelid; in addition, the conjunctiva contains several glands that secrete tears and mucus. The eyelid consists of a thin layer of skin over muscle that covers a thin plate of connective tissue (tarsal plate). The edge of the eyelid contains a row of strong protective hairs known as eyelashes as well as several glands (meibomian glands) that produce an oily secretion known as sebum. The combined actions of the tear-secreting and mucus-producing glands of the conjunctiva and the meibomian glands of the eyelid produce an essential tear film that protects the conjunctiva and cornea from damage due to drying. The eyelid spreads the tear film over the cornea during the blink reflex, helping to ensure clear vision. Moreover, the eyelid further protects the eye by closing quickly as an involuntary reaction (reflex action) to the approach of any foreign object.

The middle layer of the eye, known as the choroid, includes two involuntary muscles: the iris and the ciliary muscle. The iris, the pigmented area visible through the cornea, is a circular muscle with a hole in its center known as the pupil, which controls the amount of light entering the eye. When certain fibers in the iris contract, the pupil widens, allowing in additional light; in contrast, when other iris fibers contract, the pupil constricts, allowing in less light. The lens of the eye, which is behind the pupil, is held in place by the ciliary muscle, a circular muscle that changes the shape of the lens to make appropriate adjustments in focus. For example, the ciliary muscle contracts when the eye focuses on near objects and relaxes when the eye views distant objects.

The hollow main cavity of the eye is filled with fluids that help to ensure the proper shape of the eyeball and assist in bending light rays that fall on the retina. The fluids include the thin, watery fluid in front of the lens (aqueous humor) and the jelly-like fluid behind the lens (vitreous humor).

The retina, the innermost layer of the eye, is a complex nerve-rich membrane upon which images created by the cornea and the lens fall. More specifically, as light passes through the cornea, the pupil, the aqueous humor, the lens, and the vitreous humor, it is bent (refracted) so that it is properly focused on the retina, which contains millions of tiny nerve cells that respond to light (photoreceptors). Such nerve cells are named based upon their shapes: i.e., rods and cones. Rods are stimulated by dim light and are necessary for night vision. Cones are stimulated by brighter light and are the receptors for daytime vision. Three different types of cones respond to the colors red, blue, or green. The rods and cones convert images formed on the retina into nerve impulses that are transmitted by the optic nerve (second cranial nerve) to the brain.

The Nose and the Smell Receptors

In addition to serving as the uppermost region of the respiratory tract, the nose also functions as the special sensory organ involved in the sense of smell (olfaction). The chemical receptors necessary for olfaction are specialized nerve cell endings located in a small area of mucous membrane (nasal mucosa) lining the nasal cavities. The olfactory cells have specialized, microscopic hairs (cilia) that are stimulated by different chemicals. In response to such chemicals, the cilia generate nerve impulses that pass through the olfactory nerve (first cranial nerve) to the smell centers of the brain.

The Tongue and the Taste Receptors

The tongue is the muscular, flexible organ in the floor of the mouth. This organ-which also plays an essential role in producing speech, breaking down food during chewing (mastication), and swallowing - functions as a specialized sensory organ involved in taste.

There are approximately 10,000 microscopic chemical receptors known as taste buds that produce the nerve impulses required for taste. Although most are located on the tongue, there are also some taste buds on the roof of the mouth (palate) and the back of the throat. The taste buds surround the bases of nipple-shaped elevations (papillae) that cover the surface of the tone and other tissues. Specialized cells within the taste buds (gustatory cells) generate nerve impulses in response to dissolved chemicals within saliva. Most of these impulses pass through the facial nerve (seventh cranial nerve) and the glossopharyngeal nerve (ninth cranial nerve) to the taste center of the brain. Stimulation of the taste buds results in four types of taste sensations including sour, sweet, bitter, and salty. Other taste sensations or "flavors" result due to the combined stimulation of taste and olfactory receptors.

DESCRIPTION

Urologic

The urinary system, which consists of the two kidneys, the ureters, the bladder, and the urethra, filters waste products from the blood, returns essential nutrients back into the blood, and produces and excretes urine.

The Kidneys

The kidneys, which are located at the back of the abdominal cavity, are situated on either side of the spinal column above the waistline. The right kidney lies beneath the liver. The left kidney, which is usually slightly higher than the right, is located below the spleen.

The primary functions of the kidneys are to regulate the delicate balance of electrolytes including sodium and potassium; control the acid-base balance of the body (i.e., ensuring that the blood and other bodily fluids are neither too acidic nor alkaline); and filter soluble wastes from the blood and eliminate these waste products. More specifically, the purpose of the kidneys includes the following:

- To filter certain waste products (e.g., urea, ammonia) and excessive sodium and water from the blood

- To reabsorb particular substances and return them to the blood

- To regulate the levels of certain substances in the blood and maintain the appropriate balance between water and salt content in the body (i.e., by filtration, reabsorption, and secretion)

- To regulate blood pressure and the production and release of red blood cells. For example, cells of the juxtaglomerular apparatus of the kidneys secrete a hormone (renin) that results in the constriction of blood vessels, thereby raising blood pressure. In addition, the kidneys produce erythropoietin, a hormone that assists in stimulating and regulating the production and release of red blood cells (erythrocytes) from the bone marrow. An increase in the number of circulating red blood cells boosts the body's capacity to carry oxygen to its tissues and organs.

Urine Production and Excretion

The kidneys each contain approximately one million nephrons, the filtering units of the kidneys. Each nephron consists of two primary components, the renal corpuscle and the renal tubule, both of which are further divided into additional regions.

The top of each nephron consists of a cup-shaped structure known as Bowman's capsule. Within Bowman's capsule is a network of tiny capillaries known as a glomerulus. Together, the two structures are known as the renal corpuscle.

As blood flows through the kidneys, the fluid portion of the blood is filtered by minute pores in the blood vessels of the glomerulus and the inner layer of Bowman's capsule. The fluid then moves into the region between the inner and outer layers of Bowman's capsule and enters into the first portion of the renal tubule (proximal convoluted tubule), where most filtered substances (e.g., most of the water, glucose, and sodium) are reabsorbed into the blood via capillaries around the tubules (peritubular capillaries). Next, as fluid moves into the loop of Henle, sodium and other electrolytes are pumped out. As the fluid passes through the next portion of the renal tubule (distal convoluted tubule), additional sodium is removed in exchange for potassium. Diluted fluid from distal convoluted tubules then passes into a collecting tubule, where fluid may continue to pass through the urinary tract as dilute urine or be returned to the blood to ensure appropriate water content in the body.

Urine then drains from the collecting tubules into central collecting areas (renal pelvis) of each kidney, which are the upper portions of the ureters. The ureters are narrow muscular tubes lined by mucous membranes. Contractions of the ureters' muscular walls move small quantities of urine into the bladder, a hollow organ that gradually expands as the volume of urine increases. As the bladder nears its capacity, nerve signals are transmitted to the brain to signal that urination is necessary. When urination occurs, the circular muscle (sphincter) between the bladder and the urethra opens, allowing urine to pass out of the body. Contractions of the bladder create pressure that forces urine into the urethra and out its external opening (urinary meatus).

Glossary

A Concise Guide to Medical Terminology

This Guide is designed to help the reader decipher some unfamiliar terms used in the disorder descriptions. It is helpful to divide medical terms into their basic elements: prefix, root, and suffix. Following these examples are more than 200 commonly used medical prefixes, roots, and suffixes.

Example 1: The medical term *microcephaly* is a combination of "micr(o)," meaning small, and "cephal(o)," which means head. Therefore, microcephaly denotes an abnormally small head. In contrast, "macr(o)" means large. Thus, *macrocephaly* indicates an unusually large head.

Example 2: The word *polydactyly* includes "poly," meaning much or many, and "dactyl," which refers to fingers or toes. Thus, the medical term *polydactyly* means the presence of extra fingers or toes. Accordingly, because "brachy" means short, the word *brachydactyly* indicates abnor-mally short fingers or toes.

Example 3: The term *myositis* is a combination of "my(o)," which denotes muscle, and "itis," meaning inflamma-tion. Therefore, *myositis* means muscle inflammation. When "cardi(o)," meaning heart, is added, forming the term *myocarditis,* the meaning becomes inflammation of heart muscle.

Medical Prefixes, Roots, and Suffixes

a-	absence of, without	cerebr(o)-	brain
ab-	away from	cervic-	neck
acou-	hear	chole-	bile
aden(o)-	gland	chondr(o)-	cartilage
-algia	pain	circum-	around
andr(o)-	man	contra.	against, counter
angi(o)-	vessel	cost(o)-	rib
ankyl(o)-	bent, crooked	crani(o)-	skull
ante-	before	cry(o)-	cold
anti-	against, counter	crypt(o)-	conceal, hide
artexi(o)-	artery	cyan(o)-	blue
arthr(o)-	joint	cyst(o)-	bladder
auri-	ear	cyt(o)-	cell
aut(o)-	self	dactyl-	digit, finger or toe
bacteri(o)-	bacteria	de-	away from, down
bio-	life	dent(o)-	tooth
blast(o)-	bud, early embryonic budding	dermat(o)-	skin
blephar(o)-	eyelid	di-	two
brachi(o)-	arm	dia-	apart, through
brachy-	short	dipl(o)-	double
brady-	slow	dors(o)-	back
bronch(o)-	bronchi	dys-	abnormal, bad
bucc(o)-	cheek	-emia	blood
carcin(o)-	cancer	en-	in, on
cardi(o)-	heart	end(o)-	inside, within
-cele	hernia, protrusion, tumor	enter(o)-	intestine
cent-	one hundred	epi-	above, upon
centr(o)-	center	erythr(o)-	red
cephal(o)-	head	eso-	inside, within

esthesi(o)-	feel, perceive	mamm(o)-	breast
eu-	normal, well	mast(o)-	breast
ex-	away from, outside	medi-	middle
extra-	beyond, in addition, outside of	mega-	great, large
flav(o)-	yellow	megal(o)-	great, large
galact(o)-	milk	melan(o)-	black
gastr(o)-	stomach	mening(o)-	membrane
gen(o)-	gene or reproduction	mes(o)-	middle
gloss(o)-	tongue	meta-	after, beyond
glyc(o)-	sweet	metr(o)-	uterus
gnath(o)-	jaw	micr(o)-	small
.gram	draw, record, write	mill-	one thousand
graph(o)-	record, write	mon(o)-	only, single, sole
gynec(o)-	woman	morph(o)-	form, shape, structure
hemat(o)-	blood	myel(o)-	marrow
hemi-	half	my(o)-	muscle
hepat(o)-	liver	myx(o)-	mucus
hex-	six	narc(o)-	stupor
hidr(o)-	sweat	nas(o)-	nose
hist(o)-	tissue	necr(o)-	corpse, death
hom(o)-	common, same	nephr(o)-	kidney
hydr(o)-	water	neur(o)-	nerve
hyper-	above, beyond, excessive	nos(o)-	disease
hypn(o)-	sleep	ocul(o)-	eye
hyp(o)-	below, deficient, low	odont(o)-	tooth
hyster(o)-	uterus	-odyn(o)-	distress, pain
iatr(o)-	physician	olig(o)-	deficient, few, little
idi(o)-	distinct, separate	-oma	neoplasm, tumor
ili(o)-	intestines	omphal(o)-	navel
inter-	among, between	onc(o)-	mass, tumor
intra-	inside, within	onych(o)-	nail
ischi(o)-	hip	oo-	egg
-itis	inflammation	ophthalm(o)-	eye
kary(o)-	nucleus	oro-	mouth
kilo-	one thousand	orchi(o)-	testicle
kinet(o)-	move	osse(o)-	bone
labio-	lips	oste(o)-	bone
lact(o)-	milk	ot(o)-	ear
lapar(o)-	flank, loin	ovari(o)-	ovary
laryng(o)-	larynx	oxy-	sharp
latero-	side	pachy-	thick
leuc(o)-	white	para-	beside, beyond, resembling
leuk(o)-	white	path(o)-	disease
lien(o)-	spleen	ped(o)-	child
lingu(o)-	tongue	penia-	abnormal reduction, deficient
lip(o)-	fat	pent(a)-	five
lith(o)-	stone	per-	throughout
lymph(o)-	lymph, water	pen-	around
macr(o)-	large	phag(o)-	consume, eat
mal-	abnormal, bad	pharmaco-	drug, medicine
malac(o)-	soft	pharyng(o)-	throat

phleb(o)	vein	sial(o)	saliva
phon(o)	sound	somat(o)	body
phot(o)	light	spasm(o)	spasm
pil(o)	hair	spermat(o)	seed
-plasia	development, formation	splen(o)	spleen
platy	broad, flat	spondyl(o)	vertebra
pleur(o)	rib, side	spor(o)	spore
-pnea	breathing	steat(o)	fat
pneumat(o)	air, breathing	sten(o)	compressed, narrow
pneum(o)	air, breath, lung	stomat(o)	mouth, opening
pod(o)	foot	sub-	below, near, under
poly-	many, much	super-	above, beyond, excessive
post-	after, behind	syn-	together, with
pre-	before, in front of	tachy	fast, rapid
pro	before, in front of	tel(o)	end
proct(o)	rectum	tetra	four
pseud(o)	false	therm(o)	heat
psych(o)-	mind	thorac(o)	chest
pulmon(o)	lung	thromb(o)	clot
pyel(o)-	pelvis	-tome	instrument for cutting
pyr(o)-	fire, heat	tox(o)	poison
quadri	four	traumat(o)-	wound
rachi(o)-	spine	tri	three
re-	again, back	trich(o)	hair
ren(o)	kidneys	troph(o)	food, nourishment
retr(o)	backward, behind	-uria	urine
rheo	flow	vas(o)	vessel
rhin(o)	nose	vertebr(o)	vertebrae
sangui	blood	vesic(o)	bladder or blister
sarc(o)	flesh	xanth(o)	yellow
scler(o)	hard	xer(o)	dry
-scope	instrument for examining	zyg(o)-	junction, union
semi-	half		

Guidelines for Obtaining Additional Information and Resources

Many parents and caregivers are interested in obtaining information regarding *physicians* who specialize in certain pediatric disorders, accredited *hospitals, approved drugs or medical devices* for certain pediatric conditions, or current *clinical trials* that are investigating possible new therapies for particular diseases. In addition, some individuals may wish to have access to medical journal articles and other medical literature that may be available on their child's disorder, disease, or condition. Following are several tips that may be shared with parents and caregivers in their efforts to obtain such information and resources.

Disease-Specific Resources: Many of the disease-specific resources in this *Directory* maintain listings of physicians who are experts in a particular pediatric disorder. They may also offer information on accredited hospitals with appropriate specialty departments. In addition, many may provide information on standard therapies for certain pediatric conditions and ongoing clinical trials that are investigating possible new therapies. Some of these organizations, such as certain national voluntary health associations (NVHAs) or support groups, function as patient registries, working closely with expert physicians, researchers, and university medical centers specializing in specific pediatric disorders.

Online "Physician Finder" Services: Several professional medical associations provide searchable databases on the Internet as a public service for individuals who wish to obtain information on physicians.

Example: The *American Medical Association (AMA) Physician Select* database provides information on licensed physicians in the United States, including credential data that has been verified by medical schools, residency training programs, certifying and licensing boards, and accrediting agencies. AMA Physician Select enables online visitors to search for physicians by name, medical specialty, or geographic location. This online service is located at http://www.webapps.ama-assn.org/doctorfinder.

Example: The *American Board of Medical Specialties (ABMS) Public Education Program* offers an online physician locator and information service. This service, which lists all physicians certified by ABMS Member Boards, allows online visitors to verify board certification status, specialty, and location of physicians who are certified by one or more of the ABMS Member Boards. The ABMS also provides the *Certified/Doctor Locator Service,* which lists physicians certified by ABMS Member Boards who have subscribed to the service. Such listings include board certification(s), address, telephone number, and hospital affiliation(s). These online services may be accessed at www.abms.org.

Example: The U.S. federal government has an online service known as *healthfinder*® that serves as a Web portal or directory for those who are interested in locating current, high quality health information and resources on the Internet. The site is located at www.healthfinder.gov.

Hospital Accreditation: Individuals who are interested in learning about a particular medical facility's accreditation status may consider contacting the *Joint Commission,* which is the the United States' leading health care quality evaluator and accredits approximately 15,000 health care facilities, organizations, and programs. Accreditation is recognized as a *"Gold Seal of Approval"* indicating that the hospital meets certain standards of performance and is committed to meeting state-of-the-art performance expectations. The Joint Commission offers an online service known as *Quality Check* that enables online visitors to obtain information about an organization's accreditation, such as how it was rated during its most recent quality report. This service is located at www.qualitycheck.org. Callers may also receive information concerning a hospital's accreditation status by calling the Joint Commission, at (630) 792-5800 or visiting www.jointcommission.org.

Hospital Public Information Lines and Web Sites: Many hospitals are creating and strongly promoting special public information lines. Such help lines are often publicized within local or regional newspapers and in the introductory sections of local phone books. In addition, many hospitals are creating Web sites that: offer information on their services and programs; link to sites offered by different departments or facilities; discuss ongoing research; provide searchable physician directories; publish newsletters, various reports, press releases, and other materials; and offer a variety of additional information. These Web sites may be located by visiting various search engines and using the name of the facility as a search term. (For more information, see *Search Engines* below.)

Academic Hospitals: If children have been diagnosed with a chronic, difficult-to-treat, or relatively uncommon disorder or if they remain undiagnosed after visits to several primary care or specialist pediatricians, parents or other caregivers may wish to consider taking their children to a major academic medical center. Generally, such teaching hospitals use state-of-the-art testing techniques, have comprehensive evaluation centers, and follow multidisciplinary approaches to diagnosis and treatment. In addition, such centers are often affiliated with medical schools where clinical research is conducted.

Food and Drug Administration: Individuals who are interested in learning more about approved drug therapies or medical devices for certain pediatric disorders may wish to contact the *U. S. Food and Drug Administration (FDA)*. The FDA is the U.S. agency that enforces federal regulations to prevent the sale and distribution of dangerous or impure substances, such as unsafe foods, impure cosmetics, or unsafe or ineffective drugs or medical devices. For example, according to the FDA Modernization Act of 1997, one of the agency's primary objectives is "to promote the public health by promptly and efficiently reviewing clinical research and taking appropriate action on the marketing of regulated products in a timely manner." The agency is a branch of the U.S. Department of Health and Human Services. The FDA's Web site provides: FAQs (Frequently Asked Questions) areas; Consumer Drug Information Sheets; information on new and generic drug approvals, medical device product approvals, and drug labeling changes; health advisories; and access to MedWatch, the FDA's *Safety Information and Adverse Event Reporting Program.* MedWatch enables consumers and health care professionals to report adverse reactions to approved medical products directly to the FDA and/or the manufacturers. The primary purpose of MedWatch is to ensure the rapid identification of potential health hazards associated with approved medical products and the prompt communication of safety information to the health care and medical communities. The FDA's Web site is located at www.fda.gov/medwatch. The agency's address follows:

FDA
5600 Fishers Lane
Rockville, MD 20857
Toll-free: (888) INFO-FDA or (888) 463-6332

Clinical Research: A clinical protocol is a scientific study that evaluates the safety or effectiveness (efficacy) of a particular drug therapy or medical device in humans. Clinical studies enable researchers and physicians to determine new and more effective ways to prevent, diagnose, manage, and treat disease. Medications and treatments that are found to be safe and effective during laboratory and animal testing must then prove safe and effective in humans before they are approved for use by the general public. Participation in clinical studies may only occur if individuals volunteer and are fully informed and understanding of both the potential benefits and risks of such participation ("informed consent"). Participants may voluntarily leave a clinical study at any time.

Research on new drugs, which are known as *investigational new drug applications* or *INDS,* is conducted in three phases:

Phase I Study - The main objective of a Phase I study is to establish the *safety* of the investigational new drug. Such studies:

- may take several months

- typically involve a relatively small number of participants who are healthy volunteers

- are designed to evaluate the INDs biologic activities in the human body (e.g., absorption, metabolism, etc.) and its potential side effects as drug dosages are raised

Phase II Study - The purpose of a Phase II study is to establish the *safety and efficacy* of the investigational new drug in treating a specific disease. Such studies:

- may take from several months to a few years

- may include a relatively small number or up to several hundred patients

- usually involve randomized, double-blind trials. During such studies, one group of participants receives the drug (experimental group) and the other group is given a harmless, unmedicated substance (placebo) or a standard, well-established therapy (control group). The information concerning which patients are included in which group is hidden from both the patients and the researchers.

Phase III Study - The purpose of a Phase III study is to evaluate the overall *safety, efficacy, possible adverse effects, and benefits* of the investigational new drug in a large number of patients and to compare such therapy with the use of well-established treatments or with an untreated disease course. Such studies:

- may last for several years

- may involve hundreds or thousands of patients

- may include research teams from multiple national or international clinical centers

- typically involve randomized, double-blind trials

If an investigational new drug application successfully completes Phase III studies, the drug's sponsor may request FDA approval for marketing to the public, which is known as a *New Drug Approval* (NDA). In some cases, additional clinical research may be conducted:

Phase IV Study – The purpose of a Phase IV study may be to:

- monitor the drug's long-term efficacy

- compare the drug with other medications that have been available for longer periods

As mentioned above, disease-specific organizations and registries, support groups, and online services may serve as essential sources of information concerning clinical studies for a particular disease. There are also several additional, more general resources that promote and provide information on clinical trials:

Example: The *Warren Grant Magnuson Clinical Center,* which is part of the National Institutes of Health (NIH), is a federally funded biomedical research hospital. The Clinical Center was designed to support studies conducted by the NIH. Only individuals with conditions or disorders under NIH investigation are admitted for treatment, and all patients must be referred by their physicians. The Clinical Center's Web site includes a clinical research database that enables online visitors to search for current research studies by certain predefined parameters, such as primary disease category, or specific diagnosis, symptom, sign, or other keywords. The Clinical Center's Web site is located at www.cc.nih.gov and its Protocol Database may be accessed at http://clinicalstudies.info.nih.gov. The Clinical Center's address follows:

Department of Health and Human Services
Public Health Service
National Institutes of Health (NIH)
Warren G. Magnuson Clinical Center
Patient Recruitment and Referral Center
9000 Rockville Pike
Bethesda, MD 20892
Toll-free: (800) 411-1222
E-mail: prpl@mail.cc.nih.gov

Example: *CenterWatch, Inc.* provides a *Clinical Trials Listing Service*™ on its Web site for patients and research professionals. The site provides listings of over 7 ,000 national and international clinical trials that are searchable by geographic region and therapeutic area. Interested individuals may also sign up for CenterWatch's confidential *Patient Notification Service,* which provides notification via e-mail of future clinical trial postings in a certain therapeutic area. CenterWatch's Clinical Trials Service also provides: a listing of NIH-funded clinical research programs that are currently being conducted at the NIH's Warren Grant Magnuson Clinical Center; a general explanation of clinical trials, profiles of clinical research centers; listings of medications recently approved by the

FDA; and linkage to health-related sites for patients and patient advocates. The Clinical Trials Listing Service™ is located at www.centerwatch.com. CenterWatch's address follows:

Thompson CenterWatch, Inc.
22 Thomson Place, 47th floor
Boston, MA 02210
Phone: (617) 856-5900
Fax: (617) 856-5901
E-Mail: customerservice@ahcmedia.com

Example: The *National Cancer Institute (NCI)* offers an online service known as *CancerNet™* that provides information for patients and family members, health professionals, and researchers. The site offers: information on current clinical trials; summaries on cancer prevention, screening, treatment, and supportive care; cancer fact sheets; and linkage to the *Physician Data Query* or *PDQ® Cancer Information Service,* the NCI's cancer database. PDQ contains a registry of open and closed cancer clinical trials as well as directories of organizations, physicians, and genetic counselors who provide cancer care. CancerNet™ also provides access to *cancerTrials,* a clinical trials information center, and *CANCERLIT®,* a bibliographic database. CancerNet™ is located at http://cancer.gov. The NCI also offers a Cancer Information Service (CIS) for callers Monday through Friday from 9 a.m. to 4:30 p.m., Eastern Standard Time. The CIS may be reached at (800) 422-6237. Individuals with hearing impairment who have TTY equipment may call (800) 332-8615.

Example: *OncoLink* is an online resource on the Internet that is affiliated with the University of Pennsylvania Medical Center and the University of Pennsylvania Cancer Center. The site provides: information on cancer clinical trials; symptom management; personal experiences and psychosocial support; cancer causes, prevention, and screening; FAQs (frequently asked questions); financial issues for cancer patients; and additional topics. The site is located at www.oncolink. upenn.edu.

Search Engines. If individuals are interested in locating a particular organization's Web site but do not have its address or wish to determine what online services may be available in a certain subject area, Internet search engines are an essential resource. Search engines enable online visitors to conduct general or targeted searches for information within their areas of interest and appropriate to their needs. In addition to searching for and providing direct linkage to certain Web sites, many search engines enable users to search for e-mail discussion groups (listservs), UseNet newsgroups, FAQs (frequently asked questions), or other tools. Following is a sample listing of some of the search engines available on the Web:

- Achoo: achoo.8media.org
- Altavista: www.altavista.com
- Dogpile: www.dogpile.com
- Excite: www.excite.com
- HotBot: www.hotbot.com
- Lycos: www.lycos.com
- Metacrawler: www.metacrawler.com
- Snap.com: www.snap.com
- Yahoo: www.yahoo.com

General Medical and Professional Association Sites: Some individuals may be interested in visiting medical sites that offer general information on disease and health issues. In addition, many professional medical associations and societies have Web sites that provide access to patient and professional information, press releases, journals, clinical updates, and other areas that may be helpful to those interested in pediatric disorder topics. Following is a brief listing of such sites:

- American Academy of Family Physicians: www.aafp.org
- American Academy of Pediatrics: www.aap.org
- American Medical Association: www.ama-assn.org
- HealthAtoZ: www.HealthAtoZ.com

- HealthGate: www.healthgate.com
- John Hopkins Health Information: www.hopkinshospital.org/health_info
- Mayo Clinic Health Information: www.mayoclinic.com
- Medical Matrix: www.medmatrix.org/reg/login.asp
- Medscape: www.medscape.com
- US Pharmacopeia (information on medications): www.usp.org

Medical Journal Articles. Individuals who are interested in accessing abstracts summarizing medical journal articles may visit the National Library of Medicine's (NLM's) *PubMed.* The PubMed search service provides free access to the approximately 17 million medical journal citations within NLM's *MEDLINE.* MEDLINE is essentially the online version of *Index Medicus,* a monthly subject/author guide to articles in thousands of medical journals. Online visitors to PubMed may conduct searches for medical journal citations and abstracts by journal title and date, author, and topic. In addition to providing access to selected journal abstracts, PubMed offers links to participating online journals and enables registered users to order full-text articles for a fee. (If individuals are interested in accessing other medical journal sites, such online journals may often be located by using various search engines.) PubMed may be accessed at www.pubmed.gov. In addition, several general medical sites provide access to PubMed and enable users to order full-text journal articles for a fee.

Online Mendelian Inheritance in Man (OMIM). Individuals who wish to access comprehensive and timely medical information on genetic disorders may be interested in visiting OMIMTM or *Online Mendelian Inheritance in Man,* a database of genetic disorders and human genes. This searchable database, which is written and edited by Dr. Victor A. McKusick and colleagues at Johns Hopkins University and other locations, was developed for the Web by the National Center for Biotechnology Information (NCBI). OMIM™ contains entries on genetic diseases, clinical synopses, links to relevant MEDLINE citations, and more. OMIM™ is located at www.ncbi.nlm.nih.gov/sites/entrez?db=OMIN.

A

A&K Associates, 4408

A-T Project: Cancer Research for Childrenwith A-T Newsletter, 6975, 6993

A-TMRF Newsletter, 549

A-to-Z Health & Disease Information, 6896

AABA Newsletter, 2862

AACAP, 2408

AACAP News, 5291

AAP Education Resource Guide, 8309

AASK: Adopt A Special Kid, 7515

ABA Program Companion, 889

ABC Stories, 3413

ABC's of Finger Spelling, 3556

ABCs of AVT: Analyzing Auditory-Verbal Therapy, 3557

ABCs of AVT: Analyzing Auditory-VerbalTherapy, 3414

ABDC Newsletter, 8299

ABLEDATA, 7516

ACRMD:Lifespire, 7517

AD-IN: Attention Deficit InformationNetwork, 588

ADA Technical Assistance Program, 1360

The ADA: Questions and Answers, 6403

ADARA, 7518

ADD & Learning Disabilities, 633

ADD From A To Z-Understanding The Diagnosis & Treatment of ADD in Children & Adult, 606

ADD, Stepping Out of the Dark, 607

ADD: Helping Your Child, 634

ADHD, 698

The ADHD Book of Lists, 691

ADHD Challenge, 589

ADHD Parenting Handbook: Practical Advicefor Parents from Parents, 635

ADHD Report, 695

ADHD Survival Guide for Parents andTeachers, 636

ADHD in Schools: Assessment andIntervention Strategies, 637

ADHD in the Young Child, 638

ADHD: Handbook for Diagnosis & Treatment, 639

ADHD: What Can We Do?, 608

ADHD: What Do We Know?, 609

AEGIS, 3152

AES News, 6380

AGSA Newsletter, 7308

AHEPA Cooley's Anemia Foundation, 7017

AIDS Awareness Library, 3166

AIDS Knowledge Base, 3153

AIDS and the Education of Our Children, 3167

AIM for the Handicapped Adventures inMovement, 7519

AJAO Newsletter, 4375

ALL Kids, 114

AMOR - A Cancer Support Group forPatients & Their Families, 1170

AMT Children of Hope Foundation, 5486

APF Newsletter, 5614

APSAC Advisor, 5557

APT/HI: Auditory Perception Test for theHearing Impaired, 3558

ARC Family Connection Parent to ParentProgram, 7896

ARC Family Resource Project, 7753

ARC Suburban, 7919

ARC of East Central Iowa Pilot Parents, 7868

ARC of Morgan County, 7730

ARC of the United States, 590, 2546, 2631, 3012, 3042, 3049, 3075, 3081, 4162, 4165, 4532, 4538, 4578, 4602, 7520

ARRISE, 725

AS Support Network, 333

AS Web, 246

ASL Babies: First Signs, 3559

ASL Babies: Let's Eat, 3560

ASL Clip and Create Version 3, 3512

ASL Songs for Kids, 3513

ASL Stories: Christmas Stories, 3415

ASL Stories: Fairy Tales I, 3416

ASL Stories: Fairy Tales II, 3417

ASL Tales and Games for Kids, 3514

ASL Tales and Games for Kids 2, 3515

ASL Tales and Songs for Kids CD-1, 3516

ASL Tales and Songs for Kids CD-2, 3517

ATTAIN: Assistive Technology ThroughAction in Indiana, 7853

AUSPLAN Auditory Speech and Language, 3561

AVKO Dyslexia Research Foundation, 4434

AWARE, 7828

Aaron's Awful Allergies, 419

Abbott Northwestern Brain Tumor SupportGroup at Abbott Northwestern Hospital, 1163

Ability First, 8346

Ability First, Camp Paivika, 8347

About Children's Eyes, 8310

About Children's Vision: A Guide forParents, 8311

About Ependymoma, 1268

About Glioblastoma Multiforme andAnaplastic Astrocytoma, 1269

About Headaches, 4638

About Hydrocephalus - Book for Families, 4234

About Medulloblastoma/PNET(Medulloblastoma), 1270

About Meningioma, 1271

About Metastatic Tumors to the Brain andSpine, 1272

About Oligodendroglioma and Mixed Glioma, 1273

About Overeaters Anonymous, 2866, 5217

About Pituitary Tumors, 1274

About the American Brain Tumor Association, 1275

About.com on Sleep Disorders, 5022, 6465, 6493

AboutFace USA, 1702, 1710, 1720, 2107, 2920, 2933, 4498

Academic Acceptance of ASL, 3562

Academy for Eating Disorders (AED), 2768

Academy for Guided Imagery, 7521

Academy of Rehabilitative Audiology, 3332, 7522

Accepting CMT: The Grieving Process andYou, 1557

Access Board, 7523

Access for All: Integrating Deaf, Hard-of-Hearing and Hearing Preschoolers, 3563

Accidents of Nature, 1500

Achieving in Spite of...A Booklet on Learning Disabilities, 4949

Achondroplasia, 1, 19

Achondroplasia UK, 11

Acoustic Neuroma Association, 3190

Acoustics, Audition and Speech Reception, 3418

Acquiring Courage: Audio Cassette Programfor the Rapid Treatment of Phobias, 5430

Activity Schedules for Children withAutism, 890

Acute Gastrointestinal Infections, 20

Acute Lymphoblastic Leukemia, 77

Acute Lymphocytic Leukemia, 179

Acute Myeloid Leukemia, 134

Adam and the Magic Marble, 7178

Adaptation to the Initial Crisis, 2619

Adjustment to Long-Term Health Problems, 1327

C

E

F

H

HED Hypohidrotic Ectodermal DysplasiaFoundation & Related Disorders, 2878

HEMALOG, 4015

HIV Infection, 3132

HOPE (Helping Oncology Parents Endure)Brain Tumor Foundation of the Southwest, 1231

HYCEPH-L, 4212

Hahnemann University Lupus Study Center, 6909

Hair Club for Kids: Hair Club for Men, 90, 146, 2988

Hand Eczema, 2910

Handbook Of Autism and PervasiveDevelopmental Disorders, 919

Handbook of Childhood Impulse Disordersand ADHD: Theory and Practice, 663

Handbook of Head Truma: Acute Care toRecovery, 3308

Handbook of Headache, 4627

Handbook of Headache Disorders, 4628

The Handbook of Pediatric Audiology, 3757

Handbook of Psoriasis, 5837

Handbook of School-Based Interventions, 2426

Handbook of Scoliosis, 6277

Handi-Kids/King Solomon Foundation, 8399

Handicapped Scuba Association, 7625

Handle with Care, 7626

Handling the Young Cerebral Palsied Childat Home, 1525

Handout on Health: Scleroderma, 6239

Hands Organization, 3351

Happiness Bag Incorporated, 8376

Happy Hollow Children's Camp, 8377

Harbor Regional Center Family andProfessional Resource Center, 7769

Harold Goodglass Aphasia Research Center, 3280

Harold Talks About How He InheritedHemophilia, 4004

Harold's Secret: A Boy with Hemophilia, 4005

Harris County Health Department, 6823

Harrison's Principles of Inernal Medicine15th Edition, 7079

Harvard Eating Disorders Center, 2808

Harvard Web Forum for Spina Bifida, 6624

Having Leukemia Isn't So Bad, of Course,It Wouldn't Be My First Choice, 123

Hawaii Down Syndrome Congress, 2568

Hawaii SIDS Information & CounselingProject, 6777

Head Injuries, 3188

Head Injury Hotline, 3196, 3266

Head Injury in Children and Adolescents: AResource and Review for School, 3309

Head Trauma Sourcebook, 3310

Headache, 4635

Headache Book: Prevention & Treatmentfor All Types of Headaches, 4629

Headache Facts-What Everyone Should Know, 4642

Headache Handbook, 4643

Headache Q & A, 4644

Headache in Children-Fact Sheet, 4645

Headaches and Hydrocephalus, 4243

Headline News, 4026

The Headliner, 3320

Headlines, 3316

Heads Up Brain Tumor Support Group, 1067

Heads Up Ohio, 3317

Headstrong, 1151

Headstrong Brain Tumor Support Group, 1134

Headway, 3318

Healing Exchange Brain Trust, 1068

Healing Hearts, 4300

Healing Well, 2339

HealingWell.com, 6349

Health Answers, 541, 629, 1338, 1507, 1549, 2180, 2636, 2809, 3084, 3108, 3996, 6160, 6225, 6263, 6853, 6944, 7169, 7290, 7309, 7366, 7395

Health Insurance, 568

Health Insurance Issues and Solutions forPeople with Torette Syndrome, 7211

Health Research Project (HaRP), 37, 262, 4110, 4839, 5792

HealthCentral.com, 5819

Healthcare for Children on the AutismSpectrum, 920

Healthfinder, 4672, 4683, 6945, 7439

A Healthy Mouth for Your Baby, 7092

Hear, 3792

Hear & Listen! Talk & Sing!, 3526

Hear Center, 3381

Hear Now, 3352

The Hearing Aid Handbook: Clinician's Guide to Client Orientation, 3758

Hearing Aid Handbook: User's Guide forChildren, 3650

Hearing Alert Informational Brochures, 3812

Hearing Care for Children, 3651, 5333

Hearing Health, 3783

Hearing Impairment/Deafness, 3330

Hearing Impairments in Young Children, 3652, 5334

Hearing ImpairmentsBetter Hearing Institute, 3353

Hearing Loss, 3653

Hearing is Believing, Volume One, 3527

Hearing is Believing, Volume Three, 3528

Hearing is Believing, Volume Two, 3529

Hearing-Impaired Child, 3654

Hearing-Impaired Children and Youth withDevelopmental Disabilities, 3655

Hearing-Impaired Children in theMainstream, 3656

HearingPlanet, 3354

Heart Burn, Hiatal Hernia, andGastroesophageal Reflux Disease, 63

Heart Center Online, 305

Heart Disease, 277, 583

Heart Disease, High Blood Pressure, Strokeand Diabetes, 8319

Heart Failure Society Newsletter, 312

Heart Failure Society of America, 300

Heart and Down Syndrome, 2680

Heart of the Matter, 4287

Heart to Heart, 1909, 1930, 2049, 2073, 4284, 4304, 4307, 4309, 5155, 5174, 6010, 6029

Heart to Heart - St. Louis, 4292

Heart to Heart Fund, 4289

HeartLight, 4281

Hearts and Homes For Youth, 3355

Heights, 5434

Helen Keller Center's NationalParent Network, 7627

Helen Keller International, 7628

Helen Keller National Center, 1890, 1903, 2027, 2043, 5138, 5150, 5992, 6005

Helen Keller National Center - NorthCentral Region, 5931

Helen Keller National Center - Rocky Mountain Center, 7791

Helen Keller National Center SW Region, 1834, 1971, 5083, 5928

Helicobacter Pylori and Peptic Ulcer, 64

Help Me, I'm Sad, 2427

Help Parent Support Group Hope & Education for Loving Parents, 7792

Help with a Hidden Disease Update, 6152

Helpful Techniques to Aid the Student withTourette Syndrome, 7212

I

J

K

N

Newsline, 3795, 8306

Newsline Eight & Nine, 4032

Newslink, 969

Next Steps - Parents Reaching Parents, 7848

Nick Joins In, 6647

The Night Before Christmas told in Signedenglish, 3761

Night Terrors, 5008

Nightmares, 4984

NineLine, 7695

No Fears, No Tears, 8232

No Fears, No Tears - 13 Years Later, 8233

No Time for Jello: One Family's Experience, 1531

Nobody Knows, 1532

Nocturnal Enuresis, 5035

Non-Chew Cookbook, 127

Non-Hodgkin's Lymphoma, 5049

Non-Malignant Brain Tumor Support Group, 1168

None So Deaf - Student Text, 3699

Nonverbal Learning Disorder Syndrome, 4255

Noonan Connection, 5073

Noonan Syndrome, 5064

Noonan Syndrome Support Group, 5069

North Ameerican Spine Society, 6266

North American Riding for the Handicapped, 7696

North American Society for Childhood OnsetSchizophrenia - NACOS, 1626

North American Society for PediatricGastroenterology/Hepatology/Nutrition, 28, 256, 1761, 2976, 4092, 4096, 4656, 4854, 5273, 5905

North Carolina Library for the Blind, 1892, 2029, 5140, 5994

North Carolina SIDS Information andCounseling Program, 6811

North Carolina Speech, Hearing and Language Association, 6510

North Central Oklahoma Support Group, 517

North Dakota Comprehensive Hemophilia andThrombosis Treatment Center, 3963

North Dakota SIDS Management Program, 6812

North Pacific Epilepsy Research, 6351

North Platte Public Library, 8158

North Texas Chapter of Crohn's &Colitis Foundation of America, 2173

North Texas SIDS Information AndCounseling Program, 6824

North Texas Support Group, 527

Northeast Ohio Chapter of Crohn's &Colitis Foundation of America, 2165

Northeast Rehabilitation Health Network, 3299

Northern California Chapter of Asthma andAllergy Foundation of America, 366

Northern California Chapter of Crohn's and Colitis Foundation, 2135

Northern California Comprehensive Sickle Cell Center, 6433

Northern California Support Group, 467

Northern Colorado Area Support Group, 474

Northern Connecticut Affiliate Chapter ofCrohn's & Colitis Foundation of America, 2139

Northern Illinois Center for AdaptiveTechnology, 8117

Northern Kentucky Talking Book Library, 8137

Northern Ohio Chapter of the NationalHemophilia Foundation, 3893

Northridge Hospital: Leavey Cancer Center, 1085

Northwest Hospital Brain Tumor GroupSupport Hotline, 1241

Northwest Hospital Brain TumorSupport Group, 1240

Northwest Indiana Subregional Library forBlind and Physically Handicapped, 1863, 2000, 5112, 5966

Northwest Ohio Hemophilia Foundation, 3894

Northwest Ohio Hemophilia TreatmentCenter, 3964

Northwestern Region-Helen Keller NationalCenter, 1838, 1975, 5087, 5941

Northwestern University Asthma and AllergyDisease Center, 390

Not Just a Cancer Patient, 8234

Nothing Hurts But My Heart, 6278

Now We Can Successfully Treat the IllnessCalled Depression, 2457

Nuclear Medicine at Children's Hospital,Boston, 8275

Number Signs for Everyone: Numbering in American Sign Language, 3484

Nursery Rhymes from Mother Goose: Told in Signed English, 3700

Nursing Your Baby with Down Syndrome, 2657

Nutitional Care for Children with PWS, Infants and Toddlers, 5728

Nutrition for Early Chronic Kidney Disease, 8330

Nutrition for Later Chronic Disease, 8331

Nystagmus, 5074

Nystagmus Network, 5162

O

OCD Newsletter, 5265

OCD in Children and Adolescents: ACognitive-Behavioral Treatment Manual, 5258

OCECD, 8008

OHSU Homepage Search, 3110

Oak-Leyden Developmental Services, 757

Oakhurst, 8438

Oakland County Health Division - SIDSProject, 6794

Oakland School & Camp, 4472

Oasis, 7793

Oasis Guide to Asperger Syndrome, 346

Obesity, 5186

Obesity Online, 5201

Obesity Sourcebook, 5209

Obesity: Theory and Therapy, 2850, 5210

Obsessive Compulsive Anonymous, 5230

Obsessive Compulsive Disorder (OCD), 5248

Obsessive Compulsive Disorder General Packet, 5267

Obsessive Compulsive Disorder in Childrenand Adolescents: A Guide, 5259

Obsessive Compulsive Disorder: HelpingChildren and Adolescents, 5260

Obsessive Compulsive Foundation, 5231, 5249

Obsessive Compulsive Foundation of Metropolitan Chicago, 5234

Obsessive Compulsive Information Center, 5235

Obsessive-Compulsive Disorder, 5219

Obsessive-Compulsive Disorder in Childrenand Adolescents, 5261

Obsessive-Compulsive Disorder, A Real Illness, 5268

Oconee Regional Library, Library for theBlind and Physically Handicapped, 8110

Of Their Own-Person To Person Show, 6154

Office Integrated Social Services, 8032

Office for Fair Housing & EqualOpportunity, 7511

Office of Community Health and PreventionBureau of Early Intervention, DHR, 7849

Office of Exceptional ChildrenSouth Carolina Department of Education, 8038

Office of Special Education, 7916, 7930, 8041

Office of Special Education Administration, 8077

Office of Special Education andRehabilitative Services, 7512, 8276

Office of Special Education, StateDepartment of Education, 8045

Office of Special Education, Virginia, 8068

Office of Women's & Children's Health, 6763

Office of the Dean, University of Texas atAustin, 8049

P

Physical Therapy Intervention for Individuals With Prader-Willi Syndrome, 5741

Physician Referral and Information Line, 383

Pica Information Page, 5570

Pike Institute on Law and Disability, 7701

Pikes Peak Area Support Group, 475

Pilot Parents (PP), 7702

Pilot Parents in Anoka and Ramsey Counties, 7924

Pilot Parents of Northeast Minnesota, 7925

Pilot Parents of Southern Arizona, 7744

Pine Tree Camp Children - Adults, 8391

Pinworm (Enterobius Vermicularis), 5571

Pinworm Infection, 5578

Pioneers Division of CEC, 7703

Pittsburgh Area Brain Injury Alliance, 3255

Pittsburgh Area Brain Tumor Support Group, 1219

Pityriasis Rosea, 5579, 5585

Plain Talk About Depression, 2459

Plan for Success: Educator's Guide toStudents with Osteogenesis Imperfecta, 5302

Planetpsych, 1041, 1643, 1795, 4999, 5024, 5250, 5356, 5443, 8282

Planetree Health Information Service, 7704

Plasma Homovanillic Asid in Schhizophrenia, 1666

Platelet Disorder Support Association, 7073, 7078

Pneumonia, 5586

Police Officer Jones, 3710

Polio Connection of America, 5798

Polio Experience Network, 5799

Polio Society, 5786

Polio Survivors Association, 5787

Polydactyly, 5597, 5606

Porphyria, 5607

Porphyria Fact Sheet, 5615

Portland Public Library, 8146

Portsmouth Regional Home, 1179

Positive Exposure, 191

Positive Solutions for Life Challenges, 7940

Post Polio Awareness & Support Society ofBritish Columbia, 5800

Post Traumatic Stress Disorder Sourcebook, 5638

Post Traumatic Stress Disorder: A Guide, 5644

Post-Polio Directory, 5807

Post-Polio Health, 5809

Post-Polio Health International, 5788

Post-Traumatic Stress Disorder, 5616

Post-Traumatic Stress Disorder, A Real Illness, 5645

Posttraumatic Stress Disorder in Childrenand Adolescents, 5639

Postural Screening Program, 6296

Practical Management of Pediatric Cardiac Arrhythmias, 309

Practice Guidelines for Eating Disorders, 2853

Prader-Willi Alliance of New York, 5687, 5723

Prader-Willi Association of New England(Maine, Mass, RI, NH, VT), 5674, 5676

Prader-Willi California Foundation, 5657

Prader-Willi Colorado Association, 5658

Prader-Willi Connecticut Association, 5660

Prader-Willi Delaware Association, 5661

Prader-Willi Families of Ohio, 5693

Prader-Willi Northwest Association, 5653, 5666, 5680

Prader-Willi Northwest Association-Idaho, 5667

Prader-Willi Syndrome, 5647

Prader-Willi Syndrome - An Overview for Health Professionals, 5720

Prader-Willi Syndrome Advocates, 5671

Prader-Willi Syndrome Arizona Association, 5654

Prader-Willi Syndrome Association, 5652, 5724

Prader-Willi Syndrome is What I Have Not Who I Am!, 5730

Prader-Willi Syndrome: A Guide for Families & Professionals, 5742

Prader-Willi Syndrome: Medical Alerts, 5743

Prader-Willi Syndrome: Some Reflections onBehavior, 5744

Prader-Willi Utah Association, 5706

Precious Hearts, 4308

Precious Time: Children Living withMuscular Dystrophy, 4717

Precocious Puberty, 5748, 5757

Preemie Magazine, 5781

Preemie Ring, 5774

Preemie Twins, 5775

Preemie World, 5776

Pregnancy and Child Health Resource Centerfrom Mayo Health Oasis, 8283

Pregnancy and Exposure to Alcohol andOther Drug Use, 3024

Pregnancy and Infant Loss Center, 6757

Premature Baby-Premature Child, 5777

Prematurely Yours, 5778, 5779

Prematurity, 5758

Prenatal Diagnostic and Genetic Center, 8129, 8211

Prenatal Exposures in Schizophrenia, 1667

Prenatal Hydrocephalus-Book for Parents, 4256

Prenatal and Postnatal Growth and Development, 8509

Preparing Your Child for Surgery, 4257

Preparing Your Child for a Bone MarrowTransplant, 8333

Preparing Yourself for Spinal Surgery (For Teenagers with Severe Scoliosis), 6255

Presbyterian Hospital/Pittsburgh CancerCenter, 1220

Presbyterian-University Hospital,Pulmonary Sleep Evaluation Center, 4803

Preschool Education Programs for Childrenwith Autism, 938

Preschool Issues in Autism, 939

Preschool Motor Speech Evaluation & Intervention, 6536

Preschool Programs - Division of SpecialPopulations, 7888

Prescription Parents, 1708, 1716

Prescription for Success, 940

President's Committee on Employmentof People with Disabilities, 7513

President's Committee on MentalRetardation, 7514

Presidential Proclamation-NationalSarcoidosis Awareness Day, 6186

Preuss Foundation, 1072

Prevent Blindness America, 1968, 7705

Prevent Child Abuse America, 5503, 5542

Prevent Child Abuse California, 5543

Prevent Child Abuse Georgia, 5513

Prevent Child Abuse Illinois, 5514

Prevent Child Abuse Indiana, 5515

Prevent Child Abuse Iowa, 5516

Prevent Child Abuse New York, 5518

Prevent Child Abuse North Carolina, 5519

Preventable Childhood Infections, 5783

Preventing Antisocial Behavior:Interventions, 1803

Prevention Initiatives State Department ofEducation, 7798

Prevention Resource Guide: Pregnant,Postpartum Women and Their Infants, 3025

Primary Brain Cancer Support Group, 1131

Primary Care Needs of Children withHydrocephalus, 4258

Primary Children's Medical Center, 8212

A Primer of Brain Tumors, 1267

Prince George's County Memorial LibraryTalking Book Center, 1870, 2007, 5118, 5972

Princess Pooh, 6648

Q

R

U

V

W

Alabama

ARC of Morgan County, 7730

Alabama Chapter of the National Hemophilia Foundation, 3865

Alabama Department of Rehabilitation Services, 3913

Alabama Head Injury Foundation, 3198

Alabama Institute for the Deaf & Blind, 1832, 1969, 3379, 5081, 5925

Alabama/Northwest Florida Chapter of Crohn 's Colitis Foundation of America, 2131

Asthma and Allergy Foundation of America - Alabama Chapter, 364

Autism Society of Alabama, 761

Autism Society of North Alabama, 762

Birmingham Support Group, 462

Brain Injury Association of Alabama, 3199

Bureau of Family Health Services-Alabama C hild Death Review, 6761

Camp ASCCA/Easter Seals, 8344

Civitan International Research Center, 3395

Down Syndrome Clinic, Children's Hospital of Alabama, 2580

Early Intervention Program, 7731

Friends for Life Auburn United Methodist Church, 7732

Gregory Fleming James Cystic Fibrosis Cent er, 2225

Hemophilia Clinic - Childrens' Rehabilitation Service, 3942

Mobile Association for the Blind, 1839, 1904, 1976, 2044, 5088, 5151

Mobile Hemophilia Clinic, 3960

National Child Advocacy Center, 8007

Pediatric Brain Tumor Support Group, 1073

Sickle Cell Foundation of Greater Montgomery, 6416

Special Education Action Committee Huntsville Outreach Office, 7733

Special Education Services, 7734

Spina Bifida Association of Alabama, 6559

Statewide Technology Access & Response System for Alabamians with Disabilities, 7735

Summer Camp for Children with Muscular Dystrophy, 4747

United Cerebral Palsy of Alabama a, 1372

United Cerebral Palsy of Greater Birmingham, 1373

United Cerebral Palsy of Huntsville & Tennessee Valley, 1374

United Cerebral Palsy of Mobile, 1375

United Cerebral Palsy of Northwest Alabama, 1376

United Cerebral Palsy of West Alabama, 1377

University of Alabama - Birmingham Arthrit is Clinical Intervention Program, 6222

University of Alabama Speech and Hearing Center, 3380

Alaska

Alaska Chapter of Asthma and Allergy Found ation of America, 365

Alaska Department of Education, 7736

Assistive Technologies of Alaska, 7737

Brain Injury Association of Alaska, 3200

Brain Injury Association of Alaska - Helpline, 3201

Maternal, Child & Family Health, Early Intervention/Infant Learning Program, 7738

PARENTS, 7739

Rid Alaska of Child Abuse, 5510

SIDS Information & Counseling Program Alaska Department of Health, 6762

Turner's Syndrome Society of Alaska, 7325

United Cerebral Palsy of Alaska/PARENTS, 1378

University of Alaska, Fairbanks, 8219

Arizona

Arizona Ataxia Support Group, 463

Arizona Chapter of Crohn's & Colitis Foundation of America, 2132

Arizona Early Intervention Program Department of Economic Security, 7740

Arizona HeartLight, 4280

Arizona Sleep Disorders Center, 4760

Arizona Spina Bifida Association, 6560

Arizona Technology Access Program Institute for Human Development, 7741

Autism Society of America Greater Phoenix Chapter, 763

Autism Society of America Northern Arizona Chapter, 764

Autism Society of America Pima County Chapter, 765

Blake Foundation Children's Achievement Center, 7742

Brain Injury Association of Arizona, 3202

Brain Tumor Support Group at NovaCare Rehabilitation Institute of Tucson, 1074

Brain Tumor Support Group at Phoenix, 1075

Children's Center for Neurodevelopmental Studies, 849

Crisis Nursery, 5511

Cystic Fibrosis Center: Phoenix Children's Hospital, 2226

Division of Special Education State Department of Education, 7743

Families of SMA - Arizona Chapter, 6677

Foundation for Children with Down Syndrome, 2561

HeartLight, 4281

Injury Prevention Center, 4186

MDA Summer Camp, 4746

Mayo Clinic Scleroderma Service, 6223

National Center for Neurogenic Communicati on Disorders, 6523

Neurofibromatosis, Inc - Arizona Chapter, 4885

Office of Women's & Children's Health, 6763

Phoenix Center for Cancer and Blood Disorders, 3968

Pilot Parents of Southern Arizona, 7744

Prader-Willi Syndrome Arizona Association, 5654

Raising Special Kids, 7745

Southwest Chapter of Crohn's & Colitis Foundation of America, 2155

Southwest Human Development, 7746

Special Needs Center/Phoenix Public Library, 8090

Steele Children's Research Center, 3977

Technology Access Center of Tucson, 8091

Tourette Syndrome Association-Arizona Chap ter, 7134

Turner's Syndrome Society of Arizona, 7326

United Cerebral Palsy of Central Arizona, 1379

United Cerebral Palsy of Southern Arizona, 1380

Arkansas

Arkansas Department of Health - SIDS Information & Counseling Program, 6764

Arkansas Disability Coalition, 7747

Arkansas Easter Seals Technology Resource Center, 8092

Arkansas Regional Library for the Blind and Physically Handicapped, 1841, 1978, 5090, 5944

Arkansas Rehabilitation Research and Training Center for Deaf Persons, 3396

Autism Society of America Arkansas Chapter, 766

Brain Injury Association of Arkansas, 3203

Camp Aldersgate, 8345

Children's Tumor Foundation-Arkansas Chapt er, 4886

Children's Tumor Foundation-Arkansas Infor mation & Support, 4887

Crowley Ridge Regional Library, 8093

DD Services, Department of Human Services, 7748

Educational Services for the Visually Impaired, 1840, 1977, 5089, 5943, 8094

Epilepsy Education Association of Arkansas, 6316

FOCUS, 7749

Hemophilia Center of Arkansas, 3866, 3936

Increasing Capabilities Access Network, 7750

Library for the Blind and Handicapped, Southwest, 8095

PWSA of Arkansas, 5655

Parent to Parent Arc of Arkansas, 7751

Special Education Section State Department of Education, 7752

Spina Bifida Association of Arkansas, 6561

United Cerebral Palsy of Central Arkansas, 1381

United Cerebral Palsy of Northeast Arkansas, 1382

United Cerebral Palsy of South Arkansas, 1383

California

ARC Family Resource Project, 7753

Ability First, 8346

Ability First, Camp Paivika, 8347

All Nations Camp, 8348

Alliance for Technology Access (ATA), 8096

American Action Fund for Blind Children and Adults, 1842, 1979, 5091, 5945

American Association for Pediatric Ophthalmology and Strabismus, 1901

Assistive Technology Center Simi Valley Hospital, 8097

Ataxia Telangiectasia Medical Research Foundation, 534

Autism Research Institute, 847

Autism Society of America Coachella Valley, 767

Autism Society of America Greater Long Beach/South Bay Chapter, 768

Autism Society of America Inland Empire Chapter, 769

Autism Society of America Los Angeles Chapter, 770

Autism Society of America North California Chapter, 771

Autism Society of America North San Diego County Chapter, 772

Autism Society of America Orange County Chapter, 773

Autism Society of America San Diego Chapter, 774

Autism Society of America San Francisco Bay Chapter, 775

Autism Society of America San Gabriel Valley Chapter, 776

Autism Society of America Santa Barbara Chapter, 777

Autism Society of America Tulare County Chapter, 778

Autism Society of California, 779

Bereavement Group for Children, 6765

Blind Children's Center, 1843, 1980, 5092, 5946

Blind Childrens Center, 5927

Bloomfield, 1938, 2082, 5182, 6037

Braille Institute Desert Center, 1844, 1981, 5093, 5947

Braille Institute Sight Center, 1845, 1982, 5094, 5948

Braille Institute Youth Center, 1846, 1983, 5095, 5949

Brain Imaging Center at the University of California, Irvine, 3276

Brain Research Institute, 3273

Brain Tumor Patient & Family Support Group, 1076

Brain Tumor Support Group at Newport Beach, 1077

Brain Tumor Support Group at San Diego, 1078

Brain Tumor Support Group at San Luis Obispo, 1079

Brain Tumor Support Group at Santa Monica, 1080

Brain Tumor Support Program Cedars-Sinai Neurosurgical Inst. & Wellness Community, 1081

Brain and Spinal Injury Center (BASIC) Research at University of California, 3277

Brian Wesley Ray Cystic Fibrosis Center, 2227

CARE Family Resource Center, 7754

California Brain Injury Association, 3204

California SIDS Program, 6766

Camp Alex A. Krem, 8349

Camp Crescent Moon, 6456

Camp Joan Mier, 8350

Camp Ronald McDonald at Eagle Lake, 8351

Camp Wonder, 6241

Camp de los Ninos - Diabetes Society, 2523

Camp-A-Lot, 8352

Carolyn Kordich Family Resource Center, 7755

Center for Accessible Technology, 8098

Center for the Partially Sighted, 1902, 2038, 2470, 5149, 6004

Center for the Research and Treatment of Anorexia Nervosa, 2791

Central California Chapter of the National Hemophilia Foundation, 3867

Central California Support Group, 464

Challenged Family Resource Center, 7756

Child Sexual Abuse Treatment Program (Giar retto), 5512

Children Living with Illness, 7757

Children's Hospital & Research Center of Oakland, 2581

Children's Hospital of Los Angeles, 2228

Children's Hospital of Orange County: Depa rtment of Pulmonology - Cystic Fibrosis, 2229

Children's Hospital: Pediatric Pulmonary Center, 2230

Clearinghouse for Specialized Media and Technology (CSMT), 8099

Comfort Connection Family Resource Center, 7758

Computer Access Center, 8201

Cooley's Anemia Foundation-California, 7025

Cystic Fibrosis Center: Cedars-Sinai Medical Center, 2231

Cystic Fibrosis Center: University of California at San Francisco, 2232

Cystic Fibrosis Research, 2233

Cystic Fibrosis and Pediatric Respiratory Diseases Center, 2234

Department of Developmental Services of Early Start Program, 7759

Down Syndrome Association of Los Angeles, 2562

Early Start Family Resource Network, 7760

Easter Seal Summer Camp Programs, 8353

Enchanted Hills Camp, 8354

EpiCenter, 6328

Epilepsy Foundation of Northern California, 6317

Exceptional Family Resource Center, 7761

Exceptional Family Support, Education and Advocacy Center, 7762

Exceptional Parents, 7763

Families Caring for Families, 7764

Families of SMA - Northern California Chapter, 6678

Family First Program Alpha Resource Center, 7765

Family Focus Resource Center, 7766

Family Resource Center, 7767

Family Resource Center at Lucile Packard Children's Hospital, 1762

Federal Hemophilia Treatment Center Program of Los Angeles, 3932

Foundation for Glaucoma Research, 2040

Fragile X Association of Southern California, 3046

Fragile X Center of San Diego, 3047

Francis J. Curry National Tuberculosis Center, 7285

Fresno Brain Tumor Support Group, 1082

Glaucoma Research Foundation, 2042

Gloriana Opera Company, 8355

Greater Los Angeles/Orange County Chapter of Chron's & Colitis Foundation, 2133

Greater North Valley California Support Group, 465

Greater San Diego/Desert Chapter of Crohn's & Colitis Foundation of America, 2134

H.E.A.R.T.S. Connection Family Resource Center, 7768

Harbor Regional Center Family and Professional Resource Center, 7769

Hear Center, 3381

Helen Keller National Center SW Region, 1834, 1971, 5083, 5928

Hemophilia Association of San Diego County, 3868

Hemophilia Foundation of Northern California, 3869

Hemophilia Foundation of Southern California, 3870

Huntington Hospital Hemophilia Center, 3952

Hydrocephalus Parent Support Group, 4187

Hydrocephalus Support Group of Southern California, 4188

Inland Empire Brain Tumor Support Group, 1083

International Pemphigus Foundation, 5385

Jodi House, 3205

Junior Wheelchair Sports Camp, 8356

Kaiser Permanente Medical Center, 2235

Kern Autism Network, 780

Loma Linda University Sleep Disorders Center, 4761

Los Angeles Ataxia Support Group, 466

MATRIX: Parent Network and Family Resource Center, 7770

Matrix Parents Network and Resource Center, 7771

Memorial Miller Children's Hospital Cystic Fibrosis Center, 2236

Neurofibromatosis, Inc - California Chapter, 4888

Neuroscience Institute Brain Tumor Support Group, 1084

New Beginnings - Blind Children's Center, 1847, 1984, 5096, 5950

New Beginnings - The Blind Children's Center, 1906, 2047, 5153, 6008

Northern California Chapter of Asthma and Allergy Foundation of America, 366

Northern California Chapter of Crohn's and Colitis Foundation, 2135

Northern California Comprehensive Sickle Cell Center, 6433

Northern California Support Group, 467

Northridge Hospital: Leavey Cancer Center, 1085

Okizu Foundation Camps, 8357

Orange County Support Group, 468

Orthopaedic Biomechanics Laboratory, 1498

Orthopaedic Hospital's Hemophilia Treatment Center, 3966

PWSA of California, 5656

Pacific Southwest Regional Genetics Group, 469

Palo Alto Brain Tumor Support Group, 1086

Parents Helping Parents of San Francisco, 7772

Parents Helping Parents of Santa Clara, 7773

Pathology Department SIDS/SUDC Research Project, 6842

Peaks and Valleys Family Resource Center, 7774

Pediatric Disabilities Clinic, Down Syndrome Clinic, 2582

Peninsula Support & Education Group for Parents of Children with Brain Tumors, 1087

Prader-Willi California Foundation, 5657

Psoriasis Research Association, 5827

Pulmonary Care and Cystic Fibrosis Center, 2237

REACH - Sarcoidosis Support, 6130

Region IX Office Program Consultants for Maternal and Child Health, 6767

SMA Research Group, 6683

Sacramento Area Brain Tumor Support Group Lawrence J Ellison Ambulatory Care Ctr, 1088

Sacramento Area Hydrocephalus Group, 4189

Sacramento Center for Assistive Technology, 8100

San Diego Support Group, 470

San Fernando Valley Support Group, 471

San Francisco Brain Tumor Support Group, 1089

San Francisco Public Library for the Blind and Print Disabled, 1848, 1985, 5097, 5951

San Gabriel/Pomona Parents' Place, 7775

Santa Barbara Brain Tumor Support Group, 1090

Santa Cruz County Brain Tumor Support Group, 1091

Santa Rosa Brain Tumor Support Group, 1092

Scleroderma Research Foundation, 6221

Sickle Cell Disease Foundation of California, 6417

South Bay Brain Tumor Support Group, 1093

South Central Los Angeles Regional Center for Devlopmentally Disabled Persons, 7776

Southern California Chapter of Asthma and Allergy Foundation of America, 367

Southern California Neuropsychiatric Institute, 3278

Southern California Pediatric Brain Tumor Network, 1094

Special Connections Family Resource Center, 7777

Special Education Division State Department of Education, 7778

Spina Bifida Association of Greater Bay Area, 6562

Spina Bifida Association of Greater San Diego, 6563

Stanford CF Center, 2238

Stanford University Center for Narcolepsy, 4762

Starlight Children's Foundation, 7779

Support Group for Caregivers of Brain Tumor Patients, 1095

Support Group for Parents of Children with Brain Tumors, 1096

Support for Families of Children with Disabilities, 7780

Team Advocates for Special Kids, Anaheim, 7781

Team Advocates for Special Kids, San Diego, 7782

Team of Advocates for Special Kids, 8216

Turner's Syndrome Society Central And Northern, 7327

Turner's Syndrome Society of Southern California, 7328

UC Berkeley School of Social Welfare, 5021, 5429, 8218

UCD Hemophilia Treatment Center, 3979

UCSD Hemophilia Treatment Center, 3980

USC - Neonatology Research Units, 6846

United Cerebral Palsy of Central California, 1384

United Cerebral Palsy of Greater Sacramento, 1385

United Cerebral Palsy of Los Angeles, Ventura and Santa Barbara Counties, 1386

United Cerebral Palsy of Orange County, 1387

United Cerebral Palsy of San Diego County, 1388

United Cerebral Palsy of San Joaquin, Calaveras & Amador Counties, 1389

United Cerebral Palsy of San Luis Obispo, 1390

United Cerebral Palsy of Santa Barbara County, 1391

United Cerebral Palsy of Santa Clara & San Mateo Counties, 1392

United Cerebral Palsy of Stanislaus County Stanislaus, 1393

United Cerebral Palsy of the Golden State, 1394

United Cerebral Palsy of the Inland Empire, 1395

United Cerebral Palsy of the North Bay, 1396

University of California, San Francisco Brain Tumor Research Center, 1252

University of California, San Francisco Dermatology Drug Research, 1588, 1594, 2894, 2900, 5470, 5476

University of Southern California Comprehensive Sickle Cell Center, 6434

Variety Audio, 1849, 1986, 5098, 5952

Vital Options, 1097

Warmline Family Resource Center, 7783

Wellness Community San Francisco/East Bay, 1098

West Los Angeles Brain Tumor Support Group, 1099

Colorado

Assistive Technology Partners, 7784

Autism Society of America Colorado Chapter, 781

Autism Society of America Larimer County Chapter, 782

Autism Society of America Pikes Peak Chapter, 783

Autism Society of American Boulder County Chapter, 784

Brain Injury Association of Colorado, 3206

Brain Tumor Patient & Family Support Group, 1100

Brain Tumor Patient/Family Group, 1101

Cardiac Kids/Association of Volunteers, 4282

Children's Hospital: Academic Pediatric Surgery Department, 1752

Children's Tumor Foundation - Colorado Chapter, 4889

Colorado Consortium of Intensive Care Nurseries United Parents (UP), 7785

Colorado SIDS Program, 6768

Delta/Montrose Parent to Parent, 7786

Denver Children's Hospital, 2239

Denver Colorado Support Group, 472

Denver Early Childhood Connections, 7787

Denver Sarcoidosis Awareness Support Group, 6131

Disability Connection and RAFT, Larimer County's Early Childhood Connection, 7788

Effective Parent Project, 7789

El Groupo Vida, 7790

Helen Keller National Center - Rocky Mount ain Center, 7791

Help Parent Support Group Hope & Education for Loving Parents, 7792

Hemophilia Society of Colorado, 3871

Little People of America - Front Range Chapter, 3099

Lung Line Information Service, 382

Magic of Music and Dance, 8358

Mile High Down Syndrome Association, 2563

Mountain States Regional Genetics Services Network, 473

National Jewish Center for Immunology and Respiratory Medicine, 388

National Jewish Medical & Research Center, 389, 5590, 6149

Northern Colorado Area Support Group, 474

Oasis, 7793

PEAK Parent Center, 7794

Parent Support Group of Littleton & Auora, 7795

Parents Supporting Parents of Eagle County, 7796

Parents Supporting Parents of Garfield and Pitkin County, 7797

Pikes Peak Area Support Group, 475

Prader-Willi Colorado Association, 5658

Prevention Initiatives State Department of Education, 7798

Region VIII Office Program Consultants for Maternal and Child Health, 6769

Resources for Young Children and Families, 7799

Rocky Mountain Chapter of Crohn's & Colitis Foundation of America, 2136

Rocky Mountain Village, 8359

Speech, Language, & Hearing Center University of Colorado, 6719

Speech, Language, and Hearing Center, 6524

Spina Bifida Association of Colorado, 6564

TIES, The Children's Hospital, 8215

Turner's Syndrome Society of Rocky Mountain, 7329

United Cerebral Palsy Colorado, 1397

University of Colorado, R.F. Stolinsky Research Laboratories, 3104

Wilderness on Wheels Foundation, 7800

Connecticut

Assistive Technology Project, 7801

Autism Society of America Connecticut Chapter, 785

Brain Injury Association of Connecticut, 3207

Brain Tumor Support Group, 1102, 1103

CPAC, 7802

Central Connecticut Chapter of Crohn's & Colitis Foundation of America, 2137

Connecticut Area Support Group, 476

Connecticut Brain Tumor Support Group (Adult), 1104

Connecticut Down Syndrome Congress, 2564

Connecticut Lead Poisoning Prevention Program, 4428

Department of Mental Retardation, 7803

Division of Child & Family Studies, 7804

Families of SMA - Connecticut Chapter, 6679

Gaylord Hospital Sleep Medicine, 4763

Hemlocks Easter Seals Recreation, 1745, 6303

Hole in the Wall Gang Camp, 3187, 4053

Isola Bella, 3834

Mansfield's Holiday Hill, 8360

Marvelwood Summer, 2714

Northern Connecticut Affiliate Chapter of Crohn's & Colitis Foundation of America, 2139

PWSA of Connecticut (North Haven), 5659

Parent to Parent Network of Connecticut the Family Center, 7805

Parents Association of Connecticut Childre n with Visual Impairments (PACVI), 6088

Prader-Willi Connecticut Association, 5660

Region 1 of the National Association for Parents of the Visually Impaired, 5929

Renfrew Center of Connecticut, 2764

SIDS Program-Connecticut Department of Health, 6770

Sickle Cell Disease Association of America - Connecticut Chapter, 6418

Spina Bifida Association of Connecticut, 6565

State Department of Education, 7806

Sudden Infant Death Syndrome (SIDS) Network, 6836

TBI Support Group for Families & Survivors, 3208

Tourette Syndrome Association-Connecticut Chapter, 7135

Tourette Syndrome Clini, 7152

Turner's Syndrome Society of Connecticut, 7330

United Cerebral Palsy of Eastern Connecticut, 1398

United Cerebral Palsy of Greater Hartford, 1399

United Cerebral Palsy of Southern Connecticut, 1400

University of Connecticut Health Center, 2240

Yale Pediatric Hematology/Oncology Research Center, 3992

Yale University Cystic Fibrosis Research Center, 2241

Yale University, Behavioral Medicine Clinic, 2400

Yale University, Ribicoff Research Facilities, 2401

Delaware

Autism Society of Delaware, 786

Brain Injury Association of Delaware, 3209

Children's Beach House, 3831

Delaware Assisstive Technology Initiative (DATI), 7807

Delaware Division of Libraries for the Blind and Physically Handicapped, 1589, 2895, 5471

Department of Public Instruction, 7808

Parent Information Center of Delaware, 7809

Pediatric Brain Tumor Support Group, 1105

Prader-Willi Delaware Association, 5661

SIDS Information & Counseling - Division of Public Health, 6771

Turner's Syndrome Society of Philadelphia, 7352

United Cerebral Palsy of Delaware, 1401

District of Columbia

Advocates for Justice and Education, 7810

Autism Society of America District of Columbia Chapter, 787

Brain Research Center, 1249

Center for Auditory and Speech Sciences-Gallaudet University, 3382

Child Welfare Information Gateway, 5521

Council of Families with Visual Impairment, 1850, 1987, 5099, 5953

DC Arc, 7811

DC-EIP Services, 7812

District of Columbia Public Library/ Librarian for the Deaf Community, 3383

Division of Community Health Nursing, 6772

Gallaudet University, Cued Speech Team, 6522

Georgetown University, 6224

Georgetown University Child Development Center, 7813, 8101, 8205
Georgetown University Sleep Disorders Center, 4764
HEATH Resource Center, 8102
Hemophilia Program at Children's National Medical Center, 3943
Howard University Center for Sickle Cell Disease, 6435
Lab School of Washington, 719, 992, 4470
Laurent Clerc National Deaf Education Center-Gallaudet Universty, 3384
National Center for Education in Maternal and Child Health, 5768
National Technical Assistance Center for Children's Mental Health, 1785
Partnership for Assistive Technology, 7815
Special Education Programs, 8054
Technical Assistance Partnership for Child and Family Mental Health, 1788
United Cerebral Palsy Research and Educational Foundation, 1499
United Cerebral Palsy of Washington DC & Northern Virginia, 1402
United Cerebral Palsy of Washington DC & Northern Virginia, 1491
Volta Bureau Library, 3385
Washington DC Metropolitan Area Support Group, 1106

Florida

Alliance for Assistive Service and Technology (FAAST), 7816
Angels in the Sun Brain Tumor Support Group, 1107
Ataxia Telangiectasia Children's Project, 533
Autism Society of America Broward Chapter, 788
Autism Society of America Emerald Coast Chapter, 789
Autism Society of America Florida Chapter, 790
Autism Society of America Jacksonville Chapter, 791
Autism Society of America Manasota Chapter, 792
Autism Society of America Panhandle Chapter, 793
Autism Society of Greater Orlando, 794
Brain Injury Association of Florida, 3211
Brain Tumor Support Group, 1108
Brain Tumor Support Group at Miami, 1109
Brain Tumor Support Group at St. Petersburg, 1110
Brain Tumor Support Group at Tampa, 1111
Broward County Support Group, 477
CF & Pediatric Pulmonary Disease Center, 2242
Camp Thunderbird, 8361
Cancer Support Group for Children, 1112

Center for Independence Technology and Education, (CITE), 8103
Cerebral Palsy of Northeast Florida, 1403
Children's Medical Services Program Florida SIDS Program, 6773
Children's Tumor Foundation - Florida Chap ter, 4890
Clearwater, FL Support Group, 478
Coconut Creek Eating Disorders Support Group, 2765
Comprehensive Pediatric Hemophilia Treatment Center, 3929
Cystic Fibrosis Center - All Children's Hospital, 2243
Developmental Center, 715, 988, 4466
Dyslexia Research Institute, 2696
Early Intervention Unit, Division of Children's Medical Services, 7817
Easter Seals Camp Challenge, 8362
Epilepsy Association of Big Bend, 6318
Epilepsy Foundation of Florida, 6319
Epilepsy Services of Northeast Florida, 6320
Family Network on Disabilities, 7818
Family/Community Support Group of the Brain Injury Association of Florida, 3212
Florida Bureau of Braille and Talking Book Library Services, 1851, 1988, 5100, 5954
Florida Camp for Children and Youth, 2526
Florida Chapter of Asthma and Allergy Foundation of America, 368
Florida Chapter of Crohn's & Colitis Found ation of America, 2140
Florida Department of Education, 7819
Florida Epilepsy Services Providers Associ ation, 6321
Florida Families of Children with Visual I mpairments, 6089
Florida Hemophilia Association, 3872
Florida Ophthalmic Institute, 2039
Florida School-Deaf and Blind, 1939, 2083, 3833, 5183, 6038
Florida's Collaboration for Young Children and their Families Head State, 7820
Gold Coast Down Syndrome Organization, 2565
Goodwill Industries-Suncoast, 2566
Goodwill Industries-Suncoast: Choices for Work Program, 3213
Hemophilia Foundation of Greater Florida, 3873
Hydrocephalus Family Support Group of Central Florida, 4190
Miami Children's Hospital, Division of Pulmonology, 2244
Miami Comprehensive Hemophilia Center, 3958
NE Florida Support Group, 479
National Ophthalmic Research Institute, 2046

Neurofibromatosis Center at North Broward Medical Center, 4938
Orlando Support Group, 480
PWSA Florida Chapter, 5662
PWSA of Florida (Tampa), 5663
Pediatric Heart Foundation, 4283
Pensacola Brain Injury, 3214
Pulmonary Wellness Program, 2245
Renfrew Center of Miami, 2766
Renfrew Center of South Florida, 2767
Research & Training Center for Children's Mental Health at University of South FL, 1786
Research and Training Center for Children' Mental Health, 8213
Scleroderma Foundation Southeast Florida Chapter, 6211
Shriners Hospital for Children, 6250
South Florida Brain Tumor Association Lynn Regional Cancer Center, 1113
Spina Bifida Association of Central Florid a, 6566
Spina Bifida Association of Florida Space Coast, 6567
Spina Bifida Association of Jacksonville N emours Childrens Clinic, 6568
Spina Bifida Association of Southeast Florida, 6569
Spina Bifida Association of Tampa Bay, 6570
Suncoast Residential Training Center/Developmental Services Program, 1633
Talking Book Library, Jacksonville Public Library, 1852, 1989, 5101, 5955
Talking Book Service - Manatee County Central Library, 1853, 1990, 5102, 5956
Tampa Bay Area Brain Tumor Support Group, 1114
Tampa Support Group, 481
Tourette Syndrome Association-Florida Chap ter, 7136
Turner's Syndrome Society - Tampa Support Group, 7331
Turner's Syndrome Society of Northern Florida, 7332
Turner's Syndrome Society of South Florida, 7333
US Blind Golfers Association, 7821
United Cerebral Palsy of Central Florida, 1404
United Cerebral Palsy of East Central Florida, 1405
United Cerebral Palsy of Florida, 1406
United Cerebral Palsy of North Florida/ Tender Loving Care, 1407
United Cerebral Palsy of Northwest Florida, 1408
United Cerebral Palsy of Sarasota-Manatee, 1409
United Cerebral Palsy of South Florida, 1410
United Cerebral Palsy of Tallahassee, 1411
United Cerebral Palsy of Tampa Bay, 1412

University of Florida Hemophilia Treatment Center, 3914
University of Miami, Mailman Center for Child Development, 8104
University of Miami, Mailman Center for Child Development, 8221
VACC Camp, 8363
West Florida Regional Library, 8105

Georgia

Albany Library for the Blind and Physical Handicapped, 1854, 1991, 5103, 5957
All Ages Support Group, 1115
American SIDS Institute, 6837
Asthma and Allergy Foundation of America - Georgia Chapter, 369
Augusta-Richmond County Public Library, 8106
Autism Society of America Greater Georgia Chapter, 795
Bainbridge Subregional Library for the Blind and Physically Handicapped, 1855, 1992, 5104, 5958
Brain Injury Resource Foundation, 3215
Brain Tumor Foundation for Children, 1116
Brain Tumor Support Group, 1117
CEL Subregional Library for the Blind and Physically Handicapped, 1856, 1993, 5105, 5959
CNS Clinical Trials: Atlanta, 1764
Cancer Support Group, 1118
Children's Tumor Foundation - Georgia, 4891
Comprehensive Sickle Cell Center, 6436
Cooley's Anemia Foundation-Buffalo Chapter, 7026
DHR/Division of Public Health - Babies Can 't Wait Program, 7822
Department for Exceptional Students Georgia Department of Education, 7823
Department of Counseling and Educational Leadership-Columbus State University, 7824
Department of Pediatrics, Medical College of Georgia, 2246
Division of Birth Defects and Genetic Diseases, 8203
Down Syndrome Association of Atlanta, 2567
Egleston Cystic Fibrosis Center: Departmen t of Pediatrics, 2247
Emory Autism Resource Center, 836
Emory Eye Center - Strabismus Research, 6702
Gainesville Subregional LBPH Hall County Public Library, 8107
Georgia Ataxia Support Group, 482
Georgia Chapter of Crohn's & Colitis Foundation of America, 2141
Georgia Department of Human Resources - Center for Family Resource Planning, 6775

Georgia Department of Human Resources Children's Health Services, 6774
Georgia Perinatal Association, 5765
Greater Atlanta Area Support Group, 483
Heart to Heart, 4284
Hemophilia Foundation of Georgia, 3874
La Fayette Subregional Library for the Blind and Physically Disabled, 8108
Macon Subregional Library for the Blind and Handicapped, Washington Memorial, 8109
Macon Support Group, 484
Oconee Regional Library, Library for the Blind and Physically Handicapped, 8110
PWSA Chapter - Atlanta, 5664
PWSA of Georgia, 5665
Parent to Parent of Georgia, 7825
Parents Educating Parents and Professional for All Children (PEPPAC), 7826
Pediatric Neurodevelopmental Center at Marcus Institute, 2583
Prevent Child Abuse Georgia, 5513
Region IV Office Program Consultants For Maternal and Child Health, 6776
Rome Subregional Library for the Blind and Physically Handicapped, 8111
Sarcoidosis Support Group, 6132
Sickle Cell Foundation of Georgia, 6419
Southeast Regional Genetics Group, 485
Southeastern Brain Tumor Foundation Brain Tumor Support Group, 1119
Southeastern Region-Helen Keller National Center, 5930
Special Needs Library of NE Georgia Athens-Clarke County Regional Library, 8112
Spina Bifida Association of Georgia, 6571
Squirrel Hollow, 8364
Subregional Library for the Blind and Physically Handicapped, 8113
Tech-Able, 8114
Tools for Life Division of Rehabilitation Services, 7827
Tourette Syndrome Association-Georgia and South Carolina Chapter, 7137
United Cerebral Palsy of Georgia, 1413

Hawaii

AWARE, 7828
Aloha Special Technology Access Center, 8115
Assistive Technology Resource Centers of H awaii (ATRC), 7829
Autism Society of Hawaii, 796
Brain Injury Association of Hawaii, 3216
Brain Tumor Support Group, 1120
Camp Erdman YMCA, 8365
Federal Hemophilia Treatment Center of Hawaii, 3933
Hawaii Down Syndrome Congress, 2568
Hawaii SIDS Information & Counseling Project, 6777

Hemophilia Foundation of Hawaii, 3875
Kardiac Kids, 4285
Library for the Blind and Physically Handicapped, Hawaii State Library, 8116
NNFF Hawaii Chapter, 4892
Pacific Head Injury Association, 3217
Parents and Children Together (PACT), 7830
Prader-Willi Northwest Association, 5666
Special Education Center of Hawaii, 3218
Special Needs Branch Department of Education, 7831
United Cerebral Palsy of Hawaii, 1414
Zero-To-3 Hawaii Project, 7832

Idaho

Assistive Technology Project, 7833
Autism Society of America Treasure Valley Chapter, 797
Brain Injury Association of Idaho, 3219
Child Health Improvement Program Idaho Department of Health, 6778
Department of Education, 7834
Hemophilia Foundation of Idaho, 3876
Idaho Parents Unlimited, 7835
Idaho State Talking Book Library, 1857, 1994, 5106, 5960
Infant/Toddler Program, 7836
NNFF Idaho Chapter, 4893
Palouse Area Parent To Parent, 7837
Parent Reaching Out to Parents, 7838
Prader-Willi Northwest Association-Idaho, 5667
Treasure Valley Brain Injury Support Group, 1121
United Cerebral Palsy of Idaho, 1415

Illinois

Academy for Eating Disorders (AED), 2768
Adult Down Syndrome Center of Lutheran General Hospital, 2584
Advocate Lutheran General Children's Hospital, Pediatric Research, 2585
Archway, 7839
Assistive Technology Project, 7840
Autism Society of Illinois, 798
Brain Injury Association of Illinois, 3220
Brain Research Foundation, 1250
Brain Tumor Resource & Support Group, 1122
Brain Tumor Support Group, 1123
Brain Tumor Support Group at Northwestern Memorial Hospital, 1124
Brain Tumor Support Group at Park Ridge, 1125
Camp Discovery, 5868, 6240, 8366
Center for Digestive Disorders, 7391
Center for Narcolepsy Research at the University of Illinois at Chicago, 4810

Central DuPage Hospital Center for Digestive Disorders, 1766

Chicago Library Service for the Blind, 1858, 1995, 5107, 5961

Chicago, IL Area Ataxia Support Group, 486

Child and Family Connections, 7841

Children's Tumor Foundation - Illinois, 4894

Children's Tumor Foundation - Illinois Cha pter, 4895

Chilren's Heart Services, 4286

Citizens United for Research in Epilepsy (CURE), 6329

Communication Matters Association, 3378

Comprehensive Bleeding Disorder Center, 3927

Cooley's Anemia Foundation-Illinois, 7027

Craniofacial Center at University of Illin ois, Chicago, 2121

Crohn's & Colitis Foundation of America, 2142

Cystic Fibrosis Center: Children's Memoria l Hospital, 2248

Dermatology Information Network (DERMINFONET), 1590, 2896, 5472

Developmental Services Center, 7842

Dystonia Medical Research Foundation, 2727

Easter Seals - Timber Pointe Outdoor Center, 8367

Eating Disorders Research and Treatment Program, 2793

Family Resource Center on Disabilities, 7843

Family T.I.E.S. Network, 7844

Greater Interagency Council Parent to Parent Support Network, 7845

Heart of the Matter, 4287

Helen Keller National Center - North Central Region, 5931

Hemophilia Foundation of Illinois, 3877

Illinois State Library, Talkng Book and Braille Service, 1859, 1996, 5108, 5962

International Society for Traumatic Stress Studies, 5621

Jewish Council for Youth Services, 8368

LaRabida Children's Hospital, Down Syndrome Clinic, 2586

Leukemia Research Foundation, 7846

Loyola University Medical Center/ Department of Pediatrics, 2249

Loyola University of Children, Parmly Hearing Institute, 3386

Mid Illinois Talking Book System, 1860, 1997, 5109, 5963

Mid-Illinois Talking Book Center, 1861, 1998, 5110, 5964

National Association for Parents of the Visually Impaired, 5932

National Center for Latinos with Disabilities, 7847

National Center on Child Abuse Prevention Research, 5522

National Eye Research Foundation, 1905, 2045, 5152, 6007, 6703

National Library of Dermatologic Teaching Slides, 1591, 2897, 5473

Neurofibromatosis, Inc - Illinois/Midwest, 4896

Next Steps - Parents Reaching Parents, 7848

Northern Illinois Center for Adaptive Technology, 8117

Northwestern University Asthma and Allergy Disease Center, 390

Obsessive Compulsive Foundation of Metropo litan Chicago, 5234

Office of Community Health and Prevention Bureau of Early Intervention, DHR, 7849

Olympia, 8369

PKU Organization of Illinois, 5398

PWSA of Illinois, 5668

Parent to Parent Network, 7850

Parents Alliance Employment Project, 8118

Parents of Children with Brain Tumors (PCBT), 1127

Park Ridge, Cystic Fibrosis Center, 2250

Peacock Camp, 8370

Prevent Child Abuse Illinois, 5514

Professional Assistance Center for Education (PACE), 8119

Region 3 of the National Association for Parents of the Visually Impaired, 5933

Region V Office Program Consultants for Maternal and Child Health, 6779

Saint Francis Medical Center Specialty Clinics, CF Center, 2251

Scleroderma Foundation Chicago Chapter, 6212

Shawnee Library System, 8120

Southern IL Child and Family Connections, 7851

Southern, IL Support Group, 487

Spina Bifida Association of Illinois, 6572

State Board of Education Department of Special Education, 7852

Statewide SIDS Program - Illinois Department of Public Health, 6780

Suburban Audio Visual Service, 8121

Summer Wheelchair Sports Camp, 8371

Talking Book Center of Northwest Illinois, 1862, 1999, 5111, 5965

Touch of Nature Environmental Center, 8372

Tourette Syndrome Association-Illinois Cha pter, 7138

Tourette Syndrome Camp Organization, 7231

UIC Eye Center, 6067

United Cerebral Palsy Land of Lincoln, 1416

United Cerebral Palsy of East Central Illinois, 1417

United Cerebral Palsy of Greater Chicago, 1418

United Cerebral Palsy of Illinois, 1419

United Cerebral Palsy of Southern Illinois, 1420

United Cerebral Palsy of Will County, 1421

United Cerebral Palsy of the Blackhawk Region, 1422

University of Chicago Children's Hospital, Department of Pediatrics, 2252

University of Chicago-Department of Psychi atry, 5192

University of Illinois at Chicago Institute for Tuberculosis Research, 7286

University of Illinois at Chicago, Craniofacial Center, 2120, 2374, 3271

Indiana

ATTAIN: Assistive Technology Through Action in Indiana, 7853

Allen County Public Library, 8122

Ann Whitehill Down Syndrome Program, 2587

Assistive Technology Training and Information Center, 7854, 8123

Autism Society of Indiana, 799

Bartholomew County Public Library, 8124

Benign Brain Tumor Support Group, 1128

Brain Injury Association of Indiana, 3221

Brain Tumor Support Group, 1129

Brain Tumor Support Group at Indianapolis, 1130

Camp Isanogel, 8373

Camp Millhouse, 8374

Central Indiana Sarcoidosis Support Group, 6133

Central Indiana Support Group, 488

Children's Tumor Foundation - Indiana Affi liate, 4897

Cystic Fibrosis and Chronic Pulmonary Disease Clinic, 2253

Division of Exceptional Learners Indiana Department of Education, 7855

Down Syndrome Association of Central Indiana, 7856

Down Syndrome Association of NWI, 2569

Down Syndrome Support Association of Southern Indiana (DSSASI), 2570

Easter Seal Society, 8375

Elkhart Public Library, 8125

Family Resource Center of Southeast Indiana, 7857

First Direction, 7858

First Steps, 7859

First Steps for Families, 7860

First Steps, Early Interventions, New Horizons Rehabilitation, 7861

Future Choices, 7862

Happiness Bag Incorporated, 8376

Happy Hollow Children's Camp, 8377

Hemophilia Foundation of Indiana, 3878

Indiana Chapter of Crohn's & Colitis Found ation of America, 2143

Indiana Hemophilia and Thrombosis Center, 3953

Indiana Parent Information Network (IPIN), 7863

Indiana Resource Center for Autism, 837

Indiana State Board of Health - SIDS Project, 6781

John Warvel, 2529

Kentucky Chapter of Crohn's & Colitis Foundation of America, 2146

Kiwanis Twin Lakes Camp, 8378

Knox County Advocates, 7864

Methodist Hospital Sleep Disorders Center, 4765

MidWest Medical Center - Sleep Disorders Center, 4766

NE Indiana Support Group, 489

NEO Fight, 7865

Neurofibromatosis, Inc - Indiana, 8

Northwest Indiana Subregional Library for Blind and Physically Handicapped, 1863, 2000, 5112, 5966

Our Hearts, 4288

PWSA of Indiana, 5669

Pediatric Ophathalmology and Adult Strabis mus Service Research, 1907

Prevent Child Abuse Indiana, 5515

Primary Brain Cancer Support Group, 1131

Project Special Care, 7866

Riley Cystic Fibrosis Center, 2254

Riley Hemophilia and Thrombophilia Center, 3915

SMA Support Inc, 6680

Sleep Disorder Center, St Elizabeth Medica l Center, 4767

Sleep Disorders Center-Good Samaritan Hospital, 4768

Sleep/Wake Disorders Center-Community Heal th Network, 4769

Special Services Division - Indiana State Library, 8126

Spina Bifida Association of Central Indian a, 6573

Spina Bifida Association of Northern Indiana, 6574

Tourette Syndrome Association-Indiana Chap ter, 7139

US Rowing Assocation, 7867

United Cerebral Palsy of Greater Indiana, 1423

United Cerebral Palsy of the Wabash Valley, 1424

Worthmore Academy, 8379

Iowa

ARC of East Central Iowa Pilot Parents, 7868

Autism Society of Iowa, 800

Blank Children's Hospital: Department of P ulmonology, 2255

Brain Injury Association of Iowa, 3222

Brain Tumor Support Group, 1132

Bureau of Children, Family, and Community Services, 7869

Camp Courageous, 8380

Camp Courageous of Iowa, 8381

Camp Tanager, 8382

Center for Disabilities and Development, 1425, 1783, 2468, 2571, 2588, 2695

Children's Tumor Foundation - Iowa Chapter, 4898

Des Moines YMCA Camp, 8383

Easter Seals Camp Sunnyside, 8384

Family Educator Connection Program, 7870

Great Plains Genetic Service Network, 490

Hemophilia Treatment Center at the University of Iowa, 3945

Iowa Chapter of Crohn's Colitis Foundation of America, 2144

Iowa Library for the Blind and Physically Handicapped, 1864, 2001, 5113, 5967

Iowa Program for Assistive Technology, 7871

Iowa SIDS Program, 6782

Iowa Support Group, 491

Iowa's System of EI Services, 7872

Mercy Sleep Laboratory, 4811

PWSA of Iowa, 5670

Parent Educator Connection, 7873

Parent Educator Connection Program, 7874

Prevent Child Abuse Iowa, 5516

Quad Cities Brain Tumor Support Group, 1133

Sioux County Iowa Chapter, 492

Spina Bifida Association of Iowa, 6576

The Link, 801

Turner's Syndrome Society of Iowa/New Found Friends, 7334

University of Iowa - Wendell Johnson Speech and Hearing Clinic, 3839, 6548, 6734

University of Iowa Birth Defects and Genetic Disorders Unit, 1817, 1865, 1948, 1958, 2002, 8220

University of Iowa Hospitals & Clinics, 2256

Kansas

Assistive Technology for Kansas Project, 7875

Autism Society of Kansas, 802

CKLS Headquarters, 1866, 2003, 5114, 5968

Camp Discovery American Diabetes Association, 2521

Department of Health & Environment, 7876

Families Together, 7877

Families Together/Parent to Parent of KS, 7878

Great Plains Region-Helen Keller National Center, 5934

Headstrong Brain Tumor Support Group, 1134

Kansas Department of Health & Environment Bureau of Family Health, 6783

Kansas State Library, 8127

Kansas University Medical Center: Departme nt of Pulmonology, 2257

Manhattan Public Library, 8128

Neurofibromatosis, Inc - Kansas & Central Plains, 4899

Prenatal Diagnostic and Genetic Center, 8129, 8211

Services for the Visually Disabled, 1867, 2004, 5115, 5969

South Central Kansas Library System, 8130

Special Education Administration State Department of Education, 7879

Spina Bifida Association of Kansas, 6577

Technology Resource Solutions for People, 8131

United Cerebral Palsy of Greater Kansas City, 1426

United Cerebral Palsy of Kansas, 1427

University of Kansas Center for Research on Learning, 4446

Via Christi Specialty Clinics: Cystic Fibr osis, Adult and Pediatrics, 2258

Wesley Medical Research Institutes, 8132, 8222

Wichita Public Library, 8133

Kentucky

Assistive Technology Services Network, 7880

Autism Society of America Bluegrass Chapter, 803

Bethel Mennonite Camp, 8385

Bluegrass Technology Center, 8134

Brain Injury Association of Kentucky, 3225

Brain Injury Support Group, 1135

College of Education - Western Kentucky University, 7881

Division of Preschool Services, 7882

Easter Seal Kysoc, 8386

EnTech: Enabling Technologies of Kentuckiana, 8135

Foundation for Prader-Willi Research, 5714

Infant-Toddler Program, Division of Mental Retardation, 7883

Kentucky Department of Human Resources Bureau of Health Services, 6784

Kentucky Hemophilia Foundation, 3879

Kentucky Library for the Blind and Physically Handicapped, 1868, 2005, 5116, 5970

Life Adventure Center, 1811

Louisville Talking Book Library, 8136

NNFF of Kentucky, 4900

Parents of Children with Down Syndrome Arc of Montgomery County, 2560

Partners in Intensive Care, 7901

Patient Recruitment & Public Liaison Office Clinical Center, 7438

Prince George's County Memorial Library Talking Book Center, 1870, 2007, 5118, 5972

Raven Rock Lutheran Camp, 4600

Sarcoidosis Awareness Network, 6134

Schizophrenia Research Branch: Division of Clinical and Treatment Research, 1632

Spina Bifida Association of Chesapeake-Pot omac, 6580

Spinal Muscular Atrophy Project, 6685

Sudden Infant Death Syndrome Institute of The University of Maryland, 6845

Technology Assistance Program Maryland Rehabilitation Center, 7902

The League at Camp Greentop and The Therapeutic Recreation, 8394

Tourette Syndrome Association-Greater Wash ington, 7140

Turner's Syndrome Society of Maryland, 7337

Turner's Syndrome Society of National Capitol Area, 7361

United Cerebral Palsy of Central Maryland, 1431

United Cerebral Palsy of Prince Georges & Montgomery Counties, 1432

United Cerebral Palsy of Southern Maryland, 1433

University of Maryland Medical Center, 4813

Youth Leadership Camp, 3840

Massachusetts

Anorexia/Bulimia Care, 2770

Association of Gastrointestinal Motility Disorders, 2789

Asthma & Allergy Foundation of America New England Chapter, 371

Autism Research Foundation, 846

Autism Society of America Massachusetts Chapter, 807

Bancroft School, 2597

Baystate Medical Center, 2265

Berkshire Center, 4445

Boston Area Support Group, 498

Boston Hemophilia Center, 3921

Braille and Talking Book Library Perkins School for the Blind, 1871, 2008, 5119, 5973

Brain Center Brain Tumor Support Group, 1146

Brain Injury Association of Massachusetts, 3229

Brain Tissue Resource Center, 1248

Brain Tumor Support Group, 1141, 1147

Brain Tumor Support Group at Burlington, 1148

Brain Tumor Support Group at Worcester, 1149

Brain Tumor Survivor Support Group, 1150

Brigham and Women's Hospital, Asthma and Allergic Disease Research Center, 384

Bureau of Early Childhood Programs, 7903

Camp Joslin, 2522

Camp Paul for Exceptional Children, 8395

Camp Ramah in New England (Summer), 8396

Camp Ramah in New England (Winter), 8397

Carroll Center for the Blind, 1872, 2009, 5120, 5974

Carroll School Summer Programs, 8398

Center for Interdisciplinary Research on Immunologic Diseases, 385

Children's Happiness Foundation, 7904

Children's Hospital Boston, 2266

Children's Tumor Foundation - Northern New England, 4902

Clara Barton Camp, 2524

Community Sickle Cell Support Group, 6421

Cooley's Anemia Foundation-Massachusetts Chapter, 7029

Developmental Medicine Center, 3146

Down Syndrome Program, Children's Hospital Boston, 2592

Eagle Hill School - Summer Program, 716, 989, 4467

Early Intervention Services, 7905

Eaton-Peabody Laboratory of Auditory Physiology, 3388

Education Development Center - EDC, 7906

Family Ties at Massachusetts Department of Public Health, 7907

Federation for Children with Special Needs, 7908

Greater Boston Arc Parent Support, 7909

Handi-Kids/King Solomon Foundation, 8399

Harold Goodglass Aphasia Research Center, 3280

Headstrong, 1151

Heart to Heart Fund, 4289

Hemophilia Center of the New England Medical Center, 3941

Hydrocephalus Support Group, 4191

Long Term Survivors Support Group, 1152

Marshfield, MA Support Group, 499

Massachusetts Assistive Technology Partnership, 7910

Massachusetts Association for Parents of t he Visually Impaired (MAPVI), 6090

Massachusetts Chapter of SIDS Alliance, 6789

Massachusetts Down Syndrome Congress (MDSC), 2572

Massachusetts Easter Seals Camping Program, 8400

Massachusetts Eating Disorder Association (MEDA), 2771

Massachusetts General Hospital, 2267

Massachusetts Sudden Infant Death Syndrome, 6840

Massachusetts, New England Hemophilia Association, 3882

NNFF Massachusetts Chapter, 4903

National Association for Parents of the Visually Impaired, 1833, 1970, 5082, 5926

National Birth Defects Center, 7911

National Temporal Bone, Hearing and Balanc e Pathology Resource Registry, 3397

National Training Center for Professional AIDS Education, 3147

Neurofibromatosis, Inc - New England/North east, 4904

Neurological Support Group of St. Luke's Hospital, 1153

New England Chapter of Crohn's & Colitis Foundation of America, 2149

New England Experience, 8401

New England Region-Helen Keller National Center, 5936

New England Regional Genetics Group, 496, 8145, 8209

New England Support Group, 500

Option Institute: Son Rise Program, 808

Parent Education/Support Group, 1154

Pediatric Pulmonary Unit, 6843

Prader-Willi Association of New England (Maine, Mass, RI, NH, VT), 5674, 5676

Region I Office Program Consultants For Maternal and Child Health, 6790

Resources for Rehabilitation, 8149

Sleep Disorders Center, 6464

Sleep Disorders Unit, Beth Israel Hospital, 4771

Spina Bifida Association of Massachusetts, 6581

Support Group for Brain Tumor Patients & Family, 1155

Talking Book Library at Worcester Public Library, 8150

Tower Program at Regis College, 2715

Tufts New England Medical Center, 2268

Turner's Syndrome Society of New England, 7338

United Cerebral Palsy of Berkshire County, 1434

United Cerebral Palsy of MetroBoston, 1435

United Cerebral Palsy of the North Shore, 1436

VALT Support Group (Vital Active Life After Trauma), 3230

Worcester Public Library, 8151

Hemophilia Foundation of Minnesota and the Dakotas, 3884

Hemophilia and Thrombosis Center at the University of Minnesota Medical Center, 3948

Interagency Early Intervention Project, 7922

Knutson, 8414

Mayo Clinic and Foundation, 4696

Mayo Comprehensive Hemophilia Center, 3957

Minneapolis, MN Support Group, 503

Minnesota Cystic Fibrosis Center, 2276

Minnesota Library for the Blind & Physically Handicapped, 1883, 2020, 5131, 5985

Minnesota Sudden Infant Death Center, 6797

Minnesota/Dakotas Chapter of Crohn's & Colitis Foundation of America, 2151

Neurofibromatosis - Minnesota, 4908

Non-Malignant Brain Tumor Support Group, 1168

PACER Center, 8153

PWSA Chapter - Minnesota, 5678

Parents For Heart of Minnesota, 4291

Parents for Parents, 7923

Pilot Parents in Anoka and Ramsey Counties, 7924

Pilot Parents of Northeast Minnesota, 7925

Search Beyond Adventures, 8415

Southwestern Minnesota Support Group, 504

Spina Bifida Association of Minnesota, 6586

Star Center for Family Health, 8154

Tourette Syndrome Association-Minnesota Ch apter, 7141

Turner's Syndrome Society of Minnesota, 7341

United Cerebral Palsy of Central Minnesota, 1439

United Cerebral Palsy of Minnesota, 1440

University of Minnesota Cystic Fibrosis Center, 2277

Vinland Center, 7926

Voyageur Outward Bound School, 7927

Wilderness Inquiry, 7928

Mississippi

Autism Society of Mississippi, 811

Brain Injury Association of Mississippi, 3234

First Steps Program, 7929

Mississippi Chapter, 505

Mississippi Hemophilia Foundation, 3885

Mississippi State Department of Health and Child Health Services, 6798

Neurofibromatosis - Mississippi, 4909

Office of Special Education, 7916, 7930

Parent Partners, 7931

Project Start, 7932

Spina Bifida Association of Mississippi, 6587

Tik-A-Witha, 8416

University of Mississippi Medical Center, 2278, 2375

Missouri

AMOR - A Cancer Support Group for Patients & Their Families, 1170

Adriene Resource Center for Blind Children, 1884, 2021, 5132, 5986

Allergy and Pulmonary Medicine, 373

Assemblies of God National Center for the Blind, 1885, 2022, 5133, 5987

Assistance Technology Project, 7933

Asthma and Allergy Foundation of America - Saint Louis Chapter, 375

Asthma and Allergy Foundation of America Greater Kansas City Chapter, 374

Autism Society of America Gateway Chapter, 812

Brain Cancer Support Group at Mid-America Cancer Center, 1171

Brain Injury Association of Kansas & Greater Kansas City, 3224

Brain Injury Association of Missouri, 3235

Brain Tumor Support Group, 1157, 1169, 1172

Brain Tumor Support Group of Greater St Louis, 1173

Camp Wee-Y, 8417

Central Institute for the Deaf, 3399

Central Missouri Area Support Group, 506

Children's Mercy Hospital, Down Syndrome Clinic, 2594

Children's Mercy Hospital, University of Missouri, 2279

Children's Therapy Center, 7934

Children's Tumor Foundation - Missouri Cha pter, 4910

Council for Extended Care of Mentally Retarded Citizens, 4596

Cystic Fibrosis, Pediatric Pulmonary and Pediatric Gastrointestinal Center, 2280

Department of Elementary and Secondary Education, 7935

Disabilities Advocacy & Support Network, 7936

Down's Syndrome Medical Clinic, 2595

EDI, 2525

Family Resource Network, 7937

Gateway Hemophilia Association of Missouri, 3886

Heart to Heart - St. Louis, 4292

Hickory Hill, 2528

Hydrocephalus Support Group, 4192, 4194

Judevine Center for Autism, 839

Kansas City, Missouri Support Group, 507

Lions Den Outdoor Learning Center, 4598

Mid-America Chapter of Crohn's & Colitis F oundation of America, 2145

Missouri Gateway Hemophilia Association, 3864

Missouri Parents Act, 7938

PWSA Missouri Chapter, 5679

Parent Act, 7939

Pediatric Brain Tumor Support Network, 1174

Pediatric Epilepsy Center, 6331

Positive Solutions for Life Challenges, 7940

Prader-Willi Syndrome Advocates, 5671

Region VII Office Program Consultants for Maternal and Child Health, 6799

SIDS Resources, 6800

Saint Louis Chapter of Crohn's & Colitis Foundation of America, 2153

Saint Louis, MO Support Group, 508

Sidney R. Baer Day Camp, 8418

Spina Bifida Association of Greater Saint Louis, 6588

Springfield Area Support Group, 509

Technology Access Center, 8155

Turner's Syndrome Society of St. Louis/ West Illinois, 7342

United Cerebral Palsy of Greater Kansas City, 1441

United Cerebral Palsy of Greater St. Louis, 1442

United Cerebral Palsy of Missouri, 1443

United Cerebral Palsy of Northwest Missouri, 1444

United Services, 7941

University of Missouri-Columbia Cystic Fibrosis Center, 2281

Washington University Cystic Fibrosis Center, 2282

Whitney Library for the Blind, 8156

Wolfner Memorial Library for the Blind, 1886, 2023, 5134, 5988

Montana

Brain Injury Association of Montana, 3236

Brain Tumor Support Group, 1175

CO-TEACH/Division of Educational Research and Service, 7942

Developmental Disabilities Program, 7943

Division of Special Education, 7944

MonTECH, 7945

Montana Department of Health & Environmental Sciences, 6801

Montana State Library, 8157

Parents Let's Unite for Kids, 7946

Quality Life Concepts, 7947

Nebraska

Assistive Technology Partnership, 7948

Autism Society of Nebraska, 813

Boys Town National Research Hospital, 6521, 6545

Brain Injury Association of Nebraska, 3237

Brain Tumor Support Group at the Nebraska Medical Center, 1176

Camp Easter Seals, 8419

Floyd Rogers, 2527

Individual and Family Support Arc of Lincoln & Lancaster County, 7949

Lied Learning and Technology Center for Childhood Deafness and Vision Disorders, 3400

National Camps for Blind Children, 1940, 2084, 5184, 6039

Nebraska Chapter of the National Hemophilia Foundation, 3887

Nebraska Library Commission Talking Book & Braille Services, 1887, 2024, 5135, 5989

Nebraska Parents Center, 7950

Nebraska Regional Hemophilia Center, 3962

Nebraska SIDS Foundation, 6802

North Platte Public Library, 8158

Omaha, NE Support Group, 510

PWSA of Nebraska, 5681

Parent Assistance Network, 7951

Parent Support Group, 7952

Special Education Office State Department of Education, 7954

Spina Bifida Association of Nebraska, 6589

United Cerebral Palsy of Nebraska, 1445

University of Nebraska at Omaha Pediatric Pulmonary/Cystic Fibrosis Center, 2283

University of Nebraska, Lincoln Barkley Memorial Center, 3389

Nevada

American Academy of Somnology, 4997, 5020, 6463, 6492

Assistive Technology Collaborative, 7955

Autism Society of Northern Nevada Chapter, 814

Brain Injury Association of Northern Nevada, 3238

Brain Injury Association of Southern Nevada, 3239

Children's Lung Specialists, 2284

Children's Tumor Foundation - Nevada, 4911

Early Intervention Services Division of Child & Family Services, 7956

Educational Equity, Special Education Branch, 7957

Hemophilia and Thrombosis Center of Nevada, 3949

Las Vegas-Clark County Library District, 8159

Nevada Parent Network, 7958

Nevada Parents Encouraging Parents (PEP), 7959

Nevada State Division of Health, Maternal & Child Health, 6803

Nevada State Library and Archives, 8160

Parents Encouraging Parents, 7953, 7960

Scleroderma Foundation Nevada Chapter, 6213

Southern Nevada 'Grey Matters' Valley Hospital Medical Center, 1177

Turner's Syndrome Society of Nevada, 7343

United Cerebral Palsy of Northern Nevada, 1446

University of Nevada - Department of Speech-Language Pathology, 6526

New Hampshire

Angels of Hope, 1178

Autism Society of New Hampshire, 815

Brain Injury Association of New Hampshire, 3240

Bureau of Early Learning, 7961

Camp Allen, 8420

Camp Dartmouth-Hitchcock, 8421

Crotched Mountain School & Rehabilitation Center, 8422

Dartmouth-Hitchcock Sleep Disorders Center Dartmouth Medical Center, 4774

Division of Special Education, 7962

Families with Heart, 4293

Family Center Early Supports & Services, 7963

Hemophilia and Coagulation Programs, 3947

High Hopes Foundation of New Hampshire, 7964

Medical Genetics Clinic, 2596

NNFF of Northern New England, 4912

New England Retinoblastoma Support Group (NERSG), 6091

New Hampshire Cystic Fibrosis Care and Teaching Center, 2285

New Hampshire Families with Heart, 4294

New Hampshire SIDS Program, 6804

New Hampshire State Library, 8161

Parent Information Center, 7965

Parent to Parent of New Hampshire, 7966

Portsmouth Regional Home, 1179

Sleep/Wake Disorders Center, Hampstead Hospital, 4775

Technology Partnership Project Institute on Disability/UAP, 7967

Turner's Syndrome Society of Northern New England, 7344

New Jersey

Asthma and Allergy Foundation of America - Southeast Pennsylvania Chapter, 376

Bancroft Camp, 8423

Bancroft NeuroHealth, 3326

Blood Research Institute of Saint Michael's Medical Center, 3920

Brain Injury Association of New Jersey, 3241

Brain Tumor Support Group at Plainfield Muhlenberg Medical Center, Neuroscience, 1181

Brain Tumor Support Group of Monmouth County, 1182

CJ Foundation for SIDS, 6838

CRI Worldwide Pediatric Center for Excellence, 1765

Camp Chatterbox, 8424

Camp Merry Heart/Easter Seals Easter Seal Society, 8425

Camp Oakhurst, 8426

Camp Sun 'N Fun, 8434

Camp Vacamas, 8427

Center for Enabling Technology, 8162

Cerebral Palsy Center Summer Program, 1539

Cooley's Anemia Foundation - New Jersey Chapter, 7030

Cross Roads Outdoor Ministries, 8428

Division of Student Services, 7968

Early Intervention System, 7969

Easter Seals Camp Merry Heart, 8429

Eating Disorders Association of New Jersey, 2772

Epilepsy Foundation New Jersey, 6322

Fairlawn, NJ Support Group, 511

Family Support Center of New Jersey, 7970

Foundation for Children with Down Syndrome, 2574

Hydrocephalus Group - Children's Hospital of New Jersey, 4195

Hydrocephalus Parents Support Group, 4196

Monmouth Medical Center, Cystic Fibrosis & Pediatric Pulmonary Center, 2286

NNFF of New Jersey, 4913

National Sarcoidosis Resource Center, 6147

Nejeda, 2530

New Jersey Camp Jaycee, 4599

New Jersey Center for Outreach & Services for the Autism Community (COSAC), 816

New Jersey Center for Outreach and Services for the Autism Community(COSAC), 840

New Jersey Chapter of Crohn's & Colitis Foundation of America, 2154

New Jersey Department of Health - Child Health Program, 6805

New Jersey Institute of Technology Center for Biomedical Engineering, 3103

New Jersey Library for the Blind and Handicapped, 1888, 2025, 5136, 5990

New Jersey Medical School, 2287

New Jersey SIDS Resource Center, 6806

New Jersey Self-Help Clearinghouse, 7971

New Jersey Statewide Parent to Parent, 7972

New Jersey Support Groups, 2773

Newark Sleep Disorders Center, 4776

PWSA - New Jersey Chapter, 5683

Princeton University, Cutaneous Communication Laboratory, 3390

Renfrew Center of Northern New Jersey, 2774

Round Lake Camp, 721, 994, 4474

SE Pennsylvania Chapter of Asthma and Allergy Foundation of America, 379

Sarcoidosis Support Resource Central New Jersey, 6138

Scleroderma Foundation New Jersey Chapter, 6214

Spina Bifida Association of Bergen and Passaic Counties, 6590

Spina Bifida Association of the Tri-State Region, 6591

Statewide Parent Advocacy Network, 7973

Tourette Syndrome Association-New Jersey Chapter, 7142

Turner's Syndrome Society of New Jersey, 7345

United Cerebral Palsy of Hudson County, 1447

United Cerebral Palsy of New Jersey, 1448

United Cerebral Palsy of Northern, Central & Southern New Jersey, 1449

Young Hearts, 4295

New Mexico

Brain Injury Association of New Mexico, 3242

Dyslexia Centers, 2713

EPICS Project-SW Communication Resources, 7974

Long Term Services Division, 7975

NM Alliance for the Neurologically Impaired, 1183

New Mexico Autism Society, 817

New Mexico State Library for the Blind and Physically Handicapped, 1889, 2026, 5137, 5991

Parents Reaching Out, 7976

People Living Through Cancer, 1184

Region 5 of the National Association for Parents of the Visually Impaired, 5937

Santa Fe Mountain Center, 8430

Sickle Cell Council of New Mexico, 6422

Special Education Unit, 7977

Spina Bifida Association of New Mexico, 6592

Technology Assistance Program, 7978

Ted R. Montoya Hemophilia Program, 3978

University of New Mexico School of Medicine, 2288

New York

Advocacy Center, 7979

Advocates for Children of New York, 7980, 8431

Albany Medical College Pediatric Pulmonary & Cystic Fibrosis Center, 2289

Albany New York Regional Comprehensive Hemophilia Treatment Center, 3917

American Diabetes Association, 2520

American Foundation for AIDS Research, 3144

Arlene R Gordon Research Institute, 6003

Armond V. Mascia CF Center, 2290

Aspire of WNY, 1450

Association for Neurologically Impaired Brain Injured Children, 1295, 3325

Association for Research of Childhood Cancer, 8198

Aurora of Central New York, 7981

Autism Speaks, 848

Big Hearts for Little Hearts, 4296

Bleeding Disorders Association of Northeastern New York, 3888

Brady Institute for Traumatic Brain Injury, 3283

Brain Injury Association of New York, 3243

Brain Injury Association of New York State, 3244

Brain Tumor Support Group, 1180, 1185

Brain Tumor Support Group at South Nassau Community Hospital, 1186

Bronx Comprehensive Sickle Cell Center, 6437

Brooklyn College Speech and Hearing Center, 6509

CF & Pediatric Pulmonary Care Center, 2291

CF, Pediatric Pulmonary & GI Center, 2292

CMTA Chapter - New York (Greater), 1542

Camp Huntington, 8433

Capital Regional Sleep-Wake Disorders Center, 4777

Cardiac Kids, 4297

Cardiovascular Research Foundation, 303

Center for Family Support, 818, 1030, 1629, 2575, 4586, 4996

Center for Neural Recovery & Rehabilitation Research, 6332

Center for Sleep Medicine of the Mount Sinai Medical Center, 4778

Center for the Disabled, 1451

Center for the Study of Anorexia and Bulimia, 2792

Central New York Chapter of Crohn's & Colitis Foundation of America, 2156

Child Abuse Prevention Project: Be'ad HaYeled (For the Sake of the Child), 5517

Child Development Clinical Services, 2598

Children's Clinical Research Center, 3145

Children's Lung and Cystic Fibrosis Center, 2293

Chrissy & Friends, 6323

Columbia Presbyterian Medical Center, 4697

Columbia Presbyterian Medical Center Sleep Disorders Center, 4779

Columbia University Clinical Research Center for Muscular Dystrophy, 4698

Cooley's Anemia Foundation - Rochester, 7031

Cooley's Anemia Foundation - Staten Island, 7032

Cooley's Anemia Foundation-Buffalo, 7033

Cooley's Anemia Foundation-Long Island/Brooklyn Chapter, 7034

Cooley's Anemia Foundation-Queens, 7035

Cooley's Anemia Foundation-Suffolk Chapter, 7036

Cooley's Anemia Foundation-Westchester/Rockland Chapter, 7037

Crohn's & Colitis Foundation of America, 2177

Dana Alliance for Brain Initiatives, 3274

Depressive and Manic-Depressive Assocation of Mount Sinai, 1031, 2396

Dunnabeck at Kildonan, 2712

Early Intervention Program, 7982

Eating Disorder Council of Long Island, 2775

Epilepsy Foundation of Long Island, 6324

Facilitated Communication Institute at Syracuse University, 850

Fairfield/Westchester Chapter of Crohn's & Colitis Foundation of America, 2138

Fairfield/Westchester Chapter of Crohn's & Colitis Foundation of America, 2157

Families of SMA - Long Island NY Chapter, 6681

Freedom Camp, 8435

Friends of Karen, 7983

Genetic Network of the Empire State, 512

Goodays Brain Tumor Support Group, 1187

Gow School Summer Programs, 8436

Greater New York Chapter of Crohn's & Colitis Foundation of America, 2158

Helen Keller National Center, 1890, 1903, 2027, 2043, 5138, 5150

Helping Hearts, 4298

Hemophilia Center of Western New York, 3889, 3939

Henry Youngerman Center for Communication Disorders, 6527

Hy Feinstein Clubhouse, 3245

Hypertrophic Cardiomyopathy Program at St. Luke's-Roosevelt Hospital Center, 4267

Inspire - Cerebral Palsy Center, 1452

Institute for Basic Research in Developmental Disabilities, 841, 2599, 8163, 8206

International NF Summer Camp, 4957

International Pemphigus Foundation: New York Support Group, 5383

JGB Cassette Library International, 8164

Keren-Or Jerusalem Center for Multi-Handicapped Blind Children, 8165, 8207

Laboratory of Dermatology Research, 1592, 2898, 5474

Leukemia Society of America - Westchester/ Hudson Valley Chapter, 152

Leukemia Society of America - Western New York & Finger Lakes Chapter, 153

Long Island Adult Brain Tumor Support Group, 1188

Long Island Brain Tumor Support Group, 1189

Long Island Chapter of Crohn's & Colitis Foundation of America, 2159

Long Island College Hospital, 2294

Long Island Sarcoidosis Support, 6139

Lupus Research Institute, 6910

Making Headway Foundation-Family Support Program, 1190

Maplebrook School, 720, 993, 4471

Marist Brothers Mid-Hudson Valley Camp, 8437

Marty Lyons Foundation, 7984

Mary M Gooley Hemophilia Center of the National Hemophilia Foundation, 3890

Metro Intergroup of Overeaters Anonymous, 2776

Montifiore Medical Center, 3401

Mount Sinai Traumatic Brain Injury, 3246

NHF Camp Directory, 4054

NNFF of New York/New Jersey, 4914

NYU Rusk Institute, 4699

Nassau Library System, 8166

National Alliance for Research on Schizophrenia and Depression, 1033, 1630, 1631, 2397, 5237

National Center for the Study of Wilson's Disease, 7471

National Eating Disorder Association of Lo ng Island (NEDA-LI), 2790

National Eating Disorders Association-Long Island (NEDA-LI), 2777

National Hemophilia Foundation, 3961

New York Autism Network, 819

New York Brain Tumor Support Group, 1191

New York Chapter of Asthma and Allergy Foundation of America, 377

New York City Area Support Group, 513

New York City Information & Counseling Program for SIDS, 6807

New York City Support Group, 2778

New York Department of Education, 7985

New York Foundation for Otologic Research, 3402

New York Obesity Research Center, 2794, 5191

New York State Talking Book & Braille Library, 1891, 2028, 5139, 5993

New York Support Group, 514

New York University Medical Center Auxillary of Tisch Hospital, 4197, 4206

Oakhurst, 8438

Overeaters Anonymous Support Group, 2779

PWSA Chapter - Franklin Square, 5685

PWSA of New York, 5686

Parent Network Center, 7986

Parent to Parent of New York State, 7987

Pediatric Pulmonary Center, 2295

People Treated for Brain Tumors and Their Caregivers, 1192

People Treated for Brain Tumors and their Caregivers, 1193

Prader-Willi Alliance of New York, 5687

Prevent Child Abuse New York, 5518

Program for Children and Youth Who are Deaf or Hard of Hearing, 3838

Programs for Children with Disabilities: Ages 3 through 5, 8439

Programs for Children with Special Health Care Needs, 8440

Programs for Infants and Toddlers with Disabilities: Ages Birth Through 2, 8441

Ramapo Anchorage Camp, 8442

Region II Office Program Consultants for Maternal and Child Health, 6808

Rehabilitation Research and Training Center on Traumatic Brain Injury, 3275

Renfrew Center of New York City, 2780

Research to Prevent Blindness, 1908, 2048, 5154, 6009

Resources for Children with Special Needs, 7988

Rochester Chapter of Crohn's & Colitis Foundation of America, 2160

Rockefeller University Laboratory for Investigative Dermatology, 1593, 2899, 5475

SIDS Regional Center for Eastern New York State, 6809

SLE Lupus Foundation, 6911

SUNY Upstate Medical University Research Development, 3973

Saint Joseph's Hospital Health Center Sleep Laboratory, 4780

Saint Mary's Healthcare System for Children, 7989

Schneider Children's Hospital of Long Island, 2296

Scleroderma Foundation Tri-State, Inc (NY, NJ, CT), 6215

Sickle Cell Disease Foundation of Greater New York, 6423

Sinergia/Metropolitan Parent Center, 7990

Sleep Center, Community General Hospital, 4781

Sleep Disorders Center of Rochester, St. Mary's Hospital, 4782

Sleep Disorders Center of Western New York Millard Fillmore Hospital, 4783

Sleep Disorders Center, University Hospital, 4784

Sleep-Wake Disorders Center, Montefiore Sleep Disorders Center, 4785

Sleep-Wake Disorders Center, New York Presbyterian Hospital, 4786

Spina Bifida Association of Albany/Capital District, 6593

Spina Bifida Association of Greater Roches ter, 6594

Spina Bifida Association of Nassau County, 6595

Spina Bifida Association of Western New York, 6596

Spinal Muscular Atrophy Clinic, 6684

State University College at Plattsburgh Auditory Research Laboratory, 3403

State University Hospital/Upstate Medical Center, 2297

State University of New York Health Sciences Center, 842, 851

Stroke Rehabilitation & Traumatic Brain Injury Research, 3284

Support for Parents of Children with Brain Tumors, Siblings and Young Adults, 1194

Syncope Center at Columbia Presbyterian Medical Center, 6885

Syracuse University, Institute for Sensory Research, 3404

TRIAD Project-Advocates for Persons with Disabilities, 7991

Techspress Resource Center for Independent Living, 8167

Tourette Syndrome Association-Greater New York State Chapter, 7143

Tourette Syndrome Association-Long Island Chapter, 7144

Tourette Syndrome Association-New York Hud son Valley Chapter, 7146

Tourette Syndrome Association-Rochester Ch apter, 7147

Triangle, 8443

Turner's Syndrome Society of Central New York, 7346

Turner's Syndrome Society of Rochester, 7347

Turner's Syndrome Society of Upstate New York, 7348

UCP of Greater Suffolk, 1453

Ulster County Social Services, 7992

United Cerebral Palsy Associations of New York State, 1454

United Cerebral Palsy of Chemung County, 1455

United Cerebral Palsy of Fulton & Montgomery Counties, 1456

United Cerebral Palsy of Nassau County, 1457

United Cerebral Palsy of New York City, 1458

United Cerebral Palsy of Niagara County, 1459

United Cerebral Palsy of Putnam & Southern Dutchess Counties, 1460

United Cerebral Palsy of Queens, 1461

United Cerebral Palsy of Westchester County, 1462

United Cerebral Palsy of the North Country, 1463

United Cerebral Palsy of the Tri-Counties, 1464

United Health Services Blood Disorder Center, 3982

University of Rochester Medical Center, 2298

Upstate/Northeast New York Chapter of Crohn's & Colitis Foundation of America, 2161

VISIONS/Vacation Camp for the Blind, 1941, 2085, 5185, 6040

WNY Brain Tumor Support Group, 1195

Wagon Road, 8444

Wallace Memorial Library, 3391

Westchester Center for Eating Disorders, 2781

Western New York Area Support Group, 515

Western New York Chapter of Crohn's & Colitis Foundation of America, 2162

Western New York SIDS Center, 6810

Winthrop-University Hospital Sleep Disorders Center, 4787

North Carolina

Assistive Technology Project, Human Resources, Voc. and Rehab. Services, 7993

Autism Society of North Carolina, 820, 843

Bless Their Hearts, 4299

Bowman Grey School of Medicine-Hemophilia Diagnostic Center, 3922

Brain Injury Association of North Carolina, 3247

Brain Tumor Support Group of the Carolinas and Virginia Cancer Services, 1196

Camp Winding Gap, 8445

Carolina Computer Access Center, 8168

Carolinas Chapter of Crohn's & Colitis Foundation of America, 2163

Communications Disorders Clinic, 6528

Comprehensive Hemophilia Diagnostic and Treatment Center, 3928

Duke Brain Tumor Support Group, 1197

Duke Pediatric Brain Tumor Family Support Program, 1198

Duke University Asthma and Allergic Disease Center, 386

Duke University Comprehensive Epilepsy Center, 6333

Duke University Comprehensive Sickle Cell Center, 6438

Duke University Medical Center/ CF Center, 2299

ECAC, 7994

Eastern North Carolina Chapter (SCDAA), 6424

Exceptional Children Division, 7995

Family Support Network of North Carolina, 7996

Giddings School Special Education Division, 7814

Hemophila Foundation of North Carolina, 3891

Herpes Resource Center, 4107, 4836

Leukemia Society of America - North Carolina Chapter, 96, 154

Lipomyelomeningocele Family Support, 4198

North Carolina Library for the Blind, 1892, 2029, 5140, 5994

North Carolina SIDS Information and Counseling Program, 6811

North Carolina Speech, Hearing and Language Association, 6510

PWSA of North Carolina, 5688

Partnerships for Inclusion, 7997

Pediatric Rheumatoid Clinic, 4365

Prevent Child Abuse North Carolina, 5519

Raleigh Area Brain Tumor Support Group, 1199

Rockingham County Schools, 7998

Sarcoidosis Support Group, 6140

Sickle Cell Disease Association of the Piedmont, 6425

Sickle Cell Regional Network, 6426

South Carolina Chapter of Crohn's & Colitis Foundation of America, 2170

Spina Bifida Association of North Carolina, 6597

Talisman Programs, 8446

Talisman Summer Camps, 1812

Turner's Syndrome Society of North Carolina, 7349

UNC CF Center, 2300

United Cerebral Palsy of North Carolina, 1465

University of North Carolina Sarcoidosis Support Group, 6141

University of North Carolina at Chapel Hill, Brain Research Center, 852

Western North Carolina Brain Tumor Support Group, 1200

North Dakota

Brain Injury Association of North Dakota, 3248

Children's Hospital Merit Care Down Syndrome Service, 2600

Developmental Disabilities Unit, 7999

Interagency Program Assistive Technology, 8000

North Dakota Comprehensive Hemophilia and Thrombosis Treatment Center, 3963

North Dakota SIDS Management Program, 6812

PWSA Chapter - Bottineau, 5689

PWSA Chapter - Fraser Ltd - Fargo, 5690

PWSA of North Dakota, 5691

Saint Alexius Medical Center/CF Center, 2301

Special Education Division, 8001

Ohio

American Council of Blind Parents, 1893, 2030, 5141, 5995

Autism Society of Greater Cincinatti, 821

Autism Society of Ohio Tri-County Chapter, 822

Beech Brook, 983, 4461

Bethesda Oak Hospital, Sleep Disorders Center, 4788

Blick Clinic for Developmental Disabilities, 8169

Brain Injury Association of Ohio, 3249

Brain Tumor Support Group, 1201

Bureau of EI Services, 8002

CMTA Chapter - Ohio, 1543

Camp Allyn, 8447

Camp Nuhop, 713, 986, 4464

Case Western Research University, Bolton Brush Growth Study Center, 3100

Case Western Reserve University Cystic Fibrosis Center, 2302

Celebrating Families of Children & Adults with Special Needs, 8003

Center for Sleep & Wake Disorders, Miami Valley Hospital, 4789

Central Ohio Brain Tumor Support Group, 1202

Central Ohio Chapter of Crohn's & Colitis Foundation of America, 2164

Central Ohio Chapter of the National Hemophilia Foundation, 3892

Children's Tumor Foundation - Ohio, 4915

Cincinnati Digestive Diseases Research Development Center, 1767

Cleveland Brain Tumor Patient Network - Adult and Pediatric, 1203

Cleveland Clinic, 4199

Cleveland Clinic Foundation, Sleep Disorders Center, 4790

Cleveland Hearing and Speech Center, 6511

Cleveland Public Library, 8170

Clinical Research Center, Pediatrics, 1011

Columbus Children's Hospital, Cystic Fibrosis Center, 2303

Comprehensive Sickle Cell Center, 6439

Division of Early Childhood Education, 8004

Down Syndrome Clinic, Department of Pediatrics, 2601

Down Syndrome Clinic, Rainbow Babies and Children's Hospital, 2602

East Central Regional Office, 8005

Emanuel-Day, 3832

Family Information Network, 8006

Fragile X Alliance of Ohio, 3048

Healing Hearts, 4300

Hemophilia and Thrombosis Center: Division of Blood Disease Center, 3950

Highbrook Lodge Camp, 8448

Jane and Richard Thomas Center for Down Syndrome, 2603

Kettering Medical Center, Sleep Disorders Center, 4791

Leukemia Society of America - Central Ohio Chapter, 97, 155

Leukemia Society of America - Northern Ohio Chapter, 98, 156

Leukemia Society of America - Southern Ohio Chapter, 99, 157

Lewis H. Walker, MD, Cystic Fibrosis Center, 2304

Miami Valley Downs Syndrome Association, 2576

NNFF of Ohio, 4916

NW Ohio Sleep Disorders Center, 4792

Neuro-Oncology Support Group, 1204

Northeast Ohio Chapter of Crohn's & Colitis Foundation of America, 2165

Northern Ohio Chapter of the National Hemophilia Foundation, 3893

Northwest Ohio Hemophilia Foundation, 3894

Northwest Ohio Hemophilia Treatment Center, 3964

OCECD, 8008

Ohio Brain Injury Association, 3250

Ohio Protection and Advocacy Organization, 8009

Ohio Regional Library for the Blind and Physically Handicapped, 8171

Ohio Sleep Medicine Institute, 4793

Ohio State University Hospitals, Sleep Disorders Center, 4794

Ohio State University Laboratory of Psychobiology, 3285

Ohio Support Group, 516

Operation Liftoff of Ohio, 8010

PWSA of Ohio, 5692

Parent Project for Muscular Dystrophy Research, 4700

Pediatric Clinical Trials International, 2604

Pediatric Pulmonary Center, 2305

Perinatal and Infant Health Unit - SIDS Information and Counseling Program, 6813

Region 2 of the National Association for Parents of the Visually Impaired, 1835, 1972, 5084, 5938

Saint Vincent Medical Center, Sleep Disorders Center, 4795

Society for Rehabilitation, 8011

Southwest Ohio Brain Tumor Support Group, 1205

Southwest Ohio Chapter of Crohn's & Colitis Foundation of America, 2166

Southwestern Ohio Chapter of the National Hemophilia Foundation, 3895

Speech and Hearing Clinic, 6512

Spina Bifida Association of Canton, 6598

Spina Bifida Association of Central Ohio, 6599

Spina Bifida Association of Cincinnati, 6600

Spina Bifida Association of Greater Dayton, 6601

Spina Bifida Association of North West Ohio, 6602

Spina Bifida Association of Tri-County Ohio, 6603

Support Group for Parents of Children with a Brain Tumor, 1206

Technology Resource Center, 8172

Tourette Syndrome Association-Ohio Chapter, 7148

Tourette Syndrome Clinic, 7153

Train-Ohio Super Computer Center, 8012

Tri-State Bleeding Disorders Chapter of the National Hemophilia Foundation, 3896

Tri-State Sleep Disorders Center Center for Research in Sleep Disorders, 4814

Turner's Syndrome Society of Southwestern Ohio, 7350

United Cerebral Palsy of Central Ohio, 1466

United Cerebral Palsy of Cincinnati, 1467

United Cerebral Palsy of Greater Cleveland, 1468

University Treatment Center of University Hospitals of Cleveland, 3983

University of Cincinnati Adult Hemophilia Program, 3984

University of Cincinnati College of Medicine/Division of Pediatrics, 2306

West Central Ohio Hemophilia Center, 3991

Youngstown Hemophilia Center, 3993

Oklahoma

Autism Society of Oklahoma, 823

Brain Injury Association of Oklahoma, 3251

Leukemia Society of America - Oklahoma Chapter, 100, 158

NNFF of Oklahoma, 4917

Neuroscience Institute at Mercy Hospital, 4939

North Central Oklahoma Support Group, 517

Oklahoma ABLE Tech-Wellness Center, 8013

Oklahoma Brain Injury Camp, 3329

Oklahoma Chapter of Crohn's & Colitis Foundation of America, 2167

Oklahoma Chapter of the National Hemophilia Foundation, 3897

Oklahoma Hemophilia Foundation, 3965

Oklahoma Library for the Blind & Physically Handicapped, 8173

Oklahoma Speech Language Hearing Associati on, 6513

Oklahoma State Department of Health - Maternal and Child Health Services, 6814

PWSA of Oklahoma, 5694

Parents Reaching Out in Oklahoma, 8014

Special Education Office, 8015

Tulsa City-County Library System, 8174

Turner's Syndrome Society of Oklahoma, 7351

United Cerebral Palsy of Oklahoma, 1469

University of Oklahoma Cystic Fibrosis Center, 2307

Oregon

Asthsma and Allergy Foundation of America Oregon Chapter, 378

Autism Society of Oregon, 824

Bend Support Group, 1207

Brain Injury Association of Oregon, 3252

Brain Tumor Education & Support Group, 1208

Children's Tumor Foundation - Oregon Suppo rt Group, 4918

Early Childhood CARES Program, 8016

Early Intervention Programs, 8017

Easter Seals Oregon Camping Program, 8449

Hemophilia Foundation of Oregon, 3898

Hydrocephalus Group of Portland, 4200

Klamath Falls Support Group, 1209

Legacy Good Samaritan Hospital & Medical C enter, 4919

Leukemia Society of America - Oregon Chapter, 101, 159

Meadowood Springs Speech and Hearing Camp, 3837, 6547, 6733

Mt Hood Kiwanis Camp, 8450

Oregon Brain Injury Resource Network, 3253

Oregon Health Sciences Unit, 2308

Oregon Health Sciences University Research Center, 3405

Oregon Parent Training and Information Center, 8018

Oregon State Health Division - SIDS Information and Counseling Program, 6815

Oregon State Library, 8175

Oregon State Library, Talking Book and Braille Services, 1894, 2031, 5142, 5996

PWSA of Oregon, 5695

Pacific Northwest Regional Genetics Group, 518

Rainrock Treatment Center, 2782

Reading and Speech Clinic, 6514

Regional Resource Center on Deafness, 3392

Research and Training Center on Family Support and Children's Mental Health, 1787, 8214

SIDS Resource of Oregon, 6816

Special Education Programs, 8019

Technology Access for Life Needs Project, 8020

United Cerebral Palsy of Oregon & SW Washington, 1470

Willamette Valley Ataxia Support Group, 519

Pennsylvania

Albert Einstein Medical Center Hemophilia Program, 3918

Autism Society of America Greater Harrisburg Area Chapter, 825

Brain Injury Association of Pennsylvania, 3254

Brain Tumor Support Group, 1210

Brain Tumor Support Group at Lancaster, 1211

Brain Tumor Support Group at Philadelphia, 1212

Brain Tumor Support Group at Pittsburgh, 1213

Brain Tumor Support Group of Philadelphia Hospital of Univ. of PA Cancer Center, 1214

Brain Tumor Support Group of Pittsburgh, 1215

Brain Tumor Support Group of the Lehigh Valley, 1216

Briarwood Day Camp, 8451

Bureau of Special Education, 8021

C-Brain (Cranial Base Resource & Information Network), 1217

CF Center at The Children's Hospital of Philadelphia, 2309

CMTA Chapter - Pennsylvania, 1544

Camelot For Children, 1218

Camp Frog, 6406

Camp Lee Mar, 8452

Cardeza Foundation Hemophilia Center, 3923

Central Pennsylvania Area Support Group, 520

Children's Hospital of Philadelphia Hemophilia Program, 3926

Children's Hospital of Pittsburgh General Clinical Research Center, 2605

Children's Seashore House, 2606

Community Medical Center, Sleep Disorders Clinic, 4796

Crozer-Chester Medical Center, 4797

Cystic Fibrosis Center at Polyclinic Medical Center, 2310

Delaware Valley Chapter of the National Hemophilia Foundation, 3899

Division of Early Intervention Services, 8022

Down Syndrome Clinic, 2607

Dr. Gertrude A. Barber National Institute, 2608

Epilepsy Foundation Eastern Pennsylvania, 6325

Epilepsy Foundation of Western/Central Pen nsylvania, 6326

Fontan Friends, 4301

Free Library of Philadelphia, 8176

Geisinger Wyoming Valley Medical Center, Sleep Disorders Center, 4798

Hahnemann University Lupus Study Center, 6909

Hemophilia Center of Central Pennsylvania, 3937

Hemophilia Center of Western Pennsylvania, 3940

Hydrocephalus Association of Philadelphia, 4201

Institutes for Achievement of Human Potential, 3286

International Foundation for Genetic Research/Michael Fund, 2609

Ken-Crest Camp, 4597

Keystone Community Resources, 8453

Krancer Center for Inflammatory Bowel Disease Research, 2178

Lankenau Hospital, Sleep Disorders Center, 4799

Lehigh Valley Sickle Cell Support Group, 6427

Leukemia Society of America - Western Pennsylvania/West Virginia Chapter, 102, 160

Library for the Blind & Physically Handicapped, Leonard C. Staisey Building, 8177

Medical College of Pennsylvania, Sleep Disorders Center, 4800

Mercy Hospital of Johnstown, Sleep Disorders Center, 4801

Mid-Atlantic Regional Human Genetics Network, 521

Montgomery County Intermediate Unit #23, 8023

NF Clinic - University of Pittsburgh Child ren's Hospital, 4940

PWSA Chapter - Western Pennsylvania, 5696

PWSA of Pennsylvania, 5697

Parent Education Network, 8024

Parent to Parent ARC Allegheny, 8025

Parent to Parent of Pennsylvania, 8026

Parents Union for Public Schools, 8027

Pediatric Hemophilia Program of Pennsylvania, 3967

Pediatric Pulmonary and Cystic Fibrosis Center, 2311

Penn Center for Sleep Disorders, Hospital of the University of Pennsylvania, 4802

Penn Neurological Institute, 4701

Pennsylvania Chapter of the American Anorexia Bulimia Association, 2783

Pennsylvania Educational Network for Eating Disorders (PENED), 2784

Pennsylvania SIDS Center, 6817

Pennsylvania's Initiative on Assistive Technology, Institute on Disabilities, 8028

Pennsylvania/Delaware Valley Chapter of Crohn's & Colitis Foundation of America, 2168

Phelps School, 4473

Philadelphia Support Group, 2785

Pittsburgh Area Brain Injury Alliance, 3255

Pittsburgh Area Brain Tumor Support Group, 1219

Presbyterian Hospital/Pittsburgh Cancer Center, 1220

Presbyterian-University Hospital, Pulmonary Sleep Evaluation Center, 4803

Region III Office Program Consultants for Maternal and Child Health, 6818

Renfrew Center of Bryn Mawr, 2786

Renfrew Center of Philadelphia, 2787

Sarcoidosis Self-Help, 6142

Sickle Cell Disease Association of America , Philadelphia/Delaware Valley Chapter, 6428

Southeast Pennsylvania Support Group, 522

Spina Bifida Association Pittsburgh, 6604

Spina Bifida Association of Delaware Valley, 6605

Spina Bifida Association of Greater Pennsy lvania, 6606

Summer Experience, 8454

Support Group for Parents and Children with Brain Tumors, 1221

Temple University, Section of Auditory Research, 3406

Thomas Jefferson University Brain Injury Rehabilitation Program, 3287

Thomas Jefferson University Sleep Disorders Center, 4804

Tourette Syndrome Association-Pennsylvania Chapter, 7149

US Wheelchair Weightlifting Association, 8029

United Cerebral Palsy Central PA, 1471

United Cerebral Palsy of Northeastern Pennsylvania, 1472

United Cerebral Palsy of Northwestern Pennsylvania, 1473

United Cerebral Palsy of Pennsylvania, 1474

United Cerebral Palsy of Philadelphia & Vicinity, 1475

United Cerebral Palsy of Pittsburgh, 1476

United Cerebral Palsy of South Central Pennsylvania, 1477

United Cerebral Palsy of Southern Allegenies Region, 1478

United Cerebral Palsy of Southwestern Pennsylvania, 1479

United Cerebral Palsy of Western Pennsylvania, 1480

University of Pennsylvania Weight and Education Program, 2788

University of Pennsylvania, Depression Research Unit, 2398

University of Pittsburgh Cystic Fibrosis Center/Children's Hospital, 2312

Variety Club Camp & Development Center, 8455

W.M. Krogman Center for Research In Child Growth and Development, 3105

Wesley Woods, 8456

Western Pennsylvania Chapter of Crohn's & Colitis Foundation of America, 2169

Western Pennsylvania Chapter of The National Hemophilia Foundation, 3900

Western Psychiatric Institute & Clinic, Sleep Evaluation Center, 4805

Wills Eye Brain Tumor Support Group, 1222

Yomeca, 8457

Rhode Island

Assistive Technology Access Partnership, 8030

Autism Society of Rhode Island, 826

Brain Injury Association of Rhode Island, 3256

Brain Tumor Support Group at Providence, 1223

Central Region Early Intervention Program, 8031

Children's Neurodevelopment Center at Hasbro Children's Hospital, 2610

Hydrocephalus Association of Rhode Island, 4202

Infant Behavior, Cry and Sleep Clinic, 1768

NNFF of Rhode Island - Coventry, 4920

NNFF of Rhode Island - Warwick, 4921

Office Integrated Social Services, 8032

Rhode Island Arc, 8033

Rhode Island Department of Health, 8034

Rhode Island Department of Health National SIDS Foundation, 6819

Rhode Island Hemophilia Foundation, 3901

Rhode Island Hemostasis and Thrombosis Center, 3972

Rhode Island Hospital, Cystic Fibrosis Center, 2313

Rhode Island Parent Information Network, 8035

Rhode Island Scleroderma Support Group, 6216

Rhode Island Support Group, 523

Sleep Disorders Center of Lifespan Hospitals, 4806

Spina Bifida Association of Rhode Island, 6607

TechACCESS of Rhode Island, 8178

Turner's Syndrome Society of Rhode Island, 7353

United Cerebral Palsy of Rhode Island, 1481

South Carolina

Assistive Technology Project, 8036

Autism Society of South Carolina, 827

BabyNet, 8037

Brain Injury Alliance of South Carolina, 3257

Brain Injury Association of South Carolina, 3258

Burnt Gin Camp, 8458

CF Center/Medical University of South Carolina, 2314

Carolinas Support Group, 524

Children's Center for Cancer and Blood Disorders, 109, 167, 3849, 3925, 6432

Children's Tumor Foundation - South Carolina Chapter, 4922

Described and Captioned Media Program, 3393

Family Connection of South Carolina, 8179

Hemophilia Association of South Carolina, 3902

International Pemphigus Foundation: South Carolina Support Group, 5384

James R Clark Memorial Sickle Cell Foundation, 6429

Newberry County Memorial Hospital Brain Tumor Support Group, 1224

Office of Exceptional Children South Carolina Department of Education, 8038

PRO-Parents, 8039

PWSA - South Carolina, 5698

Region 4 of the National Association for Parents of the Visually Impaired, 1837, 1974, 5086, 5940

Sarcoidosis Support, 6143

South Carolina Brain Injury Task Force Affiliated with National Brain Injury, 3259

South Carolina Department of Health & Environmental Control - SIDS Information, 6820

South Carolina State Library, 8180

Turner's Syndrome Society of South Carolina, 7354

United Cerebral Palsy of South Carolina a, 1482

South Dakota

Autism Society of South Dakota Black Hills Chapter, 828

DakotaLink, 8040

NNFF of South Dakota - Northern Plains, 4923

Office of Special Education, 8041

Sioux Valley Hospital, South Dakota Cystic Fibrosis Center, 2315

South Dakota Center For Bleeding Disorders, 3974

South Dakota Department of Health, 6821

South Dakota Parent Connection, 8042

South Dakota State Library, 8181

Teratogen and Birth Defects Information Project, 8217

Thumpers, 4302

University Affiliated Program, School of Medicine, 8043

Tennessee

Autism Society of America East Tennessee Chapter, 829

Bill Wilkerson Center, 3407

Brain Injury Association of Tennessee, 3260

Camp Easter Seal, 8459

Camp Hickory Wood, 3328

Center for Early Childhood, 8044

Children's Tumor Foundation - Tennessee Affiliate, 4924

Down Syndrome Association of Middle Tennessee, 2577

East Tennessee Comprehensive Hemophilia Center, 3930

East Tennessee Technology Access Center, 8182

Families of SMA - Tennessee Chapter, 6682

First Regional Hemophilia Center, 3934

Leukemia & Lymphoma Society, Tennessee Chapter, 103, 161

Memphis Cystic Fibrosis Center, 2316

Memphis Regional Brain Tumor Survivors Group, 1225

Memphis State University, Center for the Communicatively Impaired, 6515

Middle Tennessee Sarcoidosis Support Group, 6144

NNFF Tennessee Chapter, 4925

Nashville Brain Tumor Support Group, 1226

Neuroscience Institute, University of Tennessee Health Science Center, 6334

Office of Special Education, State Department of Education, 8045

PWSA - Tennessee, 5699

PWSA Chapter - Nashville, 5700

PWSA of Tennessee, 5701

Pediatric Pulmonary Medicine, 2317

STEP, 8046

Saint Jude Children's Research Hospital, 8183

Sarcoidosis Center, 6148

Sarcoidosis Patient Forum, 6145

Sarcoidosis Research Institute, 6150

Spina Bifida Association of Tennessee, 6608

Technology Access Center of Middle Tennessee, 8047

Tennesse Hemophilia & Bleeding Disorders Foundation, 3903

Tennessee Chapter of Crohn's & Colitis Foundation of America, 2171

Tennessee SIDS Program, 6822

Tennessee Saving Little Hearts, 4303

Turner's Syndrome Society of Mid-South, 7355

Turner's Syndrome Society of Tennessee, 7356

United Cerebral Palsy of Middle Tennessee, 1483

United Cerebral Palsy of the Mid-South, 1484

University of Memphis Neuropsychology Lab, 3288

University of Tennessee Hemophilia Clinic, 3986

Vanderbilt Hemostasis-Thrombosis Clinic, 3989

Texas

Asthma and Allergy Foundation of America - North Texas Chapter, 380

Ataxia Telangiectasia Project, 535

Autism Society of America Greater Austin Chapter, 830

Baylor College of Medicine, 4702

Baylor College of Medicine Birth Defects Center, 8184, 8199

Baylor Comprehensive Epilepsy Center, 6335

Baylor Sleep Wellness Center, 4815

Benign Essential Blepharospasm Research Foundation, 2726

Brain Injury Association of Texas, 3261

Brain Injury Research Center of the Institute for Rehabilitation & Research, 3272

Brain Tumor Support Group at Dallas, 1227

Brain Tumor Support Group at Plano, 1228

Brain Tumor Support Group for Families of Children with Brain and Spinal Tumors, 1229

CF Center, Pulmonary Section, 2318

Callier Center for Communication Disorders, 6516

Center for Cancer and Blood Disorders, 6440

Center for Cancer and Blood Disorders at Children's Medical Center in Dallas, 3924

Central Texas Brain Tumor Support Group, 1230

Children's Association for Maxiumum Potential CAMP, 8460

Children's Cancer Research Institute, 4964, 8200

Cook-Ft. Worth Medical Center, CF Center, 2319

Cooley's Anemia Foundation - Texas, 7038

Cystic Fibrosis Care, Teaching and Research Center, 2320

Cystic Fibrosis-Lung Disease Center Santa Rosa Children's Hospital, 2321

Dallas Academy, 714, 987, 4465

Department of Assistive and Rehabilitation Services, 8048

Down Syndrome Guild of Dallas, 2578

Down Syndrome Specialty Clinic, 2611

Golden Triangle Area Support Group, 525

HOPE (Helping Oncology Parents Endure) Brain Tumor Foundation of the Southwest, 1231

Harris County Health Department, 6823

Heart to Heart, 4304

Hill School of Fort Worth, 718, 991, 4469

Houston Area Brain Tumor Network, 1232

Houston Ear Research Foundation, 3408

Houston Support Group, 526

Houston-Gulf Coast/South Texas Chapter of Crohn's & Colitis Foundation of America, 2172

Hughen Center, 8461

Hydrocephalus Association of N Texas, 4203

Institute for Rehabilitation and Research, 3289

International Pemphigus Foundation: Housto n Support Group, 5387

Jacob's Heart, 4305

Leukemia Society of America - North Texas Chapter, 104, 162

Leukemia Society of America - South/West Texas Chapter, 105, 163

Leukemia Society of America - Texas Gulf Coast Chapter, 106, 164

Lone Star Chapter of the National Hemophilia Foundation, 3904

Menninger Child & Family Program, 1784

National Phenylketonuria (PKU) Foundation, 5399

Neurofibromatosis Texas Foundation, 4926

North Texas Chapter of Crohn's & Colitis Foundation of America, 2173

North Texas SIDS Information And Counseling Program, 6824

North Texas Support Group, 527

Office of the Dean, University of Texas at Austin, 8049

PWSA Chapter - North Texas, 5702

Parent Case Management, 8050

Partners Resource Network, 8051

Project PODER, 8052

Region VI Office Program Consultants For Maternal and Child Health, 6825

Santa Rosa Medical Center, 2612

Scleroderma Foundation Texas Bluebonnet Ch apter, 6217

Shirvers Cancer Center Brain Tumor Support Group, 1233

Sickle Cell Association of Austin - Marc Thomas Chapter, 6430

Sickle Cell Association of the Texas Gulf Coast, 6431

Sleep Disorders Center for Children, 4807

Sleep Medicine Associates of Texas, 4808

South Central Region-Helen Keller National Center, 8053

South Texas Comprehensive Hemophilia and Thrombophilia Treatment Center, 3975

Southwest SIDS Research Institute, 6844

Southwestern Comprehensive Sickle Cell Cen ter, 6441

Spina Bifida Association of Austin, 6609

Spina Bifida Association of Houston-Gulf Coast, 6610

Spina Bifida Association of North Texas, 6611

Spina Bifida Association of Texas, 6612

Sweeney, 2531

Texas Assistive Technology Partnership, 8055

Texas Association on Mental Retardation, 2579

Texas Central Chapter of the National Hemophilia Foundation, 3905

Texas Department of Health - SIDS Information and Counseling Program, 6826

Texas Heart to Heart, 4306

Texas Lions Camp, 8462

Texas Perinatal Association, 5766

Texas Prader-Willi Syndrome Association, 5703

Texas State Library, 8185

Texas Tech University Speech-Language -Hearing Clinic, 6517

Tri-Services Military CF Center, 2322

Turner's Syndrome Society Resource Center, 7364

Turner's Syndrome Society of Houston, 7357

Turner's Syndrome Society of North Texas, 7358

Turner's Syndrome Society of San Antonio, 7359

UT Southwestern Medical Center at Dallas: Hematology-Oncology Research, 3981

United Cerebral Palsy of Greater Houston, 1485

United Cerebral Palsy of Metropolitan Dallas, 1486

United Cerebral Palsy of Tarrant County, 1487

United Cerebral Palsy of Texas, 1488

Univ. of Texas-Southwestern Med. Ctr. at Dallas - Clinical Ctr. for Liver Disease, 1012

University of Texas Department of Hematology Research, 3987

University of Texas Medical Branch at Galveston, Clinical Research Center, 4816

University of Texas Sleep/Wake Disorders Center, 4809

University of Texas Southwestern Medical Center/Asthma & Allergic Diseases, 392

University of Texas at Dallas, Callier Center for Communication Disorders, 6549

University of Texas, Mental Health Clinical Research Center, 2399

Vitamin C Foundation, 5816

We've Just Begun to Live Brain Tumor Support Group, 1234

West Texas Brain Tumor Support Group, 1235

Utah

Baby Watch Early Intervention Program, 8056

Brain Injury Association of Utah, 3262

Camp Kostopulos, 8463

Children's Tumor Foundation - Utah Chapter, 4927

Computer Center for Citizens with Disabilities, 8057

Early Intervention Research Institute, Developmental Center, 8204

NNFF of Utah, 4928

PWSA Chapter - Orem, 5704

PWSA Chapter - Pleasant Grove, 5705

Peer-Led Brain Tumor Support Group, 1236

Prader-Willi Utah Association, 5706

Primary Children's Medical Center, 8212

Special Education Services Unit, 8058

Spina Bifida Association of Utah, 6613

Tourette Syndrome Association-Utah Chapter, 7150

Turner's Syndrome Society of Salt Lake City, 7360

US Disabled Ski Team, 8059

United Cerebral Palsy of Utah, 1489

University of Utah, 4703

University of Utah Intermountain Cystic Fibrosis Center, 2323

Utada Camp, 2532

Utah Center for Assistive Technology, 8060

Utah Chapter of the National Hemophilia Foundation, 3906

Utah Department of Health, 6827

Utah Parent Center, 8061

Utah State Library Commission, 8186

Utah Support Group, 528

Vermont

Assistive Technology Project, 8062

Autism Society of Vermont, 831

Bennington School, 1809

Brain Injury Association of Vermont, 3263

Center on Disabilities and Community Inclusion, 8063

Family, Infant, and Toddler Project, 8064

Farm and Wilderness Camps, 8464

Heart to Heart, 4307

Medical Center Hospital of Vermont, 2324

Special Education Unit, 8065

Thorpe Camp, 8465

Vermont Department of Health - SIDS Information and Counseling Program, 6828

Vermont Department of Libraries, 8187

Vermont Parent Information Center, 8066

Vermont Regional Hemophilia Center, 3990

Virginia

Alexandria Library Talking Book Service, 1895, 2032, 5143, 5997

Arlington County Department of Libraries, 8188

Autism Society of America Northern Virginia Chapter, 832

Brain Injury Association of Virginia, 3264

Brain Injury Association of Washington DC, 3210

Brain Tumor Support Group, 1237

Camp Baker Services, 8466

Camp Easter Seal East, Camp Easter Seal West, 8467

Camp Fantastic, 8468

Camp Holiday Trails, 8469

Childhelp Children's Center of Virginia, 5520

Children's Tumor Foundation - MidAtlantic Region Chapter, 4929

Cystic Fibrosis Center/University of Virginia Health System, 2325

Cystic Fibrosis Program of the Medical College of Virginia, 2326

Division for Research (CEC-DR), 8202

Division for the Visually Handicapped, 1896, 2033, 5144, 5998

Division on Visual Impairments, 1897, 2034, 5145, 5999

ERIC Clearinghouse on Disabilities and Gifted Education, 8189

Eastern Virginia Medical Center, 2327

Fairfax County Public Library, 8190

Hemophilia Association of the Capital Area, 3907

Hemophilia Treatment Center of Tidewater Virginia, 3946

Infant & Toddler Program, 8067

Leukemia Society of America - National Capital Area Chapter, 107, 165

Makemie Woods Camp Conference Center, 8470

National Sudden Infant Death Syndrome Research Center, 6841

National Sudden Infant Death Syndrome Resource Center, 6835

Newport News Public Library System, 8191

Oakland School & Camp, 4472

Office of Special Education, Virginia, 8068

Overlook, 8471

PWSA of Maryland, Virginia & DC, 5675, 5707

Parent Educational Advocacy Training Center, 8069

Precious Hearts, 4308

Roanoke City Public Library System, 8192

Sarcoidosis Support Group, 6146

Scleroderma Foundation Greater Washington DC Chapter, 6218

Speech Simulation Research Foundation, 6518

Spina Bifida Association of the Roanoke Valley, 6614

Tidewater Center for Technology Access, 8070

Triangle D Camp for Children, 8472

Trisomy 18 Foundation, 7268

United Cerebral Palsy of Southern & Central Virginia, 1490

United Virginia Chapter of the National Hemophilia Foundation, 3908

University of Virginia Communication Disorders Program, 3394

University of Virginia General Clinical Research Center, 393

University of Virginia Hemophilia Treatment Center, 3988

Virginia Assistive Technology System, 8071

Virginia Beach Public Library, 8193

Virginia Commonwealth University Department of Neurosurgery Research, 3290

Virginia SIDS Program - Virginia Department of Health, 6829

Virginia State Library for the Visually and Physically Handicapped, 1898, 2035, 5146, 6000

Washington

Adult Brain Tumor Support Group, 1238

Autism Society of Washington, 833

Bleeding Disorders Foundation of Washington, 3909

Brain Injury Association of Washington, 3265

Brain Tumor Support Group University of Washington Medical Center, 1239

Children's Tumor Foundation - Washington Chapter, 4930

Epilepsy Foundation Northwest, 6327

Evergreen Spina Bifida Association, 6615

Head Injury Hotline, 3266

Heart to Heart, 4309

Hemophilia Foundation of Washington, 3910

Hydrocephalus Support Group of Seattle, 4204

Infant Toddler Early Intervention Program, 8072

NNFF Washington State Chapter, 4931

National Foundation for Ectodermal Dysplasias- Regional Office, 2882

National Wilms Tumor Study, 7455

Northwest Hospital Brain Tumor Group Support Hotline, 1241

Northwest Hospital Brain Tumor Support Group, 1240

Northwestern Region-Helen Keller National Center, 1838, 1975, 5087, 5941

Office of the Superintendent of Public Instruction, 8073

PWSA Chapter - Northwest Washington, 5708

PWSA of Region Northwest, 5709

PWSA of Washington, 5710

Prader-Willi Northwest Association, 5653, 5680

Puget Sound Blood Center, 3969

Region X Office Program Consultants for Maternal and Child Health, 6830

SIDS Northwest Regional Center, 6831

Scleroderma Foundation Evergreen Chapter, 6219

Scottish Rite Centers for Childhood Langua ge Disorders, 6519

Seattle Area Support Group, 529

Tourette Syndrome Association-Washington State Chapter, 7151

Turner's Syndrome Society of Inland Northwest, 7362

United Cerebral Palsy of South Puget Sound, 1492

University of Washington CF Center, 2328

University of Washington Department of Spe ech & Hearing Sciences, 6520

University of Washington Speech and Hearin g Clinic, 6529

University of Washington: Experimental Education Unit, 2613

Washington Leukemia and Lymphoma Society Alaska Chapter, 8074

Washington Library for the Blind and Physically Handicapped, 1899, 2036, 5147, 6001

Washington PAVE, 8075

Washington State Chapter of Asthma and Allergy Foundation of America, 381

Washington State Chapter of Crohn's & Colitis Foundation of America, 2174

West Virginia

Autism Services Center, 844

Autism Society of West Virginia, 834

Autism Training Center, 845

Brain Injury Association of West Virginia, 3267

Cabell County Public Library, 8194

Early Intervention Program, 8076

Hemophilia Center of West Virginia, 3938

Huntington Area Hemophilia Association, 3951

Kanawha County Public Library, 8195

Mountain Milestones Stepping Stones, 8473

Mountaineer Spina Bifida Camp, 6667

NNFF West Virginia Chapter, 4932

Neurofibromatosis - West Virginia, 4933

Office of Special Education Administration, 8077

PWSA of West Virginia, 5711

Southern West Virginia Brain Tumor Support Group, 1242

West Virginia Assistive Technology System, 8078

West Virginia Chapter, 3911

West Virginia Department of Health and Human Services, 6832

West Virginia Library Commission, 8196

West Virginia Parent Training and Information, 8079

West Virginia School for the Blind, 1900, 2037, 5148, 6002

West Virginia University Cystic Fibrosis Center, 2329

West Virginia University Mountain State Cystic Fibrosis Center, 2330

Wisconsin

American Red Cross Hemophilia Center, 3919

Appleton Support Group, 530

Autism Society of Wisconsin, 835

Birth to 3 Program, 8080

Brain Injury Association of Wisconsin, 3268

Brain Tumor Support Group, 1243

Brain Tumor Support Group at Milwaukee, 1244

Brain Tumor Support Group at Wauwatosa Froederdt Memorial Lutheran Hospital, 1245

Brown County Library, 8197

Camp Heartland, 3186

Camp Joy, 8474

Center for the Study of Bioethics, 2614

Children's Tumor Foundation - Wisconsin Ch apter, 4934

Counseling and Research Center for SIDS, 6833

Development and Training Center, 8081

Division of Community Services, 8082

Early Childhood Handicapped Prgrams, 8083

Fox Valley Hydrocephalus Support Group, 4205

GLaRGG BLuRBB, 531

Great Lakes Hemophilia Foundation, 3912

Gundersen Clinic Comprehensive Hemophilia Treatment Center, 3935

Hemophilia Outreach Center, 3916

Information Centers for Bipolar Disorders, 1032

International Bone Marrow Transplant Registry, 110

John Sierzant Brain Tumor Support Group, 1246

Kids With Heart, 4310

LODAT (Living One Day at a Time) Brain Tumor Support Group, 1247

Left Hearts, 4311

Leukemia Society of America - Wisconsin Chapter, 108, 166

Lithium Information Center, 5236

Madison, WI Area Support Group, 532

Medical College of Wisconsin Cystic Fibrosis Center, 2331

Neurofibromatosis - Wisconsin, 4935

Obsessive Compulsive Information Center, 5235

PWSA of Wisconsin, 5712

PWSA of Wisconsin - Madison, 5713

Parent Education Project of Wisconsin, 8084

Physician Referral and Information Line, 383

Regional Epilepsy Center, 6336

Research at BloodCenter of Wisconsin, 3971

Scoliosis Research Society, 6249

Spina Bifida Association of Greater Fox Valley, 6616

Spina Bifida Association of Northern Wisconsin, 6617

Spina Bifida Association of Wisconsin, 6618

Timbertop Nature Adventure Camp, 8475

Turner's Syndrome Society of Southeastern Wisconsin, 7363

United Cerebral Palsy of Greater Dane County, 1493

United Cerebral Palsy of North Central Wisconsin, 1494

United Cerebral Palsy of Southeastern Wisconsin, 1495

United Cerebral Palsy of West Central Wisconsin, 1496

University of Wisconsin Asthma and Allergic Disease Center, 394

University of Wisconsin-Madison Cystic Fibrosis/Pulmonary Center, 2332

Waisman Center - Auditory Physiology Resea rch Laboratory, 6530

WisTech, 8085

Wisconsin Association for Perinatal Care, 5767

Wisconsin Chapter of Crohn's & Colitis Foundation of America, 2175

Wisconsin Lions Camp, 8476

Wyoming

Brain Injury Association of Wyoming, 3269

Division of Developmental Disabilities, 8086

NNFF Wyoming Chapter, 4936

NNFF of Wyoming, 4937

Parent Information Center, 8087

Parent and Information Center, 8210

Special Education Unit, 8088

Wyoming Department of Health, 6834

Wyoming's New Options in Technology (WYNOT), 8089

MLNS, 4381
MPS, 4677
MSUD, 4537
Macrocephalia, 4530
Macrocephaly, 4174, 4530
Macrocephaly, benign familial, 4530
Major depressive disorder, 2381
Male Turner syndrome, 5064
Manic-depressive disorder, 1022
Manic-depressive illness, 1022
Manic-depressive psychosis, 1022
Manifest deviation, 6697
Maple syrup urine disease, 4537
Marfan syndrome, 4547
Marfan syndrome, infantile, 4547
Marfan syndrome, neonatal, 4547
Marie-Strumpell spondylitis, 239
Marker X syndrome, 3040
Martin-Bell syndrome, 3040
Maternal phenylketonuria, 5394
McCune-Albright syndrome, 4557
Measles, 5783, 6735
Meckel-Gruber syndrome, 2918
Meconium aspiration syndrome, 6041
Medulloblastoma, 1054
Megacolon, aganglionic, 4117
Megacolon, congenital aganglionic, 4117
Megalocephaly, 4530
Meningitis, 4567
Meningitis, bacterial, 4567
Meningitis, chronic, 4567
Meningitis, neonatal, 4567
Meningitis, viral, 4567
Meningocele, 6550
Meningomyelocele, 6550
Mental deficiency, 4577
Mental retardation, 4577
Mesiodens, 2368
Metachromatic leukodystrophy, 4484
Methionine, 4161
Methylcobalamin defect, 4161
Methylenetetrahydrofolate reductase, 4161
Microcephalia, 4601
Microcephalism, 4601
Microcephaly, 4601
Microdontia, 4609
Microdontism, 4609
Middle ear, inflammation of, 5321
Migraine headaches, 4616
Migraine with aura, 4616
Migraine without aura, 4616
Mild MSUD, 4537
Milk protein allergy, 4654
Miller-Dieker lissencephaly syndrome, 4496
Miller-Fisher syndrome, 3126
Minimal change nephrotic syndrome, 4863
Mixed cerebral palsy, 1357
Mixed hearing loss, 3330
Mood disturbance, 2381
Morbilli, 5783
Morphea, 6203
Movement disorders, 1687, 2716
Mucocutaneous lymph node syndrome, 4381

Mucolipidoses, 4668
Mucopolysaccharidoses, 4677
Mucoviscidosis, 2218
Mumps, 5783
Muscular dystrophy, 4689
Mycobacterium africanum, 7278
Mycobacterium bovis, 7278
Mycobacterium tuberculosis, 7278
Myelocele, 6550
Myelomeningocele, 286, 6550
Myopia, 5918

N

NB, 4958
NF1, 4878
NF2, 4878
NHL, 5049
NS, 5064
Narcolepsy, 4748
Natal teeth, 2368
Nearsightedness, 5918
Neonatal conjunctivitis, 2086
Neonatal herpes simplex, 4832
Neonatal jaundice, 4846
Neonatal opthalmia, 2086
Neonatal pemphigus vulgaris, 5372
Neonatal tetanus, 5783
Nephroblastoma, 7446
Nephrotic syndrome, 4863
Neural tube defect, 217, 2918
Neuroblastoma, 4958
Neurocardiogenic syncope, 6882
Neurofibromatosis, 4878
Neurofibromatosis type I, 4878
Neurofibromatosis type II, 4878
Neuromuscular scoliosis, 6242
Neutropenia, 4974
Neutropenia, chronic, 4974
Neutropenia, cyclic, 4974
Neutropenia, transient, 4974
Nevi, strawberry, 3841
Newborn respiratory distress, 6041
Night terrors, 5008, 6485
Nightmares, 4984
Nine-day measles, 5783
Nocturnal enuresis, 5035
Non-Hodgkin's lymphoma, 5049
Non-Hodgkin's lymphoma, Burkitt's type, 5049
Non-Hodgkin's lymphoma, SNCC type, 5049
Non-Hodgkin's lymphoma, large cell type, 5049
Non-Hodgkin's lymphoma, small noncleaved, 5049
Non-communicating hydrocephalus, 4174
Noninfectious conjunctivitis, 2086
Nonparalytic strabismus, 6697
Nontropical sprue, 1321
Noonan syndrome, 5064
Norman-Roberts lissencephaly syndrome, 4496
Nystagmus, 5074
Nystagmus, acquired, 5074
Nystagmus, congenital, 5074
Nystagmus, convergent, 5074
Nystagmus, jerky, 5074

TSD, 6928
Talipes, 1730
Tay-Sachs disease, 6928
Tay-Sachs disease, infantile type, 6928
Tay-Sachs disease, juvenile type, 6928
Teeth, 4609
Teeth, Absence of, 2368
Temporary discoloration of the teeth, 2368
Teratologic congenital dysplasia of the, 1952
Testes, ectopic, 2199
Testes, maldescended, 2199
Testes, true undescended, 2199
Tetanus, 5783
Tetralogy of Fallot, 7000
Thalassemia, 7015
Thiamine-responsive MSUD, 4537
Third and fourth pharyngeal pouch, 2533
Third degree burns, 1303
Threadworm, 5571
Three-day measles, 5783
Three-month colic, 1757
Thrombocytopenia, 7067
Thromboembolic disease, 5811
Thrombotic disorder, 5811
Thumbsucking, 7081
Tic disorder, chronic motor, 7095
Tics, 7095, 7126
Tics of childhood, transient, 7095
Tooth decay, 2368
Tourette syndrome, 5219, 7095, 7126
Toxoplasmosis, 7232
Tracheoesophageal fistula, 2971
Transposition of the great arteries, 7244
Transposition of the great vessels, 7244
Traumatic brain injury, 3188
Trigonocephaly, 2106
Trisomy 13 syndrome, 7270
Trisomy 18 mosaicism, 7260
Trisomy 18 syndrome, 7260
Trisomy 21 mosaicism, 2544
Trisomy 21 syndrome, 2544
Trisomy 21 translocation, 2544
True precocious puberty, 5748
Tuberculosis, 7278
Tuberous sclerosis, 7302
Tumor, benign, 1054
Tumor, malignant, 1054
Turner phenotype with normal chromosomes, 5064
Turner syndrome, 7318
Turricephaly, 2106
Tympanitis, 5321
Tyrosinase neg.oculocutaneous albinism, 182
Tyrosinase pos.oculocutaneous albinism, 182

U

Ulcerative colitis, 7381
Uncoordinated movements, 459
Undescended testes, 2199
Undifferentiated conduct disorder, 1772
Unilateral neviod telangiectasia, 6973
Unstable gait, 459
Urticaria pigmentosa, 7419

V

VACTERL association, 249
VSDs, 7427
Van Bogaert's encephalitis, 6735
Vasodepressor syncope, 6882
Ventricular septal defects, 7427
Vertebrae, fused, 4417
Viral gastroenteritis, 20
Viral infections of childhood, 2963
Viral pneumonia, 5586
Visual disturbances, 5918
Von Recklinghausen disease, 4878
Von Willebrand's disease, 3858

W

WAGR syndrome, 227, 7446
WBC, 7432
WD, 7463
WMS, 7432
WND, 7463
WPW, 297
WS, 7432
Waardenburg syndrome, 182
Walker-Warburg syndrome, 4496
Weber-Cockayne syndrome, 2943
Werdnig-Hoffmann disease, 6668
White matter diseases, 4484
Whooping cough, 5783
Williams syndrome, 7432
Williams-Beuren syndrome, 7432
Wilms tumor, 7446
Wilson disease, 2716, 7463
Wohlfart-Kugelberg-Welander disease, 6668
Wolff-parkinson-white syndrome, 297
Writer's cramp, 2716

X

X-linked lissencephaly, 4496
XO syndrome, 7318
XXY syndrome, 4405

Z

Zygosyndactyly, 6890

Sedgwick Press
Health Directories

The Complete Directory for People with Disabilities, 2007

A wealth of information, now in one comprehensive sourcebook. Completely updated, this edition contains more information than ever before, including thousands of new entries and enhancements to existing entries and thousands of additional web sites and e-mail addresses. This up-to-date directory is the most comprehensive resource available for people with disabilities, detailing Independent Living Centers, Rehabilitation Facilities, State & Federal Agencies, Associations, Support Groups, Periodicals & Books, Assistive Devices, Employment & Education Programs, Camps and Travel Groups. Each year, more libraries, schools, colleges, hospitals, rehabilitation centers and individuals add *The Complete Directory for People with Disabilities* to their collections, making sure that this information is readily available to the families, individuals and professionals who can benefit most from the amazing wealth of resources cataloged here.

"No other reference tool exists to meet the special needs of the disabled in one convenient resource for information." –Library Journal

1,200 pages; Softcover ISBN 1-59237-147-7, $165.00 ◆ Online Database $215.00 ◆ Online Database & Directory Combo $300.00

The Complete Directory for People with Chronic Illness, 2007/08

Thousands of hours of research have gone into this completely updated 2005/06 edition – several new chapters have been added along with thousands of new entries and enhancements to existing entries. Plus, each chronic illness chapter has been reviewed by an medical expert in the field. This widely-hailed directory is structured around the 90 most prevalent chronic illnesses – from Asthma to Cancer to Wilson's Disease – and provides a comprehensive overview of the support services and information resources available for people diagnosed with a chronic illness. Each chronic illness has its own chapter and contains a brief description in layman's language, followed by important resources for National & Local Organizations, State Agencies, Newsletters, Books & Periodicals, Libraries & Research Centers, Support Groups & Hotlines, Web Sites and much more. This directory is an important resource for health care professionals, the collections of hospital and health care libraries, as well as an invaluable tool for people with a chronic illness and their support network.

"A must purchase for all hospital and health care libraries and is strongly recommended for all public library reference departments." –ARBA

1,200 pages; Softcover ISBN 1-59237-183-3, $165.00 ◆ Online Database $215.00 ◆ Online Database & Directory Combo $300.00

The Complete Learning Disabilities Directory, 2007

The Complete Learning Disabilities Directory is the most comprehensive database of Programs, Services, Curriculum Materials, Professional Meetings & Resources, Camps, Newsletters and Support Groups for teachers, students and families concerned with learning disabilities. This information-packed directory includes information about Associations & Organizations, Schools, Colleges & Testing Materials, Government Agencies, Legal Resources and much more. For quick, easy access to information, this directory contains four indexes: Entry Name Index, Subject Index and Geographic Index. With every passing year, the field of learning disabilities attracts more attention and the network of caring, committed and knowledgeable professionals grows every day. This directory is an invaluable research tool for these parents, students and professionals.

"Due to its wealth and depth of coverage, parents, teachers and others… should find this an invaluable resource." –Booklist

900 pages; Softcover ISBN 1-59237-122-1, $145.00 ◆ Online Database $195.00 ◆ Online Database & Directory Combo $280.00

The Complete Mental Health Directory, 2006/07

This is the most comprehensive resource covering the field of behavioral health, with critical information for both the layman and the mental health professional. For the layman, this directory offers understandable descriptions of 25 Mental Health Disorders as well as detailed information on Associations, Media, Support Groups and Mental Health Facilities. For the professional, *The Complete Mental Health Directory* offers critical and comprehensive information on Managed Care Organizations, Information Systems, Government Agencies and Provider Organizations. This comprehensive volume of needed information will be widely used in any reference collection.

"… the strength of this directory is that it consolidates widely dispersed information into a single volume." –Booklist

800 pages; Softcover ISBN 1-59237-124-8, $165.00 ◆ Online Database $215.00 ◆ Online & Directory Combo $300.00

To preview any of our Directories Risk-Free for 30 days, call (800) 562-2139 or fax to (518) 789-0556

Older Americans Information Directory, 2006/07

Completely updated for 2006/07, this sixth edition has been completely revised and now contains 1,000 new listings, over 8,000 updates to existing listings and over 3,000 brand new e-mail addresses and web sites. You'll find important resources for Older Americans including National, Regional, State & Local Organizations, Government Agencies, Research Centers, Libraries & Information Centers, Legal Resources, Discount Travel Information, Continuing Education Programs, Disability Aids & Assistive Devices, Health, Print Media and Electronic Media. Three indexes: Entry Index, Subject Index and Geographic Index make it easy to find just the right source of information. This comprehensive guide to resources for Older Americans will be a welcome addition to any reference collection.

"Highly recommended for academic, public, health science and consumer libraries…" –Choice

1,200 pages; Softcover ISBN 1-59237-136-1, $165.00 ◆ Online Database $215.00 ◆ Online Database & Directory Combo $300.00

The Directory of Drug & Alcohol Residential Rehabilitation Facilities

This brand new directory is the first-ever resource to bring together, all in one place, data on the thousands of drug and alcohol residential rehabilitation facilities in the United States. *The Directory of Drug & Alcohol Residential Rehabilitation Facilities* covers over 1,000 facilities, with detailed contact information for each one, including mailing address, phone and fax numbers, email addresses and web sites, mission statement, type of treatment programs, cost, average length of stay, numbers of residents and counselors, accreditation, insurance plans accepted, type of environment, religious affiliation, education components and much more. It also contains a helpful chapter on General Resources that provides contact information for Associations, Print & Electronic Media, Support Groups and Conferences. Multiple indexes allow the user to pinpoint the facilities that meet very specific criteria. This time-saving tool is what so many counselors, parents and medical professionals have been asking for. *The Directory of Drug & Alcohol Residential Rehabilitation Facilities* will be a helpful tool in locating the right source for treatment for a wide range of individuals. This comprehensive directory will be an important acquisition for all reference collections: public and academic libraries, case managers, social workers, state agencies and many more.

"This is an excellent, much needed directory that fills an important gap…" –Booklist

300 pages; Softcover ISBN 1-59237-031-4, $135.00

Sedgwick Press
Education Directories

The Comparative Guide to American Elementary & Secondary Schools, 2007

The only guide of its kind, this award winning compilation offers a snapshot profile of every public school district in the United States serving 1,500 or more students – more than 5,900 districts are covered. Organized alphabetically by district within state, each chapter begins with a Statistical Overview of the state. Each district listing includes contact information (name, address, phone number and web site) plus Grades Served, the Numbers of Students and Teachers and the Number of Regular, Special Education, Alternative and Vocational Schools in the district along with statistics on Student/Classroom Teacher Ratios, Drop Out Rates, Ethnicity, the Numbers of Librarians and Guidance Counselors and District Expenditures per student. As an added bonus, *The Comparative Guide to American Elementary and Secondary Schools* provides important ranking tables, both by state and nationally, for each data element. For easy navigation through this wealth of information, this handbook contains a useful City Index that lists all districts that operate schools within a city. These important comparative statistics are necessary for anyone considering relocation or doing comparative research on their own district and would be a perfect acquisition for any public library or school district library.

"This straightforward guide is an easy way to find general information. Valuable for academic and large public library collections." –ARBA

2,400 pages; Softcover ISBN 1-59237-223-6, $125.00

Educators Resource Directory, 2007/08

Educators Resource Directory is a comprehensive resource that provides the educational professional with thousands of resources and statistical data for professional development. This directory saves hours of research time by providing immediate access to Associations & Organizations, Conferences & Trade Shows, Educational Research Centers, Employment Opportunities & Teaching Abroad, School Library Services, Scholarships, Financial Resources, Professional Consultants, Computer Software & Testing Resources and much more. Plus, this comprehensive directory also includes a section on Statistics and Rankings with over 100 tables, including statistics on Average Teacher Salaries, SAT/ACT scores, Revenues & Expenditures and more. These important statistics will allow the user to see how their school rates among others, make relocation decisions and so much more. For quick access to information, this directory contains four indexes: Entry & Publisher Index, Geographic Index, a Subject & Grade Index and Web Sites Index. *Educators Resource Directory* will be a well-used addition to the reference collection of any school district, education department or public library.

"Recommended for all collections that serve elementary and secondary school professionals." –Choice

1,000 pages; Softcover ISBN 1-59237-179-5, $145.00 ◆ Online Database $195.00 ◆ Online Database & Directory Combo $280.00

To preview any of our Directories Risk-Free for 30 days, call (800) 562-2139 or fax to (518) 789-0556

Sedgwick Press
Hospital & Health Plan Directories

The Comparative Guide to American Hospitals, 2007

This is the first ever resource to compare all of the nation's hospitals by 17 measures of quality in the treatment of heart attack, heart failure and pneumonia. This data is based on the Hospital Compare study, produced by Medicare, and is available in print and in a unique and user-friendly format from Grey House Publishing, along with extra contact information from Grey House's *Directory of Hospital Personnel*. *The Comparative Guide to American Hospitals* provides a snapshot profile of each of the nations 6,000 hospitals. These informative profiles illustrate how the hospital rates in 17 important areas: Heart Attack Care (% who receive Aspirin at Arrival, Aspirin at Discharge, ACE Inhibitor for LVSD, Beta Blocker at Arrival, Beta Blocker at Discharge, Thrombolytic Agent Received, PTCA Received and Adult Smoking Cessation Advice); Heart Failure (% who receive LVF Assessment, ACE Inhibitor for LVSD, Discharge Instructions, Adult Smoking Cessation Advice); and Pneumonia (% who receive Initial Antibiotic Timing, Pneumococcal Vaccination, Oxygenation Assessment, Blood Culture Performed and Adult Smoking Cessation Advice). Each profile includes the raw percentage for that hospital, the state average, the US average and data on the top hospital. For easy access to contact information, each profile includes the hospitals address, phone and fax numbers, email and web addresses, type and accreditation along with 5 top key administrations. These profiles will allow the user to quickly identify the quality of the hospital and have the necessary information at their fingertips to make contact with that hospital. Most importantly, *The Comparative Guide to American Hospitals* provides an easy-to-use Ranking Table for each of the data elements to allow the user to quickly locate the hospitals with the best level of service. This brand new title will be a must for the reference collection at all public, medical and academic libraries.

2,500 pages; Softcover ISBN 1-59237-182-5; $225.00

The Directory of Hospital Personnel, 2007

The Directory of Hospital Personnel is the best resource you can have at your fingertips when researching or marketing a product or service to the hospital market. A "Who's Who" of the hospital universe, this directory puts you in touch with over 150,000 key decision-makers. With 100% verification of data you can rest assured that you will reach the right person with just one call. Every hospital in the U.S. is profiled, listed alphabetically by city within state. Plus, three easy-to-use, cross-referenced indexes put the facts at your fingertips faster and more easily than any other directory: Hospital Name Index, Bed Size Index and Personnel Index. *The Directory of Hospital Personnel* is the only complete source for key hospital decision-makers by name. Whether you want to define or restructure sales territories… locate hospitals with the purchasing power to accept your proposals… keep track of important contacts or colleagues… or find information on which insurance plans are accepted, *The Directory of Hospital Personnel* gives you the information you need – easily, efficiently, effectively and accurately.

"Recommended for college, university and medical libraries." -ARBA

2,500 pages; Softcover ISBN 1-59237-178-7 $325.00 ◆ Online Database $545.00 ◆ Online Database & Directory Combo, $650.00

The Directory of Health Care Group Purchasing Organizations, 2006

This comprehensive directory provides the important data you need to get in touch with over 800 Group Purchasing Organizations. By providing in-depth information on this growing market and its members, *The Directory of Health Care Group Purchasing Organizations* fills a major need for the most accurate and comprehensive information on over 800 GPOs – Mailing Address, Phone & Fax Numbers, E-mail Addresses, Key Contacts, Purchasing Agents, Group Descriptions, Membership Categorization, Standard Vendor Proposal Requirements, Membership Fees & Terms, Expanded Services, Total Member Beds & Outpatient Visits represented and more. Five Indexes provide a number of ways to locate the right GPO: Alphabetical Index, Expanded Services Index, Organization Type Index, Geographic Index and Member Institution Index. With its comprehensive and detailed information on each purchasing organization, *The Directory of Health Care Group Purchasing Organizations* is the go-to source for anyone looking to target this market.

"The information is clearly arranged and easy to access…recommended for those needing this very specialized information." –ARBA

1,000 pages; Softcover ISBN 1-59237-0091-8, $325.00 ◆ Online Database, $650.00 ◆ Online Database & Directory Combo, $750.00

To preview any of our Directories Risk-Free for 30 days, call (800) 562-2139 or fax to (518) 789-0556

The HMO/PPO Directory, 2007

The HMO/PPO Directory is a comprehensive source that provides detailed information about Health Maintenance Organizations and Preferred Provider Organizations nationwide. This comprehensive directory details more information about more managed health care organizations than ever before. Over 1,100 HMOs, PPOs, Medicare Advantage Plans and affiliated companies are listed, arranged alphabetically by state. Detailed listings include Key Contact Information, Prescription Drug Benefits, Enrollment, Geographical Areas served, Affiliated Physicians & Hospitals, Federal Qualifications, Status, Year Founded, Managed Care Partners, Employer References, Fees & Payment Information and more. Plus, five years of historical information is included related to Revenues, Net Income, Medical Loss Ratios, Membership Enrollment and Number of Patient Complaints. Five easy-to-use, cross-referenced indexes will put this vast array of information at your fingertips immediately: HMO Index, PPO Index, Other Providers Index, Personnel Index and Enrollment Index. *The HMO/PPO Directory* provides the most comprehensive data on the most companies available on the market place today.

> *"Helpful to individuals requesting certain HMO/PPO issues such as co-payment costs, subscription costs and patient complaints. Individuals concerned (or those with questions) about their insurance may find this text to be of use to them." -ARBA*

600 pages; Softcover ISBN 1-59237-158-2, $325.00 ◆ Online Database, $495.00 ◆ Online Database & Directory Combo, $600.00

Medical Device Register, 2007

The only one-stop resource of every medical supplier licensed to sell products in the US. This award-winning directory offers immediate access to over 13,000 companies - and more than 65,000 products – in two information-packed volumes. This comprehensive resource saves hours of time and trouble when searching for medical equipment and supplies and the manufacturers who provide them. Volume I: The Product Directory, provides essential information for purchasing or specifying medical supplies for every medical device, supply, and diagnostic available in the US. Listings provide FDA codes & Federal Procurement Eligibility, Contact information for every manufacturer of the product along with Prices and Product Specifications. Volume 2 - Supplier Profiles, offers the most complete and important data about Suppliers, Manufacturers and Distributors. Company Profiles detail the number of employees, ownership, method of distribution, sales volume, net income, key executives detailed contact information medical products the company supplies, plus the medical specialties they cover. Four indexes provide immediate access to this wealth of information: Keyword Index, Trade Name Index, Supplier Geographical Index and OEM (Original Equipment Manufacturer) Index. Medical Device Register, 2007 is the only one-stop source for locating suppliers and products; looking for new manufacturers or hard-to-find medical devices; comparing products and companies; know who's selling what and who to buy from cost effectively. This directory has become the standard in its field and will be a welcome addition to the reference collection of any medical library, large public library, university library along with the collections that serve the medical community.

> *"A wealth of information on medical devices, medical device companies… and key personnel in the industry is provide in this comprehensive reference work... A valuable reference work, one of the best hardcopy compilations available." -Doody Publishing*

3,000 pages Two Volumes; Hardcover ISBN 1-59237-181-7; $325.00

The Directory of Independent Ambulatory Care Centers

This first edition of *The Directory of Independent Ambulatory Care Centers* provides access to detailed information that, before now, could only be found scattered in hundreds of different sources. This comprehensive and up-to-date directory pulls together a vast array of contact information for over 7,200 Ambulatory Surgery Centers, Ambulatory General and Urgent Care Clinics, and Diagnostic Imaging Centers that are not affiliated with a hospital or major medical center. Detailed listings include Mailing Address, Phone & Fax Numbers, E-mail and Web Site addresses, Contact Name and Phone Numbers of the Medical Director and other Key Executives and Purchasing Agents, Specialties & Services Offered, Year Founded, Numbers of Employees and Surgeons, Number of Operating Rooms, Number of Cases seen per year, Overnight Options, Contracted Services and much more. Listings are arranged by State, by Center Category and then alphabetically by Organization Name. Two indexes provide quick and easy access to this wealth of information: Entry Name Index and Specialty/Service Index. *The Directory of Independent Ambulatory Care Centers* is a must-have resource for anyone marketing a product or service to this important industry and will be an invaluable tool for those searching for a local care center that will meet their specific needs.

> *"Among the numerous hospital directories, no other provides information on independent ambulatory centers. A handy, well-organized resource that would be useful in medical center libraries and public libraries." –Choice*

986 pages; Softcover ISBN 1-930956-90-8, $185.00 ◆ Online Database, $365.00 ◆ Online Database & Directory Combo, $450.00

To preview any of our Directories Risk-Free for 30 days, call (800) 562-2139 or fax to (518) 789-0556

Grey House Publishing
Business Directories

The Directory of Business Information Resources, 2007

With 100% verification, over 1,000 new listings and more than 12,000 updates, this 2007 edition of *The Directory of Business Information Resources* is the most up-to-date source for contacts in over 98 business areas – from advertising and agriculture to utilities and wholesalers. This carefully researched volume details: the Associations representing each industry; the Newsletters that keep members current; the Magazines and Journals - with their "Special Issues" - that are important to the trade, the Conventions that are "must attends," Databases, Directories and Industry Web Sites that provide access to must-have marketing resources. Includes contact names, phone & fax numbers, web sites and e-mail addresses. This one-volume resource is a gold mine of information and would be a welcome addition to any reference collection.

"This is a most useful and easy-to-use addition to any researcher's library." –The Information Professionals Institute

2,500 pages; Softcover ISBN 1-59237-146-9, $195.00 ♦ Online Database $495.00

Nations of the World, 2007/08 A Political, Economic and Business Handbook

This completely revised edition covers all the nations of the world in an easy-to-use, single volume. Each nation is profiled in a single chapter that includes Key Facts, Political & Economic Issues, a Country Profile and Business Information. In this fast-changing world, it is extremely important to make sure that the most up-to-date information is included in your reference collection. This edition is just the answer. Each of the 200+ country chapters have been carefully reviewed by a political expert to make sure that the text reflects the most current information on Politics, Travel Advisories, Economics and more. You'll find such vital information as a Country Map, Population Characteristics, Inflation, Agricultural Production, Foreign Debt, Political History, Foreign Policy, Regional Insecurity, Economics, Trade & Tourism, Historical Profile, Political Systems, Ethnicity, Languages, Media, Climate, Hotels, Chambers of Commerce, Banking, Travel Information and more. Five Regional Chapters follow the main text and include a Regional Map, an Introductory Article, Key Indicators and Currencies for the Region. As an added bonus, an all-inclusive CD-ROM is available as a companion to the printed text. Noted for its sophisticated, up-to-date and reliable compilation of political, economic and business information, this brand new edition will be an important acquisition to any public, academic or special library reference collection.

"A useful addition to both general reference collections and business collections." –RUSQ

1,700 pages; Print Version Only Softcover ISBN 1-59237-177-9, $155.00

The Directory of Venture Capital & Private Equity Firms, 2007

This edition has been extensively updated and broadly expanded to offer direct access to over 2,800 Domestic and International Venture Capital Firms, including address, phone & fax numbers, e-mail addresses and web sites for both primary and branch locations. Entries include details on the firm's Mission Statement, Industry Group Preferences, Geographic Preferences, Average and Minimum Investments and Investment Criteria. You'll also find details that are available nowhere else, including the Firm's Portfolio Companies and extensive information on each of the firm's Managing Partners, such as Education, Professional Background and Directorships held, along with the Partner's E-mail Address. *The Directory of Venture Capital & Private Equity Firms* offers five important indexes: Geographic Index, Executive Name Index, Portfolio Company Index, Industry Preference Index and College & University Index. With its comprehensive coverage and detailed, extensive information on each company, *The Directory of Venture Capital & Private Equity Firms* is an important addition to any finance collection.

"The sheer number of listings, the descriptive information provided and the outstanding indexing make this directory a better value than its principal competitor, Pratt's Guide to Venture Capital Sources. Recommended for business collections in large public, academic and business libraries." –Choice

1,300 pages; Softcover ISBN 1-59237-176-0, $565.00/$450.00 Library ♦ Online Database (includes a free copy of the directory) $889.00

To preview any of our Directories Risk-Free for 30 days, call (800) 562-2139 or fax to (518) 789-0556

The Directory of Mail Order Catalogs, 2007

Published since 1981, the *Directory of Mail Order Catalogs* is the premier source of information on the mail order catalog industry. It is the source that business professionals and librarians have come to rely on for the thousands of catalog companies in the US. New for 2007, The Directory of Mail Order Catalogs has been combined with its companion volume, *The Directory of Business to Business Catalogs*, to offer all 13,000 catalog companies in one easy-to-use volume. Section I: Consumer Catalogs, covers over 9,000 consumer catalog companies in 44 different product chapters from Animals to Toys & Games. Section II: Business to Business Catalogs, details 5,000 business catalogs, everything from computers to laboratory supplies, building construction and much more. Listings contain detailed contact information including mailing address, phone & fax numbers, web sites, e-mail addresses and key contacts along with important business details such as product descriptions, employee size, years in business, sales volume, catalog size, number of catalogs mailed and more. Three indexes are included for easy access to information: Catalog & Company Name Index, Geographic Index and Product Index. *The Directory of Mail Order Catalogs*, now with its expanded business to business catalogs, is the largest and most comprehensive resource covering this billion-dollar industry. It is the standard in its field. This important resource is a useful tool for entrepreneurs searching for catalogs to pick up their product, vendors looking to expand their customer base in the catalog industry, market researchers, small businesses investigating new supply vendors, along with the library patron who is exploring the available catalogs in their areas of interest.

"This is a godsend for those looking for information." –Reference Book Review

1,700 pages; Softcover ISBN 1-59237-156-6 $350.00/$250.00 Library ✦ Online Database (includes a free copy of the directory) $495.00

Sports Market Place Directory, 2007

For over 20 years, this comprehensive, up-to-date directory has offered direct access to the Who, What, When & Where of the Sports Industry. With over 20,000 updates and enhancements, the *Sports Market Place Directory* is the most detailed, comprehensive and current sports business reference source available. In 1,800 information-packed pages, *Sports Market Place Directory* profiles contact information and key executives for: Single Sport Organizations, Professional Leagues, Multi-Sport Organizations, Disabled Sports, High School & Youth Sports, Military Sports, Olympic Organizations, Media, Sponsors, Sponsorship & Marketing Event Agencies, Event & Meeting Calendars, Professional Services, College Sports, Manufacturers & Retailers, Facilities and much more. *The Sports Market Place Directory* provides organization's contact information with detailed descriptions including: Key Contacts, physical, mailing, email and web addresses plus phone and fax numbers. Plus, nine important indexes make sure that you can find the information you're looking for quickly and easily: Entry Index, Single Sport Index, Media Index, Sponsor Index, Agency Index, Manufacturers Index, Brand Name Index, Facilities Index and Executive/Geographic Index. For over twenty years, *The Sports Market Place Directory* has assisted thousands of individuals in their pursuit of a career in the sports industry. Why not use "THE SOURCE" that top recruiters, headhunters and career placement centers use to find information on or about sports organizations and key hiring contacts.

1,800 pages; Softcover ISBN 1-59237-189-2, $225.00 ✦ Online Database $479.00

Food and Beverage Market Place, 2007

Food and Beverage Market Place is bigger and better than ever with thousands of new companies, thousands of updates to existing companies and two revised and enhanced product category indexes. This comprehensive directory profiles over 18,000 Food & Beverage Manufacturers, 12,000 Equipment & Supply Companies, 2,200 Transportation & Warehouse Companies, 2,000 Brokers & Wholesalers, 8,000 Importers & Exporters, 900 Industry Resources and hundreds of Mail Order Catalogs. Listings include detailed Contact Information, Sales Volumes, Key Contacts, Brand & Product Information, Packaging Details and much more. *Thomas Food and Beverage Market Place* is available as a three-volume printed set, a subscription-based Online Database via the Internet, on CD-ROM, as well as mailing lists and a licensable database.

"An essential purchase for those in the food industry but will also be useful in public libraries where needed. Much of the information will be difficult and time consuming to locate without this handy three-volume ready-reference source." –ARBA

8,500 pages, 3 Volume Set; Softcover ISBN 1-59237-152-3, $595.00 ✦ Online Database $795.00 ✦ Online Database & 3 Volume Set Combo, $995.00

To preview any of our Directories Risk-Free for 30 days, call (800) 562-2139 or fax to (518) 789-0556

The Grey House Homeland Security Directory, 2007

This updated edition features the latest contact information for government and private organizations involved with Homeland Security along with the latest product information and provides detailed profiles of nearly 1,000 Federal & State Organizations & Agencies and over 3,000 Officials and Key Executives involved with Homeland Security. These listings are incredibly detailed and include Mailing Address, Phone & Fax Numbers, Email Addresses & Web Sites, a complete Description of the Agency and a complete list of the Officials and Key Executives associated with the Agency. Next, *The Grey House Homeland Security Directory* provides the go-to source for Homeland Security Products & Services. This section features over 2,000 Companies that provide Consulting, Products or Services. With this Buyer's Guide at their fingertips, users can locate suppliers of everything from Training Materials to Access Controls, from Perimeter Security to BioTerrorism Countermeasures and everything in between – complete with contact information and product descriptions. A handy Product Locator Index is provided to quickly and easily locate suppliers of a particular product. Lastly, an Information Resources Section provides immediate access to contact information for hundreds of Associations, Newsletters, Magazines, Trade Shows, Databases and Directories that focus on Homeland Security. This comprehensive, information-packed resource will be a welcome tool for any company or agency that is in need of Homeland Security information and will be a necessary acquisition for the reference collection of all public libraries and large school districts.

"Compiles this information in one place and is discerning in content. A useful purchase for public and academic libraries." –Booklist

800 pages; Softcover ISBN 1-59237-151-5, $195.00 ◆ Online Database (includes a free copy of the directory) $385.00

The Grey House Transportation Security Directory & Handbook

This brand new title is the only reference of its kind that brings together current data on Transportation Security. With information on everything from Regulatory Authorities to Security Equipment, this top-flight database brings together the relevant information necessary for creating and maintaining a security plan for a wide range of transportation facilities. With this current, comprehensive directory at the ready you'll have immediate access to: Regulatory Authorities & Legislation; Information Resources; Sample Security Plans & Checklists; Contact Data for Major Airports, Seaports, Railroads, Trucking Companies and Oil Pipelines; Security Service Providers; Recommended Equipment & Product Information and more. Using the *Grey House Transportation Security Directory & Handbook*, managers will be able to quickly and easily assess their current security plans; develop contacts to create and maintain new security procedures; and source the products and services necessary to adequately maintain a secure environment. This valuable resource is a must for all Security Managers at Airports, Seaports, Railroads, Trucking Companies and Oil Pipelines.

800 pages; Softcover ISBN 1-59237-075-6, $195

The Grey House Safety & Security Directory, 2007

The Grey House Safety & Security Directory is the most comprehensive reference tool and buyer's guide for the safety and security industry. Arranged by safety topic, each chapter begins with OSHA regulations for the topic, followed by Training Articles written by top professionals in the field and Self-Inspection Checklists. Next, each topic contains Buyer's Guide sections that feature related products and services. Topics include Administration, Insurance, Loss Control & Consulting, Protective Equipment & Apparel, Noise & Vibration, Facilities Monitoring & Maintenance, Employee Health Maintenance & Ergonomics, Retail Food Services, Machine Guards, Process Guidelines & Tool Handling, Ordinary Materials Handling, Hazardous Materials Handling, Workplace Preparation & Maintenance, Electrical Lighting & Safety, Fire & Rescue and Security. The Buyer's Guide sections are carefully indexed within each topic area to ensure that you can find the supplies needed to meet OSHA's regulations. Six important indexes make finding information and product manufacturers quick and easy: Geographical Index of Manufacturers and Distributors, Company Profile Index, Brand Name Index, Product Index, Index of Web Sites and Index of Advertisers. This comprehensive, up-to-date reference will provide every tool necessary to make sure a business is in compliance with OSHA regulations and locate the products and services needed to meet those regulations.

"Presents industrial safety information for engineers, plant managers, risk managers, and construction site supervisors..." –Choice

1,500 pages, 2 Volume Set; Softcover ISBN 1-59237-160-4, $225.00

The Grey House Biometric Information Directory

The Biometric Information Directory is the only comprehensive source for current biometric industry information. This 2006 edition is the first published by Grey House. With 100% updated information, this latest edition offers a complete, current look, in both print and online form, of biometric companies and products – one of the fastest growing industries in today's economy. Detailed profiles of manufacturers of the latest biometric technology, including Finger, Voice, Face, Hand, Signature, Iris, Vein and Palm Identification systems. Data on the companies include key executives, company size and a detailed, indexed description of their product line. Plus, the Directory also includes valuable business resources, and current editorial make this edition the easiest way for the business community and consumers alike to access the largest, most current compilation of biometric industry information available on the market today. The new edition boasts increased numbers of companies, contact names and company data, with over 700 manufacturers and service providers. Information in the directory includes: Editorial on Advancements in Biometrics; Profiles of 700+ companies listed with contact information; Organizations, Trade & Educational Associations, Publications, Conferences, Trade Shows and Expositions Worldwide; Web Site Index; Biometric & Vendors Services Index by Types of Biometrics; and a Glossary of Biometric Terms. This resource will be an important source for anyone who is considering the use of a biometric product, investing in the development of biometric technology, support existing marketing and sales efforts and will be an important acquisition for the business reference collection for large public and business libraries.

800 pages; Softcover ISBN 1-59237-121-3, $225

The Rauch Guide to the US Adhesives & Sealants, Cosmetics & Toiletries, Ink, Paint, Plastics, Pulp & Paper and Rubber Industries

The Rauch Guides are known worldwide for their comprehensive marketing information. Acquired by Grey House Publishing in 2005, new updated and revised editions will be published throughout 2005 and 2006. Each Guide provides market facts and figures in a highly organized format, ideal for today's busy personnel, serving as ready-references for top executives as well as the industry newcomer. *The Rauch Guides* save time and money by organizing widely scattered information and providing estimates for important business decisions, some of which are available nowhere else. Each Guide is organized into several information-packed chapters. After a brief introduction, the ECONOMICS section provides data on industry shipments; long-term growth and forecasts; prices; company performance; employment, expenditures, and productivity; transportation and geographical patterns; packaging; foreign trade; and government regulations. Next, TECHNOLOGY & RAW MATERIALS provide market, technical, and raw material information for chemicals, equipment and related materials, including market size and leading suppliers, prices, end uses, and trends. PRODUCTS & MARKETS provide information for each major industry product, including market size and historical trends, leading suppliers, five-year forecasts, industry structure, and major end uses. For easy access, each *Guide* contains a chapter on INDUSTRY ACTIVITIES, ORGANIZATIONS & SOURCES OF INFORMATION with detailed information on meetings, exhibits, and trade shows, sources of statistical information, trade associations, technical and professional societies, and trade and technical periodicals. Next, the COMPANY DIRECTORY profiles major industry companies, both public and private. Generally several hundred companies are analyzed. Information includes complete contact information, web address, estimated total and domestic sales, product description, and recent mergers and acquisitions. Each Guide also contains several APPENDICES that provide a cross-reference of suppliers, subsidiaries and divisions. The Rauch Guides will prove to be an invaluable source of market information, company data, trends and forecasts that anyone in these fast-paced industries.

The Rauch Guide to the U.S. Paint Industry Softcover ISBN 1-59237-127-2 $595 ♦ The Rauch Guide to the U.S. Plastics Industry Softcover ISBN 1-59237-128-0 $595 ♦ The Rauch Guide to the U.S. Adhesives and Sealants Industry Softcover ISBN 1-59237-129-9 $595 ♦ The Rauch Guide to the U.S. Ink Industry Softcover ISBN 1-59237-126-4 $595 ♦ The Rauch Guide to the U.S. Rubber Industry Softcover ISBN 1-59237-130-2 $595 ♦ The Rauch Guide to the U.S. Pulp and Paper Industry Softcover ISBN 1-59237-131-0 $595 ♦ The Rauch Guide to the U.S. Cosmetic and Toiletries Industry Softcover ISBN 1-59237-132-9 $895

The Grey House Performing Arts Directory, 2007

The Grey House Performing Arts Directory is the most comprehensive resource covering the Performing Arts. This important directory provides current information on over 8,500 Dance Companies, Instrumental Music Programs, Opera Companies, Choral Groups, Theater Companies, Performing Arts Series and Performing Arts Facilities. Plus, this edition now contains a brand new section on Artist Management Groups. In addition to mailing address, phone & fax numbers, e-mail addresses and web sites, dozens of other fields of available information include mission statement, key contacts, facilities, seating capacity, season, attendance and more. This directory also provides an important Information Resources section that covers hundreds of Performing Arts Associations, Magazines, Newsletters, Trade Shows, Directories, Databases and Industry Web Sites. Five indexes provide immediate access to this wealth of information: Entry Name, Executive Name, Performance Facilities, Geographic and Information Resources. *The Grey House Performing Arts Directory* pulls together thousands of Performing Arts Organizations, Facilities and Information Resources into an easy-to-use source – this kind of comprehensiveness and extensive detail is not available in any resource on the market place today.

"Immensely useful and user-friendly ... recommended for public, academic and certain special library reference collections." –Booklist

1,500 pages; Softcover ISBN 1-59237-138-8, $185.00 ♦ Online Database $335.00

To preview any of our Directories Risk-Free for 30 days, call (800) 562-2139 or fax to (518) 789-0556

New York State Directory, 2007/08

The New York State Directory, published annually since 1983, is a comprehensive and easy-to-use guide to accessing public officials and private sector organizations and individuals who influence public policy in the state of New York. *The New York State Directory* includes important information on all New York state legislators and congressional representatives, including biographies and key committee assignments. It also includes staff rosters for all branches of New York state government and for federal agencies and departments that impact the state policy process. Following the state government section are 25 chapters covering policy areas from agriculture through veterans' affairs. Each chapter identifies the state, local and federal agencies and officials that formulate or implement policy. In addition, each chapter contains a roster of private sector experts and advocates who influence the policy process. The directory also offers appendices that include statewide party officials; chambers of commerce; lobbying organizations; public and private universities and colleges; television, radio and print media; and local government agencies and officials.

New York State Directory - 800 pages; Softcover ISBN 1-59237-190-6; $145.00
New York State Directory with Profiles of New York – 2 volumes; 1,600 pages; Softcover ISBN 1-59237-191-4; $225

Profiles of New York ♦ Profiles of Florida ♦ Profiles of Texas ♦ Profiles of Illinois ♦ Profiles of Michigan ♦ Profiles of Ohio ♦ Profiles of New Jersey ♦ Profiles of Massachusetts ♦ Profiles of Pennsylvania ♦ Profiles of Wisconsin ♦ Profiles of Connecticut ♦ Profiles of Indiana ♦ Profiles of North Carolina ♦ Profiles of Virginia ♦ Profiles of California

Packed with over 50 pieces of data that make up a complete, user-friendly profile of each state, these directories go even further by then pulling selected data and providing it in ranking list form for even easier comparisons between the 100 largest towns and cities! The careful layout gives the user an easy-to-read snapshot of every single place and county in the state, from the biggest metropolis to the smallest unincorporated hamlet. The richness of each place or county profile is astounding in its depth, from history to weather, all packed in an easy-to-navigate, compact format. No need for piles of multiple sources with this volume on your desk. Here is a look at just a few of the data sets you'll find in each profile: History, Geography, Climate, Population, Vital Statistics, Economy, Income, Taxes, Education, Housing, Health & Environment, Public Safety, Newspapers, Transportation, Presidential Election Results, Information Contacts and Chambers of Commerce. As an added bonus, there is a section on Selected Statistics, where data from the 100 largest towns and cities is arranged into easy-to-use charts. Each of 22 different data points has its own two-page spread with the cities listed in alpha order so researchers can easily compare and rank cities. A remarkable compilation that offers overviews and insights into each corner of the state, *Profiles of New York*, *Profiles of Florida* and *Profiles of Texas* go beyond Census statistics, beyond metro area coverage, beyond the 100 best places to live. Drawn from official census information, other government statistics and original research, you will have at your fingertips data that's available nowhere else in one single source. Data will be published on additional states in 2006 and 2007.

Each Profiles of… title ranges from 400-800 pages, priced at $149.00 each

Research Services Directory: Commercial & Corporate Research Centers

This Ninth Edition provides access to well over 8,000 independent Commercial Research Firms, Corporate Research Centers and Laboratories offering contract services for hands-on, basic or applied research. *Research Services Directory* covers the thousands of types of research companies, including Biotechnology & Pharmaceutical Developers, Consumer Product Research, Defense Contractors, Electronics & Software Engineers, Think Tanks, Forensic Investigators, Independent Commercial Laboratories, Information Brokers, Market & Survey Research Companies, Medical Diagnostic Facilities, Product Research & Development Firms and more. Each entry provides the company's name, mailing address, phone & fax numbers, key contacts, web site, e-mail address, as well as a company description and research and technical fields served. Four indexes provide immediate access to this wealth of information: Research Firms Index, Geographic Index, Personnel Name Index and Subject Index.

"An important source for organizations in need of information about laboratories, individuals and other facilities." –ARBA

1,400 pages; Softcover ISBN 1-59237-003-9, $395.00 ♦ Online Database (includes a free copy of the directory) $850.00

International Business and Trade Directories

Completely updated, the Third Edition of *International Business and Trade Directories* now contains more than 10,000 entries, over 2,000 more than the last edition, making this directory the most comprehensive resource of the worlds business and trade directories. Entries include content descriptions, price, publisher's name and address, web site and e-mail addresses, phone and fax numbers and editorial staff. Organized by industry group, and then by region, this resource puts over 10,000 industry-specific business and trade directories at the reader's fingertips. Three indexes are included for quick access to information: Geographic Index, Publisher Index and Title Index. Public, college and corporate libraries, as well as individuals and corporations seeking critical market information will want to add this directory to their marketing collection.

"Reasonably priced for a work of this type, this directory should appeal to larger academic, public and corporate libraries with an international focus." –Library Journal

1,800 pages; Softcover ISBN 1-930956-63-0, $225.00 ♦ Online Database (includes a free copy of the directory) $450.00

To preview any of our Directories Risk-Free for 30 days, call (800) 562-2139 or fax to (518) 789-0556

Grey House Publishing Canada
Canadian Information Resources

Canadian Almanac & Directory, 2007

The Canadian Almanac & Directory contains ten directories in one – giving you all the facts and figures you will ever need about Canada. No other single source provides users with the quality and depth of up-to-date information for all types of research. This national directory and guide gives you access to statistics, images and over 45,000 names and addresses for everything from Airlines to Zoos - updated every year. It's Ten Directories in One! Each section is a directory in itself, providing robust information on business and finance, communications, government, associations, arts and culture (museums, zoos, libraries, etc.), health, transportation, law, education, and more. Government information includes federal, provincial and territorial - and includes an easy-to-use quick index to find key information. A separate municipal government section includes every municipality in Canada, with full profiles of Canada's largest urban centers. A complete legal directory lists judges and judicial officials, court locations and law firms across the country. A wealth of general information, the Canadian Almanac & Directory also includes national statistics on population, employment, imports and exports, and more. National awards and honors are presented, along with forms of address, Commonwealth information and full color photos of Canadian symbols. Postal information, weights, measures, distances and other useful charts are also incorporated. Complete almanac information includes perpetual calendars, five-year holiday planners and astronomical information. Published continuously for 160 years, The Canadian Almanac & Directory is the best single reference source for business executives, managers and assistants; government and public affairs executives; lawyers; marketing, sales and advertising executives; researchers, editors and journalists.

Hardcover ISBN 978-1-89502-149-3; 1,600 pages; $315.00

Associations Canada, 2007

The Most Powerful Fact-Finder to Business, Trade, Professional and Consumer Organizations
Associations Canada covers Canadian organizations and international groups including industry, commercial and professional associations, registered charities, special interest and common interest organizations. This annually revised compendium provides detailed listings and abstracts for nearly 20,000 regional, national and international organizations. This popular volume provides the most comprehensive picture of Canada's non-profit sector. Detailed listings enable users to identify an organization's budget, founding date, scope of activity, licensing body, sources of funding, executive information, full address and complete contact information, just to name a few. Powerful indexes help researchers find information quickly and easily. The following indexes are included: subject, acronym, geographic, budget, executive name, conferences & conventions, mailing list, defunct and unreachable associations and registered charitable organizations. In addition to annual spending of over $1 billion on transportation and conventions alone, Canadian associations account for many millions more in pursuit of membership interests. Associations Canada provides complete access to this highly lucrative market. Associations Canada is a strong source of prospects for sales and marketing executives, tourism and convention officials, researchers, government officials - anyone who wants to locate non-profit interest groups and trade associations.

Hardcover ISBN 978-1-59237-219-5; 1,600 pages; $315.00

Financial Services Canada, 2007/08

Financial Services Canada is the only master file of current contacts and information that serves the needs of the entire financial services industry in Canada. With over 18,000 organizations and hard-to-find business information, Financial Services Canada is the most up-to-date source for names and contact numbers of industry professionals, senior executives, portfolio managers, financial advisors, agency bureaucrats and elected representatives. Financial Services Canada incorporates the latest changes in the industry to provide you with the most current details on each company, including: name, title, organization, telephone and fax numbers, e-mail and web addresses. Financial Services Canada also includes private company listings never before compiled, government agencies, association and consultant services - to ensure that you'll never miss a client or a contact. Current listings include: banks and branches, non-depository institutions, stock exchanges and brokers, investment management firms, insurance companies, major accounting and law firms, government agencies and financial associations. Powerful indexes assist researchers with locating the vital financial information they need. The following indexes are included: alphabetic, geographic, executive name, corporate web site/e-mail, government quick reference and subject. Financial Services Canada is a valuable resource for financial executives, bankers, financial planners, sales and marketing professionals, lawyers and chartered accountants, government officials, investment dealers, journalists, librarians and reference specialists.

900 pages; Hardcover ISBN 978-1-59237-221-8 $315.00

To preview any of our Directories Risk-Free for 30 days, call (800) 562-2139 or fax to (518) 789-0556

Directory of Libraries in Canada, 2007/08

The Directory of Libraries in Canada brings together almost 7,000 listings including libraries and their branches, information resource centers, archives and library associations and learning centers. The directory offers complete and comprehensive information on Canadian libraries, resource centers, business information centers, professional associations, regional library systems, archives, library schools and library technical programs. The Directory of Libraries in Canada includes important features of each library and service, including library information; personnel details, including contact names and e-mail addresses; collection information; services available to users; acquisitions budgets; and computers and automated systems. Useful information on each library's electronic access is also included, such as Internet browser, connectivity and public Internet/CD-ROM/subscription database access. The directory also provides powerful indexes for subject, location, personal name and Web site/e-mail to assist researchers with locating the crucial information they need. The Directory of Libraries in Canada is a vital reference tool for publishers, advocacy groups, students, research institutions, computer hardware suppliers, and other diverse groups that provide products and services to this unique market.

850 pages; Hardcover ISBN 978-1-59237-222-5; $315.00

Canadian Environmental Directory, 2007/08

The Canadian Environmental Directory is Canada's most complete and only national listing of environmental associations and organizations, government regulators and purchasing groups, product and service companies, special libraries, and more! The extensive Products and Services section provides detailed listings enabling users to identify the company name, address, phone, fax, e-mail, Web address, firm type, contact names (and titles), product and service information, affiliations, trade information, branch and affiliate data. The Government section gives you all the contact information you need at every government level – federal, provincial and municipal. We also include descriptions of current environmental initiatives, programs and agreements, names of environment-related acts administered by each ministry or department PLUS information and tips on who to contact and how to sell to governments in Canada. The Associations section provides complete contact information and a brief description of activities. Included are Canadian environmental organizations and international groups including industry, commercial and professional associations, registered charities, special interest and common interest organizations. All the Information you need about the Canadian environmental industry: directory of products and services, special libraries and resource, conferences, seminars and tradeshows, chronology of environmental events, law firms and major Canadian companies, The Canadian Environmental Directory is ideal for business, government, engineers and anyone conducting research on the environment.

Hardcover ISBN 978-1-59237-218-8; 900 pages; $315.00

To preview any of our Directories Risk-Free for 30 days, call (800) 562-2139 or fax to (518) 789-0556

Grey House Publishing
General Reference Titles

The Value of a Dollar 1600-1859, The Colonial Era to The Civil War

Following the format of the widely acclaimed, *The Value of a Dollar, 1860-2004*, *The Value of a Dollar 1600-1859, The Colonial Era to The Civil War* records the actual prices of thousands of items that consumers purchased from the Colonial Era to the Civil War. Our editorial department had been flooded with requests from users of our Value of a Dollar for the same type of information, just from an earlier time period. This new volume is just the answer – with pricing data from 1600 to 1859. Arranged into five-year chapters, each 5-year chapter includes a Historical Snapshot, Consumer Expenditures, Investments, Selected Income, Income/Standard Jobs, Food Basket, Standard Prices and Miscellany. There is also a section on Trends. This informative section charts the change in price over time and provides added detail on the reasons prices changed within the time period, including industry developments, changes in consumer attitudes and important historical facts. This fascinating survey will serve a wide range of research needs and will be useful in all high school, public and academic library reference collections.

600 pages; Hardcover ISBN 1-59237-094-2, $135.00

The Value of a Dollar 1860-2004, Third Edition

A guide to practical economy, *The Value of a Dollar* records the actual prices of thousands of items that consumers purchased from the Civil War to the present, along with facts about investment options and income opportunities. This brand new Third Edition boasts a brand new addition to each five-year chapter, a section on Trends. This informative section charts the change in price over time and provides added detail on the reasons prices changed within the time period, including industry developments, changes in consumer attitudes and important historical facts. Plus, a brand new chapter for 2000-2004 has been added. Each 5-year chapter includes a Historical Snapshot, Consumer Expenditures, Investments, Selected Income, Income/Standard Jobs, Food Basket, Standard Prices and Miscellany. This interesting and useful publication will be widely used in any reference collection.

"Recommended for high school, college and public libraries." –ARBA

600 pages; Hardcover ISBN 1-59237-074-8, $135.00

Working Americans 1880-1999
Volume I: The Working Class, Volume II: The Middle Class, Volume III: The Upper Class

Each of the volumes in the *Working Americans 1880-1999* series focuses on a particular class of Americans, The Working Class, The Middle Class and The Upper Class over the last 120 years. Chapters in each volume focus on one decade and profile three to five families. Family Profiles include real data on Income & Job Descriptions, Selected Prices of the Times, Annual Income, Annual Budgets, Family Finances, Life at Work, Life at Home, Life in the Community, Working Conditions, Cost of Living, Amusements and much more. Each chapter also contains an Economic Profile with Average Wages of other Professions, a selection of Typical Pricing, Key Events & Inventions, News Profiles, Articles from Local Media and Illustrations. The *Working Americans* series captures the lifestyles of each of the classes from the last twelve decades, covers a vast array of occupations and ethnic backgrounds and travels the entire nation. These interesting and useful compilations of portraits of the American Working, Middle and Upper Classes during the last 120 years will be an important addition to any high school, public or academic library reference collection.

"These interesting, unique compilations of economic and social facts, figures and graphs will support multiple research needs.
They will engage and enlighten patrons in high school, public and academic library collections." –Booklist

Volume I: The Working Class ◆ 558 pages; Hardcover ISBN 1-891482-81-5, $145.00 ◆ Volume II: The Middle Class ◆ 591 pages; Hardcover ISBN 1-891482-72-6; $145.00 ◆ Volume III: The Upper Class ◆ 567 pages; Hardcover ISBN 1-930956-38-X, $145.00

Working Americans 1880-1999 Volume IV: Their Children

This Fourth Volume in the highly successful *Working Americans 1880-1999* series focuses on American children, decade by decade from 1880 to 1999. This interesting and useful volume introduces the reader to three children in each decade, one from each of the Working, Middle and Upper classes. Like the first three volumes in the series, the individual profiles are created from interviews, diaries, statistical studies, biographies and news reports. Profiles cover a broad range of ethnic backgrounds, geographic area and lifestyles – everything from an orphan in Memphis in 1882, following the Yellow Fever epidemic of 1878 to an eleven-year-old nephew of a beer baron and owner of the New York Yankees in New York City in 1921. Chapters also contain important supplementary materials including News Features as well as information on everything from Schools to Parks, Infectious Diseases to Childhood Fears along with Entertainment, Family Life and much more to provide an informative overview of the lifestyles of children from each decade. This interesting account of what life was like for Children in the Working, Middle and Upper Classes will be a welcome addition to the reference collection of any high school, public or academic library.

600 pages; Hardcover ISBN 1-930956-35-5, $145.00

To preview any of our Directories Risk-Free for 30 days, call (800) 562-2139 or fax to (518) 789-0556

Working Americans 1880-2003 Volume V: Americans At War

Working Americans 1880-2003 Volume V: Americans At War is divided into 11 chapters, each covering a decade from 1880-2003 and examines the lives of Americans during the time of war, including declared conflicts, one-time military actions, protests, and preparations for war. Each decade includes several personal profiles, whether on the battlefield or on the homefront, that tell the stories of civilians, soldiers, and officers during the decade. The profiles examine: Life at Home; Life at Work; and Life in the Community. Each decade also includes an Economic Profile with statistical comparisons, a Historical Snapshot, News Profiles, local News Articles, and Illustrations that provide a solid historical background to the decade being examined. Profiles range widely not only geographically, but also emotionally, from that of a girl whose leg was torn off in a blast during WWI, to the boredom of being stationed in the Dakotas as the Indian Wars were drawing to a close. As in previous volumes of the *Working Americans* series, information is presented in narrative form, but hard facts and real-life situations back up each story. The basis of the profiles come from diaries, private print books, personal interviews, family histories, estate documents and magazine articles. For easy reference, *Working Americans 1880-2003 Volume V: Americans At War* includes an in-depth Subject Index. The *Working Americans* series has become an important reference for public libraries, academic libraries and high school libraries. This fifth volume will be a welcome addition to all of these types of reference collections.

600 pages; Hardcover ISBN 1-59237-024-1; $145.00
Five Volume Set (Volumes I-V), Hardcover ISBN 1-59237-034-9, $675.00

Working Americans 1880-2005 Volume VI: Women at Work

Unlike any other volume in the *Working Americans* series, this Sixth Volume, is the first to focus on a particular gender of Americans. *Volume VI: Women at Work*, traces what life was like for working women from the 1860's to the present time. Beginning with the life of a maid in 1890 and a store clerk in 1900 and ending with the life and times of the modern working women, this text captures the struggle, strengths and changing perception of the American woman at work. Each chapter focuses on one decade and profiles three to five women with real data on Income & Job Descriptions, Selected Prices of the Times, Annual Income, Annual Budgets, Family Finances, Life at Work, Life at Home, Life in the Community, Working Conditions, Cost of Living, Amusements and much more. For even broader access to the events, economics and attitude towards women throughout the past 130 years, each chapter is supplemented with News Profiles, Articles from Local Media, Illustrations, Economic Profiles, Typical Pricing, Key Events, Inventions and more. This important volume illustrates what life was like for working women over time and allows the reader to develop an understanding of the changing role of women at work. These interesting and useful compilations of portraits of women at work will be an important addition to any high school, public or academic library reference collection.

600 pages; Hardcover ISBN 1-59237-063-2; $145.00

Working Americans 1880-2005 Volume VII: Social Movements

The newest addition to the widely-successful *Working Americans* series, *Volume VII: Social Movements* explores how Americans sought and fought for change from the 1880s to the present time. Following the format of previous volumes in the Working Americans series, the text examines the lives of 34 individuals who have worked -- often behind the scenes --- to bring about change. Issues include topics as diverse as the Anti-smoking movement of 1901 to efforts by Native Americans to reassert their long lost rights. Along the way, the book will profile individuals brave enough to demand suffrage for Kansas women in 1912 or demand an end to lynching during a March on Washington in 1923. Each profile is enriched with real data on Income & Job Descriptions, Selected Prices of the Times, Annual Incomes & Budgets, Life at Work, Life at Home, Life in the Community, along with News Features, Key Events, and Illustrations. The depth of information contained in each profile allow the user to explore the private, financial and public lives of these subjects, deepening our understanding of how calls for change took place in our society. A must-purchase for the reference collections of high school libraries, public libraries and academic libraries.

600 pages; Hardcover ISBN 1-59237-101-9; $145.00
Seven Volume Set (Volumes I-VII), Hardcover ISBN 1-59237-133-7, $945.00

The Encyclopedia of Warrior Peoples & Fighting Groups

Many military groups throughout the world have excelled in their craft either by fortuitous circumstances, outstanding leadership, or intense training. This new second edition of The Encyclopedia of Warrior Peoples and Fighting Groups explores the origins and leadership of these outstanding combat forces, chronicles their conquests and accomplishments, examines the circumstances surrounding their decline or disbanding, and assesses their influence on the groups and methods of warfare that followed. This edition has been completely updated with information through 2005 and contains over 20 new entries. Readers will encounter ferocious tribes, charismatic leaders, and daring militias, from ancient times to the present, including Amazons, Buffalo Soldiers, Green Berets, Iron Brigade, Kamikazes, Peoples of the Sea, Polish Winged Hussars, Sacred Band of Thebes, Teutonic Knights, and Texas Rangers. With over 100 alphabetical entries, numerous cross-references and illustrations, a comprehensive bibliography, and index, the Encyclopedia of Warrior Peoples and Fighting Groups is a valuable resource for readers seeking insight into the bold history of distinguished fighting forces.

"This work is especially useful for high school students, undergraduates, and general readers with an interest in military history." –Library Journal

Pub. Date: May 2006; Hardcover ISBN 1-59237-116-7; $135.00

The Encyclopedia of Invasions & Conquests, From the Ancient Times to the Present

Throughout history, invasions and conquests have played a remarkable role in shaping our world and defining our boundaries, both physically and culturally. This second edition of the popular Encyclopedia of Invasions & Conquests, a comprehensive guide to over 150 invasions, conquests, battles and occupations from ancient times to the present, takes readers on a journey that includes the Roman conquest of Britain, the Portuguese colonization of Brazil, and the Iraqi invasion of Kuwait, to name a few. New articles will explore the late 20th and 21st centuries, with a specific focus on recent conflicts in Afghanistan, Kuwait, Iraq, Yugoslavia, Grenada and Chechnya. Categories of entries include countries, invasions and conquests, and individuals. In addition to covering the military aspects of invasions and conquests, entries cover some of the political, economic, and cultural aspects, for example, the effects of a conquest on the invade country's political and monetary system and in its language and religion. The entries on leaders – among them Sargon, Alexander the Great, William the Conqueror, and Adolf Hitler – deal with the people who sought to gain control, expand power, or exert religious or political influence over others through military means. Revised and updated for this second edition, entries are arranged alphabetically within historical periods. Each chapter provides a map to help readers locate key areas and geographical features, and bibliographical references appear at the end of each entry. Other useful features include cross-references, a cumulative bibliography and a comprehensive subject index. This authoritative, well-organized, lucidly written volume will prove invaluable for a variety of readers, including high school students, military historians, members of the armed forces, history buffs and hobbyists.

"Engaging writing, sensible organization, nice illustrations, interesting and obscure facts, and useful maps make this book a pleasure to read." –ARBA

Pub. Date: March 2006; Hardcover ISBN 1-59237-114-0; $135.00

Encyclopedia of Prisoners of War & Internment

This authoritative second edition provides a valuable overview of the history of prisoners of war and interned civilians, from earliest times to the present. Written by an international team of experts in the field of POW studies, this fascinating and thought-provoking volume includes entries on a wide range of subjects including the Crusades, Plains Indian Warfare, concentration camps, the two world wars, and famous POWs throughout history, as well as atrocities, escapes, and much more. Written in a clear and easily understandable style, this informative reference details over 350 entries, 30% larger than the first edition, that survey the history of prisoners of war and interned civilians from the earliest times to the present, with emphasis on the 19th and 20th centuries. Medical conditions, international law, exchanges of prisoners, organizations working on behalf of POWs, and trials associated with the treatment of captives are just some of the themes explored. Entries range from the Ardeatine Caves Massacre to Kurt Vonnegut. Entries are arranged alphabetically, plus illustrations and maps are provided for easy reference. The text also includes an introduction, bibliography, appendix of selected documents, and end-of-entry reading suggestions. This one-of-a-kind reference will be a helpful addition to the reference collections of all public libraries, high schools, and university libraries and will prove invaluable to historians and military enthusiasts.

"Thorough and detailed yet accessible to the lay reader. Of special interest to subject specialists and historians; recommended for public and academic libraries." - Library Journal

Pub. Date: March 2006; Hardcover ISBN 1-59237-120-5; $135.00

The Religious Right, A Reference Handbook

Timely and unbiased, this third edition updates and expands its examination of the religious right and its influence on our government, citizens, society, and politics. From the fight to outlaw the teaching of Darwin's theory of evolution to the struggle to outlaw abortion, the religious right is continually exerting an influence on public policy. This text explores the influence of religion on legislation and society, while examining the alignment of the religious right with the political right. A historical survey of the movement highlights the shift to "hands-on" approach to politics and the struggle to present a unified front. The coverage offers a critical historical survey of the religious right movement, focusing on its increased involvement in the political arena, attempts to forge coalitions, and notable successes and failures. The text offers complete coverage of biographies of the men and women who have advanced the cause and an up to date chronology illuminate the movement's goals, including their accomplishments and failures. This edition offers an extensive update to all sections along with several brand new entries. Two new sections complement this third edition, a chapter on legal issues and court decisions and a chapter on demographic statistics and electoral patterns. To aid in further research, The Religious Right, offers an entire section of annotated listings of print and non-print resources, as well as of organizations affiliated with the religious right, and those opposing it. Comprehensive in its scope, this work offers easy-to-read, pertinent information for those seeking to understand the religious right and its evolving role in American society. A must for libraries of all sizes, university religion departments, activists, high schools and for those interested in the evolving role of the religious right.

" Recommended for all public and academic libraries." - Library Journal

Pub. Date: November 2006; Hardcover ISBN 1-59237-113-2; $135.00

From Suffrage to the Senate, America's Political Women

From Suffrage to the Senate is a comprehensive and valuable compendium of biographies of leading women in U.S. politics, past and present, and an examination of the wide range of women's movements. Up to date through 2006, this dynamically illustrated reference work explores American women's path to political power and social equality from the struggle for the right to vote and the abolition of slavery to the first African American woman in the U.S. Senate and beyond. This new edition includes over 150 new entries and a brand new section on trends and demographics of women in politics. The in-depth coverage also traces the political heritage of the abolition, labor, suffrage, temperance, and reproductive rights movements. The alphabetically arranged entries include biographies of every woman from across the political spectrum who has served in the U.S. House and Senate, along with women in the Judiciary and the U.S. Cabinet and, new to this edition, biographies of activists and political consultants. Bibliographical references follow each entry. For easy reference, a handy chronology is provided detailing 150 years of women's history. This up-to-date reference will be a must-purchase for women's studies departments, high schools and public libraries and will be a handy resource for those researching the key players in women's politics, past and present.

"An engaging tool that would be useful in high school, public, and academic libraries looking for an overview of the political history of women in the US." –Booklist

Pub. Date: October 2006; Two Volume Set; Hardcover ISBN 1-59237-117-5; $195.00

An African Biographical Dictionary

This landmark second edition is the only biographical dictionary to bring together, in one volume, cultural, social and political leaders – both historical and contemporary – of the sub-Saharan region. Over 800 biographical sketches of prominent Africans, as well as foreigners who have affected the continent's history, are featured, 150 more than the previous edition. The wide spectrum of leaders includes religious figures, writers, politicians, scientists, entertainers, sports personalities and more. Access to these fascinating individuals is provided in a user-friendly format. The biographies are arranged alphabetically, cross-referenced and indexed. Entries include the country or countries in which the person was significant and the commonly accepted dates of birth and death. Each biographical sketch is chronologically written; entries for cultural personalities add an evaluation of their work. This information is followed by a selection of references often found in university and public libraries, including autobiographies and principal biographical works. Appendixes list each individual by country and by field of accomplishment – rulers, musicians, explorers, missionaries, businessmen, physicists – nearly thirty categories in all. Another convenient appendix lists heads of state since independence by country. Up-to-date and representative of African societies as a whole, An African Biographical Dictionary provides a wealth of vital information for students of African culture and is an indispensable reference guide for anyone interested in African affairs.

"An unquestionable convenience to have these concise, informative biographies gathered into one source, indexed, and analyzed by appendixes listing entrants by nation and occupational field." –Wilson Library Bulletin

Pub. Date: July 2006; Hardcover ISBN 1-59237-112-4; $125.00

American Environmental Leaders, From Colonial Times to the Present

A comprehensive and diverse award winning collection of biographies of the most important figures in American environmentalism. Few subjects arouse the passions the way the environment does. How will we feed an ever-increasing population and how can that food be made safe for consumption? Who decides how land is developed? How can environmental policies be made fair for everyone, including multiethnic groups, women, children, and the poor? American Environmental Leaders presents more than 350 biographies of men and women who have devoted their lives to studying, debating, and organizing these and other controversial issues over the last 200 years. In addition to the scientists who have analyzed how human actions affect nature, we are introduced to poets, landscape architects, presidents, painters, activists, even sanitation engineers, and others who have forever altered how we think about the environment. The easy to use A–Z format provides instant access to these fascinating individuals, and frequent cross references indicate others with whom individuals worked (and sometimes clashed). End of entry references provide users with a starting point for further research.

"Highly recommended for high school, academic, and public libraries needing environmental biographical information." –Library Journal/Starred Review

Two Volume Set; Hardcover ISBN 1-57607-385-8 $175.00

World Cultural Leaders of the Twentieth Century

An expansive two volume set that covers 450 worldwide cultural icons, World Cultural Leaders of the Twentieth Century includes each person's works, achievements, and professional careers in a thorough essay. Who was the originator of the term "documentary"? Which poet married the daughter of the famed novelist Thomas Mann in order to help her escape Nazi Germany? Which British writer served as an agent in Russia against the Bolsheviks before the 1917 revolution? These and many more questions are answered in this illuminating text. A handy two volume set that makes it easy to look up 450 worldwide cultural icons: novelists, poets, playwrights, painters, sculptors, architects, dancers, choreographers, actors, directors, filmmakers, singers, composers, and musicians. World Cultural Leaders of the Twentieth Century provides entries (many of them illustrated) covering the person's works, achievements, and professional career in a thorough essay and offers interesting facts and statistics. Entries are fully cross-referenced so that readers can learn how various individuals influenced others. A thorough general index completes the coverage.

"Fills a need for handy, concise information on a wide array of international cultural figures."-ARBA

Two Volume Set; Hardcover ISBN 1-57607-038-7 $175.00

To preview any of our Directories Risk-Free for 30 days, call (800) 562-2139 or fax to (518) 789-0556

Universal Reference Publications
Statistical & Demographic Reference Books

America's Top-Rated Cities, 2007

America's Top-Rated Cities provides current, comprehensive statistical information and other essential data in one easy-to-use source on the 100 "top" cities that have been cited as the best for business and living in the U.S. This handbook allows readers to see, at a glance, a concise social, business, economic, demographic and environmental profile of each city, including brief evaluative comments. In addition to detailed data on Cost of Living, Finances, Real Estate, Education, Major Employers, Media, Crime and Climate, city reports now include Housing Vacancies, Tax Audits, Bankruptcy, Presidential Election Results and more. This outstanding source of information will be widely used in any reference collection.

"The only source of its kind that brings together all of this information into one easy-to-use source. It will be beneficial to many business and public libraries." –ARBA

2,500 pages, 4 Volume Set; Softcover ISBN 1-59237-184-1, $195.00

America's Top-Rated Smaller Cities, 2006/07

A perfect companion to *America's Top-Rated Cities*, *America's Top-Rated Smaller Cities* provides current, comprehensive business and living profiles of smaller cities (population 25,000-99,999) that have been cited as the best for business and living in the United States. Sixty cities make up this 2004 edition of *America's Top-Rated Smaller Cities*, all are top-ranked by Population Growth, Median Income, Unemployment Rate and Crime Rate. City reports reflect the most current data available on a wide-range of statistics, including Employment & Earnings, Household Income, Unemployment Rate, Population Characteristics, Taxes, Cost of Living, Education, Health Care, Public Safety, Recreation, Media, Air & Water Quality and much more. Plus, each city report contains a Background of the City, and an Overview of the State Finances. *America's Top-Rated Smaller Cities* offers a reliable, one-stop source for statistical data that, before now, could only be found scattered in hundreds of sources. This volume is designed for a wide range of readers: individuals considering relocating a residence or business; professionals considering expanding their business or changing careers; general and market researchers; real estate consultants; human resource personnel; urban planners and investors.

"Provides current, comprehensive statistical information in one easy-to-use source... Recommended for public and academic libraries and specialized collections." –Library Journal

1,100 pages; Softcover ISBN 1-59237-135-3, $160.00

Profiles of America: Facts, Figures & Statistics for Every Populated Place in the United States

Profiles of America is the only source that pulls together, in one place, statistical, historical and descriptive information about every place in the United States in an easy-to-use format. This award winning reference set, now in its second edition, compiles statistics and data from over 20 different sources – the latest census information has been included along with more than nine brand new statistical topics. This Four-Volume Set details over 40,000 places, from the biggest metropolis to the smallest unincorporated hamlet, and provides statistical details and information on over 50 different topics including Geography, Climate, Population, Vital Statistics, Economy, Income, Taxes, Education, Housing, Health & Environment, Public Safety, Newspapers, Transportation, Presidential Election Results and Information Contacts or Chambers of Commerce. Profiles are arranged, for ease-of-use, by state and then by county. Each county begins with a County-Wide Overview and is followed by information for each Community in that particular county. The Community Profiles within the county are arranged alphabetically. *Profiles of America* is a virtual snapshot of America at your fingertips and a unique compilation of information that will be widely used in any reference collection.

A Library Journal Best Reference Book "An outstanding compilation." –Library Journal

10,000 pages; Four Volume Set; Softcover ISBN 1-891482-80-7, $595.00

The Comparative Guide to American Suburbs, 2007

The Comparative Guide to American Suburbs is a one-stop source for Statistics on the 2,000+ suburban communities surrounding the 50 largest metropolitan areas – their population characteristics, income levels, economy, school system and important data on how they compare to one another. Organized into 50 Metropolitan Area chapters, each chapter contains an overview of the Metropolitan Area, a detailed Map followed by a comprehensive Statistical Profile of each Suburban Community, including Contact Information, Physical Characteristics, Population Characteristics, Income, Economy, Unemployment Rate, Cost of Living, Education, Chambers of Commerce and more. Next, statistical data is sorted into Ranking Tables that rank the suburbs by twenty different criteria, including Population, Per Capita Income, Unemployment Rate, Crime Rate, Cost of Living and more. *The Comparative Guide to American Suburbs* is the best source for locating data on suburbs. Those looking to relocate, as well as those doing preliminary market research, will find this an invaluable timesaving resource.

"Public and academic libraries will find this compilation useful...The work draws together figures from many sources and will be especially helpful for job relocation decisions." – Booklist

1,700 pages; Softcover ISBN 1-59237-180-9, $130.00

To preview any of our Directories Risk-Free for 30 days, call (800) 562-2139 or fax to (518) 789-0556

The Asian Databook: Statistics for all US Counties & Cities with Over 10,000 Population

This is the first-ever resource that compiles statistics and rankings on the US Asian population. *The Asian Databook* presents over 20 statistical data points for each city and county, arranged alphabetically by state, then alphabetically by place name. Data reported for each place includes Population, Languages Spoken at Home, Foreign-Born, Educational Attainment, Income Figures, Poverty Status, Homeownership, Home Values & Rent, and more. Next, in the Rankings Section, the top 75 places are listed for each data element. These easy-to-access ranking tables allow the user to quickly determine trends and population characteristics. This kind of comparative data can not be found elsewhere, in print or on the web, in a format that's as easy-to-use or more concise. A useful resource for those searching for demographics data, career search and relocation information and also for market research. With data ranging from Ancestry to Education, *The Asian Databook* presents a useful compilation of information that will be a much-needed resource in the reference collection of any public or academic library along with the marketing collection of any company whose primary focus in on the Asian population.

1,000 pages; Softcover ISBN 1-59237-044-6 $150.00

The Hispanic Databook: Statistics for all US Counties & Cities with Over 10,000 Population

Previously published by Toucan Valley Publications, this second edition has been completely updated with figures from the latest census and has been broadly expanded to include dozens of new data elements and a brand new Rankings section. The Hispanic population in the United States has increased over 42% in the last 10 years and accounts for 12.5% of the total US population. For ease-of-use, *The Hispanic Databook* presents over 20 statistical data points for each city and county, arranged alphabetically by state, then alphabetically by place name. Data reported for each place includes Population, Languages Spoken at Home, Foreign-Born, Educational Attainment, Income Figures, Poverty Status, Homeownership, Home Values & Rent, and more. Next, in the Rankings Section, the top 75 places are listed for each data element. These easy-to-access ranking tables allow the user to quickly determine trends and population characteristics. This kind of comparative data can not be found elsewhere, in print or on the web, in a format that's as easy-to-use or more concise. A useful resource for those searching for demographics data, career search and relocation information and also for market research. With data ranging from Ancestry to Education, *The Hispanic Databook* presents a useful compilation of information that will be a much-needed resource in the reference collection of any public or academic library along with the marketing collection of any company whose primary focus in on the Hispanic population.

"This accurate, clearly presented volume of selected Hispanic demographics is recommended for large public libraries and research collections."-Library Journal

1,000 pages; Softcover ISBN 1-59237-008-X, $150.00

Ancestry in America: A Comparative Guide to Over 200 Ethnic Backgrounds

This brand new reference work pulls together thousands of comparative statistics on the Ethnic Backgrounds of all populated places in the United States with populations over 10,000. Never before has this kind of information been reported in a single volume. Section One, Statistics by Place, is made up of a list of over 200 ancestry and race categories arranged alphabetically by each of the 5,000 different places with populations over 10,000. The population number of the ancestry group in that city or town is provided along with the percent that group represents of the total population. This informative city-by-city section allows the user to quickly and easily explore the ethnic makeup of all major population bases in the United States. Section Two, Comparative Rankings, contains three tables for each ethnicity and race. In the first table, the top 150 populated places are ranked by population number for that particular ancestry group, regardless of population. In the second table, the top 150 populated places are ranked by the percent of the total population for that ancestry group. In the third table, those top 150 populated places with 10,000 population are ranked by population number for each ancestry group. These easy-to-navigate tables allow users to see ancestry population patterns and make city-by-city comparisons as well. Plus, as an added bonus with the purchase of *Ancestry in America*, a free companion CD-ROM is available that lists statistics and rankings for all of the 35,000 populated places in the United States. This brand new, information-packed resource will serve a wide-range or research requests for demographics, population characteristics, relocation information and much more. *Ancestry in America: A Comparative Guide to Over 200 Ethnic Backgrounds* will be an important acquisition to all reference collections.

"This compilation will serve a wide range of research requests for population characteristics ... it offers much more detail than other sources." –Booklist

1,500 pages; Softcover ISBN 1-59237-029-2, $225.00

The American Tally: Statistics & Comparative Rankings for U.S. Cities with Populations over 10,000

This important statistical handbook compiles, all in one place, comparative statistics on all U.S. cities and towns with a 10,000+ population. *The American Tally* provides statistical details on over 4,000 cities and towns and profiles how they compare with one another in Population Characteristics, Education, Language & Immigration, Income & Employment and Housing. Each section begins with an alphabetical listing of cities by state, allowing for quick access to both the statistics and relative rankings of any city. Next, the highest and lowest cities are listed in each statistic. These important, informative lists provide quick reference to which cities are at both extremes of the spectrum for each statistic. Unlike any other reference, *The American Tally* provides quick, easy access to comparative statistics – a must-have for any reference collection.

"A solid library reference." -Bookwatch

500 pages; Softcover ISBN 1-930956-29-0, $125.00

The Environmental Resource Handbook, 2007/08

The Environmental Resource Handbook is the most up-to-date and comprehensive source for Environmental Resources and Statistics. Section I: Resources provides detailed contact information for thousands of information sources, including Associations & Organizations, Awards & Honors, Conferences, Foundations & Grants, Environmental Health, Government Agencies, National Parks & Wildlife Refuges, Publications, Research Centers, Educational Programs, Green Product Catalogs, Consultants and much more. Section II: Statistics, provides statistics and rankings on hundreds of important topics, including Children's Environmental Index, Municipal Finances, Toxic Chemicals, Recycling, Climate, Air & Water Quality and more. This kind of up-to-date environmental data, all in one place, is not available anywhere else on the market place today. This vast compilation of resources and statistics is a must-have for all public and academic libraries as well as any organization with a primary focus on the environment.

"...the intrinsic value of the information make it worth consideration by libraries with environmental collections and environmentally concerned users." –Booklist

1,000 pages; Softcover ISBN 1-59237-195-7, $155.00 ◆ Online Database $300.00

Weather America, A Thirty-Year Summary of Statistical Weather Data and Rankings

This valuable resource provides extensive climatological data for over 4,000 National and Cooperative Weather Stations throughout the United States. *Weather America* begins with a new Major Storms section that details major storm events of the nation and a National Rankings section that details rankings for several data elements, such as Maximum Temperature and Precipitation. The main body of *Weather America* is organized into 50 state sections. Each section provides a Data Table on each Weather Station, organized alphabetically, that provides statistics on Maximum and Minimum Temperatures, Precipitation, Snowfall, Extreme Temperatures, Foggy Days, Humidity and more. State sections contain two brand new features in this edition – a City Index and a narrative Description of the climatic conditions of the state. Each section also includes a revised Map of the State that includes not only weather stations, but cities and towns.

"Best Reference Book of the Year." –Library Journal

2,013 pages; Softcover ISBN 1-891482-29-7, $175.00

Crime in America's Top-Rated Cities

This volume includes over 20 years of crime statistics in all major crime categories: violent crimes, property crimes and total crime. *Crime in America's Top-Rated Cities* is conveniently arranged by city and covers 76 top-rated cities. *Crime in America's Top-Rated Cities* offers details that compare the number of crimes and crime rates for the city, suburbs and metro area along with national crime trends for violent, property and total crimes. Also, this handbook contains important information and statistics on Anti-Crime Programs, Crime Risk, Hate Crimes, Illegal Drugs, Law Enforcement, Correctional Facilities, Death Penalty Laws and much more. A much-needed resource for people who are relocating, business professionals, general researchers, the press, law enforcement officials and students of criminal justice.

"Data is easy to access and will save hours of searching." –Global Enforcement Review

832 pages; Softcover ISBN 1-891482-84-X, $155.00